Jablonski's

DICTIONARY OF SYNDROMES & EPONYMIC DISEASES

Dedication

This book is dedicated to the memory of Claudius Francis Mayer, MD, 1899-1988--physician, scholar, bibliophile, and the last editor of the Index-Catalogue of the Library of the Surgeon General's Office.

Jablonski's

DICTIONARY OF SYNDROMES & EPONYMIC DISEASES

by Stanley Jablonski

Krieger Publishing Company
Malabar, Florida
1991

Second Edition 1991
Based on Illustrated Dictionary of Eponymic Syndromes and Diseases and Their Synonyms

Printed and Published by
KRIEGER PUBLISHING COMPANY
KRIEGER DRIVE
MALABAR, FLORIDA 32950

Printed in the United States of America.

Library of Congress Cataloging-In-Publication Data
Jablonski, Stanley.
Jablonski's dictionary of syndromes & eponymic diseases / by Stanley Jablonski. -- 2nd ed.\
p. cm.
Rev. ed. of: Illustrated dictionary of eponymic syndromes and diseases and their synonyms. c1969.
Includes bibliographical references.
ISBN 0-89464-224-3
1. Medicine--Dictionaries. 2. Eponyms--Dictionaries. 3. Eponyms--dictionaries. I. Jablonski, Stanley. Illustrated dictionary of eponymic syndromes and diseases and their synonyms. II. Title. III. Title: Dictionary of syndromes & eponymic diseases. IV. Title: Dictionary of syndromes and eponymic diseases. V. Title: Jablonski's dictionaries of syndromes and eponymic diseases.
[DNLM: 1. Dictionaries, Medical. WB 15 J13i]
R121.J24 1990
616'.003--dc20
DNLM/DLC
for Library of Congress 89-71666
CIP

10 9 8 7 6 5 4 3 2

Acknowledgments

I would like to express my thanks to the National Library of Medicine for providing me with computer-generated listings of the pertinent references extracted from the MEDLARS data base and to the individual members of the staff of the Library for their generous assistance and cooperation. I am especially grateful for the help of Dr. Maria Farkas, Eve-Marie Lacroix, Mary Hanzes, Kristine Scannell, Karen Patrias, Estelle Abrams, Lilian Scanlon, Robert Mehnert, Daniel Carangi, and Gladys Taylor and her associates at the Collection Access Section.

Dr. Robert J. Gorlin's and Professor Hans Rudolf Wiedemann's comments and suggestions are gratefully acknowledged.

In addition, I would like to offer my appreciation to Krieger Publishing Company and its staff for the years of painstaking attention necessary to make publication of this book a reality.

Publisher's Note

The development of this volume has been unique in that it required a complete data base in order to work with and manipulate the entries for cross referencing. The dictionary is designed to be an ongoing operation; the data base will allow us to issue periodic updates and supplements. We also have plans to separate many of the entries into specific disciplines so that specialists can more easily work with the output.

The time invested by Stanley Jablonski in this massive expansion of the first edition represents an encyclopedic achievement and we hope that the information in the thousands of eponyms presented will make this a valuable tool for physicians and laymen alike.

INTRODUCTION

Purpose. The purpose of this book is to gather in one volume the profusion of eponymous and noneponymous syndromes and eponymous diseases. It is hoped that this will give the reader an understanding of the entities listed and also help to unravel the difficulties in communication concerning these conditions, a problem implicit in the very proliferation of syndromes and their synonyms.

Scope. Included in the book are the names of syndromes and eponymous diseases which occur in the literature with reasonable frequency. Many terms listed are well known by their eponymic designations; some are known chiefly by their descriptive names; and others are frankly obscure or obsolete but have been included because of their rarity and the difficulty associated with their recognition. A compendium such as this, however, can never be complete, because new syndromes are constantly being created.

Alphabetization and Orthography. Terms are spelled and alphabetized in this book in accordance with the American form. For example, the diphthong has been eliminated from common terms of Greek origin. Thus, *anaemia pseudoleukaemica* is entered and alphabetized as *anemia pseudoleukemica.* In systematic names, however, the diphthong has been retained. Thus the entry will be *Spirochaeta*, not *Spirocheta*; but for the common name, it will be *spirochetosis*, not *spirochaetosis*. For guidance, cross-references are given to the variant forms.

In dealing with foreign proper names, the umlaut and other accents have been used according to the preference in the country of origin. Some accents on capital letters (È Á Ô) have been removed for technical reasons. Again, all forms of these names are listed, and cross-references are given as necessary. Complex personal names are also considered for ease of location, as noted in the following entries:

DE LANGE, CORNELIA. See LANGE, CORNELIA DE
KAPOSI, MORITZ KOHN. See KAPOSI-KOHN, MORITZ

This book has been produced by a computer data-base and therefore terms with adjoined hyphens are sequenced using the extended ASCII character set: space, hyphen, numbers (0-9), letters (A-Z). See the following entries:

protein malnutrition
protein-energy

pseudo-Volkman syndrome
pseudobulbar palsy

Format. The entry in which a syndrome is defined is selected according to common usage: for example, *Adie syndrome* over the less commonly known eponyms or noneponymic synonyms. The main entry may be an eponym in the nominative form, in accordance with the current practice, or a descriptive designation. Eponymic entries listed under personal names are supplied with biographical data as available: that is, with the full name, nationality, specialty, and dates of birth and death. Names that could not be verified are given as found in the literature; some include only unverified family names. The complete entry consists of a list of synonyms, the definition, and the bibliography. In addition, all synonyms, both eponymic and descriptive, are listed separately as cross-references. Whenever preferences of common usage could not be clearly established, an arbitrary selection was made. In no instance, however, should the selection be understood as the author's own preference. The chromosomal abnormalities are the exception, all of which have been listed under the specific chromosome: *chromosome 21 trisomy syndrome* is the main entry for the *Down Syndrome.*

Definitions. Although a few syndromes have retained their original descriptions, most definitions form a composite picture representing viewpoints of various disciplines, based on a systematic examination of current authoritative material. A typical definition includes recent information on symptoms, pathology, metabolism, etiology, inheritance, and special characteristics. Also, an effort has been made to account for differences in various classifications and to note differences and similarities in allied conditions. Unfortunately, certain definitions fall short of the typical. On some topics the literature proved too scanty to provide the desired information. Any reference to diagnosis and treatment and judgmental interpretation has been meticulously avoided. In some instances, additional information may have appeared in the literature too late to be included in this work.

Sources. Information contained in this book was obtained through a systematic analysis of journal articles selected from some 95,000 references extracted over a period of twenty years from the MEDLARS data base of the National Library of Medicine. In most instances, information thus obtained was augmented with that from current references. Only those syndromes and eponymic diseases which occurred in the literature with a regular frequency were selected, excluding most of those which appeared rarely or irregularly, as well as those in which the term *syndrome* was used facetiously or as an expression of humor. Whenever possible, each syndrome has been traced to its original description, and the title is given in the list of references following the definition. Other than original references are supplied for untraceable syndromes or when the original references were difficult to use or obtain. The titles of original works that could not be verified are transcribed as found in the available secondary sources and prefixed with an asterisk.

Illustrations. In certain instances, particularly in those involving disorders affecting several organs and systems and in those which resist verbal description, illustrations are used to enhance the definitions. The source for each illustration is given in the legend.

SYNDROME—A HISTORICAL NOTE.[1]

The word *syndrome* derives from the Greek *syn*, together, and *dromos*, a course, things running together. One of the oldest terms in the medical vocabulary, it was used in the fifth century B.C. by Hippocrates and his contemporaries as a designation for disorders which were characterized by etiologically nonspecific similar or identical sets of symptoms and were thus otherwise undefinable. Its use remained relatively constant from the time of Hippocrates well into the seventeenth century when Thomas Sydenham concluded that the meanings of both *syndrome* and *disease* were practically synonymous, thus causing *syndrome* virtually to disappear from the literature for about two centuries.

Syndrome was reintroduced late in the nineteenth century as a term for conditions marked by multiple symptoms which occur together and may involve different, apparently unrelated organs and systems. Such conditions defied the ability of physicans to construct appropriate names through the use of the conventional methods of combining prefixes, root words, and suffixes, as would be done with less complex entities. Whenever enough was known about a condition, a descriptive compound name was appended with "syndrome." When the principal elements were too complex or too numerous to be included in a single term, the syndrome was given an eponymous name; it was usually named after the physician who originally described it.

The resurrected term *syndrome* was not universally accepted nor was everyone satisfied with the way in which it was used. The *Index Catalogue*, the principal bibliographic source of the period, did not recognize syndrome as a valid concept until 1912, when only six citations were listed under the heading. Similarly, many writers found the use of the term to be inconsistent or improper. Some even suggested replacing it with a more appropriate designation, such as *syntropy* (from the Greek *syn*, together, and *tropos*, a turning, turning toward each other). By and large, however, *syndrome* proved useful as a special designation for multiple abnormalities, errors of metabolism, genetically transmitted anomalies, and other disorders of similar complexity, which were characterized mainly by clusters of similar or identical manifestations.

The method of naming syndromes came under special scrutiny in the mid-twentieth century when, following the lead of the *Nomina Anatomica*, which banished eponyms from its terminology, a series of editorial comments questioned the validity of personal names in syndrome designations. Some of the arguments against the use of eponyms include the following: excessive accumulation of syndromes under certain names; the difficulty in differentiating syndromes named after different individuals having the same surnames; an unfairness in immortalizing some lesser personalities, when more prominent ones are ignored; the obsolescence of terms; the contention that more accurate and expressive terminology is preferable; the confusion created by some eponyms; and the fact that some eponymic names do not reflect the earliest and best descriptions that exist in the literature.

The use of the possessive form in eponyms has also been criticized and it has been suggested that the nominative form is more appropriate. The campaign against the use of eponyms has resulted in a significant drop in the number of new syndromes being named after physicians, but the effort has been more than counterbalanced by the creation of new classes of eponyms. Authors are using biblical, mythological, and literary characters[2]; patients' names; geographic locations; institutions; and subjects of famous paintings. However, most authors direct their efforts at creating designations that at least in part reflect the nature of the syndrome and are self-explanatory. They usually include as much information as possible about major features of the disorders, such as the names of the organ or organs involved, the phenotype, etiology, genetic characteristics, underlying metabolic defects, or the patients' physical appearance. The clinical characteristics and the names of organs are the most frequently used elements in formulating syndrome designations. Where self-explanatory terms are difficult or impossible to formulate, the authors may resort to other creative approaches: acronyms and abbreviations; foreign terms; and a variety of imaginative designations, such as "jumping Frenchmen of Maine syndrome," "Sunday syndrome," "sundown syndrome, " "sunrise syndrome," "Chinese restaurant syndrome," and the like.

After World War II, several events determined the way the term *syndrome* is now used First, certain Russian authors appended *syndrome* to the designations of already named diseases in an apparent effort to emphasize their special, syndromic characteristics. Tuberculosis, malaria, and diabetes became "tuberculosis syndrome," "malaria syndrome," and "diabetes syndrome." The practice gradually spread to most medical publications of the world to the point where almost all diseases are frequently designated as syndromes. Somewhat later, *syndrome* emerged from its traditional role as an exclusively medical term to become an all-purpose word to denote anything strange, bizarre, unusual, or funny, whether medical, social, behavioral, or cultural. Even when used as a medical concept, the term seems to have lost much of its original specificity, being frequently applied to situations in which the words *disease*, *symptom complex*, *sign*, *manifestation*, or *sequence* would be more appropriate. Also, once a special designation for single entities, *syndrome* is now frequently used as a heading for groups of similar or related conditions. As an example, the "headache syndrome" is not a syndrome in the customary sense, but a class designation for a large group of separate neurological conditions having commonality only in their involvement of the head, neck, and throat.

---

1. Adapted in part from Jablonski, S., "Syndrome—Le mot de jour," *Am. J. Med. Genet.* (1991).
2. See Rodin, A.E., and Key, J.D. *Medicine, Literature, & Eponyms*, Krieger Publishing Co., Malabar, Florida (1989)

An immediate consequence of the expansion of the term's scope is the enormous growth of syndrome literature. In its twenty-year coverage of the literature, the second series of the *Index Catalogue* listed fewer than ten syndromes. Now more than one thousand articles dealing with some aspects of syndromes are added to the MEDLARS data base of the National Library of Medicine each month. Even considering trivialization and misuse, one cannot argue that the word is obsolete and should be discarded. On the contrary, *syndrome* is one of the most useful terms in the vocabulary because of its unique ability to identify special types of genetic disorders and multiple abnormalities associated with characteristic clusters of symptoms.

—Stanley Jablonski

Numeric Cross Reference of Syndromes

1pter deletion syndrome. See *chromosome 1pter deletion syndrome.*

1pter- syndrome. See *chromosome 1pter deletion syndrome.*

1q deletion syndrome. See *chromosome 1q deletion syndrome.*

1q duplication syndrome. See *chromosome 1q duplication syndrome.*

1q+ syndrome. See *chromosome 1q duplication syndrome.*

1q- syndrome. See *chromosome 1q deletion syndrome.*

2n/3n mosaicism. See *chromosome diploid-triploid mosaicism syndrome.*

2p duplication syndrome. See *chromosome 2p duplication syndrome.*

2p+ syndrome. See *chromosome 2p duplication syndrome.*

2q deletion syndrome. See *chromosome 2q deletion syndrome.*

2q duplication syndrome. See *chromosome 2q duplication syndrome.*

2q+ syndrome. See *chromosome 2q duplication syndrome.*

2q- syndrome. See *chromosome 2q deletion syndrome.*

3-M syndrome. See *MMM syndrome.*

3-M slender-boned dwarfism. See *MMM syndrome.*

3p duplication syndrome. See *chromosome 3p duplication syndrome.*

3p+ syndrome. See *chromosome 3p duplication syndrome.*

3pter deletion syndrome. See *chromosome 3pter deletion syndrome.*

3pter- syndrome. See *chromosome 3pter deletion syndrome.*

3q deletion syndrome. See *chromosome 3q deletion syndrome.*

3q duplication syndrome. See *chromosome 3q duplication syndrome.*

3q+ syndrome. See *chromosome 3q duplication syndrome.*

3q- syndrome. See *chromosome 3q deletion syndrome.*

4p deletion syndrome. See *chromosome 4p deletion syndrome.*

4p duplication syndrome. See *chromosome 4p duplication syndrome.*

4p+ syndrome. See *chromosome 4p duplication syndrome.*

4p- syndrome. See *chromosome 4p deletion syndrome.*

4q deletion syndrome. See *chromosome 4q deletion syndrome.*

4q duplication syndrome. See *chromosome 4q duplication syndrome.*

4q+ syndrome. See *chromosome 4q duplication syndrome.*

4q- syndrome. See *chromosome 4q deletion syndrome.*

5p deletion syndrome. See *chromosome 5p deletion syndrome.*

5p duplication syndrome. See *chromosome 5p duplication syndrome.*

5p monosomy syndrome. See *chromosome 5p deletion syndrome.*

5p+ syndrome. See *chromosome 5p duplication syndrome.*

5p- syndrome. See *chromosome 5p deletion syndrome.*

5q deletion syndrome. See *chromosome 5q deletion syndrome.*

5q duplication syndrome. See *chromosome 5q duplication syndrome.*

5q+ syndrome. See *chromosome 5q duplication syndrome.*

5q- syndrome. See *chromosome 5q deletion syndrome.*

6p duplication syndrome. See *chromosome 6p duplication syndrome.*

6p+ syndrome. See *chromosome 6p duplication syndrome.*

6q deletion syndrome. See *chromosome 6q deletion syndrome.*

6q duplication syndrome. See *chromosome 6q duplication syndrome.*

6q+ syndrome. See *chromosome 6q duplication syndrome.*

6q- syndrome. See *chromosome 6q deletion syndrome.*

7 monosomy syndrome. See *chromosome 7 monosomy syndrome.*

7p deletion syndrome. See *chromosome 7p deletion syndrome.*

7p duplication syndrome. See *chromosome 7p duplication syndrome.*

7p+ syndrome. See *chromosome 7p duplication syndrome.*

7p- syndrome. See *chromosome 7p deletion syndrome.*

7q deletion syndrome. See *chromosome 7q deletion syndrome.*

7q duplication syndrome. See *chromosome 7q duplication syndrome.*

7q+ syndrome. See *chromosome 7q duplication syndrome.*

7q- syndrome. See *chromosome 7q deletion syndrome.*

8p deletion syndrome. See *chromosome 8p deletion syndrome.*

8p duplication syndrome. See *chromosome 8p duplication syndrome.*

8p+ syndrome. See *chromosome 8p duplication syndrome.*

8p- syndrome. See *chromosome 8p deletion syndrome.*

8q deletion syndrome. See *chromosome 8q deletion syndrome.*

8q duplication syndrome. See *chromosome 8q duplication syndrome.*
8q+ syndrome. See *chromosome 8q duplication syndrome.*
8q- syndrome. See *chromosome 8q deletion syndrome.*
9p deletion syndrome. See *chromosome 9p deletion syndrome.*
9p duplication syndrome. See *chromosome 9p duplication syndrome.*
9p tetrasomy. See *chromosome 9p tetrasomy syndrome.*
9p+ syndrome. See *chromosome 9p duplication syndrome.*
9p- syndrome. See *chromosome 9p deletion syndrome.*
10p duplication syndrome. See *chromosome 10p duplication syndrome.*
10p+ syndrome. See *chromosome 10p duplication syndrome.*
10p- syndrome. See *chromosome 10p deletion syndrome.*
10q duplication syndrome. See *chromosome 10q duplication syndrome.*
10q+ syndrome. See *chromosome 10q duplication syndrome.*
10qter deletion syndrome. See *chromosome 10qter deletion syndrome.*
10qter- syndrome. See *chromosome 10qter deletion syndrome.*
11p duplication syndrome. See *chromosome 11p duplication syndrome.*
11p+ syndrome. See *chromosome 11p duplication syndrome.*
11q deletion syndrome. See *chromosome 11q deletion syndrome.*
11q duplication syndrome. See *chromosome 11q duplication syndrome.*
11q+ syndrome. See *chromosome 11q duplication syndrome.*
11q- syndrome. See *chromosome 11q deletion syndrome.*
12 mosaic tetrasomy. See *chromosome 12p tetrasomy syndrome.*
12p deletion syndrome. See *chromosome 12p deletion syndrome.*
12p duplication syndrome. See *chromosome 12 duplication syndrome.*
12p tetrasomy. See *chromosome 12p tetrasomy syndrome.*
12p+ syndrome. See *chromosome 12p duplication syndrome.*
12p- syndrome. See *chromosome 12p deletion syndrome.*
12q duplication syndrome. See *chromosome 12q duplication syndrome.*
12q+ syndrome. See *chromosome 12q duplication syndrome.*
13q deletion syndrome. See *chromosome 13q deletion syndrome.*
13q duplication syndrome. See *chromosome 13q duplication syndrome.*
13q+ syndrome. See *chromosome 13q duplication syndrome.*
13q- syndrome. See *chromosome 13q deletion syndrome.*
13q-/r(13) mosaicism. See *chromosome 13q deletion syndrome.*
14q deletion syndrome. See *chromosome 14q deletion syndrome.*
14q duplication syndrome. See *chromosome 14q duplication syndrome.*
14q+ syndrome. See *chromosome 14q duplication syndrome.*
14q- syndrome. See *chromosome 14q deletion syndrome.*
15q duplication syndrome. See *chromosome 15q duplication syndrome.*
15q+ syndrome. See *chromosome 15q duplication syndrome.*
16p duplication syndrome. See *chromosome 16p duplication syndrome.*
16p+ syndrome. See *chromosome 16p duplication syndrome.*
16q deletion syndrome. See *chromosome 16q deletion syndrome.*
16q duplication syndrome. See *chromosome 16q duplication syndrome.*
16q+ syndrome. See *chromosome 16q duplication syndrome.*
16q- syndrome. See *chromosome 16q deletion syndrome.*
17-OHDS. See *17-α-hydroxylase deficiency syndrome.*
17p deletion syndrome. See *chromosome 17p deletion syndrome.*
17p duplication syndrome. See *chromosome 17p duplication syndrome.*
17p+ syndrome. See *chromosome 17p duplication syndrome.*
17p- syndrome. See *chromosome 17p deletion syndrome.*
17q duplication syndrome. See *chromosome 17q duplication syndrome.*
17q+ syndrome. See *chromosome 17q duplication syndrome.*
18p deletion syndrome. See *chromosome 18p deletion syndrome.*
18p tetrasomy. See *chromosome 18p tetrasomy syndrome.*
18p- syndrome. See *chromosome 18p deletion syndrome.*
18pi+ syndrome. See *chromosome +18pi syndrome.*
18q deletion syndrome. See *chromosome 18q deletion syndrome.*
18q duplication syndrome. See *chromosome 18q duplication syndrome.*
18q+ syndrome. See *chromosome 18q duplication syndrome.*
18q- syndrome. See *chromosome 18q deletion syndrome.*
19q duplication syndrome. See *chromosome 19q duplication syndrome.*
19q+ syndrome. See *chromosome 19q duplication syndrome.*
20p deletion syndrome. See *chromosome 20p deletion syndrome.*
20p duplication syndrome. See *chromosome 20p duplication syndrome.*
20p+ syndrome. See *chromosome 20p duplication syndrome.*
20p- syndrome. See *chromosome 20p deletion syndrome.*
20q deletion syndrome. See *chromosome 20q deletion syndrome.*
20q duplication syndrome. See *chromosome 20q duplication syndrome.*
20q+ syndrome. See *chromosome 20q duplication syndrome.*
20q- syndrome. See *chromosome 20q deletion syndrome.*
21 deletion syndrome. See *chromosome 21 monosomy syndrome.*

21 deletion syndrome. See *chromosome 21 monosomy syndrome.*

21 trisomy. See *chromosome 21 trisomy syndrome.*

21- syndrome. See *chromosome 21 monosomy syndrome.*

21-hydroxylase deficiency (21-OHD) syndrome . See *congenital adrenal hyperplasia.*

21-OHD (21-hydroxylase deficiency) syndrome. See *congenital adrenal hyperplasia.*

21q deletion syndrome. See *chromosome 21q deletion syndrome.*

21q- syndrome. See *chromosome 21q deletion syndrome.*

22 monosomy. See *chromosome 22 monosomy syndrome.*

22 trisomy. See *chromosome 22 trisomy syndrome, and chromosome 21 trisomy syndrome.*

46,XX syndrome. See *chromosome XX syndrome.*

48,XXXX syndrome. See *chromosome XXXX syndrome.*

48,XXXY syndrome. See *chromosome XXXY syndrome.*

48,XXYY syndrome. See *chromosome XXYY syndrome.*

48,XYYY syndrome. See *chromosome XYYY syndrome.*

49,XXXX syndrome. See *chromosome XXXX syndrome.*

49,XXXXX syndrome. See *chromosome XXXXX syndrome.*

49,XXXXY syndrome. See *chromosome XXXXY syndrome.*

49,XXXYY syndrome. See *chromosome XXXYY syndrome.*

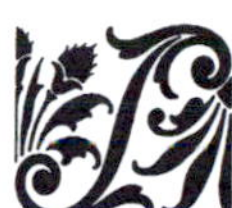

Page #	Term	Observation

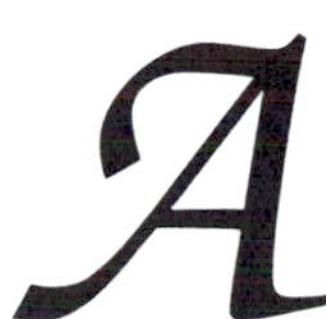

A syndrome. See *under AV (A & V) syndrome.*

AADH. See *alopecia-anosmia-deafness-hypogonadism syndrome.*

AAG (allergic angiitis and granulomatosis). See *Churg-Strauss syndrome.*

AAGENAES, O. (Norwegian physician)

Aagenaes syndrome. Synonym: *hereditary recurrent cholestasis with lymphedema.*

Recurrent cholestasis beginning in infancy, associated with lymphedema of the lower limbs in later childhood. The syndrome is believed to be transmitted as an autosomal recessive trait.

Aagenaes, O. *et al.* Hereditary recurrent intrahepatic cholestasis from birth. *Arch. Dis. Child.*, 1968, 43:646-57.

AAN (analgesic-associated nephropathy). See *analgesic nephropathy syndrome.*

AARSKOG, DAGFINN (Norwegian pediatrician)

Aarskog syndrome. Synonyms: *Aarskog-Scott syndrome (ASS), facial-digital-genital syndrome, faciogenital dysplasia, shawl scrotum syndrome.*

A syndrome combining short stature, abnormal facies, and genital and hand and foot abnormalities. Facial abnormalities usually consist of a round face with a broad forehead, hypertelorism, blepharotosis, antimongoloid slanting of the palpebral fissures, hypoplastic narrow maxilla with relative mandibular prognathism, and a broad nasal bridge with a short stubby nose and anteverted nostrils. A widow's peak is common. The hands are marked by short fingers, some interdigital webbing, simian creases, and clinodactyly of the fifth fingers. The corneae are usually enlarged. The philtrum may be long. The earlobes are thick and the upper helices malformed. The scrotum encircles the penis ventrally around the base of the penis, giving it the appearance of a shawl around the neck. Small feet, joint laxity, cervical vertebral abnormalities, pectus excavatum, inguinal hernia, pigeon-toed gait, small feet, and pes planum may be associated. The syndrome is believed to be transmitted as an X-linked trait.

Aarskog, D. A familial syndrome of short stature associated with facial dysplasia and genital anomalies. *J. Pediat.*, 1970, 77:856-61. Scott, C. I., Jr. Unusual facies, joint hypermobility, genital anomaly and short stature. A new dysmorphic syndrome. *Birth Defects*, 1971, 7:240-6.

Aarskog-Scott syndrome (ASS). See *Aarskog syndrome.*

AAS (acid aspiration syndrome). See *Mendelson syndrome.*

AAS (alcohol abstinence syndrome). See *under withdrawal syndrome.*

AASE, JON M. (American physician)

Aase syndrome. See *Aase-Smith syndrome.*

Aase-Smith syndrome. Synonyms: *Aase syndrome, anemia-triphalangeal thumb syndrome, triphalangeal thumb-hypoplastic anemia syndrome.*

A familial syndrome, originally described in two male siblings, consisting of congenital hypoplastic anemia and triphalangeal thumbs. Anemia tends to improve with age; it may be associated with leukopenia. Skeletal features of this syndrome include triphalangeal thumbs, mild radial hypoplasia, narrow shoulders, and late closure of fontanels. Mild growth retardation, hepatosplenomegaly, and cardiac defects such as ventricular septal defects, may be associated. Cleft lip and palate, retinopathy, and webbed neck were also reported. Etiology is unknown; some cases suggested recessive inheritance, while others were sporadic. Some writers consider this and the Diamond-Blackfan syndrome the same entity.

Aase, J. M., & Smith, D. W. Congenital anemia and triphalangeal thumbs: A new syndrome. *J. Pediat.*, 1969, 74:471-4.

abacterial endocarditis. See *Libman-Sacks syndrome.*

abacterial urethral syndrome. See *urethral syndrome.*

ABAZA, ALPHONSE (French physician, born 1909)

Hoet-Abaza syndrome. See *under Hoet.*

ABDERHALDEN, EMIL (Swiss physician, 1877-1950)

Abderhalden-Kaufmann-Lignac syndrome. See *cystinosis.*

abdominal cocoon syndrome. Intestinal obstruction by a cocoon-like fibrotic membrane encasing the entire small bowel.

Foo, K. T., *et al.* Unusual small intestinal obstruction in adolescent girls: The abdominal cocoon. *Brit. J. Surg.*, 1978, 65:427-30.

abdominal cutaneous nerve entrapment syndrome. Compression of the cutaneous nerves as they pass through the muscular foramina in the abdominal wall, causing abdominal pain.

Applegate, W. V. Abdominal cutaneous nerve entrapment syndrome. *Surgery*, 1972, 71:118-24.

abdominal epilepsy. See *Moore syndrome, under Moore, Matthew Thibaud.*

abdominal ischemia syndrome. Ischemia of the gastrointestinal organs due to abnormalities or disorders of branches of the abdominal aorta.

Kazanchian, P. O. O sindrome khronicheskoi abdominal'noi ishemii. *Kardiologiia, Moskva*, 1978, 18(8):43-50.

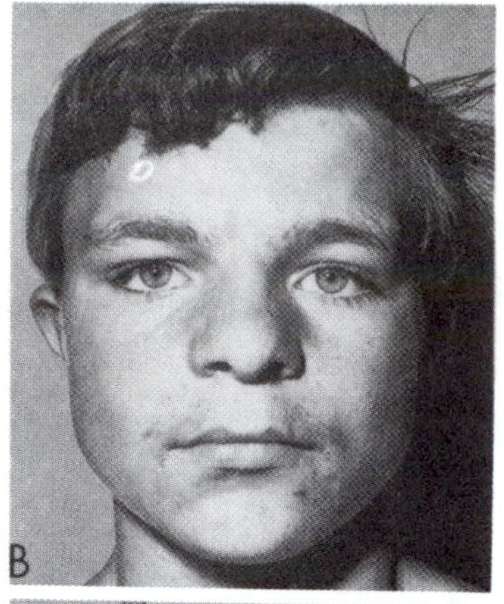

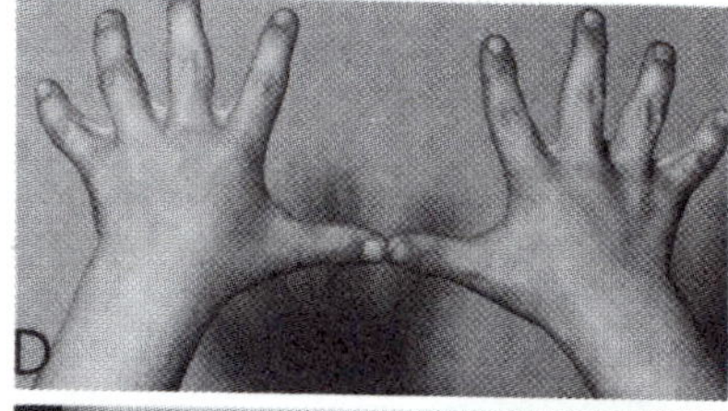

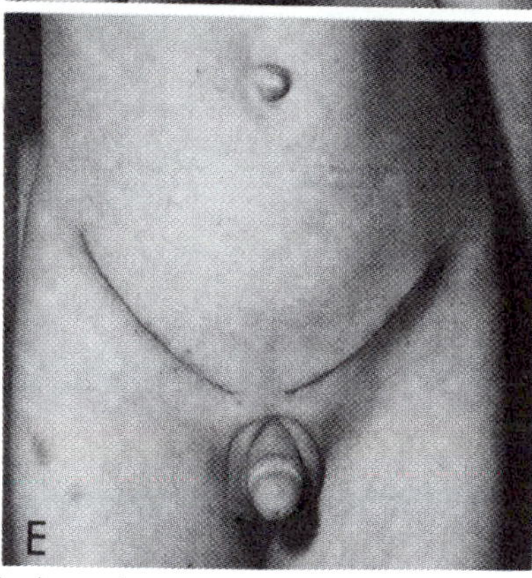

Aarskog syndrome
Furukawa, C.T., et al.: *J. Pediatr.*, 81:1117, 1972.
St. Louis: C.V. Mosby Co.

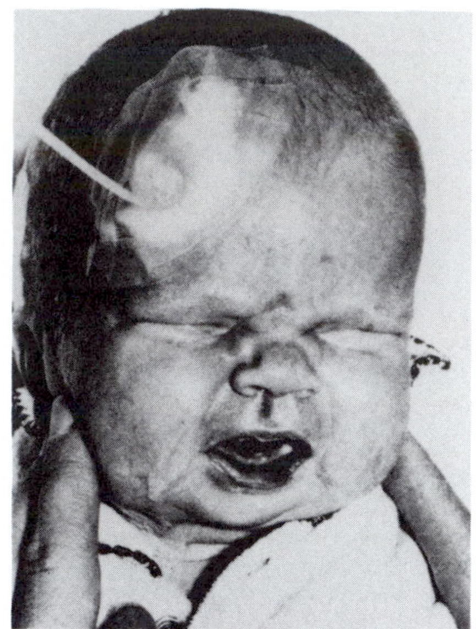

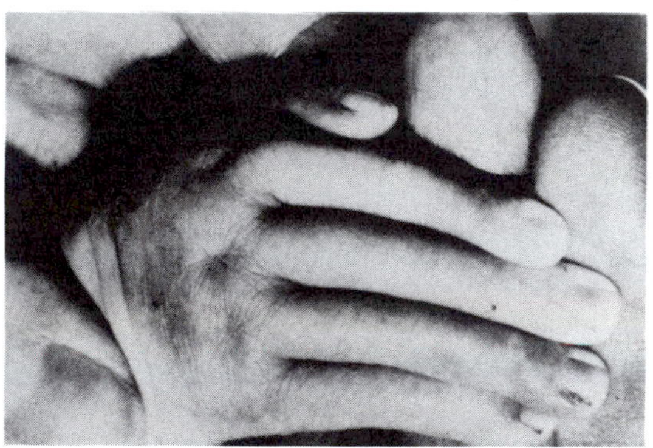

Aase-Smith syndrome
Patton, M.A., A. Sharma, & R.M. Winter: *Clinical Genetics* 28:521-525, 1985.
Munksgaard International Publishers, Copenhagen, Denmark.

abdominal muscle deficiency anomalad. See *prune belly syndrome.*

abdominal muscle deficiency syndrome. See *prune belly syndrome.*

abdominal musculature aplasia syndrome. See *prune belly syndrome.*

abdominal pain syndrome. See *acute abdominal syndrome.*

abdominal syndrome. See *acute abdominal syndrome.*

abdominal wall aplasia syndrome. See *prune belly syndrome.*

abdominothoracic syndrome. See *thoraco-abdominal syndrome.*

abducens-facial hemiplegia alternans. See *Millard-Gubler syndrome.*

ABERCROMBIE, JOHN (British physician, 1780-1844)

Abercrombie degeneration. See *amyloidosis.*

Abercrombie syndrome. See *amyloidosis.*

Abercrombie tumor. See *Hutchinson disease, under Hutchinson, Sir Robert Grieve.*

ABERFELD, D. C.

Aberfeld syndrome. See *Schwartz-Jampel syndrome, under Schwartz, Oscar.*

ABERNETHY, JOHN (British surgeon and anatomist, 1764-1831)

Abernethy sarcoma. A fatty tumor of the trunk.

Abernethy, J. *Surgical aberrations.* 1817, Vol. 2, pp. 17-30.

aberrant mongolian spot. See *Ota nevus.*

abetalipoproteinemia (ABL). See *Bassen-Kornzweig syndrome.*

abiotrophic dementia. See *Jakob-Creutzfeldt syndrome.*

ABL (abetalipoproteinemia). See *Bassen-Kornzweig syndrome.*

ablepharon-macrostomia syndrome. A congenital syndrome characterized by absent eyelids, eyebrows, eyelashes, and scalp hair; fusion defects of the mouth with an enlarged, fish-like mouth, expressionless facies, rudimentary, low-set ears; absent or rudimentary nipples; ambiguous genitalia with cryptorchism; coarse and dry skin with redundant folds; delayed speech development; and ventral hernia.

McCarthy, T. G., & West, C. Ablepharon macrostomia syndrome. *Develop. Med. Child. Neurol.*, 1977, 19:659-72.

abnormal transradiancy of one lung. See *Swyer-James syndrome, under Swyer, Paul Robert.*

abnormal weight control syndrome. See *bulimia syndrome.*

ABO erythroblastosis. See *Halbrecht syndrome.*

abortive disseminated encephalomyelitis. See *Redlich encephalitis.*

abortive type of Friedreich disease. See *Roussy-Lévy syndrome.*

ABRAMI, PIERRE (French physician, 1879-1943)

Abrami disease. See *Hayem-Widal syndrome.*

Widal-Abrami syndrome. See *Hayem-Widal syndrome.*

ABRAMOV, S. S. (Russian physician)

Abramov-Fiedler myocarditis. See *Fiedler myocarditis.*

ABRIKOSSOFF, ALEKSEI IVANOVICH. See ABRIKOSSOV, ALEKSEI IVANOVICH

ABRIKOSSOV (ABRIKOSOFF), ALEKSEI IVANOVICH (Russian physician, 1875-1955)

Abrikossoff myoblastoma. See *Abrikossov tumor.*

Abrikossoff tumor. See *Abrikossov tumor.*

Abrikossov myoblastoma. See *Abrikossov tumor.*

Abrikossov tumor. Synonyms: *Abrikossoff myoblastoma, Abrikossoff tumor, Abrikossov myoblastoma, embryonal rhabdomyoblastoma, epulis of the newborn, granular-cell myoblastoma, myoblastic myoma, myoblastoma granulare, pleomorphic-cell sarcoma, pleomorphic granular-cell sarcoma.*

A tumor of wide distribution, appearing as a firm pedunculated or sessile nodule about 0.5 to 2.0 cm in diameter. Histologically the tumor is characterized by large polyhedral cells with pale cytoplasm filled with coarse acidophilic granules. In skin tumors, strands of collagen are surrounded by small groups of tumor cells. Most of the tumors are benign and do not recur when completely excised, but some instances of malignant degeneration and metastases have been observed.

Abrikossoff, A. Über Myome, ausgehend von der quergestreiften willkurlichen Muskulatur. *Virchows Arch. Path. Anat.*, 1926, 260:215-33.

abruptio placentae. See *Couvelaire syndrome.*

ABS. See ***a**mniotic **b**and **s**yndrome.*

ABS. See ***a**ging **b**rain **s**yndrome.*

abscess without abscess syndrome. See *Borries syndrome.*

absence of abdominal muscle syndrome. See *prune belly syndrome.*

absence of septum pellucidum with porencephalia (SASPP) syndrome. A congenital abnormality consisting of absence of the septum pellucidum, porencephalia, heterotopias of the gray matter, and microgyria. Blindness due to optic atrophy, nystagmus, mental retardation, and tetraplegia are the most common clinical features.

Gruner, J. E. Sur quelques malformations cérebrales developées pendant la vie foetale. In: Heuyer, G., Feld, M., & Gruner, J., eds. *Les malformations congénitales du cerveau.* Paris, Masson, 1959, pp., 378-90. Morgan, S. A., *et al.* Absence of the septum pellucidum. Overlapping clinical syndromes. *Arch. Neurol.*, 1985, 42:769-70.

absent cervical pedicle syndrome. A rare congenital abnormality characterized by the absence of the pedicle on one side of the spine and dorsal displacement of the articular mass of the affected vertebra, the intervertebral foramen being large in the dorsoventral and axial directions. A stubby superior articular process lacks an articular surface and lies dorsal to the inferior articular process of the superjacent vertebra. The inferior articular process of the affected vertebra lies far behind the superior articular process of the subjacent vertebra. The two nerve roots passing through the enlarged intervertebral foramen may be located in a dural pouch. Associated anomalies may include spina bifida, fusion of the lamina of the superjacent vertebra, absent homolateral lamina, a small superjacent pedicle, and vertebral cleft.

van Dijk Azn, R., *et al.* The absent cervical pedicle syndrome. A case report. *Neuroradiology*, 1987, 29:69-72.

absent pulmonary valve syndrome. Synonym: *pulmonary valve agenesis syndrome.*

A congenital abnormality consisting of absence of the pulmonary valve leaflets in association with ventricular septal defect, annular pulmonary stenosis, and aneurysmal dilatation of the main and branch pulmonary arteries. Bronchial compression by the dilated pulmonary arteries causes respiratory distress. The syndrome is sometimes classified as a variant of tetralogy of Fallot because of its association with right aortic arch, annular pulmonary stenosis, and the posterior septal location of the ventricular defect.

Stafford, E. G., *et al.* Tetralogy of Fallot with absent pulmonary valve. Surgical considerations and results. *Circulation*, 1973, 48(Suppl. III):24-30. Dunnigan, A., *et al.* Absent pulmonary valve syndrome in infancy: Surgery reconsidered. *Am. J. Cardiol.*, 1981, 48:117-22.

absorptive hypercalciuria syndrome. A disorder caused by intestinal calcium hyperabsorption, the rise in the circulating calcium concentration augmenting the renal filtered load of calcium and suppressing parathyroid function. Hypercalciuria ensues from the increased renal filtered load of calcium and reduced renal tubular reabsorption. An increase in the circulating concentration of 1,25-dihydroxyvitamin D is usually associated.

Nordin, B. E., *et al.* Hypercalciuria and calcium stone disease. *Clinics Endocr. Metab.*, 1972, pp. 169-83. Pac, C. Y. C. Physiological basis for absorptive and renal hypercalciurias. *Am. J. Physiol.*, 1979, 237:415-23.

abstinence syndrome. See *withdrawal syndrome.*

ABT, ARTHUR FREDERIC (American physician, 1867-1955)

Abt-Letterer-Siwe syndrome. See *Letterer-Siwe syndrome.*

abuse dwarfism syndrome. Synonym: *child abuse dwarfism.*

A form of the child abuse syndrome characterized by reversible growth and mental retardation. See also *battered child syndrome..*

Skeels, H. M. Adult status of children with contrasting early life experience: A follow up study. *Monogr. Soc. Res. Child Develop.*, 1966, Serial 105, 31:1-65. Money, J. Growth of intelligence: Failure and catchup associated respectively with abuse and rescue in the syndrome of abuse dwarfism. *Psychoneuroendocrinology,* 1983, 8:309-19.

abused child. See *battered child syndrome.*

abused doctor. See *battered doctor syndrome.*

abused husband. See *battered spouse syndrome.*

abused parent. See *battered parent syndrome.*

abused wife. See *battered spouse syndrome.*

Ac-globulin deficiency. See *Owren syndrome (2).*

ACA (acrodermatitis chronica atrophicans). See *Herxheimer disease.*

ACA syndrome. See *anticardiolipin syndrome.*

acanthocytosis. See *Bassen-Kornzweig syndrome.*

acanthokeratolysis. See *epidermolysis bullosa syndrome.*

acantholysis bullosa. See *epidermolysis bullosa syndrome.*

acanthoma adenoides cysticum. See *Brooke epithelioma.*

acanthosis bullosa. See *epidermolysis bullosa syndrome.*

acatalasemia. See *Takahara syndrome.*

acatalasia. See *Takahara syndrome.*

accelerated skeletal maturation, Marshall-Smith type. See *Marshall-Smith syndrome, under Marshall, Richard E.*

accelerated skeletal maturation, Weaver type. See *Weaver-Smith syndrome.*

accentuated dysarthria. See *Marie anarthria, under Marie, Pierre.*

accordion abdomen. See *Alvarez syndrome.*

Accutane dysmorphic syndrome. See *fetal Accutane syndrome.*

ACD (angiokeratoma corporis diffusum). See *Fabry syndrome.*

acetaldehyde syndrome. A syndrome of facial flushing, palpitations, and hypotension following ethanol intake. Aldehyde dehydrogenase (ALDH) deficiency associated with increased blood acetaldehyde levels are believed to be the cause.

Noda, J., *et al.* Acetaldehyde syndrome after celiac plexus alcohol block. *Anesth. Analg.,* 1986, 65:1300-2.

ACH. See ***a**myotrophic **c**erebellar **h**ypoplasia syndrome.*

achalasia of cricopharyngeal sphincter syndrome. See *Asherson syndrome.*

achalasia of the urinary bladder. See *Hinman syndrome.*

achalasia-adrenal-alacrima syndrome. A familial multisystem disorder characterized by achalasia, adrenocortical insufficiency, alacrima, short stature, microcephaly, ataxia, optic atrophy, and psychomotor retardation.

Allgrove, J., *et al.* Familial glucocorticoid deficiency with achalasia of the cardia and deficient tear production. *Lancet,* 1978, 1:1284-6.

ACHARD, EMILE CHARLES (French physician, 1860-1944)

Achard syndrome. A heritable disorder of connective tissue, characterized mainly by brachycephaly, arachnodactyly, widespread dysostoses, receding lower jaw, and joint laxity of the hands and feet. Achard and Marfan syndromes are sometimes considered as the same entity, but the Achard syndrome lacks eye and heart abnormalities, subnormal subcutaneous fat content, and tall stature; elongation of the fingers are apparent, because the lengths of metacarpals and phalanges are normal in proportion to the body. The syndrome is transmitted as an autosomal dominant trait.

Achard, M. C. Arachnodactylie. *Bull. Soc. Méd. Hôp. Paris,* 1902, 19:834-43. Duncan, P. A. The Achard syndrome. *Birth Defects,* 1975, 11(6):69-73.

Achard-Thiers syndrome. Synonym: *diabetes in bearded women.*

A syndrome of facial hypertrichosis, diabetes mellitus, deep masculine voice, obesity, hypertrophy of the clitoris, and hyperplasia or adenoma of the adrenal cortex. Amenorrhea, hypertension, and osteoporosis are often present. Pathological findings include liver cirrhosis, atrophy or sclerosis of the ovaries, and an increase in the size of the islands of Langerhans. Postmenopausal women are chiefly affected.

Achard, E. C., & Thiers, J. Le virilisme pilaire et son association à l'insuffisance glycolytique (diabète des femmes à barbe). *Bull. Acad. Méd., Paris,* 1921, 86:51-66.

Marfan-Achard syndrome. See *Marfan syndrome (1), and see Achard syndrome.*

ACHENBACH, WALTER

Achenbach syndrome. Synonyms: *finger apoplexy, paroxysmal hematoma of the hand.*

Sudden appearance, either spontaneously or following strain or temperature change, of a hematoma of the size of a coin on the palmar side of the hand, associated with piercing pain and circumscribed edema.

Achenbach, W. Ematomi parossistici della mano. *Athena, Roma,* 1957, 23:187-9.

achillobursitis. See *Albert syndrome.*

achillodynia. See *Albert syndrome.*

acholuric familial jaundice. See *Minkowski-Chauffard syndrome.*

acholuric hemolytic icterus with splenomegaly. See *Hayem-Widal syndrome.*

acholuric jaundice. See *Loutit anemia.*

achondrogenesis type I. Synonyms: *anosteogenesis, Parenti disease, Parenti-Fraccaro syndrome.*

Neonatal dwarfism characterized by a short trunk, disproportionately large head, prominent abdomen, hydropic appearance, micromelia, and death in utero or shortly after birth. Radiographic signs show deficient ossification in the lumbar vertebrae and absent ossification in the sacral, pubic, and ischial bones. Type I resembles type II, except that in type I the ribs are thinner, sometimes with multiple fractures, and the long bones are more severly shortened and bowed. The condition is believed to be transmitted as an autosomal recessive trait.

Parenti, G. C. La anosteogenesi (una varietá de osteogenesi imperfetta). *Pathologica,* 1936, 28:447-62. Fraccaro, M. Contributo allo studio dell malattie del mesenchima osteopoietico l'acondrogenesi. *Fol. Hered. Path.,* 1952, 1:190-8.

achondrogenesis type II. Synonym: *Saldino syndrome.*

A form of neonatal dwarfism characterized by a short trunk, disproportionately large head, prominent abdomen, hydropic appearance, micromelia, and death in utero or shortly after birth. Radiologic signs show deficient ossification in the lumbar vertebrae and absent ossification in the sacral, pubic, and ischial bones. Type II resembles type I, except that in type I the ribs are thinner, sometimes with multiple fractures, and the long bones are more severely shortened and bowed. The condition is believed to be transmitted as an autosomal recessive trait.

Saldino, R. M. Lethal short-limbed dwarfism. *Am. J. Roentgen.*, 1971, 112:185-97.

achondrogenesis, Brazilian type. See *Grebe disease.*

achondrogenesis, Grebe type. See *Grebe disease.*

achondroplasia. Synonyms: *Kaufmann syndrome, Parrot syndrome, Parrot-Kaufmann syndrome, chondrodysplasia foetalis, chondrodystrophia foetalis, chondrodystrophic dwarfism, chondrogenesis imperfecta, fetal achondroplasia, osteochondrodystrophia foetalis.*

A common form of disproportionate short-limb dwarfism characterized by proximal segments of upper extremities being shorter than middle and distal ones. The head is proportionately large with characteristics facies marked by frontal bossing, depressed nasal bridge, and hypoplasia of the midface with narrow nasal passages. The abdomen and buttocks are usually prominent. Kyphosis at the thoraco-lumbar junction may be present. Trident hand with relatively short fingers and limited elbow extension are common. Malocclusion, anterior crowding, and crossbite are the principal dental features. Motor development is initially slow but becomes normal later during childhood. The condition is transmitted as an autosomal dominant trait.

*Parrot, J. *Les malformations achondroplasiques.* Paris, 1878. Kaufmann, E. *Untersuchungen über die sogenannte foetale Rachitis (Chondrodystrophia foetalis).* Berlin, 1892.

achondroplasia atypica. See *Silfverskiöld syndrome.*

achondroplasia with clubbed feet. See *diastrophic dwarfism syndrome.*

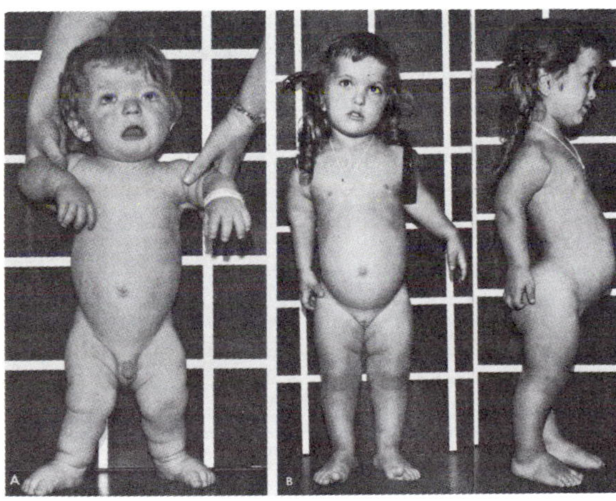

Achondroplasia
Smith, D.W.: *J. Pediatr.*, 70:504, 1967. St. Louis: C.V. Mosby Co.

ACHOO (autosomal dominant compelling helio-ophthalmic outbursts) syndrome. Synonyms: *Peroutka sneeze, photic sneeze reflex, sneezing from light exposure.*

A familial disorder, transmitted as an autosomal dominant trait with a high degree of penetrance, characterized by uncontrollable paroxysms of sneezing provoked in a reflex fashion by the sudden exposure of a dark-adapted individual to intensely bright light.

Collie, W. R., *et al.* ACHOO syndrome (autosomal dominant compelling helio-ophthalmic outburst syndrome). *Birth Defects,* 1978, 14(6B):361-3. Peroutka, S. J., & Peroutka, L. A. Autosomal dominant transmission of the "photic sneeze reflex." *N. Engl. J. Med.,* 1984, 310:599-600.

ACHOR, RICHARD WILLIAM PAUL (American physician, born 1922)

Achor-Smith syndrome. Synonym: *nutritional deficiency syndrome with hypopotassemia.*

Nutritional deficiency with pernicious anemia, sprue, and pellagra, due to potassium depletion. Severe diarrhea, renal insufficiency, muscle degeneration, achlorhydria, hypochloremic alkalosis, and hypocalcemia are also present.

Achor, R. W., & Smith, L. A. Nutritional deficiency syndrome with diarrhea resulting from hypopotassemia, muscle degeneration and renal insufficiency. Report of a case with recovery. *Proc. Mayo Clin.,* 1955, 30:207-14.

achrestic anemia. See *Wilkinson anemia, under Wilkinson, John Frederick.*

achylanemia. See *Faber syndrome.*

achylia gastrica with anemia. See *Faber syndrome.*

achylic chloranemia. See *Faber syndrome.*

acid aspiration syndrome (AAS). See *Mendelson syndrome.*

acid maltase deficiency. See *glycogen storage disease II.*

acid pulmonary aspiration. See *Mendelson syndrome.*

ACKERMAN, JAMES L. (American orthodontist)

Ackerman syndrome. A familial syndrome of pyramidal, taurodont, or fused molar roots with a single canal, hypotrichosis, full upper lip without a cupid's bow, thickened and wide philtrum, and occasional juvenile glaucoma, entropion of the eyelid, soft tissue syndactyly, hyperpigmentation and hardening of the skin over the interphalangeal joints of the fingers, and clinodactyiy of the fifth fingers.

Ackerman, J. L. Taurodont, pyramidal and fused molar roots associated with other anomalies in a kindred. *Am. J. Phys. Anthropol.,* 1973, 38:681-94.

ACKERMAN, LAUREN V. (American physician)

Ackerman carcinoma. Synonym: *verrucous carcinoma.*

Squamous carcinoma of the oral cavity, occurring predominantly in older males, most commonly seen on the buccal mucosa and lower gingiva. It is a slowly-growing, well-differentiated, verrucous tumor that tends to invade local structures, such as the mandible, soft tissues, and antrum. Generally, there are no distant metastases and local metastases are rare. Tobacco chewing is the principal etiological agent.

Ackerman, L. V. Verrucous carcinoma of the oral cavity. *Surgery,* 1948, 23:670-8.

ACKERMANN

Copeman-Ackermann syndrome. See *under Copeman.*

ACL (acromegaloid features-cutis verticis gyrata-corneal leukoma) syndrome. A hereditary syndrome, transmitted as an autosomal dominant trait, characterized by acromegaly, cutis verticis gyrata, corneal developmental leukomata, longitudinal splitting of the dermal ridges in the palms, and enlargement of the lateral half of the supraorbital arch of the frontal bone into a horn-like skin-covered projection. The corneal lesions appear as gray epithelial infiltrates over the cornea, destroying the Bowman membrane. Microscopic findings show abnormal accumulatin of granular mucopolysaccharide material and aberrant orientation of collagen fibers.

*Derbes, V. *Skin manifestations of endocrinopathies and pseudoendocrinopathies.* Presented at the American

Academy of Dermatology meeting, Chicago, 1957. Rosenthal, J. W., & Kloepper, W. An acromegaloid, cutis verticis gyrata, corneal leukoma syndrome. A new medical entity. *Arch. Ophthalmol., Chicago,* 1962, 68:722-6.

ACL (anterior cruciate ligament) insufficiency syndrome. See *anterior cruciate ligament syndrome.*

ACL syndrome. See *anterior cruciate ligament syndrome.*

ACL-deficient knee (anterior cruciate ligament-deficiency knee). See *anterior cruciate ligament syndrome.*

acne agminata. See *Barthélemy disease.*

acne decalvans. See *Quinquaud disease.*

acne scrofulosorum. See *Barthélemy disease.*

acne-myalgic-arthralgic syndrome. A syndrome of acne fulminans, myalgia, and arthralgia.

Fam, A. G., & Lester, R. Acne myalgic-arthralgic syndrome. *J. Rheumatol.,* 1981, 8:349-50.

acoustic neurinoma syndrome. See *Gardner syndrome, under Gardner, W. J*

ACPS (acrocephalopolysyndactyly). See *Carpenter syndrome, and see Sakati-Nyhan-Tisdale syndrome.*

acquired afibrinogenemia. See *disseminated intravascular coagulation syndrome.*

acquired aphasia-convulsive disorder. See *aphasia-epilepsy syndrome.*

acquired cold urticaria (ACU) syndrome. A group of disorders characterized by urticaria, angioedema, and occasional hypotension after an exposure to cold. In the primary type, there is an immediate reaction to cold stimulation in the form of wheals and/or angioedema. Persons with the secondary type show cold-induced wheals and/or angioedema, positive immediate cold-stimulation test, and the presence of a disease or another factor that causes the reaction. Cryoglobulinemia with or without neoplasms, infections such as mononucleosis or syphilis, leukocytoclastic vasculitis, and cold agglutinin disease are the usual causes of the secondary type.

Wanderer, A. A., *et al.* Clinical characteristics of cold-induced systemic reactions in acquired cold urticaria syndromes: Recommendations for prevention of this complication and a proposal for a diagnostic classificatiokn of cold urticaria. *J. Allergy Clin. Immun.,* 1986, 78:417-23.

acquired hemolytic anemia. See *Hayem-Widal syndrome.*

acquired hemolytic anemia-thrombocytopenia syndrome. See *Evans syndrome, under Evans, Robert Sherman.*

acquired hemolytic jaundice. See *Hayem-Widal syndrome.*

acquired hepatic porphyria. See *porphyria cutanea tarda syndrome.*

acquired hypofibrinogenemia. See *disseminated intravascular coagulation syndrome.*

acquired immunodeficiency syndrome (AIDS). Synonyms: *gay compromise syndrome, gay-related immunodeficiency (GRID) syndrome, sexually acquired immunodeficiency (SAID) syndrome, slim disease.*

The syndrome was originally defined by the Centers for Disease Control as the presence of a reliably diagnosed disease , such as Kaposi sarcoma, that is indicative of an underlying defect in cell-mediated immunity in previously healthy individualsin patients under 60 years of age, or a life-threatening opportunistic infection, such as *Pneumocystis carinii* pneumonia. These disorders must occur in the absence of known causes of underlying immune defects, such as medically induced immunosuppression or malignant neoplasms. After recognition of the causative virus, human immunodeficiency virus (HIV), the diagnosis is now excluded in instances when tests for the presence of the virus or antibodies are negative and number of T-helper lymphocytes is normal. In the presence of positive serologic or virologic tests for HIV, a wide variety of diseases are considered indicative of AIDS, including opportunistic infections (spergillosis, candidiasis, cryptococcosis, cytomegalovirus infection, nocardiosis, strongyloidosis, toxoplasmosis, zygomycosis, atypical mycobacterial infections, herpes simplex infections, cryptosporidiosis, and histoplasmosis), non-Hodgkin's lymphoma, chronic lymphoid interstitial pneumonia, and lymphoreticular tumors. The syndrome is caused by infection with human immunodeficiency virus (HIV), a cytopathic retrovirus previously called T-cell leukemic-lymphoma virus III (HTLV-III) and lymphadenopathy virus (LAV). Some patients with AIDS in West Africa are infected with a related retrovirus, HIV-2. Integration of viral material in the form of proviral genome in the deoxyribonucleic acid (DNA) in the host target cell takes place after the host has been infected. Once a person is infected with retroviruses, he or she becomes a permanent carrier. Target cells for the retrovirus in humans include T4 lymphocyte, the monocyte-macrophage, some cerebral and spinal cord cells, and colorectal epithelial cells. The T4 lymphocytes and monocyte-macrophage cells form the basis of the human immune system, being involved in the process of recognition and processing of antigen and production of soluble cytokines such as interferons, interleukins, and hematopoietic colony-stimulating factors; their disruption causes the body to become unable to mobilize immune defense against some pathogens. Colorectal cell infection is a factor in transmitting AIDS in the homosexual population. The range of clinical features varies from an asymptomatic carrier state to overt AIDS with fatal opportunistic infections and Kaposi's sarcoma. Several weeks after primary HIV infection, there may be an influenza-like acute illness marked by fever, myalgias, sweating, arthralgias, malaise, fatigue, and, in some cases, sore throat, adenopathy, anorexia, nausea, vomiting, skin rash, diarrhea, stiff neck, urticaria, sacral paresthesia, weight loss, abdominal cramps, and palmar and plantar desquamation. The initial symptoms last about two to four weeks. Laboratory findings include mild leukopenia and lymphopenia and some instances of T4:T8 inversion. Persistent generalized lymphadenopathy usually follows the initial symptoms. Neurological complications may include meningitis and progressive dementia. *Pneumocystis carinii* pneumonia, the most common opportunistic infection, is characterized mainly by fever, dyspnea, and hypoxemia. Kaposi's sarcoma is the usual terminal complication. It is a multifocal fulminant or indolent neoplasm that may involve different organs, most commonly affecting the skin mucous membranes, gastrointestinal organs, lymph nodes, lungs, and pleura. Some individuals do not fulfill criteria for the complete syndrome, the symptoms consisting of fever, weight loss, diarrhea, fatigue, night sweating, lymphadenopathy, and some immunological abnormalities, in the absence of opportunistic infections and neoplasms, they are known to be suffering from the *AIDS-related complex (ARC)*. Laboratory requirements for the diagnosis of ARC include depressed helper T lymphocytes; depressed helper supressor ratio; at least one of the following: leukopenia, thrombocytopenia, lymphopenia, or anemia; elevated immunoglobulins; depressed blastogenesis; and delayed cutaneous hypersensitivity. Occasionally, asymptomatic carrier state and ARC may progress to overt AIDS several years after the initial infection. The syndrome was first recognized in 1981, mainly among male homosexuals and intravenous drug abusers and later among hemophiliacs receiving transfusions of contaminated blood (*transfusion-associated acquired immunodeficiency syndrome* or *TA-AIDS*). The syndrome was also observed in Haiti and some parts of Africa. The distribution is now worldwide, involving both homosexual and heterosexual populations. The syndrome is transmitted mainly through sexual contacts, transfusion of contaminated blood, or use of contaminated syringes.

Groopman, J. E. The acquired immunodeficiency syndrome. In: Wyngaardean, J. B., & Smith, L. H. Jr., eds. *Cecil textbook of medicine.* 18th ed. Philadelphia, Saunders, 1988. pp. 1799-808. Fauci, A. S., & Lane, H. C. The acquired immunodeficiency syndrome (AIDS). In: Braunwald, E., Isselbacher, K. J., Petersdorf, R. G., Wilson, J. D., Martin, J. B., & Fauci, A. S., eds. *Harrison's principles of internal medicine.* 11th ed. New York, McGraw-Hill, 1987. pp. 1392-6.

acquired immunodeficiency-dementia complex (AIDS-dementia complex, ADC). Acquired immunodeficiency syndrome associated with dementia. The principal symptoms include motor and behavioral dysfunction with impaired memory and concentration and psychomotor slowing. Early motor deficits commonly include ataxia, leg weakness, tremor, and loss of fine-motor coordination. Behavioral disturbances are usually manifested by apathy or withdrawal and, occasionally, frank psychosis. Dementia is progressive, and in advanced stages there may be mutism, incontinence, paraplegia, and myoclonus. Histological changes are found predominantly in the white matter and subcortical structures.

Navia, B. A., *et al.* The AIDS-dementia complex. I. Clinical features. *Ann. Neur.,* 1986, 19:517-24. Navia, B. A., *et al.* The AIDS-dementia complex. II. Neuropathology. *Ann. Neur.,* 1986, 19:525-35.

acquired nevus pigmentosus et pilosus. See *Becker nevus, under Becker, Samuel William.*

acquired perforating foot ulcer. See *Bureau-Barrière syndrome.*

acquired prothrombin complex deficiency (APCD) syndrome. Synonym: *idiopathic vitamin K deficiency in infancy.*

A syndrome of bleeding, pallor, mild hepatomegaly and frequent intracranial hemorrhage occurring in breast-fed infants. Low vitamin K content of maternal milk is believed to be the cause.

Isarangkura, P. B., *et al.* Vitamin K level in maternal breast milk of infants with acquired prothrombin complex deficiency syndrome. *Southeast Asian Tropic. Med. Publ. Health,* 1983, 14:275-6.

acral ischemia syndrome. Subacute (prestasis) or acute (stasis) forms of ischemia of the extremities, differing from chronic intermittent acral ischemia (Raynaud syndrome) in that symptoms of Raynaud syndrome may be alleviated by rewarming, whereas those of acute and subacute forms of ischemia are unresponsive to warmth. Fingers and toes are most commonly affected, usually unilaterally, but in severe cases the entire foot or hand may be involved, unilaterally or bilaterally. Critical reduction of peripheral arterial pressure, pathological constriction of the arterial lumen, and high blood viscosity are the principal pathogenic mechanisms of this condition.

Hess, H. Akute und subakute akrale Ischamie-Syndrome. *NNW,* 1979, 121:517-20.

acral-renal association. See *acrorenal syndrome.*

acro-angiodermatitis. See *Favre-Chaix angiodermatitis.*

acro-asphyxia chronica hypertrohica. See *Raynaud phenomenon, under Raynaud syndrome.*

acro-osteolysis syndrome. See *Hajdu-Cheney syndrome.*

acro-osteolysis without neuropathy. See *Lamy-Maroteaux syndrome (2).*

acro-osteolysis-facial dysplasia syndrome. See *van Bogaert-Hozay syndrome.*

acro-osteopathia ulcero-mutilans. See *Bureau-Barrière syndrome.*

acro-osteopathy of the foot. See *Bureau-Barrière syndrome.*

acrocallosal syndrome (ACS). See *Schinzel syndrome (1).*

acrocephalo-synankie. See *multiple synostoses syndrome.*

acrocephalopolysyndactyly (ACPS). See *Carpenter syndrome and see Sakati-Nyhan-Tisdale syndrome.*

acrocephalospondylosyndactyly syndrome. A congenital syndrome combining features of the Apert syndrome (craniosynostosis, syndactyly, maxillary hypoplasia, parrot-beaked nose, hypertelorism, exophthalmos, strabismus, and short upper lip) with spondylothoracic dysplasia.

Wells, T. R., *et al.* Acrocephalospondylosyndactyly-a possible new syndrome: Analysis of the vertebral and intervetebral components. *Pediat. Path.,* 1990, 10:117-31.

acrocephalosyndactylism syndrome. See *Apert syndrome.*

acrocephalosyndactyly I (ACS I). See *Apert syndrome.*

acrocephalosyndactyly II (ACS II). See *Apert-Crouzon syndrome and see Saethre-Chotzen syndrome.*

acrocephalosyndactyly III (ACS III). See *Saethre-Chotzen syndrome and see Waardenburg syndrome (1).*

acrocephalosyndactyly IV (ACS IV). See *Mohr syndrome II.*

acrocephalosyndactyly IV (ACS IV). See *Pfeiffer syndrome, under Pfeiffer, Rudolf Arthur.*

acrocephalosyndactyly V (ACS V). See *Waardenburg syndrome (1).*

acrocephalosyndactyly V (ACS V). See *Summit syndrome.*

acrocephalosyndactyly V (ACS V). See *Pfeiffer syndrome, under Pfeiffer Rudolf Arthur.*

acrocephalosyndactyly VI (ACS VI). See *Pfeiffer syndrome, under Pfeiffer, Rudolf Arthur.*

acrocephaly with syndactyly. See *Apert syndrome.*

acrochondrohyperplasia. See *Marfan syndrome (1).*

acrocraniodysphalangia. See *Apert syndrome.*

acrocyanosis. See *Raynaud phenomenon, under Raynaud syndrome.*

acrodental dysostosis. See *Weyers syndrome (3).*

acrodermatitis atrophicans chronica. See *Herxheimer disease.*

acrodermatitis chronica atrophicans (ACA). See *Herxheimer disease.*

acrodermatitis continua. See *Hallopeau syndrome (2).*

acrodermatitis enteropathica. Synonyms: *Brandt syndrome, Danbolt syndrome, Danbolt-Closs syndrome.*

A zinc deficiency syndrome in infants, transmitted as an autosomal recessive trait, characterized by a triad of acral dermatitis, alopecia, and diarrhea. Onset of symptoms takes place at the time of weaning and consists of crops of vesicles which rapidly progress to pustules and crusting red scales on the face and around body orifices. Associated symptoms include failure to thrive, growth retardation, irritability, muscle wasting, depression and, occasionally, superimposed candidiasis. The syndrome is caused by the absence of the ligand essential for zinc absorption, which is present in human but not cow milk.

Brandt, T. Dermatitis in children with disturbances of the general condition and the absorption of food elements. *Acta Derm. Vener., Helsingfors*, 1936, 17:513-46. Danbolt, N., & Closs, K. Akrodermatitis enteropathica. *Acta Derm. Vener., Helsinfors*, 1942-43, 23:127-69.

acrodermatitis enteropathica-like syndrome. An acquired disorder similar to acrodermatitis enteropathica, characterized by papulosquamous and vesiculopustular lesions of periorificial areas and papulonodular to bullous lesions of the hands and feet. The vermilion border of the lips may be spared. Depression, poor wound healing, and diarrhea may be associated. The disorder is usually observed in older age groups than acrodermatitis enteropathica and is believed to occur in individuals suffering from zinc deficiency in conditions such as nephrotic syndrome or alcoholic cirrhosis, or following hyperalimentation without adequate trace metal supplement.

Carr, P. M., *et al.* Sparing of the vermilion border in an acrodermatitis enteropathica-like syndrome. *Cutis*, 1983, 31:82-3.

acrodermatitis papulosa eruptiva infantum. See *Gianotti-Crosti syndrome.*

acrodermatitis papulosa infantum. See *Gianotti-Crosti syndrome.*

acrodermatitis perstans. See *Hallopeau syndrome (2).*

acrodermatitis perstans of mild type. See *Barber dermatosis, under Barber, H. W.*

acrodermatitis verruciformis. See *Hopf keratosis.*

acrodynia. Synonyms: *Feer disease, Feer neurosis, Feer syndrome, Selter disease, Selter-Swift-Feer syndrome, Swift disease, Swift-Feer syndrome, dermatopolyneuritis, epidemic erythema, erythredema polyneuropathy, pedionalgia epidemica, pink disease, trophodermatoneurosis.*

A disease of infants and children believed to be caused by mercury poisoning. After prodromal swelling, cyanosis, and coldness of the palms and soles, there are erythemic eruptions of the fingers, toes, nose, buttocks, and cheeks (accounting for the name **pink disease**). Because of intense pruritus, the children chew on the hands and feet, which assume a raw beef appearance. Profuse sweating often produces a skin rash. Neurologic symptoms include superficial sensory loss, generalized muscle hypotonia, and paresthesia. Hypertension and tachycardia are usually present. Diarrhea and sodium and chloride loss are common. Oral symptoms may include stomatitis, spongy red gingiva, and tooth exfoliation. Restlessness, insomnia, weight loss, anorexia, conjunctivitis, photophobia, fever, leukocytosis, albuminuria, and other disorders may be associated.

Feer, E. Eine eigenartige Neurose des vegetativen Systems beim Kleinkinde. *Erg. Inn. Med.*, 1923, 24:100-22. Selter, P. Über Trophodermatoneurose. *Verh. Ges. Kinderh.*, 1903, 20:45-50. Swift, H. Erythroedema. *Lancet*, 1918, 1:611.

acrodysostosis. Synonyms: *Arkless-Graham syndrome, Maroteaux-Malamut syndrome, acrodysplasia, peripheral dysostosis-nasal hypoplasia-mental retardation (PNM) syndrome, pug nose-peripheral dysostosis syndrome.*

A syndrome of peripheral dysostosis, nasal hypoplasia, mental retardation, and peculiar facies. Facial characteristics present a flat and short nose with a low bridge and, occasionally, missing bony framework and anteverted nostrils; long philtrum; and apparent hypertelorism. Epicanthus is often present. The digits of the hands and feet are short and stubby. Intrauterine growth retardation and short stature are constant features of this syndrome. Maxillary hypoplasia and relative mandibular prognathism are frequently associated. Hypocalcemia occurs in some cases. Most reported cases have been sporadic, but dominant mode of transmission is suspected in some cases.

Maroteaux, P., & Malamut, G. L'acrodysostose. *Presse Méd.*, 1968, 76:2189-92. Arkless, R., & Graham, B. An unusual case of brachydactyly? Peripheral dysostosis? pseudopseudohypoparathyroidism? Cone epiphyses? *Am. J. Roetgen.*, 1967, 99:724-35.

acrodysplasia. See *Apert syndrome.*

acrodysplasia epiphysaria. See *Thiemann syndrome.*

acrodysplasia-exostoses syndrome. See *Langer-Giedion syndrome.*

acrodystrophic neuropathy. See *Thévenard syndrome.*

acroerythema symmetricum naeviforme. See *Lane disease, under Lane, John Edward.*

acrofacial dysostosis (AFD). See *Nager-de Reynier syndrome, and see Weyers syndrome (3).*

acrofacial syndrome. See *Weyers syndrome (3).*

acrofrontofacionasal dysostosis syndrome. A multiple congenital anomalies/mental retardation syndrome transmitted as an autosomal recessive trait. The symptoms include short stature, hypertelorism, broad notched nasal tip, cleft lip and/or palate, camptobrachypolysyndactyly, fibular hypoplasia, and foot abnomalities.

Richieri-Costa, A., *et al.* A previously undescribed autosomal recessive congenital anomalies/mental retardation (MCA/MR) syndrome with fronto-nasal dysostosis. Cleft lip/palate, limb hypoplasia, and postaxial poly-syndactyly: acro-fronto-facio-nasal dysostosis syndrome. *Am. J. Med. Genet.*, 1985, 20:631-8.

acrokeratoelastoidosis (AKE). See *Costa disease.*

acrokeratosis paraneoplastica. See *Bazex syndrome, under Bazex, A.*

acrokeratosis verruciformis. See *Hopf keratosis.*

acrokeratotic psoriasiform dermatosis. See *Bazex syndrome, under Bazex, A.*

acromegalic macrospondylitis. See *Erdheim syndrome.*

acromegalic psoriasiform dermatosis. See *Bazex syndrome, under Bazex, A.*

acromegaloid facial appearance (AFA) syndrome. A familial syndrome, transmitted as an autosomal dominant trait with variable phenotype, characterized mainly by acromegaloid facial features with thickened lips and overgrowth of the intraoral mucosa, resulting in peculiar facies marked by exaggerated rugae and frenula, thickened upper eyelids with narrow palpebral fissures (blepharophimosis), highly arched eyebrows, and bulbous nose. Associated anomalies include large and doughy hands.

Hughes, H. E., *et al.* An autosomal dominant syndrome with "acromegaloid" features and thickened oral mucosa. *J. Med. Genet.*, 1985, 22:119-25.

acromegaloid osteosis. See *pachydermoperiostosis syndrome.*

acromegaly. See *Marie syndrome (2), under Marie, Pierre.*

acromegaly-thyro-ovarian insufficiency syndrome. See *Rénon-Delille syndrome.*

acromelalgia. See *Mitchell syndrome (1).*

acromesomelic dwarfism. See *Campailla-Martinelli syndrome.*

acromicria. See *Brugsch syndrome.*

acropachia ossea. See *Marie-Bamberger syndrome, under Marie, Pierre.*

acropachyderma. See *Brugsch syndrome and see pachydermoperiostosis syndrome.*

acropachydermy with pachyperiostosis syndrome. See *pachydermoperiostosis syndrome.*

acropathia ulcerofamiliaris. See *Thévenard syndrome.*

acropathia ulceromutilans. See *Bureau-Barrière syndrome.*

acropectorovertebral dysplasia. See *F syndrome.*

acropigmentatio reticularis. See *Kitamura disease.*

acrorenal syndrome. Synonym: *acral-renal association.*

An association of malformations of the limbs and kidneys. Acral deformities include split hand and foot with oligodactyly, ectrodactyly, syndactyly, brachydactyly, and various anomalies of the carpal and tarsal bones. The associated renal anomalies consist of usually unilateral agenesis, ureter hypoplasia, duplicated collecting systems, hydronephrosis, and bladder neck obstruction. The etiology is unknown.

Dieker, H., & Opitz, J. M. Associated acral and renal malformations. *Birth Defects*, 1969, 5(3):68-77. Curran, A. S., & Curran, J. P. Associated acral and renal malformations. A new syndrome? *Pediatrics*, 1972, 49:716-25.

acroreno-ocular syndrome. A familial syndrome combining abnormalities of the limbs, kidneys, and eyes. Acral anomalies include mild to severe thumb hypoplasia and polydactyly. Urinary defects consist of mild malrotation, crossed renal ectopia, vesicoureteral reflux, and bladder diverticula. Colobomas of the eyes and optic nerve, blapharoptosis, and Duane anomaly are the principal ocular features. Dermatoglyphics are abnormal. Hypertension is usually associated. The syndrome is transmitted as an autosomal dominant trait. According to some authors, this and the Okihiro syndrome are the same entity.

Halal, F., Homsy, M., & Perreault, G. Acro-renal-ocular syndrome: autosomal dominant thumb hypoplasia, renal ectopia, and eye defects. *Am. J. Med. Genet.*, 1984, 17:753-62. Temtamy, S. A. The DR syndrome; or the Okihiro syndrome? *Am. J. Med. Genet.*, 1986, 25:173-4.

acrorenomandibular syndrome. A syndrome of severe split hand and/or foot malformation associated with renal, genital, and mandibular anomalies, combining the characteristics of the acrorenal syndrome (q.v.) with mandibular hypoplasia. The principal features of this syndrome include intrauterine growth retardation, pectus carinatum, thoracolumbar scoliosis, hemivertebrae, spina bifida occulta, large cervical spine, rib anomalies, diaphragmatic hernia, sternal defects, uterus didelphys, uterus unicornis, mullerian duct defects, polycystic kidney, small tongue, fused or aberrant frenula, peculiar facies with low-set malformed ears, syndactyly, and hypoplastic fingers and toes.

Halal, F., *et al.* Acro-renal-mandibular syndrome. *Am. J. Med. Genet.*, 1980, 5:277-84.

acrorhigosis and microangiopathic syndrome. See *Comèl acrorhigosis.*

ACS. See *acute chest syndrome.*

ACS (arocallosal syndrome). See *Schinzel syndrome (1).*

ACS I (acrocephalosyndactyly I). See *Apert syndrome.*

ACS II (acrocephalosyndactyly II). See *Apert-Crouzon syndrome and see Saethre-Chotzen syndrome.*

ACS III (acrocephalosyndactyly III). See *Saethre-Chotzen syndrome and see Wardenburg syndrome (1).*

ACS IV (acrocephalosyndactyly IV). See *Pfeiffer syndrome and see Mohr syndrome II.*

ACS V (acrocephalosyndactyly V). See *Waardenburg syndrome (1), Summit syndrome, and Pfeiffer syndrome.*

ACS VI (acrocephalosyndactyly VI). See *Pfeiffer syndrome.*

actinomycetoma. See *under Ballingall disease.*

actinomycosis. See *Rivalta disease.*

active juvenile cirrhosis. See *Waldenström hepatitis, under Waldenström, Jan Gösta.*

ACU syndrome. See *acquired cold urticaria syndrome.*

acute abdomen. See *acute abdominal syndrome.*

acute abdominal pain. See *acute abdominal syndrome.*

acute abdominal syndrome. Synonyms: *abdominal syndrome, abdominal pain syndrome, acute abdomen, acute abdominal pain, surgical abdomen.*

Sudden abdominal pain, usually associated with vomiting and constipation, that may or may not require surgery. The syndrome is caused by abdominal and thoracic disorders including appendicitis, cholecystitis, intestinal obstruction, perforated peptic ulcer, diverticulitis, and a wide variety of other disorders.

Way, L. W. Abdominal pain. In: Sleisenger, M. H., & Fordtran, J. S., eds. *Gastrointestinal disease.* 3rd ed. Philadelphia, Saunders, 1983. pp. 207-21.

acute alveolar injury. See *adult respiratory distress syndrome.*

acute articular rheumatism. See *Bouillaud disease.*

acute ascending polyradiculoneuritis. See *Guillain-Barré syndrome.*

acute ataxia. See *Wesphal-Leyden syndrome, under Westphal, Alexander Karl Otto.*

acute autoimmunohemolytic anemia. See *Donath-Landsteiner syndrome.*

acute benign erythroblastopenia. See *Gasser syndrome (2).*

acute benign hydrocephalus. See *Marie-Sée syndrome, under Marie, Julien.*

acute benign lymphoblastosis. See *Filatov disease.*

acute bone resorption. See *Gorham syndrome.*

acute central cervical spinal cord injury syndrome. See *Schneider syndrome, under Schneider, Richard C.*
acute cerebellar ataxia. See *Zappert syndrome.*
acute cerebral tremor. See *Zappert syndrome.*
acute chest syndrome (ACS). A combination of chest pain, fever, increased leukocytosis, and appearance of new shadow on chest x-rays in persons suffering from sickle cell disease.

Steinberg, B. Sickle cell anemia. *Arch. Pathol.*, 1930, 9:876-97. Charache, S., *et al.* "Acute chest syndrome" in adults with sickle cell anemia. Microbiology, treatment, and prevention. *Arch. Intern. Med.*, 1979, 139:67-9.

acute circulatory failure. See *shock syndrome.*
acute circumscribed edema. See *Quincke edema.*
acute colonic pseudo-obstruction. See *Ogilvie syndrome.*
acute coryza. See *common cold syndrome.*
acute disseminated histiocytosis X. See *Letterer-Siwe syndrome.*
acute erythremia. See *Di Guglielmo disease (1).*
acute erythremic myelosis. See *Di Guglielmo disease (1).*
acute erythroblastopenia. See *Gasser syndrome (2).*
acute erythroblastosis. See *Di Guglielmo disease (1).*
acute essential edema. See *Quincke edema.*
acute familial hemolysis. See *Bernard syndrome, under Bernard, Jean.*
acute febrile hemolytic anemia. See *Lederer anemia.*
acute febrile neutrophilic dermatosis. See *Sweet syndrome.*
acute febrile pleiochromic anemia. See *Lederer anemia.*
acute focal nephritis. See *Löhlein nephritis.*
acute glaumatocyclitic crises. See *Posner-Schlossman syndrome.*
acute glomerulonephritis. See *acute nephritis syndrome.*
acute hallucinatory mania. See *Ganser syndrome.*
acute hemorrhagic pancreatitis. See *Fitz syndrome.*
acute hydrocephalus in infants. See *Marie-Sée syndrome, under Marie, Julien.*
acute hypervitaminosis A syndrome. See *Marie-Sée syndrome, under Marie, Julien.*
acute idiopathic myocarditis. See *Fiedler myocarditis.*
acute idiopathic polyneuritis. See *Guillain-Barré syndrome.*
acute infectious adenitis. See *Filatov disease.*
acute infectious gingivostomatitis. See *Vincent infection.*
acute infectious lymphocytosis. See *Smith disease, under Smith, Carl Henry.*
acute infective polyneuritis. See *Guillain-Barré syndrome.*
acute inflammatory demyelinating polyradiculoneuropathy (AIDP). See *Guillain-Barré syndrome.*
acute intermittent porphyria (AIP). Synonyms: *Waldenström syndrome, acute porphyria, porphyria hepatica intermittens, pyrroloporphyria, Swedish porphyria.*

A hereditary disorder, transmitted as an autosomal dominant trait, characterized by abdominal pain associated with distention, constipation, and vomiting, leading to weight loss and severe emaciation. Oliguria, prerenal azotemia, and uremia may follow. Neurological symptoms are varied and may include muscle weakness, bulbar paralysis with respiratory failure, hypothalamic dysfunction with inappropriate antidiuretic hormone secretion, and peripehral neuropathy ranging from localized pain to generalized flaccid paralysis. Anxiety, depression, confusion, visual hallucinations, and other neurological complications may also occur. Many patients have hypertension, but in some cases there may be hypotension. Sinus tachycardia, fever, and leukocytosis are sometimes present. Urinary excretion of large amounts of porphobilinogen and aminolevulinic acid are the principal biochemical features. Excessive amounts of porphobilinogen are also found in the liver. In addition, there may be elevation of other urinary pyrrolic substances and fecal porphyrin. Attacks of porphyria may be induced by ingestion of several drugs, including barbiturates. The syndrome occurs most commonly in young adults; its incidence appears to be greater in Sweden than in other countries.

Waldenström, J. Studien über Porphyrie. *Acta Med. Scand.*, 1937, Suppl I82:1-254.

acute interstitial myocarditis. See *Fiedler myocarditis.*
acute lymphomatosis. See *Filatov disease.*
acute mesenteric lymphadenitis syndrome. See *Brennemann syndrome.*
acute mucocutaneous-ocular syndrome. See *Stevens-Johnson syndrome.*
acute necrotizing gingivitis. See *Vincent infection.*
acute necrotizing ulcerative gingivitis (ANUG). See *Vincent infection.*
acute nephritis syndrome. Synonym: *acute glomerulonephritis.*

Inflammatory and/or necrotizing lesions of the kidney glomeruli characterized by the abrupt onset of hematuria and proteinuria, usually associated with disorders of renal function and water and salt retention leading to hypertension and edema. Streptococcal infection and immune or autoimmune mechanisms are the frequent causes of this disorder.

Causer, W. G. Glomerular disorders. In: Wyngaarden, J. B. & Smith, L. H., Jr., eds. *Cecil textbook of medicine.* 17th ed. Philadelphia, Saunders, 1985, pp. 568-89.

acute parapsoriasis varioliformis. See *Mucha-Habermann syndrome.*
acute parenchymatous jaundice. See *Budd-Chiari syndrome.*
acute parenchymatous myositis. See *Wagner-Unverricht syndrome, under Wagner, Ernst Leberecht.*
acute plexitis. See *Guillain-Barré syndrome.*
acute polioencephalitis. See *Strümpell disease (1).*
acute polyneuritis with facial diplegia. See *Guilllain-Barré syndrome.*
acute polyneuronitis. See *Guillain-Barré syndrome.*
acute polyradiculitis. See *Guillain-Barré syndrome.*
acute porphyria. See *acute intermittent porphyria.*
acute postinfectious polyneuropathy. See *Guillain-Barré syndrome.*
acute primary diaphragmitis. See *Hedblom syndrome.*
acute primary hemorrhagic encephalitis. See *Strümpell-Lichtenstern encephalitis.*
acute retinal necrosis (ARN) syndrome. Acute necrotizing retinitis occurring in otherwise healthy persons, manifested at first by periorbital pain, episcleral injection, and diffuse uveitis. The initial symptoms are followed by vitritis, retinal vasculitis, acute retinal whitening and, ultimately, retinal detachment and lowered visual acuity and blindness. The condition may be due to infection with a variety of organisms, including *Toxoplasma*, herpes simplex virus, and cy-

tomegalovirus. Patients with the acquired immunodeficiency syndrome may show retinitis.

Urayama, A., *et al.* Unilateral acute uveitis with periarteritis an detachment. *Jpn. J. Clin. Ophthalmol.*, 1971, 25:607-19.

acute rheumatic polyarthritis. See *Bouillaud disease.*

acute serous encephalitis. See *Brown-Symmers disease, under Brown, Charles Leonard.*

acute thyrotoxic encephalopathy. See *Waldenström disease, under Waldenström, Jan Gösta.*

acute transient monocular disequilibrium. See *Halpern syndrome.*

acute ulcerative gingivitis. See *Vincent infection.*

acute ulceromembranous gingivitis. See *Vincent infection.*

acute urethral syndrome. See *urethral syndrome.*

acute vulvar ulcer. See *Lipschütz ulcer.*

AD. See *Alzheimer disease.*

AD (**A**lzheimer **d**ementia). See *Alzheimer disease.*

ADAM (**a**mniotic **d**eformity-**a**dhesion-**m**utilation) syndrome. See *amniotic band syndrome.*

ADAMANTIADES, B.

Adamantiades syndrome. See *Behçet syndrome.*

Adamantiades-Behçet syndrome. See *Behçet syndrome.*

ADAMS, FORREST H. (American physician)

Adams-Oliver syndrome. A syndrome transmitted as an autosomal dominant trait, characterized by aplasia cutis congenita of the scalp, defect of the cranium, and terminal transverse defects. Limb abnormalities range from micromelia to hypoplastic or aplastic fingers and toes with malformed toenails and fingernails, malimplantation of the toes, syndactyly, and other defects.

Adams, F. H., & Oliver, C. P. Hereditary deformities in man due to arrested development. *J. Hered.*, 1945, 36:3-7.

ADAMS, R. D. (American physician)

Bickers-Adams syndrome. See *under Bickers.*

Hakim-Adams syndrome. See *Hakim syndrome.*

pseudo-Hakim-Adams syndrome. See *under Hakim.*

ADAMS, ROBERT (Irish physician, 1791-1875)

Adams-Stokes (AS) syndrome. Synonyms: *Adams-Stokes disease, Adams-Stokes syncope, Morgagni-Adams-Stokes (MAS) syndrome, Spens syndrome, Stokes syndrome, Stokes-Adams (SA) syndrome, complete heart block.*

Sudden syncopal attacks, with or without convulsions, in severe bradycardia or prolonged asystole which accompany heart block, associated with a fall in blood pressure, paleness, and flushing with resumption of heart rate.

Morgagni, G. B. *De sedibus et causis morborum.* Lib. I. 1761, p. 70. Adams, R. Cases of diseases of the heart, accompanied with pathological observations. *Dublin Hosp. Rep.*, 1827, 4:353-453. Stokes, W. Observations on some cases of permanently slow pulse. *Dublin. Q. J. Med. Sc.*, 1846, 2:73-85. Spens, T. *History of a case in which there took place a remarkable slowness of the pulse. Medical commentaries*, Vol. 7, Edinburgh, 1792, pp. 458-65.

Adams-Stokes disease. See *Adams-Stokes syndrome.*

Adams-Stokes syncope. See *Adams-Stokes syndrome.*

Morgagni-Adams-Stokes (MAS) syndrome. See *Adams-Stokes syndrome.*

Stokes-Adams (SA) syndrome. See *Adams-Stokes syndrome.*

ADAMS, WILLIAM ELIAS (American physician, born 1923)

Kershner-Adams syndrome. See *under Kershner.*

adaptation syndrome. See *Selye syndrome.*

ADC. See *acquired immunodeficiency-dementia complex.*

ADD/HA (**a**ttention **d**eficit **d**isorder with **h**yper**a**ctivity). See *attention deficit-hyperactivity disorder.*

ADDH (**a**ttention **d**eficit **d**isorder with **h**yperactivity). See *attention deficit-hyperactivity disorder.*

Addington disease. An epidemic polio-like disease which occurred in 1955 in the Addington Hospital in Durban, South Africa, affecting about 140 persons. Encephalomyelitis and motor paresis involving one or more limbs were the most prominent symptoms. Constitutional symptoms included headache, prostration, malaise, and mild pyrexia. Emotional disorders were usually expressed as euphoria and, sometimes, mental depression, fatigability, and inability to concentrate. The course of disease was variable in both distribution of symptoms and severity, disappearing in some cases in a week or two but lingering in other instances for as long as three months.

Alexander, J. S. Observations on neuromuscular dysfunction in the Addington outbreak. *S. Afr. Med. J.*, 1956, 30:88-90.

ADDISON, THOMAS (British physician, 1793-1860)

Addison anemia. See *Addison-Biermer anemia.*

Addison crisis. Synonym: *adrenal crisis.*

The symptoms of an acute onset of Addison disease, marked by anorexia, vomiting, abdominal cramps, cyanosis, weak pulse, weak heart sound, hypotension, dehydration, hypothermia.

Addison, T. Anaemia-Disease of the supra-renal capsules. *Lond. Hosp. Gaz.*, 1849, 43:517-8.

Addison disease. Synonyms: *Addison melanoderma, Addison syndrome, morbus Addison, adrenal cortical insufficiency, adrenocortical insufficiency, bronzed disease, bronzed skin, hyperadrenocorticism, melasma suprarenale, suprarenal melasma.*

A syndrome of adrenal hypofunction, bronzed skin and mucous membranes, anemia, digestive disorders (diarrhea, anorexia, nausea, vomiting, constipation), ocular disorders (blepharoptosis, blepharitis, blepharospasm, keratoconjunctivitis, photophobia, corneal ulcers, keratitis, cataracts, and papilledema), and heart diseases. Emotional disorders, irritability, muscle weakness, salt craving, weight loss, amenorrhea, loss of libido, cramps, hypotension, vitiligo, and dehydration are usually associated. Radiological findings usually show adrenal calcification, microcardia, small kidneys, splenomegaly, bone resorption, and gallbladder diseases. Etiologic factors include lesions of the adrenal cortex by autoimmune processes, infections (such as moniliais, hepatitis, and tuberculosis), neoplasms, hemorrhage, thrombosis, trauma, adverse reactions to chemotherapy, or discontinuation of corticoid therapy. Some cases of Addison disease are isolated, but most are associated with other endocrinopathies, particularly hypoparathyroidism.

Addison, T. Anaemia-Disease of the supra-renal capsules. *London Hosp. Gaz.*, 1849, 43:517-8.

Addison disease-cerebral sclerosis syndrome. See *adrenoleukodystrophy.*

Addison keloid. Synonyms: *circumscribed scleroderma, localized scleroderma, morphea.*

A skin disease marked by pinkish patches, lines, or bands, bordered by a purplish halo.

Addison, T. On the keloid of Alibert, or on true keloid. *Med. Chir. Tr., London*, 1854, 37:27-47.

Addison melanoderma. See *Addison disease.*

Addison syndrome (1). See *Addison disease.*

Addison syndrome (2). See *Addison-Biermer anemia.*

Addison-Biermer anemia. Synonyms: *Addison anemia, Addison syndrome, Addison-Biermer syndrome, Biermer anemia, Biermer syndrome, Biermer-Ehrlich anemia, pernicious anemia, primary anemia.*

A gastric disease associated with intrinsic factor deficiency leading to vitamin B_{12} deficiency. It is characterized by faulty maturation of the erythrocytes with the formation of abnormally large megaloblastic precursors. It occurs most commonly in middle-aged individuals and is associated with weakness, pallor, shortness of breath, digital paresthesias, numbness, lack of coordination, spasticity, difficulty in walking, decreased sense of taste and smell, mental dullness, and sometimes psychoses. Gastrointestinal changes include achylia gastrica, diarrhea, and constipation. The peripheral blood may show low red cell counts, oval spherocytosis, poikilocytosis, leukopenia with hypersegmented polymorphonuclear leukocytes, thrombocytopenia, and eosinophilia. The bone marrow is usually hypercellular and shows abnormal white and red cells. Oral symptoms include glossitis, glossodynia, and glossopyrosis associated with excoriation of the tongue, chiefly of the tip and edges, and beefy red lesions characteristic of Moeller and Hunter glossitis. Periods of remission and exacerbation with parallel blood changes occur. The juvenile form of pernicious anemia includes true pernicious anemia occurring in childhood and early adolescence, congenital intrinsic factor deficiency, production of inert. intrinsic factor, and familial selective malabsorption of vitamin B_{12} (*Imerslund syndrome*).

Addison, T. Anaemia-Disease of the supra-renal capsules. *London Hosp. Gaz.*, 1849, 43:517-8. *Biermer, A. Form von progressiver perniciöser Anämie. *Korresp. Bl. Schweiz. Arzt.*, 1872, 2:15-8. Ehrlich, P. Über einen Fall von Anämie mit Bemerkungen über regenerative Veranderungen des Knochenmarks. *Charité Ann., Berlin*, 1888, 13:300-9.

Addison-Biermer syndrome. See *Addison-Biermer anemia.*

Addison-Gull syndrome. Synonyms: *Rayer syndrome, biliary xanthomatosis, fibroma lipomatodes, vitiligoidea plana, xanthelasma.*

A disorder characterized by vitiligoides of the skin, chronic jaundice, splenomgaly, and hepatomegaly.

Addison, T., & Gull, W. On certain affection of the skin. Vitiligoidea-(_) plana, (ß) tuberosa. *Guy's Hosp. Rep., London*, 1850-51, 7:265-72. *Rayer, P. F. *Traité des maladies de la peau.* 1835.

Addison-Schilder syndrome. See *adrenoleukodystrophy.*

morbus Addison. See *Addison disease.*

pseudo-Addison syndrome. See *renal salt losing syndrome.*

adducted thumbs syndrome. See *Christian syndrome (1), under Christian, Joe C.*

adductor canal compression syndrome. Synonyms: *adductor canal syndrome, adductor canal outlet syndrome.*

Arterial compression by an abnormal musculotendinous band arising from the adductor magnus muscle and lying adjacent and superior to the adductor tendon. The syndrome usually occurs in younger, otherwise healthy men and can cause loss of a limb.

Lee, B. Y., *et al.* The adductor canal syndrome. *Am. J. Surg.*, 1972, 123:617-20.

adductor canal outlet syndrome. See *adductor canal compression syndrome.*

adductor canal syndrome. See *adductor canal compression syndrome.*

adductor laryngeal paralysis syndrome. A hereditary bilateral adductor paralysis of the larynx without other abnormalities. The syndrome is believed to be transmitted as an autosomal dominant trait. The locus for this disorder is assigned to chromosome 6.

Mace, M., *et al.* Autosomal dominantly inherited adductor laryngeal paralysis-a new syndrome with a suggestion of linkage to HLA. *Clin. Genet.*, 1978, 14:265-70.

adenoacanthoma of sweat glands. See *Lever adenoacanthoma.*

adenoid epithelioma. See *Brooke epithelioma.*

adenoid squamous cell carcinoma. See *Lever adenoacanthoma.*

adenolymphoma. See *Warthin tumor.*

adenoma sebaceum disseminatum. See *Bourneville-Pringle syndrome.*

ADHD. See *attention deficit-hyperactivity disorder.*

adherence syndrome. See *Johnson syndrome, under Johnson, Lorand Victor.*

adherence syndrome of the lateral or superior rectus muscles. See *Johnson syndrome, under Johnson, Lorand Victor.*

adherent lateral syndrome. See *Johnson syndrome, under Johnson, Lorand Victor.*

adherent omentum syndrome. See *omentum adhesion syndrome.*

adhesive bursitis. See *Duplay bursitis.*

adhesive capsulitis. See *Duplay bursitis.*

ADIE, WILLIAM JOHN (British neurologist, 1886-1935)

Adie syndrome. Synonyms: *Adie-Holmes syndrome, Kehrer-Adie syndrome, Markus syndrome, Markus-Adie syndrome, Saenger syndrome, Weill syndrome, Weill-Reys syndrome, Weill-Reys-Adie syndrome, iridoplegia interna, myotonic pupil, myotonic pupillary reaction, nonluetic Argyll Robertson pupil, pseudo-Argyll Robertson syndrome, pseudotabes, pseudotabes pupillotonica, pupillotonia, tonic pupil, tonic pupil syndrome.*

A neurological phenomenon in which one or both slightly enlarged pupils respond slowly or not all to light, accompanied by slow constriction and relaxation in the change from near to distant vision, impaired accommodation, and absent tendon reflexes, particularly ankle and knee jerk. See also *Ross syndrome.*

Adie, W. J. Pseudo-Argyll Robertson pupils with absent tendon reflexes. A benign disorder simulating tabes dorsalis. *Brit. Med. J.*, 1931, 1:928-30. Holmes, G. Partial iridoplegia associated with symptoms of other diseases of the nervous system. *Tr. Ophth. Soc. U. K.*, 1931, 51:209-28. Weill, G., & Reys, L. Sur la pupillotonie. Contribution à l'étude de sa pathogénie. A propos d'un cas de réaction tonique d'une pupille a la convergence et parésie de l'accommodation avec aréflexie a la lumière chez un sujet ateint de crises tétaniformes et d'aréflexie des membres inférieurs. *Rev. Otoneurocul., Paris*, 1926, 4:433-41. Kehrer, F. Die Kuppelungen von Pupillenstörungen mit Aufhebung der Sehnenreflexe, Adie-Syndrome, Pupillotonie, Pseudotabes, konstitutionelle Areflexie. Leipzig, Thieme, 1937. *Saenger, A. Myotonische Pupillenbewegung. Zbl. Neur., 1902, 21:837. Markus, C. Notes on a peculiar pupil phenomenon in two cases of partial iridoplegia. Lancet, 1905, 2:1257.

Adie-Holmes syndrome. See *Adie syndrome.*

Kehrer-Adie syndrome. See *Adie syndrome.*

Markus-Adie syndrome. See *Adie syndrome.*

Weill-Reys-Adie syndrome. See *Adie syndrome.*

adiponecrosis a frigore. See *Haxthausen panniculitis.*

adiponecrosis subcutanea neonatorum. See *Haxthausen panniculitis.*

adiposalgia. See *Dercum syndrome.*

adiposalgia arthriticohypertonica. See *Gram syndrome.*

adiposalgia genus medialis. See *Gram syndrome.*

adipose gynandrism. See *Simpson syndrome, under Simpson, Samuel Leonard.*

adipose gynism. See *Simpson syndrome, under Simpson, Samuel Leonard.*

adiposis dolorosa. See *Dercum syndrome.*

adiposis dolorosa-arthritis genuum-hypertensio arterialis. See *Gram syndrome.*

adipositas dolorosa. See *Dercum syndrome.*

adipositas osteoporotica endocrinica. See *Cushing syndrome.*

adipositas tuberosa simplex. See *Dercum syndrome.*

adiposogenital dystrophy. See *Fröhlich syndrome, under Fröhlich, Alfred.*

ADOD (arthrodento-osteodysplasia). See *Hajdu-Cheney syndrome.*

adolescent cataract and infertility syndrome. A syndrome of cataracts and sterility in adolescent boys, associated with elevated follicle-stimulating hormone levels indicating testicular failure.

Lubinsky, M. S. Cataracts and testicular failure in three brothers. *Am. J. Med. Genet.*, 1983, 16:149-52.

adolescent kyphosis. See *Scheuermann disease.*

adolescent sexual asphyxia syndrome. See *sexual asphyxia syndrome.*

ADR. See *ataxia-deafness-retardation syndrome.*

adrenal apoplexy. See *Waterhouse-Friderichsen syndrome.*

adrenal cortical insufficiency. See *Addison disease.*

adrenal crisis. See *Addison crisis.*

adrenal hemorrhage syndrome. See *Waterhouse-Friderichsen syndrome.*

adrenal medullary neuroblastoma. See *Hutchinson disease, under Hutchinson, Sir Robert Grieve.*

adrenal virilizing syndrome. See *congenital adrenal hyperplasia.*

adrenalin-secreting neuroblastoma. See *Hutchinson disease, under Hutchinson, Sir Robert Grieve.*

adrenocortical atrophy-cerebral sclerosis syndrome. See *adrenoleukodystrophy.*

adrenogenital syndrome (AGS). See *congenital adrenal hyperplasia.*

adrenoleukodystrophy (ALD). Synonyms: *Addison disease-cerebral sclerosis syndrome, Addison-Schilder syndrome, Fanconi-Prader syndrome, Siemerling-Creutzfeldt syndrome, adrenocortical atrophy-cerebral sclerosis syndrome, adrenomyeloneuropathy, melanodermic leukodystrophy.*

A hereditary syndrome transmitted as an X-linked trait, combining the characteristics of Addison's disease and cerebral sclerosis (Schilder disease). Skin bronzing and adrenal insufficiency associated with extensive demyelination and sclerosis of the brain are the principal features. The cerebral lesions may present behavior disturbances and deteriorating mental and motor abnormalities in boys, usually seen between 5 and 15 years. The first symptoms, consisting of difficulties in learning, ataxia, or seizures, are often associated with emotional instability. In other patients, neurological symptoms may be discrete or absent, and the clinical picture is dominated by adrenal insufficiency. The course is progressive, and additional symptoms may include hemianopsia, cortical blindness, hemiparesis, aphasia, seizures, quadriplegia, and death, although some patients may survive into the fifth decade. Female carriers are unaffected, but most show hyperpigmentation. It is a metabolic disorder with accumulation of esters of cholesterol with fatty acids of abnormally long chains. It is presumed that abnormal lipid composition of myelin leads to instability, causing myelin disintegration and suggesting classification of this syndrome with demyelinating disorders or leukodystrophies.

Fanconi, A., Prader, A., *et al.* Morbus Addison mit Hirnsklerose im Kindesalter. Ein Hereditäres Syndrom mit X-chromosomaler Vererbung? *Helvet. Paediat. Acta*, 1963, 18:480-501. Siemerling, E., & Creutzfeldt, H. G. Bronzekrankheit und sklerosierende Encephalomyelitis. (Diffuse Sklerose). *Arch. Psychiat., Berlin*, 1923, 68:217-44. Addison, T. Anaemia. Disease of the supra-renal capsules. *London Hosp. Gaz.*, 1849, 43:517-8. Schilder, P. Zur Kenntnis der sogenannten diffusen Sklerose (über Encephalitis periaxialis diffusa). *Zschr. Neur.*, 1912, 10:1-60.

adrenomyeloneuropathy. See *adrenoleukodystrophy.*

ADSON, ALFRED WASHINGTON (American physician, 1887-1951)

Adson syndrome. See *cervical rib syndrome.*

Adson-Caffey syndrome. See *cervical rib syndrome.*

adult amaurotic familial idiocy. See *Kufs syndrome.*

adult ceroid lipofuscinosis. See *Kufs syndrome.*

adult cretinism. See *Gull syndrome.*

adult ganglioside lipidosis. See *Kufs syndrome.*

adult hyaline membrane disease. See *adult respiratory distress syndrome.*

adult myxedema. See *Gull syndrome.*

adult osteosclerosis. See *Albers-Schönberg syndrome.*

adult respiratory distress syndrome (ARDS). Synonyms: *acute alveolar injury, adult hyaline membrane disease, adult respiratory failure, adult respiratory insufficiency syndrome, congestive atelectasis, DaNang lung, diffuse alveolar damage (DAD), hemorrhagic atelectasis, hemorrhagic lung syndrome, hypoxic hyperventilation, post-traumatic atelectasis, post-traumatic lung failure, post-traumatic pulmonary insufficiency, progressive respiratory distress, shock lung, transplant lung, traumatic wet lung, white lung.*

An acute, life-threatening, respiratory complication of some systemic conditions, such as shock (including hemorrhagic shock); multiple transfusions; trauma, especially chest injuries, long bone fractures with the potential for fat embolism, head trauma, gunshot injuries, and crush injuries; bacterial, viral, fungal, and protozoan infections; chemical and drug intoxication; metabolic disorders, such as ketoacidosis; inhalation of toxic gases; pulmonary aspiration; heart surgery with extracorporeal perfusion; pulmonary embolism; and pulmonary edema in eclampsia and pre-eclampsia. The symptoms include at first tachycardia, tachypnea, and respiratory alkalosis, which are followed by a latent period of several hours and, subsequently, by hyperventilation, hypercapnia, labored breathing, and widening of the alveolar-arterial oxygen gradient. The next phase includes acute respiratory failure marked by tachypnea and dyspnea, decreased lung compliance, and x-ray signs (diffuse pulmonary infiltration of the alveolar type and white lung). Finally, there is hypoxemia that does not respond to therapy, intrapulmonary shunting and metabolic and respiratory acidosis. Pathological changes include diffuse damage to the alveolar wall, pulmonary edema, alveolar lining, and interstitial cells.

Ashbaugh, D. G., *et al.* Acute respiratory distress in adults. *Lancet,* 1967, 2:319-23. Taylor, R. W. The adult respiratory distress syndrome. In: Kirby, R. R., & Taylor, R. W., eds. *Respiratory failure.* Chicago, Year Book, 1986, pp. 208-44.

adult respiratory failure. See *adult respiratory distress syndrome.*

adult respiratory insufficiency syndrome. See *adult respiratory distress syndrome.*

advanced sleep phase syndrome (ASPS). A sleep-wake schedule disorder characterized by habitual sleep onset and wake time that are several hours earlier than desired.

Kamei, R., *et al.* Advanced-sleep phase syndrome studied in a time isolation facility. *Chronobiologia,* 1979, 6:115.

adynamia episodica hereditaria. See *Gamstorp syndrome.*

adynamic bowel syndrome. Congenital intestinal obstruction in newborn infants associated with decreased bowel motility, vomiting, abdominal distention, and constipation, differing from Hirschsprung disease by the absence of bowel sounds.

Kapila, L., *et al.* Chronic adynamic bowel simulating Hirschsprung's disease. *J. Pediat. Surg.,* 1975, 10:885-92.

AEC (ankyloblepharon-**e**ctodermal dysplasia-**c**left lip) syndrome. Synonym: *Hay-Wells symdrome.*

A familial syndrome of ankyloblepharon, ectodermal defects (hypotrichosis or alopecia, absent or dystrophic nails, pointed and widely spaced teeth, and partial anhidrosis), and cleft lip and palate. Supernumerary nipples, hyperpigmentation, syndactyly, photophobia, lacrimal duct atresia, and deformed ears may be associated. Inheritance is consistent with that of an autosomal dominant trait.

Hay, R. J., & Wells, R. S. The syndrome of ankyloblepharon, ectodermal defects and cleft lip and palate: An autosomal dominant condition. *Brit. J. Derm.,* 1976, 94:277-89.

AES. See ***a**uto-**e**rythrocyte **s**ensitization syndrome.*

AFA. See ***a**cromegaloid **f**acial **a**ppearance syndrome.*

AFD (acro**f**acial **d**ysostosis). See *Nager-de Reynier syndrome, and see Weyers syndrome (3).*

affectives syndrome. See *organic affective syndrome.*

afferent loop syndrome. See *postgastrectomy syndrome.*

AFRAX (autism-**fra**gile-**X**) syndrome. See *chromosome X fragility.*

African anemia. See *sickle cell anemia.*

African lymphoma. See *Burkitt lymphoma.*

African macroglobulinemia. See *Charmot syndrome.*

afterburn peripheral endocrine gland involvement syndrome. Reduction of blood testosterone and follicle-stimulating hormone following burn trauma in male patients.

Dolecek, R., *et al.* Syndrome of afterburn peripheral endocrine gland involvement. Very low plasma testosterone levels in burned male patients. *Acta Chir. Plast., Prague,* 1979, 21:114-9.

AFZELIUS, ARVID (Swedish physician)

Afzelius erythema. See *Lipschütz erythema.*

AGA (allergic **g**ranulomatosis and **a**ngiitis). See *Churg-Strauss syndrome.*

agammaglobulinemia, X-linked. See *Bruton syndrome.*

aganglionic megacolon. See *Hirschsprung syndrome.*

aganglíosis of the entire colon. See *Jirásek-Zuelzer-Wilson syndrome.*

aging brain syndrome (ABS). Neurological and psychological changes believed to be produced by aging processes in the brain, including confusion, headache, vertigo, fatigability, apprehension, irritability, lack of initiative, uncooperative behavior, emotional lability, depression, sense of failure, and difficulties in adapting to social conditions.

Passeri, M., *et al.* Studio clinico controllato sull'attivita del teprosilato di vincamina nella cosiddetta "aging brain syndrome." *Gior. Clin. Med.,* 1982, 63:874-87.

aglomerular segmental kidney hypoplasia. See *Ask-Upmark syndrome.*

aglossia-adactylia syndrome. See *Hanhart syndrome (2).*

agoraphobic syndrome. A phobic neurosis marked by a fear of being alone or in public places from which escape might be difficult or impossible or help not readily available in case of a sudden need. The condition occurs with or without attacks of panic.

Moor, W., de. The topography of agoraphobia. *Am. J. Psychother.,* 1985, 39:371-88.

AGR (aniridia-ambiguous **g**enitalia-mental **r**etardation) syndrome. Synonym: *AGR triad.*

A congenital syndrome characterized by aniridia, genitourinary anomalies (hypospadias, cryptorchism, and obstructive uropathy), mental retardation, distinctive facies (blepharoptosis, prominent nasal bridge, prominent lower lip, prominent forehead, cranial asymmetry, malformed pinnae), high and narrow palate, short neck, scoliosis, inguinal hernia, partial blindness, nystagmus, glaucoma, pale fundus or optic disk, cataracts, clinodactyly, hyperactive deep tendon reflexes, hallucal open-field patterns, and digital radial loops. The syndrome may be associated with Wilms tumor (see **aniridia-Wilms tumor syndrome).** Interstitial deletion of the short arm of chromosome 11 is a constant feature.

Riccardi, V. M., *et al.* Chromosomal imbalance in the aniridia-Wilms' tumor association: 11p interstitial deletion. *Pediatrics,* 1978, 61:604-10.

AGR triad. See *AGR syndrome.*

agranulocytic angina. See *Schultz syndrome.*

agranulocytosis. See *Schultz syndrome.*

agranulocytosis infantilis hereditaria. See *Kostmann syndrome.*

AGS (adrenogenital **s**yndrome). See *congenital adrenal hyperplasia.*

AGUECHEEK, SIR ANDREW (A shakespearean character known for his desire to please albeit frustrated by his intellectual limitations, who consumed large quantities of beef and was suspected of suffering from liver disease)

Aguecheek disease. Synonym: *meat intoxication.*

A chronic dementia in liver diseases due to intolerance of nitrogenous substances, occurring after ingestion of large amounts of proteins, in liver cirrhosis, or after portacaval shunt operation. The condition is characterized by personality changes and gradual intellectual deterioration.

Summerskill, W. H. J. Aguecheek's disease. *Lancet*, 1955, 2:288.

agyria syndrome. See *Miller-Dieker syndrome, under Miller, James Q.*

agyria-pachygyria syndrome. See *Miller-Dieker syndrome, under Miller, James Q.*

AH. See *alveolar hemorrhage syndrome.*

AHASUERUS (The Wandering Jew who was condemned to restless wandering till the Judgment Day as punishment for insulting Christ on the way to the cross)

Ahasuerus syndrome. See *Munchausen syndrome.*

AHD (**a**rterio**h**epatic **d**ysplasia) syndrome. See *Alagille syndrome.*

AHUMADA, JUAN CARLOS (Argentine physician)

Ahumada-Del Castillo syndrome. See *amenorrhea-galactorrhea syndrome.*

AICARDI, J. (French physician)

Aicardi syndrome. Synonyms: *chorioretinal anomalies-corpus callosum agenesis-infantile spasms syndrome, corpus callosum agenesis-chorioretinopathy-infantile spasms syndrome, corpus callosum agenesis-ocular anomalies-salaam seizures syndrome.*

A hereditary syndrome, probably transmitted as an X-linked dominant trait with male lethality, characterized by infantile spasms, typical bowing of the head (salaam seizures), chorioretinal lacunae, mental and motor retardation, agenesis of the the corpus callosum, and costovertebral anomalies. Ocular changes include, microphthalmia, eyelid twitching, absent pupillary reflexes, and funnel-shaped disks. Epileptic seizures, cyanosis, telangiectasia, hypotonia, craniofacial anomalies (frontal bossing, occipital flattening, plagiocephaly), cortical heterotopia, and electroencephalographic abnormalities are associated.

Aicardi, J., *et al.* A new syndrome: Spasm in flexion, callosal agenesis, ocular abnormalities. *Electroencephal. Clin. Neurophysiol.*, 1965, 19:609-10 Aicardi, J., *et al.* Le syndrome spasmes en flexion, agénésie calleuse anomalies chorio-rétiniennes. *Arch. Fr. Pediat.*, 1969, 26:1103-20.

AIDP (**a**cute **i**nflammatory **d**emyelinating **p**olyradiculoneuropathy). See *Guillain-Barré syndrome.*

AIDS. See *acquired immunodeficiency syndrome.*

AIDS-dementia complex (ADC). See *acquired immunodeficiency-dementia complex.*

AIDS-related complex (ARC). See *under acquired immunodeficiency syndrome.*

AIKENS

McLetchie-Aikens syndrome. See *under McLetchie.*

ainhoum. See *ainhum syndrome.*

ainhum syndrome. Synonyms: *ainhoum, ayun, bankokerende, dactylolysis essentialis, dactylolysis spontanea, ombaja, sukha pekla.*

A disorder, occurring chiefly in South and Central America and Africa, characterized by formation of a ring-like strip of hardened skin on the little toe at the level of the digitoplantar fold, progressing to spontaneous amputation of the digit. Most cases are essential but familial occurrence has been also reported.

Da Silva Lima, J. F. Estudio sobre o ainhum molesta ninda naeo descripta peculiará vaça etiopa, e affectado os de dos minimos dos pés. *Gaz. Med. Lisboa*, 1867, p. 321; 350; 378; 410.

AINS (**a**nterior **i**nterosseous **n**erve **s**yndrome). See *Kiloh-Nevin syndrome (1).*

AIP. See *acute intermittent porphyria.*

air freshener syndrome. A syndrome of feeling of unreality, headache, nausea, lassitude, ataxia, and tremor believed to be related to an exposure to air fresheners.

Lawson, R. H. Is there an air freshener syndrome? *Bristol Med. Chir. J.*, 1985, 100:10-3.

air leak syndrome. A disorder of newborn infants, characterized by air escape from the tracheobronchial tree. It is caused by overdistention resulting from the application of bag ventilation, high inspiratory pressure on the ventilator coupled with infant crying, or ball-valve mechanism, the airways expanding during inspiration thus allowing air to enter the alveoli around the aspirate. As the airways narrow during expiration, the aspirate blocks the passageway, preventing the air from being exhaled. The air buildup eventually ruptures the alveolar sac. The escaping air dissects toward the hilum into the mediastinum creating a pneumomediastinum.

Gregory, S. E. B. Air leak syndromes. *Neonatal Netw.*, 1987, 5:40-6.

air-fluid lock syndrome. A syndrome occurring most commonly in elderly patients with poor bowel tonus who lie in one position for prolonged periods. Fluid accumulates in dependent loops of the atonic bowel and cannot be pushed out, thus producing bowel obstruction.

Gammill, S. L. Air-fluid lock syndrome. *Radiology*, 1974, 111:27-30. Singleton, A. O., Jr., & Wilson, M. Air-fluid obstruction of the colon. *South. Med. J.*, 1967, 60:909-13.

AIRD, R. B. (American physician)

Flynn-Aird syndrome. See *under Flynn.*

airflow limitation. See *airway obstruction syndrome.*

airway interference syndrome. See *airway obstruction syndrome.*

airway obstruction syndrome. Synonyms: *airflow limitation, airway interference syndrome, bronchospastic syndrome, chronic obstructive bronchitis, chronic obstructive pulmonary disease (COPD), obstructive lung disease, obstructive pulmonary syndrome, obstructive ventilatory abnormality.*

Interference with airflow through the respiratory passages due to mechanical obstructions, such as foreign bodies, reactions of hyperreactive airways to noxious stimuli with resulting bronchospasm and mucous hypersecretion and edema, and respiratory diseases, including asthma, emphysema, and bronchitis. Alveolar hypoventilation with resulting hypoxemia, hypoxia, and hypercapnia are the early results of the obstruction. Other disorders include an increase in oxygen consumption by the respiratory muscles in their effort to overcome the obstruction; added strain on the right heart, often leading to cor pulmonale with pulmonary edema and dyspnea on exertion; and pulmonary hypertension due to the effort of pumping blood through and around the constricted vessels. Polycythemia is a compensatory reaction to hypoxemia. See also *sleep apnea syndrome* and *Pickwich syndrome*..

Burrows, B., Knudson, R. J., Quan, S. F., & Kettel, L. J. *Respiratory disorders. A pathophysiologic approach.* 2nd ed. Chicago, Year Book, 1983.

AIS (androgen-insensitivity syndrome). See *testicular feminization syndrome.*

AIS (anterior interosseous nerve syndrome). See *Kiloh-Nevin syndrome (1).*

akathisia syndrome. Motor restlessness after the administration of antipsychotic drugs.

Hodge, J. R. Akathisia: The syndrome of motor restlessness. *Am. J. Psychiat.*, 1959, 116:337-8.

AKE (acrokeratoelastoidosis). See *Costa disease.*

akinesia algera. See *Moebius syndrome (1).*

akinesia intermittens angiosclerotica. See *Determann syndrome.*

AKS (alcoholic Korsakoff syndrome). See *Korsakoff syndrome, under Korsakov.*

ALAGILLE, D. (French physician)

Alagille syndrome. Synonyms: *Watson-Miller syndrome, arteriohepatic dysplasia (AHD) syndrome, cardiovertebral syndrome, cholestasis-peripheral pulmonary stenosis syndrome, hepatic ductal hypoplasia-multiple malformations syndrome, hepatofacioneurocardiovertebral syndrome, paucity of interlobular bile ducts (PILBD).*

A congenital familial syndrome, transmitted as an autosomal dominant trait with variable penetrance, marked by intrahepatic cholestasis due to hypoplasia of the interlobular biliary duct; dysmorphic (flat) facies (prominent forehead, deep-set eyes, mild hypertelorism, straight nose, and small pointed chin), sometimes referred to as **cholestasis facies**; hoarse voice due to vocal cord nodules; and a variety of other disorders, including posterior embryotoxon, heart murmur, vertebral arch defect, growth and mental retardation, hypogonadism, portal hypertension, neonatal jaundice, pulmonary stenosis, skeletal anomalies, xanthomas, pruritus, clay-colored stools, and hepatosplenomegaly. Skeletal anomalies may include fused vertebrae, tibial exostoses, and butterfly-like vertebrae. Palmar erythema and multiple small telangiectases of the trunk, especially along the costal margins, are the main cutaneous manifestations. Serum lipid and cholesterol levels are generally high, while the serum bilirubin concentration may be normal or moderately elevated. Alkaline phospatase and, to a lesser degree, transminase levels are increased.

Alagille, D., *et al.* Hepatic ductular hypoplasia associated with characteristic facies, vertebral malformations, retarded physical, mental, and sexual development, and cardiac murmur. *J. Pediat.*, 1975, 86:63-71. Watson, G. H., & Miller, V. Arteriohepatic dysplasia. Familial pulmonary arterial stenosis with neonatal liver disease. *Arch. Dis. Child.*, 1973, 48:459-66.

ALAJOUANINE, THEOPHILE (French physician, born 1890)

Alajouanine syndrome. A congenital syndrome consisting of symmetric lesions of the sixth and seventh cranial nerves with double facial paralysis limited to lateral movements, associated with double clubfoot and convergent strabismus.

Alajouanine, T., *et al.* Quatre cas d'une affection congénitale caracteerisée par double pied bot, une double paralysie faciale et une double paralysie de la sixieme paire. *Rev. Neur., Paris,* 1930, 2:501-11.

Foix-Alajouanine syndrome. See *under Foix.*

Åland eye disease. See *Forsius-Eriksson syndrome.*

alarm reaction. See *under Selye syndrome.*

albatross syndrome. A postgastrectomy syndrome in patients with personality disorders, characterized by persistent abdominal pain without demonstrable cause, intermittent and inexplicable nausea and vomiting, continued analgesic drug dependence, and nutrition deficiencies. The affected patients fall into three groups: those with true peptic ulcer, those with salicylate addiction, and those without positive signs of ulcer but with chronic complaints.

Johnstone, F. R. C., *et al.* Post-gastrectomy problems in patients with personality defects: The "albatross" syndrome. *Canad. Med. Assoc. J.*, 1967, 96:1559-64.

ALBERS, F. H. (Dutch physician)

Taussig-Snellen-Albers syndrome. See *under Taussig.*

ALBERS-SCHÖNBERG, HEINRICH ERNST (German physician, 1865-1921)

Albers-Schönberg syndrome. Synonyms: *adult osteosclerosis, condensing disseminated osteopathy, ivory bones, late osteosclerosis, marble disease, marble bone disease, osteopetrosis with late manifestations, osteosclerosis fragilitas generalisata.*

A bone dysplasia with variable onset, characterized mainly by multiple fractures. Associated disorders usually include anemia, hepatomegaly, poor dentition, visual disorders, hearing disorders, facial paralysis, osteomyelitis of the mandible and maxilla, low blood calcium, and elevated serum phosphorus. The bones are thick, dense, and fragile with loss of trabeculae. Obtuse mandibular angle, hypoplasia of distal phalanges, "bone within bone" metacarpals, macrocephaly, frontal bossing, and bone marrow compression are usually associated. The syndrome is transmitted as an autosomal recessive trait.

Albers-Schönberg, H. E. Röntgenbilder einer seltenen Knochenerkrankung. *Münch. Med. Wschr.*, 1904, 51:365.

ALBERT, EDUARD (Austrian physician, 1841-1900)

Albert syndrome. Synonyms: *achillobursitis, achillodynia.*

Painful inflammation of the bursa located between the os calcis and the Achilles tendon.

Albert, E. Achillodynie. *Wien. Med. Presse,* 1893, 34:41-3.

ALBERT MOUCHET. See MOUCHET, ALBERT

ALBERTINI, AMBROSIUS (Swiss physician, 1894-1971)

Fanconi-Albertini-Zellweger syndrome. See *under Fanconi.*

albinism syndrome. See *NOACH syndrome.*

albinism I syndrome. Synonyms: *Garrod albinism, albinism Ty neg, oculocutaneous tyrosinase-negative albinism (OCA Ty neg), tyrosinase-negative albinism.*

A classic form of albinism, transmitted as an autosomal recessive trait, marked by total absence of pigment in the skin, hair, and eyes, and absence of pigment formation by hair roots incubated in *L*-tyrosine solution (tyrosinase test). Severe photophobia, pink to reddish skin, pigmented nevi, blue to gray eyes, severe myopia, and nystagmus are the principal clinical features of this disorder. There is a high incidence of skin neoplasms.

Garrod, A. E. Inborn errors of metabolism. *Lancet*, 1908, 2:1-7. Klein, T. P. Les diverses formes hereditaires de l'albinisme. *Bull. Acad. Suisse Sc.*, 1961, 17:351-64.

albinism II syndrome. Synonyms: *albinism Ty pos, oculocutaneous tyrosinase-positive albinism (OCA Ty pos), tyrosinase-positive albinism.*

A form of albinism, transmitted as an autosomal recessive trait, marked by decreased amounts of pigments in skin, hair, and eyes, and formation of pigment by hair roots incubated in *L*-tyrosine solution (tyrosinase test). Skin coloration varying from pink-white to cream, white to yellow or reddish hair, blue to yellow or brown eyes, initially severe but eventually improving visual acuity, moderate nystagmus and photophobia, and pigmented nevi are the principal clinical features of this syndrome.

Trevor-Roper, P. D. Marriage of two complete albinos with normally pigmented offspring. *Brit. J. Ophth.*, 1952, 36:107-10. Witkop, C. J., Jr. *et al.* Evidence for two forms of autosomal recessive albinism in man. *Proc. Soc. Intern. Cong. Hum. Genet*, Rome, Sept. 6-12, 1961, 1963, 2:1064-5.

albinism Ty neg. See *albinism I syndrome.*

albinism Ty pos. See *albinism II syndrome.*

albinism-deafness syndrome (autosomal dominant). See *Tietz syndrome.*

albinism-deafness syndrome (X-linked). See *Woolf syndrome.*

albinism-hemorrhagic diathesis syndrome. See *Hermansky-Pudlak syndrome.*

albinism-immunodeficiency syndrome. A familial syndrome, believed to be transmitted as an autosomal recessive trait, characterized by immunodeficiency, partial albinism, frequent pyogenic infections, and acute episodes of fever, neurotropenia, and thrombocytopenia. There are large clumps of pigment in the hair shafts and an accumulation of melanosomes in melanocytes. Melanocytes have few short dendritic expansions and keratinocytes are hypopigmented. Hypogammaglobulinemia in the presence of an adequate number of T and B lymphocytes is a constant feature. The affected patients are incapable of manifesting delayed skin hypersensitivity or of rejecting skin grafts.

Griscelli, C., *et al.* A syndrome associating partial albinism and immunodeficiency. *Am. J. Med.*, 1978, 65:691-702.

albinism-piebaldism syndrome. See *Woolf syndrome.*

ALBRECHT, HEINRICH (Austrian physician)

Albrecht-Arzt-Warthin tumor. See *Warthin tumor.*

ALBRIGHT, FULLER (American physician, 1900-1969)

Albright hereditary osteodystrophy. See *Albright syndrome (1).*

Albright syndrome (1). Synonyms: *Albright hereditary osteodystrophy, pseudohypoparathyroidism (PHP, PHPT), pseudohypoparathyroidism syndrome, pseudopseudohypoparathyroidism (PPHP), Seabright Bantam syndrome.*

A syndrome of uncertain etiology, occurring in two forms: (1) a hypocalcemic form with hyperphosphatemia, defective urinary excretion of adenosine-3'5'-monophosphate that is similar to hypoparathyrodism except for not responding to tubular phosphate resorption after parathyroid hormone infusion (**pseudohypoparathyroidism** or **PHP**); and (2) a normocalcemic form (**pseudopseudohypoparathyroidism** or **PPHP**). Most PHP patients exhibit short stature and obesity, whereas those with PPHP are usually taller and less obese. A characteristically rounded face is typical of PHP but it is less common in PPHP. Shortening of the fingers and toes due to abbreviation of the fourth metacarpals is the most common feature of this syndrome. Cone-shaped epiphyses of the hands and curvature of the radius with displacement of distal epiphyses and carpal bones may be associated. Mental retardation occurs in most cases of PHP and, less frequently, in PPHP. Cataracts are more common in PHP than PPHP. Enamel hypoplasia, wide root canals, and delayed tooth eruption have been noted in some PHP patients. Subcutaneous calcification of the scalp and extremities is frequent in both forms.

Albright, F., *et al.* Pseudo-hypoparathyrodism-example of "Seabright Bantam" syndrome. *Endrocrinology*, 1942, 30:92-32. Albright, F., *et al.* Pseudo-pseudohypoparathyrodism. *Tr. Assoc. Am. Physicians*, 1952, 65:337-50.

Albright syndrome (2). See *McCune-Albright syndrome.*

Albright syndrome (3). See *Lightwood-Albright syndrome.*

Albright-Butler-Bloomberg syndrome. See *hypophosphatemic familial rickets.*

Albright-Hadorn syndrome. A disorder of potassium metabolism associated with osteomalacia and paroxysmal hypokalemic muscular paralysis.

Albright, F., *et al.* Osteomalacia and late rickets. The various etiologies met in the United States with emphasis on that resulting from a specific form of renal acidosis, the therapeutic indications for each etiological sub-group, and the relationship between osteomalacia and Milkman's syndrome. *Medicine, Baltimore*, 1946, 25:399-79. Hadorn, W. Osteomalacie mit paroxysmaler hypokaliamischer Muskellahmung: ein neues Syndrom. *Schweiz. Med. Wschr.*, 1948, 78:1238-42.

Albright-McCune-Sternberg syndrome. See *McCune-Albright syndrome.*

Butler-Albright syndrome. See *Lightwood-Albright syndrome.*

Butler-Lightwood-Albright syndrome. See *Lightwood-Albright syndrome.*

Forbes-Albright syndrome. See *amenorrhea-galactorrhea syndrome.*

Fuller Albright syndrome. See *McCune-Albright syndrome.*

Klinefelter-Reifenstein-Albright syndrome. See *chromosome XXY syndrome.*

Lightwood-Albright syndrome. See *under Lightwood.*

McCune-Albright syndrome. See *under McCune.*

Morgagni-Turner-Albright syndrome. See *chromosome XO syndrome.*

Turner-Albright syndrome. See *chromosome XO syndrome.*

Weil-Albright syndrome. See *McCune-Albright syndrome.*

alcohol abstinence syndrome (AAS). See *under withdrawal syndrome.*

alcohol amnestic syndrome. See *Wernicke-Korsakoff syndrome.*

alcohol dependence syndrome. Synonym: *alcoholism.*

Chronic excessive consumpation of ethanol marked by the need of alcohol for adequate functioning, along with occasional heavy consumption and continuation of drinking despite family and social problems resulting from alcohol abuse, associated with increased ethanol tolerance or physical signs on withdrawal from alcohol. Heavy use of alcohol can result in blackouts and chronic drinking may cause a variety of clinical disorders, including peripheral neuropathy (probably due to thiamine deficiency), Wernicke and Korsakov syndromes, cerebellar degeneration, cortical disorders, permanent nervous system impairment **(alcoholic dementia)**, esophagitis, gastritis, Mallory-Weiss syndrome, intestinal hemorrhage, chronic pancreatitis, liver cirrhosis, hepatitis, anemia, folic acid deficiency, thrombocytopenia, increased heart rate and output, cardiac arrhythmias, amenorrhea, fetal alcohol syndrome, impotence, muscle diseases **(alcoholic myopathy)**, and other disorders.

Diagnostic and statistical manual of mental disorders. 3rd ed. Washington, American Psychiatric Association, 1980, pp. 167-70. Schuckit, M. A. Alcohol and alcoholism In: Braunwald, E., Isselbacher, K. J., Petersdorf, R. G., Wilson, J. D., Martin, J. B., & Fauci A. S., eds. *Harrison's principles of internal medicine.* 11th ed., New York, McGraw-Hill, 1987, pp. 2106-11.

alcohol migraine. See *under headache syndrome.*

alcohol withdrawal delirium. See *Morel disease, under Morel, Benoit Augustin.*

alcohol withdrawal syndrome (AWS). See *under withdrawal syndrome.*

alcohol-induced pseudo-Cushing syndrome. Synonyms: *Cushing-like syndrome, cushingoid syndrome, pseudo-Cushing syndrome.*

A condition produced by abuse of ethyl alcohol which is characterized by symptoms similar to those in the Cushing syndrome, including tiredness, weight gain, insomnia, confusion, depression, hallucinations, dementia, Cushing-like facies (moon face), truncal obesity, muscle weakness and wasting, easy bruising, abdominal striae, and occassional hyperpigmentation and vertebral collapse. Additionally, most patients develop hypertension, diabetes mellitus, hepatomegaly, Dupuytren contractures, swelling of the parotid glands, and peripheral neuropathy. Laboratory findings usually show macrocytosis and liver function disorders with disturbances of blood transminase levels. The syndrome is generally observed in chronic alcoholics. Alcohol withdrawal results in regression of symptoms. See also *alcohol dependence syndrome.*.

Jenkins, J. S., & Connolly, J. Adrenocortical response to ethanol in man. *Brit. Med. J.*, 1968, 2:804-5.

alcohol-liver-porphyrinuria syndrome. Hepatic porphyria with elevated urinary porphyrin levels developing in alcoholic patients with liver disease.

Doss, M. Alkoholbedingte Störungen des Porphyrinstoffwechsels. *Leber Magen Darm*, 1978, 8:278-85.

alcoholic cirrhosis. See *Laennec cirrhosis.*

alcoholic dementia. See *under alcohol dependence syndrome.*

alcoholic embryopathy. See *fetal alcohol syndrome.*

alcoholic encephalopathy. See *Wernicke syndrome.*

alcoholic hemolytic anemia-hyperlipemic syndrome. See *Zieve syndrome.*

alcoholic hyperlipemia syndrome. See *Zieve syndrome.*

alcoholic kidney. See *Formad kidney.*

alcoholic Korsakoff syndrome (AKS). See *Korsakoff syndrome, under Korsakov.*

alcoholic myopathy. See *alcohol dependence syndrome.*

alcoholic neuro-acropathy. See *Bureau-Barrière syndrome.*

alcoholic-acrodystrophic neuropathy. See *Bureau-Barrière syndrome.*

alcoholism. See *alcohol dependence syndrome.*

ALD. See *adrenoleukodystrophy.*

aldehyde syndrome. Synonym: *aldehydism.*

Increased blood acetaldehyde levels produced by oxidation of ethanol to carbon dioxide and water, whereby ethanol is oxidized in the liver first to acetaldehyde and then to acetate. The enzymes which catalyze this two-step oxidation are alcohol dehydrogenase and aldehyde dehydrogenase. High levels of blood acetaldehyde occur in persons lacking aldehyde dehydrogenase or after treatment with disulfiram. Slightly elevated concentrations of acetaldehyde in the blood may result from specific isoenzyme patterns of alcohol dehydrogeananse, aldehyde dehydrogenase and/or the induction of a microsomal ethanol-oxidizing system. Clinical symptoms of aldehyde syndrome include facial flushing, tachycardia, hypotension, headache, nausea, vomiting, muscle weakness, sleeplessness, and aversion to alcohol. The syndrome has special predilection for some racial and ethnic groups.

Wartburg, J. P., von, & Buhler, R. Biology of disease. Alcoholism and aldehydism: New biomedical concepts. *Lab. Invest.*, 1984, 50:5-15.

aldehydism. See *aldehyde syndrome.*

ALDER, ALBERT, VON (German physician, born 1888)

Alder-Reilly anomaly. Heavy azurophilic granulation of the neutrophils, eosinophils, basophils, monocytes, and lymphocytes. The disorder is inherited as an autosomal dominant trait.

Alder, A. Über konstitutionell bedingte Granulotionsveranderungen der Leukocyten. *Deut. Arch. Klin. Med.*, 1938-39, 183:372-8. Reilly, W. A. The granules in the leukocytes in gargoylism. *Am. J. Dis. Child.*, 1941, 62:489-91.

aldosterone deficiency syndrome. Insufficient aldosterone production associated with negative salt balance and hyperkalemia. Combined deficiency of mineralocorticoid and glucocorticoid hormones with features of Addison disease is associated with hypotension, hyponatremia, hyperkalemia, and azotemia. Selective low production of aldosterone is usually accompanied by renin deficiency, although normal or even high levels of plasma renin activity may occur, as in heparin therapy. Corticosterone methyoxide deficiency also is associated with normal renin activity and reduced plasm aldosterone.

Battle, D. C., & Kurtzman, N. A. Syndromes of aldosterone deficiency and excess. *Med. Clin. North Amer.*, 1983, 67:879-902.

aldosterone-producing adenoma. See *Conn syndrome.*

aldosteronism-normal blood pressure syndrome. See *Bartter syndrome.*

ALDOUS, HAROLD E. (American physician)

Woolf-Dolowitz-Aldous syndrome. See *Woolf syndrome.*

ALDRICH, ROBERT ANDERSON (American physician, born 1917)

Aldrich syndrome. See *Wiskott-Aldrich syndrome.*

Wiskott-Aldrich syndrome (WAS). See *under Wiskott.*

Wiskott-Aldrich-Huntley syndrome. See *Wiskott-Aldrich syndrome.*

ALE, G. (Italian physician)

Alè-Calò syndrome. See *Langer-Giedion syndrome.*

Aleppo boil. See *Alibert disease (2).*

aleukemic reticulosis. See *Letterer-Siwe syndrome.*

ALEXANDER, BENJAMIN (American physician, born 1909)

Alexander syndrome. Synonyms: *congenital factor VII deficiency, idiopathic hypoprothrombinemia, serum prothrombin conversion accelerator (SPCA) deficiency.*

A congenital disorder of both sexes, possibly transmitted as an autosomal recessive trait, in which deficiency of factor VII (serum prothrombin conversion accelerator) results in hemophilia-like hemorrhagic diathesis with epistaxes, deep muscular hematomas, and internal hemorrhages.

Alexander, B., *et al.* Congenital SPCA deficiency: A hitherto unrecognized coagulation defect with hemorrhage rectified by serum and serum fractions. *J. Clin. Invest.*, 1951, 30:596-608.

ALEXANDER, H. L. (American physician)

Wilson-Alexander syndrome. See *under Wilson, Keith S.*

ALEXANDER, M. K. (British pathologist)

Priest-Alexander syndrome. See *Verner-Morrison syndrome.*

ALEXANDER, W. STEWART (British physician)

Alexander disease. See *Alexander syndrome.*

Alexander syndrome. Synonyms: *Alexander disease, demyelinogenic leukodystrophy, dysmyelinogenic leukodystrophy, fibrinoid degeneration of astrocytes, fibrinoid leukodystrophy, macrocephaly with feeblemindedness and encephalopathy with peculiar deposits, megaencephaly with hyaline panneuropathy.*

A familial degenerative disease of the brain of children transmitted as an autosomal recessive trait. The **infantile type** is characterized by a rapidly progressive course, megaencephaly, psychomotor retardation, and seizures. Hydrocephalus due to obstruction of the aqueduct of Sylvius by Rosenthal fibers (hyaline, eosinophilic, and argyrophilic inclusions in astrocytes) may occur is some cases. Most children die during the preschool years; a few survive into the second decade. The **juvenile type** has a later onset and is marked by a protracted course and signs of bulbar palsy, ataxia and, sometimes, mental retardation, occurring without seizures. Rosenthal fibers are found in subapial, subependymal, and perivascular areas of the brain and, in some cases, in the brain stem and spinal cord, being most prominent in the floor of the fourth ventricle. Also found in the astrocytes are enlarged mitochondria with dense matrices and central lamellar structures. Demyelination, with loss of oligodendroglia, is usually present in areas rich in Rosenthal fibers.

Alexander, W. S. Progressive fibrinoid degeneration of fibrillary astrocytes associated with mental retardation in a hydrocephalic infant. *Brain,* 1949, 72:373-81. Rapin, I. Alexander disease. In: Rowland, L. P. ed. *Merritt's textbook of neurology.* 7th ed. Philadelphia, Lea & Febiger, 1984, pp. 441-2.

alexia without agraphia syndrome. Synonym: *pure alexia.*

A syndrome characterized by a marked impairment of reading ability with relatively well preserved spelling and writing in the absence of significant aphasia. It is usually attributed to a lesion in the dominant (often left) occipital lobe (resulting in a right homonymous hemanopia) and a concomitant lesion of the splenium of the corpus callosum.

Benson, D. f., & Geschwind, N. The alexias. In: Winken, P. J., & Bruyn, G. W. eds. *Handbook of clinical neurology.* Vol. 4. Amsterdam, North Holland, 1969. Friedman, R. B. Mechanisms of reading and spelling in a case of alexia without agraphia. *Neuropsychologia,* 1982, 20:533-45.

alexia-aphasia-apraxia syndrome. See *Bianchi syndrome.*

alexithymia. See *alexithymic behavioral syndrome.*

alexithymic behavioral syndrome. Synonym: *alexithymia.*

Inability or difficulty in describing or being aware of one's emotions or moods.

Kaplan, H. I., & Sadock, B. J., eds. *Comprehensive textbook of psychiatry.* 4th ed. Baltimore, Williams & Wilkins, 1984. pp. 2054.

ALEZZANDRINI, A. A. (Argentine physician)

Alezzandrini syndrome. A syndrome of unilteral facial vitiligo, poliosis, deafness, and tapetoretinal degeneration.

Alezzandrini, A. A. Manifestation unilatérale de dégénérescence tapéto-rétinienne, de vitiligo, de poliose, de cheveux blancs et d'hypoacousie. *Ophthalmologica, Basel,* 1964, 147: 409-19.

ALFIDI, RALPH J. (American physician)

Alfidi syndrome. Synonym: *renal-splanchnic steal.*

Occlusion of the celiac axis with resulting collateral flow from the superior mesentery artery and the right renal artery to the splanchnic bed associated with hypertension.

Alfidi, R. J., *et al.* Renal-splanchnic steal. Report of a case. *Cleveland Clin. Quart.,* 1967, 34:43-53.

algodystrophy syndrome. An association of pain and dystrophic changes in bone.

Perrigot, M., *et al.* Le syndrome algodystrophique chez l'hémiplégique. *Ann. Méd. Interne, Paris,* 1982, 133:544-8.

ALIBERT, JEAN LOUIS MARC (French physician, 1768-1837)

Alibert disease (1). Synonyms: *Alibert keloid, Hawkins keloid, cicatricial keloid, false keloid.*

A fibrocellular growth of the skin originating from a hypertrophied cicatrix. At the onset the lesion may be pinkish in color and bordered by an erythhematous halo. As it develops, its color changes to brown and the lesion may become hard and painful. Growths are often multiple, their size varying from that of a pinpoint to several centimeters in diameter. Trauma is the usual precipitating factor.

Alibert. Note sur la kéloïde. *J. Univ. Sc. Méd., Paris,* 1816, 2:207-16. Hawkins, C. H. On warty tumors in cicatrices. *London Med. Gaz.,* 1833, 13:481-2.

Alibert disease (2). Synonyms: *Borovskii disease, Aleppo boil, Baghdad boil, biskra button, chicklero ulcer, cutaneous leishmaniasis, Delhi boil, Kandahar sore, Lahore sore, leishmaniasis tropica, oriental boil, oriental sore.*

A sandfly-borne infection caused by *Leishmania tropica,* most commonly seen in countries in the Middle East, Mediterranean littoral, Africa, and South America. The infection first appears after an incubation period ranging from several weeks to several months in the form of papules on the exposed skin, followed by ulceration and scabs.

*Alibert, J. L. Sur la psyrophlyctide endémique ou pustule d'Alep. *Rev. Méd., Paris,* 1828, 3:63. *Borovskii, P. F. *Kozhnyi leishmaniaz.* Moskva, 1949.

Alibert disease (3). Synonyms: *Alibert mentagra, barber's itch, coccogenous sycosis, ficosis, folliculitis barbae, mentagra, sycosis barbae, sycosis simplex, sycosis staphylogenes.*

An inflammatory disease involving the hair follicles of the bearded region of the face. Early symptoms usually include eczema and burning sensation, followed by the appearance of painful small pustules or papules, each pierced by a hair. When neglected, the condition may become chronic and the lesions may develop crust and undergo granulomatous changes. The infection is transmitted by contaminated brushes, combs, and the like.

*Alibert, J. L. *Déscription des maladies de la peau.* Bruxelles, Wahlen, 1825, Vol. 2, p. 214.

Alibert keloid. See *Alibert disease (1).*

Alibert mentagra. See *Alibert disease (3).*

Alibert-Bazin syndrome. See *mycosis fungoides.*

ALICE IN WONDERLAND (A young girl in Lewis Carroll stories, *Alice in Wonderland* and *Looking through a looking glass*, who in her dreams sometimes imagined herself as being very tall and other times as very short, experienced feelings of depersonalization, and suffered from migraine)

Alice in Wonderland syndrome. Synonyms: *Todd syndrome, depersonalization-migraine syndrome, derealization syndrome.*

A syndrome of distorted time perception and body image, whereby the patient has a feeling that the entire body or parts of it have been altered in shape and size (metamorphosis), associated with visual hallucinations. The majority of patients have personal or family history of migraine. Associated disorders may include apraxia, agnosia, language disorders, feelings of *déjà vu* or *jamais vu*, dreamlike or trancelike states, and delirium. In Lippman's report, one of the patients stated that she felt short and wide as she walked, calling this a "tweedle dum" or "tweedle dee" feeling. Originally the syndrome was believed to be caused by psychotropic drugs but in recent cases there was no evidence of drug toxicity.

Todd, J. The syndrome of Alice in Wonderland. *Canad. Med. Assoc. J.*, 1955, 73:701-4. Lippman, C. W. Certain hallucinatiaons peculiar to migraine. *J. Nerv. Ment. Dis.*, 1952, 116:346-51.

alien hand syndrome. A disorder characterized by (1) inability to recognize the arm as one's own when held by the other arm with the eyes closed; (2) a verbally expressed feeling that movements of the arm are "not under patient's control;" and (3) personification of the arm.

Brion, S., & Jedynak, C. P. Troubles du transfert interhémisphérique (callosal disconnection), à propos de 3 observtions du tumeur du corps calleux: Le signe de la main étrangère. *Rev. Neur., Paris*, 1972, 126:257-66. Bogen, J. E. The callosal syndrome. In: Heilman, K. M., & Velenstein, E., eds. *Clinical neuropsychology*. New York, Oxford Unversity Press, 1979, pp. 308-59. Levine, D. N., & Rinn, W. E. Opticosensory ataxia and alien hand syndrome after posterior cerebral artery territory infarction. *Neurology*, 1986, 36:1094-7.

alimentary toxic oil syndrome. See *toxic oil syndrome.*

alimentary toxicosis. See *Sakamoto disease.*

alkali disease. See *Francis disease.*

alkaline reflux gastritis. See *postgastrectomy syndrome.*

alkalosis syndrome. See *milk-alkali syndrome.*

ALL-Down syndrome. An association of acute lymphoblastic leukemia (ALL) with the Down syndrome.

Krivit, W., & Good, R. A. Simultaneous occurrence of mongolism and leukemia. Report of a nationwide survey. *Am. J. Dis. Child.*, 1957, 94:289. Robinson, L. L., *et al.* Down syndrome and acute leukemia in children: A 10-year retrospective survey from Childrens Cancer Study Group. *J. Pediat.*, 1984, 105:235-42.

ALLEMANN, RICHARD (Swiss physician, 1893-1958)

Allemann syndrome. The association of familial double kidney and clubbed fingers. Facial asymmetry and degeneration of various motor nerves may also occur.

Allenmann, R. Die klinische Bedeutung familiärer Heredopathie und Mutation fur die Urologie. *Zschr. Urol.*, 1936, 641-9.

ALLEN, WILLIAM MYRON (American gynecologist)

Allen-Masters syndrome. Synonyms: *broad ligament laceration syndrome, ligamentum latum laceration syndrome, traumatic laceration of uterine support, universal joint cervix.*

Laceration of the fascial tissue layers in the broad and Mackenrodt ligaments resulting in "universal joint" type of mobility of the cervix. The cervix may be moved in any direction with minimal, if any, movement of the corpus uteri. The condition usually results from surgically traumatic or precipitate delivery or, less frequentely, from induced abortion, particularly as a result of excessive vaginal packing. Complaints include pelvic congestion and pain, menstrual disturbances, dyspareunia, fatigability, pain during intercourse, and backache.

Allen, W. M., & Masters, W. H. Traumatic laceration of uterine support. The clinical syndrome and the operative treatment. *Am. J. Obst.*, 1955, 70:500-13.

allergic angiitis and granulomatosis (AAG). See *Churg-Strauss syndrome.*

allergic cutaneous arteriolitis. See *Gougerot-Ruiter syndrome.*

allergic eczema. See *Besnier prurigo.*

allergic granulomatosis. See *Churg-Strauss syndrome.*

allergic granulomatosis and angiitis (AGA). See *Churg-Strauss syndrome.*

allergic granulomatosis of the myocardium. See *Fiedler myocarditis.*

allergic granulomatous angiitis. See *Churg-Strauss syndrome.*

allergic granulomatous vasculitis. See *Churg-Strauss syndrome.*

allergic irritability syndrome. A condition characterized by a decreased ability to concentrate, bouts of irritability, and temper tantrums that sometimes occur in association with allergic rhinitis.

Klein, G. L., *et al.* The allergic irritability syndrome: Four case reports and a position statement from the Neuroallergy Committee of the American College of Allergy. *Ann. Allergy*, 1985, 55:22-4.

allergic migraine. See *under headache syndrome.*

allergic nonthrombocytopenic purpura. See *Schönlein-Henoch purpura.*

allergic purpura. See *Schönlein-Henoch purpura.*

allergic purpura-arthralgia-gastrointestinal symptoms. See *Schönlein-Henoch purpura.*

allergic rhinitis. See *Bostock catarrh.*

allergic tension-fatigue syndrome. A neurological disorder believed to be caused by food allergy, characterized by hyperkinesia, irritability, insomnia, tiredness, sleepiness, recurrent abdominal pain, pain in the lower limbs, rings under the eyes, suborbital edema, enuresis, migraine, paleness, cough, nasal congestion, and halitosis, which occur in various combinations.

Valverde, E., *et al.* In vitro response of lymphocytes in patients with allergic tension-fatigue syndrome. *Ann. Allergy,* 1980, 45:185-8. Speer, F. The allergic tension-fatigue syndrome. *Ped. Clin. N. America,* 1954, 1:1029.

allergic vasculitis (AV). See *Gougerot-Ruiter syndrome.*

allergosis sepsiformis. See *Wissler syndrome.*

alligator baby. See *Carini syndrome.*

alligator boy. See *Carini syndrome.*

ALLINGHAM, WILLIAM (British physician, 1829-1908)

Allingham ulcer. Synonym: *fissure in ano.*

Painful ulceration and fissure of the anal mucosa.

*Allingham, W. *Fistula, haemorrhoids, painful ulcer, stricture, prolapsus, and other diseases of the rectum, their diagnosis and treatment.* London, Churchill, 1871.

ALLISON, NATHANIEL (American physician, 1876-1932)

Allison atrophy. Synonyms: *astronaut bone demineralization, nonuse bone atrophy.*

Demineralization and atrophy of bone resulting from nonuse.

Allison, N., & Brooks, B. Bone atrophy; a clinical study of the changes in bone which result from nonuse. *Arch. Surg., Chicago,* 1922, 5:499-26.

ALLISON, P. R.

Allison-Johnstone anomaly. See *Barrett syndrome.*

allopurinol hypersensitivity syndrome. A potentially fatal immunological reaction to allopurinol (4-hydroxypyrazolo[3,4-d]pyrimidine), characterized by multiple disorders such as fever, rash, kidney dysfunction, hepatocellular injury, leukocytosis, and eosinophilia.

Singer, J. Z., & Wallace, S. L. The allopurinol hypersensitivity syndrome. Unnecessary morbidity and mortality. *Arthritis Rheum.,* 1986, 29:82-7.

ALMEIDA, FLORIANO PAULO, DE. See DE ALMEIDA, FLORIANO PAULO

alopecia areata. See *Cazenave vitiligo.*

alopecia circumscripta. See *Cazenave vitiligo.*

alopecia mucinosa. See *Pinkus disease, under Pinkus, Hermann Karl Benno.*

alopecia universalis with mental retardation. See *alopecia-mental retardation syndrome.*

alopecia-anosmia-deafness-hypogonadism (AADH) syndrome. A neuroectodermal syndrome, transmitted as an autosomal dominant trait with variable expressivity, characterized by alopecia, anosmia or hyposmia, conductive deafness, microtia and/or atresia of the external auditory canal, hypogonadotrophic hypogonadism, and dental caries. Associated variable disorders may include mild facial asymmetry, mental retardation, congenital heart defect, and cleft palate.

Johnson, V. P., *et al.* A newly recognized neuroectodermal syndrome of familial alopecia, anosmia, deafness, and hypogonadism. *Am. J. Med. Genet.,* 1983, 15:497-506.

alopecia-epilepsy-oligophrenia syndrome. See *Moynahan syndrome (2).*

alopecia-hyperhidrosis-corneal dystrophy syndrome. See *Spanlang-Tappeiner syndrome.*

alopecia-mental retardation (AMR) syndrome. Synonym: *alopecia universalis with mental retardation.*

A syndrome transmitted as an autosomal recessive trait, characterized by alopecia associated with mental retardation. Deafness and convulsions may be present.

Perniola, T., *et al.* Congenital alopecia, psychomotor retardation, convulsions in two sibs of a consanguineous marriage. *J. Inherit. Metab. Dis.,* 1980, 3:49-53. Baraister, M., *et al.* A new alopecia/mental retardation syndrome. *J. Med. Genet.,* 1983, 20:64-5.

ALPERS, BERNARD JACOB (American physician, born 1900)

Alpers syndrome. Synonyms: *Christensen disease, Christensen-Krabbe disease, diffuse cortical sclerosis, familial degeneration of the cerebral gray matter in childhood, poliodysplasia cerebri, poliodystrophia cerebri progressiva, poliodystrophia cerebri progressiva infantilis, progressive cerebral degeneration in infancy, progressive infantile poliodystrophy, progressive poliodystrophy.*

A degenerative disease of the brain. In its familial form, the disorder is transmitted as an autosomal recessive trait and is characterized by seizures and diffuse myoclonus occurring in early infancy. The initial symptoms are followed by choreoathetosis; ataxia; progressive spasticity of the limbs, trunk, and cranial muscles; blindness and optic atrophy; growth retardation; microcephaly; and terminal decortication. Jaundice and fatty degeneration or cirrhosis of the liver in late stages may be due to toxic effects of anticonvulsant drugs used therapeutically. Pathological findings include degeneration of the cerebral gray matter with preservation of the white matter; loss of ganglion cells in the cerebral cortex, basal ganglia, and cerebellum; diffuse degeneration of the cerebral cortex; lipid storage in the microglia cells; and proliferation of astrocytes.

Alpers, B. J. Diffuse progressive degeneration of the gray matter of the cerebrum. *Arch. Neur., Chicago,* 1931, 25:469-505. Christensen, E., & Krabbe, K. H. Poliodystrophia cerebri progressiva (infantilis). Report of a case. *Arch. Neur., Chicago,* 1949, 61:28-43.

alpha chain disease. See *under heavy chain disease.*

alphos. See *Willan lepra.*

alpine syndrome. Synonyms: *Australian alpine syndrome, mild mountain sickness.*

A discrete clinical entity, separate from mountain sickness and hypothermia, observed in some visitors who make day trips to low altitude winter resorts. It is characterized by nausea, vomiting, headache, dizziness, drowsiness, disorientation, and a pale clammy skin. It occurs in individuals who have been fasting, within minutes of arrival at resorts of about 1500 meters of more. A similar condition was observed in young females during the premenstrual phase at about 2000 meters in the Australian Alps.

Peterson, M. J. The Australian alpine syndrome. *Aust. Fam. Physician,,* 1982, 11:737-41. Sutton, J., & Lazarus, L. Mountain sickness in the Australian Alps. *Med. J. Australia,* 1973, 1:545-6.

ALPORT, ARTHUR CECIL (British physician)

Alport syndrome (AS). Synonyms: *Dickinson syndrome, congenital hereditary hematuria, hematuria-nephropathy-deafness syndrome, hematuric familial nephropathy, hematuric hereditary nephritis, hemorrhagic familial nephritis, hereditary familial congenital hemorrhagic nephritis, hereditary nephritis, hereditary nephritis-deafness syndrome, hereditary nephropathy-deafness syndrome, progressive hereditary nephritis.*

A syndrome, transmitted as an autosomal dominant trait with probable partial sex linkage, characterized by nephropathy (nephritis, glomerulonephritis, hypertension, progressive renal failure), nerve deafness, and ocular lesions (anterior lenticonus, cataract, thinning of the lens capsule, fundus albi punctatus, retinopathy, and hyaline bodies of the optic nerve). Pathological findings consist mainly of interstitial foam cells in the kidneys. Blood and urine tests show hematuria, albuminuria, cylindruria, aminoaciduria, and increased blood urea nitrogen and creatinine.

Alport, A. C. Hereditary familial congenital haemorrhagic nephritis. *Brit. Med. J.*, 1927, 1:504-6. Dickinson, W. H. *Diseases of the kidney and urinary derangements*. London, Langmans, 1875, Part 2, p. 278.

ALS. See *amyotrophic lateral sclerosis.*

ALS-parkinsonism-dementia complex. See *amyotrophic lateral sclerosis-parkinsonism-dementia complex.*

ALS-PD complex. See *amyotrophic lateral sclerosis-parkinsonism-dementia complex.*

ALSTRÖM, CARL HENRY (Swedish physician)

Alström syndrome. Synonyms: *Alström-Hallgren syndrome, retino-otodiabetic syndrome.*

A familial syndrome, transmitted as an autosomal recessive trait, characterized by retinitis pigmentosa leading to blindness, juvenile diabetes mellitus, obesity, sensorineural deafness, and normal mental capacity. Acanthosis nigricans, hypogonadism with normal secondary sex characteristics, and kyphoscoliosis may be associated. Metabolic findings include hyperuricemia and elevated serum triglycerides and pre-ß-lipoproteins.

Alström, C. H., Hallgren, B., *et al.* Retinal degeneration combined with obesity, diabetes mellitus and neurogenous deafness. A specific syndrome (not hitherto described) distinct from the Laurence-Moon-Biedl syndrome. A clinical endocrinological and genetic examination based on a large pedigree. *Acta Psychiat. Neur. Scand.*, 1959, 34(Suppl. 129):1-35.

Alström-Hallgren syndrome. See *Alström syndrome.*

alternate inferior paralysis. See *Millard-Gubler syndrome.*

alternating bradycardia and tachycardia syndrome. See *bradycardia-tachycardia syndrome.*

alternating hypoglossal hemiplegia syndrome. See *Déjerine syndrome (2).*

ALTHERR, FRANZ (Swiss physician)

Meyenburg-Altherr-Uehlinger syndrome. See *under Meyenburg.*

von Meyenburg-Altherr-Uehlinger syndrome. See *Meyenburg-Altherr-Uehlinger syndr.*

altitude headache. See *under headache syndrome.*

altitude sickness. See *D'Acosta disease and see Monge disease.*

aluminosis. See *Shaver syndrome.*

aluminum osteomalacia. See *aluminum toxicity syndrome.*

aluminum toxicity syndrome. Synonyms: *aluminum osteomalacia, osteomalacic dialysis osteodystrophy.*

Toxic reaction to aluminum, most frequently marked by osteomalacia, fractures, and bone pain. The syndrome is usually observed in persons who are exposed to aluminum through ingestion of aluminum-containing, phosphate-binding antacids and those who are undergoing hemodialysis with the use of water-containing high concentrations of aluminum.

Platts, M., *et al.* Composition of the domestic water supply and the incidence of fractures and encephalopathy in patients on home dialysis. *Brit. Med. J.*, 1977, 657-60. Cushner, H. M., & Adams, N. D. Review: Renal osteodystrophy-pathogenesis and treatment. *Am. J. Med. Sc.*, 1986, 291:264-75.

ALVAREZ, WALTER C. (American physician)

Alvarez syndrome. Synonyms: *accordion abdomen, hysterical nongaseous abdominal bloating, pseudoileus.*

A syndrome of hysterical or neurotic abdominal bloating without any excess of gas in the digestive tract, apparently due to a contraction of muscles lining the back of the upper end of the abdominal cavity. Sometimes, in addition, there may be a relaxation of the muscles of the anterior abdominal wall with the assumption of an extremely lordotic posture.

Alvarez, W. C. Hysterical type of nongaseous abdominal bloating. *Arch. Int. Med., Chicago,* 1949, 84:217-45.

alveolar capillary block syndrome. Interference with the diffusion of oxygen across the alveolar-capillary septum in various diffuse pulmonary diseases, characterized by a reduced lung volume, maintenance of a large maximum breathing capacity, hyperventilation at rest and during exercise, normal or nearly normal arterial oxygen saturation at rest but a marked reduction of the arterial oxygen saturation after exercise, normal alveolar oxygen tension, a reduced oxygen diffusing capacity, and pulmonary artery hypertensions. The dead space-like ventilation and the venous admixture-like perfusion may be increased.

Austrian, R., *et al.* Clinical and physiologic features of some types of pulmonary disease with impairment of alveolar-capillary diffusion. The syndrome of "alveolar-capillary block." *Am. J. Med.*, 1951, 11:667-85.

alveolar hemorrhage (AH) syndrome. Synonym: *diffuse microvascular lung hemorrhage.*

A diffuse microvascular hemorrhage into the acinar portion of the lungs in immune or idiopathic conditions, most often associated with antibasement membrane antibody diseases, idiopathic pulmonary hemosiderosis, systemic lupus erythematosus, systemic vasculitis, and progressive glomerulonephritis.

Leatherman, J. W., *et al.* Alveolar hemorrhage syndromes: Diffuse microvascular lung hemorrhage in immune and idiopathic disorders. *Medicine, Baltimore,* 1984, 63:343-61.

alveolodental periostitis. See *Fauchard disease.*

alymphocytosis. See *severe mixed immunodeficiency syndrome.*

ALZHEIMER, ALOSIS (German psychiatrist, 1864-1915)

Alzheimer dementia (AD). See *Alzheimer disease.*

Alzheimer disease (AD). Synonyms: *Alzheimer dementia (AD), Alzheimer sclerosis, Alzheimer syndrome, Alzheimer-type dementia (ADT), dementia of the Alzheimer type (DAT), presenile dementia, senile dementia, senile dementia of the Alzheimer type (SDAT).*

A disabling and fatal degenerative disease of the nervous system, usually ocurring in middle-aged or older persons and very rarely in younger age groups. Onset is insidious with failure of memory for recent events and emotional changes, such as depression, anxiety, and unpredictable behavior, being the earliest symptoms. They are followed by aphasia, apraxia, space perception disorders, a shuffling gait, slow and awkward movements, and jerky muscle contractions (myoclonus), eventually leading to the late vegetative phase consisting of complete inability to think, move, or speak. Disappearance of nerve cells in the cortical and subcortical areas, leading to extensive convolutional atrophy, especially in the frontal and medial temporal regions, and corresponding enlargement of the ventricular system, are the principal features of this disease. Microscopic examination shows the presence of intracytoplasmic accumulations within neurons of filamentous material in the form of loops, coils, or tangled masses (Alzheimer neurofibrillary tangles) and intracortical foci of clustered thickened neuronal processes in the form of irregular rings around spherical deposits of amyloid fibrils (senile plaques). The reduction of cholinergic innervation is specific for this disorder. Etiology is unknown but the fact that many Down syndrome patients develop Alzheimer disease suggests a possibility of involvement of chromosome 21. Transmission as an autosomal dominant trait is suspected in some cases. Some cases are familial (*familial Alzheimer disease* or *FAD*).

Alzheimer, A. Über einen eigenartigen schweren Krankheitsprozess der Hirnrinde. *Zbl. Nervenkh.*, 1906, 25:1134; 1907, 30:177-9.

Alzheimer sclerosis. See *Alzheimer disease.*

Alzheimer syndrome. See *Alzheimer disease.*

Alzheimer-type dementia (ATD). See *Alzheimer disease.*

senile dementia of the Alzheimer type (SDAT). See *Alzheimer disease.*

amaurosis-hemiplegia syndrome. See *Espildora-Luque syndrome.*

amaurotic familial idiocy. See *Tay-Sachs syndrome, under Tay, Warren.*

ambiguospinopthalmic syndrome. See *Avellis syndrome.*

amblyopia-painful neuropathy-orogenital dermatitis syndrome. See *Strachan syndrome.*

AMBROISE TARDIEU. See TARDIEU, AMBROISE

ambulatory automatism. See *Kandinskii-Clérambault syndrome.*

ambulatory comitial automatism. See *Kandinskii-Clérambault syndrome.*

amelo-onychodyshidrotic syndrome. See *amelo-onychohypohidrotic syndrome.*

amelo-onychohypohidrotic syndrome. Synonyms: *Witkop syndrome, amelo-onychodyshidrotic syndrome, amelo-onycholiticodyshidrotic syndrome, hypohidrotic onychodental dysplasia syndrome, onychodentohypohidrotic syndrome, onycholysis-hypohidrosis-enamel hypocalcification syndrome.*

A syndrome transmitted as an autosomal dominant trait and characterized by hypocalcified and hypoplastic enamel, onycholysis, subungual hyperkeratosis, and hypotrichosis. Seborrheic dermatitis of the scalp, hypofunction of the sweat glands, and rough dry skin are usually associated.

Witkop, C. J., Jr., *et al.* Hypoplastic enamel, onycholysis, and hypohidrosis inherited as an autosomal dominant trait: A review of ectodermal dysplasia syndromes. *Oral Surg.*, 1975, 39:71-86.

amelo-onycholyticodyshidrotic syndrome. See *amelo-onychohypohidrotic syndrome.*

amelocerebrohypohidrosis syndrome. Synonyms: *Kohlschütter syndrome, epilepsy-dementia-amelogenesis imperfecta syndrome, epilepsy-mental deterioration-amelogenesis imperfecta syndrome, epilepsy-yellow teeth syndrome.*

A syndrome transmitted as an X-linked or autosomal recessive trait, characterized by severe seizures, progressive mental deterioration, muscular spasticity, hypohidrosis, and enamel hypoplasia with yellow discoloration of the teeth.

Kohlschütter, A., *et al.* Familial epilepsy and yellow teeth-a disease of the CNS associated with enamel hypoplasia. *Helv. Paediat. Acta*, 1974, 29:283-94.

amenorrhea traumatica. See *Asherman syndrome.*

amenorrhea-galactorrhea syndrome. Synonyms: *Ahumada-Del Castillo syndrome, Argonz-Del Castillo syndrome, Chiari-Frommel syndrome, Forbes-Albright syndrome, amenorrhea-hyperprolactinemia-galactorrhea syndrome, galactorrhea-amenorrhea syndrome, galactorrhea-amenorrhea-prolactinemia syndrome, hyperprolactinemia-amenorrhea-galactorrhea syndrome, hyperprolactinemic chronic anovulation syndrome, lactorrhea-amenorrhea syndrome, persistent galactorrhea-amenorrhea syndrome (PGAS).*

A disorder characterized by galactorrhea and amenorrhea. Three types are recognized: The **Chiari-Frommel syndrome** (occurring without antecedent pregnancy), the **Argonz-Del Castillo syndrome** (estrogen deficiency and decreased urinary gonadotropin levels), and the **Forbes-Albright syndrome** (occurring in the presence of pituitary prolactin-producing adenoma). Hyperprolactinemia, due to disorders of the hypothalamo-pituitary axis, occurs in some but not all instances. Other conditions contributing to the development of this syndrome include hypothyroidism, the administration of psychotrophic and antidepressive drugs, ectopic prolactin-producing tumors, acromegaly with excessive production of prolactin, the empty sella syndrome, and the use of contraceptive steroids.

Argonz, J., & Del Castillo, E. B. A syndrome characterized by estrogenic insufficiency, galactorrhea and decreased urinary gonadotropin. J. Clin. Endocr., 1953, 13:79-87. Ahumada, J. C., & Del Castillo, E. B. Sobre un caso de galactorrea y amenorrea. Bol. Soc. Obst. Gin., Buenos Aires, 1932, 11:64-72. Forbes, A. P., Henneman, P. H., Griswold, G. C., & Albright, F. Syndrome characterized by galactorrhea, amenorrhea and low urinary FSH. Comparison with acromegaly and normal lactation. J. Clin. Endocr. Metab., 1954, 14:265-71. Frommel, R. Über puerperale Atrophie des Uterus. Zschr. Geburtsh., Stuttgart, 1882, 7:305-13. Chiari, J., et al. Klinik der Geburtshilfe und Gynäkologie. Erlagen, Enke, 1855. Yen, S. S. C. Chronic anovulation. In: Yen, S. S. C., & Jaffe, R. B. eds. Reproductive endocrinology. Physiology, pathophysiology and clinical management. Philadelphia, Saunders, 1978, pp. 297-372.

amenorrhea-hyperprolactinemia-galactorrhea syndrome. See *amenorrhea-galactorrhea syndrome.*

American blastomycosis. See *Gilchrist disease.*

aminopterin embryopathy. See *fetal aminopterin syndrome.*

aminopterin fetopathy syndrome. See *fetal aminopterin syndrome.*

aminopterin syndrome. See *fetal aminopterin syndrome.*

aminopterin-like syndrome sine aminopterin (ASSA). See *fetal aminopterin-like syndrome without aminopterin.*

Amish brittle hair syndrome. See *hair-brain syndrome.*

amnestic confabulatory psychosis. See *Korsakoff syndrome, under Korsakov, Sergei Sergeevich.*

amnestic psychosis. See *Korsakoff syndrome, under Korsakov, Sergei Sergeevich.*

amnestic syndrome. See *Korsakoff syndrome, under Korsakov, Sergei Sergeevich.*

amniogenic band syndrome. See *amniotic band syndrome.*

amnion rupture sequence. See *amniotic band syndrome.*

amniotic adhesion malformation syndrome. See *amniotic band syndrome.*

amniotic band anomalad. See *amniotic band syndrome.*

amniotic band disruption complex. See *amniotic band syndrome.*

amniotic band sequence. See *amniotic band syndrome.*

amniotic band syndrome (ABS). Synonyms: *Streeter bands, Streeter dysplasia, amnion rupture sequence, amniogenic band syndrome, amniotic adhesion malformation syndrome, amniotic band anomalad, amniotic band disruption complex, amniotic band sequence, amniotic deformity-adhesion-mutilation (ADAM) syndrome, congenital amputation, congenital constricting bands, intrauterine amputation, ring constriction syndrome.*

Partial or complete ring-like constriction of fetal parts, especially the distal limbs, by amniotic tissue causing soft tissue grooves or depressions and becoming progressively more contrictive with growth to the point of amputation. Hand, foot, craniofacial, and skeletal defects are the principal features of this condition. Hand defects may include hypoplastic or absent hands or digits and other anomalies; those of the craniofacial structures include calvarial abnormalities, cleft palate, facial clefts, encephalocele, scalp rings, and other abnormalities; and those of the skeletal system consist of absent extremities and ring constrictions. According to Streeter, the primary lesions were considered to be within the developing limb mesenchyme, the other bands being a secondary phenomenon. According to more recent interpretations, the condition is due to the primary abnormality of the amnion. Three levels of involvement are recognized: partial thickness constriction of subcutaneous tissue without disability, full thickness subcutaneous tissue constriction with lymphedema, and severe deep tissue constriction, including bone, with intrauterine amputation. Autosomal recessive transmission is considered by some authors.

Streeter, G. L. Focal deficiencies in fetal tissues and their relation to intra-uterine amputations. In: *Contribution to embryology*. Vol. 22, No. 126. Publication No. 414. Carnegie Institution of Washington, 1930.

amniotic deformity-adhesion-mutilation (ADAM) syndrome. See *amniotic band syndrome.*

amphetamine withdrawal syndrome. See *under withdrawal syndrome.*

AMR. See ***a**lopecia-**m**ental **r**etardation syndrome.*

Amsterdam dwarf. See *de Lange syndrome (1), under Lange, Cornelia, de.*

Amsterdam type. See *de Lange syndrome (1), under Lange, Cornelia, de.*

amyatonia congenita. See *Oppenheim disease, under Oppenheim, Hermann.*

amylo-1,6-glucosidase deficiency. See *glycogen storage disease III.*

amyloid degeneration. See *amyloidosis.*

amyloid nephropathy. See *Ostertag syndrome.*

amyloid neuropathy type I. Synonyms: *Andrade paramyloidosis, Andrade syndrome, Corino de Andrade syndrome, Wohlwill-Andrade syndrome, Wohlwill-Corino Andrade syndrome, amyloid polyneuropathy, amyloidosis I, familial amyloid polyneuropathy, familial Portu-*

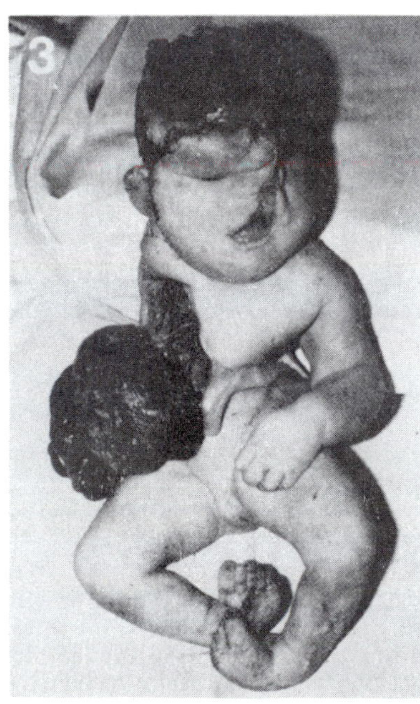

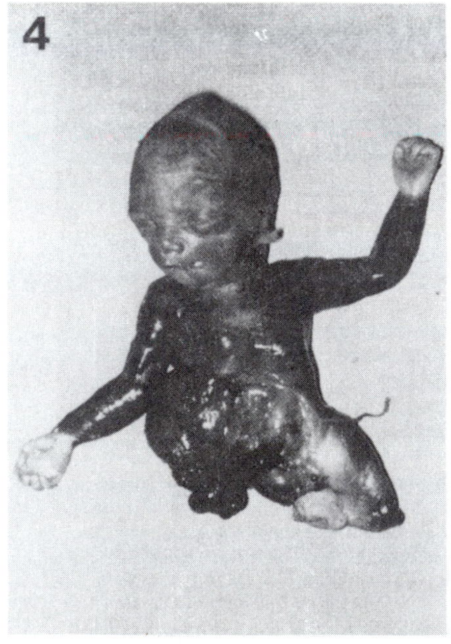

Amniotic band syndrome
Hunter, Alasdair G.W. and Blair F. Carpenter, *American Journal of Medical Genetics*, 24:691-700, 1986, Alan R. Liss Inc., New York.

guese polyneuritic amyloidosis, hereditary neuropathic amyloidosis, Portuguese neuropathic amyloid syndrome.

A hereditary form of amyloidosis, transmitted as an autosomal dominant trait, characterized by predominantly neurological symptoms. Early manifestations, having onset usually in the third or fourth decade (sometimes occurring as early as the second or as late as the sixth decade), include paresthesia and hypesthesia of the lower extremities, spreading to upper limbs, and eventually involving the trunk. They are usually followed by sensory disorders (loss of sensation of temperature, pain, vibration, and proprioception), motor disturbances (drop foot, tottering, and abnormal gait), absent deep tendon reflexes, fasciculation, trophic skin lesions, perforating ulcers, and muscle wasting. Impotence, premature menopause, orthostatic hypotension, hypohidrosis, urinary and fecal incontinence, constipation or diarrhea, anorexia, mucus in the stools, and other gastrointestinal complications are usually associated. Visual disorders include irregular pupil margins, anisocoria, delayed reaction to light, and occasional vitreous and corneal opacities and exophthalmos. In the advanced stages, there are recurrent infections, cachexia, cardiac collapse, and death, usually 7 to 12 years from the onset. Initial cases were reported in persons of Portuguese descent, but later observations indicate that this syndrome occurs. also in other ethnic groups. Pathological findings show deposition of amyloid in the visceral blood vessels, sympathetic nerves, and central nervous system.

Andrade, C. A peculiar form of peripheral neuropathy: Familial atypical generalized amyloidosis with special involvement of peripheral nerves. *Brain,* 1952, 75:408-27. Wohlwill, F. Formas atipicas da amiloidose. *Amatus Lusitatus, Lisboa,* 1942, 1:373-91.

amyloid neuropathy type II. Synonyms: *Rukavina syndrome, amyloidosis II, Indiana type amyloid neuropathy.*

A hereditary form of amyloidosis, transmitted as an autosomal dominant trait, originally reported in Indiana and Maryland. Early symptoms involve mainly the hands and consist of pain, paresthesia, numbness, weakness, and other manifestations of the carpal tunnel syndrome (q.v.). They are followed by involvement of the legs, vitreous opacities, electrocardiographic changes, hepatomegaly, splenomegaly, gastrointestinal complications, and occasional scleroderma-like lesions. Amyloid deposits in the myocardium, blood vessels, tongue, larynx, liver, spleen, adrenal glands, pancreas, lungs, prostate, and kidneys are the chief pathological findings.

Rukavina, J. G., *et al.* Familial primary systemic amyloidosis. An experimental, genetic and clinical study. *J. Invest. Derm.* 1956, 27:111-31. Falls, H. F., *et al.* Ocular manifestations of hereditary primary systemic amyloidosis. *AMA Arch. Ophth.,* 1955, 54:660-4.

amyloid neuropathy type III. Synonyms: *Van Allen syndrome, amyloidosis III, amyloidosis IV, Iowa-type amyloidosis.*

A hereditary form of amyloidosis, transmitted as an autosomal dominant trait, originally reported in Iowa in a family of Scotish-English-Irish extraction. Onset of symptoms is usually observed in the third or fourth decade with an average survival of 12 years from the onset. Loss of pain sensation is the earliest symptom. It is usually followed by muscle weakness and atrophy, diminished deep-tendon reflexes, dysenthesia, shooting pain, and other neurological disorders of the extremities, lower limbs being more severely affected than the upper ones. Associated disorders may include peptic ulcer, renal insufficiency, electrocardiographic changes, constipation or diarrhea, and, less commonly, deafness and cataracts. Amyloid deposits in the nerve roots, peripheral nerves, sympathetic ganglia, and heart are the principal pathologic changes. Laboratory findings include elevated protein levels in the cerebrospinal fluid, albuminuria, and isosthenuria.

Van Allen, M. W., *et al.* Inherited predisposition to generalized amyloidosis. Clinical and pathological studies in a family with neuropathy and peptic ulcer. *Neurology,* 1968, 19:10-25.

amyloid neuropathy type IV. Synonyms: *Meretoja syndrome, amyloidosis V, Finland-type amyloid neuropathy.*

A hereditary form of amyloidosis, transmitted as an autosomal dominant trait, characterized mainly by lattice dystrophy of the cornea, cranial neuropathy, and cutis laxa. Other ocular findings may include corneal erosions, iritis or iridocyclitis, glaucoma, and corneal anesthesia. Facial paralysis, lesions of other cranial nerves, and decreased auditory acuity, usually occurring in the fifth decade of life, are the chief neurologic features. Skin changes, appearing in middle or old age, consist of thickening and smoothing of the skin over the forehead and head; drying, lichenification, and pruritic changes of the skin of the extremities; blepharochalasia; and generalized cutis laxa and atrophy of the skin. Associated disorders include cardiac complications, arthropathy, and gastrointestinal symptoms. Intermittent proteinuria occurs in some cases. Amyloid deposition in the kidneys, blood vessels, myocardium, peripheral nerves, and central nervous system are the principal pathological findings.

Meretoja, J. Familial systemic paramyloidosis with lattice dystrophy of the cornea, progressive cranial neuropathy, skin changes and various internal symptoms. A previously unrecognized heritable syndrome. *Ann. Clin. Res.,* 1969, 1:314-24.

amyloid polyneuropathy. See *amyloid neuropathy type I.*

amyloidosis. Synonyms: *Abercrombie degeneration. Abercrombie syndrome, amyloid degeneration, amyloidosis syndrome, lardaceous disease, waxy disease.*

A pathological condition characterized by deposition of amyloid (β-pleated sheet fibrillar pathologic protein) between cells of various tissues and organs, occurring in a wide variety of acquired and hereditary disorders. See also *Lubarsch-Pick syndrome,* and *Muckle-Wells syndrome.*

Glenner, G. G., Ignaczak, T. F., & Page, D. L. The inherited systemic amyloidoses and localized amyloid deposits. In: Stanbury, J. B., Wyngaarden, J. B., Fredrickson, D. S. eds. *The metabolic basis of inherited disease.* 4th ed. New York, McGraw-Hill, 1978, pp. 1308-39. (Tables).

amyloidosis syndrome. See *amyloidosis.*

amyloidosis I. See *amyloid neuropathy type I.*

amyloidosis II. See *amyloid neuropathy type II.*

amyloidosis III See *amyloid neuropathy type III*

Classification of the systemic amyloidoses

1. Plasma cell dyscrasias with amyloidosis
   a. Plasma cell myeloma
   b. Monoclonal gammopathy
   c. Primary ("Waldenstrom's") macroglobulinemia
   d. "Heavy chain" diseases
   e. Other "lymphoid" system neoplasms

2. Agammaglobulinemia with amyloidosis

3. Chronic diseases with amyloidosis
   a. Chronic suppurative or granulomous infections (e.g., osteomyelitis, tuberculosis)
   b. Chronic inflammatory condition (e.g.,rheumatoid arthritis)
   c. Hodgkin's disease
   d. "Nonlymphoid" solid tumors (e.g., renal adenocarcinoma)

4. Heredofamilial amyloidosis
   a. Familial Mediterranean fever
   b. Amyloid polyneuropathy (e.g., Portuguese type)

Classification of the heredofamilial syndromes of amyloidosis and localized amyloid deposition

I. General hereditary amyloidosis
   A. Neuropathic forms
      1. Amyloid neuropathy Type I (Portuguese or Andrade type)
      2. Amyloid neuropathy Type II (Indiana or Rukavina type)
      3. Amyloid neuropathy Type III (Iowa or Van Allen type)
      4. Amyloid neuropathy Type IV (Finland or Meretoja type)
   B. Nonneuropathic forms
      1. Amyloid nephropathy of Ostertag
      2. Amyloidosis of familial Mediterranean fever
      3. Amyloid nephropathy with deafness,urticaria, and limb pains (Muckle-Wells syndrome)
      4. Amyloid cardiomyopathy (Denmark)
      5. Amyloid cardiomyopathy with persistent atrial standstill

II. Localized hereditary amyloid deposits
   A. Hereditary cerebral hemorrhage (Iceland)
   B. Lattice dystrophy of the cornea
   C. Hereditary amyloid deposits of the cornea
   D. Gingival hyperplasia, conjunctivitis, and mental retardation with amyloid infiltration (?)
   E. Papular cutaneous amyloid infiltration
   F. Poikilodermal cutaneous amyloid infiltration
   G. Bullous cutaneous amyloid infiltration
   H. Medullary carcinoma of the thyroid in MEA 2 with amyloid deposits

Amyloidosis
Glenner, G.G., T.F. Ignaczak & D.L. Page. "The inherited systemic amyloidoses and localized amyloid deposits. In Stanbury, J.B., J.B. Wyngaarden & D.S. Fredrickson, *The Metabolic Basis of Inherited Disease*, 4th ed. New York: McGraw-Hill, 1978, pp 1308-39 (Tables 54-3 and 54-4).

amyloidosis IV. See *amyloid neuropathy type III.*
amyloidosis V. See *amyloid neuropathy type IV.*
amyloidosis-deafness-urticaria-limb pain syndrome. See *Muckle-Wells syndrome.*
amylopectinosis. See *glycogen storage disease IV.*
amyoplasia congenita. See *arthrogryposis multiplex congenital syndrome.*
amyotrophia nuclearis progressiva. See *Aran-Duchenne syndrome.*
amyotrophic cerebellar hypoplasia (ACH) syndrome. Synonyms: *anterior horn cell disease with pontocerebellar hypoplasia, cerebellar hypoplasia in Werdnig-Hoffmann disease.*

A form of infantile spinal atrophy with lower motor neuron degeneration; cerebellar hypoplasia; atrophy of the pons, olives, and cerebellum; sclerosis of the thalamus and corpus pallidum; demyelination; laryngeal paralysis; mental retardation; progressive amyotrophy; and slow nerve conduction.

de Leon, G. A., *et al.* Amyotrophic cerebellar hypoplasia: A specific form of infantile spinal atropphy. *Acta Neuropathol., Berlin,* 1984, 63:282-6.

amyotrophic lateral sclerosis (ALS). Synonyms: *Charcot sclerosis, Charcot syndrome, Lou Gehrig disease, progressive muscular atrophy, pseudobulbar palsy.*

A degenerative disease of the nervous system characterized by early asymmetric weakness, usually of one limb, followed by fatigue, cramps, and progressive wasting and fibrillation of the muscles of the upper extremity and weakness and spasticity of the lower extremity, leading to death within three years from the onset of symptoms in about half of all cases. Pathologically, there is a loss of motor neurons in the cerebral cortex and anterior horns of the spinal cord, some motor nuclei of the brain stem being also affected. The disorder usually affects adults over 50 years of age. When occurring in younger persons, the illness appears to be transmitted an an autosomal dominant trait. Males are more frequently affected than females. The disease was named in the press after Henry Louis (Lou) Gehrig, an American baseball player who died from it in 1941.

Charcot, J. M., & Jeffroy, Deux cas d'atrophie musculaire progressive avec lésions de la substance grise et des faisaeux antérolatéraux de la moelle épinière. *Arch. Physiol. Norm. Pathol., Paris,* 1869, 2:354- 67; 629-49; 744-60.

amyotrophic lateral sclerosis-parkinsonism-dementia complex (ALS-PD complex, ALS-parkinsonism-dementia complex). Synonyms: *Groote Eylandt syndrome, Guam disease, Guam syndrome.*

An endemic neurological disorder observed in tribal aborigines in Groote Eylandt and the adjacent mainland in Australia, Guam, Saipan, islands of Micronesia, the Kii Peninsula of Honshu in Japan, coastal lowlands of West Irian, the Kuru and Fore people in New Guinea and the Arnhmem Land. The syndrome is characterized by progressive dementia, parkinsonism, and amyotrophic lateral sclerosis. A frequent feature of the condition is involvement of upper and lower neurons, sometimes resulting in teetering gait, leading to their sobriquet "bird people" among the aboriginal tribsmen, who find some resemblance to wading birds such as the heron. The syndrome is suspected of being a group of separate conditions with common etiology and pathogenesis, possibly involving environmental, pathogenic, viral, hereditary, and other factors.

Kiloh, L.G., *et al.* An endemic neurological disorder in tribal Australian aborigines. *J. Neur. Neurosurg. Psychiat.*, 1980, 43:661-8. Cawte, J. Emic accounts of a mystery illness: The Groote Eylandt syndrome. *Austral. N. Z. J. Psychiat.*, 1984, 18:179-87.

amyotrophic quadriceps syndrome. A group of disorders of of the quadriceps muscle, consisting of (1) primary muscle dystrophies (pure quadriceps myopathy, quadriceps myopathy "plus," and possibly lumbopelvifemoral myopathy), (2) metabolic muscular disorders, (3) chronic polymyositis, and (4) spinal amyotrophy localized in the quadriceps.

Serratrice, G., *et al.* Myopathie quadricipitale ou syndrome amyotrophique quadricipital. Étude nosologique à propos de 10 observations. *Rev. Neur., Paris,* 1983, 139:367-73.

amyotrophic syphilitic myelitis. See *Erb-Charcot syndrome, under Erb, Wilhelm Ernst.*

analgesia syndrome. See *congenital insensitivity to pain syndrome.*

analgesic abuse. See *analgesic syndrome.*

analgesic asthma syndrome. Asthma induced by analgesic and anti-inflammatory drugs, attributed to the inhibition of prostaglandin synthesis. In the past, the syndrome was believed to be caused almost exclusively by aspirin (acetylsalicylic acid). Now, various non-steroidal anti-inflammatory drugs with different chemical structures are known to cause bronchospasm in some hypersensitive persons.

Prickman, L. E., & Buchstein, H. F. Hypersensitivity to acetylsalicylic acid. *JAMA,* 1937, 108:445-51. Virchow, C., *et al.* Pyrazoles and analgesic asthma syndrome. *Agents Actions Suppl.*, 1986, 19:291-301.

analgesic intoxication. See *analgesic syndrome.*

analgesic nephropathy syndrome. Synonym: *analgesic-associated nephropathy (AAN).*

Chronic interstitial nephritis caused by the ingestion of large quantities of analgesic drugs, chiefly mixtures of aspirin (acetylsalicylic acid) and phenacetin. Initial symptoms are minimal, but in advanced stages they may include renal failure, renal colic, secondary infection, dysuria, hematuria, nocturia, metabolic acidosis, salt wasting, anemia, fatigue, uremia, hypertension, and azotemia. Pathological findings consist mainly of interstitial sclerosis and tubular degeneration and atrophy.

Goldberg, M. Analgesic-associated nephropathy. In: Wyngaarden, J. B., & Smith, L.H., Jr. eds. *Cecil textbook of medicine.* 17th ed. Philadelphia, Saunders, 1985. pp. 592-3. Nanra, R. S., *et al.* Analgesic nephropathy: Etiology, clinical syndrome, and clinicopathologic correlations in Australia. *Kidney Int.*, 1978, 13:79-92. *Headache cures. In: *The lone hand.*. 1907, pp. 193-5.

analgesic panaris. See *Morvan disease.*

analgesic paralysis with whitlow. See *Morvan disease.*

analgesic syndrome. Synonyms: *analgesic abuse, analgesic intoxication.*

A syndrome of toxic reactions to ingestion of large amounts of various analgesics. Asthma (see **analgesic asthma syndrome**), chronic interstitial nephritis sometimes leading to renal failure (see **analgesic nephropathy syndrome**), ischemic heart disease, hypertension, intestinal bleeding, peptic ulcer, pregnancy complications, pigmentation disorders, and mental disorders are some of the clinical forms of toxic reactions to analgesics. The condition is more common in females than males.

Nanra, R. S., *et al.* Analgesic nephropathy: Etiology, clinical syndrome, and clinicopathologic correlations in Australia. *Kidney Int.*, 1978, 13:79-92. *Headache cures. In: *The lone hand.* 1907, pp. 193-5.

analgesic-associated nephropathy (AAN). See *analgesic nephropathy syndrome.*

analphalipoproteinemia. See *Tangier disease.*

anaphylactoid purpura. See *Schönlein-Henoch purpura.*

anapolipoproteinemia C-II. See *apolipoprotein C-II deficiency syndrome.*

anarthritic rheumatoid disease. See *Forestier syndrome (1).*

ANCELL, HENRY A. (British physician, born 1802)

Ancell-Spiegler cylindroma. See *Brooke epithelioma.*

ancylostomiasis. See *Griesinger disease.*

ANDERMANN, FREDERICK (Canadian physician)

Andermann syndrome. Synonym: *Charlevoix disease.*

A familial syndrome, transmitted as an autosomal recessive trait, characterized by agenesis of the corpus callosum, mental retardation, and progressive sensimotor neuropathy. Craniofacial anomalies consist of brachycephaly, long and asymmetrical face, hypoplastic maxilla, prominent chin, low hairline, narrow forehead, high-arched palate, open mouth with protruding fissured tongue, and large ears. Skeletal defects include ulnar and radial deviation, long and tapering fingers, flexion contractures of the metacarpo-phalangeal joints, low-set thumbs, hammertoe deformity, and syndactyly of the toes. Oval optic disks, muscle hypotonia and weakness, and absent deep tendon reflexes are the associated disorders. Pneumoencephalography reveals complete agenesis of the corpus callosum; electroencephalography shows excess of slow activity and poorly regulated background without epileptogenic discharges; and electromyography demonstrates fibrillation, fasciculation, and reduced motor unit potentials. The syndrome was originally observed in children in a family from Charlevoix County and the Saguenay-Lac St-Jean area in the province of Quebec in Canada. See also *Charlevoix-Saguenay spastic ataxia.*.

Andermann, F., Andermann, E., *et al.* Familial agenesis of the corpus callosum with anterior horn disease: A syndrome of mental retardation, areflexia, and paraparesis. *Tr. Am. Neurol. Asssoc.*, 1972, 97:242-4. Larbrisseau, A., *et al.* The Andermann syndrome: Agenesis of the corpus callosum associated with mental retardation and progressive sensorimotor neuropathy. *Canad. J. Neurol. Sc.*, 1984, 11:257-61.

ANDERS, JAMES M. (American physician, 1854-1931)

Anders syndrome. See *Dercum syndrome.*

ANDERSEN, DOROTHY HANSINE (American physician, 1901-1963)

Andersen disease. See *glycogen storage disease IV.*

Andersen syndrome. See *Andersen triad.*

Andersen triad. Synonyms: *Andersen syndrome, Clarke-Hadfield syndrome, Fanconi syndrome, Glanzmann dysporia, dysporia enterobronchopancreatica congenita familiaris, pancreatic infantilism.*

A triad of cystic fibrosis of the pancreas (mucoviscidosis), celiac disease, and vitamin A deficiency.

Andersen, D. H. Cystic fibrosis of the pancreas and its relation to celiac disease. A clinical and pathological study. *Am. J. Dis. Child.*, 1938, 56:344-99. Fanconi, G. Das Coeliakiesyndrom bei angeborener zystischer Pankreasfibromatose und Bronchiektasien. *Wien. Med. Wschr.*, 1936, 86:753-6. Clarke, C., & Hadfield, G. Congenital pancreatic disease with infantilism. *Q. J. Med.*, 1923-24, 17:358-64.

Najjar-Andersen syndrome. See *glycogen storage disease IV.*

ANDERSON, L. G. (American physician)

Anderson syndrome. Synonyms: *familial osteodysplasia, Anderson type; familial osteodysplasia syndrome.*

A familial syndrome transmitted as an autosomal recessive trait, characterized by multiple bone abnormalities and peculiar facies. Craniofacial defects consist of midfacial hypoplasia, small malar prominence, prognathism, flat nasal bridge, micromaxilla, depressed zygomatic bones, calvarial thinning, brachycephaly, hypoplasia of the petrous bone, prominent eyebrows, malocclusion, and large ear lobes. Additional malformations include small and pointed spinous processes of the cervical vertebrae, scoliosis, thick cortices of the clavicles, thin ribs, thin superior pubic rami, and cortical thickening of the long bones and bones of the hands and feet. Hyperuricemia and elevated diastolic blood pressure are associated.

Anderson, L. G., *et al.* Familial osteodysplasia. *JAMA*, 1972, 220:1687-93.

familial osteodysplasia, Anderson type. See *Anderson syndrome.*

ANDERSON, WILLIAM A. (British physician, born 1842)

Anderson syndrome. See *Fabry syndrome.*

Fabry-Anderson syndrome. See *Fabry syndrome.*

Andes disease. See *Monge disease.*

ANDOGSKII (ANDOGSKY), N. (Russian physician)

Andogsky syndrome. Synonyms: *cataracta dermatogenes, cataracta syndermatotica, dermatogenic cataract.*

Bilateral stellate cataracts that begin in the anterior capsule, eventually involving the entire lens and assuming the form of total soft cataracts. The disorder occurs in adults with a history of chronic eczematous skin lesions with lichenification of the neck and flexor surfaces of the extremities. Facies leonina, keratoconjunctivitis, keratoconus, uveitis, and asthma may be associated.

Andogsky, N. Cataracta dermatogenes. Ein Beitrag zur Aetiologie der Linsentrübung. *Klin. Mbl. Augenh.*, 1914, 52:824-31.

ANDOGSKY, N. See ANDOGSKII, N.

ANDRADE, CORINO M. (Portuguese physician)

Andrade paramyloidosis. See *amyloid neuropathy type I.*

Andrade syndrome. See *amyloid neuropathy type I.*

Corino de Andrade syndrome. See *amyloid neuropathy type I.*

Wohlwill-Andrade syndrome. See *amyloid neuropathy type I.*

Wohlwill-Corino Andrade syndrome. See *amyloid neuropathy type I.*

ANDRE, M. (French physician)

André syndrome. A syndrome of peculiar facies and osseous defects. Orofacial anomalies consist of hypertelorism, antimongoloid palpebral slant, low-set ears, cleft palate, retrognathia, prominent forehead, and Robin's anomaly. Bone defects include faulty ossification of the cranial vault, broad sutures and fontanels, sinuous ribs, long and thin clavicles, flat vertebrae, abnormal bowing and hyperostosis of the long bones, and faulty ossification of the bones of hands and feet with fanned out toes and shortening of the hand bones, which appear to show almost no tubulation. The syndrome appears to be transmitted as an X-linked trait and is usually lethal within a few weeks.

André, M., *et al.* Abnormal facies, cleft palate, and generalized dysostosis: A lethal X-linked syndrome. *J. Pediat.*, 1981, 98:747-52.

ANDREWS, GEORGE CLINTON (American physician, born 1891)

Andrews bacterid. Synonyms: *Andrews disease, Andrews syndrome, pustular bacterid, recalcitrant pustular eruption.*

An eruption that usually begins as a crop of pustules on the midportion of the palms and soles, from where it spreads outward. The eruption is generally entirely pustular, but in some cases it consists of a mixture of vesicles and pustules. Fresh crops of lesions appear daily; they eventually coalesce and form a honeycomb-structure which becomes covered by adherent dry scales. The disorder usually follows a focal infection of the teeth, tonsils, or sinuses. Leukocytosis is frequent, and the affected persons have positive skin reaction to staphylococci and streptococci. The eruption usually disappears after removing the cause of infection. The presence of pustules deep in the epidermis, containing many polymorphonuclear and few epithelial cells, is the principal histologic feature. Middle-aged persons are most frequently affected.

Andrews, G. C., *et al.* Recalcitrant pustular eruption of the palms and soles. *Arch. Derm. Syph., Chicago,* 1934, 29:548-63.

Andrews disease. See *Andrews bacterid.*

Andrews syndrome. See *Andrews bacterid.*

ANDREWS, P. A. (American physician)

Christian-Andrews-Conneally-Muller syndrome. See *Christian syndrome (1), under Christian, Joe C.*

androgen receptor deficiency. See *testicular feminization syndrome.*

androgen-insensitivity (AIS). See *testicular feminization syndrome.*

androgen-resistance syndrome. See *testicular feminization syndrome.*

androgenicity-gonadal dysgenesis syndrome. See *Gordan-Overstreet syndrome.*

anemia chronica congenital aregenerativa. See *Diamond-Blackfan syndrome.*

anemia infectiosa chronica. See *Edelmann syndrome (1).*
anemia pseudoleukemica. See *Jaksch syndrome.*
anemia pseudoleukemica infantum. See *Jaksch syndrome.*
anemia splenica congenita. See *Ecklin anemia.*
anemia splenica pseudoleukemica infantum. See *Jaksch syndrome.*
anemia-triphalangeal thumb syndrome. See *Aase-Smith syndrome.*
anencephaly-spina bifida (ASB) syndrome. A lethal hereditary syndrome of anencephaly and spina bifida, transmitted as an X-linked trait.

Toriello, H. V., *et al.* Possible X-linked anencephaly and spina bifida-report of a kindred. *Am. J. Med. Genet.*, 1980, 6:119-21.

anenzymia catalasea. See *Takahara syndrome.*
anesthetic leprosy. See *Danielssen-Boeck disease.*
aneurysm of internal carotid artery. See *Jefferson syndrome.*
aneurysmal varix. See *Pott aneurysm.*
aneutrocytosis. See *Schultz syndrome.*
aneutrophilia. See *Schultz syndrome.*
ANGELMAN, HARRY (British physician)
Angelman syndrome (AS). See *happy puppet syndrome.*
ANGELUCCI, ARNALDO (Italian physician, 1854-1933)
Angelucci syndrome. Synonyms: *periodic allergic conjunctivitis, spring catarrh, spring conjunctivitis, vernal conjunctivitis.*

Conjunctivitis characteristically occurring in the spring, believed to be of allergic origin, which is associated with vasomotor lability, photophobia, lacrimation, eye itch, conjunctival congestion, watery discharge, and, sometimes, tachycardia and exitability.

Angelucci, A. Di una sindrome sconosciuta negli infermi di catarro primaverile. *Arch. Ottalm., Palermo,* 1897-98, 5:270-6.

angina agranulocytica. See *Schultz syndrome.*
angina cruris. See *Charcot syndrome (3).*
angina herpetica. See *Zahorsky syndrome (2).*
angina ludovici. See *Ludwig angina.*
angina ludwigii. See *Ludwig angina.*
angina pectoris. See *Heberden asthma.*
angina pectoris vasomotoria. See *Nothnagel syndrome (1).*
angina pectoris with normal coronary arteriogram. See *X syndrome.*
angina pectoris without coronary heart disease. See *X syndrome.*
angio-osteohypertrophy syndrome. See *Klippel-Trénaunay-Weber syndrome.*
angioblastic lymphoid hyperplasia with eosinophilia. See *Kimura disease.*
angiodermatitis pruriginosa disseminata. See *Casalá-Mosto disease.*
angiodysgenesis spinalis. See *Foix-Alajouanine syndrome.*
angiodysgenetic myelomalacia. See *Foix-Alajouanine syndrome.*
angiofollicular lymph node hyperplasia. See *Castleman disease.*
angiohemophilia. See *Willebrand-Jürgens syndrome.*
angiohypertrophic central myelitis. See *Foix-Alajouanine syndrome.*
angioid streaks. See *Knapp streaks.*
angioid streaks in cardiovascular disorders. See *Touraine syndrome, under Touraine, M. A.*
angioid streaks-pseudoxanthoma elasticum syndrome. See *pseudoxanthoma elasticum.*
angiokeratoma. See *Mibelli disease (1).*
angiokeratoma corporis diffusum (ACD). See *Fabry syndrome.*
angiokeratoma corporis diffusum universale. See *Fabry syndrome.*
angiokeratoma scrotii. See *Fordyce lesion.*
angiolymphoid hyperplasia with eosinophilia. See *Kimura disease.*
angioma capillare et venosum calcificans. See *Sturge-Weber syndrome.*
angioma corporis diffusum universale. See *Fabry syndrome.*
angioma haemorrhagicum hereditaria. See *Osler-Rendu-Weber syndrome.*
angioma pigmentosum et atrophicum. See *xeroderma pigmentosum syndrome.*
angioma serpiginosum. See *Hutchinson disease (1), under Hutchinson, Sir Jonathan.*
angiomatosis encephalofacialis. See *Sturge-Weber syndrome.*
angiomatosis meningo-oculofacialis. See *Sturge-Weber syndrome.*
angiomatosis miliaris. See *carcinoid syndrome.*
angiomatosis retinae. See *Hippel-Lindau syndrome.*
angiomatosis retinae cystica. See *Hippel-Lindau syndrome.*
angioneurotic edema. See *Quincke edema.*
angiopathia retinae juvenilis. See *Cords angiopathy, and see Eales syndrome.*
angiopathia retinae traumatica. See *Purtscher disease.*
angiopathic retinopathy. See *Purtscher disease.*
angioreticuloma cerebelli. See *Hippel-Lindau syndrome.*
angioreticulosarcomatosis. See *Kaposi sarcoma.*
angiosarcoma pigmentosum. See *Kaposi sarcoma.*
angiosclerotic intermittent akinesia. See *Determann syndrome.*
angiosclerotic intermittent dyskinesia. See *Determann syndrome.*
angiosclerotic paroxysmal myasthenia. See *Charcot syndrome (3), and see Determann syndrome.*
angiospastic acroparesthesia. See *Nothnagel acroparesthesia.*
angry back syndrome. See *excited skin syndrome.*
angular gyrus syndrome. See *Gerstmann syndrome (2).*
angularis syndrome. See *Gerstmann syndrome (2).*
angulation of the ileum. See *Lane kink, under Lane, Sir Willilam Arbuthnot.*
anhidrosis hypotrichotica. See *hypohidrotic ectodermal dysplasia syndrome.*
anhidrosis polydysplastica. See *hypohidrotic ectodermal dysplasia syndrome.*
anhidrosis-hypotrichosis-anodontia syndrome. See *hypohidrotic ectodermal dysplasia syndrome.*
anhidrosis-neurolabyrinthitis syndrome. See *Helweg-Larsen syndrome.*
anhidrotic ectodermal dysplasia. See *hypohidrotic ectodermal dysplasia syndrome.*
anhidrotic ectodermal dysplasia, autosomal recessive. Synonym: *Passarge syndrome.*

A familial syndrome, transmitted as an autosomal recessive trait, characterized by hypohidrosis, hypotrichosis, missing and conical teeth, and spoon-shaped nails. See also *hypohidrotic ectodermal dysplasia syndrome.*.

Passarge, E., *et al.* Anhidrotic ectodermal dysplasia as autosomal recessive trait in an inbred kindred. *Humangenetik,* 1966, 3:181-5.

anhidrotic hereditary ectodermal dysplasia. See *hypohidrotic ectodermal dysplasia syndrome.*

anicteric hepatitis. See *under Botkin disease.*

aniridia-ambiguous genitalia-mental retardation syndrome. See *AGR syndrome.*

aniridia-cerebellar ataxia-mental retardation syndrome. See *Gillespie syndrome (2).*

aniridia-nephroblastoma syndrome. See *aniridia-Wilms tumor syndrome.*

aniridia-Wilms tumor association (AWTA). See *aniridia-Wilms tumor syndrome.*

aniridia-Wilms tumor syndrome. Synonyms: *Brusa-Torricelli syndrome, Miller syndrome, Wilms tumor-aniridia syndrome, aniridia-nephroblastoma syndrome, aniridia-Wilms tumor association (aniridia-WT association, AWTA), oculocerebrorenal (OCR) syndrome.*

A syndrome of aniridia and nephroblastoma (Wilms tumor) associated with mental retardation, craniofacial defects, skeletal anomalies, deformed pinna, genitourinary abnormalities, hamartomas, and umbilical and inguinal hernias. Glaucoma, cataracts, microcephaly, cryptorchism, hypospadias, hemihypertrophy, and horsehoe kidney are the additional defects. The syndrome is transmitted as a genetic trait with deletion of the short arm of chromosome 11.

Miller, R. W., *et al.* Association of Wilms' tumor with aniridia, hemihypertrophy, and other congenital malformations. *N. Engl. J. Med.*, 1964, 270:922-7. Brusa, P., & Torricelli, C. Nefroblastoma di Wilms ed affezioni renali congenite nelle casistiche dell' IIPAI di Milano. *Minerva Pediat.*, 1953, 5:457-63.

aniridia-WT (aniridia-Wilms tumor) association. See *aniridia-Wilms tumor syndrome.*

anisospondylitic camptomicromelic dwarfism. See *Rolland-Desbuquois syndrome.*

ankyloblepharon-ectodermal defects-cleft lip syndrome. See *AEC syndrome.*

ankyloglossia superior. See *glossopalatine ankylosis syndrome.*

ankyloglossum superius syndrome. See *glossopalatine ankylosis syndrome.*

ankylosing hyperostosis. See *Forestier syndrome (2).*

ankylosing polyarthritis. See *Bechterew-Strümpell-Marie syndrome, under Bekhterev.*

ankylosing spondylitis (AS). See *Bechterew-Strümpell-Marie syndrome, under Bekhterev.*

ankylosing vertebral hyperostosis. See *Forestier syndrome (2).*

ankylosis-facial anomalies-pulmonary hypoplasia syndrome. A familial syndrome of multiple abnormalities, including ankylosis, facial anomalies, and pulmonary hypoplasia, identified within the symptom complex of arthrogryposis multiplex congenita. Specific defects may include intrauterine growth retardation, hydramnios, short umbilical cord, small placenta, abruptio placentae, low-set ears, hypertelorism, epicanthal folds, depressed nasal tip, muscle atrophy, arthrogryposis, clubfoot, camptodactyly, hypoplastic lungs, and cryptorchism. The syndrome is believed to transmitted as an autosomal recessive trait.

Mease, A. D., *et al.* A syndrome of ankylosis, facial anomalies and pulmonary hypoplasia secondary to fetal neuromuscular dysfunction. *Birth Defects,* 1976, 12(5):193-200.

annular constriction of the penis. See *penis tourniquet syndrome.*

annular corneal dystrophy. See *Reis-Bücklers syndrome.*

anomalous position of the popliteal artery syndrome. See *popliteal artery entrapment syndrome.*

anomalous pulmonary venous connection (APVC). See *scimitar syndrome.*

anomalous pulmonary venous return. See *scimitar syndrome.*

anonychia-ectrodactyly syndrome. Absence of the fingernails with variable absence of phalanges and metacarpals, associated with crooked fingers and toes, syndactyly, and polydactyly. The syndrome is believed to be transmitted as an autosomal dominant trait.

Charteris, F. Case of partial hereditary anonychia. *Glasgow Med. J.*, 1918, 89:207-9. Lees, D. H., *et al.* Anonychia with ectrodactyly: Clinical and linkage data. *Ann. Hum. Genet.*, 1957, 22:69-79.

anonychia-onychodystrophy syndrome. A syndrome transmitted as an autosomal dominant trait, characterized by absence or dystrophy of nails, occurring without associated anomalies.

Charteris, F. A. A case of partial hereditary anonychia. *Glasgow Med. J.*, 1918, 89:207-9. Timerman, L., *et al.* Dominant anonychia and onychodystrophy. *J. Med. Genet.*, 1969, 6:105-6.

anophthalmia-hand and foot defects-mental retardation syndrome. A syndrome of mental retardation, true anophthalmia, deformities of the fingers and toes, and orofacial abnormalities, transmitted as an X-linked recessive trait. The symptoms include a peculiar facies with a prominent forehead, a long and narrow nose with a narrow base and flared tonsils, and a wide mouth. High-arched palate, scrotal tongue, and large incisors are the main oral defects. Hand and foot abnormalities consist of wide gaps between the fourth and fifth fingers and toes, fusion of fourth and fifth metatarsal bones, clinodactyly, finger hypoplasia, short fifth phalanges, abnormal dermatoglyphics, and simian creases.

Pasllotta, R., & Dallapiccola, B. A syndrome with true anophthalmia, hand-foot defects and mental retardation. *Ophthal. Paediat. Genet.*, 1984, 4:19-24.

anophthalmos-microphthalmos-coloboma syndrome. A hereditary syndrome, transmitted as an autosomal dominant trait, characterized by anophthalmos, microphthalmos, and coloboma, frequently associated with mental ratardation.

François, J. A propos d'une familie présentant des anomalies oculaires du type colobamateux depuis le colobome unilatéral de l'iris jusqu'a l'anophthalmie bilatérale, associée au syndrome de Bardet-Biedl. *J. Génét. Hum.*, 1953, 2:203-18.

anophthalmos-syndactyly syndrome. See *Waardenburg syndrome (3).*

anorchidism. See *embryonic testicular regression syndrome.*

anorectal malformation-nephritis-nerve deafness syndrome. A familial syndrome, transmitted as an autosomal dominant trait, combining the features of Alport syndrome with abnormalities of the anus and rectum, nerve deafness, and nephritis. Imperforate anus, preauricular skin tags, enlarged pinnae, closed anoperineal fistula, neonatal hyperbilirubinemia, and sacral dermal sinus are the associated defects.

Lowe, J., *et al.* Dominant ano-recal malformation, nephritis and nerve-deafness: A possible new entity. *Clin. Genet.*, 1983, 24:191-3.

anorectal malformation-sacral bony abnormality-presacral mass (ASP) association. See *Currarino triad.*

anorectogenital elephantiasis. See *Huguier-Jersild syndrome.*

anorexia nervosa syndrome. Synonym: *anorexic syndrome.*

A disorder usually affecting previously healthy girls and young women who become emaciated as a result of voluntary starvation and dieting in an effort to control their weight. Physical examination usually shows extreme emaciation, a fine lanugo covering the body and limbs, dryness of the skin, brittle nails, cold and blue extremities, amenorrhea, low luteinizing hormone levels, low basal metabolism rate, slight hypothalamopituitary dysfunction, and moderate enlargement of the lateral and third ventricles. The condition is usually observed in white females of middle and upper social strata and very seldom in other racial and social groups. Recent findings show that young males may be also affected.

Adams, R. D., & Victor, M. *Principles of neurology.* 3rd ed. New York, McGraw-Hill, 1985, pp. 1131-4. *Diagnostic and statistical manual of mental disorders.* American Psychiatric Association. 3rd ed. Washington, 1987. pp. 65-7.

anorexic syndrome. See *anorexia nervosa syndrome.*

anosteogenesis. See *achondrogenesis type I.*

antebrachial-palmar hammer syndrome. Obstructed blood flow to the hand and fingers due to repeated blunt trauma of the ulnar and radial arteries, such as that caused by repeated impact of the hand against the ball and floor during volleyball playing. The degree of trauma may vary from a trivial hematoma to severe fragmentation of the arterial wall. The injury of the intima is likely to lead to thrombosis, whereas the damage to the media may cause aneurysm. Recurrent minor injuries may produce vasospasm.

Kokstianen, S., & Orava, S. Blunt injury of the radial and ulnar arteries in volley ball players. A report of three cases of the antebrachial-palmar hammer syndrome. *Brit. J. Sports Med.*, 1983, 17:172-6.

antecubital pterygium syndrome. A condition, originally reported in eight persons in three generations of a Mauritian family, characterized by a web extending across each cubital fossa from the distal third of the upper arm to the proximal third of the forearm. The syndrome is believed to be transmitted as an autosomal dominant trait.

Shu-Shin, M. Congenital web formation. *J. Bone Joint Surg.*, 1954, 36B:268-71.

anterior bulbar syndrome. See *Déjerine syndrome (2).*

anterior cavernous syndrome. See *under Jefferson syndrome.*

anterior chamber cleavage syndrome. A group of diseases, involving the anterior segment of the eye, which are due to faulty cleavage. The following entities are included in this group: prominent Schwalbe ring (posterior embryotoxon, posterior marginal dysplasia of Streiff, congenital hyaline membrane of Mann, peripheral refractile postcorneal rim of Graves, knob at periphery of Descemet membrane); prominent Schwalbe ring with attached iris strands-see *Axenfeld anomaly*; prominent Schwalbe ring with attached iris strands and hypoplastic anterior iris stroma (primary dysgenesis mesodermalis of the iris, dysgenesis mesodermalis corneae et iridis)-see *Rieger anomaly*; iris strands in angle and hypoplastic iris stroma (hereditary juvenile glaucoma and goniodysgenesis, congenital iris stromal hypoplasia, iridogoniodysgenesis); prominent Schwalbe ring and hypoplasia of anterior iris stroma; posterior corneal depression (posterior keratoconus, keratoconus posticus circumscriptus, posterior conical cornea); posterior corneal defect with leukoma, posterior corneal defect with leukoma and adherent iris strands (dysgenesis mesodermalis of the cornea, Hippel internal corneal ulcer, congenital leukoma with pupillary synechiae), adherent iris strands, keratolenticular contact (mesodermal dysgenesis of the cornea)-see *Peters anomaly*, corneal staphyloma (congenital anterior staphyloma); secondary mesodermal dysgenesis of the iris and cornea; and sclerocornea.

Reese, A. B., & Ellsworth, R. M. The anterior chamber cleavage syndrome. *Arch. Ophthalmol.*, 1966, 75:307-18. Waring, G. O., *et al.* Anterior chamber cleavage syndrome. A stepladder classification. *Surv. Ophthalmol.*, 1975, 20:3-27.

anterior chest wall syndrome. See *Prinzmetal angina, and see chest wall syndrome.*

anterior choroidal artery syndrome. Synonym: *Monakow syndrome.*

Contralateral hemiplegia, hemianesthesia, and hemianopsia due to rupture or occlusion of the anterior choroidal artery. Associated disorders may include blepharoptosis, pseudobulbar syndrome, and paralysis of vertical gaze.

Foix, C., *et al.* Oblitération de l'artère choroïdienne antérieure. Remollissement de son territoire cérébral. Hémiplégie, hémianesthésie, hémianopsie.. *Bull. Soc. Ophtal. Paris,* 1925, 37:221-3. Decroix, J. P., *et al.* Infarction in the territory of the anterior choroidal artery. A clinical and computerized tomographic study of 16 cases. *Brain,* 1986, 109:1071-85.

anterior cord syndrome. Compression of the anterior column of the spinal cord or lesions of the anterior spinal artery, associated with disorders of voluntary movements, pain, and absence of temperature sensation, while distal position sense, light touch, and vibratory sensation remain undisturbed.

Guttmann, L. *Spinal cord injuries. Comprehensive management and research.* 2nd ed. Oxford, Blackwell, 1976. Becker, D. P. Injury of the head and spine. In: Wyngaarden, J. B., & Smith, L. H., Jr. ed. *Cecil textbook of medicine.* 17th ed. Philadelphia, Saunders, 1985, pp. 2170-7.

anterior cruciate ligament (ACL) insufficiency syndrome. See *anterior cruciate ligament syndrome.*

anterior cruciate ligament (ACL) syndrome. Synonyms: *anterior cruciate ligament (ACL)-deficient knee, anterior cruciate ligment (ACL) insufficiency syndrome, torn anterior cruciate ligament syndrome.*

Functional instability of the knee joint due to injuries of the anterior cruciate ligament.

Feagin, J. A., Jr. The syndrome of the torn anterior cruciate ligament. *Orthop. Clin. N. America*, 1979, 10:81-

90. Andrews, J. B., & Carson, W. G., Jr., eds. Symposium on the anterior cruciate ligament. Part I. *Orthop. Clin. N. America,* 1985, 16:1-162.

anterior cruciate ligament (ACL)-deficient knee. See *anterior cruciate ligament syndrome.*

anterior horn cell disease with pontocerebellar hypoplasia. See *amyotrophic cerebellar hypoplasia syndrome.*

anterior impingement syndrome of the ankle. Pain and limitation of motion during dorsiflexion of the ankle, caused by the spur on the anterior aspect of the dorsum of the talus, occurring most commonly in ballet dancers and athletes. Repeated pull of the anterior ankle joint capsule and the impingement of the talus against the tibia in running and jumping, leading to calcific deposits along the lines of the capsular fibers, are the principal features of this disorder.

Parkes, J. C., II, *et al.* The anterior impingement syndrome of the ankle. *J. Trauma,* 1980, 20:895-8.

anterior internuclear ophthalmoplegia. See *Lhermitte syndrome.*

anterior interosseous nerve syndrome (AINS, AIS). See *Kiloh-Nevin syndrome (1).*

anterior midline syndrome. See *Zeman-King syndrome.*

anterior pituitary hyperhormonotropic syndrome. See *Zondek syndrome, under Zondek, Bernhard.*

anterior poliomyelitis. See *Heine-Medin disease.*

anterior segment traumatic syndrome. See *Frenkel syndrome.*

anterior spinal artery occlusion. See *anterior spinal artery syndrome.*

anterior spinal artery syndrome. Synonyms: *Beck syndrome, anterior spinal artery occlusion.*

Isolated occlusion of the anterior segment of the spinal artery resulting in a variety of neurological complications, including radicular paresthesia, stabbing pain and a feeling of pressure in the waist region, weakness, cramps, deafness, pain and temperature sense disorders. The prodromal symptoms usually disappear with the onset of paraplegia. The motor disorders are usually related to the level of spinal lesions; lumbar lesions produce flaccid paralysis, whereas cervical lesions result in spastic paralysis. Sphincter control and sexual disorders are usually present. Thrombosis, trauma, neoplasms, arteriosclerosis, and other spinal disorders are the most common causes of this syndrome.

Beck, K. Das Syndrom des Verschlusses der verderen Spinalarterie. *Deut. Zschr. Nervenh.,* 1951-52, 167:164-86.

anterior tarsal syndrome. See *anterior tarsal tunnel syndrome.*

anterior tarsal tunnel syndrome. Synonym: *anterior tarsal syndrome.*

A compression neuropathy of the deep peroneal nerve beneath the inferior extensor retinaculum caused by edema, fractures, subluxation, or ankle sprain. The symptoms include pain in the ankle and dorsum of the foot and paresthesia or dysesthesia in the first interdigital space.

Marinacci, A. A. Neurological syndromes of the tarsal tunnels. *Bull. Los Angeles Neurol. Soc.,* 1968, 33:90-100.

anterior thoracic wall syndrome. See *Prinzmetal angina.*

anterior tibial compartment syndrome. Synonyms: *anterior tibial syndrome, anterior tibial muscle syndrome, tibialis anterior syndrome.*

The most common of compartment syndromes (q.v.) of the lower extremity, caused by strenuous muscle activity, injuries, or arterial circulation disorders, characterized by acute onset of severe pain, swelling and tenderness of the muscles, reddening of the skin over the affected area, circulatory deficiency in the anterior tibial compartment, and ischemic necrosis.

Child, C. G.., III. Noninfective gangrene following fracture of lower leg. *Ann. Surg.,* 1942, 116:721. Greenbaum, E. I., *et al.* Value of delayed filming of the anterior bitial compartment syndrome secondary to trauma. *Radiology,* 1969, 93:373.

anterior tibial muscle syndrome. See *anterior tibial compartment syndrome.*

anterior tibial syndrome. See *anterior tibial compartment syndrome.*

antibiotic enteritis. See *Janbon syndrome.*

anticardiolipin (ACA) syndrome. Occurrence of antiphospholipid antibodies, such as anticardiolipin antibodies, in the presence of multiple venous or arterial thromboses together with thrombocytopenia or multiple abortions. Myelopathy, chorea, epilepsy, livedo reticularis, labile hypertension, migraine and other forms of headache, transient ischemia, amaurosis fugax, and hematological disorders, such as hemolytic anemia, may be associated. The syndrome most commonly occurs in lupus erythematosus patients.

Hughes, G. R. V. The anticardiolipin syndrome. *Clin. Exp. Rheumatol.,* 1985, 3:285-6. Bowie, W. E. J., *et al.* Thrombosis in SLE despite circulating anticoagulants. *J. Clin. Invest.,* 1963, 62:416.

anticholinergic intoxication. See *anticholinergic syndrome.*

anticholinergic syndrome. Synonyms: *anticholinergic intoxication, central anticholinergic syndrome.*

Toxic reactions to overdoses of anticholinergic substances characterized by fever, flushing, dilated pupils, and central nervous system disorders ranging from somnolence to delirium and coma. Specific anticholinergic may produce additional symptoms, such as extrapyramidal reactions by Benadryl (diphenhydramine hydrochloride) or cardiac arrhythmia by tricyclic antidepressants.

Kulik, A., & Willbur, R. Delirium and stereotypy from anticholinergic antiparkinson drugs. *Prog. Neuropsychopharmacol.,* 1982, 6:75-82. Feldman, M.D. The syndrome of anticholinergic intoxication. *Am. Fam. Physician,* 1986, 34(5)113-6.

antithyroid arthritis syndrome. Arthritic complications following the use of antithyroid drugs, such as propylthiouracil and methimazole, in the treatment of hyperthyroidism.

Shabitai, R., *et al.* The antithyroid arthritis syndrome reviewed. *Arthritis Rheum.,* 1984, 27:227-9.

ANTLEY, RAY M. (American physician)

Antley-Bixler syndrome. Synonyms: *multisynostotic osteodysgenesis with fractures, multisynostotic osteodysgenesis with long bone fractures, trapezoidocephaly-multiple synostoses syndrome (TMS), trapezoidoidocephaly-synostoses syndrome.*

A syndrome of bone and cartilage maldevelopment. Craniofacial defects consist mainly of craniosynostoses, brachycephaly, frontal bossing, midface hypoplasia, depressed nasal root, prominent nasal tip, choanal atresia, long philtrum, small mouth, high-arched palate, low-set ears, thick-rolled helix, marked antihelix, and underdeveloped lobule. Anomalies of the extremities include long tapering fingers, long palms, short distal phalanges with or without clubbing, camptodactyly, abnormal dermatoglyphics, bowed and fractured femora, clubfoot, talipes equinovarus, rocker bottom feet, long deformed toes, short distal phalanges, dorsal position of the phalanges, and clinocamptodactyly of the toes. Narrow chest, narrow pelvis, limited hip abduction with or without dislocation, and sacral dimple usually occur. The syndrome is transmitted as an autosomal recessive trait.

Antley, R., & Bixler, D. Trapezoidocephaly, midfacial hypoplasia and cartilage abnormalities with multiple synostoses and skeletal fractures. *Birth Defects,* 1975, 11(2):397-401.

ANTON, GABRIEL (German neurologist, 1858-1933)

Anton syndrome. See *Anton-Babinski syndrome.*

Anton-Babinski syndrome. Synonyms: *Anton syndrome, cortical blindness with denial, denial visual hallucination syndrome, hemiasomatognosia, visual anosognosia.*

Denial of blindness with resort to confabulation by blind persons.

Anton, G. Über den Ausdruck der Gemütsbewegung beim gesunden und kranken Menschen. *Psychiat. Wschr.,* 1900, 17:165-9.

ANTOPOL, WILLIAM (American physician)

Antopol disease. An inborn error of glycogen storage characterized by abnormal glycogen deposits in the heart and systemic muscles. Cardiomegaly is the principal clinical feature. Autosomal recessive transmission is suspected.

Antopol, W., *et al.* Cardiac hypertrophy caused by glycogen storage disease in a fifteen-year-old boy. *Am. Heart J.,* 1940, 20:546-56.

ANUG (acute necrotizing ulcerative gingivitis). See *Vincent infection.*

anxietas tibiarum. See *restless leg syndrome.*

AO (arthro-ophthalmopathy). See *Stickler syndrome.*

aortic arch arteritis. See *aortic arch syndrome.*

aortic arch syndrome. Synonyms: *Martorell syndrome, Martorell-Fabré syndrome, Reader-Harbitz syndrome, Takayasu arteritis, Takayasu disease, Takayasu syndrome, Takayasu-Martorell-Fabré syndrome, Takayasu-Onishi syndrome, aortic arch arteritis, arcus aortae syndrome, arteritis of aorta in young women, arteritis brachiocephalica, brachiocephalic arteritis, brachial arteritis, central aortitis, chronic subclavian-carotid obstruction syndrome, elongated coarctation of aorta, middle aortic disease, middle aortic syndrome, obliteration of supra-aortic branches, obliterative brachiocephalic arteritis syndrome, occlusion of supra-aortic trunk syndrome, prepulseless arteritis, pulseless arteritis, pulseless disease, reversed coarctation of aorta, rheumatic brachio-cephalic arteritis, stenosing aortitis, subisthmic coarction of aorta, thromboarteritis obliterans subclaviocarotica, young female arteritis syndrome.*

A syndrome of occlusion of the innominate, left subclavian, and left common carotid arteries above their origin at the aortic arch. It is a chronic relapsing disorder which may extend from childhood to late adult life, being most common in the Orient and showing predilection for young women, but also occurring in males throughout the world. The syndrome is characterized by cerebral ischemia; weak, absent, or asynchronous pulse; progeroid facial features with ulceration of the palate, nose, and ears, saddle nose, gingival atrophy, and jaw claudication; ocular disorders, including ischemia, corneal opacity, cataract, optic atrophy, retinal atrophy, iris atrophy, retinal microaneurysms, reduced retinal arterial pressure, and venous dilatations; cardiovascular disorders, such as hypertension with heart failure, aortic incompetence, angina pectoris, coarctation of the aorta, Leriche syndrome, renal hypertension, and mesenteric and celiac stenosis; fatigability; pallor; paresthesia; and potential for gangrene. Arteritis occurs in the aorta and its branches, particularly in their proximal segments, sometimes also involving pulmonary and cerebral arteries. The walls of affected arteries are thickened and their intima is wrinkled; ostial stenosis and superimposed atheromas are common. The syndrome occurs as pre-occlusive (prepulseless) and occlusive (pulseless) forms. Autoimmune mechanism has been suggested as a possible cause but the etiology remains obscure.

*Takayasu, M. Case of queer changes in central vessels of retina. *Acta Soc. Ophth. Japan.,* 1908, 12:554. Martorell, F., & Fabré Tersol, J. El sindrome de obliteración de los troncos supraaórticos. *Med. Clin. Barcelona,* 1944, 2:26-30. *Harbitz, F. Bilateral carotid arteritis. *Arch. Path. Lab. Med.,* 1926, 1:499-530.

aortic bifurcation occlusion syndrome. See *Leriche syndrome (1).*

aortic insufficiency. See *Corrigan disease.*

aortic regurgitation. See *Corrigan disease.*

aorto-iliac steal syndrome. Synonym: *mesenteric artery syndrome.*

Sudden redistribution of blood flow to the lower limbs from the mesenteric circulation with resulting fall in the arterial pressure and precipitation of arterial occlusion and mesenteric ischemia, sometimes associated with infarction and gangrene. There is an obstruction of the distal abdominal aorta below the renal arteries with diversion of the blood from the superior mesenteric circulation, through the inferior mesenteric and hypogastric arteries, to the lower extremities. In the original report, the condition was a complication of sequential lumbar sympathectomy and iliofemoral graft. See also *postcoartectomy syndrome..*

Kountz, S. L., *et al.* "Aortoiliac steal" syndrome. *Arch. Surg.,* 1966, 92:490-7. Connolly, J. E., & Stemmer, E. A. Intestinal gangrene as the result of mesenteric arterial steal. *Am. J. Surg.,* 1973, 126:197-204.

apallic syndrome. Synonyms: *Kretschmer syndrome, coma vigile, post-traumatic apallic syndrome, traumatic apallic syndrome (TAS).*

A syndrome of global aphasia, apraxia, and agnosia following severe brain injury, anoxia, or poisoning, in which patients are open-eyed, uncommunicative, and unresponsive. It is a persistent vegetative state due to the absence of function of the cerebral cortex; the lesions may involve the cortex itself, subcortical structures of the hemisphere, or the brain stem, either singly or in various combinations.

Jennett, B., & Plum, F. Persistent vegetative state after brain damage. A syndrome in search of a name. *Lancet,,* 1972, 1:734-7. Kretschmer, E. Das apallische Syndrom. *Zschr. Ges. Neurol. Psychiat.,* 1940, 169:576-9.

APCD. See *acquired prothrombin complex deficiency syndrome.*

APECED (autoimmune polyendocrinopathy-candidosis-ectodermal dystrophy) syndrome. A syndrome of hypoparathyroidism, primary adrenocortical failure, and chronic mucocutaneous candidiasis, stransmitted as an autosomal recessive trait. Associated endocrine disorders and dystrophy of the dental enamel and nails may be associated.

Perheentupa, J. Autoimmune polyendocrinopathy-candidosis-ectodermal dysplasia (APECED). In: Erikson, A. W., Forsius, H., Nevanlinna, H. R., Workman, P. L., & Norio, R. K., eds. *Population structure and genetic disorders.* New York, Academic Press, 1980, pp. 583-7.

APERT, EUGENE (French pediatrician, 1868-1940)

Apert syndactyly. See *Apert syndrome.*

Apert syndrome. Synonyms: *Apert syndactyly, acrocephalosyndactylism syndrome, acrocephalosyndactyly I (ACS I), acrocephaly with syndactyly, acrocraniodysphalangia, acrodysplasia, syndactylic oxycephaly syndrome.*

A complex of craniofacial abnormalities caused by premature craniosynostosis, usually of the coronal suture, leading to turribrachycephaly, associated with syndactyly and polydactyly. Cranial abnormalities are of the brachysphenocephalic type with high forehead, small nose, supraorbital horizontal groove, shallow orbits, antimongoloid palpebral fissures, hypoplastic maxilla, and narrow palate. Cleft palate may occur. Syndactyly is due to osseous fussion of the second and fourth fingers with a single nail and soft tissue fusion of the fourth or second to fifth, or of all toes, thus giving the hands and feet a mitten-like appearance. There may be also shortening of upper extremities, deformation of the pectoral girdle, and abnormalities of genitourinary, gastrointestinal, and cardiovascular systems. The syndrome is transmitted as an autosomal dominant trait.

Apert, E. De l'acrocéphalosyndactylie. *Bull. Soc. Méd., Paris*, 1906, 23:1310-30.

Apert-Crouzon syndrome. Synonyms: *Vogt cephalodactyly, Vogt syndrome, acrocephalosyndactyly II (ACS II).*

A syndrome combining features of the Apert syndrome with those of the Crouzon syndrome and consisting of craniosynostosis, usually of the coronal suture, flat facies, shallow orbits, hypertelorism, and fusion of the fingers with single nails and short broad thumbs, thus giving the hands a mitten-like appearance, associated with facial characteristics of Crouzon's facies. The condition is transmitted as an autosomal dominant trait. According to some authorities (e.g., McKusick), this syndrome represents an independent entity and is classified as acrocephalosyndactyly II; according to others (e.g., Spranger, Langer, and Wiedemann), this is a poorly documented disorder, whereby some cases possibly are the Apert and others Pfeiffer syndrome. The syndrome is also classified by some writers as a subset of autosomal dominant Apert syndrome (ACS I).

Vogt, A. Dyskephalie (dysostosis craniofacialis, maladie de Crouzon 1912) und eine neuartige Kombination dieser Krankheit mit Syndaktylie der 4 Extremitäten (Dyskephalodaktylie). *Klin. Monatsbl. Augenheilk.*, 1933, 90:441-54. Apert, E. De l'acrocephalosyndactylie. *Bull Soc. Méd., Paris*, 1906, 23:1310-30. McKusick, V. A. *Mendelian inheritance in man.* 5th ed., Baltimore, The Johns Hopkins Universty Press, 1978. p. 7 (No. 10130). Spranger, J. W., Langer, L. O., Jr., & Wiedemann, H. R. *Bone dysplasias*, Philadelphia, Saunders, 1974. p. 261. Wells, T. R., *et al.* acrocephalospondylosyndactyly-a possible new syndrome: Analysis of the vertebral and intervertebral components. *Pediat. Path.*, 1990, 10:117-31.

Apert-Cushing syndrome. See *Cushing syndrome.*

Cooke-Apert-Gallais syndrome. See *Cushing syndrome.*

apex of petrous bone syndrome. See *Gradenigo syndrome.*

aphasia-epilepsy syndrome. Synonym: *acquired aphasia-convulsive disorder.*

A childhood syndrome of acquired aphasia and epilepsy. Midtemporal spike activity and bilateral-synchronous bursts of spikes and slow spike-wave complexes are the principal EEG features.

Landau, W. M., & Kleffner, F. R. Syndrome of acquired aphasia with convulsive disorder in children. *Neurology,* 1957, 7:523-30. Rodriguez, I., & Niedermeyer, E. The aphasia-epilepsy syndrome in children: Electroencephalographic aspects. *Clin. Electroencephalogr.*, 1982, 13:23-35.

aphasic sensory syndrome. See *Bianchi syndrome.*

aphemia. See *Broca aphasia.*

aphthosis generalisata. See *Stevens-Johnson syndrome.*

aphthous pharyngitis. See *Zahorsky syndrome (2).*

apical dystrophy. See *brachydactyly B.*

apical dystrophy-macular coloboma syndrome. See *Sorsby syndrome (1).*

apicocostovertebral syndrome. See *Pancoast syndrome.*

aplasia axialis extracorticalis congenita. See *Pelizaeus-Merzbacher syndrome.*

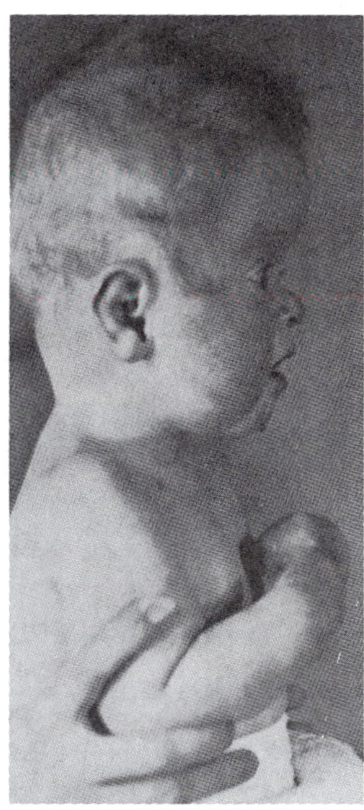

Apert syndrome
Aegerter, E. and J.A. Kirkpatrick, Jr.: *Orthopedic diseases* 3rd ed. Philadelphia: W.B. Saunders, 1968.

aplastic abdominal muscle syndrome. See *prune belly syndrome.*

aplastic anemia with congenital anomalies. See *Fanconi anemia.*

aplastic anemia-dyskeratosis congenita syndrome. See *Zinsser-Fanconi syndrome.*

aplastic anemia-paroxysmal nocturnal hemoglobinuria syndrome. Synonym: *aplastic anemia-PNH syndrome.*

An association of aplastic anemia with paroxysmal nocturnal hemoglobinuria, which may terminate in acute leukemia.

Dacie, J. V., & Lewis, S. M. Paroxysmal nocturnal haemoglinuria. Variation in clinical severity and association with bone marrow hypoplasia. *Brit. J. Haematol.*, 1961, 7:442.

aplastic anemia-PNH syndrome. See *aplastic anemia paroxysmal nocturnal hemoglobinuria syndrome.*

aplastic crisis. See *Owren syndrome (1).*

aplastic infantile funicular myelosis. See *Fanconi anemia.*

apo C2 deficiency syndrome. See *apolipoprotein C-II deficiency syndrome.*

apolipoprotein C-II deficiency syndrome. Synonyms: *anapolipoproteinemia C-II, apo C2 deficiency syndrome, hyperlipoproteinemia type IB, hyperlipoproteinemia C-II.*

A rare genetic syndrome, transmitted as an autosomal recessive trait, characterized by a deficiency of plasma apo C-II, marked elevation of plasma triglycerides and chylomicrons, and decreased low and high density lipoproteins. Clinical features include pancreatitis, exocrine and endocrine pancreatic insufficiency with diabetes mellitus, retinitis, and peripheral neuritis. Abdominal pain, xanthomas, hepatomegaly, and splenomegaly may be associated.

Breckenridge, W. C., *et al.* Hypertriglyceridemia associated with deficiency of apolipoprotein C-II. *N. Engl. J. Med.*, 1978, 298:1265-73. Baggio, G., *et al.* Apolipoprotein C-II deficiency syndrome. Clinical features, lipoprotein characterization, lipase activity, and correction of hypertriglyceridemia after apolipoprotein C-II administration in two affected patients. *J. Clin. Invest.*, 1986, 77:520-7.

apophysitis tibialis adolescentium. See *Osgood-Schlatter syndrome.*

apoplexia uteroplacentaris. See *Couvelaire syndrome.*

apoplexia uvulae. See *Bosviel syndrome.*

apostematous cheilitis. See *Baelz syndrome.*

apparent mineralocorticoid excess-cortisol metabolism defect syndrome. A metabolic syndrome characterized by failure to thrive, arterial hypertension, hypokalemia, metabolic alkalosis, suppressed plasma renin activity, and absence of abnormal secretion of mineralocorticoids. A defect in 11-beta-hydroxysteroid dehydrogenase activity resulting in low cortisone/cortisol ratio is a marker of this condition.

Ulick, S., *et al.* A syndrome of apparent mineralocorticoid excess associated with defect in the peripheral metabolism of cortisol. *J. Clin. Endocr. Metab.*, 1979, 49:7757. Batista, M. C., *et al.* Spirololactone-reversible rickets associated with 11-beta-hydroxysteroid dehydrogenase deficiency syndrome *J. Pediat.*, 1986, 109:989-93.

APPELT, H. (German pediatrician)

Appelt-Gerken-Lenz syndrome. See *Roberts syndrome.*

appendiceal syndrome. See *appendicitis syndrome.*

appendicitis syndrome. Synonym: *appendiceal syndrome.*

Inflammation of vermiform appendix that may lead to perforation and peritonitis.

Fitz, R. H. Perforating inflammation of the vermiform appendix: With special reference to its early diagnosis and treatment. *Am. J. Med. Sc.*, 1886, 92:321-46. Berry, J., Jr., & Malt, R. A. Appendicitis near its centenary. *Ann. Surg.*, 1984, 200:567-75.

appendicitis-duodenal stenosis syndrome. See *Brodin syndrome.*

APPIAN OF ALEXANDRIA (2nd century AD Greek historian)

Appian-Plutarch syndrome. Synonyms: *atropine syndrome, atropinism.*

A pathological condition caused by atropine intoxication. Side effects of therapeutic doses may cause dryness of the mouth, swallowing difficulty, thirst, pupil dilatation, loss of accommodation, photophobia, increased intra-ocular pressure, flushing, dryness of the skin, bradycardia followed by tachycardia, arrhythmias, desire to urinate with the inability to do so, constipation, vomiting, and giddiness. Toxic doses may produce tachycardia, rash, rapid or stertorous respiration, fever, restlessness, confusion, hallucinations, delirium, respiratory failure and death. The condition is named after Appian of Alexandria and Plutarch, who are said to have written about poisoning in soldiers who, driven by hunger, ate strange plants during the wars against the Parthians.

Nemery, A., *et al.* Les erreurs thérapeutiques de syndrome atrophinique (syndrome d'Appien-Plutarque). *Rev. Méd. Liège*, 1983, 38:927-9.

apple peel syndrome. Synonyms: Christmas tree deformity, maypole deformity.

A deformity consisting of a duodenal or high jejunal atresia associated with absence of the small bowel mesentery and pre-arterial arcades of the superior meseteric artery. The resulting appearance is of distal small bowel coming straight off the cecum and twisted around a marginal artery, suggesting a Christmas tree, maypole, or apple peel, hence its designations. The syndrome is transmitted as an autosomal recessive trait.

Blyth, H., & Dickinson, J. A. S. Apple peel syndrome (congenital intestinal atresia). J. Med. Genet., 1969, 6:275-7. Mishalany, H. G., & Najjar, F. B. Familial jejunal atresia. J. Pediat., 1968, 73:753-5.

APPLEBAUM, L. (German physician)

Recklinghausen-Applebaum syndrome. See *under Recklinghausen.*

approximate answers syndrome. See *Ganser syndrome.*

apraxia. See *Liepmann disease.*

aprosencephaly syndrome. See *Garcia-Lurie syndrome.*

aprosencephaly-atelencephaly syndrome. See *Garcia-Lurie syndrome.*

APVC (anomalous pulmonary venous connection). See *scimitar syndrome.*

ara-C syndrome. See *cytosine arabinose syndrome.*

arachnodactyly. See *Marfan syndrome (1).*

arachnoid fibroblastoma. See *Cushing tumor.*

ARAKAWA, TSUNEO (Japanese physician)

Arakawa syndrome (1). A formiminotransferase deficiency syndrome, transmitted as an autosomal recessive trait, characterized by mental and physical retardation, cortical atrophy, dilation of the cerebral ventricles, and abnormal EEG. Disturbed folic acid metabolism, increased urinary formiminoglutamic acid levels, and probable defect of cyclodeaminase are the additional biochemical features. Hematological changes include megaloblastic and normocytic anemias and hypersegmented neurotrophils.

Arakawa, T., *et al.* Familial occurence of formiminotransferase deficiency syndrome. *Tohoku J. Exp. Med.*, 1968, 96:211-7. Rowe, P. B. Inherited disorders of folate metabolism. In: Stanbury, J. B., Wyngaarden, J. B., & Fredrickson, D. S., eds. *The metabolic basis of inherited disease.* 4th ed. New York, McGraw-Hill, 1978, pp. 430-57.

Arakawa syndrome (2). A congenital syndrome of tetrahydrofolate methyltransferase deficiency associated with cobalamin metabolism disorders, megaloblastic anemia, vomiting, diarrhea, pallor, growth and mental retardation, hepatosplenomegaly, and neurological complications consisting of myoclonus, EEG abnormalities, and cerebral ventricular dilatation.

Arakawa, T., *et al.* Megaloblastic anemia and mental retardation associated with hyperfolicacidaemia. Probably due to N-5-methyltetrahydrofolate transferase deficiency. *Tohoku J. Exp. Med.*, 1967, 93:1-22. Rowe, P. B. Inherited disorders of folate metabolism. In: Stanbury, J. B., Wyngaarden, J. B., & Fredrickson, D. S., eds. *The metabolic basis of inherited disease.* 4th ed. New York, McGraw-Hill, 1978, pp. 430-57.

Arakawa-Higashi syndrome. Uracil-uric refractory anemia with peroxidase negative neutrophils and megaloblastic bone marrow. Neutrophils are negative to all stains for peroxidase, oxidase, succinic dehydrogenase, uracil, UMP, and UDP. The fatal outcome is due to urinary sepsis with a leukemoid blood picture. The condition was originally described in two girls aged seven and ten years.

Arakawa, T., *et al.* Uracil-uric refractory anemia with peroxidase negative neutrophils. *Tohoku J. Exp. Med.*, 1965, 87:52-76. Higashi, *et al.* A case with hematological abnormality characterized by the absence of peroxidase activity in blood polymorphonuclear leukocytes. *Tohoku J. Exp. Med.*, 1965, 87:77-93.

ARAN, FRANÇOIS ALMICAR (French physician, 1817-1861)

Aran-Duchenne syndrome. Synonyms: *Cruveilhier atrophy, Cruveilhier palsy, Duchenne-Griesinger disease, amyotrophia nuclearis progressiva, distal spinal muscular atrophy, myelopathic muscular atrophy, progressive spinal muscular atrophy, wasting palsy.*

A form of muscular atrophy which begins as weakness of small muscles of the hand, followed by stiffness, clumsiness, and cramps. The muscles supplied by the fifth cervical nerves and the extensor hallucis longus are the first ones to be affected. The wasting is progressive and eventually becomes generalized. Muscular fasciculation, simian hand (eventually becoming "cadaveric hand"), round-shouldered posture, forward droop of the head, drop foot, steppage gait, and dyspnea are the principal clinical features.

Aran, F. A. Récherches sur une maladie non encore décrite du système musculaire (atrophie musculaire progressive). *Arch. Gén. Méd., Paris,* 1850, 24:172-214. Duchenne, G. B. Étude comparée de lésions anatomique dans l'atrophie musculaire progressive et dans la paralysie générale. *lUnion Méd. Prat. Fr.*, 1853, 7:202. Cruveilhier. Sur la paralysie musculaire progressive atrophique. *Bull. Acad. Méd. Paris,* 1853, 18:490-502.

ARBUTHNOT LANE. See LANE, SIR WILLIAM ARBUTHNOT

ARC (AIDS-related complex). See *under acquired immunodeficiency syndrome.*

arcuate scotoma. See *Bjerrum scotoma.*

arcus aortae syndrome. See *aortic arch syndrome.*

ARDS. See *adult respiratory distress syndrome.*

area celsi. See *Cazenave vitiligo.*

area johnstoni. See *Cazenave vitiligo.*

AREDYLD (acrorenal field defect-ectodermal dysplasia-lipoatrophic diabetes) syndrome. A familial syndrome, transmitted as an autosomal recessive trait, characterized by lipoatrophic diabetes, unusual facies, hypotrichosis, natal teeth, enamel dysplasia, dysplastic deciduous teeth, absence of permanent teeth, low birth weight, short stature, lumbar scoliosis, renal defects, aplasia or hypoplasia of the breasts, hypoplastic and hypopigmented areolae, hyperostosis of the cranial vault, metacarpal hypoplasia, hand grasping difficulty, exertional dyspnea, absence of flexion creases, dermatoglyphic alterations, and other anomalies. Facial features include prominent forehead and bridge of the nose, apparent telecanthus, mongoloid slant of the palpebral fissures, short nasal septum, flat tip of the nose, short upper lip, flat philtrum, prominent chin, and broad intertragal incisure with hypoplastic tragus.

Pinheiro, M., *et al.* AREDYLD: A syndrome combining an acrorenal field defect, ectodermal dysplasia, lipoatrophic diabetes, and other manifestations. *Am. J. Med. Genet.*, 1983, 16:29-33.

areolar central choroiditis. See *Förster disease.*

areolar choroiditis. See *Förster choroiditis.*

argentaffinoma syndrome. See *carcinoid syndrome.*

ARGONZ, J. (Argentine physician)

Argonz-Del Castillo syndrome. See *amenorrhea-galactorrhea syndrome.*

ARGYLL ROBERTSON. See ROBERTSON, DOUGLAS MORAY COOPER LAMB ARGYLL

arhincephaly. See *holoprosencephaly syndrome.*

ARIAS, IRWIN MONROE (American physician, born 1926)

Arias syndrome. See *Crigler-Najjar syndrome.*

ARKIN, AARON (American physician, 1888-1966)

Arkin disease. See *Bayford-Autenrieth dysphagia.*

ARKLESS, RICHARD (American radiologist)

Arkless-Graham syndrome. See *acrodysostosis.*

ARLT, CARL FERDINAND, VON (Austrian physician, 1812-1887)

Arlt syndrome. See *trachoma.*

ARMANI, LUCIANO (Italian pathologist, 1839-1903)

Armani-Ebstein lesion. See *Armani-Ebstein nephropathy.*

Armani-Ebstein nephropathy. Synonyms: *Armani-Ebstein lesion, glycogen infiltration, glycogen nephrosis.*

Vacuolation of the renal tubular epithelium seen in diabetic patients who have had marked hyperglycemia and glycosuria. It is believed to be caused by reabsorption of the urinary glucose, with the accumulation of glycogen within epithelial cells of the distal portions of the proximal convoluted tubules and in the descending limbs of the loop of Henle.

Robbins, S. L., & Cotran, R. S. *Pathologic basis of disease.* 2nd ed. Philadelphia, Saunders, 1979, p. 340.

ARMENDARES, S.

Armendares syndrome. A syndrome of growth retardation, microcephaly, cranial asymmetry, craniosynostosis, small face, scant eyebrows, short nose, micrognathia, high-arched palate, blepharoptosis, epicanthus, retinitis pigmentosa, malformed ear auricles, short fifth fingers, and simian creases. The syndrome is transmitted as an autosomal recessive or X-linked recessive trait.

Armendares, S., *et al.* A newly recognized inherited syndrome of dwarfism, craniosynostosis, retinitis pigmentosa, and multiple congenital malformations. *J. Pediat.*, 1974, 85:872-3.

Armenian disease. See *Reimann periodic disease.*

ARMSTRONG (SATCHMO), LOUIS DANIEL (American jazz trumpet player, 1900-1971)

Satchmo syndrome. An overuse syndrome (q.v.) characterized by rupture of the orbicularis oris muscle, occurring among musicians who play brass or wind instruments, especially trumpeters.

Planas, J. Rupture of the orbicularis oris in trumpet players (Satchmo's syndrome). *Plast. Reconstr. Surg.*, 1982, 69:690-1.

ARN. See *acute retinal necrosis syndrome.*

ARNDT, GEORG (German physician, 1874-1929)

Arndt-Gottron scleromyxedema. See *Arndt-Gottron syndrome.*

Arndt-Gottron syndrome. Synonyms: *Arndt-Gottron scleromyxedema, lichen myxoedematous, papular mucinosis.*

A fibromucinous connective tissue disease characterized by paraproteinemia and accumulation of mucinous material in the dermis, resulting in hardening and thickening of the skin. Hematological changes include an increase of gamma-globulin and elevated hexose and hexosamine levels. Cutaneous changes appearing suddenly as reddish or grayish-brown discoloration; hardening and thickening of the skin about the neck, joint flexures, and back with formation of thick folds in the affected areas; and masklike coarse facies with difficulty in opening the mouth are usually observed. Pale reddish or whitish multiple lichenoid nodules are often found on the neck, arms, and trunk. The skin changes are believed to be caused by infiltration of paraprotein into the connective tissue and their reaction with the basic substance. Histological findings usually include deposits of abnormal material rich in acid mucopolysaccharides that are intermixed with collagen fibers, chiefly in the reticular layer of the skin and connective tissue cells, and some mast cells.

Gottron, H. A. Skleromyxödem (Eine eigenartige Erscheinungsform von Myxothesaurodermie). *Arch. Derm. Syph., Berlin,* 1954, 199:71-91. Piper, W. *et al.* Das Skleromyxödem Arndt-Gottron: eine paraproteinamische Erkrankung. *Schweiz. Med. Wschr.*, 1967, 97:829-38.

ARNETH

Arneth syndrome. A condition characterized by muffling of the palpable thrill during speech, in the presence of bronchial murmur and bronchiloquy, and caused by complete hepatization of the lung tissue.

Minerbi, C. La "sindrome polmonitica di Arneth." La vera natura fisico del fremito vocale tattile. *Atti Accad. Sc. Med. Ferrara,* 1928, 3-4:47-9.

ARNING, EDUARD (German physician, born 1855)

Arning carcinoid. Synonyms: *carcinomatosis cutis disseminata, epithelioma pagetoide, erythematoid benign epithelioma, multiple benign superficial epithelioma, multiple cutaneous carcinoid, novabasalioma, pagetoid epithelioma, superficial epitheliomatosis.*

Multiple benign, flat tumors of the skin manifested as whitish gray shiny lesions with brownish purple pigmented areas, usually seen on the face and trunk. Initial lesions are small rough spots which slowly expand. Although the tumors heal spontaneously after several years, areas around old healed lesions usually become the sites of new crops of tumors. Arning compares this tumor to carcinoid, but classifies it with basal cell carcinoma.

Arning. Einen Fall von multiplen Carcinoiden der Haut. *Arch. Derm., Berlin,* 1922, 138:458-60.

ARNOLD, JULIUS (German physician, 1835-1915)

Arnold neuralgia. Synonyms: *auriculotemporal neuralgia, recurrent laryngeal neuralgia, superior laryngeal neuralgia.*

Neuralgia of the recurrent laryngeal nerve.

Kane, C. A., & Wegner, W. Craniofacial neuralgias. In: Baker, A. B., ed. *Clinical neurology.* New York, Hoeber, 1965, Vol. 4, p. 1906.

Arnold-Chiari deformity. See *Arnold-Chiari syndrome.*

Arnold-Chiari syndrome. Synonyms: *Arnold-Chiari deformity, Chiari deformity, Chiari malformation.*

A cork-like protrusion of the cerebellar tonsils and medulla oblongata through the foramen magnum into the cervical spinal canal without displacing the lower brain stem. It may be associated with stenosis of the aqueduct of Sylvius with obstructive hydrocephalus, and atrophy of the brain tissue. Deformity of the occipital bone and cervical vertebrae, platybasia, Klippel-Feil anomaly, softening and deformity of the cranial bones, maningocele, meningomyelocele, spina bifida, nystagmus, diplopia, papilledema, adhesive arachnoiditis, hemianopia, cerebellar ataxia, lack of coordination, intention tremor, and sensory disorders are usually present.

Arnold, J. Myelocyste. Transposition von Gewebskeimen und Sympodie. *Beitr. Path. Anat.*, 1894, 16:1-28. Chiari, H. Über Veranderungen des Kleinhirns, der Pons und der Medulla oblongata, imfolge von congenitaler Hydrocephalie des Grosshirns. *Denkschr. Akad. Wiss. Wien*, 1895, 63:71.

Friedreich-Erb-Arnold syndrome. See *pachydermoperiostosis syndrome.*

arrhythmogenic right ventricular dysplasia. See *Uhl anomaly.*

ARRILLAGA, F. C. (Argentine physician)

Ayerza-Arrillaga syndrome. See *Ayerza syndrome.*

ARSACS (autosomal recessive spastic ataxia of Charlevoix-Saguenay). See *Charlevoix-Saguenay spastic ataxia.*

arterial angioneuromyoma. See *Barré-Masson syndrome, under Barré, Jean Alexandre.*

arterial mesenteric duodenal ileus. See *superior mesenteric artery syndrome.*

arterial-occlusive retinopathy and encephalopathy syndrome. A syndrome of multiple branch retinal artery occlusion and encephalopathy with behavior and memory disorders and frequent deafness.

Coppeto, J. R., *et al.* A syndrome of arterial-occlusive retinopathy and encephalopathy. *Am. J. Ophthalmol.*, 1984, 98:189-202.

arteriitis cranialis. See *Horton disease (1).*

arteriitis temporalis. See *Horton disease (1).*

arteriocapillary fibrosis. See *Gull-Sutton syndrome.*

arteriohepatic dysplasia (AHD) syndrome. See *Alagille syndrome.*

arteriolar cutaneo-gastrointestinal thrombosis. See *Degos syndrome.*

arteriolitis allergica. See *Gougerot-Ruiter syndrome.*

arteriomesenteric duodenal compression syndrome. See *superior mesenteric artery syndrome.*

arteriomesenteric duodenal ileus. See *superior mesenteric artery syndrome.*

arteriomesenteric occlusion syndrome. See *superior mesenteric artery syndrome.*

arteritis brachiocephalica. See *aortic arch syndrome.*

arteritis nodosa. See *Kussmaul-Maier syndrome.*

arteritis obliterans. See *Friedländer disease.*

arteritis of aorta in young women. See *aortic arch syndrome.*

arthralgia-purpura-weakness syndrome. Synonyms: *Peetoom-Meltzer syndrome, arthralgia-purpura-weakness-cryoglobulinemia syndrome.*

An autoimmune syndrome of arthralgia, purpura, weakness, and mixed cryoglobulinemia, the mixed cryoglobulins consisting of IgG and IgM, associated with the presence rheumatoid factor but no complement dependence. As a consequence of exposure to cold, patients may develop Raynaud phenomenon, livedo reticularis, skin ulcer, and the hyperviscosity syndrome with central nervous system dysfunction.

Meltzer, M., & Franklin, E. C. Cryoglobulin, rheumatoid factor, and connective tissue disorders. *Arthritis Rheum.*, 1967, 10:489-92. Peetoom, F., & Loghem-Langereis, E., van. Igm-IgG (beta-2M-7Sgamma) cryoglobulinaemia. An auto-immune phenomenon. *Vox Sang.*, 1965, 10:281-92. Lapes, M. J., & Davis, J. S., IV. Arthralgia-purpura-weakness-cryoglobulinemia. *Arch. Intern. Med.*, 1970, 126:287-9.

arthralgia-purpura-weakness-cryoglobulinemia syndrome. See *arthralgia-purpura-weakness syndrome.*

arthritic nodes. See *Heberden nodes.*

arthritic spirochetosis. See *Reiter syndrome.*

arthritis deformans juvenilis. See *Still syndrome.*

arthritis mutilans. See *Marie-Léri syndrome, under Marie, Pierre.*

arthritis-dermatitis syndrome. An association of arthritis with skin rash. The **gonococcal arthritis-dermatitis syndrome** is due to the dissemination of *Neisseria gonorrhoeae* via the blood and may be complicated by endocarditis, meningitis, and joint destruction. The **hepatitis-B-associated arthritis-dermatitis syndrome** is characterized by acute symmetric polyarthritis and urticaria, together with elevated liver enzymes. The erythema nodosum syndrome is sometimes associated with subcutaneous nodules and arthritis.

Graves, R. J. *A system of clinical medicine.* Dublin, Fannin, 1843. p. 564. Handsfield, H. H., *et al.* Treatment of the gonococcal arthritis-rheumatism syndrome. *Ann. Intern. Med.*, 1976, 84:661-7. Willan, R. *On cutaneous diseases.* London, Johnson, 1798. Trenholme, G. Arthritis/dermatitis syndrome. *IMJ*, 1980, 158:130-1; 179-80; 1081, 159:44-5.

arthritis-splenomegaly-leukopenia syndrome. See *Felty syndrome.*

arthro-oculosalivary syndrome. See *Sjögren syndrome under Sjögren, Henrik Samuel Conrad.*

arthro-ophthalmopathy (AO). See *Stickler syndrome.*

arthrochalasis multiplex congenita. See *Ehlers-Danlos syndrome (type 7).*

arthrodento-osteodysplasia (ADOD). See *Hajdu-Cheney syndrome.*

arthrogryposis multiplex congenita syndrome. Synonyms: *Guérin-Stern syndrome, Otto syndrome, Rocher-Sheldon syndrome, Rossi syndrome, amyoplasia congenita, arthrogryposis syndrome, arthromyodysplasia congenita, congenital arthromyodysplastic syndrome, congenital articular rigidity, congenital contractures of extremities, multiple congenital articular rigidity, multiple congenital contractures, myodysplasia fibrosa multiplex, myodysplasia fetalis deformans, myodystrophia fetalis deformans, neuro-arthromyodysplasia, pterygium universalis, pterygo-arthromyodysplasia congenita.*

A congenital syndrome of ankylosis of joints with hypoplasia of the attached musculature and multiple pterygia. The usual wrist deformities consist of flexion and ulnar deviation, sometimes in association wtih extension contractures. Carpal malalignment is followed by narrowing of the intercarpal joint spaces and fusion. Other abnormalities in the hand may include syndactyly, amputation, camptodactyly, and delayed maturation. The feet are usually abnormal, with clubfoot, vertical talus, and rocker bottom foot. The hips are dislocated and coxa valga may be present. The knees may be also dislocated or show flexion contractures. Scoliosis is common in older individuals. Infants are prone to an increased incidence of fractures. Brachycephaly, high-arched palate, and hypoplastic mandible with feeding difficulty may occur. The **myopathic type** is relatively rare and is characterized by muscle changes with fixed flexion deformities of the limbs and gross deformities of the chest and spine; the **neuropathic type** presents fixed extension or flexion deformities of the limbs; and the **distal type** affects the distal portions of the extremities. See also *multiple pterygium syndrome..*

Guérin, J. R. *Récherches sur les deformités congénitales chez les monstres.* Paris, 1880. Stern, W. G. Arthrogryposis multiplex congenita. *JAMA.*, 1923, 81:1507-10. Sheldon, W. Amyoplasia congenita (multiple congenital articular rigidity: arthrogryposis multiplex congenita). *Arch. Dis. Child.*, 1932, 7:117-36. Rossi, E. Le syndrome arthromyodysplasique congénital (contribution à l'étude de l'arthrogryposis multiplex congenita). *Helvet. Paediat. Acta*, 1947, 2:82-97. Rocher, H. L. Les raideurs articulaires congénitales multiples. *J. Méd. Bordeaux*, 1913, 43:772-80. *Otto, A. W. *Monstrorum sexcentorum descriptio anatomica.* Bratislava, 1841.

arthrogryposis syndrome. See *arthrogryposis multiplex congenita syndrome.*

arthrogryposis-like anomaly-sensorineural deafness syndrome. See *Stewart-Bergstrom syndrome, under Stewart, Janet M.*

arthrogryposis-like syndrome. See *Kuskokwin syndrome.*

arthrokatadysis. See *Otto-Chrobak syndrome.*

arthrolithiasis. See *König disease (1).*

arthromyodysplasia congenita. See *arthrogryposis multiplex congenita syndrome.*
arthropathia mutilans. See *Marie-Léri syndrome, under Marie, Pierre.*
arthropathia neurotica. See *Charcot disease.*
arthropathia tabica. See *Charcot disease.*
articular chondrocalcinosis. See *pseudogout syndrome.*
articular rheumatism. See *Bouillaud disease.*
artifactual illness. See *Munchausen syndrome.*
artisan's palsy. See *Hunt syndrome (3), under Hunt, James Ramsay.*
ARZT, L. (Austrian physician)
Albrecht-Arzt-Warthin tumor. See *Warthin tumor.*
AS. See *Angelman syndrome.*
AS. See *Alport syndrome.*
AS. See *Adams-Stokes syndrome.*
AS (ankylosing spondylitis). See *Bechterew-Strümpell-Marie syndrome, under Bekhterev.*
ASB. See *anencephaly-spina bifida syndrome.*
ASBOE-HANSEN, GUSTAV (Danish physician, born 1917)
Asboe-Hansen disease. See *Bloch-Sulzberger syndrome.*
ascending hemiplegia. See *Mills disease.*
ascending hernia. See *Birkett hernia.*
ASCHER, KARL WOLFGANG (Austrian ophthalmologist, born 1887)
Ascher syndrome. Synonym: *Laffer-Ascher syndrome.*

A combination of blepharochalasis, double lip, and nontoxic goiter.

Laffer, W. B. Blepharochalasis. Report of a case of this trophoneurosis, involving also the upper lip. *Cleveland Med. J.*, 1909, 8:131-5. *Ascher, K. W. Blepharochalasis mit Struma und Doppellippe. *Klin. Mbl. Augenhk.*, 1920, 65:86-97.

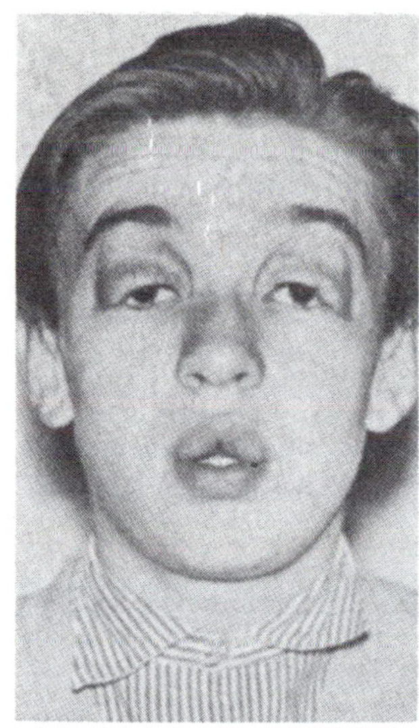

Ascher syndrome
Stehr, K., *Deut. Med. Wchnschr.*, 87:1148, 1962, Georg Thieme Verlag, Stuttgart.

Laffer-Ascher syndrome. See *Ascher syndrome.*
ascomycosis. See *Busse-Buschke disease.*
aseptic meningitis syndrome. Meningitis with fever, signs of meningeal irritation, and cerebrospinal fluid with lymphocytic cellular response from 10 to 1000 cells per cubic mm. It has multiple causes, the most common being a viral agent.

Frazier, J. J., & Kohl, S. Bacterial infection causing "aseptic maningitis syndrome." *Clin. Pediat., Philadelphia,* 1981, 20:147-8.

aseptic necrosis of the femoral head. See *Calvé-Legg-Perthes syndrome.*
aseptic necrosis of the lunate bone. See *Kienböck disease.*
ASHERMAN, JOSEPH G. (Israeli physician)
Asherman syndrome. Synonyms: *Fritsch-Asherman syndrome, amenorrhea traumatica, intrauterine adhesions (IUA), intrauterine synechiae, traumatic amenorrhea, traumatic hypomenorrhea-amenorrhea, traumatic intrauterine synechiae, traumatic intrauterine adhesions.*

Menstrual disorders (amenorrhea, cryptomenorrhea, and hypomenorrhea), habitual abortion, and secondary sterility due to intrauterine adhesions and synechiae resulting from curettage and chemical, physical, or infectious irritation.

Asherman, J. G. Amenorrhea traumatica (atretica). *J. Obst. Gyn. Brit. Emp.*, 1948, 55:23-30.

Fritsch-Asherman syndrome. See *Asherman syndrome.*
ASHERSON, N. (British physician)
Asherson syndrome. Synonym: *achalasia of cricopharyngeal sphincter syndrome.*

Achalasia of the cricopharyngeal sphincter with dysphagia (slight to severe) due to neuromuscular incoordination with failure of relaxation of the cricopharyngeal muscle in the third phase of swallowing. It is most marked for liquids, which are diverted and inhaled into the air passages, precipitating paroxysms of coughing. X-ray examination shows the delay in emptying of the hypopharynx to complete hold up with a spill over into the air passages. Fatal inhalation pneumonia may develop in severe cases.

Asherson, N. Achalasia of the cricopharyngeal sphincter. *J. Laryngol. Otol.*, 1950, 64:7747-58.

ASHLEY, R. K. (American physician)
Ashley syndrome. Synonym: *congenital metacarpotalar syndrome.*

A syndrome of unusual facies, musculoskeletal anomalies, hip dislocation, scoliosis, vertical talus, and hand abnormalities. Facial features consist of hypertelorism, micrognathia, and lack of facial expression which becomes less obvious with age. Extension deformity of the wrist and flexion deformity of the metacarpophalangeal joint and proximal interphalangeal joint give the hand a windswept abnormality. The thumb is adducted with mild to moderate ulnar deviation at the metacarptophalangeal joint. Short stature, poor wound healing, and crowding of the teeth may be associated.

Ashley, R. K., *et al.* Congenital metacarpotalar syndrome. *Ann. Acad. Med. Sinapore*, 1981, 10:434-41.

ashy dermatosis. See *Cinderella dermatosis.*
ASK-UPMARK, ERIK (Swedish physician)
Ask-Upmark kidney. See *Ask-Upmark syndrome.*
Ask-Upmark syndrome. Synonyms: *Ask-Upmark kidney, aglomerular segmental kidney hypoplasia, juvenile malignant nephrosclerosis.*

A syndrome of unilateral or bilateral segmental hypoplasia of the kidneys associated with malignant hypertension.

Ask-Upmark, E. Über juvenile maligne Nephrosclerose und ihr Verlhältnis zu Störungen in der Nierenentwicklung. *Acta Path. Microbiol. Scand.*, 1929, 7:383-45.

ASKENAZY

Askenazy syndrome. See *Meyenburg-Altherr-Uehlinger syndrome.*

Aso volcanic disease. See *Kashin-Bek disease.*

ASP (anorectal malformation-sacral bony abnormality-presacral mass) association. See *Currarino triad.*

ASPERGER, HANS (Austrian psychiatrist)

Asperger syndrome (AS). Synonym: *autistic psychopathy.*

A syndrome characterized by early childhood autism in a wide group of conditions which have in common impaired development of social interaction, communication, and imagination.

Asperger, H. Die "autistischen Psychopathen" im Kindesalter. *Arch. Psychiat. Nervenkrankh.,* 1944, 117:76-136. Wing, L. Asperger's syndrome: A clinical account. *Psychol. Med.,* 1981, 11:115-29.

asphyxiated bladder syndrome. A complication of asphyxia neonatorum, characterized by adequate urine formation and drainage to the bladder but no spontaneous voiding, resulting in bladder distention.

Ivey, H. H. The asphyxiated bladder as a cause of delayed micturition in the newborn. *J. Urol.,* 1978, 120:498-9.

asphyxiating thoracic dysplasia. See *Jeune syndrome.*

asphyxiating thoracic dystrophy. See *Jeune syndrome.*

aspiration pneumonitis. See *Mendelson syndrome.*

aspirin idiosyncrasy. See *Widal-Lermoyez syndrome.*

aspirin insensitivity. See *Samter syndrome.*

asplenia syndrome. Synonyms: *Ivemark syndrome, asplenia-cardiovascular anomalies syndrome, bilateral right-sidedness anomalad, cardiovascular anomaly-right isomerism syndrome, congenital asplenia, eusplenic heart disease, laterality anomalad, splenic agenesis syndrome.*

A syndrome of aplasia or hypoplasia of the spleen associated with complex heart defects, malposition and maldevelopment of the visceral organs, and abnormal lobation of the lungs. Bilateral trilobed lungs and bilateral eparterial bronchi are present. The liver is bilaterally symmetrical in some cases; the gallbladder tends to be located on the right side, even if the liver is isomeric. The stomach is located on the right side in about half the cases; the duodenum and pancreas usually follow the stomach. Malrotation of the jejunum and ileum is common; the colon is free, inferior to and behind the jejunum and ileum. Bilateral superior venae cavae are present in most cases; a single superior vena cava on the right side occurs in other instances. The inferior vena cava is often located on the right side, being accompanied on the contralateral side by a common hepatic vein draining the corresponding lobe of the liver. Anomalous pulmonary venous connection occurs in most cases. The great arteries are transposed in the majority of cases; the aorta being located anteriorly and the pulmonary trunk posteriorly. Stenosis or atresia of the pulmonary valve or subpulmonary region are common. The cardiac apex is often located on the right side, sometimes being associated with mesocardia. The coronary sinus is usually absent. Atrial isomerism is present in most cases. Additional cardiac defects include atrial septal anomaly, a single atrioventricular ostium, a narrow band of muscle from the posterior to the anterior wall, and a single functioning ventricle. The syndrome occurs more often in males than in females. Most affected infants die during their first year of life. The etiology is unknown. See also *polysplenia syndrome.*

Ivemark, B. I. Implications of agenesis of the spleen on the pathogenesis of cono-truncus anomalies in childhood. An analysis of the heart malformations in the splenic agensis syndrome, with fourteen new cases. *Acta Paediat., Uppsala,* 1955, 44(Suppl 104):1-110.

asplenia-cardiovascular anomalies syndrome. See *asplenia syndrome.*

ASPS. See *advanced sleep phase syndrome.*

ASS (Aarskog-Scott syndrome). See *Aarskog syndrome.*

ASSA (aminopterin-like syndrome sine aminopterin). See *fetal aminopterin-like syndrome without aminopterin.*

astasia-abasia syndrome. See *Blocq syndrome.*

asteroid bodies of the vitreous. See *Benson disease.*

asteroid hyalitis. See *Benson disease.*

asthenia crurum dolorosa. See *restless leg syndrome.*

asthenia crurum paresthetica. See *restless leg syndrome.*

asthenia universalis congenita. See *Stiller asthenia.*

asthenic bulbar paralysis. See *Erb-Goldflam syndrome, under Erb, Wilhelm Heinrich.*

asthma. See *Willis disease.*

asthma eczema. See *Besnier prurigo.*

ASTLEY, R. (British physician)

Insley-Astley syndrome. See *Weissenbacher-Zweymüller syndrome.*

astronaut bone demineralization. See *Allison atrophy.*

asymbolia for pain. See *Schilder-Stengel syndrome.*

asymmetric crying facies. See *cardiofacial syndrome.*

asymmetric rhizomelic limb shortening. See *Conradi-Hünermann syndrome.*

AT (ataxia-telangiectasia). See *Louis-Bar syndrome.*

ataxia hereditaria. See *Friedreich ataxia, under Friedreich, Nicolaus.*

ataxia hereditaria hemeralopica polyneuritiformis. See *Refsum disease.*

ataxia muscularis. See *Thomsen disease.*

ataxia teleangiectasica. See *Louis-Bar syndrome.*

ataxia-deafness-cardiomyopathy syndrome. See *Jeune-Tommasi syndrome.*

ataxia-deafness-mental retardation syndrome. See *ataxia-deafness-retardation syndrome.*

ataxia-deafness-retardation (ADR) syndrome. Synonym: *ataxia-deafness-mental retardation syndrome.*

A hereditary syndrome, transmitted as an autosomal recessive trait, characterized by progressive ataxia, hearing loss, mental retardation, and upper and lower motor neuron disorders.

Berman, W., *et al.* A new familial syndrome with ataxia, hearing loss, and mental retardation. *Arch. Neurol., Chicago,* 1973, 29:258-61.

ataxia-opsoclonus-myoclonus syndrome. See *Kingsbourne syndrome.*

ataxia-pancytopenia syndrome. A familial syndrome of cerebellar ataxia associated with fatal bone marrow hypoplasia, and, sometimes, acute myelogenous leukemia, occurring in monosomy 7.

Li, F. P., *et al.* Ataxia-pancytopenia: Syndrome of cerebellar ataxia, hypoplastics anemia, monosomy 7, and acute myelogenous leukemia. *Cancer Genet. Cytogenet.,* 1981, 4:189-96.

ataxia-telangiectasia (AT). See *Louis-Bar syndrome.*

ataxia-telangiectasia-Swiss type agammaglobulinemia syndrome. See *lymphopenic agammaglobulinemia-short limbed dwarfism syndrome.*

ataxic aphasia. See *Broca aphasia.*

ataxic nystagmus. See *Jayle-Ourgaud syndrome.*

ATD (Alzheimer-type dementia). See *Alzheimer disease.*

ateleiotic dwarfism with hypogonadism. See *Hanhart syndrome (1).*

atelencephalic microcephaly syndrome. See *Garcia-Lurie syndrome.*

ateliosis. See *Lorain-Levi syndrome.*

atelosteogenesis. See *spondylohumerofemoral hypoplasia syndrome.*

athetosis. See *Hammond syndrome.*

athetosis duplex. See *Hammond syndrome.*

athetotic dystonia. See *under Hammond syndrome.*

athletic heart syndrome. A condition marked by certain functional and morphologic cardiac adaptations brought about by isotonic and isometric athletic activities. In the isotonic athlete, the size of the left and right ventricular cavities increases, with proportional increases in septal and free-wall thickness, thus increasing the left ventricular mass. The left atrium may be dilated or hypertrophied, but the ejection fraction and myocardial contraction are unchanged. Stroke volume increases with the progress of training. In isometric athletes, septal and free-wall thickness increases, with minimal increase in left ventricular end-diastolic diameter. Left ventricular mass increases to the same degree as lean body mass. Stroke volume increases in relation to bradycardia that may develop.

Huston, T. P., *et al.* The athletic heart syndrome. *N. Engl. J. Med.*, 1985, 313:24-32.

athrepsia. See *marasmus syndrome.*

athrombocytopenic purpura. See *Glanzmann thrombasthenia.*

ATKIN, JOAN F. (American physician)

Atkin-Flaitz syndrome. An X-linked mental retardation syndrome associated with coarse facies characterized by prominent forehead and supraorbital ridges, hypertelorism, broad nasal tip with anteverted nostrils, micrognathia, and thick lips. Other anomalies may include microdontia, diastema between maxillary central incisors, palatal torus, prominent median palatal raphe, exaggerated median furrow of the tongue, macrocephaly, seizures, short stature, obesity, and short and broad hands with tapered fingers. Macrorchidism is present in postpuberal males.

Atkin, J. F., Flaitz, K., Patil, S., & Smith, W. An X-linked mental retardation syndrome. *Am. J. Med. Genet.*, 1985, 21:697-705. Opitz, J. M., Reynolds, J. F., & Spano, L. M., eds. X-linked mental retardation. *Am. J. Med. Genet.*, 1986, 23:15-6.

atlanto-axial rotary displacement. See *Grisel syndrome.*

atopic dermatitis. See *Besnier prurigo.*

atopic dermatosis. See *Besnier prurigo.*

atopic eczema. See *Besnier prurigo.*

atresia multiplex congenita. See *Weyers syndrome (1).*

atresia of the foramen of Magendie. See *Dandy-Walker syndrome.*

atresia of the foramina of Luschka and Magendie. See *Walker-Dandy syndrome.*

atrial septal defect-mitral stenosis syndrome. See *Lutembacher syndrome.*

atrio-extremital dysplasia. See *Holt-Oram syndrome.*

atriodigital dysplasia. See *Holt-Oram syndrome.*

atrophia bulborum hereditaria. See *Norrie syndrome.*

atrophia cutis idiopathica progressiva. See *Herxheimer disease.*

atrophia maculosa cutis. See *Jadassohn disease (1), under Jadassohn, Josef.*

atrophia musculorum progressiva neurotica sive neuralis. See *Charcot-Marie-Tooth syndrome.*

atrophia musculorum pseudomyopathica. See *Wohlfart-Kugelberg-Welander syndrome.*

atrophia opticocochleodentata. See *Nyssen-van Bogaert-Meyer syndrome.*

atrophic dermatitis papulosquamosa. See *Degos syndrome.*

atrophic glossitis. See *Hunter glossitis, under Hunter, William.*

atrophic ligamentous spondylitis. See *Bechterew-Strümpell-Marie syndrome, under Bekhterev.*

atrophic papulosquamous dermatitis. See *Degos syndrome.*

atrophic polychondritis. See *Meyenburg-Altherr-Uehlinger syndrome.*

atrophic red liver infarct. See *Zahn infarct.*

atrophic spondylitis. See *Bechterew-Strümpell-Marie syndrome, under Bekhterev.*

atrophoderma idiopathica progressiva. See *Pasini-Pierini syndrome.*

atropine syndrome. See *Appian-Plutarch syndrome.*

atropinism. See *Appian-Plutarch syndrome.*

attention deficit disorder with hyperactivity (ADD/HA, ADDH). See *attention deficit-hyperactivity disorder.*

attention deficit disorder-hyperactivity disorder (ADHD). Synonyms: *attention deficit disorder with hyperactivity (ADDH, ADD/HA), hyperactive behavior syndrome, hyperactive child, hyperactive child syndrome, hyperactive syndrome, hyperkinetic syndrome, hyperkinetic-minimal brain dysfunction (hyperkinetic-MBD) syndrome, minimal brain dysfunction (MBD), minimal brain dysfunction syndrome, minimal cerebral dysfunction (MCD).*

A behavioral disorder characterized by inappropriate degree of inattention, impulsiveness, and hyperactivity, usually observed in preschool children but also affecting older children and adolescents, sometimes continuing into adulthood. In young children, signs of overactivity, such as excessive climbing and running, inattention, and impulsiveness, are the principal features of this disorder. Older children and adolescents tend to be restless and are constantly fidgeting. Inattention and impulsiveness are the principal causes of failure to complete assigned tasks and instructions. Low self-esteem, mood lability, low frustration tolerance, temper outburst, and low scholastic performance are the associated disorders. In most instances, the onset of disorders takes place before the age of four years. Central nervous system disorders (cerebral palsy, epilepsy, and presence of neurotoxins), poor family environment, child abuse and neglect, and hypersensitivity to certain foods and dyes are implicated as potential causative factors.

Attention-deficit hyperactivity disorder (ADHD). In: *Diagnostic and statistical manual of mental disorders.* 3rd ed. Washington, American Psychiatric Association, 1987. pp. 50-2.

attention deficit-hyperactivity disorder. See *attention deficit disorder-hyperactivity disorder.*
atypical chondrodystrophy. See *mucopolysaccharidosis IV-A.*
atypical dystrophy-macular coloboma syndrome. See *Sorsby syndrome.*
atypical facial headache. See *Sluder neuralgia.*
atypical gingivostomatitis. See *gingivostomatitis syndrome.*
atypical mandibulofacial dysostosis. See *Weyers-Thier syndrome.*
atypical ventricular tachycardia. See *torsades de pointes syndrome.*
atypical verrucous endocarditis. See *Libman-Sacks syndrome.*
AUBINEAU, ERNEST RENE EMILE (French physician, born 1871)
Lenoble-Aubineau syndrome. See *under Lenoble.*
auditory receptive aphasia. See *Wernicke aphasia.*
auditory verbal agnosia. See *Wernicke aphasia.*
auditory vertigo. See *Ménière syndrome.*

AUDRY, CHARLES (French physician, 1865-1934)
Audry syndrome. See *pachydermoperiostosis syndrome.*
aural vertigo. See *Ménière syndrome.*
aurantiasis cutis. See *Baelz disease (2).*
auriculo-osteodysplasia syndrome. Synonyms: *Beals syndrome, oto-osteodysplasia syndrome.*

A bone dysplasia, transmitted as an autosomal dominant trait, characterized by short stature, hypoplasia of the capitellum with or without radial dislocation, broad shoulders, horizontal alignment of the clavicles, and peculiar ear shape with elongated attached lobules and small posteriorly attached lobules. Hip dislocation and short carpal areas of the wrist may occur.

Beals, R. K. Auriculo-osteodysplasia: A syndrome of multiple osseous dysplasia, ear anomaly, and short stature. *J. Bone Joint Surg.*, 1967, 49A:1541-50.

auriculotemporal and chorda tympani syndrome. See *Frey syndrome.*
auriculotemporal neuralgia. See *Arnold neuralgia.*
auriculotemporal syndrome. See *Frey syndrome.*
auro-urogenital syndrome. See *Winter syndrome.*
AUSPITZ, HEINRICH (Austrian physician, 1835-1886)
Auspitz dermatosis. See *mycosis fungoides.*
Auspitz syndrome. See *mycosis fungoides.*
AUSTIN FLINT. See FLINT, AUSTIN
Australian alpine syndrome. See *alpine syndrome.*
Austrian syndrome. A syndrome in which chronic alcoholism is associated with pneumococcal meningitis and intractable heart failure due to destruction of the mitral and aortic valves.

Ben-Yaccov, D., *et al.* Austrian syndrome. *Harefuah,* 1986, 111:367-8.

AUTENRIETH, JOHANN HERRMANN FERDINAND, VON (German physician, 1772-1835)
Bayford-Autenrieth dysphagia. See *under Bayford.*
autism-fragile X syndrome (AFRAX). See *chromosome X fragility.*
autistic psychopathy. See *Asperger syndrome.*
auto-erotic asphyxia syndrome. The act of self-asphyxiating, usually by hanging, while masturbating.

Wesselius, C. L., & Bally, R. A male with autoerotic asphyxia syndrome. *Am. J. Forens. Med. Pathol.,* 1983, 4:341-4.

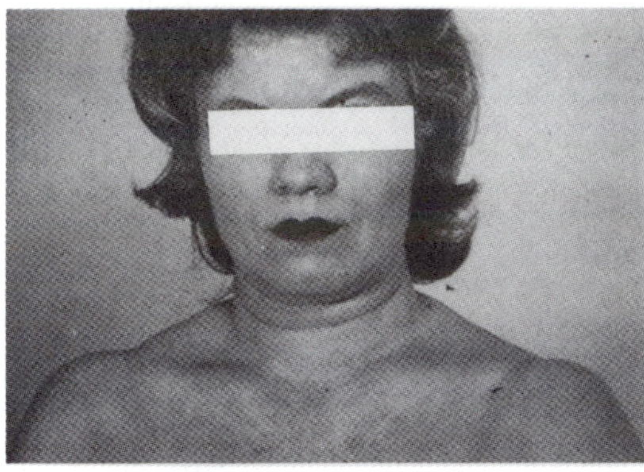

Auriculo-osteodysplasia syndrome
Beals, R.K.: *J.Bone Joint Surg.(Am.)*, 51:728,1969.

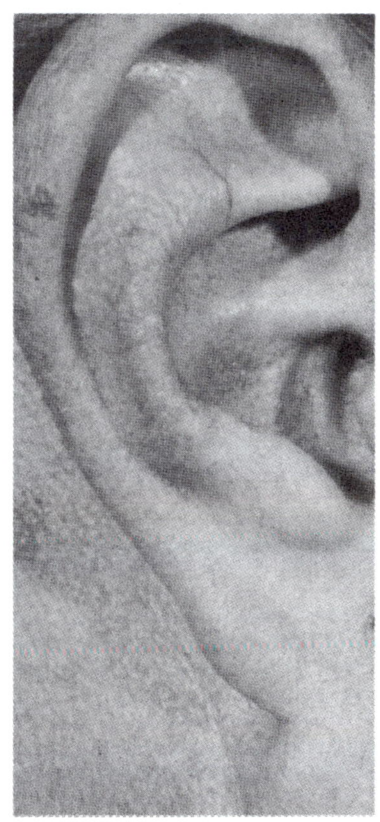

Auriculo-osteodysplasia syndrome
Beals, R.K.: *J. Bone Joint Surg. (Am.)*, 49:1541, 1967.

auto-erythrocyte sensitization (AES) syndrome. Synonyms: *Gardner-Diamond syndrome, erythrocyte sensitivity syndrome, painful ecchymotic purpura in women, psychogenic purpura.*

An auto-immune disorder, occurring most commonly in adult women, characterized by spontaneous painful purpura. The patients usually note, after a local injury, a localized aura of tingling and burning, followed by the development of raised, painful purpuric lesions which last two or three days and then resolve. Originally, the disorder was believed to be due to hypersensitivity of the patient's skin to the stroma of the red blood cells, the skin reaction being directed against the DNA and phosphatidyl serine residues of the red cell membrane. More recent findings indicate the possibility that sensitization of the erythrocytes may be an element of a psychopathological condition, purpura being a manifestation of a personalilty disorder. Also, the disorder may be a complication of lupus erythematosus.

Gardner, F. H., & Diamond, L. K. Autoerythrocyte sensitization. A form of purpura producing painful bruising following autosensitization to red blood cells in certain women. *Blood,* 1955, 10:675-90. Scott, J. P., *et al.* The autoerythrocyte sensitization syndrome as a primary manifestation of lupus erythematosus. *J. Pediat.,* 1981, 99:598-600.

autoimmune endocrine syndrome. See *polyglandular autoimmune syndrome.*

autoimmune hemolytic anemia-thrombocytopenic purpura syndrome. See *Evans syndrome, under Evans, Robert Sherman.*

autoimmune polyendocrine syndrome. See *polyglandular autoimmune syndrome.*

autoimmune polyendocrinopathy-candidosis-ectodermal dystrophy syndrome. See *APECED syndrome.*

autoimmune polyglandular syndrome. See *polyglandular autoimmune syndrome.*

autoimmune postpartum syndrome. A postpartum syndrome associated with antiphospholipid antibodies, consisting of pleural effusion, pulmonary infiltrate, and fever, observed in women with lupus anticoagulant or cardiolipin antibody, or both.

Kochenour, N. K., *et al.* A new postpartum syndrome associated with antiphospholipid antibodies. *Obstet. Gynecol.,* 1987, 69:460-8.

autoimmune thrombocytopenia-autoimmune hemolytic anemia syndrome. See *Evans syndrome, under Evans, Robert Sherman.*

automatism. See *Kandinskii-Clérambault syndrome.*

autonomic diencephalic epilepsy. See *Penfield syndrome.*

autonomic dysreflexia syndrome. Synonym: *autonomic hyperreflexia.*

A complication of cervical and upper thoracic spinal cord injuries, consisting of episodic hypertension, flushing, sweating, bradycardia, diaphoresis, anxiety, and pounding headache evoked by a variety of stimuli applied below the level of injury, such as bladder distension, pinprick to anesthetic areas, scratching of the feet, squeezing of the penis, stimulation of the rectum, enemas, accumulation of flatus, and the like.

Head, H., & Riddoch, G. The automatic bladder, excessive sweating and some other reflex conditions in gross injuries to the spinal cord. *Brain,* 1917, 40:188-263. Guttmann, L., & Whitteridge, D. Effects of bladder distention on autonomic mechanisms after spinal cord injuries. *Brain,* 1947, 70:361-404.

autonomic faciocephalalgia. See *Sluder neuralgia.*

autonomic hyperreflexia. See *autonomic dysreflexia syndrome.*

autoparalytic syndrome. Residual facial paralysis due to postoperative changes in fibers of the facial nerve.

Stennert, E. Das autoparalytische Syndrom-ein Leitsymptom der postparetischen Fazialisfunktion. *Arch. Otorhinolaryngol., Berlin,* 1982, 236:97-114.

autosomal dominant compelling helio-ophthalmic outburst syndrome. See *ACHOO syndrome.*

autosomal dominant osteosclerosis, Stanesco type. See *Stanesco syndrome.*

autosomal dominant striatonigral degeneration. See *Joseph disease, under Joseph, Antone.*

autosomal recessive spastic ataxia of Charlevoix-Saguenay (ARSACS). See *Charlevoix-Saguenay spastic ataxia.*

autotoxic cyanosis. See *Stokvis-Talma syndrome.*

autumnal catarrh. See *Bostock catarrh.*

AV (**a**llergic **v**asculitis). See *Gougerot-Ruiter syndrome.*

AV (A & V) syndrome. Ocular deviation in which the degree of esotropia or exotropia is more marked on looking either upward or downward. An A-esotropia is greater looking upward than downward and V-esotropia is greater looking downward than upward. An A-exotropia is greater looking downward than upward and V-exotropia is greater looking upward than downward.

Urist, M. J. Horizontal squint with secondary vertical deviation. *AMA Arch. Ophth.,* 1951, 46:245-67. Urist, M. J. The etiology of the so-called A and V syndromes. *Am. J. Ophth.,* 1958, 46:835-44.

AVELLIS, GEORG (German physician, 1864-1916)

Avellis hemiplegia. See *Avellis syndrome.*

Avellis syndrome. Synonyms: *Avellis hemiplegia, Avellis-Longhi syndrome, ambiguospinophthalmic syndrome, spinophthalmic tract-nucleus ambiguous syndrome, superior laryngeal nerve syndrome.*

A neurological disorder characterized by unilateral paralysis of the larynx and soft palate, with loss of the pain and temperature sense on the contralateral side, including the extremities, trunk, and neck. It usually results from occlusion of the vertebral artery in lesions of the nucleus ambiguus and pyramidal tract. Bulbar lesions and mastoiditis have been implicated. Paralysis of the soft palate produces dysphagia. In the original description, the vagus and glossopharyngeal nerves were involved; concomitant involvement of the neighboring cranial nerves was observed later.

Avellis, G. Klinische Beiträge zur halbseitigen Kehlkopflähmung. *Berliner Klin.,* 1891, No. 40:1-26.

Avellis-Longhi syndrome. See *Avellis syndrome.*

avitaminosis B_2. See *Landor-Pallister syndrome.*

avulsed retinal vessel syndrome. Recurrent vitreous hemorrhage from an avulsed retinal vessel caused by a retinal tear.

de Bustros, S., & Welch, R. B. The avulsed retinal vessel syndrome and its variants. *Ophthalmology,* 1984, 91:86-8.

AWS (**a**lcohol **w**ithdrawal **s**yndrome). See *under withdrawal syndrome.*

AWTA (**a**niridia-**W**ilms **t**umor **a**ssociation). See *aniridia-Wilms tumor syndrome.*

AXEN, OLIVER (Swedish physician)

Biörck-Axén-Thorson syndrome. See *carcinoid syndrome.*

AXENFELD, KARL THEODOR PAUL POLYKARPUS (German ophthalmologist, 1867-1930)

Axenfeld anomaly. See *Axenfeld syndrome.*

Axenfeld calcareous degeneration. Synonym: *dystrophia calcarea corneae.*

A rare condition characterized by massive deposits of calcium phosphate in superficial and central strata of the corneal parenchyma.

Axenfeld, T. Über doppelsaltige primäre progressive parenchymatöse Verkalung (Dystrophia calcarea) der

Cornea. *Klin. Mbl. Augenh.*, 1917, 69:58-65.

Axenfeld conjunctivitis. See *Morax-Axenfeld conjunctivitis.*

Axenfeld syndrome. Synonym: *Axenfeld anomaly.*

A syndrome consisiting of posterior embryotoxon, prominent Schwalbe's line, and iris adhesion to the Schwalbe's line. Glaucoma and abnormalities of the iris and anterior chamber angle may be present. The disorder is transmitted as an autosomal dominant trait. Axenfeld and Rieger syndromes are suspected as being expressions of the same gene. When associated with tooth anomalies, the disorder is known as the *Rieger syndrome.*

*Axenfeld, T. *Ber. Deut. Ophth. Ges.*, 1920, 43:301.

Axenfeld-Krukenberg spindle. See *Krukenberg spindle.*

Axenfeld-Rieger syndrome. See *Axenfeld syndrome, and see Rieger syndrome.*

Axenfeld-Schürenberg syndrome. Synonym: *cyclic oculomotor paralysis.*

Congenital oculomotor paralysis alternating with spasms, associated with blepharoptosis and mydriasis.

Axenfeld, T., & Schürenberg, E. Zur Kenntniss der angeborenen Beweglichkeitdefekte der Augen. *Klin. Mbl. Augenheilk.*, 1901, 39:64; 844.

Morax-Axenfeld conjunctivitis. See *under Morax.*

AYERZA, ABEL (Argentine physician, 1861-1918)

Ayerza syndrome. Synonyms: *Ayerza-Arrillaga syndrome, cardiopathia nigra.*

A syndrome characterized by slowly developing asthma, bronchitis, dyspnea, and cyanosis in association with polycythemia. Cardiac involvement may be present, usually in the form of dilatation and hypertrophy of the right heart. Pathologically, there are primary changes in the pulmonary artery and its branches, which are sometimes attributed to syphilis, but usually there is pulmonary atherosclerosis. Pulmonary arterial hyperplasia and stenosis, emphysema, and fibrosis may be the contributing factors. Splenomegaly, clubbing of the fingers, congestion of the liver, and heart failure are associated.

Ayerza, L. Maladie d'Ayerza, sclerose secondaire de l'artere pulmonaire (cardiaques noirs). *Sem. Med., B. Aires*, 1925, 32:43-4. *Arrillaga, R. C. *Esclerosis secundaria de la arteritis pulmonaria y su quadro clinico (cardiacos negros)*. Buenos Aires, 1912.

Ayerza-Arrillaga syndrome. See *Ayerza syndrome.*

ayun. See *ainhum syndrome.*

Azorean disease. See *Joseph disease, under Joseph, Antone.*

AZUA, JUAN, DE. See DE AZUA Y SUAREZ, JUAN

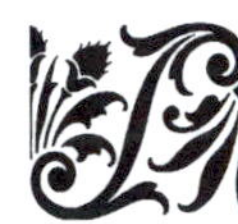

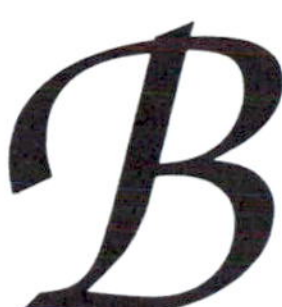

BAADER, ERNST (German physician)

Baader dermatostomatitis. See *Stevens-Johnson syndrome.*

Baader syndrome. See *Stevens-Johnson syndrome.*

BAASTRUP, CHRISTIAN INGERSLEV (Danish physician, 1885-1950)

Baastrup syndrome. Synonyms: *Michotte syndrome, diarthrosis interspinosa, kissing osteophytes, kissing spine, osteoarthrosis interspinalis.*

Mutual compression of the spinous processes of adjacent lumbar vertebrae observed in some types of degenerative diseases.

Baastrup, C. J. Proc. spin. vert. lumb. und einige zwischen diesen liegende Gelenkbildungen mit pathologischen Prozessen in dieser Region. *Fortschr. Röntgen.*, 1933, 48:430-5. Michotte, L. J. Le syndrome des épineuses. *Rev. Rhumat., Paris,* 1949, 16:249-51.

BABER, MARGARET D.

Baber syndrome. Congenital cirrhosis of the liver with clinical features similar to those found in the Fanconi syndrome and characterized by failure to thrive, abdominal distention, foul-smelling stools, rickets, and aminoaciduria with high excretion of tyrosine, serine, threonine, tryptophan, histidine, and lysine, but without increase in cystine excretion. Pathological findings include multilobular portal cirrhosis with evidence of regenerative changes and signs of adipose transformation of hepatic cells, hydronephrosis and enlargement of the kidneys with pelvic fibrosis of the kidneys, perisinusoidal fibrosis and congestion of the spleen possibly due to portal hypertension, and osteoporosis and bone changes characteristic of rickets.

Baber, M. D. A case of congenital cirrhosis of the liver with renal tubular defects akin to those in the Fanconi syndrome. *Arch. Dis. Child.,* 1956, 31:335-9.

BABINGTON, BENJAMIN GUY (British physician)

Babington disease. See *Osler-Rendu-Weber syndrome.*

BABINSKI, JOSEPH FRANÇOIS FELIX (French neurologist, 1857-1932)

Anton-Babinski syndrome. See *under Anton.*

Babinski syndrome. Synonyms: *Babinski-Vaquez syndrome, syphilitic-cardiovascular syndrome.*

The association of cardiac and arterial lesions with late syphilis.

Babinski, J. Des troubles pupillaires dans les anévrisme de l'aorte. *Bull. Soc. Hôp. Paris*, 1901, 18:1121-4.

Babinski-Fröhlich syndrome. See *Fröhlich syndrome, under Fröhlich, Alfred.*

Babinski-Froment syndrome. A neurological syndrome characterized by vasomotor and trophic disorders, diffuse amyotrophy, exaggerated tendon reflexes, and muscle contraction, whereby the affected muscles are resistant to anesthesia and are insensitive to mechanical and electrical stimuli.

*Babinski, J., & Froment, J. Troubles nerveux d'ordre reflexe. In their: *Hysterie, pithiatisme et troubles nerveux d'ordre reflexe.* Paris, Masson, 1917.

Babinski-Nageotte syndrome. Synonyms: *dorsolateral oblongata syndrome, medullary paralysis.*

Lesions of the pontobulbar or medullobulbar transitional region associated with homolateral Bernard-Horner syndrome (enophthalmos, blepharoptosis, and miosis), nystagmus, and cerebellar hemiataxia, and with contralateral hemiparesis and disturbances of sensibility.

*Babinski, J., & Nageotte, J. Hémiasynergie, latéropulsion et miosis bulbaire. *Nouv. Icon. Salpêtrière,* 1902, p. 492.

Babinski-Vaquez syndrome. See *Babinski syndrome.*

baboon syndrome. Systemic allergic contact dermatitis with diffuse erythema of the buttocks, upper inner surface of the thighs, and axillae, giving the affected person a baboon-like appearance. The disorder was originally produced by hypersensitivity to ampicillin, nickel, and mercury.

Anderson, K. E., *et al.* The baboon syndrome: Systemically-induced contact dermatitis. *Contact Dermat.,* 1984, 10:97-100.

baby bottle syndrome. Synonyms: *bottle mouth caries, nursing bottle syndrome (NBS), nursing caries.*

A form of dental caries occurring in infants who have been allowed to sleep with a nursing bottle. The high sugar content of the formula contributes to the development of dental decay.

Fass, E. N. Is bottle feeding of milk a factor in dental caries? *J. Dent. Child.,* 1962, 29:245-51.

BACCAREDDA, A. (Italian physician)

Sézary-Baccaredda syndrome. See *Sézary syndrome.*

bacillary dysentery. See *Flexner dysentery.*

BACON, SIR FRANCIS, VISCOUNT ST. ALBAN (English philosopher, died 1626)

Bacon syndrome. A syndrome based on three principal baconian notions: (1) Earth and its inhabitants exist to dominate and exploit nature. (2) Human beings and nature have been and continue to be engaged in combat and are, therefore, enemies. From ancient myth to contemporary environmentalism, human intervention has been justified by the presumed hostile actions of nature. (3) The intervention and regulation that humanity exert are derived from the mathematical constructs of repetition and predictability. Predictability is best achieved by standardizing the conditions of manipulation through mechanical routine. Physicians who follow these notions consider any means used in destroying diseases and their causes as justifiable, as long as these means are based on scientific precepts, without regard for potential damages that they may exert on nature and the environment.

Lee, R. V. Bacon's syndrome. The decline of natural history in medicine. *Am. J. Med.*, 1984, 77:972-6.

bacterial contamination syndrome. See *bacterial overgrowth syndrome.*

bacterial overgrowth syndrome. Synonyms: *bacterial contamination syndrome, contaminated small bowel syndrome (CSBS), intestinal bacterial overgrowth syndrome, small bowel bacterial overgrowth, small intestinal bacterial overgrowth syndrome.*

Proliferation of enteric microflora and bacterial overgrowth of the small intestine, usually resulting in malabsorption. Stasis of the small intestinal contents (see *blind loop syndrome*), disorders of the acid-base equilibrium in the stomach, disruption of intestinal peristalsis with resulting sweep of bacteria to the distal small intestine, secretion into the lumen of the intestine of immunoglobulins, and changes in bile salt metabolism are the principal causes of this syndrome. Proliferating bacteria generally reflect the normal bacterial population of the small intestine, *Bacteroides* and anaerobic lactobacilli being most widely distributed, also including enterobacteria, enterococci, and clostridia. Diarrhea, steatorrhea, and cobalamin malabsorption are the principal clinical features. Otherwise, the symptoms are similar to those seen in the malabsorption syndrome (q.v.).

Donaldson, R. M., Jr., & Toskes, P. P. The relation of enteric bacterial populations to gastrointestinal function and disease. In: Sleisenger, M. H., & Fordtran, J. S., eds. *Gastrointestinal disease. Pathophysiology, diagnosis, management.* 3rd ed. Philadelphia, Saunders, 1983, pp. 44-54. Greenberger, N. J., & Isselbacher, K. J. Disorders of absorption. In: Braunwald, E., Isselbacher, K. J., Petersdorf, R. G., Wilson, J. D., Martin, J. B., Fauci, A. S., eds. *Harrison's principles of internal medicine.* 11th ed. New York, McGraw-Hill, 1987, pp. 1260-76.

BADAL

Gerstmann-Badal syndrome. See *Gerstmann syndrome (2).*

BAEHR, GEORGE (American physician)

Baehr-Schiffrin disease. See *Moschcowitz syndrome.*

Brill-Baehr-Rosenthal disease. See *Brill-Symmers syndrome.*

BAELZ, ERWIN O., VON (German physician, 1849-1913)

Baelz cheilitis. See *Baelz syndrome.*

Baelz disease (1). See *Baelz syndrome.*

Baelz disease (2). Synonyms: *aurantiasis cutis, carotene jaundice, carotenoderma.*

Canary yellow, ochre, or golden pigmentation of the skin related to consumption of large amounts of carotenoids, occurring most commonly during wartime with rationing of meat, butter, and cheese, and increased consumption of carotenoid-containing fresh fruits and vegetables. Carotene deposits occur mainly in the nasolabial folds and on the sebaceous gland-rich areas of the forehead, and on the horny layer of the skin of the palms and soles. Lesser amounts are found on the upper eyelids, inner canthi, ears, malleoli, and pressure areas (the elbows and knees). Carotenoderma may be observed in some cases of diabetes mellitus.

*Kaufmann, E. Aurantiasis cutis Baelz. In: Jadassohn. ed. *Handabuch der Haut- und Geschlechtskrankheiten.* Berlin, Springer, 1933. pp. 1090-1103.

Baelz syndrome. Synonyms: *Baelz cheilitis, Baelz disease, apostematous cheilitis, cheilitis glandularis, cheilitis glandularis apostematosa, myxandenitis labialis.*

A rare disease characterized by enlargement, hardening, and finally eversion of the lip (usually the lower one) leading to exposure of the opening of the accessory salivary glands, which themselves become enlarged and sometimes nodular, appearing as small red macules with dilated follicular orifices exuding mucoid or mucopurulent fluid.

Unna, P. G. Über Erkrankungen der Schleimdrüsen des Mundes. *Mhefte. Prakt. Derm.*, 1890, 11:317-21.

BAERENSPRUNG, FRIEDRICH WEILHELM FELIX, VON (German physician, 1822-1864)

Baerensprung disease. Synonym: *Baerensprung erythrasma.*

Eczema marginatum of the thighs.

Baerensprung, F., von. *Über die Folge und dem Verlauf epidermischer Krankheiten.* Halle, Schmidt, 1954.

Baerensprung erythrasma. See *Baerensprung disease.*

BÄFVERSTEDT, BO ERIK (Swedish physician, born 1905)

Bäfverstedt syndrome. Synonyms: *Kaposi-Spiegler sarcomatosis, Spiegler-Fendt sarcoid, Spiegler-Fendt sarcomatosis, benign lymphadenosis, lymphadenosis benigna cutis, lymphocytoma benignum cutis, sarcomatosis cutis.*

A rare form of benign recurrent tumor of the lymphoreticular tissue. The lesions are pink to red to violet papules or nodules, usually occurring on the face, ear lobes, nipples, and scrotum. Pathologically, they are characterized by a thin epidermis, bands of normal dermis, and dense infiltrates in the midcutis or masses consisting of mature lymphocytes and reticulum cells.

Spiegler, E. Über die sogenante Sarkomatosis cutis. *Arch. Derm. Syph., Berlin,* 1894, 27:163-74. Fendt, H. Beiträge zur Kentnis der sogenannten Sarcoiden Geschwülste der Haut. *Arch. Derm. Syph., Berlin,* 1900, 53:213-42. Bäfverstedt, B. Über Lymphadenosis benigna cutis. Eine klinische und pathologisch-anatomische Studie. *Acta Derm. Vener., Stockholm,* 1943, 24(Suppl. 11):1-202.

Baghdad boil. See *Alibert disease (2).*

BAILLARGER, JULES GABRIEL FRANÇOIS (French neurologist, 1809-1890)

Baillarger syndrome. See *Frey syndrome.*

Frey-Baillarger syndrome. See *Frey syndrome.*

BAKER, JAMES P. (American physician)

Charcot-Weiss-Baker syndrome. See *carotid sinus syndrome.*

Weiss-Baker syndrome. See *carotid sinus syndrome.*

BAKER, WILLIAM MORRANT (British physician, 1839-1896)

Baker cyst. Synonyms: *medial gastrocnemius bursitis, popliteal bursitis, popliteal cyst, posterior hernia of the* *knee, semimenbranosus bursitis, synovial cyst of the popliteal space.*

A periarticular cyst produced by synovial fluid escaping from a joint through a natural channel or through a hernial opening in the synovial membrane. The cyst occurs most commonly in herniation of the synovial membrane of the knee joint.

Baker, W. M. The formation of abnormal synovial cysts in connection with the joints. II. *St. Bartholomew's Hosp. Rep.*, 1885, 21:177-90.

BAKWIN, HARRY (American physician)

Bakwin-Eiger syndrome. See *hyperphosphatasia-osteoctasia syndrome.*

Bakwin-Krida syndrome. See *metaphyseal dysplasia syndrome.*

balanitis circumscripta chronica. See *Zoon erythroplasia.*

balanitis plasmocellulare. See *Zoon erythroplasia.*

balanoposthitis chronica circumscripta benigna plasmocellulare. See *Zoon erythroplasia.*

bald soprano syndrome. Synonym: *prosopagnosia.*

Impaired ability to recognize faces previously familiar. The name of the syndrome was adapted from Eugene Ionesco's play, "The Bald Soprano," where the characters fail to recognize each other.

Radulescu, G. Prosopagnosia-the bald soprano syndrome. *Arch. Ophth., Chicago,* 1987, 105:32.

bald tongue. See *Möller glossitis.*

bald tongue of pernicious anemia. See *Hunter glossitis, under Hunter, William.*

balderdash syndrome. See *Ganser syndrome.*

BALDWIN, RUTH WORKMAN (American pediatrician, born 1915)

Bessman-Baldwin syndrome. See *under Bessman.*

BALESTRA, G. (Italian physician)

De Martini-Balestra syndrome. See *Burke syndrome.*

BALFOUR, GEORGE WILLIAM (British physician, 1822-1903)

Balfour disease. Synonyms: *chloroleukemia, chloroma, chloromyeloma, chlorosarcoma, green cancer.*

Tumorous masses formed by the bony infiltrates in myelogenous leukemia, which may be present in any portion of the skeleton, but are found most frequently in the skull. They are characterized by a greenish coloration due to the presence of myeloperoxidase, a green pigment with high peroxidase activity. The color is not always evident; when present, it tends to fade after exposure to air.

*Balfour, G. W. Case of peculiar disease of the skull and dura mater. *Edinburgh M. Surg. J.*, 1935, 43:319-25.

BALINT, RUDOLF (Hungarian physician)

Bálint syndrome. Synonym: *psychic paralysis of visual fixation.*

A combination of paralysis of visual fixation, optic ataxia, and impairment of visual fixation, occurring in ischemic lesions of the parieto-occipital region.

Bálint, R. Seelenlähmung des "Schauens," optische Ataxia, räumliche Störung der Aufmerksamkeit. *Mschr. Psychiat. Neur.*, 1909, 25:51-81.

ball-valve gallstone. See *Osler syndrome.*

BALLANTYNE, JOHN WILLIAM (British physician, 1861-1923)

Ballantyne syndrome (1). See *Ballantyne-Runge syndrome.*

Ballantyne syndrome (2). Synonym: *triple edema syndrome.*

A triad of maternal edema, fetal hydrops, and placentomegaly, usually caused by rhesus isoimmunization. Nonimmunological causes of this syndrome include alpha-thalassemia, feto-maternal transfusion, congenital heart disease, fetal hypoproteinemia, and various bacterial and viral infections.

Ballantyne, J. W. *The diseases and deformities of the foetus: An attempt towards a system of ante-natal pathology.* Edinburgh, Oliver & Boyd, 1892.

Ballantyne-Runge syndrome. Synonyms: *Ballantyne syndrome, Clifford syndrome, Runge syndrome, dysmaturity syndrome, placental dysfunction syndrome, postmaturity syndrome, prenatal dystrophy syndrome, prolonged gestation syndrome.*

Prolongation of gestation in a nondiabetic mother beyond the estimated time of delivery, with the birth of an infant weighing over 4500 gm.

Ballantyne, J. W. The problem of the postmature infant. *J. Obst. Gyn. Brit. Emp.*, 1902, 2:251-54. Runge, H. Über einige besondere Merkmale der übertragenen. Frucht. *Zbl. Gyn.*, 1942, 66:1202-6. Clifford, S. H. Postmaturity. *Adv. Pediat., Chicago*, 1957, vol. 9.

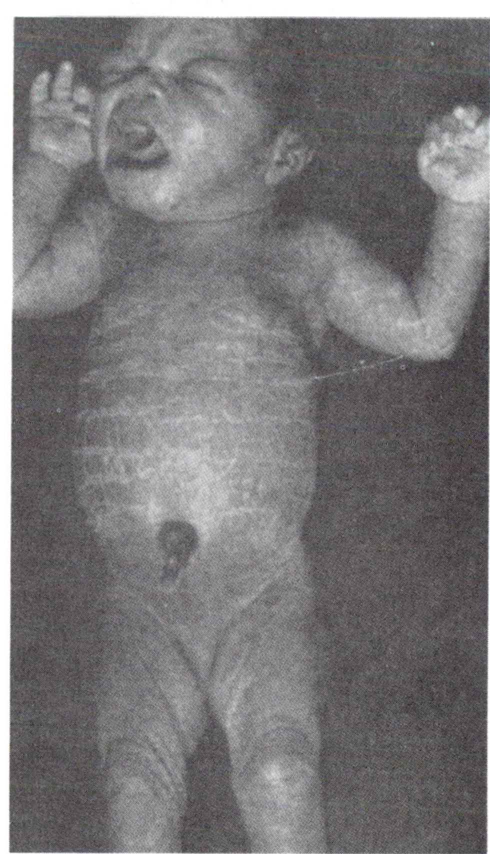

Ballantyne-Runge syndrome
Clifford, S.H., *J. Pediat.*, 44:1-13, 1954. St. Louis: C.V. Mosby Co.

BALLER, F.

Baller-Gerold syndrome. Synonym: *craniosynostosis-radial aplasia syndrome.*

A rare syndrome of oxycephaly and absent radius. Ulnar hypoplasia, epicanthal folds, dysplastic ears, steep forehead, high nasal bridge, and long philtrum are associated in some cases. Fused carpal bones, missing carpal bones, hypoplastic or absent thumb, hypoplastic or absent first metacarpal bone, and vertebral anomalies may be also present. Parental consanguinity was noted in some cases, lack of consanguinity in others, and some cases were reported as sporadic. Autosomal recessive transmission is suspected in some instances.

Baller, F. Radiusaplasie und Inzucht. *Zschr. Menschl. Vererb. Konstit. Lehre*, 1950, 29:782-90. Gerold, M. Frakturheilung bei einen seltenen Fall Kongenitaler Anomalie der oberen Gliedmassen. *Zbl. Chir.*, 1959, 84:831-4.

BALLINGALL, SIR GEORGE (British physician, 1780-1855)

Ballingall disease. Synonyms: *madura foot, maduromycosis, mycetoma, pseudoactinomycosis.*

A localized infectious (but not contagious) disease affecting chiefly exposed areas, such as bare feet **(madura foot)** and, less commonly, the legs, back, and other parts of the body. Debris of decaying vegetation introduced into the neglected open wounds are the cause of this condition. Two basic forms are recognized: one which is produced by the fungi **(eumycoma)**, and one which is caused by actinomycetes **(actinomycetoma).** The initial lesion is a painless draining nodule at a site of trauma. It is followed by the development of multiple nodules that extend deeply into subcutaneous tissues, discharging pus, and granular material formed by microbial colonies embedded in a host-derived proteinous matrix, leading to eventual formation of large granulomatous areas with purulent centers surrounded by thick, fibrous capsules. The lesions may spread to bones, joints, muscles, tendons, and nerves. Early sensation of deep itching gradually gives way to pain. In madura foot, there is tarsal bone destruction associated with plantar fibrosis, thus giving the foot a characteristic short and raised appearance with a convex sole. The syndrome occurs mainly in adult males in rural areas in subtropical zones. See also *Rivalta disease (actinomycosis).*

*Ballingall, G. *Practical observations on fever, dysentery, and liver complaints, as they occur amongst the European troops in India; with introductory remarks on the disadvantages of selecting boys for Indian military service.* Edinburgh, Brown & Constable, 1818.

ballooning mitral cusp syndrome. See *mitral valve prolapse syndrome.*

BALME, PAUL JEAN (French physician, born 1857)

Balme cough. Coughing when in the recumbent position due to nasopharyngeal obstruction.

*Balme, P. J. *De l'hypertrophie des amygdales (palatines, pharyngees, linguale).* Paris, 1888.

BALO, JOZSEF (Hungarian physician)

Baló concentric sclerosis. See *Baló syndrome.*

Baló syndrome. Synonyms: *Baló concentric sclerosis, concentric sclerosis, encephalitis periaxialis concentrica, leukoencephalitis periaxialis concentrica.*

A rare disease of the brain characterized by concentric bands of intact myelin alternating with zones of demyelination, occurring in various parts of the white matter and brainstem. The etiology is unknown.

Baló, J. Leukoencephalitis periaxialis concentrica. **Ról. Magy. Orv. Arch.*, 1927, 28:108-24. Baló, J. Encephalitis periaxialis concentrica. *Arch. Neur., Chicago,* 1928, 19:242-64.

Baltic myoclonus. See *Lafora disease.*

BAMATTER, FRED (Swiss physician)

Bamatter syndrome. See *geroderma osteodysplastica syndrome.*

Bamatter-Franceschetti-Klein-Sierro syndrome. See *geroderma osteodysplastica syndrome.*

Friderichsen-Waterhouse-Bamatter syndrome. See *Waterhouse-Friderichsen syndrome.*

BAMBERGER, EUGEN (Austrian physician, 1858-1921)

Bamberger disease. See *Marie-Bamberger syndrome, under Marie, Pierre.*

Bamberger-Pierre Marie (BPM) syndrome. See *Marie-Bamberger syndrome, under Marie, Pierre.*

Marie-Bamberger syndrome. See *under Marie, Pierre.*

Pierre Marie-Bamberger syndrome. See *Marie-Bamberger syndrome, under Marie, Pierre.*

BAMBERGER, HEINRICH, VON (Austrian physician, 1822-1888)

Bamberger albuminuria. Synonym: *hematogenic albuminuria.*

Albuminuria occurring in latter stages of severe anemia.

*Bamberger, H. Über Morbus Brighti und seine Beziehungen zu anderen Krankheiten. *Samml. Klin. Vortr., Leipzig*, 1879, No. 173, Inn. Med., No. 582, pp. 1533-68.

Bamberger disease (1). Synonyms: *palmus, saltatory spasms.*

Clonic spasms of the leg muscles, producing a peculiar jumping or springing motion.

Bamberger, H. Saltatorischer Reflekskrampf, eine merkwürdige Form von Spinal-Irritation. *Wien. Med. Wschr.*, 1859, 9:49-52; 65-7.

Bamberger disease (2). Synonym: *chronic polyserositis.*

Progressive polyserositis with effusion of fluid into the pleural and peritoneal cavities.

*Bamberger, H. Über zwei seltene Herzaffektionen mit Bezugnahme auf die Theorie des ersten Herztons. *Wien. Med. Wschr.*, 1872, 22:1-4; 25-8.

bamble disease. See *Sylvest syndrome.*

bamboo hair-erythroderma ichthyosiforme congenitum syndrome. See *Netherton syndrome.*

bamboo spine. See *Bechterew-Strümpell-Marie syndrome, under Bekhterev.*

BANERJEE, C. K.

Banerjee syndrome. See *respirator lung syndrome.*

BANG, BERNHARD LAURITS FREDERIK (Danish physician, 1848-1932)

Bang disease. See *brucellosis.*

bangungot. See *sudden unexplained death syndrome.*

banko-kerende. See *ainhum syndrome.*

BANNAYAN, GEORGE A. (American physician)

Bannayan syndrome. Synonyms: *Bannayan-Zonana syndrome, macrocephaly-hamartomas syndrome.*

A familial syndrome, transmitted as an autosomal dominant trait with male predominance of affected individuals, characterized mainly by symmetrical macrocephaly without ventricular enlargement, mild neurological dysfunction, and postnatal growth retardation. Mesodermal hamartomas are present and most patients have discrete lipomas and hemangiomas. Associated disorders may include antimongoloid palpebral fissures, high-arched palate, joint hyperextensibility, pectus excavatum, strabismus, amblyopia, drooling, mental retardation, cerebral hemorrhage, and seizures. Early speech and motor retardation are usually compensated later in life.

Bannayan, G. A. Lipomatosis, angiomatosis, and macrencephalia. *Arch. Path., Chicago,* 1971, 92:1-5. Zonana, J., *et al.* Macrocephaly with multiple lipomas and hemangiomas. *J. Pediat.,* 1976, 89:600-3. Miles, J. H., Zonana, J., *et al.* Macrocephaly with hamartomas: Bannayan-Zonana syndrome. *Am. J. Med. Genet.,* 1984, 19:225-34.

Bannayan-Zonana syndrome (BZS). See *Bannayan syndrome.*

BANNICK, EDWIN (Born 1896)

Hines-Bannick syndrome. See *under Hines.*

BANNISTER, HENRY MARTYN (American physician, 1844-1920)

Bannister disease. See *Quincke edema.*

BANNWARTH, ALFRED (German physician)

Bannwarth syndrome. Synonyms: *Garin-Bujadoux syndrome, lymphocytic meningoradiculitis (LMR), lymphocytic radiculomeningitis.*

An illness characterized by intense pain, mostly in the lumbar and cervical regions and radiating to the extremities; migrating sensory and motor disorders of the peripheral nerves; peripheral radiculopathies; and cerebrospinal fluid abnormalities in the form of lymphocytic pleocytosis indicating blood-brain barrier damage. High numbers of immunoglobulin-producing cells (IgG, IgM, and IgA) are found in the cerebrospinal fluid with normal blood immunoglobulin levels. The symptoms may include facial paralysis, abducens palsy, anorexia, tiredness, headache, diplopia, paresthesias, erythema migrans, and other disorders. The etiology is unknown, but viral infection, possibly mediated by tick bites, is suspected. See also *Lyme disease.*.

Bannwarth, A. Chronische lymphocytäre Meningitis, entzündliche Polyneuritis und "Rheumatismus." Ein Beitrag zum Problem, Allergie und Nervensystem. *Arch. Psychiat. Nervenkr.,* 1941,113:284-376. Weber, T., *et al.* Cerebrospinal fluid immunoglobulins and virus-specific antibodies in disorders affecting the facial nerve. *J. Neurol.,* 1987, 234:308-14.

BANTI, GUIDO (Italian physician, 1852-1925)

Banti disease. See *Banti syndrome.*

Banti syndrome. Synonyms: *Banti disease, Banti-Senator disease, Senator syndrome, cirrhotic splenomegaly, congestive splenomegaly, fibrocongestive splenomegaly, hepatolienal fibrosis, spleen-liver syndrome, splenic anemia.*

An association of anemia, thrombocytopenia, congestive splenomegaly, portal cirrhosis, and obstruction of splenic, portal, or intrahepatic veins, resulting in portal hypertension and ascites. Vomiting of blood, melena, flatulence, diarrhea, digestive disorders, pallor or brown skin pigmentation, weakness, and epistaxis are the principal symptoms. The syndrome occurs most frequently in females under 35 years of age.

Banti, G. Dell'anemia splenica. *Arch. Scuola Anat. Pat., Firenze,* 1883, 2:53-122. Senator, H. Über Anaemia splenica mit Ascites (Banti'sche Krankheit). *Berlin. Klin. Wschr.,* 1901, 38:1145-50.

Banti-Senator disease. See *Banti syndrome.*

BAR

Bar syndrome. Synonym: *colibacillose gravidique.*

Pain in the region of the gallbladder, ureters, and appendix, with occasional fever; the pathologic basis being cholecystitis, ureteritis, and appendicitis with bacteriuria in pregnancy.

Bar's syndrome, or colibacillose gravidique. *JAMA.,* 1945, 128:244.

BARABAS, A. P. (British physician)

Sack-Barabas syndrome. See *Ehlers-Danlos syndrome.*

BARAL, J. (Australian physician)

Reye-Morgan-Baral syndrome. See *Reye syndrome.*

BARANY, ROBERT (Hungarian physician, 1876-1936)

Bárány syndrome. Synonym: *hemicrania cerebellaris.*

A headache syndrome (q.v.) characterized by a combination of unilateral pain in the back of the head, periodic ipsilateral deafness (alternating with periods of unaffected hearing), vertigo, tinnitus, and inability to accurately point a finger, which may be corrected by induced nystagmus.

Bárány, R. Vestibularapparat und Zentralnervensystem. *Med. Klin., Berlin,* 1911, 7:1818-21.

barashek. See *burning feet syndrome.*

BARBEAU, ANDRE (Canadian physician)

Giroux-Barbeau syndrome. See *under Giroux.*

BARBER, C. GLEEN (American physician)

Blount-Barber syndrome. See *Erlacher-Blount syndrome.*

BARBER, HAROLD WORDSWORTH (British dermatologist, born 1886)

Barber dermatosis. Synonyms: *Barber disease, acrodermatitis perstans of mild type, pustular psoriasis of the extremities.*

Pustular psoriasis of the extremities, usually of the thenar and hypothenar eminences, adjacent parts of the palms, central parts of the soles, flexor surfaces of fingers and toes, lateral surfaces of the hands and feet, and around the wrists and ankles. Fresh pustules may be seen through the normal horny layers. In older patches, the lesions are exfoliated, exposing a reddened surface covered by a thick parakeratotic stratum corneum with pustules beneath, bordered by the free edge of the stripped-up normal horny layer. The pustules dry up and form brownish scabs. Lesions form in the upper rete, with formation of cavities and complete disintegration of the rete, but the pus appears to be sterile. The disorder may be observed at any age, and in many instances, the eruption is immediately preceded by acute tonsillitis or scarlet fever.

Barber, H. W. Pustular psoriasis of the extremities. *Guy's Hosp. Rep.,* 1936, 86:108-19.

Barber disease. See *Barber dermatosis.*

barber's itch. See *Alibert disease (3).*

barbiturate withdrawal syndrome. See *opioid withdrawal syndrome, under withdrawal syndrome.*

BARD

Bard syndrome. Pulmonary metastases in cancer of the stomach.

Samson, M., *et al.* Syndrome de Bard. Carcinomatose miliaire pulmonaire sécondaire à une neoplasie gastrique. *Laval Méd.,* 1962, 33:106-10.

BARD, LOUIS (French physician, 1857-1903)

Bard-Pic syndrome. Synonyms: *Courvoisier syndrome, Courvoisier-Terrier syndrome, Pic syndrome, pancreatic malignancy syndrome, pancreaticobiliary syndrome.*

A triad of obstructive jaundice, large palpable gallbladder (Courvoisier sign), and progressive cachexia, indicating the presence of cancer of the head of the pancreas.

Bard, L., & Pic, A. Contribution à l'étude clinique et anatomo-pathologique du cancer primitif du pancréas. *Rev. Méd., Paris,* 1888, 8:257-82; 363-405. Courvoisier, L. G. *Casuistisch-statistische Beiträge zur Pathologie und Chirurgie der Gellenwege.* Leipzig, Vogel, 1890, pp. 57-8.

BARDET, GEORGES (French physician, born 1885)

Bardet-Biedl syndrome. See *Laurence-Moon-Biedl syndrome.*

Laurence-Moon-Biedl-Bardet syndrome (LMBB, LMBBS). See *Laurence-Moon-Biedl syndrome.*

bare lymphocyte syndrome (BLS). A rare, severe combined immunodeficiency syndrome (q.v.) transmitted as an autosomal recessive trait, characterized by the lack of expression of histocompatibility leukocyte antigen (HLA) A, B, and C in the absence of B_2 microglobulins. The affected persons exhibit functional deficiency of both T and B cells, resulting in bacterial, viral, and fungal infections.

Shuurman, R. K.B., *et al.* Failure of lymphocyte-membrane HLA-A and B expression in two siblings with combined immunodeficiency. *Clin. Immun. Immunopath.*, 1979, 14:418-34.

BARLOW, J. B. (South African cardiologist)

Barlow syndrome. See *mitral valve prolapse syndrome.*

BARLOW, SIR THOMAS (British physician, 1819-1887)

Cheadle-Möller-Barlow disease. See *Möller-Barlow disease.*

Möller-Barlow disease. See *under Möller.*

BARNARD, R. I.

Barnard-Scholz syndrome. See *Kearns-Sayre syndrome.*

BARNARD, WILLIAM GEORGE (British physician, born 1892)

Barnard carcinoma. Synonym: *oat cell carcinoma.*

A metastatic tumor that usually forms a large mass which replaces the lymph nodes of the mediastinum and infiltrates the pericardium, while a relatively small mass occupies the hilum of the lung and involves a bronchus. Histologically, the tumor consists of small oval cells with scanty cytoplasm, which have been likened to oat grains.

Barnard, W. G. On the nature of the "oat-cell sarcoma" of the mediastinum. *J. Path. Bact., London,* 1926, 29:241-4.

BARNES, N. D. (British physician)

Barnes syndrome. Synonym: *thoracolaryngopelvic dysplasia.*

A thoracic dystrophy syndrome, transmitted as an autosomal dominant trait, characterized by thoracic dystrophy (small and rigid rigid bell-shaped thorax with small chest volume), laryngeal stenosis, normal stature with variable asymmetry, asthenic built, and small pelvis.

Barnes, N. D., *et al.* Chest reconstruction in thoracic dystrophy. *Arch. Dis. Child.*, 1971, 46:833-7.

BARR, MURRAY L. (Canadian physician)

Carr-Barr-Plunkett syndrome. See *chromosome XXXX syndrome.*

BARRAQUER, ROVIRALTA JOSE ANTONIO (Spanish physician)

Barraquer syndrome. See *Barraquer-Simons syndrome.*

Barraquer-Simons syndrome. Synonyms: *Barraquer syndrome, Holländer-Simons syndrome, Simons syndrome, lipodystrophia progressiva seu paradoxa, partial lipodystrophy of the cephalothoracic type, progressive lipodystrophy, progressive partial lipodystrophy.*

A rare, usually sporadic childhood disease of unknown etiology, characterized by a loss of subcutaneous fat from the face and trunk with normal or excessive fat deposition on the pelvic girdle and lower limbs. Most affected subjects are females and some show no other abnormality, but many develop glomerulonephritis, diabetes mellitus, hyperlipidemia, and complement deficiency.

*Barraquer, R. *Histoire clinique d'un cas d'atrophie du tissue cellulo-adipeux.* Barcelona, 1906. Simons, A. Eine seltene Trophoneurose ("Lipodystrophia progressiva"). *Zschr. Ges. Neurol. Psychiat.*, 1911, 5:29-38. Holländer, E. Über einen Fall von fortschreitendem Schwund des Fettgewebes und seinen kosmetischen Ersatz durch Menschenfett. *Münch. Med. Wschr.*, 1910, 57:1794-5.

BARRATT-BOYES, B. G.

Williams-Barratt syndrome. See *Williams syndrome, under Williams, J. C. P.*

BARRE, JEAN ALEXANDRE (French physician, born 1880)

Barré-Lieou syndrome. Synonyms: *Neri-Barré syndrome, brachialgia paresthetica nocturna, cervical migraine, neurovertebral dystonia, posterior cervical sympathetic syndrome, vertigo of cervical arthrosis.*

A syndrome, usually occurring in middle-aged or older persons, characterized by trauma or arthritic changes involving the third and fourth cervical vertebrae or cervical disk lesions with irritation of the cranial nuclei, the fifth and eighth cranial nerves being chiefly affected. Circulatory disorders with headache, pain during neck movements, vertigo, tinnitus, laryngo-pharyngeal paresthesia, facial pain and flushing, impaired vision, corneal hypesthesia, corneal ulcers, anxiety, depression, and memory and thinking disorders are the principal symptoms.

Barré, J. A. Sur un syndrome sympathique cervical postérieur et sa cause fréquente, l'arthrite cervicale. *Rev. Neur., Paris,* 1926, 1:1246-8. Lieou, Y. C. *Syndrome sympathique cervical postérieur et arthrite chronique de la colonne vertébrale cervicale (Étude clinique et radiologique).* Strassbourgh, 1928 (Thesis). Neri, V. Sindrome cerebrale del simpaticus cervicale. *Bol. Soc. Med., Bologna*, 1924, 96:382.

Barré-Masson syndrome. Synonyms: *Barré-Masson tumor, arterial angioneuromyoma, glomangioma, glomus tumor.*

A benign tumor of the glomus body, occurring as a firm, round, reddish-blue encapsulated lesion about 0.5 to 2.5 cm in diameter. The tumor may be located in various parts of the upper and lower extremities, the nail beds being its most common sites. Severe burning pain at the site of the tumor, which occurs spontaneously or is precipitated by temperature changes or touch, is the principal clinical symptom. A fear of using the extremity may cause severe atrophy of the limb from disuse.

Masson, P. Le glomus neuromyo-artériel des régions tactiles et ses tumeurs. *Lyon Méd.*, 1924, 21:257-80.

Barré-Masson tumor. See *Barré-Masson syndrome.*

Guillain-Barré syndrome. See *under Guillain.*

Guillain-Barré-Strohl syndrome. See *Guillain-Barré syndrome.*

Landry-Guillain-Barré syndrome. See *Guillain-Barré syndrome.*

Neri-Barré syndrome. See *Barré-Lieou syndrome.*

BARRETT, NORMAN RUPERT (British physician, born 1903)

Barrett esophagus. See *Barrett syndrome.*

Barrett syndrome. Synonyms: *Allison-Johnstone anomaly, Barrett esophagus, Barrett ulcer, columnar-lined esophagus, endobrachy-esophagus, gastric-lined eso-*

phagus.

A rare disorder, usually occurring in middle-aged and elderly persons, characterized by lining of the esophagus, often in its midsection, with heterotopic gastric (columnar) epithelium, in association with peptic ulcer. Accompanying disorders include hiatal hernia, dilatation of the esophago-gastric junction and stricture above the junction, esophageal ulcer and spasms, retrosternal pain, heartburn, dysphagia, vomiting, and gastrointestinal hemorrhage.

Barrett, N. R. Chronic peptic ulcer of the oesophagus and "oesophagitis." *Brit. J. Surg.*, 1950, 38:175-82. Allison, P. R., & Johnstone, A. S. The esophagus lined with gastric mucous membrane. *Thorax*, 1953, 8:87.

Barrett ulcer. See *Barrett syndrome.*

Eagle-Barrett syndrome. See *prune belly syndrome.*

BARRIERE, HENRI (French physician)

Bureau-Barrière syndrome. See *under Bureau.*

Bureau-Barrière-Thomas syndrome. See *under Bureau.*

BARRY

Barry-Perkins-Young syndrome. See *Young syndrome, under Young, Donald.*

BARRY, G. A. (British physician)

Barry and Treacher Collins syndrome. See *mandibulofacial dysostosis.*

BARSONY, THEODOR (Hungarian physician, 1887-1942)

Bársony-Polgár syndrome (1). Synonyms: *Brailsford-Bársony-Polgár syndrome, osteitis condensans ilii, osteosis condensans ilii.*

Iliosacral neuralgia associated with homologous density of the ilium seen on x-ray. The syndrome is characterized by neuralgic pain, lower back pain, restricted hip movement, and hyperesthesia of the skin in the inguinal region and thighs. Pregnancy and physical exertion tend to exacerbate the symptoms.

*Bársony, T., & Polgár, F. Ostitis condensans ilei-ein bisher nicht beschriebenes Krankheitsbild. *Fortschr. Röntgen.*, 1928, 57:663-k9.

Bársony-Polgár syndrome (2). Synonyms: *Bársony-Teschendorf syndrome, corckscrew esophagus, idiopathic diffuse esophageal spasm, segmental spasm of esophagus.*

A syndrome showing on x-ray "pearl-necklace" appearance of the esophagus due to contractions marked by alternating narrowings and dilatations that may be stationary or may form waves of peristalsis. Chest pain and dysphagia are associated. Excitable elderly individuals are most commonly affected.

Bársony, T. Funktionelle Speiseröhrendivertikel (Relaxationsdivertikel). *Wien. Klin. Wschr.*, 1926, 39:1363. Bársony, T., & Polgár, E. Symptomlose und funktionelle Speiseröhrendivertikel. *Forschr. Röntgen.*, 1927, 36:593-602. Teschendorf, W. Die Röntgenuntersuchung der Speiseröhre. *Erg. Med. Strahl.*, 1928, 3:175-88.

Bársony-Teschendorf syndrome. See *Bársony-Polgár syndrome (2).*

Brailsford-Bársony-Polgár syndrome. See *Bársony-Polgár syndrome (1).*

BARSY, A. M., DE. See DE BARSY, A. M.

BART, B. J.

Bart syndrome. See *epidermolysis bullosa syndrome.*

BART, ROBERT S. (American physician, born 1933)

Bart-Pumphrey syndrome. Synonyms: *knuckle pads syndrome, knuckle pads-leukonychia-sensineural deafness syndrome.*

A familial hereditary syndrome, transmitted as an autosomal dominant trait, consisting of knuckle pads, leukonychia, and sensineural deafness.

Bart, R. S., & Pumphrey, R. E. Knuckle pads, leukonychia and deafness. A dominant inherited syndrome. *N. Engl. J. Med.*, 1967, 276:202-7.

BARTENWERFER, KURT (German physician, 1892-1942)

Bartenwerfer syndrome. A variant of Morquio disease characterized by disproportionate dwarfism, hypertelorism, high palate, mongoloid palpebral slant, broad nose, flat vertebrae, lordoscoliosis, flat feet, hip dislocation, and epiphyseal and metaphyseal dysplasia.

Bartenwerfer, K. Destruktive Epiphysenerkrankung bei zwei Kindern von mongoloidem Aussechen. *Zschr. Orthop. Chir.*, 1924, 43:201-12.

BARTH, JEAN BAPTISTE PHILIPPE (French physician, 1806-1877)

Barth hernia. Hernia of the loops of intestine between the serosa of the abdominal wall and that of a persistent vitelline duct.

*Barth, J. B. *Observations et réflexions sur quelques cas de hernies inguinales et crurales.* Strasbourg, 1836.

BARTHELEMY, P. TOUSSAINT (French physician, born 1850)

Barthélemy disease. Synonyms: *acne agminata, acne scrofulosorum, papular and nodular tuberculid, tuberculosis papulonecrotica.*

A cutaneous manifestation of tuberculosis characterized by papulonecrotic lesions of the face (acnitis), hands, and trunk. In the early stages, the lesions are colorless; later they become bluish or brownish red. Suppuration and pustules may develop, followed by crusting, ulceration, and cicatrization. The lesions are transient but recur at regular intervals.

Barthélemy. De l'acinitis ou d'une variété speciale de folliculites et périfolliculites généralisées et disséminées. *Ann. Derm. Syph., Paris,* 1891, 2:2-38.

BARTHOLIN (BARTHOLINUS), THOMAS (Danish anatomist, 1616-1680)

Bartholin-Patau syndrome. See *chromosome 13 trisomy syndrome.*

BARTON, JOHN RHEA (American physician, 1794-1871)

Barton fracture. Anterior and posterior marginal fracture dislocations of the distal radius. In the original description, Barton delineated only the posterior marginal fracture.

Barton, J. R. Views and treatment of an important injury of the wrist. *Med. Exam., Philadelphia,* 1838, 1:365-8.

Bartonella bacilliformis anemia. See *Carrión disease.*

Bartonella fever. See *Carrión disease.*

BÄRTSCHI-ROCHAIX, WERNER (Swiss physician, born 1911)

Bärtschi-Rochaix syndrome. Synonyms: *cerebral artery compression syndrome, cervical migraine syndrome, cervical vertigo syndrome, cervico-encephalic syndrome, vertebral artery compression syndrome.*

A complex of symptoms, closely related to the Barré-Lieou syndrome, consisting of headache, paresthesia, scotoma, stiffness of the neck, pain on pressure of the cervical vertebrae, and vertigo due to traumatic cerebral artery compression.

Bärtschi-Rochaix, W. *Migraine cervicale (das encephale Syndrom nach Halswirbeltrauma).* Berne, Huber, 1949.

BARTSOCAS, CHRISTOS S. (Greek physician)

Bartsocas-Papas syndrome. A severe autosomal recessive form of the popliteal pterygium syndrome in children of consanguineous parents, characterized by low birth weight, microcephaly ankyloblepharon, corneal ulcers, filiform bands between the jaws, cleft palate and lip, hypoplastic nose, low-set ears, lanugo, absent thumb, syndactyly of the fingers and toes, pes equinovarus, bilateral popliteal pterygium, hypoplastic nails, genital abnormalities, and bone abnormalities of the hands and feet.

Bartsocas, C. S., & Papas, C. V. Popliteal pterygium syndrome. Evidence of severe autosomal recessive form. *J. Med. Genet.*, 1972, 9:222-6.

BARTTER, FREDERIC CROSBY (American physician, born 1914)

Bartter syndrome (BS). Synonyms: *aldosteronism-normal blood pressure syndrome, hypokalemic alkalosis, juxtaglomerular hyperplasia syndrome.*

A syndrome of hyperplasia of the juxtaglomerular apparatus with secondary hypokalemia and hyperchloremic alkalosis; increased concentration of renin, angiotensin II, and aldosterone; high urinary prostaglandin E and kallikrein; and elevated plasma bradykinin-in the absence of edema and with normal blood pressure. Growth retardation is frequently associated. The syndrome is transmitted as an autosomal recessive trait.

Bartter, F. C., *et al.* Hyperplasia of the juxtaglomerular complex with hyperaldosteronism and hypokalemic alkalosis. A new syndrome. *Am. J. Med.*, 1962, 33:811-28.

factitious Bartter syndrome. Synonym: *pseudo-Bartter syndrome.*

A metabolic disorder with symptoms mimicking the Bartter syndrome (hypertrophy of the juxtaglomerular apparatus, hyperaldosteronism, and normal blood pressure) associated with increased serum urate levels due to surreptitious diuretic abuse.

Jiménez, M. L., *et al.* Hyperuricemia as possible diagnostic aid to factitious Bartter's syndrome. *Adv. Exp. Med. Biol.*, 1986, 1195(Pt A):351-6.

pseudo-Bartter syndrome. See *factitious Bartter syndrome.*

Schwartz-Bartter syndrome. See *inappropriate antidiuretic hormone secretion syndrome.*

basal cell carcinoma. See *Krompecher tumor.*

basal cell nevus syndrome (BCNS). See *nevoid basal cell carcinoma syndrome.*

basal encephalocele-hypothalamic and pituitary dysfunction syndrome. A syndrome of hypothalamo-pituitary dysfunction and congenital herniation of the brain through the base of the skull (basal encephalocele) associated with growth hormone deficiency. In the original report, out of three patients, one had diabetes insipidus, two had hypogonadotropic hypogonadism, one had elevated prolactin level, and two were euthyroid.

Lieblich, J. M., *et al.* The syndrome of basal encephalocele and hypothalamic-pituitary dysfunction. *Ann. Intern. Med.*, 1978, 89:910-6.

BASAN, MARIANNE (German physician)

Basan syndrome. A form of ectodermal dysplasia, transmitted as an autosomal dominant trait, characterized by hypohidrosis, thick and short fingernails and toenails with longitudinal ridging, simian creases, and absence of fingerprint patterns. See also *Jorgenson syndrome.*

Basan, M. Ektodermale Dysplasie. Fehlendes Papillarmuster, Nagelveränderungen un Vierfingerfurche. *Arch. Klin. Exp. Derm., Berlin,* 1965, 222:546-57.

BASEDOW, CARL ADOLF, VON (German physician, 1799-1854)

Basedow disease. Synonyms: *Begbie disease, Flajani-Basedow syndrome, Graves disease, Marsh disease, Parry syndrome, exophthalmic goiter.*

A triad of hyperthyroidism, goiter, and exophthalmos. The symptoms include cardiac arrhythmias, increased pulse rate, weight loss in the presence of increased appetite, intolerance to heat, elevated basal metabolism rate, sweating, apprehension, weakness, elevated protein-bound iodine level, tremor, increased bowel activity, eyelid retraction, and stare. Thyrotoxic heart disease may develop in severe cases, complicated by congestive heart failure. In addition, the patients may have a dermatologic condition, pretibial myxedema. Emotional problems, and long-acting thyroid stimulator (LATS), thyroid-stimulating immunoglobulin (TSI), and autoimmune mechanisms have been suggested as potential causative factors, but the etiology is unknown.

Basedow, von. Exophthalmos durch Hypertrophie des Zellgewebes in der Augenhöle. *Wschr. Ges. Heilk.*, 1840, p. 197-204; 220-8. Flajani, G. *Sopra un tumore freddo nell'anteriore parte del collo. Collezione d'osservazioni e reflessioni di chirurgia.* Roma, 1802. *Graves, R. J. New observed affection of the thyroid gland in females. *London Med. Surg. J.*, 1835, p. 516-7. *Parry, C. H. Diseases of the heart. Enlargement of the thyroid gland in connection with enlargement or palpitation of the heart. In his: *Collected works.* London, vol. 1, pp. 11-28. Begbie, J. Anemia and its consequences; enlargement of the thyroid gland and eyeballs. Anemia and goitre, are they related? *Month. J. Med. Sc.*, 1849, 9:495-508. Marsh, H. Dilatation of the cavities of the heart. Englargement of the thyroid gland. *Dublin J. Med. Sc.*, 1842, 20:471-4. (Abstr).

Flajani-Basedow syndrome. See *Basedow disease.*

bashful bladder syndrome (BBS). Inability of a male to initiate urination when in the company of others.

Beary, J., III, & Gilbert, S. Coping with the "bashful bladder" syndrome. *Lancet,* 1981, 1:1429-30.

basofrontal syndrome. See *Kennedy syndrome.*

basophil adenoma. See *Cushing syndrome.*

BASS, HAROLD H. (American physician)

Bass syndrome. Synonym: *brachymesodactylia-nail dysplasia syndrome.*

A syndrome, transmitted as an autosomal dominant trait, characterized by nail dysplasia and brachymesodactyly and marked by absence of the middle phalanges in fingers and lateral four toes and duplication of distal phalanges of the thumbs.

Bass, H. N. Familial absence of middle phalanges with nail dysplasia: A new syndrome. *Pediatrics*, 1968, 42:318-23.

BASSEN, FRANK ALBERT (American physician, born 1903)

Bassen-Kornzweig syndrome. Synonyms: *abetalipoproteinemia (ABL), acanthocytosis, beta-lipoprotein deficiency, familial hypolipoproteinemia.*

A hereditary syndrome, transmitted as an autosomal recessive trait, characterized by the presence of acanthocytes (burr-cell malformation of the erythrocytes), hence the synonym **acanthocytosis** (sometimes written **acanthrocytosis**), retinitis pigmentosa, degenerative changes in the central nervous system involving the cerebellum and long tracts, ataxia, areflexia, demyelination, defective intestinal lipid absorption with low serum cholesterol level, absent serum β-lipoproteins, intestinal malabsorption, amaurosis, retarded growth, and steatorrhea. Blepharoptosis, nystagmus, external ophthalmoplegia, optic atrophy, epicanthus, cataract, and macular degeneration are the additional ocular defects. Most cases occur in children of Jewish extraction.

Bassen, F. A., & Kornzweig, A. L. Malformation of the erythrocytes in case of atypical retinitis pigmentosa. *Blood*, 1950, 5:381-7.

BASTIAN, HENRY CHARLON (British physician, 1837-1915)

Bastian aphasia. See *Wernicke aphasia.*

BATEMAN, THOMAS (British physician, 1778-1821)

Bateman disease. See *Bateman purpura.*

Bateman purpura. Synonyms: *Bateman disease, Bateman syndrome, purpura senilis.*

Purpura with petechiae and hematomas along the veins of the extremities, seen in elderly individuals suffering from severe malnutrition, associated with atrophy of the skin and depletion of subcutaneous adipose tissue.

Basegra, A. La porpora senile di Bateman. *Rass. Med.*, 1954, 31:109-10.

Bateman syndrome (1). Synonyms: *epithelioma contagiosum, molluscum contagiosum, molluscum epitheliale, molluscum sebaceum.*

An infectious disease of the skin caused by agents of the poxvirus group. The disorder occurs chiefly in children and may affect any part of the body. The lesions are characterized by hyperplasia and degeneration of the epithelium of the skin and mucous membranes, presenting pinhead- to pea-sized, pearly white, umbilicate nodules that exude waxy material. Transmission is by direct contact with the lesions, through sexual intercourse, and through fomites. Histologically, the lesions are marked by large, cytoplasmic, viral inclusions (molluscum bodies) in the epithelial cells.

Bateman, T. *Delineation of cutaneous diseases: exhibiting the characteristic appearances of the principal general and species comprised in the classification of the late Dr. Willan; and completing the series of engravings begun by that author.* London, Longman, 1817.

Bateman syndrome (2). See *Bateman purpura.*

BATTEN, FREDERIC EUSTACE (British physician, 1865-1918)

Batten disease (1). See *myotonic dystrophy syndrome.*

Batten disease (2). See *Stock-Spielmeyer-Vogt syndrome.*

Batten-Mayou syndrome. See *Stock-Spielmeyer-Vogt syndrome.*

Curschmann-Batten-Steinert syndrome. See *myotonic dystrophy syndrome.*

Rossolimo-Curschmann-Batten-Steinert syndrome. See *myotonic dystrophy syndrome.*

battered babe. See *battered child syndrome.*

battered child syndrome. Synonyms: *Ambroise Tardieu syndrome, Caffey syndrome, Caffey-Kempe syndrome, Silverman syndrome, abused child, battered babe, battered infant, child abuse, maltreatment syndrome of children, parent-infant traumatic stress syndrome, shaken baby syndrome (SBS), shaken child syndrome, whiplash shaken infant syndrome.*

Intentional injury inflicted on infants and young children, usually by a parent, less commonly a parent-substitute, and sometimes strangers. It includes trauma by the use of heat and water, as well as mechanical injury. Fractures, often multiple but inflicted at different times, and subdural hematomas are the most common types of injuries. The skin may show scratches and scars, which give an impression of healing burns, and numerous ecchymoses on various parts of the body. Oral examination may show lesions of the anterior pillar of the fauces and loss of tissue from the vault of the palate. The nose is often broken, giving it a flat appearance, such as seen in boxers. The principal radiographic signs include metaphyseal fragmentations and traumatic involucrums (external cortical thickenings) of the shafts of unfractured and otherwise healthy bones and trauma of the growing bones, such as metaphyseal cupping, traumatic bowing of the ends of the diaphyses due to metaphyseal infractions, and ectopic ossification of accessory epiphyseal centers in injured cartilaginous epiphyses, in which ossification centers do not normallly develop. Exophthalmos with orbital hemorrhage, lid hematoma and edema, glaucoma, hyphema, vitreous hemorrhage, retinal exudates and hemorrhage (Berlin edema), choroidal atrophy, retinal detachment, and papilledema are the typical ocular features. The **whiplash shaken infant syndrome** involves vigorous manual shaking of the infant by the extremities or shoulders, with whiplash-induced intracranial and intra-ocular bleeding, but with no external signs of head trauma. The **Munchausen syndrome by proxy** is considered a form of the battered child syndrome. See also *pseudobattered child syndrome* and *abuse dwarfism syndrome.*

Caffey, J. The parent-infant traumatic stress syndrome: (Caffey-Kempe syndrome), (battered babe syndrome). *Am. J. Roentgen.*, 1972, 114:218-29. Tardieu, A. Étude médico-legale sur les services et mauvais traitment exerces sur des enfants. *Ann. Hyg. Publ. Méd. Legal.*, 1860, 13:361-98. Kempe, H. C., *et al.* The battered child syndrome. *JAMA.*, 1962, 181:17-24. Silverman, F. N. Unrecognized trauma in infants, the battered child syndrome, and the syndrome of Ambroise Tardieu. *Radiology* 1972, 104:337-53.

battered doctor syndrome. Synonyms: *abused doctor, doctor bashing, malpractice stress syndrome.*

Criticism and verbal abuse of physicians by individuals and, more commonly, the media, frequently based on incomplete or false information, thus placing the medical profession on the defensive and creating public anxiety about the quallity of health care. In an extended definition, frivolous and unreasonable malpractice litigations are also a form of doctor abuse (the malpractice stress syndrome).

The "battered doctor" syndrome. *Austral. Fam. Physician*, 1979, 8:1140.

battered husband syndrome. See *battered spouse syndrome.*

battered infant. See *battered child syndrome.*

battered parent syndrome. Synonyms: *abused parent, parent abuse.*

A syndrome of family violence, wherein parents are subjected to actual physical assault or verbal or nonverbal threats of physical harm. The term includes parricide.

Harbin, H. T., & Madden, D. J. Battered parent: A new syndrome. *Am. J. Psychiat.*, 1979, 136:1288-91.

battered root syndrome. Reappearance after surgical treatment of sciatica of pain with radicular distribution, which is exacerbated by motion, the Valsalva maneuver, certain postures, or jugular compression. The pain is usually constant, often described as burning or as ice cold or aching. Its distribution down the anterolateral aspect of the thigh, in front of the knee, or down the shin suggests L4 involvement. L5 root lesions often produce pain on the lateral aspect of the leg and the lateral malleolus, dorsum of the foot, and middle toes or hallux. S1 pain usually radiates to the posterior thigh and calf, the lateral border of the foot, and the little toe. Other symptoms may include hyperesthetic skin, a slight increase in sweating, and a decrease of skin temperature over the affected areas. Reflex and motor disorders are usually present.

Bertrand, G. The "battered" root problem. *Orthop. Clin. N. America*, 1975, 6:305-10.

battered spouse syndrome. Synonyms: *abused husband, abused wife, battered husband syndrome, battered wife syndrome, battered woman syndrome, husband abuse, husband beating, abuse, spousal abuse, spouse beating, marital violence, wife abuse, wife beating.*

A syndrome of family violence where one partner in an ongoing relationship, whether or not partners are married, is subjected to actual physical assault, including sexual assault, or verbal or nonverbal threats of physical harm. Emotional abuse is included in the scope of this syndrome by some authors. See also *burnt wife syndrome.*

Sadoff, R. L. Violence in families: An overview. *Bull Am. Acad. Psychiat. Law*, 1976, 4:292-6. Goldberg, W. G., & Tomianovich, M. C. Domestic violence victims in the emergency department. New findings. *JAMA*, 1984, 251:3259-64. Frazer, M. Domestic violence. A medicolegal review. *J. Forens. Sc.*, 1986, 31:1409-19.

battered wife. See *battered spouse syndrome.*

battered woman syndrome. See *battered spouse syndrome.*

BAUMGARTEN, PAUL CLEMENS, VON (German pathologist, 1848-1928)

Baumgarten cirrhosis. See *Cruveilhier-Baumgarten syndrome.*

Cruveilhier-Baumgarten cirrhosis. See *Cruveilhier-Baumgarten syndrome.*

Cruveilhier-Baumgarten syndrome. See *under Cruveilhier.*

Pégot-Cruveilhier-Baumgarten syndrome. See *Cruveilhier-Baumgarten syndrome.*

bauxite workers' disease. See *Shaver syndrome.*

BAVCP. See ***b**ilateral **a**bductor **v**ocal **c**ord **p**aralysis syndrome.*

BAYER, JOSEPH F. (American physician)

Braun-Bayer syndrome. See *under Braun.*

BAYFORD, DAVID (British physician)

Bayford-Autenrieth dysphagia. Synonym: *Arkin disease.*

Dysphagia lusoria resulting from compression of the esophagus by an aberrant right subclavian artery. Autenrieth, & Pfeiderer. De Dysphagia lusoria. *Arch. Physiol., Halle*, 1807, 7:145-88. Bayford, D. An account on a singular case of obstructed deglutition. *Mem. Med. Soc. London*, 1789, 1:271-82.

BAYLE, ANTOINE LAURENT JESSE (French physician, 1799-1858)

Bayle disease. Synonyms: *dementia paralytica, general paralysis, general paresis, paralysis generalisata progressiva, paralysis of the insane, paralytic dementia, progressive paralysis.*

A severe form of neurosyphilis involving the neurons and blood vessels of the meninges. The symptoms usually become evident 2 to 30 years after the primary syphilitic lesion and include at first progressive simple dementia, followed by manic symptoms, megalomania, impaired memory, faulty judgement, disturbed affect (depression or euphoria), paranoid behavior, lack of insight into the nature of illness, and fine or coarse tremor often affecting facial muscles and tongue. General paresis is a constant feature of this syndrome. Associated symptoms may include abnormal pupillary responses (including Argyll Robertson pupil), impassive facies, slurred or dysarthric speech, exaggerated stretch and extensor palmar reflexes, convulsions, and stroke due to cerebral vasculitis. The cerebrospinal fluid is always abnormal, containing increased numbers of mononuclear cells, elevated total proteins, and high gamma-globulin concentrations. At autopsy, the brain is shrunken, the meninges are cloudy and thickened, and the cerebral cortex is atrophied. When left untreated, the disease is usually fatal within 3 years.

*Bayle, A. L. *Recherches sur la maladie mentale.* Paris, 1822 (Thesis).

BAZEX, A. (French physician)

Bazex syndrome. Synonyms: *acrokeratosis paraneoplastica, acrokeratotic psoriasiform dermatosis, acromegalic psoriasiform dermatosis, paraneoplastic acrokeratosis, psoriasiform acrokeratotic dermatosis.*

Symmetrical dermatosis with erythematous eruption, which accompanies neoplasms of the respiratory system, tongue, and esophagus. Skin lesions usually involve the hands, feet, ears, and nose, later spreading to the cheeks, elbows, knees, and, finally, the trunk. Acanthosis nigricans may be associated. Ungual involvement is characterized by subungual hyperkeratosis, flaky nail surfaces, and, sometimes, shedding of the nails. There may be erythematous scaling eruption, fissuring, and suppuration of the distal digits of the fingers.

Bazex, A., *et al.* Syndrome para-néoplasique à type d'hyperkératose des extrémites. Guérison après le traitement de l'épithéliome larynge. *Bull. Soc. Fr. Derm. Syph.*, 1965, 72:182.

BAZEX, J. (French physician)

Bazex syndrome. See *telangiectasia-alopecia syndrome.*

BAZIN, ANTOINE PIERRE ERNEST (French physician, 1807-1877)

Alibert-Bazin syndrome. See *mycosis fungoides.*

Bazin disease. Synonyms: *Bazin malady, erythema induratum, scrofulous ulcers of the legs, nodular vasculitis, tuberculosis cutis indurativa, tuberculosis indurativa cutanea et subcutanea.*

An erythrocyanotic disorder, characterized by symmetrical indurated cutaneous nodules of the calves, occurring most commonly in adolescent girls and menopausal women, also observed with lesser frequency in women of all ages and some males. The nodules usually persist for a few months and then become absorbed, leaving atrophic scars. During the evolution of nodules, the skin assumes a dusky or bluish color. Cutis marmorata may develop. The condition is most prevalent in early spring and winter. Initially, it was considered a form of skin tuberculosis. In a more recent literature, some cases have been observed in tuberculin-positive patients, while others appear to be unrelated to tuberculosis.

*Bazin. *Leçons sur la scrofule.* Paris, 1861. Hutchinson, J. Scrofulous ulcers of the legs (Bazin's malady), *Arch. Surg., London,* 1894, 5:31-42; 97-114.

Bazin malady. See *Bazin disease.*

BBB syndrome. See *hypertelorism-hypospadias syndrome (2).*

BBBG syndrome. See *hypospadias-dysphagia syndrome, and see hypertelorism-hypospadias syndrome.*

BBS. See *bashful bladder syndrome.*

BCDL (Brachmann-Cornelia de Lange) syndrome. See *de Lange syndrome (1), under Lange, Cornelia, de.*

BCKD (branched chain α-keto acid dehydrogenase) deficiency. See *maple syrup urine disease.*

BCNS (basal cell nevus syndrome). See *nevoid basal cell carcinoma syndrome.*

BCS. See *Budd-Chiari syndrome.*

BD. See *Byler disease.*

BD (Betçet disease). See *Behçet syndrom.*

BD (Briquet disorder). See *Briquet syndrome (1), under Briquet, Pierre.*

BD syndrome. A multiple abnormalities/mental retardation syndrome consisting of a prominent forehead, midface hypoplasia, mandibular prognathism, apparent midline cleft of the mandible, absence of the lower central incisors, eye abnormalities, malformed ears, growth retardation, cerebral palsy, and immobilization.

Neuhäuser, G., *et al.* Studies of malformation syndromes of man. XXXVIII. The BD syndrome. A "new" multiple congenital anomalies/mental retardation syndrome with athetoid cerebral palsy. *Zschr. Kinderheilk.,* 1975, 120:191-8.

beaded hairs. See *Sabouraud syndrome.*

BEAL (French physician)

Béal conjunctivitis. Synonym: *Béal syndrome.*

A transient form of acute follicular conjunctivitis characterized by a rapid onset, mild clinical course, resolution within 2 weeks, and association with preauricular adenitis.

*Béal, *Ann. Ocul., Paris,* 1907, 137:1. *Ostler, H. B. Acute follicular conjunctivitis of epizootic origin. *Arch. Ophthal.,* 1969, 82:587.

Béal syndrome. See *Béal conjunctivitis.*

BEALS, RODNEY K. (American orthopedic surgeon)

Beals syndrome (1). See *congenital contractural arachnodactyly syndrome.*

Beals syndrome (2). See *auriculo-osteodysplasia syndrome.*

Beals-Hecht syndrome. See *congenital contractural arachnodactyly syndrome.*

Hecht-Beals-Wilson syndrome. See *trismus-pseudocamptodactyly syndrome.*

BEAN, WILLIAM BENNETT (American physician)

Bean syndrome. See *blue rubber bleb nevus syndrome.*

BEARD, GEORGE MILLER (American physician)

Beard disease. See *Beard syndrome.*

Beard syndrome. Synonyms: *Beard disease, nervous exhaustion.*

Unexplained exhaustion with abnormal fatigability, lassitude, insomnia, back pain, nervousness, anxiety, depression, headache, difficulty in concentrating, reduced sexual impulse, and lack of appetite. DSM-III classifies this disorder with neurasthenia and dysthymia (depressive neurosis), but some authors associate it with the chronic fatigue syndrome (q.v.).

*Beard, G. M. Neurasthenia or nervous exhaustion. *Boston Med. Surg. J.,* 1869, 80:217-21. *Diagnostic and statistical manual of mental disorders.* Washington, American Psychiatric Association, 1980, p. 230.

BEARE, J. MARTIN (physician in Belfast)

Beare syndrome. A syndrome, transmitted as an autosomal dominant trait, characterized by pili torti, fragile nails, and mental retardation.

Beare, J. M. Congenital pilar defect showing features of pili torti. *Brit. J. Derm.,* 1952, 64:366-72.

BEARN, ALEXANDER GORDON (American physician, born 1923)

Bearn-Kunkel syndrome. Synonyms: *Bearn-Kunkel-Slater syndrome, Kunkel syndrome, chronic active lupoid hepatitis (CALH), hypergammaglobulinemic hepatitis, lupoid hepatitis, plasma-cell hepatitis.*

A liver disease seen in young women, which is characterized by liver cirrhosis with extreme hypergammaglobulinemia and an increase of plasma cells. It begins at about puberty as amenorrhea, acne, hirsutism, moon facies, and obesity, with consecutive hepatomegaly and splenomegaly. Hypergammaglobulinemia, painful joints, spider telangiectasia, esophageal varices, fever, respiratory and cardiovascular disorders, and liver pain are the late symptoms. In a few instances, LE cells and rheumatic nodules have been observed. This disease and Waldenström hepatitis are considered by some writers as the same entity.

Bearn, A. G., Kunkel, H. G., & Slater, R. J. The problem of chronic liver disease in young women. *Am. J. Med.,* 1956, 21:3-15.

Bearn-Kunkel-Slater syndrome. See *Bearn-Kunkel syndrome.*

BEAU, HONORE SIMON (French physician, 1806-1865)

Beau syndrome. Cardiac insufficiency and asystole.

Beau. Recherches d'anatomie pathologique sur une forme particulière de dilatation et d'hypertrophie due coeur. *Arch. Gén. Méd., Paris,* 1836, 425-47.

BECHTEREW, VLADIMIR MIKHAILOVICH. See BEKHTEREV, VLADIMIR MIKHAILOVICH

BECK, CLAUDE SCHAEFFER (American physician, born 1894)

Beck triad. In cardiac compression, a triad of a high venous pressure, a low arterial pressure, and a small quiet heart, reportedly described by Beck.

BECK, E. V. See BEK, E. V

BECK, KARL (German physician)

Beck syndrome. See *anterior spinal artery syndrome.*

BECK, SOMA CORNELIUS (German physician, born 1872)

Beck disease. See *Beck-Ibrahim syndrome.*

Beck-Ibrahim syndrome. Synonyms: *Beck disease, Ibrahim disease, erythema mycoticum infantile.*

An erythematous, desquamative skin disease of the perineal and perigenital regions of newborn infants, marked by mulitple pustules filled with *Candida albicans* positive pus.

*Beck, S. Über das Erythema mycoticum infantile. *Derm. Stud. Unna Fortschr.*, 1910, 1:494. Ibrahim, J. Über eine Soormykose der Haut im frühen Säugligsalter. *Arch. Kinderh.*, 1911, 55:91-101.

BECKER, PETER EMIL (German geneticist, born 1908)

Becker dystrophy. See *Becker muscular dystrophy.*

Becker muscular dystrophy (BMD). Synonyms: *Becker dystrophy; Becker progressive muscular dystrophy; Becker-Kiener muscular dystrophy; Becker-Kiener syndrome; Duchenne-Becker muscular dystrophy, Becker type; muscular dystrophy, Becker type; progressive tardive muscular dystrophy.*

Muscular dystrophy, transmitted as an X-linked trait, having an onset in the second and third decades of life and survival to a relatively advanced age. The calves are usually abnormally enlarged. Color blindness is common. The serum creatinine concentration is elevated.

Becker, P. E. Eine neue chromosomale Muskeldystrophie. *Acta Psychiat. Neur. Scand.*, 1955, 193:427.

Becker progressive muscular dystrophy. See *Becker muscular dystrophy.*

Becker-Kiener muscular dystrophy. See *Becker muscular dystrophy.*

Becker-Kiener syndrome. See *Becker muscular dystrophy.*

Duchenne-Becker muscular dystrophy. See *Becker muscular dystrophy.*

muscular dystrophy, Becker type. See *Becker muscular dystrophy.*

BECKER, SAMUEL WILLIAM (American physician, born 1894)

Becker nevus. Synonyms: *acquired nevus pigmentosus et pilosus, pigmented hairy epidermal nevus, unilateral melanosis and hypertrichosis.*

Acquired unilateral macular melanosis, appearing late in the first decade of life, followed by the growth of coarse, long, dark hair at puberty.

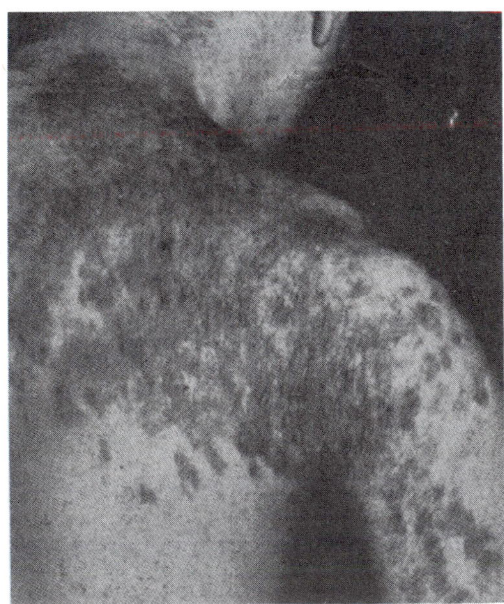

Becker nevus
Becker, S.W., *Arch. Derm. & Syph.*, 60:156, 1949, American Academy of Dermatology.

Becker, S. W. Concurrent melanosis and hypertrichosis in distribution of nevus unius lateris. *Arch. Derm., Chicago,* 1949, 60:155-60.

BECKWITH, JOHN BRUCE (American physician, born 1933)

Beckwith syndrome. See *Beckwith-Wiedemann syndrome.*

Beckwith-Wiedemann syndrome (BW, BWS). Synonyms: *Beckwith syndrome, Wiedemann syndrome, Wiedemann-Beckwith syndrome (WBS), Wiedemann-Beckwith-Combs syndrome, exophthalmos-macroglossia-gigantism (EMG) syndrome, familial macroglossia-omphalocele syndrome, macroglossia-omphalocele syndrome, macroglossia-omphalocele-visceromegaly syndrome.*

A congenital syndrome characterized by macroglossia, omphalocele or other umbilical abnormalities, cytomegaly of the fetal adrenal cortex, noncystic renal hyperplasia with medullary dysplasia, pancreatic hyperplasia, hypoglycemia, Leydig cell hyperplasia, and, often, increased birth weight. Hypoglycemia may be severe, but lasts only 1 to 4 months and responds to steroid therapy. Postnatally, somatic gigantism with increased bone age is seen. Some patients develop hemihypertrophy, and there appears to be an increased risk of adrenal carcinoma, Wilms' tumor, or other intra-abdominal neoplasms. Maxillary hypoplasia and relative mandibular prognathism are common. Asymmetric earlobes and pits, facial nevus flammeus, umbilical hernia, hepatomegaly, and intestinal malrotation are frequently associated. Mental retardation may occur. Most cases are sporadic, but autosomal recessive and dominant cases have been reported.

Beckwith, J. B. *Extreme cytomegaly of the adrenal fetal cortex. omphalocele, hyperplasia of kidneys and pancreas, and Leydig-cell hyperplasia: another syndrome?* Presented at Annual Meeting of Western Society for Pediatric Research, Los Angeles, Nov. 11, 1963. Wiedemann, H. R. Complexe malformatif familial avec hernie ombilicale et macroglossie; un "syndrome nouveau?" *J. Génét. Hum.*, 1964, 13:223-32. Combs, J. T., *et al.* A new syndrome of neonatal hypoglycemia. *N. Engl. J. M.*, 1966, 275:236-43.

Wiedemann-Beckwith syndrome (WBS). See *Beckwith-Wiedemann syndrome.*

Wiedemann-Beckwith-Combs syndrome. See *Beckwith-Wiedemann syndrome.*

BECLARD, PIERRE AUGUSTIN (French anatomist, 1785-1825)

Béclard hernia. Femoral hernia through the saphenous opening.

Béclard, P. A. *Éléments d'anatomie générale. Ou description de tous les gendres d'organes qui composent the corps humain.* Paris, Bechet, 1827.

BEDNAR, ALOIS (Physician in Vienna, 1816-1888)

Bednar aphthae. Symmetric excoriation of the hard palate over the pterygoid plates in infants, thought to be due to the pressure of the nipple against the palate during nursing, or sucking of the thumb and foreign objects.

Bednar, A. *Die Krankheiten der Neugeborenen und Säuglinge vom clinischen und pathologisch-anatomischen Standpunkt.* Wien. Gerold, 1850-1853.

Bednar-Parrot disease. See *Parrot syndrome (1).*

BEEMER, FRITS A. (Dutch physician)

Beemer syndrome. Synonyms: *Beemer type; short rib*

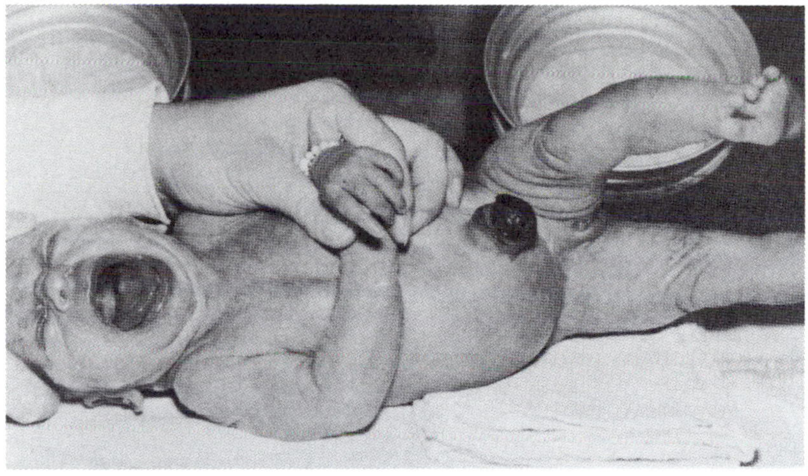

Beckwith-Wiedemann syndrome
Courtesy of J.B. Beckwith.

syndrome, Beemer type; short rib-polydactyly syndrome, Beemer type.

A congenital syndrome, transmitted as an autosomal recessive trait, characterized by hydrops, ascites, median cleft of the upper lip, narrow chest, protuberant abdomen, and short and bowed limbs. Additional defects include brachydactyly, malformed ears, omphalocele, and intestinal malrotation. The syndrome was originally reported in two unrelated infants who died shortly after birth.

Beemer, F. A., *et al.* A new short rib syndrome. Report of two cases. *Am. J. Med. Genet.*, 1983, 14:115-23.

Beemer type. See *Beemer syndrome.*

short rib syndrome, Beemer type. See *Beemer syndrome.*

beer-drinker syndrome. Synonym: *hypo-osmolality in beer drinkers.*

A disease of persons consuming large quantities of beer and little food, who, because of low osmolar production, cannot produce sufficiently dilute urine to excrete the high fluid intake. The symptoms include fatigue, dizziness, and weakness. The biochemical changes are hyponatremia and hypokalemia.

Hilden, T., & Svendsen, T. L. Electrolyte disturbances in beer drinkers. A specific "hypo-osmolality syndrome." *Lancet*, 1975, 2:245-6.

BEGBIE, JAMES (British physician, 1798-1869)

Begbie disease (1). See *Basedow disease.*

Begbie disease (2). See *Bergeron disease.*

BEGUEZ CESAR, ANTONIO (Cuban physician)

Béguez César-Steinbrinck-Chédiak-Higashi syndrome. See *Chédiak-Higashi syndrome.*

BEHÇET, HALUSHI (Turkish dermatologist, 1889-1948)

Adamantiades-Behçet syndrome. See *Behçet syndrome.*

Behçet aphthae. See *Behçet syndrome.*

Behçet disease (BD). See *Behçet syndrome.*

Behçet syndrome (BS). Synonyms: *Adamantiades syndrome, Adamantiades-Behçet syndrome, Behçet aphthae, Behçet disease (BD), Behçet triple symptom, Gilbert syndrome, Gilbert-Behçet syndrome, Halushi Behçet syndrome, Touraine syndrome, cutaneomucouveal syndrome, dermatostomato-ophthalmic syndrome, generalized aphthosis, genito-oral aphthosis with uveitis and hypopyon, hypopyon recidivans, iridocyclitis recidivans, iridocyclitis recidivans purulenta, iridocyclitis septica, iridocyclitis with hypopyon, iritis septica, oculobuccogenital syndrome.*

A disorder with onset between the ages of 10 and 45 years, which consists of relapsing ulcerations of the mucous membranes of the mouth and pharynx, ulceration of the genitalia, and uveitis with hypopyon. In the early stages, mild iritis is the only symptom, but thrombosis of the central retinal vein and thrombophlebitis of the dural sinus and thigh and calf veins are often associated. Oral lesions consist chiefly of aphthae of the lips, tongue, gingivae, buccal mucosa, or palate. Genital lesions are generally larger than those of the mouth and appear on the penis, scrotum, and vulva, sometimes leading to fenestration of the labia majora. The perineum may be involved. Skin lesions are varied and consist of pyoderma, pustules, impetigo folliculitis, furuncles, or simple ulcers. The blood picture shows moderate leukocytosis and increased sedimentation rate. The disorder is chronic and may become fatal when the nervous system is involved. Autoimmune etiology is suspected.

Behçet, H. Über rezidiverende Aphthöse durch ein Virus verursachte Geschwüre am Mund, am Auge und am den Genitalien. *Dermatol. Wschr.*, 1937, 105:1152-7. Adamantiades, B. Sur un cas d'iritis à hypopyon recidivant. *Ann. Ocul., Paris*, 1931, 168:271-8. Gilbert, W. Über eine chronische Verlaufsform der metastatischen Ophthalmie ("Ophthalmia lenta"). *Arch. Augenhk.*, 1925, 96:119-30. Touraine, A. L'aphthose. Donnes récentes et synthèse. *Presse Méd.*, 1955, 63:1493-5.

Behçet triple symptom. See *Behçet syndrome.*

Gilbert-Behçet syndrome. See *Behçet syndrome.*

Halushi Behçet syndrome. See *Behçet syndrome.*

BEHR, CARL (German ophthalmologist, born 1876)

Behr disease. See *Behr syndrome (1).*

Behr syndrome (1). Synonyms: *Behr disease, central tapetoretinal degeneration.*

Familial macular degeneration, occurring in adult and presenile forms, which is marked by central atrophic chorioretinitis with pigmentary degenerative changes and peripheral retinal lesions.

Behr, C. Die Heredodegeneration der Makula. *Klin. Mbl. Augenh.*, 1920, 65:465-505.

Behr syndrome (2). Synonyms: *infantile optic atrophy-ataxia syndrome, optic atrophy-ataxia syndrome.*

A hereditary familial syndrome of ocular and neurologic disorders, transmitted as an autosomal recessive trait, characterized by optic atrophy, nystagmus, scotoma, progressive temporal nerve atrophy, bilateral retrobulbar neuritis, ataxia, increased tendon reflexes, Babinski sign, incoordination, spastic gait, mental deficiency, bladder sphincter insufficiency, and muscle hypertonia. The syndrome begins in infancy and progresses slowly, eventually becoming static.

Behr, C. Die komplizierte, hereditär-familiäre Optikusatrophie des Kindesalters: Ein bisher nich beschriebener Symptomkomplex. *Klin. Mb. Augenheilk.*, 1909, 47:138-60.

BEIGEL, HERMANN (German physician, 1830-1879)

Beigel disease. Synonyms: *Chignon disease, Paxton disease, piedra, tinea nodosa, trichomycosis nodosa, trichomycosis nodularis.*

A fungal disease of the hair, with stony nodules along the shafts. *Piedraia hortai* causes white piedra; *Trichosporum beigelii* causes black piedra.

Beigel, H. Über Auftreibung und Bersten der Haare, eine eigentümliche Erkrankung des Haarschaftes. *S. B. Math. Naturwiss. Class.*, 1855, 17:612-7. Paxton, F. V. On a diseased condition of the hairs of the axilla, probably of a parasitic origin. *J. Cutan. Med., London*, 1869, 3:133-6.

BEIGHTON, PETER (Physician in South Africa)

Sallis-Beighton syndrome. See *digitotalar dysmorphism syndrome.*

BEK (BECK), E. V. (Russian physician)

Bek disease. See *Kashin-Bek disease.*

Kaschin-Beck disease. See *Kashin-Bek disease.*

Kashin-Bek disease. See *under Kashin.*

BEKHTEREV (BECHTEREW) VLADIMIR MIKHAILOVICH (Russian physician 1857-1927)

Bechterew nystagmus. Synonyms: *Bekhterev nystagmus, compensatory nystagmus.*

Nystagmus that develops after the destruction of the labyrinth. When one labyrinth is destroyed, nystagmus develops and gradually disappears. Then, when the other labyrinth is destroyed, compensatory nystagmus develops as though the first labyrinth were still intact.

Bechterew, W., von. Durchschneidung des Nervus acusticus. *Arch. Ges. Physiol.*, 1883, 30:312.

Bechterew syndrome. See *Bechterew-Strümpell-Marie syndrome.*

Bechterew-Strümpell-Marie syndrome. Synonyms: *Bechterew syndrome, Bekhterev syndrome, Marie disease, Marie-Strümpell disease, Pierre Marie disease, ankylosing polyarthritis, ankylosing spondylitis (AS), atrophic ligamentous spondylitis, atrophic spondylitis, bamboo spine, fibrosis ankylopoietica dorsi, infectious spondylitis, juvenile-adolescent spondylitis, ossifying ligamentous spondylitis, pelvospondylitis ossificans, poker back, rheumatismal ossifying pelvispondylitis, rheumatoid spondylitis, rhizomelic spondylosis, spondylitis adolescens, spondylitis ankyloarthrica, spondylitis atrophica ligamentosa, spondylitis deformans, spondylitis ossificans ligamentosa, syndesmitis ossificans.*

A progressive chronic disease characterized by arthritis of the posterior intervertebral, costovertebral, and sacroiliac joints; chronic proliferative changes in the joint capsules and intervertebral ligaments; and ossification of the intervertebral disks and the overlying intervertebral ligament. Early symptoms include insidious discomfort and morning stiffness that seem to improve with exercise, low back pain, and muscle spasms. They are followed by stiffening of the joints and ligaments, distortion of posture, decreased chest expansion with breathing difficulty, and, eventually, fusion of the spine and formation of bony bridges (syndesmophytes). Extraskeletal changes may include uveitis, chronic infiltrative and fibrotic pulmonary complications, aortic incompetence, cardiomegaly, amyloidosis, and mild anemia. Increased erythrocyte sedimentation rate, elevated immunoglobulin A levels, presence of immune complexes, and increased serum creatine kinase and alkaline phosphatase are the principal laboratory findings. Histopathological changes consist mainly of intimal cell hyperplasia and lymphocyte and plasma cell infiltrates, most findings being similar to those in rheumatoid arthritis. It was once believed that the disease affects mainly young males between the ages of 15 and 40 years; recent findings indicate about equal sex distribution. The disorder is transmitted as an autosomal dominant trait with reduced penetrance.

Bekhterev, V. M. Oderevenelost' pozvonochnika s iskrivleniem ego, kak osobaia form zabolevaniia. *Vrach, S. Petersburg*, 1892, 13:899-903. Strümpell, A. Bemerkung über die chronische ankylosirende Entzündung der Wirbelsäule und der Hüftgelenke. *Deut. Zschr. Nervenh.*, 1897, 11:338-42. Marie, P. Sur spondylose rhizomelique, *Rev. Méd., Paris*, 1898, 18:285-315.

Bekhterev nystagmus. See *Bechterew nystagmus.*

Bekhterev syndrome. See *Bechterew-Strümpell-Marie syndrome.*

BELL, J. A. (British physician)

Martin-Bell syndrome (MBS). See *chromosome X fragility.*

Martin-Bell-Renpenning syndrome. See *chromosome X fragility.*

BELL, JULIA (British scientist, born 1879)

Bell brachydactyly. Abnormal shortness of fingers and toes classified as Bell's brachydactyly A-1, A-2, A-3, B, C, D, and E. See under *brachydactyly.*

BELL, LUTHER VOSE (American physician, 1806-1862)

Bell delirium. See *Bell mania.*

Bell disease. See *Bell mania.*

Bell mania. Synonyms: *Bell delirium, Bell disease, Stauder syndrome, confusocatatonia, deadly catatonia, delirium aigu, exhaustion death, exhaustion syndrome, fatal catatonia, hypertoxic schizophrenia, lethal catatonia, mortal catatonia, pernicious catatonia.*

A syndrome of hyperactivity, delusions, hallucinations, and frequent episodes of fever followed in a few days to months by death. After a sudden onset, the patient becomes increasingly restless, wildly excited, and destructive. Some develop stupor, muscular rigidity, and severe exhaustion and dehydration leading to death. The condition was once classified with schizophrenia but most modern writers attribute it to an encephalopathy.

Bell, L. V. On a form of disease resembling some advanced stages of mania and fever, but so contradistinguished from any ordinarily observed or described combination of symptoms, as to render it probable that it may be an overlooked and hitherto unrecorded malady. *Am. J. Insanity,* 1849, 6:97-127. Stauder, K. H. Die todliche Katatonia. *Arch. Psychiat. Nervenkr.,* 1934, 102:614-34.

BELL, SIR CHARLES (British physician, 1774-1842)

Bell palsy (BP). Synonym: *refrigeration palsy.*

Peripheral, usually unilateral, idiopathic facial paralysis with a mild onset, characterized by pain and swelling behind the ears and pain and stiffness of the neck. Exacerbation of pain, excessive lacrimation, vertigo, fever, tinnitus, impaired hearing, distorted speech, and paralysis appear within a few hours. In severe cases, the affected side of the face becomes immobile, the labiofacial fold is erased, the mouth is drawn toward the unaffected side, the forehead cannot be wrinkled, the upper eyelid cannot be closed, whistling becomes impossible, and the sense of taste becomes distorted. Spontaneous recovery occurs in most cases within 2 weeks. Adults are most commonly affected, especially after an exposure to draft or cold, although cold in itself is not considered to be the etiologic factor. The *Mona Lisa syndrome* (q.v.) is considered to be related to Bell's palsy.

Bell, C. On the nerves; giving an account of some experiments on their structure and functions, which lead to a new arrangement of the system. *Philos. Tr. R. Soc. London,* 1821, 111:398-424.

BENCE JONES, HENRY (British physician, 1814-1875)

Bence Jones albuminuria. See *Bence Jones proteinuria.*

Bence Jones disease. See *Bence Jones proteinuria.*

Bence Jones proteinuria. Synonyms: *Bence Jones albuminuria, Bence Jones disease, Bradshaw albumosuria, light chain disease, myelopathic albumosuria.*

The presence of Bence Jones protein (a heat-sensitive abnormal protein, or paraprotein, formed by a single clone of plasma cells as the result of production of abnormally large numbers of light chains without the corresponding number of heavy chains) in the urine, usually but not exclusively observed in multiple myeloma. It is commonly associated with reduction of serum immunoglobulins, pulmonary infections, osteolytic lesions, fractures, and renal insufficiency due to intralobular deposits of light chain proteins, with consequent atrophy.

Bence Jones, H. On a new substance occurring in the urine of a patient with mollities ossium. *Philos. Tr. R. Soc. London,* 1848, 138:55-62. Bradshaw, T. R. The recognition of myelopathic albumose in the urine. *Brit. Med., J.,* 1906, 2:1442-5.

BENCZE, J. (Hungarian physician)

Bencze syndrome. Synonym: *hemifacial hyperplasia-strabismus syndrome.*

A congenital syndrome, transmitted as an autosomal dominant trait, characterized by hemifacial hyperplasia, esotropia, amblyopia, and submucous cleft palate.

Bencze, J., *et al.* Dominant inheritance of hemifacial hyperplasia associated with strabismus. *Oral Surg.,* 1973, 35:489-501.

BENEDIKT, MORITZ (Austrian physician, 1835-1920)

Benedikt syndrome. Synonyms: *tegmental mesencephalic paralysis, tegmental syndrome.*

A syndrome characterized by lesions of the inferior nucleus ruber with obstructive ipsilateral oculomotor paralysis; contralateral hyperkinesia, tremor of the upper extremities, and paralysis; and ipsilateral ataxia. The oculomotor paralysis involves associated movements of convergence, elevation, and depression of the eyes.

Benedikt, M. Tremblement avec paralysie croisée du moteur oculaire commun. *Bull. Méd., Paris,* 1889, 3:547-8.

Bengal splenomegaly. See *tropical splenomegaly syndrome.*

benign calcifying epithelioma. See *Malherbe epithelioma.*

benign chondroblastoma. See *Codman tumor.*

benign congenital hypotonia. See *Oppenheim disease, under Oppenheim, Hermann.*

benign cystic disease of the breast. See *Cheatle disease.*

benign cystic multiple adenoma. See *Brooke epithelioma.*

benign cystic multiple epithelioma. See *Brooke epithelioma.*

benign essential granulocytopenia. See *Vahlquist-Gasser syndrome.*

benign inguinal lymphogranulomatosis. See *Durand-Nicolas-Favre disease, under Durand, J.*

benign inoculation lymphoreticulosis. See *cat scratch disease.*

benign intracranial hypertension. See *pseudotumor cerebri syndrome.*

benign juvenile malanoma. See *Spitz nevus.*

benign lymphadenosis. See *Bäfverstedt syndrome.*

benign lymphoepithelial lesion of the parotid gland. See *Godwin tumor.*

benign mesenchymal melanoma. See *Jadassohn-Tièche nevus, under Jadassohn, Josef.*

benign mucosal pemphigoid. See *Lortat-Jacob disease.*

benign paroxysmal ocular hypertension. See *Posner-Schlossman syndrome.*

benign paroxysmal peritonitis. See *Reimann periodic disease.*

benign paroxysmal vertigo (BPV, BVP) syndrome. A syndrome of unknown etiology, occurring mainly in young children, characterized by attacks of vertigo, which last from a few minutes to a couple of days. The attacks occur while the patients may be in any position (erect, recumbent, or sitting); the affected child clutches on objects or holds to a another person, being unable to move or change position without assistance. Associated symmptoms may include pallor, sweating, vomiting, and nystagmus.

Basser, L. S. Benign paroxysmal vertigo in children. *Brain,* 1964, 87:141.

benign pemphigoid. See *Brunsting disease.*

benign polycythemia. See *Gaisböck disease.*

benign recurrent aseptic meningitis. See *Mollaret meningitis.*

benign recurrent cholestasis. See *Summerskill-Walshe syndrome.*

benign recurrent endothelial-leukocytic meningitis. See *Mollaret meningitis.*

benign recurrent intrahepatic cholestasis. See *Summerskill-Walshe syndrome.*

benign recurrent vertigo syndrome. See *Ménière syndrome.*

benign reticulosis. See *cat scratch disease.*

benign symmetrical lipomatosis. See *Madelung syndrome, and see Touraine-Renault syndrome, under Touraine, A.*

benign unconjugated hyperbilirubinemia. See *Gilbert syndrome, under Gilbert, Nicolas Augustin.*

BENJAMIN, E. (German physician)

Benjamin anemia. See *Benjamin syndrome.*

Benjamin syndrome. Synonym: *Benjamin anemia.*

A combination of hypochromic anemia, hypoplastic bone deformities, growth and mental retardation, dental caries, proportionately small extremities, megalocephaly, and, less frequently, heart murmur, epicanthus, external ear deformities, genital infantilism, and splenic tumors.

Benjamin, E. Über eine selbständige Form der Anämie im frühen Kindesalter. *Verh. Deut. Ges. Kinderh.*, 1911, p. 119-24.

BENNET

Bennet syndrome. A combination of erythroblastic anemia, osteoporosis, and steatorrhea in children, reportedly described by Bennet.

BENNETT, EDWARD HALLARAN (Irish physician, 1837-1907)

Bennett fracture. Synonyms: *Bennett fracture-luxation, boxer's fracture, stave of the thumb.*

A longitudinal fracture of the first metacarpal bone running into the carpometacarpal joint and complicated by subluxation.

*Bennett, E. H. Fractures of the metacarpal bones of the thumb. *Dublin, J. M. Sc.*, 1882, 73:72.

Bennett fracture-luxation. See *Bennett fracture.*

BENNETT, JOHN HUGHES (British physician, 1812-1875)

Bennett disease. Synonym: *leukemia.*

A malignant, frequently fatal disease of the blood-forming organs, characterized by proliferation of immature leukocytes and their infiltration in the bone marrow, lymph nodes, liver, spleen, and other tissues. The etiology is unknown but chronic exposure to radiations and to some drugs and chemicals and infection with certain viruses are known to have leukemogenic effects. Chromosomal defects found consistently in leukemic patients suggest a possible genetic factor. Leukemia is classified clinically on the basis of (1) duration and character of the disease-acute or chronic; (2) the type of cell involved-myeloid (myelogenous), lymphoid (lymphogenous), or monocytic; (3) increase or nonincrease in the number of abnormal cells in the blood-leukemic or aleukemic (subleukemic). See also *Jaksch syndrome (pseudoleukemia infantum)*, and see *myelodysplastic syndrome..*

*Bennett, J. H. Case of hypertrophy of the spleen and liver, in which death took place from suppuration of the blood. *Edinburgh M. Sc. J.*, 1845, 64:413-23.

BENSAUDE, RAOUL (French physician)

Launois-Bensaude syndrome. See *Madelung syndrome.*

Madelung-Launois-Bensaude syndrome. See *Madelung syndrome.*

BENSIMON, JOSEPH R. (Canadian physician)

Robinson-Miller-Bensimon syndrome. See *Robinson syndrome, under Robinson, Geoffrey C.*

BENSON, ALFRED HUGH (Irish ophthalmologist, 1852-1912)

Benson disease. Synonyms: *asteroid bodies of the vitreous, asteroid hyalitis, snowball opacities of the vitreous.*

The presence in an otherwise normal vitreous of small, solid, and stellate, spherical, or disk-shaped bodies arranged without any apparent order. They are creamy, flat-white, or shiny when viewed with the ophthalmoscope, but sparkle brightly under the slit-lamp.

Benson, A. H. A case of "monocular asteroid hyalitis." *Tr. Ophth. Soc. U. K.*, 1894, 14:101-4.

BERANT, N.

Berant syndrome. See *under Berant, W.*

BERANT, W.

Berant syndrome. A syndrome of craniosynostosis and radioulnar synostosis transmitted as an autosomal dominant trait.

Berant, W., & Berant, N. Radioulnar synostosis and craniosynostosis syndromes. *Birth Defects*, 1973, 11(2):137-89.

BERARDINELLI, WALDEMAR (Argentine physician, 1903-1956)

Berardinelli syndrome. See *Berardinelli-Seip syndrome.*

Berardinelli-Seip syndrome. Synonyms: *Berardinelli syndrome, Berardinelli-Seip-Lawrence syndrome, Lawrence syndrome, Seip syndrome, congenital lipodystrophy, generalized lipodystrophy, lipoatrophic diabetes.*

The concurrence of generalized loss of body fat, insulin-resistant diabetes mellitus, and hepatomegaly. The syndrome occurs in acquired and congenital forms, the inherited form being transmitted as an autosomal recessive trait. A loss of subcutaneous fat causes muscles to appear enlarged and the veins to stand out. Female patients usually develop a male body build. Associated disorders include accelerated growth and maturation, enlarged hands and feet, enlarged phallus or clitoris, coarse pigmented skin, acanthosis nigricans, hirsutism with curly hair, excess fat and glycogen in the liver, liver cirrhosis, hyperlipidemia, cardiomegaly, corneal opacity, and hyperproteinemia. Mental retardation and renal complications may occur.

Berardinelli, W. An undiagnosed endocrinometabolic syndrome: Report of 2 cases. *J. Clin. Endocr. Metab.*, 1954, 14:193-204. Seip, M., & Trygstad, O. Generalized lipodystrophy. *Arch. Dis. Child.*, 1963, 38:447-53. Lawrence, R. D. Lipodystrophy and hepatomegaly with diabetes, lipaemia, and other metabolic disturbances. A case throwing new light on the action of insulin. *Lancet*, 1946, 1:724-31; 773-5.

Berardinelli-Seip-Lawrence syndrome. See *Berardinelli-Seip syndrome.*

BERCONSKY, I. (Argentine physician)

Cossio-Berconsky syndrome. See *Cossio syndrome.*

BERDON, WALTER E. (American physician)

Berdon syndrome. See *megacystis-microcolon-intestinal hypoperistalsis syndrome.*

BERENBERG, WILLIAM (American physician, born 1915)

Neuhauser-Berenberg syndrome. See *under Neuhauser.*

bergamot dermatitis. See *Freund dermatitis, under Freund, Emanuel.*

BERGEMEISTER

Bergemeister papilla. A congenital abnormality of the vitreous manifested as a preretinal or papillary veil produced by an occluded persistent hyaloid artery surrounded by glial tissue.

Hogan, M. J., & Zimmermann, L. E. *Ophthalmic pathology. An atlas and textbook.* 2nd ed. Philadelphia, Saunders, 1962, p. 641.

Bergen syndrome. Synonyms: *facies leprosa, nasal leprosy.*

Bergen syndrome I (facies leprosa, nasal leprosy) is a type of leprosy which is characterized by atrophy of the anterior nasal spine; atrophy and recession of the maxillary alveolar process, which is confined to the incisor region and begins centrally at the prosthion, resulting in lossening and/or loss of corresponding teeth; and endonasal inflammatory changes. **Bergen syndrome II** is characterized by changes in the superior maxillary process associated with loosening and/or loss of the frontal incisors. The disease was discovered in the city of Bergen in Norway, hence its name.

Möller-Christensen, V. Changes in the anterior nasal spine and the alveolar process of the maxillae in leprosy. A clinical examination. *Internat. J. Leprosy,* 1974, 42:431-5.

BERGER, J. (French physician)

Berger nephropathy. See *Berger syndrome.*

Berger syndrome. Synonyms: *Berger nephropathy, Berger-Hinglais syndrome, IgA disease, IgA nephropathy, IgG-IgA nephritis, immunoglobulin A nephropathy, mesangial IgA/IgG nephropathy.*

A renal syndrome characterized by glomerulonephritis associated with hematuria, mesangial IgA deposits, and a variety of glomerular lesions. Male children and young adults are most frequently affected. Hematuria and a viral upper respiratory tract infection, the earliest symptoms, are followed by flu-like symptoms, gastrointestinal problems, or other prodromal disorders. Associated complaints include mild fever, malaise, muscle pain, dysuria, and loin pain. Acute nephritic syndrome, edema, and hypertension occur in some instances. Renal failure usually takes place within 6 months and many patients face death unless they are placed on renal dialysis. Immune deposits in the mesangium of the glomeruli consist mainly of IgA and less frequently IgG and C3. The syndrome is now regarded as a form of the Henoch-Schönlein syndrome.

Berger, J., & Hinglais, N. Les dépôts intercapillaires d'IgA-IgG. *J. Nephrol., Paris,* 1968, 74:694-5.

Berger-Hinglais syndrome. See *Berger syndrome.*

BERGER, OSKAR (German physician, 1845-1908)

Berger paresthesia. Paresthesia of the lower extremities accompanied by weakness but without any objective symptoms.

Berger, Über eine eigenthümliche Form von Paraesthesie. *Bresl. Arztl. Zachr.,* 1879, 1:60-1.

BERGERON, ETIENNE JULES (French physician, 1817-1900)

Bergeron chorea. See *Bergeron disease.*

Bergeron disease. Synonyms: *Begbie disease, Bergeron chorea, Dubini disease, Dubini syndrome, Guertin syndrome, chorea electrica, electric chorea, electrolepsy, hysterical chorea.*

A disease of childhood characterized by violent rhythmic spasms, but with a short and benign course, suspected of being of hysterical etiology. The disease was named by Berland in honor of his professor, Étienne Jules Bergeron. This disorder has clinical characteristics similar to those in Henoch's chorea.

*Berland, R. *Treatment par le tartre stibié d'une forme de chorée dite électrique.* Poitiers, 1880. *Begbie, J. Remarks on rheumatism and chorea; their relation and treatment. *Month. J. Med. Sc.* 1847, 7:740-54. Guertin, A. *D'une névrose convulsive et rythmique déjà nommée for de chorée dite électrique.* Paris, 1881. *Dubini, A. Primi cenni sulla elettrica. *Ann. Univ. Med., Milano,* 1846, 117:5-50.

BERGH, A. A. HIJAMS, VAN DEN (Dutch physician, 1861-1943)

van den Bergh disease. See *Stokvis-Talma syndrome.*

BERGMANN, GUSTAV, VON (German physician, 1878-1955)

Bergmann syndrome. Synonyms: *von Bergmann syndrome, epiphrenal syndrome, gastrocardial symptom complex, hiatus hernia syndrome.*

A congenital or acquired condition in which part of the stomach protrudes above the diaphragm. Pressure exerted on the thoracic organs produces dysphagia, tachycardia, hiccups with a feeling of discomfort, and pain in the cardiac region simulating angina pectoris or cardiospasm. See also *Roemheld syndrome.*

Bergmann, G., von. Das "epiphrenale Syndrom," seine Beziehungen zur Angina pectoris und zum Kardiospasmus. *Deut. Med. Wschr.,* 1932, 58:605-9.

von Bergmann syndrome. See *Bergmann syndrome.*

BERGSTRAND, HILDING (Swedish physician, born 1886)

Bergstrand disease. Synonym: *osteoid osteoma.*

A well-defined benign tumor, usually found in the shafts of the long bones, appearing as a small, grayish red nodule composed of vascularized fibrous tissue and osteoid or calcified, poorly developed bone spicules. Male adolescents and young adults are most commonly affected.

Bergstrand, H. Über eine eigenartige, wohrscheinlich bisher nicht beschriebene osteoblastische Krankheit in den longen Knochen der Hand und des Fusses. *Acta. Radiol., Stockholm,* 1930, 11:596-613.

BERGSTROM, LAVONNE (American physician)

Rosenberg-Bergstrom syndrome. See *under Rosenberg, Alan L.*

Stewart-Bergstrom syndrome. See *under Stewart, Janet M.*

BERK, M. E. (South African physician)

Berk-Tabatznik syndrome. A syndrome of congenital cervical kyphosis, due to multiple hemivertebrae, associated with short distal phalanges, optic atrophy with nystagmus, small optic disks, tilting of the atlas, conical odontoid process, and other vertebral abnormalities. In the original report, the patient was the only affected member of her family.

Berk, M. E., & Tabatznik, B. Cervical kyphosis from posterior hemivertebrae with brachyphalangy and congenital optic atrophy. *J. Bone Joint Surg.,* 1961, 43B:77-86.

BERLIN, CHAIM (Israeli physician)

Berlin syndrome. A familial multiple abnormality syndrome characterized by short stature bordering on dwarfism; slender build; hyperflexibility of the fingers; sparse eyebrows; saddle nose; small moustache; thick lips with telangiectases; epicanthal folds; pale, dry, thin, pliable skin; generalized mottled dyschromia consisting of various degrees of hyper- and hypopigmentation; anetopoikiloderma-like lesions; atrophic scars caused by pyoderma; hyperkeratosis palmaris et plantaris with hyperhidrosis; hypofunction of the sebaceous glands; dark, dry, and abundant hair with a tendency to premature graying; delayed dentition; hypodontia; genital infantilism, hypospadias, and testicular atrophy in males, but normal sexual development in females; and mental retardation. The syndrome is transmitted as an autosomal recessive trait.

Berlin, C. Congenital generalized melanoleucoderma associated with hypodontia, hypotrichosis, stunted growth and mental retardation occurring in two brothers and two sisters. *Dermolologica, Basel,* 1961, 123:227-43.

BERLIN, RUDOLF (German ophthalmologist, 1833-1897)

Berlin disease (1). Synonyms: *Berlin edema, commotio retinae, traumatic edema of the retina.*

Perimacular edema of the retina caused by a blunt trauma of the eye, frequently followed by retinal detachment.

Berlin, R. Zur sogenennten Commotio retinae. *Klin. Mbl. Augenh.,* 1873, 11:43-78.

Berlin disease (2). Synonyms: *canalis opticus syndrome, optic canal syndrome.*

Posttraumatic blindness in which optic nerve lesions are caused by extra-ocular injuries.

*Berlin, R. Über Sehstörungen nach Verletzung durch stumpfe Gewalt. *Klin. Mbl. Augenheilk.,* 1978, vol. 17.

Berlin edema. See *Berlin disease (1).*

berloque dermatitis. See *Freund dermatitis, under Freund, Emanuel.*

BERNARD, CLAUDE (French physiologist, 1813-1878)

Bernard syndrome. See *Horner syndrome.*

Bernard-Horner syndrome. See *Horner syndrome.*

Claude Bernard syndrome. See *Horner syndrome.*

Claude Bernard-Horner syndrome. See *Horner syndrome.*

BERNARD, JEAN (French physician, born 1907)

Bernard syndrome. Synonym: *acute familial hemolysis.*

A familial syndrome characterized by a sudden attack of acute anemia, jaundice, hemoglobinuria, and severe hemolysis. Generalized malaise, fever, abdominal pain, vomiting, and arthralgia may precede the onset of acute symptoms.

Bernard, J. L'hémolyse aiguë familiale. *Sang,* 1950, 21:206-90.

Bernard-Soulier syndrome (BSS). Synonyms: *congenital thrombocytic dystrophy, giant platelet syndrome, hereditary giant platelet syndrome (HGPS), Montreal platelet syndrome (MPS), platelet glycoprotein Ib deficiency.*

A familial bleeding disorder, transmitted as an autosomal recessive trait, characterized by unusually large platelets with dense condensation of granules and associated with prolonged bleeding time and abnormal prothrombin consumption. A defect in the platelet membrane, due to decreased levels of glycoprotein I (GP Ib and GP Ig), is believed to the cause of this condition. Potentially fatal hemorrhage (bleeding from the skin, muscles and visceral organs, epistaxis, and menorrhagia) is the principal clinical characteristic of this disorder.

Bernard, J., & Soulier, J. P. Sur une nouvelle variété de dystrophie thrombocytaire hémorragipare congénitale. *Sem. Hôp. Paris,* 1948, 24:3217-23.

BERNDORFER, ALFRED (Hungarian physician)

Berndorfer syndrome. A syndrome of facial and limb abnormalities consisting of cleft palate and harelip associated with cleft hand and feet. The etiology is unknown.

Berndorfer, A. Gesichtsspalten gemeinsam mit Hand- und Fusssspalten. *Zschr. Orthop.,* 1970, 107:344-54.

BERNHARDT, MARTIN (German neurologist, 1844-1915)

Bernhardt disease. See *Rot-Bernhardt syndrome, under Rot, Vladimir Karlovich.*

Bernhardt paralysis. See *Rot-Bernhardt syndrome, under Rot, Vladimir Karlovich.*

Rot-Bernhardt syndrome. See *under Rot, Vladimir Karlovich.*

Roth-Bernhardt syndrome. See *Rot-Bernhardt syndrome, under Rot, Vladimir Karlovich.*

Vulpian-Bernhardt syndrome. See *under Vulpian.*

BERNHEIM

Bernheim syndrome. Synonym: *right ventricle obstruction-failure syndrome.*

Hypertrophy of the left ventricle with bulging of the interventricular septum into the right ventricle resulting in stenosis or obstruction of the blood flow and right heart failure.

Bernheim. De l'asystolie veineuse dans l'hypertrophie du coeur gauche par sténose concomitante du ventricule droit. *Rev. Méd., Paris,* 1910, 30:785-90.

BERNHEIMER (Austrian physician)

Bernheimer-Seitelberger syndrome. See *gangliosidosis G_{M2} type III.*

BERNUTH, FRITZ, VON (German physician)

Bernuth syndrome. Synonym: *sporadic hemophilia.*

A sporadic form of hemophilia.

Bernuth, F., von. Über Kapillarbeobachtungen bei Hämophilie und anderen hämorrhagischen Diathesen. *Deut. Arch. Klin. Med.,* 1926, 152:321-30.

BERRY, GEORGE ANDREAS (British physician, 1853-1929)

Berry syndrome. See *mandibulofacial dysostosis.*

Berry-Treacher Collins syndrome. See *mandibulofacial dysostosis.*

berserker-blind rage syndrome. A dissociative disorder characterized by violent overreaction to physical, verbal, or visual stimuli; amnesia during the actual period of violence; abnormally great strength; and specifically target-oriented violence.

Simón, A. The berserker/blind rage syndrome as a potentially new diagnostic category for the DSM-III. *Psychol. Rep.,* 1987, 60:131-5.

BERTOLOTTI, MARIO (Italian physician, born 1876)

Bertolotti-Garcin syndrome. See *Garcin syndrome.*

BERTRAND, IVAN GEORGES (French neurologist)

Canavan-van Bogaert-Bertrand syndrome. See *Canavan syndrome.*

van Bogaert-Bertrand syndrome. See *Canavan syndrome.*

BESNIER, ERNEST (French dermatologist, 1831-1909)

Besnier disease. See *Besnier prurigo.*

Besnier prurigo. Synonyms: *Besnier disease, allergic eczema, asthma eczema, atopic dermatitis, atopic dermatosis, atopic eczema, eczema pruriginosum allergicum, exudative and diathetic eczema, exudative eczematoid, generalized neurodermatitis, infantile eczema, neurodermatitis disseminata, prurigo-asthma syndrome, prurigo eczematodes allergicum.*

A skin disease which usually begins in infancy as lichenification of the face, scalp, and cubital and popliteal areas, followed by severe pruritus, eczema, erythema, exudations, excoriation, and crusting, frequently in association with eosinophilia, asthma, and hay fever. The course may be marked by a quiescent period with the subsequent appearance of atopic dermatitis. In some instances the eczema appears to be a manifestation of food allergy. Infants from families with a history of allergic disorders seem to be most susceptible, and genetic transmission is suspected.

Besnier, E. Première note et observations préliminaires pour sevir d'introduction à l'étude des prurigos diathésiques (dermatites multiformes prurigineuses chroniques exacerbantes et paroxystiques du type du prurigo de Hebra). *Ann. Derm. Syph., Paris,* 1892, 3:634-48.

Besnier-Boeck sarcoid. See *Besnier-Boeck-Schaumann syndrome.*

Besnier-Boeck-Schaumann syndrome. Synonyms: *Besnier-Boeck sarcoid, Besnier-Tennesson syndrome, Boeck disease, Boeck lupoid, Boeck miliary lupoid, Boeck sarcoid, Hutchinson-Boeck disease, Hutchinson-Boeck granulomatosis, Jüngling disease, Moeller-Boeck syndrome, Schaumann disease, granulomatosis benigna, lymphogranulomatosis benigna.*

A benign systemic granulomatous disease of young adults that usually involves the liver, spleen, lymph nodes, skin, and lungs. Typically, the lesion is a tubercle with little or no necrosis. Systemic lesions usually include paratracheal and hilar adenopathy, intrapulmonary adenopathy, parenchymatous lung lesions, pulmonary fibrosis, pneumothorax, mycetoma, cor pulmonale, compression of the esophagus by the lymph nodes, lytic lesions of the phalanges and long bones, subperiosteal new bone formation of the long bones, arthritis, kidney enlargement due to sarcoid granulomas, nodular lymphoid hyperplasia of the small intestine, antral and pyloric stiffening and constriction, peptic ulcer, mucosal abnormality of the gastrointestsinal system, and ectasia with progressive destruction of the salivary ducts. Ocular complications usually include orbital granulomas, lacrimal gland adenopathy, glaucoma, uveitis, iris nodules, keratitis, cataract, and optic nerve atrophy. Fever, weight loss, dyspnea, cough, low-grade anemia, elevated serum globulins hypercalcemia, and hypercalciuria are the common symptoms.

Besnier, E. Lupus pernio de la face: Synovite fongeuses (scrofulotuberculeuses). *Ann. Derm. Syph., Paris,* 1889, 10:333-6. Boeck, C. P. Multipelt benignt hud-sarcoid. *Norsk. Mag. Laegevid.,* 1889, 60:1321-34. Schaumann, J. Étude sur le lupus pernio et ses rapports avec les sarcoides et la tuberculose. *Ann. Derm. Syph., Paris,* 1916-17, 6:357-73. Hutchinson, J. *Illustrations of chronical surgery.* London, 1877. ec. 42.

Besnier-Tennesson syndrome. See *Besnier-Boeck-Schaumann syndrome.*

Kaposi-Besnier-Libman-Sacks syndrome. See *Libman-Sacks syndrome.*

Tarral-Besnier disease. See *Kaposi disease (2).*

BESSMAN, SAMUEL PAUL (American physician, born 1921)

Bessman-Baldwin syndrome. Synonyms: *imidazole syndrome, late cerebromacular degeneration.*

Excretion of large amounts of carnosine, anserine, histidine, and 1-methyl-histidine in persons with cerebromacular degeneration and blindness. The syndrome is transmitted as an autosomal recessive trait. In the original report, neurological disorders (including convulsions and mental deterioration) and retinitis pigmentosa with considerable loss of vision were observed in five patients in three families.

Bessman, S. P., & Baldwin, R. Imidazole aminoaciduria in cerebromacular degeneration. *Science,* 1962, 135:789-91.

BEST, FRANZ (German ophthalmologist, 1878-1920)

Best disease. See *Best macular degeneration.*

Best macular degeneration. Synonyms: *Best disease, Best syndrome, hereditary vitelliform macular degeneration, hereditary vitelliruptive macular degeneration, polymorphic macular degeneration of Braley, polymorphic vitelline macular degeneration, vitelliruptive macular dystrophy, vitelliform macular dystrophy.*

A yellow, orange, or pink lesion of the macula lutea, resembling the yolk of a poached egg, which is later absorbed, leaving atrophic scars. Complications include hemorrhage, serous exudates, hyperopia, esotropia, strabismus, and amblyopia. The disorder is transmitted as an autosomal dominant trait with variable expressivity.

Best F. Über eine hereditäre Makulaaffektion: Beitrage zur Veterbungslehre. *Zschr. Augenheilk.,* 1905, 13:199-212. Braley, A. E., Spivey, B. E. Hereditary vitelline macular degeneration, A Clinical and functional evaluation of a new pedigree with variable expressivity and dominant inheritance. *Arch. Ophth.,* 1964, 72:743-52.

Best syndrome. See *Best macular degeneration.*

beta-lipoprotein deficiency. See *Bassen-Kornzweig syndrome.*

BEUERMANN, CHARLES LUCIEN, DE (French physician, 1851-1923)

Beuermann disease. See *Schenck disease.*

Beuermann-Gougerot disease. See *Schenck disease.*

BEUREN, ALOIS J.

Beuren syndrome. See *Williams syndrome, under Williams, J. C. P.*

Williams-Beuren syndrome. See *Williams syndrome, under Williams, J. C. P.*

BEZOLD, FRIEDRICH (German physician, 1842-1908)

Bezold abscess. See *Bezold disease.*

Bezold disease. Synonym: *Bezold abscess.*

Otitis media complicated by rupture of the tympanic membrane and escape of pus into (1) the adjacent area, particularly the digastric groove of the sternomastoid muscle, resulting in mastoiditis (known as **Bezold mastoiditis**); (2) the back of the neck, occasionally involving the vertebrae; and, less frequently, (3) the thoracic cavity, leading to death. The symptoms include severe pain in the affected areas, otorrhea, and edema of the glottis.

Bezold, F. Ein neuer Weg für Ausbreitung eitriger Entzündung aus den Räumen des Mittelohrs aus die Nachbarschaft und die in diesem Falle eizuschlagende Therapie. *Deut. Med. Wschr.,* 1881, 7:381-5.

Bezold mastoiditis. See *under Bezold disease.*

BF. See *brain fag syndrome.*

BFL (Börjeson-Forssman-Lehman) syndrome. See *Börjeson syndrome.*

BFLS (Börjeson-Forssman-Lehmann **syndrome**). See *Börjeson syndrome.*

BIANCHI, LEONARDO (Italian psychiatrist, 1848-1927)

Bianchi syndrome. Synonyms: *alexia-aphasia-apraxia syndrome, aphasic sensory syndrome, parietal syndrome.*

A combination of alexia, aphasia, apraxia, and right hand and foot hemianesthesia in lesions of the right parietal lobe.

Bianchi, L. La sindrome parietale, *Med. Ital.*, 1911, 9:187; 243; 333.

BIANCO, I. (Italian physician)

Silvestroni-Bianco syndrome. See *under Silvestroni.*

BIASOTTI, ALFREDO (Argentine physiologist, born 1903)

Houssay-Biasotti syndrome. See *Houssay syndrome.*

BIBER, HUGO (Swiss ophthalmologist, 1864-1918)

Biber-Haab-Dimmer syndrome. Synonyms: *Haab-Dimmer syndrome, dystrophia corneae reticulata, lattice corneal dystrophy.*

A localized form of amyloidosis manifested by progressive corneal opacity with distinct borders and a network of lattice-like branching filaments. Round spots may be scattered throughout the cornea, but the intervening spaces are clear, and there may be extracellular deposits of amyloid material. The disorder is transmitted as an autosomal dominant trait.

*Biber, H. *Über einige seltenere Hornhauterkrankungen.* Zurich, 1890. *Haab, O. Die gittrige Keratitis. *Zschr. Augenh.*, 1899, 2:235-46. *Dimmer, F. Über oberflächliche gittrige Hornhauttrübung. *Zschr. Augenh.*, 1899, 2:354.

BICKEL

Bickel-Bing-Harboe syndrome. See *Bing-Neel syndrome, under Bing, Jens.*

BICKERS, D. S. (American physician)

Bickers-Adams syndrome. Synonym: *X-linked hydrocephalus.*

A hereditary syndrome characterized by stenosis of the aqueduct of Sylvius with hydrocephalus, mental retardation, flexion of the thumb over the palm and spasticity, affecting chiefly the lower extremities. Associated disorders may include asymmetric coarse facies, fusion of the thalamus, small pons, absence of the septum pellucidum, hypoplasia of the corticospinal tracts, and porencephalic cysts. The syndrome is transmitted as a X-linked recessive trait.

Bickers, D. S., & Adams, R. D. Hereditary stenosis of the aqueduct of Sylvius as a cause of congenital hydrocephalus. *Brain*, 1949, 72:246-62.

BICKERSTAFF, E. R. (British physician)

Bickerstaff encephalitis. Synonym: *brain stem encephalitis.*

A syndrome consisting of prodromal malaise followed by a downward progression of midbrain disturbances with almost complete supression of all functions related to brain stem innervation, but without cardiac or respiratory disorders. Clinically, the syndrome is manifested by drowsiness, headache, defective conjugate movements, diplopia, and nystagmus. Most cases are associated with ophthalmoplegia, deafness, and palsy of the fifth cranial nerve. Palsy of the seventh cranial nerve is almost always present. Herpes simplex virus is suspected as a pathogenic agent.

Bickerstaff, E. R., & Cloake, R. C. P. Mesencephalitis and rhombencephalitis. *Brit. Med. J.*, 1951, 2:77-81.

BIDS (**b**rittle hair, **i**ntellectual impairment, **d**ecreased fertility, **s**hort stature) **syndrome.** See *hair-brain syndrome.*

BIEDL, ARTHUR (Prague endocrinologist, 1869-1933)

Bardet-Biedl syndrome. See *Laurence-Moon-Biedl syndrome.*

Laurence-Biedl syndrome. See *Laurence-Moon-Biedl syndrome.*

Laurence-Moon-Biedl syndrome. See *under Laurence.*

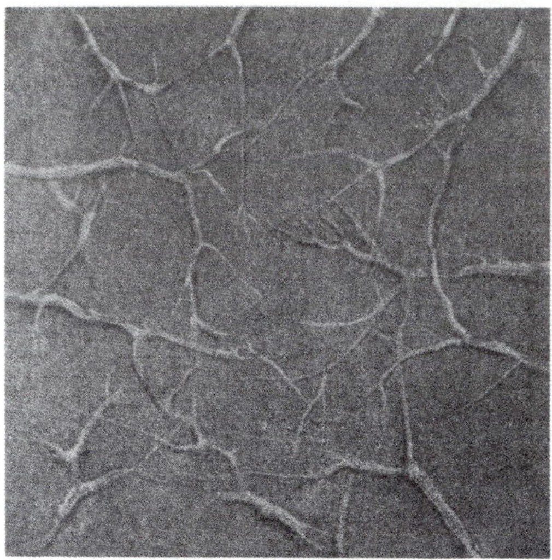

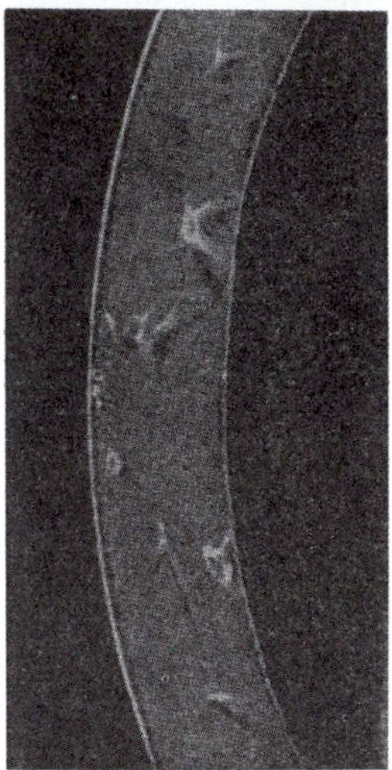

Biber-Haab-Dimmer syndrome
Francois, Jules, *Heredity in Ophthalmology*, St. Louis: C.V. Mosby Co., 1961.

Laurence-Moon-Biedl-Bardet syndrome (LMBB, LMBBS). See *Laurence-Moon-Biedl syndrome.*

BIELSCHOWSKY, ALFRED (German ophthalmologist, 1871-1040)

Bielschowsky disease. Synonym: *dissociated vertical divergence.*

A temporary loss of vertical comitancy of the eyes, as the elevating centers of the eyes are unable to work harmoniously.

Bedrassian, E. H. *The eye. A clinical and basic science book.* Springfield, Illinois, Thomas, 1958, p. 290.

Bielschowsky-Lutz-Cogan syndrome. Synonym: *internuclear ophthalmoplegia.*

Unilateral or bilateral paralysis of the internal rectus muscle during conjugate movement of the eye, associated with contralateral nystagmus in the maximally abducted eye. It is secondary to interruption of the medial longitudinal fasciculus connecting the nuclei of third, fourth, and sixth cranial nerves, especially those fibers which connect the abducens nucleus with

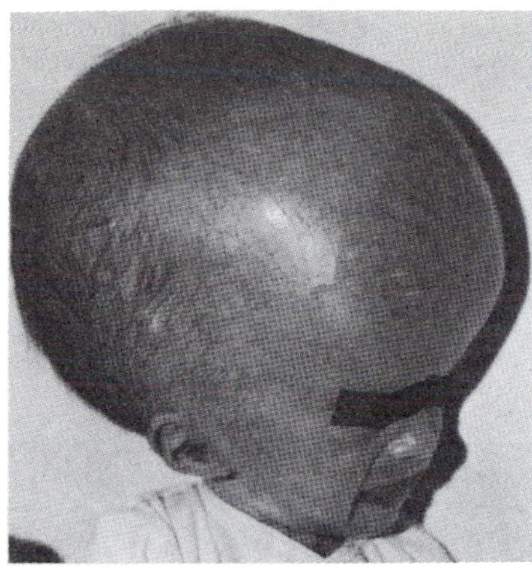

Bickers-Adams syndrome
Courtesy of Dr. John M. Opitz, Helena, Montana.

the subnucleus of the internal rectus muscle and coordinate their activity during conjugate lateral movement.

Bielschowsky, A. Die Innervation der Musculi recti interni als Seitenwender. *Berl. Deut. Ophth. Ges.*, 1902, 30:164-71. Lutz, A. Über einseitige Ophthalmoplegia internuclearis anterior. (Beschreibung eines neuen Falls in Verbindung mit heterolateraler Herabsetzung des automatischen Blinzelreflexes und Verlust der Reaktionsfähigkeit der homolateralen vertikelen Bogengäng). *Graefes Arch. Ophth.*, 1924-25, 115:695-717. *Cogan, D. G., *et al.* Unilateral internuclear ophthalmoplegia: Report of eight clinical cases with one postmortem study. *Arch. Ophth., Chicago,* 1950, 44:783-96.

Rot-Bielschowsky syndrome. See *under Rot, Vladimir Karlovich.*

Roth-Bielschowsky syndrome. See *Rot-Bielschowsky syndrome, under Rot, Vladimir Karlovich.*

BIELSCHOWSKY, MAX (German neurologist, 1869-1940)

Bielschowsky amaurotic idiocy. See *gangliosidosis G_{M2} type III.*

Bielschowsky syndrome. See *gangliosidosis G_{M2} type III.*

Dollinger-Bielschowsky syndrome. See *gangliosidosis G_{M2} type III.*

Jansky-Bielschowsky syndrome. See *gangliosidosis G_{M2} type III.*

Scholz-Bielschowsky-Henneberg syndrome. See *metachromatic leukodystrophy.*

BIEMOND, A. (Dutch physician)

Biemond syndrome (1). Synonym: *brachydactyly-nystagmus-cerbellar ataxia syndrome.*

A syndrome of nystagmus, cerebellar ataxia, and shortening of the fourth metacarpal bone, associated with mental deficiency and strabismus. The syndrome is believed to be transmitted as an autosomal dominant trait.

Biemond, A. Brachydactylie, nystagmus en cerebellaire ataxie als familiar syndrome. *Ned. Tijdschr. Geneesk.*, 1934, 78:1423-31.

Biemond syndrome (2). A condition combining coloboma of the iris, mental retardation, obesity, hypogonadism, and postaxial polydactyly. Hydrocephalus and hypospadias may also occur. The syndrome is believed to be transmitted as an autosomal recessive trait.

Biemond, A. Het syndrome van Laurence-Biedl en een annverwant, nieuw syndrome. *Ned. Tijdschr. Geneesk.*, 1934, 78:1801-14.

Biemond syndrome (3). Synonym: *congenital familial analgesia.*

A form of the congenital insensitivity to pain syndrome (q.v.) characterized by the absence of pain sensation, diminished touch and temperature sense, and absent tendon reflexes. Pathological findings show defects in posterior root ganglia, gasserian ganglion, posterior roots, posterior horns, and the spinal gray matter and posterior columns. The syndrome is transmitted as an autosomal recessive trait.

*Biemond, A. Investigation of the brain in a case of congenital and familial analgesia. *Proc. 11th Internat. Cong. Neuropath., London*, Sept. 1955.

Biemond syndrome (4). Synonym: *posterior column ataxia.*

Ataxia due to degeneration of the posterior column and large fibers of the dorsal roots, and loss of Purkinje cells in the cerebellum. The disorder is transmitted as an autosomal dominant trait.

Biemond, A. Les degenerations spino-cerebelleuses. *Folia Psychiat. Neerl.*, 1951, 54:216-23.

Biemond syndrome (5). Synonym: *myopathia distalis juvenilis hereditaria.*

A familial form of symmetrical paresis and atrophy of the distal muscles of extremities. It is a relatively benign condition having its onset at the age of 5 to 15 years and progressing to the age of 50 years, when it becomes stationary. The syndrome is transmitted as an autosomal dominant trait.

Biemond, A. Myopathia distalis juvenilis hereditaria. *Acta Psychiat. Neur. Scand.*, 1955, 30:25-38.

BIER, AUGUST (German physician)

Bier spots. See *Marshall-White syndrome, under Marshall, Wallace.*

BIERMER, MICHAEL ANTON (German physician, 1827-1892)

Addison-Biermer anemia. See *under Addison.*

Addison-Biermer syndrome. See *Addison-Biermer anemia.*

Biermer anemia. See *Addison-Biermer anemia.*

Biermer syndrome. See *Addison-Biermer anemia.*

Biermer-Ehrlich anemia. See *Addison-Biermer anemia.*

pseudo-Biermer anemia. See *Gerbasi anemia.*

BIETTI, GIAMBATTISTA (Italian ophthalmologist, born 1907)

Bietti dystrophy. Synonyms: *Bietti keratopathy, Bietti tapetoretinal degeneration, climatic droplet keratopathy (CDK), dystrophia marginalis crystallinea, marginal corneal dystrophy, marginal crystalline dystrophy.*

Retinitis punctata albescens associated with marginal crystalline degeneration of the cornea, transmitted as an autosomal recessive trait, and characterized by an opacification at the level of Bowman membrane. It is particularly common in areas of bright sunlight. Climatic and environmental conditions appear to be the contributing factors.

Bietti, G. B. Su alcune forme atipiche o rare di degenerazione retinica. *Boll. Ocul.*, 1937, 16:1159-1239.

Bietti keratopathy. See *Bietti dystrophy.*

Bietti syndrome. Xerosis conjunctivae with iridopupillary anomalies.

*Bietti, G. B. *Studi sussaresi.* 1943, 21:3. Bietti, G. B. Iridopupillare Anomalien und Xerosis conjunctivae. *Klin. Mbl. Augenheilk.*, 1963, 143:321-31.

Bietti tapetoretinal degeneration. See *Bietti dystrophy.*

big jaw. See *Rivalta disease.*

BIGNAMI, AMICO (Italian physician, 1862-1929)

Marchiafava-Bignami disease (MBD). See *Marchiafava-Bignami syndrome.*

Marchiafava-Bignami syndrome. See *under Marchiafava.*

bilateral abductor vocal cord paralysis syndrome (BAVCP). A syndrome characterized by airway obstruction (with normal voice), hypothyroidism, hypoparathyroidism, and psychiatric manifestations, such as anxiety and depression, occurring as a post-thyroidectomy complication.

Holinger, L. D., Holinger, P. C., & Holinger, P. H. Etiology of bilateral vocal cord paralysis. A review of 389 cases. *Ann. Otol. Rhinol. Laryngol.*, 1976, 85:428-36. Holinger, P. C., *et al.* Vocal cord paralysis and psychopathology. Data and clinical issues. *Arch.Otolaryngol., Chicago,* 1981, 107:33-6.

bilateral anterior opercular syndrome. See *Foix-Chavany-Marie syndrome.*

bilateral congenital melanosis of the cornea. See *Krukenberg spindle.*

bilateral facial agenesis. See *mandibulofacial dysostosis.*

bilateral hilar adnopathy syndrome. See *Löfgren syndrome.*

bilateral hilar lymphoma syndrome. See *Löfgren syndrome.*

bilateral polycystic ovarian syndrome. See *polycystic ovary syndrome.*

bilateral renal agenesis (BRA) syndrome. See *Potter syndrome (1), under Potter, Edith Louise.*

bilateral right-sidedness anomalad. See *asplenia syndrome.*

bilateral symmetrical intracerebral calcifications. See *Fahr syndrome.*

bile nephrosis. See *hepatorenal syndrome.*

bile plug syndrome. Synonyms: *bile sludge syndrome, cholestatic jaundice of newborn, infantile obstructive jaundice, inspissated bile syndrome.*

Obstruction of the bile ducts in newborn infants by thickened bile, resulting in jaundice, liver enlargement, and anemia. Some authors differentiate the **bile plug syndrome**, which causes extrahepatic biliary cholestasis, from the **inspissatated bile syndrome**, which causes predominantly hepatocellular disorders.

Patterson, D. Y., *et al.* Prolonged obstructive jaundice in infancy. I. General survey of 156 cases. *Pediatrics*, 1952, 10:243-52. Bernstein, J., *et al.* Bile-plug syndrome: A correctable cause of obstructive jaundice in infants. *Pediatrics*, 1969, 43:273.

bile sludge syndrome. See *bile plug syndrome.*

biliary cirrhosis. See *Hanot cirrhosis.*

biliary xanthomatosis. See *Addison-Gull syndrome.*

bilious vomiting syndrome. See *postgastrectomy syndrome.*

billowing mitral valve syndrome. See *mitral valve prolapse syndrome.*

BILLROTH, CHRISTIAN ALBERT THEODOR (German surgeon, 1829-1894)

Billroth disease (1). Synonyms: *cephalohydrocele traumatica, spurious meningocele.*

Accumulation of cerebrospinal fluid under the scalp in children, associated with skull fracture and tear of the arachnoid.

Billroth, T. Ein Fall von Meningocele spuria cum fistula ventriculi cerebri. *Arch. Klin. Chir., Berlin,* 1862, 3:398-412.

Billroth disease (2). Malignant lymphoma.

Billroth, T. Neue Beobachtungen über die feinere Structur pathologisch veränderter Lymphdrüsen. *Arch. Path. Anat., Berlin,* 1861, 21:423-43.

BINDER, K. H. (German dentist)

Binder syndrome. Synonyms: *dysostosis maxillonasalis, maxillonasal dysostosis, maxillonasal dysplasia, nasomaxillary hypoplasia.*

A syndrome of hypoplasia of the maxillary and nasal bones. Flattening of the nasal spine, apparent elongation of the nose, absence of the angle between the frontal bone and nasal spine, small alae and openings with characteristic semilunar shape, and recession of perinasal structures are the principal nasal anomalies. Maxillary hypoplasia is associated with narrowing of the upper dental arch, gothic palate, and malocclusion.

Binder, K. H. Dysostosis maxillo-nasalis, ein arhinencephaler Missbildungskomplex. *Deut. Zahnärztl. Zschr.*, 1962, 17:438-44.

BING, JENS

Bickel-Bing-Harboe syndrome. See *Bing-Neel syndrome.*

Bing-Neel syndrome. Synonyms: *Bickel-Bing-Harboe syndrome, macroglobulinemia-neuropsychiatric syndrome, neuropsychiatric macrohyperglobulinemia syndrome.*

Macroglobulinemia associated with diffuse slowing of retinal and cerebral circulation, anorexia, emaciation, irritability, episodic confusion, personality changes, mental deterioration, coma, and sometimes stroke. Subacute or chronic neuropathy, either asymmetric in a multiple nerve trunk involvement, or symmetric and distal in distribution, may occur. Laboratory and postmortem findings may include myelitis, polyradiculitis, high erythrocyte sedimentation rate, positive formol-gel reaction, and extensive pathological changes in the central nervous system..

Bing, J., & Neel, A. V. Two cases of hyperglobulinaemia with affection of the central nervous system on a toxi-infectious basis. (Myelitis, polyradiculitis, spinal-fluid changes). *Acta Med. Scand.*, 1936, 88:492-506.

BING, RICHARD JOHN (American physician, born 1909)

Bing erythroprosopalgia. See *Horton neuralgia.*

Bing syndrome. See *Horton neuralgia.*

Bing-Horton syndrome. See *Horton neuralgia.*

Taussig-Bing anomaly. See *Taussig-Bing syndrome.*

Taussig-Bing complex. See *Taussig-Bing syndrome.*

Taussig-Bing heart. See *Taussig-Bing syndrome.*

Taussig-Bing malformation. See *Taussig-Bing syndrome.*

Taussig-Bing syndrome. See *under Taussig.*

binge eating syndrome. See *bulimia syndrome.*

binge-purge syndrome. See *bulimia syndrome.*

BINSWANGER, OTTO (German physician, 1852-1929)

Binswanger dementia. See *Binswanger disease.*

Binswanger disease. Synonyms: *Binswanger dementia,*

Binswanger encephalitis, Binswanger encephalopathy, chronic progressive subcortical encephalopathy, encephalitis subcorticalis chronica, encephalomalacia subcorticalis chronica arteriosclerotica, lacunar dementia, presenile dementia, progressive subcortical arteriosclerotic encephalopathy, progressive subcortical encephalitis, subcortical arteriosclerotic encephalopathy, subcortical paraplegia, subcortical vascular paraplegia.

A progressive arteriosclerotic disorder, occurring mostly during the fifth or sixth decade, manifested by diffuse neurological and mental aberrations, which include uncertain gait, urinary incontinence, parkinsonian features, pseudobulbar palsy, memory disorders, emotional instability, paranoia, hallucinations, speech disorders, convulsions, and dementia. Demyelination of the subcortical white matter with complete sparing of the gray cortex is the main pathological feature of this syndrome. High resolution computed tomography scan shows decreased density of frontal and periventricular white matter, ventricular dilation, and lacunar infarcts. Small artery lipohyalinosis is the cause of the lacunae and the leukoencephalopathy.

Binswanger, O. Die Abgrenzung der allgemeinen progressiven Paralyse. *Berlin. Klin. Wschr.*, 1894, 31:1103-5; 1180-6. Binswanger, O., & Alzheimer, A. Die arteriosklerotische Atrophie des Gehirns. *Allg. Zshchr. Psychiat.*, 1895, 51:809.

Binswanger encephalitis. See *Binswanger disease.*

Binswanger encephalopathy. See *Binswanger disease.*

BIOCHI

Senior-Biochi syndrome. See *Senior syndrome (1).*

BIÖRCK, GUNNAR (Swedish physician)

Biörck-Axén-Thorson syndrome. See *carcinoid syndrome.*

Biörck-Thorson syndrome. See *carcinoid syndrome.*

BIRCH-HIRSCHFELD, FELIX VICTOR (German physician, 1842-1899)

Birch-Hirschfeld tumor. See *Wilms tumor.*

bird fancier lung. See *pigeon breeder syndrome.*

bird fancier lung syndrome. See *pigeon breeder syndrome.*

bird-headed dwarfism. See *Seckel syndrome.*

birdlike face syndrome. See *Seckel syndrome.*

birdlike facies. See *Hallermann-Streiff syndrome.*

birdshot retinochoroidopathy syndrome. An ocular condition characterized by a white, painless eye with minimal anterior segment inflammation, particulate debris in the anterior and posterior vitreous, and profuse retinal vascular leakage causing edema and retinal and macular disorders with resulting decreased visual acuity.

Byan, S. J., & Maumenee, A. E. Birdshort retinochoroidopathy. *Am. J. Ophthalmol.*, 1980, 89:31-45.

BIRKETT, JOHN (British physician, 1815-1904)

Birkett hernia. Synonyms: *ascending hernia, intermuscular hernia, intraparietal hernia,.*

Intraparietal inguinal hernia, including hernias in which the sac extends into either the anterior or the inferior wall.

Birkett, J. Description of a case of a intra-parietal inguinal hernia, with reference to cases which were probably of a similar kind. *Guy's Hosp. Rep.*, 1861, 7:270-91.

BIRT, ARTHUR R. (Canadian physician)

Birt-Hogg-Dubé syndrome. A dermatological syndrome, apparently transmitted as an autosomal dominant trait, characterized by an eruption of dome-shaped papules of the head, chest, back, and arms, frequently with acrochordons. The lesions consist of multiple follicular tumors (fibrofolliculomas and trichodiscomas), representing benign proliferations of mesodermal and ectodermal components of the pilar system.

Birt, A. R., Hogg, G. R., & Dubé, W. J. Hereditary multiple fibrofolliculomas with trichodiscomas and acrochordons. *Arch. Dermatol., Chicago,* 1977, 113:1674-7.

BIS. See *bone cement implantation syndrome.*

BIS (building illness syndrome). See *sick building syndrome.*

biskra button. See *Alibert disease (2).*

BITOT, PIERRE A. (French physician, 1822-1888)

Bitôt patches. See *Bitôt spots.*

Bitôt spots. Synonyms: *Bitôt patches, xerosis conjunctivae, xerosis corneae.*

Small, gray, or white, cheeselike, foamy patches or film of the corneal epithelium, caused by a deficiency of vitamin A, which may result in nyctalopia and keratomalacia.

Bitôt. Mémoire sur une lésion conjonctivale non encore décrite, coincidant avec l'héméralopie. *Gaz. Hebd. Méd., Paris,* 1863, 10:284-8.

BIXLER, DAVID (American dentist and geneticist, born 1929)

Antley-Bixler syndrome. See *under Antley.*

Bixler syndrome. See *hypertelorism-microtia-clefting syndrome.*

bizarre vertebral anomalies syndrome. See *spondylothoracic dysplasia.*

BJERRUM, JANNIK PETERSON (Danish physician, 1851-1920)

Bjerrum scotoma. Synonym: *arcuate scotoma.*

A progressive form of scotoma seen in glaucoma, with the development of a sickle-shaped defect extending from the blind spot around the macular region and ending on the nasal side. Contraction of peripheral fields progresses to total blindness.

*Bjerrum, J. P. *Vejledning i anvendelsen af ojespejlet.* Copenhagen, Priors, 1890.

BJÖRNSTAD, R. (Swedish physician)

Björnstad syndrome. Synonym: *pili torti-deafness syndrome.*

An association of twisted hair with sensorineural deafness probably transmitted as an autosomal recessive trait. The severity of deafness is directly related to the degree of hair loss.

Björnstad, R. Pili torti and sensori-neural loss of hearing. *Proc. 17th Meeting. Northern Dermatological Society,* Copenhagen, May, 1965.

BK (B-K) mole syndrome. See *dysplastic nevus syndrome.*

BL. See *Burkitt lymphoma.*

black baby. See *fetal PCB syndrome.*

black liver-jaundice syndrome. See *Dubin-Johnson syndrome.*

black thyroid syndrome. Coal-black discoloration of the thyroid gland, usually due to the administration of minocycline, some instances being associated with hypothyrodism and follicular adenoma. Some rare cases are idiopathic. Abnormal accumulation of neu-

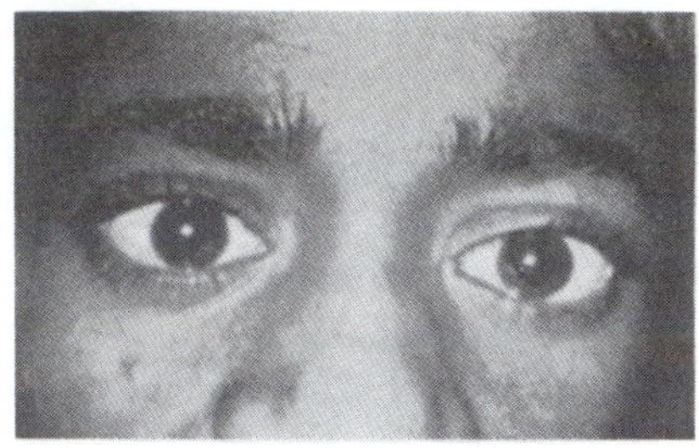

Bitôt spots
Scheie, H.G. & D.M. Albert: *Adler's Textbook of Ophthalmology*, 8th ed. Philadelphia: W.B. Saunders Co., 1968.

romelanin (a melanin pigment) in the thyroid gland is believed to be the cause of this syndrome. Accumulation of the pigment increases with normal aging processes and is further accelerated by the administration of minocycline.

Attwood, H. D., & Dennett, X. A black thyroid and minocycline treatment. *Brit. Med. J.*, 1976, 2:1109-10. Landas, S. K., *et al.* Black thyroid syndrome: Exaggeration of a normal process? *Am. J. Clin. Pathol.*, 1986, 85:411-8.

BLACKFAN, KENNETH D. (American physician, 1883-1941)

Diamond-Blackfan anemia (DBA). See *Diamond-Blackfan syndrome.*

Diamond-Blackfan syndrome. See *under Diamond.*

Josephs-Diamond-Blackfan anemia. See *Diamond-Blackfan syndrome.*

Josephs-Diamond-Blackfan syndrome. See *Diamond-Blackfan syndrome.*

bladder immaturity syndrome. Synonym: *urinary bladder immaturity syndrome.*

Urinary incontinence in young girls, characterized by diurnal or nocturnal urine leakage, sometimes associated with urinary tract infection.

Averous, M. Le syndrome d'immaturité vésicale. A propos de 1,097 observations. *J. Urol., Paris,* 1985, 91:257-67.

bladder neck obstruction. See *Marion disease.*

BLANC, EMILE (French physician, 1901-1952)

Bonnet-Dechaume-Blanc syndrome. See *under Bonnet, Paul.*

BLAND, EDWARD FRANKLIN (American cardiologist, born 1901)

Bland-White-Garland syndrome. Anomalous origin of the left coronary artery from the pulmonary artery that may be associated with enlargement of the heart as a result of hypertrophy and dilation of the left ventricle and degenerative changes in the ventricular wall supplied by the malposed vessel. The symptoms include failure to thrive, dyspnea, tachypnea, precordial pain, sweating, pallor, and crying after feeding and exertion. Most untreated infants die within two years.

Bland, E. F., White, P. D., & Garland, H. Congenital anomalies of the coronary arteries. Report of an unusual case associated with cardiac hypertrophy. *Am Heart J.*, 1932-33, 8:787-801.

blastomycetic dermatitis. See *Gilchrist disease.*

blastomycosis purulenta profunda. See *Busse-Buschke disease.*

BLATIN, MARC (French physician, born 1878)

Blatin syndrome. Synonym: *hydatid fremitus.*

Tremulous impulse or thrill over a large intra-abdominal hydatid cyst, reportedly described by Blatin.

bleeder's disease A. See *hemophilia.*

BLEGVAD, OLAF (Danish physician, 1888-1961)

Blegvad-Haxthausen syndrome. An association of atrophy of the skin, zonular cataract, osteogenesis imperfecta, and blue sclera.

Blegvad, O., & Haxthausen, H. Blaa sclerae og tendens til knoglebrud med pletformet hudatrofi og zonular katarakt. *Hospitalstidende,* 1921, 64:609-16.

BLENCKE, AUGUST (German orthopedic surgeon, 1868-1937)

Blencke syndrome. Synonyms: *epiphysitis calcanei, metaphyseal osteodystrophy of the calcaneum, metaepiphyseal osteodystrophy of the os calcis, osteitis deformans calcanei, osteochondrosis calcanei, osteodystrophia metaepiphysaria calcanei.*

Epiphyseal ischemic necrosis resulting in metaphyseal osteodystrophy of the calcaneum.

Toniolo, G. Perche non puo esistere una osteodistrofia metafisaria del calcagno. *Radiol. Clin., Basel,* 1950, 19:81-94.

blenorrhagic balantiform keratoderma with oral involvement. See *Reiter syndrome.*

blepharochalasis syndrome. Relaxation of the skin of the eyelids associated with eyelid deformities characterized by blepharoptosis and prolapse of the orbital fat and lacrimal gland. Some patients develop blepharophimosis secondary to the dehiscence of the canthal tendons. In this stage, the tendons still adhere to the periosteum of the orbital rims and loss of fixation occurs at the distal attachment between the tendons and the eyelid tissue, resulting in a horizontally shortened palpebral fissure and a rounded deformity of the lateral canthal angle.

Custer, P. L., *et al.* Blepharochalasis syndrome. *Am. J. Ophthalmol.*, 1985, 15L424-8.

blepharonasofacial syndrome. A familial syndrome, transmitted as an autosomal dominant trait, characterized by telecanthus, lateral displacement and stenosis of the lacrimal puncta, bulky nose with a broad bridge, masklike facies, midfacial hypoplasia, longitudinal cheek furrows, trapezoidal upper lip, hyperextensible joints, positive Babinski reflex, poor coordination, torsion dystonia, syndactyly of the fingers, and mental retardation.

Pashayan, H. A family with blepharo-naso-facial malformations. *Am. J. Dis. Child.*, 1973, 125:389-93.

blepharophimosis congenita. See *blepharophimosis syndrome.*

blepharophimosis syndrome. Synonyms: *blepharophimosis congenita, familial blepharophimosis.*

A hereditary syndrome, transmitted as an autosomal dominant trait, marked by inverted inner canthi with abnormal narrowness of the palpebral fissures, blepharoptosis, low nasal bridge, and hypoplasia and fibrosis of the levator palpebrae muscle. Muscle hypotonia, strabimus, and malformed ears may be associated.

Vignes. Epicanthus héréditaire. *Rev. Gen. Ophthal., Paris,* 1889, 8:438. Briggs, H. H. Hereditary congenital ptosis with report of 64 cases conforming to the mendelian rule of dominance. *Am. J. Opthal.*, 1919, 2:408-17.

blepharophimosis-ptosis-epicanthus inversus syndrome (BPEI). See *blepharoptosis-blepharophimosis-epicanthus inversus-telecanthus syndrome.*

blepharoptosis-blepharophimosis-epicanthus inversus-telecanthus syndrome. Synonym: *blepharophimosis-ptosis-epicanthus inversus syndrome (BPEI).*

A syndrome of blepharoptosis, blepharophimosis, epicanthus inversus, telecanthus, amenorrhea, and infertility. The clinical findings include lateral displacement of the lower punctum, medial displacement of the upper punctum, canalicular stenosis, elongation of the horizontal canaliculi, punctal reduplication, posterior ectopia of the lower puncta, and aplasia of the upper puncta.

Kohn, R., & Romano, P. E. Blepharoptosis, blepharophimosis, epicanthus inversus, and telecanthus-A syndrome with no name. *Am. J. Ophth.*, 1971, 72:625-32. Kohn, R. Additional lacrimal findings in the syndrome of blepharoptosis, blepharophimosis, epicanthus inversus, and telecanthus. *J. Pediat. Ophth. Strabismus*, 1983, 20:98-100.

blepharospasm-oromandibular dystonia syndrome. See *Meige syndrome (2).*

BLESOVSKY, A. (British physician)

Blesovsky syndrome. Synonym: *folded lung.*

A condition characterized by lung folding which may occur in association with larger pleural plaques or grossly thickened pleural membrane.

Blesovsky, A. The folded lung. *Brit. J. Dis. Chest*, 1966, 60:19-22.

BLESSIG, ROBERT (German physician, 1830-1878)

Blessig-Iwanoff cyst. See *Blessig-Iwanoff disease.*

Blessig-Iwanoff disease. Synonyms: *Blessig-Iwanoff cyst, peripheral cystoid degeneration of the retina.*

Degeneration of the nonfunctioning zone of the retina, characterized by microcysts behind the dentate process of the retina at the ora serrata. These cysts increase in size and coalesce, extending almost to the inner and outer limiting membrane and, eventually, giving rise to retinoschisis.

Hogan, M. J., & Zimmerman, L. E. *Ophthalmic pathology. An atlas and textbook.* 2nd ed. Philadelphia, Saunders, 1962, pp. 550-2.

blighted ovum syndrome. Abnormal development of the trophoblastic anlagen leading to gross fetal abnormalities or to the death of the fetus. Pathologic examination of the aborted tissue does not reveal any recognizable fetal parts.

Schweditsch, M. O., *et al.* Hormonal considerations in early normal pregnancy and blighted ovum syndrome. *Fertil. Steril.*, 1979, 31:252-7.

blind headache. See *migraine under headache syndrome.*

blind loop malabsorption syndrome. See *blind loop syndrome.*

blind loop syndrome. Synonyms: *blind loop malabsorption syndrome, blind pouch syndrome, dead loop syndrome, excluded loop syndrome, intestinal stasis syndrome, stagnant loop syndrome (SLS).*

Formation of a loop or pouch in the small intestine which is disconnected from the main flow of the gastrointestinal tract or which will accept intestinal contents without allowing them to egress. The syndrome may be a complication of surgical procedures, such as side-to-side or end-to-side ileotransverse colostomy; multiple intestinal strictures, as when occurring in diffuse granulomatous ileojejunitis and tuberculosis or after x-irradiation; jejunal diverticula with pocket formation; and fistulae involving the stomach, small intestine, and colon. Proliferation of enteric microflora, with resulting bacterial overgrowth (see *bacterial overgrowth syndrome*) and malabsorption (see *malabsorption syndrome*) are usually associated with stasis of intestinal contents. The symptoms vary depending on the nature of the bowel condition; they may include weight loss, malnutrition, growth retardation, cramps, abdominal distention, diarrhea, steatorrhea, and vitamin deficiencies. Achlorhydria and megaloblastic anemia may occur. See also *Lane syndrome.*

*White, W. H. On the pathology and prognosis of pernicious anemia. *Guy's Hosp. Rep.*, 1890, 32:149. *Barker, W. H., & Hummel, L. E. Macrocytic anemia in association with intestinal stricture and anastomoses. *Bull. Johns Hopkins Hosp.*, 1939, 46:215. Hughes, J. M. Blind loop syndrome associated with growth retardation. *Gastroenterology*, 1974, 67:338-40.

blind pouch syndrome. See *blind loop syndrome.*

blind spot syndrome. Synonyms: *Swan syndrome, squint syndrome.*

An ophthalmological disorder characterized by esotrophia accompanied by occasional diplopia and confusion of images, blind spot of deviating eye consistently overlying fixation area, good vision in each eye, normal correspondence, and good fusional potential.

Swan, K. C. A squint syndrome. *Arch. Ophth., Chicago*, 1947, 37:149-54.

blinding filariasis. See *Robles disease.*

BLIZZARD, ROBERT (American physician)

Johanson-Blizzard syndrome (JBS). See *under Johanson, Ann.*

BLOCH

Bloch-Miescher syndrome. See *Miescher syndrome (2).*

BLOCH, B.

Bloch-Stauffer dyshormonal dermatosis. See *Rothmund-Thomson syndrome.*

BLOCH, BRUNO (Swiss physician, 1878-1933)

Bloch-Siemens syndrome. See *Bloch-Sulzberger syndrome.*

Bloch-Sulzberger melanoblastosis. See *Bloch-Sulzberger syndrome.*

Bloch-Sulzberger syndrome. Synonyms: *Asboe-Hansen disease, Bloch-Siemens syndrome, Bloch-Sulzberger melanoblastosis, Siemens-Bloch pigmented dermatosis, incontinentia pigmenti (IP), melanoblastosis cutis linearis sive systematisata, melanosis corii degenerativa, nevus pigmentosus systematicus.*

A congenital disorder which occurs mostly in females as an X-linked dominant trait and is usually lethal to males. Its principal features consist of verrucous, pigmented macular lesions of the skin and lesions of the eyes, nails, teeth, central nervous system, and hair. Patches of vesicles may be present at birth, but they are replaced by crops of violaceous papules and inflammatory lesions. The inflammatory stage may pass directly to the pigmented stage, or it may blend into a warty or papillomatous phase with subsequent development of pigmented macules. Pigmented areas have strikingly bizzare configurations in flecks, whorls, spider forms, lines, and patches which do not follow the lines of cleavage or distribution of nerves or blood vessels. Chocolate-brown, gray-brown, or slate-colored macules may persist unchanged or may fade, leaving normal depigmented skin. The hair is thin, alopecia of the scalp is frequent, and the nails may be dystrophic. Eye abnormalities usually include strabismus, cataracts, optic atrophy, myopia, blue sclerae, nystagmus, microphthalmia, and ophthalmia. Dental abnormalities consist of delayed tooth eruption, pegged or conical crowned teeth, and malformed teeth, affecting both the primary and permanent dentitions. The central nervous system complications consist of mental. retardation, microcephaly, spastic paralysis, epilepsy, and hydrocephalus. Retarded growth, hearing disorders, hemivertebrae, syndactyly, hemiatrophy, supernumerary ribs, patent ductus arteriosus, supernumerary nipples, unilateral breast aplasia, and urachal cysts may be associated.

Bloch, B. Eigentümliche, bisher nicht beschriebene Pigmentaffektion (Incontinentia pigmenti). *Schweiz, Med. Wschr.*, 1926, 7:404-5. Sulzberger, M. B. Über eine bisher nicht beschriebene congenitale Pigmentanomalie (Incontinentia pigmenti). *Arch. Derm. Syph., Berlin*, 1928, 154:19-32. Siemens, H. W. Die Melanosis corri degenerativa, eine neue Pigmentdermatose. *Arch. Derm. Syph., Berlin*, 1929, 157:382-91. Asboe-Hansen, G. Bullous keratogenous and pigmentary dermatitis wih blood eosinophilia in newborn girls. *Arch. Derm Syph., Chicago*, 1953, 67:152-7.

Siemens-Bloch pigmented dermatosis. See *Bloch-Sulzberger syndrome.*

BLOCQ, PAUL OSCAR (French physician, 1860-1896)

Blocq syndrome. Synonyms: *astasia-abasia syndrome, hysterical dysbasia, stasibasiphobia.*

Hysterical inability to stand up or walk, or fear of standing or walking.

*Blocq, P. O. Sur une affection caractérisée par de l'astasie et de l'abasie. *Arch. Neur., Paris*, 1888, 15:24-51; 187-211.

BLODI, FREDERICK C. (American ophthalmologist)

Reese-Blodi syndrome. See *Reese syndrome.*

blood hyperviscosity syndrome. See *hyperviscosity syndrome.*

BLOODGOOD, JOSEPH COLT (American physician, 1866-1935)

Bloodgood disease. See *Cheatle disease.*

BLOOM, DAVID (American dermatologist)

Bloom syndrome (BS). Synonyms: *Bloom-Torre-Machacek syndrome, congenital telangiectatic erythema-stunted growth syndrome.*

A syndrome transmitted as an autosomal recessive trait, in which telangiectatic erythema of the face, sensitivity to sunlight, and dwarfism are the cardinal features. Disproportionate microcephaly, narrow facial features, and, sometimes, a prominent nose and ears, receding mandible, and dolichocephaly are the principal craniofacial characteristics. Skin eruption appears as erythematous telangiectatic spots, plaques, or patches, or as scattered macular lesions; sun exposure usually causes exacerbation. The birth weight is low and slow growth becomes evident early. Associated defects may include conjunctivitis, lichen pilaris, hypertrichosis, café-au-lait spots, cheilitis, ichthyosis, acanthosis nigricans, pilonidal cysts, syndactyly, absence of toes, clinodactyly, short lower extremities, pes equinus, absence of upper incisors, hypospadias, cryptorchism, and other anomalies. Leukemias, lymphomas, and other neoplastic conditions are frequently associated.

Bloom, D. Congenital telangiectatic erythema resembling lupus erythematosus in dwarfs. Probably a syndrome entity. *Am. J. Dis. Child.*, 1954, 88:754-8. Torre, D. P. (presented for J. Cramer) Primordial dwarfism; discoid lupus erythematosus. *Arch. Derm., Chicago*, 1954, 69:511-3.

Bloom-Torre-Machacek syndrome. See *Bloom syndrome.*

BLOOMBERG, ESTHER (American physician)

Albright-Butler-Bloomberg syndrome. See *hypophosphatemic familial rickets.*

BLOUNT, WALTER PUTNAM

Blount syndrome. See *Erlacher-Blount syndrome.*

Blount-Barber syndrome. See *Erlacher-Blount syndrome.*

Erlacher-Blount syndrome. See *under Erlacher.*

BLS. See ***b**are **l**ymphocyte **s**yndrome.*

blubber finger. See *seal finger syndrome.*

blue and bloated syndrome. Chronic obstructive pulmonary disease in overweight patients with cor pulmonale, chronic bronchitis, emphysema, and productive cough. Sleep hypoxemia with a reduction in baseline saturation during sleep may cause severe oxygen desaturation.

DeMarco, F. J., Jr., *et al.* Oxygen desaturation during sleep as a determinant of the "blue and bloated" syndrome. *Chest*, 1981, 79:621-5.

blue baby. See *Fallot tetralogy.*

blue diaper syndrome. Familial hypercalcemia with nephrocalcinosis and indicanuria, transmitted as an autosomal recessive trait, caused by poor absorption of the amino acid tryptophan from the gastrointestinal tract. Gastrointestinal bacteria convert tryptophan to indole, which is absorbed, oxidized, sulfated, and excreted in the urine as indican which, in turn, is oxidized to indigo blue on exposure to air, thus causing blue discoloration of the urine.

Drummond, K. N., *et al.* The blue diaper syndrome: Familial hypercalcemia with nephrocalcinosis and indicanuria. A new familial disease, with definition of the metabolic abnormality. *Am. J. Med.*, 1964, 37:928-48.

blue digit syndrome. Synonym: *blue toe syndrome.*

Digital ischemia due to microembolization from a proximal source, as when microemboli are dislodged from a focal ulcerating plaque. A painful, cool, cyanotic digit in the presence a well perfused warm leg is the chief manifestation.

Crane, C. Atherothrombotic embolization to lower extremities in atherosclerosis. *Arch. Surg.*, 1967, 94:96-100. Lee, B. Y., *et al.* Blue digit syndrome: Urgent indication for digital salvage. *Am. J. Surg.*, 1984, 147:418-22.

blue dome cyst. See *Cheatle disease.*

blue edema. See *Charcot edema.*

blue jeans syndrome. A form of compartment syndrome caused by shrinking of tight wet blue jeans in which the patient had slept, leading to severe ischemia and disability.

Mathiesen, B., & Reumert, T. Blue jeans syndrome. *Ugersk. Laeger*, 1981, 143:1333.

blue neuronevus. See *Jadassohn-Tièche nevus, under Jadassohn, Josef.*

blue nevus. See *Jadassohn-Tièche nevus, under Jadassohn, Josef.*

blue rubber bleb nevus syndrome (BRBN, BRBNS). Synonyms: *Bean syndrome, cutaneo-intestinal cavernous hemangioma.*

The association of soft, erectile, rubbery, bluish hemangiomas of the skin with hemangiomas of the gastrointestinal tract; some of the larger tumors resemble nipples. Complications may include gastrointestinal bleeding (leading to iron-deficiency anemia), amputation of extremities, ocular lesions, intussusception, and orthopedic disorders. Nocturnal pain and regional hyperhidrosis may occur. The lesions are usually present in infants and children with only a few cases having been reported in adults. Most cases are sporadic, although autosomal dominant inheritance has been reported.

Bean, W. B. *Vascular spider and related lesions of the skin.* Springfield, Illinois, Thomas, 1958.

blue toe syndrome. See *blue digit syndrome.*

Blueberry syndrome. A syndrome characterized by lack of speech, low frustration tolerance, and aggressive response to invasion of personal space. Onset follows a normal pre- and perinatal period, with no evidence of brain damage or emotional disorders. There is mental retardation secondary to language deficits. The syndrome was named after the Blueberry Treatment Centers in Brooklyn, N. Y.

Levinson, B. M. The Blueberry syndrome. *Psychol. Rep.,* 1980, 46:47-52.

blueberry muffin baby. See *blueberry muffin syndrome.*

blueberry muffin syndrome. Synonym: *blueberry muffin baby.*

A syndrome of newborn infants characterized by hemorrhagic purpuric eruption and thrombocytopenia due to in utero infection with rubella. The lesions are 2 to 10 mm in diameter, deep blue or purple macules or papules, which gradually disappear over the course of 4 to 6 weeks. The term *blueberry muffin baby* refers to infants with neuroblastoma and subcutaneous metastases.

Banatvala, J. E., *et al.* Rubella syndrome and thrombocytopenic purpura in newborn infants. Clinical and virologic observations. *N. Engl. J. Med.,* 1965, 273:474-8. Brough, A. J., *et al.* Dermal erythropoiesis in neonatal infants. A manifestation of intra-uterine viral disease. *Pediatrics,* 1967, 40:627-35. Shown, T. E., & Durfee, M. F. Blueberry muffin baby: Neonatal neuroblastoma with subcutaneous metastases. *J. Urol.,* 1970, 104:193-5.

BLUEFARB, SAMUEL M. (American physician)

Bluefarb-Stewart syndrome. Synonyms: *Kaposi-like angiodermatitis, pseudo-Kaposi angiodermatitis, pseudo-Kaposi stasis dermatitis.*

Angiomatous stasis dermatitis, usually of one leg or foot, arising from a congenital arteriovenous malformation, which morphologically and histologically resembles Kaposi disease.

Bluefarb, S. M., & Adams, L. A. Arteriovenous malformation with angiodermatitis. Stasis dermatitis simulating Kaposi's disease. *Arch. Derm., Chicago,* 1967, 96:176-81. *Stewart, W. M. Fausse angiosarcomatose de Kaposi par fistules artério-veinulaires multiples. *Bull. Soc. Fr. Derm. Syph.,* 1967, 74:664-5.

BLUM, PAUL (French physician, 1878-1933)

Gougerot-Blum syndrome. See *under Gougerot, Henri.*

BLUMER, GEORGE (American physician, 1858-1940)

Blumer shelf. Synonym: *rectal shelf.*

Cancer or inflammatory infiltration in the Douglas pouch, forming a shelflike structure.

Blumer, G. The rectal shelf. A neglected rectal sign of value in the diagnosis and prognosis of obscure malignant and inflammatory diseases within the abdomen. *Albany Med. Ann.,* 1909, 30:361-6.

BMD. See *Becker muscular dystrophy.*

boba. See *Charlouis disease.*

bobble-head doll syndrome. Nodding of the head similar to that seen in a bobble-head doll, occurring in third ventricle dilatation from a cyst or hydrocephalus in aqueduct stenosis, associated with tremor of the trunk and extremities and macrocephaly.

Benton, J. W., *et al.* The bobble-head doll syndrome: Report of a unique truncal tremor associated with third ventricle cyst and hydrocephalus in children. *Neurology,* 1966, 16:725-9.

BOCHDALEK, VINCENT ALEXANDER (Anatomist in Prague, 1801-1883)

Bochdalek hernia. Synonyms: *congenital posterolateral diaphragmatic hernia, foramen of Bochdalek hernia.*

Congenital diaphragmatic hernia, with extrusion of bowel and visceral contents into the thorax, due to failure of closure of the foramen of Bochdalek (the pleuroperitoneal hiatus).

*Bochdalek, V. A. Einige Bemerkungen über die Enstehung des angeborenen zerchfellbruches: Als Beitrag zur pathologischen Anatomie der Hernien. *Vjrschr. Prakt. Heilk., Prag,* 1848, 3:89-97.

BOCKHART, MAX (German physician)

Bockhart impetigo. Synonym: *superficial pustular perifolliculitis.*

A superficial folliculitis, usually caused by *Staphyloccus aureus* infection, characterized by small purulent pustules at the pilosebaceous glands, affecting chiefly the scalp and extremities.

*Bockhart, M. Über die Aetiologie und Therapie der Impetigo, des Furunkels und der Sykosis. *Mschr. Prakt. Derm.,* 1887, 6:450-71.

BODECHTEL, GUSTAV (German physician, born 1899)

Bodechtel-Guttmann disease. See *van Bogaert encephalitis.*

BODER, ELENA (American physician)

Boder-Sedgwick syndrome. See *Louis-Bar syndrome.*

BODIAN, MARTIN (British physician)

Shwachman-Bodian syndrome. See *Shwachman syndrome.*

body packer syndrome. Synonym: *cocaine body packer syndrome.*

Ingestion of multiple small packages, usually containing drugs (in one case, 147 cocaine-filled condoms were found in the stomach), for the purpose of transporting contraband. Acute, frequently fatal poisoning may occur when the package breaks or its contents leach into the gastrointestinal system. The term *body stuffer syndrome* refers to the condition resulting from ingestion of drugs to conceal them when confronted by police, and *mini-packer* pertains to a person who had swallowed a single bag of cocaine to avoid police detection.

Mebane, L. C., & DeVito, J. J. Cocaine intoxication: A unique case. *J. Fla. Med. Assoc.,* 1975, 62:119-20. Roberts, J. R., *et al.* The bodystuffer syndrome: A clandestine form of drug overdose. *Am. J. Emerg. Med.,* 1986, 4:24-7.

body stuffer syndrome. See *under body packer syndrome.*

BOECK, CAESAR PETER MOELLER. See MOELLER-BOECK, CAESAR PETER

BOECK, KARL WILHELM (Norwegian physician, 1808-1875)

Boeck itch. See *Boeck scabies.*

Boeck scabies. Synonyms: *Boeck itch, Norwegian itch, Norwegian scabies, scabies crustosa norvegica, scabies norvegica Boeckii.*

A severe form of scabies with crusting, itching, scaling, and suppuration of the fingers, face, and scalp, as well as other parts of the body, observed in infestation with an immense number of mites under the skin.

Boeck, C. W. Om den spedalski sygdom. Elephantiasis graecorum. *Norsk. Mag. Laegevid,* 1842, 4:129; 127-8.

Danielssen-Boeck disease. See *under Danielssen.*

scabies norvergica boeckii. See *Boeck scabies.*

BOERHAVE, HERMANN (Dutch physician, 1668-1738)

Boerhave syndrome. Synonym: *spontaneous rupture of the esophagus.*

Spontaneous rupture of all layers of the esophagus accompanied by vomiting, epigastric and chest pain, subcutaneous emphysema, rapid respiration, and dysphagia.

Boerhave, H. *Atrocis, néc descripti prius, morbi historia: Secundum medicae artis leges descripta.* Boustestenina, 1774.

BOFFA, M. C. (French physician)

Soulier-Boffa syndrome. See *under Soulier.*

BOGAERT, LUDO, VAN. See VAN BOGAERT, LUDO

BOGDAN, ALADAR (Hungarian physician)

Bogdán-Buday disease. The development of abscesses of the liver and possibly of the lungs, spleen, and joints following extrahepatic injuries. The abscesses are unrelated to wound infection.

Bogdán, A. Eine bisher unbekannte Infektionskrankheit bei Verwundeten. *Med. Klin., Berlin,* 1916, 12:383-6. Buday, K. Endemisch auftretende Leberabszesse bei Verwundeten werursacht durch einen anaeroben Bacillus. *Zbl. Bakt.,* 1915-16, 77:453-69.

BOGORAD, F. A. (Russian physician)

Bogorad syndrome. See *gustatory lacrimation syndrome.*

BOHMANN

Walter-Bohmann syndrome. See *postcholecystectomy syndrome.*

BOLTSHAUSER

Joubert-Boltshauser syndrome. See *Joubert syndrome.*

BOMFORD, R. R. (British physician)

Bomford-Rhoads anemia. See *Davidson anemia.*

bone cement implantation syndrome (BIS). Postoperative complications after implantation of endoprostheses with bone cement, consisting mainly of circulatory disorders and pulmonary embolism. An abrupt decrease or, less commonly, increase in the blood pressure are the the first symptoms. Occasional hypoxemia and heart arrest may follow.

Rinecker, H. New clinico-pathophysiological studies on the bone cement implantation syndrome. *Arch. Orthop. Traum. Surg.,* 1980, 97:263-74.

BONFILS, EMILE ADOLPHE (French physician)

Bonfils disease. See *Hodgkin disease.*

BONGIOVANNI, ALFRED M. (American physician)

Bongiovanni-Eisenmenger syndrome. A chronic liver illness of unknown etiology with clinical features of hyperadrenalism and characterized by elevated glycogen level and storage. The syndrome was originally observed in a group of young women.

Bongiovanni, A. M., & Eisenmenger, W. J. Adrenal cortical metabolism in chronic liver disease. *J. Clin. Endocr.,* 1951, 11:152-72.

BONNET, CHARLES (French physician, 1720-1793)

Bonnet syndrome. Synonym: *Charles Bonnet syndrome.*

Visual hallucinations in old age that are not associated with any mental disorder.

*Bonnet, C. *Essai analytique sur les facultés de l'âme.* 2nd ed. Copenhagen, 1769. Vol. 2, pp. 176-8.

Charles Bonnet syndrome. See *Bonnet syndrome.*

BONNET, PAUL (French physician)

Bonnet syndrome (1). See *Bonnet-Dechaume-Blanc syndrome.*

Bonnet syndrome (2). Synonym: *trigeminosympathetic neuralgia.*

Sudden trigeminal neuralgia associated with the Bernard-Horner syndrome and vasomotor disorders in the area supplied by the trigeminal nerve.

Bonnet, P. Les syndromes trigeminosympathiques. *Arch. Opht., Paris,* 1956, 16:361-79.

Bonnet-Dechaume-Blanc syndrome. Synonyms: *Bonnet syndrome, Wyburn-Mason syndrome, cerebroretinal arteriovenous aneurysm, neuroretino-angiomatosis.*

Arteriovenous malformations of the fundus oculi, sometimes in association with involvement of the brain and ipsilateral periocular nevus flammeus. Three types are recognized: **Type 1** is marked by an arteriolar or capillary plexus interposed between the artery and vein, usually occurring without vascular compensation, arteriovenous malformations of the face and brain, or visual disorders. **Type 2** is characterized by the direct arteriovenous communication accompanied by vascular decompensation ranging from mild edema to exudation and hemorrhage and occasional cerebrovascular malformations. **Type 3** consists of large-caliber intertwined anastomosing channels in which the vessels undergo sheathing and sclerosis and the retina shows exudation, hemorrhage, and pigmentary migration. Mild proptosis, orbital enlargement, conjunctival hyperemia, unilateral loss of visual acuity, and a cranial bruit are common. Contralateral corticospinal tract dysfunction, seizures, and nystagmus may also be present. Some authors use the term **Wyburn-Mason syndrome** only for the third type.

Bonnet, P., Dechaume, J., & Blanc, E. L'anévrysme cirsoïde de la rétine (anévrysme racemeux). Ses relations avec l'anévrysme crisoïde de la face et avec l'anévrysme cirsoïde du cerveau. *J. Méd., Lyon,* 1937, p. 163-78. Wyburn-Mason, R. Arterio-venous aneurysm of midbrain and retina, facial naevi and mental changes. *Brain,* 1943, 66:163-203.

BONNEVIE, KRISTINE (Norwegian zoologist, 1872-1950)

Bonnevie-Ullrich syndrome. Synonyms: *pterygium colli syndrome, pterygolymphangiectasia syndrome.*

A congenital syndrome, possibly transmitted as either an X-linked or autosomal dominant trait, characterized by pterygium colli, lymphedema of the hands and feet, hypoplasia of the bones and muscles, syndactyly, laxity of the skin, dystrophy of the nails, disorders of the cranial nerves, and short stature. The syndrome is similar to the Klippel-Feil and Noonan syndromes. See also *multiple pterygium syndrome.*

Bonnevie, K. Embryological analysis of gene manifestation in Little and Bogg's abnormal mouse tribe. *J. Exp. Zool.,* 1934, 67:443-520. Ullrich, O. Über typische Kombinationsbilder mulitpler Abortungen. *Zschr. Kinderh.,* 1930, 49:271-6.

BONNIER, PIERRE (French physician, 1861-1918)

Bonnier syndrome. Synonym: *Deiter nucleus syndrome.*

Lesions of the Deiter nucleus or vestibular apparatus associated with vertigo, pallor, somnolence, tachycardia, trigeminal neuralgia, locomotor weakness, and a sense of apprehension.

Bonnier, P. Un nouveau syndrome bulbaire. *Presse Méd.*, 1903, 11:174-7; 861-2.

BÖÖK, JAN ARVID (Swedish geneticist)

Böök syndrome. Synonyms: *PHC (premolar hypodontia-hyperhidrosis-canities prematura) syndrome, premolar aplasia-hyperhidrosis-canities syndrome.*

A syndrome, transmitted as an autosomal dominant trait with complete penetrance, characterized by diffuse whitening of the hair early in life, hyperhidrosis, and absence of one or more premolar teeth with corresponding retention of their deciduous precursors.

Böök, J. A. Total premolar aplasia, canities prematura and hyperhidrosis. *8th Internat. Congress of Genetics*, Stockholm, 1948. Böök, J. A. Clinical and genetical studies of hypodontia. I. Premolar aplasia, hyperhidrosis, and canities prematura: A new hereditary syndrome in man. *Am. J. Hum. Genet.*, 1950, 2240-63.

BOR. See *branchio-otorenal syndrome.*

BORDA, J. M. (Argentine physician)

Borda syndrome. A syndrome of keratodermal genodermatosis associated with hydrocystomas, miliary cysts, xanthelasma, dental dysplasia, onychodysplasia, and basal cell epithelioma.

*Borda, J. M., & Abulafia, J. Queratosis displásicas. *Arch. Argent. Derm.*, 1971, 21:1-81.

borderline syndrome. A psychiatric syndrome characterized by anger as the main or only affect, sometimes with defect in affectional relationship, absence of indication of self-identity, and depressive loneliness. Four subgroups are identified: (1) the psychotic border, characterized by inappropriate and negativistic behavior and affect toward others; (2) the borderline syndrome characterized by negativistic and chaotic feelings and behavior, contradictory behavior, and a strong potential for acting out; (3) the adaptive, affectless, defended person, characterized by superficially adaptive but affectively deficient interactions; and (4) the border with the neuroses, which presents clinging depression.

*Grinker, R. R., Werble, B., & Drye, R. *The borderline syndrome.* New York, 1968. Kernberg, O. F. Neurosis, psychosis, and the borderline states. In: Kaplan, H. I., & Sadock, B. J. *Comprehensive textbook of psychiatry.* 4th ed. Williams & Wilkins, Baltimore, 1985. vol. I, pp. 621-30.

BÖRJESON, MATS GUNNAR (Swedish physician, born 1922)

Börjeson syndrome. Synonyms: *Börjeson-Forssman-Lehmann syndrome (BFL, BFLS), mental deficiency-epilepsy-endocrine disorders syndrome.*

A familial syndrome, transmitted as an X-linked trait, characterized by a variety of clinical symptoms, including characteristic facies (prominent supraorbital ridges, deep-set eyes, blepharoptosis, relative microcephaly, large ears, protruding tongue, round fat face), mental retardation, epilepsy, abundant abdominal fat, dwarfism, kyphosis, short neck, muscle hypotonia, narrow palpebral fissures, and hypogonadism.

Börjeson, M., Forssman, H., & Lehmann, O. An X-linked, recessively inherited syndrome characterized by grave mental deficiency, epilepsy, and endocrine disorder. *Acta Med. Scand.*, 1962, 171:13-21.

Börjeson-Forssman-Lehmann syndrome (BFL, BFLS). See *Börjeson syndrome.*

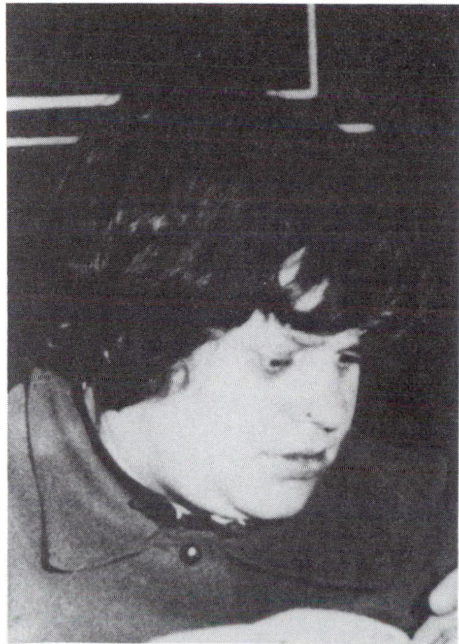

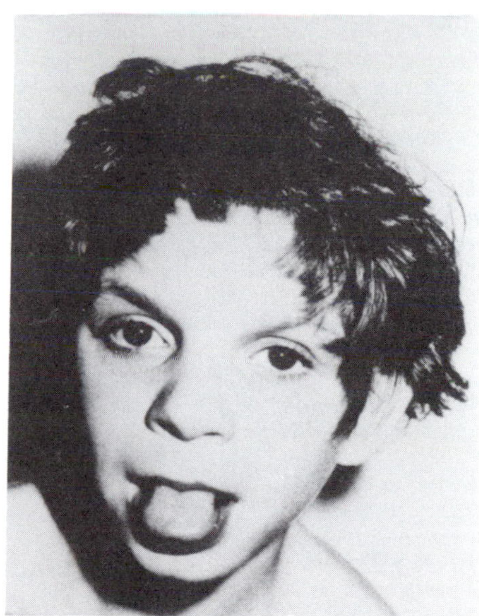

Börjeson syndrome
Dereymaeker, A.M., J.P. Fryns, M. Hoefnagels, G. Heremans, J. Marien & H. van den Berghe, *Clinical Genetics* 29:317-320, 1986, Munksgaard International Publishers, Copenhagen, Denmark.

Bornholm disease. See *Sylvest syndrome.*

Bornholm syndrome. See *Sylvest syndrome.*

BOROVSKII, P. F. (Russian physician)

Borovskii disease. See *Alibert disease (2).*

BORRIES, T. (Danish physician)

Borries syndrome. Synonyms: *abscess without abscess syndrome, neurologic-spinal fluid dissociation syndrome.*

Nonsuppurative localized encephalitis with changes in the cerebrospinal fluid suggesting abscess of the brain. Headache, fever, nausea, vomiting, listnessness, blurred vision, diplopia, and other symptoms are the principal symptoms.

*Borries, T. Otogene Encephalitis. *Zschr. Ges. Neur. Psychiat.*, 1921, 70:93-101.

BORST, MAXIMILIAN (German pathologist, 1869-1946)

Borst-Jadassohn epithelioma. Synonym: *intraepidermal acanthoma.*

Superficial basal cell epithelioma in which multiple sharply defined foci of basal cell epithelioma are embedded in the acanthotic epidermis.

Borst, M. Über die Möglichkeit einer ausgedehnten intraepidermalen Ausbreitung des Hautkrebses. *Verh. Deut. Path. Ges.*, 1904, 7:118-23. Jadassohn, J. Demonstration von seltenen Hautepitheliomen. *Beitr. Klin. Chir.*, 1926, 136:345-8.

BOSCH, HERNANDEZ JUAN (Spanish physician)

Gardner-Bosch syndrome. See *Gardner syndrome, under Gardner, Eldon John.*

BOSCH, MILLARES JUAN (Spanish physician)

Gardner-Bosch syndrome. See *Gardner syndrome, under Gardner, Eldon John.*

BOSTOCK, JOHN (British physician, 1773-1846)

Bostock catarrh. Synonyms: *allergic rhinitis, autumnal catarrh, catarrhus estivus, hay asthma, hay fever, pollenosis, vasomotor rhinitis.*

A seasonal (hay fever) or non-seasonal (perennial) form of hypersensitivity marked by rhinitis, conjunctivitis, and, often, asthmatic symptoms, brought on by exposure to specific antigens, such as pollen and fungi. Histamine and other mediators are released after contact with the allergen, leading to nasal congestion, rhinorrhea, sneezing, lacrimation, and itching of the nose, pharynx, and eyes. Large numbers of eosinophils are found in nasal secretions. The condition is considered to be a type IV (IgE-mediated) allergic reaction.

Bostock, J. Case of a periodical affection of the eyes and chest. *Med. Chir. Tr., London,* 1819, 10:161-5.

BOSVIEL, J. (French physician)

Bosviel syndrome. Synonyms: *Bosviel-Martin syndrome, Martin syndrome, apoplexia uvulae, staphylohematoma.*

Hemorrhage from a ruptured uvular hematoma.

Bosviel, J. Apoplexie d'un pilier amygdalien. *Ann. Mal. Oreil. Lar.*, 1911, p. 125-6. Martin, A. Über das Staphylhaematoma. *Neue Med. Chir. Ztg.*, 1846, p. 225-7.

Bosviel-Martin syndrome. See *Bosviel syndrome.*

BOTCAZO

Dide-Botcazo syndrome. See *under Dide.*

BOTKIN, SERGEI PETROVICH (Russian physician, 1832-1889)

Botkin disease. Synonyms: *anicteric hepatitis, catarrhal jaundice, epidemic hepatitis, epidemic jaundice, hepatitis A, hepatitis epidemica, infectious hepatitis, infective hepatitis, virus A hepatitis.*

A viral disease usually transmitted by a fecal-oral route. Epidemics occur most commonly in institutions that house small children, owing to ingestion of contaminated beverages and food, such as drinking water, milk, or shellfish; poor hygienic conditions being the contributing factor. It is characterized by hepatitis with or without jaundice (**anicteric hepatitis**) and liver necrosis. In young patients, the course is usually mild and often unaccompanied by jaundice; in older persons, it has frequently an acute or subacute course and is complicated by jaundice and liver necrosis.

Botkina bolezn'. *Bol'shaia meditsinskaia entsiklopediia.* Moskva. 1958, Vol. 4, pp. 239-58.

bottle mouth caries. See *baby bottle syndrome.*

BOU. See *branchio-otoureteral syndrome.*

bouba. See *Charlouis disease.*

BOUCHARD, CHARLES JACQUES (French physician, 1837-1915)

Bouchard disease (1). Insufficiency of the gastric muscles resulting from dilation of the stomach.

Bouchard. Du role pathogénique de la dilatation de l'estomas et des relations cliniques de cette maladie avec divers accidents morbides. *Bull. Soc. Méd. Hôp., Paris,* 1884, 1:226-40.

Bouchard disease (2). See *Heberden nodes.*

Heberden-Bouchard disease. See *Heberden nodes.*

BOUILLAUD, JEAN BAPTISTE (French physician, 1796-1881)

Bouillaud disease. Synonyms: *Sokolskii-Bouillaud disease, Sokolsky-Bouillaud disease, acute articular rheumatism, acute rheumatic polyarthritis, articular rheumatism, endocarditis rheumatica, rheumapyra, rheumatismus cordis, rheumarthritis, rheumatic fever, rheumatopyra.*

A systemic inflammatory disease, considered to be a collagen disease, characterized by acute attacks of fever spaced by remissions. The symptoms include carditis, chorea, subacute nodules, and erythema marginatum. Other findings include arthralgia, elevated erythrocyte sedimentation rate, elevated C-reactive protein, leukocytosis, and prolonged P-R interval on the electrocardiogram. Onset may follow scarlet fever, streptococcal sore throat, and tonsillitis, infection with the group A streptococci being considered the principal etiological factor. Serious complications include cardiac lesions characterized by Aschoff bodies, a collection of cells and leukocytes in the interstitial tissue, fibrosis, inflammatory reaction, thickening of the mural endocardium, and valvulitis often associated with fibrous scarring and stenosis. Subcutaneous nodules (large fibroid areas), fibrosis and scarring of the synovia, joint capsules, tendons, fasciae, and muscle sheaths; acute inflammatory exudative changes in the blood vessels; and pneumonia may be associated.

Bouillaud, B. *Traité clinique du rheumatisme articulaire.* Paris, 1832. Sokolskii, G. I. O revmatizme myshechnoi tkani serdtsa (rheumatismus cordis). *Uchen. Zap. Imp. Mosk. Univ.*, 1838, No. 12:568.

Sokolskii-Bouillaud disease. See *Bouillaud disease.*

Sokolsky-Bouillaud disease. See *Bouillaud disease.*

BOURNEVILLE, DESIRE MAGLOIRE (French physician, 1840-1909)

Bourneville disease. See *Bourneville-Pringle syndrome.*

Bourneville syndrome. See *Bourneville-Pringle syndrome.*

Bourneville-Brissaud disease. See *Bourneville-Pringle syndrome.*

Bourneville-Pringle syndrome. Synonyms: *Bourneville disease, Bourneville syndrome, Bourneville-Brissaud disease, Pringle disease, adenoma sebaceum, epiploia, neurinomatosis centralis, neurinomatosis universalis, neurospongioblastosis diffusa, phacomatosis, sclerosis tuberosa, spongioblastosis circumscripta, tuberose sclerosis, tuberous sclerosis.*

A triad of epilepsy, mental retardation, and cutaneous angiofibromas transmitted as an autosomal dominant trait with variable expressivity. Cutaneous angiofibromas (adenoma sebaceum) of the face become evident in childhood, mainly over the nose, cheeks, nasolabial furrows, and chin, and spread at puberty. Soft polypoid fibromatous masses over the dorsal area of the trunk and scalp and beneath the nails (subungual fibromas), and less commonly, round, flat plaques (shagreen patches) in the lumbar areas are associated. Characteristic leukodermic areas and café-au-lait spots are usually present. Smooth, hard, potato-like masses (tuberous sclerosis), located on the brain tissue, are the principal lesions of the central nervous system. Intracranial calcifications are often associated. Ocular manifestations usually consist of retinal tumors (phacomas) and epicanthus. Thickened calvaria, exostoses of the frontal bone, and increased density of the cranium occur in most cases. The phalanges may show cyst-like foci and periosteal reaction.

Bourneville, D. M. Sclérose tubéreuse des circonvolutions cérébrales, idiotie et epilepsie hemiplegique. *Arch. Neur., Paris*, 1880, 1:81-91. Pringle, J. J. A case of congenital adenoma sebaceum. *Brit. J. Derm.*, 1890, 2:1-14.

BOUVERET, LEON (French physician, 1850-1926)

Bouveret syndrome (1). Synonyms: *gallstone ileus, gastric outlet syndrome.*

Gastric outlet obstruction caused by a large gallstone impacted in the duodenal bulb.

Nielsen, S. M., & Nielsen, P. T. Gastric retention caused by gallstones (Bouveret's syndrome). *Acta Chir. Scand.*, 1983, 149:207-8.

Bouveret syndrome (2). Synonyms: *Bouveret-Hoffmann syndrome, essential paroxysmal tachycardia, paroxysmal atrial tachycardia, paroxysmal junctional tachycardia, paroxysmal supraventricular tachycardia (PSVT).*

An excessively rapid action of the heart that is typically abrupt in onset and termination. The condition sometimes complicates various heart diseases, occasionally occurring in apparently normal persons. Palpitations and, less frequently, light-headedness, shortness of breath, weakness, and polyuria are the typical symptoms.

Bouveret, L. De la tachycardie essentielle paroxystique. *Rev. Méd., Paris*, 1889, 9:753-93; 837-55.

Bouveret-Hoffmann syndrome. See *Bouveret syndrome (2).*

BOUVRAIN, Y. (French physician)

Sézary-Bouvrain syndrome. See *Sézary syndrome.*

bowel bypass syndrome. Synonyms: *bowel-associated dermatosis-arthritis syndrome, bowel bypass syndrome without bowel bypass, dermato-arthritis syndrome, intestinal bypass dermatosis-arthritis syndrome.*

An episodic illness that occurs in as many as 20 percent of patients who have undergone a jejunoileal bypass operation for morbid obesity. Onset of symptoms may range from a few days to several years after the operation. The symptoms usually consist of a flu-like illness, fever, chills, malaise, pain in the muscles, tendinitis, polyarthralgia, and inflammatory skin eruption on the extremities and trunk. The cutaneous lesions begin as erythematous macules, about 2 to 4 mm in diameter, and progress through an urticarial stage to become vesiculopapular eruption. Erythema nodosum may occur on the legs. The illness lasts 2 to 6 days and then recurs in about 1 to 6 weeks. Bacterial overgrowth in a blind loop of the bowel is believed to produce immune complexes which, in turn, enter the circulation and cause this syndrome. A similar condition may occur in association with various gastrointestinal diseases, without jejunoileal bypass, hence the term **bowel bypass syndrome without bowel bypass**.

Shagrin, J. W., *et al.* Polyarthritis in obese patients with intestinal bypass. *Ann. Intern. Med.*, 1971, 75:377-80. Ely, P. H. The bowel bypass syndrome: A response to bacterial peptidoglycans. *Am. J. Acad. Dermatol.*, 1980, 2:473-87. Jorizzo, J. L., *et al.* Bowel-bypass syndrome without bowel bypass: Bowel-associated dermatosis-arthritis syndrome. *Arch. Intern. Med.*, 1983, 143:457-61.

bowel bypass syndrome without bowel bypass. See *under bowel bypass syndrome.*

bowel-associated dermatosis-arthritis syndrome. See *bowel bypass syndrome.*

BOWEN, JOHN TEMPLETON (American physician, 1857-1941)

Bowen dermatosis. See *Bowen disease.*

Bowen disease. Synonyms: *Bowen dermatosis, Bowen epithelioma, Bowen-Darier disease, dermatosis precancerosa, precancerous dermatitis.*

A cutaneous and mucosal neoplastic lesion considered by some writers as being a premalignant tumor and by others a laterally spreading, superficial, intraepithelial carcinoma. Typically, it appears as a white, red, and ulcerated, or a leukoplakic lesion, or less commonly, a velvety or granular tumor. The floor of the mouth, tongue, lips, and buccal mucosa are the most commonly affected sites. The condition occurs more frequently in males than in females. Queyrat's erythroplasia and Bowen's disease are considered to be variants of carcinoma in situ.

Bowen, J. T. Precancerous dermatoses: A study of 2 cases of chronic atypical epithelial prolifertion. *J. Cutan. Dis.*, 1912, 30:241:55.

Bowen epithelioma. See *Bowen disease.*

Bowen-Darier disease. See *Bowen disease.*

BOWEN, PETER

Bowen Hutterite syndrome. See *Bowen-Conradi syndrome.*

Bowen-Conradi syndrome. Synonym: *Bowen Hutterite syndrome.*

A highly lethal syndrome, transmitted as an autosomal recessive trait, characterized by proportionate intrauterine growth retardation, cryptorchidism, microcephaly, micrognathia, a prominant nose, rocker-bottom feet, limited joint movement, clinodactyly, cloudy corneae, abnormal tubulation of the long bones, and failure to thrive. Most patients die in the first year of life. First cases of this syndrome were reported in the Hutterites, a highly inbred religious isolate that practices communal farming in several Midwestern states and Canadian prairie provinces.

Bowen, P., & Conradi, G. J. Syndrome of skeletal and genitourinary anomalies with unusual facies and failure to thrive in Hutterite sibs. *Birth Defects*, 1976, 12(6):101-8.

bowler's finger syndrome. Synonym: *bowler's thumb.*

A stress disorder seen in bowlers, characterized by a soft tissue mass at the base of the thumb web and painful, stiff interphalangeal joints of the first, third, and fourth fingers.

Howell, A. E., & Leach, R. E. Bowler's thumb-perineural fibrosis of the digital nerve. *J. Bone Joint Surg.*, 1970, 52(A):379-81.

bowler's thumb. See *bowler's finger syndrome.*

boxer's fracture. See *Bennett fracture, under Bennett, Edward Hallaran.*

BOYD, JULIAN DEIGH (American physician, born 1894)

Boyd-Stearns syndrome. A Fanconi-like syndrome characterized by rickets that begins during infancy, dwarfism, hypophosphatemia that is resistant to the usual antirachitic therapy, osteoporosis, and malnutrition, associated with various metabolic disorders, including glycosuria, acidosis, albuminuria, and hypochloremia. Polyuria and polydipsia (with urine of normal specific gravity) and kidney lesions may be present.

Boyd, J. D. & Stearns, G. Late rickets resembling the Fanconi syndrome. *Am. J. Dis. Child.*, 1941, 61:1012-22.

BOYER, ALEXIS, DE (French surgeon, 1757-1833)

Boyer cyst. A painless and gradual englargement of the subhyoid bursa.

Boyer, A., de. *Traité complet d'anatomie, ou description de toutes les parties du corps humain. Paris,* Migneret, 1803-9.

BOZZOLO, CAMILLO (Italian physician, 1845-1920)

Kahler-Bozzolo disease. See *Kahler disease.*

BP. See ***B**ell **p**alsy, under Bell, Sir Charles.*

BPD (bronchopulmonary dysplasia). See *Wilson-Mikity syndrome, under Wilson, Miriam Geisendorfer, and see respirator lung syndrome*

BPEI (blepharophimosis-ptosis-epicanthus inversus) syndrome. See *blepharoptosis-blepharophimosis-epicanthus inversus-telecanthus syndrome.*

BPM (Bamberger-Pierre Marie) syndrome. See *Marie-Bamberger syndrome, under Marie, Pierre.*

BPV. See ***b**enign **p**aroxysmal **v**ertigo syndrome.*

BRA (bilateral renal agenesis) syndrome. See *Potter syndrome (1), under Potter, Edith Louise.*

brachial arteritis. See *aortic arch syndrome.*

brachial paresthesia during sleep. See *Wartenberg disease (1).*

brachialgia paresthetica. See *Wartenberg disease (1).*

brachialgia paresthetica nocturna. See *Barré-Lieou syndrome, and see Wartenberg disease (1).*

brachialgia statica paresthetica. See *Wartenberg disease (1).*

brachiocephalic arteritis. See *aortic arch syndrome.*

BRACHMANN, W. (German physician)

Brachmann-Cornelia de Lange (BCDL) syndrome. See *de Lange syndrome (1), under Lange, Cornelia, de.*

Brachmann-de Lange syndrome. See *de Lange syndrome (1), under Lange, Cornelia, de.*

brachycamptodactyly syndrome. Synonym: *camptobrachydactyly.*

Brachydactyly involving both hands and feet, associated with flexion contractures of the fingers. Occasional anomalies include syndactyly, polydactyly, septate vagina, and urinary incontinence. The syndrome is transmitted as an autosomal dominant trait with variable expressivity and complete penetrance.

Edwards, J. A., & Gale, R. P. Camptobrachydactyly: A new autosomal dominant trait with two probable homozygotes. *Am. J. Hum. Genet.*, 1972, 24:464-74.

brachydactyly A-1. Synonyms: *Bell brachydactyly A-1, Farabee brachydactyly.*

A type of brachydactyly that is confined mainly to the middle phalanges, which may be fused to the terminal phalanges, although in severe cases all of the fingers and toes may be involved. Shortening of the proximal phalanges of the thumb and of the great toe may be associated. The disorder is transmitted as an autosomal dominant trait.

Farabee, W. C. *Hereditary and sexual influence in meristic variation. A study of digital malformations in man.* Harvard University Thesis, 1903. Bell, J. On brachydactyly and symphalangism. In: Penrose, L. S., ed. *The treasury of human inheritance.* University Press, Cambridge, 1951, 5(pt 1):1-31.

brachydactyly A-2. Synonyms: *Bell brachydactyly A-2, Mohr-Wriedt brachydactyly, brachymesophalangy 2, delta phalanx.*

A rare condition characterized by a short rudimentary middle phalanx of the second finger, which may be triangular (hence the synonym **delta phalanx**), resulting in radial deviation. Syndactyly is sometimes associated. The disorder is transmitted as an autosomal dominant trait.

Mohr, O. L., & Wriedt, C. *A new type of hereditary brachyphalangy in man.* Carnegie Inst. of Washington (Publication 295). Washington, 1919, pp. 5-64. Bell, J. On brachydactyly and symphalangism. In: Penrose, L. S., ed. *The treasury of human inheritance.* University Press, Cambridge, 1951, 5(pt 1):1-31.

brachydactyly A-3. Synonyms: *Bell brachydactyly 3, brachydactyly-clinodactyly syndrome, brachymesophalangy 5, clinomicrodactyly, crooked little fingers.*

The most common form of brachydactyly, characterized by shortening of the middle phalanx of the fifth finger. Rhomboid shape of the rudimentary middle phalanx results in radial curvature of the fifth finger or clinodactly. The disorder is inherited as an autosomal dominant trait with 50 to 60 percent penetrance.

Birkbeck, J. A. The origin of clinodactyly and brachymesophalangy of the fifth finger. *Aust. Paediad. J.*, 1975, 11:218-24. Bell, J. On brachydactyly and symphalangism. In: Penrose, L. S., ed. *The treasury of human inheritance.* University Press, Cambridge, 1951, 5(pt 1):1-31.

brachydactyly A-4. Synonym: *Temtamy brachydactyly.*

Brachymesophalangy affecting mainly the second and fifth digits with the fourth digit, when affected, showing an abnormally shaped middle phalanx leading to radial deviation of the distal phalanx. Absence of the middle phalanges of the lateral four toes is usually associated. The disorder is transmitted as an autosomal dominant trait.

Temtamy, S. A. *Genetic factors in hand malformations.* Johns Hopkins University Thesis, 1966.

brachydactyly A-5. Absence of middle phalanges associated with nail dysplasia and duplication of the terminal phalanx of the thumb. The disorder is transmitted as an autosomal dominant trait.

Bass, H. N. Familial absence of middle phalanges with new dysplasia: A new syndrome. *Pediatrics*, 1968, 42:318-23.

brachydactyly B. Synonyms: *Bell brachydactyly B, apical dystrophy.*

A type brachydactyly, characterized by rudimentary or absent terminal phalanges of fingers and toes, transmitted as an autosomal dominant trait.

MacArthur, J. W., & McCullough, E. Apical dystrophy: An inherited defect of hands and feet. *Hum. Biol.* 1932, 4:179-207. Bell, J. On brachydactyly and symphalangism. In: Penrose, L. S., ed. *The treasury of human inheritance.* University Press, Cambridge, 1951, 5(pt 1):1-31.

brachydactyly C. Synonym: *Bell brachydactyly C.*

A type of brachydactyly, in which the anomaly varies from one finger to another, the distinguishing feature being a defect of the middle and proximal phalanges of some digits, associated with relatively normal terminal phalanges. The thumbs may be normal. The disorder is transmitted as an autosomal dominant trait.

Bell, J. On brachydactyly and symphalangism. In: Penrose, L. S., ed. *The treasury of human inheritance.* University Press, Cambridge, 1951, 5(pt 1):1-31.

brachydactyly D. Synonyms: *Bell brachydactyly D, murderer's thumb, petter's thumb, stub thumb.*

Brachydactyly characterized by a short and broad distal phalanx of the thumb. Shortness of the fourth toe and fourth and fifth metacarpals (brachydactyly E) may be associated. The disorder is transmitted as an autosomal dominant trait with incomplete penetrance.

Breitenbecher, J. K. Hereditary shortness of thumbs. *J. Hered.*, 1923, 14:15-22. Bell, J. On brachydactyly and symphalangism. In: Penrose. L. S., ed. *The treasury of human inheritance.* University Press, Cambridge, 1951, 5(pt 1):1-31.

brachydactyly E. Synonym: *Bell brachydactyly E.*

A type in which the third, fourth, and fifth metacarpals and metatarsals are shortened.

Bell, J. On brachydactyly and symphalangism. In: Penrose, L. S., ed. *The treasure of human inheritance.* University Press, Cambridge, 1951, 5(pt 1):1-31.

brachydactyly type 6. See *Osebold-Remondini syndrome.*

brachydactyly-clinodactyly syndrome. See *brachydactyly A-3.*

brachydactyly-nystagmus-cerebellar ataxia syndrome. See *Biemond syndrome (1).*

brachydactyly-spherophakia syndrome. See *Weill-Marchesani syndrome, under Weill, G.*

brachymesodactylia-nail dysplasia syndrome. See *Bass syndrome.*

brachymesomelia-renal syndrome. A syndrome of upper arm mesomelia, glomerulocystic renal dysplasia, craniofacial abnormalities (oxobrachycephaly without molding, depressed nasal bridge, small pelpebral fissures with complete medial epicanthal folds, micrognathia, and low-set ears with folded transverse upper helices and prominent lobules), corneal opacities, a simian line, and possible heart defect. The syndrome, transmitted as an autosomal dominant trait, was originally reported in a Japanese infant who died in the newborn period.

Langer, L. O., *et al.* Brachymesomelia-renal syndrome. *Am. J. Med. Genet.*, 1983, 15:57-65.

brachymesophalangy 2. See *brachydactyly A-2.*

brachymesophalangy 5. See *brachydactyly A-3.*

brachymetacarpalia-cataract-mesiodens syndrome. See *Nance-Horan syndrome.*

brachymorphism and ectopia lentis syndrome. See *Weill-Marchesani syndrome, under Weill, Georges.*

BRADBURY, SAMUEL (American physician)

Bradbury-Eggleston syndrome. Synonyms: *chronic idiopathic orthostatic hypotension, idiopathic orthostatic hypotension (IOH), primary autonomic insufficiency.*

A disorder, usually occurring in older males in the summer months during early morning hours, characterized by postural hypotension associated with dizziness, visual disturbances, and presyncope or syncope on standing up or following physical exertion. Slow unchanging pulse rate, inability to perspire, and lowered basal metabolism rate are usually associated. The syndrome is due primarily to impaired peripheral vasoconstriction, acceleration of heart rate and maintenance of cardiac output in response to the assumption of the upright position. Depletion of the sympathetic nerve endings and their inability to take up norepinephrine is believed to be the cause.

Bradbury, S., & Eggleston, C. Postural hypotension. A report of three cases. *Am. Heart J.*, 1925, 1:73-86.

BRADLEY, W. H. (British physician)

Bradley disease. See *Spencer disease.*

BRADSHAW, THOMAS ROBERT (British, physician, 1857-1927)

Bradshaw albumosuria. See *Bence Jones proteinuria.*

brady-tachy syndrome. See *bradycardia-tachycardia syndrome.*

bradycardia-hypotension syndrome. Toxic reactions to therapeutic doses of nitroglycerin, consisting of bradycardia and hypotension.

ssNoer, J. Poisonous symptoms from nitroglycerin. *Ther. Gaz.*, 1887, 3:459. Sprague, H. B., & White, P. D. Nitroglycerin collapse-a potential danger in therapy. Report of three cases. *Med. Clin N. Am.*, 1933, 16:895-8. Come, P. C., & Pitt, B. Nitroglycerin-induced severe hypotension and bradycardia in patients with acute myocardial infarction. *Circulation,* 1976, 54:624-8.

bradycardia-tachycardia syndrome. Synonyms: *Laslett syndrome, Short syndrome, alternating bradycardia and tachycardia syndrome, brady-tachy syndrome, tachycardia-bradycardia syndrome.*

A form of the sick sinus syndrome (q.v.) characterized by recurrent episodes of supraventricular tachyarrhythmias in patients with sinus bradycardia or other bradyarrhythmias. The disorder is a complication of some forms of thromboembolism and myocardial infarction.

Laslett, E. E. Syncopal attacks, associated with prolonged arrest of the whole heart. *Q. J. Med.*, 1909, 2:347-55. Short, D. S. The syndrome of alternating bradycardia and tachycardia. *Brit. Heart J.*, 1954, 16:208-14.

BRAHAM, R. L. (Canadian dentist)

Braham syndrome. A syndrome of progeroid skin appearance, dilated veins, open large anterior fontanels, increased density of the bones, large ears, syndactyly of the fingers and toes with occasional symphalangism, hyperflexible joints, atresia of the choanae, central notching of the vertebrae, enamel hypoplasia, thickened clavicles, ribs, and diaphyses of the long bones, and increased density of the cranium and mandible. See also *Camurati-Engelmann syndrome.*

Braham, R. L. Multiple congenital abnormalities with diaphyseal dysplasia (Camurati-Engelmann's syndrome). Report of a case. *Oral Surg.*, 1969, 27:20-6.

BRAHMACHARI, UPENDRA NATH (Indian physician)

Brahmachari leishmanoid. Synonym: *dermal leishmanoid.*

A cutaneous form of leishmaniasis characterized by multiple infections of the skin by *Leishmania donovani* and observed in individuals who had previously suffered from kala-azar and were subsequently cured.

Brahmachari, U. N. Chemotherapy of antimonial compounds in kala-azar infection; dermal leishmanoid with positive flagellate culture from the peripheral blood. *Cal-*

cutta Med. J., 1925-27, 21:401-4.

BRAID, JAMES (British physician, 1795-1860)

Braid strabismus. Induction of hypnosis by turning the eyes simultaneously upward and inward.

Braid, J. *Observations on trance; or human hypernation.* London, Churchill, 1850.

BRAILSFORD, JAMES FREDERIC (British radiologist)

Brailsford-Bársony-Polgár syndrome. See *Bársony-Polgár syndrome (1).*

Morquio-Brailsford syndrome. See *mucopolysaccharidosis IV-A.*

brain fag (BF) syndrome. A complex of symptoms, originally reported among students, teachers, and other white collar workers in Africa. The symptoms include inability to concentrate or retain studied information, paresthesias, headache and other forms of poorly defined pain, unhappy facial expression, irritability, agitation, nervousness, sleep disorders, perspiration, tremor, loss of weight, respiratory problems, sensation disorders, blurring of vision, and tinnitus. The syndrome is considered by some authors as a form of anxiety neurosis or depressive neurosis.

Prince, R. H. The brain fag syndrome in Nigerian students. *J. Ment. Sc.*, 1960, 106:559-70.

brain stem encephalitis. See *Bickerstaff encephalitis.*

BRALEY, A. E. (American ophthalmologist)

polymorphic macular degeneration of Braley. See *Best macular degeneration.*

branched chain alpha-keto acid dehydrogenase deficiency (BCKD). See *maple syrup urine disease.*

branched chain ketoaciduria. See *maple syrup urine disease.*

brancher deficiency. See *glycogen storage disease IV.*

branchial arches syndrome. See *oculo-auriculovertebral dysplasia.*

branchio-otorenal (BOR) syndrome. Synonym: *branchio-otorenal dysplasia.*

An autosomal dominant disorder manifested by various combinations of preauricular pits, branchial fistulae or cysts, lacrimal duct stenosis, hearing loss, structural defects of the outer, middle, or inner ear, and renal dysplasia. Associated defects include asthenic habitus, long narrow facies, constricted palate, deep overbite, and myopia. Hearing loss may be due to Mondini type cochlear defect and stapes fixation.

Melnick, M., *et al.* Autosomal dominant branchiootorenal dysplasia. *Birth Defects*, 1975, 11(5):121-8.

branchio-otorenal dysplasia. See *branchio-otorenal syndrome.*

branchio-otoureteral syndrome (BOU, BOUU). A familial syndrome, transmitted as an autosomal dominant trait, characterized by sensorineural hearing loss, preauricular pits or tags, and duplication of the ureters or bifid renal pelvices.

Fraser, F. C., *et al.* Autosomal dominant duplication of the renal collecting system, hearing loss, and external ear anomalies: A new syndrome? *Am. J. Med. Genet.*, 1983, 14:473-8.

branchioskeletogenital (BSG) syndrome. See *Elsahy-Waters syndrome.*

BRANDT, THORE EDVARD (Swedish dermatologist, born 1901)

Brandt syndrome. See *acrodermatitis enteropathica.*

BRAS, GERRIT (Indonesian physician)

Stuart-Bras disease. See *under Stuart, Kenneth Lamont.*

BRAUER

Brauer disease. See *Fischer syndrome, under Fischer, Heinrich F.*

Buschke-Fischer-Brauer syndrome. See *Fischer syndrome, under Fischer, Heinrich F.*

BRAUER, AUGUST (German physician, born 1883)

Brauer syndrome. Synonyms: *focal facial dermal dysplasia, hereditary symmetrical aplastic nevi of the temples.*

Hereditary focal pigmented nevi of the forehead and chin, associated with either the absence of eyelashes or double rows of eyelashes and aplasia of the sweat glands in the lesions, transmitted as an autosomal dominant trait.

Brauer, A. Hereditärer symmetrischer systematisierter Naevus aplasticus bei 38 Personen. *Derm. Wschr.*, 1929, 89:1163-8.

Brauer syndrome. See *Unna-Thost syndrome, under Unna, Paul Gerson.*

BRAUN, FREDERICK C., JR. (American physician)

Braun-Bayer syndrome. A familial syndrome, probably transmitted as an autosomal recessive or X-linked dominant trait, characterized by nephrosis, deafness, urinary tract anomalies, bifid uvula, and brachytelephalangy. Digital defects consist of short and bifid distal phalanges of thumbs and great toes. Ureterovesical obstruction with nonfunctional kidney and duplication of the renal pelvis are the urinary anomalies. Deafness is conductive, without malformations of the middle ear.

Braun, F. C., Jr., & Bayer, J. F. Familial nephrosis associated with deafness and congenital urinary tract anomalies in siblings. *J. Pediat.*, 1962, 60:33-41.

BRAUN-FALCO, OTTO (German physician)

Marghescu and Braun-Falco syndrome. See *under Marghescu.*

BRAVAIS, LOUIS F. (French physician)

Bravais-Jackson epilepsy. See *Jackson epilepsy, under Jackson, John Huglings.*

Brazilian blastomycosis. See *Lutz-Splendore-de Almeida syndrome, under Lutz, Adolfo.*

Brazilian trypanosomiasis. See *Chagas disease.*

BRBN. See ***b**lue **r**ubber **b**leb **n**evus syndrome.*

BRBNS. See ***b**lue **r**ubber **b**leb **n**evus **s**yndrome.*

breakdance back syndrome. Low back pain with difficulty in bending due to injuries sustained while break dancing.

Norman, R. A., & Grodin, M. A. Injuries from break dancing. *Am. Fam. Physician,* 1984, 30(4):109-12.

breaststroke swimmer's knee syndrome. Synonym: *breaststroker's knee.*

An overuse syndrome (q.v.) in breaststroke swimmers, characterized by medial pain in the knee joint.

Kennedy, J. C., & Hawkins, R. J. Breaststroker's knee. *Phys. Sportsmed.*, 1974, 2:33-8.

breaststroker's knee. See *breaststroke swimmer's knee syndrome.*

BREDA, ACHILLE (Padua physician, 1850-1933)

Breda disease. See *Charlouis disease.*

BREEN, WILLIAM (American physician)

Cross-McKusick-Breen syndrome. See *Cross syndrome.*

BREISKY, AUGUST (German physician, 1832-1889)

Breisky disease. Synonyms: *kraurosis vulvae, leukokraurosis.*

An atrophic, progressive disease of the vulva affecting women of advanced age or younger ones who have undergone artificial menopause. Vulvar edema is an early symptom, followed by atrophy of the labia minora, clitoris, frenulum, and labia majora stenosis of the vaginal orifice. In advanced stages, the perineum and the gluteal area may be involved, and leukoplakia may also occur. Hormonal imbalance, associated with menopause, chronic irritation, and nutritional deficiency, especially lack of vitamin A, have been suspected of being the etiologic factors.

Breisky, A. Die Krankheiten der Vagina. *Hand. Allg. Spec. Chir.*, 1879, 4:1-256.

BRENNEMANN, JOSEPH (American physician, 1872-1944)

Brennemann syndrome. Synonyms: *acute mesenteric lymphadenitis syndrome, mesenteric lymphadenitis-upper respiratory tract infection syndrome.*

A pathological condition affecting young children, characterized by mesenteric and retroperitoneal lymphadenitis with abdominal pain, fever, vomiting, and nausea, following upper respiratory tract infection, usually of the throat.

Brennemann, J. "The abdominal pain of throat infection in children" and appendicitis. *JAMA*, 1927, 89:2183-6.

BRENNER, FRITZ (German physician, born 1877)

Brenner tumor. Synonyms: *Orthmann tumor, brenneroma, oophoroma folliculare.*

A rarely malignant ovarian tumor of follicular origin, usually occurring in elderly women. The tumors are characterized by the presence of islands of stratified epithelial cells. Lumina in some foci may be filled with a globular mass resembling degenerating ova in follicles undergoing atresia.

Brenner, F. Das Oophoroma folliculare. *Frankf. Zschr. Path.*, 1907, 1:150-71. Orthmann, E. G. Über die Entstehungsweisen der Sacrosalpingen und Tubo-Ovarialcysten. *Arch. Path. Anat., Berlin,* 1899, 155:220-34.

brenneroma. See *Brenner tumor.*

BRENTANO

Brentano syndrome. A disorder of muscle glycogen metabolism during pregnancy, with depletion of liver glycogen and creatinuria, said to have been first reported by Brentano.

BRESCHET

Breschet-Gorham syndrome. See *Gorham syndrome.*

BRET, J. (French physician)

Bret syndrome. See *Swyer-James syndrome, under Swyer, Paul Robert.*

BRETONNEAU, PIERRE FIDELE (French physician, 1778-1862)

Bretonneau angina. See *Bretonneau disease.*

Bretonneau disease. Synonyms: *Bretonneau angina, diphtheria, diphtherial tonsillitis, diphtheric croup, diphtheritis, malignant angina.*

An acute, contagious disease usually affecting young children, transmitted by direct contact and caused by the bacillus *Corynebacterium diphtheriae.* After an incubation period of 2 to 5 days, the symptoms include fever, prostration, myocarditis, headache, vomiting, and restlessness. Diphtheritic membranes, which are patchy, grayish, thick pseudomembranes, usually of the tonsils, present the principal symptom. Bronchopneumonia, paralysis, and cardiac failure may be associated. Polymorphonuclear leukocytosis is the chief hematological symptom. See also *Epstein syndrome (pseudodiphtheria).*

Bretonneau, P. F. *Des inflammations spéciales du tissue muqueux, et en particulier de la diphtherite, ou inflammation pelliculaire.* Paris, Crevot, 1826.

BREUS, CARL (Austrian physician, 1852-1914)

Breus mole. Synonyms: *hematomole, subchorial hematoma mole, subchorial thrombohematoma.*

A malformation of the ovum consisting of a tuberous subchorional hematoma of the decidua.

Breus, C. *Das tuberöse subchoriale Hämatom der Decidua; eine typische Form bei Molenschwangershaft.* Leipzig, Deuticke, 1892.

BRIC (benign recurrent intrahepatic cholestasis). See *Summerskill-Walshe syndrome.*

BRIDGES, ROBERT A. (American physician)

Bridges-Good syndrome. See *chronic granulomatous disease of childhood.*

BRIGHT, RICHARD (British physician, 1789-1858)

Bright disease. A group of nonsuppurative inflammatory or degenerative kidney diseases characterized by proteinuria and hematuria and sometimes by edema, hypertension, and nitrogen retention.

Bright. Cases and observations illustrative of renal disease accompanied with the secretion of albuminous urine. *Guy's Hosp. Rep., London,* 1836, 1338-400.

BRILL, NATHAN EDWIN (American physician, 1860-1925)

Brill disease. Synonyms: *Brill-Zinsser disease, recrudescent typhus.*

Recrudescence in a patient with a history of typhus. The disease is caused by the bacterium *Rickettsia prowazekii* which is indistinguishable from strains causing primary epidemic typhus. According to Zinsser, rickettsiae remain viable in the body of the host and recrudescence can occur years after the initial illness.

Brill, N. E. An acute infectious disease of unknown origin. A clinical study based on 221 cases. *Am. J. M. Sc.*, 1910, 139:484-502. Zinsser, M. Rats, lice and history. *Boston Atlantic Monthly Press,* 1935.

Brill-Baehr-Rosenthal disease. See *Brill-Symmers syndrome.*

Brill-Symmers syndrome. Synonyms: *Brill-Baehr-Rosenthal disease, Symmers syndrome, follicular lymphadenopathy with splenomegaly, follicular lymphoma, follicular reticulosis, generalized follicle hyperplasia of lymph nodes and spleen, giant follicle hyperplasia, giant follicle lymphoma, giant follicle lymphosarcoma, giant follicular lymphadenopathy, giant follicular lymphoblastoma, lyphoblastoma gigantofollicularis, macrofollicular lymphoblastoma.*

A lymphoma characterized by the combined proliferation of lymphoblasts and reticulum cells within lymphoid follicles, resulting in an increase in the number and size of germinal follicles. The course is initially benign but there is often malignant transformation. It may occur at any age (middle-aged individuals being most commonly affected), beginning insidiously with painless enlargement of superficial lymph nodes which are followed by splenomegaly, fever, debility, weight loss, and anemia.

Brill, N. E., Baehr, G., & Rosenthal, N. Generalized giant lymph follicle hyperplasia of lymph nodes and spleen. A hitherto undescribed type. *JAMA,* 1925, 84:668-71. Symmers, D. Follicular lymphadenopathy with splenomegaly. A newly recognized disease of the lymphatic system. *Arch. Path., Chicago,* 1927, 3:816-20.

Brill-Zinsser disease. See *Brill disease.*
Lederer-Brill syndrome. See Lederer anemia.

BRINTON, WILLIAM (British physician, 1823-1867)
Brinton disease. Synonyms: *cirrhosis of the stomach, cirrhotic gastritis, fibromatosis ventriculi, gastric sclerosis, hypertrophic gastritis, leather bottle stomach, linitis gastrica.*

Hypertrophy and carcinomatous changes of the mucous and submucous tissues of the stomach with thickening and hardening of the gastric wall, which give it the appearance of a leather bottle.

Brinton, W. Cirrhotic inflammation of plastic linitis of the stomach-suppurative linitis-tumours-hypertrophy-atrophy-dilatation from obstruction, destruction, injury, paralysis-secondary inflammation. In his: The diseases of the stomach, with an introduction on its anatomy and physiology. London, Churchill, 1859, pp. 310-56.

BRION, ALBERT (physician in Strasburg, born 1876)
Brion-Kayser disease. See *Schottmüller disease.*
BRIQUET, ALBERT (French physician, born 1876)
Briquet gangrene. Pulmonary gangrene in bronchiectasis.

Briquet. Mémoire sur un mode de gangrène du poumon, dépendant de la mortification des extrémités dilatées de bronches. *Arch. Gén. Méd., Paris,* 1841, 11:5-23.

BRIQUET, PIERRE (French physician, 1796-1881)
Briquet ataxia. Hysterical ataxia with anesthesia of the skin and leg muscles.

Briquet, P. *Traité clinique et thérapeutique de l'hystérie.* Paris, Baillière, 1859, p. 297.

Briquet disorder (BD). See *Briquet syndrome (1).*
Briquet syndrome (1). Synonyms: *Briquet disorder (BD), classic hysteria, female hysteria, hysteria, somatization disorder (SD).*

A disorder characterized by multiple somatic complaints, without any apparent physical cause, for which patients seek constant medical attention. The symmptoms usually begin in the teens and, rarely, in the twenties. Associated disorders may include anxiety, depression, antisocial behavior, interpersonal and marital difficulties, and hallucinations. Menstrual disorders are usually the earliest manifestations. Headache, abdominal pain, and other physical symptoms may follow.

Briquet, P. *Traité clinique et thérapeutique de l'hystérie.* Paris, Baillière, 1859. *Diagnostic and statistical manual of mental disorders.* 3rd ed. Washington, American Psychiatric Association, 1987, pp. 261-4.

Briquet syndrome (2). Hysterical paralysis of the diaphragm with aphonia and apnea.

Briquet, P. *Traité clinique et thérapeutique de l'hystérie.* Paris, Baillière, 1859, p. 475.

BRISSAUD, EDOUARD (French physician, 1855-1909)
Bourneville-Brissaud disease. See *Bourneville-Pringle syndrome.*
Brissaud disease. See *Gilles de la Tourette syndrome.*
Brissaud hemicraniosis. See *Brissaud-Sicard syndrome.*
Brissaud infantilism. Synonyms: *Brissaud-Meige syndrome, congenital goiter, congenital hypothyroidism, congenital myxedema, cretinism, dysthyroidal infantilism, infantile myxedema.*

A congenital disease of infants and children, caused by deficiency of thyroid hormone owing to insufficiency or lack of the thyroid gland, characterized by mental deficiency, dwarfism with disproportionately long trunk in relation to legs, epiphyseal dysgenesis, large head, delayed closure of the fontanelles, broad nose with wide flaring nostrils, open mouth, coarse facies, puffy lips, deep husky voice, constipation, and protruding abdomen. Oral symptoms include delayed dentition, delayed shedding of the primary dentition, underdeveloped jaws, especially the mandible, and a tongue enlarged by edema, protruding and leading to malocclusion.

Brissaud, E. L'infantilisme vrai. *Nov. Icon. Salpêtrière,* 1907, 20:1-17.

Brissaud syndrome. See *Brissaud-Sicard syndrome.*
Brissaud-Marie syndrome. Synonyms: *conversion hysteria, conversion reaction, conversion symptoms, hysterical glossolabial paralysis.*

A condition characterized by symptoms such as amnesia, paralysis, blindness, aphonia, and the like, which mimic neurological diseases, occurring without any physical cause.

*Brissaud, E., & Marie, P. De la déviation faciale dans l'hémiplegie hystérique. *Pro Méd.,* 1887, 5:84.

Brissaud-Meige syndrome. See *Brissaud infantilism.*
Brissaud-Sicard syndrome. Synonyms: *Brissaud hemicraniosis, Brissaud syndrome.*

Facial hemispasm associated with contralateral paralysis of the extremities, due to lesions of the pons.

Brissaud, & Sicard, J. A. L'hémispasme facial alterne. *Presse Méd.,* 1908, 16:234-6.

BRISTOWE, JOHN SYER (British physician)
Bristowe syndrome. Synonym: *corpus callosum tumor syndrome.*

A syndrome caused by tumors of the corpus callosum and characterized by ideomotor apraxia, hemiplegia, and mental disorders.

Bristowe, J. S. Cases of tumour of the corpus callosum. *Brain,* 1884, 7:315-33.

brittle bone disease. See *osteogenesis imperfecta syndrome (dominant form).*
brittle cornea syndrome. A triad of red hair, blue sclerae, and brittle corneae. The syndrome is transmitted as an autosomal recessive trait and was reported in Tunisian Jewish families.

Ticho, U., *et al.* Brittle cornea, blue sclera, and red hair syndrome (the brittle cornea syndrome). *Brit. J. Ophth.,* 1980, 64:175-7.

brittle hair syndrome (BIDS). See *hair-brain syndrome.*
brittle hair-mental deficit syndrome. See *Sabinas syndrome.*
broad ligament laceration syndrome. See *Allen-Masters syndrome, under Allen, William Myron.*
broad thumb-mental retardation syndrome. See *Rubinstein-Taybi syndrome.*
BROADBENT, SIR WILLIAM HENRY (British physician, 1835-1907)
Broadbent apoplexy. See *Broadbent syndrome.*
Broadbent syndrome. Synonyms: *Broadbent apoplexy, ingravescent apoplexy.*

Cerebral hemorrhage which begins outside the ventricles but progesses until it breaks into the ventricles.

*Broadbent, W. H. On ingravescent apoplexy. *Med. Chir. Soc., London,* 1876, 8:103-8.

BROBERGER, O.
Broberger-Zetterström syndrome. Idiopathic hypoglycemia in children without an increase in urinary excretion of adrenalin.

Broberger, O., Jungner, I., & Zetterström, R. Studies in spontaneous hypoglycemia in childhood. Failure to increase the epinephrine secretion in insulin-induced hypoglycemia. *J. Pediat.*, 1959, 55:713-9.

BROCA, PIERRE PAUL (French physician, 1824-1880)

Broca aphasia. Synonyms: *aphemia, ataxic aphasia, expressive aphasia, motor aphasia, verbal aphasia.*

Aphasia in which the patient is able to utter only a few simple words and is unable to write, even though he knows what he wishes to say. Lesions of the third frontal convolution and the lower part of the precentral convolution of the dominant hemisphere, with possible involvement of some adjoining areas, are believed to be the cause. Some cases are accompanied by hemiplegia due to independent capsular lesions. Extension of the lesion into the adjacent premotor cortex may cause an associated motor apraxia.

Broca, P. Remarques sur le siège de la faculté de language articulé, suivi d'une observation d'aphémie (perte de la parole). *Bull. Soc. Anat., Paris,* 1861, 36:330-57.

BROCK, D. R. (American physician)

Brock-Suckow polyposis. Obliterative arteriolar sclerosis of the colon associated with multiple colonic mucosal polypoid structures that exhibit ischemic necrosis. In the original description, the patient had diabetes mellitus.

Brock, D. R., & Suckow, E. E. Obliterative arteriolar sclerosis of the colon with focal mucosal necrosis. *Gastroenterology,* 1963, 44:190-4.

BROCK, RUSSEL CLAUDE (British physician, born 1903)

Brock syndrome. See *middle lobe syndrome.*

Brock-Graham syndrome. See *middle lobe syndrome.*

BROCKS, ERIC R. (American scientist)

Townes-Brocks syndrome. See *Townes syndrome.*

BROCQ, ANNE JEAN LOUIS (French dermatologist, 1856-1928)

Brocq disease (1). Synonyms: *Vidal disease, lichen chronicus circumscriptus, lichen simplex chronicus, lichenification, neurodermatitis circumscripta, pruritus with lichenification.*

A skin disease marked by localized and circumscribed patches of thickened skin with lichenification that results from repetitive rubbing and scratching subsequent to pruritogenic stimuli. A papular form may occur in the nuchal area in women and in the anogenital area in both sexes. In the early stages, the skin acquires a dusky pinkish tint and a granular mottled apppearance; later it becomes thickened and furrowed, and scaling is usually present. Histological findings include hyperkertosis, parakeratosis, acanthosis, and papillomatosis, and infiltrations containing lymphocytes and eosinophils may be found in the upper cutis.

Vidal, E. Du lichen (lichen, prurigo, strophulus). *Ann. Derm. Syph., Paris,* 1886, 7:133-54.

Brocq disease (2). Synonyms: *guttate parapsoriasis, parakeratosis psoriasiformis, pityriasis lichenoides chronica.*

A chronic form of pityriasis lichenoides that may begin de novo or evolve from the acute form. It is characterized by finely scaling, slightly raised, circumscribed plaques or small, brown, scaling papules which also appear as a smooth and glistening eruption that may reveal mica-like scales on scratching. The lesions, usually a few millimeters in diameter, are arranged in a retiform pattern. Histopathological findings show psoriasiform epidermal hyperplasia and a sparse infiltrate containing histiocytes and lymphocytes about vessels of the cutis.

Brocq, L. Les parapsoriasis. *Ann. Derm. Syph., Paris,* 1902, 3:313-5; 433-68.

Brocq disease (3). Synonyms: *erythrose peribuccale pigmentaire, erythrosis pigmentosa faciei.*

A combination of erythema and diffuse brownish pigmentation of the perioral region, often extending to other parts of the face; it develops in apparently normal females at puberty and disappears and reappears during the menstrual cycle. A photosensitive substance in cosmetics is the suspected cause.

Ormsby, O. S., & Ebert, M. H. Erythrose péribuccale pigmentaire de Brocq. *Arch. Derm., Chicago,* 1931, 23:429-38.

Brocq pseudopelade. A slowly progressive scarring disease of the scalp characterized by multiple smooth lesions, 0.5 to 2.0 cm in diameter, with atrophic centers and sharp margins. The condition is considered to be a form of slowly progressive alopecia areata, representing advanced stages of some skin diseases, such as lichen planus or lupus erythematosus.

Gay Prieto, J. Pseudopelade of Brocq: Its relationship to some forms of cicatricial alopecias and to lichen planus. *J. Derm. Invest.,* 1965, 24:323-35.

Brocq-Debré-Lyell syndrome. See *toxic epidermal necrolysis.*

Brocq-Duhring disease. See *Duhring disease.*

Brocq-Pautrier glossitis. See *Brocq-Pautrier syndrome.*

Brocq-Pautrier syndrome. Synonyms: *Brocq-Pautrier glossitis, glossitis rhombica mediana, median rhomboid glossitis, tuberculum rhombicum medianum glossis.*

A congenital disorder of noninflammatory origin, characterized by a somewhat rhomboid reddish, smooth, and shiny lesion with some opalescent spots, occurring at about the middle third of circumvallate papillae of the tongue.

Brocq, L., & Pautrier, L. M. Glossite losangique médiane de la face dorsale de la langue. *Ann. Derm. Syph., Paris,* 1914-15, 5:1-48.

BRODIE, SIR BENJAMIN COLLINS (British physician, 1783-1862)

Brodie abscess. A bone abscess, occurring as a puss-filled cavity surrounded by a wall of dense fibrous tissue, usually found in the metaphyses of the long bones. It consists of necrotic debris and inflammatory cells, sometimes being sterile but, in some instances, acting as a reservoir for the bacteria, leading to the development of osteomyelitis.

Brodie, B. C. An account of some cases of chronic abscess of the tibia. *Med. Chir. Tr., London,* 1832, 17:239-49.

Brodie disease (1). Hysterical pseudofracture of the spine.

Brodie, B. C. *Lectures illustrative of certain local nervous affections.* London, Longman, 1837.

Brodie disease (2). See *Brodie knee.*

Brodie knee. Synonym: *Brodie disease.*

Chronic synovitis of the knee joint.

Brodie, B. C. Pathological researches respecting the diseases of the joints. *Med. Chir. Tr., London,* 1813, 4:207-77.

Brodie pile. A mass of inflamed anal mucosa at the lower end of a fissure in ano.

Brodie, B. C. Lectures on diseases of the rectum. III. Preternatural contraction of the sphincter ani. *London, Med. Gaz.*, 1835, 16:26-31.

BRODIN, M. (French physician)

Brodin syndrome. Synonym: *appendicitis-duodenal stenosis syndrome.*

Duodenal stenosis caused by lymphadenitis associated with appendicitis.

Brodin, M. L'appendicite chronique. Son diagnostic par la palpation abdominale en position verticale et son retentissement duodénal avec arrêt ou "genu inferius" mis en évidence par l'étude radiologique de la traversée digestive. *Presse Méd.*, 1941, 49:619-21.

BRODY, IRWIN A. (American physician)

Brody syndrome. A muscle function disorder, characterized by painless contractures occurring with exercise, caused by a deficiency of $CA2^{+}$-adenosine triphosphatase in sarcoplasmic reticulum.

Brody, I. A. Muscle contracture induced by exercise. A syndrome attributable to decreased relaxing factor. *N. Engl. Med. J.*, 1969, 281:187-92.

BROESICKE, GUSTAV (German anatomist, born 1853)

Treitz-Broesicke hernia. See *Treitz hernia.*

BROMBERG, YEHUDA M. (Israeli physician)

Zondek-Bromberg-Rozin syndrome. See *Zondek syndrome, under Zondek, Bernhard.*

bronchial carcinoma-myasthenia syndrome. See *Eaton-Lambert syndrome, under Eaton, Lealdes McKendree.*

bronchial irritability syndrome. A cluster of abnormalities, consisting of nocturnal dyspnea, prolonged morning discomfort, and low PC>20, associated with bronchial hyperreactivity to histamine.

Mortagy, A. K., *et al.* Respirtory symptoms and bronchial reactivity: Identification of a syndrome and its relation to asthma. *Brit. Med. J. (Clin. Res.)*, 1986, 293:525-9.

bronchiectasis-lymphedema-yellow nail syndrome. See *yellow nail syndrome.*

bronchopulmonary dysplasia (BPD). See *respirator lung syndrome.*

bronchopulmonary dysplasia (BPD). See *Wilson-Mikity syndrome, under Wilson, Miriam Geisendorfer.*

bronchospastic syndrome. See *airway obstruction syndrome.*

bronchospirochetosis. See *Castellani bronchitis.*

bronze baby syndrome. A gray-brown discloration of the skin of neonates who are undergoing phototherapy for hyperbilirubinemia.

Kopelman, A. E., *et al.* The "bronze" baby syndrome: A complication of phototherapy. *J. Pediat.*, 1972, 81:466-72.

bronze diabetes. See *Recklinghausen-Applebaum disease.*

bronze diabetes. See *Troisier-Hanot-Chauffard syndrome.*

bronzed diabetes. See *Recklinghausen-Applebaum disease.*

bronzed disease. See *Addison disease.*

bronzed disease of the newborn. See *Winckel-Charrin syndrome.*

bronzed skin. See *Addison disease.*

BROOKE, HENRY AMBROSE GRUNDY (British physician, 1858-1919)

Brooke disease. See *Brooke epithelioma.*

Brooke epithelioma. Synonyms: *Ancell-Spiegler cylindroma, Brooke disease, Brooke syndrome, Brooke tumor, Brooke-Fordyce disease, Brooke-Fordyce trichoepithelioma, Brooke-Spiegler syndrome, acanthoma adenoides, adenoid epithelioma, cystic adenoid epithelioma, disseminated embryonic lichenoid eruption, epithelioma adenoides cysticum (EAC), hereditary benign cystic epitheliomas, multiple benign cystic epitheliomas, multiple benign epitheliomas of the scalp, nevi epitheliomatosi cystici, nevus follicularis, nevus trichoepitheliomatosus adenoides cysticum, tomato tumor, trichoepithelioma papulosum multiplex, turban tumor.*

A familial, usually benign skin disease, transmitted as an autosomal dominant trait, in which masses of basal cells in the corium originate from the basal cell layer of the epidermis and hair follicle. The lesions form firm, flesh-colored, translucent papules with slight surface telangiectasia; small lesions may coalesce to form a solid sheet tumor. In some forms of the disease, the lesions are confined to the eyelids, with a symmetrical distribution of virtually hundreds of lesions, although solitary lesions sometimes occur. In other cases, the lesions vary in size from that of a pea to that of a large tomato, some multiple lesions resembling bunches of grapes, often covering the entire scalp like a turban. The tumors usually appear near puberty and become stationary after enlarging for several years. Regression and, rarely, malignant degeneration may occur.

Spiegler, E. Über Endotheliome der Haut. *Arch. Derm. Syph., Berlin*, 1899, 50:163-76. *Ancell, H. History of a remarkable case of tumours developed on the head and face. *Med. Chir. Tr.*, 1842, 25:227. Brooke, H. G. Epithelioma adenoides cysticum. *Brit. J. Derm.*, 1892, 4:269-86. Fordyce, J. A. Multiple benign cystic epithelioma of the skin. *J. Cutan. Dis.*, 1892, 10:459-73.

Brooke syndrome. See *Brooke epithelioma.*

Brooke tumor. See *Brooke epithelioma.*

Brooke-Fordyce disease. See *Brooke epithelioma.*

Brooke-Fordyce trichoepithelioma. See *Brooke epithelioma.*

Brooke-Spiegler syndrome. See *Brooke epithelioma.*

Morrow-Brooke syndrome. See *under Morrow.*

BROWN, C. H.

Brown-Vialetto-van Laere syndrome. Synonyms: *pontobulbar palsy with deafness, pontobulbar palsy with neurosensory deafness.*

A rare, often familial disorder characterized by bilateral nerve deafness followed by or associated with various neurological disorders, including involvement of the motor components of the seventh, ninth, twelfth, and, less frequently, third, fifth, and sixth cranial nerves. Spinal motor neurons are affected in some instances. The condition is progressive, having its onset in childhood. Familial cases are believed to be transmitted as an autosomal recessive trait. Associated symptoms may include mental retardation, microcephaly, epileptic fits, auditory hallucinations, ataxia, retinitis pigmentosa, and respiratory disorders.

*Brown, C. H. Infantile amyotrophic lateral sclerosis of the family type. *J. Nerv. Ment. Dis.*, 1894, 21:707-16. Vialetto, E. Contributo alla forma ereditaria della paralisi bulbare progressiva. *Riv. Sper. Freniat.*, 1936, 40:1-24. Laere, J., van. Paralysie bulbo-pontile chronique progressive familiale avec surdité. Un cas de syndrome de Klippel-Trenaunay das la même fratrie-Problèmes diagnostiques et génétiques. *Rev. Neur., Paris*, 1966, 115:289-95. Gallai, V., *et al.* Ponto-bulbar palsy with deafness (Brown-Vialetto-van Laere syndrome). *J. Neurol. Sc.*, 1981, 50:259-75.

BROWN, CHARLES LEONARD (American physician, born 1899)

Brown-Symmers disease. Synonym: *acute serous encephalitis.*

A rapidly fatal form of encephalitis in children, marked by a sudden onset of symptoms, which include irritability, lack of appetite, vomiting, diarrhea, sore throat, fever, respiratory difficulties, blepharoptosis, strabimus, nystagmus, papilledema, retraction of the angle of the mouth, muscular twitching, rigidity of the neck and jaws, coma, hemiplegia, and convulsions. Pathologically, the disease is characterized by extreme enlargement of the brain with splotch-like hemorrhages, flattening of the convolutions, obliteration of the sulci, and softening of the brain tissue. On section, the tissue is pinkish, and microscopic findings include hyperemia and edema of the subarachnoid space, engorgement of the blood vessels, perivascular and pericellular edema with or without vacuolation of the ground substance, capillary crowding with erythrocytes, and apparent emptiness around the blood vessels in edematous areas. In some sites, numerous glia cells are present, representing areas of edema, but giving an appearance of vacuoles.

Brown, C. L., & Symmers, D. Acute serous encephalitis. A newly recognized disease of children. *Am. J. Dis. Child.*, 1925, 29:174-81.

BROWN, GEORGE ELGIE (American physician, 1885-1935)

Horton-Magath-Brown syndrome. See *Horton disease (1).*

Nygaard-Brown syndrome. See *under Nygaard.*

BROWN, H. W. (American ophthalmologist)

Brown syndrome. Synonyms: *superior oblique tendon sheath syndrome, tendon sheath adherence syndrome.*

Fibrosis and shortening of the superior oblique tendon and attachment of the tendon sheath to the trochlea, resulting in restriction of eye movements, associated with bilateral blepharoptosis, backward head tilt, widening of the palpebral fissures with attempted upward gaze, and choroidal coloboma.

*Brown, H. W. *Strabismus. Symposium I.* St. Louis, Mosby, 1950, pp. 205-36.

BROWN, JASON W. (American physician)

Brown syndrome. Synonym: *neural crest syndrome.*

A syndrome, occurring in persons with blond hair, blue or blue-green eyes, and fair complexion, characterized by congenital analgesia with loss of deep and/or superficial pain sensitivity, anhidrosis, autonomic dysfunction, aplasia of the dental enamel, meningeal thickening and cystic changes, mild mental retardation, and hyporeflexia. The autonomic dysfunction is manifested by pupillary abnormalities ranging from partial to complete Horner syndrome, neurogenic anhidrosis with otherwise normal sweat glands, and vasomotor instability with abnormal vanillylamandelic and homovanillic acid urine assays. An abnormality in the differentiation of the neural crest is suggested as the main cause of this syndrome.

Brown, J. W., & Podosin, R. A syndrome of the neural crest. *Arch. Neur., Chicago*, 1966, 15:294-301.

BROWN, S. I. (American ophthalmologist)

Brown-McLean syndrome. A syndrome of peripheral corneal edema after cataract extraction, associated with discerete orange punctate pigmentation of the endothelial surface of the edematous areas. Severe myopia is a frequent complication.

*Brown, S. I., & McLean, J. M. Peripheral corneal edema after cataract extraction. A new clinical entity. *Tr. Am. Acad. Ophth. Otolaryng.*, 1969, 73:465.

brown bowel syndrome (BBS). Synonym: *brown intestine.*

A rare disease characterized by malabsorption and accumulation of lipofuscin in the smooth muscle cells of the muscularis externa of the small intestine.

Fox, B. Lipofuscinosis of the gastrointestinal tract in man. *J. Clin. Path.*, 1968, 20:806-13. Foster, C. S. The brown bowel syndrome: A possible smooth muscle mitochondrial myopathy? *Histopathology*, 1979, 3:1-17.

brown intestine. See *brown bowel syndrome.*

BROWN KELLY. See KELLY, ADAM BROWN

brown pulmonary induration. See *Ceelen-Gellerstedt syndrome.*

brown spot syndrome. See *McCune-Albright syndrome.*

BROWN-SEQUARD, CHARLES EDOUARD (French physician, 1817-1894)

Brown-Séquard hemiplegia. See *Brown-Séquard syndrome.*

Brown-Séquard syndrome. Synonyms: *Brown-Séquard hemiplegia, hemiparaplegic syndrome, hemiplegia et hemiparaplegia spinalis, spinal hemiparaplegia.*

Unilateral lesion of the spinal cord (inflammation, tumor, truma, or other type) associated with ipsilateral motor paralysis; loss of vibratory, joint, and tendon sensation; decreased tactile discrimination; and contralateral anesthesia and loss of temperature sense.

Brown-Séquard, C. E. De la transmission croisée des impressions sensitives par la moelle épinière. *C. Rend. Soc. Biol.*, 1850, 2:33-4.

BRUCE, SIR DAVID (British physician, 1855-1931)

Bruce septicemia. See *brucellosis.*

brucellosis. Synonyms: *Bang disease, Bruce septicemia, Cyprus fever, febris melitensis, febris undulans, Gilbraltar fever, goat fever, Malta fever, Mediterranean fever, melitensis septicemia, melitococcosis, mountain fever, Neapolitan fever, rock fever, undulant fever.*

Infection with *Brucella* (*B. suis* in swine, *B. melitensis* in goats, and *B. abortus* in cattle), which is transmissible to man and involves primarily the reticuloendothelial system. After an incubation period of 5 to 21 days, the disease is manifested in man by the sudden onset of undulant fever, generalized pain, chills, sweating, constipation, and anemia. In most instances, patients recover within 3 months, but in chronic forms the infection may persist over a period of several years. Five types of human infection have been delineated: (1) the **intermittent type** with shifting articular rheumatism, weakness, night sweating, and body temperature near normal in the morning but rising to 101 to 104ºF in the evening; (2) the **ambulatory type** with symptoms similar to those of the intermittent type, but to a milder degree; (3) the **undulant type**, generally due to *B. melitensis*, characterized by step-like increases in the temperature from day-to-tay to a maximum, and, after a time, gradual decrease in temperature and possibly successive repetition of events; (4) the **malignant type**, almost always due to *B. melitensis*, in which the temperature is high and sustained with extreme hyperpyrexia before death; and (5) the **atypical chronic type** which may take the form of muscular stiffness, gastric disturbances, and neurological symptoms.

Bang, B. Die Aetiologie des seuchenhaften ("infectiösen") Verwerfens. *Zschr. Tiermed.*, 1897, 1:241-78. Bruce, D. Note on the discovery of a microorganism in Malta fever. *Practitioner, London*, 1887, 39:161-70.

BRUCK, ALFRED (German physician, born 1865)

Bruck disease. Multiple fractures associated with joint ankylosis and muscle atrophy.

Bruck, A. Über eine seltene Form von Erkrankung der Knochen und Gelenke. *Deut. Med. Wschr.*, 1897, 23:152-5.

BRUCK, F. (German physician)

Bruck-de Lange syndrome. See *de Lange syndrome (2), under Lange, Cornelia, de.*

BRUEGHEL, PIETER, THE ELDER (Flemish painter, c. 1525-1569)

Brueghel syndrome. See *Meige syndrome (2).*

BRUGSCH, THEODOR (German physician, 1878-1963)

Brugsch syndrome. Synonyms: *acromicria, acropachyderma, dystrophia osteogenitalis, pachydermoperiostosis, pseudoacromegaly.*

A syndrome of thickening and folding of the skin with increased sebaceous secretion, giving the face a peculiar, despair-like appearance; periostitis with periosteal ossification of the limbs, fingers, and toes with thickening of the bones; thickening of the skin of the hands and feet; clubbing of the toes; hyperhidrosis; gynecomastia; and facial and pubic hypotrichosis. The syndrome is suspected of being transmitted as an autosomal dominant trait. This disorder differs from the pachydermoperiostosis syndrome by the absence of acromegaly.

Brugsch, T. Akromikrie oder Dystrophia osteogenitalis. *Med. Klin., Berlin*, 1927, 23:81-2.

BRÜNAUER, STEFAN ROBERT (German physician)

Brünauer syndrome. See *Unna-Thost syndrome, under Unna, Paul Gerson.*

BRUNHES, J. (French physician)

Chavany-Brunhes syndrome. See *under Chavany.*

BRUNS

Bruns-Garland syndrome. Synonyms: *diabetic amyotrophy, diabetic myelopathy, proximal diabetic neuropathy, subacute proximal diabetic neuropathy.*

A diabetic neuropathy characterized by subacute, progressive proximal weakness and wasting of muscles, especially of the lower extremities. Originally, some patients were thought to have signs of spinal cord involvement, hence the synonym **diabetic myelopathy.** Older males are most commonly affected.

Chokroverty, S., *et al.* Bruns-Garland syndrome of diabetic amyotrophy. *Tr. Am. Neur. Assoc.*, 1977, 102:173-7.

BRUNS, LUDWIG (German physician, 1858-1916)

Bruns syndrome. Synonym: *postural changes-brain tumor syndrome.*

Vertigo, vomiting, headache, and visual disturbances due to an obstruction in the flow of the cerebrospinal fluid during changes of posture of the head. Cysts and cysticercosis of the fourth ventricle and tumors of the midline of the cerebellum and third ventricle are the principal causes of this disorder.

Bruns. Neuropathologische Demonstrationen. *Neurol. Zbl.*, 1902, 21:561-7.

BRUNSTING, LOUIS A. (American physician, born 1900)

Brunsting disease. Synonyms: *Brunsting-Perry syndrome, benign pemphigoid, cicatricial pemphigoid, localized cicatricial pemphigoid, parapemphigus.*

A persistent eruption of grouped pruritic vesicles confined to one or more circumscribed plaques about the head or neck, extending through a succession of flares and resulting in cicatricial scarring. Allergic incidents, particularly urticaria and asthma, are usually associated. The disorder was originally observed in males of middle or older ages.

Brunsting, L. A., & Perry, H. O. Benign pemphgoid? A report of seven cases with chronic, scarring herpetiform plaques about the head and neck. *Arch. Derm., Chicago*, 1957, 75:489-501.

Brunsting-Perry syndrome. See *Brunsting disease.*

BRUSA, P. (Italian physician)

Brusa-Torricelli syndrome. See *aniridia-Wilms tumor syndrome.*

BRUSHFIELD, THOMAS (British physician)

Brushfield spots. Synonym: *mongolian spots.*

Pigmented spots on the iris seen in the Down syndrome (see *chromosome 21 trisomy*).

Brushfield, T. Mongolism. *Brit. J. Child. Dis.*, 1924, 21:241-58.

Brushfield-Wyatt syndrome. A syndrome of mental retardation, extensive unilateral port-wine nevus, contralateral hemiplegia, homonymous hemianopia, and cerebral angioma, considered by some writers to be a variant of the Sturge-Weber syndrome.

Brushfield, T., & Wyatt, W. Hemiplegia associated with extensive naevus and mental defect. *Brit. J. Child. Dis.*, 1927, 24:98-106.

BRUTON, OGDEN CARR (American physician, born 1908)

Bruton agammaglobulinemia. See *Bruton syndrome.*

Bruton syndrome. Synonyms: *Bruton agammaglobulinemia, Bruton-Gitlin syndrome, congenital hypogammaglobulinemia, infantile X-linked agammaglobulinemia, X-linked agammaglobulinemia.*

A congenital form of agammaglobulinemia, transmitted as an X-linked trait, characterized by susceptibility to bacterial but not viral infections and symptoms similar to those seen in rheumatoid arthritis. After a normal infancy, the affected children contract infection by pyogenic bacteria, mainly staphylococci, pneumocci, streptocci, and *Haemophilus pneumoniae*, and develop purulent sinusitis, pneumonia, septicemia, meningitis, furunculosis, and other types of infection. If left untreated, patients die of pulmonary complications of bronchiectasis. Associated disorders may include *Pneumocystis carinii* superinfection, joint enlargement, edema, ligneous muscle induration, muscle weakness, rash over the extensor surfaces of the joints, neurological complications, hemolytic anemia, drug eruptions, atopic eczema, poison ivy dermatitis, allergic rhinitis, and asthma.

Bruton, O. C. Agammaglobulinemia. *Pediatrics*, 1952, 9:722-8. Gitlin, D., & Craig, J. M. The thymus and other lymphoid tissues in congenital agammaglobulinemia. *Pediatrics*, 1963, 32:517-30.

Bruton-Gitlin syndrome. See *Bruton syndrome.*

BS. See ***B**loom **s**yndrome.*

BS. See ***B**artter **s**yndrome.*

BS. See ***B**ehçet **s**yndrome.*

BSG (branchioskeletogenital) syndrome. See *Elsahy-Waters syndrome.*

BSS. See *Bernard-Soulier syndrome, under Bernard, Jean.*
bubbly lung syndrome. See *Wilson-Mikity syndrome, under Wilson, Miriam Geisendorfer.*
buccal neuralgia. See *Sluder neuralgia.*
buccolinguomasticatory syndrome. See *tardive dyskinesia syndrome.*
BUCHEM, FRANCIS STEVEN PETER, VAN (Dutch physician)
van Buchem syndrome. Synonyms: *chronic hyperphosphatasemia; craniofacial cortical hyperostosis; endosteal hyperostosis, recessive type; hyperostosis corticalis generalisata familiaris; hyperphosphatasemia tarda.*

An autosomal recessive disorder characterized by thickening and osteosclerosis of the base of the skull, calvaria, mandible, clavicles, and ribs, and hyperplasia of the diaphyseal cortex, often associated with elevated blood alkaline phosphatase. Onset of symptoms is at puberty. Stenosis of the cranial foramina may produce facial paralysis, and thickening of the base of the skull may cause optic atrophy and hearing disorders.

Buchem, F. S. P., van, *et al.* An uncommon familial systemic disease of the skeleton: hyperostosis corticalis generalisata famialis. *Acta Radiol., Stockholm*, 1955, 44:109-20.

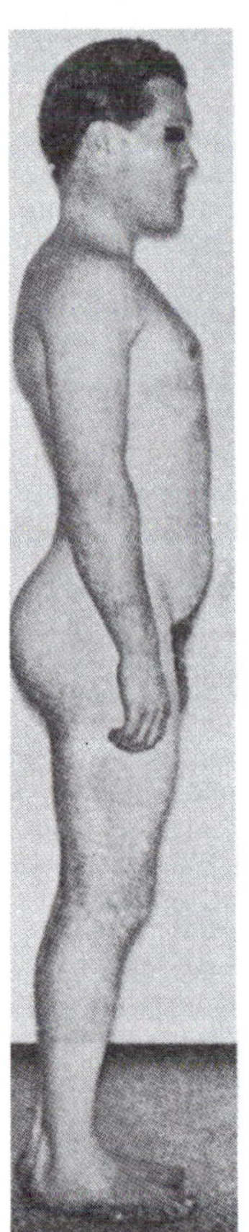
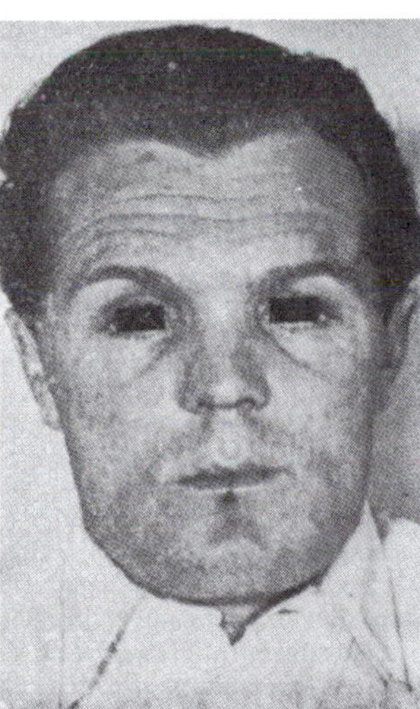

van Buchem syndrome
Robin, P.: *Dynamic Classification of Bone Dysplasias.* Chicago, Year Book Medical Publishers, 1964.

BUCKHARDT, W. (Swiss physician)
Buckhardt dermatitis. Synonym: *vernal photodermatosis.*

An eruption on the external ear margin, consisting of red papules and vesicles similar to those seen in erythema exudativum multiforme, after exposure to sunlight during the spring. The eruption disappears without a trace in about 15 hours.

Burckhardt, W. Über eine im Frühling, besonders on de Ohren, outftretende. *Dermatologica, Basel*, 1942, 86:85-91.

BÜCKLERS, MAX (German ophthalmologist, 1895-1969)
Bücklers dystrophy. See *Reis-Bücklers syndrome.*
Reis-Bücklers syndrome. See *under Reis.*
BUCKLEY, REBECCA, H. (American physician)
Buckley syndrome. See *Job syndrome.*
BUCY, PAUL CLANCY (American neurologist, born 1904)
Klüver-Bucy syndrome (KBS). See *under Klüver.*
Klüver-Bucy-Terzian syndrome. See *Klüver-Bucy syndrome.*
BUDAY, K. (Hungarian physician)
Bogdán-Buday syndrome. See *under Bogdán.*
BUDD, GEORGE (British physician, 1808-1882)
Budd cirrhosis. Chronic hepatomegaly believed to be caused by intestinal intoxication.

Budd, G. *On diseases of the liver.* London, Churchill, 1845.

Budd disease. See *Budd-Chiari syndrome.*
Budd jaundice. See *Budd-Chiari syndrome.*
Budd-Chiari syndrome (BCS). Synonyms: *Bud disease, Budd jaundice, Chiari disease, Chiari syndrome, Rokitansky disease, von Rokitansky disease, acute parenchymatous jaundice, hepatic vein thrombosis.*

A rare disorder resulting from obstruction of the blood from the the liver, caused by a tumor or thrombus, characterized by congestion most pronounced around the terminal hepatic venules, cell necrosis, and a scant inflammatory reaction. Major clinical manifestations include hepatomegaly, pain in the right upper abdominal quadrant, and ascites. Associated disorders usually include jaundice, hematemesis, leg edema, esophageal varices, thrombophlebitis of the inferior vena cava, and portal hypertension. Polycythemia and nocturnal paroxysmal hemoglobinuria are usually associated. Use of oral contraceptives is believed to increase the tendency to develop this syndrome.

Budd, G. *On diseases of the liver. London*, Churchill, 1945. Chiari, H. Erfahrungen über Infarktbildungen in der Leber des Menschen. *Zschr. Heilk.*, 1898, 19:475-512. Rokitansky, K. *Handbuch der pathologischen Anatomie.* Wien, Braumüller, 1842-46, Vol. 3, pp. 269-313.

BÜDINGER, KONRAD (Austrian physician, 1867-1944)
Büdinger-Läwen syndrome. See *Büdinger-Ludloff-Läwen syndrome.*
Büdinger-Ludloff-Läwen syndrome. Synonyms: *Büdinger-Läwen syndrome, Haglund-Läwen-Fründ syndrome, chondromalacia patellae, chondromalacia posttraumatica patellae, chondropathia patellae, chondrosis of the patella, osteopathia patellae, traumatic chondritis of the patella.*

Traumatic separation of the cartilage of the patella with fissures.

*Büdinger, K. Über die Ablösung von Gelenkteilen und verwandte Prozesse. *Deut. Zschr. Chir.*, 1906, 84:311-65. Ludloff, K. Zur Pathologie des Kniegelenkes. *Verh. Deut. Ges. Chir.*, 1910, 39:223-5. Läwen, A. Knorpelresektion bei fissuraler Knorpeldegeneration der Patella-eine Frühoperation der Arthritis deformans. *Beitr. Klin.*

Chir., 1925, 134:265-307. Haglund, P. Die hintere Patellarkontusion. *Zbl. Chir.*, 1926, 53:1757. *Fründ, H. Traumatische Chondropathie der Patella, ein selbstandiges Krankheitsbild. *Zbl. Chir.*, 1926, 53:707.

BUERGER, LEO (American physician, 1879-1943)

Buerger disease. See *Buerger syndrome.*

Buerger syndrome. Synonyms: *Buerger disease, Winiwater-Buerger syndrome, presenile gangrene, thromboangiitis obliterans.*

A chronic inflammatory, obliterative disease of the peripheral vessels, chiefly of the radial and ulnar arteries, sometimes also involving the arteries of the lower limbs. Males over 40 years of age are mainly affected, the disease being very rare in women. Inflammation and fibrosis usually spread beyond the vessels to adjacent nerves. A migrating superficial thrombophlebitis, gangrene of a digit or extremity, and intermittent claudication are frequently present. Central nervous system involvement may include focal lesions of the cerebral cortex with resulting paralysis, sensory disorders, convulsions, aphasia, hemianopsia, personality changes, and mental deterioration. Tobacco sensitivity is believed to be the cause.

Buerger, L. Thrombo-angiitis obliterans: A study of the vascular lesions leading to presenile spontaneous gangrene. *Am. J. Med.*, 1908, 136:567-80. Winiwarter, F., von. Über eine eigentümliche Form von Endarteriitis und Endophlebitis mit Gangrän des Fusses. *Arch. Klin. Chir., Berlin*, 1878-79, 23:202-25.

Winiwarter-Buerger syndrome. See *Buerger syndrome.*

BUHL, LUDWIG, VON (German physician, 1816-1880)

Buhl disease. Acute sepsis in newborn infants, associated with hemorrhage into the skin, mucous membrane, navel, and intestine, complicated by cyanosis and jaundice.

Buhl. L. Die acute Fettdegeneration der Neugeborenen. In: Hecker, C., & Buhl, L. eds. *Klinik der Geburstekunde. Beobachtungen und Untersuchungen aus der Gebärnstalt zu München.* Leipzig, Engelmann, 1861, Vol. 1, pp. 296-300.

building illness syndrome (BIS). See *sick building syndrome.*

BUJADOUX

Garin-Bujadoux syndrome. See *Bannwarth syndrome.*

bulbospinal paralysis. See *Erb-Goldflam syndrome, under Erb, Wilhelm Heinrich.*

bulbus retractus syndrome. See *Stilling-Türk-Duane syndrome.*

bulimarexia. See *bulimia syndrome.*

bulimia. See *bulimia syndrome.*

bulimia nervosa. See *bulimia syndrome.*

bulimia syndrome. Synonyms: *abnormal weight control syndrome, binge eating syndrome, binge-purge syndrome, bulimarexia, bulimia, bulimia nervosa, bulimia-vomiting syndrome, dietary chaos syndrome.*

An eating disorder characterized by massive binge eating, followed by induced vomiting or diarrhea with laxatives. Binge eating may alternate with strict dieting and fasting or exercise in order to control weight. The disorder is more common in adolescent and young adult females than other groups. See also *sorcerer's apprentice syndrome..*

Johnson, C., *et al.* The syndrome of bulimia. Review and synthesis. *Psychiat. Clin. N. Am.*, 1984, 7:247-73.

bulimia-vomiting syndrome. See *bulimia syndrome.*

bulldog syndrome. See *Simpson syndrome, under Simpson, J. L.*

bullous malignant erythema multiforme. See *Stevens-Johnson syndrome.*

bullous recurrent eruption. See *epidermolysis bullosa syndrome.*

BUREAU, YVES (French physician)

Bureau syndrome. See *Bureau-Barrière-Thomas syndrome.*

Bureau-Barrière syndrome. Synonyms: *acquired perforating foot ulcer, acro-osteopathia ulceromutilans, acro-osteopathy of the foot, alcoholic-acrodystrophic neuropathy, alcoholic neuro-acropathy, sporadic acropathia ulceromutilans, sporadic ulcerating and mutilating acropathy (SUMA), ulcero-mutilating acropathy.*

A syndrome of sporadic mutilating acro-osteolysis and perforating ulcers of the feet, associated with dysproteinemia and moderate thrombocytopenia. High serum immunoglobulin A levels are constant. The condition appears to be exacerbated by an exposure to cold. Some authors suspect an exposure to vinyl chloride vapors as the etiologic factor; others consider alcoholism as the principal causative agent.

Bureau, Y., Barrière, H., *et al.* Acropathies ulcéro-mutilantes pseudo-syringomyéliques non familiales des membres inférieurs. (A propos de vingt-trois observations). *Presse Méd.*, 1957, 65:2127-32.

Bureau-Barrière-Thomas syndrome. Synonym: *Bureau syndrome.*

A familial form of keratosis palmaris and plantaris, transmitted as an autosomal recessive trait, characterized by sharply defined keratosis of the palms and soles, bone hypertrophy with diminished osseous density and enlargement of the terminal phalanges (hippocratic fingers and toes), hourglass nails, and hyperhidrosis of the palms and soles.

Bureau, Y., Barrière, H., & Thomas, M. Hippocratisme digital congénital palmo-plantaire et troubles osseux. *Ann. Derm. Syph., Paris*, 1959, 86:611-22. Rauch,H. J., & Neumayer, K. Bureau-Barrière-Thomas-Syndrom. Eine seltene hereditäre Palmoplantarkeratose mit assozüerten Symptomen. *Zschr. Hautkr.*, 1981, 56:102-8.

BURFORD, THOMAS H. (American physician)

Graham-Burford-Mayer syndrome. See *middle lobe syndrome.*

BÜRGER, MAX (German physician, born 1885)

Bürger-Grütz syndrome. Synonyms: *essential familial hyperlipemia, familial hyperchylomicronemia, familial hyperlipoproteinemia, fat-induced hyperlipemia, hepatosplenomegalic lipidosis, hypercholesterinemic xanthomatosis, hyperlipoproteinemia type I, hyperlipoproteinemia type IA, idiopathic hyperlipemia, idiopathic lipoidosis, lipoprotein lipase deficiency, retention hyperlipemia.*

A rare familial disorder, transmitted as an autosomal recessive trait, characterized by hyperchylomicronemia which gives the blood serum a milky appearance, causes lipid deposits in the reticuloendothelial cells, and produces xathomas. The symptoms include abdominal pain, eruptive xanthomas of the skin, hepatosplenomegaly, and occasional lipemia retinalis. Hyperchylomicronemia appears after consuming foods with a normal fat content and disappears on fat-free diets. Lipoprotein lipase deficiency is responsible for a defective metabolism of dietary fats. See also *Harbitz-Müller disease.*

Bürger, M., & Grütz, O. Über hepatosplenomegale Lipoidose mit xanthomatösen Veränderungen in Haut und Schleimhaut. *Arch. Derm. Syph., Berlin*, 1932, 166:542-75.

BURGIO, G. R.

Burgio pseudodiastrophic dwarfism syndrome. Synonyms: *pseudodiastrophic dwarfism, Burgio type; pseudodiastrophic dysplasia, Burgio type.*

A hereditary form of bone dysplasia, assumed to be transmitted as an autosomal recessive trait, characterized by short-limb dwarfism, brevicollis, clubfoot, joint contractures and dislocations, cleft palate, and characteristic facies. Facial features include large ear auricles, flat nose, hypertelorism, micrognathia, and full cheeks. Radiography of the limbs shows shortening of the long bones, hypoplasia of the scapulae, malformed ilia, hypoplasia of the cervical vertebrae, platyspondylitis of the lower vertebrae, and widening of the intervertebral spaces. See also *diastrophic dwarfism syndrome.*

Burgio, G. R., *et al.* Nanisme pseudiastrophique. Étude de deux soeurs nouveau-nées. *Arch. Fr. Pédiat.*, 1974, 31:681.

BURKE, RICHARD M. (American physician, born 1903)

Burke syndrome. Synonyms: *De Martini-Balestra syndrome, cotton candy lung, idiopathic pulmonary atrophy, progressive pulmonary dystrophy, solitary lobar atrophy, vanishing lung.*

Progressive vanishing of pulmonary x-ray markings in advanced pulmonary emphysema. See also *Swyer-James syndrome.*

Burke, R. M. Vanishing lungs: A case report of bullous emphysema. *Radiology*, 1937, 28:367-l71. De Martini, A., & Balestra, C. Sindromi di rarefazione del tessuto polmonare con particolare riguardo all atrofia polmonare idiopatica. *Minerva Med.*, 1951, 2:917-26.

BURKITT, DENNIS (British physician)

Burkitt lymphoma (BL). Synonyms: *Burkitt sarcoma, Burkitt syndrome, Burkitt tumor, African lymphoma.*

A unique form of lymphoma, usually of the retroperitoneal and jaw areas, which also may involve the kidneys, liver, ovaries, adrenal glands, thyroid gland, testes, and gastrointestinal tract. It is usually found in areas of the world up to 1500 meters above sea level where the temperature never falls below 12ºC and the annual rain fall is at least 60 cm, principally in central Africa, New Guinea, and Colombia. Viruses, especially the Epstein-Barr virus, are the suspected pathogens. The jaw tumor usually orignates in the alveolar process, growing rapidly and producing gross deformity and displacement and exfoliation of the teeth. It usually extends through the periosteum and invades surrounding soft tissue, but the skin remains normal. Typically, the lesion presents as a soft, grayish, fleshy mass composed of cells lying intermediately between immature lymphocytes and reticulum cells, with a spattering of large phagocytic histiocytic cells, producing the so-called "starry-sky" effect.

Burkitt, D. A. sarcoma involving the jaws in African children. *Brit. J. Surg.*, 1958, 46:218-23.

Burkitt sarcoma. See *Burkitt lymphoma.*

Burkitt syndrome. See *Burkitt lymphoma.*

Burkitt tumor. See *Burkitt lymphoma.*

burn-induced immunodeficiency syndrome. Suppression of immune processes after thermal injury. Decreased T-cell number, immunosuppression induced by monocytes and prostaglandin, T-suppressor cell activation, helper cell dysfunction and a deficiency in the production of interleukin-2, and changes in peripheral blood lymphocyte phenotype with a decreased number and percentage of IgM-Fc binding T-lymphocytes are the suspected causes.

Antonacci, A. C., *et al.* Flow cytometric analysis of lymphocyte subpopulations after thermal injury in human beings. *Surg. Gyn. Obst.*, 1984, 159:1-8.

BURNETT, CHARLES HOYT (American physician, born 1913)

Burnett syndrome. See *milk-alkali syndrome.*

BURNIER, R. (American physician)

Burnier syndrome. Synonym: *hypophyseal nanism.*

Dwarfing, optic atrophy, and adiposogenital dystrophy due to decreased functioning of the anterior pituitary as a result of compression exerted by a slow-growing tumor. See also *Lorain-Levi syndrome,* and *Fröhlich syndrome.*

Burnier, R. A new hypophysial syndrome-hypophysial nanism. *Ann. Ophth., St. Louis*, 1912, 21:263-73.

burning feet syndrome. Synonyms: *Gopalan syndrome, barashek, burning feet, chacaleh, electric feet syndrome, electric foot, lightning foot, nutritional melalgia, painful feet syndrome.*

Severe burning and aching of the feet associated with hyperesthesia, raised skin temperature, and vasomotor changes. Ocular complications may include scotoma and amblyopia. Deficiencies of vitamin B and proteins and possibly a toxic factor in old polished rice are considered as potential etiologic factors.

Gopalan, C. The "burning-feet" syndrome. *Indian Med. Gaz.*, 1946, 81:22-6.

burning hand syndrome. Burning dysesthesias and paresthesias in the hands frequently associated with cervical fracture dislocations and, sometimes, occurring in the absence of cervical spine abnormalities.

Maroon, J. C. Burning hands in football spinal cord injuries. *JAMA*, 1977, 238:2049-51.

burnout syndrome. Synonyms: *occupational stress syndrome, professional stress syndrome.*

A condition precipitated by overwhelming stress associated with job-related severe physical and/or mental trauma. The symptoms include loss of efficiency, interest, and initiative; inability to maintain work performance in times of stress; insomnia; fatigability; headache; gastrointestinal disorders; depression; lability of mood; irritability; decreased frustration tolerance; and, frequently, use of drugs and self-medication.

Freudenberger, H. J. The staff burnout syndrome in alternative institutions. *Psychother. Res. Pract.*, 1975, 12:73-82.

BURNS, F. S.

Burns syndrome. Synonym: *oculo-auriculocutaneous syndrome.*

A triad of congenital ichthyosis, deafness, and keratitis.

*Burns, F. S. A case of generalized congenital erythroderma. *J. Cutan. Dis.*, 1915, 32:255. Legrand, J., *et al.* Un syndrome rare oculo-auriculo-cutané (syndrome de Burns). *J. Fr. Ophtalmol.*, 1982, 5:441-5.

burnt wife syndrome. Killing or torture, sometimes by burning, of Hindu wives by their husbands or in-laws for failing to provide appropriate dowries. See also *battered spouse syndrome.*

Das Gupta, S. M., & Tripathi, C. G. Burnt wife syndrome. *Ann. Acad. Med. Singapore,* 1984, 13:37-42.

bursitis calcarea. See *Duplay bursitis.*

bursitis chronica subdeltoidea. See *Duplay bursitis.*

BURY, JUDSON SYKES (British physician, 1852-1944)

Bury disease. Synonym: *erythema elevatum diutinum.*

Erythema characterized by painless, pinkish to purplish nodules formed by the coalescing of irregular elevations, plaques, or nodular tumors, and most frequently affecting the extensor suffaces of the extremities, palms, soles, and ears. Polyarthritis may be associated. The disorder occurs most commonly in middle-aged males. Albuminuria is the main hematological feature.

Bury, J. S. A case of erythema with remarkable nodular thickening and induration of the skin, associated with intermittent albuminuria. *Illust. Med. News, London,* 1889, 3:145-8.

BUSACCA, ARCHIMEDE (Italian physician, born 1893)

Busacca floccule. See *Busacca nodule.*

Busacca nodule. Synonym: *Busacca floccule.*

Nodules appearing on the anterior mesodermal layers of the iris.

Busacca, A. Anatomische und klinische Beobachtungen der Papillarsaumknötchen (Koeppeschen Knötchen) bei Iridozyklitis. *Klin. Mbl. Augenh.,* 1932, 88:14-40.

BUSBY

Busby syndrome. See *Rowley-Rosenberg syndrome.*

BUSCHKE, ABRAHAM (German dermatologist, 1868-1943)

Buschke disease (1). Synonym: *scleroderma adultorum.*

A skin disorder characterized by hard nonpitting edema, usually preceded by a febrile disease such as streptococcal infection, influenza, mumps, or tuberculous lymphadenitis. The process usually begins in the deep layers of the cutis on the posterior or lateral aspects of the neck and spreads to the face, anterior neck, shoulders, upper arms, and chest. The normal markings are smoothed out, giving the skin a shiny or waxy appearance, resulting in masklike facies. Pleural effusions, pericardial effusions, tongue involvement, dysphagia, esophageal lesions, difficulty in opening the mouth, reversible ECG changes, restricted eye movement, and muscle weakness and tenderness may be associated. Collagen bundles in the corium are thickened. After a period of 1 to 6 months, the lesions disappear without sequelae.

Buschke. Verhandlungen der Berliner Dermatologischen Gessellschaft. *Arch. Derm. Syph., Berlin,* 1900, 53:383-6.

Buschke disease (2). See *Busse-Buschke disease.*

Buschke disease (3). See *Madelung syndrome.*

Buschke-Fischer syndrome. See *Fischer syndrome, under Fischer, Heinrich F.*

Buschke-Fischer-Brauer syndrome. See *Fischer syndrome, under Fischer, Heinrich F.*

Buschke-Loewenstein tumor. Synonyms: *giant condyloma of the penis, giant condyloma acuminatum of the penis, pseudotumor of the penis.*

A large warty tumor that usually originates in the preputial sac and penetrates deeply into the penile substance, destroying the corpora cavernosa and forming urethrocutaneous fistulae and ulcers. There may be malignant degeneration.

Loewenstein, L. W. Carcinoma-like condylomata acuminata of the penis. *Med. Clin. N. Am.,* 1939, 23:789-95.

Buschke-Ollendorff syndrome. Synonyms: *dermatofibrosis lenticularis disseminata, dermatofibrosis lenticularis disseminata with osteopoikilosis, disseminated dermatofibrosis with osteopoikilosis.*

A rare skin disease, transmitted as an autosomal dominant trait with high penetrance and variability of expression, characterized by a flesh-colored or slightly yellowish eruption distributed symmetrically on the trunk and extremities. The lesions may vary from isolated discrete nodules to disseminated papules with a cobblestone appearance. Foci of dense bone seen on x-rays are the principal symptoms of osteopoikilosis. Accumulation of basophilic elastic fibers (elastin) in the dermis is the chief histopathological feature.

Buschke, A., & Ollendorff, H. Ein Fall von Dermatofibrosis lenticularis disseminata und Osteopathia condensans disseminata. *Derm. Wschr.,* 1928, 86:257-62.

Busse-Buschke disease. See *under Busse.*

BUSQUET, PAUL (French physician, 1866-1930)

Busquet disease. Synonym: *metatarsal periostitis.*

Osteoperiostitis of the metatarsal bones with exostoses to the dorsum of the foot. The symptoms include pain of the foot during walking.

Busquet, P. De l'ostéo-périostite ossifiante des metatarsiens. *Rev. Chir., Paris,* 1897, 17:1065-99.

BUSSE, OTTO (German physician, 1867-1922)

Busse-Buschke disease. Synonyms: *Buschke disease, ascomycosis, blastomycosis purulenta profunda, cryptococcosis, European blastomycosis, Torula meningitis, torulopsis, torulosis.*

A subacute or chronic *Crytococcus neoformans* infection, chiefly affecting the central nervous system. It usually begins as a mild respiratory infection or granulomatous dermatitis, which may be followed by fever, visual disorders, stiffness of the neck, headache, vomiting, convulsions, and other symptoms and complications of meningoencephalitis. The pulmonary lesions may occur alone or in combination with central nervous system infections. The cutaneous lesions usually appear as verrucoid granuloma, superficial acneiform lesions, or diffuse subcutaneous nodules which form draining sinuses and scars. Infrequently, there may be granulomatous and ulcerative lesions of the nasopharynx; the vaginal, conjunctival, and oral mucosa may be involved in rare instances. Soft, verrucous, dark-violet lesions may be found on the tonsils, tongue, and lips, resulting in necrosis and secondary ulcerating nodules.

*Buschke, A. Über eine durch Coccidien hervorgerufene Krankheit des Menschen. *Deut. Med. Wschr.,* 1895, 21: No. 14, p. v.

busulfan toxicity syndrome. Synonyms: *bulsulphan toxicity syndrome, Myleran toxicity syndrome.*

A syndrome of diffuse pulmonary interstitial fibrosis, cutaneous pigmentation, and symptoms resembling adrenal cortical insufficiency caused by therapeutic doses of busulfan. Fatigue, weakness, weight loss, anorexia, and nausea are the common symptoms.

Kyle, R. A., *et al.* A syndrome resembling adrenal cortical insufficiency associated with long term busulfan (Myleran) therapy. *Blood,* 1961, 18:497-510.

busulphan toxicity syndrome. See *busulfan toxicity syndrome.*

BUTLER, ALLAN MACY (American physician)

Albright-Butler-Bloomberg syndrome. See *hypophosphatemic familial rickets.*

Butler-Albright syndrome. See *Lightwood-Allbright syndrome.*

Butler-Lightwood-Albright syndrome. See *Lightwood-Albright syndrome.*

BVP. See ***b**enign **p**aroxysmal **v**ertigo.*

BW. See ***B**eckwith-**W**iedemann syndrome.*

BWS. See ***B**eckwith-**W**iedemann **s**yndrome.*

BYLER

Byler disease (BD). Synonyms: *familial intrahepatic cholestasis, familial progressive intrahepatic cholestasis, fatal familial cholestasis, progressive intrahepatic cholestasis.*

A condition originally observed in Amish sibships. The children were affected by a hepatic disorder characterized by early onset of loose foul-smelling stools, jaundice, hepatosplenomegaly, and dwarfism, culminating in death between the ages of 17 months and 8 years in four of six cases. The biochemical changes included hyperbilirubinemia, serum alkaline phosphatase elevation, hypoprothrombinemia responsive to parenteral vitamin K, and normal to low serum cholesterol. Intrahepatic cholestasis and early fibrosis were seen in some biopsy specimens and intracellular encapsulated reticular-like material was detected by electron microscopy. The syndrome was transmitted as an autosomal recessive trait.

Clayton, R. J., *et al.* Byler's disease: fatal familial intrahepatic cholestasis in an Amish kindred. *J. Pediat.,* 1965, 67:1025-8.

BYWATERS, ERIC GEORGE LAPTHORNE (British physician)

Bywaters syndrome. See *crush syndrome.*

BZS (Bannayan-Zonana syndrome). See *Bannayan syndrome.*

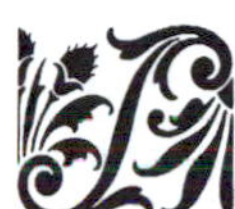

Page #	Term	Observation

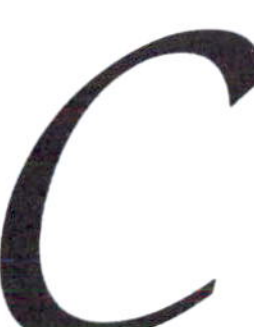

C syndrome. See *Optiz trigonocephaly syndrome.*

CACCHI, ROBERTO (Italian physician)

Cacchi-Ricci syndrome. Synonyms: *cystic disease of the renal pyramids, medullary polycystic kidney, precalyceal tubular ectasia, sponge kidney.*

A congenital cystic disease of the pyramids with multiple small cysts in the medulla, giving the kidneys a spongy appearance.

Cacchi, R., & Ricci, V. Sur une rare maladie kystique multiple des pyramides rénales, le "rein en éponge." *J. Urol. Med., Paris,* 1949, 55:497-519.

CACCHIONE, ALDO (Italian phychiatrist)

De Sanctis-Cacchione (DSC) syndrome. See *under De Sanctis.*

cachetic aphthae. See *Riga-Fede disease.*

cachexia strumipriva. See *Gull syndrome.*

cachexic retinitis. See *Pick retinitis, under Pick, Ludwig.*

CAD (congenital abduction deficiency). See *Stilling-Türk-Duane syndrome.*

caecal slap syndrome. See *cecal slap syndrome.*

CAENIS (A mythological character who refused to marry anyone and, after being raped by Neptune, requested not to be a woman and thus prevent the risk of being traumatized again).

Caenis syndrome. Female genital self-mutilation associated with dysorexia and the hysterical personality.

Goldney, R. D., & Simpson, I. G. Female self-mutilation, dysorexia and the hysterical personality: The Caenis syndrome. *Canad. Psychiat. Assoc. J.,* 1975, 20:435-41.

café coronary syndrome. Synonym: *foreign body airway obstruction.*

Obstruction of the upper respiratory tract by food particles, frequently resulting in sudden death.

Haugen, R. K. The cafe coronary. Sudden death in restaurants. *JAMA,* 1963, 186:142-3.

caffeine withdrawal syndrome. See *under withdrawal syndrome.*

CAFFEY, I. R. (American physician)

Adson-Caffey syndrome. See *cervical rib syndrome.*

CAFFEY, JOHN (American physician, 1895-1966)

Caffey pseudo-Hurler syndrome. See *gangliosidosis* G_{M1} *type I.*

Caffey syndrome (1). See *Caffey-Silverman syndrome.*

Caffey syndrome (2). See *battered child syndrome.*

Caffey-Kempe syndrome. See *battered child syndrome.*

Caffey-Silverman syndrome. Synonyms: *Caffey syndrome, Caffey-Smyth syndrome, De Toni-Caffey syndrome, De Toni-Caffey-Silverman syndrome, Roske-De Toni-Caffey-Silverman syndrome, Roske-De Toni-Caffey-Smyth syndrome, fetoinfantile regressive periosteochondral hyperosteogenesis, hyperosteogenesis periosteoenchondralis progressiva, hyperostosis corticalis infantilis, hyperplastic periostosis, infantile cortical hyperostosis, polyosteopathia deformans regressiva, regressive periosteal enchondral hyperosteogenesis, subperiosteal cortical hyperostosis.*

Cortical hyperostoses in infants under 6 months of age, involving several bones at the same time, usually the mandible and, less commonly, the clavicle, tibia, ulna, femur, ribs, humerus, and fibula. The disorder is usually associated with bilateral swelling of the affected tissues, irritability, fever, and roentgenographic signs of cortical resorption with widening of the medullary canal, diaphyseal expansion, and longitudinal overgrowth and bowing deformities of long bones. Puffy jaws and cheeks give the face a characteristic appearance. Dysphagia, pleurisy, leukocytosis, high erythrocyte sedimentation rate, and excess of blood alkaline phosphatase are common. The ocular signs may include edema around the orbits, proptosis, and conjunctivitis. The syndrome is believed to be transmitted as an autosomal dominant trait.

Caffey, J., & Silverman, W. A. Infantile cortical hyperostoses. Preliminary report of a new syndrome. *Am. J. Roentgen.,* 1945, 54:1-16. Roske, G. Eine eigenartige Knochenerkrankung im Säuglingsalter. *Mschr. Kinderh.,* 1930, 47:385-400. Smyth, F. S., & Silverman, W. Periosteal reaction, fever, and irritability in young infants. A new syndrome? *Am. J. Dis. Child.,* 1946, 71:333-50. Faure, C., *et al.* Predominant or exclusive orbital and facial involvement in infantile cortical hyperostosis, De Toni-Caffey disease. *Pediat. Radiol.,* 1977, 6:103-6.

Caffey-Smyth syndrome. See *Caffey-Silverman syndrome.*

De Toni-Caffey syndrome. See *Caffey-Silverman syndrome.*

De Toni-Caffey-Silverman syndrome. See *Caffey-Silverman syndrome.*

Kenny-Caffey syndrome. See *Kenny syndrome.*

Roske-De Toni-Caffey-Silverman syndrome. See *Caffey-Silverman syndrome.*

Roske-De Toni-Caffey-Smyth syndrome. See *Caffey-Silverman syndrome.*

CAGLAR, M. (American physician)

Wohlmann-Caglar syndrome. See *under Wohlmann.*

CAH. See *congenital adrenal hyperplasia.*

CAHS (central alveolar hypoventilation syndrome). See *Ondine curse.*

calamity syndrome. See *Roth syndrome, under Roth, Martin.*

calcific aortic stenosis-gastrointestinal bleeding syndrome. Calcific aortic stenosis associated with bleeding from the gastrointestinal tract in elderly persons. The bleeding has been attributed to minute mucosal vascular lesions usually found on the right colon.

Heyde, E. C. Gastrointestinal bleeding in aortic stenosis. *N. Engl. J. Med.*, 1958, 259:196.

calcified aortic plug syndrome. A complication of atherosclerosis characterized by calcified, mass-like, obstructing lesions producing a functional coarctation of the aorta, involving both the thoracic and abdominal segments. Upper limb hypertension is the presenting symptom.

Walter, J. F., *et al.* Calcified aortic plug syndrome. *J. Canad. Assoc. Radiol.*, 1981, 32:155-8.

calcifying collagenolysis. See *Teutschländer syndrome.*

calcifying giant-cell tumor. See *Codman tumor.*

calcinosis circumscripta. See *Profichet disease.*

calcinosis cutis-Raynaud phenomenon-esophageal dysfunction-sclerodactyly-telangiectasia syndrome. See *CREST syndrome.*

calcinosis cutis-scleroderma syndrome. See *Thibierge-Weissenbach syndrome.*

calcinosis infantum. See *Lightwood-Albright syndrome.*

calcinosis interstitialis universalis. See *Teutschländer syndrome.*

calcinosis lipogranulomatosa progradiens. See *Teutschländer syndrome.*

calcinosis multiplex lipogranulomatosa. See *Teutschländer syndrome.*

calcinosis-Raynaud phenomenon-sclerodactyly-telangiectasia syndrome. See *CRST syndrome.*

calcium gout. See *pseudogout syndrome.*

calcium pyrophosphate dihydrate deposition syndrome. See *pseudogout syndrome.*

calf hypertension. See *compartment syndrome.*

CALH (chronic active lupoid hepatitis). See *Bearn-Kunkel syndrome.*

callosal demyelinating encephalopathy. See *Marchiafava-Bignami syndrome.*

CALO, S. (Italian physician)

Alè-Calò syndrome. See *Langer-Giedion syndrome.*

calvarial hyperostosis. See *Morgagni-Stewart-Morel syndrome.*

CALVE, JACQUES (French physician, 1875-1954)

Calvé syndrome. Synonyms: *infantile osteochondritis, infantile pseudospondylitis, osteochondritis of the vertebral body, osteochondritis vertebralis infantilis, platyspondylia, vertebra plana, vertebra plana osteonecrotica, vertebral osteochondritis.*

Flattening of the vertebral bodies in children probably caused by a diminished blood supply and resulting in fragmentation and collapse of the affected vertebrae. Eosinophilic granuloma may be the cause.

Calvé, J. Sur une affection particulière de la colonne vertébrale chez l'enfant simulant le mal de Pott. Ostéochondrite vertébrale infantile. *J. Radiol. Eléctr.*, 1925, 9:22-7.

Calvé-Legg-Perthes syndrome. Synonyms: *Calvé-Perthes disease, Legg disease, Maydl disease, Perthes disease, Perthes-Calvé-Legg-Waldenström syndrome, Waldenström syndrome, aseptic necrosis of the femoral head, coxa plana, coxalgia infantilis seu infantilis, malum coxae, osteoarthritis coxae, osteochondrosis deformans juvenilis coxae, osteochondropathia deformans juvenilis coxae, osteochondrosis deformans coxae juvenilis, osteochondrosis of capitular epiphysis of femur, pseudocoxalgia.*

Aseptic necrosis of the epiphysis of the femoral head, probably due to a diminished blood supply. The disease progresses from necrosis through revascularization, mottling, and fragmentation of the epiphysis to reossification and flattening of the head of the femur. The sporadic type is unilateral in most instances, and boys are more frequently affected than girls. The hereditary type is transmitted as an autosomal dominant trait, and there is equal susceptibility of the sexes and a greater proportion of bilateral involvement.

Calvé, F. Sur une forme particulière de pseudocoxalgie greffée. Sur une déformation caractéristique de l'extrémité supérieure du femur. Rev. *Chir., Paris,* 1910, 42:54-84. Legg, A. T. On obscure affection of the hip-joint. *Boston Med. & S. J.*, 1910, 162:202-4. Perthes, G. C. Über Arthritis deformans juvenilis. *Deut. Zschr. Chir.*, 1910, 107: 111-59. Waldenström, H. Der obere tuberkulöse Cullumherd. *Zschr. Orthop. Chir.*, 1909, 24:487-512.

Calvé-Perthes disease. See *Calvé-Legg-Perthes syndrome.*

Perthes-Calvé-Legg-Waldenström syndrome. See *Calvé-Legg-Perthes syndrome.*

CAMERA, UGO (Italian physician)

Camera syndrome. Synonym: *neuralgic lumbosciatic osteopathy syndrome.*

Vertebral and paravertebral lumbosciatic neuralgiform osteopathy caused by inflammatory lesions involving the lower lumbar spine and the sacrum.

Bertola, L., & Pedrocca, A. Osteopathie nevralgiformi lumbosciatalgiche a localizzazioni vertebrali e paravertebrali (sindrome del Camera). *Minerva Ortop.*, 1953, 4:215-8.

camp dizziness. See *Strachan syndrome.*

camp eyes. See *Obal syndrome.*

camp fever. See *Hildenbrand disease.*

CAMPAILLA, E. (Italian physician)

Campailla-Martinelli syndrome. Synonym: *acromesomelic dwarfism.*

A familial form of mesomelic dwarfism, transmitted as an autosomal recessive trait, in which the forearms, hands, and feet are primarily involved. The metacarpals, metatarsals, and phalanges are especially short; the radius is curved with a frequently dislocated head; the phalanges are almost square; and the tubular bones of the hands and feet are dysplastic.

Campailla, E., & Martinelli, B. Deficit staturale con micromesomelia. *Minerva Ortop.*, 1971, 22:180-4.

CAMPBELL, PETER E. (Australian physician)

Williams-Campbell syndrome. See *under Williams, Howard.*

campomelia syndrome. See *campomelic syndrome.*

campomelic dwarfism syndrome. See *campomelic syndrome.*

campomelic syndrome. Synonyms: *campomelia syndrome, campomelic dwarfism syndrome, campomelique syndrome, camptomelic syndrome, camptomelic dwarfism syndrome.*

A disorder of the newborn, characterized by congenital bowing and angulation of the long bones,

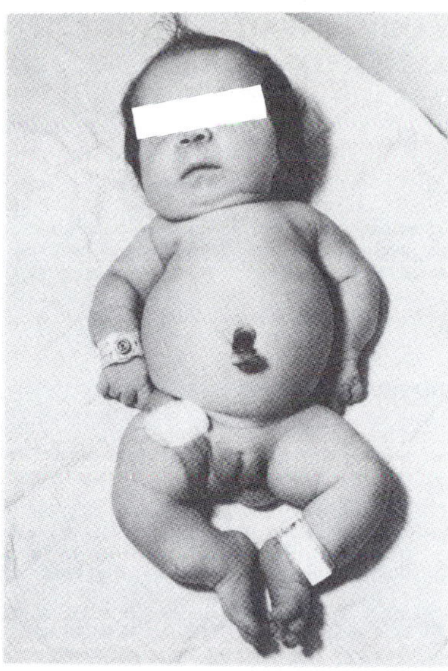

Campomelic syndrome
Hoefnagel, D., Dartmouth Medical School & D. Hoefnagel et al.: *Lancet*, 1:1068, 1972.

associated with skeletal, neurological, and other defects. Most patients die during the neonatal period from respiratory distress, and those who survive into early infancy experience feeding difficulty, failure to thrive, and apnea. Camptomelia is the principal clinical feature of this syndrome. Associated anomalies include prenatal growth deficiency, short and flat vertebrae, hypoplastic scapulae, small thoracic cage, thin and short clavicles, kyphoscoliosis, small iliac wings, wide pelvic outlet, tracheobronchiomalacia, cellular disorganization of the brain, large brain, and peculiar facies marked by a flat small face with a low nasal bridge and micrognathia. In addition to bowing, the extremities show cortical thickening of the concave borders and dimpling over the convex area, short fibulae, and pes equinovarus. Etiology is unknown.

Bound, J. P., *et al.* Congenital anterior angulation of the tibia. *Arch. Dis. Child.*, 1952, 27:179-84. Spranger, J., *et al.* Increasing frequency of a syndrome of multiple osseous defects? *Lancet*, 1970, 2:716. Maroteaux, P., *et al.* Le syndrome campomelique. *Presse Méd.*, 1971, 79:1157-62. Caffey, J. P. Prematal bowing and thickening tubular bones, with multiple cutaneous dimples in arms and legs. A congenital syndrome of mechanical origin. *Am. J. Dis, Child.*, 1947, 74:543-62.

campomelique syndrome. See *campomelic syndrome.*

camptobrachydactyly. See *brachycamptodactyly syndrome.*

camptodactyly syndrome. Synonyms: *campylodactyly, congenital finger contractures, flexed fingers, hammer finger, streblomicrodactyly.*

A hand deformity characterized by permanent flexion of one or more fingers (the little finger being most frequently affected), located usually at the proximal interphalangeal joint, probably due to a fascial abnormality and contracture of the flexor digitorum sublimis. The disorder is a component of several syndromes and is transmitted as an autosomal dominant trait with variable penetrance. The term **streblomicrodactyly** is generally used to mean camptodactyly of the fifth finger.

Landouzy, L. Camptodactylie: Stigmata organique precoce du neuroarthritisme. *Presse Méd.*, 1906, 14:251. Anderson, W. Contractions of the fingers and toes; their varieties, pathology, and treatment. *Lancet*, 1891, 2:107-1-5; 107-11; 161-3.

camptodactyly-ankyloses-facial anomalies-pulmomary hypoplasia syndrome. See *Pena-Shokeir syndrome (1).*

camptodactyly-arthropathy-pericarditis (CAP) syndrome. A familial syndrome of constrictive pericarditis, arthritis of large joints, and flexion contractures of the fingers.

Martínez-Lavín, M., *et al.* A familial syndrome of pericarditis, arthritis, and camptodactyly. *N. Engl. J. Med.*, 1983, 309:224-5. Laxer, R. M., *et al.* The camptodactyly-arthropathy-pericarditis syndrome: Case report and literature review. *Arthr. Rheum.*, 1986, 29:439-44.

camptodactyly-ectodermal dysplasia-sensorineural hearing loss syndrome. See *Mikaelian syndrome.*

camptodactyly-muscular hypoplasia syndrome. See *Tel Hashomer camptodactyly syndrome.*

camptodactyly-sensorineural hearing loss syndrome. See *Stewart-Bergstrom syndrome, under Stewart, Janet M.*

camptomelic dwarfism syndrome. See *campomelic syndrome.*

camptomelic syndrome. See *campomelic syndrome.*

campylodactyly. See *camptodactyly syndrome.*

CAMURATI, MARIO (Italian physician, 1896-1948)

Camurati-Engelmann syndrome. Synonyms: *Engelmann disease, diaphyseal dysplasia, diaphyseal sclerosis, osteopathia hyperostotica scleroticans multiplex infantilis, periostitis hyperplastica, polystotic infantilia, progressive diaphyseal dysplasia.*

A progressive developmental disorder characterized by hyperostoses, osteosclerosis, and muscular dystrophy. The major clinical findings consist of reduction of muscle mass and subcutaneous fat, failure to thrive, leg pain, muscular weakness, abnormal gait, and occasional thickening of the diaphyseal portion of the long bones, lumbar lordosis, scoliosis, knock knees, and shortness of stature in childhood. Radiographic findings usually include cortical thickening and sclerosis of the diaphyses of the long bones by both endosteal and periosteal proliferation and sclerosis of the basilar portion of the skull. Hyperostosis of the calvaria sometimes occurs. The syndrome is transmitted as an autosomal dominant trait with variability of expression and occasional complete lack of penetrance. See also *Braham syndrome..*

Camurati, M. Di un raro caso di osteite simmetrica ereditaria degli arti inferiori. *Chir. Org. Mov., Bologna*, 1922, 6:662-5. Engelmann, G. Ein Fall von Osteopathia hypeostotica (scleroticans) multiplex infantilis. *Fortschr. Roentgenstr.*, 1929. 39:1101-6.

CANADA, WILMA JEANNE (American physician)

Cronkhite-Canada (CC) syndrome. See *under Cronkhite.*

Canadair syndrome. See *water-skier colon.*

CAÑADELL, J. M. (Spanish physician)

Vilanova-Cañadell syndrome. See *under Vilanova.*

CANALE, VIRGINIA C. (American physician)

Canale-Smith syndrome. Synonyms: *chronic lymphadenopathy simulating malignant lymphoma, chronic pseudomalignant immunoproliferation.*

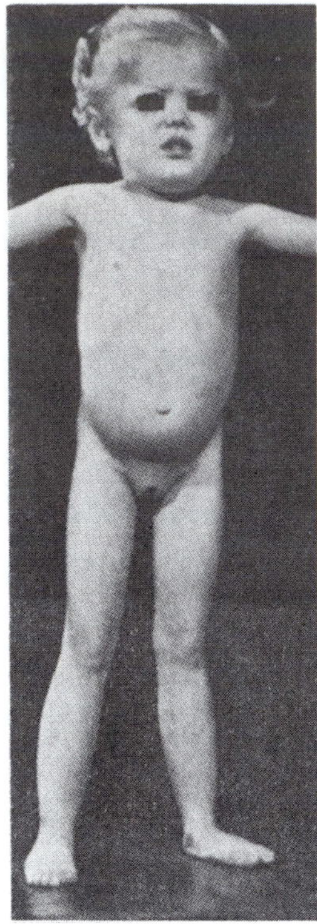
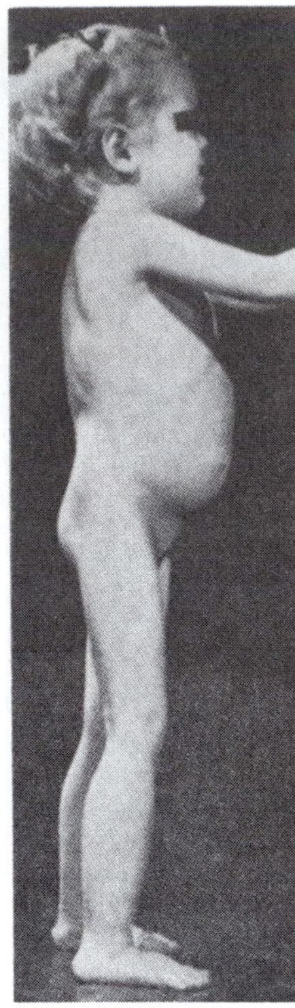

Camurati-Engelmann syndrome
Rubin, P.: *Dynamic Classification of Bone Dysplasias.* Chicago: Year Book Medical Publishers, 1964.

A chronic immunological syndrome in infants, characterized by generalized lymphadenopathy, γ-globulin disorders with manifestations of an autoimmune disease, variable lymph node histology, and response to immunosupressive drugs. The syndrome simulates malignant lymphoma.

Canale, V. C., & Smith, C. H. Chronic lymphadenopathy simulating malignant lymphoma. *J. Pediat.*, 1967, 70:891-9.

canalis opticus syndrome. See *Berlin disease (2), under Berlin, Rudolf.*

CANAVAN, MYRTELLE MAY (American neurologist, born 1879)

Canavan sclerosis. See *Canavan syndrome.*

Canavan syndrome. Synonyms: *Canavan sclerosis, Canavan-van Bogaert-Bertrand syndrome, van Bogaert-Bertrand syndrome, cerebral white matter spongy degeneration, encephalopathia spongiotica, familial idiocy with spongy degeneration, familial spongy degeneration, hereditary spongy dystrophy, infantile spongy degeneration, spongy degeneration of the nervous system, spongy degeneration of the white matter.*

A hereditary disease of the nervous system, transmitted as an autosomal recessive trait, in which onset is early and death occurs within 18 months. The clinical picture is one of mental retardation; muscle hypotonia, especially of the neck, with drooping of the head; macrocephaly; progressive visual deterioration leading to complete blindness and optic atrophy; spasticity of the limbs and development of decerebrate posturing of the extremities; feeding difficulty; and hearing disorders. The syndrome appears to have predilection for persons of Jewish origin. The affected individuals tend to have blond hair and light complexion, in contrast to the darker hair and complexion of their normal siblings. Computed tomography shows a decreased attenuation of the cerebral and cerebellar white matter in an enlarged brain with relatively normal ventricles. Histological findings show spongy degeneration and vacuolation of the white matter, a paucity of myelin and myelin breakdown products, and absence of glial or vascular reaction. Additional findings include loss of Purkinje cells and hyperplasia of Alzheimer type II astrocytes in the cerebral cortex and basal ganglia.

Canavan, M. M. Schilder's encephalitis periaxialis diffusa. Report of a case in a child aged sixteen and one-half months. *Arch. Neur., Chicago,* 1931, 25:299-308. van Bogaert, L., & Bertrand, I. Sur une idiotie familiale avec dégénérescence spongieuse du névraxe. (Note préliminaire). *Acta Neur. Psychiat. Belg.,* 1949, 49:572-87.

Canavan-van Bogaert-Bertrand syndrome. See *Canavan syndrome.*

cancellous exostoses. See *multiple cartilaginous exostoses syndrome.*

cancer family syndrome (CFS). See *under hereditary nonpolyposis colorectal cancer syndrome.*

cancer-associated myasthenic syndrome. See *Eaton-Lambert syndrome, under Eaton, Lealdes McKendree.*

cancer-associated retinopathy (CAR) syndrome. Synonym: *paraneoplastic retinopathy.*

Vision loss secondary to retinal degeneration in extra-ocular cancer. Interference with normal function of the retina by cancer cells and autoimmune mechanisms are suspected as the causative agents.

Sawyer, R. A., *et al.* Blindness caused by photoreceptor degeneration as a remote effect of cancer. *Am. J. Ophth.,* 1976, 81:606-13.

cancer-prone syndrome. A condition in which there is predisposition for the development of cancer, as in xeroderma pigmentosum.

Arlett, C. F., & Cole, J. Mutation studies in cells established from human cancer-prone syndromes. *Prog. Clin. Biol. Res.,* 1986, 209A:237-44.

Candida endocrinopathy syndrome. See *candidiasis-endocrinopathy syndrome.*

candidiasis-endocrinopathy syndrome. Synonyms: *Candida endocrinopathy syndrome, endocrine-candidosis syndrome.*

An association of superficial candidiasis with Addison disease, juvenile hypoparathyroidism, and keratoconjunctivitis. Additional disorders may include a celiac-like condition, malabsorption, liver diseases, achlorhydria, pernicious anemia, Hashimoto syndrome, and pulmonary infiltrates. Candidiasis is usually the first to appear, normally before the age of 6 years. It is followed by hypoparathyroidism and adrenocortical insufficiency. Tetany is the usual manifestation of hypoparathyroidism. Lassitude, anorexia, weakness, hypotension, pigmentation of the skin and mucous membrane and low sodium and high potassium levels are the common symptoms. Death from adrenal crisis may follow. The skin is dry and the hair is brittle and and thin. The fingernails at the site of infection are dystrophied and brittle. Cerebrospinal hypertension, papilledema, seizures, mental retardation, and paresthesia are the principal neurological complications. Other disorders may include photophobia, cataracts, hoarseness, laryngospasm, wheezing, and creamy-white plaques of the lips, tongue, oral mucosa, palate, and larynx. Delayed hypersensitivity to *Candida albicans* is a constant feature. Autosomal recessive transmission is suspected.

Collins-Williams, C. Idiopathic hypoparathyroid with papilledema in a boy of 6 years. Report of a case associated with moniliasis and celiac syndrome and brief review of the literature. *Pediatrics*, 1950, 5:998-1007. *Lehner, T. Classification and clinicopathological features of *Candida* infections in the mouth. In: Winner, H. I., & Hurley, R., eds. *Symposium on Candida Infections*. Livingstone, Edinburgh, 1966, p. 119.

canicola fever. See *leptospirosis.*

CANNON, A. BENSON (American dermatologist, born 1888)

Cannon nevus. See *white sponge nevus.*

Cannon syndrome. See *white sponge nevus.*

CANTRELL, JAMES R. (American physician)

Cantrell syndrome. See *thoraco-abdominal syndrome.*

Cantrell-Haller-Ravitch syndrome. See *thoraco-abdominal syndrome.*

CANTU, JOSE MARIA

Cantú syndrome. See *faciocardiomelic dysplasia.*

cao gio. See *pseudobattered child syndrome.*

CAP. See *camptodactyly-arthropathy-pericarditis syndrome.*

CAPDEPONT, CHARLES (French dentist, 1867-1917)

Capdepont syndrome. See *dentinogenesis imperfecta.*

Capdepont teeth. See *dentinogenesis imperfecta.*

Capdepont-Hodge syndrome. See *dentinogenesis imperfecta.*

Stainton-Capdepont syndrome. See *dentinogenesis imperfecta.*

CAPGRAS, JOSEPH (French physician, 1873-1950)

Capgras delusion. See *Capgras syndrome.*

Capgras illusion. See *Capgras syndrome.*

Capgras phenomenon. See *Capgras syndrome.*

Capgras symptom. See *Capgras syndrome.*

Capgras syndrome. Synonyms: *Capgras delusion, Capgras illusion, Capgras phenomenon, Capgras symptom, delusional misidentification, illusion of doubles, illusion of negative doubles, misidentification syndrome, nonrecognition syndrome, phantom double syndrome, subjective doubles syndrome.*

A mental disorder in which the patient recognizes the appearance of a person confronting him but fails to identify that person, steadfastly asserting that it is a double.

Capgras, J., & Reboul-Lachaux, J. L'illusion des "sosies" dans un délire systématisé chronique. *Ann. Méd. Psychol., Paris*, 1923, (series 13):81-186.

capillarotoxic purpura. See *Schönlein-Henoch purpura.*

capillary angiomas. See *De Morgan spots.*

capillary escape syndrome. See *capillary leak syndrome.*

capillary leak syndrome. Synonyms: *capillary escape syndrome, systemic capillary leak syndrome (SCLS).*

Increased systemic capillary permeability with transcapillary escape of albumin and monoclonal IgG and complement alterations, resulting in generalized angioedema and hypovolemic shock. The symptoms include stiff and painful muscles, gastric pain, fatigability, sweating, dizziness, hypotension, and seizures. Infection and physical effort are the precipitating factors.

Clarkson, B., *et al.* Cyclic edema and shock due to increased capillary permeability. *Am. J. Med.*, 1960, 29:193. Löfdahl, C. G., *et al.* Systemic capillary leak syndrome with monoclonal IgG and complement alterations. A case report of an episodic syndrome. *Acta Med. Scand.*, 1979, 206:405-412.

CAPLAN, ANTHONY (British physician)

Caplan syndrome. Synonyms: *Caplan-Colinet syndrome, rheumatoid arthritis-pneumoconiosis syndrome, rheumatoid lung silicosis, rheumatoid pneumoconiosis, rheumatoid-pneumoconiosis syndrome, silicoarthritis.*

In persons exposed to fibrogenic dust, a combination of rheumatoid arthritis and pneumoconiosis marked by painful swelling of the joints, cough, dyspnea, hemoptysis, and radiographic signs of multiple well-defined round opacities of both lungs. Pulmonary granulomas with central necrosis, thickened alveolar septa, and presence of epithelioid and giant cells are the principal pathological features. At the onset of arthritis, the lung opacities may appear suddenly and increase rapidly in size and number, or they may develop in patients already suffering from rheumatoid arthritis.

Caplan, A. Certain unusual radiological appearances in the chest of coal-miners suffering from rheumatoid arthritis. *Thorax, London*, 1953, 8:29-37. Colinet, E. Polyarthrite chronique évolutive et silicose pulmonaire. *Acta Physiother. Rheum. Belge*, 1953, 8:37-41.

Caplan-Colinet syndrome. See *Caplan syndrome.*

CAR syndrome. See *cancer-associated retinopathy syndrome.*

carbamyl phosphate synthetase (CPS) deficiency. See under *hyperammonemic syndrome.*

carbonic anhydrase II deficiency. See *Guibaud-Vainsel syndrome.*

carcinoembryonic antigen (CEA) family syndrome. Presence of the carcinoembryonic antigen (CEA), a tumor-specific antigen in human colonic carcinomata, in the blood plasma of retinoblastoma patients. High plasma CEA levels in asymptomatic family members indicates a risk for malignancy or a genetic predisposition for malignancy.

Felberg, N. T., *et al.* CEA family syndrome. Abnormal carcinoembryonic antigen (CEA) levels in asymptomatic retinoblastoma family members. *Cancer*, 1976, 37:1397-402.

carcinogenetic thromboembolism. See *Trousseau syndrome.*

carcinogenic thrombophlebitis. See *Trousseau syndrome.*

carcinoid syndrome (CS). Synonyms: *Biörck-Axén-Thorsen syndrome, Biörck-Thorsen syndrome, Cassidy syndrome, Cassidy-Scholte syndrome, Hedinger syndrome, Scholte syndrome, Steiner-Voerner syndrome, angiomatosis miliaris, argentaffinoma syndrome, carcinoidosis, flush syndrome, intestinal carcinoid syndrome, malignant carcinoid syndrome, metastatic carcinoid syndrome.*

A carcinoid tumor (argentaffinoma), usually of the ileum and less frequently the stomach, bile duct, duodenum, pancreas, lungs and ovary, with metastases to the liver, which causes overproduction of serotonin and its metabolite 5-hydroxyindoleacetic acid (5-HIAA). The symptoms include episodic flushing, usually beginning in the face and spreading to the trunk and, sometimes, extremities; telangiectases of the face; increased heart rate; hypertension; headache; intestinal hypermobility with diarrhea and abdominal pain; pleural, peritoneal, and retroperitoneal fibrosis; right endocardial fibrosis associated with pulmonary stenosis, tricuspid insufficiency, and heart failure; and bronchial constriction with asthma-like wheezing and respiratory distress. The syndrome is usually sporadic but some familial cases are transmitted as an autosomal dominant trait.

Cassidy, M. A. Abdominal carcinomatosis with probable adrenal involvement. *Proc. Roy. Soc. Med., London,* 1930-31, 24:139-41. Biörck, G., Axén, O., & Thorsen, A. Unusual cyanosis in a boy with congenital pulmonary stenosis and tricuspid insufficiency. Fatal outcome after angiocardiography. *Am. Heart J.,* 1952, 44:143-8. Steiner, L., & Voerner, H. Angiomatosis miliaris. "Eine idiopathische Gefässerkrankung." *Deut. Arch. Klin. Med.,* 1909, 96:105-16. Scholte, A. J. Ein Fall von Angioma teleangiectaticum cutis mit chronischer Endocarditis und malignen Dünndarmcarcinoid. *Beitr. Path. Anat., Jena,* 1930, 86:440-3. Isler, P., & Hedinger, C. Metastasierendes Dünndarmcarcinoid mit schweren, vorwiegend das rechte Herz betreffenden Klappenfehlern und Pulmonalstenose; ein eigenartiger Symptomkomplex. *Schweiz. Med. Wschr.,* 1953, 83:4-7.

carcinoidosis. See *carcinoid syndrome.*

carcinoma in situ. See *Bowen disease, and see Queyrat erythroplasia.*

carcinoma simplex of the nipple. See *mammary Paget disease, under Paget.*

carcinoma unknown primary (CUP) syndrome. A malignancy with metastases but without any evidence of a primary tumor.

Nissenblatt, M. J. The CUP syndrome (carcinoma unknown primary). *Cancer Treat. Rev.,* 1981, 8:211-24.

carcinoma-disseminated thrombocytopenic purpura syndrome. See *Jarcho syndrome.*

carcinomatosis cutis disseminata. See *Arning carcinoid.*

CARDARELLI (Italian physician)

Cardarelli aphthae. See *Riga-Fede disease.*

Cardarelli disease. See *Riga-Fede disease.*

cardiac anxiety syndrome. See *Da Costa syndrome, under Da Costa, Jacob Mendez.*

cardiac asthma. See *Heberden asthma.*

cardiac ballet. See *torsades de pointes syndrome.*

cardiac cyanosis. See *Fallot tetralogy.*

cardiac glycogenosis. See *glycogen storage disease II.*

cardiac hypochondriasis. See *Da Costa syndrome, under Da Costa, Jacob Mendez.*

cardiac neurosis. See *Da Costa syndrome, under Da Costa, Jacob Mendez.*

cardiac phobia. See *Da Costa syndrome, under Da Costa, Jacob Mendez.*

cardiac syncope after swallowing. See *swallowing syncope syndrome.*

cardiac syncope after vomiting. See *swallowing syncope syndrome.*

cardiac-limb syndrome. See *Holt-Oram syndrome.*

cardiasthenia. See *Da Costa syndrome, under Da Costa, Jacob Mendez.*

cardio-acrofascial syndrome. Synonym: *Rabenhorst syndrome.*

An inherited syndrome, probably transmitted as an autosomal dominant trait, of facial abnormalities, cardiac defect, pulmonary stenosis, and multiple minor anomalies of the hands and feet. Facial abnormalities include a narrow face with a high and narrow nose and a prominent septum, slight mongoloid slant of the palpebral fissures, microstomia, prognathism, adherent ear lobes, high arched palate, and dolichocephaly. Restricted mobility at the distal interphalangeal joints with hypoplasia of the corresponding articular folds, simian creases, and syndactyly of the second and third toes are the principal limb defects.

Grosse, F. R. The Rabenhorst syndrome. A cardio-acrofascial syndrome. *Zschr. Kinderheilk.,* 1974, 117:109-14.

cardio-auditory syndrome. See *long QT syndrome.*

cardio-esophageal relaxation syndrome. See *Neuhauser-Berenberg syndrome.*

cardio-inhibitory carotid sinus syndrome. See *carotid sinus syndrome.*

cardio-osseous syndrome. See *Holt-Oram syndrome.*

cardiocutaneous syndrome. See *LEOPARD syndrome, and see Da Costa syndrome, under Da Costa, Jacob Mendez.*

cardiofacial syndrome. Synonyms: *Cayler syndrome, asymmetric crying facies.*

A syndrome of unilateral facial weakness which may be associated with heart defects. The face appears symmetric at rest, the mouth being pulled downward to one side when crying owing to unilateral partial weakness involving the lip depressor muscle (depressor anguli oris). Cardiovascular abnormalities may include a wide variety of defects, such as patent ductus arteriosus, pulmonary stenosis, and atrial, ventricular, or septal defects. Various abnormalities of the central nervous system, bones, gastrointestinal system, and other organs may be associated. Microcephaly and mental retardation may be present.

Cayler, G. G. Cardiofacial syndrome. Congenital heart disease and facial weakness, a hitherto unrecogenized association. *Arch. Dis. Child.,* 1969, 44:69-75.

cardiofaciocutaneous (CFC) syndrome. A multiple congenital anomalies/mental retardation syndrome characterized by congenital heart defect, characteristic facies, ectodermal abnormalities, and growth failure. Cardiac defects are variable, the most common being pulmonic stenosis and atrial septal defect. Typical facial characteristics include a high forehead with bitemporal constriction, hypoplasia of supraorbital ridges, antimongoloid slant of the palpebral fissures, depressed nasal bridge, and posteriorly angulated ears with prominent helices. The hair is usually sparse and friable. Skin changes vary from patchy hyperkeratosis to a severe generalized ichthyosis-like condition. The etiology is unknown.

Reynolds, J. F., *et al.* New multiple congenital anomalies/mental retardation syndrome with cardio-facio-cutaneous involvement-The CFC syndrome. *Am. J. Med. Genet.,* 1986, 25:413-27.

cardiomegalia glycogenica diffusa. See *glycogen storage disease II.*

cardiomegaly-laryngeal paralysis syndrome. See *Ortner syndrome.*

cardiomelic syndrome. See *Holt-Oram syndrome.*

cardiopathia nigra. See *Ayerza syndrome.*

cardioptosis. See *Rummo disease, under Rummo, Gaetano.*

cardiopulmonary obesity syndrome. See *Pickwick syndrome.*

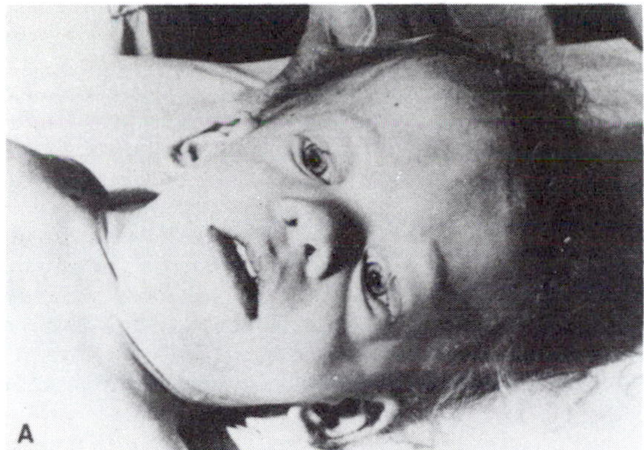

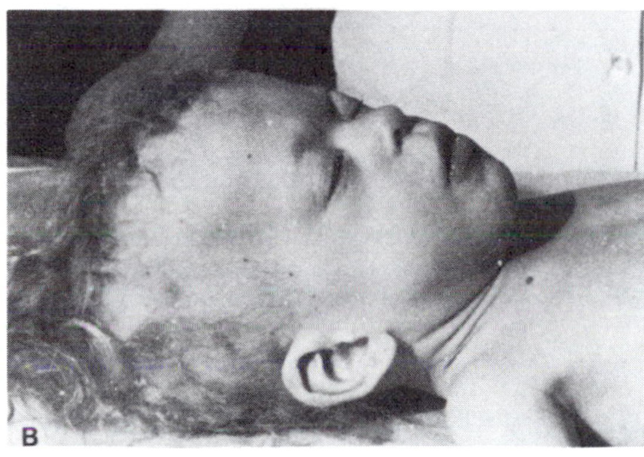

Cardiofaciocutaneous syndrome
Reynolds, James F., Giovanni Neri, Jurgen P. Hermann, Bruce Blumberg, James G. Coldwell, Paul V. Miles, & John M. Opitz, *American Journal of Medical Genetics* 25:413-427, 1986. New York: Alan R. Liss.

cardiorespiratory syndrome of obesity in child. See *Prader-Willi syndrome.*

cardiorespiratory-obesity syndrome. See *Pickwick syndrome.*

cardiotuberculous cirrhosis of the liver. See *Hutinel cirrhosis.*

cardiovascular anomaly-left isomerism syndrome. See *polysplenia syndrome.*

cardiovascular anomaly-right isomerism syndrome. See *asplenia syndrome.*

cardiovasorenal syndrome. See *Fabry syndrome.*

cardiovertebral syndrome. See *Alagille syndrome.*

cardiovocal syndrome. See *Ortner syndrome.*

careotrypanosis. See *Chagas disease.*

CARINI, ANTONINO (Italian physician, 1872-1950)

Carini syndrome. Synonyms: *Seeligmann syndrome, alligator baby, alligator boy, collodion baby, collodion skin, congenital ichthyosiform erythroderma, ichthyosis congenita, ichthyosis sebacea, lamellar desquamation of the newborn, lamellar exfoliation of the newborn, lamellar ichthyosis.*

A skin disease of newborn infants characterized by encasement of the body in a collodion membrane, a shiny, rigid scale made up of a thickened stratum corneum saturated with water. Evaporation of water causes the membrane to crack with eventual formation of fissures and shedding of the membrane, exposing red skin underneath. Some infants have a bullous form of X-linked ichtyosis but most are affected with lamellar ichthyosis. See also *ichthyosis congenita syndrome..*

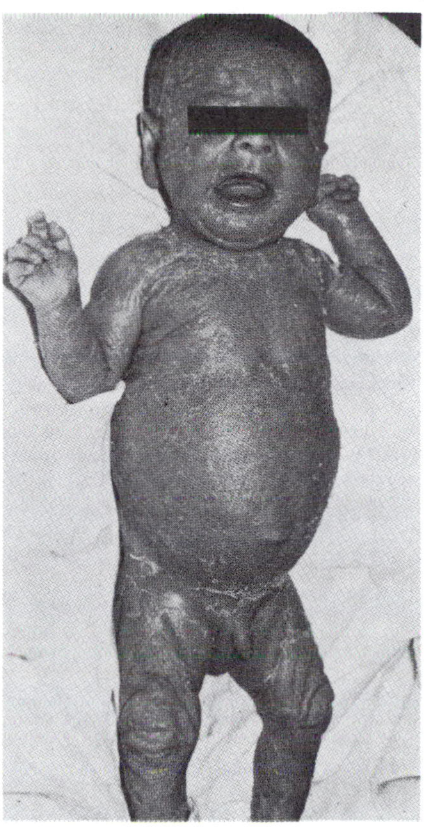

Carini syndrome
Andrews, G.C. & A.N. Domonkos: *Diseases of the skin.,* 5th ed. Philadelphia, W.B. Sanders Co., 1963.

Carini, A. Di una forma della cosidetta "ittiosi sebacea" (ittiosi lamellare). *Gior. Ital. Mal. Vener.,* 1895, 36:82-8.
*Seeligmann, E. *De epidermis imprimis neonatorum desquamatione.* Berlin, 1841. (Thesis).

CARL SMITH. See SMITH, CARL HENRY

CARNEY, J. A. (American physician)

Carney syndrome. See *Carney triad.*

Carney triad. Synonym: *Carney syndrome.*

The triad of pulmonary chondroma, extra-adrenal paraganglioma, and gastric leiomyosarcoma.

Carney, J. A. The triad of gastric epithelioid leiomyosarcoma, functioning extra-adrenal paraganglioma, and pulmonary chondroma. *Cancer,* 1979, 43:374-82.

CAROL, WILLEM LAMBERTUS LEONARD (Dutch physician, 1879-1945)

Godfried-Prick-Carol-Prakken syndrome. See *under Godfried.*

CAROLI, JAQUES (French physician, born 1902)

Caroli disease. See *Caroli syndrome (1).*

Caroli syndrome (1). Synonyms: *Caroli disease, valvular gallbladder.*

Plication of the neck of the gallbladder, causing painful biliary dyskinesia and hypertonia.

Caroli, J., *et al.* La coudure douloureuse intermittente du col de la vésicule. Variété fréquentes des dyskinésie biliaires pures. Démonstration radiomanometrique. *Sem. Hôp., Paris,* 1948, 24:526-31.

Caroli syndrome (2). Synonyms: *congenital cystic degeneration of bile ducts, congenital cystic dilatation of intrahepatic bile ducts, congenital dilatation of great intrahepatic ducts, congenital dilatation of intrahepatic bile ducts, congenital dilatation of intrahepatic segmentary bile ducts, congenital intrahepatic cysts of bile ducts, congenital saccular dilatation of hepatic bile ducts, cystic intrahepatic bile duct dilatation, focal dilatation of intrahepatic bile ducts, intrahepatic bile duct cysts, segmental saccular dilatation of intrahepatic bile ducts.*

A congenital disease characterized by cystic dilatation of intrahepatic bile ducts, complicated by formation of gallstones, cholangitis, and liver abscesses. Associated disorders may include portal hypertension, liver cirrhosis, splenomegaly, and cysts of other organs, such as the spleen, kidneys, and pancreas. Infection with gram-negative bacteria is a frequent fatal complication.

Caroli, J., & Corcos, V. *Maladies des voies biliaires intrahépatiques segmentaires.* Paris, Masson, 1964.

Caroli triad. The triad of arthritis, excruciating headache, and urticaria preceding icteric hepatitis.

Caroli, J., & Ferroir, J. L'urticaire et l'ictère catarrhal. *Bull. Mém. Soc. Méd. Hop. Paris,* 1935, Pt I:604-9.

carotene jaundice. See *Baelz disease (2).*

carotenoderma. See *Baelz disease (2).*

carotid pain. See *Hilger syndrome.*

carotid sinus hypersensitivity syndrome. See *carotid sinus syndrome.*

carotid sinus syncope. See *carotid sinus syndrome.*

carotid sinus syndrome (CSS). Synonyms: *Charcot-Weiss-Baker syndrome, Weiss-Baker syndrome, cardio-inhibitory carotid sinus, carotid sinus hypersensitivity syndrome, carotid sinus syncope, hyperactive carotid sinus syndrome, tight collar syndrome, vagal syncope, vasovagal syndrome.*

Fall in the arterial pressure and cardiac arrest, caused by strong pressure on the neck over the bifurcation of the carotid arteries, which cause the excitation of baroreceptors of the carotid sinuses. In most cases, there is escape of the ventricles of the heart from the vagal inhibition with restoration of normal heart beat; in some cases, the ventricles fail to escape and the patient dies of heart arrest. Elderly persons, especially those with calcified atherosclerotic plaques in the carotid arteries, are most susceptible. The attacks may also be produced by a sudden turn of the head, wearing a tight collar, or carotid neoplasms.

Charcot, J. M. *Leçons sur les maladies du système nerveux faites a la Salpétrière.* Paris, 1872-73. Weiss, S., & Baker, J. The carotid sinus reflex in health and disease. Its role in the causation of fainting and convulsions. *Medicine,* 1933, 12:197-354.

carotid steal syndrome. Diversion of blood flow from the distal portion of the common carotid artery after carotid-subclavian bypass surgery.

Dumanian, A. V., *et al.* The surgical treatment of the subclavian steal syndrome. *J. Thorac. Cardiovasc. Surg.,* 1965, 50:22-5. Sergeant, P., *et al.* The true value of the carotid steal syndrome after the carotid subclavian bypass. *Acta Chir. Belg.,* 1980, 79:9-14.

carotidodynia. See *Hilger syndrome.*

carotidynia. See *Hilger syndrome.*

carpal entrapment syndrome. See *carpal tunnel syndrome.*

carpal tunnel syndrome (CTS). Synonyms: *Guyon tunnel syndrome, carpal entrapment syndrome.*

Compression of the median nerve as it passes within the tissue of the flexor retinaculum in the carpal tunnel at the wrist, causing numbness, tingling, burning sensation, and pain of the hands and fingers, sometimes extending as far as the forearm, or even the shoulder and neck. Radial fingers are most commonly affected but other digits may be also involved. The symptoms are most prominent at night or after prolonged inactivity but they may also recur at other times. The syndrome is observed most frequently in middle-aged females but it may also occur in younger women and in males. Predisposing factors include gout, tenosynovitis, rheumatoid arthritis, osteoarthritis, old fractures, pregnancy, myxedema, acromegaly, carpal ligament lesions in amyloidosis, and hemodialysis. In younger persons, the syndrome may be associated with excessive straining when using the hand. The syndrome may occur when the nerve is compressed within the loge of Guyon in the burned patient.

*Marie, P., & Foix, C. Atrophie isolée de l'éminence thénar d'origine névritique, röle due legament anulaire antérior du carpe dans la pathogénie de la lésion. *Rev. Neur., Paris,* 1913 26:647-9.

CARPENTER, GEORGE (British physician)

Carpenter syndrome. Synonym: *acrocephalopoysyndactyly (ACPS).*

A congenital syndrome consisting of soft-tissue syndactyly, especially of the third and fourth fingers, syndactyly of the toes, brachymesophalangy, preaxial polydactyly, coxa valga, pes varus, mental retardation, hypogonadism, mild obesity, hernia, and congenital heart defects. Craniofacial abnormalities usually include turricephaly with premature synostosis of cranial sutures, flat nasal bridge, and dystopia canthorum, which may occur asymmetrically. The hands are usually short with short stubby fingers. The syndrome is transmitted as an autosomal recessive trait.

Carpenter, G. Two sisters showing malformations of the skull and other congenital abnormalities. *Rep. Soc. Study Dis. Child., London,* 1900-1, 1:110-8.

carpotarsal osteolysis syndrome (dominant and sporadic forms). Synonyms: *essential multifocal osteolysis, phantom bone, tarsocarpal acro-osteolysis with or without nephropathy, vanishing bone disease.*

A rare bone disease in early childhood which begins as an arthritic episode and progresses to involve multiple peripheral joints, eventually becoming relatively silent, but causing disability in adults. As the disease progresses, there is a marked decrease in adult height with muscle weakness and hypotonia, shortening and cavus foot deformities, asymmetric and sporadic involvement of the joints, and a generally painless course, except for recurrent arthritic episodes. X-ray findings show progressive osteolysis, usually in the carpal and tarsal bones, sometimes involving the distal ends of the radius, ulna, and tibia. Associated disorders may include skull abnormalities, scoliosis, micrognathia, plantar cysts, and flexion contractures of the elbows, knees, and hips. Nephropathy with proteinuria may occur. Some cases are transmitted as an autosomal dominant trait and others are sporadic.

Froelich, & Corret. Ostéolyse du carpe. *Rev. Méd Nancy,* 1937, 65:696. Erickson, C. M., *et al.* Carpal-tarsal osteolysis. *J. Pediat.,* 1978, 93:779-82.

carpotarsal osteolysis syndrome (recessive form). Synonyms: *Winchester syndrome, Winchester-Grossman syndrome, pseudorheumatoid arthritis.*

A hereditary syndrome, transmitted as an autosomal recessive trait, characterized by short stature, joint contractures, corneal opacities, coarse facies, carpo-tarsal osteolysis, osteoporosis, kyphoscoliosis and intra- and peri-articular joint lesions simulating rheumatoid arthritis. Radiological findings show thinning of the long bones, pelvic malformations, osteolysis of the femoral heads, wide thin ribs, expanded clavicle, resorption of distal phalanges, bulging of the midshafts of the phalanges, delayed closure of the fontanels, flat mandibular condyles, and delayed tooth eruption. The syndrome was originally believed to be a mucopolysaccharidosis; more recent findings indicate that this is a nonlysosomal connective tissue disease.

Winchester, P., Grossman, H., *et al.* A new acid mucopolysaccharidosis with skeletal deformities simulating rheumatoid arthritis. *Am. J. Roentgen.,* 1969, 106:121-8.

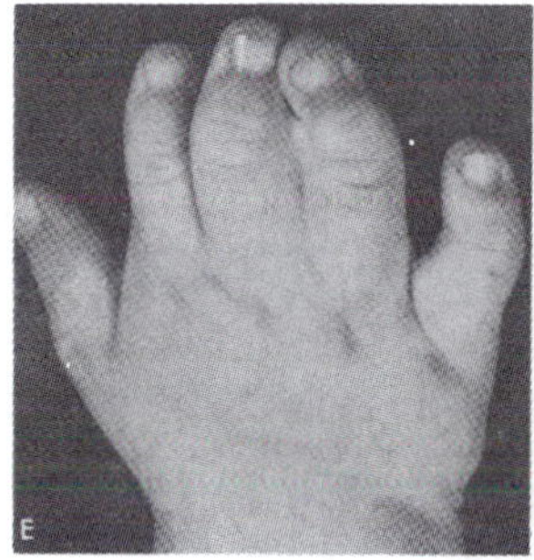

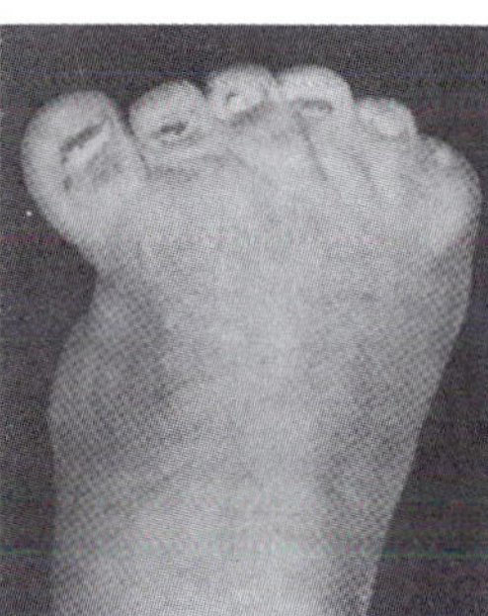

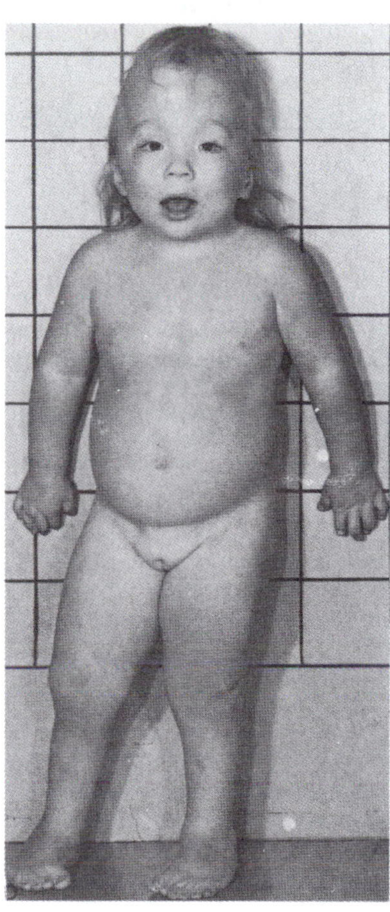

Carpenter syndrome
Temtamy, S.A.: *J. Pediatr.* 69:111, 1966. St. Louis: C.V. Mosby Co.

carpus carvus. See *Madelung deformity.*

CARR, DAVID H. (Canadian physician)

Carr-Barr-Plunkett syndrome. See *chromosome XXXX syndrome.*

CARRARO, ARTURO (Italian physician)

Carraro syndrome. A familial syndrome of deafmutism, shortening of the calves, foot deformities, and hypoplasia of the tibiae, believed to be transmitted as an autosomal recessive trait.

Carraro, A. Assenza congenita della tibia e sordomutismo in quatro fratelli. *Chir. Organi Mov.,* 1931, 16:429-38. Wendler, H., & Schwarz, R. Carraro-Syndrom. *ROEFO,* 1980, 133:43-6.

CARRION, DANIEL A. (Medical student in Peru who inoculated himself with *Bartonella bacilliformis* and died of the disease, 1850-1885)

Carrión disease. Synonyms: *Carrión fever, Bartonella bacilliformis anemia, Oroya fever, Peruvian wart, verruga peruana.*

An infectious disease caused by *Bartonella bacilliformis* and transmitted by the biting flies *Phlebotomus noguchi* and *P. verrucarum.* The infection is endemic in parts of Peru, Colombia, and Ecuador at altitudes of 600 to 3700 meters. Two forms are recognized: the mild form **(verruga peruana)** and the severe form

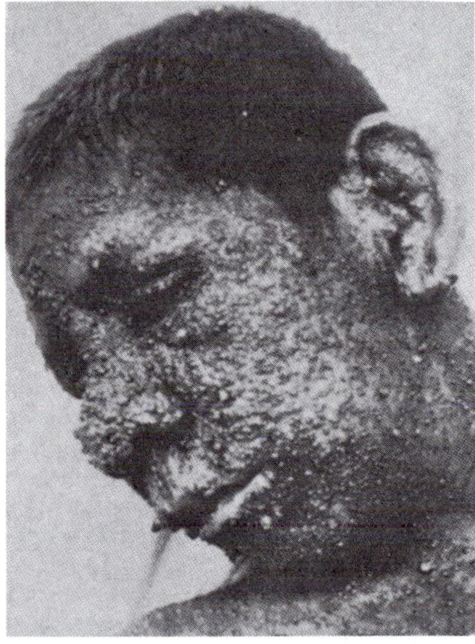

Carrión disease
Andrews, G.C. & A.N. Domonkos: *Diseases of the Skin* 5th ed. Philadelphia, W.B. Saunders Co., 1963.

(**Oroya fever**). The mild form is characterized by mild anemia and either miliary or nodular eruptions. The miliary lesions are cherry-red, varying in size from that of a pinhead to that of a pea, and affect the face and extremities. The nodular lesions begin in the subcutaneous tissue of the elbows and knees, eventually become ulcerated, and reach 1 to 2 cm in diameter. The nodular type may develop into the malar type, in which the lesions, which reach the size of a small apple, are covered by thin bluish skin and form bleeding ulcerated masses. The severe form is characterized by acute fever, pernicious anemia, and muscular pain and weakness. A few patients who survive this stage develop cherry-red lesions.

Odriazola, E. La erupción en la enfermedad de Carrión (verruga peruana). *Monit. Med., Lima*, 1895, 10:309-11.

Carrión fever. See *Carrión disease.*

CARSON, NINA A. J. (Irish physician)

Carson-Neill syndrome. See *homocystinuria syndrome.*

CARTEAUD, ALEXANDRE (French physician, born 1897)

Gougerot-Carteaud papillomatosis. See *Gougerot-Carteaud syndrome, under Gougerot, Henri.*

Gougerot-Carteaud syndrome. See *under Gougerot, Henri.*

cartilage-containing giant-cell tumor. See *Codman tumor.*

cartilage-hair hypoplasia syndrome. See *McKusick metaphyseal chondrodysplasia syndrome.*

CASAL, GASPAR (Spanish physician, 1691-1759)

Casal necklace. Necklace-like erythema and pigmentation around the neck in pellagra.

Casal, G. *Historia natural, y medica de el Principado de Asturias.* Madrid, Martin, 1762.

CASALA, AUGUSTO M. (Argentine physician)

Casalá-Mosto disease. Synonyms: *Doucas-Kapetanakis disease, Loewenthal purpura, angiodermatitis pruriginosa disseminata, eczematid-like purpura, itching purpura.*

A form of purpura characterized by the presence of small reddish punctiform maculae on the lower extremities, extending to the entire body within several weeks. Pruritus, residual yellowish pigmentation, and pityriasis-like scaling are the secondary features. The disease usually occurs during the spring and summer, chiefly in males.

Casalá, A. M., & Mosto, S. J. Angiodermatitis pruriginosa disseminaata: "Eczematid-like purpura" (Doucas C. & Kapetanakis); "itching purpura" (Loewenthal). *Arch. Argent. Derm.*, 1955, 5:209-16. Doucas, C., & Kapetanakis, J. Eczematid-like purpura. *Dermatologica, Basel*, 1953, 106:86-95. Loewenthal, L. J. Itching purpura. *Brit. J. Derm.*, 1954, 66:95-103.

CASS, JOHN W. (American physician)

Meigs-Cass syndrome. See *Meigs syndrome.*

CASSIDY, MAURICE A. (British physician)

Cassidy syndrome. See *carcinoid syndrome.*

Cassidy-Scholte syndrome. See *carcinoid syndrome.*

CASSIRER, RICHARD (German physician, 1868-1925)

Cassirer syndrome. See *Raynaud phenomenon, under Raynaud syndrome.*

Crocq-Cassirer syndrome. See *Raynaud phenomenon, under Raynaud syndrome.*

cast syndrome. Synonyms: *plaster cast syndrome, spinal traction syndrome, vascular compression of the duodenum.*

Compressive obstruction of the transverse or ascending portion of the duodenum by the superior mesenteric artery after the application of a body cast. The obstruction may lead to acute gastric dilatation and ileus of the duodenum with nausea, pernicous vomiting, hypovolemia, hypokalemia, dehydration, metabolic alkalosis, oliguria, abdominal distention, rupture of the stomach, shock, and death. The disorder occurs in wearers of surgical corsets and as a complication of skeletal traction in the treatment of scoliosis and kyphosis, whereby the angle of origin of the superior mesenteric artery from the abdominal aorta is altered, thus causing obstruction of the duodenum.

Willett, A. Fatal vomiting, following the application of the plaster-of-Paris bandage in a case of spinal curvature. *St. Barts Hosp. Rep.*, 1878, 14:333-5. Dorph, M. H. The cast syndrome: Review of the literature and report of a case. *N. Engl. J. Med.*, 1950, 243:440.

CASTELLANI, SIR ALDO (Italian-born physician in England, 1877-1971)

Castellani bronchitis. Synonyms: *Castellani disease, bronchospirochetosis, hemorrhagic bronchitis.*

Spirochaeta bronchialis bronchitis with hemoptysis.

Castellani, A. Observations on the fungi found in tropical bronchomycosis. *Lancet*, 1912, 1:13-5.

Castellani disease. See *Castellani bronchitis.*

Castellani syndrome. A peculiar form of febrile hepatosplenomegaly with arthritis, characterized by slow onset, malaise, fever, and joint pain. The fever is usually undulating, resembling that in Bang disease, but it may be irregular, intermittent, or remittent. The spleen and liver are hard and enlarged, often reaching the transverse umbilical line. The disease is usually observed in middle-aged males.

Castellani, A. A note on a peculiar febrile hepatosplenomegaly with arthritis. *J. Trop. Med. Hyg., London*, 1935, 38:229-30.

CASTLEMAN, BENJAMIN (American physician, born 1906)

Castleman angiofollicular hyperplasia. See *Castleman disease.*

Castleman disease. Synonyms: *Castleman angiofollicular hyperplasia, Castleman lymphadenopathy, angiofollicular lymph node hyperplasia, giant lymph node hyperplasia (GLNH), giant lymphoid hyperplasia of the mediastinum, lymphoid angio-follicular hyperplasia.*

A pathological condition characterized by large, benign, hyperplastic lymph nodes. In the original report, the condition was asymptomatic, but the more recent literature indicates that the lesions may be associated with various clinical manifestations. The more common hyaline vascular subtype is characterized by minimal symptoms and small hyaline vascular follicles and interfollicular capillary proliferations. Plasma cells are often present. The plasma cell subtype is often associated with fever, anemia, hyperglobulinemia, and, occasionally, nephrotic syndrome, lymphoproliferative disorders, plasmacytoma, and Kaposi sarcoma. Histologically, the lymph nodes in the plasma cell variant contain large follicles with inconspicuous hyaline vascular changes and sheets of plasma cells within the paracortical and interfollicular zones. Immunological findings consist mainly of the presence of a polyclonal population of cytoplasmic Ig-producing cells. The clumps of plasma cells also contain IgM and IgA.

Castleman, B., *et al.* Localised mediastinal lymph node hyperplasia resembling thymoma. *Cancer,* 1956, 46:822-30. Martin, J. M. E., *et al.* Giant lymph node hyperplasia (Castleman disease) of hyaline vascular type. Clinical heterogeneity with immunohistologic uniformity. *Am. J. Clin. Path.,* 1985, 84:439-46.

Castleman lymphadenopathy. See *Castleman disease.*

Castleman lymphoma. See *Castleman tumor.*

Castleman tumor. Synonym: *Castleman lymphoma.*

Mediastinal lymph node hyperplasia resembling thymoma and characterized by the germinal center formation and marked capillary proliferation. The condition is believed to be neither neoplastic nor thymic in origin.

Castleman, B., *et al.* Localized mediastinal lymph node hyperplasia resembling thymoma. *Cancer,* 1956, 9:822-30.

Rosen-Castleman-Liebow syndrome. See *under Rosen.*

CASTROVIEJO

Castroviejo syndrome. See *Urretz-Zavalia syndrome.*

cat cry syndrome. See *chromosome 5p deletion syndrome.*

cat eye syndrome. Synonyms: *Schmid-Fraccaro syndrome, coloboma-anal atresia syndrome.*

An association of iridal and choroidal coloboma (giving the appearance of cat eyes), anal atresia, auricular anomalies, and genitourinary defects. Congenital heart disease is often associated. Additional anomalies usually include mental and growth retardation, hypertelorism, antimongoloid palpebral slant, cleft palate, preauricular skin tags or sinuses, low-set and malformed ears, microphthalmia, strabismus, epicanthus, depressed nasal bridge, hip dislocation, long and slender thumbs, skeletal anomalies, renal abnormalities, and seizures. Tricuspid atresia, anomalous pulmonary vein return, hypoplasia of the inferior vena cava, tetralogy of Fallot, and atrial septal defect are the most common cardiovascular anomalies. Most patients show an extra small chromosome 22 (trisomy 22), but a few have normal chromosome complements.

Haab, O. Beitrage zu den angeborenen Fehlern des Auges. *Graefes Arch. Klin. Ophth.,* 1878, 24:257-62. Schachnmann, G., *et al.* Chromosomes in coloboma and anal atresia. *Lancet,* 1965, 2:290. Schmid, W. Pericentric inversions (report of two malformation cases suggestive of parental inversion heterozygosity). *J. Genet. Hum.,* 1967, 16:89-96.

cat scratch disease (CSD). Synonyms: *Debré syndrome, Debré-Mollaret syndrome, Foshay-Mollaret syndrome, Petzetakis disease, benign inoculation lymphoreticulosis, benign reticulosis, cat scratch fever, felinosis, inoculation adenitis, inoculation lymphoreticulosis, lymphoreticulosis benigna, morbus Petzetakis, nonbacterial regional lymphadenitis.*

An acute infectious disease, occurring most commonly in young children, characterized by tender regional lymphadenopathy, sterile suppurative papules at the site of inoculation, fever, nausea, and malaise taking place 1 to several weeks after being scratched or bitten by a cat. Most cases are benign and self limiting, but lymphadenopathy may persist for several months after other symptoms disappear. Encephalitis is a rare complication. Laboratory findings include eosinophilia, elevated erythrocyte sedimentation rate, leukocytosis, and tuberculin-like reaction. Cat scratch disease, when associated with ocular granuloma or conjunctivitis, is known as the *Parinaud oculoglandular syndrome.*

Debré, R., *et al.* La maladie des griffes de chat. *Bull. Méd. Soc. Hôp. Paris,* 1950. 66:76-9. *Petzetakis, M. Monoadénite subaiguë multiple de nature inconue. *Soc. Méd. Athènes,* 1935, 16:229. Mollaret, P., *et al.* La découverte du virus de la lymphoréticulose bénign d'inoculation. II. Inoculation expérimentale ou singe et coloration. *Presse Méd., Paris,* 1951, 59:701-4.

cat scratch fever. See *cat scratch disease.*

cat scratch-oculoglandular syndrome. See *Parinaud oculoglandular syndrome.*

catalase deficiency. See *Takahara syndrome.*

catalepsy of awakening. See *Rosenthal disease, under Rosenthal, Curt.*

cataract-mental retardation-hypogonadism syndrome. Synonym: *Martsolf syndrome.*

A familial syndrome, transmitted as an autosomal recessive trait, characterized by mental retardation, short stature, brachycephaly, cataract, hypogonadism, hypertelorism, low nasal bridge, maxillary retrusion, prognathism, short philtrum, pouting mouth, malocclusion, furrowed tongue, sparse facial hair, low hairline, flat and broad sternum, prominent nipples, broad fingertips, ulnar deviation of fingers, finger joint laxity, short palms and abnormal finger/palm ratio, excess of palmar creases, abnormal toenails, talipes valgus, and short ulna. The syndrome appears to occur mainly in

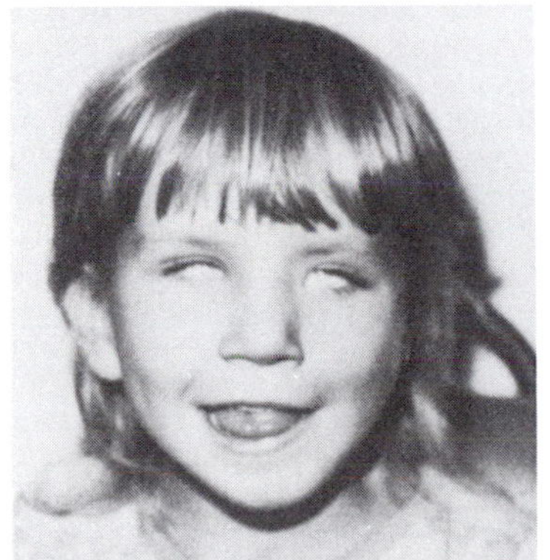

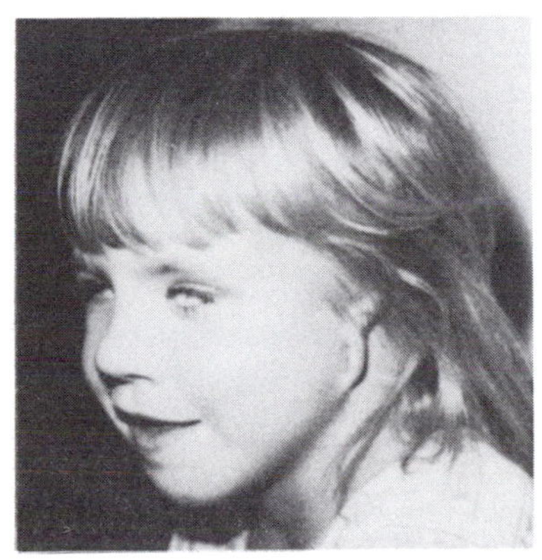

Cat eye syndrome
Ing, Paul S., Mark S. Lubinsky, Shelley D. Smith, Ellen Golden, Warren G. Sanger, & Alessandra M.V. Duncan, *American Journal of Medical Genetics* 26:621-628, 1987. New York: Alan R. Liss Inc.

patients of Jewish descent.

Martsolf, J. T., *et al.* Severe mental retardation, cataracts, short stature and primary hypogonadism in two brothers. *Am. J. Med. Genet.*, 1978, 1:291-9. Sanchez, J. M., *et al.* Two brothers with Martsolf's syndrome.. *Med. Genet.*, 1985, 22:308-10.

cataract-oligophrenia syndrome. See *Marinesco-Sjögren syndrome, under Marinescu, Gheorghe.*

cataract-progressive sensorineural hearing loss syndrome. A syndrome of progressive sensorineural hearing loss and cataracts, transmitted as an autosomal dominant trait.

Nadol, J. B., Jr., & Burgess, B. Cochleosaccular degeneration of the inner ear and progressive cataracts inherited as an autosomal dominant trait. *Laryngoscope*, 1982, 92:1028-37.

cataracta dermatogenes. See *Andogsky syndrome.*
cataracta syndermatotica. See *Andogsky syndrome.*
catarrhal jaundice. See *Botkin disease.*
catarrhal rhinitis. See *common cold syndrome.*
catarrhus estivus. See *Bostock catarrh.*
CATEL, W.
Catel-Manzke syndrome. See *palatodigital syndrome.*
CATTAN, ROGER (French physician)
Siegal-Cattan-Mamou disease. See *Reimann periodic disease.*
CAUCHOIS
Cauchois-Eppinger-Frugoni syndrome. See *Frugoni syndrome.*
caudal dysplasia syndrome (CDS). See *caudal regression syndrome.*

caudal regression syndrome. Synonyms: *Duhamel anomalad, Duhamel syndrome, caudal dysplasia syndrome (CDS), mermaid syndrome, phocomelic diabetic embryopathy, sacral agenesis syndrome, sacral dysplasia syndrome, sacrococcygeal agenesis syndrome, sirenomelia, symmelia, sympodia.*

Aplasia or hypoplasia of the caudal vertebrae associated with defects of the corresponding segments of the spinal cord and hypoplasia or aplasia of the pelvis and lower limbs. There is a shortening, narrowing, or malformation of the lower trunk with disproportionate shortness of stature, flattening of the buttocks with dimpling, and, in the most severe cases, "mermaid" configuration of the lower extremities, hence the synonyms **mermaid syndrome** and **sirenomelia**. Various other abnormalities may be associated, including imperforate anus, hypoplasia and weakness of the lower limbs, hip dislocation, knee and hip contractures, pes equinovarus, pelvic muscle paralysis, neurogenic bladder, bowel dysfunction, fused iliac bones, femoral hypoplasia, and other defects and disorders. Irregular autosomal dominant inheritance is suspected in some cases, but most instances are attributed to maternal diabetes, thus accounting for the synonym **phocomelic diabetic embryopathy**.

Duhamel, B. From the mermaid to anal inperforation: The syndrome of caudal regression. *Arch. Dis. Child., Chicago*, 1961, 36:152. Smith, D. W., *et al.* Monozygotic twinning and the Duhamel anomalad (imperforate anus to sirenomelia): A nonrandom association between two aberrations in morphogenesis. *Birth Defects*, 1976, 12(5):53-63.

caudolateral pontine syndrome. A syndrome associated with compromised circulation through the anterior inferior cerebellar artery. The symptoms may include ipsilateral paresthesia in the area supplied by the trigeminal nerve, cerebellar ataxia, Horner syndrome, hypoacusis, vertigo, contralateral sensitivity and hemiparesis, uveal and pharyngeal myoarrhythmias, nausea, headache, impaired conciousness, organic psychosyndrome, and peripheral facial paresis.

Perneczky, A., *et al.* The relationship between caudolateral pontine syndrome and the anterior inferior cerebellar artery. *Acta Neurochir.*, 1981, 58:245-57.

causalgia. See *reflex sympathetic dystrophy syndrome.*

CAVALLAZZI, C. (Italian physician)
Cavallazi syndrome. See *craniomandibular dermatodysostosis.*
CAVARE, C.
Cavaré-Romberg syndrome. See *Westphal syndrome, under Westphal, Karl Friedrich Otto.*
Cavaré-Romberg-Westphal syndrome. See *Westphal syndrome, under Westphal, Karl Friedrich Otto.*
Cavaré-Westphal syndrome. See *Westphal syndrome, under Westphal, Karl Friedrich Otto.*
cavernitis fibrosa. See *Peyronie disease.*
cavernous angioma of the spinal cord. See *Foix-Alajouanine syndrome.*
cavernous hemangioma-thrombocytopenia syndrome. See *Kasabach-Merritt syndrome.*
cavernous optic atrophy. See *Schnabel atrophy.*
cavernous sinopharyngeal tumor syndrome. See *Godtfredsen syndrome.*

cavernous sinus syndrome. Synonyms: *Foix syndrome, lateral wall of the cavernous sinus syndrome, thrombosis of cavernous sinus syndrome.*

Ophthalmoplegia and paralysis of the third, fourth, fifth, and sixth cranial nerves, with bulging and edema of the eyelids, secondary to intracranial aneurysms or thrombosis of the cavernous or lateral sinuses, sometimes associated with trigeminal neuralgia.

Foix, C. Syndrome de la paroi externe du sinus caverneux (ophthalmoplégie unilatérale à marche rapidement progressive. Algie du territoire de l'ophthalmique). Amélioration considerable par traitement radiothérapique. *Rev. Neur., Paris*, 1922, 38:827-32.

cavernous sinus-nasopharyngeal tumor syndrome. See *Godtfredsen syndrome.*

CAYLER, GLEN G. (American physician)
Cayler syndrome. See *cardiofacial syndrome.*
CAZENAVE, PIERRE LOUIS ALPHEE (French physician, 1795-1877)
Cazenave disease (1). See *lupus erythematosus.*
Cazenave disease (2). See *pemphigus foliaceus.*
Cazenave vitiligo. Synonyms: *alopecia areata, alopecia circumscripta, area Johnstoni, pelade, porrigo decalvans, tinea declavans.*

Loss of hair in circumscribed patches reportedly first described by Cazenave.

CBS (cystathionine beta-synthase) deficiency. See *homocystinuria syndrome.*
CC. See *Cronkhite-Canada syndrome.*
CCHS (congenital central hypoventilation syndrome). See *Ondine curse.*
CCM. See *cerebrocostomandibular syndrome.*
CCMS. See *cerebrocostomandibular syndrome.*
CD. See *Crohn disease.*
CDK (climatic droplet keratopathy). See *Bietti dystrophy.*

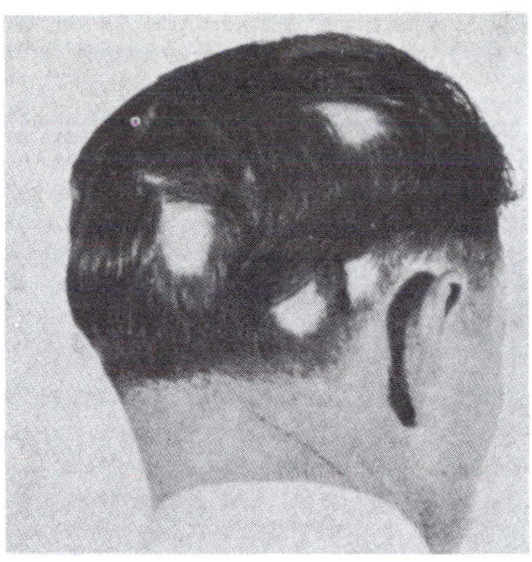

Cazenave vitiligo
Andrews, G.C. & A.N. Domonkos: *Diseases of the Skin* 5th ed. Philadelphia: W.B. Saunders Co., 1963.

CDS (caudal **d**ysplasia **s**yndrome**).** See *caudal regression syndrome.*

CEA family syndrome. See *carcinoembryonic antigen family syndrome.*

cecal (caecal) slap syndrome. Slapping of the cecum against the fixed anterior abdominal wall, occurring in runners at the time when the foot hits the ground and the muscles of the wall tighten and there is a brief check in momentum. The symptoms include lower abdominal discomfort with a tender cecum, nausea, and diarrhea.

Porter, A. M. W. Marathon running and the caecal slap syndrome. *Brit. J. Sports Med.*, 1982, 16:178.

CED (chondro**e**ctodermal **d**ysplasia**).** See *Ellis-van Creveld syndrome.*

CEELEN, WILHELM (German physician, 1884-1964)

Ceelen-Gellerstedt syndrome. Synonyms: *brown pulmonary induration, essential brown induration of the lung, hemosiderosis of the lung, idiopathic pulmonary hemosiderosis (IPH).*

A rare lung disease occurring chiefly in infants and children, sometimes also observed in adults. Pulmonary changes consist of siderosis, intersitital fibrosis, and capillary hemorrhage in association with hypochromic anemia. Hepatomegaly and splenomegaly may occur. Fever, cyanosis, episodes of cough, dyspnea, hemoptysis, and abdominal pain are the principal clinical symptoms, and cor pulmonale is a frequent complication. Clubbing of the fingers is sometimes present.

Ceelen, W. Die Kreislaufstörungen der Lungen. In: Henke, F., & Lubarsch, O., eds. *Handbuch der speziellen pathologischen Anatomie und Histologie.* Berlin, Springer, 1931. Gellerstedt, N. Über die "essentielle" anämisierende Form der braunen Lungeninduration. *Acta Path. Microb. Scand.*, 1939, 16:386-400.

celiac disease. Synonyms: *Gee disease, Gee-Herter disease, Gee-Herter-Heubner disease, Gee-Thaysen disease, Herter infantilism, Heubner-Herter disease, celiac sprue, celiac syndrome, gluten-induced enteropathy, gluten-sensitive enteropathy, idiopathic steatorrhea, intestinal infantilism, morbus celiacus, morbus coeliacus, nontropical sprue.*

A gastrointestinal disease of both children and adults, caused by an inborn error of protein metabolism with secondary intestinal malabsorption disorders. In the infantile form, the manifestations typically begin after weaning and the introduction of cereals in the diet. The symptoms may include diarrhea with bulky foul-smelling stools and steatorrhea, abdominal distention, failure to gain weight, growth retardation, dehydration, acidosis, and oral symptoms. Vomiting and diarrhea are the early complaints, other symptoms appearing later. Ingestion of gluten exacerbates the condition. Commonly, the symptoms disappear in later childhood and adolescence, despite continued malabsorption. In the adult form, the symptoms appear in the third to sixth decades and may present a wide spectrum of disorders, ranging from mild to severe, and consisting of discomfort, diarrhea, anemia, foul-smelling stools, bleeding tendency, hypocalcemia, iron deficiency, folate deficiency, defective bone development, malnutrition, muscle wasting, edema, hypotension, abdominal bloating, clubbing of the fingers, and pigmentation disorders. The oral symptoms may include glossitis, atrophy of the filiform papillae with persistence of the fungiform papillae on the atrophic surface, burning sensation, and sometimes, painful vesicular erosion. Intestinal biopsy shows villus atrophy. Dilatation of the proximal loops of the small intestine and coarsening of the jejunal folds are the principal radiographic characteristics. Some authors suggest autosomal dominant inheritance; others discount a possibility of mendelian inheritance. See also *malabsorption syndrome.*

Herter, C. A. *On infantilism from chronic intestinal infection.* New York, Macmillan, 1908. *Heubner, O. J. Über schwere Verdauungsinsuffizienz beim Kinde jenseits des Säuglingsalters. *Jb. Kinderh.*, 1909, 70:667. Thaysen, E. T. The "coeliac affection"-idiopathic steatorrhea. *Lancet,* 1929, 1:1086-9. Gee, S. On the coeliac affection. *St. Bartholomew Hosp. Rep., London,* 1888, 24:17-20.

celiac sprue. See *celiac disease.*

celiac syndrome. See *celiac disease.*

celluloradiculoneuritis. See *Guillain-Barré syndrome.*

cementoperiostitis. See *Fauchard disease.*

central alveolar hypoventilation syndrome (CAHS). See *Ondine curse.*

central angiospastic retinopathy. See *Masuda-Kitahara disease.*

central anticholinergic syndrome. See *anticholinergic syndrome.*

central aortitis. See *aortic arch syndrome.*

central cloudy dystrophy. See *François dystrophy (1).*

central cord syndrome. Central injury of the spinal cord, whereby the lesion located just above the concussive blow extends from the central gray matter into the medial part of the white matter of the cord. Lower motor neuron changes are primarily associated with spasticity in the legs; weaker symptoms may occur in the arms. The symptoms vary with the extent of injury in the posterior and anterolateral columns, consisting mainly of reduced pain and temperature sensations and urinary retention incontinence.

Becker, D. P. Injury to the head and spine. In: Wyngaarden, J. B., & Smith, L. H., Jr., eds. *Cecil textbook of medicine.* 17th ed. Philadelphia, Saunders, 1985, pp. 2170-7. Guttmann, L. *Spinal cord injuries. Management and research.* 2nd ed. Oxford, Blackwell, 1976.

central core disease. See *Shy-Magee syndrome.*
central hematomyelia. See *Minor disease.*
central hypoventilation syndrome (CHS). See *under hypoventilation syndrome.*
central neurofibromatosis. See *Wishart disease.*
central sleep apnea syndrome. See *under sleep apnea syndrome.*
central tapetoretinal degeneration. See *Behr syndrome (1).*
centronuclear myopathy. See *Shy-Magee syndrome.*
CEP. See *congenital erythropoietic porphyria.*
CEP (chronic eosinophilic pneumonia). See *pulmonary infiltration with eosinophilia syndrome.*
cephalalgia pharyngotympanica. See *Legal disease.*
cephalgia. See *headache syndrome.*
cephalic zoster syndrome. See *Hunt syndrome (2), under Hunt, James Ramsay.*
cephalo-oculocutaneous telangiectasis. See *Louis-Bar syndrome.*
cephalohydrocele traumatica. See *Billroth disease (1).*
cephalopolysyndactyly syndrome. See *Greig syndrome.*
ceramide trihexosidosis. See *Fabry syndrome.*
cerebellar ataxia. See *Zappert syndrome.*
cerebellar degeneration-slow eye movement syndrome. See *Wadia-Swami syndrome.*
cerebellar hereditary ataxia. See *Marie syndrome (1), under Marie, Pierre.*
cerebellar hypoplasia in Werdnig-Hoffmann disease. See *amyotrophic cerebellar hypoplasia syndrome.*
cerebello-olivary degeneration. See *Holmes disease, under Holmes, Gordon Morgan.*
cerebelloretinal hemangioblastomatosis. See *Hippel-Lindau syndrome.*
cerebral amyloidosis with spongiform encephalopathy. See *Gerstmann syndrome (1).*
cerebral artery compression syndrome. See *Bärtschi-Rochaix syndrome.*
cerebral beriberi. See *Wernicke syndrome.*
cerebral cholesterinosis. See *van Bogaert-Scherer-Epstein syndrome.*

cerebral diplegia. See *Little disease, under Little, William John.*
cerebral disconnection syndrome. See *disconnection syndrome.*
cerebral gigantism. See *Sotos syndrome.*
cerebral hyponatremia. See *cerebral salt wasting syndrome.*
cerebral idiopathic nonarteriosclerotic calcification. See *Fahr syndrome.*
cerebral infantile paralysis. See *Strümpell disease (1).*
cerebral peduncle syndrome. See *Leyden paralysis (1).*
cerebral pseudosclerosis. See *Wilson disease, under Wilson, Samual Alexander Kinnier.*

cerebral salt wasting syndrome. Synonym: *cerebral hyponatremia.*

A syndrome combining features of the renal salt losing syndrome (q.v.), inappropriate secretion of antidiuretic hormone, and brain disease. It is marked by a decrease in body sodium levels, and is often accompanied by hyponatremia under conditions of normal sodium intake. It is being unresponsive to standard doses of mineralocorticoids, and therein differs from the inappropriate antidiuretic hormone secretion syndrome (q.v.).

Peters, J. P., *et al.* Salt-wasting syndrome associated with cerebral disease. *Tr. Am. Tr. Assoc. Am. Physicians,* 1950, 63:57-64.

cerebral spastic paralysis. See *Little disease, under Little, William John.*
cerebral symmetric calcification. See *Fahr syndrome.*
cerebral vasomotor syndrome. See *Friedmann syndrome (1), under Friedmann, Max.*
cerebral white matter spongy degeneration. See *Canavan syndrome.*
cerebro-arthrodigital syndrome. Synonym: *cerebrodigital syndrome.*

A congenital syndrome of arthromyodysplasia associated with sacral agenesis, brain malformation, and digital hypoplasia. The symptoms include intrauterine growth retardation, central nervous system malformations (mainly hydrocephaly or microcephaly), sacral and coccygeal agenesis, digital hypoplasia, muscle hypoplasia, joint contractures, short stature, lack of tubular bone modeling, lung hypoplasia, short perineum, piloinidal sinus, and excessive short tissue mass. Toxic agents such as ergotamine and diazoxide are suspected as etiologic factors.

Spranger, J. W., *et al.* Cerebrodigital syndrome: A newly recognized formal genesis syndrome in three patients with apparent arthromyodysplasia and sacral agenesis, brain malformation and digital hypoplasia. *Am. J. Med. Genet.,* 1980, 5:13-24.

cerebro-ocular dysgenesis. See *Walker-Warburg syndrome, under Walker, Arthur Earl.*
cerebro-ocular dysplasia-muscular dystrophy syndrome (COD-MD). See *cerebro-oculomuscular syndrome.*
cerebro-oculofacioskeletal (COFS) syndrome. Synonym: *Pena-Shokeir syndrome.*

A familial syndrome (with some cases of parental consanguinity) transmitted as an autosomal recessive trait, characterized mainly by microcephaly, muscle hypotonia, failure to thrive, arthrogryposis, eye defects, peculiar facies (prominent nose, large ears, overhanging upper lip, micrognathia), widely spaced nipples, kyphoscoliosis, and osteoporosis.

Pena, S. D. J., & Shokeir, M. H. K. Autosomal recessive cerebro-oculo-facio-skeletal (COFS) syndrome. *Clin. Genet.,* 1974, 5:285-93.

cerebro-oculomuscular syndrome (COMS). Synonym: *cerebro-ocular dysplasia-muscular dystrophy (COD-MD) syndrome.*

A triad of brain, eye, and muscle abnormalities. Cerebellar or cerebral agyria-micropolygyria, cortical disorganization, glial mesodermal proliferation in the leptomeninges, neuronal heterotopias, hypoplasia of the nerve tracts, hydrocephalus, and occasional encephalocele are the principal neurological features. Ocular defects include microphthalmia, cataract, immature anterior chamber angle, retinal dysplasia with or without retinal detachment, persistent hyperplastic primary vitreous, optic nerve hypoplasia, and coloboma. Skeletal muscle disorders consist of fiber splitting, variable fiber size, and endomysial fibrosis. The syndrome is similar to Walker-Warburg, Fukuyama, and Santavuori syndromes (q.v.).

Heggie, P., *et al.* Cerebro-ocular dysplasia-muscular dystrophy syndrome. *Arch. Ophth.,* 1987, 105:520-4.

cerebrocardiac syndrome. See *Krishaber disease.*

cerebrocostomandibular syndrome (CCM, CCMS). Synonyms: *Smith-Theiler-Schachenmann syndrome, rib gap defect with micrognathia.*

A hereditary developmental disorder, transmitted as an autosomal recessive trait, characterized chiefly by costovertebral malformations (segmentation of the ribs and fusion of their dorsal ends to the vertebral bodies with a bell-shaped thorax), mental deficiency, and orofacial defects, mainly micrognathia, short hard palate with a central hole, absent soft palate, absent uvula, and glossoptosis. Collapsed tracheal cartilage, microcephaly, delayed myelination, redundant skin, and elbow hypoplasia may be associated. Additional disorders may include pterygium colli, fusion of the vertebrae to each other, scoliosis, hemivertebrae, renal ectopy, deafness, and limb abnormalities. Neonatal respiratory distress and barking cough are frequently observed. Possible teratogenic etiology is considered by some writers. The syndrome is potentially lethal in the neonatal period.

Smith, D. W., Theiler, K., & Schachenmann, G. Rib-gap defect with micrognathia, malformed tracheal cartilage, and redundant skin: A new pattern of defective development. *J. Pediat.*, 1966, 69:799-803. McNicholl, B., *et al.* Cerebro-costo-mandibular syndrome. A new familial developmental disorder. *Arch. Dis. Child.*, 1970, 45:421-4. Silverman, F. N., *et al.* Cerebro-costo-mandibular syndrome. *J. Pediat.*, 1980, 97:406-16.

cerebrocutaneous angiomatosis. See *Sturge-Weber syndrome.*

cerebrodigital syndrome. See *cerebro-arthrodigital syndrome.*

cerebrofaciothoracic dysplasia syndrome. A multiple abnormalilty-mental retardation syndrome, probably transmitted as an autosomal recesssiuve trait, characterized by peculiar facies (narrow forehead, bushy eyebrows, synophrys, hypertelorism, broad nose, wide philtrum, triangular mouth, maxillary hypoplasia, low hairline, brachycephaly), short neck, and multiple osseous abnormalities involving upper thoracic and cervical vertebrae and upper ribs.

Pascual-Castroviejo, I., *et al.* Cerebro-facio-thoracic dysplasia: Report of three cases. *Dev. Med. Child. Neur.*, 1975, 17:343-51.

cerebrohepatorenal syndrome (CHR, CHRS). See *Zellweger syndrome.*

cerebromacular degeneration. See *Stock-Spielmeyer-Vogt syndrome.*

cerebromacular dystrophy. See *Stock-Spielmeyer-Vogt syndrome.*

cerebropathia psychica toxemica. See *Korsakoff syndrome, under Korsakov, Sergei Sergeevich.*

cerebroretinal arteriovenous aneurysm. See *Bonnet-Dechaume-Blanc syndrome, under Bonnet, Paul.*

cerebroretinal syndrome. See *Hippel-Lindau syndrome.*

cerebroside lipidosis. See *Gaucher disease.*

cerebrospinal cholesterinosis. See *van Bogaert-Scherer-Epstein syndrome.*

cerebrotendinous xanthomatosis (CTX). See *van Bogaert-Scherer-Epstein syndrome.*

cerebrovascular familial idiopathic calcification. See *Fahr syndrome.*

ceroid storage disease. See *Landing-Oppenheimer syndrome.*

CERTONCINY, A. (French physician)

Forestier-Certonciny syndrome. See *Forestier syndrome (1).*

CERVENKA, JAROSLAV

Cervenka syndrome. A syndrome of myopia, hyaloderoretinal degeneration, cleft palate, and flattening of the midface. Genua valga, hip joint deformity, hypospadias, and mental retardation are sometimes associated. The syndrome is transmitted as an autosomal dominant trait.

Cohen, M. M., Jr., Knobloch, W. H., & Gorlin, R. J. A dominantly inherited syndrome of hyaloideoretinal degeneration, cleft palate and maxillary hypoplasia (Cervenka syndrome). *Birth Defects*, 1971, 7(7):83-6.

cervical hydrocele. See *Maunoir hydrodele.*

cervical lipomatosis. See *Madelung syndrome.*

cervical migraine. See *Barré-Lieou syndrome.*

cervical migraine syndrome. See *Bärtschi-Rochaix syndrome.*

cervical rib syndrome. Synonyms: *Adson syndrome, Adson-Caffey syndrome, Coote-Hanauld syndrome.*

A form of the thoracic outlet syndrome (q.v.) in which there is a compression of the nerves and vessels in the outlet of the thorax and the costoclavicular area or between the clavicle and the first rib due to angulation of the brachial plexus over a cervical rib (a supernumerary rib from the costal portion of the seventh cervical vertebra and extending into the posterior triangle of the neck or the thoracic outlet), with resulting pain (involving the chest wall, shoulder, arm, and hand), paresthesia, numbness, skin color changes, claudication, diminished pulse, lowered blood pressure on the affected side, and wasting and weakness of the muscles of the hand and forearm.

Adson, A. W., & Caffey, I. R. Cervical rib. A new method of approach for relief of symptoms by division of the scalenus anticus. *Ann. Surg.*, 1927, 85:839-57. *Grüber, W. Über die Halstrippen des Menschen mit vergleichenden anatomischen Bemerkungen. *Mem. Acad. Imp. Sc., St. Petersburg,* 1869, 13: *Hanauld. *Communications to the Royal Academy of Sciences in 1740*, Amsterdam, 1744. Coote, H. Pressure on the axillary vessels and nerve by an exostosis from a cervical rib. Interference with the circulation of the arm. Removal of the rib and exostosis. Recovery. *Med. Times Gaz.*, 1861, 2:108.

cervical sympathetic paralysis syndrome. See *Horner syndrome.*

cervical vertigo syndrome. See *Bärtschi-Rochaix syndrome.*

cervico-encephalic syndrome. See *Bärtschi-Rochaix syndrome.*

cervico-oculo-acoustic dysplasia. See *Wildervanck syndrome (1).*

cervico-oculo-acoustic dystrophy. See *Wildervanck syndrome (1).*

cervico-oculo-acoustic syndrome. See *Wildervanck syndrome (1).*

cervico-oculo-acusticus syndrome. See *Wildervanck syndrome (1).*

cervico-oculofacial dysmorphia. See *Wildervanck syndrome (1).*

cervico-oculofacial syndrome. See *Wildervanck syndrome (1).*

cervicodermorenogenital dysplasia. See *Goeminne syndrome.*

cervicolinguomasticatory syndrome. See *tardive dyskinesia syndrome.*

cervicothoracic outlet compression syndrome. See *thoracic outlet syndrome.*

CES. See *cat eye syndrome.*

CESTAN, ETIENNE JACQUES MARIE RAYMOND (French Physician, 1872-1932)

Céstan paralysis. See *Céstan-Chenais syndrome.*

Céstan-Chenais syndrome. Synonym: *Céstan paralysis.*

Thrombosis of the vertebral artery below the point of origin of the posterior inferior cerebellar artery, characterized by unilateral paralysis of the soft palate and vocal cords, ipsilateral ocular signs (enophthalmos, blepharoptosis, nystagmus, and miosis), contralateral hemiplegia, ataxia, and diminution of touch and proprioceptive senses.

Céstan, E. J., & Chenais, J. Du myosis dans certains lésions bulbaires en foyer (hémiplégia du type Avellis associée au syndrome oculaire sympathique). *Gaz. Hôp., Paris*, 1903, 76:1229-33.

Céstan-LeJonne syndrome. See *Emery-Dreifuss syndrome.*

Raymond-Céstan syndrome. See *under Raymond.*

CFC. See *cardiofaciocutaneous syndrome.*

CFDS (craniofacial dyssynostosis). See *craniosynostosis-craniofacial dysostosis syndrome.*

CFS (cancer family syndrome). See *under hereditary nonpolyposis colorectal cancer syndrome.*

chacaleh. See *burning feet syndrome.*

CHAGAS, CARLOS (Brazilian physician, 1879-1934)

Chagas disease. Synonyms: *Chagas-Cruz disease, Chagas-Mazza disease, Brazilian trypanosomiasis, careotrypanosis, South American trypanosomiasis.*

An infectious insect-borne disease that is endemic in the interior of Brazil and affects man and the armadillo; it is caused by *Trypanosoma cruzi*. Onset is usually in the first decade, involving one eye or, less frequently, the skin, with consecutive intermittent fever, edema, lymph node hypertrophy, subcutaneous nodules, and cardiac lesions. Cardiopathy may be latent in the acute form, but in the chronic form it is the conspicuous symptom.

Chagas, C. Nova tripanozomiaze humana. *Mem. Inst. Oswaldo Cruz*, 1909, 1:159-218.

Chagas-Cruz disease. See *Chagas disease.*

Chagas-Mazza disease. See *Chagas disease.*

CHAIX, ACHILLE (French physician, born 1875)

Favre-Chaix angiodermatitis. See *under Favre.*

Favre-Chaix syndrome. See *Favre-Chaix angiodermatitis.*

chalazion. See *meibomian cyst.*

chalazoderma. See *cutis laxa syndrome.*

chalodermia. See *cutis laxa syndrome.*

CHAMPION, R. H.

Sneddon-Champion syndrome. See *Sneddon syndrome (2).*

CHAMPION, RANDELL (British physician)

Champion-Cregan-Klein syndrome. See *popliteal pterygium syndrome.*

CHANARIN, I. (British physician)

Chanarin-Dorfman syndrome. Synonym: *ichthyosiform dermatosis with systemic lipidosis.*

Neurocutaneous lipidosis, transmitted as an autosomal recessive trait, marked by ichthyosiform dermatosis, electromyographic abnormality, and accumulation of lipids in the granulocytes and monocytes. Associated disorders may include impaired scotopic and photopic function of the eyes, nystagmus, ataxia, areflexia, defective visual acuity, neurosensory deafness, electrocardiographic changes, fatty liver, and muscular disorders. Biochemical changes include hyperglycemia, glycosuria, high protein level in the cerebrospinal fluid, and elevated serum glutamate oxaloacetate transmaminase. The syndrome is most common in persons of the Mid-Eastern and Mediterranean extraction.

Chanarin, I., *et al.* Neural lipid storage disease: A new disorder of lipid metabolism. *Brit. Med. J.*, 1975, 1:553-5. Dorfman, M. L., *et al.* Ichthyosiform dermatosis with systemic lipidosis, *Arch. Derm., Chicago*, 1974, 110:261-6.

CHANCE, G. O. (British physician)

Chance fracture. Synonyms: *distraction fracture of the lumbar spine, flexion fracture of the spine, fulcrum fracture of the lumbar spine.*

A horizontal fracture of the lumbar spine, affecting the posterior vertebral arch and ending in an upward curve which usually reaches the upper surface of the body of the vertebra just in front of the neural foramen. It occurs most commonly during automobile collisions while wearing seat belts.

Chance, G. Q. Note on a type of flexion fracture of the spine. *Brit. J. Radiol.*, 1948, 21:452-3. Van Tiggelen, R., *et al.* Chance's fracture. *J. Belge Radiol.*, 1985, 68:63-5.

chancroid. See *Ducrey disease.*

CHANDLER, FREMONT AUGUSTUS (American orthopedic surgeon, 1893-1954)

Chandler syndrome. Synonyms: *idiopathic necrosis of femoral head, primary idiopathic nontraumatic necrosis of femoral head, osteochondritis dissecans of femoral head.*

Idiopathic, usually bilateral aseptic necrosis of the femur, appearing most often in early middle age. The disease is manifested by pain of the hip and occasionally of the knee area and by avascular necrosis of the bone and bone marrow of the femoral head.

Chandler, F. A. Aseptic necrosis of the head of the femur. *Wisconsin Med. J.*, 1936, 35:583-618.

CHANDLER, PAUL A. (American ophthalmologist)

Chandler syndrome. A syndrome of atrophy of the stroma of the iris, corneal dystrophy with edema, peripheral anterior synechiae, and glaucoma. A prominent feature and the presenting symptom is edema of the cornea with normal or slightly increased intraocular pressure. Males and females are equally affected.

Chandler, P. A. Atrophy of the stroma of the iris, endothelial dystrophy, corneal edema, and glaucoma. *Tr. Am. Ophth. Soc.*, 1955, 53:75-89.

CHANDS (curly hair-ankyloblepharon-nail dysplasia syndrome). A rare form of ectodermal dysplasia characterized by curly hair that does not grow past shoulder length, dysplastic nails, ankyloblepharon at birth, and ataxia. The syndrome is transmitted as an autosomal recessive trait.

Baughman, F. A. CHANDS: The curly hair-ankyloblepharon-nail dysplasia syndrome. *Birth Defects*, 1971, 7(8):100-2. Toriello, H. V., *et al.* Re-evaluation of CHANDS. *J. Med. Genet.*, 1979, 16:316-7.

CHAPPLE, CHARLES CULLODEN (American pediatrician, born 1903)

Chapple syndrome (1). Synonym: *duosyndrome of the laryngeal nerve.*

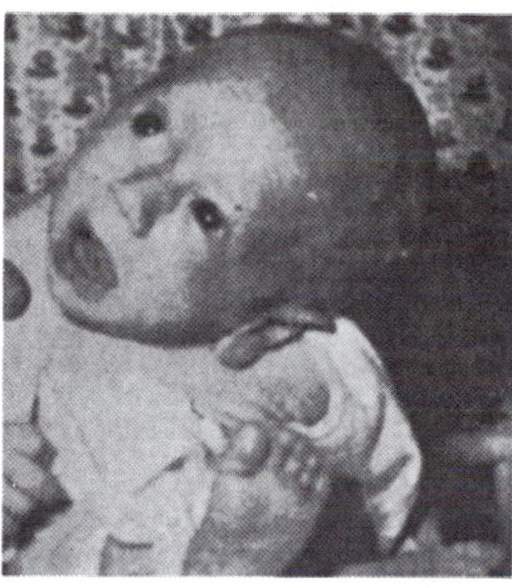

Chapple syndrome (2)
Nelson, W.E. (Ed.), *Textbook of Pediatrics* 9th ed.Philadelphia: W.B. Saunders Co., 1969.

In the newborn, a unilateral facial weakness or paralysis associated with comparable weakness or paralysis of the vocal cord and/or the muscles of deglutition (parts innervated by the recurrent or superior laryngeal nerve) on the opposite side. This condition is caused by lateral flexion of the head in utero, which holds the thyroid cartilage against the hyoid or cricoid bones with consequent pressure on the laryngeal nerve or its blood supply.

Chapple, C. C. A duosyndrome of the laryngeal nerve. *AMA J. Dis. Child.*, 1956, 91:14-8.

Chapple syndrome (2). Synonyms: *Sally syndrome, genu recurvatum-uterine retroversion-dysmenorrhea syndrome.*

A congenital syndrome of back-bent knees, uterine retroversion, and dysmenorrhea. Abnormal intrauterine position of the fetus appears to be the cause.

Chapple, C. C. Genu recurvatum, uterine retroversion and dysmenorrhea. Relation to fetal position. *Clin. Pediat.*, 1971, 10:6-8.

CHARCOT, JEAN MARTIN (French physician, 1825-1893)

Charcot arthrosis. See *Charcot disease.*

Charcot disease. Synonyms: *Charcot arthrosis, Charcot joint, Charcot syndrome, arthropathia neurotica, arthropathia tabica, neuroarthropathy, neuropathic arthritis, neuropathic arthropathy, tabetic osteoarthropathy.*

A progressive degenerative disease of the joints resulting from neurological disorders, including tabes dorsalis, diabetic neuropathy, alcoholic neuropathy, or syringomyelia. Degeneration of the cartilage, hypertrophic changes, effusions into the joints, intra-articular fractures and loose bodies, dislocations, knock knees, bone fragmentation, and osteophytic formations are among the usual findings. The condition is constantly aggravated by the loss of pain in and hypermobility of the joints, which deprive the affected organ of natural protection from injuries.

Charcot, J. M. Sur quelques arthropathies qui paraissent dépendre d'une lésion du cerveau ou de la moelle épinière. *Arch. Physiol., Paris*, 1868, 1:161-78; 379-400.

Charcot edema. Synonym: *blue edema.*

Edema with a bluish appearance of the extremities, seen in hysterical paralysis.

Guinon, G. L'oedème bleu de hystériques. *Progr. Méd., Paris*, 1890, 12:259-64.

Charcot fever. Fever resulting from impacted gallstones.

Charcot, J. M., & Gombault. Note sur les oblitérations du foie consecutives à la ligature du canal cholédoque. *Arch. Physiol. Norm. Path.*, 1876, 8:272-99.

Charcot joint. See *Charcot disease.*

Charcot sclerosis. See *amyotrophic lateral sclerosis.*

Charcot syndrome (1). See *amyotrophic lateral sclerosis.*

Charcot syndrome (2). See *Charcot disease.*

Charcot syndrome (3). Synonyms: *angina cruris, angiosclerotic paroxysmal myasthenia, claudicatio intermittens, gangrena spontanea chirurgigorum, intermittent claudication, intermittent limping syndrome, myasthenia paroxysmalis angiosclerotic.*

A disorder that usually involves the legs and less frequently the arms. Pain, cramps, discomfort, tension, and weakness, most commonly appearing after a physical effort and disappearing after rest, are its chief features. The condition is symptomatic of a variety of vascular diseases, including Buerger disease.

Charcot, Sur la claudication intermittente observée dans un cas d'oblitération de l'une des artères iliaques primitives. *C. Rend. Soc. Biol.*, 1858, 5(part 2):225-58.

Charcot triad. A triad of intention tremor, nystagmus, and scanning speech in multiple sclerosis.

Charcot, M. Diagnostic des formes frustes de la sclérose en plaque. *Progr. Méd., Paris*, 1879, 7:97-9.

Charcot vertigo. Synonyms: *ictus laryngis, laryngeal syncope, laryngeal vertigo.*

A rare condition in which vertigo or syncope, caused by an attack of coughing, results in laryngeal spasm or closure of the glottis.

Charcot, J. M. Du vertige laryngé. *Progr. Méd., Paris*, 1879, 17:317-9.

Charcot-Marie syndrome. See *Charcot-Marie-Tooth syndrome.*

Charcot-Marie-Tooth disease (CMTD). See *Charcot-Marie-Tooth syndrome.*

Charcot-Marie-Tooth syndrome (CMTS). Synonyms: *Charcot-Marie syndrome, Charcot-Marie-Tooth disease (CMTD), Charcot-Marie-Tooth-Hoffmann syndrome, Tooth muscular atrophy, atrophia musculorum progressiva neurotica sive neuralis, hereditary motor and sensory neuropathy I (HMSN I), neuropathic muscular atrophy, peroneal muscle atrophy.*

A hereditary syndrome which begins with atrophy of the peroneal muscle and advances insidiously to involve other distal muscles of the leg and arm, associated with pathological changes in the anterior horn cells, posterior columns, peripheral nerves, dorsal root ganglia, and other parts of the spinal cord. Dropfoot, pes equinovarus, paresthesia, cyanosis, bone atrophy, and perforating ulcer may occur. Optic atrophy is sometimes present. The syndrome usually begins in children and adolescents and progresses slowly. It is transmitted as an autosomal dominant or recessive trait in some families and as an X-linked trait in others.

Charcot, J. M., & Marie, P. Sur une forme particulière d'atrophie musculaire progressive, souvent familiale, débutant par les pieds et les jambes et atteignant plus tard

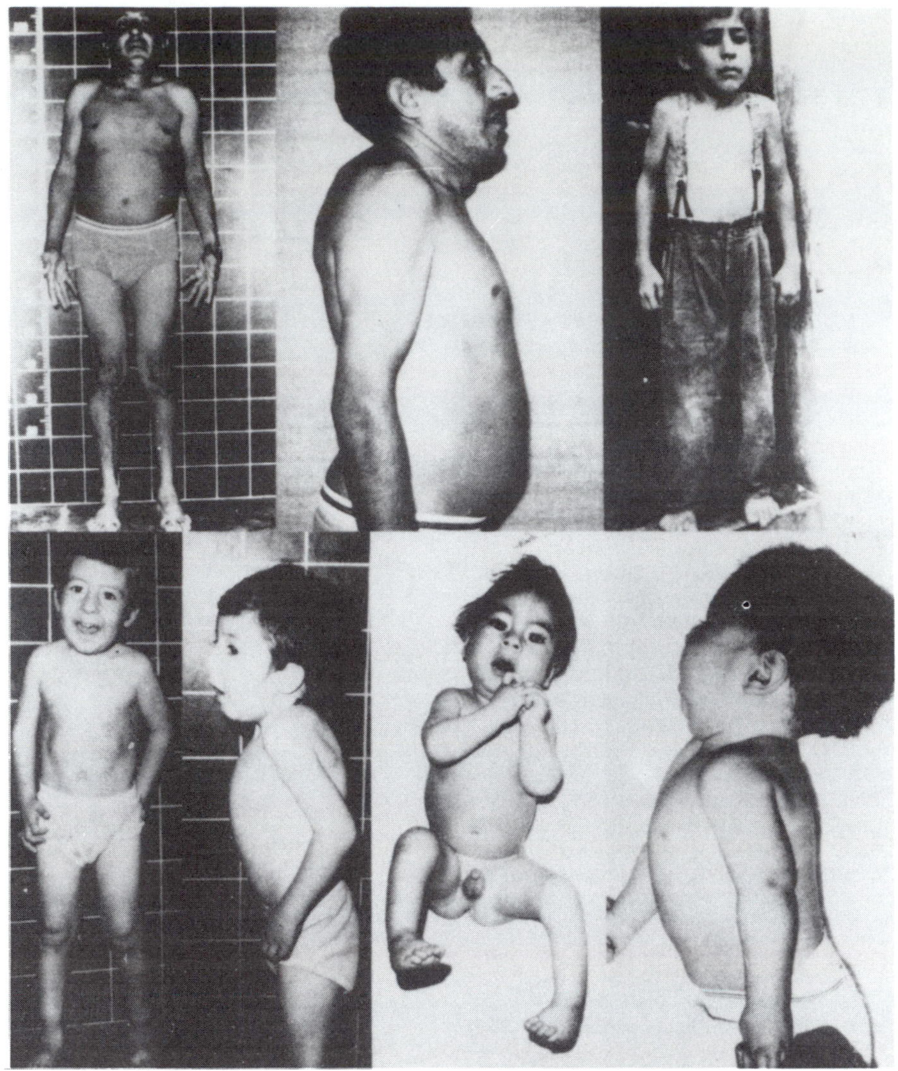

Charcot-Marie-Tooth syndrome
Ruiz, C., F. Rivas, G. Ramirez-Casillas, R. Vazquez-Santana, B. Mendoza-Chalita, A. Feria-Velasco, G. Tapia-Arizmendi, & J.M. Cantu: *Clinical Genetics* 31:109-113, 1987, Munksgaard International Publishers, Copenhagen, Denmark.

les mains. *Rev. Méd., Paris*, 1886, 6:97138. *Tooth, H. H. *The peroneal type of progressive muscular atrophy.* London, 1886. Hoffman, J. Weitere Beiträg zur Lehre von der hereditären progressiven spinalen Muskelatrophie im Kindesalter nebst Bemerkungen uber den fortschreitenden Muskelschwund im Allgemeinen. *Deut. Schr. Nervenh.*, 1897, 10:292-20.

Charcot-Marie-Tooth-Hoffmann syndrome. See *Charcot-Marie-Tooth syndrome.*

Charcot-Weiss-Baker syndrome. See *carotid sinus syndrome.*

Erb-Charcot syndrome. See *under Erb.*

Souques-Charcot geroderma. See *under Souques.*

CHARGE (coloboma-heart disease-atresia of choanae-retarded mental development and growth-genital hypoplasia-ear abnormalities-deafness) syndrome. Synonym: *CHARGE association.*

An association of choanal atresia with multiple abnormalities. Coloboma usually involves the choroid, iris, and optic nerve. A wide variety of heart defects may occur, including tetralogy of Fallot, septal defect, valvular stenosis, and other anomalies. Choanal atresia may be unilateral or bilateral. Most affected patients exhibit mental and growth retardation. Hypogenitalism may be present in some cases. In many instances, deafness is not due to ear malformations, but to recurrent episodes of otitis. Additional anomalies may include cleft lip and palate, tracheo-esophageal fistulae and atresia, renal abnormalities, and dysmorphic facial features, including dysplastic and low-set ears, antimongoloid palpebral slant, and anteverted nostrils. Etiology is unkown.

Hall, B. D. Choanal atresia and associated multiple anomalies. *J. Pediat.*, 1979, 95:395-8. Pagon, R. A., *et al.* Coloboma, congenital heart disease, and choanal atresia with multiple anomalies: CHARGE association. *J. Pediat.*, 1981, 99:223-7.

CHARGE association. See *CHARGE syndrome.*

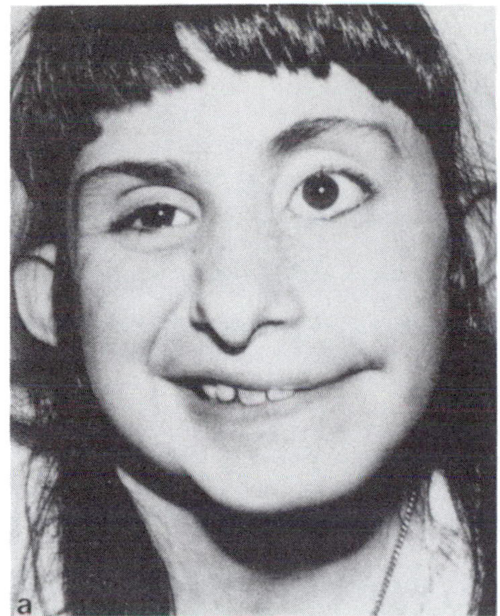

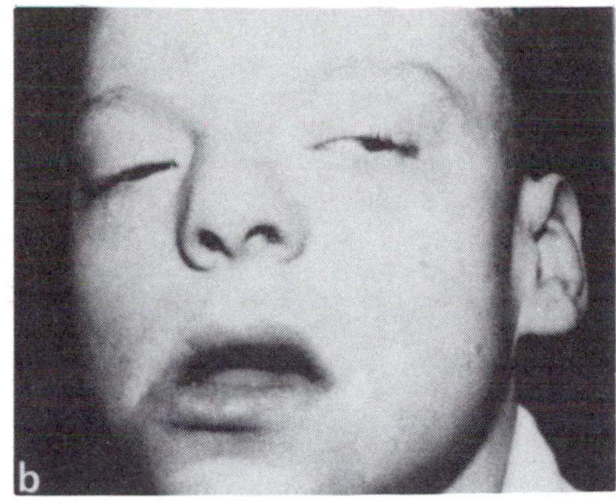

CHARGE
Davenport, Sandra L.H., Margaret A. Hefner, & Joyce A. Mitchell: *Clinical Genetics* 29:298-310, 1986, Munksgaard International Publishers, Copenhagen, Denmark.

CHARLES BONNET. See BONNET, CHARLES

CHARLET, HENRI (French physician, born 1884)

Nicolas-Moutot-Charlet syndrome. See *under Nicolas.*

Charlevoix disease. See *Andermann syndrome.*

Charlevoix-Saguenay spastic ataxia. Synonym: *autosomal recessive spastic ataxia of Charlevoix-Saguenay (ARSACS).*

Spastic ataxia, transmitted as an autosomal recessive trait, first observed in the Charlevoix-Saguenay region of Quebec in Canada. The syndrome is characterized by spasticity, dysarthria, distal muscle wasting, foot deformities, truncal ataxia, absence of sensory evoked potentials in the lower limbs, retinal striations similar to those in Leber atrophy, and frequent mitral valve prolapse. Biochemically, many cases show impaired pyruvate oxidation, others have hyperbilirubinemia, and some have low serum ß-lipoproteins and high-density lipoproteins. The syndrome is believed to have originated from a couple who lived in Quebec City about 1650. See also *Andermann syndrome.*

Bouchard, J. P., *et al.* Autosomal recessive spastic ataxia of Charlevoix-Saguenay. *Canad. J. Neur. Sc.,* 1978, 5:61-9.

CHARLIN, CARLOS (Chilean ophthalmologist, born 1886)

Charlin syndrome. Synonyms: *ciliary neuralgia, nasociliary neuralgia, neuralgia nasociliaris, supraorbital neuralgia.*

A unilateral nasociliary nerve disorder characterized by paroxysmal congestion of the anterior segment of the eye (with superficial keratitis and serous iritis), rhinorrhea, and neuralgia at the inner angle of the eye at the side of the frontal nerve.

Charlin, C. La sindrome del nervo nasale. *Boll. Ocul., Firenze,* 1931, 10:921-36.

CHARLOUIS, M. (Dutch physician in Java)

Charlouis disease. Synonyms: *Breda disease, boba, bouba, frambesia, parangi, pian, polypapilloma tropicum, tonga, yaws.*

An infectious disease caused by *Treponema pertennue* and characterized by raspberry-like lesions of the skin. Endemic in certain tropical areas, it may begin in childhood. The primary lesions, known as *mother yaws,* are formed by fusion of several papules into larger lesions covered by an amber-yellow crust; these disappear after a few months, leaving atrophic and depigmented areas. In the second stage the lesions are irregularly disseminated small reddish papules, which leave furfuraceous patches. The tertiary lesions are characterized by gummatous nodules with deep ulcers.

*Charlouis, M. Über Polypapilloma tropicum (Frambesia). *Vjersch. Derm. Syph.,* 1881, pp. 431-66. Breda, A. Beitrag zum klinischen und bacteriologischen Studium der brasilianischen Framboesie oder "Boubas." *Arch. Derm. Syph., Berlin,* 1895, 33:3-18.

CHARMOT, GUY DENIS (French physician, born 1914)

Charmot syndrome. Synonyms: *African macroglobulinemia, macroglobulinemic splenomegaly.*

Macroglobulinemia associated with splenomegaly, originally observed in a group of adults in the Congo. Emaciation, asthenia, anemia, erythroblastosis of the bone marrow, subclinical jaundice, and abdominal pain were the chief symptoms. Histological studies revealed hypertrophy of the reticuloendothelial system and lymphatic infiltration of the liver and bone marrow. A parasitic infection was suspected as a possible cause.

Charmot, G., *et al.* Un nouvel aspect des splénomégalies en Afrique Noire. Le syndrome splénomégalie avec macroglobulinémie. *Presse Méd.,* 1959, 67:11-2.

CHARRIN, SALOMON (French physician)

Winckel-Charrin syndrome. See *under Winckel.*

CHASLIN, PHILIPPE (French physician, born 1857)

Chaslin syndrome. Synonym: *neuroglial sclerosis.*

Sclerotic changes of the brain in epilepsy, characterized by densification of the horizontal glial fibers found in the tangential layers beneath the pial surface.

Chaslin. Note sur l'anatomie pathologique de l'épilepsie dite essentielle. La sclérose névroglique. *C. Rend. Soc. Biol., Paris,* 1889, 1:169-71.

CHASSAIGNAC, CHARLES MARIE EDOUARD (French physician, 1805-1879)

Chassaignac paralysis. In infants, a painful disorder of the arms resembling paralysis, caused by excessive stretching of the muscles.

Chassaignac. De la paralysie douloureuse dess jeunes enfants. *Arch. Gén. Méd., Paris,* 1856, 7:653-69.

CHAUDHRY, ANAND P. (American dentist, born 1922)

Gorlin-Chaudhry-Moss syndrome. See *under Gorlin.*

CHAUFFARD, ANATOLE MARIE EMILE (French physician, 1855-1932)

Chauffard-Ramon syndrome. See *Still syndrome.*

Chauffard-Still syndrome. See *Still syndrome.*

Hanot-Chauffard syndrome. See *Troisier-Hanot-Chauffard syndrome.*

Minkowski-Chauffard syndrome. See *under Minkowski.*

Minkowski-Chauffard-Gänsslen syndrome. See *Minkowski-Chauffard syndrome.*

Still-Chauffard-Felty syndrome. See *Still syndrome, and see Felty syndrome.*

Troisier-Hanot-Chauffard syndrome. See *under Troisier.*

CHAVANY, JEAN ALFRED EMILE (French neurologist, 1892-1959)

Chavany-Brunhes syndrome. Synonym: *falx cerebri calcification syndrome.*

A syndrome of unknown etiology marked by persistent headache and psychoneurotic disorders associated with calcification of the falx cerebri. Attacks of headache may be precipitated by fatigue, emotional stress, or maintaining a fixed position of the head for long periods. The mental disorders vary in form and severity.

Chavany, J. A., & Brunhes, J. Syndromes céphalgique et psychonévrotique avec calcifications de faux du cerveau. *Rev. Neur., Paris,* 1938, 69:113-31.

Foix-Chavany syndrome. See *Foix-Chavany-Marie syndrome.*

Foix-Chavany-Marie syndrome (FCMS). See *under Foix.*

Putti-Chavany syndrome. See *under Putti.*

CHEADLE, WALTER BUTLER (British physician, 1836-1910)

Cheadle disease. See *Möller-Barlow disease.*

Cheadle-Möller-Barlow disease. See *Möller-Barlow disease.*

CHEATLE, SIR GEORGE LENTHAL (British physician, born 1865)

Cheatle disease. Synonyms: *Bloodgood disease, Cooper disease, Reclus syndrome, Reclus-Schimmelbusch disease, Schimmelbusch disease, Tillaux-Phocas disease, benign cystic disease of the breast, blue dome cyst, chronic cystic mastitis, cystadenoma, cystadenoma mammae, cystic disease of the mammary gland, cystic fibroadenomatosis, cystiphorous desquamative epithelial hyperplasia, fibroadenomatosis cystica, hydrocystoma mammae, mastitis chronica cystica, mastopathia chronica cystica, senile parenchymatous hypertrophy of the breast.*

A disease of the female breast characterized by brown to blue cysts up to 5 cm in diameter that are filled with fluid showing through a smooth membranous lining. The fluid may be clear and serous, thick and greenish, or cream-like. The cysts are usually multifocal and often bilateral. Histologically, there is dysplasia of the mammary tissue, epithelial and stromal hyperplasia, and cystic formation. The large cysts are acinous in origin; duct cysts are always small. Menopausal hyperplasia of the ductal epithelium and cystic dilatation of the ducts are the cause.

Reclus, P. La maladie kystique des mamelles. *Bull. Soc. Anat., Paris,* 1883, 8:428-33. Bloodgood, J. C. The pathology of chronic cystic mastitis of the female breast, with special consideration of the blue-dome cyst. *Arch. Surg., Chicago,* 1921, 3:445-42. Schimmelbusch, C. Das Cystadenom der Mamma. *Arch. Klin. Chir., Berlin,* 1892, 44:117-34. Cheatle, G. L., & Cutler, M. Cystipharous desquamative epithelial hyperplasia. (Chronic cystic mastitis, "maladie kystique des mammelles" or Reclus disease, benign cystic disease, senile parenchymatous hypertrophy [Bloodgood]-Schimmelbusch's disease, fibroadenomatosis cystica [Semb.]. In their: *Tumours of the breast. Their pathology, symptoms, diagnosis and treatment.* London, Arnold, 1931.

checkrein shoulder. See *Duplay bursitis.*

CHEDIAK, MOISES (Cuban physician)

Béguez César-Steinbrinck-Chédiak-Higashi syndrome. See *Chédiak-Higashi syndrome.*

Chédiak anomaly. See *Chédiak-Higashi syndrome.*

Chédiak disease. See *Chédiak-Higashi syndrome.*

Chédiak-Higashi syndrome (CHS). Synonyms: *Béguez César-Steinbrinck-Chédiak-Higashi syndrome, Chédiak anomaly, Chédiak disease, Chédiak-Steinbrinck syndrome, Steinbrinck anomaly, constitutional granular gigantism.*

A rare hereditary syndrome occurring in infants, characterized by defective pigmentation, abnormal granulation of leukocytes, susceptibility to infections, and early death. Photophobia and albinism are usually associated. It is a disorder of giant lysosomal inclusion bodies in all circulating granulocytes and other cells. The blood shows anemia, neutropenia, and thrombocytopenia. Progressive neuropathy with muscle weakness may occur. Oral aphthae and gingivitis are frequently present. The syndrome is transmitted as an autosomal recessive trait.

Chédiak, M Nouvelle anomalie leucocytaire de caractère constitutionel et familial. *Rev. Hémat., Paris,* 1952, 7:362-7. Higashi, O. Congenital gigantism of peroxidase granules. The first case ever reported of qualitative abnormity of peroxidase. *Tohoku J. Exp. Med.,* 1953-54, 59:315-32. Béguez César, A. Neutropenia cronica maligna familial con granulaciones atipicas de los leucocitos. *Bol. Soc. Cubana Pediat.,* 1943, 15:900-22. Steinbrinck, E. Über eine neue Granulationanomalie der Leukocyten. *Deut. Arch. Klin. Med.,* 1948, 193:577-81.

Chédiak-Higashi-like syndrome (1). See *pseudo-Chédiak-Higashi syndrome (1).*

Chédiak-Higashi-like syndrome (2). See *Griscelli syndrome.*

Chédiak-Steinbrinck syndrome. See *Chédiak-Higashi syndrome.*

pseudo-Chédiak-Higashi syndrome (1). Synonym: *Chédiak-Higashi-like syndrome.*

A disease evolving from pancytopenia with normocellular bone marrow to a myeloblastic leukemia, occurring in a patient with a myelodysplastic syndrome.

Gallardo, R., & Kranwinkel, R. N. Pseudo-Chédiak-Higashi anomaly. *Am. J. Clin. Path.*, 1985, 83:127-9.

pseudo-Chédiak-Higashi syndrome (2). See *Griscelli syndrome.*

cheilitis glandularis. See *Baelz syndrome, and see Melkersson-Rosenthal syndrome.*

cheilitis glandularis apostematosa. See *Baelz syndrome.*

cheilitis granulomatosa. See *Melkersson-Rossenthal syndrome.*

cheilitis-glossitis-gingivitis syndrome. See *gingivostomatitis syndrome.*

cheiralgia paresthetica. See *Wartenberg disease (2).*

cheiro-oral syndrome (COS). A sensory disorder limited to the hands or fingers with ipsilateral involvement of the corner of the mouth. In the past, the disorder was attributed to parietal and thalamic lesions, but later findings indicate a possibility of lesions in other parts of the brain.

Sittig, O. Klinische Beiträge zur Lehre von der Localisation der sensiblen Rindenzenten. *Prag. Med. Wschr.*, 1914, 45:548-50. Garcin, R., & Lapresle, J. Syndrome sensitif de type thalamique et à topographie cheiro-orale par lésion localisée du thalamus. *Rev. Neur., Paris*, 1954, 90:124-9. Ten Holter, J., & Tijssen, C. Cheiro-oral syndrome: Does it have a specific localizing value? *Eur. Neurol.*, 1988, 28:326-30.

cheirolumbar dysostosis. Synonym: *Wackenheim syndrome.*

An association of brachycheiry (brachyphalangy, branchymetacarpy, brachymetacarpophalangy) and stenosis of the lumbar spinal canal without other skeletal anomalies. Low back pain and sciatica are the principal clinical signs.

Wackenheim, A. Une dysostose cheiro-lombaire (brachymetacarpophalangie et dysostose sténosante de l'arc vertebral postérieur). *J. Radiol. Electrol.*, 1978, 59:563-6.

chemical porphyria. See *porphyria cutanea tarda syndrome.*

CHENAIS, L. (French physician)

Céstan-Chenais syndrome. See *under Céstan.*

CHENANTAIS, J., JR. (French physician)

Malherbe-Chenantais epithelioma. See *Malherbe epithelioma.*

CHENEY, WILLIAM D. (American radiologist)

Cheney syndrome. See *Hajdu-Cheney syndrome.*

Hajdu-Cheney syndrome. See *under Hajdu.*

CHERNOGUBOV (TSCHERNOGUBOW) (Russian physician)

Chernogubov syndrome. See *Ehlers-Danlos syndrome.*

cherry angiomas. See *De Morgan spots.*

cherry red spot-myoclonus syndrome. Synonym: *sialidosis I.*

A familial syndrome of progressive ataxia and visual failure, due to bilateral macular cherry red spots and cataracts starting early in the third decade of life. Large amounts of sialylated oligosaccharides are found in the urine, and cultured skin fibroblasts show deficiency of sialidase (neuraminidase). The syndrome is believed to be transmitted as an autosomal recessive trait.

O'Brien, J. S. The cherry-red spot-myoclonus syndrome: A newly recognized inherited lysosomal storage disease due to acid neuraminidase deficiency. *Clin. Genet.*, 1978, 14:55-60.

cherry-red epiglottitis. See *Kleinschmidt syndrome.*

cherubism. Synonyms: *Jones disease, Jones syndrome, cherubism syndrome, disseminated fibrous jaw dysplasia, familial fibrous jaw dysplasia, familial fibrous swelling of jaw, familial multilocular cystic jaw disease, fibrous jaw dysplasia.*

A familial bone disease, transmitted as an autosomal dominant trait, characterized by fullness of the cheeks, producing a typical chubby face (suggestive of a cherub), associated with a white line on the sclera beneath the iris, swelling of the submandibular region, wide alveolar ridges, a narrow V-shaped palate, premature shedding of deciduous teeth, defective permanent dentition, absence of many teeth, and displacement and lack of eruption of some teeth. Multinucleate giant cells of the osteolytic type, small hemorrhages, scattered deposits of granular hemosiderin, spindle cell fibroblasts, dilated capillary-like blood spaces lined with endothelium, lacunar absorption and replacement of the connective tissue in the cortical bone, replacement of the medulla and most of the cortex by dysplastic bone tissue, and collagenous intercellular deposits are the principal pathological findings. The disorder occurs in early childhood and is considered to be a form of fibrous bone dysplasia with partial shift of the osteolytic phase of bone metamorphosis. See also *Ramon syndrome..*

Jones, W.A. Familial multilocular cystic disease of the jaw. *Am. J. Cancer*, 1933, 17:946-50.

cherubism syndrome. See *cherubism.*

cherubism-gingival fibromatosis-epilepsy-mental deficiency syndrome. See *Ramon syndrome.*

Cheshire cat syndrome. A situation in which a disease is diagnosed on the basis of less than all the required clinical characteristics, or *forme sine* with only one or a few of the criteria present. It is named after the Cheshire cat, a cat who disappeared while his grin remained, a character in *Alice in Wonderland* by Lewis Carroll.

Bywaters, E. G. L. The Cheshire cat syndrome. *Postgrad. Med. J.*, 1968, 44:19-22. Rodin, A. E., & Key, J. D. *Encyclopedia of medical eponyms derived from literary characters.* Krieger, Melbourne, Fla., 1989.

chest cold. See *common cold syndrome.*

chest wall syndrome. Synonym: *anterior chest wall syndrome.*

A syndrome of chest pain in the presence of normal coronary arteries and no objective evidence of heart disease. The syndrome includes the Tietze syndrome (q.v.), costochondritis, and the precordial catch syndrome (q.v.). See also *Prinzmetal angina,* and *Heberden asthma.*

Epstein, S. E., *et al.* Chest wall syndrome, a common cause of unexplained cardiac pain. *JAMA* 1979, 241:2793-7. Calabro, J. J., *et al.* Classification of anterior chest wall syndrome. *JAMA* 1980, 243:1420-1.

CHESTER, W.

Erdheim-Chester syndrome. See *under Erdheim.*

Chester porphyria. A familial disorder, transmitted as an autosomal dominant trait, originally reported in Chester, U. K. Patients presented suffering from neurovisceral dysfunction, but none had cutanenous photosensitivity. Biochemically, the excretion of heme precursors varied between individuals; some had a pattern typical of acute intermittent porphyria, others showed that of variegate porphyria, and some had an intermediate pattern. There was a dual enzyme deficiency, with reduced activity of both porphobilinogen deaminase and protoporphyrinogen oxidase.

McColl, K. E. L., *et al.* Chester porphyria: Biochemical studies of a new form of acute porphyria. *Lancet,* 1985, 2:796-9.

CHEVALLIER

Chevallier glossitis. Synonym: *posterior triangular glossitis.*

A disease occurring in gastritis and other inflammatory diseases of the gastrointestinal system, characterized by triangular lesions on the posterior third of the tongue. The lesions are glossy red with nipple-like structures, often forming clusters of isolated small plaques with well-defined borders. The course is transitory, but the lesions usually recur with exacerbation of gastrointestinal disorders.

Gallina, L. Contributo allo studio della glossite triangolare posteriore di Chevallier. *Rass. Internaz. Stomat. Prat.,* 1968, 19:423-7.

CHEVASSU, MAURICE (French physician, born 1877)

Chevassu tumor. Synonym: *seminoma.*

A germ-cell tumor, usually affecting men over the age of 30 years, that arises in the testes, sometimes also occurring in other parts of the body, such as the retroperitoneum and mediastinum. Histologically, it is the counterpart of the dysgerminoma in the female.

*Chevassu, M. *Tumeurs du testicle.* Paris, 1906 (Thesis).

CHEYNE, GEORGE (British physician, 1671-1743)

Cheyne disease. Synonyms: *English malady, hypochondria, hypochondriasis.*

Morbid anxiety about one's health.

Cheyne, G. *The English malady; or, a treatise of nervous diseases of all kinds as spleen, vapours, lowness of spirits, hypochondrical and hysterical distempers, etc.* London, Powell, 1733.

CHEYNE, JOHN (British physician, 1777-1836)

Cheyne-Stokes respiration (CSR). A respiratory pattern characterized by alternating periods of apnea and hyperpnea, occurring in conditions such as congestive heart failure, brain damage, and chronic hypoxia. It may also occur in normal persons at high altitude, especially during sleep.

Cheyne, J. A case of apoplexy in which the fleshy part of the heart was converted into fat. *Dublin Hosp. Rep.,* 1818, 2:216-23. Stokes, W. *The diseases of the heart and aorta.* Dublin, Hodges & Smith, 1854, pp. 320-7.

CHIARI, HANS (German physician, 1851-1916)

Arnold-Chiari deformity. See *Arnold-Chiari syndrome.*

Arnold-Chiari syndrome. See *under Arnold.*

Budd-Chiari syndrome (BCS). See *under Budd.*

Chiari deformity. See *Arnold-Chiari syndrome.*

Chiari disease. See *Budd-Chiari syndrome.*

Chiari malformation (1). See *Arnold-Chiari syndrome.*

Chiari malformation (2). Synonym: *Chiari syndrome.*

Downward displacement of parts of the elongated inferior cerebellar vermis together with the lower brain stem into an enlarged cervical spinal canal. The rhomboid fossa is elongated, and there is a kinking of the medulla oblongata in the area of its transition to the cervical spinal cord. Additional features include hypoplasia of the tentorium cerebelli, low insertion, and an abnormally large tentorial notch. It is associated with spina bifida cystica.

Chiari, H. Über Veränderungen des Kleinhirns, des Pons und der Medulla oblongata infolge von congenitaler hydrocephalie des Grosshirns. *Denkschr. Kaiserl. Akad. Wissensch., Math. Naturw. Klasse.* 1896, 63:71-116.

Chiari malformation (3). Synonym: *Chiari syndrome.*

Total displacement of the severely hypoplastic cerebellum into the occipitocervical space.

Chiari, H. Über Veränderungen des Grosshirns. *Deut. Med. Wschr.,* 1891, 17:1172-5. Chiari, H. Über Veränderungen des Kleinhirns, des Pons und der Medulla oblongata infolge von congenitaler Hydrocephalie des Grosshirns. *Denkschr. Kaiserl. Akad. Wissensch., Math. Naturw. Klasse,* 1896, 63:71-116. Schmitt, H. P. Syndrome of primary transtentorial cerebellar displacement-"inverse Chiari II syndrome." *Neuropaediatrie,* 1978, 9:268-76.

Chiari malformation (4). Synonym: *Chiari syndrome.*

Displacement of a hypoplastic cerebellum into the posterior cranial fossa.

Chiari, H. Über Veränderungen des Grosshirns. *Deut. Med. Wschr.,* 1891, 17:1172-5. Chiari, H. Über Veränderungen des Kleinhirns, des Pons und der Medulla oblongata infolge von congenitaler Hydrocephalie des Grosshirns. *Denkschr. Kaiserl. Akad. Wissensch., Math. Naturw. Klasse,* 1896, 63:71-116. Schmitt, H. P. Syndrome of primary transtentorial cerebellar displacement-"inverse Chiari type II syndrome." *Neuropaediatrie,* 1978, 9:268-76.

Chiari syndrome (1). See *Budd-Chiari syndrome.*

Chiari syndrome (2). See *Chiari malformation (2).*

Chiari syndrome (3). See *Chiari malformation (3).*

Chiari syndrome (4). See *Chiari malformation (4).*

inverse Chiari syndrome. See *primary transtentorial cerebellar displacement syndrome.*

CHIARI, JOHANN BAPTIST (Austrian physician, 1817-1854)

Chiari-Frommel syndrome. See *amenorrhea-galactorrhea syndrome.*

chiclero ulcer. See *Alibert disease (2).*

CHIGNON

Chignon disease. See *Beigel disease.*

CHILAIDITI, DEMETRIOS (Radiologist in Vienna, born 1883)

Chilaiditi anomaly. See *Chilaiditi syndrome.*

Chilaiditi syndrome. Synonyms: *Chilaiditi anomaly, interpositio hepatodiaphragmatica, subphrenic displacement of the colon, subphrenic interposition syndrome.*

Interposition of a portion of the colon or, less frequently, the small intestine between the liver and the diaphragm, caused by congenital anomalies of the calciform ligament of the diaphragm. The symptoms usually include abdominal pain, vomiting, anorexia, constipation, flatulence, and air swallowing.

Chilaiditi, D. Zur Frage der Hepatoptose im Anschluss an Fälle von temporarer partieller Leberverlagerung. *Fortschr. Röntgen.,* 1910-11, 16:173-208.

CHILD (congenital **h**emidysplasia with **i**chthyosiform erythroderma and **l**imb **d**efects) **syndrome.** A disorder of skin cornification marked by unilateral erythema and scaling, with a distinct demarcation in the middle of the trunk, that is either present at birth or develops during the first weeks of life. Ipsilateral limb defects may vary from hypoplasia of some fingers to complete absence of an extremity. In addition, ipsilateral hypoplasia of other parts of the skeleton, defects of the brain and the viscera, and occasional ipsilateral punctate epiphyseal calcification may occur. The syndrome is suspected of being transmitted as an X-linked dominant trait lethal in hemizygous males.

Happle, R., *et al.* The CHILD syndrome. Congenital hemidysplasia with ichthyosiform erythroderma and limb defects. *Eur. J. Pediat.*, 1980, 134:27-33.

child abuse. See *battered child syndrome.*

child abuse dwarfism. See *abuse dwarfism syndrome.*

childhood dementia. See *Heller syndrome, under Heller, Theodor O.*

childhood psychosis. See *Heller syndrome, under Heller, Theodor O.*

childhood schizophrenia. See *Heller syndrome, under Heller, Theodor O.*

Chinese headache. See *Chinese restaurant syndrome.*

Chinese restaurant syndrome. Synonyms: *Kwok quease, Chinese headache, duck-sauce headache, post-sinocibal syndrome, sin-cib-syn.*

A syndrome with onset of symptoms 15 to 20 minutes after consumption of food heavily seasoned with monosodium glutamate; it is characterized by headaches that are severe, pulsatile, and associated with flushing, precordial pain with tingling, angor animi, burning sensation in the back and neck, and infraorbital pressure and tightness.

Kwok, R. H. M. Chinese-restaurant syndrome. *N. Engl. J. Med.*, 1968, 278:796.

chiralgia paresthetica. See *Wartenberg disease (2).*

chloroleukemia. See *Balfour disease.*

chloroma. See *Balfour disease.*

chloromyeloma. See *Balfour disease.*

chlorosarcoma. See *Balfour disease.*

chocolate cyst. See *Sampson cyst.*

chocolate migraine. See *under headache syndrome.*

cholangiolitic biliary cirrhosis. See *Hanot cirrhosis.*

cholecystohepatic flexure adhesions. See *Verbrycke syndrome.*

choledocho-cholecystoenterostomy sump syndrome. See *sump syndrome.*

cholemia familiaris simplex. See *Gilbert syndrome, under Gilbert, Nicolas Augustin.*

cholemic nephrosis. See *hepatorenal syndrome.*

cholera infantum. See *Sakamoto disease.*

cholera-like diarrhea. See *Verner-Morrison syndrome.*

choleriform enteritis. See *Janbon syndrome.*

choleriform syndrome. See *Janbon syndrome.*

cholestasis-peripheral pulmonary stenosis syndrome. See *Alagille syndrome.*

cholestatic jaundice of newborn. See *bile plug syndrome.*

cholestenalosis. See *van Bogaert-Scherer-Epstein syndrome.*

cholesterol granulomatosis. See *Hand-Schüller-Christian syndrome.*

chondral dysplasia. See *multiple cartilaginous exostoses syndrome.*

chondro-osseous dystrophy with punctate epiphyseal dysplasia. See *Conradi-Hünermann syndrome, under Conradi, Erich.*

chondro-osteodystrophy. See *mucopolysaccharidosis IV-A.*

chondroangiopathia calcarea seu punctata. See *Conradi-Hünermann syndrome, under Conradi, Erich.*

chondroangiopathia punctata. See *Conradi-Hünermann syndrome, under Conradi, Erich.*

chondrocalcinosis articularis hereditaria. See *pseudogout syndrome.*

chondrocalcinosis idiopathica. See *pseudogout syndrome.*

chondrocalciosynovitis syndrome. See *pseudogout syndrome.*

chondrodermatitis helicis. See *Winkler disease.*

chondrodermatitis nodularis chronica helicis. See *Winkler disease.*

chondrodynia costosternalis. See *Tietze syndrome.*

chondrodysplasia. See *Ollier syndrome.*

chondrodysplasia calcificans congenita. See *Conradi-Hünermann syndrome, under Conradi, Erich.*

chondrodysplasia ectodermica. See *Ellis-van Creveld syndrome.*

chondrodysplasia epiphysialis punctata. See *Conradi-Hünermann syndrome, under Conradi, Erich.*

chondrodysplasia foetalis. See *achondroplasia.*

chondrodysplasia punctata syndrome, X-linked. See *X-linked dominant chondrodysplasia punctata syndrome.*

chondrodysplasia punctata, dominant type. See *Conradi-Hünermann syndrome, under Conradi, Erich.*

chondrodysplasia punctata, recessive type. See *Spranger syndrome (1).*

chondrodysplasia punctata, rhizomelic type. See *Spranger syndrome (1).*

chondrodysplasia punctata, X-linked dominant type. Synonym: *X-linked dominant chondrodysplasia punctata syndrome.*

Chondrodysplasia, trasmitted as an X-linked dominant trait, characterized by cutaneous, skeletal, and ocular disorders, occurring in asymmetric patterns. Skeletal anomalies include shortening of the long bones, dysplasia and contractures of the joints, asymmetry of the facial bones, and occasional hexadactyly. Radiological findings show stippling (punctate calcifications) occurring in the epiphyses of the long bones and other parts of the skeleton. Congenital ichthyosiform erythroderma with patchy hyperkeratosis is the principal dermatological feature. Alopecia and occasional brittle and twisted hair and sparse eyelashes and eyebrows are associated. Ocular complications consist of cataracts. Facial features include depressed nose with a broad root, slight antimongoloid palpebral slant, and asymmetry. Additional anomalies include striated pigmentation, flat split nails, and short stature. See also *X-linked dominant chondrodysplasia punctata syndrome.*

Manzke, H., Christophers, E., & Wiedemann, H. R. Dominant sex-linked inherited chondrodysplasia punctata: A distinct type of chondrodysplasia punctata. *Clin. Genet.*, 1980, 17:107. Happle, R. X-linked dominant chondrodysplasia punctata. Review of literature and report of a case. *Hum. Genet.*, 1979, 53:65-73.

chondrodysplasia spondylometaphysaria, Kozlowski type. See *Kozlowski spondylometaphyseal dysplasia syndrome, see under Kozlowski, Kazimierz S.*

chondrodysplasia tridermica. See *Ellis-van Creveld syndrome.*

chondrodysplasia-angiomatosis syndrome. See *Maffucci syndrome.*

chondrodysplasia-hemangioma syndrome. See *Maffucci syndrome.*

chondrodystrophia calcarea. See *Conradi-Hünermann syndrome, under Conradi, Erich.*
chondrodystrophia calcificans. See *Conradi-Hünermann syndrome, under Conradi, Erich.*
chondrodystrophia calcificans congenita. See *Conradi-Hünermann syndrome, under Conradi, Erich.*
chondrodystrophia foetalis. See *achondroplasia.*
chondrodystrophia foetalis hypoplastica. See *Conradi-Hünermann syndrome, under Conradi, Erich.*
chondrodystrophia hypoplastica calcinosa. See *Conradi-Hünermann syndrome, under Conradi, Erich.*
chondrodystrophia myotonica. See *Schwartz-Jampel syndrome, under Schwartz, Oscar.*
chondrodystrophia punctata. See *Conradi-Hünermann syndrome, under Conradi, Erich.*
chondrodystrophia tarda. See *mucopolysaccharidosis IV-A.*
chondrodystrophic dwarfism. See *achondroplasia.*
chondrodystrophic myotonia. See *Schwartz-Jampel syndrome, under Schwartz, Oscar.*
chondrodystrophy with angiomatosis. See *Maffucci syndrome.*
chondrodystrophy with vascular hamartoma. See *Maffucci syndrome.*
chondroectodermal dysplasia (CED). See *Ellis-van Creveld syndrome.*
chondrogenesis imperfecta. See *achondroplasia.*
chondrohypoplasia. See *hypochondroplasia syndrome.*
chondrolytic perichondritis. See *Meyenburg-Altherr-Uehlinger syndrome.*
chondromalacia patellae. See *Büdinger-Ludloff-Läwen syndrome.*
chondromalacia post-traumatica patellae. See *Büdinger-Ludloff-Läwen syndrome.*
chondromalacic arthritis. See *Meyenburg-Altherr-Uehlinger syndrome.*
chondromatous giant-cell tumor. See *Codman tumor.*
chondropathia calcificans. See *Conradi-Hünermann syndrome.*
chondropathia hypertrophica transitoria ischiopubica. See *Van Neck disease.*
chondropathia patellae. See *Büdinger-Ludloff-Läwen syndrome.*
chondropathia punctata. See *Conradi-Hünermann syndrome.*
chondropathia tuberosa. See *Tietze syndrome.*
chondrosis of the patella. See *Büdinger-Ludloff-Läwen syndrome.*
chorea chronica progressiva. See *Huntington chorea.*
chorea chronica progressiva hereditaria. See *Huntington chorea.*
chorea electrica. See *Bergeron disease, and see Henoch chorea.*
chorea fibrillaris. See *Morvan chorea.*
chorea gravidarum. See *under Sydenham chorea.*
chorea infectiosa. See *Sydenham chorea.*
chorea laryngis. See *Schroetter chorea.*
chorea minor. See *Sydenham chorea.*
chorea rheumatica. See *Sydenham chorea.*
chorea St. Viti. See *Sydenham chorea.*
chorea variabilis. See *Gilles de la Tourette syndrome.*
choreoacanthocytosis. See *Levine-Critchley syndrome.*
choreoathetosis-mental retardation syndrome. See *Schimke syndrome.*
choriogenic gynecomastia. See *Gilbert syndrome, under Gilbert, Judson Bennett.*
chorioretinal anomalies-corpus callosum agenesis-infantile spasms syndrome. See *Aicardi syndrome.*
chorioretinitis centralis serosa. See *Masuda-Kitahara disease.*
chorioretinopathia post-traumatica. See *Siegrist-Hutchinson syndrome.*
chorioretinopathy-pituitary dysfunction (CPD) syndrome. Synonyms: *congenital trichomegaly, trichomegalia congenita.*

A congenital syndrome characterized by severe early-onset chorioretinal degeneration, hypothalamo-pituitary dysfunction, growth and mental retardation, sexual infantilism, trichosis, and mild hypothyroidism. The etiology is unknown.

Oliver, G. L., & McFarlane, D. C. Congenital trichomegaly: With associated pigmentary degeneration of the retina, dwarfism, and mental retardation. *Arch. Ophth., Chicago,* 1965, 74:169-71.

choroiditis guttata senilis. See *Hutchinson disease (2), under Hutchinson, Sir Jonathan.*
CHOTZEN, F. (German psychiatrist)
Chotzen syndrome. See *Saethre-Chotzen syndrome.*
Saethre-Chotzen syndrome. See *under Saethre.*
CHR (**c**erebro**h**epato**r**enal) syndrome. See *Zellweger syndrome.*
CHRIST, JOSEF (German dentist, 1871-1948)
Christ-Siemens-Touraine (CST) syndrome. See *hypohidrotic ectodermal dysplasia syndrome.*
Christ-Siemens-Weech syndrome. See *hypohidrotic ectodermal dysplasia syndrome.*
CHRISTENSEN, ERNA (Danish physician, 1906-1967)
Christensen disease. See *Alpers syndrome.*
Christensen-Krabbe disease. See *Alpers syndrome.*
CHRISTIAN, HENRY ASBURY (American physician, 1876-1951)
Christian syndrome. See *Hand-Schüller-Christian syndrome.*
Hand-Schüller-Christian (HSC) syndrome. See *under Hand.*
Pfeifer-Weber-Christian disease. See *Weber-Christian syndrome, under Weber, Frederic Parkes.*
Schüller-Christian disease. See *Hand-Schüller-Christian syndrome.*
Weber-Christian disease (WCD). See *Weber-Christian syndrome, under Weber, Frederick Parkes.*
Weber-Christian syndrome. See *under Weber, Frederick Parkes.*
CHRISTIAN, JOE C. (American geneticist)
Christian brachydactyly syndrome. Synonym: *dominant preaxial brachydactyly.*

A familial syndrome of mental retardation, brachydactyly, hallux varus, and adducted thumbs, transmitted as an autosomal dominant trait.

Christian, J. C., *et al.* Dominant preaxial brachydactyly with hallus varus and thumb adduction. *Am. J. Hum. Genet.*, 1972, 24:694-701.

Christian syndrome (1). Synonyms: *Christian-Andrews-Conneally-Muller syndrome, adducted thumbs syndrome, craniosynostosis-arthrogryposis-cleft palate syndrome.*

A syndrome of craniosynostosis, arthrogryposis, and cleft palate associated with microcephaly, prominent occiput, hypertelorism, antimongoloid palpebral fissures, ophthalmoplegia, abnormal ear placement, and bifid uvula. Also associated are adducted thumbs, camptodactyly of other digits, limited extension of elbows and knees, talipes equinovarus, and pectus excavatum. Dysphagia, laryngomalacia, and muscle fibrillation occur in some cases. Neurological complications include dysmyelination with glial proliferation in white matter. The syndrome is transmitted as an autosomal recessive trait. It was first reported in three siblings in an Amish kindred.

Christian, J. C., Andrews, P. A., Conneally, P. M., & Muller, J. The adducted thumbs syndrome. An autosomal recessive disease with arthrogryposis, dysmyelination, craniosynostosis, and cleft palate. *Clin. Genet.*, 1971, 2:95-103.

Christian syndrome (2). A familial syndrome of short stature, ridging of the metopic sutures, fusion of cervical vertebrae, thoracic hemivertebrae, scoliosis, sacral hypoplasia, and short middle phalanges. Glucose intolerance, imperforate anus, and abducens palsies are observed in some cases. The syndrome is transmitted as an X-linked trait.

Christian, J. C., *et al.* X-linked skeletal dysplasia with mental retardation. *Clin. Genet.*, 1977, 11:128-36.

Christian-Andrews-Conneally-Muller syndrome. See *Christian syndrome (1).*

CHRISTMAS

Christmas disease. Synonyms: *factor IX deficiency, hemophilia II, hemophilia B (HEMB), hemophiloid state C, hereditary plasma thromboplastin component (PTC) deficiency, plasma thromboplastin component (PTC) deficiency, plasma thromboplastin factor-B (PTF-B) deficiency.*

A genetically determined blood coagulation disorder, similar to but somewhat milder than hemophilia A, caused by a deficiency of factor IX (Christmas factor, named after the family name of the first patient in whom the disease was studied in detail), and transmitted as an X-linked recessive trait through female carriers. It occurs most frequently in males, but the incidence in females is somewhat greater than in hemophilia A. The severity varies from family to family but is about equal in different members of the same family. The symptoms are similar to those in hemophilia A and include oozing of the blood from many sites, especially in the oral cavity, which may persist for several days or weeks, and hematomas, especially of the tongue and floor of the mouth. Minor surgery, such as tooth extraction and tonsillectomy, may produce massive bleeding.

Biggs, R., *et al.* Christmas disease: A condition previously mistaken for haemophilia. *Brit. Med. J.*, 1952, 2:1378. Hougie, C. Hemophilia and related conditions-congenital deficiencies of prothrombin (factor II), factor V, and factors VII to XII. In: Williams, W. J., Beutler, E., Erslev, A. J., & Lichtman, M. A., eds. *Hematology*, 3rd ed. McGraw-Hill, New York, 1983, pp. 1381-99.

Christmas tree deformity. See *apple peel syndrome.*

CHROBAK, RUDOLF (Austrian physician, 1843-1910)

Otto-Chrobak syndrome. See *under Otto.*

chromatophore nevus. See *Naegeli syndrome, under Naegeli, Oskar.*

chromatophoroma. See *Jadassohn-Tièche nevus, under Jadassohn, Josef.*

chromosome 1pter deletion syndrome. Synonyms: *1pter- syndrome, 1pter deletion syndrome, del(1pter) syndrome, monosomy 1pter, partial monosomy 1pter syndrome.*

Deletion of the terminal portion of the short arm of chromosome 1 associated with characteristic facies (wide fontanels, low-set posteriorly rotated ears, flat nasal bridge, bulbous nasal tip, cleft and thin lip), clinodactyly, and heart defect.

Yunis, e., *et al.* Monosomy 1pter. *Hum. Genet.*, 1981, 56:279-82. Desangles, F., *et al.* Monosomie 1pter translocation familiale (1;9p). *Ann. Génét., Paris*, 1983, 26:53-5.

chromosome 1q deletion syndrome. Synonyms: *1q- syndrome, 1q deletion syndrome, del(1q) syndrome, monosomy 5q, partial monosomy 1q syndrome.*

Deletion of the long arm of chromosome 1 characterized by psychomotor retardation and multiple abnormalities. Craniofacial anomalies include microcephaly, brachycephaly, round face, small fontanels, oblique palpebral fissures, epicanthal folds, apparent hypertelorism, short and broad nose, smooth and long philtrum, cupid's bow, thin vermilion border of the lips, down-turned corners of the mouth, microretrognathia, low-set malformed ears, and abnormal palate. Other associated abnormalities may include strabismus, short neck, and variable heart, genital, hand, and foot deformities. Occasionally, single kidney, hernia, kyphosis, cervical rib, spina bifida, agenesis of the corpus callosum, accessory spleen, and encephalocele may occur.

Mankinen, C. B., *et al.* Terminal (1)(q43) long arm deletion of chromosome No. 1 in three-year-old female. *Birth Defects*, 1976, 11(5):132-6. Johnson, V. P., *et al.* Deletion of the distal long arm of chromosome 1: A definable syndrome. *Am. J. Med. Genet.*, 1985, 22:685-94.

chromosome 1q duplication syndrome. Synonyms: *1q+ syndrome, 1q duplication syndrome, chromosome 1q trisomy syndrome, dup(1q) syndrome, duplication 1q syndrome, partial trisomy 1q syndrome, trisomy 1q.*

Duplication of the long arm of chromosome 1 due to translocation, associated with psychomotor retardation, macrocephaly, trigonocephaly, coloboma, hypertelorism, antimongoloid palpebal slant, microphthalmia, synophrys, long philtrum, small mouth, high-arched palate, cleft palate, low-set malformed ears, widely set nipples, dysplastic nails, hypertrichosis, muscle hypotonia, and various anomalies of the heart, central nervous system, kidneys, and biliary tract.

Bonfante, A., *et al.* Partial trisomy of the long arm of chromosome 1 due to a familial translocation t(1;10)(q32;q26). *Hum. Genet.*, 1978, 45:339-43. Gagnon, J. A., *et al.* Apparition de novo d'une trisomie 1q partielle en mosaïque par translocation 1;9. *Ann. Génét., Paris*, 1984, 27:33-7.

chromosome 1q trisomy syndrome. See *chromosome 1q duplication syndrome.*

chromosome 2 ring syndrome. Synonyms: *r(2) ring syndrome, ring chromosome 2.*

A syndrome in which both ends of chromosome 2 have been lost (deletion) and the two broken ends have reunited to form a ring-shaped figure. It is associated with growth and mental retardation and variable multiple malformations, including craniofacial abnormalities (microcephaly, bulging metopic suture, flat occiput, arched eyebrows, mongoloid palpebral slant, epicanthus, flat nasal bridge, long philtrum, micrognathia, low-set ears), short neck, widely spaced nipples, hypogenitalism, hypospadias with bifid scro-

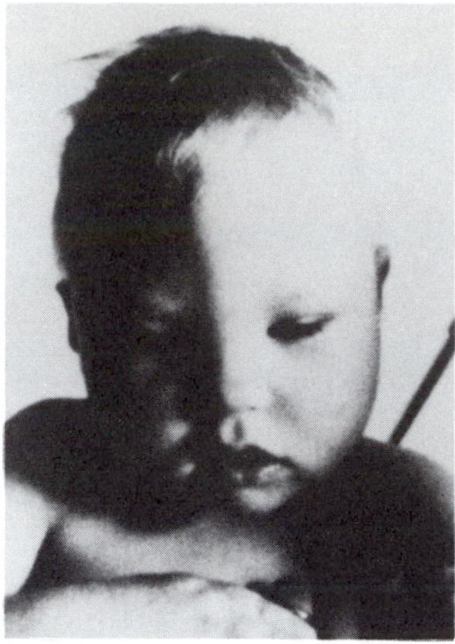
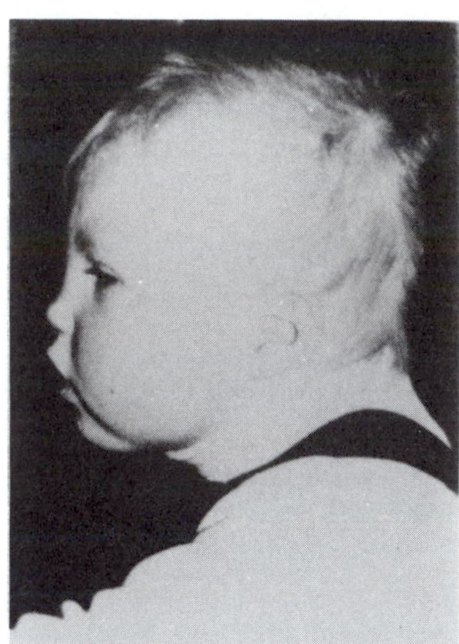

Chromosome 1q deletion syndrome
Manouvrier-Hanu, S., R. Walbaum, & C. Gayot, *American Journal of Medical Genetics* 25:599-600 1986. New York: Alan R. Liss Inc.

tum, inguinal hernia, clinodactyly, foot deformities, lymphedema of the hands and feet, cutis laxa, joint laxity, skeletal abnormalities, retinal dystrophy, and heart defect.

Garau, A., *et al.* In tema di patologia autosomica: sindrome plurimalformativa con cromosoma ad anello del gruppo A. *Clin. Pediat., Parma,* 1973, 55:84-95. Maraschio, P., *et al.* Three cases of ring chromosome 2, one derived from a paternal 2/6 translocation. *Hum. Genet.,* 1979, 48:157-67.

chromosome 2p duplication syndrome. Synonyms: *2p+ syndrome, 2p duplication syndrome, chromosome 2p trisomy syndrome, dup(2p) syndrome, duplication 2p syndrome, partrial trisomy 2p syndrome, trisomy 2p.*

Duplication of the short arm of chromosome 2 with mental and growth retardation accompanied by multiple abnormalities. Craniofacial abnormalities include prominent forehead, frontal upsweep of hair, hypertelorism, epicanthal folds, maxillary hypoplasia, short nose with prominent tip (pug nose), broad alveolar ridges, narrow palate, blepharoptosis, and hydrocephalus. Strabismus, dacryostenosis, and myopia are the ocular features. Skeletal anomalies consist of pectus excavatum, long and narrow trunk, dolichostenomelia, long fingers and toes, hyperextensible fingers, widely spaced toes, flat feet, overlapping fingers, scoliosis, congenital hip dislocation, dysplastic pubic bone, hemivertebrae, and 11 pairs of ribs. Genital anomalies include shawl scrotum, hypoplastic external genitalia, ovarian dysplasia, cryptorchism, and hypospadias. Other abnormalities include simian creases, hypoplastic kidneys, heart defect, and cerebellar dysplasia.

Francke, U., & Jones, K. L. The 2p partial trisomy syndrome. *Am. J. Dis. Child.,* 1976, 91:934-8.

chromosome 2p trisomy syndrome. See *chromosome 2p duplication syndrome.*

chromosome 2q deletion syndrome. Synonyms: *2q- syndrome, 2q deletion syndrome, del(2q) syndrome, monosomy 2q, partial monosomy 2q syndrome.*

Deletion of the long arm of chromosome 2 characterized by mental retardation and multiple abnormalities. Craniofacial anomalies consist of microretrognathia, small face, small and upturned nose with depressed root, low-set malformed ears, antimongoloid palpebral slant, blepharoptosis, high-arched palate, cleft palate, and defective dentition. Microphthalmia and cataract are the ocular features. Associated defects and disorders include failure to thrive, growth retardation, unresponsiveness to stimuli, delayed speech, short and webbed neck, scoliosis, flexion deformity of the fingers (overlapping of the second over the third and fifth over the fourth fingers), abnormal flexion creases of the palms, long fingers and toes, clefts between the first and second toes, short metatarsal bones, prominent calcanei, heart and lung abnormalities, cystic gonads, and anemia. The clinical picture varies, depending on the segment involved in the deletion, the most severe malformations occurring with deletion of segment 2 (q22-q31).

German, J., & Chaganti, R. S. R.. Mapping human autosomes, assignment of the MN locus to a specific segment in the long arm of chromosome No. 2. *Science,* 1973, 182:1261-2. Shabtal, F., *et al.* Partial monosomy of chromosome 2. Delineable syndrome of deletion 2 (q23-q31). *Ann. Génét., Paris,* 1982, 25:156-8.

chromosome 2q duplication syndrome. Synonyms: *2q+ syndrome, 2q duplication syndrome, chromosome 2q trisomy syndrome, dup(2q) syndrome, duplication 2q syndrome, partial trisomy 2q syndrome, trisomy 2q.*

Duplication of the long arm of chromosome 2 characterized by the phenotype consisting of psychomotor retardation, peculiar facies (microcephaly, square face, prominent forehead, prominent glabellar region, hypertelorism, antimongoloid palpebral slant, broad and flat nasal bridge, upturned nostrils, long and flat philtrum, micrognathia, and low-set dysplastic ears), nystagmus, short neck, clinodactyly, brachymesophalangy of the fifth digit, malformed feet, persistence of infantile reflexes, muscle hypotonia and hypotrophy, vitium cordis, urinary tract anomalies, genital anomalies, intestinal anomalies, skin anomalies, dry skin, feeding difficulty, and generalized dystrophia.

Warren, R. J., *et al.* Inherited partial trisomy 2: 46,XX,1,p+,t(1;2)(p36;q31). *Birth Defects,* 1975, 11(5):177-9. Dallapiccola, B., *et al.* Trisomy 2q. *Acta Genet. Med. Gamel.,* 1975, 24:307-10.

chromosome 2q trisomy syndrome. See *chromosome 2q duplication syndrome.*

chromosome 3p duplication syndrome. Synonyms: *3p+ syndrome, 3p duplication syndrome, chromosome 3p trisomy syndrome, dup(3p) syndrome, duplication 3p syndrome, partial trisomy 3p syndrome, trisomy 3p.*

A syndrome of duplication of the short arm of chromosome 3, exhibiting mental retardation, low birth weight, short stature, hypotonia, characteristic facies (square face, microcephaly, brachycephaly, frontal bossing, temporal indentation, epicanthal folds, hypertelorism and/or telecanthus, short nose with a large tip and prominent philtrum, everted lips, downturned corners of the mouth, cleft lip and/or palate, malformed auricles, retrognathia), congenital heart defect (usually septal defects), strabismus, hypoplastic penis, hypospadias, renal abnormalities, seizures, and gastrointestinal defect. The syndrome is often fatal within the first six months of life.

Walter, S., *et al.* A new translocation syndrome (3/B). *N. Engl. J. Med.,* 1966, 275:290-8. Charrow, J., *et al.* Duplication 3p syndrome. *Am. J. Med. Genet.,* 1981, 8:431-6.

chromosome 3p trisomy syndrome. See *chromosome 3p duplication syndrome.*

chromosome 3pter deletion syndrome. Synonyms: *3pter- syndrome, 3pter deletion syndrome, del(3pter) syndrome, monosomy 3pter syndrome, partial monosomy 3pter syndrome.*

Deletion of the terminal portion of the short arm of chromosome 3 associated with mental retardation and multiple abnormalities. Facial characteristics may include a triangular face, flat occiput, abnormal nose (prominent, flat or broad nose with anteverted nostrils and prominent bridge), low-set ears, hypertelorism, epicanthal folds, blepharoptosis, and synophrys or bushy eyebrows. Associated abnormalities usually consist of growth retardation, widely spaced nipples, heart murmur, cardiovascular defect, renal anomalies (pelvic kidney, cystic kidney, and renal hypoplasia), and scoliosis.

Verjaal, M., & De Nef, J. A patient with a partial deletion of the short arm of chromosome 3. *Am. J. Dis. Child.,* 1978, 132:43-5. Reifen, R., *et al.* Partial deletion of the short arm of chromosome 3: Further delineation of the 3p25-3pter syndrome. *Clin. Genet.,* 1986, 30:127-30.

chromosome 3q deletion syndrome. Synonyms: *3q- syndrome, 3q deletion syndrome, del(3q) syndrome, monosomy 3q, partial monosomy 3q.*

Deletion of the long arm of chromosome 3. The phenotype is poorly defined, characteristic facies being the most significant feature (microcephaly, bony defects in the parietal occipital area, scaphocephalic skull, widow's peak, high forehead with dilated veins, flared eyebrows, synophrys, epicanthic folds, telecan-

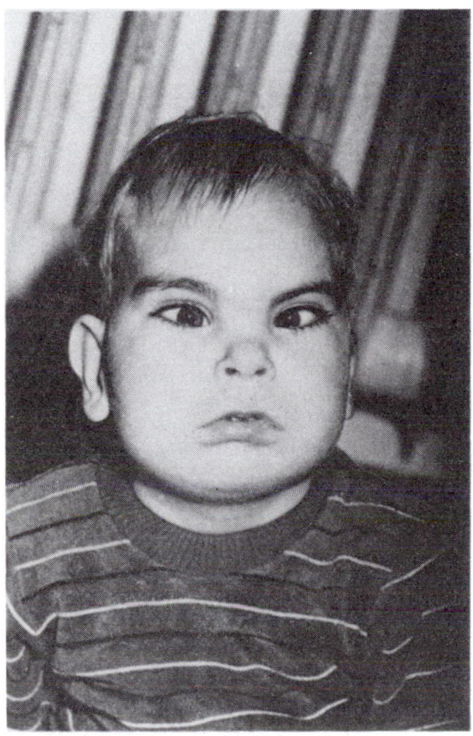

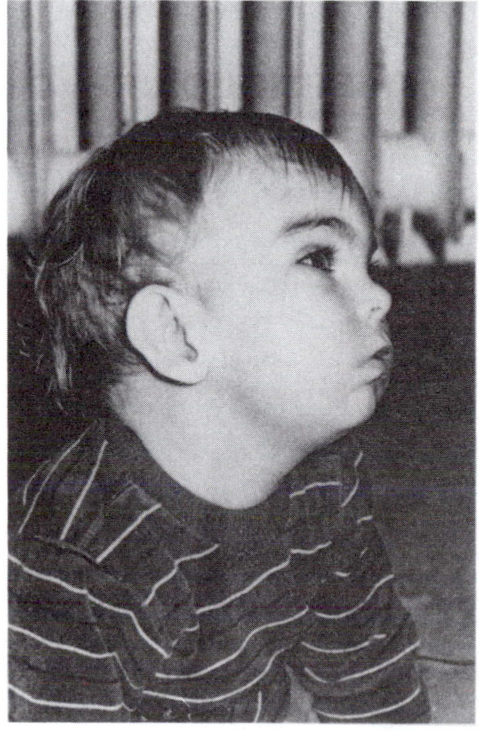

Chromosome 3q duplication syndrome
Tranebjaerg, Lisbeth, Ulla Britt Baekmark, Margrethe Dyhr- Nielsen, & Sven Kreiborg, *Clinical Genetics,* 32:137-143, 1987, Munksgaard International Publishers, Copenhagen, Denmark.

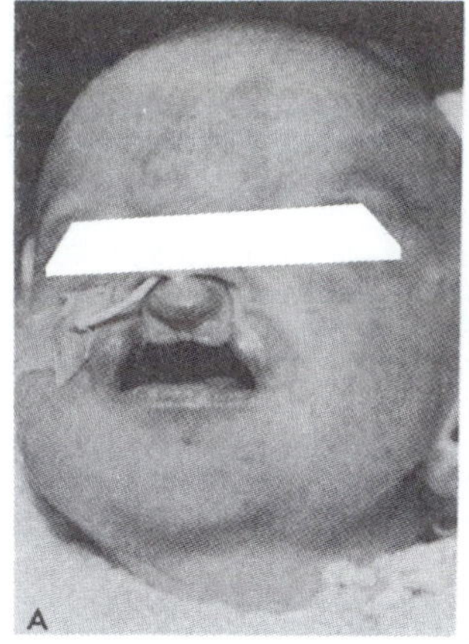

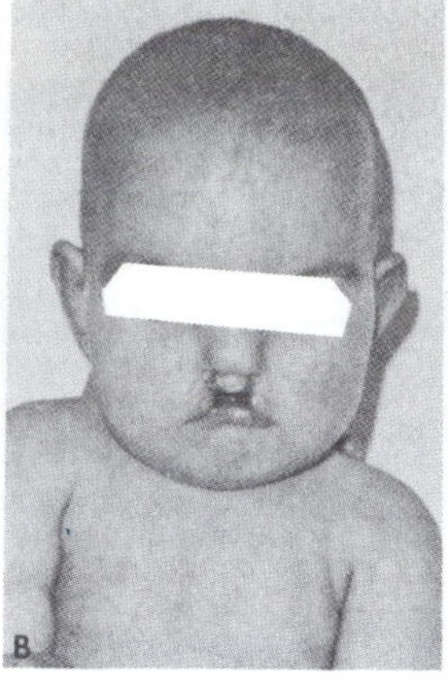

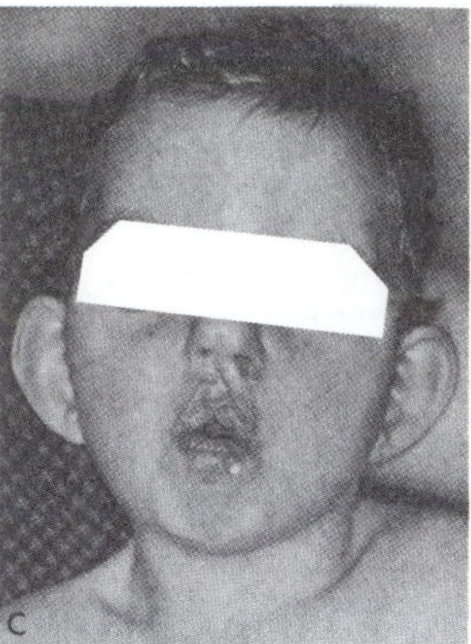

Chromosome 4p deletion syndrome (Wolf-Hirschhorn syndrome)
Wolf, U., & Reinwein, H.: *Z. Kinderheilkd.* 98:235, 1967. New York: Springer-Verlag.

thus, strabismus, hypoplastic nose with anteverted nostrils, long philltrum, narrow tongue with a pointed tip, narrow and pointed mandible, flattened maxilla, bow-shaped thin lips, asymmetric malformed ears). Associated anomalies may include short neck, ventricular septal defect, umbilical hernia, hyperactive reflexes and hypertonia, asymmetry of the lower limbs, limited joint movement, abnormal dermatoglyphics, and delayed development.

Martsolf, J. T., & Ray, M. Interstitial deletion of the long arm of chromosome 3. *Ann. Génét., Paris,* 1983, 26:98-99.

chromosome 3q duplication syndrome. Synonyms: *3q+ syndrome, 3q duplication syndrome, chromosome 3q trisomy syndrome, dup(3q) syndrome, duplication 3q syndrome, partial trisomy 3q syndrome, trisomy 3q.*

Duplication of the long arm of chromosome 3 characterized by multiple abnormalities similar to those seen in de Lange syndrome (1) (q.v.). Craniofacial anomalies include abnormal shape of the head, synophrys, broad nasal root, anteverted nostrils, downturned corners of the mouth, malformed ears, hirsutism, maxillary prognathism, upslanting palpebral fissures, long upper lip, highly arched palate, and cleft palate. Other defects may include short or webbed neck, abnormal chest, heart defect (mainly septal defects), omphalocele, urogenital abnormalities, clinodactyly or camptodactyly, hypoplastic nails, simian creases, talipes, and brain anomalies with seizures. Most patients die during the first year; those who survive usually develop severe growth and mental retardation.

Falek, U., *et al.* Familial de Lange syndrome with chromosome abnormalities. *Pediatrics,* 1966, 37:92-101. Wilson, G. N., *et al.* Further delineation of the dup(3q) syndrome. *Am. J. Med. Genet.,* 1985, 22:117-23.

chromosome 3q trisomy syndrome. See *chromosome 3q duplication syndrome.*

chromosome 4p deletion syndrome. Synonyms: *Wolf syndrome, Wolf-Hirschhorn syndrome, 4p deletion syndrome, 4p- syndrome, 4p deletion syndrome, del(4p) syndrome, monosomy 4p, partial monosmmy 4p.*

A relatively rare syndrome of partial deletion of the short arm of chromosome 4, characterized by psychomotor and growth retardation and multiple abnormalities. A low birth-weight, hypotonia, and seizures are usually present at birth. They are associated with craniofacial abnormalities, including microcephaly, cranial asymmetry, prominent glabella, ocular hypertelorism, antimongoloid palpebral slant, blepharoptosis, low-set deformed ears with preauricular dimples and sinuses and narrow external canals, and a short philtrum. Down-turned corners of the mouth, cleft palate or lip, and micrognathia are the most prominent oral defects. Bony anomalies may consist of late ossification of pelvic and metacarpal bones, synostoses, fusion or bony structures, hip dislocation, pseudoepiphyses in the metacarpals, clinodactyly and shortness of the fifth middle phalanges. Urogenital and cardiovascular anomalies, simian creases, dermal ridges, strabismus, hydrocephalus, and other defects may also be present. Life expectancy is low, about one-third of all affected infants dying within the first 2 years of life.

Wolf, U., *et al.* Defizienz an den kurzen Armen eines Chromosoms Nr 4. *Humangenetik,* 1965, 1:397-413. Hirschhorn, K., *et al.* Deletion of short arms of chromosome 4-5 in a child with defects of midline fusion. *Humangenetik,* 1965, 1:479-82.

chromosome 4p duplication syndrome. Synonyms: *4p+ syndrome, 4p duplication syndrome, chromosome 4p trisomy syndrome, dup(4p) syndrome, duplication 4p syndrome, partial trisomy 4p syndrome, trisomy 4p.*

Duplication of the short arm of chromosome 4 associated with variable clinical manifestations. The symptoms may include growth and mental retardation, seizures, microcephaly, triangular and asymmetric face, prominent glabella, synophrys, low anterior hairline, hypotelorism, ocular refraction errors, long eyelashes, bulbous nose, depressed nasal bridge, broad nasal root, malformed ear auricles, high-arched palate, prominent central incisors, malocclusion, prominent chin, short neck, widely spaced nipples, scoliosis, contractures, excess digital whorls, long and slender hands and feet, genu valgum, pes planus, small phallus, hypoplastic scrotum, hypospadias, and cryptorchism.

Wilson, M. G., *et al.* Inherited pericentric inversion fo chromosome No. 4. *Am. J. Med. Genet.,* 1970, 22:679-90. Reynolds,. J. F., *et al.* Trisomy 4p in four relatives: Variability and lack of distinctive features in phenotypic expression. *Clin. Genet.*, 1983, 24:365-74.

chromosome 4p trisomy syndrome. See *chromosome 4p duplication syndrome.*

chromosome 4q deletion syndrome. Synonyms: *4q- syndrome, 4q deletion syndrome, del(4q) syndrome, monosomy 4q, partial monosomy 4q syndrome.*

Deletion of the long arm of chromosome 4 associated with mental retardation, growth retardation, craniofacial abnormalities (asymmetric head, upward palpebral slant, epicanthic folds, hypertelorism, depressed or flat bridge of the nose, short philtrum, upturned nose, low-set malformed ears, cleft lip and/or cleft palate, retromicrognathia), hand and foot anomalies (syndactyly of fingers and toes, overriding of fingers and toes, abnormal implantation of fingers and toes, clinodactyly of fingers and toes, poorly developed flexion creases of fifth finger, transverse palmar creases), widely spaced hypoplastic nipples, hypospadias, small scrotum, feeding difficulty, cyanosis, and heart and kidney abnormalities. Most patients die in infancy.

Ockey, C. H., *et al.* A large deletion of the long arm of chromosome No. 4 in a child with limb abnormalities. *Arch. Dis. Child.*, 1967, 428-34. Yu, C. W., *et al.* Terminal deletion of the long arm of chromosome 4. Report of a case of 46,XY,del(4)(q31) and review of 4q- syndrome. *Ann. Génét., Paris,* 1981, 24:158-61.

chromosome 4q duplication syndrome. Synonyms: *4q+ syndrome, 4q duplication syndrome, chromosome 4q trisomy syndrome, dup(4q) syndrome, duplication 4q syndrome, partial trisomy 4q syndrome, trisomy 4q.*

Duplication of the long arm of chromosome 4 associated with mental retardation and variable multiple abnormalities, including craniofacial malformations (microcephaly, epicanthal folds, depressed or wide nasal bridge, micrognathia, sloping forehead, antimongoloid palpebral slant, short philtrum, downturned corners of the mouth, malformed or low-set ears), low birth weight, muscle hypotonia, umbilical or inguinal hernia, cryptorchism, and different abnormalities of the heart, urinary system, hands, and feet.

Hoehn, H., *et al.* Aneusomie de recombinaison: Rearrangement between paternal chromosomes 4 and 18 yielding offspring with features of the 18q- syndrome. Ann. Génét., Paris, 1971, 14:187-92. Fonatsch, C., et al. Partial trisomy 4q and partial monosomy 18q as a consequence of paternal balanced translocation t(4q-;18q+). 1974, 25:227-33. Bofante, A., et al. Partial trisomy 4q: Two cases resulting from a familial translocation t(4;18)(q27;p11). Hum. Genet., 1979, 52:85-90.

chromosome 4q trisomy syndrome. See *chromosome 4q duplication syndrome.*

chromosome 5p deletion syndrome. Synonyms: *Lejeune syndrome, 5p- syndrome, 5p deletion syndrome, cat cry syndrome, cri-du-chat syndrome, del(5p) syndrome, monosomy 5p, partial monosomy 5p syndrome.*

A syndrome of partial deletion of the short arm of chromosome 5, bands 5p14 and 5p15 being missing. It is characterized by severe mental deficiency, growth retardation, multiple abnormalities, and a peculiar crying sound resembling that of a suffering kitten (hence the synonym *crying cat syndrome*), that disappears within weeks or months after birth. Birth weight is usually less than 2500 g, and the affected infants are hypotonic and fail to thrive. Craniofacial abnormalities usually include microcephaly, round face, hypertelorism, antimongoloid palpebral slant, epicanthus, large frontal sinuses, broad nasal bones, and low-set ears. Hypertelorism and facial roundness usually disappear with age, and the face becomes thin with a short philtrum. Most patients attain an adult height of about 124 to 168 cm. Orodental abnormalities may consist of mild micrognathia, malocclusion, and, sometimes, harelip and cleft palate. Premature graying of the hair, strabismus, preauricular skin tags, musculoskeletal anomalies, flat feet, shortening of the metacarpals, and other defects may be associated.

Lejeune, J., *et al.* Trois cas de délétion de bras court d'un chromosome 5. *C. Rend. Acad. Sc., Paris*, 1963, 257:3098-3102.

chromosome 5p duplication syndrome. Synonyms: *5p+ syndrome, 5p duplication syndrome, chromosome 5p trisomy syndrome, dup(5p) syndrome, duplication 5p syndrome, partial trisomy 5p syndrome, trisomy 5p.*

Partial trisomy of the short arm of chromosome 5 associated with severe mental retardation and multiple congenital abnormalities, including postnatal growth retardation, dolichocephaly, prominent occiput, hypotonia, respiratory and/or crying difficulty, seizures, clubfoot, pectus excavatum, umbilical and/or inguinal hernia, accessory spleen, and ureterorenal abnormalities. Death usually takes place between the ages of 1 month to 6 years.

Lejeune, J., *et al.* Ségrégation familiale d'une translocation 5-13 déterminant une monosomie et une trisomie partielles du bras court du chromosome 5: Maladie du "cri du chat" et sa "réciproque." *C. Rend. Acad. Sc., Paris,* 1964, 258:5767-70. Opitz, J. M., & Patau, K. A partial trisomy 5p syndrome. *Birth Defects,* 1975, 11(5):191-200.

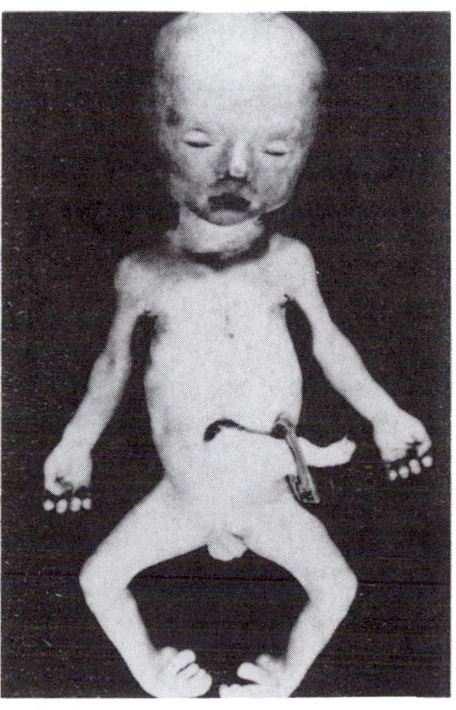

Chromosome 5p duplication syndrome
Kleczkowska, A., J.P. Fryns, Ph. Moerman, K. Vandenberghe & H. Van den Berghe, *Clinical Genetics* 32:49-56, 1987, Munksgaard International Publishers, Copenhagen, Denmark.

chromosome 5p trisomy syndrome. See *chromosome 5p duplication syndrome.*

chromosome 5q deletion syndrome. Synonyms: *5q- syndrome, 5q deletion syndrome, del(5q) syndrome, monosomy 5q, partial monosomy 5q syndrome.*

Deletion of the long arm of chromosome 5 characterized by psychomotor retardation and multiple abnormalities. Craniofacial anomalies include frontal bossing, retromicrognathia, hypertelorism, blepharophimosis, epicanthal folds, flat nasal bridge, anteverted nostrils, large philtrum, low-set malformed ears, and cleft palate. Other disorders include failure to thrive, muscle hypotonia or hypertonia, short neck, bone and joint abnormalities, heart defect, heart murmur, urogenital and anal malformations, and abnormal dermatoglyphics or flexion creases.

Stoll, C., *et al.* Interstitial deletion of the long arm fo chromosome 5 in a deformed boy: 46,XY,del(q13q15) *J. Med. Genet.,* 1980, 17:486-7. Felding, I., & Kristoffersson, U. A child with interstitial deletion of chromosome No. 5. *Hereditas,* 1980, 93:337-9.

chromosome 5q duplication syndrome. Synonyms: *5q+ syndrome, 5q duplication syndrome, chromosome 5q trisomy syndrome, dup(5q) syndrome, duplication 5q syndrome, partial trisomy 5q syndrome, trisomy 5q.*

Duplication of the long arm of chromosome 5 associated with psychomotor retardation, microcephaly, receding forehead, antimongoloid slant of the palpebral fissures, epicanthus, hypertelorism, long upper lip, microstomia, carp mouth, micrognathia, dysplastic ears, brachydactyly, preaxial polydactyly, short extremities, diaphragmatic and other hernias, heart defect, and accessory spleen.

Bartsch-Sandhoff, M., & Liersch, R. Partial duplication 5q syndrome: Phenotypic similarity in two sisters with identical karyotype (partial duplication 5q33 to 5qter and partial deficiency 8p23-pter). *Ann. Génét., Paris,* 1977, 20:281-4. Osztovics, M., & Kiss, P. Trisomy 5q15-q31 due to maternal insertion, ins(6;5)(q21;q15q31). *Acta Paediat. Acad. Sc. Hung.,* 1982, 23:231-7.

chromosome 5q trisomy syndrome. See *chromosome 5q duplication syndrome.*

chromosome 6 ring syndrome. Synonyms: *r(6) syndrome, ring chromosome 6 syndrome.*

A syndrome in which both ends of chromosome 6 have been lost (deletion) and the two broken ends have reunited to form a ring-shaped figure. Intrauterine and postnatal growth retardation, mental retardation, and facial abnormalities are the most frequent manifestations. Eye anomalies usually include glaucoma, megalocornea, microphthalmos, embrytoxon, strabismus, aniridia, and albinoid fundi. Epicanthal folds, microcephaly, micrognathia, low-set ears, hypertelorism, and bird-like head give the affected infants a peculiar facial appearance. Associated defects may include central nervous system malformations, convulsions, and hydrocephalus.

Moore, C. M., *et al.* Developmental abnormalities associated with ring chromosome 6. *J. Med. Genet.,* 1973, 10:299-303. Shitayad, D. *et al.* Ring chromosome 6. *Am. J. Med. Genet.,* 1987, 26:145-51.

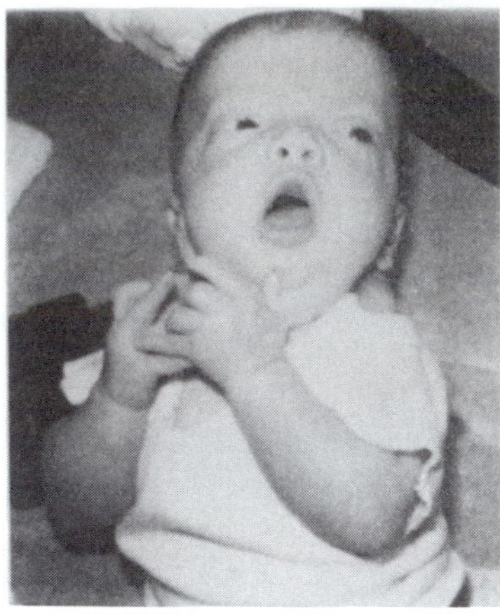

Chromosome 6 ring syndrome
Chitayat, D., S.Y.E. Hahm, M.A. Iqbal, & H.M. Nitowsky, *American Journal of Medical Genetics* 26:145-151, 1987. New York: Alan R. Liss, Inc.

chromosome 6p duplication syndrome. Synonyms: *6p+ syndrome, 6p duplication syndrome, chromosome 6p trisomy syndrome, dup(6p) syndrome, duplication 6p syndrome, partial trisomy 6p, trisomy 6p.*

Duplication of the short arm of chromosome 6 characterized by peculiar facies (frontal bossing, hypotelorism, and midfacial hypoplasia), low birth-weight, cardiovascular abnormalities, small kidneys, and psychomotor retardation. Additional defects include anomalies of the brain and skull (microcephaly, shortened basisphenoid/occiput, small cranial fossa, steep orbital roof, absence of the bulbs, and rudimentary olfactory tract), interventricular septal defect, right ventricular hypertrophy, absence of the uterus and vagina, hypoplastic ovaries, common mesentery, double extensors indicis bellies, and absence of the palmaris brevis and peroneus tertius muscles.

Turleau, C., *et al.* La trisomie 6p partielle. *Ann. Génét., Paris,* 1978, 21:88-91. Smith, B. S., & Petterson, J. C. An anatomical study of a duplication 6p based on two sibs. *Am. J. Med. Genet.,* 1985, 20:649-63.

chromosome 6p trisomy syndrome. See *chromosome 6p duplication syndrome.*

chromosome 6q deletion syndrome. Synonyms: *6q- syndrome, 6q deletion syndrome del(6q) syndrome, deletion 6q syndrome, monosomy 6q, partial monosomy 6q syndrome.*

Deletion of the long arm of the chromosome 6 characterized by multiple abnormalities, including short stature, mental retardation, dolichocephaly, characteristic facies (facial asymmetry, upslanting palpebral fissures, epicanthus, long philtrum, thin upper lip, malformed ears), brevicollis, vertebral anomalies, heart defect, deformed feet (wide spaces between the first and second toes, flat feet, pes valgus), umbilical hernia, and simian creases. Associated abnormalities may include tracheo-esophageal fistula, ectopic kidney, clinodactyly, hiatus or inguinal hernia, lacrimal duct atresia, small nails, long great toes, cleft palate, protrusion of the glabella, mandibular prognathism, and excessive keloid formation.

McNeal, R. M., *et al.* Congenital anomalies including VATER association in a patient with a del(6)q deletion. *J. Pediat.,* 1977, 91:957-60. Yamamoto, Y., *et al.* Deletion of proximal 6q: A clinical report and review of the literature. *Am. J. Med. Genet.,* 1986, 25:467-71.

chromosome 6q duplication syndrome. Synonyms: *6q+ syndrome, 6q duplication syndrome, chromosome*

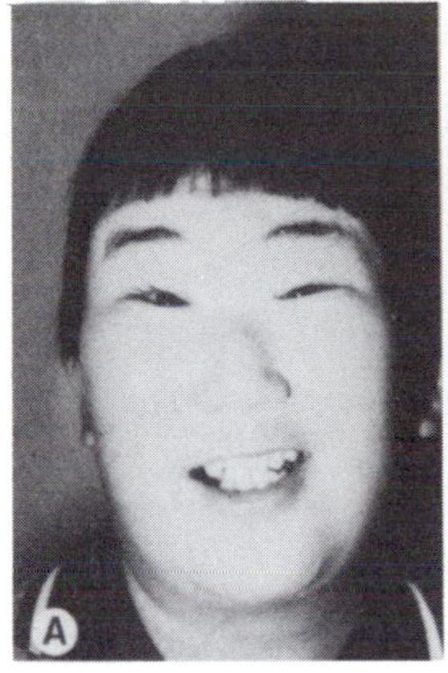
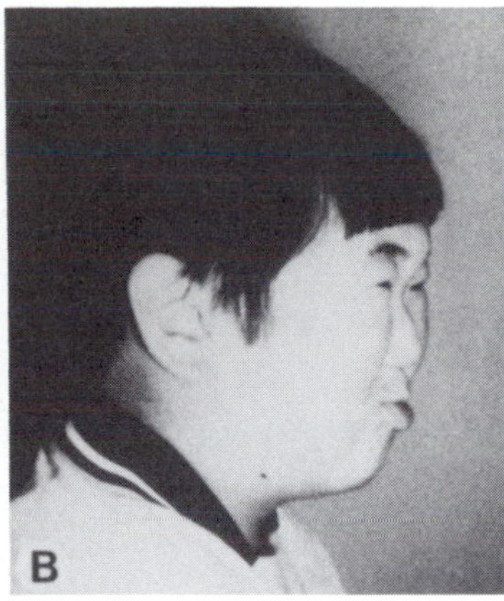
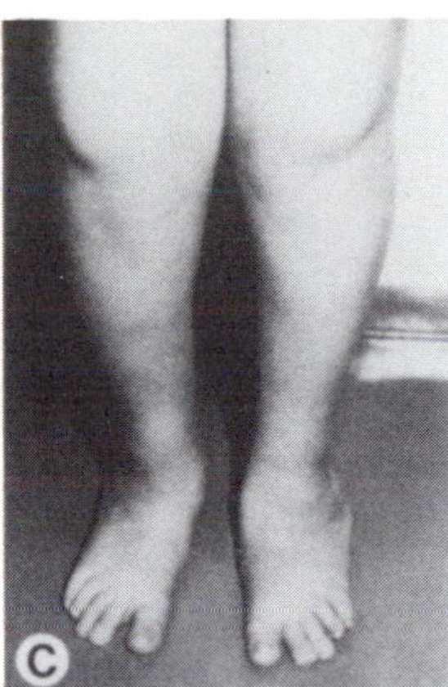

Chromosome 6q deletion syndrome
Yamamoto, Yoshifumi, Noriko Okamoto, Hirohiko Shiraishi, Masayoshi Yanagisawa & Shigehiko Kamoshita, *American Journal of Medical Genetics* 25:467-471, 1986. New York: Alan R. Liss, Inc.

6q trisomy syndrome, dup(6q) syndrome, duplication 6q syndrome, partial trisomy 6q, trisomy 6q.

Duplication of the long arm of chromosome 6. The phenotype is characterized by mental and growth retardation, craniofacial abnormalities (microcephaly, acrocephaly, flat facies, prominent forehead, extended nasal septum, flat nasal bridge, micrognathia, antimongoloid palpebral slant, high-arched palate, carp mouth, low-set ears), strabismus, dental abnormalities, short webbed neck, pectus excavatum, flexion deformity, club foot, scoliosis, syndactyly, clinodactyly, abnormal palmar creases, and feeding difficulty.

Chen, H. M., *et al.* Familial partial trisomy 6q resulting from inherited ins(5;6)(q33;q15q27). *Clin. Genet.*, 1976, 9:631-7. Tipton, R. E., *et al.* Duplication 6q syndrome. *am. J. Med. Genet.*, 1979, 3:325-30.

chromosome 6q trisomy syndrome. See *chromosome 6q duplication syndrome.*

chromosome 7 monosomy syndrome. Synonyms: *7 monosomy, monosomy 7, monosomy C.*

The absence of one chromosome of one pair in an otherwise diploid cell of chromosome 7, which is frequently present in preleukemia and is responsible for an increased susceptibility to bacterial infections.

Nowell, P., & Finan, J. Chromosome studies in leukemia. IV. Myeloproliferative versus cytogeanic studies. *Cancer*, 1978, 42:2254. Gyger, M., *et al.* Childhood monosomy 7 syndrome. *Am. J. Hemat.*, 1982, 13:329-34.

chromosome 7 ring syndrome. Synonyms: *r(7) syndrome, ring chromosome 7 syndrome.*

A syndrome in which both ends of chromosome 7 have been lost (deletion) and the two broken ends have reunited to form a ring-shaped figure. It is characterized mainly by short stature and multiple pigmented nevi suggestive of hamartoma. The phenotypic expression varies and may include craniofacial, oral, ocular, and other anomalies. Craniofacial abnormalities usually consist of microcephaly, craniosynostosis, facial asymmetry, antimongoloid palpebral slant, proptosis, epicanthic folds, and hypertelorism. Microcornea, cataract, and strabismus are the principal ocular features. Delayed dentition, high-arched palate, and gingival hypertrophy are the oral symptoms. Other defects include sacral dimple, pectus excavatum, widely spaced nipples, microphallus, and cryptorchism. Most infants have normal intelligence, but some suffer from mental retardation.

Zachai, E. H., & Breg, W. R. Ring chromosome 7 with variable phenotypic expression. *Cytogen. Cell Genet.*, 1973, 12:40-8. Nakano, S., & Miyamoto, N. A ring C7 chromosome in a mentally and physically retarded male with various somatic abnormalities. *Jpn. J. Hum. Genet.*, 1977, 22:33-41. DeLozier, C. D., et al. A fourth case of ring chromosome 7. Clin. Genet., 1982, 22:90-8.

chromosome 7 trisomy syndrome. Synonym: *trisomy 7.*

The presence of an additional (third) chromosome on an otherwise diploid chromosome 7. Most cases terminate in spontaneous abortion. Those infants who survive the gestational period die shortly after birth. They usually exhibit the features of the Potter syndrome (q.v.), including ocular abnormalities, low-set posteriorly rotated ears, flat nasal bridge, micrognathia, cleft palate, prominent occiput, redundant skin, abnormal dermatoglyphics, vertebral anomalies, hyperextensible joints, clinodactyly, club foot, genu recurvatum, pulmonary hypoplasia, abnormal genitalia, muscle hypotonia, renal agenesis, polycystic kidney, and hydronephrosis.

Blair, J. D. Trisomy C and cystic dysplasia of kidneys, liver, and pancreas. *Birth Defects*, 1976, 12:139-49. Boué, J., *et al.* Identification of C trisomies in human abortuses. *J. Med. Genet.*, 1975, 12:265-8. Yunis, E., *et al.* Full trisomy 7 and Potter syndrome. *Hum. Genet.*, 1980, 54:13-8.

chromosome 7p deletion syndrome. Synonyms: *7p-syndrome, 7p deletion syndrome, del(7p) syndrome, monosomy 7p, partial monosomy 7p syndrome.*

Deletion of the short arm of chromosome 7 associated with multiple abnormalities, including craniofacial malformations (flattened occiput, prominent forehead, median bony protrusions of the forehead, craniosynostosis), epicanthal folds, eyelid-axis displacement, short eyelid axis, hypertelorism or hypotelorism, exo-

chromosome 7p

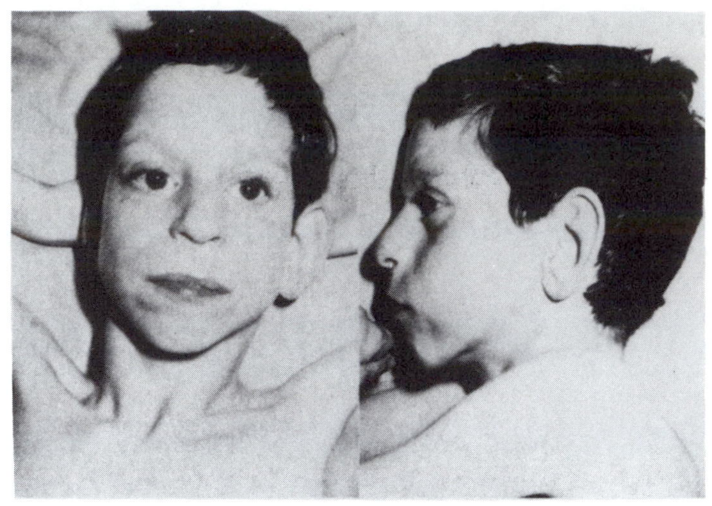

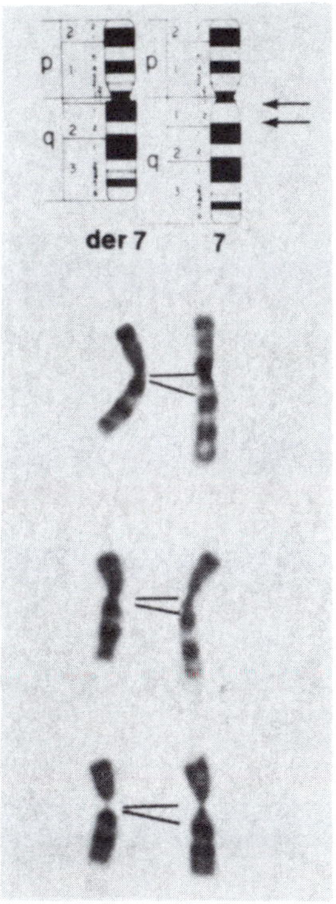

Chromosome 7q deletion syndrome
Frydman, Moshe, Julia Steinberger, Fiorella Shabtai, & Reuben Steinherz, *American Journal of Medical Genetics* 25:245-249, 1986. New York: Alan R. Liss, Inc.

phthalmos, blepharoptosis, saddle nose, low-set posteriorly rotated small ears, high-arched palate, cleft palate, hand abnormalities (limited motion, abnormal thumb insertion, clinodactyly, overlapping fingers), foot abnormalities, anal atresia with fistula, simian creases, and various heart, kidney, and genital abnormalities. Mental retardation may occur.

McPherson, E., *et al.* Chromosome 7 short arm deletion and craniosynostosis, a 7p- syndrome. *Hum. Genet.*, 1976, 35:117-23. Schömig-Spingler, M., *et al.* Chromosome 7 short arm deletion, 7p21 to pter. *Hum. Genet.*, 1986, 74:323-5.

chromosome 7p duplication syndrome. Synonyms: *7p+ syndrome, 7p duplication syndrome, chromosome 7p trisomy syndrome, dup(7p) syndrome, duplication 7p syndrome, partial trisomy 7p syndrome, trisomy 7p.*

Duplication of the short arm of chromosome 7 associated with growth and mental retardation, dolichocephaly, delayed fontanel closure or ossification, hypertelorism, antimongoloid palpebral slant, high-arched palate, micrognathia, large smooth ears, muscle hypertrophy, osteoarticular abnormalities, and joint dimples. Additional abnormalities may include epicanthus, broad or double fingers, and brain and heart anomalies.

Eriksson, B., *et al.* Unusual chromosome mosaic (46,XX/46,XX,Cp+) in a girl with multiple malformations. *Ann. Génét., Paris,* 1968, 11:6-10. Cantú, J. M., *et al.* Trisomy 7p due to a mosaic normal/dir dup(7)(p13 to p22). Syndrome delineation, critical segment assignment, and comment on duplication. *Ann. Génét., Paris,* 1985, 28:254-7.

chromosome 7p trisomy syndrome. See *chromosome 7p duplication syndrome.*

chromosome 7q deletion syndrome. Synonyms: *7q- syndrome, 7q deletion syndrome, del(7q) syndrome, monosomy 7q, partial monosomy 7q syndrome.*

Deletion of the long arm of chromosome 7 characterized by mental retardation and multiple developmental abnormalities. Craniofacial defects consist mainly of microcephaly, brachycephaly, eye abnormalities (enophthalmos, exophthalmos, esotropia, exotropia, optic nerve atrophy, blue sclera, hypermetropia, glaucoma, and retinochoroidal colobomata), peculiar facial characteristics (flat and broad nasal bridge, bulbous nasal tip, prominent forehead, cleft lip and/or palate, malformed ears, upslanted palpebral fissures), low birthweight, genital disorders (micropenis, cryptorchism, small testes, hypospadias), abnormal palmar creases, chest abnormalities (pectus excavatum, short sternum, and widely spaced nipples), and clinodactyly. Some cases may show additional defects, including muscle atonia, feeding problems, micrognathia, large mouth, hypertelorism, abnormal EEG, seizures, skin laxity, hernia, brachydactyly, syndactyly, overriding toes, joint hyperextensibility, tappering fingers, frequent infections, and heart defect. Most cases have terminal deletions of 7q, but some are interstitial deletions 7q.

Grouchy, J., de, *et al.* A case of ?6p- chromosomal aberration. *Am. J. Dis. Child.,* 1968, 115:93-9. Grouchy, J., de, *et al.* Tentative localization of Hageman (factor XII) locus on 7q, probably the 7q35 band. *Humangenetik,* 1974, 24:197-200. Young, R. S., *et al.* Terminal and interstitial deletions of the long arm of chromosome 7: A review with five new cases. *Am. J. Med. Genet.,* 1984, 17:437-50.

chromosome 7q duplication syndrome. Synonyms: *7q+ syndrome, 7q duplication syndrome, chromosome 7q trisomy syndrome, dup(7q) syndrome, duplication 7q syndrome, partial trisomy 7q syndrome, trisomy 7q.*

Partial duplication of the long arm of chromosome 7 characterized by low birth weight, growth and mental retardation, cleft palate, microretrognathia, small nose, downward slant of the palpebral fissures, hypertelorism, deeply set eyes, and facial asymmetry. Less frequent symptoms include transverse palmar creases, muscle hypo- or hypertonia, frontal bossing, coloboma of the iris, exophthalmos, cataract, hypertelorism, low-set ears, short neck, pterygium colli, scoliosis, and vertebral anomalies. The phenotype is variable, depending on the segment of the chromosome involved.

Carpentier, S., *et al.* Trisomie partielle 7q par translocation familiale t(7;12)(q22;q24). *Ann. Génét., Paris* 1972, 15:283-6.

chromosome 7q trisomy syndrome. See *chromosome 7q duplication syndrome.*

chromosome 8 trisomy syndrome. Synonyms: *Warkany syndrome, chromosome C trisomy, trisomy 8, trisomy C syndrome.*

Triplication of chromosome 8, associated with mental retardation and multiple abnormalities. The most frequently occurring anomalies include abnormal toe posture, everted lower lip, peculiar facies, micrognathia, cleft lip and palate, abnormal nipples, limited thumb abduction, clumsiness, sacral dimples, rib anomalies, dermatoglyphic and skin abnormalities, limited supination and pronation, muscular atrophy, spina bifida occulta, abnormal ears, slender pelvis, abnormal cry, prominent forehead, clinodactyly, renal defects, abnormal scapulae, hip abnormalities, contractures, camptodactyly, scoliosis, long fingers, ocular abnormalities, hypertelorism, strabismus, absent patellae, cryptorchism, narrow shoulders, abnormal sternum, short or webbed neck, abnormal nails, and other anomalies.. Trisomy is usually partial; total trisomy is believed to be lethal. Trisomy 8 is often due to translocation of the distal segment of the long arm.

Warkany, J., *et al.* Mental retardation, absence of patellae, other malformations with chromosomal mosaicism. *J. Pediat.,* 1962, 61-803-12. Riccardi, V. M. Trisomy 8: An international study of 70 patients. *Birth Defects,* 1977, 13(3C):171-84. Pfeiffer, R. A., *et al.* Chromosomenanomalien in den Blutzellen eines Kindes mit multiple Abartungen. *Klin. Wschr.,* 1962, 40:1058-67.

chromosome 8p deletion syndrome. Synonyms: *8p- syndrome, 8p deletion syndrome, del(8p) syndrome, monosomy 8p, partial monosomy 8 syndrome.*

A syndrome characterized by deletion of the short arm of chromosome 8, associated with mental retardation, growth retardation, peculiar facies, widely-set nipples, and cardiac defects. Craniofacial anomalies usually consist of microcephaly, narrow forehead, prominent occiput, narrow palpebral fissures, epicanthus, short stubby nose, thin mouth, abnormal palate, retrognathia, and dysplastic ears.

Lubs, H. A., & Lubs, M. L. New cytogenetic technics applied to a series of children with mental retardation. In: Casperson, T.,& Zech, L. eds. *Chromosome identification technique and application in biology and medicine.* Nobel Symposia 23, New York, Academic Press, 1973, p. 241-50.

chromosome 8p duplication syndrome. Synonyms:

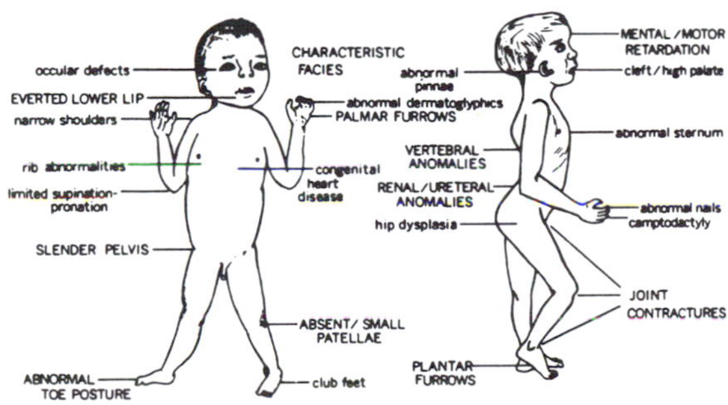

Chromosome 8 trisomy syndrome
Riccardi, V.M.: Trisomy 8: An international study of 70 patients. In Bergsma, D., Lowry, R.B. (eds): *Natural History of Specific Birth Defects.* New York: Alan R. Liss, Inc. for the National Foundation - March of Dimes BD:OAS XIII(3C):171-184, 1977. New York: Alan R. Liss, Inc., with permission.

8p+ syndrome, 8p duplication syndrome, chromosome 8p trisomy syndrome, dup(8p) syndrome, duplication 8p syndrome, partial trisomy 8p syndrome, trisomy 8p.

Duplication of the short arm of chromosome 8 characterized by multiple abnormalities, including mental and growth retardation, seizures, hypertelorism, antimongoloid slant of palpebral fissures, strabismus, depressed nasal bridge, malocclusion, high arched palate, cleft lip and/or palate, mandibular prognathism, large mouth, malformed ears, heart defect, diaphragmatic hernia, microphallus, cryptorchism, joint abnormalities, hypoplastic toenails, abnormal dermatoglyphics, simian creases, Sydney line, and single creases of the fingers.

Yanagisawa, S. Partial trisomy 8: Further observation on a familial C/G translocation chromosome identified by the Q-staining method. *J. Ment. Defic. Res.*, 1973, 17:28-32.

chromosome 8p trisomy syndrome. See *chromosome 8p duplication syndrome.*

chromosome 8q deletion syndrome. Synonyms: *8q- syndrome, 8q deletion syndrome, del(8q) syndrome, deletion 8q syndrome, monosomy 8q, partial monosomy 8q syndrome.*

Deletion of the long arm of chromosome 8 characterized by growth and psychomotor retardation, craniofacial anomalies (hypertelorism, deep-set eyes, antimongoloid palpebral slant, depressed nasal bridge, round tip of the nose, microretrognathia, low-set malformed ears, prominant forehead, carp mouth), hypoplastic thumbs, inguinal hernia, and sacral dimples. Associated defects may include short neck, congenital cardiac abnormalities, genital anomalies, altered muscle tone, and hirsutism.

Dallapicola, B., *et al.* Deletion of the long arm of chromosome 8 resulting from a de novo translocation t(4;8)(q13;q213). *Hum. Genet.*, 1977, 38:125-30. Beighle, C., *et al.* Small structural changes of chromosome 8. Two cases with evidence for deletion. *Hum. Genet.*, 1977, 38:113-21. Taysi, K., *et al.* Presumptive long arm deletion of chromosome 8: A new syndrome? *Hum. Genet.*, 1979, 51:49-53.

chromosome 8q duplication syndrome. Synonyms: *8q+ syndrome, 8q duplication syndrome, chromosome 8q trisomy syndrome, dup(8q) syndrome, duplication 8q syndrome, partial trisomy 8q syndrome, trisomy 8q.*

Duplication of the long arm of chromosome 8 characterized by mental and growth retardation with multiple abnormalities. Craniofacial anomalies may include a wide face, hypertelorism, blepharoptosis, microcephaly, broad nose, low-set large ears, retrognathia, micrognathia, cleft palate, high-arched palate, short oral frenula, and bifid tongue. Frequently associated defects and disorders consist of seizures, recurrent infections, nevi of the head and neck, short neck, short thorax, pectus excavatum, heart defect, widely spaced nipples, kidney malformations, genital abnormalities, malformed spine, clinodactyly, short phalanges, distal radial triradius, abnormal toe position, pes equinus, limited joint movement, and simian creases.

Fryns, J. P., *et al.* Partial trisomy 8: Trisomy of the distal part of the long arm of chromosome number 8+(8q2) in severely retarded girl. *Humangenetik,* 1974, 24:241-6. Fujimoto, A., *et al.* Familial inversion of chromosome No. 8: An affected child and carrier fetus. *Humangenetik,* 1975, 27:67-73.

chromosome 8q trisomy syndrome. See *chromosome 8q duplication syndrome.*

chromosome 9 ring syndrome. Synonyms: *r(9) syndrome, ring chromosome 9.*

A congenital syndrome in which both ends of chromosome 9 have been lost (deletion) and the two broken ends have reunited to form a ring-shaped figure. Associated abnormalities include psychomotor retardation, microcephaly, trigonocephaly, hypertrichosis, exophthalmos, mongoloid palpebral slant, anteverted nares, long philtrum, cryptorchism, hypospadias, and various osseous and cardiac anomalies.

Jacobsen, P., *et al.* A ring chromosome diagnosed by quinacrine fluorescence as No. 9 in a mentally retarded girl. *Clin. Genet.*, 1973, 4:434-41. Portnoi, M. F., *et al.* Une nouvelle observation de chromosome 9 en anneau. *Ann. Génét., Paris,* 1982, 25:164-7.

chromosome 9 trisomy syndrome. Synonym: *trisomy 9.*

A syndrome of triplication of chromosome 9, characterized mainly by microcephaly, low-set and malformed ears, micrognathia, broad nose with bulbous tip, brain abnormalities, congenital heart defects, hand and foot abnormalities, joint dislocation, cryptorchism, microphallus, growth retardation, hypotonia, and motor retardation. Less frequent anomalies include dolichocephaly, presence of a third fontanel, narrow temples, occipital bossing, facial asymmetry, enophthalmos, narrow palpebral fissures, epicanthus, mongoloid palpebral slant, hypertelorism or hypotelorism, high-arched palate, cleft lip and palate, thin upper lip, maxillary prognathism, low hairline, short or webbed neck, shield chest, widely spaced nipples, umbilical hernia, kyphoscoliosis, renal cysts, hydronephrosis, absent or abnormal toes, and hypoplastic scrotum. Most affected patients die during infancy or childhood.

Feingold, M., & Atkins, L. A case of trisomy 9. *J. Med. Genet.*, 1973, 10:184-7. Kurnick, J., *et al.* Trisomy 9: Predominence of cardiovascular, liver, brain, and skeletal anomalies in the first diagnosed case. *Hum. Path.*, 1974, 5:223-32.

chromosome 9p deletion syndrome. Synonyms: *9p- syndrome, 9p deletion syndrome, del(9p) syndrome, monosomy 9p, partial monosomy 9p syndrome.*

A syndrome characterized by partial deletion of the short arm of chromosome 9 and associated with mental retardation, craniofacial anomalies, dermatoglyphic abnormalities, short and webbed neck, widely set nipples, cardiac murmurs, long fingers, and square nails. Craniofacial defects include trigonecephaly, mongoloid palpebral slant, epicanthus, flat nasal bridge, anteverted nostrils, long philtrum, low-set ears, abnormal ear lobules, high-arched palate, micrognathia, and low hairline.

Elliott, D., *et al.* C-G group chromosome abnormality (?10p-). Occurrence in a child with multiple malformations. *Am. J. Dis. Child.*, 1970, 119:72-3. Alfi, O., *et al.* Deletion of the short arm of chromosome 9(46,9p-): A new deletion syndrome. *Ann. Genet.*, Paris, 1973, 16:17-22.

chromosome 9p duplication syndrome. Synonyms: *Rethoré syndrome, 9p+ syndrome, 9p duplication syndrome, chromosome 9p trisomy syndrome, dup(9p) syndrome, duplication 9p syndrome, partial trisomy 9p, trisomy 9p.*

A syndrome characterized by duplication of the

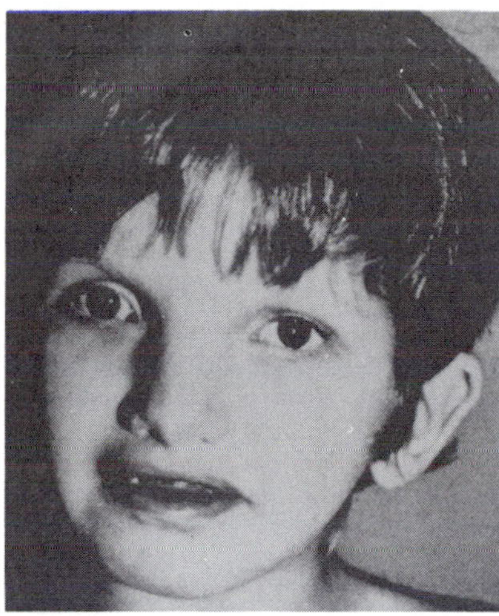
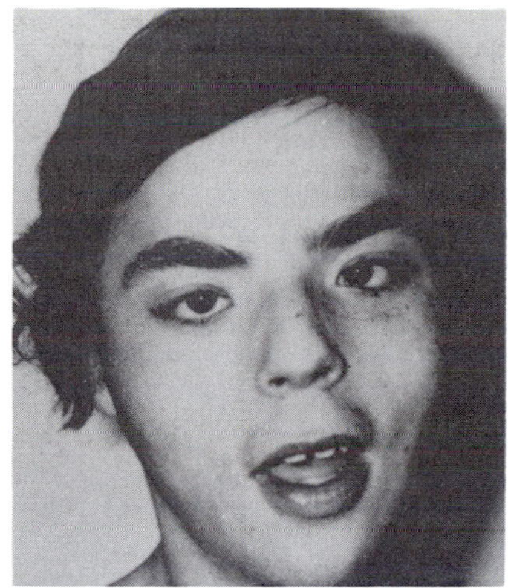

Chromosome 9p duplication syndrome
Fryns, J.P, "Chromosomal anomalies and autosomal syndromes." In Evers-Kiebooms, G., J-J. Cassiman, H. Van den Berghe, G. d'Ydewalle (eds): *Genetic Risk, Risk Perception, and Decision Making.* New York: Alan R. Liss, Inc., for the March of Dimes Birth Defects Foundation BD:OAS 23(2):7-32, 1987. New York: Alan R. Liss, Inc., with permission.

short arm of chromosome 9. The phenotype is marked chiefly by craniofacial malformations, mental retardation, hand anomalies, and dermatoglyphic abnormalities. A small cranium, large anterior fontanel, small sunken eyes, acentric displacement of pupils, epicanthus, strabimus, eye retraction problems, antimongoloid palpebral slant, hypertelorism, large nose, protruding ears, down-turning mouth, short upper lip, and outward-turning of the lower lip are the principal craniofacial features. Small hands with short digits, frequent clinodactyly, and shortening of the fifth fingers are usually associated. There is hypoplasia of the phalanges; the distal phalanges of the thumbs are often triangular and short. Delayed skeletal maturation and ossification are a constant feature. Associated defects may include funnel chest, widely spaced nipples, diastasis, lordosis, scoliosis, and subacromial and coccygeal dimples.

Rethoré, M. O., *et al.* Sur quatre cas de trisomie pour le bras court du chromosome 9. Individualisation d'une nouvelle entité morbide. *Ann. Genet., Paris*, 1970, 13:217-32.

chromosome 9p tetrasomy syndrome. Synonyms: *9p tetrasomy, tetrasomy 9p.*

Tetrasomy of the short arm of chromosome 9 associated with psychomotor retardation and variable multiple abnormalities. Anomalies of the head and face usually consist of open sutures and fontanels, hydrocephalus, microcephaly, antimongoloid palpebral slant, hypertelorism, strabismus, enophthalmos, epicanthus, bulbous beaked nose, protruding malformed ears, cleft lip, cleft palate, down-slanting mouth, and microretrognathia. Less commonly occurring defects include short neck, widely spaced nipples, cryptorchism, onychodysplasia, single palmar crease, absence of fusion of the triradius, and clinodactyly of the fifth finger. Cardiac, skeletal, and renal anomalies may occur.

Ghymers, D., *et al.* Tétrasomie partielle du chromosome 9, à l'état de mosaïque, chez un enfant porteur de malformation multiples. *Humangenetik*, 1973; 20:273-82.

chromosome 9p trisomy syndrome. See *chromosome 9p duplication syndrome.*

chromosome 9q duplication syndrome. Synonyms: *9q+ syndrome, 9q duplication syndrome, chromosome 9q trisomy syndrome, dup(9q) syndrome, duplication 9q syndrome, partial trisomy 9q, trisomy 9q.*

A familial syndrome characterized by duplication of the long arm of chromosome 9. The main features of this syndrome include mental retardation, microcephaly, prominent forehead, hypertelorism, enophthalmos, prominent nose, hypoplastic phalanges and nails, clinodactyly, absence of the C triradius, and simian creases. Additional anomalies, depending on the length of the segment of the long arm involved, include dolichocephaly, deep-set small eyes, small mouth, microretrognathia, large ears, short neck with redundant skin, long fingers and toes, flexed fingers, limited joint movement, congenital heart malformations, hypoplastic genitalia, failure to thrive, and early death.

Turleau, C., *et al.* Partial trisomy 9q: A new syndrome. *Hum. Genet.*, 1975, 29:233-42.

chromosome 9q trisomy syndrome. See *chromosome 9q duplication syndrome.*

chromosome 10 ring syndrome. Synonyms: *r(10) syndrome, ring chromosome 10 syndrome.*

A syndrome in which both ends of chromosome 10 have been lost (deletion) and the two broken ends have reunited to form a ring-shaped figure. The associated abnormalities include growth and mental retardation, microcephaly, hypertelorism, strabismus, large bridge of the nose, stubby nose, pointed chin, cryptorchism, and hydronephrosis.

Lansky, S., *et al.* Physical retardation associated with ring chromosome mosaicism: 46,r(10)/45,XX. *J. Med. Genet.*, 1977, 14:61-80.

chromosome 10 trisomy mosaicism syndrome. Synonym: *trisomy 10 mosaicism.*

The presence of an additional (third) chromosome

in an otherwise diploid chromosome 10 with mosaicism, characterized by early feeding difficulty, failure to thrive, high and prominent forehead, hypertelorism, mongoloid slant of the palpebral fissures, blepharophimosis, low-set dysplastic and large ears, high-arched palate, retrognathia, short neck, and long and slender trunk. Other abnormalities may include palmar and plantar furrows, sacral dimple, cryptorchism, inguinal hernia, arthrogryposis, joint hypermobility, convulsions, mental retardation, and heart defect. Most patients die in infancy.

Higurashi, M., *et al.* Two cases of trisomy C6-12 mosaicism and multiple congenital malformations. *J. Med. Genet.*,1969, 6:429-34. Nakagome, Y., *et al.* Trisomy 10 with mosaicism. A clinical and cytogenic entity. *Jpn. J. Hum. Genet.*,1972, 18:216-9.

chromosome 10p deletion syndrome. Synonyms: *10p- syndrome, 10p deletion syndrome, del(10p) syndrome, monosomy 10p syndrome, partial monosomy 10p.*

Deletion of the short arm of chromosome 10 characterized by mental and growth retardation, brachycephaly, microcephaly, trigonocephaly, mongoloid or antimongoloid slant of the palpebral fissures, hypertelorism, epicanthal folds, blepharoptosis, strabismus, dysplastic nose, cleft palate, high-arched palate, microdontia, crowded teeth, micrognathia, small low-set posteriorly rotated ears, widely-set nipples, pyloric stenosis, cryptorchism, abnormal dermatoglyphics, thoracic asymmetry, and minor abnormalities of the hands and feet. The phenotype is variable.

Shokeir, M. H. K., *et al.* Deletion of the short arm of chromosome No. 10. *J. Med. Genet.*, 1975, 12:99-113. Francke, U., *et al.* 10p-: A new autosomal deletion syndrome? *Birth Defects*, 1975, 11(5):207-12.

chromosome 10p duplication syndrome. Synonyms: *10p+ syndrome, 10p duplication syndrome, chromosome 10p trisomy syndrome, dup(10p) syndrome, duplication 10p syndrome, partial trisomy 10p syndrome, trisomy 10p.*

Duplication of the short arm of chromosome 10 characterized by growth and mental retardation, hypotonia, microsomia, dolichocephaly, wide sagittal sutures, high prominent forehead, long face, microphthalmia, coloboma, hypertelorism, mongoloid slant of the palpebral fissures, arched eyebrows, wide or prominent nasal root, anteverted nostrils, turtle-like mouth, cleft lip or palate, long philtrum, low-set posteriorly rotated ears, micrognathia, and various renal, cardiovascular, genital, and skeletal abnormalities.

Pfeiffer, R. A. Analyse einer reziproken Translokation zwischen den Chromosomen C(10) und D1. *Kinderheilk.*, 1967, 98:51-62. Yunis, E., *et al.* Trisomy 10p. *Ann. Génét.*, 1976, 19:57-60.

chromosome 10p trisomy syndrome. See *chromosome 10p duplication syndrome.*

chromosome 10q duplication syndrome. Synonyms: *10q+ syndrome, 10q duplication, chromosome 10q trisomy syndrome, dup(10q) syndrome, duplication 10q syndrome, partial trisomy 10q syndrome, trisomy 10q.*

Duplication of the long arm of chromosome 18 associated with peculiar facies (microcephaly, prominent forehead, flat and round face, arched eyebrows, hypertelorism, blepharophimosis, antimongoloid palpebral slant, blepharoptosis, microphthalmia, small nose, depressed nasal bridge, bow-shaped mouth, prominent upper lip, high-arched palate, cleft palate, micrognathia, and malformed low-set ears), skeletal anomalies (osteoporosis, scoliosis, rib abnormalities, foot deformity, webbing of fingers and toes, and camptodactyly), mental retardation, severe hypotrophy, abnormal muscle tone, short neck, heart defects, hypolobulation of the lungs, hypoplasia of the kidneys and collecting system, inguinal hernia, cryptorchism, deep plantar furrows, and simian creases.

Yunis, J. J. & Sanchez, O. A new syndrome resulting from partial trisomy of the distal third of the long arm of chromosome 10. *J. Pediat.*, 1974, 84:567-70. Taysi, K., *et al.* Partial trisomy 10q in three unrelated patients. *Ann. Génét., Paris,* 1983, 26:79-95.

chromosome 10q trisomy syndrome. See *chromosome 10q duplication syndrome.*

chromosome 10qter deletion syndrome. Synonyms: *10qter- syndrome, 10qter deletion syndrome, del(10qter) syndrome, monosomy 10qter, partial monosomy 10qter syndrome.*

Deletion of the terminal portion of the long arm of chromosome 10 manifested by mental retardation, short stature, and multiple abnormalities. Craniofacial abnormalities may include microcephaly, brachycephaly, triangular face, low forehead, hypertelorism, absent eyebrows at lateral margins, scant lower eyelashes, downward or upward slanting of the palpebral fissures, prominent nasal bridge, small nose, anteverted nostrils, low-set malformed and rotated ears, and microgenia. Associated disorders and defects may consist of respiratory distress, muscle hypotonia, strabismus, short neck, flexion contractures, syndactyly, clinodactyly, heart defect, and hernias.

Lewandowski, R. C., Jr., *et al.* Partial deletion of 10q. *Hum. Genet.*, 1978, 42:339-43.

chromosome 11 ring syndrome. Synonyms: *r(11) syndrome, ring chromosome 11 syndrome.*

Chromosome 11 in which both ends have been lost (deletion) and the two broken ends have reunited to form a ring-shaped figure, associated with growth and mental retardation, microcephaly, trigonocephaly, short and low nasal root, mongoloid or antimongoloid palpebral slant, low-set ears, digital anomalies, telangiectases, café-au-lait spots, and heart defect. Occasional abnormalities may include hypertelorism, epicanthus, strabismus, high and narrow palate, micrognathia, simian creases, and muscle hypertonia. Females are affected more frequently than males.

Valente, M., *et al.* Ring 11 chromosome 46,XX,r(11)(p15q25). *Hum. Genet.*, 1977, 36:345-50. Palka, G., *et al.* Ring chromosome 11. A case report and review of the literature. *Ann. Génét., Paris,* 1986, 29:55-8.

chromosome 11p duplication syndrome. Synonyms: *11p+ syndrome, 11p duplication syndrome, chromosome 11p trisomy syndrome, dup(11p) syndrome, duplication 11p syndrome, partial trisomy 11p syndrome, trisomy 11p.*

Duplication of the short arm of chromosome 11 associated with polyhydramnios, a large-for-gestational-age infant, growth and mental retardation, soft and lax skin, hyperextensible joints, muscle hypotonia, low-set ears, hypertelorism, strabimus, nystagmus, epicantahic folds, wide and flat nasal bridge, macroglossia, cleft palate, cleft lip, overlapping toes, a weak suck, crying, broad and full cheeks, and heart defect.

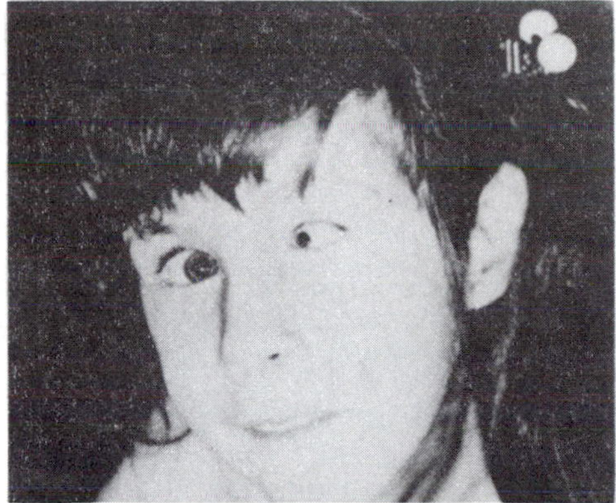

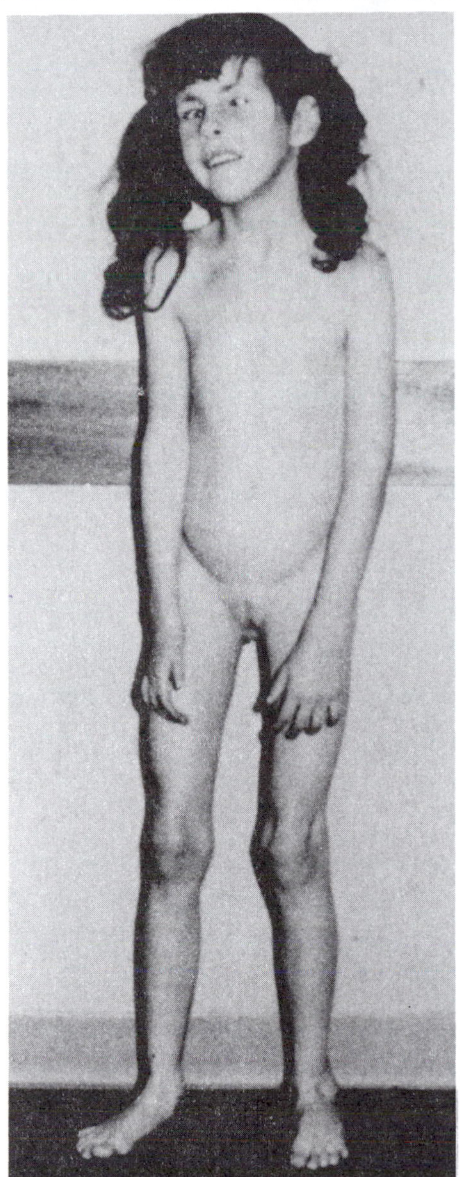

Chromosome 10q duplication syndrome
Fryns, J.P., A. Kleczkowska, L. Igodt-Ameye & H. Van den Berghe, *Clinical Genetics* 32:61-65, 1987, Munksgaard International Publishers, Copenhagen, Denmark.

Francke, U. Quinacrine mustard fluorescence of human chromosomes: Characterization of unusual translocations. *Am. J. Hum. Genet.*, 1972, 24:189-213. Aleck, K., *et al.* Partial trisomy 11p with interatrial septal aneurysm. Case report and literature review. *Ann. Génét., Paris*, 1985, 28:102-6.

chromosome 11p trisomy syndrome. See *chromosome 11p duplication syndrome.*

chromosome 11q deletion syndrome. Synonyms: *Jacobsen syndrome, 11q- syndrome, 11q deletion syndrome, del(11q) syndrome, monosomy 11q, partial monosomy 11q syndrome.*

Deletion of the long arm of chromosome 11 associated with characteristic facies (narrow and protruding forehead, hypertelorism, blepharoptosis, epicanthic folds, mongoloid or antimongoloid palpebral fissures, strabismus, broad nasal root, short nasal bridge, upturned nasal tip, carp mouth, retrognathia, posteriorly rotated and malformed ears with prominent anthelices), growth retardation, mental retardation, short digits, simian creases, foot abnormalities, coloboma of the iris, heart defect, pyloric stenosis, inguinal hernia, hypospadias, cryptorchism, and respiratory infection.

Jacobsen, P., *et al.* An (11;21) translocation in four generations with chromosome 11 abnormalities in the offspring. A clinical, cytogenetical, and gene marker study. *Hum. Genet.*, 1973, 23:568-85.

chromosome 11q duplication syndrome. Synonyms: *11q+ syndrome, 11q duplication syndrome, chromosome 11q trisomy syndrome, dup(11q) syndrome, duplication 11q syndrome, partial trisomy 11q syndrome, trisomy 11q.*

Partial duplication of the long arm of chromosome 11, characterized by growth and mental retardation, brachycephaly, microcephaly, flat occiput and forehead, short nose, long philtrum, high-arched palate, cleft palate, microretrognathia, retracted lower lip, low-set posteriorly rotated ears, pre-auricular fistula, cutis laxa, clavicular defects, hip dislocation, muscle hypotonia, talipes equinovarus, and urogenital malformations. The phenotype may vary.

Tusques, J., *et al.* Trisomie partielle llq identifiée grace à l'étude en "denaturation ménagée" par la chaleur, de la translocation équilibrée paternelle. *Ann. Genet., Paris,* 1972, 15:167-72.

chromosome 11q trisomy syndrome. See *chromosome 11q duplication syndrome.*

chromosome 12 mosaic tetrasomy. See *chromosome 12p tetrasomy syndrome.*

chromosome 12 ring syndrome. Synonyms: *r(12) syndrome, ring chromosome 12 syndrome.*

Chromosome 12 in which both ends have been lost (deletion) and the two broken ends have reunited to form a ring-shaped figure, associated with retarded psychomotor development, characteristic facies (low-set cupped ears and low hairline), high-arched palate, short neck, clinodactyly, and single crease on the fifth finger.

Scribanu, N., *et al.* The syndrome of ring chromosome 12. *Am. J. Med. Genet.*, 1980, 5:165-70.

chromosome 12 tetrasomy. See *chromosome 12p tetrasomy syndrome.*

chromosome 12 trisomy mosaicism syndrome. Synonyms: *dup(12) mosaicism, mosaic trisomy 12, trisomy 12 mosaicism.*

Mosaic trisomy of chromosome 12. The disorder is frequently lethal, but in liveborn infants it is characterized by mental retardation and mutiple abnormalities. Craniofacial anomalies include high and/or prominent forehead, skull deformities, flat and/or broad face, hypertelorism, epicanthus, nystagmus, flat short nose with a broad bridge, low-set ears, prominent anthelix, highly arched palate, thick lower lip, and micrognathia. Associated abnormalities consist of brevicollis, excess skin folds on the neck, short or malformed sternum, clinodactyly, short fingers and toes, clinodactyly, increased spaces between the first and second toes, foot deformity, muscle hypotonia, simian creases, heart defect, and kidney abnormalities.

Patil, S. R., *et al.* First report of mosaic trisomy 12 in a liveborn individual. *Am. J. Med. Genet.*, 1983, 14:453-60.

chromosome 12p deletion syndrome. Synonyms: *12p- syndrome, 12p deletion syndrome, del(12p) syndrome, monosomy 12p, partial monosomy 12p syndromes.*

Deletion of the short arm of chromosome 12 associated with variable phenotypes, mental retardation, microcephaly, and micrognathia being the most constant features. Associated symptoms may include narrow prominent occiput, high forehead, flat midface, hypertelorism, synophrys, epicanthal folds, antimongoloid palpebral slant, sclerocornea, blue sclera, strabismus, optic atrophy, low-set malformed ears, prominent or flat nasal bridge, bulbous and upturned tip of the nose, pit at the base of the nasal septum, choanal atresia, retarded dentition, crowded teeth, malocclusion, tooth agenesis, enamel hypoplasia, high-arched or narrow palate, mandibular retrognathia, short neck with redundant skin, widely set nipples, asymmetric thorax, pectus excavatum, coarctation of the aorta, ventricular septal defect, aortic stenosis, absent right pulmonary artery, atrial septal defect, inguinal hernia, omphalocele, small penis, cryptorchism, joint contractures, hypotonic or spastic muscle tone, camptodactyly, low-set thumbs, clinodactyly, brachydactyly, ulnar finger deviation, hypoplastic toe nails, abnormal dermatoglyphics, seizures, and multiple fractures.

Malpuech, G., *et al.* Une observation de deletion partielle du bras court du chromosome 12. *Lyon Méd.*, 1975, 233:275-9. Tenconi, R., *et al.* Partial deletion of the short arm of chromosome 12(p11:13). *Ann. Génét., Paris,* 1975, 95-8. Orye, E., & Craen, M. Short arm deletion of chromosome 12. *Humangenetik,* 1975, 28:335-42. Kivlin, J. D., *et al.* Phenotypic variation in del(12p) syndrome. *Am. J. Med. Genet.*, 1985, 22:769-79.

chromosome 12p duplication syndrome. Synonyms: *12p+ syndrome, 12p duplication syndrome, chromosome 12p trisomy syndrome, dup(12p) syndrome, duplication 12p syndrome, partial trisomy 12p syndrome, trisomy 12p.*

Duplication of the short arm of chromosome 12 characterized by psychomotor retardation, muscle hypotonia, peculiar facies (prominent cheeks, epicanthic folds, broad eyebrows, broad and flat nasal bridge with short and narrow nose, anteverted nostrils, long philtrum, broad and prominent lower lip, low-set ears with broad helices, prominent anthelices, and deep concha), brevicollis, simian creases, genu valgum, increased space between first and second toe, hyporeflexia of the knees and ankles, and retarded bone age. Additional symptoms may include seizures, Brushfield spots, congenital heart defect, flexion anomalies of the fingers and toes, hexadactyly, abnormal teeth, hyperkeratotic and supernumerary nipples, severe mental retardation, hexadactyly of the toes, enlarged tongue, rectus diastasis, and umbilical hernia. The break point of chromosome 12 almost always takes place in 12p11.

Armendares, S., *et al.* The 12p trisomy syndrome. *Ann. Génét., Paris,* 1975, 18:89-94. Rethoré, M. O., *et al.* Augmentation de l'activité la LDH-B chez un garçon trisomique 12p par malségrégation d'une translocation maternelle t(12:14)(q12:p11). *Ann. Génét., Paris,* 1975, 18:81-7.

chromosome 12p mosaic tetrasomy. See *chromosome 12p tetrasomy syndrome.*

chromosome 12p tetrasomy syndrome. Synonyms: *Killian syndrome, Pallister mosaic syndrome, Pallister syndrome, Pallister tetrasomy syndrome, Pallister-Killian syndrome, Teschler-Nicola and Killian syndrome, chromosome 12p mosaic tetrasomy, chromosome 12 mosaic tetrasomy, 12 mosaic tetrasomy, tetrasomy 12.*

Tetrasomy of the short arm of chromosome 12. It is a multiple anomaly/mental retardation syndrome characterized at birth by brachycephaly, large flattened face with puffy eyelids, small nose with indented nares, down-turned nares, loosely helical ears, flat occiput with excess of skin, supernumerary nipples, sacral dimple, short limbs and fingers, proximal insertion of the thumbs, and large big toe. Pigmentation disorders, delayed dentition, and abnormal distribution of hair usually follow. The extra chromosome resembles chromosome 20. The appearance of band R suggests the fusion of two 12p chromosomes. The condition was once interpreted as tetrasomy 21.

Pallister, P. D.., *et al.* The Pallister mosaic syndrome. *Birth Defects,* 1977, 13(3B):103-10. *Killian, W., & Teschler-Nicola, M. Case report 72: Mental retardation, unusual facial appearance, abnormal hair. *Synd. Ident.*, 1981, 7:6-7.

chromosome 12p trisomy syndrome. See *chromosome 12p duplication syndrome.*

chromosome 12q duplication syndrome. Synonyms: *12q+ syndrome, 12q duplication syndrome, chromosome 12q trisomy syndrome, dup(12q) syndrome,*

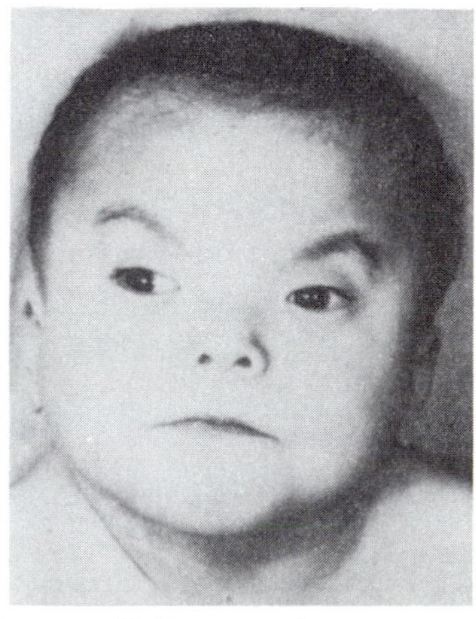

Chromosome 12p tetrasomy syndrome
Kawashima, Dr. Hiroko: *Am. J. Med. Gens.* 27:285-289, 1987. New York: Alan R. Liss.

duplication 12q syndrome, partial trisomy 12q, trisomy 12q.

Deletion of the long arm of chromosome 12 associated with mental retardation and multiple abnormalities. The phenotype consists of retarded growth and development, dolichocephaly, brain anomaly, hypertelorism, flat and/or broad nasal bridge, micrognathia, down-turned mouth, low-set ears, poor lobulation of the ears, loose skin at the nape, short neck, simian creases, hip subluxation, pes planovalgus, widely set nipples, sacral dimple, cryptorchism, and heart defect with murmur.

Hobolth, N., *et al.* Partial trisomy 12 in a mentally retarded boy and translocation (12;21) in his mother. *J. Med. Genet.,* 1974, 11:299-303. Hemminng, L., & Brown, R. Partial trisomy 12q associated with a familial translocation. *Clin. Genet.,* 1979, 16:25-8.

chromosome 12q trisomy syndrome. See *chromosome 12q duplication syndrome.*

chromosome 13 ring syndrome. Synonyms: *chromosome D13 ring syndrome, D13 ring syndrome, r(13) syndrome, ring chromosome 13 syndrome.*

A syndrome in which both ends of chromosome 13 been lost (deletion) and the two broken ends have been reunited to form a ring-shaped figure, associated with mental retardation and multiple abnormalities, including microcephaly, hypertelorism, broad and prominant nasal bridge, large or low-set malformed ears, and high-arched palate. Less frequently occurring anomalies may include protruding premaxilla, micrognathia, heart murmur, head and foot abnormalities, renal defect, genital anomalies, iris coloboma, corpus callosum agenesis, skeletal malformations, webbed neck, rocker-bottom feet, widely spaced nipples, anteriorly placed anus, perineal fistula, and small anterior fontanel.

Wang, H. C., *et al.* Ring chromosomes in human beings. *Nature,* 1962, 195:733-4. McCandless, A., & Walker, S. D13 ring chromosome syndrome. *Arch. Dis. Child.,* 1976, 51:449. Martin, N. J., *et al.* The right chromosome 13 syndrome. *Hum. Genet.,* 1982, 61:18-23.

chromosome 13 trisomy syndrome. Synonyms: *Bartholin-Patau syndrome, Patau syndrome, trisomy 13. Formerly called trisomy 13-15, trisomy D1.*

Trisomy 13 caused usually by primary nondisjunction and, occasionally, translocation and mosaicism. Birth weight is about 2500 g; life expectancy is seldom more than 10 years, most infants dying during the first 3 months of life. The syndrome is characterized by multiple abnormalities of the head, brain, ears, eyes, cardiovascular system, spleen, reproductive system, pancreas, and other organs. Microcephaly, sloping forehead, wide sagittal suture and fontanelles, arhinencephaly, cebocephaly, premaxillary agenesis, microphthalmia, single umbilical artery, umbilical hernia, hyperconvex narrow fingernails, narrow distal phalanges, polydactyly, capillary hemangiomas, and scalp defects are the common anomalies. Orofacial defects may include micrognathia and cleft lip and palate. Breath-holding spells, seizures, mental retardation, hypertonicity, deafness, and feeding difficulties are the most common symptoms. Hematological features may include the presence of large amounts of fetal hemoglobin in the blood and sessile and pedunculated nuclear projections in neutrophilic leukocytes.

Patau, K., *et al.* Multiple congenital anomaly caused by an extra autosome. *Lancet,* 1960, I:790-3. Bartholinus, T. *Historiarum anatomicarum rariorum centuria III et IV. Ejusdem cura accessere observationes anatomicae... Petri Pavi Hafniae.* Sumtibus Petri Haubold Bibl., 1657, p. 95.

chromosome 13q deletion syndrome. Synonyms: *Orbeli syndrome, 13q- syndrome, 13q deletion syndrome, del(13q) syndrome, monosomy 13q, partial monosomy 13q syndrome.*

Breakage of the long arm of the chromosome 13 sometimes associated with reunion at both ends of the chromosome to form ring chromosome 13, (see *chromosome 13 ring syndrome*), with resulting ring chromosome 13 mosaicism [13q-/r(13) mosaicism]. Peculiar facies, mental retardation, eye defects, and hand abnormalities are the principal characteristics of an otherwise variable phenotype. Facial anomalies consist chiefly of hypertelorism, prominent nasal bridge, blepharoptosis, epicanthus, microphthalmos, coloboma, prominent maxilla, micrognathia, large and low-set ears, and retinoblastoma. The neck is usually short and webbed. Growth deficiency, hypospadias, cryptorchism, hip dislocation, and vertebral anoma-

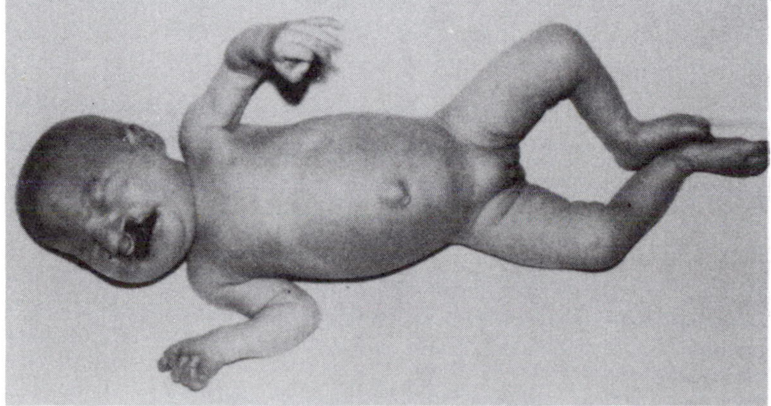

Chromosome 13 trisomy syndrome
Fryns, J.P.: Chromosomal Anomalies and Autosomal Syndromes. In Evers-Kiebooms G., J-J Cassiman, H. Van den Berghe, G. d'Ydewalle, (eds.): "Genetic Risk, Risk Perception, and Decision Making." New York: Alan R. Liss, Inc. for the March of Dimes Birth Defects Foundation BD:OAS 23(2):7-32, 1987, with permission.

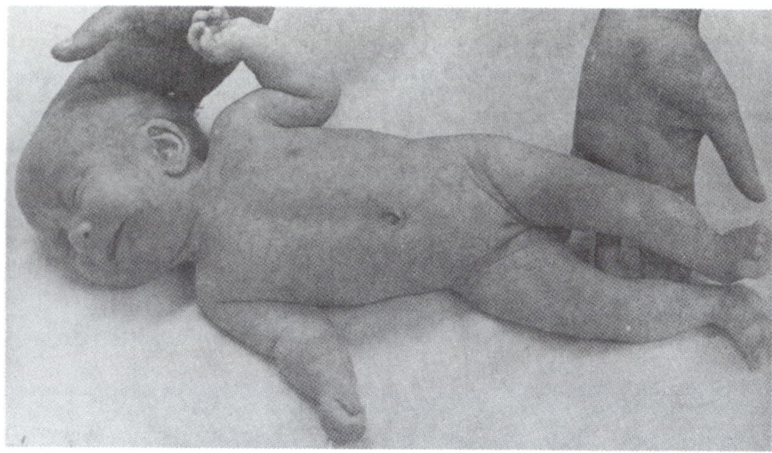

Chromosome 13q deletion syndrome
Courtesy of Dr. M. Jansch, St. Joseph's Hospital, Fort Wayne, Indiana.

lies are generally associated. Hand abnormalities may consist of thumb hypoplasia, synostosis between the fourth and fifth metacarpals, short fifth middle phalanges, short fifth digits, and deviations of the phalanges.

Lele, K.P., *et al.* Chromosome deletion in a case of retinoblastoma. *Ann. Hum. Genet.*, 1963, 27:171-4. Allderdice, P. W., *et al.* The 13q deletion syndrome. *Am. J. Hum. Genet.*, 1969, 21:499-512. Orbeli, D. J., *et al.* The syndrome associated with the partial D-monosomy. Case report and review. *Humangenetik,* 1971, 13:296-308.

chromosome 13q duplication syndrome. Synonyms: *13q+ syndrome, 13q duplication syndrome, chromosome 13q trisomy syndrome, dup(13q) syndrome, duplication 13q syndrome, partial trisomy 13q syndrome, trisomy 13q.*

Duplication of the long arm of chromosome 13 associated with multiple abnormalities. The phenotypic expression of proximal and distal 13q trisomy consists of psychomotor retardation, long curly eyelashes, long philtrum, muscle hypotonia, thin upper lip, hypertelorism, frontal bossing, malformed low-set ears, hyperactivity, dental anomalies, cryptorchism, polydactyly, clinodactyly, microcephaly, simian creases, depressed nasal bridge, increased number of nuclear projections on neutrophils, heart defect, narrow high-arched palate, persistent fetal hemoglobin, cleft palate, hemangioma, broad nasal bridge, and bushy eyebrows. Most common phenotypic characteristics in all cases of partial trisomy 13q consist of psychomotor retardation, low-set malformed ears, hypertelorism, thin upper lip, long philtrum, wide and depressed nasal bridge, microcephaly, and frontal bossing.

Noel, B., *et al.* Partial deletions and trisomies of chromosome 13; mapping of bands associated with particular malformations. *Clin. Genet.,* 1976, 9:593-602. Schinzel, A., & Schmid, W. Different forms of incomplete trisomy 13. Mosaicism and partial trisomy for the proximal and distal long arm. *Hum. Genet.,* 1974, 22:287-98. Rogers, J. F. Clinical delineation of proximal and distal partial trisomy 13. *Clin. Genet.,* 1984, 25:221-9.

chromosome 13q trisomy syndrome. See *chromosome 13q duplication syndrome.*

chromosome 14 ring syndrome. Synonyms: *r(14) syndrome, ring chromosome 14 syndrome.*

A syndrome in which both ends of chromosome 14 have been lost (deletion) and the two broken ends have reunited to form a ring-shaped figure, associated with moderate craniofacial dysmorphism (flat occiput, epicanthal folds, downward slanting of the palpebral fissures, flat nasal bridge, upturned nostrils, large low-set ears), short neck, seizures, mental retardation, abnormal retinal pigmentation, and recurrent respiratory infection. Focal cerebral atrophy is the cause of neurological complications.

Gilderkrantz, S., *et al.* Le syndrome Dr. Étude d'un nouveau cas (46,XX,14r). *Ann. Génét., Paris,* 1971, 14:23-31.

chromosome 14 trisomy syndrome. Synonyms: *trisomy 14, trisomy D14 syndrome.*

Trisomy of chromosome 14 characterized mainly by growth and mental retardation, prominent forehead, wide nasal bridge, hypertelorism, low-set ears, micrognathia, congenital heart defect, and, less commonly, cleft palate, evanescent translucent film over the eyes, and asymmetry of the body. Upslant of the palpebral fissures, capillary hemangioma of the forehead, upturned nose, and anteriorly positioned anus may be associated.

Murken, J., *et al.* Trisomie D bei einem 2 1/2 jahringen Madchen (47,XX,14+). *Humangenetik,* 1970, 10:254-68.

chromosome 14q deletion syndrome. Synonyms: *14q- syndrome, 14q deletion syndrome, del(14q) syndrome, monosomy 14q, partial monosomy 14q syndrome.*

Deletion of the long arm of chromosome 14 associated with multiple abnormalities, including characteristic facies (round face, frontal hypertrichosis, thick eyebrows, horizontal narrow palpebral fissures, short bulbous nose with a flat root, micrognathia, brachycephaly, dolichocepaly), pes equinovarus, cleft uvula, high-arched palate, atrial septal defect, inguinal hernia, small penis, cryptorchism, and frequent respiratory infections.

Nielsen, J., *et al.* Deletion 14q and pericentric inversion 14. *J. Med. Genet.,* 1978, 15:236-8. Yamamoto, Y., *et al.* Deletion 14q(q24.3 to q32.1) syndrome: Significance of peculiar facial appearance in its diagnosis, and deletion mapping of Pi(alpha-1-antitrypsin). *Hum. Genet.*, 1986, 74:190-2.

chromosome 14q duplication syndrome. Synonyms: *14q+ syndrome, 14q duplication syndrome, chromosome 14q trisomy syndrome, dup(14q) syndrome, duplication 14q syndrome, partial trisomy 14q, trisomy 14q.*

Duplication of the long arm of chromosome 14 characterized by growth retardation, delayed motor development, mental retardation, microcephaly, large mouth, blepharophimosis, antimongoloid palpebral slant, large nose, cleft palate, high-arched palate, deep-seated malformed ears, short neck, cryptorchidism, pes equinovarus, abnormal palmar creases, and arches on fingerprints.

Short, E. M., *et al.* A case of partial 14 trisomy 47,XY,(14q-)+ and translocation t(9p+;14q-). *J. Med. Genet.*, 1972, 9:367-73. Simpson, J., & Zellweger, H. Partial trisomy 14q and parental translocation of No. 14 chromosome. Report of a case and review of the literature. *J. Med. Genet.*, 1977, 14:124-7.

chromosome 14q trisomy syndrome. See *chromosome 14q duplication syndrome.*

chromosome 15 ring syndrome. Synonyms: *r(15) syndrome, ring chromosome 15 syndrome.*

Chromosome 15 in which both ends have been lost (deletion) and the two broken ends have reunited to form a ring-shaped figure, associated with growth and mental retardation, small hands and feet, and peculiar facies with triangular face, micrognathia, short neck, hypertelorism, and progeroid appearance. Brachymesophalangy, clinodactyly, finger malposition, cardiac defects, and skin pigmentation disorders may occur.

Jacobsen, P. A ring chromosome in the 13-15 group associated with microcephalic dwarfism, mental retardation and emotional immaturity. Hereditas, 1966, 55:188-91.

chromosome 15q duplication syndrome. Synonyms: *15q+ syndrome, 15q duplication syndrome, chromosome 15q trisomy syndrome, dup(15q) syndrome, duplication 15q syndrome, partial trisomy 15q syndrome, trisomy 15q.*

Duplication of the long arm of chromosome 15 associated with microcephaly, facial asymmetry, prominent occiput, antimongoloid palpebral slant, blepharoptosis, high-arched palate, low-set ears, prominent nose, preauricular pits, long philtrum, downturned mouth, midline crease in the lower lip, puffy cheeks, and micrognathia. Associated disorders consist of mental retardation, growth retardation, heart defect, seizures, muscle hypotonia, torticollis, pectus excavatum, scoliosis, short neck with or without vertebral anomalies, cryptorchism, and hyperextensible thumbs.

Fujimoto, A., *et al.* Inherited partial duplication of chromosome 15. *J. Med. Genet.*, 1974, 11:287-91. García-Cruz, D., *et al.* Trisomy 15q23-qter due to a de novo t(11;15)(q25;q223) and assignment of the critical segment. Ann. Génét., Paris, 1985, 28:192-6.

chromosome 15q trisomy syndrome. See *chromosome 15q duplication syndrome.*

chromosome 16p duplication syndrome. Synonyms: *16p+ syndrome, 16p duplication syndrome, chromosome 16p trisomy syndrome, dup(16p) syndrome, duplication 16p syndrome, partial trisomy 16p syndrome, trisomy 16p.*

Duplication of the short arm of chromosome 16 characterized by mental retardation and multiple abnormalities. Head and neck abnormalities may include microcephaly, absence of the eyebrows and eyelashes, low-set ears, palatognathoschisis, micrognathia, and webbed neck. Associated abnormalities and disorders may consist of retarded psychomotor development, weak cry, agenesis of the thumbs, overlapping fingers, muscle hypertonia, tetralogy of Fallot, defective atrial septum, single umbilical artery, and sacral dimple and/or coccygeal sinus. Most patients die in infancy.

Roberts, S. H., & Duckett, D. P. Trisomy 16p in a liveborn infant and a review of partial and full trisomy 16. *J. Med. Genet.*, 1978, 15:375-81. Leschot, N. J., *et al.* Five familial cases with a trisomy 16p syndrome due to translocation. *Clin. Genet.*, 1979, 16:205-14.

chromosome 16p trisomy syndrome. See *chromosome 16p duplication syndrome.*

chromosome 16q deletion syndrome. Synonyms: *16q- syndrome, 16q deletion syndrome, del(16q) syndrome, monosomy 16q, partial monosomy 16q syndrome.*

Deletion of the long arm of chromosome 16 characterized by delayed growth and development, feeding difficulty, hypotonia of the abdominal muscles, high forehead, prominent metopic suture, large anterior fontanels with or without diastasis of the cranial sutures, hydrocephalus, narrow palpebral fissures, low-set folded ears, micrognathia, short neck, narrow thorax, skeletal anomalies, and cardiac, renal, intestinal, and other anomalies. Most patients die during childhood, but some may survive into adolescence.

Fryns, J. P., *et al.* Partial monosomy of the long arm of chromosome 16 in a malformed newborn: Karyotype 46,XX,del(16)(q21). *Hum. Genet.*, 1977, 38:343-6.

chromosome 16q duplication syndrome. Synonyms: *16q+ syndrome, 16q duplication syndrome, chromosome 16q trisomy syndrome, dup(16q) syndrome, duplication 16q syndrome, partial trisomy 16q syndrome, trisomy 16q.*

Duplication of the long arm of chromosome 16. Because of different secondary chromosome arrangements, the phenotypic expression is variable. The symptoms may include low birth-weight, muscle hypotonia, failure to thrive, absence of the suck reflex, slender sternum, asymmetric skull, high and prominent forehead with frontal bossing, small and narrow palpebral fissures with antimongoloid slanting, periorbital edema, horizontal crease under the lower eyelid, clinodactyly and short middle phalanges of the hands and feet, sclerosis in the tufts of the distal phalanges of the hand, metatarsus adductus deformities of the feet, and occasional abnormalities of the external genitalia. Most patients die early in infancy.

Boué, J., Boué, A., & Lazar, P. The epidemiology of human spontaneous abortions with chromosomal anomalies. In: Blandeau, R. J., ed. *Biology and pathology of aging gametes. International symposium. Seattle, 1973.* Basel, Karger, pp. 330-48. Schimckel, R., *et al.* 16q Trisomy in a family with a balanced 15/16 translocation. *Birth Defects*, 1975, 11(5):229-36.

chromosome 16q trisomy syndrome. See *chromosome 16q duplication syndrome.*

chromosome 17 ring syndrome. Synonyms: *r(17) syndrome, ring chromosome 17 syndrome.*

Chromosome 17 in which both ends have been lost (deletion) and the broken ends have reunited to form a ring-shaped figure. The phenotype is variable, consisting of psychomotor retardation, craniofacial abnormalities (microcephaly, slanted forehead, depressed nasal bridge, anteverted nostrils, malformed ears, epicanthus, hypertelorism), short stature, muscle hypotonia, café-au-lait spots, fundoscopic abnormalities, strabismus, dermatoglyphic abnormalities (transverse hypothenar creases and ulnar loops), clinodactyly, and genital abnormalities.

Petit, P., & Koulischer, L. Étude d'une mosaique 46,XX/46,XX,17r. *Ann. Génét., Paris,* 1971, 14:55-8. Carpenter, N. J., *et al.* An infant with ring 17 chromosome and unusual dermatoglyphs: A new syndrome? *J. Med. Genet.,* 1981, 18:234-6.

chromosome 17p deletion syndrome. Synonyms: *17p- syndrome, 17p deletion syndrome, del(17p) syndrome, monosomy 17p, partial monosomy 17p syndrome.*

Deletion of the short arm of chromosome 17 characterized by a varied phenotype. The symptoms may include mental retardation, growth retardation, microcephaly, muscle hypotonia, esotropia, prognathism, short philtrum, enamel hypoplasia, heart defect, facial cleft, and other anomalies. Partial monosomy 17p13 was reported to be associated with the Miller-Dieker syndrome (q.v.).

Smith, A. C. M., *et al.* Deletion of the short arm in two patients with facial clefts and congenital heart disease. *Am. J. Hum. Genet.,* 1982, 34:146A. Patil, S. R., & Bartley, J. A. Interstitial deletion of the short arm of chromosome l7. *Hum. Genet.,* 1984, 67:237-8.

chromosome 17p duplication syndrome. Synonyms: *17p+ syndrome, 17p duplication syndrome, chromosome 17p trisomy syndrome, dup(17p) syndrome, duplication 17p syndrome, partial trisomy 17p syndrome, trisomy 17p.*

Duplication of the short arm of chromosome 17 associated with mental retardation and multiple abnormalities. Intra-uterine growth retardation, failure to thrive, single umbilical artery, polyhydramnios, and psychomotor retardation are the early symptoms. Craniofacial features include characteristic facies (prominent occiput, high-arched palate, malformed low-set ears, micrognathia, hypertelorism, narrow palpebral fissures, microphthalmia with small pupils, and broad nasal bridge), microcephaly, and hydrocephalus. Associated defects and disorders consist of seizures, widely set nipples, inguinal and hiatal hernia, cryptorchism, kidney abnormalities, heart defect, flexion deformity of the fingers, adduction deformity of the thumbs, long tapered fingers, simian creases, distal palmar axial triradius, and short neck with redundant skin.

Latta, E., & Hoo, J. Trisomy of the short arm of chromosome 17. *Hum. Genet.,* 1974, 34:199-206. Feldman, G. M., *et al.* Brief clinical report: The dup(17p) syndrome. *Am. J. Med. Genet.,* 1982, 11:299-304.

chromosome 17p trisomy syndrome. See *chromosome 17p duplication syndrome.*

chromosome 17q duplication syndrome. Synonyms: *17q+ syndrome, 17q duplication syndrome, chromosome 17q trisomy syndrome, dup(17q) syndrome, duplication 17q syndrome, partial trisomy 17q, trisomy 17q.*

Duplication of the long arm of chromosome 17 associated with psychomotor retardation and multiple abnormalities. Craniofacial anomalies may include microcephaly, plagiocephaly, frontal bossing, temporal retraction, facial asymmetry, widow's peak, hypertelorism, antimongoloid palpebral slant, epicanthal folds, flat nasal bridge, wide mouth with thin upper lip, downturned corners of the mouth, cleft lip and palate, micrognathia, and low-set and posteriorly rotated malformed ears. Long thin fingers, postaxial polydactyly of the hands and feet, overlapping toes, syndactyly of the fingers and toes, plexus adductus deformity of the thumbs, excessive laxity of the joints, and proximal shortness are the major defects of the limbs. Associated abnormalities may consist of pectus carinatum, cavernous hemangiomas, and various cardiac, renal, and neurological defects.

Berberich, M., *et al.* Duplication (partial trisomy) of the distal long arm of chromosome 17: A new clinically recognizable chromosome disorder. *Birth Defects,* 1978, 14(6C):287-95. Fryns, J., *et al.* Partial trisomy 17q. *Hum. Genet.,* 1979, 49:361-4. Bridge, J., *et al.* Partial duplication of distal 17q. *Am. J. Med. Genet.,* 1985, 22:229-35.

chromosome 17q trisomy syndrome. See *chromosome 17q duplication syndrome.*

chromosome 18 ring syndrome. Synonyms: *r(18) syndrome, ring chromosome 18 syndrome.*

Chromosome 18 in which both ends have been lost (deletion) and the broken ends have reunited to form a ring-shaped figure, associated mainly with mental retardation, microcephaly, muscle hypotonia, and low birth weight. Additional malformations and disorders may include encephalopathy, seizures, hypertelorism, epicanthus, carp mouth, low-set ears, short fingers, tapering fingers, high-set thumbs, abnormal flexion of the fingers, clubfoot, and other defects.

Lejeune, J. Modèle théorique de la répartition des duplications et des déficiences dans les chromosomes en anneau. *C. Rend. Acad. Sc.,* 1967, 264:2588-90. Grouchy, J., de. The 18p-, 18q- and 18r syndromes. *Birth Defects,* 1969, 5(5):74-87.

chromosome 18 trisomy syndrome. Synonyms: *Edwards syndrome, trisomy 18, trisomy 18 syndrome, Formerly called trisomy 16-18, trisomy E.*

A syndrome characterized by the presence of an extra chromosome 18, associated with double trisomies, translocation, and mosaicism. Out of more than 130 different abnormalities occurring with this syndrome, the following are the most common: Perinatal mortality, whereby mean survival time is about 70 days (134 days for females and 15 days for males); altered gestational time, about one-third of newborn infants (weighing about 2300 gm) being premature and one third, postmature; fetal abnormalities consisting of polyhydramnios, small placenta, and single umbilical artery; craniofacial defects consisting of prominent occiput, scaphocephaly, and cleft lip and palate; neurological disorders consisting of mental deficiency, hypertonicity, and diminished response to sound; musculo-skeletal defects consisting of hypoplasia of skeletal muscles, foot deformities with short and dorsiflexed great toes, ulnar deviation of some or all of the fingers, short sternum, and reduced number of ossification centers; dermatological anomalies consisting of dermatoglyphic abnormalities, hypoplasia of subcutaneous tissue, loose skin, mild hirsutism, cutis marmorata, small nipples, and onychodysplasia; and

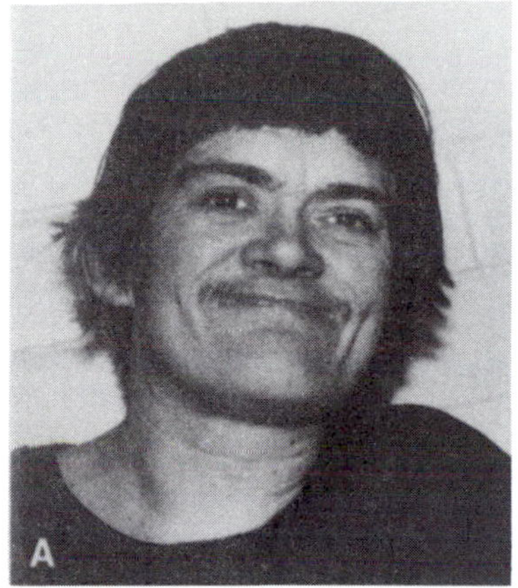
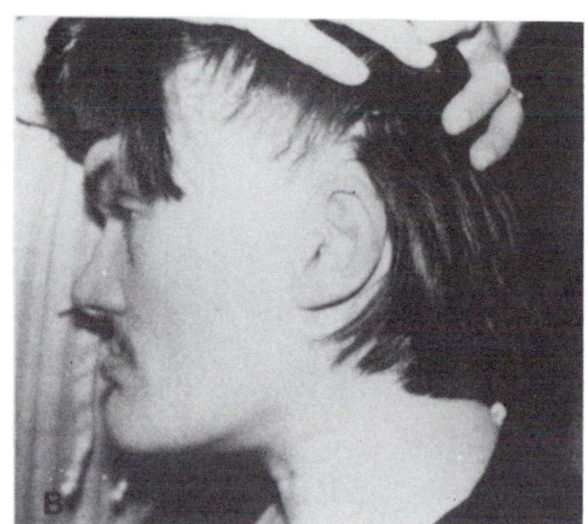

Chromosome 17p deletion syndrome
Stratton, Robert F., William B. Dobyns, Frank Greenberg, Jeanne B. Desana, Charleen Moore, George Fidone, Gretchen H. Runge, Paula Feldman, Gurbax S. Sekhon, Richard M. Pauli & David H. Ledbetter, *American Journal of Medical Genetics*, 24:421-432, 1986. New York: Alan R. Liss, Inc.

cardiovascular disorders consisting of ventricular and auricular septal defects and patent ductus arteriosus. Inguinal or umbilical hernia. Meckel diverticulum, cryptorchidism, and a wide variety of renal, cardiac, genital, and other abnormalities may be associated.

Edwards, J. H., *et al*. A new trisomic syndrome. *Lancet*, 1960, 1:787-90. Patau, K., *et al*. Multiple congenital anomaly caused by autosome. *Lancet*, 1960, 1:790-3.

chromosome 18p deletion syndrome. Synonyms: *de Grouchy syndrome, 18p- syndrome, 18p deletion syndrome, del(18p) syndrome, monosomy 18p, partial monosomy 18p syndrome.*

Deletion of the short arm of a chromosome 18 with interstitial or terminal deletions, unequal interchromatid exchange, or reciprocal translocation, associated with a variable phenotype. The most commonly occurring anomalies include mental retardation, low birth weight, retarded somatic growth, microcephaly, midfacial dysplasia, dermatoglyphic abnormalities, brachydactyly, and clinodactyly of the fifth fingers. Orofacial manifestations may consist of hypertelorism, epicanthal folds, strabismus, blepharoptosis, low-set malformed ears, broad and short nose, carp mouth, small mandible, short neck, and low hairline. Lymphedema of the hands and feet, shield chest, widely spaced nipples, holoprosocephaly, pectus excavatum, and muscular hypotonia may be associated. There is 2:1 female sex predilection; maternal age is generally advanced..

Grouchy, J., de, *et al*. Dysmorphie complexe avec oligophrénie: délétion des bras courts d'un chromosome 17-18. *C. Rend. Seances Acad. Sc.*, 1963, 256:1028-9.

chromosome 18p tetrasomy syndrome. Synonyms: *18p tetrasomy syndrome, tetrasomy 18p.*

Tetrasomy of the short arm of chromosome 18 associated with normal or abnormal birth weight, mental retardation, signs of lesions of the pyramidal tract (muscle hypotonia, increased deep tendon reflexes, Babinski sign), asthenic body habitus, characteristic facies (microdolichocephaly, pinched nose, low-set dysplastic ears, high-arched palate, small triangular mouth, micrognathia), narrow shoulders and thorax, scoliosis, and, occasional absence of distal flexion creases of the fingers, kidney deformities, and immunological deficiency. The clinical picture changes as the patient becomes older; spasticity, abnormal gait, facial asymmetry, osteoarticular abnormalities, de-

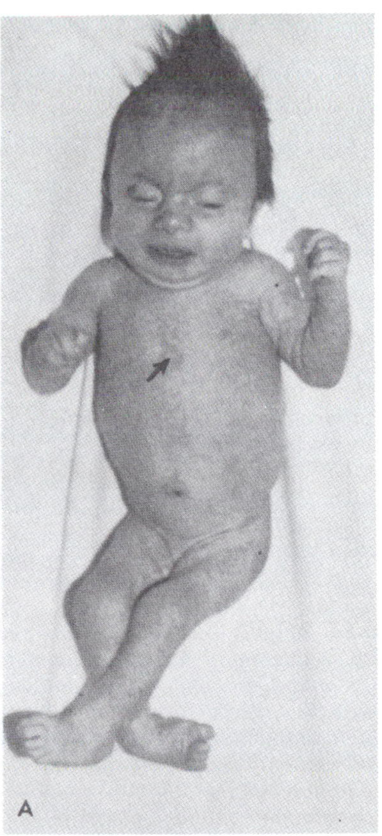

Chromosome 18 trisomy syndrome
Smith, D.W., *Am. J. Obstet. Gynecol.* 90:1055, 1964. St. Louis: C. V. Mosby Company.

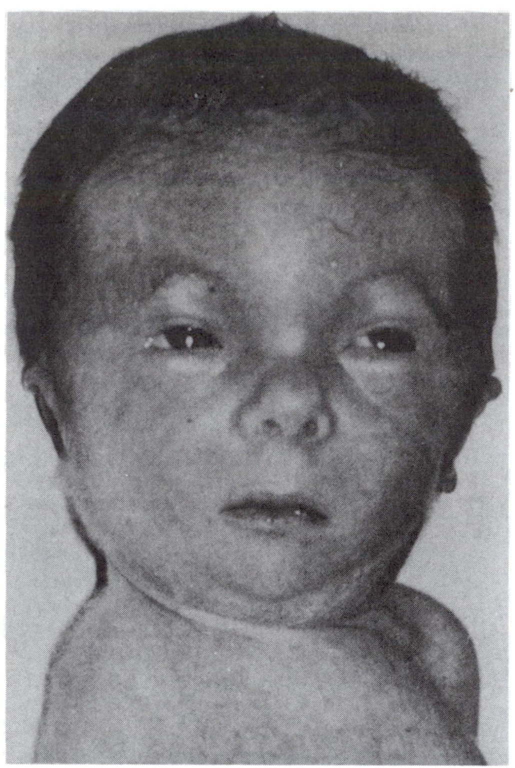

Chromosome 18 trisomy syndrome
Fryns, J.P., Chromosomal anomalies and autosomal syndromes. In Evers-Kiebooms G., J-J. Cassiman, H. Van den Berghe, G. d'Ydewalle (eds): *Genetic Risk, Risk Perception, and Decision Making*. New York: Alan R. Liss, Inc., for the March of Dimes Birth Defects Foundation BD:OAS 23(2):7-32, 1987, with permission.

layed speech, irritability, and destructive behavior are frequently observed in adult patients.

Froland, A., *et al.* Multiple anomalies associated with an additional metacentric chromosome. *Cytogenetics*, 1963, 2:99-106. Balicek, P., *et al.* An isochromosome of the short arm of the No. 18 chromosome in a mentally retarded girl. *Clin. Genet.*, 1976, 9:192-6. Rivera, H., *et al.* Tetrasomy 18p: A distinctive syndrome. *Ann. Génét., Paris*, 1984, 27:187-9. Fryns, J. P., *et al.* 18p tetrasomy. Further evidence for a distinctive clinical syndrome. *Ann. Génét., Paris*, 1985, 28:111-2.

chromosome +18pi syndrome. Synonyms: *+18pi syndrome, supernumerary isochromosome 18 syndrome.*

A supernumerary metacentric chromosome 18 associated with multiple anomalies. The principal characteristics of this disorder include advanced parental age, early feeding difficulty and vomiting, psychomotor retardation, narrow face, pinched nose, narrow high-arched palate, small triangular mouth, low-set ears, dolichocephaly, absence of flexion creases on fingers, pes equinovalgus, poor muscle development, long slim limbs, upper motor neuron lesions of lower limbs, frail body habitus, small head, and retinal coloboma. Radiological symptoms consist of metacarpal and metatarsal pseudoepiphyses, poorly mineralized bones, rib abnormalities, coxa valga, small iliac wings, radioulnar synostoses, and hip subluxation.

Abbo, G., & Zellweger, H. The syndrome of the metacentric microchromosome. *Helv. Paediat. Acta*, 1970, 25:83-94. Condron, C. J., *et al.* The supernumerary isochromosome 18 syndrome (+18pi). *Birth Defects*, 1974, 10(10):36-42.

chromosome 18q deletion syndrome. Synonyms: *18q- syndrome, 18q deletion syndrome, del(18q) syndrome, monosomy 18q, partial monosomy 18q syndrome.*

Deletion of the long arm of a chromosome 18 associated with a distinct phenotype. The principal anomalies include mental retardation, midface aplasia, carp mouth, malformed ears, mandibular prognathism, tapering fingers, and dermatoglyphic abnormalities. Associated defects may include hypotonia, seizures, skin dimples, supernumerary ribs, cardiovascular defects, microphallus, and hypoplasia of the labiae and clitoris. Additional orofacial manifestations may consist of deeply set eyes, glaucoma, strabismus, nystagmus, tapetoretinal degeneration, optic atrophy, short nose, ear canal atresia, cleft lip, and cleft palate. Fusiform fingers, implanted thumbs, relatively long palms, and short first metarpals are the main hand defects. The voice is often husky.

Grouchy, J., de, *et al.* Délétion partielle des bras longs du chromosome 18. *Path. Biol., Paris,* 1964, 12:579-82.

chromosome 18q duplication syndrome. Synonyms: *18q+ syndrome, 18q duplication syndrome, chromosome 18q trisomy syndrome, dup(18q) syndrome, duplication 18q syndrome, partial trisomy 18q syndrome, trisomy 18q.*

Duplication of the long arm of the chromosome 18 with features similar to those of trisomy 18. Craniofacial dysmorphisms consist mainly of bird-like facies, small mouth, prominent occiput, narrow palpebral fissures, slightly antimongoloid palpebral slant, low-set malformed ears, and retrognathia. Associated disorders may include mental retardation, clenched hands, short sternum, hypoplastic ribs, vertebral deformities, congenital hip dislocation, protruding calcaneus, dorsiflexion of the big toes, hypoplastic nails, pseudohermaphroditism, polycystic or ectopic kidneys, and cardiovascular defects, including coarctation of the aorta and patent ductus arteriosus.

Lejeune, J., *et al.* Sur un cas 47;XY(?18q-)+. *Ann. Génét., Paris*, 1970, 13:47-51. Bass, H. N., *et al.* 47,XX,+der(l8), t(9;18)(p24;q21)mat: A distinct partial trisomy 18q syndrome. *J. Med. Genet.*, 1978, 15:391-403. Turleau, C., *et al.* Trisomy 18q. Trisomy mapping of chromosome 18 revisited. *Clin. Genet.*, 1980, 18:20-26.

chromosome 18q trisomy syndrome. See *chromosome 18q duplication syndrome.*

chromosome 19 trisomy syndrome. Synonym: *trisomy 19.*

Mosaic trisomy 19 characterized by prenatal hydramnios, head edema, abdominal ascites, postnatal hydrops, epicanthal fold, hypertelorism, flat nasal bridge, short nose, small mouth, low-set malformed ears, narrow meati, short neck with redundant skin, short chest, protuberant abdomen, mild shortening of the proximal parts of the extemities, spoon nails, simian creases, and clubfeet.

Chen, H., *et al.* Mosaic trisomy 19 syndrome. *Ann. Génét., Paris,* 1981, 24:32-3.

chromosome 19q duplication syndrome. Synonyms: *19q+ syndrome, 19q duplication syndrome, chromosome 19q trisomy syndrome, dup(19q) syndrome,*

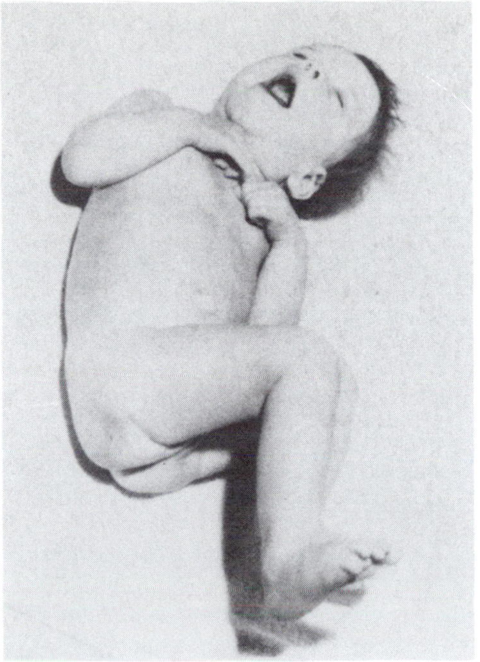

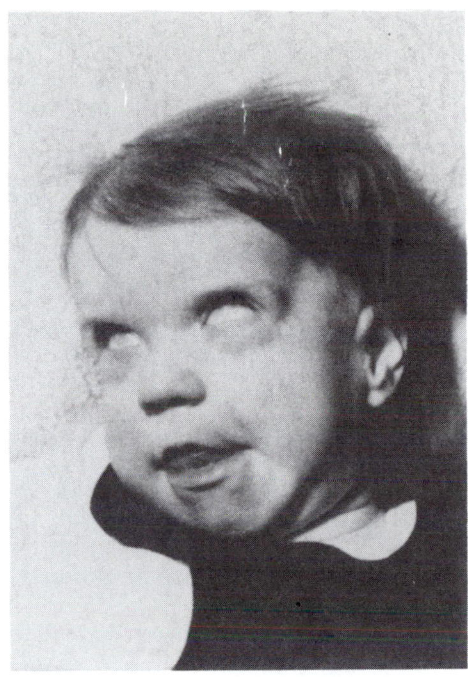

Chromosome 18q deletion syndrome
Felding, I., U. Kristoffersson, H. Sjostrom, & O. Noren, *Clinical Genetics,* 31:206-210, 1987, Munksgaard Internatioal Publishers, Copenhagen, Denmark.

duplication 19q syndrome, partial trisomy 19q, trisomy 19q.

Duplication of the long arm of chromosome 19. Common clinical characteristics include low birth weight, microcephaly, widened fontanel, flat facies, hypertelorism, flat nasal bridge, short nose, low-set malformed ears, narrow meati, short neck with redundant skin, and spoon-shaped nails.

Lange, M., & Alfi, O. Trisomy 19q. *Ann. Génét., Paris,* 1976, 19:17-21. Schmid, W. Trisomy for the distal third of the long arm of chromosome 19 in brother and sister. *Hum. Genet.,* 1979, 46:263-70.

chromosome 19q trisomy syndrome. See *chromosome 19q duplication syndrome.*

chromosome 20 trisomy syndrome. Synonym: *trisomy 20.*

The presence of an additional (third) chromosome in an otherwise diploid chromosome 20. The condition is frequently lethal; a few infants who are liveborn present mental and growth retardation, speech disorders, lethargy, seizures, microcephaly, genital abnormalities with hypogonadism, pigmentary dysplasia of the skin with pigmented moles and nevi, dermatoglyphic abnormalities, kyphoscoliosis, sacral dimple, cataract, miosis, keratoconus, thoracic protuberance, hip dislocation, asymmetric breasts with supernumerary nipples, hypoactive atrophic musculature, deep tendon reflexes, and coarse facies (particularly telecanthus, hypertelorism, broad nose with comedones at the tip, hirsute forehead, synophrys, broad eyebrows and ectopic eyelashes, mongoloid palpebral slant, ear abnormalities, macrostomia, macroglossia, and widely spaced teeth).

Pallister, P. D., *et al.* Trisomy 20 syndrome in man. *Lancet,* 1976, 1:431.

chromosome 20p deletion syndrome. Synonyms: *20p- syndrome, 20p deletion syndrome, del(20p) syndrome, monosomy 20p, partial monosomy 20p syndrome.*

Deletion of the short arm of chromosome 20 associated with low birth-weight, flat facies, down-turned corners of the mouth, low bridge of the nose, long philtrum, short neck, small folded ears, chest deformity, kyphoscoliosis, heart defect, aplastic or hypoplastic ribs, rachischisis, and seizures.

Kazlousek, D. K., & Thérien, S. Deletion of short arm of chromosome 20. *Hum. Genet.,* 1976, 34:89-92. García-Cruz, D., *et al.* Monosomy 20p due to a de novo del(20)(p12.2). Clinical and radiological delineation of the syndrome. *Ann. Génét., Paris,* 1985, 28:231-4.

chromosome 20p duplication syndrome. Synonyms: *20p+ syndrome, 20p duplication syndrome, chromosome 20p trisomy syndrome, dup(20p) syndrome, duplication 20p syndrome, partial trisomy 20p syndrome, trisomy 20p.*

Duplication of the short arm of chromosome 20 with translocation, characterized by psychomotor retardation, speech disorders, poor coordination, coarse hair, characteristic facies (round face with prominent cheeks, occipital flattening, retrognathia, epicanthal folds, up-slanting palpebral fissures, short nose with up-turned tip and large nostrils), abnormal dermatoglyphics, and dental abnormalities. Unless complicated by cardiac, renal, and central nervous system abnormalities, the syndrome is compatible with life.

Carrel, R. E., *et al.* Partial F trisomy associated with familial F/13 translocation identified by parental chromosome studies. *J. Pediat.,* 1971, 78:664-72. Archidiacono, N., *et al.* Trisomy 20p from maternal t(3:20) translocation. *J. Med. Genet.,* 1979, 16:229-32.

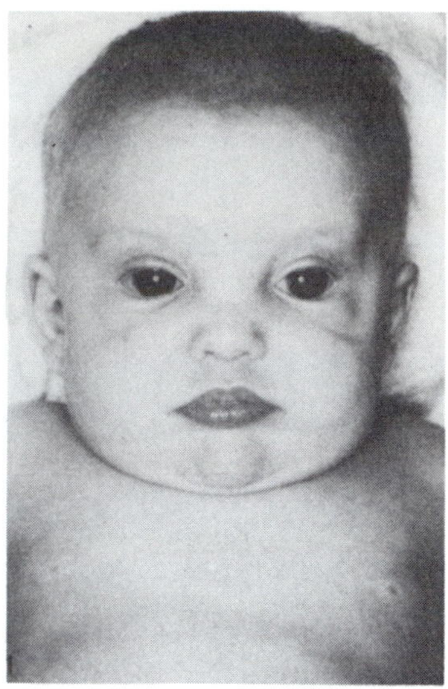

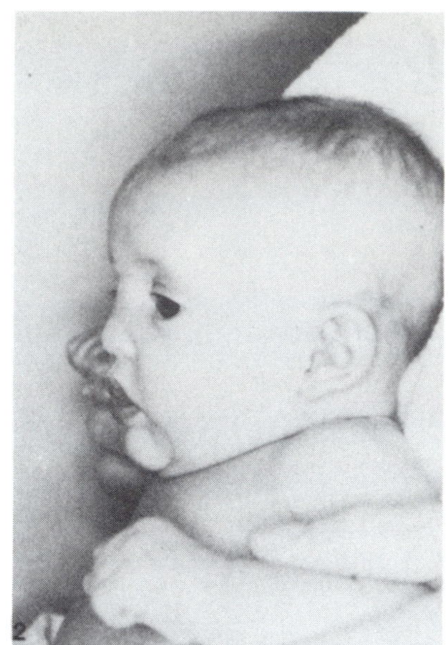

Chromosome 20p deletion syndrome
Byrne, J.L.B., M.J.E. Harrod, J.M. Friedman & P.N. Howard- Peebles, *American Journal of Medical Genetics,* 24:673-678 1986. New York: Alan R. Liss.

chromosome 20p trisomy syndrome. See *chromosome 20p duplication syndrome.*

chromosome 20q deletion syndrome. Synonyms: *20q- syndrome, 20q deletion syndrome, del(20q) syndrome, monosomy 20q, partial monosomy 20q syndrome.*

Deletion of the long arm of chromosome 20 associated with mental retardation, epilepsy, upward palpebral slant, long philtrum, hypoplastic nasal bridge, bulbous nose, microretrognathia, and aplasia of the middle phalanges of the fingers and toes.

Fraisse, J., *et al.* Un nouveau syndrome: del(20)(q13 to qter), Localisation segmentaire de gène de l'adénosine déaminase (ADA). *Ann. Génét., Paris,* 1981, 24:216-9.

chromosome 20q duplication syndrome. Synonyms: *20q+ syndrome, 20q duplication syndrome, chromosome 20q trisomy syndrome, dup(20q) syndrome, duplication 20q syndrome, partial trisomy 20q syndrome, trisomy 20q.*

Duplication of the long arm of chromosome 20 associated with brachycephaly, low-set posteriorly rotated ears, epicanthus, microphthalmia, anteverted nostrils, chin dimple, short neck, heart defect, heart murmur, clinodactyly, camptodactyly, and large toes.

Sanchez, O., *et al.* Partial trisomy 20 (20q13) and partial trisomy 21 (21pter-21q21.3). *J. Med. Genet.,* 1977, 14:459-62. Pawlowitzki, I. H., *et al.* Trisomy 20q due to maternal t(6;20) translocation. First case. *Clin. Genet.,* 1979, 15:167-70.

chromosome 20q trisomy syndrome. See *chromosome 20q duplication syndrome.*

chromosome 21 monosomy syndrome. Synonyms: *21- syndrome, 21 deletion syndrome, chromosome G monosomy, del(21) syndrome, G deletion syndrome, monosomy 21 syndrome,.*

The absence of one chromosome of one pair in an otherwise diploid chromosome 21, characterized by the phenotype consisting of mental retardation, agenesis of the corpus callosum, intrauterine growth retardation, failure to thrive, peculiar facies (broad base of the nose, large nose, carp mouth, high-arched palate, cleft lip and/or cleft palate, micrognathia, low-set large ears, antimongoloid palpebral slant, microcephaly), restricted joint movement, flexion deformity, malposition of fingers and toes, muscle hypertonicity, abnormal dermatoglyphics, and cardiac defects. The affected patients seldom survive past the neonatal period.

Richmond, H. G., *et al.* A "G" deletion syndrome antimongolism. *Acta Paediat. Scand.,* 1973, 62:216-20. Gripenberg, U., *et al.* A 45,XX,21-child. Attempt at a cytological and clinical interpretation of the karyotype. *J. Med. Genet.,* 1972, 9:110-5. Thornburn, M. J., & Johnson, B. E. Apparent monosomy of G autosome in a Jamaican infant. *J. Med. Genet.,* 1966, 3:290-2.

chromosome 21 ring syndrome. Synonyms: *r(21) syndrome, ring chromosome 21 syndrome.*

Chromosome 21 in which both ends have been lost (deletion) and the broken ends have reunited to form a ring-shaped figure, associated with variable phenotypes. Mild cases are characterized by nonexistent or minimal symptoms, such as slight mental retardation which improves with age, and azoospermia. The symptoms in patients with severe forms of ring chromosome 21 ring and chromosome 21 mosaics may include psychomotor retardation, muscle hypertonia, prominant occiput, microcephaly, large protuberant ears, antimongoloid palpebral slant, broad and prominent nasal bridge, cleft palate, micrognathia, and hypospadias. Acute leukemia may be associated with some cases.

Richer, C. L., *et al.* Analysis of banding patterns in a case of ring chromosome 21. *Am. J. Med. Genet.,* 1981, 10:323-31. Kleczkowska, A., & Fryns, J. Ring chromo-

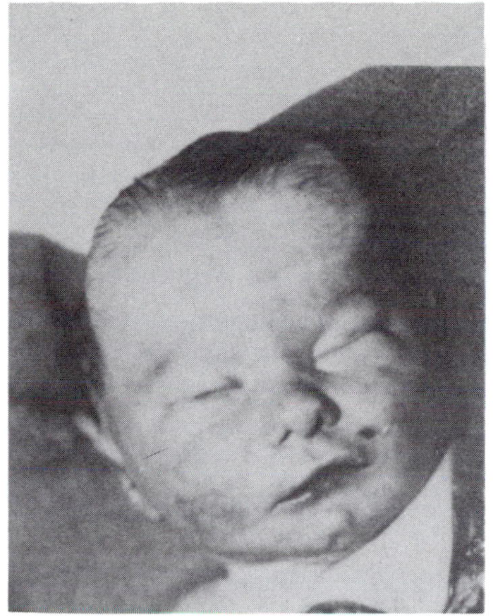

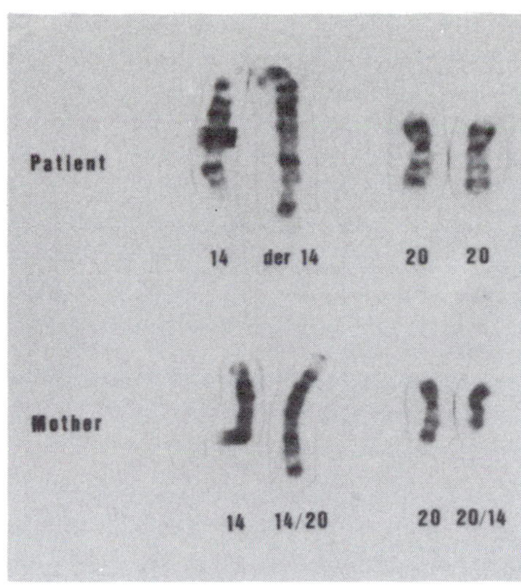

Chromosome 20q duplication syndrome
Sax, Christina M., Joann N. Bodurtha, & Judith A. Brown, *Clinical Genetics*, 30:462-465, 1986, Munksgaard International Publishers, Copenhagen, Denmark.

some 21 in a normal female. *Ann. Génét., Paris,* 1984, 27:126-8.

chromosome 21 trisomy syndrome. Synonyms: *Down syndrome, Langdon Down disease, 21 trisomy, congenital acromicria syndrome, morbus Down. Formerly called mongoloid idiocy, mongolism, 22 trisomy, chromosome 22 trisomy, trisomy G.*

The presence of an extra chromosome 21, usually caused by nondisjunction and, rarely, by translocation. The most common defects consist of mental retardation, short stature, and small skull with a flat occiput, epicanthus, broad flat face, small nose, small ears, small mandible, and slanting palpebral fissures (mongoloid facies), giving patients a peculiar facial appearance. Other orofacial abnormalities include a large, fissured, and protruding tongue, high-arched palate, small maxilla, thick lower lip, delayed dentition, malformed teeth, malocclusion, enamel hypoplasia, and microdontia. Ocular symptoms usually consist of hypotelorism, blue or gray irides, Brushfield spots, and cataracts later in life. Defects of the reproductive system include a small penis, hypogonadism, straight silky pubic hair, delayed puberty, early menopause, large labia majora, and small labia minora. Clinodactyly and simian creases are constant. Associated defects may include loops on finger tips, rib aplasia, intestinal stenosis, dysplastic pelvis, wide spacing of big toes, megacolon, liver and portal system abnormalities, and cardiovascular defects, such as tetralogy of Fallot, ventricular septal defect, and atrioventricular defects. The syndrome occurs most commonly in children of mothers over 35 years of age. The affected children give an appearance of being happy and affectionate; their physical development is usually retarded. Muscular hypotonia creates an impression of floppiness. Predisposition to infections, acute leukemia, and Alzheimer disease later in life may be associated.

Down, J. L. Marriages of consanguinity in relation to degeneration of race. *London Hosp. Clin. Lect. Rep.*, 1866, 3:224-36. Down, J. L. Observations on an ethnic classification of idiots. *London Hosp. Clin. Lect Rep.*, 1866, 3:259-62.

chromosome 21q deletion syndrome. Synonyms: *21q- syndrome, 21q deletion syndrome, del(21q) syndrome, monosomy 21q, partial monosomy 21q syndrome.*

Deletion of the long arm of chromosome 21, characterized by mental and growth retardation, muscle hypertonia, nail dysplasia, cryptorchism, hypospadias, inguinal hernia, pyloric stenosis, thrombocytopenia, eosinophilia, and hypogammoglobulinemia. Facial and oral manifestations include microcephaly, large and poorly developed low-set ears, antimongoloid palpebral slant, blepharochalasis, high-arched palate, cleft lip and palate, and micrognathia. Dermatoglyphic abnormalities may occur.

Mikkelsen, M., & Vestermark, S. Karyotype 45,XX,-21/46,XX,21q- in an infant with symptoms of the G-deletion of syndrome. *J. Med. Genet.*, 1974, 11:389-93.

chromosome 22 monosomy syndrome. Synonyms: *22 monosomy, monosomy 22.*

Absence of one chromosome of one pair in an otherwise diploid cell of chromosome 22 associated with psychomotor retardation, muscle hypotonia, large ears, epicanthus, synophrys, and cutaneous syndactyly between all the fingers.

Moghe, M. S., *et al.* Monosomy 22 with mosaicism. *J. Med. Genet.*, 1981, 18:71-3.

chromosome 22 ring syndrome. Synonyms: *r(22) syndrome, ring chromosome 22 syndrome.*

Chromosome 22 in which both ends have been lost (deletion) and the broken ends have reunited to form a ring-shaped form, associated with variable phenotypes; mental retardation, doe's eye anomaly, and disturbed equilibrium being its principal features.

Hunter, A. G. W., *et al.* Phenotype correlations in patients

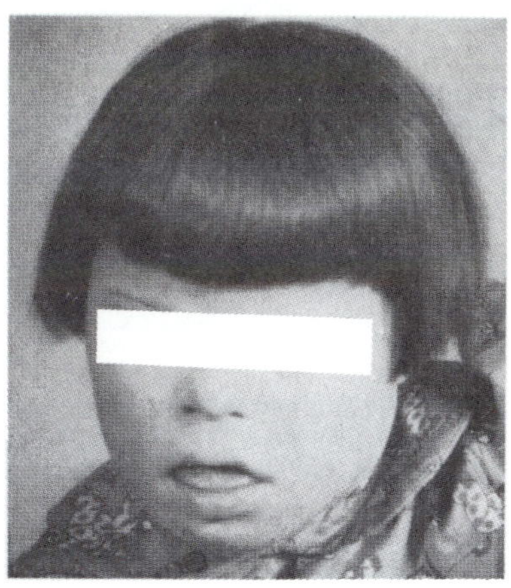

Chromosome 21 trisomy syndrome
Nelson, W.E. (ed.): *Textbook of Pediatrics.* 8th ed. Philadelphia: W.B. Saunders Co.

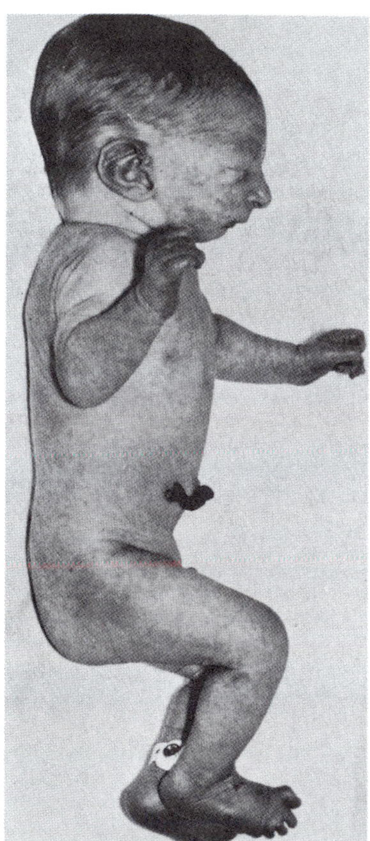

Chromosome 21q deletion syndrome
Reisman, L.E., *Lancet,* 1:394, 1966, London, England.

with ring chromosome 22. *Clin. Genet.,* 1977, 12:239-49. Rethoré, M. O., *et al.* Le syndrome r(22). A propos de 4 nouvelles observations. *Ann. Génét., Paris,* 1976, 19:111-7.

chromosome 22 trisomy syndrome. Synonym: *trisomy 22.*

Trisomy of the chromosome 22 characterized chiefly by mental retardation, growth retardation, microphallus, cryptorchism, congenital heart defects, cleft palate, cleft uvula, long philtrum, long and beaked nose, and peculiar facies marked by microcephaly, low-set and malformed ears, and micrognathia. Less commonly occurring defects may include preauricular skin tags and/or sinus, muscle hypotonia, finger-like thumb, long slender fingers, congenital hip dislocation, antimongoloid palpebral slant, strabismus, and hypoplastic or low-set nipples. In older literature, chromosome 22 was sometimes identified with the Down syndrome (chromosome 21 trisomy).

Uchida, I. A., *et al.* Familial occurrence of trisomy 22. *Am. J. Hum. Genet.,* 1968, 20:107-18.

chromosome C trisomy. See *chromosome 8 trisomy syndrome.*

chromosome D13 ring syndrome. See *chromosome 13 ring syndrome.*

chromosome diploid-triploid mosaicism syndrome. Synonyms: *2n/3n mosaicism, diploid-triploid mosaicism.*

A syndrome of diploidy (the state of having two full sets of homologous chromosomes), triploidy (the presence of three haploid, or 69, sets of chromosomes), and mosaicism (the presence of two or more cell lines that are karyotypically or genotypically distinct and are derived from a single zygote). It is characterized by respiratory distress, feeding difficulty, growth and mental retardation, retarded bone age, muscle hypotonia, seizures, asymmetry of facial and body structures, dolichocephaly, prominent forehead, micrognathia, low-set malformed ears, ambiguous genitalia, small phallus, hypospadias, cryptorchism, disproportionate length of the legs, muscle atrophy of the extremities, flexion deformity, clubfoot, clinodactyly, syndactyly, and transverse palmar creases.

Dewald, G., *et al.* A diploid-triploid human mosaic with cytogenic evidence of double fertilization. *Clin. Genet.,* 1975, 8:149-60. Ferrier, P., *et al.* Congenital asymmetry associated with diploid-triploid mosaicism and large satellites. *Lancet,* 1964, 1:80-2.

chromosome fra(X)(q28) syndrome. See *chromosome X fragility.*

chromosome G trisomy. See *chromosome 21 trisomy.*

chromosome tetraploidy syndrome. Synonym: *tetraploidy syndrome.*

A condition characterized by the presence of four sets of chromosomes, usually observed in spontaneous abortion, live-born infants with tetraploid cell line having been reported infrequently. Major clinical manifestations include microcephaly, microphthalmia/anophthalmia, beaked nose, low-set hypoplastic ears, prominent forehead with narrow biparietal diameter, flexion deformities or malpositioning of the extremities, cryptorchism, mild genital ambiguity, meningomyelocele, microgyria of the brain, hypoplasia or aplasia of the optic and olfactory tracts, and rudimentary pituitary gland. Abnormalities sometimes associated with tetraploidy include hypertelorism, short palpebral fissures, high-arched or cleft palate, micrognathia, arachnodactyly, hypotonia, congenital heart defect, and Arnold-Chiari malformation.

Kohn, G., *et al.* tetraploid-diploid mosaicism in a surviving infant. *Pediat. Res.,* 1967, 1:461-9. Scarbrough, P. R., *et al.* Tetraploidy: A report of three live-born infants. *Am. J. Med. Genet.,* 1984, 19:29-37.

chromosome triploidy syndrome. Synonyms: *fetal triploidy syndrome, infantile triploidy syndrome, triploidy syndrome.*

A syndrome characterized by the presence of three haploid sets of chromosome (69) and associated with multiple abnormalities, including intrauterine growth retardation, large posterior fontanel, dysplastic cranial bones, ocular abnormalities with hypertelorism, cleft palate, macroglossia, congenital heart defects, syndactyly of the third and fourth fingers, abnormal dermatoglyphics, genital anomalies (hypospadias, microphallus, cryptorchism), polyhydramnios, and abnormally large placenta with hydatiform changes. Most cases terminate in spontaneous abortion; a small number of infants who survive die within several days of weeks after birth.

Niebuhr, E. Triploidy in man. *Hum. Genet.*, 1974, 21:103-25. Wertelecki, W., *et al.* The clinical syndrome of triploidy. *Obst. Gyn.*, 1976, 47:69-76. Bernard, R., *et al.* Triploidie chromosomique chez un nouveau-née polymorphe. *Ann. Génét., Paris,* 1967, 10:70.

chromosome X fragility. Synonyms: *Escalante syndrome, Martin-Bell syndrome (MBS), Martin-Bell-Renpenning syndrome, Renpenning syndrome, autism-fragile-X (AFRAX) syndrome, fra(X) syndrome, fra(X)(q27) syndrome, fra(X)(q27-28) syndrome, fra(X)(28) syndrome, fragile X-mental retardation syndrome, fragile-X syndrome (FXS), fragile Xq syndrome, macro-orchidism-marker X (MOMX) syndrome, mar(X) syndrome, marker X syndrome.*

An X-linked mental retardation syndrome characterized by a cytogenic marker, a fragile site localized on the long arm of X chromosome at the band 27 or 28. Its principal clinical features consist of enlarged testes, abnormal speech pattern, large ears, long face, high-arched palate, and malocclusion. Attention problems and autism are the chief behavioral and emotional disorders. Additional abnormalities may include lordosis, heart defect, pectus excavatum, flat feet, shortening of the tubular bones of the hands, and joint laxity. Renpenning's cases (short stature, moderate microcephaly, neurological disorders) were reported in a Dutch Mennonite pedigree from Alberta and Saskatchewan.

Martin, J. P., & Bell, J. A. A pedigree of mental defect showing sex linkage. *J. Neur. Neurosurg. Psychol.*, 1943, 6:154-7. Optiz, J. M., Reynolds, J. F., & Spano, L. M., eds. X-linked mental retardation 2. *Am. J. Med. Genet.*, 1986, 23:1-735. Renpenning, H., *et al.* Familial sex-linked mental retardation. *Canad. Med. Assoc. J.*, 1962, 87:954-6. *Escalante, J. A. *Estudio genético da deficiencia mental.* Sao Paulo, 1971 (Thesis). Escalante, J. A., *et al.* Severe sex-linked mental retardation. *Proc. II Cong. Internat. Study Ment. Defic.*, Warsaw, 1970, p. 745. Gilberg, C. V., *et al.* Folic acid as an adjunct in the treatment of children with autism-fragile X syndrome (AFRAX). *Dev. Child Neurol.*, 1986, 28:624-7.

chromosome X pentasomy. See *chromosome XXXXX syndrome.*

chromosome XO syndrome. Synonyms: *Morgagni-Turner syndrome, Morgagni-Turner-Albright syndrome, Shereshevskii-Turner syndrome, Turner syndrome (TS), Turner-Albright syndrome, Ullrich-Turner syndrome, genital dwarfism, gonadal agenesis syndrome, gonadal dysgenesis syndrome, ovarian dwarfism, ovarian short stature syndrome, primary ovarian insufficiency,*

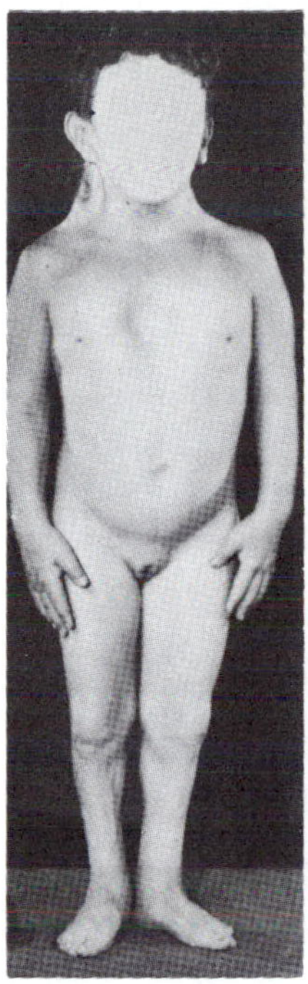
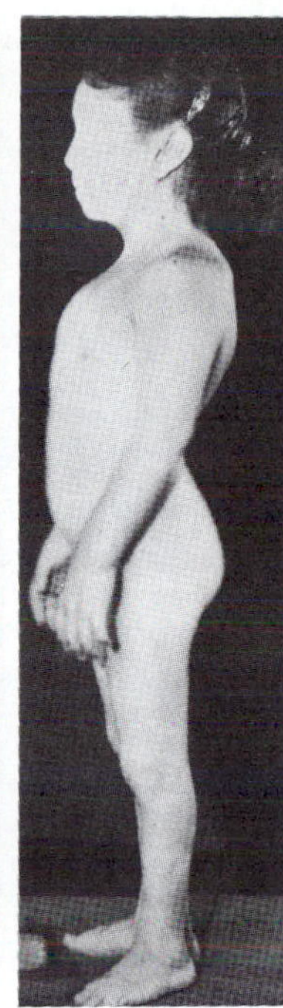

Chromosome XO syndrome
Federman, D.D.: *Abnormal Sexual Development.* Philadelphia: W.B. Saunders Co., 1967.

pseudonuchal infantilism, pterygonuchal infantilism, XO syndrome.

A syndrome in which the affected patients have only 45 chromosomes, the loss of one of the X chromosomes producing an XO chromosome constitution. Typical features are short stature; infantile development of the vagina, uterus, and breast; dysgenesis of the ovaries; pterygium colli and apparent short neck; cubitus valgus or other anomaly of the elbow; low hairline; transient edema and puffiness of the fingers and toes; broad chest with widely spaced nipples, which may be hypoplastic, inverted, or both; mild pectus excavatum; characteristic facies with narrow maxilla, micromandible, inner canthal folds, and anomalous auricles of the ears; bone dysplasia; finger abnormalities, especially short fourth metacarpal and metatarsal bones and marrow, hyperconvex and/or deep set nails; knee anomalies such as tibial exostosis; loose skin, especially about the neck; renal disorders, most commonly horseshoe kidneys, double or cleft renal pelvis, and other defects; perceptive hearing impairment; and sometimes, premature dentition, short dental roots, microdontia, strabismus, blue sclerae, cataracts, mental retardation, idiopathic hypertension, asymmetry of the facial and cranial bones and alveolar processes, pigmented nevi, coarctation of the aorta, and other anomalies.

*Morgagni, G. B. *Epistola anatomica medica.* 1768, XLVII, Art. 20. Turner, H. H. A syndrome of infantilism, congenital webbed neck, and cubitus valgus. *Endocrinology*, 1938, 23:566-74. Albright, F., *et al.* A syndrome characterized by primary ovarian insufficiency and decreased stature. Report of eleven cases, with a digression on hormonal control of axillary and pubic hair. *Am. J. Med, Sc.*, 1942, 204-625-48. Shereshevskii, N. A. A syndrome of endocrine origin. *Am. Rev. Sov. Med.*, 1943, 1:337. Ullrich, O. Über typische Kombinationsbilder multipler Abartungen. *Zschr. Kinderh.*, 1930, 49:271-6.

chromosome XO/XY syndrome. Synonyms: *XO/XY mosaicism, XO/XY syndrome.*

A chromosomal disorder with a variable phenotype, characterized mainly by ambiguous genitalia. Some patients exhibit some stigmata of the Turner syndrome, some have a female phenotype (with streak gonads), some have a male phenotype (with bilateral cryptorchism), and some have unambiguous genitalia. Those with ambiguous genitalia always have a uterus and many have one streak gonad and one testis, while some have two streak gonads, bilateral testes, or no gonads at all. Only about 2 percent are true hermaphrodites. Seminoma or gonadoblastoma may occur in cases of ambiguous genitalia.

Van Campenhout, J., *et al.* The phenotype and gonadal histology in XO/XY mosaic individuals: Report of two personal cases. *J. Obstet. Gynaec. Brit. Commonw.*, 1969, 76:631-9.

chromosome XX syndrome. Synonyms: *male XX syndrome, sex reversal syndrome, XX male sydrome, XX syndrome, 46,XX syndrome.*

A variant of the Klinefelter syndrome, characterized mainly by small testes, sterility, hypotrichosis, hypogenitalism, elevated gonadotropin level, and low plasma testosterone level. Associated anomalies may include gynecomastia and hypoplastic penis and scrotum. The affected males have 46 chromosomes and an extra chromosome X, but lack the chromosome Y.

de la Chapelle, A., *et al.* XX sex chromosomes in a human male. First case. *Acta Med. Scand.* 1960, Suppl 412:25-38.

chromosome XX/XXY syndrome. Synonyms: *XX/XXY mosaic, XX/XXY syndrome.*

A relatively mild variant of the Klinefelter (XXY) syndrome characterized by an XX/XXY mosaic. The affected males may show hypotrichosis, small testes, small penis, sterility, gynecomastia, high gonadotropin level, and low testosterone level.

Gordon, D. L., *et al.* Pathologic testicular findings in Klinefelter syndrome. *Arch. Int. Med.*, 1972, 130:726-9.

Ferguson-Smith, M. A. Phenotypic aspects of sex chromosome aberrations. *Birth Defects*, 1969, 5(5):3-9.

chromosome XXX syndrome. Synonyms: *super female, triple-X syndrome, triple-X chromosome syndrome, trisomy X, X trisomy, XXX syndrome.*

A condition characterized by the presence of three X (female) chromosomes. The syndrome does not exhibit a distinctive phenotype, about one-fourth being physically and mentally normal, one-fourth having some type of congenital deformity but without any constant pattern, one-fourth having a mildly retarded development, and one-fourth being borderline between normal and defective. Sexual disorders in triple-X females vary from amenorrhea and sterility to mild menstrual disorders. Clinodactyly and radioulnar synostosis have been reported in some cases.

Jacobs, P. A., *et al.* Evidence for the existence of the human "super female." *Lancet*, 1959, 2:423-5.

chromosome XXXX syndrome. Synonyms: *Carr-Barr-Plunkett syndrome, 48,XXXX syndrome, XXXX syndrome.*

A genetic syndrome characterized by four X chromosomes (48,XXXX). The symptoms include mental deficiency and variable abnormalities, including midfacial hypoplasia, hypertelorism, epicanthic folds, micrognathia, clinodactyly, radioulnar synostosis, narrow shoulder girdle, and occasional webbed neck and amenorrhea or irregular menses. Behavioral disorders may be associated.

Carr, D. H., *et al.* An XXXX sex chromosome complex in two mentally retarded females. *Canad. Med. Assoc. J.*, 1961, 84:131-7.

chromosome XXXXX syndrome. Synonyms: *49,XXXXX syndrome, chromosome X pentasomy, pentasomy X syndrome, penta-X syndrome, quintuple-X syndrome, XXXXX syndrome.*

A hereditary syndrome characterized by the presence of five X chromosomes (49,XXXXX). The symptoms include low birth weight, failure to thrive, small head, short stature, mental or psychomotor retardation, peculiar facies (flat nasal bridge, mongoloid palpebral slant, malformed ears, thick and everted lips, micrognathia, prognathism), cleft palate, malocclusion, dental abnormalities, short neck, low hairline, congenital heart defect, radioulnar synostosis with elbow abnormality, camptodactyly, clinodactyly, joint hyperflexion or dislocation, talipes, micromelia, metatarsus varus, genu valgum, delayed bone maturation, dermal ridge hypoplasia of the fingers, renal hypoplasia, small uterus, and abnormal ovaries.

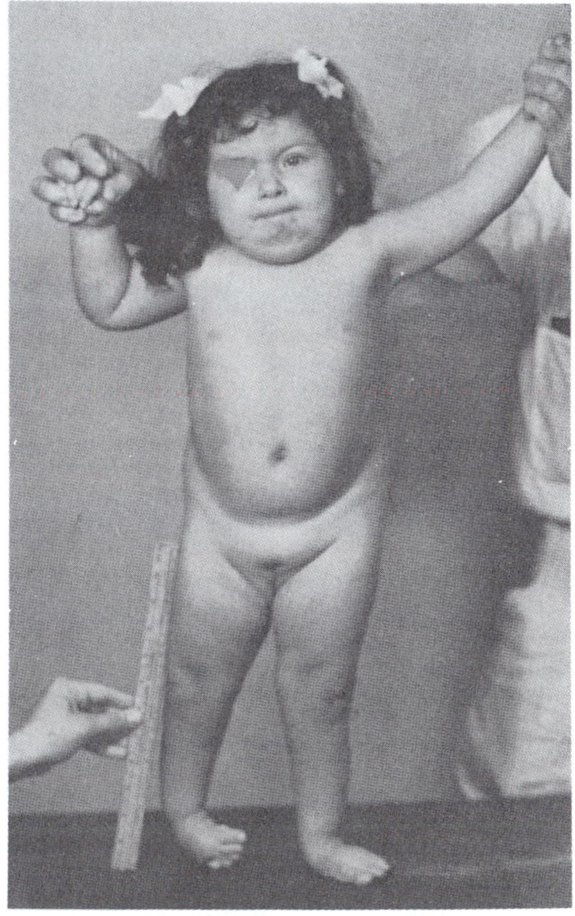

Chromosome XXXXX syndrome
Brody, J., et al.: *J. Pediatr.* 70:105, 1961. St. Louis: C.V. Mosby Co.

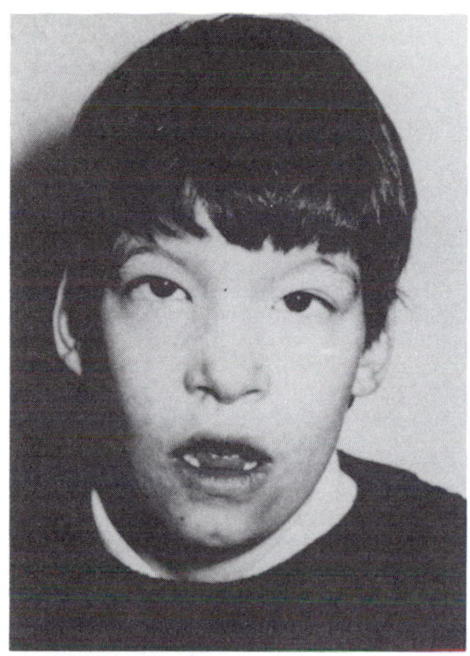

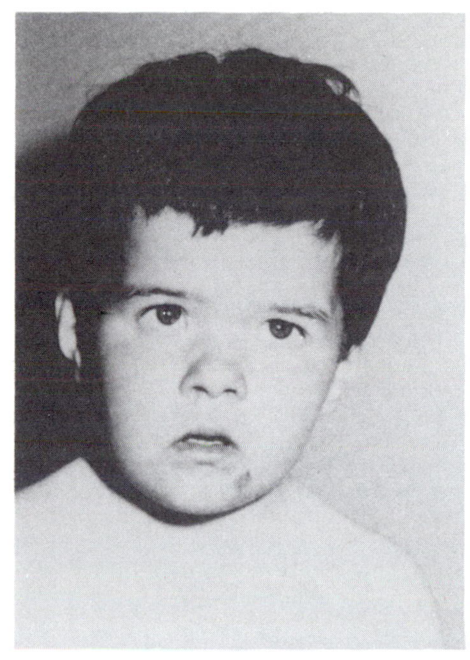

Chromosome XXXXY syndrome
Borghgraef, M., J.P. Frynes, E. Smeets, J. Marien & H. van den Berghe, *Clinical Genetics* 33:419-434, 1988. Munksgaard International Publishers, Copenhagen, Denmark.

Kesaree, N., & Wolley, P. V., Jr. A phenotypic female with 49 chromosomes, presumably XXXXX. *J. Pediat.*, 1963, 63:1099-103. Funderburk, S. J., *et al.* Pentasomy X: Report of patient and studies of X-inactivation. *Am. J. Med. Genet.*, 1981, 8:27-33.

chromosome XXXXY syndrome. Synonyms: *49,XXXXY syndrome, XXXXY aneuploidy syndrome, XXXXY syndrome.*

A variant of the Klinefelter (XXY) syndrome characterized by severe mental retardation, hypotonia, small penis, cryptorchism, hypospadias, small testes, and various bone defects. Orofacial anomalies include microcephaly, ocular hypertelorism, myopia, strabismus, mongoloid palpebral slant, epicanthus, and poorly developed pinnae. The round face at birth disappears with age and is replaced by retarded midfacial growth with dish face and relative mandibular prognathism. Short neck with redundant skin on the posterior part and mild webbing usually occur. The limbs may exhibit limited pronation at the elbows, radioulnar synostoses, clinodactyly of the fifth fingers, coxa valga, genua valga, and pes planus. The affected males have chromosomes with three extra X group chromosomes.

Fracaro, M., *et al.* A child with 49 chromosomes. *Lancet*, 1960, 2:899-902.

chromosome XXXY syndrome. Synonyms: *48,XXXY syndrome, XXXY syndrome.*

A variant of the Klinefelter (XXY) syndrome characterized chiefly by mental retardation, tall stature, and small testes. Associated defects may include gynecomastia, hypertelorism, epicanthal folds, strabismus, prognathism, pterygium colli, microphallus, radioulnar synostoses, and clinodactyly. The affected males have 48 chromosomes and an extra two X chromosomes.

Ferguson-Smith, M. A., *et al.* Primary amentia and microorchidism associated with an XXXY sex chromosome constitution. *Lancet*, 1960, 2:184-7.

chromosome XXXYY syndrome. Synonyms: *49,XXXYY syndrome, XXXYY syndrome.*

A chromosomal abnormality marked by mental retardation, hypogenitalism, tall stature, prognathism, cryptorchism, small penis, and, less commmonly, prominent cheek bones, hypotrichosis, strabismus, apparent short neck, gynecomastia, and thoracic scoliosis. The affected males have three X and two Y chromosomes (49,XXXYY).

Bray, P., & Josephine, A. An XXXYY sex chromosome anomaly. Report of a mentally deficient male. *JAMA*, 1963, 184:179-82.

chromosome XXY syndrome. Synonyms: *Klinefelter syndrome (KS), Klinefelter-Reifenstein-Albright syndrome, gynecomastia-aspermatogenesis syndrome, medullary gonadal dysgenesis, primary microorchidism, puberal seminiferous tubule failure, sclerosing tubular degeneration, seminiferous tubule dysgenesis, XXY syndrome.*

A hereditary syndrome characterized chiefly by dull mentality and/or behavioral problems associated with hypogenitalism and hypogonadism. The affected children tend to have small penises and testes with inadequate testosterone production and elevated gonadotropin level, long limbs, and relatively slim and tall statures. Without testosterone therapy, they may become obese as adults. Sterility with hyalinization and fibrosis of the seminiferous tubules are usually associated. Occasional abnormalities may include cryptorchism, hypospadias, ataxia, scoliosis during adolescence, and diabetes mellitus during adulthood. The classic form of the Klinefelter syndrome is the XXY

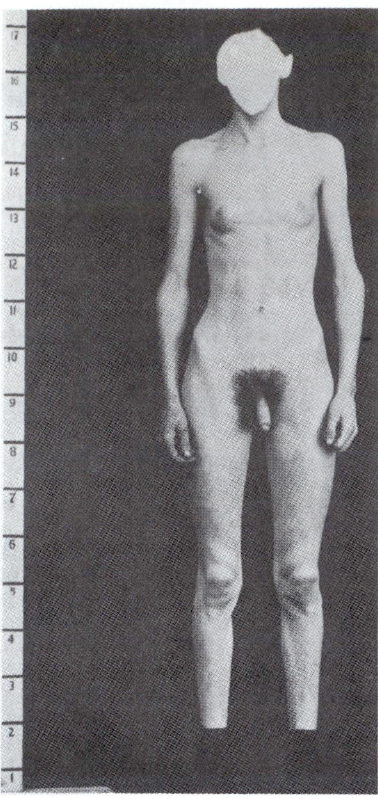

Chromosome XXY syndrome
Federman, D.D.: *Abnormal Sexual Development.* Philadelphia: W.B. Saunders Co., 1967.

syndrome, but variants, such as XXYY, XXXY, XXXXY syndromes and mosaic patterns, such as XXX/XY, also exist.

Klinefelter, H. F., Jr., Reifenstein, E. C., Jr., & Albright, F. Syndrome characterized by gynecomastia, aspermatogenesis without A-leydigism, and increased excretion of follicle-stimulating hormone. *J. Clin. Endocr.*, 1942, 2:615-27.

chromosome XXYY syndrome. Synonyms: *48,XXYY syndrome, XXYY syndrome.*

A variant of the Klinefelter (XXY) syndrome. Characteristics of both disorders are similar, except for tall stature, aggressiveness, and mental retardation which are more severe in the XXYY syndrome. Otherwise, the phenotype is quite similar and is characterized chiefly by small firm testes, eunuchoid habitus, sparse body hair, genecomastia, elevated gonadotropin level, and low urinary 17-ketosteroids. The affected males have 48 chromosomes and extra X and Y chromosomes (48,XXYY).

Muldal, S., & Ockey, C. H. The "double male": A new chromosome constitution in Klinefelter's syndrome. *Lancet*, 1960, 2:492-3.

chromosome XY female syndrome. Synonyms: *Swyer syndrome, chromosome XY gonadal dysgenesis, XY female syndrome, XY gonadal dysgenesis (GDXY).*

A syndrome of familial gonadal dysgenesis in females who have 46,XY chromosome constitution. The affected young females appear to be normal except for underdeveloped secondary sexual characteristics at puberty and amenorrhea. H-Y positive and H-Y negative forms are recognized. Many patients develop ovarian neoplasms in streak gonads, usually gonadoblastoma or germinoma. The syndrome is transmitted as an X-linked trait.

Swyer, G. I. M. Male pseudohermaphroditism: A hitherto undescribed form. *Brit. Med. J.*, 1955, 2:709-12.

chromosome XY gonadal dysgenesis. See *chromosome XY female syndrome.*

chromosome XYY syndrome. Synonyms: *chromosome YY syndrome, double male syndrome, super male, YY syndrome.*

A syndrome associated with the presence of an extra Y chromosome in males and characterized by a long body, muscle weakness, a high bridge of the nose, acne vulgaris, mild facial asymmetry with mandibular deformities, mild pectus excavatum, mild scapular winging, long ears, bony chin points, and occasional radioulnar synostosis. The affected patient may have mild mental retardation and exhibit explosive behavior with a propensity to destroy property rather than violence against others.

Sandberg, A. A., *et al.* An XYY human male. *Lancet*, 1961, 2:488-9. Muldal, S., & Ockey, C. H. The "double male." New chromosome constitution in Klinefelter's syndrome. *Lancet*, 1960, 2:492.

chromosome XYYY syndrome. Synonyms: *48,XYYY syndrome, XYYY syndrome.*

A polysomic syndrome with 48,XYYY chromosomal constitution and variable phenotype, consisting chiefly of psychomotor retardation or low normal intelligence, aggressive behavior, cryptorchism, testicular hypotrophy, predisposition to pulmonary infections, inguinal hernia, pulmonary stenosis, simian creases, hypotrichosis, acne vulgaris, and dental hypoplasia.

Townes, P. L., *et al.* A patient with 48 chromosomes (XYYY). *Lancet*, 1965, 1:1041-3. Ridler, M., *et al.* An adult with XYYY sex chromosomes. *Clin. Genet.*, 1973, 4:69-71.

chromosome XYYYY syndrome. Synonyms: *tetrasomy Y syndrome, XYYYY syndrome.*

A polysomic syndrome with four Y (XYYYY) chromosomes and variable phenotype characterized by mental retardation, cataract, facial asymmetry, clinodactyly of the fifth fingers, brachymesophalangy, and radioulnar synostosis. The external genitalia, although normal at birth, may remain undeveloped at the time of puberty. Motor retardation, prominent upper lip, epicanthus, micrognathia, low-set ears scoliosis, and other defects may be associated.

Berghe, H., van den, *et al.* A male with 4 Y-chromosomes. *J. Clin. Endrocr. Metab.*, 1968, 28:1370-2.

chromosome YY syndrome. See *chromosome XYY syndrome.*

chronic active lupoid hepatitis (CALH). See *Bearn-Kunkel syndrome.*

chronic aorto-iliac occlusion. See *Leriche syndrome (1).*

chronic atrophic lichenoid dermatitis. See *Hallopeau syndrome (1).*

chronic benign infantile granulocytopenia. See *Vahlquist-Gasser syndrome.*

chronic chlorosis. See *Faber syndrome.*

chronic constitutional granulocytopenia. See *Vahlquist-Gasser syndrome.*

chronic cystic mastitis. See *Cheatle disease.*

chronic disseminated histiocytosis X. See *Hand-Schüller-Christian syndrome.*

chronic eosinophilic pneumonia (CEP). See *pulmonary infiltration with eosinophilia syndrome.*

chronic erythroblastopenia. See *Diamond-Blackfan syndrome.*

chronic erythrocyte aplasia. See *Diamond-Blackfan syndrome.*

chronic factitious disease. See *Munchausen syndrome.*

chronic factitious disorder with physical symptoms. See *Munchausen syndrome.*

chronic familial erythremia. See *Cooley anemia.*

chronic familial methemoglobinemia. See *Hörlein-Weber disease.*

chronic fatigue syndrome (CFS). Synonyms: *fatigue-dysphoria syndrome, postinfective chronic fatigue syndrome (PICFS), postviral asthenia syndrome, postviral fatigue syndrome, postviral syndrome, yuppie (young urban professional) disease.*

A chronic disorder characterized by debilitating fatigue of longer than 6 month duration. The symptoms include low-grade fever, chills, pharyngitis, myalgias, cervical adenopathy, arthralgia, new headaches unlike any in the past, prolonged exhaustion after exercise and a self-perpetuating cycle of avoidance of exercise, mental disorders (e.g., faulty memory, irritability, confusion, inability to concentrate, and depression), sleep disorders, and hypersensitivity to bright light, the symptoms being similar to those seen in fibromyalgia. In most patients, onset starts suddenly as an acute flu-like illness. Lymphocytosis, monocytosis, elevated liver enzyme levels, varying levels of antithyroid antibodies, hypergammaglobulinemia, low levels of antinuclear antibodies, and decreased cytolytic activity of natural killer cells are the principal laboratory findings in some patients, indicating a prior viral infection, particularly Epstein-Barr virus or human herpesvirus infection. However, some studies indicate that there is no relationship between this syndrome and viral infections. See also *Beard syndrome.*

Wessely, S., *et al.* Management of chronic (post-viral) fatigue syndrome. *J. Roy. Coll. Gen. Pract.,* 1989, 39(318):26-9. Komaroff, A. L., & Goldenberg, D. The chronic fatigue syndrome: Definition, current studies and lessons for fibromyalgia research. *J. Rheum. Suppl.,* 1989, 19:23-7.

chronic follicular keratoconjunctivitis. See *trachoma.*

chronic granulomatous disease of childhood. Synonyms: *Bridges-Good syndrome, Quie syndrome, fatal granulomatous disease of childhood, neutrophil dysfunction syndrome.*

An inherited disease with onset of symptoms in the first 2 years of life, which is transmitted as an X-linked recessive trait and is frequently fatal. The most common features of this syndrome consist of protracted fever, purulent granulomatous or eczematoid skin lesions, lymphadenopathy, hepatosplenomegaly, draining lymph nodes, pneumonia, chronic rhinitis, osteomyelitis affecting mainly the small bones of the hands and feet, and diarrhea. Ulcerative stomatitis and conjunctivitis may be present. Female carriers have a high incidence of discoid or systemic lupus erythematosus, but only a few women develop this disease. *Staphylococcus aureus, Serratia marcescens, Pseudomonas, Candida,* and *Aspergillus* are the principal organisms isolated in this disorder. Polymorphonuclear leukocytes, although able to digest bacteria, lack the ability to kill them in patients suffering from this condition. See also *Job syndrome.*

Quie, P. G., *et al.* Defective polymorphonuclear-leukocyte function and chronic granulomatous disease in two female children. *N. Engl. J. Med.,* 1968, 278:976-80. Bridges, R. A., *et al.* A fatal granulomatous disease of childhood. The clinical, pathological, and laboratory features of a new syndrome. *AMA J. Dis. Child.,* 1959, 97:387-404. Good, R. A., *et al.* Fatal (chronic) granulomatous disease of childhood: A hereditary defect of leukocyte function. *Semin. Hematol.,* 1969, 5:215-54 Gold, R. H., *et al.* Roentgenographic features of the neutrophil dysfunction syndrome. *Radiology,* 1969, 92:1045-54.

chronic hereditary trophedema. See *Meige syndrome (1).*

chronic hypercorticism of rheumatoid arthritis. See *Slocumb syndrome.*

chronic hyperphosphatasemia. See *van Buchem syndrome, under Buchem, Francis Steven Peter, van.*

chronic hyperphosphatasia. See *hyperphosphatasia-osteoclasia syndrome.*

chronic hypertrophic gastritis. See *Ménétrier syndrome.*

chronic hypochromic anemia. See *Faber syndrome.*

chronic idiopathic hyperphosphatasia. See *hyperphosphatasia-osteoclasia syndrome.*

chronic idiopathic jaundice. See *Rotor syndrome.*

chronic idiopathic orthostatic hypotension. See *Bradbury-Eggleston syndrome.*

chronic infantile cerebral sclerosis. See *Pelizaeus-Merzbacher syndrome.*

chronic intermittent juvenile jaundice. See *Gilbert syndrome, under Gilbert, Nicolas Augustin.*

chronic lingual papillitis. See *Möller glossitis.*

chronic lymphadenopathy simulating malignant lymphoma. See *Canale-Smith syndrome.*

chronic microcytic anemia. See *Faber syndrome.*

chronic mountain sickness. See *Monge disease.*

chronic mucocutaneous candidiasis syndrome. Inherited mucocutaneous candidiasis, transmitted as an autosomal dominant trait, characterized by early onset, mild mucocutaneous eruption, increased susceptibility to bacterial infections, hyperkeratosis follicularis, alopecia universalis, keratoconjunctivitis with loss of vision, diarrhea in infancy, T and B cell abnormalities, and possible hypoadrenalism.

Okamoto, G. A., *et al.* A new syndrome of chronic mucocutaneous candidiasis. *Birth Defects,* 1977, 13(3B):117-25.

chronic necrotic stomatitis. See *Sutton disease, under Sutton, Richard Lighburn, Jr.*

chronic nonspecific suppurative pneumonitis. See *Kershner-Adams syndrome.*

chronic nonsuppurative destructive cholangitis (CNDC). See *primary biliary cirrhosis syndrome.*

chronic nutritional hypochromic anemia. See *Faber syndrome.*

chronic obstructive bronchitis. See *airway obstruction syndrome.*

chronic obstructive pseudoemphysema. See *Swyer-James syndrome, under Swyer, Paul Robert.*

chronic obstructive pulmonary disease (COPD). See *airway obstruction syndrome.*

chronic osteopathy-hyperphosphatasia syndrome. See *hyperphophatasia-osteoctasia syndrome.*

chronic overdrainage syndrome. See *slit-ventricle syndrome.*

chronic overuse. See *overuse syndrome.*

chronic paroxysmal hemicrania. See *Sjaastad syndrome.*

chronic polyserositis. See *Bamberger disease (2), under Bamberger, Heinrich, von.*

chronic postrheumatic arthritis. See *Jaccoud syndrome.*

chronic postrheumatic fever arthropathy. See *Jaccoud syndrome.*

chronic progressive ophthalmoplegia. See *Graefe syndrome.*

chronic progressive subcortical encephalopathy. See *Binswager disease.*

chronic pseudomalignant immunoproliferation. See *Canale-Smith syndrome.*

chronic recurrent acantholysis. See *Hailey-Hailey disease, under Hailey, William Howard.*

chronic serpiginous ulcer. See *Mooren ulcer.*

chronic sinopulmonary infection-infertility syndrome. See *Young syndrome, under Young, Donald.*

chronic subclavian-carotid obstruction syndrome. See *aortic arch syndrome.*

chronic superficial glossitis. See *Möller glossitis.*

chronic suppurative pericementitis. See *Fauchard disease.*

chronic tactile hallucinosis. See *Ekbom syndrome (2).*

chronic vasoconstrictor spots. See *Marshall-White syndrome, under Marshall, Wallace.*

CHRS (cerebrohepatorenal syndrome). See *Zellweger syndrome.*

CHS. See *Chédiak-Higashi syndrome.*

CHS (central hypoventilation syndrome). See *under hypoventilation syndrome.*

CHS (congenital hypoventilation syndrome). See *Ondine curse.*

chubby puffer syndrome. A respiratory disorder in obese prepubescent males, which resembles adult pickwickian syndrome (q.v.), and the symptoms of which have been attributed to primary alveolar hypoventilation.

Hobson, J. A. Sleep and its disorders. In: Wyngaarden, J. B., & Smith, L. H., Jr., eds. *Cecil textbook of medicine.* 17th ed. Philadelphia, Saunders, 1985, pp. 1986-91.

CHURG, JACOB (American physician)

Churg-Strauss syndrome (CSS). Synonyms: *Churg-Strauss vasculitis, Strauss-Churg-Zak syndrome, allergic angiitis and granulomatosis (AAG), allergic granulomtosis, allergic granulomatosis and angiitis (AGA), allergic granulomatous angiitis, allergic granulomatous vasculitis.*

Granulomatous vasculitis of multiple organs, occurring in individuals with an allergic background, characterized by fever, leukocytosis, eosinophilia, and frequent Loeffler-like pulmonary infiltrations. The syndrome is usually associated with cardiac, pulmonary, gastrointestinal, and cutaneous symptoms (nodular, hemorrhagic, and erythema multiforme-like lesions). Typically, it begins with allergic rhinitis, often with nasal polyposis and sinusitis, and asthma. The systemic form resembles polyarteritis nodosa. Severe renal complications are uncommon.

Churg, J., & Strauss, L. Allergic granulomatosis, allergic angiitis, and periarteritis nodosa. *Am. J. Path.,* 1951, 27:277-94.

Churg-Strauss vasculitis. See *Churg-Strauss syndrome.*

Strauss-Churg-Zak syndrome. See *Churg-Strauss syndrome.*

Wegener-Churg-Klinger syndrome. See *Wegener granulomatosis.*

CHURILOV (Russian physician)

Churilov disease. See *hemorrhagic fever with renal syndrome.*

CHUTORIAN, ABE (American physician)

Rosenberg-Chutorian syndrome. See *under Rosenberg, Roger N.*

chylomicronemia syndrome. A condition characterized by plasma triglyceride levels in excess of 2000 mg per deciliter. The symptoms may include abdominal pain, pancreatitis, chest pain, impaired recent memory, paresthesias of the extremities simulating carpal tunnel syndrome, lipemia retinalis, hepatomegaly, splenomegaly, and eruptive xanthomas. Congenital lipoprotein lipase metabolism disorders with faulty plasma triglyceride removal and the interaction of an acquired and a genetic form of hypertriglyceridemia are the common causes. Diabetes mellitus with familial hypertriglyceridemia or familial combined hyperlidemia may be associated.

Brunzell, J. D. The hyperlipoproteinemias. In: Wyngaarden, J. B., & Smith, L. H., Jr., eds. *Cecil textbook of medicine.* 18th ed. Philadelphia, Saunders, 1988, pp. 1137-45.

cicatricial keloid. See *Alibert disease (1).*

cicatricial pemphigoid. See *Brunsting disease.*

ciliary neuralgia. See *Charlin syndrome.*

CINDERELLA (A heroine of a fairy tale, who is oppressed by a malevolent stepmother)

Cinderella complex. An unconscious desire to be taken care of by others, based primarily on a fear of being independent.

Dowling, C. *The Cinderella complex. Women's hidden fear of independence.* New York, Summit Books, 1981. Rodin, A. E., & Key, J. D. *Encyclopedia of medical eponyms derived from literary characters.* Melbourne, Fl., Krieger, 1989.

Cinderella dermatosis. Synonyms: *ashy dermatosis, erythema dyschromicum perstans, dermatosis cinicienta, erythema chromicum figuratum melanodermicum.*

A skin disease characterized by ash-colored macules of various sizes with shading of grayish pigment, usually found on the scalp, palms, and toes. Histologically, the lesions are marked by follicular hyperkeratosis, low melanin levels, vacuolation of epidermal cells, degenerative changes in the basal stratum of the skin, and perivascular infiltrates. The disorder was named after Cinderella who sat by the fireplace in the ashes after finishing her tasks.

Ramirez, C. O. The ashy dermatosis (erythema dyschromicum perstans)-epidemiological study and report of 139 cases. *Cutis,* 1967, 3:244-7. Rodin, A. E., & Key, J. D. *Encyclopedia of medical eponyms derived from literary characters.* Melbourne, Fl., Krieger, 1989.

Cinderella syndrome. False accusation by adopted children of being mistreated or neglected by their adoptive mothers.

Goodwin, J., *et al.* Cinderella syndrome: Children who simulate neglect. *Am. J. Psychiat.,* 1980, 137:1223-5. Rodin, A. E., & Key, J. D. *Encyclopedia of medical eponyms derives from literary characters.* Melbourne, Fl., Krieger, 1989.

Cinderella's stepmother syndrome. Overcompensation by a stepmother in an effort to find acceptance in a new family situation. The presenting clinical picture is similar to that of depressive illness and consists of preoccupation with position in the family, feeling of anxiety, rejection, ineffectiveness, guilt, hostility, exhaustion, and loss of self-esteem.

Morrison, K., & Thompson-Guppy, A. Cinderella's stepmother syndrome. *Canad. J. Psychiat.*, 1985, 30:521-9.

circulatory migraine. See *under headache syndrome.*

circumscribed precancerous melanosis. See *Hutchinson freckle, under Hutchinson, Sir Jonathan.*

circumscribed scleroderma. See *Addison keloid.*

cirrhosis gastroenterorrhagica seu hemorrhagica. See *Maixner cirrhosis.*

cirrhosis of the stomach. See *Brinton disease.*

cirrhosis of young women. See *Waldenström hepatitis, under Waldenström, Jan Gösta.*

cirrhotic gastritis. See *Brinton disease.*

cirrhotic splenomegaly. See *Banti syndrome.*

cisternal block syndrome. See *Zange-Kindler syndrome.*

CITELLI, SALVATORE (Italian physician, 1875-1947)

Citelli syndrome. Loss of the power of concentration and drowsiness or insomnia often associated with intelligence disorders, seen in children with upper respiratory obstruction due to adenoids or paranasal sinus infection.

Citelli, S. Vegetazioni adenoidi e sordomutismo. *Boll. Mal Orecchio Gola Naso,* 1904, 22:141-50.

CIUFFINI

Ciuffini-Pancoast syndrome. See *Pancoast syndrome.*

CIVATTE, ACHILLE (French physician, 1877-1956)

Civatte disease. Synonym: *reticulated pigmented poikiloderma.*

Poikiloderma of the face and neck, affecting most often menopausal women, characterized by an irregular reticulated network of symmetrical patches of pigmented and atrophic lesions which are reddish brown and covered by small scales. It progresses from initial erythema, to edema and pruritus, pigmentation around the hair follicles, dryness of the skin, desquamation, and occasionally, follicular keratosis. The syndrome is considered to be identical with Riehl melanosis. (q.v.).

Civatte, A. Poikilodermie reticulée pigmentaire du visage et du cou. *Ann. Derm. Syph., Paris,* 1923, 4:605-20.

CJD (Creutzfeldt-Jakob disease). See *Jakob-Creutzfeldt syndrome.*

clams. See *Rivalta disease.*

CLARKE, CECIL (British physician)

Clarke-Hadfield syndrome. See *Andersen triad.*

CLARKE, SIR CHARLES MANSFIELD (British physician, 1782-1857)

Clarke ulcer. Ulceration of the neck of the uterus.

Clarke, C. M. *Observations on those diseases of females which are attended by discharges.* London, Longman, 1814-21.

classic hysteria. See *Briquet syndrome (1), under Briquet, Pierre.*

classic polyarteritis nodosa. See *Kussmaul-Maier syndrome.*

classical granulomatosis. See *Wegener granulomatosis.*

CLAUDE, HENRI (French physician, 1869-1945)

Claude syndrome. See *inferior nucleus ruber syndrome.*

Claude-Loyez syndrome. See *inferior nucleus ruber syndrome.*

CLAUDE BERNARD. See BERNARD, CLAUDE

claudicatio intermittens. See *Charcot syndrome (3).*

claudicatio intermittens spinalis. See *Verbiest syndrome.*

claudicatio venosa intermittens. See *Paget-Schroetter syndrome.*

CLAUSEN, J. (Danish physician)

Dyggve-Melchior-Clausen dwarfism. See *Dyggve-Melchior-Clausen syndrome.*

Dyggve-Melchior-Clausen syndrome (DMC, DMCS). See *under Dyggve.*

CLAUSSEN, O. (Norwegian physician)

Mohr-Claussen syndrome. See *orofaciodigital syndrome II.*

clay shoveler disease. See *Schmitt syndrome.*

clay shoveler fracture. See *Schmitt syndrome.*

CLC. See *Clerc-Lévy-Cristesco syndrome.*

cleidocranial digital dysostosis. See *cleidocranial dysostosis.*

cleidocranial dysostosis. Synonyms: *Marie-Sainton syndrome, Scheuthauer-Marie syndrome, Scheuthauer-Marie-Sainton syndrome, cleidocranial dysplasia, cleidocranial digital dysostosis, dysostosis cleidocranialis, dysostosis cleidocraniodigitalis, dysostosis cleidocraniopelvina, dysostosis generalisata, mutational dysostosis, osteodental dysplasia, pelvicocleidocranial dysostosis.*

A syndrome inherited as an autosomal dominant trait, marked by aplasia or hypoplasia of the clavicle with a remarkable range of shoulder movements and delayed ossification of the skull with excessively large fontanels and delayed closing of the sutures. The fontanels may remain open until adulthood, but the sutures often close with interposition of wormian bones. Large bosses of the frontal, parietal, and occipital regions give the skull a large globular shape with a small face. Other abnormalities may include hypoplasia of the facial bones, absence of paranasal sinuses, high-arched palate, cleft palate, hip dislocation, underdeveloped pelvis, and various osseous defects. The maxilla is smaller than normal in relation to the mandible. The lacrimal and zygomatic bones may be hypoplastic. Delayed tooth eruption, short, thin and deformed roots, absence of cementum on the roots of permanent teeth, and the presence of unerupted supernumerary teeth are usually associated. Less frequently occurring defects include funnel chest, narrow pelvis, abnormal gait, joint hypermobility, muscle hypotonia, short distal phalanges, and hypoplastic nails.

Marie, P., & Sainton, R. Observation d'hydrocéphalie héréditaire (père et fils), par vice de dévelopment du crâne et du cerveau. *Bull. Mem. Soc. Méd. Hôp. Paris*, 1897, 14:706-12. Scheuthauer, G. Kombination rudimentarer Schulselbeine mit Anomalien des Schädels bei erwachsenen Menschen. *Allg. Wien. Med. Ztg.*, 1871, 16:293-5.

cleidocranial dysplasia. See cleidocranial dysostosis.

CLEJAT, CHARLES PHILIPPE ANTOINE (French physician, born 1880)

Petges-Cléjat syndrome. See *under Petges.*

CLEMENT

Müller-Ribbing-Clément syndrome. See *multiple epiphyseal dysplasia I.*

CLERAMBAULT, GAETAN HENRI ALFRED EDOUARD LEON MARIE GATIAN, DE (French psychiatrist, 1872-1934)

Clérambault syndrome. Synonyms: *de Clérambault syndrome, Simenon syndrome, erotic delusion, erotomania, paranoia erotica, psychose passionelle.*

A condition in which a woman has delusions that a man, usually of a higher social and economic status, is madly in love with her, sometimes resulting in pursuing, even harassing, the unsuspecting object of her fantasies. The delusion usually concerns idealized love rather than sexual attraction.

Clérambault, G. G. Les psychoses passionelles. In his: *Oevre psychiatrique.* Paris, Presses Universitaires de France, 1942. Simenon, G. Monsieur Lundi. In his: *Nouvelle enquêtes de Maigret.* Paris, Presses Univ. de France, 1944.

Kandinskii-Clérambault complex. See *Kandinskii-Clérambault syndrome.*

Kandinskii-Clérambault syndrome. See *under Kandinskii.*

CLERC, ANTONIN (French physician, 1871-1954)

Clerc-Lévy-Cristesco (CLC) syndrome. Synonyms: *Lown-Ganong-Levine syndrome, short PR-normal QRS syndrome.*

A combination of short P-R interval and normal QRS complex on the electrotrocardiogram in paroxysmal tachycardia.

Lown, B., Ganong, W. F., & Levine, S. A. The syndrome of short P-R interval, normal QRS complex and paroxysmal rapid heart action. *Circulation,* 1952, 5:693-706. Clerc, A., Lévy, R., & Cristesco, C. A. A propos du raccourcissement permanent de l'espace P-R de l'électrocardiogramme sans déformation du complexe ventriculaire. *Arch. Mal. Coeur,* 1938, 31:569-82.

CLERET, M. (French physician)

Launois-Cléret syndrome. See *Fröhlich syndrome, under Fröhlich, Alfred.*

click syndrome. See *mitral valve prolapse syndrome.*

click-murmur syndrome. See *mitral valve prolapse syndrome.*

clicking rib syndrome. See *slipping rib syndrome.*

CLIFFORD, STEWART HILTON (American physician, born 1900)

Clifford syndrome. See *Ballantyne-Runge syndrome.*

climacteric keratosis. See *Haxthausen syndrome.*

climacteric keratosis palmaris et plantaris. See *Haxthausen syndrome.*

climacteric syndrome (CS). Synonym: *menopasual syndrome.*

A complex of symptoms experienced by menopausal women, including hot flushes, cold sweats, weight gain, flooding, arthritic pains, headache, cold hands and feet, numbness and tingling, sore breasts, constipation, diarrhea, paresthesia, tiredness, arrhythmias, dizziness, scotoma, irritability, depression, excitability, forgetfulness, sleep disorders, concentration difficulty, feeling of suffocation, and anxiety.

Greene, J. G. *The social and psychological origins of the climacteric syndrome.* Aldershot, Gower, 1984. 247 pp.

climatic bubo. See *Durand-Nicolas-Favre disease, under Durand, J.*

climatic droplet keratopathy. See *Bietti dystrophy.*

climatic droplet keratopathy (CDK). See *Bietti dystrophy.*

clinomicrodactyly. See *brachydactyly A-3.*

CLODIUS, LEO (American physician)

Walker-Clodius syndrome. See *EEC syndrome.*

CLOQUET, JULES GERMAIN (French physician, 1790-1883)

Cloquet hernia. Synonyms: *crural hernia, femoral hernia.*

Hernia of the femoral canal.

*Cloquet, J. G. *Recherches anatomiques sur les hernies de l'abdomen.* Paris, 1817 (Thesis).

CLOSS, KARL (Norwegian physician)

Danbolt-Closs syndrome. See *acrodermatitis enteropathica.*

cloudy central corneal dystrophy. See *François dystrophy (1).*

CLOUGH, MILDRED C. (American hematologist)

Clough-Richter syndrome. See *cryopathic hemolytic syndrome.*

CLOUSTON, H. R. (Canadian physician)

Clouston syndrome. Synonym: *hidrotic ectodermal dysplasia.*

A syndrome of dyskeratosis of the palms and soles, hypoplasia or dysplasia of the nails, hypotrichosis or alopecia, strabismus, and skin hyperpigmentation, especially over the knuckles, elbows, areaolae, axillae, and pubic area. Short stature, mental deficiency, and cataracts may be associated. The syndrome is transmitted as an autosomal dominant trait.

Clouston, H. R. The major forms of hereditary ectodermal dysplasia (with an autopsy and biopsies on the anhidrotic type). *Canad. Med. Assoc. J.,* 1939, 40:1-7. Clouston, H. R. A hereditary ectodermal dystrophy. *Canad. Med. Assoc. J.,* 1929, 21:18-31.

cloverleaf skull. See *Holtermüller-Wiedemann syndrome.*

CLP (cleft lip and palate)-lip pits syndrome. See *van der Woude syndrome.*

CLS. See *Coffin-Lowry syndrome.*

CLS (Cornelia de Lange syndrome). See *de Lange syndrome (1), under Lange, Cornelia, de.*

clubbed fingers. See *Marie-Bamberger syndrome, under Marie, Pierre.*

cluster headache. See *Horton neuralgia.*

CLUTTON, HENRY HUGH (British physician, 1850-1909)

Clutton joint. See *Clutton syndrome.*

Clutton syndrome. Synonym: *Clutton joint.*

Painless symmetrical hydrathrosis, especially of the knee joint, in congenital syphilis.

Clutton, H. H. Symmetrical synovitis of the knee in hereditary syphilis. *Lancet,* 1886, 1:391-3.

clyers. See *Rivalta disease.*

CMTC (cutis marmorata teleangiectatica congenita). See *Lohuizen disease.*

CMTD (Charcot-Marie-Tooth disease). See *Charcot-Marie-Tooth syndrome.*

CMTS. See *Charcot-Marie-Tooth syndrome.*

CNDC (chronic nonsuppurative destructive cholangitis). See *primary biliary cirrhosis syndrome.*

coastal erysipelas. See *Robles disease.*

COATS, GEORGE (British ophthalmologist, 1876-1915)

Coats retinitis. See *Coats syndrome.*

Coats ring. A white ring of lipoid material in Bowman's membrane of the cornea, below the epithelium.

*Coats, G. Forms of retinal disease with massive exudation. *Ophth. Hosp. Rep.,* 1908, 17:440-525.

Coats syndrome. Synonyms: *Coats retinitis, exudative*

retinitis, exudative retinopathy, retinal telangiectasia, retinitis hemorrhagica externa.

A disease occurring predominantly in male children, characterized by exudative retinitis and telangiectasias of the retina, conjuctiva, face, nail beds, and breasts. There is retinal hemorrhage and slow progression to retinal detachment, cataract, atrophy, or glaucoma. The pathological findings include retinal hemorrhage penetrating into the subretinal space; subretinal fibrous tissue; cystic retinal degeneration; vascular anomalies, such as dilation, hyaline thickening, endothelial proliferation, and thrombosis; and subretinal accumulation of foam cells.

*Coats, G. Forms of retinal disease with massive exudation. *Ophth. Hosp. Rep.*, 1908, 17:440-525.

COBB, STANLEY (American physician)

Cobb syndrome. Synonyms: *cutaneomeningospinal angiomatosis, metameric angiomatosis, segmental skin hemangioma-spinal meninges hemangioma syndrome.*

Segmental cutaneous hemangioma of the thorax associated with hemangioma of the spinal meninges in corresponding segments. Symptoms of spinal cord compression, vertebral or renal angiomas, and kyphoscoliosis may occur.

Cobb, S. Haemangioma of the spinal cord associated with skin naevi at the same metamere. *Ann. Surg.*, 1915, 62:641-9.

Coca-Cola baby. See *fetal PCB syndrome.*

cocaine body packer syndrome. See *body packer syndrome.*

coccogenous sycosis. See *Alibert disease (3).*

coccygodynia. See *levator syndrome.*

cochlear hydrops. See *Ménière syndrome.*

COCKAYNE, EDWARD ALFRED (British physician, 1880-1956)

Cockayne syndrome (CS). Synonyms: *Neill-Dingwall syndrome, progeria-like syndrome, progeroid nanism.*

An autosomal recessively inherited syndrome characterized by dwarfism, kyphosis, ankylosis, disproportionately long extremities with large hands and feet, cold blue extremities, mental deficiency, hypersensitivity of the skin to sunlight with pigmentation and scarring, retinal pigmentary degeneration, optic atrophy, cataract, partial deafness, unsteady gait, thickened skull, dental caries appearing during the second year of life after an apparently normal infancy, lack of subcutaneous fat of the face, prognathism, sunken eyes, and thin nose giving the patient a prematurely old appearance. Associated disorders may include joint movement limitation, flattening of the vertebrae, hepatomegaly, albuminuria, intracranial calcification, marble epiphyses in digits, and short second toes. Death may be due to atherosclerosis.

Cockayne, E. A. Dwarfism with retinal atrophy and deafness. *Arch. Dis. Child.*, 1946, 21:52. Cockayne, E. A. Dwarfism with retinal atrophy and deafness. *Arch. Dis. Child.*, 1936, 11:148. Neill, C. & Dingwall, M. M. A syndrome resembling progeria. A review of two cases. *Arch. Dis. Child.*, 1950, 25:213-21.

Cockayne-Touraine syndrome. See *epidermolysis bullosa syndrome.*

Weber-Cockayne syndrome. See *epidermolysis bullosa syndrome.*

COCKETT, F. B. (British physician)

Cockett syndrome. Synonym: *iliac vein compression.*

Compression of the iliac vein by the iliac artery at the pelvic inlet level, leading to thrombosis and lower limb dysfunction.

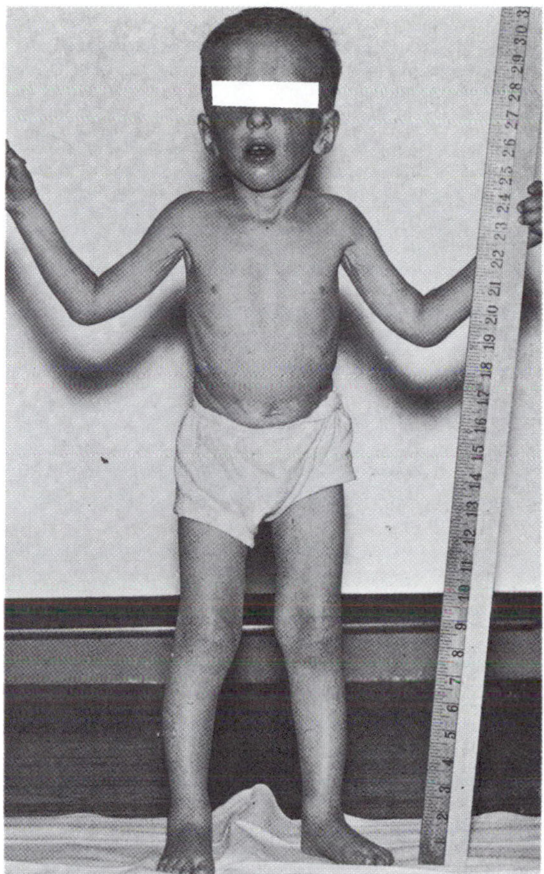

Cockayne syndrome
Windmiller, J. *Am. J. Dis. Child*, 105:204, 1963.

Cockett, F. B., *et al.* Iliac vein compression. Its relation to iliofemoral thrombosis and post thrombotic syndrome. *Brit. Med. J.*, 1967, 2:14-9.

cocktail party syndrome. A language disorder in mentally retarded but educable children who have the ability to learn words and to talk, without knowing what they are talking about. They love to chatter, but think illogically.

Tew, B. The "cocktail party syndrome" in children with hydrocephalus and spina bifida. *Brit. J. Disord. Communication*, 1979, 14:89-101.

COD-MD (**c**erebro-**o**cular **d**ysplasia-**m**uscular**d**ystrophy) syndrome. See *cerebro-oculomuscular syndrome.*

CODMAN, ERNEST AMORY (American physician, 1869-1940)

Codman tumor. Synonyms: *benign chondroblastoma, calcifying giant-cell tumor, cartilage-containing giant-cell tumor, chondromatous giant-cell tumor.*

A benign tumor of the cartilage and cartilage-forming connective tissue, usually affecting the femur, tibia, and humerus, and, less frequently, the pelvic bones, hands, and feet. Foci of necrosis and calcification with the presence of round or polyhedral cells and giant multinucleated cells are the principal pathological features. The lesions, which seldom undergo malignant degeneration, are usually observed in adolescent and young adult males.

Codman, E. A. Epiphyseal chondromatous giant cell tumors of the upper end of the humerus. *Surg. Gyn. Obst.*, 1931, 32:543-8.

COFFIN, GRANGE S. (American physician)

Coffin syndrome (1). See *Coffin-Lowry syndrome.*

Coffin syndrome (2). Synonym: *lean spastic dwarfism.*

A familial syndrome of unknown etiology characterized by retarded growth, mental retardation, slender habitus, joint laxity, spastic tetraplegia, convulsions, predisposition to infections, retarded bone age, and characteristic facies with prominent eyes and forehead, infantile lips, and low-set simplified external ears. Cleft palate and tetralogy of Fallot occur in some cases.

Coffin, G. S. A syndrome of retarded development with characteristic appearance. *Am. J. Dis. Child.*, 1968, 115: 698-702.

Coffin-Lowry syndrome (CLS). Synonyms: *Coffin syndrome, Coffin-Siris-Wegienka syndrome, soft hands syndrome.*

A familial syndrome of mental and growth deficiency, pectus carinatum, lax ligaments, vertebral anomalies, and peculiar facies characterized by frontal bossing, hypertelorism, antimongoloid palpebral fissures, maxillary hypoplasia, mandibular prognathism, thick nasal septum, bulbous nose, large low-set ears, and crowded teeth. Thoracolumbar scoliosis and anterior superior vertebral defects are the principal spinal anomalies. Large soft hands with tapering fingers, tufted drumstick and short distal phalanges and flat feet characterize limb abnormalities. Occasional defects include thick calvarium, hypoplastic sinuses, and simian creases. X-linked semidominant inheritance is suspected.

Coffin, G. S., Siris, E., & Wegienka, L. C. Mental retardation with osteocartilaginous anomalies. *Am. J. Dis. Child.*, 1966, ll2:205-13. Lowry, B., *et al.* A new dominant gene mental retardation syndrome. *Am. J. Dis. Child.*, 1971, 121:496-500.

Coffin-Siris syndrome. Synonyms: *dwarfism-onychodysplasia syndrome, fifth digit syndrome.*

Mental and growth deficiency, nail hypoplasia or absence (usually of the fifth finger or toes), short distal phalanges, hypotonia, feeding difficulty during infancy, and coarse facies (bushy eyebrows, long eyelashes, scant scalp hair, full lips, microcephaly) are the principal features of this syndrome. Occassional abnormalities include congenital heart defects, small patella, coxa valga, lax joints, radial dislocation, blepharoptosis, hypotelorism, preauricular skin tags, hemangioma, cryptorchism, hernia, short sternum, short forearm, vertebral anomalies, cleft palate, and the Dandy-Walker anomaly. Most reported cases have been sporadic.

Coffin, G. S., & Siris, E. Mental retardation with absent fingernail and terminal phalanx. *Am. J. Dis. Child.*, 1970, 119:433-9.

Coffin-Siris-Wegienka syndrome. See *Coffin-Lowry syndrome.*

COFS. See *cerebro-oculofacioskeletal syndrome.*

COGAN, DAVID GLENDENNING (American ophthalmologist, born 1908)

Bielschowsky-Lutz-Cogan syndrome. See *under Bielschowsky, Alfred.*

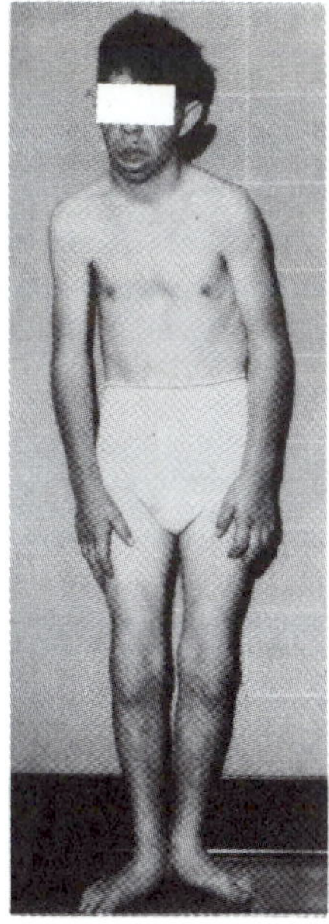

Coffin-Lowry syndrome
Courtsey of S. Myhre, Rainier Training School, Buckley, Washington.

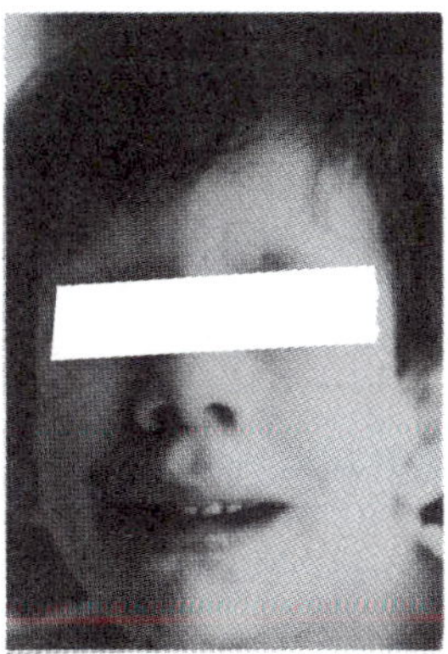

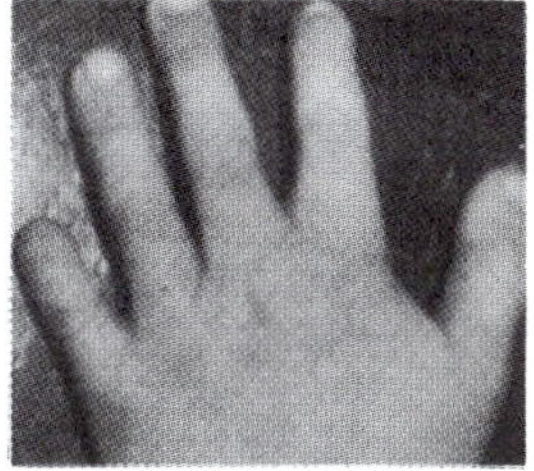

Coffin-Siris syndrome
Coffin, G.S. & Siris, E.: *American Journal of Disease of Children,* 119:433, 1970, Chicago, IL.

Cogan dystrophy. Synonyms: *maplike epithelial dystrophy, microcystic dystrophy of the corneal epithelium, microscopic cystic epithelial dystrophy.*

Maplike corneal dystrophy characterized by grayish white, discrete, but sometimes confluent spheres measuring usually 0.1 to 0.5 mm in diameter and situated in the superficial portion of the cornea. The larger opacities may be comma-shaped or irregular, up to 1 mm in length. They are most common in the pupillary areas, where they may cause slight reduction in visual acuity. The surface of the cornea is usually smooth; rarely does the condition show evidence of exfoliation or give rise to foreign body sensation. The disorder occurs spontaneously and symmetrically in both eyes, and the opacities appear and disappear spontaneously without residual scarring. Histological examination shows microcysts within the epithelium. In the original report, the patients were five adult women in otherwise good health.

Cogan, D. G., *et al.* Microcystic dystrophy of the corneal epithelium. *Tr. Am. Ophth. Soc.*, 1964, 62:213-25.

Cogan syndrome (1). Synonyms: *keratitis-deafness syndrome, nonsyphilitic interstitial keratitis.*

Interstitial keratitis associated with vestibuloauditory symptoms. The disease is characterized by the abrupt onset of vertigo, tinnitus, and deafness, with pain in the eyes, ciliary injection, and reduced vision. The vertigo subsides, usually as total deafness supervenes. The ocular signs are characterized by patchy infiltration of the deep corneal stroma with minimal intraocular reaction.

Cogan, D. G. Syndrome of nonsyphilitic interstitial keratitis and vestibuloauditory symptoms. *Arch. Ophth., Chicago*, 1945, 33:144-9.

Cogan syndrome (2). Synonyms: *congenital oculomotor apraxia syndrome, conjugate gaze paralysis syndrome.*

A presumably congenital form of oculomotor apraxia (probably transmitted as an autosomal recessive trait) in which there is an absence of voluntary movement of the eyes side-to-side, although full random movements may be retained , and in which fixation of gaze is accomplished by jerky spasmodic compensatory overshooting of the head. Rotation of the head results in an involuntary and maintained deviation in the direction opposite to that of rotation.

Cogan, D. G. A type of congenital ocular motor apraxia presenting jerky head movements. *Am. J. Ophth.*, 1953, 36:433-41.

Cogan-Reese syndrome. A syndrome of unilateral glaucoma in the eyes with multiple anterior synechiae, multiple nodules of the iris, and ectopic Desmecet membrane. Associated disorders may include corneal edema, stromal iris atrophy, iris pigment epithelial atrophy, ectropion uveae, and ectopic pupil.

Cogan, D. G., & Reese, A. B. A syndrome of iris nodules, ectopic Descemets membrane, and unilateral glaucoma. *Documenta Ophth.*, 1969, 26:424-33.

COHEN, M. MICHAEL, JR. (American oral pathologist)

Cohen syndrome. Facial, oral, ocular, and spinal abnormalities associated with hypotonia, mental deficiency, and obesity. Orofacial anomalies consist mainly of microcephaly, antimongoloid palpebral slant, maxillary hypoplasia, short philtrum, open mouth, prominent maxillary incisors, micrognathia, high-arched palate, and crowded teeth. Mottled retina, strabismus, myopia, microphthalmia, and coloboma are the principal ocular features. The feet and hands are narrow, with cubitus valgus, genua valga, hyperextensible joints, simian creases, shortening of metacarpals and metatarsals, and some instances of syndactyly. Lumbar lordosis and thoracic scoliosis are associated. The patients are obese, hypotonic, and mentally deficient. The condition is probably inherited as an autosomal recessive trait.

Cohen, M. M., Jr., *et al.* A new syndrome with hypotonia, obesity, mental deficiency, and facial, oral, ocular, and limb anomalies. *J. Pediat.*, 1973, 83:280-4.

Gorlin-Cohen syndrome. See *frontometaphyseal dysplasia.*

COHN, MAX (German physician)

Pyle-Cohn syndrome. See *metaphyseal dysplasia syndrome.*

COIF (**c**ongenital **o**nychodysplasia of the **i**ndex **f**inger) syndrome. See *Iso-Kikuchi syndrome.*

Cola baby. See *fetal PCB syndrome.*

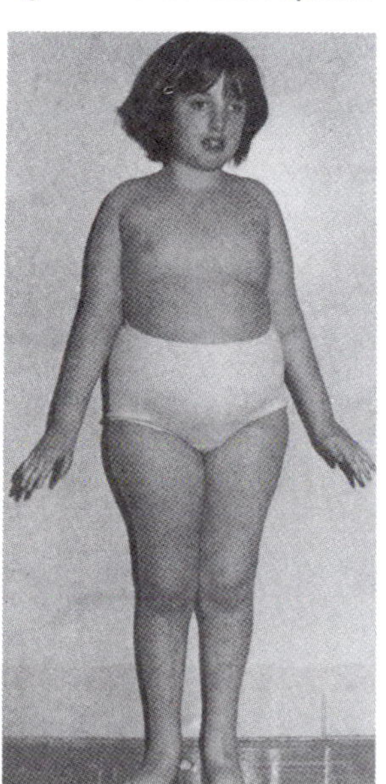

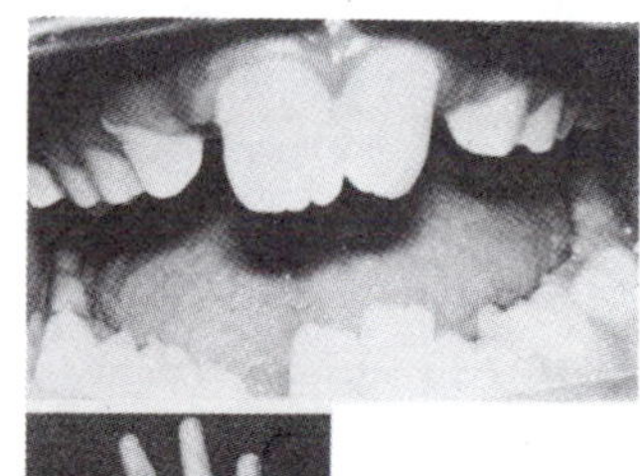

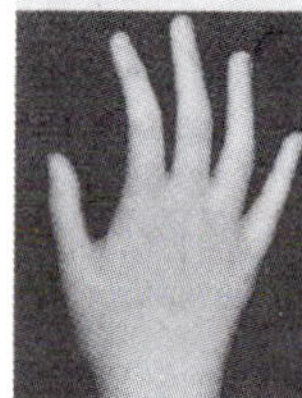

Cohen syndrome
Cohen, M.M., Jr.: *J. Pediatr.*, 83:280, 1973. St. Louis, C.V. Mosby Co.

cold agglutinin disease. See *cryopathic hemolytic syndrome.*

cold agglutinin syndrome. See *cryopathic hemolytic syndrome.*

cold hemagglutinin syndrome. See *cryopathic hemolytic syndrome.*

cold hypersensitivity syndrome. See *familial cold urticaria syndrome.*

cold panniculitis. See *Haxthausen panniculitis.*

cold urticaria syndrome. See *acquired cold urticaria syndrome.*

COLE, HAROLD NEWTON (American dermatologist, 1884-1966)

Cole syndrome. See *Zinsser-Engman-Cole syndrome.*

Cole-Rauschkolb-Toomey syndrome. See *Zinsser-Engman-Cole syndrome.*

Zinsser-Engman-Cole syndrome. See *under Zinsser.*

COLEMAN, CLAUDE C. (American physician, 1879-1953)

Coleman syndrome. Synonyms: *Coleman-Meredith syndrome, occipital-cervical-shoulder girdle syndrome, post-traumatic occipital-cervical shoulder girdle syndrome.*

Injury of the cervical spine associated with injuries of the head and shoulder.

Coleman, C. C., & Meredith, J. M. Treatment of fracture-dislocation of the spine associated with cord injury. *JAMA*, 1938, 111:2168-72.

Coleman-Meredith syndrome. See *Coleman syndrome.*

colibacillose gravidique. See *Bar syndrome.*

COLINET, E. (Belgian physician)

Caplan-Colinet syndrome. See *Caplan syndrome.*

COLLES, ABRAHAM (Irish physician, 1773-1843)

Colles fracture. Fracture of the lower end of the radius with posterior displacement of the lower fragment. Complications may include residual deformity, loss of mobility, median and ulnar nerve injury, shoulder-hand syndrome, and rupture of the extensor pollicis longus tendon. This injury is encountered in patients of either sex and in all age groups, but it is most common in postmenopausal women, osteoporosis being the predisposing factor.

Colles, A. On the fracture of the carpal extremity of the radius. *Edinburgh Med. Surg. J.*, 1814, 10:182-6.

reverse Colles fracture. See *Smith fracture, under Smith, Robert William.*

COLLET, FREDERIC JUSTIN (French physician, born 1870)

Collet syndrome. See *Collet-Sicard syndrome.*

Collet-Sicard syndrome. Synonyms: *Collet syndrome, Sicard syndrome, glossolaryngoscapulopharyngeal hemiplegia, lacerocondylar space syndrome, pharyngolaryngeal paralysis syndrome, posterior intercondylar space syndrome.*

A variant of the Villaret syndrome (q.v.), unaccompanied by the Horner syndrome, in which involvement of the ninth, tenth, eleventh, and twelfth cranial nerves produces paralysis of the vocal cords, palate, trapezius muscle, and sternocleidomastoid muscle; secondary loss of the sense of taste in the back of the tongue; and anesthesia of the larynx, pharynx, and soft palate.

Collet, Sur un nouveau syndrome paralytique pharyngo-laryngé par blesure du guerre (hémiplegie glosso-laryngo-scapulo-pharyngée). *Lyon Méd.* 1915, 124:121-9. Sicard, J. A. Syndrome du carrefour condylo-déchiré postérieur (type pur de paralysie de quatre derniers nerfs craniens). *Marseilles Méd.*, 1917, pp. 385-97.

COLLIER, JAMES STANSFIELD (British physician, 1870-1935)

Collier syndrome. Synonym: *orbital periostitis.*

Orbital periostitis or fibrosis associated with unilateral orbital pain, slight proptosis, tenderness over the eyeball, and paralysis of the first, fourth, and third cranial nerves and the first and second division of the sensory component of the fifth cranial nerve.

Cheah, J. S., & Ransome, G. A. Collier's syndrome (orbital periostitis). *Med. J. Australia*, 1970, 1:277-8.

COLLINS, EDWARD TREACHER (British physician, 1862-1919)

Berry-Treacher Collins syndrome. See *mandibulofacial dysostosis.*

Treacher Collins syndrome. See *mandibulofacial dysostosis.*

collodion baby. See *Carini syndrome.*

collodion skin. See *Carini syndrome.*

coloboma-anal atresia syndrome. See *cat eye syndrome.*

colonic aganglíosis. See *Hirschsprung syndrome.*

colonic inertia-rectal obstruction syndrome. See *Lane syndrome, under Lane, Sir William Arbuthnot.*

colonic neurosis. See *irritable bowel syndrome.*

colonic polyposis-malignant central nervous system tumor syndrome. See *Turcot syndrome.*

colonic pseudo-obstruction. See *Ogilvie syndrome.*

columnar-lined esophagus. See *Barrett syndrome.*

coma vigile. See *apallic syndrome.*

combat fatigue. See *post-traumatic stress syndrome.*

COMBS, J. T. (American physician)

Wiedemann-Beckwith-Combs syndrome. See *Beckwith-Wiedemann syndrome.*

COMEL, M. (Italian physician)

Comèl acrorhigosis. Synonym: *acrorhigosis and microangiopathic syndrome.*

Acral hypothermia of the extremities due to a vascular disorder, with a sensation of having on a "cold stocking" or "cold glove," reported by Comèl at the International Congress of Dermatology in Budapest in 1935.

Mian, E. U. Akrorhigose und mikroangiopatische Syndrome (Angiolopathien). *Zbl. Phleb.*, 1966, 4:182-4.

Rille-Comèl disease. See *under Rille.*

COMLY, HUNTER HALL (American physician, born 1919)

Comly syndrome. Synonym: *well-water methemoglobinemia.*

Methemoglobinemia caused by drinking water from a well containing high concentrations of nitrates, sometimes occurring in infants fed formulas prepared with such water. When ingested, nitrates are converted by bacteria to nitrites, the nitrite ion being absorbed into the blood and oxidizing hemoglobin to methemoglobin. Except for cyanosis and chocolate brown blood, the condition is usually asymptomatic. However, in severe cases in which methemoglobin concentrations are greater than 60 to 70 %, there may be collapse, coma, and death.

Comly, H. H. Cyanosis in infants caused by nitrates in well water. *JAMA*, 1945, 129:112-6.

command automatism. See *Kandinskii-Clérambault syndrome.*

commissural syndrome. See *under disconnection syndrome.*

common cold syndrome. Synonym: *acute coryza.*

A general term for a symptom complex of a viral infection of the upper respiratory tract, marked by congestion of the nasal mucosa, profuse nasal discharge, sneezing, sore or dry throat, malaise, postnasal discharge, headache, cough, feverishness, chilliness, burning eyes, and muscle aching. Fever is usually absent. Rhinoviruses comprise the largest single etiologic group, but picornaviruses, enteroviruses (poliovirus, coxsackievirus, and echovirus), influenza and parainfluenza, and other viruses are sometimes associated. The terms **catarrhal rhinitis, chest cold, head cold, laryngitis,** and **pharyngitis** are sometimes used to designate the principal anatomic sites of infection.

Kapikian, A. Z. The common cold. In: Wyngaarden, J. B., & Smith, L. H., Jr., eds. *Cecil textbook of medicine.* 17th ed. Philadelphia, Saunders, 1985, pp. 1691-5.

commotio retinae. See *Berlin disease (1), under Berlin, Rudolf.*

compartment syndrome. Synonyms: *Volkmann ischemia, anterior tibial syndrome, calf hypertension, compartmental syndrome, exercise ischemia, exercise myopathy, impending ischemic contracture, medial tibial syndrome, muscle compartment syndrome, rhabdomyosis, traumatic tension ischemia in muscles, vascular compartment syndrome.*

A vascular disorder in which increased pressure within a limited space compromises the circulation and function of tissues within that space, marked by the presence of a limiting envelope within which increased pressure produces reduced circulation that results in abnormalities of neuromuscular function. Common locations include the arm (deltoid and biceps muscles), forearm (dorsal and volar areas), hand (interosseous muscle), buttocks (gluteal muscle), thigh (quadriceps muscle), and leg (anterior, lateral, superficial posterior, and deep posterior areas). Compartment syndrome may occur after the use of medical antishock trousers (MAST) in injuries of lower extremities, when it is called the **MAST-associated compartment syndrome (MACS).** See also *Volkmann contracture.*

Volkmann, R., von. Die ischämischen Muskellähmungen und Kontrakturen. *Zbl. Chir.*, 1881, 8:801-3. Matsen, F. A., III. *Compartmental syndromes.* New York, Grune & Stratton, 1980, 162 pp. Aprahamian, C., *et al.* MAST-associated compartment syndrome: A review. *J. Trauma,* 1989, 29:549-55.

compartmental syndrome. See *compartment syndrome.*

compensatory nystagmus. See *Bechterew nystagmus, under Bekhterev, Vladimir Mikhailovich.*

complete dextroposition of the aorta. See *Taussig-Bing syndrome.*

complete heart block. See *Adams-Stokes syndrome, under Adams, Robert.*

complete transposition of the aorta and levoposition of the pulmonary artery. See *Taussig-Bing syndrome.*

compound Hurler-Scheie disease. See *mucopolysaccharidosis I-H/S.*

compression neuropathy of the lower limb. See *wasted leg syndrome.*

compression syndrome. See *crush syndrome.*

compulsive binge eating. See *bulimia syndrome.*

compulsive tic. See *Gilles de la Tourette syndrome.*

COMS. See *cerebro-oculomuscular syndrome.*

CONCATO, LUIGI MARIA (Italian physician, 1825-1882)

Concato disease. Tuberculous inflammation of the serous membranes.

Concato, L. M. Sulla poliorromennite scrofolosa o tisi dell sierose. *Gior. Ingern, Sc. Med., Napoli,* 1881, 3:1037-53.

concentration camp survivor syndrome. Synonyms: *concentration camp syndrome, KZ (Konzentrationslager) syndrome, survivor syndrome.*

A form of the post-traumatic stress syndrome (q.v.) in persons who have survived persecution, starvation, torture, and other forms of abuse in concentration camps. The symptoms include recurrent and intrusive recollection of the event or series of events; recurrent dreams of the event; a sense or reliving the experience, including hallucinations, illusions, or flashbacks; distress on exposure to situations which may symbolize the event or bring back the memories of it; efforts to avoid thoughts of traumatic experiences; psychogenic amnesia; diminished interest in current activities; feeling of estrangement from the society; inability to develop loving relationships; lack of interest in the future; sleep disorders; difficulty in expressing feelings of anger; difficulty in concentrating; hypervigilance; exaggerated startle response; and abnormal physiological reactions to situations or objects that resemble or symbolize the traumatic experience.

Niederland, W. G. The problem of the survivor. *J. Hillside Hosp.*, 1961, 10:233-47. *Diagnostic and statistical manual of mental disorders.* 3rd ed. Washington, American Psychiatric Association, 1987, pp. 247-50.

concentration camp syndrome. See *concentration camp survivor syndrome.*

concentric sclerosis. See *Baló syndrome.*

condensing disseminated osteopathy. See *Albers-Schönberg syndrome.*

conditioned hyperirritability and para-allergy. See *excited skin syndrome.*

CONDORELLI, LUIGI (Italian physician)

Condorelli disease. A condition characterized by acro-osteodystrophy, amenorrhea, and parathyroid disorders.

Condorelli, L. L'acro-steo-distrofia ipogenitalica da disparatiroidismo. *Clin. Nuova,* 1945, 1:15-24.

conductive deafness-stapes fixation syndrome. See *Nance syndrome.*

condylomatosis pemphigoides maligna. See *Neumann syndrome (2), under Neumann, Isidor Elder von Heilwart.*

cone-shaped epiphyses-nephropathy-retinitis pigmentosa syndrome. A familial syndrome of cone epiphyses of the middle phalanges of the hands and feet, nephrophthisis, retinitis pigmentosa, and cerebellar ataxia. Additional defects include flattened capital femoral epiphyses, wide femoral neck, and sclerosis of the metaphyses.

Meier, D. A., *et al.* Familial nephropathy with retinitis pigmentosa: A new oculorenal syndrome in adults. *Am. J. Med.*, 1965, 39:58. Saldino, R. M., *et al.* Cone-shaped epiphyses (CSE) in siblings with hereditary renal disease and retinitis pigmentosa. *Radiology,* 1971, 98:39.

confluent and reticulated papillomatosis. See *Gougerot-Carteaud syndrome, under Gougerot, Henri.*

confusocatatonia. See *Bell mania, under Bell, Luther Vos.*

congenital abducens-facial paralysis. See *Moebius syndrome (1).*

congenital abduction deficiency (CAD). See *Stilling-Türk-Duane syndrome.*

congenital acromicria syndrome. See *chromosome 21 trisomy syndrome.*

congenital adrenal hyperplasia (CAH). Synonyms: *Debré-Fibiger syndrome, de Crecchio syndrome, Fibiger-Debré-von Gierke syndrome, Gallais syndrome, Pirie syndrome, Wilkins disease, adrenal virilizing syndrome, adrenogenital syndrome (AGS), female pseudohermaphroditism, 21-hydroxylase deficiency syndrome (21-OHD syndrome), macrogenitosomia praecox, pseudosexual precocity, salt losing syndrome, suprarenal genital syndrome, suprarenal pseudohermaphroditism-virilism-hirsutism syndrome, virilizing adrenocrotical hyperplasia.*

An inborn error of metabolism, characterized by a deficiency of enzymes involved in the production of adrenocorticosteroid hormones, chiefly cortisol and aldosterone, and hormone precursors, such as deoxycorticosterone and androgens, in asssociation with adrenal hyperplasia. Three principal biochemically distinct types are recognized: (1) The **virilizing type** is the most common and is caused by 21-hydroxylase deficiency, occurring as hypertensive or nonhypertensive subtypes. (2) **Mixed adrenal hyperplasia** caused by 3-hydroxysteroid hydrogenase deficiency, usually occurring as a salt-losing subtype (see also *renal salt losing syndrome.*) (3) **Nonvirilizing adrenal hyperplasia** caused by 17-hydroxylase deficiency (occuring as a hypertensive type), 20,22-desmolase deficiency (occuring often as a salt-losing subtype), and 17,20-desmolase deficiency. In females, excessive secretion of androgens results in virilism, which becomes apparent at birth. Associated disorders include masculinization of the external genitalia, hypertrophy of the clitoris, and its ventral binding with fusion of the labioscrotal folds conceals the introitus, giving affected girls the appearance of males with bilateral cryptorchism and hypospadias; because of labioscrotal fusion, the urethra resembles a phallus. This form is sometimes referred to as **female pseudohermaphroditism.** Hirsutism, seborrhea, clitoral enlargement, and deepening of the voice appear later in life. Failure of normal sexual development and menstruation are usually noted at puberty. In males, the symptoms include rapid development of the penis and sexual characteristics, accelerated growth, acne, deepening of the voice, frequent erections, and excessive muscular development, but the testes remain infantile and affected males are sterile. This type is sometimes referred to as **macrogenitosomia praecox** and **pseudosexual precocity.** In both sexes, early rapid growth and somatic maturation are associated with premature epiphyseal maturation and closure of the epiphyses, resulting in paradoxical dwarfism in adults who were tall for their ages as children. In the classic form, virilization begins in the second month of gestational life; in the nonclassic form, it begins after birth. Salt wasting is a feature in the classical form. Levels of precursor hormones are less markedly elevated in nonclassical than in the classical type. All forms are transmitted as an autosomal recessive trait. Some synonyms of this syndrome are also used to designate the Cushing syndrome.

*de Crecchio, L. *Sopra un caso di apparenze virili in una donna.* II. Morgagni, 1865, 7, 151. *Gallais, A. *Le syndrome génito-surrénal; étude anatomo-clinique,* 1912 (Thesis). Debré, R., & Semelaigne, G. Hypertrophie considerable des capsules surrénales chez un nourrisson mort a 10 mois sans avoir augmenté de poids depuis sa naissance. *Bull. Soc. Pediat, Paris,* 1925, 23:270-1. Fibiger, J. Beitrage zur Kenntnis des weiblichen Scheinzwittertums. *Virchows Arch. Path.,* 1905, 181:1-51. Pirie, G. R. A study of hyper-adrenalism, its influence in producing congenital pyloric hypertrophy and subsequent obstruction, *Lancet,* 1919, 2:513-5. Gierke, E., von. Über Interrenalismus und interrenale Intoxikation. *Verh. Deut. Path. Ges.,* 1928, 23:449-56. Bongiovanni, A. M. Congenital adrenal hyperplasia and related conditions. In: Stanbury, J. B., Wyngaarden, J. B., & Fredrickson, D. S., eds. *The metabolic basis of inherited disease.* 4th ed. New York, MacGraw-Hill, 1978, pp. 868-93. Wilkins, L. *et al.,* The supression of androgen secretion in a case of congenital adrenal hyperplasia. Preliminary report. *Bull. Johns Hopkins Hosp.,* 1950, 86:249-52. New, M. I., & Speiser, P. W. Genetics of adrenal steroid 21-hydroxylase deficiency. *Endocr. Rev.,* 1986, 7:331-459.

congenital afibrinogenemia. See *Rabe-Salomon syndrome.*

congenital agranulocytosis. See *Kostmann syndrome.*

congenital aleukia. See *Vaal-Seynhaeve syndrome.*

congenital amputation. See *anmiotic band syndrome.*

congenital analgia. See *congenital insensitivity to pain syndrome.*

congenital anosmia-hypogonadoptropic hypogonadism syndrome. See *olfactogenital syndrome.*

congenital aplastic anemia. See *Fanconi anemia.*

congenital aregenerative anemia. See *Diamond-Blackfan syndrome.*

congenital arthromyodysplastic syndrome. See *arthrogryposis multiplex congenita syndrome.*

congenital asplenia. See *asplenia syndrome.*

congenital asymmetry. See *Curtius syndrome (1).*

congenital atonic pseudoparalysis. See *Oppenheim disease, under Oppenheim, Hermann.*

congenital atonic sclerotic muscular dystrophy. See *Ullrich syndrome.*

congenital autonomic dysfunction syndrome. See *Riley-Day syndrome, under Riley, Conrad Milton.*

congenital brevicollis. See *Klippel-Feil syndrome.*

congenital bulbar paralysis. See *Moebius syndrome (1).*

congenital cataracts-microcornea syndrome, X-linked. See *Nance-Horan syndrome.*

congenital central alveolar hypoventilation syndrome. See *Ondine curse.*

congenital central corneal leukoma. See *Peters anomaly.*

congenital central hypoventilation syndrome (CCHS). See *Ondine curse.*

congenital cerebellar ataxia. See *Marie syndrome (1), under Marie, Pierre.*

congenital chorea. See *Vogt syndrome, under Vogt, Cécille.*

congenital constrictive bands. See *amniotic band syndrome.*

congenital contractural arachnodactyly syndrome. Synonyms: *Beals syndrome, Beals-Hecht syndrome.*

A heritable disorder of connective tissue combining features of Marfan's syndrome with arthrogryposis.

The principal features of this syndrome include multiple congenital joint contractures, arachnodactyly, dolichostenomelia, kyphoscoliosis, and crumpled ears. It is transmitted as an autosomal dominant trait.

Beals, R. K., & Hecht, F. Congenital contractural arachnodactyly. A heritable disorder of connective tissue. *J. Bone Joint Surg.*, 1971, 53A:987-93.

congenital contractures of extremities. See *arthrogryposis multiplex congenita syndrome.*

congenital cutaneous dystrophy. See *Rothmund-Thomson syndrome.*

congenital cystic degeneration of intrahepatic bile ducts. See *Caroli syndrome (2).*

congenital cystic dilatation of intrahepatic bile ducts. See *Caroli syndrome (2).*

congenital deafness-split hands and feet syndrome. See *Wildervanck syndrome (4).*

congenital dilatation of great intrahepatic ducts. See *Caroli syndrome (2).*

congenital dilatation of intrahepatic bile ducts. See *Caroli syndrome (2).*

congenital dilatation of intrahepatic segmentary bile ducts. See *Caroli syndrome (2).*

congenital dyserythropoietic anemia type II. See *HEMPAS syndrome.*

congenital dyskeratosis. See *Zinsser-Engman-Cole syndrome.*

congenital ectodermosis. See *Sturge-Weber syndrome.*

congenital encephalo-ophthalmic dysplasia. See *Krause syndrome.*

congenital endothelial corneal dystrophy. See *Fuchs dystrophy.*

congenital epulis. See *Neumann syndrome, under Neumann, Ernst.*

congenital erythroid hypoplasia. See *Diamond-Blackfan syndrome.*

congenital erythropoietic porphyria (CEP). Synonyms: *Günther disease, congenital photosensitive porphyria, erythropoietic porphyria, haematoporphyria congenita, porphyria erythropoetica.*

A rare syndrome, transmitted as an autosomal recessive trait, characterized at first by moderate to severe cutaneous photosensitivity and pinkish red urine, which are usually present in infancy. Skin lesions consist of vesicles, bullae, erosions, hypertrichosis or lanugo hair, hypermelanosis, and excessive sensitivity to injuries. Later symptoms include scarring with atrophy, cicatrizing alopecia, sclerodermoid changes, and mutilation of the hands, ears, face, and nose. Associated disorders may include hemolytic anemia, erythrodontia, splenomegaly, ulcerations of the sclera, and fluorescent erythrocytes. The presence of porphyrins in the erythrocytes, plasma and skin is believed to be the main cause of photosensitivity. Most of the urinary porphyrins are of the type I isomer, but there usually also is an increase in uroporphyrin III. The feces contain large amounts of coproporphyrins.

Günther, H. Die Hamatoporphyrie. *Deut. Arch. Klin. Med.*, 1912, 105:89-146.

congenital facial diplegia. See *Moebius syndrome (1).*

congenital facial paralysis. See *Moebius syndrome (1).*

congenital factor VII deficiency. See *Alexander syndrome, under Alexander, Benjamin.*

congenital familial analgesia. See *Biemond syndrome (3).*

congenital familial cholemia. See *Gilbert syndrome, under Gilbert, Nicolas Augustin.*

congenital fascial dystrophy syndrome. See *stiff skin syndrome.*

congenital finger contractures. See *camptodactyly syndrome.*

congenital generalized dropsy. See *Schridde syndrome.*

congenital German measles. See *congenital rubella syndrome.*

congenital gingival hyperplasia-hypertrichosis syndrome. See *gingival fibromatosis-hypertrichosis syndrome.*

congenital goiter. See *Brissaud infantilism.*

congenital hemidysplasia with ichthyosiform erythroderma and limb defects. See *CHILD syndrome.*

congenital hemihypertrophy. See *Curtius syndrome (1).*

congenital hemolytic anemia. See *Minkowski-Chauffard syndrome.*

congenital hemolytic icterus. See *Minkowski-Chauffard syndrome.*

congenital hemorrhagic thrombocytic dystrophy. See *Glanzmann thrombasthenia.*

congenital hereditary hematuria. See *Alport syndrome.*

congenital hereditary hypotrichosis. See *Unna syndrome, under Unna, Marie.*

congenital high scapula. See *Sprengel deformity.*

congenital hyperchloremic acidosis syndrome. See *Lightwood-Albright syndrome.*

congenital hypertrophy of the bladder neck. See *Marion disease.*

congenital hypofibrinogenemia. See *Rabe-Salomon syndrome.*

congenital hypogammaglobulinemia. See *Bruton syndrome.*

congenital hypoplastic anemia. See *Diamond-Blackfan syndrome.*

congenital hypothalamic hamartoblastoma. See *Hall syndrome, under Hall, J. G.*

congenital hypothyroidism. See *Brissaud infantilism.*

congenital hypoventilation syndrome (CHS). See *Ondine curse.*

congenital ichthyosiform erythroderma. See *Carini syndrome.*

congenital idiopathic hypertrophy of the heart. See *Kugel-Stoloff syndrome.*

congenital idiopathic methemoglobinemia. See *Gibson disease, under Gibson, Quentin Howieson.*

congenital indifference to pain. See *congenital insensitivity to pain syndrome.*

congenital insensitivity to pain syndrome. Synonyms: *analgesia syndrome, congenital analgia, congenital indifference to pain, congenital pure analgesia.*

A syndrome characterized by complete indifference to pain, resulting in soft and hard tissue injury. Scarring of the face and mutilation of the lips, arms, and legs are the main features. Self-induced amputation of the fingers is frequent, and other disorders may include osteomyelitis, aseptic necrosis, fractures, Charcot joint, and spontaneous resorption of toes and fingers. Dental caries with the absence of toothache may lead to loss of teeth. The syndrome is suspected of being transmitted as an autosomal recessive trait. See also *Biemond syndrome (3).*

Dearborn, B. A case of congenital pure analgesia. *J. Nerv. Ment. Dis.*, 1931, 75:612-5.

congenital insensitivity to pain with anhidrosis. See *Swanson syndrome.*

congenital intrahepatic cysts of bile ducts. See *Caroli syndrome (2).*

congenital keratoma of the palms and soles. See *Unna-Thost syndrome, under Unna, Paul Gerson.*

congenital labile factor deficiency with syndactyly. See *De Vries syndrome.*

congenital leukokeratosis. See *white sponge nevus.*

congenital lipodystrophy. See *Berardinelli-Seip syndrome.*

congenital lipomatosis of pancreas. See *Shwachman syndrome.*

congenital lymphedema. See *Nonne-Milroy syndrome, and see Meige syndrome (1).*

congenital macrogingivae-hypertrichosis syndrome. See *gingival fibromatosis-hypertrichosis syndrome.*

congenital megacolon. See *Hirschsprung syndrome.*

congenital mesodermal dystrophy. See *Marfan syndrome (1).*

congenital metacarpotalar syndrome. See *Ashley syndrome.*

congenital microangiopathic hemolytic anemia. See *Schulman-Upshaw syndrome.*

congenital microspherocytic hemolytic anemia. See *Minkowski-Chauffard syndrome.*

congenital muscular dystrophy. See *Thomsen disease.*

congenital muscular hypertrophy-cerebral syndrome. See *de Lange syndrome (2), under Lange, Cornelia, de.*

congenital myoblastoma of the newborn. See *Neumann syndrome, under Neumann, Ernst.*

congenital myotonic dystrophy. See *myotonic dystrophy syndrome.*

congenital myxedema. See *Brissaud infantilism.*

congenital neuroectodermal dysplasia. See *Sturge-Weber syndrome.*

congenital neurogenic ileus. See *Jirásek-Zuelzer-Wilson syndrome.*

congenital nonhemolytic jaundice. See *Crigler-Najjar syndrome.*

congenital nonhemolytic jaundice with kernicterus. See *Crigler-Najjar syndrome.*

congenital nonspherocytic hemolytic anemia. See *Crosby syndrome, under Crosby, William H.*

congenital nuclear agenesis. See *Moebius syndrome (1).*

congenital nuclear aplasia. See *Moebius syndrome (1).*

congenital oculofacial paralysis. See *Moebius syndrome (1).*

congenital oculomotor apraxia syndrome. See *Cogan syndrome (2).*

congenital onychodysplasia of the index finger (COIF) syndrome. See *Iso-Kikuchi syndrome.*

congenital optic atrophy. See *Thompson syndrome, under Thompson, A. Hugh.*

congenital osseous torticollis syndrome. See *Klippel-Feil syndrome.*

congenital osteosclerosis. See *Koszewski syndrome.*

congenital pain asymbolia-auditory imperception syndrome. See *Osuntokun syndrome.*

congenital pain insensitivity. See *congenital insensitivity to pain syndrome.*

congenital pancytopenia. See *Fanconi anemia.*

congenital panleukia syndrome. See *Vaal-Seynhaeve syndrome.*

congenital paralysis of the sixth and seventh nerves. See *Moebius syndrome (1).*

congenital paramyotonia. See *Eulenburg disease.*

congenital photosensitive porphyria. See *congenital erythropoietic porphyria.*

congenital pigmentary dystrophy. See *Leschke syndrome.*

congenital poikiloderma atrophicans vasculare. See *Rothmund-Thomson syndrome.*

congenital poikiloderma-juvenile cataracts syndrome. See *Rothmund-Thomson syndrome.*

congenital polycystic disease. See *Potter syndrome (2), under Potter, Edith Louise.*

congenital posterolateral diaphragmatic hernia. See *Bochdalek hernia.*

congenital progressive oculo-acoustico-cerebral degeneration. See *Norrie syndrome.*

congenital pseudohydrocephalic progeroid syndrome. See *Wiedemann-Rautenstrauch syndrome.*

congenital pure analgesia. See *congenital insensitivity to pain syndrome.*

congenital pure red cell aplasia. See *Diamond-Blackfan syndrome.*

congenital rubella syndrome (CRS). Synonyms: *congenital German measles, embryopathia rubeolaris, embryopathia rubeolosa, postrubella syndrome, rubella embryopathy, rubella syndrome, rubeola syndrome, rubeolar embryopathy.*

A syndrome occurring in newborn infants of mothers infected with the rubella virus (an RNA virus in the togavirus family) during the first trimester of pregnancy. Some infants are stillborn; others show multiple abnormalities, including low birth-weight, thrombocytopenic purpura, hepatosplenomegaly, cataract, microphthalmia, retinopathy, deafness, heart defect, obstructive jaundice, osteolytic metaphyseal lesions, interstitial pneumonia, retarded growth, and mental deficiency. Additional disorders may include glaucoma, corneal opacity, chorioretinitis, and strabismus. Heart defect usually consists of patent ductus arteriosus, pulmonary artery stenosis, and septal defect. Radiological features generally include radiolucency and sclerosis in the metaphyses of the long bones (celery stalk), poor mineralization of the provisional zones of calcification, coarse trabeculae, some instances of fractures, large anterior fontanels, hypoplasia and occlusion of the aorta and its branches, and left ventricular anerurysm. Occasional anomalies may include kidney diseases, hemolytic anemia, delayed tooth eruption, hypospadias, cryptorchism, and dermatoglyphic abnormalities. Congenital rubella with retinopathy is known as the **Gregg syndrome.** See also *Zahorsky syndrome I (pseudorubella).*

Ray, C. G. Rubella ("German measles") and other viral exanthems. In: Braunwald, E., Isselbacher, K. J., Petersdorf, R. G., Wilson, J. D., Martin, J. B., & Fauci, A. S., eds. *Harrison's principles of internal medicine.* 11th ed. New York, McGraw-Hill, 1987, pp. 684-6. Gregg, N. M. Congenital cataract following German measles in the mother. *Tr. Ophth. Soc. Australia,* 1941, 3:35-46. Gilles, W. E. Hypoplasia of the iris stroma in Gregg's syndrome unaccompanied by catarct but with deafness, rubella retinopathy and onset of glaucoma in adult or adolescent life. *Austral. J. Ophth.,* 1980, 8:189-92.

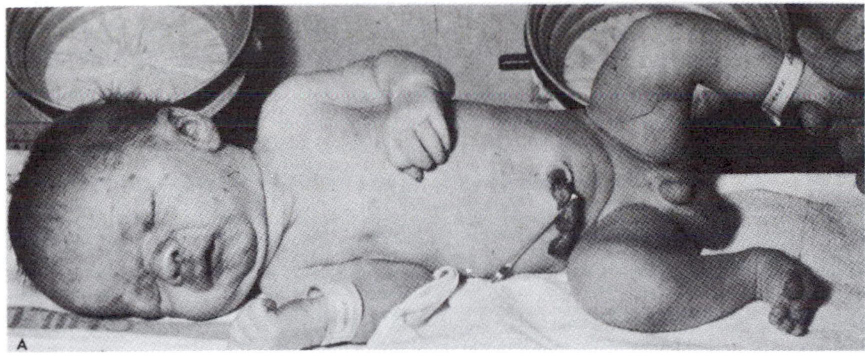

Congential rubella syndrome
Smith, D.W.: *J. Pediatr.*, 70:517, 1967., St. Louis, MO.

congenital saccular dilatation of hepatic bile ducts. See *Caroli syndrome (2).*

congenital sensory neuropathy syndrome. Synonym: *recessive hereditary sensory neuropathy.*

A familial neurological syndrome, transmsitted as an autosomal recessive trait, characterized by congenital sensory neuropathy involving all modalities of sensation. The lack of pain sensation in the limbs results in traumatic tissue damage with recurrent ulcers, local suppuration, and osteomyelitis. Nerve biopsy shows absence of myelinated nerve fibers with little evidence of degenerative changes.

Murray, T. J. Congenital sensory neuropathy. *Brain,* 1973, 96:387-94. Jedrzejowska, T. J., & Milczarek, H. Recessive hereditary sensory neuropathy. *J. Neurol. Sc.,* 1976, 29:371-87.

congenital sensory neuropathy with anhidrosis. See *Swanson syndrome.*

congenital spastic diplegia. See *Little disease, under Little, William John.*

congenital suprabulbar paresis. See *Worster-Drough syndrome.*

congenital synostosis of cervicothoracic vertebrae syndrome. See *Klippel-Feil syndrome.*

congenital syphilitic paralysis. See *Dennie-Marfan syndrome.*

congenital talus luxation. See *Volkmann deformity.*

congenital telangiectatic erythema-stunted growth syndrome. See *Bloom syndrome.*

congenital thrombocytic dystrophy. See *Bernard-Soulier syndrome, under Bernard, Jean.*

congenital trichomegaly. See *chorioretinopathy-pituitary dysfunction syndrome.*

congenital trigeminal anesthesia syndrome (CTA). A rare congenital neurological disorder consisting of a stable deficit involving all or part of the sensory function of the fifth cranial nerve.

Rosenberg, M. L. Congenital trigeminal anaesthesia. A review and classification. *Brain,* 1984, 107:1073-82.

congenital varicella syndrome. A disease in infants whose mothers have been infected with the varicella-zoster virus, usually between the 8th and 19th week of pregnancy. It is characterized by involvement of the limbs (consisting mainly of hypoplasia and paralysis with muscle atrophy and hypoplastic and missing fingers), Horner syndrome, ocular disorders (chorioretinitis, cataract, and optic atrophy), cicatricial skin lesions, and central nervous system complications (seizures, encephalitis, cortical atrophy, and mental retardation). Entry of the virus into fetal brachial or lumbar plexus causes limb defects; invasion of the cervical sympathetic nerves produces Horner syndrome; and infection of the brain results in encephalitis.

Williamson, A. The varicella-zoster virus in the etiology of severe congenital defects. *Clin. Pediat.,* 1975, 14:553-9.

congenital vitamin B_{12} malabsorption syndrome. See *Imerslund-Gräsbeck syndrome.*

congenital warfarin syndrome. See *fetal warfarin syndrome.*

congenital webbed neck syndrome. See *Klippel-Feil syndrome.*

congestion headache. See *under headache syndrome.*

congestion-fibrosis syndrome. See *Taylor syndrome, under Taylor, Howard Canning, Jr.*

congestive atelectasis. See *adult respiratory distress syndrome.*

congestive dysmenorrhea syndrome. See *Taylor syndrome, under Taylor, Howard Canning, Jr.*

congestive fibrosplenomegaly. See *Frugoni syndrome.*

congestive splenomegaly. See *Banti syndrome.*

conjugate gaze paralysis syndrome. See *Cogan syndrome (2).*

conjunctivitis et cheilostomatitis pseudomembranacea exanthematodes. See *Stevens-Johnson syndrome.*

conjunctivitis et stomatitis pseudomembranacea. See *Stevens-Johnson syndrome.*

conjunctivitis meibomiana. See *Elschnig conjunctivitis.*

conjunctivitis necroticans infectiosa. See *Pascheff conjunctivitis.*

conjunctivo-urethrosynovial syndrome. See *Reiter syndrome.*

conjunctivoglandular syndrome. See *Parinaud oculoglandular syndrome.*

CONN, JEROME W. (American physician, born 1907)

Conn adenoma. See *Conn syndrome.*

Conn syndrome. Synonyms: *Conn adenoma, Conn-Louis syndrome, aldosterone-producing adenoma, potassium-losing nephritis, primary aldosteronism, primary hyperaldosteronis.*

An endocrine disease characterized by adenoma, carcinoma, or hyperplasia of the zona glomerulosa of the adrenal cortex, resulting in excessive production of aldosterone and leading to sodium retention and hydrogen loss. Associated features include hypertension (sometimes causing myocardial infarction), stroke, renal damage with proteinuria and urinary calculi, muscle weakness, tetany, polyuria, polydipsia, arrhythmia, carbohydrate intolerance, and resistance to vasopressin.

Conn, J. W. Primary aldosteronism, a new clinical syndrome. *J. Lab. Clin. Med.*, 1955, 45:3-17.

Conn-Louis syndrome. See *Conn syndrome.*

connatal cutis laxa syndrome. See *cutis laxa syndrome.*

CONNEALLY, P. M. (American physician)

Christian-Andrews-Conneally-Muller syndrome. See *Christian syndrome (1), under Christian, Joe C.*

CONRADI, ERICH (German physician, born 1882)

Conradi syndrome. See *Conradi-Hünermann syndrome.*

Conradi-Hünermann syndrome. Synonyms: *Conradi syndrome; Hünermann syndrome; asymmetric rhizomelic limb shortening; chondroangiopathia calcarea seu punctata; chondroangiopathia punctata; chondrodysplasia calcificans congenita; chondrodysplasia punctata, dominant type; chondrodysplasia epiphysialis punctata; chondrodystrophia calcarea; chondrodystrophia punctata, dominant type; chondrodystrophia calcificans; chondrodystrophia calcificans congenita; chondrodystrophia foetalis hypoplastica; chondrodystrophia hypoplastica calcinosa; chondrodystrophia calcificans; chondropathia punctata; dysplasia epiphysealis congenita; dysplasia epiphysialis punctata; multiple epiphyseal dysplasia (MED); punctate epiphyseal dysplasia; stipled epiphyses.*

A rare bone disorder of infants, which is characterized by punctate or stippled changes most marked in the epiphyses of long bones, carpal and tarsal regions, processes of the vertebrae, and ischiopubic bones. Associated abnormalities may include a flat face with depressed nasal bridge, asymmetric shortening of long bones, scoliosis developing during the first year of life, ichthysiform skin changes, alopecia, joint contractures, and various skeletal changes. Irregular deformities of the vertebral bodies may occur. Some infants may be stillborn or may die during the first weeks of life. In less severely affected infants, life expectancy and mental development may be normal. The syndrome is transmitted as an autosomal dominant trait with variability of expression. See also *multiple epiphyseal dysplasia.*

Conradi, E. Vorzeitiges Auftreten von Knochenund eigenartigen Verkalkungskernen bei Chondrodystrophia foetalis hypoplastica. *Jahrb. Kinderh.*, 1914, 80:86-97. Hünermann, C. Chondrodystrophia calcificans congenita als abortive Form der Chondrodystrophie. *Zschr. Kinderh.*, 1931, 51:1-19.

CONRADI, GERHARD J.

Bowen-Conradi syndrome. See *under Bowen, Peter.*

constitutional afibrinogenemia. See *Rabe-Salomon syndrome.*

constitutional aplastic anemia. See *Fanconi anemia.*

constitutional arterial narrowing. See *small blood vessel syndrome.*

constitutional familial leukopenia. See *Gänsslen disease.*

constitutional familial neutropenia. See *Gänsslen disease.*

constitutional granular gigantism. See *Chédiak-Higashi syndrome.*

constitutional hemolytic anemia. See *Minkowski-Chauffard syndrome.*

constitutional hemolytic jaundice. See *Minkowski-Chauffard syndrome.*

constitutional hepatic dysfunction. See *Gilbert syndrome, under Gilbert, Nicolas Augustin.*

constitutional hyperbilirubinemia. See *Gilbert syndrome, under Gilbert, Nicolas Augustin.*

constitutional hyperbilirubinemia syndrome. See *Dubin-Johnson syndrome.*

constitutional liver dysfunction. See *Gilbert syndrome, under Gilbert, Nicolas Augustin.*

constitutional microcythemic anemia. See *Rietti-Greppi-Micheli syndrome.*

constitutional microcytic anemia. See *Silvestroni-Bianco syndrome.*

constitutional thrombopathy. See *Willebrand-Jürgens syndrome.*

constrictive fibrous endocarditis. See *Löffler endocarditis.*

constructive apraxia. See *Mayer-Gross apraxia.*

consumption coagulopathy. See *disseminated intravascular coagulation syndrome.*

contact urticaria syndrome (CUS). Synonyms: *immediate reativities syndrome, syndrome of immediate reactivities (SIR).*

Wheal, flare reaction of the skin, or angioedema occurring within 1 hour after contact is made with a toxic substance, although a variant, **delayed-onset contact urticaria**, may be observed 4 to 6 hours after the exposure. **Nonimmunologic contact urticaria (NICU)** is caused by substances which induce histamine release without involving immunologic processes. These include biogenic polymers produced by some plants (such as nettles), certain animals (such as caterpillars and jellyfish), and various drugs (such as nicotinates, dimethyl sulfoxide, and others). **Immunologic contact urticaria (ICU)** is due to histamine release through allergic mechanisms, or antigen release of biologically active materials from mast cells or basophilic leukocytes sensitized with specific IgE antibody. Some cases of contact urticaria are elicited by chemical substances with undetermined modes of action.

Maibach, H. I., & Johnson, H. L. Contact urticaria syndrome. Contact urticaria to diethyltoluamide. *Arch. Derm., Chicago,* 1975, 111:726-30. von Krogh, G., & Maibach, H. I. The contact urticaria syndrome-an update review. *J. Am. Acad. Derm.*, 1981, 5:328-42. Fisher, A. A. *Contact dermatitis.* 2nd ed. Philadelphia, Lea & Febiger, 1973, pp. 283-6. Burdick, A. E., & Mathias, C. G. The contact urticaria syndrome. *Derm. Clinics,* 1985, 3:71-84.

contaminated small bowel syndrome (CSBS). See *bacterial overgrowth syndrome.*

CONTARINI, FRANCESCO (Died 1625)

Contarini condition. Synonym: *Contarini syndrome.*

Bilateral pleural effusions in leukemic and cancer patients, said to be similar to those observed in Contarini, the 95th Doge of Venice, who died after a long illness with fever, emaciation, cough, orthopnea, foul-smelling sputum, and arrhythmia. The autopsy report stated that his chest cavity contained about 5 lb of watery matter, the flaccid right part of the lung appeared to be full of mucous fluid, and the left lung had turned entirely into a whitish gore. Hydrothorax due to cardiac failure and lung abscess are the suspected causes.

Kutty, C. P. K., & Verkey, B. "Contarini's condition": Bilateral pleural effusions with markedly different characteristics. *Chest*, 1978, 74:679-90. Lawton, F., *et al.* Co-existing chylous and serous pleural effusions associated with ovarian cancer: A case report of Contarini's syndrome. *Eur. J. Surg. Oncol.*, 1985, 11:177-8.

Contarini syndrome. See *Contarini condition.*

CONTINO, ANTONINO (Italian ophthalmologist, 1878-1951)

Contino epithelioma. A rapidly developing papilloma of the anterior segment of the eye, involving the limbus corneae and the cornea.

Contino, A. Neue Beobachtungen und Untersuchungen über die Papillome des Limbus und der Hornhaut. *Arch. Augenh.*, 1911, 68:366-413.

Contino glaucoma. Glaucoma characterized by thickening of the anterior chamber, partial dilatation of the pupil, and congestive changes in the iris.

Contino, A. Del glaucoma anterior emorragico. *Ann. Ottalm.*, 1936, 64:433-6.

continual skin peeling syndrome. Synonyms: *continuous skin peeling syndrome, deciduous skin, familial continual skin peeling syndrome, keratolysis exfoliativa congenita, peeling skin syndrome, skin shedding.*

A rare, usually familial, skin disease, transmitted as an autosomal recessive trait, characterized by generalized, noninflammatory exfoliation of the stratum corneum. Histologically, there is a separation of corneocytes above the granular cell layer, the plasma membrane of the peeling cell remaining adherent to the underlying cell while the upper part of the cell exfoliates.

Fox, H. Skin shedding (keratolysis exfoliativa congenita). *Arch. Derm. Syph., Chicago,* 1921, 3:202.

continuous epilepsy. See *Kozhevnikov syndrome.*

continuous skin peeling syndrome. See *continual skin peeling syndrome.*

conversion hysteria. See *Brissaud-Marie syndrome.*

conversion reaction. See *Brissaud-Marie syndrome.*

conversion symptoms. See *Brissaud-Marie syndrome.*

COOKE, ARTHUR CARLETON (British physician)

Cooke-Apert-Gallais syndrome. See *Cushing syndrome.*

Cooke-Gallais syndrome. See *Cushing syndrome.*

COOLEY, THOMAS BENTON (American physician, 1871-1945)

Cooley anemia. Synonyms: *Cooley anemia syndrome, Cooley disease, Cooley syndrome, Cooley-Lee syndrome, Dameshek syndrome, chronic familial erythremia, erythroblastic anemia, hereditary leptocytosis, Mediterranean anemia, Mediterranean disease, primary erythroblastic anemia, target cell anemia, target-oval cell syndrome, thalassemia major, thalassemic syndrome.*

Hereditary hemolytic anemia, which is the homozygous form of beta-thalassemia, occurring in infancy, usually in persons of the Mediterranean extraction. It is characterized by the absence or low levels of β-chain, an excess of α-chain, and continued high production of γ-chain with elevated Hb F. The affected infants are normal at first but, by the age of 6 to 9 months (or the time when the switch from Hb F to Hb A is completed and there is β-globin production deficiency), they develop faulty erythropoiesis with anemia and hypertrophy of the bone marrow, spleen, and liver with hepatosplenomegaly. The condition is associated with pallor, retarded growth, fever, inadequate food intake, dyspnea, weakness, numbness and tingling of the extremities, and edema. Other symptoms include petechiae, purpura, and hematoma with nasal, oral, and gastrointestinal bleeding, and gingival and pharyngeal ulcers. Blood examination shows hypochromia, microcytosis, poikilocytosis, target cells, ovalocytosis, Cabot rings, Howell-Jolly bodies, nuclear fragments, siderocytosis, anisochromia, anisocytosis, and normoblastosis. The bone marrow is composed of yellowish material containing fat, fibrous tissues, and lymphocytes. Extravasation of blood may occur.

*Cooley, T. B., & Lee, P. Series of cases of splenomegaly in children with anemia and peculiar bone changes. *Tr. Am. Pediat. Soc.*, 1925, 37:29. Dameshek, W. "Target cell" anemia. Anerythroblastic type of Colley's erythroblastic anemia. *Am. J. Med. Sc.*, 1940, 200:445-54.

Cooley anemia syndrome. See *Cooley anemia.*

Cooley disease. See *Cooley anemia.*

Cooley syndrome. See *Cooley anemia.*

Cooley-Lee syndrome. See *Cooley anemia.*

Coombs-positive hemolytic anemia-immune thrombocytopenia syndrome. See *Evans syndrome, under Evans, Robert Sherman.*

COOPER, SIR ASTLEY PASTON (British physician, 1769-1841)

Cooper disease (1). See *Cheatle disease.*

Cooper disease (2). See *Reclus disease.*

Cooper hernia. Retroperitoneal hernia.

*Cooper, A. *The anatomy and surgical treatment of abdominal hernia.* London, 1827.

Cooper neuralgia. Synonyms: *irritable breast, mastodynia, neuralgia mammalis.*

Irritability and neuralgia of the breast.

Cooper, A. *Illustrations of the diseases of the breast.* London. Longman, 1829.

Cooper syndrome. See *scalenus anticus syndrome.*

Cooper testis. Irritable testicular neuralgia.

Cooper, A. *Observations on the structure and diseases of the testis.* London, Longman, 1830.

COOPERMAN, H. N. (American dentist)

Cooperman-Miura syndrome. Synonym: *uvula-tongue malposture.*

A syndrome of irritation of the dorsum of the tongue and uvula, retrusion of the mandible, narrowing of the respiratory pathways, and malocclusion. Mandibular retrusion is said to cause the tongue and the uvula to impinge on one another, thereby causing irritation. Associated symptoms include respiratory disorders, headache, facial pain, and temporomandibular joint dysfunction.

*Cooperman, H. N. New approach to the establishing the plane of occlusion and freeway space in dentures. *Dent. Digest*, 1965, 71:202. *Cooperman, H. N., Miura, N., *et al.* Uvula tongue malposture. A new approach in Costen's syndrome. *Dent. Diamond, Tokyo,* 1977. 2:127-9.

COOTE, HOLMES (British physician, 1817-72)

Coote-Hanauld syndrome. See *cervical rib syndrome.*

COPD (chronic obstructive pulmonary disease). See *airway obstruction syndrome.*

COPE, C. L.

Cope syndrome. See *milk-alkali syndrome.*

COPELAND, MURRAY M. (American physician)

Geschickter-Copeland tumor. See *Geschickter tumor.*

COPEMAN
Copeman-Ackermann syndrome. Synonym: *painful lumbar sclerolipoma.*
Lipoma characterized by painful hard subcutaneous nodules of the lumbosacral region and the sacroiliac joint, considered variously as a form of cellulitis, fat hernia, fibrositis, and manifestation of the Weber-Christian syndrome. The syndrome reportedly was described by Copeman and Ackermann in 1944.
Baciu, C., *et al.* Bolestivy lumbalni sklerolipom (syndrom Copemanuv-Ackermannuv). *Acta. Chir. Orthop. Traum. Cech.*, 1968, 35:429-32.
copper deficiency syndrome. See *kinky hair syndrome, and see neonatal copper deficiency syndrome.*
coprolalia-compulsive tic syndrome. See *Gilles de la Tourette syndrome.*
CORBEEL, L. (Belgian physician)
Denys-Corbeel syndrome. See *under Denys.*
cord contraction syndrome. See *tethered conus syndrome.*
cord phlebitis of the chest wall. See *Mondor disease (1).*
cord traction syndrome. See *tethered conus syndrome.*
CORDA, L. (Italian physician)
Silvestrini-Corda syndrome. See *under Silvestrini.*
CORDS, RICHARD (German ophthalmologist, born 1881)
Cords angiopathy. Synonym: *angiopathia retinae juvenilis.*
Juvenile tuberculous phlebitis or thrombosis of the vena contralis retinae. Pathologically, there are round cell infitrations in the wall of the vein and edema in the surrounding tissue. Spreading infiltration may result in occlusion of the vessel and, eventually, in reduction of the visual field and atrophy of the optic nerve.
Cords, R. Papillitis und Glaukom. Zugleich ein Beitrag zur juvenilen Phlebitis der Zentralvene. *Graefes Arch. Ophth.*, 1921, 105:916-63.

CORI, GERTY THERESA (American biochemist, 1896-1955)
Cori disease. See *glycogen storage disease III.*
CORINO DE ANDRADE. See ANDRADE, CORINO M.
corkscrew esophagus. See *Bársony-Polgár syndrome (2).*
cornea farinata. See *Vogt cornea, under Vogt, Alfred.*
cornea guttata. See *Fuchs dystrophy, and see Vogt degeneration, under Vogt, Alfred.*
cornea verticillata. See *Fleischer dystrophy (1).*
corneal leukomas in ichthyosis. See *KID syndrome.*
corneal melting syndrome. See *Mooren ulcer.*
corneal opacity-cranioskeletal dysostosis syndrome. See *Helmholz-Harrington syndrome.*

CORNELIA DE LANGE. See LANGE, CORNELIA, DE
CORNIL, LUCIEN (French physician, 1888-1952)
Lhermitte-Cornil-Quesnel syndrome. See *under Lhermitte.*
Roussy-Cornil syndrome. See *under Roussy.*
CORNO, RENZO (Italian physician)
Corno disease. A familial form of Sprengel's deformity.
Corno, R. Scapola alta congenita a carattere familiare. *Clin. Pediat., Bologna*, 1956, 38:948-52.
coronary steal syndrome. Synonym: myocardial steal.
Diversion of the coronary blood flow, thereby producing myocardial ischemia.
Braunwald, E. *Heart disease. A textbook of cardiovascular medicine.* Philadelphia, Saunders, 1980, pp. 1288-9.
coronary-subclavian steal syndrome. Reversal of blood flow in the internal mammary and vertebral arteries, complicating internal mammary artery graft for coronary artery bypass, taking place after proximal subclavian artery stenosis.
Harjola, P. T., & Valle, M. The importance of aortic arch or subclavian angiography before coronary reconstruction. *Chest*, 1974, 66:436-8. Niemiera, M. L., *et al.* Retrograde internal mammary artery flow and resistant angina pectoris: Clues to the coronary-subclavian steal syndrome. Cathet. Cardiovasc. Diagn., 1986, 12:93-5.
corpus callosum agenesis-chorioretinopathy-infantile spasms syndrome. See *Aicardi syndrome.*
corpus callosum agenesis-ocular anomalies-salaam seizure syndrome. See Aicardi syndrome.
corpus callosum degeneration. See *Marchiafava-Bignami syndrome.*
corpus callosum tumor syndrome. See *Bristowe syndrome.*
corpus luteum persistens. See *Halban syndrome.*
corpus striatum syndrome. See *Hunt paralysis, under Hunt, James Ramsay.*
CORRIGAN, SIR DOMINIC JOHN (Dublin physician, 1802-1880)
Corrigan cirrhosis. See *Hamman-Rich syndrome.*
Corrigan disease. Synonyms: *aortic insufficiency, aortic regurgitation.*
Insufficiency of the aortic valve with backflow of the blood through the incompetent valve.
Corrigan, D. J. On permanent patency of the mouth of the aorta, or inadequacy of the aortic valves. *Edinburgh Med. Surg. J.*, 1832, 37:225-45.
cortical blindness with denial. See *Anton-Babinski syndrome.*
cortical cerebellar degeneration. See *olivopontocerebellar atrophy.*
cortical epilepsy. See *Jackson epilepsy.*
cortical hyperostosis with syndactyly. See *sclerosteosis syndrome.*
cortical sensory aphasia. See *Wernicke aphasia.*
cortical word deafness. See *Wernicke aphasia.*
corticopallidospinal degeneration. See *Jakob-Creutzfeldt syndrome.*
corticostriatal-spinal degeneration. See *Jakob-Creutzfeldt syndrome.*
CORVISART DE MARETS, BARON JEAN NICHOLAS, DE (French physician, 1755-1821)
Corvisart complex. Synonym: *Corvisart disease.*
An association of right-sided aortic arch with Fallot tetralogy.
Corvisart, J. N. *Traité des mal du coeur.* Paris, 1814, Vol. 2, p. 680.
Corvisart disease (1). See *Corvisart complex.*
Corvisart disease (2). Chronic hypertrophic myocarditis.
Corvisart, J. N., de. *Essai sur les maladies et les lésions organiques du coeur et des gros voisseaux, extrait des leçons cliniques*. Paris, Migneret, 1806.

COS. See *cheiro-oral syndrome.*
COSSIO, P. (Argentine physician)
Cossio syndrome. Synonym: *Cossio-Berconsky syndrome.*
An association of congenital interventricular septal defect and pericarditis.
Cossio, P., & Berconsky, I. Communicatión interauricular

y sinfisis pericardiaca, *Rev. Argent. Cardiol.*, 1936-37, 3:360-6.

Cossio-Berconsky syndrome. See *Cossio syndrome.*

COSTA, O. G. (Brazilian physician)

Costa disease. Synonym: *acrokeratoelastoidosis (AKE).*

A familial skin disease, transmitted as an autosomal dominant trait, characterized by punctate keratoderma of the palms and soles, sometimes extending to the dorsal surfaces of the hands and feet. The lesions are nodular skin-colored to yellow hyperkeratotic papules with disorganized elastic fibers.

Costa, O. G. Acrokeratoelastoidosis: A hitherto undescribed skin disease. *Dermatologica, Basel*, 1953, 107:164-7.

costal chondritis. See *Tietze syndrome.*

costal junction syndrome. See *Tietze syndrome.*

COSTELLO, J. M. (British physician)

Costello-Dent syndrome. Synonym: *hypo-hyperparathyroidism.*

A syndrome combining the symptoms of hyperparathyroidism (osteitis fibrosa generalisata) with those of mild tetany due to idiopathic hypoparathyroidism.

Costello, J. M., & Dent, C. E. Hypo-hyperparathyroidism. *Arch. Dis. Child.*, 1963, 38:397-407.

COSTEN, JAMES BRAY (American otorhinolaryngologist, born 1895)

Costen syndrome. See *temporamandibular joint syndrome.*

costobrachial syndrome. See *costoclavicular compression syndrome.*

costochondral junction syndrome. See *Tietze syndrome.*

costochondritis. See *Tietze syndrome.*

costoclavicular compression syndrome. Synonyms: *Falconer-Weddell syndrome, costobrachial syndrome, costoclavicular syndrome, military posture syndrome.*

Intermittent compression of the subclavian artery and vein between the clavicle and first thoracic rib with backward and downward shoulder position (as in standing at attention), associated with paresthesia, weakness, and vascular disorders of the upper limbs.

Falconer, M. A., & Weddell, G. Costoclavicular compression of the subclavian artery and vein. Relation to the scalenus anticus syndrome. *Lancet*, 1943, 2:539-43.

costoclavicular syndrome. See *costoclavicular compression syndrome.*

costovertebral dysplasia. See *spondylothoracic dysplasia.*

costovertebral segmentation anomalies syndrome. See *spondylothoracic dysplasia.*

costovertebral segmentation defect with mesomelia. See *COVESDEM syndrome.*

costovertebral syndrome. See *spondylothoracic dysplasia.*

costovertebral syndrome. See *Erdheim syndrome.*

cot death. See *sudden infant death syndrome.*

COTARD, JULES (French physician, 1840-1887)

Cotard syndrome. A syndrome of mental depression, suicidal tendencies, and ideas of negation, the patient being convinced that he no longer has a body.

Cotard, J. Du délire hypochondriaque dans une forme grave de la mélancolie anxieuse. *Ann. Méd. Psych., Paris*, 1880, 4:168-74.

COTE, G. B.

Côté-Katsantoni syndrome. A familial syndrome characterized by a low birth weight, ichthyosis, dental caries, short and splitting hair, onychodysplasia, clinodactyly, osteosclerosis, neutrophilia, abnormal immunologlobulins, growth retardation, and mental retardation.

*Côté, G. B., & Katsantoni, A. Osteosclerosis and ectodermal dysplasia. In: Papadatos, C. J., & Bartosocas, C. S., eds. *Skeletal dysplasia.* New York, Liss, 1982, pp. 161-2. Blau, E. B. Ectodermal dysplasia, osteosclerosis, atrial septal defect, malabsorption, neutropenia, growth and mental retardation: The Côté-Katsantoni syndrome? *Am. J. Med. Genet.*, 1987, 26:729-32.

COTTON, FREDERIC JAY (American physician, 1869-1938)

Cotton fracture. Synonym: *fender fracture of the tibia.*

A fracture of the outer side of the tibial head produced by abduction of the leg that is forcible enough to smash the external tuberosity against the fulcrum of the outer condyle of the femur, usually caused by the impact of an automobile fender.

Cotton, F. J., & Berg, R. "Fender fracture" of the tibia at the knee. *N. Engl. J. Med.*, 1929, 201:989-95.

cotton candy lung. See *Burke syndrome.*

COTUGNO, DOMENICO (Italian physician, 1736-1822)

Cotugno syndrome. Synonyms: *ischias, malum cotunnii, sciatica.*

Neuralgia along the distribution of the sciatic nerve, including the posterior aspect of the thigh, postero- and antero-lateral aspects of the leg, and into the foot, sometimes associated with paresthesia and weakness. Lesions of the fifth lumbar and first sacral nerve roots, such as as those caused by hernia of the lumbosacral disk, arthritis, spondylosis, spinal neoplasms, vertebral fractures or dislocations, and various injuries, are the most frequent causes. See also *Putti syndrome.*

*Cotugno, D. *De ischiade nervoso commentarius.* Napoli, Fratres Simonis, 1764.

coumadin syndrome. See *fetal warfarin syndrome.*

COURVOISIER, LUDWIG GEORG (Basel physician, 1843-1918)

Courvoisier syndrome. See *Bard-Pic syndrome, under Bard, Louis.*

Courvoisier-Terrier syndrome. See *Bard-Pic syndrome, under Bard, Louis.*

COUTO, MIGUEL (Brazilian physician, 1864-1934)

Couto disease. Fatty degeneration of the visceral organs.

Couto, M. Da polysteatase visceral curavel. *Arch. Brasil. Med.*, 1914, 4:475-83.

couvade syndrome. A syndrome in which the expectant father suffers from psychogenic symptoms related to his wife's pregnancy. The most common symptoms include weight gain, nausea, vomiting, bloating, toothache, anorexia, and unspecified aches and pains. The term "couvade" is derived from the French verb *couver*, which means to brood or hatch.

Bogren, L. Y. Couvade. *Acta Psychiat. Scand.*, 1983, 68:55-65.

COUVELAIRE, ALEXANDRE (French physician, 1873-1948)

Couvelaire syndrome. Synonyms: *Couvelaire uterus, abruptio placentae, apoplexia uteroplacentaris, uteroplacental apoplexy.*

The premature separation of a normally implanted placenta in association with disruption of the uterine musculature, hemorrhage, and anemia. Albuminuria, azotemia, and shock may be associated.

Couveilaire, A. Traitement chirurgical des hemorrhagies utéroplacentaires avec décollement du placenta normalement inséré. *Ann. Gyn. Obst., Paris,* 1911, 8:591-608.

Couvelaire uterus. See *Couvelaire syndrome.*

COVESDEM (costovertebral segmentation defect with mesomelia) syndrome. A disorder characterized by segmentation defect of most thoracic vertebrae, mesomelia affecting more severely upper than lower limbs, and peculiar facies characterized by hypertelorism, depressed nasal bridge, large upper lip, constantly open mouth, and peg-like teeth. In the original report, the disorder was observed in two sibs of consanguineous parents. The syndrome is believed to transmitted as an autosomal recessive trait.

Wadia, R. S., *et al.* Recessively inherited constovertebral segmentation defect with mesomelia and peculiar facies (COVESDEM syndrome). *J. Med. Genet.*, 1978, 15:123-7.

COWDEN

Cowden syndrome. Synonyms: *mulitple hamartoma syndrome, multiple hamartoma and neoplasia syndrome.*

A syndrome of disseminated polyposis of the gastrointestinal tract, scattered from the mouth to the anus; orocutaneous hamartomas and benign or malignant tumors of the skin, thyroid, and breasts; occasional giant virginal hypertrophy of the breasts; hypertrichosis; and characteristic adenoid facies. Lichenoid and papillomatous lesions of the pinnae and lateral cervical, periorbital, nasal, perioral, dorsal hand, and forearm areas are the principal cutaneous manifestations. Histologically, the tumors are compatible with tricholemmomas. Macrogingiva, hypoplasia of the mandible and maxilla, high-arched palate, hypoplasia of the soft palate and uvula, microstomia, papillomatosis of the lips and pharynx, and scrotal tongue are the main orofacial features. Hypertrichosis usually intensifies after the menarche. Hydronephrosis occurs in some cases. The syndrome is believed to be transmitted as an autosomal dominant trait. Cowden is the family name of the propositus.

Lloyd, K. M., & Dennis, M. Cowden's disease. A possible new symptom complex with multiple system involvement. *Ann. Int. Med.*, 1963, 58:136-42.

coxa plana. See *Calvé-Legg-Perthes syndrome.*

coxalgia fugax. See *observation hip syndrome.*

coxalgia infantilis seu juvenilis. See *Calvé-Legg-Perthes syndrome.*

coxitis fugax. See *observation hip syndrome.*

coxitis serosa seu simplex. See *observation hip syndrome.*

coxo-auricular syndrome. A hereditary syndrome of shortness of stature, malformed middle or external ear (microtia) with hearing loss, hip dislocation, and skeletal changes. The syndrome is believed to be transmsitted as an autosomal dominant or X-linked trait that is lethal in males.

Duca, D., & Ciovirnache, M. A previously unreported dominantly inherited syndrome of shortness of stature, ear malformations and hip dislocation: The coxoauricular syndrome-autosomal or X-linked male-lethal. *Am. J. Med. Genet.,* 1981, 8:173-80.

COYLE SHEA. See SHEA, M. COYLE, JR

CPD. See *chorioretinopathy-pituitary dysfunction syndrome.*

CPPD (calcium pyrophosphate dihydrate) crystal deposition syndrome. See *pseudogout syndrome.*

CPS (carbamyl phosphate synthetase) deficiency. See *under hyperammonemic syndrome.*

crab dermatitis. See *Rosenbach erysipeloid, under Rosenbach, Anton Julius Friedrich.*

CRAIK

Craik blindness. Temporary blindness caused by external pressure applied to the eye.

Schapero, M., Cline, & Hofstetter, H. W. *Dictionary of visual science.* Philadelphia, Chilton, 1968.

cramp neurosis. See *Wernicke cramp.*

CRANDALL, BARBARA F. (American physician)

Crandall syndrome. Synonym: *deafness-alopecia-hypogonadism syndrome.*

An association of Björnstad syndrome (pili torti, sensorineural deafness, and alopecia), hypogonadism, and deficiency of luteinizing and growth hormones. The normal stature indicates a possibility that growth hormone deficiency has late onset. The syndrome appears to be inherited as an autosomal recessive trait.

Crandall, B. F., *et al.* A familial syndrome of deafness, alopecia, and hypogonadism. *J. Pediat.,* 1973, 82:461-5.

cranial arteritis. See *Horton disease (1), under Horton, Bayard Taylor.*

cranio-ectodermal dysplasia syndrome. Synonyms: *Levin syndrome, Sensenbrenner syndrome, Sensenbrenner-Dorst-Owens syndrome.*

A syndrome of dolichocephaly, tendency toward premature closure of the sagittal suture, antimongoloid palpebral slant, epicanthal folds, full cheeks, everted lip, multiple oral frenula, mildly low-arched palate, microdontia with enamel defect, posteriorly rotated low-set ears with deficient cartilage, a small short thorax with pectus excavatum, abnormal dermatoglyphics, sparse slow-growing hair, disproportionate shortening of the fibulae and the middle and distal phalanges of the toes and fingers, and flattened epiphyses. The syndrome is transmitted as an autosomal recessive trait.

Sensenbrenner, J. A., Dorst, J. P., & Owens, R. P. New syndrome of skeletal, dental and hair abnormalities. *Birth Defects*, 1975, 11(2):372-9. Levin, L. S., *et al.* A heritable syndrome of craniosynostosis, short thin hair, dental abnormalities, and short limbs: Cranioectodermal dysplasia. *J. Pediat.*, 1977, 90:55-61.

craniocarpotarsal dysplasia. See *Freeman-Sheldon syndrome.*

craniocarpotarsal dystrophy. See *Freeman-Sheldon syndrome.*

craniodiaphyseal dysplasia syndrome. A syndrome, probably transmitted as an autosomal recessive trait, characterized by progressive hyperostosis and sclerosis, especially involving the skull and facial bones with widening of the interorbital distance and flattening of the nasal area. Associated defects usually include small stature, mental retardation, seizures, failure of vision, deafness, absence of sexual maturity, and nasal obstruction. Roentgenologically, there are moderate thickening and sclerosis of the ribs and clavicles, and diaphyseal thickening, mostly in the metacarpals and proximal phalanges.

Halliday, J. A rare case of bone dystrophy. *Brit. J. Surg.*, 1949-50, 37:52-63. De Souza, O. Leontiasis ossea. *Porto Alegre Faculdade de Med. Rev. Dos. Cursos*, 1927 13:47-54.

craniofacial cortical hyperostosis. See *van Buchem syndrome, under Buchem, Francis Steven Peter, van.*

craniofacial dysjunction. See *Le Fort fracture III.*

craniofacial dysostosis. Synonyms: *Crouzon disease, Crouzon syndrome, dysostosis craniofacialis, dysostosis craniofacialis hereditaria, dysostosis cranio-orbitofacialis.*

A syndrome characterized by premature craniosynostosis, midface hypoplasia, and shallow orbits. The principal craniofacial symptoms include parrot-beaked nose, relative mandibular prognathism, short upper lip, protruding lower lip, and hypertelorism. Brachycephaly, scaphocephaly, and trefoil skull may be associated. Exophthalmos, strabismus, nystagmus, spontaneous luxation of the globes, megalocornea, ectopia lentis, iris colobomata, and corectopia are the chief ophthalmological symptoms. Atresia of the auditory meatus is the principal ear defect. Orodental complicions include malocclusion, crowding of the upper teeth, V-shaped dental arch, high-arched palate, bifid uvula, oligodontia, and macrodontia. Autosomal dominant transmission is the most constant feature of this syndrome but some cases have had a negative family history.

Crouzon, O. Dysostose cranio-faciale héréditaire. *Bull. Soc. Méd. Hôp., Paris*, 1912, 33:545-55.

craniofacial dysostosis with diaphyseal hyperplasia. See *Stanesco syndrome.*

craniofacial dyssynostosis (CFDS). See *craniosynostosis-craniofacial dysostosis syndrome.*

craniohypophyseal xanthoma. See *Hand-Schüller-Christian syndrome.*

craniomandibular dermatodysostosis. Synonyms: *Cavallazzi syndrome, Young syndrome, mandibuloacral dysplasia.*

A syndrome of mandibular hypoplasia, delayed closure of the cranial sutures, presence of wormian bones, narrow shoulders, dysplastic clavicles, abbreviated terminal club-shaped phalanges, acro-osteolysis, stiff joints, fat deposits over the abdomen, skin atrophy of the hand and feet with mottled brown rash of the trunk, prominent eyes, sharp nose, short stature, calcium deposits in the scalp, elbows and fingertips, abnormal modeling of the femur and humerus, inability to open the mouth widely, crowding of the lower teeth, and absence of cellular cementum in the tooth roots.

Cavallazzi, C., *et al.* Su di caso di disostosi cleido-cranica. *Riv. Clin. Pediat.*, 1960, 65:312-26. Danks, D. M., *et al.* Craniomandibular dermatodysostosis. *Birth Defects*, 1974, 10(1):99-105. Young, L. W., *et al.* New syndrome manifested by mandibular hypoplasia, acroosteolysis, stiff joints, and cutaneous atrophy (mandibuloacral dysplasia) in two unrelated boys. *Birth Defects*, 1971, 7(7):291-2.

craniometaphyseal dysplasia syndrome. A rare congenital disorder, transmitted as an autosomal dominant trait with variability of expression, characterized by enlargement and increased density of the craniofacial bony structures together with metaphyseal abnormalities of the long bones. Major facial abnormalities consist of a thick bony wedge over the bridge of the nose and glabella, hypertelorism, wide alveolar ridges, and stenosis of the nasal passages with resultant mouth breathing. Hearing loss, occasional impairment of vision, and facial paralysis may be associated. Principal radiographic features consist of hyperostosis of the frontal and occipital bones, sclerosis of the base of the skull, and hyperostosis of the facial bones and

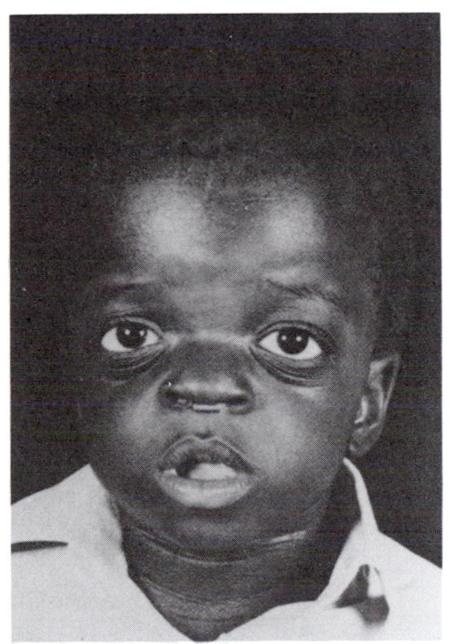

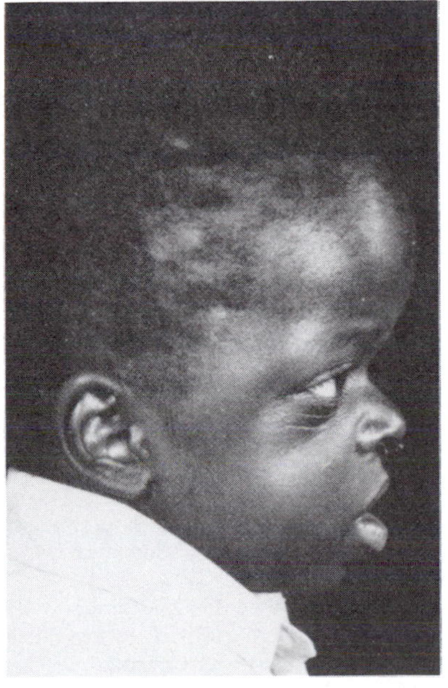

Craniofacial dysostosis
Suslak, L., B.Glista, G.B. Gertzman, L. Lieberman, R.A.Schwartz & F. Desposito: "Crouzon syndrome with periapical cemental dysplasia and acanthosis nigricans: The pleiotropic effect of a single gene?" In Shprintzen, R.J., N.W. Paul, (eds): *Diagnostic Accuracy: Effect on Treatment Planning.* New York: Alan R. Liss, Inc., for the March of Dimes Birth Defects Foundation BD:OAS 21(2):127-134, 1985, with permission.

the mandible. In children, there may be club-shaped metaphyseal widening of the tubular bones with transition between the splayed and normal metaphyses. The term **Pyle disease** (see *metaphyseal dysplasia syndrome*) is sometimes used to designate this syndrome.

Spranger, J., *et al.* Die kraniometaphysare Dysplasie. *Zschr. Kinderheilkh.*, 1965, 93:64-79. Gorlin, E., *et al.* Genetic craniotubular bone dysplasias and hyperostoses. A critical analysis. *Birth Defects*, 1969, 5(4):79-95. Holt, J. F. The evolution of craniometaphyseal dysplasia. *Ann. Radiol., Paris*, 1966, 9:209-24.

craniosynostosis-arthrogryposis-cleft palate syndrome. See *Christian syndrome (1), under Christian, Joe C.*

craniosynostosis-craniofacial dysostosis syndrome. Synonym: *craniofacial dyssynostosis (CFDS).*

A syndrome of shortness of stature, craniosynostosis, and craniofacial dysostosis involving the lambdoid suture and the posterior part of the sagittal suture and structures of the base of the skull, causing scaphocephaly with prominent forehead and small, narrow occiput. Mental retardation, hydrocephalus, and agenesis of the corpus callosum are associated in some cases. In the original report, the disorder occurred in two sisters and five cases were sporadic, four of seven patients being of Spanish, Mexican, Puerto Rican, or Cuban ancestry. Observation of two sisters suggests autosomal recessive inheritance.

Neuhauser, G., Kaveggia, E. G., & Opitz, J. M. Studies of malformation syndromes of man. XXXIX: A craniosynostosis-craniofacial dysostosis syndrome with mental retardation and other malformations: "Craniofacial dyssynostosis." *Eur. J. Pediatr.* 1976, 123(1):15-28.

craniosynostosis-fibular aplasia syndrome. See *Lowry syndrome (1).*

craniosynostosis-radial aplasia syndrome. See *Baller-Gerold syndrome.*

craniosynostosis-syndactyly-obesity syndrome. See *Summitt syndrome.*

craw-craw. See *Robles disease.*

crazy back. See *excited skin syndrome.*

CREGAN, J. C. F. (British physician)

Champion-Cregan-Klein syndrome. See *popliteal pterygium syndrome.*

CREST (**c**alcinosis cutis-**R**aynaud phenomenon-**e**sophageal dysfunction-**s**lerodactyly-**t**elangiectasia) syndrome. A variant of sceroderma characterized by calcinosis cutis, Raynaud phenomenon, esophageal dysfunction, sclerodactyly, and telangiectasia. The vascular lesions are most apparent on the surface of the skin, particularly the face, upper trunk, and hands, and also occurring on the lips, oral mucosa, and gastrointestinal tract. Gastrointestinal hemorrhage, pulmonary hypertension, biliary cirrhosis, and the Sjögren syndrome may be associated. Antibodies to centromeric chromatin (anticentromere antibodies) are found in most cases.

Eisen, A., Uitto, J. J., & Bauer, E. A. Scleroderma. In: Fitzpatric, T. B., Eisen, A. Z., Wolff, K., Freedberg, I. M., & Austen, K. F., eds. *Dermatology in general medicine.* 3rd ed. New York, McGraw-Hill, 1987, pp. 1841-52.

cretinism. See *Brissaud infantilism.*

cretinism-muscular hypertrophy syndrome. See *Debré-Semelaigne syndrome.*

CREUTZFELDT, HANS GERHARD (German physician, 1885-1964)

Creutzfeldt-Jakob disease (CJD). See *Jakob-Creutzfeldt syndrome.*

Jakob-Creutzfeldt syndrome. See *under Jakob.*

Siemerling-Creutzfeldt syndrome. See *adrenoleukodystrophy.*

CREVELD, SIMON, VAN (Dutch pediatrician, 1894-1971)

Ellis-van Creveld (EVC) syndrome. See *under Ellis.*

van Creveld-von Gierke syndrome. See *glycogen storage disease I.*

CREYX, MAURICE (French physician)

Creyx-Lévy syndrome. Synonyms: *ophthalmorhinostomatohygrosis, reverse Gougerot-Sjögren syndrome, reverse Sjögren syndrome.*

A reverse form of the Gougerot-Sjögren syndrome (see *Sjögren syndrome,* under *Sjögren, Henrik Samuel Conrad),* in which xerosis is replaced by hypersecretion, in association with chlorhydria, chemical changes of the saliva, chloride metabolism disorders, insensitivity to belladonna, and cervical vertebral calcification.

Creyx, M., & Lévy, J. Syndrome d'ophthalmo-rhino-stomato-xérose, dit de "Gougerot-Sjögren," syndrome d'ophthalmo-rhino-stomato-hygrose. *Bull. Soc. Méd. Hôp. Paris,* 1948, 64:1123-8.

cri-du-chat syndrome. See *chromosome 5p deletion syndrome.*

crib death. See *sudden infant death syndrome.*

CRIGLER, JOHN FIELDING, JR. (American physician, born 1919)

Crigler-Najjar syndrome. Synonyms: *Arias syndrome, congenital nonhemolytic jaundice, congenital nonhemolytic jaundice with kernicterus.*

A familial form of hyperbilirubinemia, transmitted as an autosomal dominant trait with incomplete penetrance and varied expressivity, characterized by kernicterus with neurological complications and jaundice of the skin, sclera, and mucous membrane. Partial defect of bilirubin conjugation is believed to be the cause. A deficiency of glucuronide formation was demonstrated by Arias in an anicteric father of two jaundiced children with a defect of hepatic glucuronyl transferase activity.

Crigler, J. F., & Najjar, V. A. Congenital familial nonhemolytic jaundice with kernicterus. *Pediatrics,* 1952, 10:169-80. Arias, I. M. Chronic unconjugated hyperbilirubinemia without overt signs of hemolysis in adolescents and adults. *J. Clin. Invest.,* 1962, 41:2233-45. Schmid, R., & McDonagh, A. F. Hyperbilirubinemia. In: Stanbury, J. B., Wyngaarden, J. B., & Fredrickson, D. S., eds. *The metabolic basis of inherited disease.* 4th ed. New York, McGraw-Hill, 1978, pp. 1221-57.

CRISTESCO, C. (French physician)

Clerc-Lévy-Cristesco (CLC) syndrome. See *under Clerc.*

CRISWICK, V. G. (American ophthalmologist)

Criswick-Schepens syndrome. Synonym: *familial exudative vitreoretinopathy (FEVR).*

A familial eye disease, transmitted as an autosomal trait, with symptoms similar to those in retrolental fibroplasia. The condition is usually observed in otherwise healthy children, and is characterized by slowly progressive ocular changes with posterior vitreous detachment, traction on the retina in all quadrants, snowflake opacities in the vitreous body, heterotopia of the macula with temporal traction, subretinal and intraretinal exudates occurring at the periphery, localized retinal detachment, often forming a broad fold extending temporally from the disc, occasional retinal breaks and degenerative changes, and new retinal vessels in scattered areas, which are subject to recurrent hemorrhage.

Criswick, V. G., & Schepens, C. L. Familial exudative vitreoretinopathy. *Am. J. Ophth.*, 1969, 68:578-95.

CRITCHLEY

Critchley syndrome. See *Kleine-Levin syndrome.*

Kleine-Levin-Critchley syndrome. See *Kleine-Levin syndrome.*

CRITCHLEY, E. M. R. (British physician)

Levine-Critchley syndrome. See *under Levine, Irving M.*

CROCKER, ALLEN C. (American physician)

Crocker syndrome. See *Niemann-Pick syndrome.*

CROCKER, HENRY RADCLIFFE (British physician)

Crocker disease. Synonym: *dermatitis repens.*

A form of spreading dermatitis occurring almost exclusively on the upper extremities. Vesicles and bullae usually appear on the fingers at the site of trivial injury, rupture, and leave bright red surfaces oozing a clear or slightly turbid fluid. The borders of the denuded areas are bound by sodden and irregular collars of the epidermis, which are elevated by subjacent fluid. The process advances by peripheral detachment of the epidermis, exudation, or development of new vesicles and bullae.

Crocker, H. R. *Diseases of the skin. Their description, pathology, diagnosis, and treatment.* London, Lewis, 1888, pp. 128-30.

crocodile shagreen. See *Vogt degeneration, under Vogt, Alfred.*

crocodile tears syndrome. See *gustatory lacrimation syndrome.*

CROCQ, JEAN B. (Belgian physician, 1868-1925)

Crocq disease. See *Raynaud phenomenon, under Raynaud syndrome.*

Crocq-Cassirer syndrome. See *Raynaud phenomenon, under Raynaud syndrome.*

CROHN, BURRILL BERNARD (American physician, born 1884)

Crohn colitis. See *Crohn disease.*

Crohn disease (CD). Synonyms: *Crohn colitis, Crohn-Lesniowski disease, enteritis regionalis, regional enteritis, regional ileitis, segmental enteritis, segmental ileitis, terminal ileitis.*

A subacute and chronic inflammatory disease, originally believed to be limited to the terminal ileum, but subsequently recognized as involving other parts of the intestine, especially the distal ileum, colon, and anorectal region. Abdominal pain and cramps may indicate narrowing of the lumen and partial obstruction of the intestine. Diarrhea and fever are often associated. In children, the disorder is often characterized by weight loss, growth retardation, and delayed sexual maturation. Oral lesions usually include granulomatous lesions similar to those present in the intestine, having a coarsely nodular or cobblestone mucosal surface, miliary ulceration, and linear fissures, with a patchy distribution. Swelling of the underlying submucosal connective tissue, proliferation of sulci with formation of ridges, and aphthous ulcer or glossitis may be associated. Some patients develop painful perirectal or perianal fistulae and purulent drainage. Arthritis, ankylosing spondylitis, and erythema nodusum may precede or occur in conjunction with other symptoms. The involved bowel is usually thickened with hyperemic lesions, serosal fibrin deposition, and formation of adhesions between the loops; the adjacent mesentery is thickened with fat migrating into the serosal part of the intestine. Fistulae between the adjoining loops, sometimes communicating with the stomach, gallbladder, and other organs, are common. The inflammatory process involves all layers of the intestine and consists of infiltration of lymphocytes, histiocytes, and plasma cells. Focal granulomas may be found in some cases.

Crohn, B. B., *et al.* Regional ileitis. A pathologic and clinical entity. *JAMA*, 1932, 99:1323-9. Lesniowski, A. Przyczynek do chirurgii kiszek. *Medycyna*, 1903, 31:460-4; 483-9; 514-8.

Crohn-Lesniowski disease. See *Crohn disease.*

CRONKHITE, LEONARD W., JR. (American physician)

Cronkhite-Canada (CC) syndrome. Synonyms: *diffuse gastrointestinal polyposis with ectodermal changes, polyposis-skin pigmentation-alopecia-fingernail changes.*

A rare, usually sporadic, syndrome characterized by generalized gastrointestinal polyposis associated with ectodermal defects, such as nail atrophy, alopecia, excessive pigmentation of the skin, and, sometimes, intussusception and carcinoma of the colon. Protein-losing enteropathy, malabsorption, and deficiency of blood calcium, potassium, and magnesium may also occur. Gastrointestinal complaints such as nausea, vomiting, and diarrhea are the common symptoms.

Cronkhite, L. W., Jr., & Canada, W. J. Generalized gastrointestinal polyposis. An unusual syndrome of polyposis, pigmentation, alopecia, and onychotrophia. *N. Engl. J. Med.*, 1955, 252:1011-5.

crooked little fingers. See *brachydactyly A-3.*

CROSBY, WILLIAM H. (American physician)

Crosby syndrome. Synonyms: *Zuelzer-Kaplan syndrome, congenital nonspherocytic hemolytic anemia, familial nonspherocytic hemolytic anemia, hereditary nonspherocytic hemolytic anemia (HNSHA).*

A hereditary form of hemolytic anemia caused by enzyme disorders, hemoglobinopathies, or defects in membrane structure. Jaundice, splenomegaly, and cholelithiasis are its main clinical characteristics. Enzyme disorders, transmitted as an autosomal recessive trait, include deficiencies of hexokinase, glucose phosphate isomerase, phosphofructokinase (with muscle glycogen storage disease), aldolase (with liver glycogen storage disorder and possible mental retardation), triosephosphate isomerase (with neuromuscular disease), diphosphoglycerate mutase (with polycythemia), pyruvate kinase, γ-glutamyl cysteine synthetase (in drug- or infection-induced hemolysis), glutathione sythetase (in drug- or infection-induced hemolysis with neurological disorders), pyrimidine-5'-nucleotidase (with occasional mental retardation), and adenylate kinase NADH-diaphorase (with methemoglobinemia and occasional mental retardation). Enzyme deficiencies transmitted as an X-linked trait include glucose-6-phosphate dehydrogenase deficiency (in drug- or infection-induced hemolysis or favism) and phosphoglycerate kinase deficiency (with mild behavioral disorders). Increased activity of adenosine deaminase, decreased activity adenosine deaminase (with immunodeficiency), and 5-oxoprolinuria are transmitted as an autosomal recessive trait.

Crosby, W. H. Hereditary nonspherocytic hemolytic anemia. *Blood,* 1950, 5:233-53. Beutler, E. Hereditary nonspherocytic hemolytic anemia-pyruvate kinase deficiency and other abnormalities. In: Williams, W. J., Beutler, E., Erslev, A. J., & Lichtman, M. A., eds. *Hematology*. 3rd ed. McGraw-Hill, New York, 1983, pp. 574-82. Kaplan, E., & Zuelzer, W. W. Familial nonspherocytic hemolytic anemia. *Blood,* 1950, 5:1811-21.

CROSS, HAROLD E. (American physician)

Cross syndrome. Synonyms: *Cross-McKusick-Breen syndrome, oculocerebral hypopigmentation syndrome.*

An oculocerebral syndrome characterized by gingival fibromatosis, hypopigmentation, microphthalmia, mental retardation, athetoid movements, and spasticity. Microphthalmia and cloudy corneae are present at birth, and spasticity and mental retardation appear by the third month of life. A high-arched palate and constriction of the maxillary arch, growth retardation, coarse nystagmus, and cryptorchism are frequently associated. Autosomal recessive inheritance is suspected.

Cross, H. E., McKusick, V. A., & Breen, W. A new oculocerebral syndrome with hypopigmentation. *J. Pediat.*, 1967, 70:398-406.

Cross-McKusick syndrome. See *Troyer syndrome.*

Cross-McKusick-Breen syndrome. See *Cross syndrome.*

CROSTI, A. (Italian physician)

Crosti reticulosis. A form of well-defined, slowly growing lymphomas with malignant development.

Crosti, A. Micosi fungoide e reticolo-istiocitomi cutanei maligni. *Minerva Derm.,* 1951, 26:3-11.

CROSTI, AGOSTINO (Italian physician, born 1896)

Gianotti-Crosti syndrome (GCS). See *under Gianotti.*

CROUZON, OCTAVE (French physician, 1874-1938)

Apert-Crouzon syndrome. See *under Apert.*

Crouzon disease. See *craniofacial dysostosis.*

Crouzon syndrome. See *craniofacial dysostosis.*

CROW, R. S. (British physician)

Crow-Fukase syndrome. See *POEMS syndrome.*

CRS. See *caudal regression syndrome, and see congenital rubella syndrome.*

CRST (calcinosis-Raynaud phenomenon-sclerodactyly-telangiectasia) syndrome. A syndrome combining calcinosis, the Raynaud phenomenon, sclerodactyly, and telangiectasia. Individual features of this syndrome occur at various times in a patient's life, seldom before puberty. The Raynaud phenomenon is the first to appear. It is marked by paresthesia, blueness of the extremities, and often, ischemic changes at the fingertips. Scleroderma involves chiefly the fingers, but may also present in other parts of the body. The calcinosis is usually subcutaneous or in the dermis. Telangiectasia is generally found on the cheeks, nose, oral mucosa, hands, and upper trunk. Associated disorders may include liver cirrhosis, collagen diseases such as lupus erythematosus, dermatomyositis, rheumatoid arthritus, and other conditions. The etiology is not known. The term is sometimes used in the literature as a synonym for the Thibierge-Weissenbach syndrome.

Winterbauer, R. H. Multiple telangiectasia, Raynaud's phenomenon, sclerodactyly, and subcutaneous calcinosis: A syndrome mimicking hereditary hemorrhagic gelangiectasia. *Bull. Johns Hopkins Hosp.,* 1964, 114:361-83.

CRUCHET, JEAN RENE (French physician)

Cruchet disease. Synonyms: *torticollis, wryneck.*

Twisting of the neck with an abnormal position of the head due to contraction of the cervical muscles.

Cruchet, J. R. *Traité des torticolis spasmodiques.* Paris, 1907.

cruciate geniculate ganglion neuralgia. See *Reichert syndrome, under Reichert, Frederick Leet.*

crural hernia. See *Cloquet hernia.*

crush injury. See *crush syndrome.*

crush syndrome. Synonyms: *Bywaters syndrome, compression syndrome, crush injury, myorenal syndrome, traumatic rhabdomyolysis.*

Acute tubular necrosis with anuria or oliguria, uremia, and myoglobinuria caused by excessive amounts of the products of tissue breakdown in the circulation, resulting from crushing of the soft tissue. The same type of acute renal failure may be produced by poisons, burns, ischemia, and other shock-causing conditions. The syndrome was first observed in air raid victims in World War II. See also *Young-Paxson syndrome.*.

Bywaters, E. G. L., & Beall, D. Crush injuries with impair ment of renal function. *Brit. Med. J.,* 1941, 1:427-32.

CRUVEILHIER, JEAN (French pathologist, 1791-1873)

Cruveilhier atrophy. See *Aran-Duchenne syndrome.*

Cruveilhier palsy. See *Aran-Duchenne syndrome.*

Cruveilhier ulcer. Simple gastric ulcer.

Cruveilhier, J. *Anatomie pathologique du corps humain.* Paris, Bailliére, 1829-35, Vol. 1, livr. 10; 1835-42, vol. 2, livr. XXX.

Cruveilhier-Baumgarten cirrhosis. See *Cruveilhier-Baumgarten syndrome.*

Cruveilhier-Baumgarten syndrome. Synonyms: *Baumgarten cirrhosis, Cruveilhier-Baumgarten cirrhosis, Pégot-Cruveilhier-Baumgarten syndrome.*

Cirrhosis of the liver with intrahepatic portal obstruction and hypertension, patency of the umbilical vein, esophageal varices, abdominal distention, prominent periumbilical and thoraco-abdominal veins, venous thrill or murmur, and congestive splenomegaly. Anemia, leukopenia, and thrombocytopenia are the principal hematological features.

Cruveilhier, J. Maladie des veines. In his: *Anatomie pathologique de corps humain*. Vol. 1. Paris, Bailliére, 1829-1835, p. 16. Baumgarten, P., von. *Über vollständiges, Offenbleiben der Vena umbilicalis; zuglich ein Beitrag zur Frage des Morbus Banti, in Baumgartens Arbeiten*. Leipzig, 1907, pp. 93-110. Pégot. Tumeur variqueuse avec anomalie du système veineux et persistance de la veine ombilicale, développement des veines souscutaneés abdominales. *Bull. Soc. Anat. Paris,* 1833, 44:57. Pégot. Anomalie veineuse. *Bull. Soc. Anat. Paris,* 1833, 8:108.

Pégot-Cruveilhier-Baumgarten syndrome. See *Cruveilhier-Baumgarten syndrome.*

CRUZ, OSWALDO (Brazilian physician, 1871-1917)

Chagas-Cruz disease. See *Chagas disease.*

crying cat syndrome. See *chromosome 5p deletion syndrome.*

cryoglobulinemia. See *cryopathic hemolytic syndrome.*

cryopathic hemolytic syndrome. Synonyms: *Clough-Richter syndrome, cold agglutinin disease, cold aggluti-*

nin syndrome, cold hemagglutinin syndrome, cryoglobulinemia.

A chronic autoimmune hemolytic disease in which exposure to cool temperatures (below 37ºC) causes autoantibodies to agglutinate human red cells. Hemolytic anemia, episodic hemoglobinuria, acrocyanosis, and peripheral vasomotor disturbances are the principal clinical features. The syndrome may occur as the primary (idiopathic) form, usually in middle-aged individuals, or as the secondary from, generally in adolescents and young adults, as a complicaion of *Mycoplasma pneumoniae* infection or infectious mononucleosis, and, in older persons, as a complication of malignant lymphoproliferative disorders.

Landsteiner, K. Über Beziehungen zwischen dem Blutserum und den Körperzellen. *Münch. Med. Wschr.*, 1903, 50:1812. Clough, M. C., & Richter, I. M. A study of an autoagglutinin occurring in a human serum. *Johns Hopkins Hosp. Rep.*, 1918, 29:86-93. Packman, C. H., & Leddy, J. P. Cryopathic hemolytic syndromes. In: Williams, W. J., Beutler, E., Erslev, A. J., & Lichtman, M. A., eds. *Hematology.* 3rd ed. New York, McGraw-Hill, 1983, pp. 642-7.

cryptococcosis. See *Busse-Buschke disease.*
cryptodontic brachymetacarpalia. See *Gorlin-Sedano syndrome.*
cryptogenic infantile cyanosis. See *Wilkinson syndrome, under Wilkinson, Scott J.*
cryptogenic polycythemia. See *Vaquez-Osler syndrome.*
cryptophthalmos syndrome. See *Fraser syndrome, under Fraser, G. R.*
cryptophthalmos-syndactyly syndrome. See *Fraser syndrome, under Fraser, G. R.*
crystal synovitis. See *pseudogout syndrome.*
crystalline corneal degeneration. See *Schnyder dystrophy, under Schnyder, W.*
CS. See ***c**arcinoid **s**yndrome.*
CS. See ***C**ushing **s**yndrome.*
CS. See ***c**limacteric **s**yndrome.*
CS. See ***C**ockayne **s**yndrome.*
CSBS (**c**ontaminated **s**mall **b**owel **s**yndrome). See *bacterial overgrowth syndrome.*
CSD. See ***c**at **s**cratch **d**isease.*
CSF. See ***c**hronic **f**atigue **s**yndrome.*
CSILLAG, J.
Csillag disease. See *Hallopeau syndrome (1).*
CSR. See ***C**heyne-**S**tokes **r**espiration, under Cheyne, John.*
CSS. See ***C**hurg-**S**trauss **s**yndrome.*
CSS. See ***c**arotid-**s**inus **s**yndrome.*
CSS. See ***c**avernous **s**inus **s**yndrome.*
CST (**C**hrist-**S**iemens-**T**ouraine) **syndrome.** See *hypohidrotic ectodermal dysplasia syndrome.*
CTA. See ***c**ongenital **t**rigeminal **a**nesthesia syndrome.*
CTS. See ***c**arpal **t**unnel **s**yndrome.*
CTX (**c**erebro**t**endinous **x**anthomatosis). See *van Bogaert-Scherer-Epstein syndrome.*
cubital tunnel syndrome. See *Kiloh-Nevin syndrome (1).*
CUP syndrome. See ***c**arcinoma **u**nknown **p**rimary syndrome.*

CURLING, THOMAS BLIZARD (British physician, 1801-1888)
Curling ulcer. A form of the stress ulcer syndrome (q.v.) characterized by a duodenal ulcer associated with severe burns on the surface of the body.

Curling, T. B. On acute ulceration of duodenum in case of burn. *Med. Chir. Tr., London*, 1842, 25:260-81.

CURRARINO, GUIDO (American radiologist)
Currarino triad. Synonym: *ASP (**a**norectal malformation-**s**acral bony abnormality-**p**resacral mass) association.*

A triad of congenital malformations consisting of anorectal malformations (anal stenosis, anal ectopia, and imperforate anus), sacral abnormality (crescentic bony defect and malsegmentation), and presacral anomaly (anterior meningocele, teratoma, and enteric cyst) occurring singly or in combinations.

Currarino, G., *et al.* Triad of anorectal, sacral and presacral anomalies. *AJR*, 1981, 137:395-8. Kennedy, R. L. J. An unusual rectal polyp: Anterior sacral meningocele. *Surg. Gyn. Obst.*, 1926, 43:803-4.

current escape syndrome. See *electrical leak syndrome.*
current loss syndrome. See *electrical leak syndrome.*
CURRY, CYNTHIA J. R. (American physician)
Curry-Hall syndrome. See *Weyers syndrome (3).*
CURSCHMANN, HANS (German physician, 1875-1950)
Curschmann-Batten-Steinert syndrome. See *myotonic dystrophy syndrome.*
Curschmann-Steinert syndrome. See *myotonic dystrophy syndrome.*
Rossolimo-Curschmann-Batten-Steinert syndrome. See *myotonic dystrophy syndrome.*
CURTH, HELEN. See OLLENDORFF-CURTH, HELEN
CURTIS, ARTHUR H. (American physician)
Fitz-Hugh and Curtis syndrome. See *Fitz-Hugh syndrome.*

CURTIUS, FRIEDRICH (German physician, 1896-1975)
Curtius syndrome (1). Synonyms: *Steiner syndrome, congenital asymmetry, congenital hemihypertrophy, ectodermal dysplasia with ocular malformations, hemiacrosomia, hemifacial hypertrophy, hemigigantism, hemimacrosomia, lateral asymmetry, partial gigantism, unilateral gigantism, unilateral hypertrophy.*

A form of hypertrophy which may involve a single small part of the body, such as a finger; a whole system, such as the nervous system, the muscular system, the skeletal system, or the vascular system; or half of the body with enlargement of several systems. Associated disorders may include mental retardation, ocular disorders (hypertelorism, sparse eyelashes, nystagmus, deficient tearing, cataract, tapetoretinal degeneration, and coloboma), cutaneous lesions (hemangiomas, café-au-lait spots, telangiectasia, and nevi), adrenal cortex tumors, Wilms tumor, kidney defects (sponge kidney), hepatoblastoma, and other disorders. Some authors use the synonym **Steiner syndrome** only when schizophrenia is present.

Curtius, F. Kongenitaler partieller Reisenwuchs mit endokrinen Störungen. *Deut. Arch. Klin. Med.*, 1925, 147:310-9.

Curtius syndrome (2). Synonyms: *Curtius-Krüger syndrome, dysfunctio pluriglandularis dolorosa, vasomotor ataxia.*

An association of ovarian insufficiency (marked by menstruation disorders), leukorrhea, habitual constipation, and vasomotor disorders (mainly acrocyanosis, hyperhidrosis, migraine, erythema, angina pectoris, vertigo, and occasional syncope).

Curtius, F., & Krüger, K. H. *Das vegetativ-endokrine Syndrom der Frau.* München, Urbach & Schwarzenberg, 1952.

Curtius-Krüger syndrome. See *Curtius syndrome (2).*
CUS. See ***c**ontact **u**rticaria **s**yndrome.*

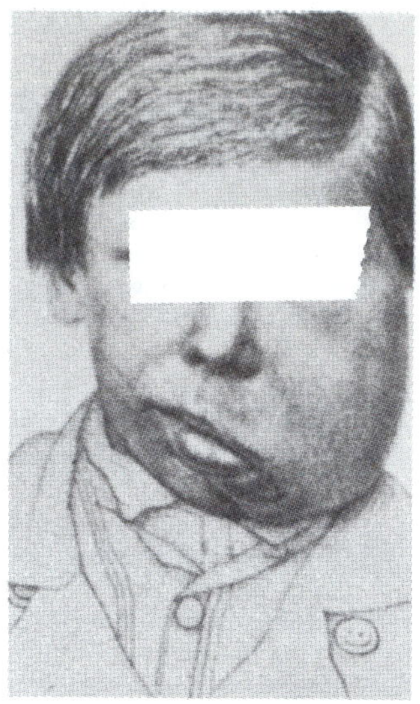

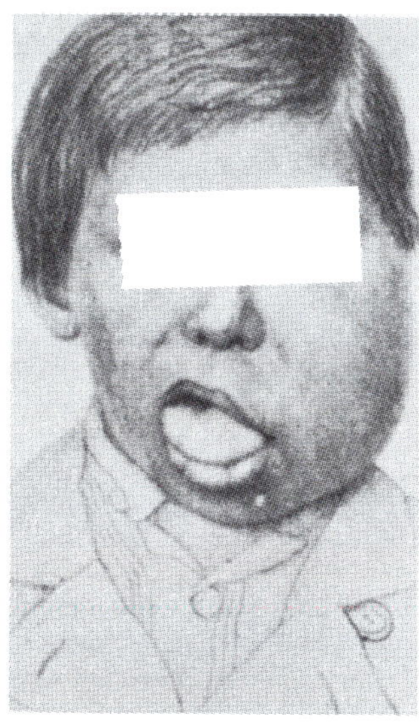

Curtius syndrome (1)
Passauer, O., *Virchows Arch. Path. Anat.*, 37:410, 1866.

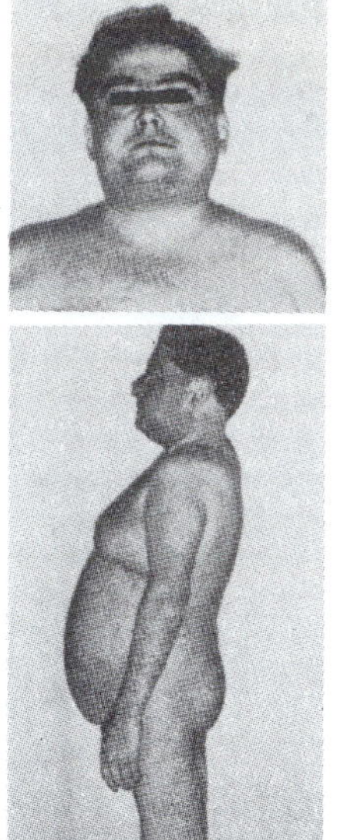

Cushing syndrome
Molinatti, G.M., F. Cammanni, & M. Tedeschin, *Journal of Clinical Endocrinology*, 19:1145, 1959.

CUSHING, HARVEY WILLIAMS (American neurosurgeon, 1869-1939)

alcohol-induced pseudo-Cushing syndrome. See *under* ***alcohol.***

Cushing basophilism. See *Cushing syndrome.*

Cushing disease. Traditionally, the term was used in connection with a condition caused by adrenocorticotropic hormone (ACTH) producing tumors of the anterior pituitary gland, but currently some writers use it to denote any disorder produced by hypersecretion of pituitary ACTH, whether or not a tumor is present. The symptoms are similar to those seen in the *Cushing syndrome* (q.v.) and include central adiposity, muscle weakness, fatigability, purplish striae, hypertension, amenorrhea, osteoporosis, depression, confusion, and psychotic disorders.

Cushing, H. W. The basophil adenomas of the pituitary body and their clinical manifestions (pituitary basophilism). *Bull. Johns Hopkins Hosp.*, 1932, 50:137-95.

Cushing medulloblastoma. Synonyms: *glioma sarcomatodes, medulloblastoma cerebelli, neurospongioblastoma, neurospongioma.*

A pinkish to grayish solid malignant neoplasm that arises in the cerebellum and consists of spongioblastic and neuroblastic cells.

Bailey, P., & Cushing, H. W. Medulloblastoma cerebelli; a common type of midcerebellar glioma in childhood. *Arch. Neur. Psychiat.*, 1925, 14:192-225.

Cushing symphalangism. See *symphalangism syndrome.*

Cushing syndrome (CS). Synonyms: *Cooke-Apert-Gallais syndrome, Cooke-Gallais syndrome, Cushing basophilism, Gallais syndrome, Itsenko-Cushing syndrome, adipositas osteoporotica endocrinica, basophil adenoma, hypercorticism, hypercortisolism, hypophyseal basophilism, hypophyseal basophilic adenoma, pituitary basophilism.*

A syndrome of obesity, hypertension, fatigability, weakness, amenorrhea, hirsutism, purplish abdominal striae, edema, glycosuria, and osteoporosis associated with a basophilic tumor of the pituitary gland. An excessive production of cortisol by the adrenal cortex is the cause. Rupture of dermal collagen fibers are manifested by cutaneous striae and easy bruisability. Osteoporosis is the cause of pathological fractures and occasional collapse of vertebral bodies. Impaired glucose tolerance is due to increased liver gluconeogenesis and insulin resistance (diabetes mellitus occurs in some cases). Deposition of fatty tissue causes the development of moon (cushingoid) facies, buffalo hump, truncal obesity, and occasional episternal fatty tumors. The face has a plethoric appearance. Hypertension, emotional disorders, depression, confusion, and psychotic changes are frequently associated. Increased androgen secretion causes acne, hirsutism, and oligomenorrhea in women. Hyperplasia of the adrenal cortices, the main etiologic factor, is caused by overproduction of ACTH due to hypothalamo-pituitary disorders, ACTH-producing pituitary adenomas, ectopic ACTH or corticotropin-releasing hormone (CRH) producing tumors, adrenal nodular hyperplasia adenoma or carcinoma of the adrenals, and iatrogenic causes, including prolonged use of ACTH or glucocorticoids. Some synonyms of this syndrome are used also to designate *congenital adrenal hyperplasia* (q.v.).

Cushing, H. W. The basophil adenomas of the pituitary body and their clinical manifestations (pituitary basophilism). *Bull. Johns Hopkins Hosp.*, 1932, 50:137-95. *Itsenko, N. M. *K klinike, patogenezu tsentral'nykh vegetativnykh sindromov v sviazi s ucheniem o mezhutochno-gipofizarnoi sisteme.* Voronezh, 1946. Apert, E. Dystrophies en relation avec des lésions de capsules surrénales. Hirsutisme et progenia. *Bull. Soc. Pédiat., Paris,* 1910, 12:501. *Gallais. *Le syndrome génitosurrénal, étude anatomo-clinique.* Paris, 1912.

Cushing tumor. Synonyms: *arachnoid fibroblastoma, dural endothelioma, leptomeningioma, meningoblastoma, meningioma.*

A slow-growing, benign, solid, nodular tumor varying in size from that of a pea to that of an orange, which arises from the arachnoidal villi and frequently invades the adjacent dura mater and skull bones. The tumor is most frequently observed in patients 40 to 70 years of age.

Cushing, H. The meningiomas (dural endotheliomas): Their source, and favoured seats of origin. *Brain.* 1922, 5:282-316.

Cushing-like syndrome. See *alcohol-induced pseudo-Cushing syndrome.*

Itsenko-Cushing syndrome. See *Cushing syndrome.*

pre-Cushing syndrome. The presence of adrenal hormonally active tumors without clinical symptoms of the Cushing syndrome.

Beierwaltes, W. H., *et al.* Imaging functional nodules of the adrenal glands with 131I-19-iodocholessterol. *J. Nucl. Med.*, 1974, 15:246-51. Charbonnel, B., *et al.* Does the corticoadrenal adenoma with "preCushing syndrome" exist? *J. Nucl. Med.*, 1981, 22:1059-61.

pseudo-Cushing syndrome. See *alcohol-induced pseudo-Cushing syndrome.*

Rokitansky-Cushing ulcer. See *under Rokitansky.*

CUSHING, HARVEY WILLILAMS (American neurosurgeon, 1869-1939)

Apert-Cushing syndrome. See *Cushing syndrome.*

cushingoid syndrome. See *alcohol-induced pseudo-Cushing syndrome.*

cutaneo-intestinal cavernous hemangioma. See *blue rubber bleb syndrome.*

cutaneo-intestinal mortal syndrome. See *Degos syndrome.*

cutaneocerebral angioma. See *Sturge-Weber syndrome.*

cutaneomeningospinal angiomatosis. See *Cobb syndrome.*

cutaneomuco-intestinal syndrome. See *Degos syndrome.*

cutaneomuco-oculo-epithelial syndrome. See *Stevens-Johnson syndrome.*

cutaneomuco-uveal syndrome. See *Behçet syndrome.*

cutaneomucous proteinosis. See *Urbach-Wiethe syndrome.*

cutaneous allergic vasculitis. See *Gougerot-Ruiter syndrome.*

cutaneous angioneurosis. See *Quincke edema.*

cutaneous dyschondroplasia-dyschromia syndrome. See *Maffucci syndrome.*

cutaneous leishmaniasis. See *Alibert disease (2).*

cutaneous lentiginosis with atrial myxoma syndrome. Synonyms: *LAMB (lentigines-atrial myxoma-mucocutaneous myxomas-blue nevi) syndrome, NAME (nevi-trial myxoma-myxoid neurofibromatosis-ephelides) syndrome.*

A syndrome of unknown etiology characterized by the association of cutaneous lentigines and atrial myxomas. Cutaneous pigmented nevi, myxoid neurofibromas, mammary fibroadenomas, arterial aneurysm of the central nervous system, cerebral embolism, and cardiac abnormalities (heart conduction defects, coarctation of the aorta, hypertrophic obstructive cardiomyopathy, and cardiac rhabdomyosarcoma) are usually associated.

Rhodes, A. R., *et al.* Mucocutaneous lentigines, cardiomucocutaneous myxomas, and multiple blue nevi: The LAMB syndrome. *J. Am. Acad. Dermat.*, 1984, 10:72-82. Rees, J. R. *et al.* Lentiginosis and left atrial myxoma. *Brit. Heart J.*, 1973, 35:874-6.

cutaneous papillomatosis. See *Gougerot-Carteaud syndrome, undera Gougerot, Henri.*

cutaneous T-cell lymphoma. See *mycosis fungoides.*

cutis elastica syndrome. See *Ehlers-Danlos syndrome.*

cutis hyperelastica. See *Ehlers-Danlos syndrome.*

cutis hyperelastica dermatorrhexis. See *Ehlers-Danlos syndrome.*

cutis laxa. See *Ehlers-Danlos syndrome.*

cutis laxa syndrome. Synonyms: *chalaxoderma, chalodermia, connatal cutis laxa syndrome, dermatochalasis connata, dermatolysis, dermatomegaly, generalized elastolysis, primary elastolysis.*

A rare congenital disorder of connective tissue in which the skin hangs loosely in redundant folds, giving the face a peculiar bloodhound-like, old appearance (churchillian facies). The skin is not hyperplastic and there is no fragility, which is a feature in the *Ehlers-Danlos syndrome* (q.v.). Additional symptoms include blepharoptosis, ectropion, emphysema, right ventricular heart enlargement, bundle branch block, cor pulmonale, tortuous blood vessels, diverticula of the gastrointestinal and urogenital tracts, gastric ulcer, esophageal dilatation, dilatation and tortuosity of the

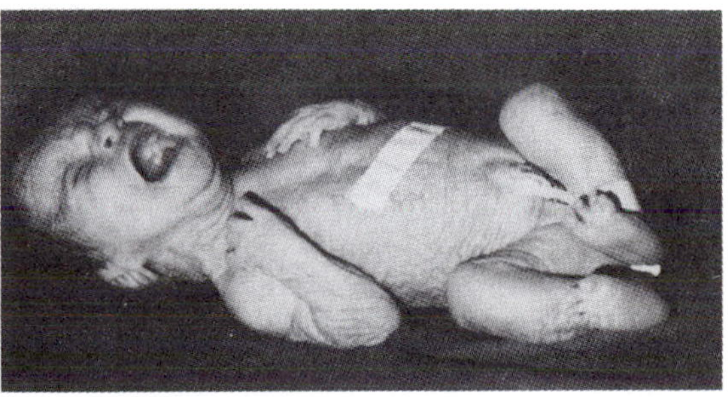

Cutis laxa-growth deficiency syndrome
Reisner, S.H., et al.: *Acta Paediatrica Scandinavica*, 60:357, 1971.

ureters, hernias, hip dislocation, muscle hypotonia, growth retardation, deep voice, mental retardation, and other defects. The syndrome may be transmitted as an autosomal recessive or, less commonly, as an autosomal dominant trait. Some sporadic cases also have been reported.

*Variot, & Cailliau. Peau ridée senile chez un enfant de deux ans. Agénésie des réseux élastique du derme. *Bull. Soc. Méd. Hôp. Paris*, 1919, 43:989-94. Goltz, R. W., & Hulr, A. M. Generalized elastolysis (cutis laxa) and Ehlers-Danlos syndrome (cutis hyperelastica). *South. Med. J.*, 1965, 58:848-54.

cutis laxa-growth deficiency syndrome. A syndrome of cutis laxa and growth deficiency, probably transmitted as an autosomal recessive trait, associated with congenital hip dislocation, joint laxity, and, sometimes, large fontanels, low-set ears, coloboma of the macula lutea, and slow progress of disease processes.

Reisner, S. H., *et al.* Cutis laxa associated with severe intrauterine growth retardation and congenital dislocation of the hip. *Acta Paediat. Scand.*, 1971, 60:357. Swith, D. W. *Recognizable patterns of malformation. Genetic, embryologic and clinical aspects.* 2nd ed. Philadelphia, Saunders, 1976, p. 358.

cutis marmorata teleangiectatica (CMTC). See *Lohuizen disease.*

cutis verticis gyrata. See *pachydermoperiostosis syndrome.*

cutis verticis gyrata-mental retardation syndrome. A syndrome, transmitted as an autosomal recessive trait, characterized by furrowing of the face, forehead, and scalp and mental retardation. Associated disorders include microcephaly with asymmetric skull and small cerebellum, cerebral palsy, epilepsy, and eye defects.

McDowall, T. W. Case of abnormal development of the scalp. *J. Ment. Sc.*, 1893, 39:62-4. Akesson, H. O. Cutis verticis gyrata and mental deficiency in Sweden. I. Epidemiological and clinical aspects. *Acta Med. Scnad.*, 1964, 175:115-27.

cyclic albuminuria. See *Pavy disease.*

cyclic glaucoma. See *Posner-Schlossman syndrome.*

cyclic oculomotor paralysis. See *Axenfeld-Schürenberg syndrome.*

cyclical edema syndrome. Synonym: *idiopathic cyclic edema.*

Periodic edema in women, occurring on assuming the standing position and disappearing on lying down. Associated disorders may include headache, oliguria, dyspnea, constipation, thirst, asthenia, and hypotension. Exacerbation may occur during the premenstrual period. Hyperaldosteronism is suspected as the etiologic factor.

Mach, R. S., *et al.* Oedème idiopathique par rétention solique avec hyperaldostéronurie. *Bull. Mem. Soc. Méd. Hôp. Paris*, 1955, 71:726-32.

cyclokeratitis. See *Dalrymple disease.*

cyclopism. See *Fraser syndrome, under Fraser, G. R.*

Cyprus fever. See *brucellosis.*

CYRIAX, EDWARD F. (British orthopedic surgeon)

Cyriax syndrome. See *slipping rib syndrome.*

cystadenoma. See *Cheatle disease.*

cystadenoma mammae. See *Cheatle disease.*

cystathionine beta-synthase (CBS) deficiency. See *homocystinuria syndrome.*

cystic adenoid epithelioma. See *Brooke epithelioma.*

cystic disease of the mammary gland. See *Cheatle disease.*

cystic disease of the renal pyramids. See *Cacchi-Ricci syndrome.*

cystic fibroadenomatosis. See *Cheatle disease.*

cystic intrahepatic bile duct dilatation. See *Caroli syndrome (2).*

cystic papillary adenoma. See *Warthin tumor.*

cystine diathesis. See *cystinosis.*

cystine storage disease. See *cystinosis.*

cystine storage-aminoaciduria-dwarfism syndrome. See *cystinosis.*

cystinosis. Synonyms: *Abderhalden-Kaufmann-Lignac syndrome, De Toni-Fanconi syndrome, Fanconi syndrome, Fanconi-De Toni-Debré syndrome, Lignac disease, Lignac-Fanconi syndrome, Lignac-Fanconi-Debré syndrome, cystine diathesis, cystine storage-aminoaciduria-dwarfism syndrome, cystine storage disease, familial cystine diathesis, nephrotic-glycosuric dwarfism with hypophosphatemic rickets.*

An inherited error of metabolism, transmitted as an autosomal recessive trait, characterized by free (nonprotein) cystine in lysosomes of the cornea, conjunctiva, bone marrow, lymph nodes, leukocytes, and internal organs. In the **nephropathic form**, faulty water reabsorption (due to renal tubular disorders) is the first manifestation. It occurs during the first 6 months of life and is followed by polyuria, polydipsia, dehydration, and recurrent fever. By the age of 1 year, there are additional symptoms, including failure to thrive; growth retardation; rickets; acidosis; increased urinary levels of cystine, glucose, amino acids, phosphate, and potassium; and frequent weakness, prostration, cardiac failure, and death. X-ray findings show frontal bossing, genu valgum, thickening of the wrists and ankles, rachitic rose, Harrison groove, and broad and frayed epiphyses similar to those seen in rickets. Most affected children have blond hair and fair complexion and are resistant to sunlight and tanning but suffer from photophobia. Ocular changes include opacities of the cornea and conjunctiva and peripheral retinopathy. The **early form** is manifested by onset at the age of 5 years and deposition of cystine crystals in the cornea, bone marrow, and leukocytes in the absence of renal dysfunction and retinopathy. The **intermediate (late onset or adolescent)** form is marked by a later onset and a progressive course of glomerular insufficiency with deposition of crystals in the bone marrow, cornea, conjunctiva, leukocytes, and skin fibroblasts in association with mild forms of photophobia, retinopathy, and growth retardation. The precise classification of cystinosis is still unsettled. Some authors use the term **Fanconi syndrome** as a synonym for cystinosis, whereas others restrict its use to the nephropathic type. Also, a condition characterized by an association of rickets and stunted growth with glycosuria and albuminuria, and one marked by spontaneous fractures in dwarfed children associated with low levels of serum phosphate, acidosis, albuminuria, and glycosuria **(De Toni-Fanconi, Fanconi,** and **Fanconi-De Toni-Debré syndromes)** are considered by some authors as separate entities, but are treated by others as clinical expressions of the same condition.

Fanconi, G. Der frühinfantile nephrotisch-glycosurische Zwergwuchs mit hypophosphatämischer Rachitis. *Jahrb.*

Kinderh., 1936, 147:299-318. Abderhalden, E. Familiäre Cystindiathese. *Hoppe Seyler Zschr. Physiol. Chem.*, 1903, 38:557-61. De Toni, G. Remarks on the relations between renal rickets (renal dwarfism) and renal diabetes. *Acta Paediat., Uppsala*, 1933, 16:479-84. Lignac, G. O. Über Störung des Cystinstoffwechsels bei Kindern. *Deut. Arch. Klin. Med.*, 1924, 145:139-50. Debré, R., *et al.* Rachitisme tardif coexistant avec une néphrite chronique et une glycosurie. *Arch. Méd. Enf., Paris*, 1934, 37:597-606. Schneider, J. A., *et al.* Cystinosis and the Fanconi syndrome. In: Stanbury, J. B., Wyngaarden, J. B., & Frederickson, D. S., eds. *The metabolic basis of inherited disease.* 4th ed. New York, McGraw-Hill, 1978, pp. 1660-82.

cystiphorous desquamative epithelial hyperplasia. See *Cheatle disease.*

cytomegalia infantum. See *Wyatt disease, under Wyatt, John Poyner.*

cytomegalic inclusion disease. See *Wyatt disease, under Wyatt, John Poyner.*

cytosine arabinose syndrome. Synonym: *ara-C syndrome.*

A complex of symptoms following the use of cytosine arabinose, including fever, myalgias, joint and bone pain, and less commonly, chest pain, maculopapular rash, and conjunctivitis. Other complicatations may include ara-C lung (noncardiogenic pulmonary edema), pancreatitis, peritonitis, pericarditis, and central nervous system (especially cerebellar) disorders.

Castleberry, R. P., *et al.* The cytosine arabinose (ara-C) syndrome. *Med. Pediat. Oncol.*, 1981, 9:257-64.

CZERMAK

Hippel-Czermak syndrome. See *Hippel-Lindau syndrome.*

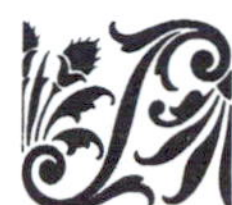

Page #	Term	Observation

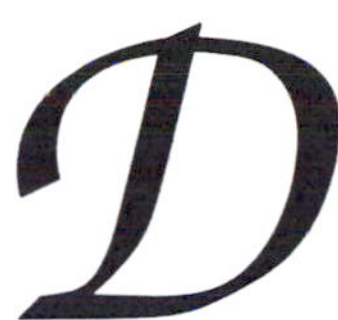

D13 ring syndrome. See *chromosome 13 ring syndrome.*

D fever. See *Dutton fever.*

D'ACOSTA, JOSE (Spanish Jesuit missionary in Peru, 1539-1600)

D'Acosta disease. Synonyms: *altitude sickness, mountain climber's disease.*

An acute form of mountain sickness which occurs shortly after reaching high altitudes, and is characterized by anoxia from diminished oxygen intake, difficulty in breathing coordination, muscle tonus defect, hyperventilation, color vision and light adaptation disorders, fatigue, dizziness, headache, nausea, vomiting, insomnia, prostration, and impaired mental capacity and judgment.

*D'Acosta, J. Efecto estraño que hace en ciertas tierras de Indios el aire, lo viento que corre. Forms Lib. 3. Chap. 9. In his: *Historia natural y moral de las Indias.* Sevilla, Juan de Leon, 1590.

DA COSTA, JACOB MENDEZ (American physician, 1833-1900)

Da Costa disease. See *Da Costa syndrome.*

Da Costa syndrome. Synonyms: *Da Costa disease, cardiac anxiety syndrome, cardiac neurosis, cardiac phobia, cardiasthenia, effort syndrome, irritable heart, nervous heart, neurocirculatory asthenia, neurocirculatory dystonia (NCD), soldier's heart.*

A disorder combining effort fatigue, dyspnea, chest pain, palpitation, and dizziness, originally attributed to physical or emotional stress, but subsequently also associated with conditions such as mitral valve prolapse and autonomic hyperactivity. The terms **cardiac phobia** and **cardiac neurosis** are sometimes used for cardiac anxiety which is unrelated to an endogenous depression or other psychotic disorders; functional cardiovascular symptoms associated with fear of suffering from undiagnosed cardiac disease are termed **cardiac hypochondriasis** by some authors. The disorder was frequently observed in Civil War and World War I soldiers.

Da Costa, J. M. On irritable heart; a clinical study of a form of functional cardiac disorder and its consequences. *Am. J. Med.,* 1871, 61:17-52. Maier, W., *et al.* The cardiac anxiety syndrome-subtype of panic attack. *Eur. Arch. Psychiat. Neur. Sc.,* 1985, 235-52.

DA COSTA, MENDES SAMUEL. See MENDES DA COSTA, SAMUEL

DABNEY, WILLIAM CECIL (American physician, 1849-1894)

Dabney grippe. See *Sylvest syndrome.*

DACIE, SIR JOHN V. (British physician)

Dacie syndrome. Synonyms: *nontropical idiopathic splenomegaly, primary hypersplenic pancytopenia, primary hypersplenism, simple splenic hyperplasia.*

A syndrome of massive splenomegaly of unknown etiology with symptoms of hypersplenism. The blood picture is characterized by leukopenia, neutropenia, thrombocytopenia, and reticulocytosis. The affected persons are anemic and some have auto-antibodies against red cells and agammaglobulinemia. Congestive changes and lymphoid hyperplasia of the spleen are the principal histological features. Some patients develop non-Hodgkin lymphomas.

Dacie, J. V., *et al.* 'Non-tropical idiopathic splenomegaly' ('primary hypersplenism'): A review of ten cases and their relationship to malignant lymphomas. *Brit. J. Haemat.,* 1969, 17:317-33.

dacryosialadenopathia atrophicans. See *Sjögren syndrome under Sjögren, Henrik Samuel Conrad.*

dacryosialoadenopathy. See *Sjögren syndrome under Sjögren, Henrik Samuel Conrad.*

dacryosialocheilopathy. See *Sjögren syndrome under Sjögren, Henrik Samuel Conrad.*

dactylitis. See *under sickle cell anemia.*

dactylolysis essentialis. See *ainhum syndrome.*

dactylolysis spontanea. See *ainhum syndrome.*

DAD (**d**iffuse **a**lveolar **d**amage). See *adult respiratory distress syndrome.*

DAENTL, DONNA L. (American physician)

Daentl syndrome. See *femoral hypoplasia-unusual facies syndrome.*

DAGNINI, GUIDO (Italian physician)

Scaglietti-Dagnini syndrome. See *Erdheim syndrome.*

DALEN, JOHAN ALBIN (Swedish ophthalmologist, born 1866)

Dalén-Fuchs nodules. See *Dalén-Fuchs spots.*

Dalén-Fuchs spots. Small depigmented areas in the retina which remain after the disappearance of white-grayish nodules (**Dalén-Fuchs nodules**) seen in sympathetic choroiditis.

*Dalén, A. Zur Kenntnis der sogenannten Choroiditis sympathetica. Mitteilungen Augenklin. *Carolin. Med. Chir. Inst., Stockholm,* 1904, 6:1-21. Fuchs, E. Über sympathisierende Entzündung (nebst Bemerkungen über seröse traumatische Iritis). *Graefes Arch. Ophth.,* 1905, 61:365-456.

DALRYMPLE, JOHN (British ophthalmologist, 1804-1852)

Dalrymple disease. Synonym: *cyclokeratitis.*

Inflammation of the ciliary body and cornea.

*Dalrymple, J. *Pathology of the human eye.* London, Churchill, 1852.

DAMESHEK, WILLIAM (American physician, born 1900)

Dameshek syndrome. See *Cooley anemia.*

Estren-Dameshek syndrome. See *under Estren.*

DAMOCLES (A courtier of Dyonysus, tyrant of Syracuse, who was seated at a banquet with a sword suspended over his head by a single hair, that he might learn of his own insecurity)

Damocles syndrome. A feeling of uncertainty hanging over the heads of survivors of childhood cancer.

Koocher, G. P., & O'Malley, J. E. *The Damocles syndrome: Psychosocial consequences of surviving childhood cancer.* McGraw-Hill, New York, 1981.

DANA, CHARLES LOOMIS (American physician, 1852-1935)

Dana syndrome. Synonyms: *Lichtheim syndrome, Putnam disease, Putnam-Dana syndrome, dorsolateral degenerative myelopathy, funicular myelitis, funicular myelosis, funicular sclerosis, neuroanemic syndrome, posterolateral sclerosis, subacute combined degeneration of the spinal cord, subacute combined sclerosis.*

A neurological disease characterized by degenerative changes in the white matter of the spinal cord associated with pernicious anemia. The disease usually begins insidiously with weakness, fatigue, and dyspnea on exertion. Other symptoms may include paralysis of the legs and arms, myalgia, edema of the feet and ankles, numbness and tingling in the distal portions of the extremities, glossitis, headache, malaise, peculiar gait, recurrent mental disorders, and hallucinations. Myocardial damage may occur. Degenerative changes, small hemorrhagic foci, and demyelinated zones in the anterior funiculi are most frequently found in the posterior and lateral columns of the spinal cord. The brain and peripheral nerves may be involved in some cases.

Dana, C. L. The degenerative diseases of the spinal cord, with the description of a new type. *J. Nerv. Ment. Dis.*, 1891, 18:205-16. Putnam, J. J. A group of cases of system sclerosis of the spinal cord, associated with diffuse collateral degeneration; occurring in enfeebled persons past middle life, and especially in women; studied with particular reference to etiology. *J. Nerv. Ment. Dis.*, 1891, 18:69-110. Lichtheim. Zur Kenntnis der perniciösen Anämie. *Verh. Deut. Ges. Inn. Med.*, 1887, pp. 84-96.

Putnam-Dana syndrome. See *Dana syndrome.*

DANAIDS (Mythological daughters of Danaüs, one of Io's descendants, who dwelt by the Nile. As a punishment for killing their husbands, they were condemned to bail out the sea with leaking jars)

Danaïd syndrome. Synonyms: *Stanley syndrome, Sisyphus complex.*

A condition characterized by overestimating one's own abilities while underestimating the size and degree of difficulty of the job ahead, resulting in a mental state similar to that experienced by the Danaïd sisters, who discovered that they were not up to the task and that the ocean was as large and deep as ever, even though they were bailing it out with all their might. The malady is most common among medical lexicographers, who seem to be unable to learn that the size, rapid growth, and complexity of medical terminology make it unconquerable.

Stanley, J. Personal communication.

DaNang lung. See *adult respiratory distress syndrome.*

DaNang syndrome. See *posttraumatic stress syndrome.*

DANBOLT, NIELS CHRISTIAN (Norwegian dermatologist)

Danbolt syndrome. See *acrodermatitis enteropathica.*

Danbolt-Closs syndrome. See *acrodermatitis enteropathica.*

dancing eye syndrome. See *Kingsbourne syndrome.*

dancing eye and dancing feet syndrome. See *Kingsbourne syndrome.*

dancing eye syndrome with myoclonic ataxia. See *Kingsbourne syndrome.*

dancing eyeball syndrome. See *Kingsbourne syndrome.*

DANDY, WALTER EDWARD (American physician, 1886-1946)

Dandy syndrome. Bilaterally absent vestibular function, occurring in two basic forms: a compensated type, without oscillopsia, and a decompensated type, with oscillopsia. The two principal symptoms include visual jumbling of objects, occurring when the patient is in motion and disappearing when he is at rest, and dysequilibrium, occurring when walking in the dark. The majority of patients have mild to moderate sensorineural hearing loss. Vascular lesions secondary to infections, neoplasm, and toxic reactions to some ototoxic drugs are the cause. In the original report, the syndrome occurred after bilateral division of the vestibular nerves in Ménière's disease.

Dandy, W. E. The surgical treatment of Ménière's disease. *Surg. Gynec. Obst.*, 1941, 72:421-5.

Dandy-Walker anomaly. See *Dandy-Walker syndrome.*

Dandy-Walker cyst. See *Dandy-Walker syndrome.*

Dandy-Walker syndrome (DWS). Synonyms: *Dandy-Walker anomaly, Dandy-Walker cyst, atresia of the foramen of Magendie, atresia of the foramina of Luschka and Magendie.*

Partial or complete absence of the cerebellar vermis, hydrocephalus, and posterior fossa cyst continuous with the fourth ventricle. A cystlike structure, representing the dilated fourth ventricle, expands in the midline, causing the occipital bone to bulge posteriorly and to dislodge the tentorium and torcula upward. Absent or poorly developed corpus callosum and dilatation of the aqueduct and third and lateral ventricles may be present. Atresia of the foramina of Magendie and Luschka causes congenital hydrocephalus. Complications may include papilledema, blepharoptosis, and sixth cranial nerve paralysis.

Dandy, W. E. The diagnosis and treatment of hydrocephalus due to occlusion of the foramina of Magendie and Luschka. *Surg. Gyn. Obst.*, 1921, 32:112-24.

Dandy-Walker-like syndrome. A familial syndrome, transmitted as an autosomal recessive trait, combining characteristics of the Dandy-Walker syndrome (malformation of the posterior fossa, high insertion of confluent sinus, hydrocephalus, cerebellar hypoplasia, cerebellar vermis aplasia, enlarged subarachnoid spaces and cisterna magna) with other abnormalities, including cranial anomalies (microcephaly, large fontanelles, wide cranial sutures, bulging forehead, prominent occiput, foramina parietalia), characteristic facies (hypertelorism, down-slanting palpebral fissures, depressed nasal bridge, low-set ears), narrow palate, bifid uvula, short stature, hypoplastic nipples, slightly

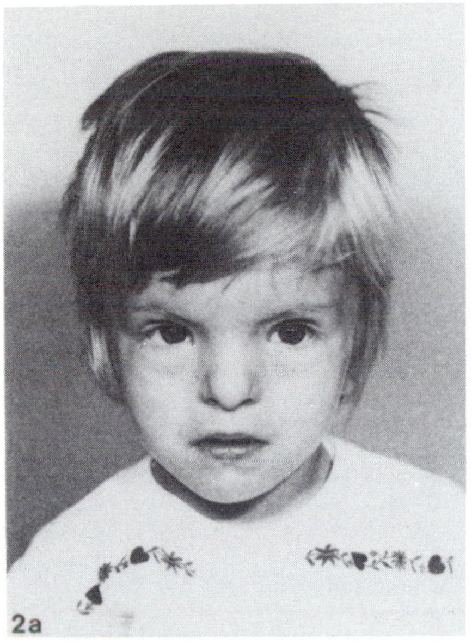

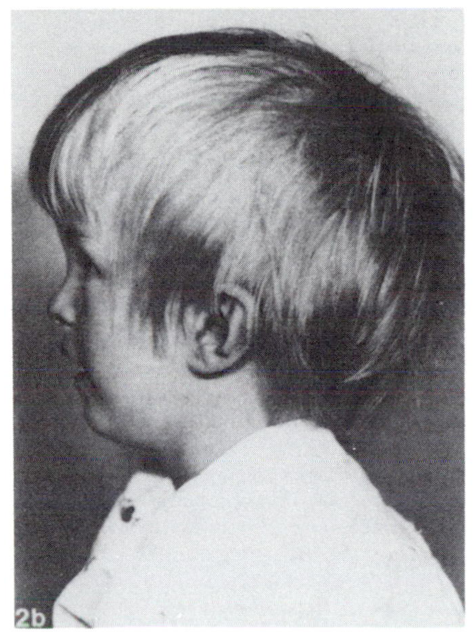

Dandy-Walker syndrome
Ritscher, Daniel, Albert Schinzel, Eugen Boltshauser, Jakob Briner, Urs Arbenz & Peter Sigg, *American Journal of Medical Genetics* 26:481-491 1987. New York: Alan R. Liss Inc.

gaping vulva, eleven pairs of ribs, abnormal palmar creases, atrioventricular defect, and mental retardation.

Ritscher, D., *et al.* Dandy-Walker (like) malformation, atrio-ventricular septal defect and a similar pattern of minor anomlies in 2 sisters: A new syndrome? *Am. J. Med. Genet.*, 1987, 26:481-91.

DANIELSSEN, DANIEL CORNELIUS (Norwegian physician, 1815-1894)

Danielssen-Boeck disease. Synonyms: *anesthetic leprosy, lepra tuberoanesthetica.*

A type of leprosy which is marked by hyperesthesia followed by anesthesia, paralysis, ulcers, gangrene, and mutilation. See also *Hansen disease..*

*Danielssen, D. C., & Boeck, C. W. *Om spedalskheden.* Christiania, 1847.

DANIS, P. (Swiss ophthalmologist)

Maeder-Danis dystrophy. See *under Maeder.*

DANKS, D. M. (Australian physician)

Pitt-Rogers-Danks syndrome. See *Pitt syndrome.*

DANLOS, HENRI ALEXANDRE (French physician, 1844-1912)

Danlos syndrome. See *Ehlers-Danlos syndrome.*

Ehlers-Danlos syndrome (ED, EDS). See *under Ehlers.*

Meekeren-Ehlers-Danlos syndrome. See *Ehlers-Danlos syndrome.*

DARIER, JEAN FERDINAND (French dermatologist, 1856-1938)

Bowen-Darier disease. See *Bowen disease, under Bowen, John Templeton.*

Darier disease (1). Synonyms: *Darier syndrome, Darier-White disease, Lutz-Darier syndrome, White disease, dyskeratosis follicularis, dyskeratosis follicularis vegetans, keratosis follicularis, keratosis vegetans, psorospermosis.*

A disease of the skin, transmitted as an autosomal dominant trait, usually beginning by the end of the first or during the second decade of life and rarely in infants. It presents flesh-colored papules which soon are covered by a yellowish to tan scaly crust covering the seborrheic areas of the body (the chest, ears, nasolabial folds, scalp, and groin). On removing the lesion, a porelike opening is revealed. Eventually, the lesions coalesce into large, sometimes thick plaques to form hypertrophic, warty, foul-smelling masses. Flat warty papules may occur on the dorsa of the feet and hands, and punctate keratoses may be seen on the palms and soles. The nails are usually fragile and, after breaking off, show V-shaped scalloping and subungual thickening. Alopecia is a frequent complication. Mucous membranes of the palate, gingivae, uvula, larynx, pharynx, and rectum may also be involved. The condition tends to be aggravated by sunlight.

Darier, J. Psorospermose folliculaire végétante. Étude anatomo-pathologique d'une affection cutanée non décrite ou comprise dans le groupe des acnés sebacées, cornées, hypertophiantes, des kératoses (ichthyoses) folliculaires, etc. *Ann. Derm. Syph., Paris,* 1889, 10:597-612. White, J. C. A case of keratosis (ichthyosis) follicularis. *J. Cutan. Dis.,* 1889, 7:201-9.

Darier disease (2). See *erythema annulare centrifugum.*

Darier erythema. See *erythema annulare centrifugum.*

Darier syndrome. See *Darier disease (1).*

Darier-Ferrand dermatofibrosarcoma. Synonyms: *dermatofibrosarcoma protuberans, progressive recurrent dermatofibroma.*

A rare, slowly-growing fibroblastic tumor of the skin on the trunk and, less frequently, the extremities, that usually begins as a single small nodule or multiple nodules which coalesce to form a thick, hard plaque. Ulceration occurs in most instances. Histologically, the lesion consists of spindle-shaped, fibrolast-like cells. Metastases are uncommon. Females are affected more frequently than males.

Darrier, J., & Ferrand, M. Dermato-fibromes progressifs et récidivantes our fibro-sarcomes de la peau. *Ann. Derm. Syph., Paris,* 1924, 5:545-62.

Darier-Grönblad-Strandberg syndrome. See *pseudoxanthoma elasticum.*

Darier-Roussy sarcoid. Synonyms: *subcutaneous nodular sarcoidosis, subcutaneous sarcoidosis.*

A rare cutaneous expression of systemic sarcoidosis characterized by subcutaneous nodules, chiefly on the extremities, which show the typical histological appearance of sarcoidosis. It may be associated with the early benign hilar adenopathy syndrome of sarcoidosis or with the later stages of progressive sarcoidosis. In the past, the term had been used for various forms of granulomatous panniculitis, including sarcoidosis.

Darier, & Roussy. Un cas de tumeurs bénigne multiples (sarcoides souscutanées ou tuberulides nodulares hypodermiques). *Bull. Soc. Fr. Derm.,* 1904, 15:54-9.

Darier-White disease. See *Darier disease (1).*

Lutz-Darier syndrome. See *Darier disease (1).*

DARLING, SAMUEL TAYLOR (American physician, 1872-1925)

Darling disease. See *histoplasmosis.*

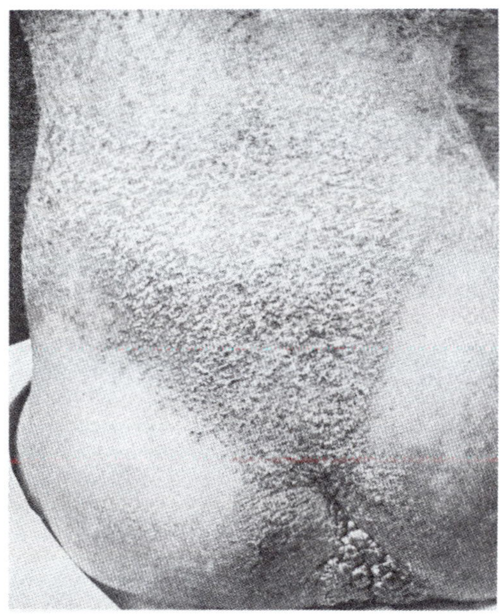

Darier disease (1)
Andrew, G.C. & A.W. Domonkos: *Diseases of the skin.* 5th ed. Philadelphia, W.B. Saunders Co., 1963.

DAT (dementia of the Alzheimer type). See *Alzheimer disease.*

DAVID, JEAN PIERRE (French physician, 1737-1784)

David disease. See *Pott disease.*

DAVID, W. WALTER (German physician, born 1890)

David disease. Synonym: *purpura feminarum typica.*

A disease of women, believed to be caused by a deficiency of ovarian hormone, and marked by hemorrhage from the gums and mucous membranes.

David. W. Über "Purpura"-Erkrankungen bei Frauen. *Med. Klin., Berlin,* 1926, 22:1755-6.

DAVIDENKOV (DAVIDENKOV), S. (Russian physician)

Davidenkov syndrome. See *scapuloperoneal syndrome.*

DAVIDOFF, L. M.

Dyke-Davidoff-Masson (DDM) syndrome. See *under Dyke, C. G.*

DAVIDSON, L. S. (British physician)

Davidson anemia. Synonyms: *Bomford-Rhoads anemia, refractory anemia.*

A group of anemias that are refractory to any therapy other than blood transfusion.

Davidson, L. S., *et al.* Studies on refratory anaemia. I. The technique and interpretation of sternal puncture biopsies. Classification. *Edinburgh M. J.,* 1943, 50:226-36. Bomford, R. R., & Rhoads, C. P. Refractory anaemia. I. Clinical and pathological aspects. *Q. J. Med., Oxford,* 1941, 10:175-234.

DAVIES, H. E. F. (British physician)

Wrong-Davies syndrome. See *under Wrong.*

DAVIES, J. N. P.

Davies disease. Synonym: *endomyocardial fibrosis.*

An acquired, progressive, and frequently fatal disease of children and young adults in Uganda. It is characterized by broad, thick scars of the mural endocardium and a sudden or insidious failure of one or both ventricles followed by death. Pathologically, there are endocardial lesions at the apex of the right ventricle, the posterior wall of the left ventricle, or the apex of the left ventricle. The connective tissue, especially of the endocardium, is swollen with acid mucopolysaccharide and covered with fibrin. In advanced stages, the lesions become hard white scars composed of collagen and elastica.

Davies, J. N. P. Endocardial fibrosis in Africans. *East. Afr. Med. J.,* 1948, 25:10-4.

DAVIES-COLLEY, R. (British physician)

Davies-Colley syndrome. See *slipping rib syndrome.*

DAWSON, J. B. (American physician)

Dawson encephalitis. See *van Bogaert encephalitis.*

DAY, RICHARD LAWRENCE (American physician, born 1905)

Riley-Day syndrome. See *under Riley, Conrad Milton.*

DBA (Diamond-Blackfan anemia). See *Diamond-Blackfan syndrome.*

DC. See ***D**upuytren **c**ontracture.*

DC (dyskeratosis congenita). See *Zinsser-Engman-Cole syndrome.*

DCM (dyssynergia cerebellaris myoclonica). See *Hunt syndrome (1).*

DD (dyssegmental dwarfism; dyssegmental dysplasia). See *Rolland-Desbuquois syndrome, and see Silverman syndrome (2).*

DDD. See ***D**owling-**D**egos **d**isease.*

DDM. See *Dyke-Davidoff-Masson syndrome, under Dyke, C. G.*

DE. See ***d**ialysis **e**ncephalopathy syndrome.*

DE ALMEIDA, FLORIANO PAULO (Brazilian physician)

de Almeida disease. See *Lutz-Splendore-de Almeida syndrome, under Lutz, Alfredo.*

Lutz-Splendore-de Almeida syndrome. See *under Lutz, Adolfo.*

DE AZUA Y SUAREZ, JUAN (Spanish dermatologist, 1859-1922)

Azua pseudoepithelioma. See *De Azua pseudoepithelioma.*

De Azua pseudoepithelioma. Synonyms: *Azua pseudoepithelioma, pyodermitis chronica vegetans.*

A blastomycosislike form of pyoderma, giving the histological picture of epithelioma.

De Azua, J., & Sada y Pons, C. Pseudo-épithéliomas cutanés. *Ann. Derm. Syph., Paris,* 1903, 4:745-6.

DE BARSY, A. M. (Belgian physician)

De Barsy syndrome. See *De Barsy-Moens-Dierckx syndrome.*

De Barsy-Moens-Dierckx syndrome. Synonym: *De Barsy syndrome.*

A congenital progeroid syndrome of mental retardation, shortness of stature, and multiple abnormalities, associated with degenerative changes of the elastic tissues of the skin and cornea, motor retardation, muscle hypotonia, brisk tendon reflexes, and intermittent abnormal eye movements. The skin is lax and wrinkled (especially of the neck and axillary regions), dry, inelastic, and translucent, showing superficial blood vessels. The skull is microcephalic and asymmetric, with frontal bossing, open fontanelles and sutures, and hypertelorism. The mouth is small with thin lips. The corneae are cloudy. The hands are small and malformed in a claw-like position.

De Barsy, A. M., Moens, E., & Dierckx, L. Dwarfism, oligophrenia and degeneration of the elastic tissue in skin and cornea. A new syndrome? *Helvet. Paediat. Acta,* 1968, 23:305-13.

DE BEUERMANN, CHARLES LUCIEN. See BEUERMANN, CHARLES, LUCIEN, DE

DE BOYER, ALEXIS. See BOYER, ALEXIS, DE

DE CLERAMBAULT, G. G. See CLERAMBAULT, GAETAN HENRI ALFRED EDOUARD LEON MARIE GATIAN, DE

DE CORVISART. See CORVISART DE MARETS, BARON JEAN NICHOLAS, DE

DE CRECCHIO, L. (Italian anatomist)

de Crecchio syndrome. See *congenital adrenal hyperplasia.*

DE GIMARD, MARTIN JULES LOUIS ALEXANDRE. See MARTIN DE GIMARD, JULES LOUIS ALEXANDRE

DE GROUCHY, JEAN. See GROUCHY, JEAN, DE

DE KLEYN, A. See KLEYN, A., DE

DE LA PEYRONIE, FRANÇOIS. See PEYRONIE, FRANÇOIS, DE LA

DE LANGE, CORNELIA. See LANGE, CORNELIA DE

DE MARTINI, A. (Italian physician)

De Martini-Balestra syndrome. See *Burke syndrome.*

DE MORGAN, CAMPBELL (British physician, 1811-1876)

De Morgan spots. Synonyms: *capillary angiomas, cherry angiomas, ruby spots, senile angiomas.*

Bright red angiomas, about 2 to 6 mm in diameter, containing numerous vascular loops. They are caused by telangiectatic vascular disorders and may be found on the trunk and, sometimes, other parts of the body, usually in middle-aged or elderly persons.

De Morgan, C. *The origin of cancer: Considered with reference to the treatment of the disease.* London, Churchill, 1872.

DE MORSIER, GEORGES. See MORSIER, GEORGES, DE

DE POZZI, SAMUEL JEAN. See POZZI, SAMUEL JEAN, DE

DE QUERVAIN, FRITZ. See QUERVAIN, FRITZ, DE

DE REYNIER, JEAN PIERRE. See REYNIER, JEAN PIERRE, DE

DE SANCTIS, CARLO (Italian psychiatrist)

De Sanctis-Cacchione (DSC) syndrome. Synonyms: *idiotia xerodermica, xeroderma pigmentosum with neurologic manifestations, xerodermic idiocy.*

A multiple abnormality syndrome, transmitted as an autosomal recessive trait, characterized by xeroderma pigmentosum, microcephaly, mental retardation, growth retardation, and gonadal hypoplasia. Many affected infants exhibit acute sun sensitivity. The skin appears normal at birth, but erythema of the exposed parts usually occurs within a few months, followed by freckles, atrophy, pigmentation, dryness, scaling, and telangiectasia. Photophobia, lacrimation, conjunctivitis, pigmentation, and telangiectasia are the common ocular findings. Most affected patients develop cutaneous neoplasms resulting in death during adolescence. Basal cell carcinoma, squamous cell carcinoma, and melanoma are the most frequent tumors.

De Sanctis, C., & Cacchione, A. L'idiozia xerodermica. *Riv. Sper. Freniat.,* 1932, 56:269-92.

DE TONI, GIOVANNI (Italian pediatrician, 1896-1973)

De Toni-Caffey syndrome. See *Caffey-Silverman syndrome.*

De Toni-Caffey-Silverman syndrome. See *Caffey-Silverman syndrome.*

De Toni-Fanconi syndrome. See *cystinosis.*

Fanconi-De Toni-Debré syndrome. See *cystinosis.*

Roske-De Toni-Caffey-Silverman syndrome. See *Caffey-Silverman syndrome.*

Roske-De Toni-Caffey-Smyth syndrome. See *Caffey-Silverman syndrome.*

DE VAAL, O. M. See VAAL, O. M., DE

DE VRIES, ANDRE (Israeli physician)

De Vries syndrome. Synonyms: *congenital labile factor deficiency with syndactyly, familial congenital labile factor deficiency with syndactyly.*

A familial congenital condition, observed in both sexes, characterized by factor V deficiency associated with a tendency to bleed and syndactyly.

De Vries, A., *et al.* Familial congenital labile factor deficiency with syndactylism. Investigation on the mode of action of the labile factor. *Acta Haemat., Basel,* 1951, 5:129-42.

de-afferented state. See *locked-in syndrome.*

dead loop syndrome. See *blind loop syndrome.*

deadly catatonia. See *Bell mania, under Bell, Luther Vos.*

deafmutism-goiter-euthyroidism syndrome. See *Refetoff syndrome.*

deafness-alopecia-hypogonadism syndrome. See *Crandall syndrome.*

deafness-ear pits syndrome. See *Wildervanck syndrome (3).*

deafness-goiter syndrome. See *Pendred syndrome.*

deafness-keratopachyderma-digital constriction syndrome. See *Vohwinkel syndrome.*

deafness-ocular albinism syndrome. See *ocular albinism-sensorineural deafness syndrome.*

deafness-onychodystrophy-osteodystrophy-retardation syndrome. See *DOOR syndrome.*

deafness-perilymphatic gusher syndrome. See *Nance syndrome.*

deafness-piebaldism syndrome. See *Woolf syndrome.*

deafness-strabismus-symphalangism syndrome. See *symphalangism syndrome.*

deafness-symphalangism syndrome. See *facio-audio-symphalangism syndrome.*

DEBLER, K. (German physician)

Debler anemia. Synonym: *familial hemolytic anemia.*

A familial form of hemolytic anemia with onset in infancy, characterized by hepatosplenomegaly, growth retardation, gastrointestinal disorders, and occasional fever and porphyrinuria. The hematological findings include severe hypochromic anemia, decreased resistance of erythrocytes, presence in the blood of nucleated erythrocytes, erythroblastosis, reticulocytosis, anisocytosis, and microcytosis.

Debler, K. Familiäre hämolytische Anämie. *Zschr. Kinderh.,* 1939, 61:198-205.

DEBOVE, GEORGES MAURICE (French physician, 1845-1920)

Débove disease. Essential splenomegaly.

Débove, G. M., & Cruhl, I. La splénomegalie primitive. *Bull. Soc. Méd. Hôp. Paris,* 1892, 9:596-613.

debrancher deficiency syndrome. See *glycogen storage disease III.*

DEBRAY

Looser-Debray-Milkman syndrome. See *Milkman syndrome.*

DEBRE, ROBERT (French physician, 1882-1978)

Brocq-Debré-Lyell syndrome. See *toxic epidermal necrolysis.*

Debré syndrome (1). See *cat scratch disease.*

Debré syndrome (2). Synonyms: *glucoadipositas hepatomegalica, hepatomegalic glucoadiposity, polycoric hepatomegaly, polycoric hypertrophy.*

A disease of small children characterized by an accumulation of reserve material in the liver cells and hepatomegaly, caused by a disorder of carbohydrate and, indirectly, lipid metabolism.

Debré, R. Les polycories. *Presse Méd.,* 1935, 43:801-3.

Debré-Fibiger syndrome. See *congenital adrenal hyperplasia.*

Debré-Julien Marie syndrome (1 and 2). See *Debré-Marie syndrome (1 and 2).*

Debré-Lamy-Lyell syndrome. See *toxic epidermal necrolysis.*

Debré-Marie syndrome (1). Synonyms: *Debré-Julien Marie syndrome, infectious edematous polyneuritis, neuroedematous syndrome.*

A pathological condition characterized by initial fever followed by edema and polyneuritis involving all four extremities. Drooping of the hands and feet, walking difficulty, and amyotrophy are the main symptoms. There are no disorders of electrical conductivity, and the cerebrospinal fluid is apparently normal.

Marie, J., *et al.* Sur un syndrome neuro-oedemateux épidémique décrit avec M. Robert Debré. *Bull. Mem. Soc. Méd. Hôp. Paris,* 1941-42, 57:304-15.

Debré-Marie syndrome (2). Synonym: *Debré-Julien Marie syndrome.*

Dwarfism, genital infantilism, and disorders of water metabolism marked by excessive hydrophilia of the body, oligodypsia, oliguria, retarded water elimination, and high density of urine.

Debré, R., & Marie, J. Nanisme avec hypertrophie des organes génitaux, oligodypsie et hyperhydrophilie. *Bull. Mem. Soc. Méd. Hôp. Paris,* 1938-39. 54:1347-58.

Debré-Mollaret syndrome. See *cat scratch disease.*

Debré-Semelaigne syndrome. Synonyms: *Kocher-Debré-Semelaigne (KDS) syndrome, cretinism-muscular hypertrophy syndrome, hypothyroid myopathy, hypothyroidism-large muscle syndrome, infantile myxedema-muscular hypertrophy syndrome, myopathy-myxedema syndrome, myxedema-muscular hypertrophy syndrome, myxedema-myotonic dystrophy syndrome.*

Apparent muscular hypertrophy in hypothyroid children giving them the "herculean" (prize-fighter, athletic, or pseudo-athletic) appearance. Associated disorders may include retarded physical and mental development, delayed dentition, coarse hair, peculiar facies, painful movement, clumsy gait, macroglossia with dysarthria, and increased muscle mass. Absence of painful spasms and pseudomyotonia is the major point of difference from the Hoffmann syndrome (see under *Hoffmann, Johann*).

Debré, R., & Semelaigne, G. Hypertrophie musculaire généralisée du petit enfant. *Bull. Soc. Pediat., Paris,* 1934, 32:699-706. Kocher, T. Zur Verhütung des Cretinismus und cretinoider Zustande nach neueren Forschungen. *Deut. Zschr. Chir.,* 1892, 34:556-626.

Fanconi-De Toni-Debré syndrome. See *cystinosis.*

Fibiger-Debré-von Gierke syndrome. See *congenital adrenal hyperplasia.*

Kocher-Debré-Semelaigne (KDS) syndrome. See *Debré-Semelaigne syndrome.*

Lignac-Fanconi-Debré syndrome. See *cystinosis.*

DECHAUME, JEAN (French physician, 1896-1968)

Bonnet-Dechaume-Blanc syndrome. See *under Bonnet, Paul.*

deciduous skin. See *continual skin peeling syndrome.*

deep gyrate erythema. See *erythema annulare centrifugum.*

deep punctate dystrophy of the cornea with ichthyosis. See *Franceschetti syndrome (1).*

deer fly fever. See *Francis disease.*

DEF (**d**ysplasie **e**ctodermique, **f**ente labiale et/ou palatine) **syndrome.** A hereditary syndrome, probably transmitted as an autosomal dominant trait, characterized by ectodermal dysplasia and cleft lip and/or palate, sometimes associated with hair dysplasia (scrubbing-brush hair).

Bonafé, J. L., *et al.* Association "dysplasie ectodermique-division palatine-cheveux-chiendent." Sa place dans les syndromes dysmorphiques à type de "D.E.F." (dysplasie ectodermique, fente labiale et/ou palatine). *Ann. Derm. Vener., Paris,* 1979, 106:898-93.

defective abdominal wall syndrome. See *prune belly syndrome.*

defibrination syndrome. See *disseminated intravascular coagulation syndrome.*

deficiency dermatosis. See *Stryker-Halbeisen syndrome.*

degeneracy. See *Nordau disease.*

degeneratio cristallinea corneae hereditaria. See *Schnyder dystrophy, under Schnyder, W.*

degeneratio hyaloidea granuliformis corneae. See *Kozlowski degeneration, under Kozlowski, Bogumil.*

degeneratio hyaloideo-retinalis hereditaria. See *Wagner syndrome, under Wagner, H.*

degenerative chorea. See *Huntington chorea.*

DEGOS, ROBERT (French dermatologist, born 1904)

Degos syndrome. Synonyms: *Degos-Delort-Tricot syndrome, Köhlmeier syndrome, Köhlmeier-Degos syndrome, arteriolar cutaneogastrointestinal thrombosis, atrophic dermatitis papulosquamosa, atrophic papu-*

losquamous dermatitis, cutaneointestinal mortal syndrome, cutaneomuco-intestinal syndrome, dermatitis papulosquamosa atrophicans, fatal cutaneointestinal syndrome, malignant atrophic papulosis, malignant papulosis atrophicans, malignant papulosis with atrophy, papulosis atrophicans maligna, thromboangiitis cutaneo-intestinalis disseminata.

Malignant atrophic papulosis usually occurring in males as pathognomonic skin lesions followed by acute abdominal episodes, bowel perforation, peritonitis, and death. Some patients may lack gastrointestinal symptoms and present mainly the central nervous system manifestations (headache, paresthesia, weakness, and rapid deterioration followed by death) and the cutaneous lesions (pale rose edematous papules which become umbilicated and form white centers, progressing to ulceration, hemorrhage, and scab formation). Histological findings show thrombosis of the blood vessels of the skin and intestinal mucosa and hyaline degeneration and necrobiosis of the cutaneous appendages. Mucosal necrosis, ulceration, and exudates are usually observed in the intestine. There is little inflammation. Progressive cerebral and cerebellar atrophy and multiple cerebral infarcts and/or thrombosis of small arteries may occur. Ocular complications usually include atrophic skin of the eyelids, intermittent diplopia, conjunctival atrophy, telangiectases of the conjunctiva, peripheral choroiditis, and papilledema.

Degos, R., Delort, J., & Tricot, R. Dermatite papulosquameuse atrophiante. *Ann. Derm. Syph., Paris*, 1942, 2:148-50; 281. Köhlmeier, W. Multiple Hautnekrosen bei Thrombangiitis obliterans. *Arch. Derm., Berlin*, 1940-41, 181:783-92.

Degos-Delort-Tricot syndrome. See *Degos syndrome.*

Dowling-Degos disease (DDD). See *under Dowling.*

Köhlmeier-Degos syndrome. See *Degos syndrome.*

DEGROOT, LESLIE J. (American physician)

Refetoff-DeWind-DeGroot syndrome. See *Refetoff syndrome.*

DEITERS, OTTO FRIEDRICH CARL (German anatomist, 1834-1863)

Deiters nucleus syndrome. See *Bonnier syndrome.*

DEJEAN, M. C. (French physician)

Dejean syndrome. See *orbital floor syndrome.*

DEJERINE, JOSEPH JULES (French neurologist, 1849-1917)

Déjerine disease. See *Déjerine-Sottas syndrome.*

Déjerine syndrome (1). Synonyms: *diphtheric neuritis, diphtheric polyneuritis, neuritis multiplex atactica, neurotabes periphérica.*

Polyneuritis secondary to an infection with *Corynebacterium diphtheriae.*.

Déjerine, J. Sur un cas de paraplégie par névrites périphériques chez une ataxique morphiomane. (Contribution à l'étude de la névrite péripherique). *C. Rend. Soc. Biol. Paris,* 1887, 4:137-43.

Déjerine syndrome (2). Synonyms: *alternating hypoglossal hemiplegia syndrome, anterior bulbar syndrome, pyramid-bulbar syndrome, pyramid-hypoglossal syndrome.*

Hemorrhage or thrombosis of the anterior spinal artery producing ipsilateral paralysis of the tongue, contralateral pyramidal paralysis of the arm and leg, and occasional contralateral loss of the proprioceptive and tactile senses.

Gorlin, R. J., Pindborg, J. J., & Cohen, N. M., Jr. *Syndromes of the head and neck.* 2nd ed. New York, McGraw-Hill, 1976, p. 200.

Déjerine-Roussy syndrome. Synonyms: *posterior thalamic syndrome, retrolenticular syndrome, thalamic hyperesthetic anesthesia, thalamic syndrome, thalamic pain syndrome.*

Posterolateral thalamic lesions, such as infarcts or hemorrhage, associated with contralateral pain. It is at first characterized by hemianesthesia, which is followed by a gradual return of sensory function and, in turn, by pain. In some cases, there may be spontaneous recovery and the pain ceases, but, more commonly, it continues with little sensory loss, involving mostly the face or arm.

Déjerine, J., & Roussy, G. Le syndrome thalamique. *Rev. Neur., Paris,* 1906, 14:521-32.

Déjerine-Sottas syndrome. Synonyms: *Déjerine disease, Gombault degeneration, Gombault neuritis, hypertrophic interstitial neuritis, hypertrophic interstitial polyneuritis, hypertrophic interstitial neuropathy, hypertrophic interstitial radiculoneuropathy, hypertrophic neuritis syndrome, progressive hypertrophic interstitial neuritis.*

A slowly progressive hereditary form of hypertrophic neuritis transmitted as an autosomal dominant trait. After onset during childhood or adolescence, the early symptoms include numbness, paresthesia, cramps, and lancinating pain in the extremities. They are followed by symmetrical muscle weakness and atrophy with secondary claw hands and talipes equinovarus, the affected muscles showing decreased responsiveness to electric stimulation. Kyphoscoliosis, muscle fasciculation, and arthropathies may occur. Pathological findings include diffuse thickening of the nerve trunks, hypertrophy of the Schwann sheath with concentric lamination, degeneration of the myelin of the peripheral nerves, degeneration of the axis cylinders, degeneration of the posterior columns, and thickening of the spinal roots. Ocular complications include myosis, nystagmus, anisocoria, papillotonia, and optic atrophy.

Déjerine, J. J., & Sottas, J. Sur la névrite interstitielle hypertrophique et progressive de l'enfant; affection souvent familiale et à début infantile, caractérisée par une atrophie musculaire des extré- mities, avec troubles marqués de la sensibilité et ataxie des mouvements et relevant d'une névrite interstitielle hypertrophique a marche ascendante avec lésions médullaires consécutives. *C. Rend. Soc. Biol.,* 1890, 2:43-53. Combault. Contribution à l'étude anatomique de la névrite parenchymateuse subaiguë out chronique. Névrite segmentaire périaxiale. *Arch. Neur., Paris,* 1880, 1:11-38.

Déjerine-Thomas syndrome. See *olivopontocerebellar atrophy.*

Erb-Landouzy-Déjerine syndrome. See *Landouzy-Déjerine syndrome.*

Landouzy-Déjerine dystrophy. See *Landouzy-Déjerine syndrome.*

Landouzy-Déjerine syndrome. See *under Landouzy.*

DEJERINE-KLUMPKE, AUGUSTA (French neurologist, 1859-1927)

Déjerine-Klumpke paralysis. See *Déjerine-Klumpke syndrome.*

Déjerine-Klumpke syndrome. Synonyms: *Déjerine-Klumpke paralysis, Klumpke palsy, Klumpke paraly-*

sis, lower brachial plexus palsy, lower radicular syndrome.

Paralysis of the area supplied by the ulnar nerve and the inner head of the median nerve, resulting from injuries (including birth injuries, particularly in breech delivery) of the lower primary trunk or the eight cervical and first thoracic roots. There is weakness and wasting of small muscles of the hand and the inner forearm. Paralysis of the cervical sympathetic nerves with Horner's syndrome may be associated.

Déjerine-Klumpke, A. Contribution á l'étude de paralysies radiculaires du plexus brachial. Paralysies radiculaires totales. Paralysies radiculaires inférieures. De la participation des filets sympathiques oculo-pupillaires dans ces paralysies. *Rev. Méd., Paris,* 1885, 5:591-616; 739-90.

Klumpke palsy. See *Déjerine-Klumpke syndrome.*

Klumpke paralysis. See *Déjerine-Klumpke syndrome.*

DEL CASTILLO, E. B. (Argentine physician)

Ahumada-Del Castillo syndrome. See *amenorrhea-galactorrhea syndrome.*

Argonz-Del Castillo syndrome. See *amenorrhea-galactorrhea syndrome.*

Del Castillo syndrome. See *Sertoli cell only syndrome.*

del(1pter) syndrome. See *chromosome 1pter deletion syndrome.*

del(1q) syndrome. See *chromosome 1q deletion syndrome.*

del(2q) syndrome. See *chromosome 2q deletion syndrome.*

del(3pter) syndrome. See *chromosome 3pter deletion syndrome.*

del(3q) syndrome. See *chromosome 3q deletion syndrome.*

del(4p) syndrome. See *chromosome 4p deletion syndrome.*

del(4q) syndrome. See *chromosome 4q deletion syndrome.*

del(5p) syndrome. See *chromosome 5p deletion syndrome.*

del(5q) syndrome. See *chromosome 5q deletion syndrome.*

del(6q) syndrome. See *chromosome 6q deletion syndrome.*

del(7p) syndrome. See *chromosome 7p deletion syndrome.*

del(7q) syndrome. See *chromosome 7q deletion syndrome.*

del(8p) syndrome. See *chromosome 8p deletion syndrome.*

del(8q) syndrome. See *chromosome 8q deletion syndrome.*

del(9p) syndrome. See *chromosome 9p deletion syndrome.*

del(10p) syndrome. See *chromosome 10p deletion syndrome.*

del(10qter) syndrome. See *chromosome 10qter deletion syndrome.*

del(11q) syndrome. See *chromosome 11q deletion syndrome.*

del[(11)(q23)] syndrome. See *chromosome 11q deletion syndrome.*

del(12p) syndrome. See *chromosome 12p deletion syndrome.*

del(13q) syndrome. See *chromosome 13q deletion syndrome.*

del(14q) syndrome. See *chromosome 14q deletion syndrome.*

del(16q) syndrome. See *chromosome 16q deletion syndrome.*

del(17p) syndrome. See *chromosome 17p deletion syndrome.*

del(18p) syndrome. See *chromosome 18p deletion syndrome.*

del(18q) syndrome. See *chromosome 18q deletion syndrome.*

del(20p) syndrome. See *chromosome 20p deletion syndrome.*

del(20q) syndrome. See *chromosome 20q deletion syndrome.*

del(21) syndrome. See *chromosome 21 monosomy syndrome.*

del(21q) syndrome. See *chromosome 21q deletion syndrome.*

DELAYE, J. B. (French physician)

Delaye syndrome. Incomplete partial paralysis said to occur in the insane.

*Delaye, J. B. *Considérations sur une espèce de paralysie qui affecte particulièrement les aliènés.* Paris, 1824 (Thesis).

delayed cerebellar ataxic syndrome. See *olivopontocerebellar atrophy.*

delayed cold-induced urticaria syndrome. A familial form of urticaria, transmitted as an autosomal dominant trait, characterized by a delayed cutaneous response to cold, taking place 9 to 18 hours after the exposure.

Soter, N. A., *et al.* Delayed cold-induced urticaria: A dominantly inherited disorder. *J. Allergy Clin. Immun.,* 1977, 59:294-7.

delayed cortical cerebellar atrophy. See *olivopontocerebellar atrophy.*

delayed psychomotor awakening. See *Rosenthal disease, under Rosenthal, Curt.*

delayed repolarization arrhythmia. See *torsades de pointes syndrome.*

deletion 1pter syndrome. See *chromosome 1pter deletion syndrome.*

deletion 2q syndrome. See *chromosome 2q deletion syndrome.*

deletion 3pter syndrome. See *chromosome 3pter deletion syndrome.*

deletion 3q syndrome. See *chromosome 3q deletion syndrome.*

deletion 5p syndrome. See *chromosome 5p deletion syndrome.*

deletion 6q syndrome. See *chromosome 6q deletion syndrome.*

deletion 7p syndrome. See *chromosome 7p deletion syndrome.*

deletion 7q syndrome. See *chromosome 7q deletion syndrome.*

deletion 8p syndrome. See *chromosome 8p deletion syndrome.*

deletion 8q syndrome. See *chromosome 8q deletion syndrome.*

deletion 9p deletion syndrome. See *chromosome 9p deletion syndrome.*

deletion 10p syndrome. See *chromosome 10p deletion syndrome.*

deletion 10pter syndrome. See *chromosome 10pter deletion syndrome.*

deletion 11q syndrome. See *chromosome 11q deletion syndrome.*
deletion 12p syndrome. See *chromosome 12p deletion syndrome.*
deletion 13q syndrome. See *chromosome 13q deletion syndrome.*
deletion 14q syndrome. See *chromosome 14q deletion syndrome.*
deletion 16q syndrome. See *chromosome 16q deletion syndrome.*
deletion 17p syndrome. See *chromosome 17p deletion syndrome.*
deletion 18p syndrome. See *chromosome 18p deletion syndrome.*
deletion 18q syndrome. See *chromosome 18q deletion syndrome.*
deletion 20p syndrome. See *chromosome 20p syndrome.*
deletion 20q syndrome. See *chromosome 20q deletion syndrome.*
Delhi boil. See *Alibert disease (2).*
DELILLE, ARTHUR (French physician)
Rénon-Delille syndrome. See *under Rénon.*
delirium aigu. See *Bell mania, under Bell, Luther Vos.*
delirium alcoholicum. See *Morel disease, under Morel, Benoit Augustin.*
delirium syndrome. A mental disorder marked by a clouded state of consciousness and difficulty in sustaining attention to both external and internal stimuli, sensory misperceptions, and a disordered stream of thought. Principal features of this syndrome include disorientation, illusions, delusions, hallucinations, impaired memory, disturbances of affect, psychomotor disorders, and autonomic dysfunction. Associated disturbances consist mostly of anxiety, fear, depression, irritability, anger, euphoria, apathy, and sleep-wakefulness disorders. Systemic infections, alcohol and drug addiction, reactions to drugs, metabolic disorders (hypoxia, hypercarbia, ionic imbalance, hepatic and renal diseases), thiamine deficiency, postoperative complications, intoxications, substance withdrawal reactions, hypertensive encephalopathy, seizures, and focal lesions of the right parietal lobe and inferomedial surface of the occipital lobe are the principal causes. Elderly persons are most frequently affected.

Diagnostic and statistical manual of mental disorders. 3rd ed. Washington,D. C., American Psychiatric Association, 1980, pp. 104-7. Wells, C. E. Organic syndromes: Delirium. In: Kaplan, H. I., & Sadock, B. J., eds. *Comprehensive textbook of psychiatry.* 4th ed. Baltimore, Williams & Wilkins, 1985, pp. 838-51.

delirium tremens (DT). See *Morel disease, under Morel, Benoit Augustin.*

DELITALE (Italian physician)
Delitale-Valtancoli syndrome. See *Van Neck disease.*
DELORT, J. (French physician)
Degos-Delort-Tricot syndrome. See *Degos syndrome.*
delta phalanx. See *brachydactly A-2.*
delusional syndrome. See *organic delusional syndrome.*
delusional ectoparasitosis. See *Ekbom syndrome (2).*
delusional misidentification syndrome. See *Capgras syndrome.*
delusions of parasitosis. See *Ekbom syndrome (2).*
delusions of skin infestation. See *Ekbom syndrome (2).*

DEMARQUAY, JEAN N. (French physician, 1811-1875)
Demarquay-Richet syndrome. See *van der Woude syndrome.*
dementia syndrome. An organic brain syndrome characterized by a loss of intellectual abilities, involving impairment of memory, orientation, and cognition and interferring with one's normal social functioning. Illusions or hallucinations, incoherent speech, sleep-wakefulness disorders, and psychomotor disorders are the principal symptoms. Etiololgic factors include tertiary neurosyphilis, tuberculosis of the central nervous system, fungal meningitis, encephalitis, Jakob-Creutzfeld disease, brain injuries, subdural hematoma, pernicious anemia, folic acid deficiency, hypothyroidism, bromide intoxication, vascular diseases of the brain, hydrocephalus, Huntington chorea, multiple sclerosis, Parkinson disease, cerebral anoxia, and hypoglycemia.

Diagnostic and statistical manual of mental disorders. 3rd ed., Washington, D. C., American Psychiatric Association, 1980, pp. 107-12. Wells, C. E. Organic syndromes: Dementia. In: Kaplan, H. I., & Sadock, B. J., eds. *Comprehensive textbook of psychiatry.* 4th ed. Baltimore, Williams & Wilkins, 1985, pp. 851-70.

dementia infantilis. See *Heller syndrome, under Heller, Theodor O.*
dementia of the Alzheimer type (DAT). See *Alzheimer disease.*
dementia paralytica. See *Bayle disease.*
dementia-cortical presenile degeneration syndrome. See *Heidenhain syndrome.*
DEMONS, ALBERT JEAN OCTAVE (French physician, 1842-1920)
Demons-Meigs syndrome. See *Meigs syndrome.*
DEMPSEY, MARY JOSEPH, SISTER (American Catholic nun, 1856-1929)
Sister Joseph nodule. See *Sister Mary Joseph nodule.*
Sister Mary Joseph nodule. Metastatic nodule of the umbilicus in intra-abdominal neoplasms, named in honor of Sister Mary Joseph who assisted Dr. William Mayo in surgery and who was the first to draw his attention to the nodule. Sometimes incorrectly called *Sister Joseph nodule.*

Bailey, H. *Demonstration of physical signs in clinical surgery.* 11th ed. Baltimore, Williams & Wilkins, 1949, p. 227. Key, J. D. *et al.* Sister Mary Joseph's nodule and its relationship to diagnosis of carcinoma of the umbilicus. *Minnesota Med.,* 1976, 59:561-6.

demyelinogenic leukodystrophy. See *Alexander syndrome, under Alexander, W. Stewart.*
DEMYER, WILLIAM (American physician)
DeMyer syndrome. See *median cleft face syndrome.*
DEN (**d**ermatitis **e**xfoliativa **n**eonatorum). See *staphylococcal scalded skin syndrome.*
denial visual hallucination syndrome. See *Anton-Babinski syndrome.*

DENNIE, CHARLES CLAYTON (American physician, born 1884)
Dennie-Marfan syndrome. Synonyms: *Marfan syndrome, congenital syphilitic paralysis, paralysis-congenital syphilis syndrome.*

Incomplete flaccid paralysis of the lower extremities and mental retardation in children with congenital syphilis. Epilepsy, cataract, and nystagmus may occur.

Dennie, C. C. Partial paralysis of the lower extremities in children, accompanied by backward mental development. *Am. J. Syph.*, 1929, 13:157-63. Marfan, A. B. Paraplégie spasmodique avec troubles cérébraux d'origine hérédo-syphilitique chez les grands enfants. *Rev. Fr. Pédiat.*, 1936, 12:1-16.

DENNY-BROWN, D. (British neurologist)

Denny-Brown syndrome (1). See *Thévenard syndrome.*

Denny-Brown syndrome (2). Primary degeneration of the dorsal root ganglion cells with primary degeneration of the muscles in association with bronchogenic carcinoma.

Denny-Brown, G. Primary sensory neuropathy with muscular changes by carcinoma. *J. Neurol. Neurosurg. Psychiat., London,* 1948, 2:73-87.

DENT, CHARLES ENRIQUE (British physician)

Costello-Dent syndrome. See *under Costello.*

Dent-Friedman syndrome. Synonyms: *juvenile idiopathic osteoporosis, juvenile osteoporosis.*

Osteoporosis of children and adolescents, characterized chiefly by bone fragility, pain in the lumbar spine and leg joints, multiple fractures (often malunited), lumbosacral kyphosis, protuberant sternum, and occasional loosejointedness. Negative calcium balance occurs in most cases. The etiology is unknown.

Dent, C. E., & Friedman, M. Idiopathic juvenile osteoporosis. *Quart. J. Med.*, 1965, 34:177-210.

dental headache. See *under headache syndrome.*

dentate cerebellar ataxia. See *Hunt syndrome (1), under Hunt, James Ramsay.*

dentatorubral atrophy. See *Hunt syndrome (1), under Hunt, James Ramsay.*

dentes de Chiaie. See *Spira disease.*

dentinogenesis hypoplastica hereditaria. See *dentinogenesis imperfecta.*

dentinogenesis imperfecta. Synonyms: *Capdepont syndrome, Capdepont teeth, Capdepont-Hodge syndrome, Fargin-Fayolle syndrome, Stainton syndrome, Stainton-Capdepont syndrome, dentinogenesis hypoplastica hereditaria, hereditary dark teeth, hereditary opalescent dentin, hereditary opalescent teeth, odontogenesis imperfecta.*

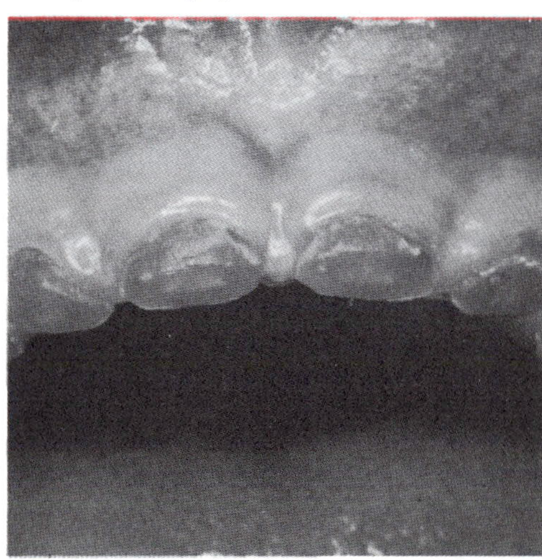

Dentinogenesis imperfecta
Robbins, S.L.: *Pathology.* 3rd. Ed. Philadelphia: W.B. Saunders Co.

A hereditary disorder of tooth development, transmitted as an autosomal dominant trait, characterized by discoloration of the teeth (ranging from dusky blue to brownish), poorly formed dentin with an abnormally low mineral content, obliteration of the pulp canal, and normal enamel. The teeth usually wear down rapidly, leaving short, brown stumps.

Capdepont, C. Dystrophie dentaire non encore décrite a type héréditaire et familial. *Rev. Stomat., Paris,* 1905, 12:550-61. *Stainton, C. W. Crownless teeth. *Dent. Cosmos,* 1892, 34:978-81. *Hodge, H. C. Correlated clinical and structural study of hereditary opalescent dentin. *J. Dent. Res.*, 1936, 15-516.

dentobronchitis. See *Veeneklaas syndrome.*

dentopulmonary syndrome. See *Veeneklaas syndrome.*

DENYS, P. (Belgian physician)

Denys-Corbeel syndrome. A familial syndrome of dwarfism, mental retardation, buphthalmos, renal acidosis, hypokaliuria, and gastric achlorhydria. Dysfunction of the proximal renal tubules is suspected as the cause.

Denys, P., & Corbeel, L. Acidose rénale, hypokaliémie, nanisme et syndrome oculo-cérébral. *Ann. Paediat., Basel,* 1964, 203:313-27.

depersonalization-migraine syndrome. See *Alice in Wonderland syndrome.*

depletion syndrome. See *villous adenoma depletion syndrome.*

depressive neurosis. See *Beard syndrome.*

DERCUM, FRANCIS XAVIER (American physician, 1856-1931)

Dercum syndrome. Synonyms: *Anders syndrome, adiposalgia, adiposis dolorosa, adipositas dolorosa, adipositas tuberosa simplex, fibrolipomatosis dolorosa, lipalgia, lipomatosis dolorosa, neurolipomatosis.*

Paresthesia, tenderness, and pain, usually observed in postmenopausal women, believed to be caused by subcutaneous deposits of fat, thus producing pressure exerted on the cutaneous nerves. Emotional and mental problems may be associated.

*Dercum, F. X. A subcutaneous connective tissue dystrophy of the arms and back, associated with symptoms resembling myxoedema. *Univ. Med. Gaz., Philadelphia,* 1888-89, 1:140-50.

derealization. See *Alice in Wonderland syndrome.*

dermal leishmanoid. See *Brahmachari leishmanoid.*

dermal melanocytoma. See *Jadassohn-Tièche nevus, under Jadassohn, Josef.*

dermatite bulleuse muco-synéchiante et atrophiante. See *Lortat-Jacob disease.*

dermatitis atrophicans diffusa progressiva. See *Herxheimer disease.*

dermatitis atrophicans maculosa lipoides diabetica. See *Oppenheim-Urbach syndrome, under Oppenheim, M.*

dermatitis blastomycetica. See *Gilchrist disease.*

dermatitis bullosa hereditaria. See *epidermolysis bullosa syndrome.*

dermatitis chronica atrophicans. See *Herxheimer disease.*

dermatitis erysipelatosa. See *staphylococcal scalded skin syndrome.*

dermatitis exfoliativa generalisata. See *Leiner dermatitis.*

dermatitis exfoliativa generalisata subacuta. See *Wilson disease (1), under Wilson, Sir William Erasmus.*
dermatitis exfoliativa infantum. See *staphylococcal scalded skin syndrome.*
dermatitis exfoliativa neonatorum (DEN). See *staphylococcal scalded skin syndrome.*
dermatitis herpetiformis. See *Duhring disease.*
dermatitis infectiosa eczematoides. See *Engman disease.*
dermatitis lichenoidea chronica. See *Hallopeau syndrome (1).*
dermatitis lichenoidea chronica atrophicans. See *Hallopeau syndrome (1).*
dermatitis lichenoides purpurica pigmentosa. See *Gougerot-Blum syndrome, under Gougerot, Henri.*
dermatitis multiformis. See *Duhring disease.*
dermatitis neurotica. See *Duhring disease.*
dermatitis nodularis non-necroticans. See *Gougerot-Ruiter syndrome.*
dermatitis papulosquamosa atrophicans. See *Degos syndrome.*
dermatitis polymorpha dolorosa. See *Duhring disease.*
dermatitis pruriginosa. See *Duhring disease.*
dermatitis pustularis. See *Hallopeau syndrome (3).*
dermatitis pustulosa subcornealis. See *Sneddon-Wilkinson syndrome.*
dermatitis repens. See *Crocker disease, under Crocker, Henry Radcliffe.*
dermatitis seborrhoides. See *Unna disease, under Unna, Paul Gerson.*
dermatitis trophoneurotica. See *Duhring disease.*
dermatitis vegetans. See *Hallopeau syndrome (3).*
dermato-arthritis syndrome. See *bowel bypass syndrome.*
dermatochalasis connata. See *cutis laxa syndrome.*
dermatofibrosarcoma protuberans. See *Darier-Ferrand dermatofibrosarcoma.*
dermatofibrosis lenticularis disseminata. See *Buschke-Ollendorff syndrome.*
dermatofibrosis lenticularis disseminata with osteopoikilosis. See *Buschke-Ollendorff syndrome.*
dermatogenic cataract. See *Andogsky syndrome.*
dermatomegaly. See *cutis laxa syndrome.*
dermatomyositis. See *Wagner-Unverricht syndrome, under Wagner, Ernst Leberecht.*
dermatomyositis syndrome. See *Wagner-Unverricht syndrome, under Wagner, Ernst Leberecht.*
dermatopolyneuritis. See *acrodynia.*
dermatorrhexis with dermatochalasis and arthrochalasis. See *Ehlers-Danlos syndrome.*
dermatosis cenicienta. See *Cinderella dermatosis.*
dermatosis precancerosa. See *Bowen disease, under Bowen, John Templeton.*
dermatosis pustulosa subcornealis. See *Sneddon-Wilkinson syndrome.*
dermatostomatitis. See *Stevens-Johnson syndrome.*
dermatostomato-ophthalmic syndrome. See *Behçet syndrome.*
dermochondrocorneal dystrophy. See *François syndrome (2).*
dermoepidermal nevus. See *Hutchinson freckle, under Hutchinson, Sir Jonathan.*
dermopathic lymphadenopathy. See *Pautrier-Woringer syndrome.*
DERRY, DAVID M. (Canadian physician)
Derry syndrome. See *gangliosidosis G_{M1} type II.*
DES. See *dialysis enncephalopathy syndrome.*
DES. See *disequilibrium syndrome.*
DES (diethylstilbestrol) syndrome. Benign vaginal adenosis or adenocarcinoma in young women exposed to diethylstilbestrol.

Fetherston, W. C. Squamous neoplasia of vagina related to DES syndrome. *Am. J. Obst. Gyn.*, 1975, 122:176-81.

DES (dysequilibrium syndrome. See *Halpern syndrome.*
DESBUQUOIS, G. (French physician)
Rolland-Desbuquois (RD) syndrome. See *under Rolland.*
desquamative inflammatory vaginitis. See *Gardner vaginitis, under Gardner, Herman L.*
DESTOMBES
Destombes-Rosai-Dorfman syndrome. See *Rosai-Dorfman syndrome.*
DETERMANN, HERMANN (German physician, born 1865)
Determann syndrome. Synonyms: *akinesia intermittens angiosclerotica, angiosclerotic intermittent akinesia, angiosclerotic intermittent dyskinesia, angiosclerotic paroxysmal myasthenia, dyskinesia intermittens angiosclerotica, dyskinesia intermittens angiopastica.*

Intermittent myasthenia of various muscles secondary to arteriosclerosis.

Determann. "Intermittierendes Hinken" eines Armes, der Zunge und der Beine (Dyskinesia intermittens angiosclerotica). *Deut. Zschr. Nervenh.*, 1905, 29:152-62.

detrussor-sphincter dyssynergia. See *Hinman syndrome.*
DEUTSCHLÄNDER, CARL ERNST WILHELM (German physician, 1872-1942)
Deutschländer disease. Synonym: *march foot.*

A painful swelling of the foot, frequently associated with fractures of a metatarsal bone resulting from excessive strain, as in prolonged marching.

Deutschländer, C. W. Über entzündliche Mittelfussgeschwülste. *Arch. Klin. Chir., Berlin,* 1921, 118:530-49.

DEVERGIE, MARIE GUILLAUME (French physician, 1798-1879)
Devergie disease. See *Kaposi disease (2).*
DEVIC, EUGENE (French physician, 1869-1930)
Devic syndrome. Synonyms: *Devic-Gault syndrome, disseminated myelitis with optic neuritis, myelitis with optic neuritis, neuromyelitis optica, neuroptic myelitis, neuro-opticomyelitis, ophthalmo-encephalomyelopathy, opthalmoneuromyelitis, optic encephalomyelitis, optic myelitis, optic neuromyelitis, optic neuromyelopathic multiple sclerosis, optic neuromyelopathy.*

A partial or complete transverse myelopathy and optic neuritis frequently associated with paraplegia and progressive blindness. Accumulation of fat-containing phagocytes, proliferation of astrocytes, increased protein levels of the cerebrospinal fluid, and demyelinating lesions of the occipital white matter may be associated. The disorder sometimes occurs as a complication of multiple sclerosis, acute disseminated encephalomyelitis, systemic lupus erythematosus, or sarcoidosis. When associated with multiple sclerosis, its clinical and pathological features are indistinguishable from those of multiple sclerosis.

*Devic, M. E. Myélite aiguë dorso-lombaire avec névrite optique. Autopsie. *Cong. Fr. Méd., Lyon,* 1894, 1:434-9.
*Gault, F. *De la neuromyélite optique aiguë.* Lyon, 1894. (Thesis).

Devic-Gault syndrome. See *Devic syndrome.*
devil's clutch. See *Sylvest syndrome.*
devil's grip. See *Sylvest syndrome.*
DEWALD, R. L.
Solomon-Fretzin-Dewald syndrome. See *epidermal nevus syndrome.*
DEWIND, LOREN T. (American physician)
Refetoff-DeWind-DeGroot syndrome. See *Refetoff syndrome.*
DGS. See *DiGeorge syndrome.*
DHTR (dihydrotestosterone receptor) deficiency. See *testicular feminization syndrome.*
DI GUGLIELMO, GIOVANNI (Italian hematologist, 1886-1961)
Di Guglielmo disease (1). Synonyms: *Di Guglielmo syndrome, acute erythremia, acute erythremic myelosis, acute erythroblastosis, erythremic myelosis, erythroleukemia, malignant erythroblastosis, myelosis erythremica.*

A variant of acute myeloblastic leukemia developing in three basic phases: (1) erythremic myelosis, (2) erythroleukemia, and (3) acute myelogenous leukemia. The first stage, known as **erythremic myelosis**, is marked by characteristic blood changes with anemia and bizarre red cell morphology (anisocytosis, poikilocytosis, anisochromia, nucleated red cells, and erythroid bone marrow hyperplasia). The erythroblasts in the bone marrow have giant and multinucleated forms, nuclear budding, and nuclear fragmentation. The erythropoietic phase may be protracted or may evolve into one which resembles erythroleukemia and is characterized by the prominence of the myeloblasts in the bone marrow, amegakaryocytic thrombocytdopenia, and impairment of granulopoiesis. In the following stage, the condition evolves into acute myelogenous leukemia with the replacement of marrow by leukemic blast cells. The course is sometimes variable, ranging from idiopathic refractory anemia (preleukemia) through erythroleukemia.

Di Guglielmo, G. Eritremie acute. *Boll. Soc. Med. Chir.*, 1926, 1:665-73. Henderson, E. S. Acute myelogenous leukemia. In: Williams, W. J., Beutler, E., Erslev, A. J., & Lichtman, M. A., eds. *Hematology,* 3rd ed. New York, McGraw-Hill, 1983, pp. 239-53.

Di Guglielmo disease (2). See *Mortensen disease.*
Di Guglielmo syndrome. See *Di Guglielmo disease (1).*
DI MAURO, SALVATORE (American physician)
Di Mauro disease. Carnitine palmityl transferase deficiency with recurrent attacks of myoglobinuria as the only symptom.

Di Mauro, S., *et al.* Disorders of lipid metabolism in muscle. *Muscle Nerve,* 1980, 3:369-88.

DI SAIA, P. J.
Di Saia syndrome. See *fetal warfarin syndrome.*
diabetes in bearded women. See *Achard-Thiers syndrome, under Achard, Emile Charles.*
diabetes insipidus and mellitus with optic atrophy and deafness (DIDMOAD). Synonyms: *Wolfram syndrome, diabetes insipidus-diabetes mellitus-optic atrophy (DIDMO) syndrome.*

A familial syndrome, transmitted as an autosomal recessive trait, characterized by juvenile diabetes mellitus, diabetes insipidus, optic atrophy, neurosensory hearing loss, autonomic dysfunction, hypothalamo-pituitary disorders, and hyperalanineuria.

Wolfram, D. J. Diabetes mellitus and simple optic atrophy among siblings: Report of four cases. *Proc. Staff. Meet. Mayo Clin.,* 1938, 13:715-8. Niemeyer, G., & Marquardt, J. L. Retinal function in an unique syndrome of optic atrophy, juvenile diabetes mellitus, diabetes insipidus, neurosensory hearing loss, autonomic dysfunction, and hyperalanineuria. *Invest. Ophth.,* 1972, 11:617-24.

diabetes insipidus-diabetes mellitus-optic atrophy (DIDMO) syndrome. See *diabetes insipidus and mellitus with optic atrophy and deafness.*
diabetes mellitus. See *diabetic syndrome.*
diabetes mellitus-hypertension-nephrosis syndrome. See *Kimmelstiel-Wilson syndrome.*
diabetes mellitus-optic atrophy (DMOA) syndrome. A syndrome of insulin-dependent juvenile diabetes mellitus and optic atrophy. Associated disorders may include hypoacusis, vestibular disorders with nystagmus, hypogonadism, delayed sexual maturation, amenorrhea, congenital cataracts, tetralogy of Fallot, hydronephrosis, Klinefelter disease, and aminoaciduria. Some cases are familial and parental consanguinity is frequent.

Graefe, A., von. Über die mit Diabetes vorkommenden Sehgstörungen. *Arch. Ophth., Berlin,* 1858, 4:230-4. Babel, J. Association d'un diabète juvénile insulino-dépendant et d'atrophie optique (syndrome DMOA). *Rev. Méd. Suisse Rom.,* 1980, 100:337-41.

diabetes-dwarfism-obesity syndrome. See *Mauriac syndrome, under Mauriac, Leonard Pierre.*
diabetes-hemochromatosis syndrome. See *Troisier-Hanot-Chauffard syndrome.*
diabetes-nephrosis syndrome. See *Kimmelstiel-Wilson syndrome.*

diabetic syndrome. Synonym: *diabetes mellitus.*

A metabolic disease caused by deficiency of insulin in disorders of the beta-cells of the islands of Langerhans of the pancreas, manifested by faulty utilization of carbohydates and compensatory catabolism of proteins and fats to supply the energy needs of the body, which result in hyperglycemia, ketosis, and glycosuria. Several types of diabetes mellitus are recognized: (1) Primary diabetes consists of insulin-dependent diabetes mellitus type 1 and non-insulin-dependent diabetes mellitus type 2 (non-obese non-insulin-dependent diabetes mellitus, obese non-insulin-dependent diabetes mellitus, and maturity-onset diabetes mellitus); and (2) diabetes mellitus secondary to pancreatic diseases, hormonal abnormalities, drug- or chemical-induced, insulin receptor abnormalities, and inherited diseases. Vascular changes, including arteriosclerosis and degenerative vascular disorders, affecting the kidneys, eyes, heart, and nervous system, frequently leading to blindness, neuritis, congestive heart failure, and hypertension, are usually associated. The symptoms include accelerated aging, weakness, lassitude, loss of of weight, and specific odor due to ketosis. Diabetes mellitus is a component of several syndromes.

Dobson, M. Experiments and observations on the urine in diabetes. *Med. Observ. Inquiries,* 1776, 5:298. Foster, D. W. Diabetes mellitus. In: Braunwald, E., Isselbacher, K. J., Petersdorf, R. G., Wilson, J. D., Martin, J. B., & Fauci, A. S., eds. *Harrison's principles of internal medicine.* 11th ed. New York, McGraw-Hill, 1987, pp. 1778-97. Renold, A. E., *et al.* Diabetes mellitus. In: Stanbury, J. B., Wyngaarden, J. B., & Fredrickson, D. S., eds. *The meta-*

bolic basis of inherited disease. New York, McGraw-Hill, 1978. pp. 80-109.

diabetic amyotrophy. See *Bruns-Garland syndrome.*

diabetic dwarfism. See *Mauriac syndrome, under Mauriac, Leonard Pierre.*

diabetic glomerulohyalinosis. See *Kimmelstiel-Wilson syndrome.*

diabetic glomerulosclerosis. See *Kimmelstiel-Wilson syndrome.*

diabetic myelopathy. See *Bruns-Garland syndrome.*

diabetic nephroangiopathy. See *Kimmelstiel-Wilson syndrome.*

diabetic neuropathic cachexia. See *Ellenberg syndrome.*

diabetic stiff joint syndrome. See *Rosenbloom-Frias syndrome.*

diacyclothrombopathy. See *Glanzmann thrombasthenia.*

dialysis dementia. See *dialysis encephalopathy syndrome.*

dialysis disequilibrium. See *disequilibrium syndrome.*

dialysis encephalopathy (DE). See *dialysis encephalopathy syndrome.*

dialysis encephalopathy syndrome (DES). Synonyms: *dialysis dementia, dialysis encephalopathy (DE), progressive dialysis encephalopathy (PDE).*

A progressive disease of the central nervous system, occurring during or immediately after chronic dialysis. It is characterized by speech and motor disorders, dementia, and seizures. Early symptoms, consisting of a hesitant stuttering dysarthria, dysphasia, and sometimes apraxia of speech, are followed by myoclonic facial and generalized jerks, seizures, personality changes, psychotic behavior, intellectual decline, and EEG abnormalities. Initially, the symptoms are intermittent, but in time they become progressively more severe and frequent, eventually becoming permanent. Most patients die in about six months, but some may linger for several years. Pathological findings consist of minute cavitations in the upper layers of the cerebral cortex, the left hemisphere usually being more severely affected than the right one. Presence of excessive amounts of aluminum in the cerebral gray matter suggests the possibility of aluminum intoxication. See also the *disequilibrium syndrome.*

Alfrey, A. C., *et al.* Syndrome of dyspraxia and multifocal seizures associated with chronic hemodialysis. *Tr. Am. Soc. Artif. Intern. Organs,* 1972, 18:257-61.

dialysis osteomalacia syndrome. Severe osteomalacia with spontaneous fractures complicating chronic hemodialysis.

Cameron, E. C., *et al.* Hemodialysis patients with a unique mineralization defect unresponsive to 1,25-dihydroxycholecalciferol. Dialysis osteomalacia syndrome. *Contrib. Nephrol.,* 1980, 18:162-71.

dialyzer hypersensitivity syndrome. Anaphylactic reactions in patients dialyzed on artificial kidneys. The symptoms include respiratory distress; wheezing; nausea; flushing; urticaria; pruritus; choking; conjunctival injection; fever; chills; hypotension; back, chest, and abdominal pain; and, sometimes, cardiopulmonary arrest and death. Ethylene oxide, a substance used to dry sterilize artificial kidneys, is the suspected allergen.

Hoy, W., & Cestero, R. Eosinophilia in maintenance hemodialysis patients. *J. Dial.,* 1979, 3:73-87. Caruana, R. J., *et al.* Dialyzer hypersensitivity syndrome: Possible role of allergy to ethylene oxide. Report of 4 cases and review of the literature. *Am. J. Nephrol.,* 1985, 5:271-4.

DIAMOND, LOUIS KLEIN (American physician, born 1902)

Diamond-Blackfan anemia (DBA). See *Diamond-Blackfan syndrome.*

Diamond-Blackfan syndrome. Synonyms: *Diamond-Blackfan anemia, Josephs-Diamond-Blackfan anemia (DBA), Josephs-Diamond-Blackfan syndrome, anemia chronica congenita aregenerativa, chronic erythroblastopenia, chronic erythrocyte aplasia, congenital aregenerative anemia, congenital erythroid hypoplasia, congenital hypoplastic anemia, congenital pure red cell aplasia, erythroblastophthisis, erythrocyte hypoplasia, erythrogenesis imperfecta, erythrophthisis, hereditary red cell aplasia, hypoplastic anemia of childhood, primary red cell aplasia, pure red cell anemia.*

A rare normocytic and normochromic aplastic or hypoplastic anemia of young infants, resulting from defective erythropoiesis and lack of regenerative capacity with gross deficiency of nucleated erythrocytes in the bone marrow, normal platelet count, and mild leukopenia. The course is progressive and blood transfusions may be necessary, which may lead to siderosis. Complications may include growth retardation, failure of sexual maturation, and portal hypertension. Skeletal abnormalities, such as triphalangeal thumb, are sometimes associated. Spontaneous remissions are infrequent and, when they occur, may be only temporary. The condition is believed to be transmitted as an autosomal recessive trait. Diamond-Blackfan and Aase-Smith syndromes are considered by some writers to be the same entity.

Josephs, H. W. Anemia of infancy and early childhood. *Medicine,* 1936, 15:307-451. Diamond, L. K., & Blackfan, K. D. Hypoplastic anemia. *Am. J. Dis. Child.,* 1938, 56:464-7.

Gardner-Diamond syndrome. See *auto-erythrocyte sensitization syndrome.*

Josephs-Diamond-Blackfan anemia. See *Diamond-Blackfan syndrome.*

Josephs-Diamond-Blackfan syndrome. See *Diamond-Blackfan syndrome.*

Shwachman-Diamond syndrome. See *Shwachman syndrome.*

Shwachman-Diamond-Oski-Khaw syndrome. See *Shwachman syndrome.*

diaphragmatic chorea. See *Schroetter chorea.*

diaphyseal aclasis. See *multiple cartilaginous exostoses syndrome.*

diaphyseal dysplasia. See *Camurati-Engelmann syndrome.*

diaphyseal sclerosis. See *Camurati-Engelmann syndrome.*

diarrheogenic syndrome. See *Verner-Morrison syndrome.*

diarthrosis interspinosa. See *Baastrup syndrome.*

diastrophic dwarfism syndrome. Synonyms: *Lamy-Maroteaux syndrome, achondroplasia with clubbed feet, diastrophic dysplasia, diastrophic nanism syndrome.*

An autosomal recessive syndrome characterized by prenatal micromelic dwarfism; progressive kyphoscoliosis; multiple joint contractures, especially of the shoulders, elbows, interphalangeal joints, and hips; proximally set hypermobile thumbs; bilateral talipes equinovarus; soft cystic masses on the ear auricles; and, in some cases, cleft palate. Associated abnormalities may include thick pectinate strands at the root of the iris, micrognathia, cryptorchism, and inguinal hernia. Radiological manifestations consist of shortening and thickening of the long bones, flattened and distorted epiphyses, widened and deformed metaphyses, synostosis of the proximal interphalangeal joints, accelerated carpal development with secondary centers of the metacarpals, metatarsals, and phalanges retarded in appearance. See also *Burgio pseudodiastrophic dwarfism syndrome.*

Lamy, M., & Maroteaux, P. Le nanisme diastrophique. *Presse Méd.*, 1960, 68:1977-80.

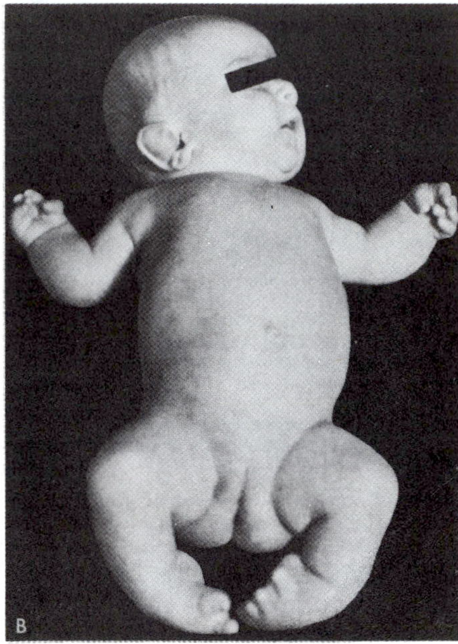

Diastrophic dwarfism syndrome
Langer, L.O.: *Am. J. Roentgenol. Radium Ther. Nucl. Med.* 93:399, 1965. Baltimore, Williams & Wilkins.

diastrophic dysplasia. See *diastrophic dwarfism syndrome.*

diastrophic nanism syndrome. See *diastrophic dwarfism syndrome.*

DIC. See ***d**isseminated **i**ntravascular **c**oagulation syndrome.*

DICKINSON, WILLIAM HOWSHIP (British physician, 1832-1913)

Dickinson syndrome. See *Alport syndrome.*

DIDE

Dide-Botcazo syndrome. A syndrome of visual disorders, spatial agnosia, and amnesia (due to bilateral calcarine lesions); involvement of the occipital lobe, and encephalomalacia resulting from cerebrovascular disorders. The disorder reportedly was first described by Dide and Botcazo.

Pauly, R., et al. Syndrome de Dide et Botcazo. *Rev. Neur., Paris,* 1967, 116:164-6.

DIDMO (diabetes **i**nsipidus-**d**iabetes **m**ellitus-**o**ptic atrophy) syndrome. See *diabetes insipidus and mellitus with optic atrophy and deafness.*

DIDMOAD. See ***d**iabetes **i**nsipidus and **m**ellitus with **o**ptic **a**trophy and **d**eafness.*

DIEKER, H. (American physician)

Miller-Dieker syndrome (MDS). See *under Miller, James Q.*

diencephalia infantilitis. See *diencephalic syndrome.*

diencephalic cachexia. See *diencephalic syndrome.*

diencephalic syndrome. Synonyms: *Russell syndrome, diencephalia infantilitis, diencephalic cachexia, diencephalic syndrome of emaciation, diencephalic syndrome of infancy.*

A neoplasm in the region of the anterior hypothalamus, most commonly a glioma, associated with progressive emaciation in spite of normal or increased food intake, subcutaneous lipodystrophy, pseudoanemic pallor, hyperkinesis, increased cheerfulness or euphoria, exceptional alertness, accelerated growth with acromegaloid features, hypotension, hypoglycemia, increased intracranial pressure with widening of the cranial sutures, hydrocephalus, and, frequently, emesis, tremor, and excessive sweating.

Russell, A. A diencephalic syndrome of emaciation in infancy and childhood. *Arch. Dis. Child., London,* 1951, 26:274.

diencephalic syndrome of emaciation. See *diencephalic syndrome.*

diencephalic syndrome of infancy. See *diencephalic syndrome.*

DIERCKX, L. (Belgian physician)

De Barsy-Moens-Dierckx syndrome. See *under De Barsy.*

dietary chaos syndrome. See *bulimia syndrome.*

diethylstilbestrol syndrome. See *DES syndrome.*

DIETL, JOZEF (Polish physician, 1804-1878)

Dietl crisis. An attack of acute urethral colic with severe pain, hypotension, oliguria, and vomiting in patients with nephroptosis (floating kidney) precipitated by assuming the upright position.

Dietl. Nerki wedrujace i ich uwiezienie. *Przegl. Lek., Kraków,* 1864, 3:225-7; 223-5; 241-4.

DIETLEN, HANS (German physician, 1879-1955)

Dietlen syndrome. A syndrome of cardiac flutter and diaphragmatic tension on inspiration associated with specific roentgenological signs in patients with cardiopericardial and cardiodiaphragmatic adhesions and adhesions at the apex of the heart.

Dietlen, H. *Herz und Gefässe im Röntgenbild. Ein Lehrbuch.* Leipzig, Barth, 1923.

DIEULAFOY, GEORGES (French physician, 1839-1911)

Dieulafoy erosion. Synonym: *Dieulafoy syndrome.*

Simple mucosal erosion causing upper gastrointestinal hemorrhage. A single bleeding point consists of a bare artery located in the folds of the upper third of the stomach.

Diaulafoy, G. Ulcérations gastriques. *Sem. Méd. Paris,* 1900, p. 263.

diffuse alveolar damage (DAD). See *adult respiratory distress syndrome.*

diffuse angiokeratosis. See *Fabry syndrome.*

diffuse cerebellar hypertrophy. See *Lhermitte-Duclos disease.*

diffuse cortical sclerosis. See *Alpers syndrome.*

diffuse corticomeningeal angiomatosis. See *van Bogaert-Divry syndrome.*

diffuse fasciitis with eosinophilia. See *Shulman syndrome, under Shulman, L. E.*

diffuse gastric polyadenoma. See *Ménétrier syndrome.*

diffuse gastrointestinal polyposis with ectodermal changes. See *Cronkhite-Canada syndrome.*

diffuse globoid body sclerosis. See *Krabbe disease.*

diffuse globoid cell cerebral sclerosis. See *Krabbe disease.*

diffuse idiopathic interstitial pulmonary fibrosis. See *Hamman-Rich syndrome.*

diffuse idiopathic skeletal hyperostosis (DISH). See *Forestier syndrome (2).*

diffuse interstitial pulmonary fibrosis. See *Hamman-Rich syndrome.*

diffuse intravascular coagulation. See *disseminated intravascular coagulation syndrome.*

diffuse mesenchymal hepatitis with nodular lymphomatosis. See *Hanot-Kiener syndrome.*

diffuse microvascular lung hemorrhage. See *alveolar hemorrhage syndrome.*

diffuse perichondritis. See *Meyenburg-Altherr-Uehlinger syndrome.*

diffuse sclerosing alveolitis. See *Hamman-Rich syndrome.*

diffuse sclerosing encephalitis. See *van Bogaert encephalitis.*

diffuse sclerosis with meningeal angiomatosis. See *van Bogaert-Divry syndrome.*

DIGEORGE, ANGELO MARIO (American physician, born 1921)

DiGeorge anomalad. See *DiGeorge syndrome.*

DiGeorge syndrome (DGS). Synonyms: *DiGeorge anomalad, familial third and fourth pharyngeal pouch syndrome, pharyngeal pouch syndrome, third and fourth pharyngeal pouch syndrome, thymic aplasia syndrome, thymic and parathyroid agenesis syndrome.*

A congenital developmental defect of derivatives of the third and fourth pharyngeal pouches, almost invariably associated with agenesis or hypoplasia of the parathyroids, cardiovascular anomalies, and immunodeficiency. Most infants die within the first few months of life. The symptoms include hypocalcemic seizures, frequent infections, aortic arch defects, ventricular septal defect, patent ductus arteriosus, tetralogy of Fallot, and peculiar facies consisting of hypertelorism, malformed ears, short philtrum, and antimongoloid palpebral slant. Dental features are similar to those in hypoparathyroidism, including delayed dentition, tooth retention, enamel defects, dentinal hypoplasia, and incomplete root formation. Immunological findings show normal to severely decreased lymphocyte count, percent T-cell, total T-cells, and T-lymphocyte function. Mental retardation, esophageal atresia, choanal atresia, imperforate anus, and diaphragmatic hernia may occur in some cases. The syndrome is twice as common in males as in females. Most cases are sporadic.

DiGeorge, A. M. A new concept of the cellular basis of immunity. *J. Pediat.*, 1965, 67:907-8.

digital hippocratism. See *Marie-Bamberger syndrome, under Marie, Pierre.*

digital neuroma. See *Morton neuralgia, under Morton, Thomas George.*

digital osteoarthropathy. See *Thiemann syndrome.*

digital vibration (DV) syndrome. See *vibration syndrome.*

digito-atrial dysplasia. See *Holt-Oram syndrome.*

digitorenocerebral (DRC) syndrome. A familial syndrome, transmitted as an autosomal recessive trait, characterized by brachydactyly due to absence of distal phalanges and nails of all fingers and toes, cystic dysplasia of the kidneys, and dilated right ventricle of the brain. In the original report, associated disorders included coarse facies with a short and wide nose, full lips, bushy hair, and low-set malformed ears; high and narrow palate; gingival hyperplasia; mental retardation; muscle hypotonia; perinatal cyanosis and breathing difficulty; precordial systolic murmur; convulsions; optic atrophy with blindness; and absent stem-evoked brain potentials.

Eronen, M., *et al.* New syndrome: A digito-reno-cerebral syndrome. *Am.. J. Med. Genet.*, 1985, 22:281-5.

digitotalar dysmorphism syndrome. Synonyms: *Sallis-Beighton syndrome, ulnar drift syndrome.*

A syndrome, originally described in 14 persons of both sexes in 5 generations, characterized by flexion deformities, abnormal dermatoglyphics, and ulnar deviation of the fingers, the thumb being held in an abnormal position by soft tissue webs. Rocker-bottom feet due to vertical talus are associated. The syndrome is believed to be transmitted as an autosomal dominant trait.

Sallis, J. G., & Beighton, P. Dominantly inherited digitotalar dysmorphism. *J. Bone Joint Surg.*, 1972, 54B:509-15.

dihydropteridine reductase deficiency. See *under phenylketonuria.*

dihydrotestosterone receptor (DHTR) deficiency. See *testicular feminization syndrome.*

dik kop disease. See *thick skull syndrome.*

Dilantin syndrome. See *fetal hydantoin syndrome.*

DIMITRI, VINCENTE (Austrian dermatologist in Argentina, 1885-1955)

Parkes Weber-Dimitri syndrome. See *Sturge-Weber syndrome.*

Sturge-Weber-Dimitri syndrome. See *Sturge-Weber syndrome.*

Weber-Dimitri syndrome. See *Sturge-Weber syndrome.*

DIMMER, FRIEDRICH (German ophthalmologist, 1855-1926)

Biber-Haab-Dimmer syndrome. See *under Biber.*

Dimmer keratitis. Synonyms: *keratitis nummularis, nummular keratitis.*

A usually bilateral, sporadic form of keratitis that is not accompanied by conjunctivitis. Pain, photophobia, excessive lacrimation, and discoid infiltrations in the superficial corneal layers are the chief features. The disease usually follows a minor injury of the eye and progresses slowly. See also *Sanders syndrome..*

Dimmer, F. Über eine der Keratitis nummularis nahestehende Hornhautentzündung. *Zschr. Augenh.*, 1905, 13:621-35.

Haab-Dimmer syndrome. See *Biber-Haab-Dimmer syndrome.*

DINGWALL, MARY M. (British pediatrician)

Neill-Dingwall syndrome. See *Cockayne syndrome.*

DIOGENES (A Greek philosopher and probably the founder of Cynicism, c. 412 B.C.-c. 323 B.C.)

Diogenes syndrome. A condition usually observed in the elderly, characterized by gross self-neglect, lack of self-consciousness about personal habits, untidiness, and hoarding of rubbish. It appears to be unrelated to the socioeconomic status of the person, who is often aloof, suspicious, emotionally labile, aggressive, group dependent, and reality distorting. Multiple nutritional deficiencies are usually associated. The syndrome was named after Diogenes, a Greek philosopher known for his bizarre behavior, who gave up all comforts of life and possesssions and lived in an empty wooden tub in order to prove his views and to discredit the social conditions of his times.

Clark, A. N. G., *et al.* Diogenes syndrome. A clinical study of gross neglect in old age. *Lancet*, 1975, I:366-8.

diphtheria. See *Bretonneau disease.*
diphtherial tonsillitis. See *Bretonneau disease.*
diphtheric croup. See *Bretonneau disease.*
diphtheritic neuritis. See *Déjerine syndrome (1).*
diphtheritic polyneuritis. See *Déjerine syndrome (1).*
diphtheritis. See *Bretonneau disease.*
diphtheroid subglossitis. See *Riga-Fede disease.*
diplegia spastica infantilis. See *Little disease, under Little, William John.*
diplobacillary conjunctivitis. See *Morax-Axenfeld conjunctivitis.*
diploid-tripoid mosaicism. See *chromosome diploid-triploid mosaicism syndrome.*
disappearing bone disease. See *Gorham syndrome.*
disappearing limy bile. See *limy bile syndrome.*
disconnection syndrome. Synonyms: *Geschwind syndrome, cerebral disconnection syndrome, disconnexion syndrome, interhemispheric disconnection syndrome.*

A group of disorders resulting from interruption of connections between the two cerebral hemispheres. When taking place in the corpus callosum or adjacent white matter, the condition is referred to as the **commissural syndrome**; when occurring between different parts of one hemisphere, it is known as the **intrahemispheric disconnection syndrome**.

Geschwind, N. The clinical syndromes of cortical disconnections. In: Williams, D., ed. *Modern trends in neurology.* vol. 5. London, Butterworth, 1970. p. 29. Adams, R. D., & Victor, M. *Principles of neurology.* 3rd ed. New York, McGraw-Hill, 1985, pp. 347-50.

disconnexion syndrome. See *disconnection syndrome.*
discontinuation syndrome. Potentially fatal complications after abrupt cessation of antihypertensive therapy, consisting of enhanced sympathetic activity, severe hypertension, and cardiovascular disorders. Predisposing factors include ischemic heart disease, severe hypertension, and renovascular or high renin hypertension. The symptoms include restlessness, anxiety, tachycardia, abdominal cramps, insomnia, headache, exacerbation of angina pectoris, vivid dreams, malaise, tremor, diaphoresis, salivation, hiccups, and facial flushing. Myocardial infarction and hypertensive encephalopathy may occur. The syndrome is most frequent after the use of antiadrenergic and beta-adrenergic blocking agents or combinations of different antihypertensive drugs.

Houston, M. C. Abrupt discontinuation of antihypertensive therapy. *South Med. J.*, 1981, 74:1112-23.

disease of Hapsburgs. See *hemophilia A.*
disease of kings. See *hemophilia A.*
disequilibrium syndrome (DES). Synonyms: *dialysis disequilibrium, hemodialysis disequilbrium.*

Complications of hemodialysis or peritoneal dialysis, occurring in the third or fourth hour of dialysis and lasting for several hours. The symptoms include headache, nausea, muscle cramps, irritability, agitation, drowsiness, and convulsions. Originally, the syndrome was believed to be due to the rapid lowering of serum urea, leaving the brain with a higher concentration of urea than the serum, thus resulting in a shift of water into the brain to equalize the osmotic gradient (the **reverse urea syndrome**). It is now believed that there is a shift of water into the brain similar to that in water intoxication and the inappropriate antidiuretic hormone secretion syndrome (q.v.). Not to be confused with the *Halpern (dysequilibrium) syndrome.* See also *dialysis encephalopathy syndrome.*

*Merrill, J. P. *Proceedings of First International Congress of Nephrology.* Geneve, Evian, p. 346. *Rosen, S. M., *et al.* Haemodialysis disequilibrium. *Brit. Med. J.*, 1964, 2:672-5.

DISH (diffuse **i**diopathic **s**keletal **h**yperostosis). See *Forestier syndrome (2).*
disklike atelectasis. See *Fleischner syndrome.*

DISNEY, WALTER ELIAS (American motion picture producer and cartoonist, 1901-1966)
Walt Disney dwarf. See *geroderma osteodysplastica syndrome.*
disseminated arteriolar-capillary platelet thrombosis. See *Moschcowitz syndrome.*
disseminated dermatofibrosis with osteopoikilosis. See *Buschke-Ollendorff syndrome.*
disseminated embryonic lichenoid eruption. See *Brooke epithelioma.*
disseminated epidemic cerebrospinal meningitis. See *Redlich encephalitis.*
disseminated fibrin thromboembolism. See *disseminated intravascular coagulation syndrome.*
disseminated fibrous jaw dysplasia. See *cherubism.*
disseminated intravascular coagulation (DIC) syndrome. Synonyms: *acquired afibrinogenemia, acquired hypofibrinogenemia, consumption coagulopathy, defibrination syndrome, diffuse intravascular coagulation, disseminated fibrin thromboembolism, fibrinolytic thromboembolism, hemorrhagic diathesis-acute progranulocytic leukemia syndrome, microangiopathic hemolytic anemia syndrome, thrombosis-fibrinolysis-thrombocytopenia syndrome, thrombotic thrombocytopenic purpura.*

A blood coagulation disorder, caused by a diffuse deposition of fibrin within the blood vessels, accompanied by formation of microthrombi, most commonly in the kidneys, lungs, spleen, adrenals, heart, brain, and liver. The disorder is most frequently associated with obstetrical complications, disseminated tumors, massive trauma, and bacterial sepsis. It is generally produced by endotoxins, immune or inflammatory reactions, and extrinsic coagulation factors. The severity of symptoms vary, multiple hemorrhages, especially from surgical incisions, venipuncture, and catheter sites, being the most common features. Associated symptoms may include acrocyanosis, thrombosis, and pregangrenous changes. Thrombocytopenia, prolonged prothrombin and partial prothrombin time, reduced fibrinogen levels, and elevated fibrin degradation products due to secondary fibrinolysis are the principal laboratory findings.

Miale, J. B. Diffuse intravascular coagulation (DIC). In his: *Laboratory medicine. Hematology.* St. Louis, Mosby, 1982. pp. 843-7. Barraud, S. Über extremitätengangrän im Jugendlichen alter nach Infektionskrankheiten. *Deut. Zschr. Chir.*, 1904, 74:237-97.

disseminated lipogranulomatosis. See *Farber disease.*

disseminated myelitis with optic neuritis. See *Devic syndrome.*

dissociated vertical divergence. See *Bielschowsky disease, under Bielschowsky, Alfred.*

distal arthrogryposis type IIa. See *Gordon syndrome, under Gordon, Hymie.*

distal late hereditary myopathy. See *Gowers syndrome (1).*

distal spinal muscular atrophy. See *Aran-Duchenne syndrome.*

distichiasis-lymphedema syndrome. A syndrome of double rows of eyelashes and lymphedema of the limbs, especially below the knees, occasionally associated with vertebral anomalies, epidural cysts, ectropion of the lower lids, epicanthus, and pterygium colli. The syndrome is transmitted as an autosomal dominant trait.

Falls, H. S., & Dertesz, E. D. A new syndrome combining pterygium colli with developmental anomalies of the eyelids and lymphatics of the lower extremities. *Tr. Am. Ophth. Soc.*, 1964, 62:248-75.

distorted limb dwarfism. See *parastremmatic dwarfism syndrome.*

distraction fracture of the spine. See *Chance fracture.*

diverticular hernia. See *Littre hernia.*

DIVRY, PAUL (Belgian physician, born 1889)

van Bogaert-Divry syndrome. See *under van Bogaert.*

DIXON, FRANK J. (American physician)

Dixon-Moore seminoma. See *Dixon-Moore tumor.*

Dixon-Moore tumor. Synonyms: *Dixon-Moore seminoma, extragonadal seminoma.*

A retroperitoneal metastatic form of seminoma, believed to originate in germ cells left behind during the migration of the yolk sac to the gonads in early stages of embryonic development.

Dixon, F. J., & Moore, R. A. Testicular tumors. A clinicopathological study. *Cancer,* 1953, 6:427-54.

DJS. See ***D****ubin-****J****ohnson* ***s****yndrome.*

DLUHOSOVA, O. (Czech physician)

Hornová-Dluhosová syndrome. See *under Hornová.*

DMC. See ***D****yggve-****M****elchior-****C****lausen syndrome.*

DMCS. See ***D****yggve-****M****elchior-****C****lausen* ***s****yndrome.*

DMD. See ***D****uchenne* ***m****uscular* ***d****ystrophy.*

DMOA. See ***d****iabetes* ***m****ellitus-****o****ptic* ***a****trophy syndrome.*

DMS (dysmyelopoietic syndrome). See *myelodysplastic syndrome.*

DNS. See ***d****ysplastic* ***n****evus* ***s****yndrome.*

DOAN, CHARLES A. (American physician)

Wiseman-Doan syndrome. See *under Wiseman.*

DOBRIN, ROBERT S. (American physician)

Dobrin syndrome. A syndrome of acute eosinophilic interstitial nephritis, renal failure, bone marrow and lymph node granulomas, and anterior uveitis.

Dobrin, R. S. Acute eosinophilic interstitial nephritis and renal failure with bone marrow-lymph node granulomas and anterior uveitis. A new syndrome. *Am. J. Med.*, 1975, 59:325-33.

doctor bashing. See *battered doctor syndrome.*

DOEGE, KARL HERMAN (American physician, born 1892)

Doege-Potter syndrome. Synonyms: *hypoglycemia-mesenchymal tumor syndrome, mesenchymal hypoglycemic tumor, paraneoplastic hypoglycemia-malignant histiocytoma syndrome, primary hypoglycemic mesenchymal tumor.*

Paraneoplastic hypoglycemia associated with an extrapancreatic mesenchymal tumor.

Doege, K. H. Fibro-sarcoma of the mediastinum. *Ann. Surg.*, 1930, 92:955-60. Potter, R. P. Intrathoracic tumors. Case report. *Radiology,* 1930, 14:60-1.

DOHI

Dohi acropigmentation. A familial skin disease characterized by hyperpigmented and hypopigmented macules.

Mosher, D. B., *et al.* Disorders of pigmentation. Fitzpatrick, T. B., Eisen, A. Z., Wolff, K., Freedberg, I. M., & Austen, K. F., eds. *Dermatology in general medicine.* 3rd ed. New York, 1987, pp. 794-876.

DÖHLE, KARL GOTTFRIED PAUL (German pathologist, 1855-1928)

Heller-Döhle disease. See *under Heller, Arnold Ludwig Gotthilf.*

Heller-Döhle mesoaortitis. See *Heller-Döhle disease, under Heller, Arnold Ludwig Gotthilf.*

dolichostenomelia. See *Marfan syndrome (1).*

DOLLINGER, A. (German physician)

Dollinger-Bielschowsky syndrome. See *gangliosidosis G_{M2} type III.*

dolor faciei fothergilli. See *trigeminal neuralgia.*

DOLOWITZ, DAVID A. (American physician)

Woolf-Dolowitz-Aldous syndrome. See *Woolf syndrome.*

dominant acro-osteolysis. See *Lamy-Maroteaux syndrome (2).*

dominant fundus dystrophy. See *Sorsby disease.*

dominant preaxial brachydactyly. See *Christian brachydactyly syndrome, under Christian, Joe C.*

dominant spinal pontine atrophy. See *Marie syndrome (1), under Marie, Pierre.*

DONATH, JULIUS (German physician, 1870-1950)

Donath-Landsteiner syndrome. Synonyms: *acute autoimmunohemolytic anemia, paroxysmal cold hemoglobinuria, paroxysmal hemoglobinuria a frigore.*

Hemoglobinuria characterized by the sudden passage of dark brownish to black urine following exposure to cold, often associated with leg pain, abdominal cramps, malaise, chills, fever, vasomotor disorders, pallor, and blanching of the ears and lips. It is believed to be due to the presence of autohemolysins in the blood which causes the erythrocytes to unite at low temperatures and to hemolyse when the blood is rewarmed. The condition was originally observed in patients with syphilis, but it is also seen in the absence of syphilis and in patients recovering from viral infections.

Donath, J., & Landsteiner, K. Über paroxysmale Hämoglobinurie. *Münch. Med. Wschr.,* 1904, 51:1590-3.

DONOHUE, WILLIAM LESLIE (Canadian physician, born 1906)

Donohue syndrome. Synonyms: *Donohue-Uchida syndrome, dysendocrinism, leprechaunism.*

A syndrome of familial, congenital lipodystrophy, probably transmitted as an autosomal recessive trait, consisting of marked lack of adipose tissue, insulin resistance, intrauterine dwarfism, retarded bone maturation, and grotesque facies characterized by small face, prominent eyes, wide nostrils, thick lips, and large ears. Large phallus, breast hyperplasia in females, Leydig cell hyperplasia in males, follicular development with cystic ovary, increased pituitary gonadotropins, islets of Langerhans hyperplasia, hir-

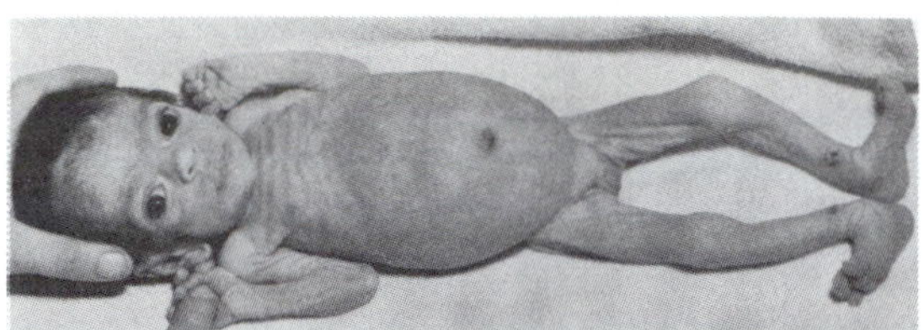

Donohue syndrome
Donohue, W.L. & Uchida, I: *J. Pediat.*, 45:505, 1954.

sutism, iron deposition in the liver, and motor and mental retardation may be associated. See also *Patterson syndrome (leprehaunism)*.

Donohue, W. L., Uchida, I. Leprechaunism. A euphemism for a rare familial disorder. *J. Pediat.*, 1954, 45:505-19.

Donohue-Uchida syndrome. See *Donohue syndrome.*

DOOR (**d**eafness-**o**nychodystrophy-**o**steodystrophy-**r**etardation) **syndrome.** Synonym: *Feinmesser-Zelig syndrome.*

A syndrome of congenital sensorineural deafness associated with bony anomalies, mainly triphalangeal thumb, biphalangeal digits of the fingers and toes, dystrophic terminal phalanges of some fingers and toes, and absence or hypoplasia of the nails of some fingers and toes. The osteodystrophy is confined mainly to the tumbs and fingers. In addition, there is mental retardation and the dermatoglyphics are characterized by the presence of 10 arches and elevation of the ATD angles. Autosomal dominant and recessive transmission, as well as sporadic cases, have been reported.

Feinmesser, M., & Zelig, S. Congenital deafness associated with onychodystrophy. *Arch. Otolar.*, 1961, 74:507-8. Cantwell R. J. Congenital sensori-neural deafness associated with onycho-osteo-dystrophy and mental retardation (D.O.O.R syndrome). *Humangenetik*, 1975, 26:261-5.

DORFMAN, MAURICE L. (Israeli physician)

Chanarin-Dorfman syndrome. See *under Chanarin.*

DORFMAN, RONALD F.

Destombes-Rosai-Dorfman syndrome. See *Rosai-Dorfman syndrome.*

Rosai-Dorfman syndrome. See *under Rosai.*

DÖRING, GERHARD (German neurologist, born 1909)

Pette-Döring encephalitis. See *under Pette.*

dorsolateral degenerative myelopathy. See *Dana syndrome.*

dorsolateral medullary syndrome. See *Wallenberg syndrome.*

dorsolateral oblongata syndrome. See *Babinski-Nageotte syndrome.*

DORST, J. P. (American physician)

Sensenbrenner-Dorst-Owens syndrome. See *cranioectodermal dysplasia syndrome.*

double athetosis syndrome. See *Vogt syndrome, under Vogt, Cécille.*

double male syndrome. See *chromosome XXY syndrome.*

double-entrapment radial tunnel syndrome. See *under radial tunnel syndrome.*

DOUCAS, CHRISTOPHE (Greek dermatologist, born 1890)

Doucas-Kapetanakis disease. See *Casalá-Mosto disease.*

DOWLING, G. B. (British physician)

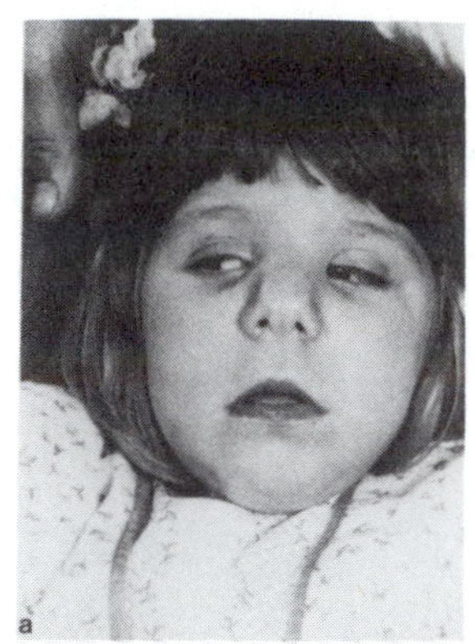

a

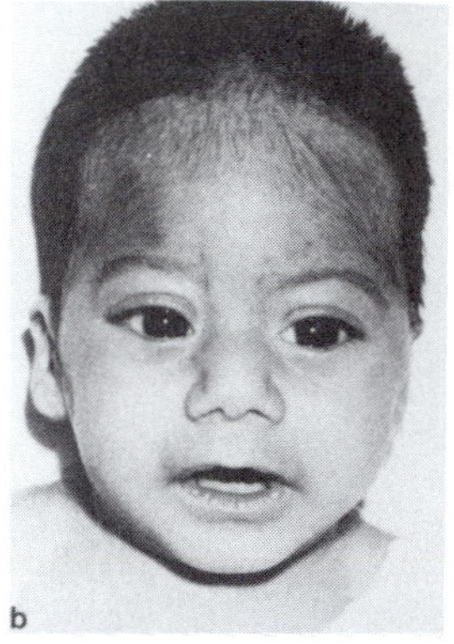

b

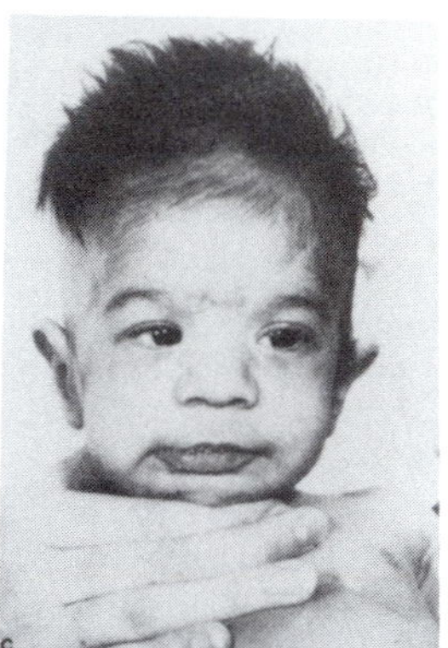

c

DOOR syndrome
Patton, M.A. S. Krywawych, R.M. Winter, D.P. Breton & M. Baraitser, *American Journal of Medical Genetics* 26:207-215 1987. New York: Alan R. Liss, Inc.

Dowling-Degos disease (DDD). Synonym: *reticular pigmented anomaly of the flexures.*

A benign form of reticular pigmentation of skin flexures with pitted scars around the mouth, scattered comedolike lesions on the nape, and verrucous lesions of the trunk. It begins on the axillae and groin, spreading to other areas, including the intergluteal and inframammary folds, neck, trunk, and arms. Pigmented, filiform, epidermal projections, involving the follicular infundibulum and epidermis, are the principal histological findings. The melanocytes are hyperactive but otherwise normal. Melanin concentrations are found mainly in the keratinocytes. The disorder affects both sexes and has a familial occurrence, usually appearing in early adult life.

Dowling, G., & Freudenthal, W. A case of acanthosis nigricans. *Brit. J. Derm. Syph.*, 1938, 50:467-71. Degos, R., & Ossipowski, B. Dermatose pigmentaire reticulée de plis. Discussion de l'acanthosis nigricans. *Ann. Derm. Syph., Paris,* 1954, 81:147-51. Mosher, D. B., *et al.* Disorders of pigmentation. In: Fitzpatrick, T. B., Eisen, A. Z., Wolff, K., Freedberg, I. M., & Austen, K. F., eds. *Dermatology in general medicine.* 3rd ed. New York, McGraw-Hill, 1987, pp. 795-876.

DOWN, JOHN LANGDON HAYDON (English physician, 1828-1891)

ALL-Down syndrome. See *under "A".*

Down syndrome. See *chromosome 21 trisomy syndrome.*

Langdon Down disease. See *chromosome 21 trisomy syndrome.*

morbus Down. See *chromosome 21 trisomy syndrome.*

DOYNE, ROBERT WALTER (British ophthalmologist, 1857-1896)

Doyne choroiditis. Synonyms: *familial honeycomb choroiditis, honeycomb degeneration of the retina.*

A familial disease of the eye, transmitted as an autosomal dominant trait, characterized by small round white spots on the posterior pole of the eye, including the macula and optic disc, progressing to form a mosaic pattern.

Doyne, R. W. A peculiar condition of choroiditis occurring in several members of the same family. *Tr. Ophth. Soc. U. K.*, 1899, 19:71.

Doyne iritis. Synonyms: *guttate iritis, iritis guttata.*

Iritis characterized by precipitates seen as small round gray masses on the anterior surface of the iris.

Duke-Elder, S., & Leigh, A. G. *Systems of ophthalmology.* London, Kimpton, 1965, Vol. 8, p. 721.

DR (Duane-radial ray) syndrome. See *Okihiro syndrome.*

DRAGER, GLENN A. (American physician)

Shy-Drager syndrome (SDS). See *under Shy.*

DRASH, ALLAN (American physician)

Drash syndrome. Synonyms: *glomerulonephritis-male pseudohermaphroditism-nephroblastoma syndrome, male pseudohermaphroditism-nephritis-Wilms tumor syndrome, nephropathy-male pseudohermaphroditism-Wilms tumor syndrome, pseudohermaphroditism-glomerulopathy-Wilms tumor syndrome.*

A syndrome of nephropathy with diffuse mesangial sclerosis of early onset, Wilms tumor, male pseudohermaphroditism, and hypertension. Typically, the patients show the 46,XY karyotype with nearly normal female external genitalia, mixed gonadal dysgenesis, and severe androgen receptor deficiency.

Drash, A., *et al.* A syndrome of pseaudohermaphroditism, Wilms' tumor, hypertension, and degenerative renal disease. *J. Pediat.*, 1970, 76:585-93. Turleau, C., *et al.* Partial androgen receptor deficiency and mixed gonadal dysgenesis in Drash syndrome. *Hum. Genet.*, 1987, 75:81-3.

DRC. See *digitorenocerebral syndrome.*

DREIER

Dreier syndrome. See *Still syndrome.*

DREIFUSS, F. E.

Dreifuss syndrome. See *Emery-Dreifuss syndrome.*

Dreifuss-Emery-Hogan syndrome. See *Emery-Dreifuss syndrome.*

Emery-Dreifuss muscular dystrophy (EMD). See *Emery-Dreifuss syndrome.*

Emery-Dreifuss syndrome (EDS). See *under Emery.*

drepanocytic anemia. See *sickle cell anemia.*

DRESBACH, MELVIN (American physician, 1874-1946)

Dresbach anemia. Synonyms: *Dresbach syndrome, elliptocytosis, hereditary elliptocytosis, hereditary ovalocytosis, ovalocytosis.*

A hereditary hematological disorder, transmitted as an autosomal dominant trait, characterized by the presence of elliptical erythrocytes in the blood. Five subgroups are recognized: (1) A mild form with little or no hemolysis, (2) a mild form with transient poikilocytosis in infants, (3) elliptocytosis with sporadic hemolysis, (4) elliptocytosis with hemolysis and spherocytosis, and (5) homozygous elliptocytosis with severe hemolysis associated with butting and fragmentation of the erythrocytes.

Dresbach, M. Elliptical human red corpuscles. *Science*, 1904, 19:469-70. Cooper, R. A. Hereditary elliptocytosis and related disorders. In: Williams, W. J., Beutler, E., Erslev, A. J., & Lichtman, M. A., eds. *Hematology.* 3rd ed. New York, McGraw-Hill, 1983, pp. 553-6.

Dresbach syndrome. See *Dresbach anemia.*

DRESCHER, EDWARD (Polish physician)

Murray-Puretic-Drescher syndrome. See *Murray syndrome.*

DRESSLER, D. R. (German physician)

Dressler syndrome. Synonyms: *Harley disease, intermittent hemoglobinuria, paroxysmal hemoglobinuria, periodic hemoglobinuria.*

Intermittent hemoglobinuria observed in hemolytic disorders.

Dressler. Ein Fall von intermittiender Albuminurie und Chromaturie. *Arch. Path. Anat., Berlin*, 1854, 6:264-6. Harley, G. On intermittent haematuria with remarks upon its pathology and treatment. *Med. Chir. Tr., London*, 1865, 48:161-84.

DRESSLER, WILLIAM (American physician)

Dressler syndrome. See *postmyocardial infarction syndrome.*

DREYFUS, JULES R. (Swiss physician)

Dreyfus syndrome. Synonyms: *platyspondylia generalisata, platyspondylia vera generalisata.*

Congenital flattening of the vertebrae followed by kyphoscoliosis, ankylosis of the spine, short neck, relative dwarfsim, hypermobility of joints, muscle weakness and atonia, and protruding abdomen.

Dreyfus, J. R. Über ein neues mit allgemeiner wahrer oder scheinbarer Breitwirbligkeit (Platyspondylia vera aut spuria generalisata) einhergehendes Syndrom. *Jahr. Kinderh.*, 1938, 150:42-54.

drug withdrawal syndrome. See *withdrawal syndrome.*

dry eye syndrome. A group of eye diseases (including the Sjögren syndrome) consisting of secretory deficiencies which involve major or accessory lacrimal glands and/or their secretory ducts, and mucin deficiency of the conjunctival tissues, or their combination. Pathologically, the condition is characterized by the loss of conjunctival goblet cells, abnormal enlargement of non-goblet epithelial cells, increase of cellular stratification, and keratinization. During the progress of disease, normal secretory conjunctival mucosa evolves into a nonsecretory keratinized epithelium, the process being referred to as squamous metaplasia.

Tseng, S. C. G. Topical retinoid treatment for dry eye disorders. *Tr. Ophth. Soc. U. K.*, 1985, 104:489-95.

dry syndrome. See *Sjögren syndrome, under Sjögren, Henrik Samuel Conrad.*

DS (dumping syndrome). See *postgastrectomy syndrome.*

DSC. See *de Sanctis-Cacchione syndrome.*

DT (delirium tremens). See *Morel disease, under Morel, Benoit Augustin.*

DU PAN, C. MARTIN (Swiss orthopedic surgeon)

Du Pan syndrome. A syndrome of symmetric fibular aplasia and complex brachydactyly. Radial deviation of the thumbs, shortening of the metacarpal bones, small carpal bones, trapezoid middle phalanx of the index finger, complete absence of the fibula, tibiotarsal dislocation, and short and laterally deviated toes are the principal features of this syndrome. Autosomal recessive inheritance has been suggested.

Du Pan, C. M. Absence congénitale du péroné sans déformation du tibia. Curieuses déformations congénitales des mains. *Rev. Orthop., Paris*, 1924, 11:227-34.

DU PETIT, FRANÇOIS POURFOUR. See PETIT, FRANÇOIS POURFOUR, DU

DUANE, ALEXANDER (American ophthalmologist, 1858-1926)

Duane syndrome. See *Stilling-Türk-Duane syndrome.*

Duane radial dysplasia syndrome. See *Stilling-Türk-Duane syndrome.*

Duane retraction syndrome. See *Stilling-Türk-Duane syndrome.*

Duane-radial ray (DR) syndrome. See *Okihiro syndrome.*

Stilling-Türk-Duane syndrome. See *under Stilling.*

DUBE, W. JAMES (Canadian physician)

Birt-Hogg-Dubé syndrome. See *under Birt.*

DUBIN, ISIDORE NATHAN (American physician, born 1913)

Dubin-Johnson syndrome (DJS). Synonyms: *Dubin-Johnson-Sprinz syndrome, Dubin-Sprinz syndrome, black liver-jaundice syndrome, constitutional hyperbilirubinemia syndrome, hyperbilirubinemia II, icterus-hepatic pigmentation syndrome.*

A liver disease, transmitted as an autosomal recessive trait with reduced penetrance, characterized by hyperbilirubinemia, prolonged retention of sulfobromophthalein, and deposition of a melanin or melanin-like substance in liver cells, causing the liver to become black. Associated disorders usually include mild abdominal pain, hepatomegaly, episodes of jaundice, fatigability, and dark urine.

Dubin, I. N., & Johnson, F. B. Chronic idiopathic jaundice with unidentified pigment in liver cells. A new clinicopathologic entity with a report of 12 cases. *Medicine*, 1954, 33:155-97. Sprinz, H., & Nelson, R. S. Persistent nonhemolytic hyperbilirubinemia associated with lipochrome-like pigment in liver cells; Report of four cases. *Ann. Int. Med.*, 1954, 41:952-62.

Dubin-Johnson-Sprinz syndrome. See *Dubin-Johnson syndrome.*

Dubin-Sprinz syndrome. See *Dubin-Johnson syndrome.*

DUBINI, ANGELO (Italian physician, 1813-1902)

Dubini disease. See *Bergeron disease.*

Dubini syndrome. See *Bergeron disease.*

DUBOIS, PAUL (French physician, 1795-1871)

Dubois abscess. Synonym: *Dubois disease.*

Abscess of the thymus in congenital syphilis.

Dubois, P. Du diagnostic de la syphilis considerée comme une des causes possibles de la mort du foetus. *Gaz. Méd., Paris,* 1850, 25:392-85.

Dubois disease. See *Dubois abscess.*

DUBOWITZ, VICTOR (British physician)

Dubowitz syndrome (1). Synonym: *dwarfism-eczema-peculiar facies syndrome.*

A rare, autosomal, recessively inherited syndrome of intrauterine dwarfism, mild mental retardation, high-pitched voice, and characteristic facies. Craniofacial features include microcephaly, shallow supraorbital ridges with high nasal bridge, high forehead, hypertelorism, blepharophimosis, blepharoptosis, slight mongoloid or antimongoloid palpebral slant, micrognathia, and prominent low-set ears. Skeletal defects consist of a slightly retarded bone age, periosteal hyperostosis of the long bones, rib anomalies, metatarsus varus, pes planus, and pes planovalgus. Polydactyly and clinodactyly have been noted in some cases. Eczematous skin eruption, especially of the face and extremities, sparse scalp hair, rhinorrhea, and serous otitis may occur. Mental retardation and behavioral problems with hyperactivity, short attention span, and shyness occur in most cases, but some patients have normal intelligence. Other anomalies include cleft palate, high-arched palate, bifid uvula, delayed dentition, and dental caries.

Dubowitz, V. Familial low birthweight dwarfism with an unusual facies and a skin eruption. *J. Med. Genet.*, 1965, 2:12-7.

Dubowitz syndrome (2). See *rigid spine syndrome.*

DUBREUIL-CHAMBARDEL, L. (French dentist)

Dubreuil-Chambardel syndrome. Dental caries of the incisors, in most instances only the upper ones, sometimes associated with alopecia.

Dubreuil-Chambardel, L. De la carie précoce des quatre incisives supérieures. *Congress de Stomatologie,* Paris, 1911.

DUBREUILH, M. W. (French physician)

Dubreuilh melanosis. See *Hutchinson freckle, under Hutchinson, Sir Jonathan.*

DUCHENNE, GUILLAUME BENJAMIN AMAND. See DUCHENNE DE BOULOGNE, GUILLAUME BENJAMIN AMAND

DUCHENNE DE BOULOGNE, GUILLAUME BENJAMIN AMAND (French physician, 1806-1875)

Aran-Duchenne syndrome. See *under Aran.*

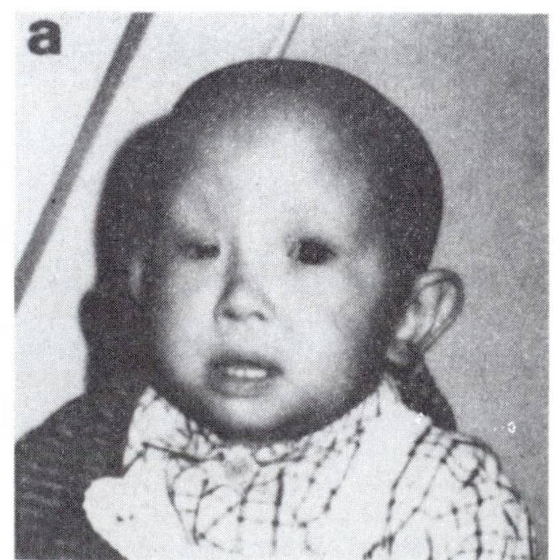

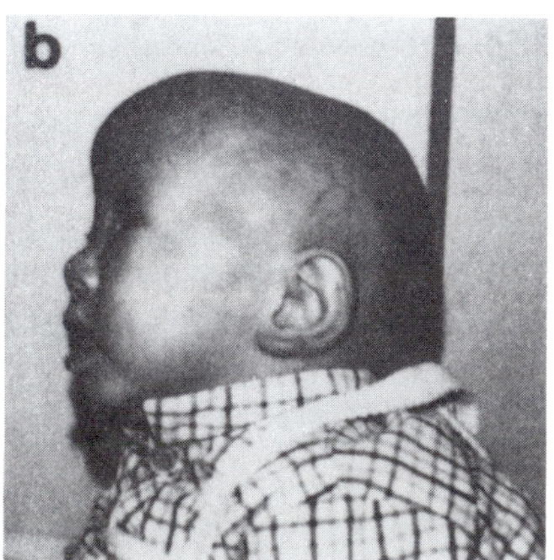

Dubowitz syndrome (1)
Kondo, I., K. Takeda, K. Kuwajima & T. Hirano, *Clinical Genetics,* 31:389-392, 1987. Munksgaard International Publishers, Copenhagen, Denmark.

Duchenne de Boulogne muscular dystrophy. See *Duchenne muscular dystrophy.*

Duchenne disease. See *locomotor ataxia.*

Duchenne dystrophy. See *Duchenne muscular dystrophy.*

Duchenne muscular dystrophy (DMD). Synonyms: *Duchenne dystrophy; Duchenne myodystrophy; Duchenne progressive muscular dystrophy; Duchenne pseudohypertrophic muscular dystrophy; Duchenne syndrome; Duchenne de Boulogne muscular dystrophy; Duchenne-Griesinger syndrome; progressive muscular dystrophy, Duchenne type; pseudohypertrophic muscular dystrophy; pseudohypertrophic progressive muscular dystrophy, Duchenne type.*

A genetically determined pseudohypertrophic form of progressive muscular dystrophy which occurs predominantly in boys and is transmitted as an X-linked recessive trait. Onset usually takes place between the ages of 2 and 6 years, beginning with atrophic changes in the muscles of the pectoral girdle and trunk and extending to the extremities. As their size increases, the muscles become firm and resilient, but their strength diminishes and, eventually, atrophy ensues. Inability to rise to an upright position without turning to the side, waddling gait, and progressive weakness are the characteristic features. Usually the limbs become flaccid and loose; shortening and contractures may occur. Kyphoscoliosis, pes equinus, loss of tendon reflexes, bone demineralization, and cardiac failure are frequent. The blood shows an increase of enzymes, notably aldolase and creatine phosphokinase. Orofacial features include involvement of the masticatory, facial, ocular, laryngeal, and pharyngeal muscles in the late stages. Few patients survive past the second decade of life.

Duchenne. Recherches sur la paralysie musculaire pseudohypertrophique ou paralysie myo-sclérosique. *Arch. Gén. Méd., Paris*, 1868, 11:5-25; 179-209; 305-21; 421-43; 522-88. Griesinger, W. Über Muskelhypertrophie. *Arch. Heilk.*, 1865, 6:1-13.

Duchenne myodystrophy. See *Duchenne muscular dystrophy.*

Duchenne paralysis. Synonyms: *Duchenne syndrome, Fazio-Londe paralysis, glossolabiolaryngeal paralysis, glossolabiopharyngeal paralysis, progressive bulbar paralysis.*

A chronic, progressive bulbar paralysis, usually occurring during the sixth and seventh decades, which may represent early manifestations of amyotrophic lateral sclerosis. Motor nuclei of the medulla oblongata and, often, the pons and midbrain, are the first organs affected; the hypoglossal nerve is usually the first one to be involved and atrophy and fasciculation of the tongue are the early signs. Involvement of the vagus nerve is followed by dysphagia, pseudosialorrhea, dysarthria, and thickened nasal speech. Atrophy and fasciculation of the palatal and pharyngeal muscles may follow. Involvement of the facial and trigeminal nerves leads to paralysis of the muscles of facial expression and mastication. The accessory nerve may be also affected.

Duchenne, G. B. Paralysie musculaire progressive de lalangue, du voile, du palais et des lèvres, affection non encore décrite comme espèce morbide distincte. *Arch. Gen. Méd., Paris*, 1860, 16:283-96. Fazio, M. Ereditarietà della paralisi bulbare progressiva. *Rif. Med.*, 1892, 8:327. *Londe, P. Paralysie bulbaire progressive infantile et familiale. *Rev. Méd., Paris*, 1894, 14:212-54.

Duchenne progressive muscular dystrophy. See *Duchenne muscular dystrophy.*

Duchenne syndrome (1). See *Duchenne paralysis.*

Duchenne syndrome (2). See *Duchenne muscular dystrophy.*

Duchenne syndrome (3). See *locomotor ataxia.*

Duchenne-Becker muscular dystrophy. See *Becker muscular dystrophy.*

Duchenne-Erb paralysis. See *Duchenne-Erb syndrome.*

Duchenne-Erb syndrome. Synonyms: *Duchenne-Erb paralysis, Erb palsy, upper arm type of brachial palsy, upper radicular syndrome.*

A birth injury manifested as flaccid paralysis of the arm and shoulder muscles, mainly the deltoid, biceps, brachialis, and supinator longus muscles and, less frequently, the supinator brevis, infraspinatus, and subcapularis muscles, caused by lesions of the fourth, fifth, and sixth cervical roots.

Duchenne, G. B. *De l'électrisation localisée et de son application à la pathologie et à la thérapeutique.* Paris, Bailliere, 1855. *Erb. W. Über eine eigentümliche Lokalisation von Lähmung im Plexus brachialis. *Verh. Naturhist. Med. Verein, Heidelberg*, 1874, 2:130-7.

Duchenne-Griesinger disease. See *Duchenne muscular dystrophy.*

Duchenne-Griesinger syndrome. See *Duchenne muscular dystrophy.*

progressive muscular dystrophy, Duchenne type. See *Duchenne muscular dystrophy.*

duck-sauce headache. See *Chinese restaurant syndrome.*

DUCLOS, P. (French physician)

Lhermitte-Duclos disease. See *under Lhermitte.*

DUCREY, AUGOSTO (Italian physician, 1860-1940)

Ducrey disease. Synonyms: *chancroid, soft chancre, ulcus molle.*

Infection of the genitalia with *Haemophilus ducreyi*, characterized by the presence of soft pustules which rupture and form small bleeding and suppurative ulcers of the prepuce, glans, or frenum in males and the vulva, urethra, and portio in women. The infection is usually transmitted by sexual contact.

*Ducrey, A. Il virus dell'ulcera venerea. *Gazz. Internaz. Med.* Chir., 1889, 11:44.

DUDLEY, HOMER DANIEL (American physician, 1877-1950)

Dudley-Klingenstein syndrome. Synonym: *jejunal neoplasm syndrome.*

Tumors of the small intestine with melena and ulcerlike symptoms.

Dudley, H. D. Vascular tumors of the small intestine with symptoms simulating peptic ulcer. *Surg. Clin. N. America,* 1934, 14:1331-7. Klingenstein, P. Benign neoplasm of the small intestine complicated by severe hemorrhage. Report of two cases; operative intervention and recovery. *J. Mount Sinai Hosp. New York,* 1938, 4:972-9.

DUHAMEL, B.

Duhamel anomalad. See *caudal regression syndrome.*

Duhamel syndrome. See *caudal regression syndrome.*

DUHRING, LOUIS ADOLPHUS (American dermatologist, 1845-1913)

Brocq-Duhring disease. See *Duhring disease.*

Duhring disease. Synonyms: *Brocq-Duhring disease, dermatitis herpetiformis, dermatitis multiformis, der-*

matitis neurotica, dermatitis polymorpha dolorosa, dermatitis pruriginosa, dermatitis trophoneurotica, herpes circinatus bullosus, herpes gestationis, hydroa herpetiformis, hydroa pruriginosa, pemphigus circinatus.

A blistering skin disease characterized by a symmetrical distribution of vesicles, bullae, or pustules, usually on the buttocks, shoulders, elbows, and knees, and sometimes scalp, face, and ears. The buccal mucosa, gingival tissue under dentures, and borders of the tongue are the common sites, and glossodynia and glossopyrosis are the usual symptoms of oral involvement. The lesions may appear in various forms, as erythematous, pseudovesicular, pruritic, or erosive. The areas predisposed to trauma are most frequently affected. Histologically, the lesions consist of microabscesses in the connective tissue papillae. Extravasated erythrocytes in the submucosal tissue and at the epithelial-connective tissue junctions are the cause of purpuric puncta. Granular deposits of IgA are usually found in the skin and oral mucosa.

Duhring, L. A. Dermatitis herpetiformis. *JAMA,* 1884, 3:225-9. Brocq, L. De la dermatite herpétiforme de Duhring. *Ann. Derm. Syph., Paris,* 1888, 9:1-20.

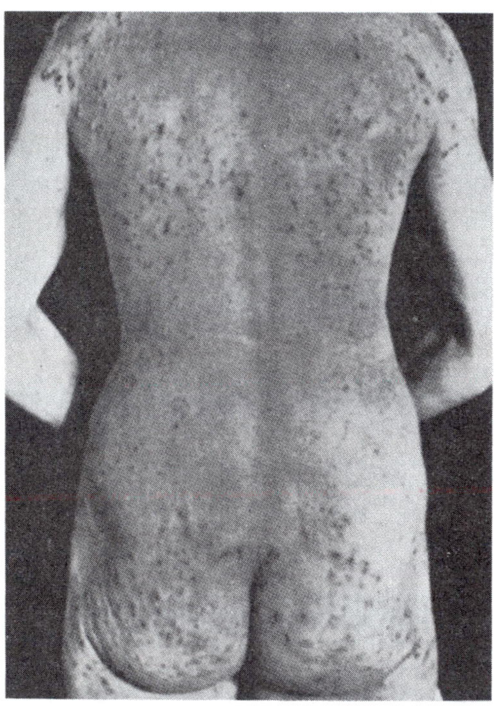

Duhring disease
Andrews, G.C. & A.N. Domonkos: *Diseases of the skin.* Philadelphia: W.B. Saunders Co.

Duhring pruritus. Synonyms: *pruritus hiemalis, winter itch.*

A form of pruritus that occurs chiefly during the winter. Cold water, some soaps, and wool appear to be the precipitating factors.

*Duhring, L. A. Pruritus hiemalis-an undescribed form of pruritus. *Philadelphia Med. Times,* 1874, 4:225-30.

Duhring-Sneddon-Wilkinson syndrome. See *Sneddon-Wilkinson syndrome.*

DUKES, CLEMENT (British physician, 1845-1925)

Dukes disease. Synonyms: *Dukes-Filatov disease, fourth disease, parascalatina.*

An infectious disease of childhood, usually occurring during the spring or summer, and characterized by an exanthematous skin eruption associated with slight fever, following an incubation period of 9 to 21 days.

Dukes, C. On the confusion of two different diseases under the name of rubeola (rose-rash). *Lancet,* 1900, 2:89-94. Filatov, N. *Lektsii ob ostrykh infektsionnykh bolezniiakh detei.* Moskva, 1887, Vol. 2, p. 113.

DÜMLING

Werter-Dümling disease. See *under Werter.*

dumping syndrome (DS). See *postgastrectomy syndrome.*

DUNCAN

Duncan syndrome. A familial syndrome, transmitted as an X-linked recessive trait, characterized by cancer associated with immunodeficiency. The peripheral blood picture is similar to that in infectious mononucleosis, consisting of mature lymphocytes, macrophages, and mature plasma cells. The disease is associated with lymphoma but the maturity and heterogeneity of the peripheral white cells distinguish it from leukemia, leukosarcoma, and sarcoma. The syndrome is named after the surname of the affected family in the original report.

Another familial cancer added to lengthening list. *JAMA,* 1976, 235:2066.

DUNGY, CLAIBOURNE I. (American pediatrician)

McKusick-Dungy-Kaufman syndrome. See *McKusick-Kaufman syndrome.*

DUNNIGAN, M. G. (British physician)

Dunnigan syndrome. See *Köbberling-Dunnigan syndrome.*

Köbberling-Dunningan syndrome. See *under Köbberling.*

duodenal stasis syndrome. See *superior mesenteric artery syndrome.*

duodenal vascular compression syndrome. See *superior mesenteric artery syndrome.*

duodenojejunal hernia. See *Treitz hernia.*

duosyndrome of the laryngeal nerve. See *Chapple syndrome (1).*

dup(1q) syndrome. See *chromosome 1q duplication syndrome.*

dup(2p) syndrome. See *chromosome 2p duplication syndrome.*

dup(2q) syndrome. See *chromosome 2q duplication syndrome.*

dup(3p) syndrome. See *chromosome 3p duplication syndrome.*

dup(3q) syndrome. See *chromosome 3q duplication syndrome.*

dup(4p) syndrome. See *chromosome 4p duplication syndrome.*

dup(4q) syndrome. See *chromosome 4q duplication syndrome.*

dup(5p) syndrome. See *chromosome 5p duplication syndrome.*

dup(5q) syndrome. See *chromosome 5q duplication syndrome.*

dup(6p) syndrome. See *chromosome 6p duplication syndrome.*

dup(6q) syndrome. See *chromosome 6q duplication syndrome.*

dup(7p) syndrome. See *chromosome 7p duplication syndrome.*

dup(7q) syndrome. See *chromosome 7q duplication syndrome.*

dup(8p) syndrome. See *chromosome 8p duplication syndrome.*

dup(8q) syndrome. See *chromosome 8q duplication syndrome.*

dup(10p) syndrome. See *chromosome 10p duplication syndrome.*

dup(10q) syndrome. See *chromosome 10q duplication syndrome.*

dup(11p) syndrome. See *chromosome 11p duplication syndrome.*

dup(11q) syndrome. See *chromosome 11q duplication syndrome.*

dup(12) mosaicism. See *chromosome 12 trisomy mosaicism syndrome.*

dup(12p) syndrome. See *chromosome 12p duplication syndrome.*

dup(12q) syndrome. See *chromosome 12q duplication syndrome.*

dup(13q) syndrome. See *chromosome 13q duplication syndrome.*

dup(14q) syndrome. See *chromosome 14q duplication syndrome.*

dup(15q) syndrome. See *chromosome 15q duplication syndrome.*

dup(16p) syndrome. See *chromosome 16p duplication syndrome.*

dup(16q) syndrome. See *chromosome 16q duplication syndrome.*

dup(17p) syndrome. See *chromosome 17p duplication syndrome.*

dup(17q) syndrome. See *chromosome 17q duplication syndrome.*

dup(18q) syndrome. See *chromosome 18q duplication syndrome.*

dup(19q) syndrome. See *chromosome 19q duplication syndrome.*

dup(20p) syndrome. See *chromosome 20p duplication syndrome.*

dup(20q) syndrome. See *chromosome 20q duplication syndrome.*

DUPLAY, EMANUEL SIMON (French physician, 1836-1924)

Duplay bursitis. Synonyms: *Duplay disease, adhesive bursitis, adhesive capsulitis, bursitis calcarea, bursitis chronica subdeltoidea, checkrein shoulder, frozen shoulder, periarthritis humeroscapularis, periarthritis of the shoulder, peritendinitis calcarea, peritendinitis of the shoulder, scapulohumeral periarthritis, subacromial bursitis, subdeltoid bursitis.*

Scapulohumeral periarthritis, frequently bilateral, associated with calcifying lesions of the subacromial bursa and resulting in severe pain and limitation of motion of the shoulder joint. The condition occurs most frequently in middle life, more often in women than men.

Duplay, E. S. De la péri-arthrite scapulo-humérale et des raideurs de l'épaule qui en sont la conséquence. *Arch. Gén. Méd., Paris,* 1872, 20:513-42. Codman, E. A. *The shoulder rupture of the supraspinatus tendon and other lesions in or about the subcromial bursa.* Boston, Thomas Todd, 1934, p. 216.

Duplay disease. See *Duplay bursitis.*

Duplay fibroma. A benign fibroma of the breast.

Duplay, E. S. Des tumeurs dites bénignes du sein. *Lancette Fr.,* 1878, 51:602-3.

duplication 1q syndrome. See *chromosome 1q duplication syndrome.*

duplication 2q syndrome. See *chromosome 2q duplication syndrome.*

duplication 3p syndrome. See *chromosome 3p duplication syndrome.*

duplication 3q syndrome. See *chromosome 3q duplication syndrome.*

duplication 4p syndrome. See *chromosome 4p duplication syndrome.*

duplication 4q syndrome. See *chromosome 4q duplication syndrome.*

duplication 5p syndrome. See *chromosome 5p duplication syndrome.*

duplication 5q syndrome. See *chromosome 5q duplication syndrome.*

duplication 6p syndrome. See *chromosome 6p duplication syndrome.*

duplication 6q syndrome. See *chromosome 6q duplication syndrome.*

duplication 7p syndrome. See *chromosome 7p duplication syndrome.*

duplication 7q syndrome. See *chromosome 7q duplication syndrome.*

duplication 8p syndrome. See *chromosome 8p duplication syndrome.*

duplication 8q syndrome. See *chromosome 8q duplication syndrome.*

duplication 10p syndrome. See *chromosome 10p duplication syndrome.*

duplication 10q syndrome. See *chromosome 10q duplication syndrome.*

duplication 11p syndrome. See *chromosome 11p duplication syndrome.*

duplication 11q syndrome. See *chromosome 11q duplication syndrome.*

duplication 12 mosaicism. See *chromosome 12 trisomy mosaicism syndrome.*

duplication 12p syndrome. See *chromosome 12p duplication syndrome.*

duplication 12q syndrome. See *chromosome 12q duplication syndrome.*

duplication 13q syndrome. See *chromosome 13q duplication syndrome.*

duplication 14q syndrome. See *chromosome 14q duplication syndrome.*

duplication 15q syndrome. See *chromosome 15q duplication syndrome.*

duplication 16q syndrome. See *chromosome 16q duplication syndrome.*

duplication 17p syndrome. See *chromosome 17p duplication syndrome.*

duplication 17q syndrome. See *chromosome 17q duplication syndrome.*

duplication 18q syndrome. See *chromosome 18q duplication syndrome.*

duplication 19q syndrome. See *chromosome 19q duplication syndrome.*

duplication 20p syndrome. See *chromosome 20p duplication syndrome.*

DUPONT, A. (Belgian physician)

Dupont-Vandaele syndrome. See *Woringer-Kolopp, under Woringer, Frederic.*

DUPRE, ERNEST (French physician, 1862-1921)

Dupré syndrome. Synonyms: *pseudomeningitis, serous meningitis, toxic encephalopathy.*

Meningeal irritation that may follow extracerebral infections.

*Dupré, L. Le méningisme. *Cong. Fr. Méd.*, 1985, 1:411-23.

DUPUY

Dupuy syndrome. See *Frey syndrome.*

DUPUYTREN, BARON GUILLAUME (French surgeon, 1777-1835)

Dupuytren abscess. Abscess of the right iliac fossa.

Dupuytren, G. Abcés developpé dans le petit bassin. *Rev. Méd. Fr. Étr.*, 1829, 33:367-8.

Dupuytren contracture (DC). Synonym: *palmar fibromatosis.*

Flexion deformity of the fingers at their proximal interphalangeal joints due to thickening and shortening of the palmar fascia. The lesion may begin as a single painless nodule of the palmar surface, usually of the right hand, with other nodules appearing later to form bands of thickened tissue on the palmar fascia. All the digits, including the thumb, can be affected, but particularly the ring and little finger. In rare cases, similar contractures may occur on the plantar fascia of the foot. The disorder occurs most commonly in males of northern European extraction, usually between the ages of 40 and 60 years, but females and other age groups can be also affected. It is a familial disorder with probable autosomal dominant inheritance with variable penetrance.

*Dupuytren G. De la rétraction des doigts par suite d'une affection de l'aponéurose palmaire. Operation chirurgicale, qui convient dans le case. *J. Univ. Hebd. Méd. Chir. Prat., Paris*, 1833, 5:271-3.

Dupuytren fracture. See *Pott fracture.*

Dupuytren phlegmon. Phlegmon in the anterolateral part of the neck.

Ragnetta, D. M. Du phlegmon large du cou et de son traitement. *Bull. Gen. Ther., Paris*, 1833, 5:271-3.

Dupuytren-Nélaton disease. See *Nélaton disease.*

dural endothelioma. See *Cushing tumor.*

DURAND, J. (French physician)

Durand disease. See *Durand-Nicholas-Favre disease.*

Durand-Nicolas-Favre disease. Synonyms: *Durand disease, Frei bubo, Frei disease, Nicolas-Favre disease, benign inguinal lymphogranulomatosis, climatic bubo, fifth venereal disease, lymphogranuloma inguinale, lymphogranuloma tropicum, lymphogranuloma venereum (LGV), lymphoma inguinale, lymphomatosis inguinalis suppurativa subacuta, lymphopathia venerea, Miyagawanella lymphogranulomatosis, poradenitis inguinalis, poradenitis nostras, suppurative inguinal adenitis, tropical bubo, venereal lymphogranuloma.*

Chlamydia trichomatis infection, usually occurring in tropical and subtropical climates as a sexually-transmitted disease, sometimes also observed in nonvenereal forms. The initial lesions are infiltrated papules or small erosions at the site of contact, which become matted with ovoid firm lobulated swellings covered by adherent erythematous skin. In some instances, the nodes produce linear depressions parallel to the inguinal ligament. The initial lesions progress to lymphadenitis, discharging sinuses, elephantiasis in males, and occasional rectal stricture in females. When transmitted by the genito-oral contact, the initial lesions progress to lymphadenitis and inflammation of the oral tissues, obliteration of the lymphatic vessels, discharging sinuses, and hyperplastic cicatrization. Associated complaints include fever, chills, headache, nausea, weight loss, and, sometimes, generalized rash, meningitis, erythema nodosum, erythema multiforme, urticaria, and scarlatinous eruption. The oculoglandular syndrome may develop (see *Parinaud oculoglandular syndrome*).

Durand, N. J., & Favre. Lymphogranulomatose inguinale subaiguë d'origine génitale probable, peut-être vénérienne. *Bull. Soc. Méd. Hôp. Paris,* 1913, 35:274-88. Frei, W. Eine neue Hautreaktion bei "Lymphogranuloma inguinale." *Klin. Wschr.*, 1925, 4:2148-9.

DURAND, PAUL (Italian physician)

Durand disease. A viral infection of humans and animals characterized by fever, cough, nausea, and hematemesis.

Durand, P. Virus filtrant pathogéne pour l'homme et les animaux de laboratoire, et à affinités méningée et pulmonaire. I. *Arch. Inst. Pasteur, Tunis,* 1940, 29:179-227.

Durand-Zunin syndrome. An association of agenesis of the septum pellucidum with status dysraphicus, lacunar skull, clubfoot, hydrocephalus, spina bifida, and other abnormalities.

Durand, P., & Zunin, C. Associazione de agenesia del setto pellucido, cranio lacunare, spina bifida, e altri segni malformativi. *Minerva Pediat.*, 1955, 7:1249-56.

DURANTE, GUSTAVE (French physician, 1865-1934)

Porak-Durante syndrome. See *osteogenesis imperfecta syndrome (recessive form).*

DURET, HENRI (French physician, 1849-1921)

Duret hemorrhage. Brainstem hemorrhage.

Duret, H. *Traumatismes cranio-cérébraux.* Paris, Librairie Félix Alcan, 1919.

DUROZIEZ, PAUL LOUIS (French physician, 1826-1897)

Duroziez disease. Congenital mitral stenosis.

Duroziez, P. L. Du rétrécissement mitral pur. *Arch. Gen. Méd., Paris,* 1877, 30:32-54; 184-97.

DUSARD

Dusard syndrome. A familial hematological syndrome characterized by congenital dysfibrinogenemia with defective fibrin lysis and thrombotic and phlebitic complicataions. The syndrome was named after the family Dusard.

Soria, J., *et al.* A new type of congenital dysfibrinogenaemia with defective fibrin lysis-usard syndrome: Possible relation to thrombosis. *Brit. J. Haemat.*, 1983, 53:575-86.

Dutch-Kentucky syndrome. See *trismus-pseudocamptodactyly syndrome.*

DUTTON, JOSEPH EVERETT (British physician, 1877-1905)

Dutton disease. Synonym: *trypanosomiasis.*

An infection with any member of the genus *Trypanosoma.*

Dutton, J. E., & Bruce, D. Preliminary note upon a *Trypanosoma* occurring in the blood of man. *Thompson Yates Lab. Rep., Liverpool,* 1902, 4:455-68.

Dutton fever. Synonym: *D fever.*

Tick-borne relapsing fever caused by *Borrelia duttoni* infection.

Dutton, J. E., & Todd, J. L. The nature of tick fever in the eastern part of the Congo Free State, with notes on the distribution and bionomics of the tick. *Brit. Med. J.*, 1905, 2:1259-60.

DV (digital vibration) syndrome. See *vibration syndrome.*

dwarfism-congenital anterior bowing of legs. See *Weismann-Netter syndrome.*

dwarfism-congenital medullary stenosis syndrome. See *Kenny syndrome.*

dwarfism-eczema-peculiar facies syndrome. See *Dubowitz syndrome (1).*

dwarfism-ichthyosiform erythroderma-mental deficiency syndrome. See *Rud syndrome.*

dwarfism-onychodysplasia syndrome. See *Coffin-Siris syndrome.*

dwarfism-septo-optic dysplasia syndrome. See *septo-optic dysplasia.*

DWS. See *Dandy-Walker syndrome.*

DYGGVE, H. V. (Danish physician)

Dyggve-Melchior-Clausen dwarfism. See *Dyggve-Melchior-Clausen syndrome.*

Dyggve-Melchior-Clausen syndrome (DMC, DMCS). Synonyms: *Dyggve-Melchior-Clausen dwarfism, Smith-McCort dwarfism.*

A short-trunk type dwarfism-mental retardation syndrome associated with protrusion of the sternum, lumbar lordosis and scoliosis, small hands and feet, and mild clawing of the fingers. Major radiographic features consist of flattening of the vertebral bodies in infancy (persisting into adult life) and notching in superior and inferior plates of the vertebral bodies, shortening of the tubular bones with irregular epiphyseal and metaphyseal ossification, and short and broad ilia with hypoplasia of the basilar portions and lacelike appearance of the iliac crests. The syndrome is transmitted as an autosomal trait. Dyggve-Melchior-Clausen syndrome without mental retardation is referred to as *Smith-McCort dwarfism.*

Dyggve, H. V., Melchior, J. C., & Clausen, J. Morguio-Ullrich's disease. An inborn error of metabolism. *Arch. Dis. Child.*, 1962, 37:525-34. Smith, R., & McCort, J. J. Osteochondrodystrophy (Morquio-Brailsford type). Occurrence in three siblings. *California Med.*, 1958, 88:55-9. Spranger, J. *et al.*, Heterogeneity of Dyggve-Melchior-Clausen dwarfism. *Hum. Genet.*, 1976, 33:279-87.

DYKE, C. G.

Dyke-Davidoff-Masson (DDM) syndrome. Cerebral hemiatrophy with homolateral hypertrophy of the calvaria and frontal sinuses (resulting in facial asymmetry) and elevation of the sphenoid wing and petrous ridge, in association with contralateral hemiplegia, mental retardation, and impaired speech.

Dyke, C. G., Davidoff, L. M. & Masson, C. B. Cerebral hemiatrophy with homolateral hypertrophy of the skull and sinuses. *Surg. Gyn. Obstet.*, 1933, 57:588-600.

DYKE, SIDNEY CAMPBELL (British physician, born 1886)

Dyke-Young syndrome. Synonym: *macrocytic hemolytic anemia.*

Macrocytic hemolytic anemia with increased erythrocyte fragility.

Dyke, S. C., & Young, F. Macrocytic hemolytic anaemia associated with increased red cell fragility. *Lancet*, 1938, 2:817-21.

dysbasia lordotica progressiva. See *Ziehen-Oppenheim syndrome.*

dyscalculia and right-left disorientation. See *Gerstmann syndrome (2).*

dyscephalia mandibulo-oculo-facialis. See *Hallermann-Streiff syndrome.*

dyscephalia oculo-mandibulo-facialis. See *Hallermann-Streiff syndrome.*

dyscephaly-congenital cataract-hypotrichosis syndrome. See *Hallermann-Streiff syndrome.*

dyschondrodysplasia-angiomatosis syndrome. See *Maffucci syndrome.*

dyschondroplasia. See *Ollier syndrome.*

dyschondroplasia with hemangioma. See *Maffucci syndrome.*

dyschondrosteosis. See *Léri-Weill syndrome, under Léri, André.*

dyschromia irido-cutanea et dysplasia auditiva. See *Waardenburg syndrome (2).*

dyscranio-pygo-phalangia. See *Ullrich-Feichtiger syndrome.*

dysencephalia splanchnocystica. See *Meckel syndrome, under Meckel, Johann Friedrich, Jr.*

dysendocrinism. See *Donohue syndrome.*

dysequilibrium syndrome (DES). See *Halpern syndrome.*

dysfunctio pluriglandularis dolorosa. See *Curtius syndrome (2).*

dysfunctional bladder. See *Hinman syndrome.*

dysfunctional lazy bladder syndrome. See *Hinman syndrome.*

dysgenesis iridodentalis. See *Weyers syndrome (2).*

dysgenesis mesodermalis corneae. See *Peters anomaly.*

dysgenesis mesodermalis corneae et iridis. See *Rieger syndrome.*

dysgenesis mesodermalis corneae et iridis with oligodontia. See *Weyers syndrome (2).*

dysgenesis mesostromalis anterior. See *Rieger syndrome.*

dyshemopoiesis. See *myelodysplastic syndrome.*

dyshemopoietic anemia. See *myelodysplastic syndrome.*

dyshemopoietic syndrome. See *myelodysplastic syndrome.*

dyskeratoid dermatosis. See *Hailey-Hailey disease, under Hailey, William Howard.*

dyskeratosis bullosa hereditaria. See *Hailey-Hailey disease, under Hailey, William Howard.*

dyskeratosis congenita. See *Zinsser-Engman-Cole syndrome.*

dyskeratosis follicularis. See *Darier disease (1).*

dyskeratosis follicularis vegetans. See *Darier disease (1).*

dyskinesia intermittens angiosclerotica. See *Determann syndrome.*

dyskinesia intermittens angiospastica. See *Determann syndrome.*

dysmaturity syndrome. See *Ballantyne-Runge syndrome.*

dysmelia syndrome. See *Wiedemann syndrome (1).*

dysmorpho-dystrophia mesodermalis congenita. See *Weill-Marchesani syndrome, under Weill, Georges.*

dysmyelinogenic leukodystrophy. See *Alexander syndrome, under Alexander, W. Stewart.*

dysmyelopoiesis. See *myelodysplastic syndrome.*

dysmyelopoietic syndrome (DMS). See *myelodysplastic syndrome.*

dysosteosclerosis syndrome. A bone dysplasia transmitted as an autosomal recessive trait, and characterized chiefly by osteosclerosis and platyspondyly. The affected children are usually short and suffer from bone fragility, dental anomalies (lack of permanent teeth and enamel hypoplasia) and, occasionally, optic atrophy, bulbar paralysis, and macular skin atrophy. Radiological findings include thickening and sclerosis of the calvarium and base of the skull; absent pneumatization of the mastoids and paranasal sinuses; sclerosis of the ribs, clavicles, scapulae, and pelvic bones; hypoplasia of the ilia; flattening, sclerosis, and wedging of the vertebrae; wide metaphyseal flare of the tubular bones; sclerosis of the epiphyses, metaphyses, and central parts of the tubular bones; and cortical thinning and radiolucency of the submetaphyseal parts of the tubular bones.

*Roy, M., *et al.* Un nouveau syndrome osseux avec anomalies cutanée et troubles neurologiques. *Arch. Fr. Pédiat.*, 1968, 25:983. Spranger, J., *et al.* Die Dysosteosklerose-eine Sonderform der generalisierten Osteosklerose. *Fortschr. Roentgen.*, 1968, 109:504-12.

dysostosis cleidocranialis. See *cleidocranial dysostosis.*

dysostosis cleidocraniodigitalis. See *cleidocranial dysostosis.*

dysostosis cleidocraniopelvina. See *cleidocranial dysostosis.*

dysostosis cranio-orbitofacialis. See *craniofacial dysostosis.*

dysostosis craniofacialis. See *craniofacial dysostosis.*

dysostosis craniofacialis hereditaria. See *craniofacial dysostosis.*

dysostosis craniofacialis *with hypertelorism syndrome.* *See Saethre-Chotzen syndrome.*

dysostosis enchondralis epiphysaria. *See multiple epiphyseal dysplasia I.*

dysostosis enchondralis metaepiphysaria. See *mucopolysaccharidosis IV-A.*

dysostosis enchondralis polyepiphysaria. See *multiple epiphyseal dysplasia I.*

dysostosis enchondralis, Schmid type. See *Schmid metaphyseal chondrodysplasia syndrome, under Schmid, Franz.*

dysostosis epiphysealis multiplex. See *multiple epiphyseal dysplasia I.*

dysostosis generalisata. See *cleidocranial dysostosis.*

dysostosis mandibularis. See *Nager-de Reynier syndrome.*

dysostosis maxillo-nasalis. See *Binder syndrome.*

dysostosis maxillofacialis. See *maxillofacial dysostosis syndrome.*

dysostosis metaphysaria, Jansen type. See *Jansen metaphyseal chondrodysplasia syndrome.*

dysostosis metaphysaria, Murk Jansen type. See *Jansen metaphyseal chondrodysplasia syndrome.*

dysostosis spondylometaphysaria, Kozlowski type. See *Kozlowski spondylometaphyseal dysplasia syndrome, under Kozlowski, Kazimierz S.*

dysostosis zygomatico-maxillo-mandibulo-facialis. See *Wildervanck syndrome (2).*

dysostotic idiocy. See *mucopolysaccharidosis I-H.*

dysphagia-dysphonia syndrome. See *Jackson-MacKenzie syndrome, under Jackson, John Hughlings.*

dysplasia dentofacialis. See *Weyers-Fülling syndrome.*

dysplasia epiphysealis capitis femoris. See *Meyer syndrome, under Meyer, J.*

dysplasia epiphysealis congenita. See *Conradi-Hünermann syndrome, under Conradi, Erich.*

dysplasia epiphysealis hemimelica. See *Trevor syndrome.*

dysplasia epiphysealis multiplex. See *multiple epiphyseal dysplasia I.*

dysplasia epiphysialis punctata. See *Conradi-Hünermann syndrome, under Conradi, Erich.*

dysplasia linguofacialis. See *orofaciodigital syndrome I.*

dysplasia marginalis posterior. See *Rieger syndrome.*

dysplasia oculoauricularis. See *oculo-auriculovertebral dysplasia.*

dysplasia oculodentodigitalis. See *oculodentodigital syndrome.*

dysplasia oculovertebralis. See *Weyers-Thier syndrome.*

dysplasia renofacialis. See *Potter syndrome (1), under Potter, Edith Louise.*

dysplasia spondyloepiphysaria congenita. See *spondyloepiphyseal dysplasia congenita.*

dysplasia spondyloepiphysaria tarda. See *spondyloepiphyseal dysplasia tarda.*

dysplasia spondylometaphysaria, Kozlowski type. See *Kozlowski spondylometaphyseal dysplasia syndrome, under Kozlowski, Kazimierz S.*

dysplasia spondylothoracica. See *spondylothoracic dysplasia.*

dysplastic nevus syndrome (DNS). Synonyms: *BK (B-K) mole syndrome, expanded and activated melanocyte syndrome, familial atypical multiple mole melanoma (FAMMM), large atypical mole syndrome.*

A melanocyte abnormality, transmitted as an autosomal dominant trait, that may progress to melanoma. The nevi, usually occurring in groups of several to 100 or more, present discolored, irregular, frequently angulated, predominantly macular lesions, sometimes with central papules. Their color is usually tan, brown, or pink, often with areas of depigmentation; focal black areas suggest a malignant melanoma. They are usually distributed on the back and trunk and, occasionally, on the scalp, breasts, and buttocks. Onset is late in childhood or adolescence, new nevi often appearing through adulthood. Nuclear dysplasia of melanocytes, marked by pleomorphism, hyperchromatism, and irregularities in nuclear membranes, in association with dermal lymphocytic host response and lamellar fibroplasia, are the principal pathological features of this disorder.

Kraemer, K. N. Heritable diseases with increased sensitivity to cellular injury. In: Fitzpatrick, T. B., Eisen, A. Z., Wolff, K., Freedberg, I. M., & Austen, K. F., eds. *Dermatology in general medicine.* 3rd ed. New York, McGraw-Hill, 1987, Vol. 2, pp. 1791-811.

dysporia enterobronchopancreatica congenita familiaris. See *Andersen triad.*

dyssegmental dwarfism (DD), Rolland-Desbuquoid type. See *Rolland-Desbuquois syndrome.*

dyssegmental dwarfism (DD), Silverman type. See *Silverman syndrome (2).*

dyssegmental dysplasia (DD), Rolland-Desbuquoid type. See *Rolland-Desbuquois syndrome.*

dyssegmental dysplasia (DD), Silverman type. See *Silverman syndrome (2).*

dyssynergia cerebellaris myoclonica (DCM). See *Hunt syndrome (1), under Hunt, James Ramsay.*

dyssynergia cerebellaris progressiva. See *Hunt syndrome (1), under Hunt, James Ramsay.*

dystelephalangy. See *Kirner deformity.*

dysthymia. See *Beard syndrome.*

dysthyroidal infantilism. See *Brissaud infantilism.*
dystonia musculorum deformans. See *Ziehen-Oppenheim syndrome.*
dystopia canthi medialis lateroversa. See *Waardenburg syndrome (2).*
dystopia canthorum. See *Greig ocular hypertelorism syndrome.*
dystrophia adiposogenitalis. See *Fröhlich syndrome, under Fröhlich, Alfred.*
dystrophia brevicollis congenita. See *Nielsen syndrome, under Nielsen, Herman.*
dystrophia bullosa atrophicans congenita. See *Hallopeau-Siemens syndrome.*
dystrophia bullosa congenita. See *Hallopeau-Siemens syndrome.*
dystrophia calcarea corneae. See *Axenfeld calcareous degeneration.*
dystrophia corneae reticulata. See *Biber-Haab-Dimmer syndrome.*
dystrophia cornealis posterior polymorpha. See *Schlichting dystrophy.*
dystrophia cutis spinosa congenita. See *Hallopeau-Siemens syndrome.*
dystrophia dermochondrocornealis familiaris. See *François syndrome (2).*
dystrophia epithelialis corneae. See *Fuchs dystrophy.*
dystrophia filiformis profunda corneae. See *Maeder-Danis dystrophy.*
dystrophia hyaliniforms lamellosa corneae. See *Koeppe disease (2).*
dystrophia marginalis crystallinea. See *Bietti dystrophy.*
dystrophia mesodermalis congenita. See *Ehlers-Danlos syndrome, and see Weill-Marchesani syndrome, under Weill, Georges.*
dystrophia mesodermalis hypoplastica. See *Weill-Marchesani syndrome, under Weill, Georges.*
dystrophia musculorum progressiva. See *Erb syndrome (1), under Erb, Wilhelm Heinrich.*
dystrophia musculorum retrahens. See *Emery-Dreifuss syndrome.*
dystrophia myotonica. See *myotonic dystrophy syndrome.*
dystrophia myotonica familiaris. See *myotonic dystrophy syndrome.*
dystrophia osteochondralis polyepiphysaria. See *multiple epiphyseal dysplasia I.*
dystrophia osteogenitalis. See *Brugsch syndrome.*
dystrophia periostalis hyperplastica familiaris. See *Dzerzhinskii syndrome.*
dystrophia pigmentosa. See *Leschke syndrome.*
dystrophia punctiformis profunda corneae with congenital ichthyosis. See *Franceschetti syndrome (1).*
dystrophia unguium mediana canaliformis. See *Heller disease, under Heller, Julius.*
dystrophic metalipoid calcinosis. See *Teutschländer syndrome.*
dystrophic osteoarthropathy. See *Lucherini syndrome.*
dysuria-frequency syndrome. See *urethral syndrome.*

DZERZHINSKII (DZIERZYNSKY) V.V. (Russian physician)
Dzerzhinskii syndrome. Synonyms: *Dzierzynsky syndrome, dystrophia periostalis hyperplastica familiaris.*

An apparently hereditary form of craniomandibulofacial dysostosis marked by acrocephaly, scaphocephaly, lordotic curvature at the base of the skull, peculiar facies, protruding and straight nose, premature closure of cranial sutures, thickening of the skull, and thick phalanges, clavicles, and sternum.

Dzierzynsky, W. Dystrophia periostalic hyperplastica familiaris. *Zbl. Ges. Neur.*, 1913, 20:547.

Dzierzynsky syndrome. See *Dzerzhinskii syndrome.*
DZIERZYNSKY, W. See DZERZHINSKII, V. V.

Page #	Term	Observation

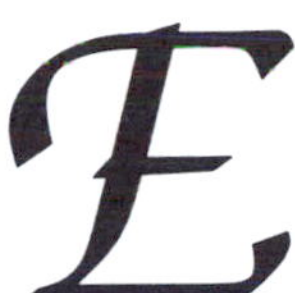

EAC. See *erythema annulare centrifugum.*

EAC (epithelioma adenoides cysticum). See *Brooke epithelioma.*

EAGLE, J. F., JR.

Eagle-Barrett syndrome. See *prune belly syndrome.*

EAGLE, WATT WEEMS (American physician, born 1898)

Eagle syndrome. Synonyms: *hyoid syndrome, styloid elongation syndrome, stylohoid syndrome, styloid syndrome, styloid process syndrome, styloid process-carotid artery syndrome, styloid-stylohyoid syndrome.*

Elongation or calcification of the styloid process, resulting in two clinically distinct types: **Type 1** chiefly affects persons over 30 years of age, usually after tonsillectomy, with the symptoms presenting a dull, nagging pain in the pharyngeal region, which may become stabbing and is aggravated by the act of swallowing. Deglutition disorders and the sensation of a foreign body are usually associated, leading the patient to believe that the surgical wound failed to heal. The constrictor muscles of the upper part of the esophagus and hypopharynx are primarily affected, but pain may be referred to the ear. **Type 2** (called **styloid process-carotid artery syndrome)** is caused by pressure exerted by the elongated and medially or laterally deviated process on the carotid artery, resulting in irritation of the sympathetic nerve fibers. Pain below the level of the eyes and along the routes supplied by the external carotid; pain in the parietal region and along the ophthalmic artery indicate impairment of the internal carotid.

Eagle, W. W. Symptomatic elongated styloid process. Report of two cases of styloid process-carotid artery syndrome with operation. *Arch. Otolaryng., Chicago*, 1949, 49:490-503.

EALES, HENRY (British ophthalmologist, 1852-1913)

Eales disease. See *Eales syndrome.*

Eales syndrome. Synonyms: *Eales disease, angiopathia retinae juvenilis, periphlebitis retinae, retinitis proliferans.*

A noninflammatory disorder of the peripheral retinal vessels characterized by frequently bilateral periphlebitis, avascular peripheral areas, microaneurysms, rope ladder-like capillary dilatations, tortuosity of adjacent vessels, and spontaneous chorioretinal scars. Neovascularization, hemorrhage, vascular obliteration, and vascular sheathing may be associated. Neurological complications may include vascular lesions of the brain and demyelination of the optic nerve. Epistaxis and constipation may occur.

Eales, H. Cases of retinal hemorrhage, asociated with epistaxis and constipation. *Birningham Med. Rev.*, 1880, 9:262-73.

EATON, LEALDES (LEE) MCKENDREE (American physician, 1905-1958)

Eaton-Lambert myasthenic syndrome. See *Eaton-Lambert syndrome.*

Eaton-Lambert syndrome (ELS). Synonyms: *Eaton-Lambert myasthenic syndrome, Eaton-Lambert-Rooke syndrome, Lambert-Eaton myasthenic syndrome (LEMS, LES), bronchial carcinoma-myasthenia syndrome, cancer-associated myasthenic syndrome, myasthenic syndrome of Eaton and Lambert.*

Myasthenia associated with bronchial cancer (usually small-cell carcinoma).

Lambert, E. H., Eaton, L. M., & Rooke, E. D. Defect of neuromuscular conduction associated with malignant neoplasms. *Am. J. Physiol.*, 1956, 187:612-3.

Eaton-Lambert-Rooke syndrome. See *Eaton-Lambert syndrome.*

Lambert-Eaton myasthenic syndrome (LEMS, LES). See *Eaton-Lambert syndrome.*

myasthenic syndrome of Eaton and Lambert (MSEL). See *Eaton-Lambert syndrome.*

EATON, MONROE DAVIS (American bacteriologist, born 1904)

Eaton agent pneumonia. See *Eaton pneumonia.*

Eaton pneumonia. Synonyms: *Eaton agent pneumonia, pleuropneumonia-like organism pneumonia.*

Primary atypical pneumonia caused by *Mycoplasma pneumoniae* (Eaton agent).

Eaton, M. D., *et al.* Studies on the etiology of primary atypical pneumonia. A filtrable agent transmissible to cotton rats, hamsters, and chick embryos. *J. Exper. Med.*, 1944, 79:649-68.

eau de cologne dermatitis. See *Freund dermatitis, under Freund, Emanuel.*

EB. See *epidermolysis bullosa syndrome.*

EBDH (epidermolysis bullosa dystrophica Hallopeau-Siemens). See *Hallopeau-Siemens syndrome.*

EBERTH, CARL JOSEPH (German physician, 1835-1926)

Eberth disease. Synonyms: *enteric fever, typhoid fever, typhus abdominalis.*

A contagious disease caused by ingestion of food or water contaminated with *Salmonella (Eberthella) typhi* or, occasionally, other species of salmonellae. The disease lasts about 4 weeks after the incubation of 7 to 14 days. Early symptoms consist mainly of the triad of fever, headache, and abdominal pain, usually of the right lower quadrant. They are followed by splenomegaly and a rash (rose spots), consisting of deeply red macules, 2 to 4 mm in diameter, which erupt in clusters on the upper anterior abdomen and thorax. During the second week, the symptoms include a marked deterioration in the mental state, delirium, coma, cough, and epistaxis. The third week is usually marked by further deterioration of the mental state, extreme toxemia, greenish pea-soup diarrhea, and intestinal hemorrhage. Additional complaints may include weight loss, a dry and brown tongue (baked tongue), suppurative pneumonia, renal pain, pyuria, hematuria, cholecystitis, jaundice, hepatitis, nerve deafness, conjunctivitis, keratitis, optic neuritis, and osteomyelitis. Severe cases may be complicated by intestingal ulcers, abscess formation, massive hemorrhage, and fatal intestinal perforation. Recovering patients shed the organism in their feces for periods up to 3 months after the onset.

Eberth, C. J. Die Organismen in den Organen bei Typhus abdominalis. *Arch. Path., Berlin,* 1880, 81:58-74. Gorbach, S. L. Typhoid fever. In: Wyngaarden, J. B., & Smith, L. H., Jr., eds. *Cecil textbook of medicine.* 17th ed. Philadelphia, Saunders, 1985, pp. 1587-9.

EBSTEIN, WILHELM (German physician, 1836-1912)

Armani-Ebstein lesion. See *Armani-Ebstein nephropathy.*

Armani-Ebstein nephropathy. See *under Armani.*

Ebstein anomaly. Synonym: *Ebstein syndrome.*

Downward displacement of a deformed tricuspid valve into the right ventricle with attachment of the septal and posterior leaflets to the wall of the ventricle and normal attachment of the anterior leaflets to the anulus fibrosus. The portion of the ventricle above the valve is incorporated into the right atrium, the right ventricle being small and the right atrium grossly enlarged. The valve may not be competent. Cardiac arrhythmias, especially extrasystoles and paroxysmal tachycardia, dyspnea, cyanosis, fatigability, and sudden death are the common features. The clinical course varies, depending on the degree of anomaly; some patients die in infancy, others may survive to advanced age.

Ebstein, W. Über einen sehr seltenen Fall von Insufficenz der Valvula tricuspidalis bedingt durch eine angeborene hochgradige Missbildung derselben. *Arch. Anat. Physiol., Leipzig,* 1866:238-53.

Ebstein disease. Hyaline degeneration and necrosis of the epithelial cells of the renal tubules in diabetes mellitus.

Ebstein, W. Über Drüsenepithelnekrosen beim Diabetes mellitus mit besonderer Berücksichtigung des diabetischen Coma. *Deut. Arch. Klin. Med.,* 1880-81, 28:143-242.

Ebstein syndrome. See *Ebstein anomaly.*

Pel-Ebstein disease. See *Hodgkin disease.*

eccentro-osteochondrodysplasia. See *mucopolysaccharidosis IV-A.*

eccentrochondrodysplasia. See *mucopolysaccharidosis IV A.*

eccrine poroma. See *Pinkus tumor, under Pinkus, Hermann Karl Benno.*

echolic folliculitis. See *Grindon disease.*

ECKLIN, THEOPHIL (Swiss physician)

Ecklin anemia. Synonym: *anemia splenica congenita.*

A usually fatal form of normoblastic myelocytic anemia of newborn infants, characterized by splenomegaly, hepatomegaly, low hemoglobin level, reticulocytosis, erythroblastosis, leukocytosis, and jaundice without hemolysis.

Ecklin, T. Ein Fall von Anämie bei einem Neugeborenen. *Mschr. Kinderh.,* 1918-19, 15:425-36.

eclampsia nutants. See *West syndrome.*

ECONOMO, CONSTANTIN, VON (Austrian physician, 1876-1931)

Economo disease. Synonyms: *von Economo disease, encephalitis lethargica, lethargic encephalitis, sleeping sickness.*

A disease of the central nervous system thought to be caused by a virus, and marked mainly by pronounced somnolence (lethargy) and ophthalmoplegia. The condition first occurred during and about 10 years after World War I and is now considered to be extinct. Clonic or choreiform movements, rigidity, delirium, headache stupor, dizziness, fatigability, confusion, hemiplegia, hearing and visual disturbances, cortical sensory loss, aphasia, coma, reversal of sleep rhythm, and a number of other disorders were associated. Inflammatory lesions of the brain stem, basal ganglia, cerebellum, cerebral cortex, and spinal cord were believed to be the causative factors. Most patients recovering from Economo disease developed parkinsonism and personality changes. Lymphocytic pleocytosis and elevated protein levels in the cerebrospinal fluid were found in some patients. The causative virus was never identified. Redlich suspected that this disorder and Redlich encephalitis were variants of the same entity.

Economo, C., von Encephalitis lethargica. *Wien. Klin. Wschr.,* 1917, 30:581-5.

von Economo disease. See *Economo disease.*

ECP. See *ectrodactyly-cleft palate syndrome.*

ectodermal dysplasia with ocular malformations. See *Curtius syndrome (1).*

ectodermal dysplasia, Robinson type. See *Robinson syndrome, under Robinson, Geoffrey C.*

ectodermal dysplasia-ectrodactyly-macular dystrophy (EEM) syndrome. A familial syndrome, probably transmitted as an autosomal recessive trait, characterized by ectodermal dysplasia, ectrodactyly, syndactyly or cleft hand, and macular dystrophy.

Ohdo, S., *et al.* Association of ectodermal dysplasia, ectrodactyly, and macular dystrophy: The EEM syndrome. *J. Med. Genet.,* 1983, 20:52-7.

ectodermosis erosiva pluriorificialis. See *Stevens-Johnson syndrome.*

ectoneurodermal hamartoma. See *Sturge-Weber syndrome.*

ectopic ACTH syndrome. The presence of adrenocorticotropic hormone (ACTH) in both the tumor and blood of patients with nonpituitary tumors in association with symptoms of the Cushing syndrome. Clinical features include weakness, hypertension, cushingoid appearance, peripheral edema, personality disorders, and hyperpigmentation. Biochemical features consist of an increase in urinary free cortisol, hypokalemia, and elevated ACTH. Bronchial oat cell carcinoma is the most frequent cause. Other tumors implicated in the production of ectopic ACTH include carcinoid tumors (usually of the bronchi) and tumors of the thymus, stomach, appendix, pancreas, ileum, ovaries, and other organs.

Liddle, G. W., *et al.* Normal and abnormal regulation of corticotropin secretion in man. *Rec. Prog. Horm. Res.*, 1962, 18:125-66. Christy, N. P. Adrencorticotropic activity in the plasma of patients with Cushing's syndrome associated with pulmonary neoplasms. *Lancet*, 1961, 1:85-6.

ectopic cloaca. See *OEIS complex.*

ectopic ventricular tachycardia. See *torsades de pointes syndrome.*

ectrodactyly-cleft palate (ECP) syndrome. A familial syndrome, transmitted as an autosomal dominant trait, consisting of ectrodactyly and cleft palate.

Opitz, J. M., *et al.* The ECP syndrome, another autosomal dominant case of monodactylous ectrodactyly. *Eur. J. Pediat.*, 1980, 133:217-20.

ectrodactyly-ectodermal dysplasia-clefting syndrome. See *EEC syndrome.*

ectromelia-ichthyosis syndrome. Synonym: *unilateral ectromelia-ichthyosis syndrome.*

An association of unilateral ichthyosiform erythema and ipsilateral aplastic or hypoplastic bone lesions of the limbs, including hypoplasia of the pelvic bones, rib anomalies, and absent or hypoplastic phalanges or monodactyly. Congenital heart defect may occur.

Rossman, R. E., *et al.* Unilateral ichthyosiform erythroderma. *Arch. Derm., Chicago*, 1963, 88:567-71.

eczema exfoliativum. See *Wilson disease (1), under Wilson, Sir Willilam Erasmus.*

eczema herpeticum. See *Kaposi varicelliform eruption.*

eczema herpetiformis. See *Kaposi varicelliform eruption.*

eczema pruriginosum allergicum. See *Besnier prurigo.*

eczema seborrheicum. See *Unna disease, under Unna, Paul Gerson.*

eczema universale seborrheicum. See *Leiner dermatitis.*

eczema vaccinatum. See *Kaposi varicelliform eruption.*

eczema verrucosum callosum. See *Hyde syndrome.*

eczema-thrombocytopenia syndrome. See *Wiskott-Aldrich syndrome.*

eczema-thrombocytopenia-diarrhea syndrome. See *Wiskott-Aldrich syndrome.*

eczema-thrombocytopenia-immunodeficiency syndrome. See *Wiskott-Aldrich syndrome.*

eczematid-like purpura. See *Casalá-Mosto disease.*

EDDOWES, ALFRED (British physician, 1850-1946)

Eddowes syndrome. See *osteogenesis imperfecta syndrome (dominant form).*

Spurway-Eddowes syndrome. See *osteogenesis imperfecta syndrome (dominant form).*

EDELMANN, ADOLF (Polish physician, 1885-1939)

Edelmann anemia. See *Edelmann syndrome (1).*

Edelmann syndrome (1). Synonyms: *Edelmann anemia, anemia infectiosa chronica.*

A form of chronic infectious anemia.

Edelmann, A. Über Anaemia infectiosa chronica und ihre Aetiologie. *Wien. Klin. Wschr.*, 1925, 38:268-9.

Edelmann syndrome (2). Synonym: *pancreaticohepatic syndrome.*

Chronic pancreatitis with secondary involvement of the nervous system and skin and lesions of the brain and spinal cord, with mental symptoms similar to those of the Korsakov syndrome, polyneuritis, cachexia, and atrophic changes of the skin with diffuse gray pigmentation and follicular hyperkeratosis. Edelmann attributed this syndrome to escape of pancreatic juice into the blood.

Edelmann, A. Über ein bisher nicht beachtetes pankreatohepatisches Syndrom, bedingt durch Übertritt des Pankreassaftes in die Blutbahn. *Wien. Klin. Wschr.*, 1936, 49:1336-9.

edema cutis circumscriptum. See *Quincke edema.*

edematous necrosis of the pancreas. See *Zoepffel edema.*

edematous pancreatitis. See *Zoepffel edema.*

Edinburgh malformation syndrome. Synonym: *typus edinburgensis.*

A familial syndrome, transmitted as an autosomal dominant trait, characterized by peculiar facies, true or apparent hydrocephalus, psychomotor retardation, failure to thrive, and death in the first month of life. Neonatal hyperbilirubinemia and advanced bone age may occur.

Habel, A. "Typus edinburgensis?" *Pediatrics*, 1974, 53:425-30.

EDS. See *Emery-Dreifuss syndrome.*

EDWARDS, J. H. (British physician)

Edwards syndrome. See *chromosome 18 trisomy syndrome.*

EEC (ectrodactyly-ectodermal dysplasia-clefting) syndrome. Synonyms: *Rüdiger syndrome, Walker-Clodius syndrome, lobster-claw defect with ectodermal defects syndrome, odontotrichomelic hypohidrotic dysplasia, split hand-cleft lip/palate and ectodermal (SCE) dysplasia.*

A syndrome of cleft deformity of the hands and feet, nasolacrimal duct obstruction, and cleft lip and palate, which often are observed in incomplete forms. Hand deformities may occur as oligodactyly, monodactyly, absent carpal bones or their hypoplasia and fusion, sometimes in association with clinodactyly and syndactyly. Foot deformities are parallel with those of the hands. Absent lacrimal puncta, tearing, blepharitis, dacryocystitis, keratoconjunctivitis, and photophobia are the principal ocular findings. The skin may show albinoid changes, hypohidrosis, absence of sebaceous glands, pigmented nevi, and sparse eyebrows, eyelashes, and scalp hair (hypotrichosis). The nails may be dysplastic. Microcephaly and mental retardation are often associated. Kidney aplasia, hydronephrosis, and hydroureter are the chief urological complications. Orodental abnormalities usually include anodontia, oligodontia, lack of permanent teeth, enamel hypoplasia, xerostomia, and furrowed tongue. The syndrome is transmitted as an autosomal dominant trait with incomplete penetrance and variable expressivity.

Rüdiger, R. A., *et al.* E. Association of ectrodactyly, ectodermal dysplasia and cleft lip/palate. The EEC syndrome. *Am. J. Dis. Child.*, 1970, 120:160-3. Walker, J. C., & Clodius, L. The syndromes of cleft lip, cleft palate, and lobster-claw deformities of hands and feet. *Plast. Recostr. Surg.*, 1963, 32:627-36.

EEM syndrome. See *ectodermal dysplasia-ectrodactyly-macular dystrophy syndrome.*

EFAS (embryofetal alcohol syndrome). See *fetal alcohol syndrome.*

EFE (endocardial fibroelastosis). See *Weinberg-Himelfarb syndrome.*

effort syndrome. See *Da Costa syndrome, under Da Costa, Jacob Mendez.*

effort thrombosis. See *Paget-Schroetter syndrome.*

EGGLESTON, CARY (American physician, born 1884)

Bradbury-Eggleston syndrome. See *under Bradbury.*
Egyptian chlorosis. See *Griesinger disease.*
Egyptian ophthalmia. See *trachoma.*
EHF (**e**pidemic **h**emorrhagic **f**ever). See *hemorrhagic fever with renal syndrome.*
EHLERS, EDVARD (Danish dermatologist, 1863-1937)
Ehlers-Danlos syndrome (ED, EDS). Synonyms: *Chernogubov syndrome, Meekeren-Ehlers-Danlos syndrome, Sack syndrome, Sack-Barabas syndrome, arthrochalasia multiplex congenita, cutis elastica syndrome, cutis hyperelastica, cutis hyperelastica dermatorrhexis, cutis laxa, dermatorrhexis with dermatochalasis and arthrochalasis, dystrophia mesodermalis congenita, elastic skin, fibrodysplasia elastica, fibrodysplasia elastica generalisata.*

A syndrome characterized chiefly by hyperextensibility of the joints and skin and poor wound healing. The most consistently associated orofacial features include narrow maxillae, lop ears, epicanthal folds, wide nasal bridge, recurrent temporomandibular joint subluxation, and fragile and easily bruised oral mucosa. The skin has a velvety appearance and is hyperelastic, especially over the major joints, with poor wound healing and resulting pigmented papyraceous scars. Molluscoid or raisinlike pseudotumors, usually of the heels and over the major joints, are frequent. Dislocations, pes planus, talipes, kyphoscoliosis, thoracic asymmetry, and inguinal and umbilical hernias may occur. Occasional ocular abnormalities may include blue sclera, myopia, microcornea, keratoconus, glaucoma, and retinal detachment. Small irregular teeth and partial anodontia are the chief dental features. The most common vascular defects consist of ecchymoses and dissecting aneurysm of the aorta. Musculoskeletal anomalies may include a weak hand clasp, genu recurvatum, and recurrent joint dislocations. Prematurity due to early rupture of fetal membranes is common.

Ehlers, E. Neigung zu Hämorrhagien in der Haut, Lockerung mehrerer Artikulationen. *Derm. Zschr.*, 1901, 8:173-4. Danlos, H. Un cas de cutis laxa avec tumeurs por contusion chronique de coudes et des genoux (xanthoma juvenile pseudo-diabetique de MM. Hallopeau et Mace de Lepinay). *Bull Soc. Fr. Derm. Syph.*, 1908, 19:70-2. Sack, G. Status dysvascularis, ein Fall von besonderer Zerreisslichkeit der Blutgefässe. *Deut. Arch. Klin. Med.*, 1935-36, 178:663-9. Barabas, A. P. Heterogeneity of the Ehlers-Danlos syndrome: Description of three clinical types and a hypothesis to explain the basic defect(s). *Brit. Med. J.*, 1967, 2:612-3. *Tschernogubow. Über einen Fall von Cutis laxa. *Mtschr. Prakt. Dermatol.*, 1892, 14:76. Meekeren, J. A., van. De dilatabilitate extraordinaria cutis. *Observationes Medicochirurgicae*. Chapter 32, Amsterdam, 1682.

Meekeren-Ehlers-Danlos syndrome. See *Ehlers-Danlos syndrome.*
EHRENFRIED, ALBERT (American physician, 1880-1951)
Ehrenfried disease. See *multiple cartilaginous exostoses syndrome.*
EHRET, HEINRICH (German physician, born 1870)
Ehret paralyis. See *Ehret syndrome.*
Ehret syndrome. Synonym: *Ehret paralysis.*

Paralysis developing after a painful but not damaging injury, as a result of which the patient assumes the least painful static position, resulting in muscular atrophy and contractures. The paralysis persists even after the cause is completely removed.

Ehret, H. Über eine functionelle Lähmungsform der Peronealmuskeln traumatischen Ursprunges. *Arch. Unfallh. Stuttgart,* 1898, 3:32-56.

EHRLICH, PAUL (German pharmacologist, 1854-1915)
Biermer-Ehrlich anemia. See *Addison-Biermer anemia.*
EICHHORST, HERMANN LUDWIG (Swiss physician, 1849-1921)
Eichhorst disease. Synonyms: *Eichhorst neuritis, neuritis fascians.*

A form of neuritis in which both the nerve sheath and the interstitial tissue of the muscle are affected.

*Eichhorst, H. L. Über *Nervendegeneration und Nervenregeneration.* Königsberg, Longrien, 1873.

Eichhorst neuritis. See *Eichhorst disease.*
EIGER, MARVIN S. (American physician)
Bakwin-Eiger syndrome. See *hyperphosphatasia-osteoctasia syndrome.*
EISENLOHR, CARL (German physician, 1847-1896)
Eisenlohr syndrome. Weakness and numbness of the

	Type	Clinical Features	Genetics	Biochemical Defect
I.	gravis	Classic features, all severe	Autosomal dominant	Unknown
II.	mitis	Classic features, all mild	Autosomal dominant	Unknown
III.	benign hypermobile	Generalized marked joint hypermobility without skeletal deformity, skin features minimal	Autosomal dominant	Unknown
IV.	ecchymotic, arterial, (Sack-Barabas syndrome)	Severe bruisability, very thin skin, rupture of bowel, rupture of large arteries, minimal joint laxity (for example, limited to fingers)	Autosomal recessive	Deficient synthesis of type III collagen
V.	X-linked	Stretchable skin striking, joint hypermobility minimal, skin fragility and bruisability variable	X-linked recessive	Deficiency of lysyl oxidase
VI.	ocular	Scoliosis severe, skin features moderate, blindness from retinal detachment or ocular rupture	Autosomal recessive	Deficiency of procollagen lysyl hydroxylase
VII.	arthrochalasis multiplex congenita	Short stature, severe joint laxity with congenital dislocations, moderate skin stretchability and bruisability	Autosomal recessive	Deficiency of procollagen protease (or peptidase)

(Adapted from: McKusick, V.A., & Martin, G.R. Molecular defects in collagen. *Ann. Intern. Med.*, 1975, 82:585-6.)

extremities, dysarthria, and paralysis of the lips, tongue, and palate.

Eisenlohr, C. Über einen eigentümlichen Symptomkomplex bei Abdominaltyphus. *Deut. Med. Wschr.*, 1892, 19:122-3.

EISENMENGER, VICTOR (Austrian physician, 1864-1934)

Eisenmenger complex. See *Eisenmenger syndrome.*

Eisenmenger syndrome. Synonym: *Eisenmenger complex.*

A congenital heart disease. Anatomically, it consists of a ventricular septal defect, overriding aorta, right ventricular hypertrophy, and a normal or dilated pulmonary artery. Physiologically, it is marked by a ventricular septal defect associated with right-to-left shunt and high pulmonary vascular resistance. The early symptoms include dyspnea, feeding difficulty, fatigue, and failure to thrive. Increased cyanosis, squatting, angina pectoris, episodes of syncope, clubbing, and polycythemia appear later in childhood.

Eisenmenger, V. Die angeborenen Defekte der Kommerscheidewand des Herzen. *Zschr. Klin. Med.*, 1897, 32(Suppl):1-28.

EISENMENGER, WILLIAM J. (American physician)

Bongiovanni-Eisenmenger syndrome. See *under Bongiovanni.*

EKBOM, KARL AXEL (Swedish physician)

Ekbom syndrome (1). See *restless leg syndrome.*

Ekbom syndrome (2). Synonyms: *chronic tactile hallucinosis, delusional ectoparasitosis, delusions of parasitosis, delusions of skin infestation.*

A delusional syndrome, occurring most commonly in middle-aged and elderly female schizophrenics, in which the patient imagines the symptoms of parasitic infestation of the skin, most often of the outer rectal area.

Ekbom, K. Praeseniler Dermat-zooenwahn. *Acta Psychiat. Scand.*, 1938, 13:227-59.

Wittmaack-Ekbom syndrome. See *restless leg syndrome.*

EKMAN, OLOF JACOB (Swedish physician, 1764-1839)

Ekman syndrome. See *osteogenesis imperfecta syndrome (dominant form).*

Ekman-Lobstein syndrome. See *osteogenesis imperfecta syndrome (dominant form).*

EKV (erythrokeratodermia variabilis). See *Mendes Da Costa syndrome.*

EL-TEMTAMY, SAMIA ALI. See TEMTAMY, SAMIA ALI

elasteidosis cutanea nodularis. See *Favre-Racouchot disease.*

elasteidosis cutis cystica et comedonica. See *Favre-Racouchot disease.*

elastic skin. See *Ehlers-Danlos syndrome.*

elastica disease. See *pseudoxanthoma elasticum.*

elastoidosis cutanea nodularis. See *Favre-Racouchot disease.*

elastoidosis cutis cystica et comedonica. See *Favre-Racouchot disease.*

elastoma intrapapillare perforans verruciforme. See *Lutz-Miescher syndrome, under Lutz, Wilhelm.*

elastorrhexis generalisata. See *pseudoxanthoma elasticum.*

elastosis dystrophica. See *pseudoxanthoma elasticum.*

elastosis perforans serpiginosa (EPS). See *Lutz-Miescher syndrome, under Lutz, Wilhelm.*

ELDRIDGE, ROSWELL (American physician)

Strasburger-Hawkins-Eldridge syndrome. See *symphalangism syndrome.*

Strasburger-Hawkins-Eldridge-Hargrave-McKusick syndrome. See *symphalangism syndrome.*

electric chorea. See *Bergeron disease, and see Henoch chorea.*

electric feet syndrome. See *burning feet syndrome.*

electric foot. See *burning feet syndrome.*

electrical leak syndrome. Synonyms: *current escape syndrome, current loss syndrome, shunt syndrome.*

Cardiac disorders caused by an improperly functioning implanted artificial pacemaker. A faulty contact, breakage in the wiring, or a defect in the insulation, including axis change with an increase of the amplitude of the stimulation spikes that may be associated with ectopic stimulation of the pectoralis muscle, are the main causes.

Fontaine, G.,. *et al.* Le syndrome de fuite électrique chez les porteurs de pacemaker. *Arch. Mal. Coeur,* 1972, 65:190-8. Green, G. D., *et al.* Detection of faults in implanted cardiac pacemakers. *Brit. Heart J.,* 1969, 31:707-10.

electrolepsy. See *Bergeron disease, and see Henoch chorea.*

elephantiasis congenita hereditaria. See *Nonne-Milroy syndrome.*

elephantiasis genitoanorectalis. See *Huguier-Jersild syndrome.*

elephantiasis genitorectalis. See *Huguier-Jersild syndrome.*

elephantiasis gingivae-hypertrichosis syndrome. See *gingival fibromatosis-hypertrichosis syndrome.*

elephantiasis graecorum. See *Hansen disease.*

elfin facies. See *Williams syndrome, under Williams, J. C. P.*

elfin facies syndrome. See *Williams syndrome, under Williams, J. C. P.*

ELLENBERG, MAX (American physician)

Ellenberg syndrome. Synonym: *diabetic neuropathic cachexia.*

A syndrome of diabetes mellitus associated with bilateral symmetrical peripheral neuropathy. The two principal symptoms are profound weight loss and pain. In the original report the patients, males in the sixth decade, had severe emotional disturbances, anorexia, impotence, mild diabetes, simultaneous onset of nephropathy and diabetes, absence of other specific diabetic complications, and spontaneous recovery in about one year.

Ellenberg, M. Diabetic neuropatahic cachexia. *Diabetes,* 1974, 23:418-23.

ELLINGSON, F. THOMAS (American physician)

Ellingson syndrome. See *uveitis-glaucoma-hyphema syndrome.*

elliptocytosis. See *Dresbach anemia.*

ELLIS, RICHARD WHITE BERNHARD (British pediatrician, 1902-1966)

Ellis-Sheldon syndrome. See *mucopolysaccharidosis I-H.*

Ellis-van Creveld (EVC) syndrome. Synonyms: *chondrodysplasia ectodermica, chondroectodermal dysplasia (CED), mesoectodermal dysplasia, polydactyly-chondrodystrophy syndrome.*

A syndrome of disproportionate short-limb dwarfism with distal shortening of extremities, hexadactyly of the fingers and occasionally the toes, hypoplastic nails, short upper lip connected by frenula to the alveolar ridge, defective dentition (oligodontia, natal teeth, small teeth, and delayed dentition), and frequent cardiac defects (atrial septum defect or single atrium). Associated abnormalities may include scant or fine hair, mental retardation, cryptorchism, epispadias, and talipes equinovalgus. The syndrome is transmitted as an autosomal recessive trait. Some authors suggest that there are many overlapping features of renohepatopancreatic dysplasia and Ellis-van Creveld and Jeune syndromes, which indicate that these three conditions may be parts of a disease spectrum rather than being distinct entities.

Ellis, R. W., & van Creveld, S. A syndrome characterized by ectodermal dysplasia, polydactyly, chondro-dysplasia and congenital morbus cordis. Report of three cases. *Arch. Dis. Child., London*, 1940, 15:65-84. Brueton, L. A., *et al.* Ellis-van Creveld syndrome, Jeune syndrome, and renal-hepatic-pancreatic dysplasia: Separate entities or disease spectrum? *J. Med. Genet.*, 1990, 27:252-5.

ELLISON, EDWIN HOMER (American physician, 1918-1970)

pseudo-Zollinger-Ellison syndrome (Ps-ZES). See *under Zollinger.*

Strom-Zollinger-Ellison syndrome. See *Zollinger-Ellison-syndrome.*

Zollinger-Ellison syndrome (ZE, ZES). See *under Zollinger.*

elongated coarctation of aorta. See *aortic arch syndrome.*

ELS. See ***E**aton-**L**ambert **s**yndrome, under Eaton, Lealdes McKendree.*

ELSAHY, NABIL I. (Canadian physician)

Elsahy-Waters syndrome. Synonyms: *branchioskeletogenital (BSG) syndrome, hypertelorism-hypospadias syndrome.*

A familial syndrome, probably transmitted as an autosomal recessive trait or possibly an X-linked trait, consisting of the triad of branchial arch abnormalities, bone defects, and genital anomalies. Brachycephaly, midfacial hypoplasia, mandibular prognathism, hypertelorism, strabismus, nystagmus, blepharoptosis, and broad nasal bridge with a wide nasal tip and flared alae are the principal orofacial features. Associated disorders include seizures, mental retardation, pectus excavatum, hypospadias, fused second and third cervical vertebrae, and oral anomalies, including cleft palate, bifid uvula, multiple jaw cysts, dysplastic dentin, dental caries, malocclusion, and dentigerous cysts. See also *hypertelorism-hypospadias syndrome.*

Elsahy, N. I., & Waters, W. R. The branchio-skeleto-genital syndrome. A new hereditary syndrome. *Plast. Reconstr. Surg.*, 1971, 48:542-50.

ELSBERG, C. A. (American physician)

Elsberg syndrome. Acute urinary retention in women. The condition is associated with bilateral involvement of the sacral nerve roots, accompanied by sphincter disturbances and an increased cell count and elevated protein content in the cerebrospinal fluid, due to polyradiculitis of the cauda equina caused by local pressure from a tumor or an infection of viral origin, as in genital herpes.

*Elsberg, C. A. Experiences in spinal surgery. Observations upon 60 laminectomies in spinal diseases. *Surg. Gyn. Obst.*, 1931, 16:117. Hemrika, D. J., *et al.* Elsberg syndrome: A neurologic basis for acute urinary retention in patients with genital herpes. *Obst. Gyn.*, 1986, 68(3 Suppl):37S-39S.

ELSCHNIG, ANTON (Austrian ophthalmologist, 1863-1939)

Elschnig conjunctivitis. Synonym: *conjunctivitis meibomiana.*

Chronic conjunctivitis associated with hyperplasia of the tarsal glands and frothy secretions.

Elschnig, A. Beitrag zur Aetiologie und Therapie der chronischen Conjunctivitis. *Deut. Med. Wschr.*, 1908, 34:1133-5.

Elschnig spots. Isolated black flecks surrounded by bright yellow or red halos in hypertensive retinopathy.

Elschnig, A. Die diagnostische und prognostische Bedeutung der Netzhauterkrankungen bei Nephritis. *Wien. Med. Wschr.*, 1904, 54:445-50; 494-8.

Elschnig syndrome. A combination of deformities consisting of extension of the palpebral fissure laterally, displacement of the lateral canthus outward and downward, and ectropion of the lower eyelid and of the lateral canthus. Hypertelorism, cleft palate, and cleft lip are frequently associated.

Elschnig, A. Zur Kenntnis der Anomalien der Lidspaltenform. *Klin. Mbl. Augenh.*, 1912, 50:17-30.

Koerber-Salus-Elschnig syndrome. See *under Koerber.*

ELSNER, CHRISTOPH FRIEDRICH (German physician, 1749-1820)

Elsner asthma. See *Heberden asthma.*

embolic nonsuppurative focal nephritis. See *Löhlein nephritis.*

embryofetal alcohol syndrome (EFAS). See *fetal alcohol syndrome.*

embryoma. See *Wilms tumor.*

embryonal adenosarcoma. See *Wilms tumor.*

embryonal carcinosarcoma. See *Wilms tumor.*

embryonal mixed tumor. See *Wilms tumor.*

embryonal rhabdomyoblastoma. See *Abrikossov tumor.*

embryonal sarcoma. See *Wilms tumor.*

embryonic testicular regression syndrome. Synonyms: *anorchidism, familial anorchia syndrome, fetal testicular regression syndrome, chromosome XY gonadal dysgenesis, XY gonadal dysgenesis.*

A familial syndrome of bilateral or unilateral anorchia due to regression of the embryonic testis, transmitted as an X-linked trait with variable phenotypic expression. The syndrome is usually observed in 46,XY males and may be associated with mental retardation, eunuchoid body proportions, infantile type of external genitalia, low blood testosterone levels, and elevated levels of LH and FSH.

Pérez-Palacios, G., *et al.* Anorchia and persistent müllerian duct: a variant of the embryonic testicular regression syndrome. *J. Clin. Endocr.*, 1978, 47:812-7. Sarto, G. E., & Opitz, J. M. The XY gonadal dysgenesis syndrome. *J. Med. Genet.*, 1973, 10:288-93.

embryopathia alcoholica. See *fetal alcohol syndrome.*

embryopathia rubeolaris. See *congenital rubella syndrome.*

embryopathia rubeolosa. See *congenital rubella syndrome.*

EMD (Emery-Dreifuss **m**uscular **d**ystrophy). See *Emery-Dreifuss syndrome.*

EMERY, ALAN E. H. (British physician)

Dreifuss-Emery-Hogan syndrome. See *Emery-Dreifuss syndrome.*

Emery-Dreifuss muscular dystrophy (EMD). See *Emery-Dreifuss syndrome.*

Emery-Dreifuss syndrome (EDS). Synonyms: *Céstan-LeJonne syndrome, Dreifuss syndrome, Dreifuss-Emery-Hogan syndrome, Emery-Dreifuss muscular dystrophy (EMD), dystrophia musculorum retrahens, myopathia sclerosans limitans, scapulohumerodistal muscular dystrophy, tardive muscular dystrophy.*

A rare X-linked muscular dystrophy with onset in childhood and a slowly progressive course. Contractures of the elbow, ankle, and spine are the principal musculoskeletal characteristics. Muscle weakness first involves the lower limbs at the age of 4 to 5 years, causing the affected children to walk on their toes. Waddling gait, lumbar lordosis, and weakness of the shoulder girdle become apparent during adolescence. Mild pectus excavatum may be present. Cardiac complications include atrial rhythm and conduction disorders, which range fromn PR prolongation to P waves to permanent atrial paralysis and complete, frequently fatal heart block, usually before the age of 55 years.

Emery, A. E. H., & Dreifuss, F. E. Unusual type of benign X-linked muscular dystrophy. *J. Neur. Neurosurg. Psychiat.*, 1966, 29:338-42. Céstan, R., & LeJonne, N. J. Une myopathie avec rétractions familiales. *Nouv. Icon. Salpêtrière,* 1902, 15:38-52. Dreifuss, F. E., & Hogan, G. R. Survival in X-chromosomal muscular dystrophy. *Neurology,* 1961, 11:734-7.

Emery-Nelson syndrome. A syndrome of short stature; nonprogressive contractures of the digits consisting of flexion contractures of the first three metacarpophalangeal joints, extension deformitites of the interphalangeal joints of the thumb, and clawed toes; peculiar facies characterized by flat malar region, high forehead, and long philtrum; dry and coarse hair; and thin and shiny skin. The syndrome is believed to be transmitted as either an autosomal dominant or an X-linked dominant trait.

Emery, A. E. H., & Nelson, M. M. A familial syndrome of short stature, deformities of the hands and feet, and an unusual facies. *J. Med. Genet.*, 1970, 7:379-82.

EMG (**e**xophthalmos-**m**acroglossia-**g**igantism). See *Beckwith-Wiedemann syndrome.*

empty sella syndrome (ESS). A disorder characterized by incomplete or vestigial diaphragma sellae and flattening of the pituitary gland, whereby the pituitary fossa appears to be empty. The sella turcica forms an extension of the subarachnoid space and is partially or completely filled with cerebrospinal fluid; on pneumoencephalography, the space is filled with air. The presenting symptoms are nonspecific, consisting mostly of nasal cerebrospinal fluid discharge and headache. The amenorrhea-galactorrhea syndrome is frequently associated.

Busch, W. Die morphologie der Sella turcica und ihre Beziehungen zur Hypophyse. *Arch. Path. Anat.*, 1951, 320:437-40.

EN (**e**pidemic **n**ephritis). See *hemorrhagic fever with renal syndrome.*

encephalitis lethargica. See *Economo disease.*

encephalitis periaxialis concentrica. See *Baló syndrome.*

encephalitis periaxialis diffusa. See *Schilder disease.*

encephalitis subcorticalis chronica. See *Binswager disease.*

encephalo-ophthalmic syndrome. See *Krause syndrome.*

encephalocraniocutaneous lipomatosis syndrome. A rare congenital syndrome of macrocephaly, possibly associated with hydrocephalus; soft tissue tumors of the cranium and eyes, including the conjunctiva, sclera, cornea, and eyelids; focal cerebral seizures; mental retardation; unilateral porencephalic cysts communicating with the ventricular system; and cerebral hemiatrophy.

Haberland, C., & Perou. Encephalocraniocutaneous lipomatosis. *Arch. Neur.*, 1970, 22:144. Sanchez, N. P., *et al.* Encephalocraniocutaneous lipomatosis: A new neurocutaneous syndrome. *Brit. J. Dermat.*, 1981, 104:89-96.

encephalofacial angiomatosis. See *Sturge-Weber syndrome.*

encephalofacial neuroangiomatosis. See *Sturge-Weber syndrome.*

encephalomalacia subcorticalis chronica arteriosclerotica. See *Binswager disease.*

encephalomyelitis funicularis infectiosa. See *Redlich encephalitis.*

encephalomyeloradiculoneuritis. See *Guillain-Barré syndrome.*

encephalopathia spongiotica. See *Canavan syndrome.*

encephalotrigeminal angiomatosis. See *Sturge-Weber syndrome.*

encephalotrigeminal syndrome. See *Sturge-Weber syndrome.*

enchondromatosis. See *Ollier syndrome.*

enchondromatosis with hemangiomata. See *Maffucci syndrome.*

encysted rectum. See *Gross disease, under Gross, Samuel David.*

endarteritis obliterans. See *Friedländer disease.*

endemic myalgia. See *Sylvest syndrome.*

endemic paralytic vertigo. See *Gerlier disease.*

endemic polyarthritis. See *Kashin-Bek disease.*

endobrachy-esophagus. See *Barrett syndrome.*

endocardial dysplasia. See *Weinberg-Himelfarb syndrome.*

endocardial fibroelastosis (EFE). See *Weinberg-Himelfarb syndrome.*

endocarditis fibroplastica with eosinophilia. See *Löffler endocarditis.*

endocarditis parietalis fibroplastica. See *Löffler endocarditis.*

endocarditis rheumatica. See *Bouillaud disease.*

endocrine adenoma-peptic ulcer syndrome. See *multiple endocrine neoplasia I syndrome.*

endocrine candidosis syndrome. See *candidiasis-endocrinopathy syndrome.*

endocrine deficiency-hepatic cirrhosis syndrome. See *Silvestrini-Corda syndrome.*

endocrine headache. See *under headache syndrome.*

endocrine hypertensive syndrome. See *Schroeder syndrome (1).*

endolymphatic hydrops. See *Ménière syndrome.*

endometrial cyst. See *Sampson cyst.*

endomyocardial fibrosis. See *Davies disease, under Davies, J. N. P.*

endophlebitis of the thoraco-epigastric veins. See *Mondor disease (1).*

endosteal hyperostosis (recessive type). See *van Buchem syndrome, under Buchem, Francis Steven Peter, van.*
endothelial myeloma. See *Ewing sarcoma.*
endothelial sarcoma. See *Ewing sarcoma.*
endothelial-epithelial corneal dystrophy. See *Fuchs dystrophy.*
energetic-dynamic heart insufficiency. See *Hegglin syndrome.*

ENGEL
Engel syndrome. Synonyms: *laurel fever, privet cough.*
Anaphylactic edema of the lungs in association with eosinophilia and severe cough caused by pollen.
Duroux, A. Les infiltrats labiles non tuberculeux des poumons. *Sem. Hôp. Paris,* 1950, 26:4955-66.
ENGEL, GERHARD (German physician)
Engel-von Recklinghausen disease. See *Recklinghausen disease (2).*
ENGLEMANN, GUIDO (German physician, born 1876)
Camurati-Engelmann syndrome. See *under Camurati.*
Engelmann disease. See *Camurati-Engelmann syndrome.*
English disease. See *Glisson disease.*
English malady. See *Cheyne disease, under Cheyne, George.*
ENGMAN, MARTIN FEENEY (American physician, born 1869)
Engman disease. Synonym: *dermatitis infectiosa eczematoides.*
Dermatitis characterized by erythematous, crusted, scaling lesions and weeping spots. The individual lesions expand and coalesce, forming large patches with vesicles and pustules at the borders. *Staphylococcus aureus,* other staphylococci, and streptococci are the etiologic agents. Trauma, ulcers, insect bites, and irritation may be the precipitating factors.
Engman, M. F. An infectious form of an eczematoid dermatitis. *Am. Med.,* 1902, 4:769-73.
Engman syndrome. See *Zinsser-Engman-Cole syndrome.*
Zinsser-Engman-Cole syndrome. See *under Zinsser.*
ENL. See *erythema nodosum leprosum syndrome.*
ENSLIN (German ophthalmologist)
Enslin syndrome. Synonym: *Enslin triad.*
A triad of tower skull due to premature ossification of the coronal suture, adenoid hypertrophy, and exophthalmos. Associated with the triad may be greenish white discoloration of the papilla, papillary edema, peripapillary pigmentary atrophy, neuroretinitis, optic nerve atrophy, amaurosis, amblyopia, strabismus, nystagmus, hyperemia and tortuosity of the retinal veins, constriction of the retinal arteries, and mydriasis with insensitivity to light.
Enslin. Augenveränderungen bei Turmschädel, besonders die Schnervenerkrankung. *Graefes Arch. Ophth.,* 1904, 58:151-201.
Enslin triad. See *Enslin syndrome.*
enteric fever. See *Eberth disease.*
enteritis regionalis. See *Crohn disease.*
enterogenic cyanosis. See *Stokvis-Talma syndrome.*
enteroptosis. See *Glénard syndrome.*
eosinophilic cellulitis. See *Wells syndrome, under Wells, G. C.*
eosinophilic fasciitis. See *Shulman syndrome, under Shulman, L. E.*
eosinophilic infiltration with flame figures. See *Wells syndrome, under Wells, G. C.*
eosinophilic lung. See *pulmonary infiltration with eosinophilia syndrome.*
eosinophilic lymphofolliculosis of the skin. See *Kimura disease.*
eosinophilic myocarditis. See *Fiedler myocarditis.*
eosinophilic myositis. See *Shulman syndrome, under Shulman, L. E.*
eosinophilic pneumonia. See *pulmonary infiltration with eosinophilia syndrome.*
eosinophilic pneumonitis. See *pulmonary infiltration with eosinophilia syndrome.*
eosinophilic pneumopathy. See *pulmonary infiltration with eosinophilia syndrome.*
eosinophilic pulmonary infiltrate. See *pulmonary infiltration with eosinophilia syndrome.*
eosinophilic pulmonary syndrome. See *pulmonary infiltration with eosinophilia syndrome.*
eosinophilic pustular folliculitis. See *Ofuji syndrome.*
eosinophilic pustulosis. See *Ofuji syndrome.*
eosinophilic-monocytic fever. See *Frugoni disease.*
epidemic erythema. See *acrodynia.*
epidemic exfoliative dermatitis. See *Savill disease.*
epidemic hemorrhagic fever (EHF). See *hemorrhagic fever with renal syndrome.*
epidemic hepatitis. See *Botkin disease.*
epidemic jaundice. See *Botkin disease.*
epidemic keratoconjunctivitis. See *Fuchs syndrome (2).*
epidemic louse-borne typhus. See *Hildenbrand disease.*
epidemic mesonephritis. See *hemorrhagic fever with renal syndrome.*
epidemic myalgia. See *Sylvest syndrome.*
epidemic nephritis (EN). See *hemorrhagic fever with renal syndrome.*
epidemic nephrosonephritis. See *hemorrhagic fever with renal syndrome.*
epidemic neurolabyrinthitis. See *Pedersen syndrome.*
epidemic pleurodynia. See *Sylvest syndrome.*
epidemic spirochetal jaundice. See *leptospirosis.*
epidemic superficial keratitis. See *Fuchs syndrome (2).*
epidemic toxic syndrome. See *toxic oil syndrome.*
epidemic vertigo. See *Pedersen syndrome.*
epidemic vomiting. See *Spencer disease.*
epidermal nevus syndrome. Synonyms: *Feuerstein-Mims syndrome, Schimmelpenning-Feuerstein-Mims syndrome, Solomon syndrome, Solomon-Fretzin-Dewald syndrome, linear nevus sebaceous syndrome, linear sebaceous nevus syndrome, linear verrucous epidermal nevus, nevus sebaceous of Feuerstein and Mims, nevus sebaceous linearis, skin-eye-brain syndrome.*
A congenital syndrome of anomalies affecting multiple body systems, especially the skin, skeleton, eyes, and central nervous system. The nevi are generally present at birth and subsequently undergo pigmentary and verrucous changes, having special predilection for the face and scalp. Focal epilepsy, defects of the the aorta, lesions of the ribs, cleft palate, and ocular lesions, including coloboma of the iris and retina and lipodermoids of the conjunctiva and cornea, may be associated. Additional disorders may include hemimacrocephaly, mental retardation, hypophosphatemic rickets, and osteomalacia.
Feuerstein, R. C., & Mims, L. C. Linear nevus sebaceus with convulsions and mental retardation. *Am. J. Dis. Child.,* 1962, 104:675-9. Solomon, L. L., Fretzin, D. F., &

Dewald, R. L. The epidermal nevus syndrome. *Arch. Derm., Chicago*, 1968, 97:273-85. Schimmelpenning, G. W. Klinischer Beitrag zur Symptomatologie der Phakomatosen. *Fortschr. Röntgen.*, 1957, 87:716-20.

epidermodysplasia verruciformis. See *Lewandowski-Lutz syndrome.*

epidermoid cyst. See *Middeldorpf tumor.*

epidermolysis acuta toxica. See *toxic epidermal necrolysis.*

epidermolysis bullosa (EB) syndrome. Synonyms: *Bart syndrome, Cockayne-Touraine syndrome, Fox disease, Goldscheider disease, Herlitz syndrome, Köbner syndrome, Weber-Cockayne syndrome, acanthokeratolysis, acantholysis bullosa, acanthosis bullosa, bullous recurrent eruption, dermatitis bullosa hereditaria, epidermolysis dystrophica, epidermolysis hereditaria tarda, keratolysis bullosa congenita, pemphigus hereditarius.*

A hereditary skin disease characterized by bullous and vesicular eruptions precipitated by minor trauma or heat, with some types arising spontaneously. Several types are recognized: **Epidermolysis bullosa simplex** occurs at the time when the infant begins to crawl, and involves sites of friction on the feet, hands, and neck, rarely the ankles, knees, trunk, and elbows. The condition usually improves after puberty and there are no residual scars. This type is transmitted as an autosomal dominant trait. Most classifications separate the generalized type (**Köbner syndrome**) from the type in which only the hands and feet are involved (**Weber-Cockayne syndrome**). **Dominant dystrophic (hypertrophic) epidermolysis bullosa (Cockayne-Touraine syndrome**) is characterized by flat, pink, scarring bullae of the ankles, knees, hands, elbows, and feet, sometimes associated with milia. Nail dystrophy and hyperhidrosis are present in most cases. The lesions appear early in infancy and some improvement occurs with age. **Recessive dystrophic epidermolysis bullosa** is marked by bullae erupting shortly after birth at sites of pressure or trauma or appearing spontaneously. Ruptured bullae peel off, exposing raw painful surfaces, which may become infected, leaving keloid scars and causing contractures, growth disorders, dwarfism, and clawhand. The Nikolsky sign is often present. Associated disorders may include nail dystrophy, hyperhidrosis of the palms and soles, hypotrichosis, blepharitis, symblepharon, conjunctivitis, corneal opacity, hoarseness, dysphagia, esophageal stenosis, mental retardation, and clawlike fingers. **Epidermolysis bullosa lethalis (Herlitz syndrome)** is characterized by neonatal onset and death within the first 3 months of life. Vesicles, usually hemorrhaging, appear at the base of the fingernails soon after birth, causing the nails to shed. The trunk, umbilicus, face, and scalp are involved shortly after. This type is transmitted as an autosomal recessive trait.

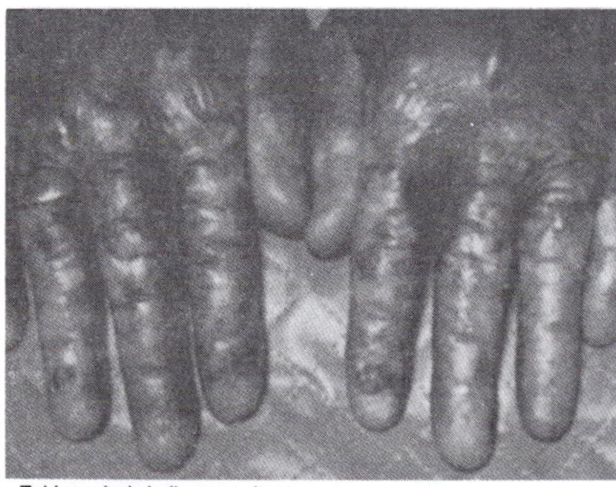

Epidermolysis bullosa syndrome
Pillsbury, D.M., W.B. Shelley, & A.M. Kilgman, *Dermatology*. Philadelphia: W.B. Saunders Co., 1956.

Cockayne, E. A. Recurrent bullous eruption of the feet. *Brit. J. Derm. Syph.*, 1938, 50:358-62. Fox, W. T. Notes on unusual or rare forms of skin diseases. IV. Congenital ulceration of the skin (two cases) with pemphigus eruption and arrest of development generally. *Lancet*, 1879, 1:766-7. Goldscheider, A. Hereditäre Neigung zu Blasenbildung. *Mhfte Prakt. Derm.*, 1882,1:163-74. Köbner, H. Hereditäre Anlage zur Blasenbildung (Epidermolysis bullosa hereditaria). *Deut. Med. Wschr.*, 1886, 2:21-2. Bart, B. Epidermolysis bullosa with congenital localized absence of skin. *Arch. Derm., Chicago*, 1970, 101:78-81. Touraine, A. *L'hérédité en medicine*. Paris, Masson, 1955. Weber, F. P. Recurrent bullous eruptions of the feet in a child. *Proc. R. Soc. Med., London*, 1926, 19:72. Herlitz, L. G. Kongenitaler, nichtsyphilitischer Pemphigus. *Acta Paediat.*, 1937, 17:315-71.

epidermolysis bullosa dystrophica. See *Hallopeau-Siemens syndrome.*

epidermolysis bullosa dystrophica Hallopeau-Siemens (EBDH). See *Hallopeau-Siemens syndrome.*

epidermolysis bullosa hereditaria dystrophica polydysplastica. See *Hallopeau-Siemens syndrome.*

epidermolysis bullosa polydysplastica. See *Hallopeau-Siemens syndrome.*

epidermolysis combustiformis. See *toxic epidermal necrolysis.*

epidermolysis dystrophica. See *epidermolysis bullosa syndrome.*

epidermolysis hereditaria tarda. See *epidermolysis bullosa syndrome.*

epidermolysis necroticans combustiformis. See *toxic epidermal necrolysis.*

epidermolysis toxica. See *toxic epidermal necrolysis.*

epidermotropic cutaneous reticulosis. See *Woringer-Kolopp syndrome, under Woringer, Frederic.*

epidural ascending spinal paralysis. See *Spiller syndrome.*

epilepsia partialis continua. See *Kozhevnikov syndrome.*

epilepsia partialis continua corticalis. See *Kozhevnikov syndrome.*

epilepsy-dementia-amelogenesis imperfecta syndrome. See *amelocerebrohypohidrosis syndrome.*

epilepsy-mental deterioration-amelogenesis imperfecta syndrome. See *amelocerebrohypohidrosis syndrome.*

epilepsy-telangiectasia syndrome. A familial syndrome, transmitted as an autosomal recessive trait, characterized by mental retardation, epilepsy, palpebral conjunctival telangiectasia, peculiar facies (low hairline on the forehead, anteverted nostrils, long philtrum, irregularly implanted teeth, small chin, and large ears), short fifth finger, and diminished serum immunoglobulin A (IgA) levels.

Aguilar, L., *et al.* A new syndrome characterized by mental retardation, epilepsy, palpebral conjunctival telangiectasias and IgA deficiency. *Clin. Genet.*, 1978, 13:154-8.

epilepsy-yellow teeth syndrome. See *amelocerebrohypohidrosis syndrome.*

epileptiform neuralgia. See *trigeminal neuralgia.*

epiphrenal syndrome. See *Bergmann syndrome.*

epiphyseal acrodysplasia. See *Thiemann syndrome.*

epiphyseal dysplasia. See *multiple epiphyseal dysplasia I.*

epiphyseal necrosis of the capitellum humeri. See *Panner disease (2).*

epiphyseal osteochondromatosis. See *Trevor syndrome.*

epiphyseal syndrome. See *Pellizzi syndrome.*

epiphysitis calcanei. See *Blencke syndrome.*

epiphysitis of the tibial tuberosity. See *Osgood-Schlatter syndrome.*

epiploia. See *Bourneville-Pringle syndrome.*

episcleritis metastatica furunculiformis. See *Kramer disease.*

epithelial and endothelial dystrophy of the cornea. See *Fuchs dystrophy.*

epithelial cell disease. See *Munk disease.*

epithelial erosion syndrome. See *Franceschetti dystrophy.*

epithelial punctate keratitis. See *Koeppe disease (1).*

epithelioid cell nevus. See *Spitz nevus.*

epithelioma adenoides cysticum (EAC). See *Brooke epithelioma.*

epithelioma basocellulare. See *Krompecher tumor.*

epithelioma calcificans. See *Malherbe epithelioma.*

epithelioma contagiosum. See *Bateman syndrome (1).*

epithelioma pagetoide. See *Arning carcinoid.*

EPPINGER, HANS (Austrian physician, 1879-1946)

Cauchois-Eppinger-Frugoni syndrome. See *Frugoni syndrome.*

EPS (**e**lastosis **p**erforans **s**erpiginosa). See *Lutz-Miescher syndrome, under Lutz, Wilhelm.*

EPSTEIN, ALBERT ARTHUR (American physician, born 1880)

Epstein syndrome. See *nephrotic syndrome.*

EPSTEIN, ALOIS (pediatrician in Prague, 1849-1918)

Epstein syndrome. Synonym: *pseudodiphtheria.*

The development of pseudomembranes on the soft palate in children. See also *Bretonneau disease (diphtheria).*

*Epstein, A. Über septische Erkrankungen der Schleimhäute bei Kindern. *Prag. Med. Wschr.*, 1879, 4:329-133; 341-4.

EPSTEIN, C. J. (Amearican physician)

Epstein syndrome. See *Epstein triad.*

Epstein triad. Synonyms: *Epstein syndrome, hereditary macrothrombocytopathia-deafness-nephritis syndrome.*

A syndrome transmitted as an autosomal dominant trait, an X-linked trait, or a new mutation, consisting of macrothrombocytopenia, progressive sensorineural hearing loss, and nephritis. The symptoms include macrocytothrombocytopathic thrombocytopenia, bleeding tendency, and renal dysfunction. Blood tests show giant platelets with defective aggregation and adenine nucleotide release, impaired platelet factor-3, and ultrastructural abnormalities in both platelets and megakaryocytes.

Epstein, C. J., *et al.* Hereditary macrothrombocytopenia, nephritis and deafness. *Am. J. Med.*, 1972, 52:299-310.

EPSTEIN, E. (German physician)

Epstein syndrome. See *Mortensen syndrome.*

Epstein-Goedel syndrome. See *Mortensen disease.*

EPSTEIN, EMIL (Austrian biochemist)

van Bogaert-Scherer-Epstein syndrome. See *under van Bogaert.*

epulis congenita. See *Neumann syndrome, under Neumann, Ernst.*

epulis of the newborn. See *Abrikossov tumor, and see Neumann syndrome, under Neumann, Ernst.*

ERASMUS, L. D. (South African physician)

Erasmus syndrome. Synonym: *scleroderma-silicosis syndrome.*

Scleroderma associated with silicosis. Cytoxic effects of silicon dioxide and autoimmune mechanisms are the suspected etiologic factors.

Erasmus, L. D. Scleroderma in gold-miners on the Witwatersrand with particular reference to pulmonary manifestations. *So. Afr. J. Lab. Clin. Med.*, 1957, 3:209-31.

ERB, WERNER (German physician)

Rotter-Erb syndrome. See *under Rotter.*

ERB, WILHELM HEINRICH (German physician, 1840-1921)

Duchenne-Erb paralysis. See *Duchenne-Erb syndrome.*

Duchenne-Erb syndrome. See *under Duchenne de Boulogne.*

Erb disease. See *Erb-Charcot syndrome.*

Erb dystrophy. See *Erb syndrome (1).*

Erb palsy. See *Duchenne-Erb syndrome.*

Erb paralysis. See *Erb-Charcot syndrome.*

Erb syndrome (1). Synonyms: *Erb dystrophy, dystrophia musculorum progressiva, juvenile muscular dystrophy, limb-girdle dystrophy.*

A slowly progressive form of muscular dystrophy usually occurring in adolescence or early adulthood. The muscles of the thoracic girdle are the the first ones to be affected with resultant difficulty in raising the hands above the the head. The deltoid and erector spinae muscles become involved later, and eventually the muscles of the trunk, pelvic girdle, and thighs also become affected.

Erb, W. Über die "juvenile Form" der progressiven Muskelatrophie, ihre Beziehungen zur sogenannten Pseudohypertrophie der Muskeln. *Deut. Arch. Klin. Med.*, 1884, 34:467-519.

Erb syndrome (2). See *Erb-Goldflam syndrome.*

Erb-Charcot syndrome. Synonyms: *Erb disease, Erb paralysis, Strümpell disease, amyotrophic syphilitic myelitis, spastic paraplegia, spastic spinal paralysis, spastic tabes dorsalis, syphilitic poliomyelitis, vascular syphilis of the spinal cord.*

Spinal syphilis with paresthesia, spastic weakness, tiredness of the legs associated with pain, sphincter disorders, exaggerated deep reflexes, muscle atrophy, sensory disorders, and paraplegia. Several forms are known: meningomyelitis with involvement of the leptomeninges and nerve roots of the spinal cord, pachymeningitis with thickening of the dura mater, and the vascular form (**Erb syndrome**) in which endarteritis of the spinal cord results in slow degeneration of the lateral columns.

Charcot, M. Du tabes dorsal spasmodique. *Progr. Méd., Paris*, 4:737-8; 773-5; 793-5. Erb, W. H. Über die spastische Spinalparalyse (Tabes dorsalis spasmodique, Charcot). *Arch. Path. Anat., Berlin*, 1877, 70:241-67; 293-328. *Strümpell, A., von. Über eine bestimmte Form der primären kombinierten Systemerkrankungen des Rückenmarks. *Arch. Psychiat., Berlin*, 1868, 17:217.

Erb-Goldflam disease. See *Erb-Goldflam syndrome.*

Erb-Goldflam syndrome. Synonyms: *Erb syndrome, Erb-Goldflam disease, Erb-Oppenheim-Goldflam syndrome, Hoppe-Goldflam syndrome, asthenic bulbar paralysis, bulbospinal paralysis, myasthenia gravis, myasthenia gravis pseudoparalytica.*

A disorder occurring in both sexes at any age, but affecting most commonly middle-aged women. It is due to the presence of circulating antibodies to acetylcholine receptor (AChR) and faulty synaptic transmission at the myoneural junction, resulting in muscle weakness, fatigability, and paralysis. The voluntary muscles of the face, larynx, and throat are affected initially, but other muscles also become involved. Difficulty in mastication and swallowing toward the end of a meal, ptosis, diplopia, slurred speech, and weak voice after prolonged talking, inability to close the mouth, weakness of the leg muscles after a walk, dyspnea, hyperventilation, and repetitive movements are the principal symptoms. Initially, the symptoms may last for short periods, then disappear, to return a few weeks later, becoming more pronounced. Mastication and swallowing difficulty may lead to weight loss. Weakness of neck muscles occurs in advanced stages. Death usually takes place within 2 years.

Erb, W. Zur Casuistik der bulbären Lähmungen. *Arch. Psychiat., Berlin*, 1879, 9:325-50. Goldflam, S. Über einen scheinbar heilbaren bulbär-paralytischen Symptomenkomplex mit Beteiligung der Extremitäten. *Deut. Zschr. Nervenh.*, 1893, 4:312-52. Hoppe, H. H. Ein Beitrag zur Kenntniss der Bulbärparalyse. *Berlin. Klin. Wschr.*, 1892, 29:332-6.

Erb-Landouzy-Déjerine syndrome. See *Landouzy-Déjerine syndrome.*

Erb-Oppenheim-Goldflam syndrome. See *Erb-Goldflam syndrome.*

Friedreich-Erb-Arnold syndrome. See *pachydermoperiostosis syndrome.*

Gänsslen-Erb syndrome. See *Minkowski-Chauffard syndrome.*

Nievergelt-Erb syndrome. See *Nievergelt syndrome.*

ERDHEIM, JAKOB (Austrian physician, 1874-1937)

Erdheim disease. See *Gsell-Erdheim syndrome.*

Erdheim syndrome. Synonyms: *Scaglietti-Dagnini syndrome, acromegalic spondylitis, costovertebral syndrome.*

Acromegaly with bone and cartilage hypertrophy of the clavicle, vertebral bodies, and intervertebral disks, resulting in pain, kyphosis, and restricted movement.

Erdheim, J. Über Wirbersäulenveränderungen bei Akromegalie. *Virchows Arch. Path. Anat.*, 1931, 281:197-296. Scaglietti, O., & Dagnani, G. Sul quadro radiografico della alterazioni acromegaliche dei corpi vertebrali secondo Erdheim. *Radiol. Fis. Med., Bologna*, 1935, 2:251-64.

Erdheim-Chester syndrome. A rare histiocytic disorder with variable clinical manifestations which range from asymptomatic to fatal multisystem involvement. Typically, the syndrome presents a lipid (cholesterol) granulomatosis in which cholesterol-laden foam cells are the primary aggregates involving bones, kidneys, heart, and lungs.

Chester, W. Über lipogranulomatose. *Virchow Arch. Path. Anat. Physiol.*, 1930, 279:561-602. Jaffe, H. L. *Metabolic, degenerative and inflammatory diseases of bone.* Philadelphia, Lea & Febiger, 1972, pp. 535-41.

Gsell-Erdheim syndrome. See *under Gsell.*

ERIKSSON, ALDUR W. (Finnish human geneticist)

Forsius-Eriksson ocular albinism. See *Forsius-Eriksson syndrome.*

Forsius-Eriksson syndrome. See *under Forsius.*

ERLACHER, PHILIP (German physician)

Erlacher-Blount syndrome. Synonyms: *Blount syndrome, Blount-Barber syndrome, nonrachitic bowleg in children, osteochondritis deformans tibiae, osteochondrosis deformans tibiae, subepiphyseal osteochondropathy, tibia vara.*

Osteochondrosis of the medial side of the proximal tibial epiphyses resulting in abrupt angulation into varus with back-knee and internal rotation of the leg. In the infantile type, the deformity appears before the age of 8 years and is usually bilateral; otherwise there is normal development, except for some overweight. The bowing is evident as an abrupt angulation with the apex laterally, just below the knee. The changes may appear as a developmental exaggeration with sloping epiphysis and beaklike recurving metaphysis. In the adolescent type, a similar deformity may occur on one side after the age of 8 years. The familial infantile type (Blount) is transmitted as an autosomal recessive trait.

Erlacher, P. Deformierende Prozesse der Epiphysengegend bei Kindern. *Arch. Orthop., München*, 1922, 20:81-96. Blount, W. P. Tibia vara. Osteochondrosis deformans tibiae. *J. Bone Joint Surg.*, 1937, 19:1-29. Barber, C. G. Osteochondrosis deformans tibiae. Nonrachitic bow legs in children. *Am. J. Dis. Child.*, 1942, 64:831-42.

erotic delusion. See *Clérambault syndrome.*

erotomania. See *Clérambault syndrome.*

eruptive papulous dermatitis of the extremities. See *Gianotti-Crosti syndrome.*

erysipeloid. See *Rosenbach erysipeloid, under Rosenbach, Anton Julius Friedrich.*

erythema annulare centrifugum (EAC). Synonyms: *Darier disease, Darier erythema.*

Figurate erythema beginning as one or more erythematous or urticaria-like papules which enlarge in a centrifugal fashion to form arcuate, ringed, or polycyclic figures. The lesions spread to form large rings with clear central depressed areas. In time, the eruption disappears, often to be replaced by a new crop. Two subtypes are recognized: **Deep gyrate erythema** which is marked by firm indurate borders and absence of scales and pruritus, and **superficial gyrate erythema**, which is characterized by indistinct borders, scales and pruritus.

Darier, J. De l'érythème annulaire centrifuge (érythème papulo-circiné migrateuse et chronique) et de quelques éruptions analogues. *Ann. Derm. Syph., Paris*, 1916-17, 6:57-8.

erythema bullosum vegetans. See *Neumann syndrome (2), under Neumann, Isidor Elder von Heilwart.*

erythema chromicum figuratum melanodermicum. See *Cinderella dermatosis.*

erythema chronicum migrans. See *Lipschütz erythema.*

erythema dyschromicum perstans. See *Cinderella dermatosis.*

erythema elevatum diutinum. See *Bury disease.*

erythema gyratum repens. Synonym: *Gammel syndrome.*

A paraneoplastic disorder characterized by the presence of scaling erythematous lesions in association with a wide variety of internal neoplasms, including tumors of the lungs, stomach, bladder, prostate, and other organs. The lesions cover the skin, forming bizarre patterns resembling the grain in wood (cypress burl).

Gammel, J. A. Erythema gyratum repens. Skin manifestations in patient with carcinoma of breast. *Arch. Derm., Chicago,* 1952, 66:494-505.

erythema induratum. See *Bazin disease.*

erythema infectiosum. See *Sticker disease.*

erythema multiforme. See *Stevens-Johnson syndrome.*

erythema multiforme exudativum. See *Stevens-Johnson syndrome.*

erythema mycoticum infantile. See *Beck-Ibrahim syndrome, under Beck, Soma Cornelius.*

erythema nodosum syndrome. A nonspecific cutaneous hypersensitivity reaction to a variety of antigens, consisting of inflammatory, spontaneously regressing nodular lesions over the extensor surfaces of the lower extremities. The condition may be associated with a wide range of diseases, including sarcoidosis, streptococcal and other bacterial infections, fungal infections, viral and chlamydial infections, reaction to some drugs (sulfonamides, oral contraceptives, bromides), ulcerative colitis, Crohn disease, lymphoma, leukemia, radiation therapy, and Behçet syndrome. When associated with arthritis, the condition is a component of the arthritis-dermatitis syndrome.

Willan, R. *On cutaneous diseases.* London, Johnson, 1798. Bondi, E. E., & Lazarus, G. S. Panniculitis. In: Fitzpatrick,T. B., Eisen, A. Z., Woff, K., Freedberg, I. M., & Austen, K. F., eds. *Dermatology in general medicine.* 3rd ed. New York, McGraw-Hill, 1987, pp. 1131-48.

erythema nodosum leprosum (ENL) syndrome. Erythema nodosum occurring in patients with lepromatous leprosy in association with fever, arthralgia, neuritic pain, iritis, orchitis, hepatosplenomegaly, lymphadenopathy, hematuria, and proteinuria. Sulfone therapy, infection, physical or mental stress, and reaction to extreme climatic conditions are the principal precipitating factors.

Dutta, R. K. Clofazimine and dapsone; a combination therapy in erythema nodosum leprosum syndrome. *Lepr. India,* 1980, 52:252-9.

erythema nodosum syphiliticum. See *Mauriac syndrome, under Mauriac, Charles Marie Tamarelle.*

erythema palmaris hereditaria. See *Lane disease, under Lane, John Edward.*

erythema palmoplantare. See *Lane disease, under Lane, John Edward.*

erythema perstans solare. See *Hutchinson prurigo, under Hutchinson, Sir Jonathan.*

erythematoid benign epithelioma. See *Arning carcinoid.*

erythredema polyneuropathy. See *acrodynia.*

erythremia. See *Vaquez-Osler syndrome.*

erythremic myelosis. See *Di Guglielmo disease (1).*

erythroblastic anemia. See *Cooley anemia.*

erythroblastophthisis. See *Diamond-Blackfan syndrome.*

erythrocyte hypoplasia. See *Diamond-Blackfan syndrome.*

erythrocyte sensitization syndrome. See *auto-erythrocyte sensitization syndrome.*

erythrocytosis megalosplenica. See *Vaquez-Osler syndrome.*

erythroderma congenitum symmetricum progressiva. See *Mendes Da Costa syndrome.*

erythroderma ichthyosiforme congenitum-trichorhexis nodosa syndrome. See *Netherton syndrome.*

erythroderma-macrocytic anemia syndrome. See *Stryker-Halbeisen syndrome.*

erythrodermia bullosa with epidermolysis. See *toxic epidermal necrolysis.*

erythrodermia desquamativa in infants. See *Leiner dermatitis.*

erythrogenesis imperfecta. See *Diamond-Blackfan syndrome.*

erythrokeratodermia figurata variabilis. See *Mendes Da Costa syndrome.*

erythrokeratodermia variabilis (EKV). See *Mendes Da Costa syndrome.*

erythroleukemia. See *Di Guglielmo disease (1).*

erythromelalgia. See *Mitchell syndrome (1).*

erythromelalgia of the head. See *Horton neuralgia.*

erythromelia. See *Herxheimer disease.*

erythrophthisis. See *Diamond-Blackfan syndrome.*

erythroplakia. See *Queyrat erythroplasia.*

erythropoietic uroporphyria. See *congenital erythropoietic porphyria.*

erythroprosalgia. See *Horton neuralgia.*

erythrose péribuccale pigmentaire. See *Brocq disease (3).*

erythrosis pigmentata faciei. See *Brocq disease (3).*

erythrothermia. See *Mitchell syndrome (1).*

ESCALANTE, J. A. (Brazilian scientist)

Escalante syndrome. See *chromosome X fragility.*

ESCAMILLA, ROBERTO FRANCISCO (Mexican-born American physician, born 1905)

Escamilla-Lisser syndrome. Synonyms: *Escamilla-Lisser-Shepardson syndrome, internal myxedema.*

Hypothyroidism in adults, associated with ascites, anemia, menorrhagia, carotinemia, and atony of the heart, intestine, and bladder.

Escamilla, R. F., Lisser, H., & Shepardson, H. C. Internal myxedema: Report of a case showing ascites, cardiac, intestinal and bladder atony, menorrhagia, secondary anemia, and associated carotinemia. *Ann. Int. Med.,* 1935, 9:297-316.

Escamilla-Lisser-Shepardson syndrome. See *Escamilla-Lisser syndrome.*

ESCAT, ETIENNE (French physician, 1865-1948)

Escat phlegmon. A juxtatonsillar, odontogenic, periosteal abscess, described by Escat in 1908.

Kolf, J., & & Duc, P. A propos de phlegmons d'Escat. *Actual. Odontostomat., Paris,* 1967, 21:483-91.

ESCOBAR, VICTOR (American physician)

Escobar syndrome. See *multiple pterygium syndrome.*

ESPILDORA-LUQUE, CRISTOBAL (Chilean ophthalmologist)

Espildora-Luque syndrome. Synonyms: *amaurosis-hemiplegia syndrome, ophthalmic-sylvian syndrome.*

Blindness in one eye associated with contralateral hemiplegia due to an embolism of the ophthalmic artery, causing reflex spasm of the sylvian artery on the same side.

Espildora-Luque, C. Sindrome oftalmico-silviano (ceguera monocular hemiplejia alterna). *Arch. Oft. Hisp. Amer.,* 1934, 34:616-21.

ESS. See *empty sella syndrome.*
essential athrombopenic purpura. See *Schönlein-Henoch purpura.*
essential benign granulocytopenia. See *Vahlquist-Gasser syndrome.*
essential brown induration of the lung. See *Ceelen-Gellerstedt syndrome.*
essential familial hypercholesterolemia. See *Harbitz-Müller disease.*
essential familial hypercholesterolemic xanthomatosis. See *Harbitz-Müller disease.*
essential familial hyperlipemia. See *Bürger-Grütz syndrome.*
essential gangrene of the scrotum. See *Fournier disease.*
essential granulomatous macrocheilitis. See *Melkersson-Rosenthal syndrome.*
essential hemorrhagic thrombocythemia. See *Mortensen disease.*
essential hypochromic anemia. See *Faber syndrome.*
essential hypoproteinemia. See *protein-losing gastroenteropathy.*
essential lipoid histiocytosis. See *Niemann-Pick syndrome.*
essential lymphocytophthisis. See *severe mixed immunodeficiency syndrome.*
essential multifocal osteolysis. See *carpo-tarsal osteolysis syndrome (dominant and sporadic forms).*
essential paroxysmal tachycardia. See *Bouveret syndrome (2).*
essential pulmonary hemosiderosis. See *Ceelen-Gellerstedt syndrome.*
essential thrombocythemia. See *Mortensen disease.*
essential thrombocytopenia. See *Werlhof disease.*
essential thrombophilia. See *Nygaard-Brown syndrome.*
ESTERLY, N. B. (American physician)
Esterly-McKusick syndrome. See *stiff skin syndrome.*
ESTREN, SOLOMON (American physician, born 1918)
Estren-Dameshek syndrome. A familial form of hypoplastic anemia, transmitted as an autosomal recessive trait, characterized by pancytopenia, pallor, weakness, and a bleeding tendency.

Estren, S., & Dameshek, W. Familial hypoplastic anemia of childhood. Report of 8 cases in two families with beneficial effect of splenectomy in one case. *Am. J. Dis. Child.,* 1947, 73:671-87.

état marbré. See *Vogt syndrome, under Vogt, Cécille.*
ethanol abstinence syndrome. See *under withdrawal syndrome.*
etiocholanone fever. See *Reimann periodic disease.*
EULENBURG, ALBERT (German physician, 1840-1917)
Eulenburg disease. Synonyms: *congenital paramyotonia, myotonia congenita intermittens, paramyotonia congenita.*

A hereditary disease, transmitted as an autosomal dominant trait. The symptoms, present from infancy and precipitated by exposure to cold, consist of myotonia of the pharyngeal, orofacial, and distal muscles. Facial grimacing, closing of the eyelids, and clenching of the hands may be produced by brief cold exposures; longer exposures result in severe flaccid weakness of the extremities with abolition of deep reflexes.

*Eulenburg, A. Über eine familiäre, durch 6 Generationen verfolgbare Form kongenitaler Paramyotonie. *Zbl. Neur.,* 1886, 5:265.

eumycoma. See *under Ballingall disease.*
European blastomycosis. See *Busse-Buschke disease.*
eusplenic heart disease. See *asplenia syndrome.*
euthyroid hyperthyroxinemia. See *high T_4 syndrome.*
euthyroid sick syndrome. See *low T_3 syndrome.*
EVANS, ROBERT SHERMAN (American physician, born 1912)
Evans syndrome. Synonyms: *Fisher-Evans syndrome, acquired hemolytic anemia-thrombocytopenia syndrome, autoimmune hemolytic anemia-thrombocytopenic purpura syndrome, autoimmune thrombocytopenia-autoimmune hemolytic anemia syndrome, Coombs-positive hemolytic anemia-immune thrombocytopenia syndrome, thrombocytopenic purpura-acquired hemolytic anemia syndrome.*

The association of autoimmune thrombocytopenia and warm antibody autoimmune hemolytic anemia in Coombs positive patients.

Evans, R. S., *et al.* Primary thrombocytopenic purpura and hemolytic anemia. Evidence for a common etiology. *Arch. Int. Med., Chicago,* 1951, 87:48-65. Fisher, J. A. The cryptogenic acquired haemolytic anaemias. *Quart. J. Med.,* 1947, 16:245-62.

Fisher-Evans syndrome. See *Evans syndrome.*

EVANS, WILLIAM (British physician, born 1895)
Evans disease. Synonym: *familial cardiomegaly.*

A familial form of heart enlargement characterized by an irregular pulse resulting from extrasystole, paroxysmal tachycardia, atrial fibrillation, or the Morgagni-Adams-Stokes syndrome. The heart sounds are normally clear, and there is either splitting of the second sound or triple heart rhythm from the addition of the third heart sound. The ECG shows exceptionally wide QRS complexes and inverted T waves. Pathological examination shows fibrosis associated with hypertrophy of the remaining fibers of the myocardium, and glycogen may be present. Intracardiac thrombosis is common. Death may occur suddenly.

Evans, W. Familial cardiomegaly. *Brit. Heart J.,* 1949, 11:68-82.

Evans and Lloyd-Thomas syndrome. Synonym: *suspended heart syndrome.*

A peculiar radiological picture of the heart in the presence of chest pain and depressed S-T segment in the ECG. In the anterior view, the heart appears normal but, during inspiration, the left cardiophrenic junction moves toward the middle and the angle narrows correspondingly; on the right side, the cleavage between the right atrium and the diaphragm uncovers the inferior vena cava. In the right oblique view, the heart and the diaphragm separate during inspiration and bring the inferior vena cava into view as it crosses the gap. In the left oblique view, the heart is lifted during inspiration above the depressed diaphragmatic platform, to which it appears to be anchored centrally by the inferior vena cava.

Evans, W., & Lloyd-Thomas, H. G. The syndrome of suspended heart. *Brit. Heart J.,* 1957, 19:159-63.

EVC. See *Ellis-van Creveld syndrome.*
evolutive tubular nephropathy. See *Lightwood-Albright syndrome.*
EWING, JAMES (American pathologist, 1866-1943)
Ewing angioendothelioma. See *Ewing sarcoma.*
Ewing endothelial sarcoma. See *Ewing sarcoma.*
Ewing sarcoma. Synonyms: *Ewing angioendothelioma, Ewing endothelial sarcoma, Ewing tumor, endothelial*

myeloma, endothelial sarcoma, omoblastoma, round-cell sarcoma.

A primary malignant tumor of bone, usually with a poor prognosis never exhibiting osteoblastic properties, affecting children, adolescents, and young adults. It is composed of compact, uniform cells with large, round, or ovoid nuclei containing scattered chromatin. Mitotic changes are common; small vascular channels may be present. Long bones are the most common site; the skull, clavicle, ribs, and shoulder and pelvic girdles may be involved. The jaws are frequently affected, with pain, swelling, facial neuralgia, and lip paresthesia being the early symptoms. A low-grade fever and high white blood may be present.

Ewing, J. Further report on endothelial endothelioma of bone. *Proc. N. Y. Path. Soc.*, 1924, 24:93-101.

Ewing tumor. See *Ewing sarcoma.*

exanthema subitum. See *Zahorsky syndrome (1).*

excitable colon syndrome. See *irritable bowel syndrome.*

excited skin syndrome (ESS). Synonyms: *angry back syndrome, conditioned hyperirritability and para-allergy, crazy back, metallergic and parallergic reactions, rogue positive reactions, skin fatigue, spillover, status eczematicus.*

Skin hyperirritability induced by a concomitant allergic dermatitis on any part of the body, which is responsible for nonreproducible false-positive test and results in battery patch testing for allergic contact dermatitis.

Zambusch, L., von. Über die behandlung des Ekzems. *Münch. Med. Wschr.*, 1921, 68:40l. Mitchell, J. C. The angry back syndrome: Eczema creates eczema. *Contact Dermatitis*, 1975, 1:193-4.

excluded loop syndrome. See *blind loop syndrome.*

exercise ischemia. See *compartment syndrome.*

exercise myopathy. See *compartment syndrome.*

exercise-induced anaphylaxis syndrome. A syndrome occuring after exercise or some forms of athletic activities, characterized by potentially life-threatening symptoms similar to anaphylactic reactions. Prodromal manifestations include nausea, pruritus, fatigue, feeling of warmth, erythema, angioedema, urticaria, flushing, and vertigo, which are followed by gastrointestinal disorders, choking, wheezing, headache, rhinitis, respiratory distress, and collapse.

Sheffer, A. L., & Austen, K. F. Exercise-induced anaphylaxis. *J. Allergy Clin. Immunol.*, 1980, 66:106-11.

exertional headache. See *under headache syndrome.*

exfoliative acute catarrhal conjunctivitis. See *Widmark conjunctivitis.*

exfoliative dermatitis. See *Wilson disease (1), under Wilson, Sir William Erasmus.*

exfoliative dermatitis of the newborn. See *staphylococcal scalded skin syndrome.*

exhaustion death. See *Bell mania, under Bell, Luther Vos.*

exhaustion syndrome. See *Bell mania, under Bell, Luther Vos.*

exophthalmia normometabolica hereditaria. See *Sforzini syndrome.*

exophthalmic goiter. See *Basedow disease.*

exostosis cartilaginea multiplex. See *multiple cartilaginous exostoses syndrome.*

exostosis luxurians. See *fibrodysplasia ossificans progressiva.*

exostosis multiplex cartilaginea. See *multiple cartilaginous exostoses syndrome.*

exostotic dysplasia. See *multiple cartilaginous exostoses syndrome.*

expanded and activated melanocyte syndrome. See *dysplastic nevus syndrome.*

expressive aphasia. See *Broca aphasia.*

exstrophia splanchnica. See *OEIS complex.*

exstrophy of the cloaca. See *OEIS complex.*

extensor indicis proprius syndrome. A condition manifested by dorsal wrist pain localized over the extensor indicis proprius musculotendinous junction and the tendons of the extensor digitorum communis, within the fourth dorsal compartment. The pain is caused by an extension of the bulky musculotendinous portion of the extensor indicis proprius into the rigid confines of the fourth dorsal compartment of the wrist.

Ritter, M. A., & Inglis, A. E. The extensor indicis proprius syndrome. *J. Bone Joint Surg.*, 1969, 51A:1645-8.

external chondromatosis syndrome. See *multiple cartilaginous exostoses syndrome.*

external ophthalmoplegia-retinitis pigmentosa-heart block syndrome. See *Kearns-Sayre syndrome.*

extra-articular rheumatism. See *fibrositis-fibromyalgia syndrome.*

extracortical axial aplasia. See *Pelizaeus-Merzbacher syndrome.*

extracranial headache. See *under headache syndrome.*

extragonadal seminoma. See *Dixon-Moore tumor.*

extramammary Paget disease. See *under Paget.*

extrarenal kidney syndrome. See *Nonnenbruch syndrome.*

extrarenal oliguria. See *Nonnenbruch syndrome.*

extrasacral dermal melanosis. See *Ota nevus.*

extremity osteochondrodystrophy syndrome. See *Silfverskiöld syndrome.*

extrinsic allergic alveolitis. See *Ramazzini syndrome.*

exudative and diathetic eczema. See *Besnier prurigo.*

exudative discoid and lichenoid dermatosis. See *Sulzberger-Garbe syndrome.*

exudative eczematoid. See *Besnier prurigo.*

exudative enteropathy. See *protein-losing gastroenteropathy.*

exudative retinitis. See *Coats syndrome.*

exudative retinopathy. See *Coats syndrome.*

exudative vaginitis. See *Gardner vaginitis, under Gardner, Herman L.*

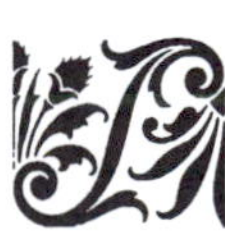

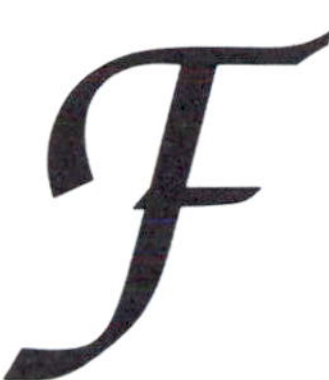

F syndrome. Synonym: *F-form of acropectorovertebral dysplasia.*

A form of skeletal dysplasia involving chiefly the hands, feet, sternum, and the lumbosacral spine. Its principal features include prominence of the sternum, with or without pectus excavatum, spina bifida occulata, carpal and tarsal synostoses, deformities of the first and second fingers frequently with syndactyly, hypoplasia and synostoses of the metatarsal bones, postaxial polydactyly of the toes, and webbing of adjacent toes. In the original report, eight persons in four generations of a kindred (of the surname F, hence the name of the syndrome) were affected. The syndrome is inherited as an autosomal dominant trait. Male-to-male transmission was noted.

Grosse, F. R., Herrmann, J., & Opitz, J. M. The F-form of acropectoro-vertebral dysplasia: The F-syndrome. *Birth Defects*, 1969, 5(3):48-63.

F-form of acro-pectoro-vertebral dysplasia. See *F syndrome.*

FA. See *Fanconi anemia.*

FA. See *Friedreich ataxia, under Friedreich, Nicolaus.*

FABER, KNUD HELGE (Danish physician, 1862-1956)

Faber anemia. See *Faber syndrome.*

Faber syndrome. Synonyms: *Faber anemia, Hayem-Faber syndrome, Kaznelson syndrome, Knud Faber syndrome, Witts anemia, achylanemia, achylia gastrica with anemia, achylic chloranemia, chronic chlorosis, chronic hypochromic anemia, chronic microcytic anemia, chronic nutritional hypochromic anemia, essential hypochromic anemia, hypochromic-achlorhydric anemia, idiopathic hypochromic anemia, idiopathic hypochronemia, late chlorosis of Hayem, simple achlorhydric acid anemia.*

Iron-deficiency anemia with a low corpuscular concentration of hemoglobin, characterized by small, pale-red erythrocytes, and associated with achlorhydria, glossalgia, koilonychia, pallor, fatigability, and premature graying of the hair. In the past, the disorder was usually observed in middle-aged women as a complication of hemorrhagic disorders; now it is relatively rare.

Faber, K. Achylia gastrica mit Anämie. *Med. Klin.*, 1909, 5:1310-12. Witts, L. J. Achlorhydria and anaemia. *Practitioner, London*, 1930, 124:348-57.

Hayem-Faber syndrome. See *Faber syndrome.*

Knud Faber syndrome. See *Faber syndrome.*

FABRE TERSOL, J. (Spanish physician)

Martorell-Fabré syndrome. See *aortic arch syndrome.*

Takayasu-Martorell-Fabré syndrome. See *aortic arch syndrome.*

FABRY, JOHANNES (German physician, 1860-1930)

Fabry disease. See *Fabry syndrome.*

Fabry syndrome. Synonyms: *Anderson syndrome, Fabry disease, Fabry-Anderson syndrome, Ruiter-Pompen syndrome, Ruiter-Pompen-Wyers syndrome, Sweeley-Klionsky disease, alpha-galactosidase A (GLA) deficiency, angiokeratoma corporis diffusum (ACD), angiokeratoma corporis diffusum universale, angioma corporis diffusum universale, cardiovasorenal syndrome, ceramide trihexosidosis, diffuse angiokeratosis, glycolipid lipidosis, hereditary dystopic lipoidosis, thesaurismosis hereditaria, thesaurismosis hereditaria lipoidica, thesaurismosis lipoidica.*

An X-linked syndrome, with complete penetrance and variable clinical expressivity in hemizygous males, caused by progressive accumulation of trihexosyl ceramide (galactosylglucosyl ceramide) in body tissues secondary to a deficiency of α-galactosidase, trihexylceramide galactosyl hydrolase. Telangiectases that do not blanch with pressure and appear in clusters of macular to papular punctate lesions (angiokeratoma corporis diffusum) are the principal cutaneous manifestations. They usually appear in childhood over the iliosacral area, scrotum, posterior thorax, thighs, buttocks, and umbilicus and progressively increase with age. Frontal bossing, mandibular prognathism, and lower macrocheilia may be associated. Ocular disorders include aneurysmal dilatation and tortuosity of conjunctival and retinal vessels and corneal opacity. Proteinuria, isothenuria, and azotemia develop later in life due to progressive renal insufficiency. Hypertension, left ventricular hypertrophy, and myocardial infarct may follow. Uremia may cause death. The oral mucosa usually shows lesions which are similar to those of the skin, except that they are smaller. Seizures, headache, dizziness and hemiplegia are the principal neurological symptoms. Attacks of burning pain of the hands and feet, nausea, vomiting, diarrhea, lymphedema of the legs, hypohidrosis, and dyspnea are common.

Fabry, J. Ein Beitrag zur Kenntnis der Purpura haemorrhagica nodularis (Purpura papulosa haemorrhagica Hebrae). *Arch. Derm. Syph., Berlin*, 1898, 43:187-200. Anderson, W. A case of "angeio-keratoma." *Brit. J. Derm.*, 1898, 10:113-7. Pompen, A., Ruiter, M., & Wyers, H. J. Angiokeratoma corporis diffusum (universale) Fabry, as a sign of an unknown internal disease; two autopsy reports. *Acta Med. Scand.*, 1947, 128:234-55. Sweeley, C. C., &

Klionsky, B. Fabry disease: Classification as a sphingolipidosis and partial characterization of a novel glycolipid. *J. Biol. Chem.*, 1963, 238:3148-50.

Fabry-Anderson syndrome. See *Fabry syndrome.*

FACES (unique **f**acies-**a**norexia-**c**achexia-**e**ye and **s**kin lesions) **syndrome.** A syndrome characterized by a unique facial appearance, a high-pitched nasal voice, severe muscle wasting, multiple lentigines, and café-au-lait spots. Principal facial features consist of anteverted nares, bifid tip of the nose, and short palate. Ocular disorders include blepharoptosis, retinitis pigmentosa, and xanthelasma. Musculoskeletal defects are syndactyly of the fingers and toes, severe generalized muscle wasting, and atrophy of the temporal and interosseous muscles. Pectus excavatum, chest asymmetry, genu varum, pes planus, and thyroid anomalies may be associated. The syndrome was originally described in a mother and two daughters of Jewish Yemenite ancestry.

Friedman, E., and Goodman, R. M. The "FACES" syndrome: A new syndrome with unique facies, anorexia, cachexia, and eye and skin lesions. *J. Craniofac. Genet. Develop. Biol.*, 1984, 4:227-31.

facial hemiatrophy. See *Romberg syndrome (2).*

facial hemihypertrophy. See *Friedreich disease (2), under Friedreich, Nicolaus.*

facial sympathalgia. See *Sluder neuralgia.*

facial trophoneurosis. See *Romberg syndrome (2).*

facial vagosympathetic algia. See *Horton neuralgia.*

facial-digital-genital syndrome. See *Aarskog syndrome.*

faciei morbus nervorum crucians. See *trigeminal neuralgia.*

facies leprosa. See *Bergen syndrome.*

facio-audio-symphalangism syndrome. Synonyms: *Herrmann syndrome, deafnesss-symphalangism syndrome, multiple synostoses-brachydactyly syndrome, symphalangism-brachydactyly syndrome, WL syndrome, WL symphalangism-brachydactyly syndrome.*

A familial camptodactyly syndrome, transmitted as an autosomal dominant trait, associated with dysplasia and synostoses of the elbow; synostoses of the fingers, wrist, and foot with short middle phalanges; craniofacial anomalies; conductive hearing loss; strabismus; and other defects. Head abnormalities consist mainly of low-set ears, broad and hemicylindrical nose, narrow upper lip, and asymmetrical mouth. Upper extremity defects include short arms, brachydactyly, clinodactyly, symphalangism of the second, third, and fourth fingers, cutaneous syndactyly, hypoplasia or aplasia of the distal phalanges, abnormal dermatoglyphics, and hypoplasia of the thenar and hypothenar muscles. Lower extremity anomalies are shortness of the legs and feet, genu valgum, pes planovalgus, a large gap between the hallux and other toes, aplastic or hypoplastic nails, and proximal symphalangism of the second, third, and fourth toes. Pectus excavatum and anterior sloping of the shoulder are usually present. See also *symphalangism syndrome.*

Herrmann, J. Symphalangism and brachydactyly syndrome: Report of the WL symphalangism-brachydactyly syndrome: Review of the literature and classification. *Birth Defects*, 1974, 10(5):23-53. Hurvitz, S. A., *et al.* The facio-audio-symphalangism syndrome: A report of a case and review of the literature. *Clin. Genet.*, 1985, 28:61-8.

facio-auriculovertebral anomalad. See *oculo-auriculovertebral dysplasia.*

faciobuccolinguomasticatory dyskinesia. See *tardive dyskinesia syndrome.*

faciocardiomelic dysplasia. Synonyms: *Cantú syndrome, lethal faciocardiomelic dysplasia.*

A lethal autosomal recessive disorder characterized by mesoacromelic dwarfism, facial dysplasia, and cardiac defects. Associated anomalies include low birth weight, microretrognathia, microstomia, microglossia, hydramnios, delayed bone age, epicanthal folds, ear abnormalities, glossoptosis, webbed neck, radial and ulnar hypoplasia, radial deviation of the hands, simian creases, thumb hypoplasia, fifth finger hypoplasia with clinodactyly, fibular and tibial hypoplasia, talipes with hypoplastic heels, and wide gap between first and second toes.

Cantú, J. M., *et al.* Lethal faciocardiomelic dysplasia-a new autosomal recessive disorder. *Birth Defects*, 1975, 11(5):91-8.

faciocardiorenal syndrome. A familial syndrome, transmitted as an autosomal recessive trait, marked by horseshoe-shaped kidneys, heart defects, mental retardation, and peculiar facies. Heart defects consist of conduction disorders, functional murmur, left ventricular filling defect, enlargement of the left ventricle, and pulmonary congestion. Poorly developed musculature, tight heel cords, limitation of motion in ankles and knees, and waddling gait are the principal neuromuscular disorders. Orofacial abnormalities include malar hypoplasia, broad nasal root, prominent antigonial notch of the mandible, poorly developed philtrum, hypoplastic vermillion border, maldeveloped alae nasi, prominent and flexible ears, plagiocephaly, cleft palate, and hypodontia. Associated disorders include cryptorchism, hypoplastic testes, unusual dermatoglyphics, decrease in muscle mass, pigmented nevi, broad toes with hypoplastic nails, finger abnormalities (clinodactyly of the thumbs, hypoplastic nails, symphalangism, joint anomalies), respiratory disorders at birth, bronchopneumonia, cyanosis, and abnormal EEG.

Eastman, J. R., & Bixler, D. Facio-cardio-renal syndrome: A newly delineated recessive disorder. *Clin. Genet.*, 1977, 11:424-30.

faciogenital dysplasia. See *Aarskog syndrome.*

faciogenitopopliteal syndrome. See *popliteal pterygium syndrome.*

facioscapulmohumeral muscular dystrophy (FSHD). See *Landouzy-Déjerine syndrome.*

factitious Bartter syndrome. See *under Bartter.*

factitious disease. See *Munchausen syndrome.*

factitious syndrome. See *Munchausen syndrome.*

factor IX deficiency. See *Christmas disease.*

factor V deficiency. See *Owren syndrome (2).*

factor X deficiency. See *Stuart-Prower factor deficiency.*

factor XI deficiency. See *Rosenthal disease, under Rosenthal, Robert Louis.*

factor XII deficiency. See *Hageman factor deficiency.*

FACWA (**f**amilial **a**myotrophic **c**horea **w**ith **a**canthocytosis) **syndrome.** A rare progressive neurological disorder that begins in midlife and is characterized by seizures, buccolingual dyskinesia, facial tics, dysarthria, choreiform movements, areflexia, muscle atrophy, and a pes cavus deformity. Laboratory findings include acanthocytosis and elevated serum creatine kinase. Degeneration of the basal ganglia and denervation atrophy of the muscles are the principal pathological features. The syndrome is familial but the mode of transmission is unknown.

Gross, K. B., *et al.* Familial amyotrophic chorea with acanthocytosis. New clinical and laboratory investigations. *Arch. Neur., Chicago,* 1985, 42:753-6.

FAD (familial Alzheimer disease). See *under Alzheimer disease.*

FAHR, THEODOR (German physician, 1877-1945)

Fahr disease. See *Fahr syndrome.*

Fahr syndrome. Synonyms: *Fahr disease, Fahr triad, bilateral symmetrical intracerebral calcification, cerebral idiopathic nonarteriosclerotic calcification, cerebral symmetric calcification, cerebrovascular familial idiopathic calcification, idiopathic familial brain calcification, idiopathic familial cerebrovascular ferrocalcinosis, symmetrical calcification of basal cerebral ganglia (SCBG).*

A rare idiopathic familial cerebrovascular disorder characterized by punctate areas of calcification, usually symmetrical calcium deposits distributed in parts of the gray and dentate nuclei with occasional involvement of the adjacent tissues. There is special predilection for the capillaries, precapillaries, and other small vessels of the deep cortical layers and the lenticular nuclei of the cerebellum, with the greatest density of deposits occurring in the basal ganglia. The symptoms include mental and growth retardation, seizures, athetosis, and dystonia. Parathyroid dysfunction and hypercalcemia are considered as the etiologic factors. The term **Fahr triad** consists of symmetrical calcificiation of the basal ganglia, neuropsychiatric symptoms, and hypofunction of the parathyroid gland.

Fahr, T. Idiopatische Verkalkung der Hirngefässe. *Zbl. Allg. Path.*, 1930-31, 50:129-33.

Fahr triad. See *under Fahr syndrome.*

failure of respiratory center automaticity. See *Ondine curse.*

FAIRBANK, SIR THOMAS (British physician)

Fairbank disease. See *Trevor syndrome.*

Fairbank syndrome (1). A syndrome characterized by short stature, short stubby hands and fingers, turribrachycephaly with supraorbital depression, exophthalmia, short legs, limited extension of the knees and elbows, lumbar lordosis, digital impressions in the calvaria, enlarged sella turcica, conical epiphyses, and cystic changes in the femoral metaphyses.

*Fairbank, T. Acrocephaly with abnormalities of the extremities. In his: *An atlas of general affections of the skeleton*. Livingstone, Edinburgh, 1951, case 84. Gorlin, R. J., Pindborg, J. J., & Cohen, M. M., Jr. *Syndromes of the head and neck*. 2nd ed., McGraw-Hill, New York, 1976, p. 232.

Fairbank syndrome (2). See *multiple epiphyseal dysplasia I.*

FALCONER, MURRAY ALEXANDER (New Zealand-born physician in England, born 1910)

Falconer-Weddell syndrome. See *costoclavicular compression syndrome.*

FALLOT, ETIENNE LOUIS ARTHUR (French physician, 1850-1911)

Fallot tetrad. See *Fallot tetralogy.*

Fallot tetralogy. Synonyms: *Fallot tetrad, blue baby, cardiac cyanosis, morbus ceruleus.*

A congenital heart defect with pulmonary stenosis, ventricular septal defect, dextroposition of the aorta, and right ventricular hypertrophy. The symptoms include cyanosis, feeding difficulty, failure to thrive, dyspnea or fatigability on exertion, squatting, polycythemia, and digital clubbing. Systolic murmur, systolic thrill, and a weak or absent pulmonic second sound are the principal cardiac signs. See also *absent pulmonary valve syndrome.*

Fallot, E. L. Contribution à l'anatomie pathologique de la maladie bleue (cyanose cardiaque). *Marseille Méd.*, 1888, 25:77-93; 138-58; 207-23; 370-86; 341-54; 403-20.

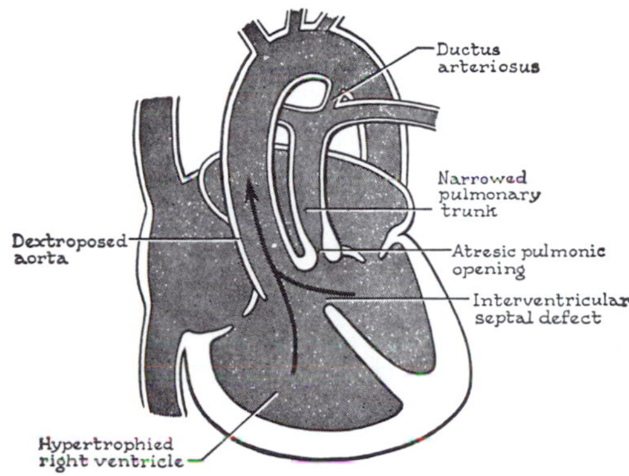

Fallot tetralogy
Robbins, S.L.: *Pathology,* 3rd ed. Philadelphia: W.B. Saunders Co., 1967.

FALLS, HAROLD FRANCIS (American physician, born 1909)

Rundles-Falls syndrome. See *under Rundles.*

false colonic obstruction. See *Ogilvie syndrome.*

false keloid. See *Alibert disease (1).*

false shift to the left. See *Pelger-Huët anomaly.*

FALTA, WILHELM (Austrian physician, 1875-1950)

Falta syndrome. Synonyms: *Gougerot syndrome, pluriglandular insufficiency syndrome.*

Polyglandular insufficiency, usually combining hypofunction of the anterior pituitary gland with myxedema and, less frequently, Addison's disease. Thyropituitary, thyrogonadal, and thyroadrenal variants may also occur.

*Falta, W. *Die Erkrankungen der Blutdrüsen.* 2nd ed. Berlin, 1928.

falx cerebri calcification syndrome. See *Chavany-Brunhes syndrome.*

familial acrogeria. See *Gottron syndrome (1).*

familial acropathia ulceromutilans. See *Thévenard syndrome.*

familial amyloid polyneuropathy. See *amyloid neuropathy type I.*

familial amyotrophic chorea with acanthocytosis. See *FACWA syndrome.*

familial anorchia syndrome. See *embryonic testicular regression syndrome.*

familial aplastic anemia with congenital defects. See *Fanconi anemia.*

familial ataxia. See *Friedreich ataxia, under Friedreich, Nicolaus.*

familial ataxia-hypogonadism syndrome. See *Richards-Rundle syndrome.*

familial atypical multiple mole melanoma (FAMMM). See *dysplastic nevus syndrome.*

familial benign chronic pemphigus. See *Hailey-Hailey disease, under Hailey, William Howard.*

familial benign hypercalcemia. See *familial hypercalcemia-hypocalciuria syndrome.*

familial benign pemphigus. See *Hailey-Hailey disease, under Hailey, William Howard.*

familial blepharophimosis. See *blepharophimosis syndrome.*

familial cardiomegaly. See *Evans disease, under Evans, William.*

familial centrolobar sclerosis. See *Pelizaeus-Merzbacher.*

familial cholemia. See *Gilbert syndrome, under Gilbert, Nicolas Augustin.*

familial cholesterolemia. See *Harbitz-Müller disease.*

familial chronic atrophic polychondritis. See *Meyenburg-Altherr-Uehlinger syndrome.*

familial chronic infantile diffuse sclerosis. See *Pelizaeus-Merzbacher syndrome.*

familial chronic pemphigus. See *Hailey-Hailey disease, under Hailey, William Howard.*

familial cirrhosis with deposition of abnormal glycogen. See *glycogen storage disease IV.*

familial claw foot with absent tendon jerks. See *Roussy-Lévy syndrome.*

familial cold urticaria syndrome. Synonym: *cold hypersensitivity syndrome.*

A familial form of urticaria, transmitted as an autosomal dominant trait, precipitated by environmental rather than local cooling, and characterized by burning urticarial wheals, chills, fever, headache, arthralgia, swelling of the joints, and amyloidosis.

Witherspoon, F. G., *et al.* Familial urticaria due to cold. *Arch. Derm. Syph., Chicago,* 1948, 58:52-5.

familial congenital alopecia-epilepsy-mental retardation-unusual EEG syndrome. See *Moynahan syndrome (2).*

familial congenital labile factor deficiency with syndactyly. See *De Vries syndrome.*

familial constitutional panmyelopathy. See *Fanconi anemia.*

familial continual skin peeling syndrome. See *continual skin peeling syndrome.*

familial cystine diathesis. See *cystinosis.*

familial degeneration of the cerebral gray matter in childhood. See *Alpers syndrome.*

familial dwarfism-stiff joints syndrome. See *Moore-Federman syndrome under Moore, W. T.*

familial dysautonomia I. See *Riley-Day syndrome, under Riley, Conrad Milton.*

familial dysautonomia II. See *Swanson syndrome.*

familial dysplastic osteopathy. See *Mankowsky syndrome.*

familial endocrine osteochondropathy. See *Lucherini-Giacobini syndrome.*

familial eosinophilia. See *Zuelzer syndrome.*

familial erythrophagocytic lymphohistiocytosis. See *Omenn syndrome.*

familial exudative vitreoretinopathy (FEVR). See *Criswick-Schepens syndrome.*

familial fibrous jaw dysplasia. See *cherubism.*

familial fibrous swelling of jaw. See *cherubism.*

familial granular dystrophy of the cornea. See *Groenouw dystrophy (1).*

familial HDL (high-density lipoprotein) deficiency. See *Tangier disease.*

familial hemolytic anemia. See *Debler anemia.*

familial hemolytic jaundice. See *Minkowski-Chauffard syndrome.*

familial hemophagocytic reticulosis. See *Omenn syndrome.*

familial hemorrhagic telangiectasia. See *Osler-Rendu-Weber syndrome.*

familial high-density lipoprotein (HDL) deficiency. See *Tangier disease.*

familial histiocytic reticulosis. See *Omenn syndrome.*

familial honeycomb choroiditis. See *Doyne choroiditis.*

familial hypercalcemia-hypocalciuria (FHH) syndrome. Synonyms: *familial benign hypercalcemia, familial hypocalciuric hypercalcemia, hypercalcemia-hypocalciuria syndrome, hypocalciuria-hypercalcemia syndrome.*

A familial metabolic syndrome of hypercalcemia and hypocalciuria, transmitted as an autosomal dominant trait. The majority of cases are asymptomatic; increased renal tubular calcium reabsorption and normal functioning of the parathyroid glands in the face of hypercalcemia being the main features.

Foley, T. P., *et al.* Familial benign hypercalcemia. *J. Pediat.,* 1972, 81:1060-7.

familial hyperchylomicronemia. See *Bürger-Grütz syndrome.*

familial hyperlipoproteinemia. See *Bürger-Grütz syndrome.*

familial hypertrichosis cubiti. See *hairy elbows syndrome.*

familial hypocalciuric hypercalcemia. See *familial hypercalcemia-hypocalciuria syndrome.*

familial hypolipidemia. See *Hooft syndrome.*

familial hypolipoproteinemia. See *Bassen-Kornzweig syndrome.*

familial hypophosphatemia. See *hypophosphatemic familial rickets.*

familial idiocy with spongy degeneration of the neuraxis. See *Canavan syndrome.*

familial infantile diffuse brain sclerosis. See *Krabbe disease.*

familial intermittent adynamia. See *Hamstorn syndrome.*

familial intrahepatic cholestasis. See *Byler disease.*

familial joint dislocation. See *under Ehlers-Danlos syndrome.*

familial joint instability syndrome. A familial syndrome, transmitted as an autosomal dominant trait with high penetrance, characterized by joint laxity frequently complicated by dislocation of major joints.

Horton, W. A., *et al.* Familial joint instability syndrome. *Am. J. Med. Genet.,* 1980, 6:221-8.

familial juvenile macular degeneration. See *Stargardt syndrome.*

familial juvenile nephrophthisis (FJN). Synonyms: *Fanconi syndrome, idiopathic parenchymatous contracted kidney, nephrophthisis.*

An autosomal recessive disease which may exist as an isolated nephropathy or in combination with involvement of other organs. The first symptoms include polydipsia, polyuria, and nycturia, which become evident at the age of 2 to 3 years. They are followed by low blood glucose and high electrolyte levels and, later, by signs of glomerular failure marked by increased urinary nitrogen and blood phosphorus. Low blood calcium levels, growth retardation, and osteodystrophy indicate parathyroid involvement. Other metabolic disorders include a low alkaline reserve and low urinary ammonia excretion. Neurological problems may include mental retardation, seizures, and cerebellar ataxia. Fever may be present. Pathological findings show progressive degeneration of the kidney parenchyma with hyaline changes in the proximal tubules and basal membranes. The collecting tubules are usually atrophied but, on occasion, they may be hypertrophied. The anterior pituitary may show eosinophilia, and adenomatous hyperplasia may be found in the parathyroid gland. The bones show fibroid degeneration with excessive production of osteoid tissue. Most affected persons die in 4 to 15 years from the onset.

Fanconi, G., *et al.* Die familiäre juvenile Nephrophthise (die idiopatische parenchymatose Schrumpfniere). *Helv. Paediat. Acta*, 1951, 6:1-49.

familial macroglossia-omphalocele syndrome. See *Beckwith-Wiedemann syndrome.*

familial Mediterranean fever (FMF). See *Reimann periodic disease.*

familial metaphyseal dysplasia. See *metaphyseal dysplasia syndrome.*

familial multilocular cystic jaw disease. See *cherubism.*

familial neurovascular dystrophy. See *Thévenard syndrome.*

familial neutropenia. See *Gänsslen disease.*

familial nonhemolytic jaundice. See *Gilbert syndrome, under Gilbert, Nicolas Augustin.*

familial nonhemolytic nonobstructive jaundice. See *Gilbert syndrome, under Gilbert, Nicolas Augustin.*

familial nonspherocytic hemolytic anemia. See *Crosby syndrome, under Crosby, William.*

familial opposable triphalangeal thumb-big toe duplication syndrome. See *triphalangeal thumb-big toe duplication syndrome.*

familial osseous dystrophy. See *mucopolysaccharidosis IV A.*

familial osteoctasia-macrocranium syndrome. See *hyperphosphatasia-osteoctasia syndrome.*

familial osteodysplasia syndrome. See *Anderson syndrome, under Anderson, L. G.*

familial osteodysplasia, Anderson type. See *Anderson syndrome, under Anderson, L. G.*

familial paroxysmal choreoathetosis. See *Mount-Reback syndrome.*

familial paroxysmal dystonic choreoathetosis. See *Mount-Reback syndrome.*

familial paroxysmal paralysis. See *Westphal syndrome, under Westphal, Karl Friedrich Otto.*

familial paroxysmal polyserositis. See *Reimann periodic disease.*

familial partial lipodystrophy. See *Köbberling-Dunnigan syndrome.*

familial perforating ulcer of the foot. See *Thévenard syndrome.*

familial polysyndactyly-craniofacial anomalies syndrome. See *Hootnick-Holmes syndrome.*

familial Portuguese polyneuritic amyloidosis. See *amyloid neuropathy type I.*

familial primary xanthomatosis with adrenal calcification. See *Wolman syndrome.*

familial progressive cerebral sclerosis. See *metachromatic leukodystrophy.*

familial progressive intrahepatic cholestasis. See *Byler disease.*

familial pterygium syndrome. See *multiple pterygium syndrome.*

familial recurrent polyserositis. See *Reimann periodic disease.*

familial reticuloendotheliosis with eosinophilia. See *Omenn syndrome.*

familial selective vitamin B_{12} malabsorption syndrome. See *Imerslund-Gräsbeck syndrome.*

familial spastic paraplegia. See *Strümpell-Lorrain disease.*

familial spherocytosis. See *Minkowski-Chauffard syndrome.*

familial spinal muscular atrophy. See *Werdnig-Hoffmann syndrome.*

familial splenic anemia. See *Gaucher disease.*

familial spongy degeneration. See *Canavan syndrome.*

familial third and fourth pharyngeal pouch syndrome. See *DiGeorge syndrome.*

familial Turner syndrome. See *Noonan syndrome.*

familial visceral amyloidosis. See *Ostertag syndrome.*

familial white folded dysplasia. See *white sponge nevus.*

family periodic paralysis. See *Westphal syndrome, under Westphal, Karl Friedrich Otto.*

FAMMM (**f**amilial **a**typical **m**ultiple **m**ole **m**elanoma). See *dysplastic nevus syndrome.*

FANCONI, A. (Swiss physician)

Fanconi-Prader syndrome. See *adrenoleukodystrophy.*

FANCONI, GUIDO (Swiss physician, 1892-1979)

De Toni-Fanconi syndrome. See *cystinosis.*

Fanconi anemia (FA). Synonyms: *Fanconi pancytopenia (FP) syndrome, Fanconi panmyelopathy, Fanconi refractory anemia, Fanconi syndrome, aplastic anemia with congenital anomalies, aplastic infantile funicular myelosis, congenital pancytopenia, congenital aplastic anemia, constitutional aplastic anemia, familial aplastic anemia with congenital defects, familial constitutional panmyelopathy, pancytopenia-dysmelia syndrome.*

A familial syndrome, originally described in three male siblings, consisting of pancytopenia, hyperpigmentation, small stature, small skull, and multiple congenital abnormalities. The pancytopenia is characterized by hypoplasia of erythropoietic, myeloid, and megakaryocytic bone marrow elements, and is usually progressive. Thumb abnormalities may include polydactyly, bifid thumb, absent or hypoplastic first metacarpal, and hypoplasia or absence of the thumb. A wide spectrum of symptoms may be associated, including mental retardation, blepharoptosis, strabismus, nystagmus, microphthalmos, auricular defects, deafness, osteoporosis, aplasia of the radius, syndactyly, hip dislocation, heart defects, hypospadias, hypogonadism, leukemia, splenic hypoplasia, kidney anomalies, and a number of other abnormalities. The syndrome is believed to be transmitted an an autosomal recessive trait.

Fanconi, G. Familiäre, infantile perniciosaähliche Anämie. (Perniziöses Blutbild und Konstitution.) *Jahrb. Kinder.*, 1927, 117:257-80.

Fanconi pancytopenia (FP) syndrome. See *Fanconi anemia.*

Fanconi panmyelopathy. See *Fanconi anemia.*

Fanconi refractory anemia. See *Fanconi anemia.*

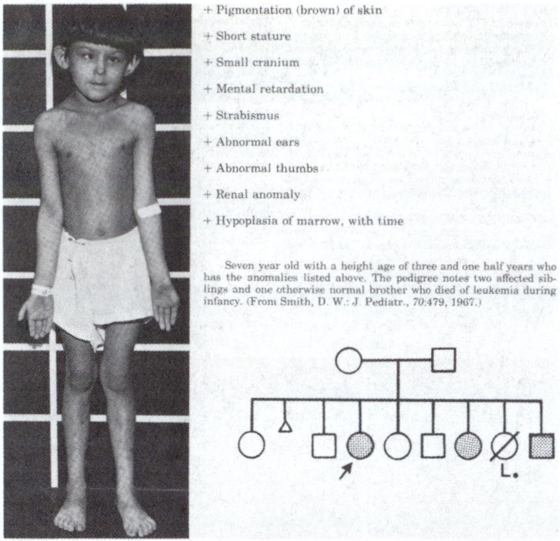

Fanconi anemia
Smith, D.W.: *J. Pediatr.*, 70:479, 1967. St. Louis: C.V. Mosby Co.

Fanconi syndrome (FS) (1). See *familial juvenile nephrophthisis.*

Fanconi syndrome (FS) (2). See *cystinosis.*

Fanconi syndrome (FS) (3). See *Andersen triad.*

Fanconi syndrome (FS) (4). See *Fanconi anemia.*

Fanconi-Albertini-Zellweger syndrome. Synonym: *osteopathia acidotica pseudorachitica.*

A syndrome of congenital heart defect, pachycephalia, calcification of the falx cerebri, peculiar facies, microdontia, albuminuria, leukocytosis and casts in the urine, metabolic acidosis, osteoporosis with spontaneous fractures, curving of the long bones, anemia, cerebrospinal fluid changes, and growth retardation.

Fanconi, G., Albertini, A., & Zellweger, H. Osteopathia acidotica pseudorachitica. *Helv. Paediat. Acta,* 1948, 2:95-112.

Fanconi-De Toni-Debré syndrome. See *cystinosis.*

Fanconi-Hegglin syndrome. Synonyms: *seropositive nonsyphilitic pneumopathy, Wassermann-positive pneumonia, Wassermann-positive pulmonary infiltration.*

Pneumonia with perihilar infiltrations and a positive Wassermann reaction in nonsyphilitic patients.

Fanconi, G. Die pseudoluetische, subakute hilifugale Bronchopneumonie des heruntergekommenen Kindes. *Schweiz. Med. Wschr.,* 1936, 66:821-6. Hegglin, R. Das Wassermann-positive Lungeninfiltrat. *Helv. Med. Acta,* 1940-4l, 7:497-527.

Fanconi-Schlesinger syndrome. See *Williams syndrome, under Williams, J. C. P.*

Fanconi-Turler syndrome. A congenital, probably familial, syndrome marked by cerebellar ataxia associated with uncoordinated eye movements, nystagmus, and mental retardation. In all three originally described cases, the pneumoencephalographic examination showed signs of atrophy of the cerebellum and, probably, of the brain stem, and the EEG indicated involvement of the cerebral cortex. One infant was born to consanguineous parents, and two were delivered following complicated labor.

Fanconi, G., & Turler, U. Kongenitale Kleinhirnatrophie mit supranuclearen Storungen der Motilitat der Augenmuskeln. *Helv. Paediat. Acta,* 1951, 6:475-83.

Lignac-Fanconi syndrome. See *cystinosis.*

Lignac-Fanconi-Debré syndrome. See *cystinosis.*

Prader-Labhart-Willi-Fanconi syndrome. See *Prader-Willi syndrome.*

Wissler-Fanconi syndrome. See *Wissler syndrome.*

Zinsser-Fanconi syndrome. See *under Zinsser.*

far eastern hemorrhagic fever. See *hemorrhagic fever with renal syndrome.*

far out syndrome. Compression of the spinal nerve far laterally, even beyond the foramen, occurring in elderly individuals with scoliosis, and in younger persons with isthmic spondylolisthesis.

Wiltse, L. L., *et al.* Alar transverse process impingement of the L5 spinal nerve: The far out syndrome. *Spine,* 1984, 9:31-41.

FARABEE, WILLIAM CURTIS (American anthropologist, 1865-1925)

Farabee brachydactyly. See *brachydactyly A-1.*

FARBER, SIDNEY (American pediatrician)

Farber disease. Synonyms: *Farber lipogranulomatosis, Farber-Uzman syndrome, disseminated lipogranulomatosis.*

A form of lipid metabolism disorder recognizable at birth or shortly after, and characterized by a hoarse cry, feeding difficulty, irritability, mental retardation, muscle hypotonia, periarticular swelling with poor mobility, and fatal respiratory failure. The soft tissue nodules may appear as soft swellings or as extensive, discrete nodules. Massive bony demineralization and articular erosion may be associated. The carpus may have an appearance similar to that in juvenile rheumatoid arthritis. Histologically, the lesions are granulomatous and there is an excess of ceramide in the cytoplasm and mast cells.

Farber, S. A lipid metabolism disorder-disseminated "lipogranulomatosis"-a syndrome with similarity to, and important difference from Niemann-Pick and Hand-Schüller-Christian disease. *Am J. Dis. Child.*, 1952, 84:499-500. Farber, S., Cohen, J., & Uzman, L. L. Lipogranulomatosis: A new lipo-glyco-protein "storage" disease. *J. Mt. Sinai Hosp.* 1957, 24:816-37.

Farber lipogranulomatosis. See *Farber disease.*

Farber-Uzman syndrome. See *Farber disease.*

FARGIN-FAYOLLE, PAUL (French dentist, born 1876)

Fargin-Fayolle syndrome. See *dentinogenesis imperfecta.*

farmer's lung. See *Ramazzini syndrome.*

FAS. See ***f**etal **a**lcohol **s**yndrome.*

fasciitis with eosinophilia. See *Shulman syndrome, under Shulman, L. E.*

fat embolism syndrome (FES). Synonym: *post-traumatic fat embolism syndrome.*

Formation of fat emboli in the pulmonary vessels, usually after long bone fractures, characterized by an initial asymptomatic period that is followed by tachycardia, pyrexia, cerebral symptoms (restlessness, disorientation, drowsiness, confusion, and occasional coma), petechiae, hypoxia, retinal changes, jaundice, renal changes, dyspnea, tachypnea, hemoptysis, and pulmonary alveolar and interstitial opacities on x-ray examination. Anemia, hypocalcemia, elevated serum

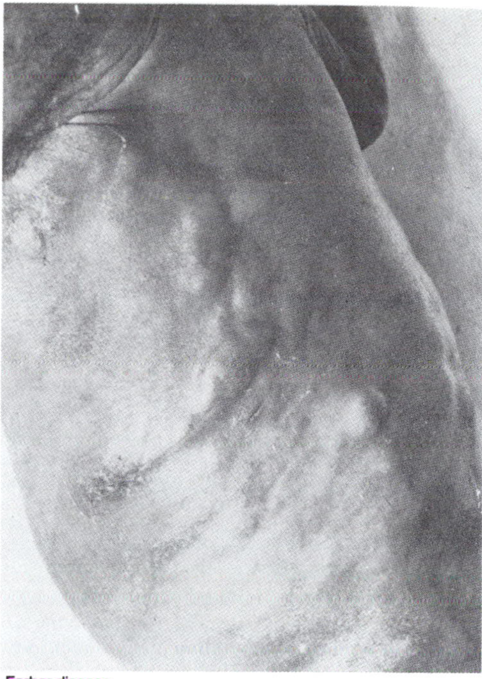

Farber disease
Nelson, W.E. (ed.): *Textbook of Pediatrics*, 8th ed. Philadelphia: W.B. Saunders Co., 1964.

lipase, low hemoglobin level, elevated erythrocyte sedimentation rate, thrombocytopenia, and the presence of fat globules in the sputum, urine, and blood are usually associated. The syndrome is sometimes classified as the acute type, with embolization of the cerebral or coronary arteries leading to death; the classic type, with chest x-ray findings ranging from a normal pattern or patchy densities to linear streaks radiating from the hilar region, sometimes accompanied by pulmonary edema; and a type which is considered a variant of the adult respiratory distress syndrome. Fat embolism may also occur after muscle injuries, severe burns, hemorrhagic pancreatitis, fatty liver secondary to poisoning, extracorporeal circulation, total hip replacement, and administration of corticosteroids. Pathological changes consist mainly of the presence of fat emboli in the lung capillaries.

*Carrara, M. Über die Fettembolie der Lungen in ihren Beziehungen zur gerichtlichen Medizin. *Friedreichs Bl. Gerrichtl. Med.*, 1898, 49:241. Alho, A. Clinical manifestations of fat embolism syndrome. *Arch. Orthop. Traum. Surg.*, 1978, 93:153-8. Worthley, L. I. G., & Fisher, M. M. The fat embolism syndrome treated with oxygen, diuretics, sodium restriction and spontaneous ventilation. *Anaesth. Intens. Care*, 1979, 7:136-42. Gossling, H. R., & Donohue, T. A. The fat embolism syndrome. *JAMA*, 1979, 241:2740-2.

fat Joe's folly. See *Pickwick syndrome.*

fat-induced hyperlipemia. See *Bürger-Grütz syndrome.*

fatal catatonia. See *Bell mania, under Bell, Luther Vos.*

fatal cutaneointestinal syndrome. See *Degos syndrome.*

fatal familial cholestasis. See *Byler disease.*

fatal granulomatous disease of childhood. See *chronic granulomatous disease of childhood.*

fatal subacute myocarditis. See *Fiedler myocarditis.*

fatigue syndrome. See *chronic fatigue syndrome.*

fatigue-dysphoria syndrome. See *chronic fatigue syndrome.*

fatty liver-encephalopathy syndrome. See *Reye syndrome.*

fatty neck. See *Madelung syndrome.*

fatty nutritional cirrhosis. See *Laennec cirrhosis.*

FAUCHARD, PIERRE (French dentist, 1678-1761)

Fauchard disease. Synonyms: *Riggs disease, alveolodental periostitis, cementoperiostitis, chronic suppurative pericementitis, gingivitis expulsiva, gingivopericementitis, marginal periodontitis, paradontitis, periodontitis simplex, primary periodontitis, pyorrhea, pyorrhea alveolaris, schmutz pyorrhea, simple periodontitis.*

An inflammatory periodontal disease which begins as a simple marginal gingivitis, and is caused by calculus, impacted food debris, materia alba, or irritation by fillings. Minute ulcerations of the crevicular epithelium are the initial symptoms. If left untreated, the inflammation will migrate along the tooth toward the apex, producing periodontal pockets and destruction of the periodontal and alveolar structures (periodontoclasia and alveoloclasia), causing the teeth to become loose. Swelling, edema, hyperemia, and bleeding of the gingivae, detachment of the tissue from the tooth structure and recession of soft tissue, expulsion of suppurative material on pressure from periodontal pockets, and halitosis are the principal symptoms. The condition is observed most frequently among adults and elderly persons, but it also occurs in children.

Fauchard, P. *Le chirurgien dentiste, ou traité des dents.* Paris, Mariette, 1746. Riggs, J. M. Suppurative inflammation of the gums, and absorption of the gums and alveolar process. *Penn. J. Dent. Sc.*, 1876, 3:99-104.

FAUVEL, SULPICE ANTOINE (French physician, 1813-1884)

Fauvel granules. Multiple peribronchial abscesses.

Fauvel, S. A. *Recherches sur la bronchite capillaire, purulente et pseudo-membraneuse (catarrhe suffocant, croup bronchique), chez les enfants.* Paris, Rignoux, 1840.

FAVRE, MAURICE JULES (French physician, 1876-1954)

Durand-Nicolas-Favre disease. See *under Durand, J.*

Favre disease (1). See *Favre-Chaix angiodermatitis.*

Favre disease (2). See *Favre-Goldman syndrome.*

Favre hyaloideoretinal degeneration. See *Favre-Goldman syndrome.*

Favre-Chaix angiodermatitis. Synonyms: *Favre disease, Favre-Chaix syndrome, acro-angiodermatitis.*

Angiodermatitis of the foot due to chronic venous insufficiency, associated with peculiar purple maculae and plaques with central ulcers. The lesions, usually located on the extensor side of the toes or on the foot, may vary in size from that of a pinpoint to that of the hand. Histological examination shows proliferation of small vessels, fibroblasts, purpura, and hemosiderin in the stratum papillae. The disorder is most frequently observed during the fourth decade.

*Favre, M. *Nouvelle pratique dermatologique.* Paris, 1941, p. 413. *Chaix, A. *La dermite pigmentée et purpurique des membres inférieurs Lésions pré-erosive des ulcères dits variqueux.* Lyon, 1926 (Thesis).

Favre-Chaix syndrome. See *Favre-Chaix angiodermatitis.*

Favre-Goldman syndrome. Synonyms: *Favre disease, Favre hyaloideoretinal degeneration, retinoschisis with early hemerolopia.*

A familial eye disease, transmitted as an autosomal recessive trait, characterized by early onset of night blindness, pigmentary dystrophy of the retina, degenerative changes in the retina with liquefaction and the presence of microfibrillar strands, retinoschisis, lens opacities, and electroretinographic abnormalities.

Favre, M. A propos de deux cas de denerescence hyaloideoretinienne. *Ophthalmologica, Basel,* 1958, 135:604-9.

Favre-Racouchot disease. Synonyms: *elasteidosis cutanea nodularis, elasteidosis cutis cystica et comedonica, elastoidosis cutanea nodularis, elastoidosis cutis et comedonica, nodular elastoidosis.*

A skin disease characterized by yellowish nodules with dilated hair sacs, atrophic sebaceous glands, cystic formations, and comedones superimposed on the furrowed and wrinkled skin beneath. Histological findings show thick compact skin and loss of elastic and connective fibers from the papillary region and from around the nerves and blood vessels. The face, neck, and back are most commonly affected. Chronic exposure to sunlight is the cause.

Favre, M., & Racouchot, J. L'elastéidose cutanée nodulaire à kystes et à comédons. *Ann. Derm. Syph., Paris,* 1951, 78:681-702.

Nicolas-Favre disease. See *Durand-Nicolas-Favre disease, under Durand, J.*

FAZIO, M. (Italian physician)

Fazio-Londe paralysis. See *Duchenne paralysis.*

FCMD (**F**ukuyama type **c**ongenital **m**uscular **d**ystrophy). See *Fukuyama syndrome.*

FCMS. See ***F**oix-**C**havany-**M**arie **s**yndrome.*

FDH (**f**ocal **d**ermal **h**ypoplasia) **syndrome.** See *Goltz syndrome.*

feather hair. See *Miescher trichofolliculoma.*

febrile neutrophilic dermatosis. See *Sweet syndrome.*

febrile polyneuritis. See *Guillain-Barré syndrome.*

febris eosinophilica monocytaria. See *Magrassi-Leonardi syndrome.*

febris melitensis. See *brucellosis.*

febris periodica hyperergica. See *Wissler syndrome.*

febris quintana. See *Werner-His disease, under Werner, Heinrich.*

febris undulans. See *brucellosis.*

febris uveoparotidea subchronica. See *Heerfordt syndrome.*

FEDE, FRANCESCO (Italian physician, 1832-1913)

Fede disease. See *Riga-Fede disease.*

Riga-Fede disease. See *under Riga.*

FEDERMAN, D. D.

Moore-Federman syndrome. See *under Moore, W. T.*

FEER-SULZER, EMIL (Swiss physician, 1864-1955)

Feer disease. See *acrodynia.*

Feer neurosis. See *acrodynia.*

Feer syndrome. See *acrodynia.*

Selter-Swift-Feer syndrome. See *acrodynia.*

Swift-Feer syndrome. See *acrodynia.*

FEGELER, FERDINAND (German physician)

Fegeler syndrome. Synonym: *post-traumatic nevus flammeus.*

A port wine nevus of the part of the face that is supplied by the trigeminal nerve, associated with ipsilateral weakness and hyperesthesia of the arm and leg, following a head injury. Damage of the spinal cord and the cervical autonomic nerves that results in vasomotor disorders is the probable cause.

Fegeler, F. Naevus flammeus im Trigeminusgebiet nach Trauma im Rahmen eines posttraumatisch-vegetativen Syndroms. *Arch. Derm. Syph., Berlin,* 1949-50, 188:416-22.

FEHR, OSKAR (German ophthalmologist, born 1871)

Fehr dystrophy. See *Groenouw dystrophy (2).*

FEICHTIGER, H. (German physician)

Ullrich-Feichtiger syndrome. See *under Ullrich.*

FEIL, ANDRE (French neurologist, born 1889)

Klippel-Feil anomalad. See *Klippel-Feil syndrome.*

Klippel-Feil syndrome. See *under Klippel.*

FEINMESSER, MOSHE (Israeli physician)

Feinmesser-Zelig syndrome. See *DOOR syndrome.*

FELDMAN, HARRY ALFRED (American physician, born 1914)

Sabin-Feldman syndrome. See *under Sabin.*

FELDMAN, SAMUEL (Polish-born American dermatologist, 1877-1947)

Graham Little-Lassueur-Feldman syndrome. See *Little syndrome, under Little, Ernest Gordon Graham.*

FELDSTEIN, ERNEST (French physician, born 1888)

Klippel-Feldstein syndrome. See *under Klippel.*

felinosis. See *cat scratch disease.*

FELTY, AUGUSTUS ROI (American physician, born 1895)

Felty syndrome (FS). Synonyms: *Still-Chauffard-Felty syndrome, arthritis-splenomegaly-leukopenia syndrome, neutropenic hypersplenism-arthritis syndrome, primary splenic neutropenia with arthritis syndrome, rheumatoid arthritis-hypersplenism syndrome, rheumatoid arthritis-splenomegaly-leukopenia syndrome.*

A syndrome of rheumatoid arthritis, splenomegaly, and leukopenia, occurring in association with granulocytopenia, lymphadenopathy, and anemia. The rheumatoid factor is almost always present. Ocular changes may include keratoconjunctivitis sicca, episcleritis, hypopyon ulcer, and scleromalacia. Nonspecific inflammatory oral lesions are commonly present. The symptoms usually include anorexia, weight loss, general malaise, bronchitis, pallor, brown pigmentation of exposed surfaces, joint pain, pain in the upper left quadrant of the abdomen, and recurrent infections.

Felty, A. R. Chronic arthritis in the adult, associated with splenomegaly and leucopenia. A report of 5 cases of an unusual clinical syndrome. *Bull. Johns Hopkins Hosp.,* 1924, 35:16-20.

Still-Chauffard-Felty syndrome. See *Still syndrome, and see Felty syndrome.*

female facial melanosis. See *Riehl melanosis.*

female hysteria. See *Briquet syndrome (1), under Briquet, Pierre.*

female pseudo-Turner syndrome. See *Noonan syndrome.*

female pseudohermaphroditism. See *congenital adrenal hyperplasia.*

female urethral syndrome. See *urethral syndrome.*

femoral arteriovenous hyperostomia. See *Pratesi syndrome.*

femoral hernia. See *Cloquet hernia.*

femoral hypoplasia-unusual facies syndrome (FH-UFS). Synonyms: *Daentl syndrome, femoral-facial syndrome.*

An association of facial and femoral abnormalities. Facial defects consist of a short nose with hypoplastic alae, long philtrum, thin upper lip, micrognathia, cleft palate, and antimongoloid palpebral slant. Hypoplastic or aplastic femora and fibulae may be associated with hypoplasia of the humeri, restricted elbow movement, and club feet. Additional anomalies may include hypoplastic acetabula, constricted iliac base, large obturator foramina, spinal abnormalities, posterior tapering of the ribs, short metatarsal bones, astigmatism, esotropia, inguinal hernia, and cryptorchism. Short-limbed dwarfism is due to femoral hypoplasia. The etiology is unknown.

Franz, C. H., & O'Rahilly, R. Congenital skeletal limb deficiencies. *J. Bone Joint Surg.*, 1961, 43(B):1202. Kucera, V. J., *et al.* Missbildungen der Beine und der kaudalen Wirbelsaule bei Kindern diabetischer Mütter. *Deut. Med. Wschr.*, 1965, 90:902-5. Daentl, D. L. *et al.* Femoral hypoplasia-unusual facies syndrome. *J. Pediat.*, 1975, 86:107-11.

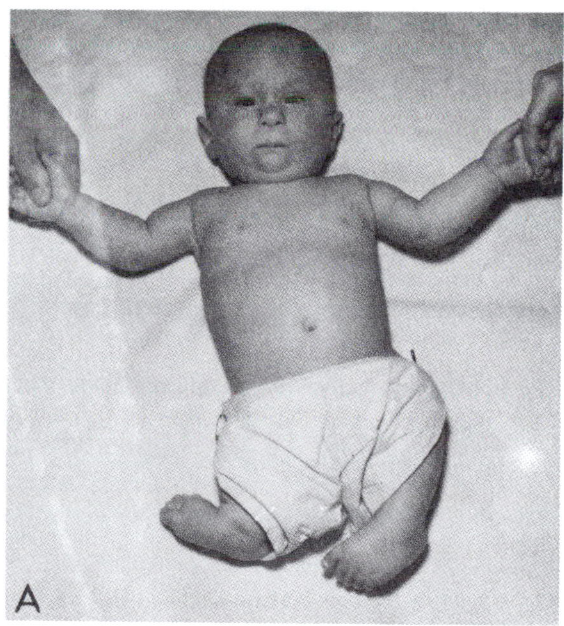

Femoral hypoplasia-unusual faciess
Daentl, D.L., et al.: *J. Pediatr.*, 86:107, 1975. St. Louis: C.V. Mosby Co.

femoral-facial syndrome. See *femoral hypoplasia-unusual facies syndrome.*

femur-fibula-ulna (FFU) syndrome. Synonym: *proximal focal femoral deficiency (PFFD).*

An association of femoral defects with arm anomalies, including amelia, peromelia at the lower end of the humerus, humeroradial synostosis, and defects of the ulna at the ulnar rays. The etiology is unknown.

Lenz, W. D. Bone defects of the limbs-an overview. *Birth Defects,* 1969, 5(3):1-6. Kuhne, D., *et al.* Defekt von Femur und Fibula mit Amelie, Peromelie oder ulnaren Strahldefekten der Arme. Ein Syndrom. *Humangenetik,* 1967, 3:244-63. Aitken, G. T. *Proximal femoral focal deficiency, a congenital anomaly.* A symposium. National Academy of Science. Washington, D. C., 1969.

fender fracture of the tibia. See *Cotton fracture.*

FENDT, HEINRICH (German physician)

Spiegler-Fendt sarcoid. See *Bäfverstedt syndrome.*

Spiegler-Fendt sarcomatosis. See *Bäfverstedt syndrome.*

FENWICK, EDWIN HURRY (British physician, 1856-1944)

Fenwick ulcer. Chronic ulcer of the bladder, beginning as a superficial lesion manifested by painful hematuria, with consecutive cystitis, encrustation over the surface of the ulcer, and, ultimately, destruction of the muscular layer. The condition occurs predominantly in young, apparently healthy males as a solitary ulcer and, less frequently, in women as a double ulcer.

Fenwick, E. H. The clinical significance of the simple solitary ulcer of the urinary bladder. *Lancet,* 1896, 1:1133-5.

FENWICK, SAMUEL (British physician, 1821-1902)

Fenwick disease. Idiopathic atrophic gastritis in a patient with pernicious anemia.

Fenwick, S. *On atrophy of the stomach and on the nervous affections of the digestive organs.* London, Churchill, 1880.

FERE

Fere-Langmead lipomatosis. A form of plantar lipomatosis reportedly described by Fere and Langmead.

FERGUSON SMITH. See SMITH, JOHN FERGUSON

FERNAND WIDAL. See WIDAL, M. FERNAND

FERRAND, MARCEL (French physician, 1878-1940)

Darier-Ferrand dermatofibrosarcoma. See *under Darier.*

FERRANINI, A. (Italian physician)

Rummo-Ferranini syndrome. See *under Rummo.*

fertile eunuch syndrome. See *Pasqualini syndrome.*

FES. See *fat embolism syndrome.*

fetal Accutane syndrome. Synonyms: *Accutane dysmorphic syndrome, isotretinoin embryopathy.*

A teratogenic syndrome caused by oral administration of Accutane (isotretinoin, 13-*cis*-retinoic aid) in pregnancy. The abnormalities include rudimentary external ears, absent or imperforate auditory canals, triangular microcephalic skull, cleft palate, depressed midface, and anomalies of the brain, jaw, and heart. The affected infants have large occiputs with narrowing of the frontal bone. Heart defects usually include overriding aorta, interrupted or hypoplastic aortic arch, and atrial and septal defect. Associated anomalies may include microphthalmia, abnormal orbits, decreased muscle tone, micromelia, and abnormal origin of the subclavian arteries.

Willhite, C. C., *et al.* Isotretinoin-induced craniofacial malformations in humans and hamsters. *J. Craniofac. Genet. Develop. Biol.,* 1986, Suppl. 2:193-209.

fetal achondroplasia. See *achondroplasia.*

fetal alcohol syndrome (FAS). Synonyms: *alcoholic embryopathy, embryofetal alcohol syndrome (EFAS), embryopathia alcoholica.*

A syndrome of infants born to alcoholic mothers, characterized by variable abnormalities, including growth deficiency, mental retardation, motor deficiency, microcephaly, short palpebral fissures, maxillary hypoplasia, heart murmur (disappearing by one year of age), joint anomalies, and abnormal palmar creases. Blepharoptosis, strabismus, cleft palate, perinatal hirsutism, capillary hemangioma, hypoplasia of the labia majora, pilonidal sinus, nail hypoplasia, limitation of joint movement, clinodactyly, and hypoplastic digits are usually associated.

Jones, K. L., & Smith, D. W. Recognition of the fetal alcohol syndrome in early infancy. *Lancet*, 1973, 2:999-1001.

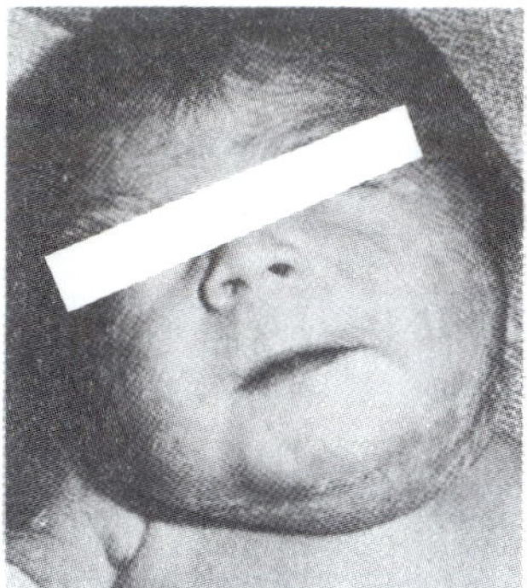

Fetal alcohol syndrome
Jones, K.L., & Smith, D.W.: *Lancet*. London, 2:999, 1973.

fetal aminopterin syndrome. Synonyms: *aminopterin embryopathy, aminopterin fetopathy syndrome, aminopterin syndrome, fetal methotrexate syndrome.*

A syndrome of variable anomalies in infants after failed use of aminopterin (methotrexate) as an abortifacient agent. The abnormalities include growth and mental deficiency; cranial dysplasia; abnormal facies, including broad nasal bridge, shallow supraorbital ridge, low-set ears, epicanthus, hypertelorism, micrognathia, protruding eyes, and upsweep of hair on the forehead; myopia; cleft palate; and various limb defects, such as micromelia or mesomelia, talipes equinovarus, synostosis, hip dislocation, short thumbs, and syndactyly. Radiological features may include skull ossification disorder, multiple wormian bones, cranium bifidum, aberrant longitudinal suture in the parietal bone, and other defects.

Thiersch, J. B. Therapeutic abortions with a folic acid antagonists, 4-aminopteroylglutamic acid (4-amino-P.G.A.) administered by the oral route. *Am. J. Obstet. Gyn.*, 1952, 63:1298. Shaw, E. B., *et al.* Aminopterin-induced fetal malformation. Survival of infant after attempted abortion. *Am. J. Dis. Child.*, 1968, 115:477.

fetal aminopterin-like syndrome without aminopterin. Synonym: *aminopterin-like syndrome sine aminopterin (ASSA).*

A syndrome with clinical features similar to those produced by aminopterin in early pregnancy, but without any evidence of maternal exposure to the substance. The principal characteristic traits include ossification defects of the cranium, temporal recession of hairline with upswept frontal hair pattern, hypertelorism, prominent nasal root, low-set anteriorly rotated ears, limited elbow movement, variable digital defects, simian creases, short stature, and psychomotor retardation. Autosomal recessive inheritance is suspected.

Fraser, F. C., *et al.* An aminopterin-like syndrome without aminopterin (ASSA). *Clin. Genet.*, 1987, 32:28-34.

fetal anticoagulant embryopathy. See *fetal warfarin syndrome.*

fetal Dilantin syndrome. See *fetal hydantoin syndrome.*

fetal endocardial fibroelastosis. See *Weinberg-Himelfarb syndrome.*

fetal endocarditis. See *Weinberg-Himelfarb syndrome.*

fetal face syndrome. See *Robinow syndrome.*

fetal folic acid antagonist syndrome. See *fetal aminopterin syndrome.*

fetal gigantism-renal hamartomas-nephroblastomosis syndrome. See *Perlman syndrome.*

fetal hydantoin syndrome (FHS). Synonyms: *Meadow syndrome, Dilantin syndrome, fetal Dilantin syndrome, hydantoin syndrome.*

A syndrome occurring in infants whose mothers received anticonvulsant hydantoin (Dilantin, phenytoin) therapy during pregnancy, consisting of mental retardation, growth retardation, wide fontanels, metopic ridging, hypertelorism, broad depressed nasal bridge, low-set deformed ears, cleft lip, cleft palate, broad alveolar ridge, brevicollis, rib defects, widely spaced nipples, umbilical hernia, inguinal hernia, piloinidal sinus, coarse hair, hirsutism, low hairline, abnormal palmar creases, aplasia or hypoplasia of the distal phalanges with nail hypoplasia and short fingers, polyhyperphalangism, clubfoot, and supernumerary phalangeal epiphyses. Microcephaly, brachycephaly, mongoloid palpebral slant, heart defects, eye abnormalities, genital malformations, and a number of other anomalies may occur.

Meadow, S. R. Anticonvulsant drugs and congenital abnormalities. *Lancet*, 1968, 2:1296.

fetal methotrexate syndrome. See *fetal aminopterin syndrome.*

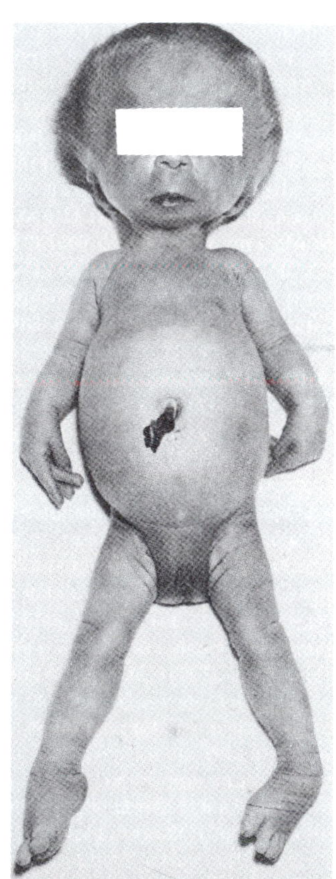

Fetal aminopterin syndrome
Warkany, J., et al.: *Am. J. Dis. Child.* 97:274, 1959. Chicago: American Medical Association.

fetal PCB syndrome (FPS). Synonyms: *black baby, Cola baby, Coca-Cola baby, fetal yusho (PCB-contaminated oil poisoning), neonatal yusho (PCB-contaminated oil poisoning), PCB-induced fetopathy yusho.*

A toxic condition of infants born to mothers who were exposed to PCB (polychlorinated biphenyl) during pregnancy. The manifestations consist of dark brown pigmentation of the skin and mucous membranes (hence the synonyms *black baby, Cola baby* and *Coca-Cola baby*), gingival hyperplasia, exophthalmic edematous eyes, premature tooth eruption, abnormal skull calcification, rocker-botton feet, and low birth weight. Altered calcium metabolism is the suspected mechanism. The syndrome occurred in western Japan during the 1968 mass poisoning due to ingestion of PCB-contaminated cooking rice oil.

*Kikuchi, M., An autopsy case of stillborn of chlorobiphenyls poisoning. *Fukuoka Acta Med.*, 1969, 60:489-95. *Kusuka, M. Yusho and females. *Sanka to Fujinka*, 1971, 38:1063-72. Yamashita, F., & Hayashi, M. Fetal PCB syndrome: Clinical features, intrauterine growth retardation and possible alteration in calcium metabolism. *Environ. Health Persp.*, 1985, 59:41-5.

fetal polycystic disease. See *Potter syndrome (2), under Potter, Edith Louise.*

fetal ricin syndrome. Synonym: *ricin syndrome.*

A congenital syndrome of growth retardation, convulsions, craniofacial malformations, absence deformity of the limbs, and vertebral segmentation defect in infants born to mothers who have taken castor oil seeds (*Ricinus communis*) orally for contraceptive purposes. Enlarged skull, occipital bulge, hypertelorism, flat nasal bridge with a rounded top and broad base, low-set ears with prominent anthelices and antitragus and unfolded upper helices, wide-open mouth, and high-arched palate are the principal craniofacial features.

El Mauhoub, M., *et al.* "Ricin syndrome." A possible new teratogenic syndrome associated with ingestion of castor oil seed in early pregnancy: a case report. *Ann. Trop. Paediat.*, 1983, 3:57-61.

fetal testicular regression syndrome. See *embryonic testicular regression syndrome.*

fetal thalidomide syndrome. See *Wiedemann syndrome (1).*

fetal tobacco syndrome (FTS). Adverse effects of maternal smoking of tobacco during pregnancy on infant's health. Birth weight deficit, abruptio placentae, bleeding during pregnancy, premature rupture of membranes, fetal death, and sudden infant death syndrome have been attributed to smoking during pregnancy.

Simpson, W. J. Preliminary report on cigarette smoking and the incidence of prematurity. *Am. J. Obst. Gyn.*, 1957, 73:808-15. Nieburg, P., *et al.* The fetal tobacco syndrome. *JAMA*, 1985, 253:2998-9.

fetal transfusion syndrome. See *twin transfusion syndrome.*

fetal trimethadione syndrome. Synonyms: *German syndrome, paramethadione syndrome, tridione syndrome, trimethadione embryopathy, trimethadione syndrome.*

A syndrome of infants whose mothers received trimethadione or paramethadione during pregnancy, consisting of growth retardation, speech disorders, V-shaped eyebrows, epicanthus, low-set ears with anteriorly folded helices, broad and low nasal bridge, prominent forehead, synophrys, strabismus, blepharoptosis, epicanthus, cleft lip, cleft palate, high-arched palate, micrognathia, heart septum defects, tetralogy of Fallot, hypospadias, hypertrophy of the clitoris, and simian creases. Microcephaly and inguinal hernia may occur.

German, J., *et al.* Trimethadione and human teratogenesis. *Teratology*, 1970, 3:349-61.

fetal triploidy syndrome. See *chromosome triploidy syndrome.*

fetal warfarin embryopathy. See *fetal warfarin syndrome.*

fetal warfarin syndrome. Synonyms: *Di Saia syndrome, congenital warfarin syndrome, coumadin syndrome, fetal anticoagulant syndrome, fetal warfarin syndrome, foetal warfarin syndrome, warfarin embryopathy, warfarin syndrome.*

A complex of fetal abnormalities caused by the use of anticoagulants (such as warfarin) during pregnancy, including growth and mental retardation, muscle hypotonia, convulsions, optic atrophy, hypoplastic nose with low nasal bridge, airway obstruction, feeding difficulty, failure to thrive, punctate epiphyses, hypoplasia and shortening of digits, calcific stippling in uncalcified epiphyses, and other bone defects similar to those in chondrodysplasia punctata.

Di Saia, P. J. Pregnancy and delivery of a patient with Stan-Edwards mitral valve prosthesis. Report of a case. *Obstet. Gynec.*, 1966, 28:469-71.

fetal yusho (PCB-contaminated oil poisoning). See *fetal PCB syndrome.*

fetofetal transfusion. See *twin transfusion syndrome.*

fetoinfantile regressive periosteoenchondral hyperosteogenesis. See *Caffey-Silverman syndrome.*

fetomaternal transfusion syndrome. Transplacental passage of fetal blood into the maternal circulation resulting in iron deficiency and hypochromic and microcytic anemia in the newborn. Massive fetomaternal hemorrhage near term may cause hemorrhagic anemia, shock, or hydrops fetalis in the newborn infant. See also *twin transfusion syndrome.*

Wiener, A. S. Diagnosis and treatment of anemia of the newborn caused by occult placental hemorrhage. *Am. J. Obst. Gyn.*, 1948, 56:717-22.

fetoplacental anasarca. See *Schridde syndrome.*

FEUERSTEIN, FRICHARD C. (American physician)

Feuerstein-Mims syndrome. See *epidermal nevus syndrome.*

Feuerstein-Mims syndrome with resistant rickets. See *hypophosphatemic rickets-osteomalacia-linear nevus sebaceous syndrome.*

linear nevus sebaceus of Feuerstein and Mims. See *epidermal nevus syndrome.*

nevus sebaceus of Feuerstein and Mims. See *epidermal nevus syndrome.*

Schimmelpenning-Feuerstein-Mims syndrome. See *epidermal nevus syndrome.*

fever-stomatitis-ophthalmia syndrome. See *Stevens-Johnson syndrome.*

FEVR (familial exudative vitreoretinopathy). See *Criswick-Schepens syndrome.*

FEVRE, MARCEL PAUL LUIS EDMOND (French orthopedic surgeon, born 1897)

Fèvre-Languepin syndrome. See *popliteal pterygium syndrome.*

FEYRTER, FRIEDRICH (Austrian physician, born 1895)
Feyrter disease. Diffuse pulmonary plasmocytosis in premature infants.
Feyrter, F. Über die pathologische Anatomie der Lungenveränderungen beim Keuchhusten. *Frankf. Zschr. Path.*, 1927, 35:213-55.
Pospischill-Feyrter aphthoid. See *Pospischill-Feyrter disease.*
Pospischill-Feyrter disease. See *under Pospischill.*
FFU. See *femur-fibula-ulna syndrome.*
FG syndrome. A multiple congenital anomalies/mental retardation syndrome transmitted as an X-linked trait. Mental retardation, characteristic personality, peculiar facies, megalencephaly, joint contractures and/or camptodactyly, broad thumbs and/or halluces, imperforate anus/sacral dimples, and sensorineural hearing loss are its principal features. The abbreviation "FG" stands for the surnames of patients in whom the syndrome was first reported.
Opitz, J. M., & Kaveggia, E. G. The FG syndrome. An X-linked recessive syndrome of multiple congenital anomalies and mental retardation. *Kinderheilk.*, 1974, 117:1-18.
FH-UFS. See ***f**emoral **h**ypoplasia-**u**nusual **f**acies **s**yndrome.*
FHC. See ***F**uchs **h**eterochromic **c**yclitis.*
FHH. See ***f**amilial **h**ypercalcemia-**h**ypocalciuria syndrome.*
FHI (**F**uchs **h**eterochromic **i**ridocyclitis). See *Fuchs heterochromic cyclitis.*
FHS. See ***f**etal **h**ydantoin **s**yndrome.*
FIBIGER, JOHANNES ANDREAS GRIB (Danish physician, 1867-1928)
Debré-Fibiger syndrome. See *congenital adrenal hyperplasia.*
Fibiger-Debré-von Gierke syndrome. See *congenital adrenal hyperplasia.*
fibrillary chorea. See *Morvan chorea.*
fibrinoid degeneration of astrocytes. See *Alexander syndrome, under Alexander, W. Stewart.*
fibrinoid leukodystrophy. See *Alexander syndrome, under Alexander, W. Stewart.*
fibrinolytic thromboembolism. See *disseminated intravascular coagulation syndrome.*
fibroadenomatosis cystica. See *Cheatle disease.*
fibrocellulitis progressiva ossificans. See *fibrodysplasia ossificans progressiva.*
fibrochondrogenesis. See *Lazzaroni-Fossati syndrome.*
fibrocongestive splenomegaly. See *Banti syndrome.*
fibrocystic disease (of bone). See *Jaffe-Lichtenstein syndrome.*
fibrodysplasia elastica. See *Ehlers-Danlos syndrome.*
fibrodysplasia elastica generalisata. See *Ehlers-Danlos syndrome.*
fibrodysplasia ossificans congenita. See *fibrodysplasia ossificans progressiva.*
fibrodysplasia ossificans multiplex progressiva. See *fibrodysplasia ossificans progressiva.*
fibrodysplasia ossificans progressiva (FOP). Synonyms: *Guy Patin syndrome, Muenchmeyer syndrome, Münchmeyer syndrome, Patin syndrome, exostosis luxurians, fibrocellulitis progressiva ossificans, fibrodysplasia ossificans congenita, fibrodysplasia ossificans multiplex progressiva, fibrositis ossificans, hyperplasia fascialis ossificans, hyperplasia fascialis progressiva, interstitial ossifying myositis, myo-ossificatio progressiva multiplex, myopathia osteoplastica, myositis ossificans multiplex progressiva, myositis ossificans progressiva, osteoma multiplex intramusculare, polyossificatio congenita progressiva.*

A connective tissue disorder characterized by progressive ossification adjacent to striated muscle. Swelling and pain, mostly around the paravertebral areas, shoulder, and arms, are the early symptoms, which usually take place in young children. Hypoplasia of the great toe and sometimes the thumb is usually present at birth. Widened medullary space, often having a ground-glass appearance, radiolucency appearing as punched-out lesions, advanced bone maturation, and fibrous bone dysplasia may be seen on x-rays.
Illingworth, R. S. Myositis ossificans progressiva (Münchmeyer disease). *Arch. Dis. Child., Chicago*, 1971, 46:264. *Münchmeyer, E. Über Myositis ossificans progressiva. *Zschr. Ration. Med.*, 1869, 34:1. McKusick, V. A. *Mendelian inheritance in man.* 7th ed. Baltimore, Johns Hopkins Univ. Press, 1986, No. 13510.

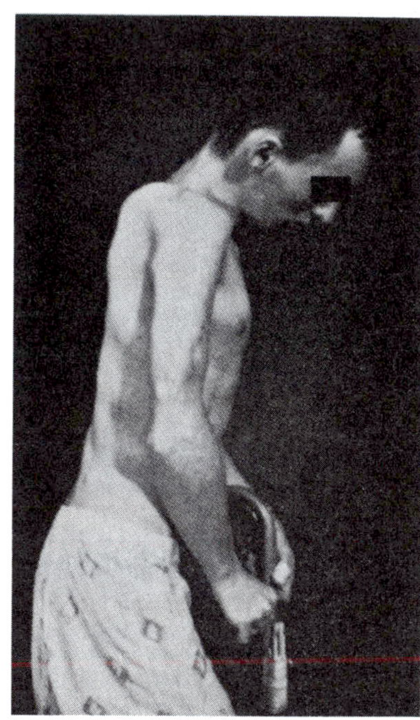

Fibrodysplasia ossificans progressiva (Munchmeyer's syndrome)
Aegerter E., & J.A. Kirkpatrick, Jr.: *Orthopedic diseases*, 3rd ed. Philadelphia: W.B. Saunders Co., 1968.

fibroid phthisis. See *Hamman-Rich syndrome.*
fibrolipomatosis dolorosa. See *Dercum syndrome.*
fibroma lipomatodes. See *Addison-Gull syndrome.*
fibromatosis gingivae-hypertrichosis syndrome. See *gingival fibromatosis-hypertrichosis syndrome.*
fibromatosis hyalinica multiplex juvenilis. See *Murray syndrome.*
fibromatosis ventriculi. See *Brinton disease.*
fibromyalgia syndrome (FMS). See *fibrositis-fibromyalgia syndrome.*
fibromyeloid medullary reticulosis. See *Hodgkin disease.*

fibroplastic endocarditis. See *Löffler endocarditis.*
fibroplastic endomyocarditis. See *Löffler endocarditis.*
fibroplastic parietal endocarditis with eosinophilia. See *Löffler endocarditis.*

fibrosarcoma ovarii mucocellulare carcinomatodes. See *Krukenberg tumor.*

fibrosing lung disease. See *Hamman-Rich syndrome.*

fibrosis ankylopoietica dorsi. See *Bechterew-Strümpell-Marie syndrome, under Bekhterev.*

fibrositis ossificans. See *fibrodysplasia ossificans progressiva.*

fibrositis syndrome. See *fibrositis-fibromyalgia syndrome.*

fibrositis-fibromyalgia syndrome. Synonyms: *extra-articular rheumatism, fibromyalgia syndrome, fibrosis syndrome, muscle pain syndrome, muscular rheumatism, myofascial pain syndrome, neurasthenia syndrome, primary fibromyalgia syndrome (PFS), rheumatic pain modulation disorder (RPMD), primary fibromyalgia syndrome (PFS).*

A syndrome of musculoskeletal pain and aching, with pain of the joints, axial skeleton, and muscles and neurovascular disorders being the chief complaints, all patients having multiple areas of local tenderness (tender points). Additionally, there are sleep disorders, morning stiffness, fatigue, subjective swelling, paresthesias, and numbness. Headache and irritable bowel syndrome are frequently associated. The syndrome is usually observed between the ages of 40 and 60 years with an at least five female to one male ratio. See also *Forestier syndrome (1),* and *myofascial trigger point syndrome.*

Cowers, W. R. A lecture on lombago: Its lesson and analogues. *Brit. Med. J.,* 1904, 1:117-21. Stockman, R. The causes, pathology, and treatment of chronic rheumatism. *Edinburgh Med. J.,* 1904, 15:107-16. Bennett, R. M., ed. The fibrositis/fibromyalgia syndrome. Current issues and perspectives. *Am. J. Med.,* 1986, 81(3A):1-115.

fibrous bone dysplasia. See *Jaffe-Lichtenstein syndrome.*

fibrous cavernitis. See *Peyronie disease.*

fibrous jaw dysplasia. See *cherubism.*

fibrous osteoma. See *Jaffe-Lichtenstein syndrome.*

fibrous sclerosis of the penis. See *Peyronie disease.*

FICKLER, A.

Fickler-Winkler syndrome. See *OPCA II, under olivopontocerebellar atrophy.*

olivopontocerebellar atrophy (OPCA), Fickler-Winkler type. See *OPCA II, under olivopontocerebellar atrophy.*

ficosis. See *Alibert disease (3).*

FIEDLER, CARL LUDWIG ALFRED (German physician, 1835-1921)

Abramov-Fiedler myocarditis. See *Fiedler myocarditis.*

Fiedler cardiomyopathy. See *Fiedler myocarditis.*

Fiedler myocarditis. Synonyms: *Abramov-Fiedler myocarditis, Fiedler cardiomyopathy, Fiedler syndrome, acute idiopathic myocarditis, acute interstitial myocarditis, allergic granulomatosis of the myocardium, eosinophilic myocarditis, fatal subacute myocarditis, giant-cell granulomatous myocarditis, granulomatous myocarditis, idiopathic granulomatous myocarditis, isolated granulomatous myocarditis, isolated myocarditis, pernicious myocarditis, specific giant-cell myocarditis, specific productive myocarditis.*

A rare, idiopathic, and frequently fatal form of myocarditis that is not accompanied by endocarditis or pericarditis. Two pathological types are recognized. The more common of the two is characterized by inflammatory interstitial reactions associated with infiltration by leukocytes. Second, the granulomatous type, is marked by large foci containing lymphocytes, macrophages, and, sometimes, multinucleated giant-cells. The disease may occur at any age. When associated with extensive eosinophilic infiltrations, the disorder is known as the *Rheinhard myocarditis.*

Fiedler, A. Über akute interstitielle Myokaraditis. *Zbl. Inn. Med.,* 1900, 21:212-3. Abramov, S. S. K kazuistike pervichnykh miokarditov. *Med. Obzor.,* 1897, 48:889-98.

Fiedler syndrome. See *Fiedler myocarditis.*

FIESSINGER, NÖEL (French physician, 1881-1946)

Fiessinger-Leroy syndrome. See *Reiter syndrome.*

Fiessinger-Leroy-Reiter syndrome. See *Reiter syndrome.*

Fiessinger-Rendu syndrome. See *Stevens-Johnson syndrome.*

fifth digit syndrome. See *Coffin-Siris syndrome.*

fifth eruptive disease. See *Sticker disease.*

fifth venereal disease. See *Durand-Nicolas-Favre disease, under Durand, J.*

FILATOV, NIL FEDOROVICH (Russian physician, 1847-1902)

Filatov disease. Synonyms: *Pfeiffer disease, Türk lymphomatosis, acute benign lymphoblastosis, acute infectious adenitis, acute lymphocytosis, glandular fever, infectious mononucleosis, monocytic angina.*

An acute infectious disease caused by the Epstein-Barr virus and characterized by a triad of fever, lymphadenopathy, and pharyngitis with the transient appearance of heterophil antibodies and atypical lymphocytosis. Malaise, anorexia, and chills are the prodromal symptoms. They are followed by pharyngitis, fever, and lymphadenopathy. Complications may include autoimmune hemolytic anemia, thrombocytopenia, granulocytopenia, splenic rupture, encephalitis, cranial nerve palsy (including Bell palsy), meningoencephalitis, Guillain-Barré syndrome, seizures, mononeuritis multiplex, transverse myelitis, psychoses, hepatitis, pericarditis, myocarditis, airway obstruction, and interstitial pneumonia.

Filatov, N. *Lektsii ob ostrykh infektsionnykh bolezniakh u detei.* Moskva, 1887. *Pfeiffer, E. Brüsenfieber. *Jahr. Kinderh.,* 1889, 29:257-64. *Türk, W. *Vorlesungen über klinische Haematologie.* 1904, Vol. 2. Schooley, R. T. Epstein-Barr virus infections, including infectious mononucleosis. In: Braunwald, E., Isselbacher, K. J., Petersdorf, R. G., Wilson, J. D., Martin, J. B., & Fauci, A. S., eds. *Harrison's principles of internal medicine.* 11th ed. New York, McGraw-Hill, 1987, pp. 699-703.

Filatov spots. See *Koplik spots.*

filiform corneal dystrophy. See *Maeder-Danis dystrophy.*

FILIPPI, G. (Italian physician)

Filippi syndrome. A familial syndrome, transmitted as an autosomal recessive trait, characterized by growth and mental retardation, unusual facies (slightly protruding forehead and prominent and broad root of the nose with diminished alar flare), microcephaly, bilateral syndactyly of the third and fourth fingers, clinodactyly of the fifth fingers, bilateral syndactyly of the second, third, and fourth toes, cryptorchism, and speech disorders.

Filippi, G. Unusual facial appearance, microcephaly, growth and mental retardation, and syndactyly. A new syndrome? *Am. J. Med. Genet.,* 1985, 22:821-4.

filum terminale syndrome. See *tethered conus syndrome.*

FINCHER, EDGAR F. (American physician)

Fincher syndrome. Cauda equina tumors associated with spinal subarachnoid hemorrhage. Low back pain followed by headache are the principal symptoms. Ependymoma is the most common tumor.

Fincher, E. F. Spontaneous subarachnoid hemorrhage in intradural tumors of the lumbar sac. A clinical syndrome. *J. Neurosurg.*, 1951, 8:576-84.

FINEMAN, ROBERT M. (American physician)

Smith-Fineman-Myers syndrome. See *under Smith, Richard D.*

finger agnosia. See *Gerstmann syndrome (2).*

finger apoplexy. See *Achenbach syndrome.*

finger osteochondropathy. See *Thiemann syndrome.*

Finland-type amyloid neuropathy. See *amyloid neuropathy type IV.*

first and second branchial arch syndrome. See *oculoauriculovertebral dysplasia.*

FISCHER, HEINRICH F. (German physician)

Buschke-Fischer syndrome. See *Fischer syndrome.*

Buschke-Fischer-Brauer syndrome. See *Fischer syndrome, under Fischer, Heinrich F.*

Fischer syndrome. Synonyms: *Brauer disease, Buschke-Fischer syndrome, Buschke-Fischer-Brauer syndrome.*

A syndrome, transmitted as an autosomal dominant trait, characterized by keratosis palmaris et plantaris, hair hypoplasia, onycholysis, onychogryposis, hyperhidrosis of the hands and feet, occasional clubbing of the distal phalanges of the toes and fingers, progeria, apathy, mental retardation, edema of the eyelids, and xeroderma.

Fischer, H. Familiär hereditäres Vorkommen von Keratoma palmare et plantare, Nagelveränderungen, Haaranomalien und Verdickungen der Endglieder der Finger und Zehen in 5 Generationen. (Die Beziehungen dieser Veränderungen zur inneren Sekretion). *Derm. Zschr., Berlin,* 1921, 32-33:114-42.

fish-odor syndrome. Synonym: *trimethylaminuria.*

A rotten fish odor due to the presence of triethylamine (TMA) in sweat, urine, and breath. Ingestion of foods containing trimethylamine precursors, including milk and choline-containing foods such as eggs, liver, soy beans, meat, wheat germ, yeast, and lecithin, causes the odor.

Humbert, J. R., *et al.* Trimethylaminuria: The fish odor syndrome. *Lancet,* 1970, 2:770-1.

FISHER, J. A. (British physician)

Fisher-Evans syndrome. See *Evans syndrome, under Evans, Robert S.*

FISHER, MILLER (American physician)

Fisher syndrome (FS). Synonyms: *Miller Fisher syndrome, ophthalmoplegia-ataxia-areflexia syndrome.*

A variant of the Guillain-Barré syndrome, characterizead by total external ophthalmoplegia, ataxia, and loss of tendon reflexes. Early symptoms include fever, headache, and pneumonia. They are followed by facial paralysis, diplopia, external ophthalmoplegia, and paresthesia of the arms and trunk.

Fisher, M. An unusual variant of idiopathic polyneuritis (syndrome of ophthalmoplegia, ataxia and areflexia). *N. Engl. J. Med.,* 1956, 255:57-65.

Miller Fisher syndrome. See *Fisher syndrome.*

fissure in ano. See *Allingham ulcer.*

FITZ, REGINALD HEBER (American physician, 1843-1913)

Fitz syndrome. Synonym: *acute hemorrhagic pancreatitis.*

A series of symptoms seen in acute pancreatitis, consisting of sudden, severe attacks of epigastric pain, in most cases followed by nausea, vomiting, tenderness, and tympanites. There is prostration, frequent collapse, low grade-fever, and a feeble pulse. Constipation for several days is the rule, but diarrhea sometimes occurs.

Fitz, R. H. Acute pancreatitis. A consideration of pancreatic hemorrhage, hemorrhagic, suppurative, and gangrenous pancreatitis, and of disseminated fat-necrosis. *Boston Med. S. J.,* 1889, 181-7; 205-7; 299-35.

FITZ-HUGH, THOMAS, JR. (American physician, born 1894)

Fitz-Hugh and Curtis syndrome. See *Fitz-Hugh syndrome.*

Fitz-Hugh syndrome. Synonyms: *Fitz-Hugh and Curtis syndrome, Stojano subcostal syndrome, Stojano syndrome, gonococcal perihepatitis, gonococcal peritonitis of the upper abdomen, subcostal syndrome.*

Gonococcal peritonitis of the upper abdomen in persons with a history of gonorrheal infection. Affected patients most commonly have a sudden onset of sharp pain in the right upper quadrant of the abdomen. The pain is pleuritic in nature and may be referred to the right shoulder, bilateral involvement being uncommon. An antecedent history of pelvic inflammatory disease is common, but a latent or subclinical gonoccocal infection may have been present. In advanced stages, there may be violin-string adhesions between the anterior surface of the liver and the anterior abdominal wall.

Fitz-Hugh, T., Jr. Acute gonococcic peritonitis of the right upper quadrant in women. *JAMA,* 1934, 102:2094-6. Curtis, A. H. A cause of adhesions in the right upper quadrant. *JAMA,* 1930, 94:1221-2. Stojano, C. La reacción frenica en ginecologia. *Sem. Med. B. Aires,* 1920, 27:243-8.

FITZSIMMONS, J. S. (British physician)

Fitzsimmons syndrome. A familial syndrome, transmsitted as an X-linked trait, characterized by mental retardation, spasticity in the lower limbs (spastic paraplegia), pes cavus, bilateral foot deformity with abnormal gait, and hyperkeratosis palmaris et plantaris.

Fitzsimmons, J. S., *et al.* Four brothers with mental retardation, spastic paraplegia and palmoplantar hyperkeratosis. A new syndrome? *Clin. Genet.,* 1983, 23:329-35.

five-day fever. See *Werner-His disease, under Werner, Heinrich.*

five-year burp syndrome. Recurrent gastrointestinal disorders in which burping is the most common symptom.

Wright, J. T. The five-year burp syndrome. *Lancet,* 1986, 1:1320.

FJN. See *familial juvenile nephrophthisis.*

FKS (Foster Kennedy syndrome). See *Kennedy syndrome.*

FLAITZ, KATHERINE (American physician)

Atkin-Flaitz syndrome. See *under Atkin.*

FLAJANI, GIUSEPPE (Italian physician, 1741-1808)

Flajani-Basedow syndrome. See *Basedow disease.*

flat chest syndrome. See *straight back syndrome.*

FLATAU, EDWARD (Polish physician, 1869-1932)
Redlich-Flatau syndrome. See *Redlich encephalitis.*
FLECK, L. (Polish physician)
Fleck syndrome. Synonym: *leukergy.*

The aggregation of leukocytes into cytologically similar groups in pregnancy and in fever, inflammation, epilepsy, anaphylactic shock, cerebral edema, cerebrovascular disorders, and other pathological conditions.

Fleck, L. Technika i tematyka leukergii. *Pol. Tygod. Lek.*, 1951, 6:866-9.

FLEGEL, H. (German physician)
Flegel disease. Synonym: *hyperkeratosis lenticularis perstans (HLP).*

A rare skin disease, probably transmitted as an autosomal dominant trait, characterized by inflammatory keratotic papules of the extremities.

Flegel, H. Hyperkaratosis lenticularis perstans. *Hautarzt*, 1958, 9:362.

FLEISCHER, BRUNO (German ophthalmologist, 1848-1904)
Fleischer dystrophy (1). Synonyms: *cornea verticillata, vortex corneal dystrophy.*

Corneal dystrophy characterized by multiple brown punctate lesions on Bowman's membrane, spreading toward the center of the cornea in a whirlpool-like manner.

Fleischer, B. Über eine eigenartige bisher nicht bekannte Hornhauttrübung (ein Hinweis auf die normale Struktur der Hornhout?). *Graefes Arch. Ophth.*, 1910, 77:136-40.

Fleischer dystrophy (2). See *Groenouw dystrophy (1).*
Fleischer line. See *Fleischer ring.*
Fleischer ring. Synonym: *Fleischer line.*

A pigmented greenish or brownish thin line forming an incomplete ring around the base of the cone of the cornea in keratoconus, probably due to deposits of iron (hemosiderin). Pathologically, the Fleischer ring is similar to the Stocker line and the Hudson-Stahl ring. A tear in the Bowman membrane is the suspected cause of all three conditions.

Fleischer, B. Über Keratokonus und eigenartige Pigmentbildung in der Kornea. *Münch. Med. Wschr.*, 1906, 53:625-6.

Fleischer-Strümpell ring. See *Kayser-Fleischer ring, under Kayser, Bernhard.*
Groenouw-Fleischer dystrophy. See *Groenouw dystrophy (1).*
Kayser-Fleischer ring. See *under Kayser, Bernhard.*
FLEISCHNER, FELIX (German physician, born 1893)
Fleischner syndrome. Synonyms: *disklike atelectasis, horizontal linear atelectasis, lamelliform atelectatic foci, linear atelectasis, platelike atelectasis, reflex atelectasis.*

A radiological symptom seen in various intra-thoracic and intra-abdominal diseases, consisting of the appearance over the hypotonic diaphragm of linear shadows corresponding to areas of atelectasis. The atelectatic areas are discoid in form and are located in the lower third of one or both lungs.

Fleischner, F. Plattenförmige Atelektasen in den Unterlappen der Lunge. *Fortsch. Geb. Röntgen.*, 1936, 54:315-21.

Thiemann-Fleischner disease. See *Thiemann syndrome.*
FLEISHER, THOMAS A. (American physician)
Fleisher syndrome. Synonym: *growth hormone deficiency-hypogammaglobulinemia syndrome.*

A familial syndrome, transmitted as an X-linked trait, characterized by growth hormone and immunological deficiencies, with absent specific antibody production in vivo and impaired immunoglobulin production in vitro, in association with a lack of B lymphocytes. Clinical features include short stature, delayed bone maturation, retarded puberty, and recurrent respiratory infections.

Fleisher, T. A., *et al.* X-linked hypogammaglobulinemia and isolated growth hormone deficiency. *N. Engl. J. Med.*, 1980, 302:1329-34.

flexed fingers. See *camptodactyly syndrome.*
flexion fracture of the spine. See *Chance fracture.*
flexion spasm. See *West syndrome.*

FLEXNER, SIMON (American physician, 1863-1946)
Flexner disease. See *Flexner dysentery.*
Flexner dysentery. Synonyms: *Flexner disease, bacillary dysentery, Japanese disease, Shigella dysentery.*

A gastrointestinal disorder marked by intestinal inflammation and attended by pain and frequent stools, caused by infection with bacteria of the genus *Shigella* (usually *S. sonnei* and *S. dysenteriae*), and transmitted by food and water contaminated by fecal material. The disease is characterized by the sudden onset of abdominal cramps, fever, and diarrhea with mucus and blood in the stools. The lesions generally are confined to the terminal ileum and colon, and intestinal ulcers are usually present.

Flexner, S. On the etiology of tropical dysentery. *Bull. Johns Hopkins Hosp.*, 1900, 11:231-42.

flexura lienalis syndrome. See *splenic flexure syndrome.*
FLINT, AUSTIN (American physician, 1812-1886)
Austin Flint murmur. See *Flint murmur.*
Flint murmur. Synonym: *Austin Flint murmur.*

An atypical, rumbling, diastolic murmur starting in mid-diastole or presystole, or both, often noted in severe aortic insufficiency.

Flint, A. On cardiac murmurs. *Am. J. Med. Sc.*, 1862, 44:29-54.

Floating Harbor syndrome. A congenital syndrome characterized by growth retardation, language development retardation with aphasia, pseudoarthrosislike anomaly of the clavicle, short neck, small hands with short stubby fingers, clinodactyly, incurved toes, limited extension of elbows, and triangular face with wide forehead, hypoplastic maxilla, micrognathia, mandibular overbite, large nose, broad nasal base, deep-set eyes, narrow palate, hypertrophy of the maxillary alveolar ridge, and low-set posteriorly-rotated ears. The intelligence appears to be normal. The syndrome was named after the Boston Floating Harbor General Hospital.

Leisti, J., *et al.* The Floating-Harbor syndrome. *Birth Defects*, 1975, 11(5):305.

floppy baby syndrome. See *floppy infant syndrome.*
floppy eyelid syndrome. A syndrome of a loose upper eyelid that readily everts on elevating the lid, a soft rubbery tarsus that can be folded on itself, and a diffuse papillary conjunctivitis. The syndrome is most commonly observed in obese persons.

Culbertson, W. W., & Ostler, H. B. The floppy eyelid syndrome. *Am. J. Ophth.*, 1981, 92:568-75.

floppy infant syndrome. Synonym: *floppy baby syndrome.*

A condition in newborn and young infants characterized by hypotonia and muscle weakness. Lethargy, diminished suck, weakness, feeble cry, and diminished spontaneous activity with loss of head control are the principal symptoms. The syndrome may occur after maternal use of benzodiazepines in pregnancy, in infantile botulism, in neonatal radiculoneuropathy, and as a complication of other diseases.

Dubowitz, V. "The floppy infant." *Clinics in developmental medicine*. No. 31. London, Heinemann Medical, 1969.
Gilmartin, R. C., *et al.* Familial fatal neonatal radiculoneuropathy. *Birth Defects,* 1977, 13(3B):95-101.

floppy valve syndrome. See *mitral valve prolapse syndrome.*

floriform cataract. See *Koby cataract.*

floury cornea. See *Vogt cornea, under Vogt, Alfred.*

flowing hyperostosis. See *Léri syndrome (1).*

flowing periostitis. See *Léri syndrome (1).*

fluorosis. See *Spira disease.*

flush syndrome. See *carcinoid syndrome.*

FLYNN, P. (American physician)

Flynn-Aird syndrome. A familial neuroectodermal syndrome, transmitted as an autosomal dominant trait, characterized by abnormalities of the nervous system, eyes, ears, skin, teeth, and bones. Progressive sensorineural deafness, cataracts, retinitis pigmentosa, myopia, ataxia, peripheral neuritis, mental deficiency, high cerebrospinal fluid protein levels, skin ulcers and atrophy, alopecia, dental caries, joint stiffness, and cystic bone changes are the principal symptoms.

Flynn, P., & Aird, R. B. A neuroectodermal syndrome of dominant inheritance. *J. Neurol. Sc.,* 1965, 2:161-82.

FMD. See *frontometaphyseal dysplasia.*

FMF (familial Mediterranean fever). See *Reimann periodic disease.*

FMS (fibromyalgia syndrome). See *fibrositis-fibromyalgia syndrome.*

focal dermal hypoplasia (FDH) syndrome. See *Goltz syndrome.*

focal dilatation of intrahepatic bile ducts. See *Caroli syndrome (2).*

focal embolic nephritis. See *Löhlein nephritis.*

focal epilepsy. See *Jackson epilepsy.*

focal epithelial hyperplasia. See *Heck disease.*

focal facial dermal dysplasia. See *Brauer syndrome, under Brauer, August.*

focal glomerulonephritis. See *Löhlein nephritis.*

focal thrombotic glomerulonephritis. See *Löhlein nephritis.*

foetal alcohol syndrome. See *fetal alcohol syndrome.*

foetal warfarin syndrome. See *fetal warfarin syndrome.*

FOIX, CHARLES (French physician, 1882-1927)

Foix syndrome. See *cavernous sinus syndrome.*

Foix-Alajouanine syndrome. Synonyms: *angiodysgenesis spinalis, angiodysgenetic myelomalacia, angiohypertrophic central myelitis, cavernous angioma of the spinal cord, myelitis necroticans, myelopathia necroticans, subacute necrotizing myelitis.*

A disease of the spinal cord characterized by softening of the gray matter with obliterative sclerosis of the small vessels and thickening of the walls of the large vessels supplying the spinal cord. Degeneration of the parenchyma is secondary to ischemia and causes paraplegia and amyotrophy. The symptoms include spasticity of the lower extremities, dissociated sensory changes, and loss of sphincter control. Death takes place within 1 to 2 years.

Foix, C., & Alajouanine, T. La myélite nécrotique subaiguë. Myélite centrale angéio-hypertrophique à évolution progressive. Paraplégie amyotrophique lentement ascendante, d'abord spasmodique, puis flasque. *Rev. Neur., Paris,* 1926, 2:1-42.

Foix-Chavany syndrome. See *Foix-Chavany-Marie syndrome.*

Foix-Chavany-Marie syndrome (FCMS). Synonyms: *Foix-Chavany syndrome, bilateral anterior opercular syndrome.*

Facio-pharyngo-glosso-mastictory diplegia resulting from bilateral anterior opercular infarction. The symptoms include linguo-bucco-facial apraxia with facial weakness, drooling, palatal and lingual speech disorders, masticatory problems, and jaw jerks.

Foix, C., Chavany, J. A., & Marie, J. Diplégie facio-linguo-masticatrice d'origine sous-corticale sans paralysie des membres (contribution à l'étude de la localisation des centres de la face et du membre supérieur). *Rev. Neur., Paris,* 1926, 33:214-9.

Schilder-Foix disease. See *under Schilder.*

folded lung. See *Blesovsky syndrome.*

follicular lymphadenopathy with splenomegaly. See *Brill-Symmers syndrome.*

follicular lymphoma. See *Brill-Symmers syndrome.*

follicular mucinosis. See *Pinkus disease, under Pinkus, Hermann Karl Benno.*

follicular reticulosis. See *Brill-Symmers syndrome.*

folliculitis barbae. See *Alibert disease (3).*

folliculitis decalvans. See *Little syndrome, under Little, Ernest Gordon Graham.*

folliculitis decalvans et atrophicans. See *Little syndrome, under Little, Ernest Gordon Graham.*

folliculitis pustulosa eosinophilica. See *Ofuji syndrome.*

FOLLING, IVAR ASBJORN (Norwegian physiologist, born 1888)

Følling syndrome. See *phenylketonuria.*

FONG, EDWARD EVERETT (American physician, born 1912)

Fong syndrome. See *nail-patella syndrome.*

Österreicher-Fong syndrome. See *nail-patella syndrome.*

FOP. See *fibrodysplasia ossificans progressiva.*

foramen of Bochdalek hernia. See *Bochdalek hernia.*

FORBES, ANNE P. (American physician)

Forbes-Albright syndrome. See *amenorrhea-galactorrhea syndrome.*

FORBES, GILBERT BURNETT (American physician, born 1915)

Forbes disease. See *glycogen storage disease III.*

FORDYCE, JOHN ADDISON (American physician, 1858-1925)

Brooke-Fordyce disease. See *Brooke epithelioma.*

Brooke-Fordyce trichoepithelioma. See *Brooke epithelioma.*

Fordyce angiokeratoma. See *Fordyce lesion.*

Fordyce disease. Synonyms: *Fordyce spots, pseudocolloid of the lips.*

Ectopic sebaceous glands found on the lips and gums and in the mucosa of the cheeks in the form of yellowish-white milia.

Fordyce, J. A peculiar affection of the mucous membrane of the lips and the oral cavity. *J. Cutan. Dis., N. Y.,* 1896, 14:413-9.

Fordyce lesion. Synonyms: *Fordyce angiokeratoma, angiokeratoma scrotii, phlebectasia of the scrotum.*

A disorder, normally observed in patients over 50 years of age, characterized by multiple, spherical, reddish to black, elevated lesions rarely over 4 mm in diameter, which usually follow the course of the scrotal veins. The lesions are divided by irregular septa into cavernous spaces filled with blood.

Fordyce, J. A. Angiokeratoma of the scrotum. *Tr. Am. Derm. Assoc,* 1896:5-11.

Fordyce spots. See *Fordyce disease.*

Fox-Fordyce disease. See *under Fox, George Henry.*

forefoot eczema. See *wet and dry foot syndrome.*

foreign body airway obstruction. See *cafe coronary syndrome.*

FORESTIER, JACQUES (French physician, born 1890)

Forestier syndrome (1). Synonyms: *Forestier-Certonciny syndrome, anarthritic rheumatoid disease, humeroscapular periarthrosis, inflammatory rhizomelic rheumatism, periextra-articular rheumatism, polymyalgia rheumatica (PMR), rhizomelic pseudopolyarthritis, senile gout, senile rheumatic gout.*

A disease occurring predominantly in older people and affecting women twice as often as men. Onset may be sudden or gradual; the initial symptoms are usually generalized and include malaise, fatigue, fever, morning stiffness, loss of weight, anorexia, and emotional lability. Myalgia, the dominant symptom, is usually localized in the neck and shoulder muscles, although the pelvic girdle and other muscles may be involved. Elevated erythrocyte sedimentation rate is the principal hematological feature. Nonhemolytic anemia with or without other clinical symptoms may occur. Some patients have an associated temporal arteritis with headache and blindness. Biopsy of asymptomatic temporal arteries may show giant cell arteritis-like changes. Joint scintigram usually shows synovitis. A rapid response to corticosteroid therapy is the positive diagnostic criterion. The condition is considered by some to be a variant or prodromal phase of Horton disease (1). Other writers consider this syndrome an independent entity, possibly linked to rheumatoid arthritis. The etiology is unknown. See also *fibrositis-fibromyalgia syndrome.*

Forestier, J., & Certonciny. Pseudopolyarthrite rhizomelique. *Rev. Rhum., Paris,* 1953, 20:854-62.

Forestier syndrome (2). Synonyms: *Forestier and Rotés-Querol syndrome, ankylosing hyperostosis, ankylosing vertebral hyperostosis, diffuse idiopathic skeletal hyperostosis (DISH), senile ankylosing hyperostosis of the spine, spondylorheostosis, spondylosis hyperostotica, vertebral ankylosing hyperostosis.*

An ankylosing disease of the spine in middle-aged and elderly persons, characterized by spinal rigidity and the presence of hyperostoses, mainly from the dorsal region, but sometimes extending from the upper part of the sacrum. The symptoms include aching spinal stiffness with relative preservation of function. Elbow and heel pain and dysphagia may be associated. Typical radiographic findings include ossification of the ligaments, periarticular osteophytosis, and bone formation at sites of spinal and extraspinal ligaments and tendon attachments, mainly in the pelvis, calcaneus, tarsal bones, ulnar olecranon, and patella.

Forestier, J., & Rotés-Querol, J. Senile ankylosing hyperostosis of the spine. *Ann. Rheum. Dis., London,* 1950, 9:321-30.

Forestier and Rotés-Querol syndrome. See *Forestier syndrome (2).*

Forestier-Certonciny syndrome. See *Forestier syndrome (1).*

FORMAD, HENRY F. (American physician, 1847-1892)

Formad kidney. Synonyms: *alcoholic kidney, pig-backed kidney.*

An enlarged and deformed kidney seen in alcoholics.

Formad, H. F. The "pig-backed" or alcoholic kidney of drunkards. A contribution to the post-mortem diagnosis of alcoholism. *Tr. Assoc. Am. Phys., Philadelphia,* 1886, 1:225-36.

forme fruste of Hurler syndrome. See *mucopolysaccharidosis I-S.*

formicophilia. See *His syndrome.*

FORNEY, WILLIAM R. (American physician)

Forney-Robinson-Pascoe syndrome. A familial syndrome, transmitted as an autosomal dominant trait, characterized by mitral insufficiency, conductive deafness due to malformation of the stapes, bone abnormalities consisting of fusion of cervical vertebrae and carpal bones, freckles of the face and iris, and short stature.

Forney, W. R., Robinson, S. J., & Pascoe, D. J. Congenital heart disease, deafness and skeletal malformations: A new syndrome? *J. Pediat.,* 1968, 68:14-26.

FORSIUS, HENRIK (Finnish physician)

Forsius-Eriksson ocular albinism. See *Forsius-Eriksson syndrome.*

Forsius-Eriksson syndrome. Synonyms: *Åland disease, Forsius-Eriksson ocular albinism.*

A familial form of ocular albinism, transmitted as an X-linked trait, associated with foveal hypoplasia, visual disorders, nystagmus, myopia, astigmatism, and color blindness. Female carriers exhibit slight color discrimination disorders and nystagmus. The syndrome was first observed on the Åland Islands in the Sea of Bothnia (the Baltic Sea).

Forsius, H., & Eriksson, A. W. Ein neues Augensyndrom mit X-chromosomaler Transmission. Eine Sippe mit Fundusalbinismus, Foveahypoplasie, Nystagmus, Myopie, Astigmatismus und Dyschromatopsie. *Klin. Mbl. Augenheilk.,* 1964, 144:447-57.

FORSSELL, JARL (Finnish physician, 1912-1964)

Forssell syndrome. Synonyms: *nephrogenic erythrocytosis, nephrogenic polycythemia.*

Polycythemia associated with various types of kidney diseases.

Forssell, J. Polycytemi vid hypernefrom. *Nordisk Med.,* 1946, 30:1415-9.

FORSSMAN, HANS AXEL (Swedish physician, born 1912)

Börjeson-Forssman-Lehmann syndrome (BFL, BFLS). See *Börjeson syndrome.*

FÖRSTER, CARL FRIEDRICH RICHARD (German ophthalmologist, 1825-1902)

Förster choroiditis. See *Förster disease.*

Förster disease. Synonyms: *Förster choroiditis, areolar central choroiditis, areolar choroiditis.*

A form of disseminated choroiditis that is associated with secondary or, occasionally, congenital syphilis, and is characterized by spots which are black at first, but become white in the centers with black rings around them as they enlarge. The lesions progress eccentrically from the macula toward the periphery of the retina.

Walsh, F. B. *Clinical neuro-ophthalmology*. Baltimore, 1957, p. 558.

Fort Bragg fever. See *leptospirosis.*

FOSHAY, LEE (American physician, born 1896)

Foshay-Mollaret syndrome. See *cat scratch disease.*

FOSTER KENNEDY. See KENNEDY, ROBERT FOSTER

FOTHERGILL, JOHN (British physician, 1712-1780)

Fothergill disease. Synonym: *scarlatina anginosa.*

Scarlet fever with severe throat involvement.

*Fothergill, J. *An account of the sore throat attended with ulcers. A disease which hath of late years appeared in this city, and the parts adjacent*. London, Davis, 1748.

FOTHERGILL, SAMUEL (British physician)

dolor faciei fothergilli. See *trigeminal neuralgia.*

Fothergill neuralgia. See *trigeminal neuralgia.*

Fothergill syndrome. See *trigeminal neuralgia.*

FOTOPOULOS, D. (Physician in Germany)

Fotopoulos syndrome. Chronic chorea associated with spinal amyotrophy of the scapular girdle.

Fotopoulos, D. Huntington Chorea und chronisch-progressive Muskelatrophie. *Psychiat. Neur. Med. Psychol., Leipzig,* 1966, 18:63-70.

FOUNTAIN, R. B. (British physician)

Fountain syndrome. A familial syndrome, transmitted as an autosomal recessive trait, characterized by mental retardation, congenital deafness due to inner ear anomalies, broad and stubby hands and feet, hyperkyphosis, generalized seizures, and coarse facies with swelling of the subcutaneous tissue, especially of the cheeks and lips.

Fountain, R. B. Familial bone abnormalities, deaf mutism, mental retardation, and skin granuloma. *Proc. Roy. Soc. Med.,* 1974, 67:878-9. Fryns, J. P., *et al.* Mental retardation, deafness, skeletal abnormalities, and coarse face with full lips: Confirmation of the Fountain syndrome. *Am. J. Med. Genet.,* 1987, 26:551-5.

Fountain syndrome
Fryns, Jean-Pierre, Annemie Dereymaeker, Margot Hoefnagels, & Herman Van den Berghe, *American Journal of Medical Genetics* 26:551-555, 1987. New York: Alan R. Liss, Inc.

FOURNIER, JEAN ALFRED (French physician, 1832-1914)

Fournier disease. Synonyms: *Fournier gangrene, Fournier syndrome, essential gangrene of the scrotum, gangrene of the scrotum, gas gangrene of the scrotum, idiopathic gangrene of the male genitalia, idiopathic gangrene of the scrotum, necrotizing fasciitis of the male genitalia, necrotizing infection of the scrotum, perineal necrotizing fasciitis, spontaneous fulminating gangrene of the scrotum, streptococcal gangrene.*

A spontaneous life-threatening form of fulminating gangrene most commonly confined to the male genitalia. It is characterized by the explosive onset of severe pain, edema, swelling, and inflammatory reaction that occur in persons in apparently good health and in the absense of obvious causes of gangrene. There is a rapid development of necrosis with sloughing of tissues of the scrotum and penis, involving the whole thickness of the scrotal skin, but not the underlying testes. The disorder may occur in persons suffering from diabetes mellitus and streptococal infections.

Orfuss, A. J., & Michaelides, P. Fournier's gangrene. *Arch. Derm., Chicago*, 1964, 90:440-1.

Fournier gangrene. See *Fournier disease.*

Fournier syndrome. See *Fournier disease.*

Fournier tibia. Fusiform thickening and anterior bowing of the tibia in congenital syphilis.

Fournier, J. *La syphilis héréditaire tardive*. Paris, Rueff, 1886.

FOVILLE, ACHILLE LOUIS FRANÇOIS (French physician, 1831-1887)

Foville syndrome. Synonyms: *hemiplegia abducentofacialis alternans, hemiplegia alternans inferior, hemiplegia alternans inferior pontina, peduncular syndrome, pontine tegmentum syndrome.*

A syndrome in which, in addition to loss of outward movement of one eye due to abducens and facial paralysis with contralateral hemiplegia (Millard-Gubler syndrome), there is a loss in the inward movement of the other eye in attempting to look toward the side of the lesion.

Foville, A. Note sur une paralysie peu connue des certains muscles de l'oeil, et la liaison avec quelques points de l'anatomie et la physiologie de la protubérance annulaire. *Bull. Soc. Anat., Paris*, 1858, 33:393-414.

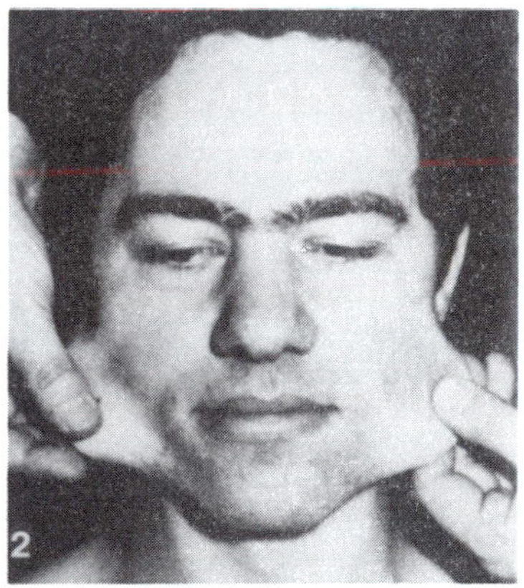

Foville-Wilson syndrome. Impaired lateral convergenceconsisting of paralysis of abduction, preserved convergence, and dissociated monocular nystagmus of theabducted eye in association with disseminated sclerosis.

Foville, A. Note sur une paralysie peu connue des certain muscles de l'oeil, et la liaison avec quelques points de l'anatomie et la physiologie de la protubérance annulaire.

Bull. Soc. Anat., Paris, 1858, 393 33:393-414. Wilson, S. A. Case of disseminated sclerosis, with weakness of each internal rectus and nystagmus, an lateral deviation limited to the outer eye. *Brain*, 1906, 29:298.

FOX, GEORGE HENRY (American physician, 1846-1937)

Fox-Fordyce disease. A lichenoid eruption characterized by small dry papules and pruritus of the axillary region, also affecting the nipple areolae, the pubes, and the sternal region. Most cases are seen in women 13 to 35 years of age. Spontaneous improvement has been noted during pregnancy.

Fox, G. H., & Fordyce, J. A. Two cases of rare papular disease affecting the axillary region. *J. Cutan. Dis.*, 1902, 20:1-5.

FOX, WILLIAM TILBURY (British dermatologist, 1836-1879)

Fox disease. See *epidermolysis bullosa syndrome.*

Fox impetigo. Synonyms: *impetigo contagiosa streptogenes, impetigo parasitaria, impetigo simplex, impetigo vulgaris, porrigo.*

An infectious skin disease of children, marked by superficial vesicular or pustular lesions which become encrusted and exudative and then heal without scarring. It is often associated with acute glomerulonephritis.

Fox, W. T. On impetigo contagiosa, or porrigo. *Brit. Med. J.*, 1864, 1:467-9; 607-9.

FP (Fanconi pancytopenia). See *Fanconi anemia.*

FPS. See *fetal PCB syndrome.*

FRACCARO, M. (Italian physician)

Parenti-Fraccaro syndrome. See *achondrogenesis type I.*

Schmid-Fraccaro syndrome. See *cat eye syndrome.*

FRAENKEL, ALBERT. See FRÄNKEL, ALBERT

fragile X syndrome (FXS). See *chromosome X fragility.*

fragile X-linked mental retardation syndrome. See *chromosome X fragility.*

fragile Xq syndrome. See *chromosome X fragility.*

fragilitas oculi syndrome. A syndrome, transmitted as an autosomal recessive trait, characterized by corneal fragility, keratoglobus, blue sclerae, and joint hyperextensibility. Red hair, buphthalmos, dental defects, spontaneous fractures, and hernia may be associated.

Badtke, G. Über einen eigenartigen Fall von Keratokonus und blauen Skleren bei Geschwistern. *Klin. Mbl. Augenh.*, 1941, 106:585-92. Stein, R., *et al.*, Brittle cornea. A familial trait associated with blue sclera. *Am. J. Ophth.*, 1968, 66:67-9.

fragilitas ossium. See *osteogenesis imperfecta syndrome (recessive & dominant forms).*

FRALEY, ELWIN E. (American physician)

Fraley syndrome. Synonym: *upper calyx renovascular obstruction.*

Intrarenal vascular obstruction of the upper calyceal infundibulum. Hematuria and nephralgia are the main symptoms. Complications may include urinary tract infection and lithiasis.

Fraley, E. E. Vascular obstruction of superior infundibulum causing nephralgia. A new syndrome. *N. Engl. J. Med.*, 1966, 275:1403-9.

frambesia. See *Charlouis disease.*

FRANCESCHETTI, ADOLPHE (Swiss ophthalmologist, 1896-1968)

Bamatter-Franceschetti-Klein-Sierro syndrome. See *geroderma osteodysplastica syndrome.*

Franceschetti disease. Synonym: *fundus flavimaculatus.*

A form of retinal dystrophy characterized by multiple yellow or yellow white lesions of the retina, identical to those seen in tapetoretinal degeneration.

*Franceschetti, A., François, J., & Babel, J. *Les hérédo-dégénérescences chorio-rétiniennes*. Paris, 1963, Vol. 1, pp. 426-36; 441-6.

Franceschetti dystrophy. Synonyms: *Franceschetti-Kaufman dystrophy, Kaufman dystrophy, epithelial erosion syndrome, metaherpetic keratitis.*

A familial form of corneal epithelial dystrophy characterized by recurrent erosions of the cornea that become evident at the age of 4 to 6 years, usually following a minor injury. The symptoms are most severe immediately after awakening. Franceschetti theorized that dystrophic epithelium adheres to the eyelids during sleep and that fragments become detached when the eyes are opened. The frequency of attacks diminishes with age, and after the age of 50 years they become quite rare. The disorder is believed to be transmitted as an autosomal dominant trait.

Franceschetti, A. Hereditäre rezidivierende Erosion der Hornhaut. *Zschr. Augenh.*, 1928, 66:309-16. Kaufman, H. E. Epithelial erosion syndrome: Metaherpetic keratitis. *Am. J. Ophth.*, 1964, 57:983-7.

Franceschetti syndrome (1). Synonyms: *deep punctate dystrophy of the cornea with ichthyosis, dystrophia punctiformis profunda corneae with congenital ichthyosis.*

Dystrophy of the deep layers of the cornea, near the Descemet membrane, in association with ichthyosis. Corneal lesions form minute whitish spots with filaments or rod-shaped formations.

Franceschetti, A., & Maeder, G. Dystrophie profonde de la cornee dans un cas d'ichtyose congenitale. *Bull. Soc. Fr. Opht.*, 1954, 67:146-9.

Franceschetti syndrome (2). See *mandibulofacial dysostosis.*

Franceschetti-Jadassohn syndrome. See *Naegeli syndrome, under Naegeli, Oskar.*

Franceschetti-Kaufman dystrophy. See *Franceschetti dystrophy.*

Franceschetti-Klein-Wildervanck syndrome. See *Wildervanck syndrome (1).*

Franceschetti-Zwahlen syndrome. See *mandibulofacial dysostosis.*

Franceschetti-Zwahlen-Klein syndrome. See *mandibulofacial dysostosis.*

Naegeli-Franceschetti-Jadassohn syndrome. See *Naegeli syndrome, under Naegeli, Oskar.*

Wildervanck-Waardenburg-Francheschetti-Klein syndrome. See *Wildervanck syndrome (1).*

FRANCIS, EDWARD (American physician, 1872-1957)

Francis disease. Synonyms: *Ohara disease, alkali disease, deer fly fever, Pohvant Valley plague, rabbit fever, tularemia, yato-byo.*

An infectious disease caused by *Pasteurella (Francisella) tularensis*, which may be transmitted to man from animals (chiefly rabbits) by contact with diseased or dead animals, bites of infected ticks or deer flies, ingestion of contaminated food or water, or inhalation of aerosolized bacteria. The symptoms consist of the sudden onset of chills, fever, pain (including headache), prostration, vomiting, and sweating. The **ulceroglandular form**, the most common type, is characterized by a papule at the site of inoculation, which becomes necrotic, forming a depressed lesion with a central ulcer surrounded by an indurated border. Later, the regional lymph nodes become affected and may break down. Less common forms include the **glandular variant**, in which the lymph nodes are affected but there is no local lesion, and the **oculoglandular variant**, in which there is ulceration of the conjunctiva, swelling of the eyelids, and involvement of the lymph nodes. In the **Japanese form (Ohara disease, yato-byo)**, the primary lesion is often a small ulcer of the thumb or ocular and tonsillar lesions. The oculoglandular and glandular forms appear to occur mostly in Japan.

Francis, E. Tularemia. *Pub. Health Rep., Washington, D. C.,*, 1921, 36:1731-53. Ohara, S. Studies on yato-byo (Ohara's disease, tularemia in Japan). *Jpn. J. Exp. Med.*, 1954, 24:69-79; 1955, 25:7014.

FRANÇOIS, JULES (Belgian ophthalmologist)

François dyscephalia. See *Hallermann-Streiff syndrome.*

François dyscephalic syndrome. See *Hallermann-Streiff syndrome.*

François dystrophy (1). Synonyms: *central cloudy dystrophy, cloudy central corneal dystrophy.*

A familial form of parenchymatous, bilateral dystrophy of the central third of the cornea, characterized by small, grayish snowflakelike patches covering the pupillary areas. The lesions show no definite structure or limits, being more dense, thick, and numerous near the Descemet membrane and becoming fewer toward the anterior surface and toward the periphery. They may occupy all the layers of the parenchyma up to the Bowman membrane, or they may be limited to the deep layers.

François, J. Une nouvelle dystrophie hérédo-familiare de la cornée. *J. Génét. Hum.*, 1956, 5:189-96.

François dystrophy (2). Synonym: *speckled corneal dystrophy.*

Corneal dystrophy characterized by minute punctate opacities found in all layers of the cornea, which may be detected with the use of slit lamp. The lesions vary in size, form, and degree of opacity, but are identical in both eyes. The anterior limiting membranes are always intact. The disorder is congenital and nonprogressive, and appears to be transmitted as an autosomal dominant trait.

François, J. *Heredity in ophthalmology*. St. Louis, Mosby, 1961, pp. 310-2.

François syndrome (1). Synonym: *Jules François syndrome.*

A syndrome of dyscephaly, skin atrophy, dental abnormalities, nanism, hypotrichosis, microphthalmia, and congenital cataract.

François, J. Syndrome with congenital cataract. *Am. J. Ophth.*, 1961, 52:207-38.

François syndrome (2). Synonyms: *Jules François syndrome, dermochondrocorneal dystrophy, dystrophia dermochondrocornealis familiaris, idiopathic carpotarsal osteolysis of François syndrome.*

A familial syndrome, transmitted as an autosomal recessive trait, characterized by corneal dystrophy with minute punctate opacities in all layers, osteochondral dystrophy of the extremities, and cutaneous xanthomas. Osseous changes are detectable during the first decade and consist of defective endochondral ossification with progressive carpotarsal osteolysis, shortening of the wrist and ankle, ulnar deviation with micromelia, clawhand, and short pes cavus. Nephropathy and proteinuria may occur.

François, J. Dystrophie dermo-chondro-cornéenne familiale. *Ann. Ocul., Paris*, 1949, 182:409-42.

Hallermann-Streiff-François syndrome. See *Hallermann-Streiff syndrome.*

idiopathic carpotarsal osteolysis of François syndrome. See *François syndrome (2).*

Jules François syndrome. See *François syndrome (1 and 2).*

FRANKE, GUSTAV (German physician, born 1878)

Franke syndrome. See *Franke triad.*

Franke triad. Synonym: *Franke syndrome.*

A triad of palatal abnormalities, deviation of the nasal septum, and enlarged adenoids. Associated with the triad may be respiration through the mouth, dry lips, and susceptibility to infection.

Franke, G. *Über Wachstum und Verbildungen des Kiefers und der Nasenscheidewand auf Grund vergleichender Kiefer-Messungen und experimenteller Untersuchungen über Knochenwachstum*. Leipzig, Kabitzsch, 1921.

FRÄNKEL (FRAENKEL), ALBERT (German physician, 1848-1916)

Fränkel disease. Synonym: *indurative pneumonia.*

Chronic lobar pneumonia with hardening of the fibrous exudate and proliferation of the interstitial tissue. See also *Hamman-Rich syndrome.*

Fraenkel, A. Klinische und anatomische Mitteilungen über indurative Lungenentzündung. *Deut. Med. Wschr.*, 1895, 21:153-6; 177-80; 190-5.

FRANKL-HOCHWART, LOTHAR, VON (Austrian physician, 1862-1914)

Frankl-Hochwart disease. See *Frankl-Hochwart syndrome (1).*

Frankl-Hochwart syndrome (1). Synonyms: *Frankl-Hochwart disease, polyneuritis cerebralis menieriformis, polyneuritis cranialis menieriformis.*

Cochlear, vestibular, facial, and trigeminal lesions in syphilis, reportedly described by Frankl-Hochwart.

Frankl-Hochwart syndrome (2). Synonym: *pineal-neurologic-ophthalmic syndrome.*

A syndrome of limitation of the upward gaze, papilledema, concentric field constriction, bilateral deafness, ataxia, and hypopituitarism.

*Tassman. *The eye manifestations of internal diseases.* St. Louis, Mosby, 1951.

FRANKLIN, E. C. (American physician)

Franklin disease. See *under heavy chain disease.*

FRANZ, CARL AUGUST OTTO (German physician, born 1870)

Franz syndrome. Cessation of thrill after ligation of the vein proximal to an arteriovenous fistula.

Franz, C. A. Klinische und experimentelle Beiträge betreffend das Aneurysma arteriovenosum. *Arch. Klin. Chir., Berlin.*, 1905, 75:572-622.

FRASER, F. CLARKE (Canadian physician)

Hunter-Fraser syndrome. See *under Hunter, Alasdair G. W.*

FRASER, G. R. (British geneticist)

Fraser syndrome. Synonyms: *cryptophthalmos syndrome, cryptophthalmos-syndactyly syndrome, cyclopism.*

An association of cryptophthalmos with a wide range of congenital abnormalities, consisting mostly of orofacial defects (cleft lip, cleft palate, hypoplastic notched nares, malformed ears, high-arched palate, hypertelorism, hair growth on the lateral forehead extending to the lateral eyebrow), laryngeal stenosis, syndactyly, decreased number of digits, renal dysgenesis, and hypogenitalism (hypospadias, cryptorchism, bicornuate uterus, vaginal atresia). Less commonly occurring defects may include lacrimal duct abnormalities, widely spaced nipples, umbilical anomaly, primitive mesentery, small bowel, malformed fallopian tubes, fusion of the labia, enlargement of the clitoris, and other anomalies. About half of the affected patients are stillborn. The syndrome is believed to be transmitted as an autosomal recessive trait.

Fraser, G. R. Our genetical "load." A review of some aspects of genetical variation. *Ann. Hum. Genet.*, 1962, 25:387-415. Zehender, W. Eine Missgeburt mit hautüberwachsenen Augen oder Kryptophthalmus. *Klin. Monatsbl. Augenheilkd.*, 1872, 10:225-34.

ffra(X) (fragile-X syndrome). See *chromosome X fragility*.

fra(X)(q27) syndrome. See *chromosome X fragility*.

fra(X)(q27-28) syndrome. See *chromosome X fragility*.

fra(X)(q28) chromosome syndrome. See *chromosome X fragility*.

FREDERICK

Frederick syndrome. Auricular fibrillation associated with complete atrioventricular block.

Taikh, Ia. I. *et al.* Dva sluchaia ostro razvivshegosia sindroma Frederika. *Ter. Arkh., Moskva*, 1964, 36(7):109-11.

FREEMAN, E. A. (British orthopedic surgeon)

Freeman-Sheldon syndrome (FSS). Synonyms: *craniocarpotarsal dysplasia, craniocarpotarsal dystrophy, whistling face syndrome (WFS), whistling face-windmill vane hand syndrome, windmill-vane fingers syndrome.*

An association of cranial, hand, and foot malformations characterized chiefly by a stiff, immobile, flat midface, long philtrum, hypertelorism, sunken eyes, and small puckered mouth as in whistling. The skull is usually small and compressed frontodorsally but broadened in the frontal plane. Ocular symptoms include blepharoptosis, convergent strabismus, epicanthus, and occasional antimongoloid palpebral slant. Musculoskeletal defects consist of growth retardation, flexion contractures of the fingers (the thumbs being especially involved), ulnar deviation of the fingers, and talipes equinovarus. A small nose with narrow nostrils, scoliosis, spina bifida occulta, inguinal hernia, high-arched palate, and microglossia are the associated abnormalities. Most cases are sporadic, but trans-

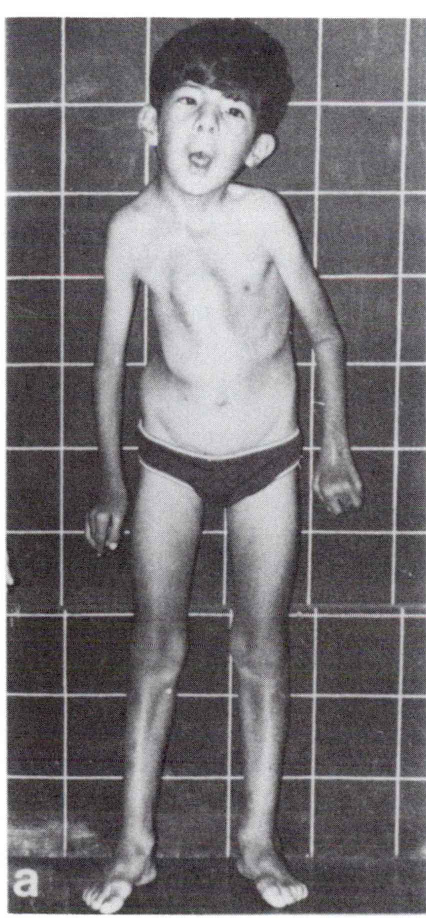

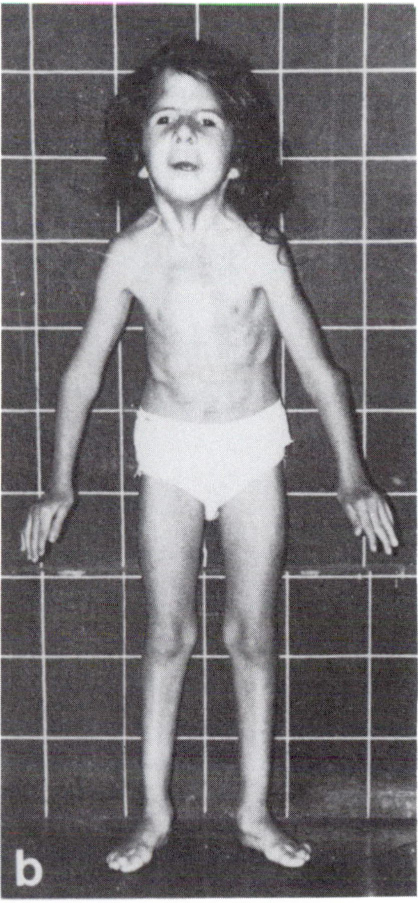

Freeman-Sheldon syndrome
Sanchez, Jose Maria & Catalina Patrick Kaminker, *American Journal of Medical Genetics*, 25:507-511, 1986, New York: Alan R. Liss, Inc.

mission as an autosomal dominant trait is suspected in some instances. See also *windmill-vane camptodactyly/ichthyosis syndrome.*

Freeman, E. A., & Sheldon, J. H. Cranio-carpo-tarsal dystrophy. An undescribed congenital malformation. *Arch. Dis. Child.*, 1938, 13:277-83.

FREI, WILHELM SIEGMUND (German physician, 1885-1943)

Frei bubo. See *Durand-Nicolas-Favre disease, under Durand, J.*

Frei disease. See *Durand-Nicolas-Favre disease, under Durand, J.*

FREIBERG, ALBERT HENRY (American physician, 1874-1947)

Freiberg infraction. See *Köhler disease (2).*

Freiberg-Köhler disease. See *Köhler disease (2).*

FREIRE-MAIA, N. (Brazilian physician)

Freire-Maia syndrome. Synonym: *odontotrichomelic syndrome.*

A tetramelic deficiency syndrome, transmitted as an autosomal recessive trait, marked by shortness of the limbs, hypotrichosis, deformed auricles, abnormal dentition, hypoplastic nipples and areolae, hypoplastic nails, hypogonadism, thyroid enlargement, growth retardation, cleft lip, mental retardation, and EEG and ECG abnormalities. Disorders of amino acid metabolism (tyrosine and/or tryptophan) are the principal biochemical features.

Freire-Maia, N. A newly recognized genetic syndrome of tetramelic deficiencies, ectodermal dysplasia, deformed ears, and other abnormalities. *Am. J. Hum. Genet.*, 1970, 22:370-7.

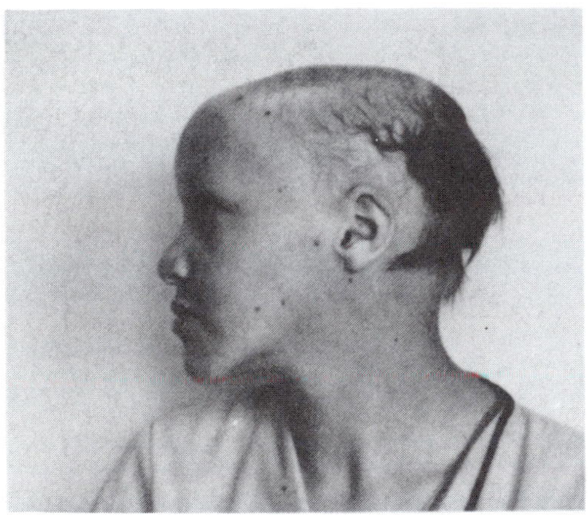

Freire-Maia syndrome
Freire-Maia, N. & M. Pinheiro: Selected Conditions with Ectodermal Dysplasia. In Salinas, C.F., J.M. Opitz, N.W. Paul (eds.): "Recent Advances in Ectodermal Dysplasias." New York: Alan R. Liss, Inc. for the March of Dimes Birth Defects Foundation BD:OAS 24(2):109-121, 1988, with permission.

FREMEREY-DOHNA, H. (German physician)

Ullrich and Fremerey-Dohna syndrome. See *Hallermann-Streiff syndrome.*

FRENKEL, HENRI (French ophthalmologist, 1864-1934)

Frenkel syndrome. Synonyms: *anterior segment traumatic syndrome, ocular contusion syndrome.*

A post-traumatic syndrome following injury of the anterior segment of the eye and consisting of D-shaped mydriasis and iridoplegia, subluxation of the lens, iridodialysis, hyphema, punctate opacities, retrolental pigment particles, and peripheral pigment disorders resembling atypical retinitis pigmentosa.

Frenkel, H. Sur la valeur médico-légale du syndrome traumatique du segment antérieur. *Arch. Opht., Paris*, 1931, 48:5-27.

frequency incontinence. See *urge incontinence syndrome.*

frequency-urgency syndrome. See *urge incontinence syndrome.*

FRETZIN, D. F.

Solomon-Fretzin-Dewald syndrome. See *epidermal nevus syndrome.*

FREUND, EMANUEL (Austrian physician, born 1869)

Freund dermatitis. Synonyms: *bergamot dermatitis, berloque dermatitis, eau de cologne dermatitis, photodermatitis pigmentaria.*

A form of photodermatitis characterized by erythema, usually appearing at the site of application of toilet water or other cosmetic preparations. Spots of erythema develop into well-defined dark brown pigmented areas after exposure to sunlight. Bergamot oil in cosmetics is believed to be the cause.

Freund, E. Über bisher noch nicht beschriebene künstliche Hautverfärbungen. *Derm. Wschr.*, 1916, 62-63:931-3.

FREUND, WILLIAM ALEXANDER (German physician, 1833-1918)

Freund anomaly. Shortening of the first rib.

*Freund, W. A. *Über primäre Thoraxanomalien.* Berlin, Karger, 1906.

FREY, LUCIE (Polish-born physician in France)

Frey syndrome. Synonyms: *Baillarger syndrome, Dupuy syndrome, Frey-Baillarger syndrome, Madame Frey syndrome, auriculotemporal syndrome, auriculotemporal and chorda tympani syndrome, gustatory sweating, gustatory sweating and flushing, unilateral sweat.*

Gustatory sweating, flushing, and a feeling of warmth in the area of sensory distribution of the auriculotemporal nerve, following an injury or surgery in the vicinity of the parotid gland. The symptoms are triggered by the eating of foods that produce strong salivary stimulation. Misdirected nerve fiber regeneration is considered to be the cause. See also *gustatory lacrimation syndrome.*

Frey, L. Le syndrome du nerf auriculo-temporal. *Rev. Neur., Paris*, 1923, 2:97-104. *Baillarger. Mémoire sur l'obliteration du canal du sténon. *Gaz. Med., Paris*, 1853, 23:194-7. *Dupuy. Sur enlèvement des ganglions gutturaux des nerfs trisplanchniques sur des chevaux. *J. Med. Chir. Pharm.*, 1816, 37:340-50.

Frey-Baillarger syndrome. See *Frey syndrome.*

FRIAS, JAIME L. (Chilean physician)

Opitz-Frias syndrome. See *hypospadias-dysphagia syndrome.*

Rosenbloom-Frias syndrome. See *under Rosenbloom.*

FRIDERICHSEN, CARL (Danish pediatrician, born 1886)

Friderichsen-Waterhouse-Bamatter syndrome. See *Waterhouse-Friderichsen syndrome.*

Marchand-Waterhouse-Friderichsen syndrome. See *Waterhouse-Friderichsen syndrome.*

Waterhouse-Friderichsen syndrome. See *under Waterhouse.*

FRIEDENWALD

Friedenwald syndrome. A condition characterized by lifting of a ptosed eyelid on turning the eyes to the right, opening the mouth wide, and sticking out the tongue.

Beauvieux, J. Quelques aspects de syncinésie oculaires.

Concours Méd., 1952, 74:369-72.

FRIEDLÄNDER, KARL (German physician, 1847-1887)

Friedländer bacillus pneumonia. See *Friedländer pneumonia.*

Friedländer disease. Synonyms: *arteritis obliterans, endarteritis obliterans.*

Narrowing of the small arteries caused by an increase in fibrous tissue of the intima.

*Friedländer, K. Über Arteritis obliterans. *Zbl. Med. Wiss.*, 1876, 14:65-70.

Friedländer pneumonia. Synonyms: *Friedländer bacillus pneumonia, Klebsiella pneumonia.*

Acute infectious pneumonia caused by the Friedländer bacillus *(Klebsiella pneumoniae)* and characterized by the sudden onset of productive cough, pleuritic chest pain, and true rigors. Early prostration, fever, dyspnea, frequent cyanosis, and tachycardia are usually associated. In some instances, there may be early epigastric pain and vomiting. Occasionally, a nondescript upper respiratory infection may precede the acute onset. The sputum is usually grayish-green and blood tinged. Radiographic findings include massive lobar consolidation, lobular involvement, lung abscesses, and parenchymal fibrosis. Rapid destruction of lung tissue with suppuration or fibrosis, followed by necrosis complicate some cases. Other complications may include pleural effusion, pneumothorax, and, somtimes, massive pulmonary gangrene.

Friedlaender, C. Über die Schizomyceten bei der acute fibrosen Pneumonia. *Virchows Arch. Path.*, 1882, 87:319-24.

FRIEDMAN, ARNOLD PHINEAS (American physician, born 1909)

Friedman-Roy syndrome. An association of mental deficiency, strabismus, extensor plantar reflexes, speech defects, and clubfoot, originally observed in a family of six (mother and five children). The mother had internal strabismus and a positive Oppenheim reflex. EEG of the mother and children were similar. The parents of the affected children were cousins.

Friedman, A. P., & Roy, J. E. An unusual familial syndrome. *J. Nerv. Ment. Dis.*, 1944, 99:42-4.

FRIEDMAN, M. (British physician)

Dent-Friedman syndrome. See *under Dent.*

FRIEDMANN, MAX (German physician, 1858-1925)

Friedmann disease. See *Friedmann syndrome (3).*

Friedmann syndrome (1). Synonym: *cerebral vasomotor syndrome.*

A progressive form of subacute post-traumatic encephalitis associated with vasomotor disorders of the brain.

*Friedmann, M. *Zur pathologischen Anatomie der multiplen chronischen Enzephalitis*. Wien, 1883.

Friedmann syndrome (2). Synonym: *pyknolepsy.*

A form of petit mal epilepsy that occurs in children.

*Friedmann, M. *Zur Kenntnis der nichtepileptischen Absenzen im Kindesalter. Vortrag gehalten auf der Naturforscherversammlung*. Karlsrube, 1911.

Friedmann syndrome (3). Synonym: *Friedmann disease.*

Recurrent spastic paralysis in children, resulting from congenital syphilis.

Friedmann, M. Über recidivierende (wahrscheinlich luetische) sogen. spastische Spinalparalyse im Kindesalter. *Deut. Zschr. Nervenh.*, 1893, 3:182-206.

FRIEDREICH, NICOLAUS (German physician, 1826-1882)

abortive type of Friedreich disease. See *Roussy-Lévy syndrome.*

Friedreich ataxia (FA). Synonyms: *Friedreich disease, Friedreich syndrome, ataxia hereditaria, familial ataxia, hereditary ataxia, spinal hereditary ataxia, spinocerebellar heredoataxia.*

A rare spinocerebellar degeneration, appearing before adolescence, which involves the dorsal columns, pyramidal tracts, and, less severely, the cerebellum and medulla oblongata. The symptoms include lack of coordination, dysarthria, nystagmus, diminished or absent tendon reflexes, the Babinski sign, position and vibratory sense disorders, tremor, hypotonia, dysmetria, asynergia, and choreiform movements. Associated disorders may include kyphoscoliosis, pes cavus, hammer toe, and heart enlargement. The syndrome is trasmitted as autosomal recessive trait.

Friedreich, N. Über degenerative Atrophie der spinalen Hinterstränge. *Arch. Path. Anat., Berlin,* 1863, 391-419; 433-59.

Friedreich disease (1). Synonyms: *hereditary essential myoclonus, paramyoclonus multiplex, polyclonia.*

A hereditary disease characterized by sudden, brief muscle contractions affecting mainly the proximal muscles of the extremities, which may be aggravated by excitement and disappear during sleep. The condition is transmitted as an autosomal dominant trait.

Friedreich, N. Paramyoclonus multiplex. *Arch. Path. Anat., Berlin*, 1881, 86:421-30.

Friedreich disease (2). Synonym: *facial hemihypertrophy.*

Facial hemihypertrophy involving the eyelids, cheeks, lips, facial bones, tongue, ears, and tonsils. It may occur alone or in generalized hemihypertrophy.

Abbott, K. H. The vegetative nervous system. In: Baker, A. B., ed. *Clinical neurology.* 1965, Vol. 4, p. 2067.

Friedreich disease (3). See *Friedreich ataxia.*

Friedreich syndrome. See *Friedreich ataxia.*

Friedreich-Erb-Arnold syndrome. See *pachydermoperiostosis syndrome.*

FRIEDRICH, H. (German physician)

Friedrich syndrome. A rare form of aseptic epiphyseal necrosis of the sternal ends of the clavicles.

Friedrich, H. Über ein noch nicht beschriebenes, der Perthesschen Enkrankung analoges Krankheitsbild des sternalen Klavikelendes. *Deut. Zschr. Chir.*, 1924, 187:385-98.

FRIESS

Friess-Pierrou syndrome. Filariasis associated with eosinophilia, adenopathies, and pneumopathies. The condition was originally observed in French soldiers returning from Indochina.

Jalet, J. Le syndrome de Friess-Pierrou (eosinophilie, adénopathie, pneumopathie d'origine filarienne). *J. Radiol. Electr.*, 1954, 35:202-4.

FRIMODT-MÖLLER, C. (Danish physician)

Frimodt-Möller syndrome. See *tropical eosinophilia syndrome.*

FRITSCH, HEINRICH (German physician, 1844-1915)

Fritsch-Asherman syndrome. See *Asherman syndrome.*

FROEHLICH, ALFRED. See FRÖLICH, ALFRED

FROEHLICH, F. See FRÖHLICH, F.

FRÖHLICH (FROEHLICH), ALFRED (Austrian physician, 1871-1953)

Babinski-Fröhlich syndrome. See *Fröhlich syndrome.*

Fröhlich disease. See *Fröhlich syndrome.*

Fröhlich obesity. See *Fröhlich syndrome.*

Fröhlich syndrome. Synonyms: *Babinski-Fröhlich syndrome, Fröhlich disease, Fröhlich obesity, Launois-Cléret syndrome, adiposogenital dystrophy, dystrophia adiposogenitalis, hypophyseal syndrome, hypophyseothalamic syndrome.*

Obesity and sexual infantilism due to lesions of the hypothalamus secondary to neoplasms, especially craniopharyngioma, and to injuries and other diseases of the pituitary gland or perihypothalamic structures. Obesity or the breast region, lower abdomen, and genitalia, associated with a small penis embedded in adipose tissue, cryptorchism, beardless face, and high-pitched voice after adolescence give males a feminine appearance. In females, there is accumulation of fatty tissue over the underdeveloped mammary glandular tissue and lower abdomen, associated with genital hypoplasia. Ocular changes include hemianopsia, scotoma, faulty dark adaptation, and papilledema. See also *Burnier syndrome,* and *Lorain-Levi syndrome.*

Fröhlich, A. Ein Fall von Tumor der Hypophysis cerebri ohne Akromegalie. *Wien. Klin. Rdschr.*, 1901, 15:883-6; 906-8. Babinski, J. Tumeur du corps pituitaire sans acromégalie et avec arrët de développement des organes génitaux. *Rev. Neur., Paris*, 1900, 8:531-5. Launois, P. E., & Cléret, M. Le syndrome hypophysaire adiposogénital. *Gaz. Hôp. Paris*, 1910, 83:57-64; 83-6.

FRÖHLICH (FROEHLICH), F.

Fröhlich syndrome. See *prune belly syndrome.*

FROIN, GEORGES (French physician, born 1874)

Froin syndrome. Synonyms: *Lépine-Froin syndrome, Nonne compression syndrome, Nonne-Froin syndrome, loculation syndrome, spinal block syndrome.*

A disorder of the cerebrospinal fluid marked by xanthochromia, excessive amounts of globulin, and spontaneous massive coagulation of the fluid, resulting from blockage of the spinal canal due to intramedullary tumors, tuberculous meningitis, Pott disease, meningomyelitis, and pachymeningitis.

Froin, G. Inflammations méningées avec réactions chromatique, fibrineuse et cytologique du liquide céphalorachidien. *Gaz. Hôp. Paris*, 1903, 76:1005-6. Nonne, M. Über das Vorkommen von starker Phase I-Reaktion bein fehlender Lymphozytose bei 6 Fällen von Rückenmarkstumor. *Deut. Zschr. Nervenh.*, 1910, 40:161-7.

Lépine-Froin syndrome. See *Froin syndrome.*

Nonne-Froin syndrome. See *Froin syndrome.*

FROMENT, J. (French physician)

Babinski-Froment syndrome. See *under Babinski.*

FROMMEL, RICHARD JULIUS ERNST (German physician, 1854-1912)

Chiari-Frommel syndrome. See *amenorrhea-galactorrhea syndrome.*

frontal apraxia. See *Hartmann apraxia.*

frontodigital syndrome. See *Greig syndrome.*

frontofacionasal dysostosis. See *frontofacionasal dysplasia.*

frontofacionasal dysplasia. Synonyms: *frontofacionasal dysostosis, frontofacionasal syndrome.*

A familial syndrome, transmitted as an autosomal recessive trait, marked by encephalocele, hypertelorism, midfacial hypoplasia, hypoplasia of the frontal bone, malformed eyes, absent inner eyelashes, irregular S-shaped palpebral fissures, deformed nostrils, hypoplastic nasal wing, cleft lip, clefts of the premaxilla, cleft palate and uvula and, less commonly, brachycephaly, cranium bifidum occultum, frontal lipoma, widow's peak, blepharophimosis, lagophthalmos, eyelid coloboma, limbic dermoid of the eye, telecanthus, cataracts, microphthalmia, microcornea, and coloboma of the iris. Frontofacionasal dysplasia and median cleft face syndrome are believed by some to be the same entity.

Gallop, T. R. Fronto-facio-nasal dysostosis-a new autosomal recessive syndrome. *Am. J. Med. Genet.*, 1981, 10:409-12.

frontofacionasal syndrome. See *frontofacionasal dysplasia.*

frontometaphyseal dysplasia (FMD). Synonyms: *Gorlin syndrome, Gorlin-Cohen syndrome, Gorlin-Holt syndrome.*

A congenital syndrome of tooth, bone, and connective tissue abnormalities of unknown etiology. Pronounced supraorbital ridge, wide nasal bridge, and mandibular hypoplasia with a small pointed chin give the patient a striking facial appearance. Orodental abnormalities include malocclusion, missing permanent teeth, retained deciduous teeth, and bifid uvula. Associated defects include wasting of muscles of the arms and legs, restricted joint mobility, thin fingers, clinodactyly, and deafness.

Gorlin, R. J., & Cohen, M. M., Jr. Frontometaphyseal dysplasia. A new syndrome. *Am. J. Dis. Child.*, 1969, 118:487-94. Holt, J. F., *et al.* Frontometaphyseal dysplasia. *Radiol. Clin. N. Am.*, 1972, 10:225-43.

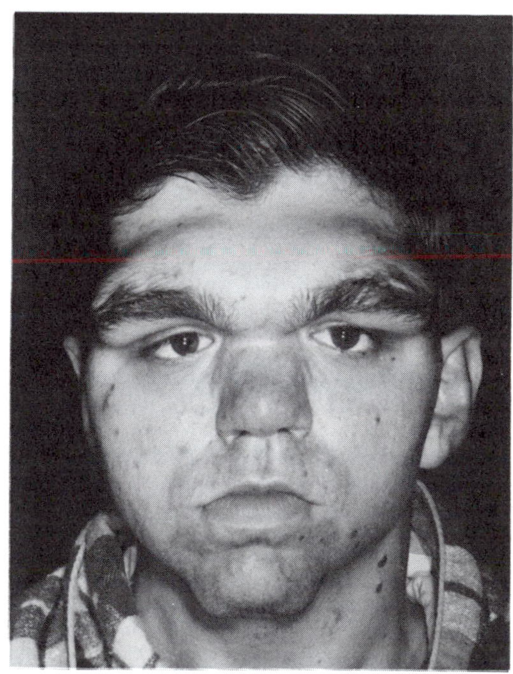

Frontometaphyseal dysplasia
Courtesy of Dr. Robert J. Gorlin, Minneapolis, MN.

frontonasal dysplasia. See *median cleft face syndrome.*

frontonasal dysplasia anomalad. See *median cleft face syndrome.*

FRORIEP, ROBERT (German physician, 1804-1861)

Froriep disease. Synonyms: *Froriep induration, Froriep rheumatism, myositis fibrosa.*

Abnormal formation of conective tissue within muscle.

Froriep, R. *Die rheumatische Schwiele.* Weimar, 1843.

Froriep induration. See *Froriep disease.*

Froriep rheumatism. See *Froriep disease.*

frosted cataract. See *Vogt cataract, under Vogt, Alfred.*

frozen shoulder. See *Duplay bursitis.*

frozen shoulder syndrome. See *Duplay bursitis.*

FRUGONI, CESARE (Italian physician, born 1881)

Cauchois-Eppinger-Frugoni syndrome. See *Frugoni syndrome.*

Frugoni disease. Synonyms: *eosinophilic-monocytic fever, infectious eosinophilia.*

Infectious eosinophilia associated with arthralgia, respiratory involvement, gastrointestinal manifestations, and asthenia, reportedly described by Frugoni.

Frugoni syndrome. Synonyms: *Cauchois-Eppinger-Frugoni syndrome, congestive fibrosplenomegaly, thrombophlebitic splenomegaly.*

Chronic splenomegaly due to portal thrombophlebitis and thrombosis of the splenic vein, associated with gastrointestinal hemorrhage, recurrent ascites, esophageal varices, anemia, leukopenia, and thrombopenia.

Greppi, E. Die hepatolienalen Syndrome im Lichte neuerer Erkenntnisse, Jahre nach Eppinger. *Schweiz. Med. Wschr.*, 1956, 86:1087-91.

FRÜND, H. (German physician)

Haglund-Läwen-Fründ syndrome. See *Büdinger-Ludloff-Läwen syndrome.*

FRYNS, J. P. (Belgian physician)

Fryns syndrome. A lethal autosomal recessive disorder marked by corneal clouding, camptodactyly, nail hypoplasia, lung hypoplasia, diaphragmatic defects, genital abnormalities, and characteristic facies marked by small eyes, micrognathia, anteverted nares, and cleft lip or palate. Hepatomegaly and renal abnormalities may occur.

Fryns, J. P., *et al.* A new lethal syndrome with cloudy corneae, diaphragmatic defects and distal limb deformities. *Hum. Genet.*, 1979, 50:65-70.

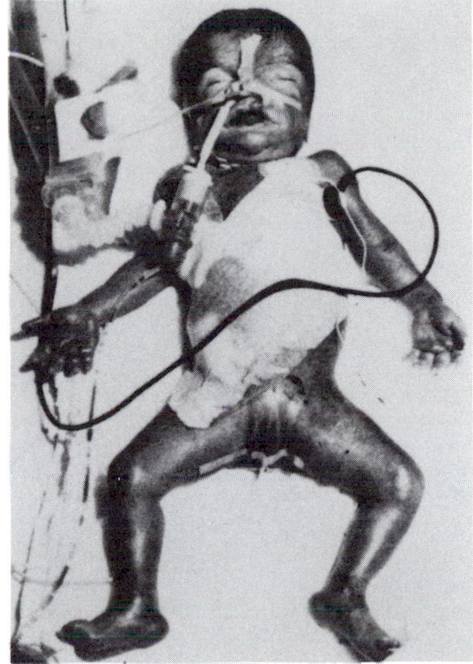

Fryns syndrome
Meinecke, P. & J.P. Fryns, *Clinical Genetics* 28:516-520, 1985. Munksgaard International Publishers, Copenhagen, Denmark.

FS. See *Fisher syndrome, under Fisher, Miller.*

FS. See *Felty syndrome.*

FS 1 (Fanconi syndrome 1). See *familial juvenile nephrophthisis.*

FS 2 (Fanconi syndrome 2). See *cystinosis.*

FS 3 (Fanconi syndrome 3). See *Andersen triad.*

FS 4 (Fanconi syndrome 4). See *Fanconi anemia.*

FSHD (facioscapulohumeral muscular dystrophy). See *Landouzy-Déjerine syndrome.*

FSS. See *Freeman-Sheldon syndrome.*

FTS. See *fetal tobacco syndrome.*

FUCHS, ERNST (German ophthalmologist, 1851-1930)

Dalén-Fuchs nodules. See *Dalén-Fuchs spots.*

Dalén-Fuchs spots. See *under Dalén.*

Fuchs atrophy. Peripheral atrophy of the optic nerve.

Fuchs, E. Die periphere Atrophie des Sehnerven. *Graefes Arch. Ophth.*, 1885, 31:177-200.

Fuchs combined dystrophy. See *Fuchs dystrophy.*

Fuchs corneal dystrophy. See *Fuchs dystrophy.*

Fuchs dellen. See *Fuchs dimples.*

Fuchs dimples. Synonym: *Fuchs dellen.*

Shallow, saucerlike depressions on the surface of the cornea.

Fuchs, E. Über Dellen in der Hornhaut. *Graefes Arch. Ophth.*, 1911, 78:82-92.

Fuchs dystrophy. Synonyms: *Fuchs combined dystrophy, Fuchs corneal dystrophy, Fuchs endothelial dystrophy, Fuchs syndrome, Fuchs-Kraupa syndrome, Kraupa syndrome, congenital endothelial corneal dystrophy, cornea guttata, dystrophia epithelialis corneae, endothelial-epithelial corneal dystrophy, epithelial and endothelial dystrophy of the cornea.*

Bilateral, epithelial and endothelial corneal dystrophy that begins as epithelial edema with clouding of the stroma, followed by formation of vesicles and bullae, erosion, pain, photophobia, blurring of vision, and vacularization and scarring of the cornea. The etiology is unknown. Autosomal dominant inheritance with a greater expression in the female is suspected.

Fuchs, E. Dystrophia epithelialis corneae. *Graefes Arch. Ophth.*, 1910, 76:478-508. *Kraupa, E. Pigmentierungen der Hornhauthinterfläche bei "Dystrophia epithelialis (Fuchs)." *Zschr. Augenh.*, 1920, 44:247.

Fuchs endothelial dystrophy. See *Fuchs dystrophy.*

Fuchs heterochromia. See *Fuchs heterochromic cyclitis.*

Fuchs heterochromic cyclitis (FHC). Synonyms: *Fuchs heterochromia, Fuchs heterochromic iridocyclitis, Fuchs syndrome, Fuchs uveitis syndrome, heterochromia cyclica, heterochromia iridis, heterochromic cyclitis, iridocyclitis heterochromica.*

The concurrence of heterochromia, uveitis, cataract, and glaucoma. Cyclitis is usually unilateral and is associated with depigmentation and atrophy of the iris, secondary cataract, vitreous opacities, mild uveitis, and discrete keratic precipitates. Glaucoma and ipsilateral hemiatrophy may occur.

*Fuchs, E. Über Komplikationen der Heterochromie. *Zschr.*

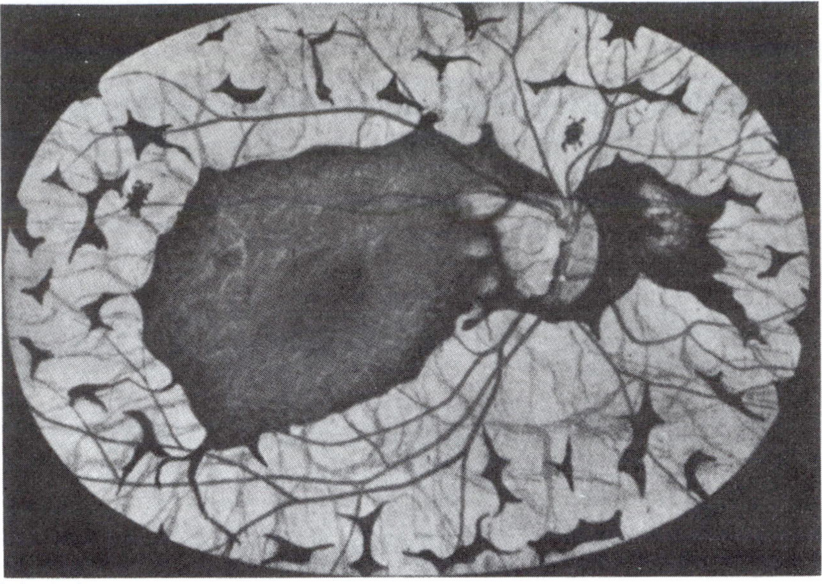

Fuchs atrophy
Francois, Jules: *Heredity in Ophthalmology*. St. Louis: C.V. Mosby Co., 1961

Augenh., 1906, 15:191.

Fuchs heterochromic iridocyclitis (FHI). See *Fuchs heterochromic cyclitis.*

Fuchs keratitis. Synonym: *superficial marginal keratitis.*

A rare form of keratitis of the middle-aged and elderly, characterized by bilateral bands of superficial infiltrates around the corneal margins, while the central portions remain clear. A ring ulcer may develop in later stages. The etiology is obscure.

Fuchs, E. *Lehrbuch der Augenheildunde*. Wien, Deuticke, 1893.

Fuchs spot. A small black spot on the fundus oculi in high myopia, occurring after macular hemorrhage.

Bender, M. B. Neuroophthalmology. In: Baker, A. B., ed. *Clinical neurology*. 2nd ed. New York, Hoeber, 1965.

Fuchs syndrome (1). See *Stevens-Johnson syndrome.*

Fuchs syndrome (2). Synonyms: *epidemic keratoconjunctivitis, epidemic superficial keratitis, keratitis punctata superficialis, superficial punctate keratitis.*

Keratitis secondary to conjunctivitis, characterized by punctate opacities scattered in the superficial layers of the cornea. The lesions are grayish to white, round, flat macules that may persist for three to six months and occasionally longer.

Fuchs, E. Keratitis punctata superficialis. *Wien. Klin. Wschr*., 1889, 2:837.

Fuchs syndrome (3). See *Fuchs heterochromic cyclitis.*

Fuchs syndrome (4). See *Fuchs dystrophy.*

Fuchs uveitis syndrome. See *Fuchs heterochromic cyclitis.*

Fuchs-Kraupa syndrome. See *Fuchs dystrophy.*

FUKASE, MASAICHI (Japanese physician)

Crow-Fukase syndrome. See *POEMS syndrome.*

FUKUYAMA, YUKIO (Japanese physician)

Fukuyama syndrome. Synonym: *Fukuyama type congenital muscular dystrophy (FCMD).*

A syndrome, transmitted as an autosomal recessive trait, characterized by congenital progressive muscular dystrophy and brain disorders. Muscular disorders consist of early-onset generalized involvement of the muscles, the proximal muscles being most severely affected; involvement of the facial muscles with resulting peculiar facial characteristics; joint contractures; muscle hypotonia and hypokinesis; pseudohypertrophy of the skeletal muscles occurring in some cases; and the inability of most patients to walk or stand up. Neuropathological disorders include dilatation of the ventricles and exterior liquor spaces; Dandy-Walker malformation; hypodensity of the white matter; agyria, pachygyria, and microgyria of the cerebral cortex; absence of cortical lamination; cytological abnormalities; frontal adhesions of the cerebral hemispheres; stenosis of the aqueduct of Sylvius; pial thickening; micropolygyria of the cerebellum; hypoplasia of the pyramidal tracts; and heterotopias in the brain stem and basal meninges. Associated disorders include mental retardation, delayed speech, and asymmetric skull. Earlier cases of this syndrome were reported exclusively in Japanese infants, but the later literature indictes its occurrence in other ethnic groups.

Fukuyama, Y., *et al.* A peculiar form of congenital progressive muscular dystrophy. Report of fifteen cases. *Paediat. Univer. Tokyo,* 1960, 4:5-8.

Fukuyama type congenital muscular dystrophy (FCMD). See *Fukuyama syndrome.*

fulcrum fracture of the lumbar spine. See *Chance fracture.*

FULLER ALBRIGHT. See ALBRIGHT, FULLER

FÜLLING, GEORG (German physician)

Weyers-Fülling syndrome. See *under Weyers.*

fulminant meningococcemia. See *Waterhouse-Friderichsen syndrome.*

fulminant thrombotic thrombopenic purpura. See *Moschcowitz syndrome.*

fulminating purpuric meningococcemia. See *Waterhouse-Friderichsen syndrome.*

functional dysautonomia. See *Riley-Day syndrome, under Riley, Conrad M.*

functional hypoglycemic syndrome. See *Harris syndrome, under Harris, Seale.*

functional renal failure. See *hepatorenal syndrome.*
fundus albipunctatus cum hemeralopia. See *Lauber disease.*
fundus albipunctatus-hemerolopia-xerosis syndrome. See *Uyemura syndrome.*
fundus flavimaculatus. See *Franceschetti disease.*
fundus punctatus albescens. See *Lauber disease.*
funicular myelitis. See *Dana syndrome.*
funicular myelosis. See *Dana syndrome.*
funicular sclerosis. See *Dana syndrome.*

FÜRMAIER, A.

Fürmaier syndrome. A syndrome of femorolumbar rigidity with difficulty in flexing the lumbar spine forward and thoracic scoliosis. Irritation of the lumbosacral nerve roots due to a compression by a tumor or posttraumatic cicatricial formation is the cause.

*Fürmaier, A. Der Symptomen Komplex der Hüftlendenstrecksteife. *Chirurg,* 1947, 17/18:563-9.

FURST, WILLIAM (American physician)

Furst-Ostrum syndrome. Synonym: *platybasia-cervical synostosis-Sprengel deformity syndrome.*

Platybasia associated with congenital synostosis of the neck and Sprengel deformity.

Furst, W., & Ostrum, H. W. Platybasia, Klippel-Feil syndrome and Sprengel's deformity. *Am. J. Roentgen.,* 1942, 47:588-90.

furunculus atonicus. See *Lewandowski periporitis.*
fusospirillary marginal gingivitis. See *Vincent infection.*
fusospirillosis. See *Vincent infection.*
fusospirochetal gingivitis. See *Vincent infection.*
FXS (fragile-**X** syndrome). See *chromosome X fragility.*

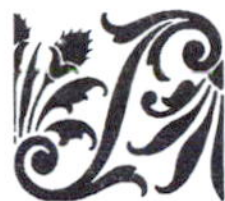

Page #	Term	Observation

G syndrome. See *hypospadias-dysphagia syndrome.*
G deletion syndrome. See *chromosome 21 monosomy syndrome.*
GABLER, HEDDA (The title character in an Ibsen play.)
Hedda Gabler syndrome. Suicide in pregnancy.

Goodwin, J., & Harris, D. Suicide in pregnancy: The Hedda Gabler syndrome. *Suicide Life Threat. Behav.*, 1979, 9:105-15.

GAISBÖCK, FELIX (Austrian physician, 1868-1955)
Gaisböck disease. Synonyms: *Gaisböck syndrome, benign polycythemia, hypertonic polycythemia, polycythemia hypertonica, polycythemia rubra hypertonica, pseudopolycythemia, relative polycythemia, spurious polycythemia, stress erythrocytosis, stress polycythemia.*

According to Gaisböck, this syndrome consists of plethora without splenomegaly, leukocytosis, or thrombocytosis. In modern usage, the term denotes a condition characterized by chronic elevation of venous hematocrit in the presence of a normal measured red cell mass, with or without associated cardiovascular disease or other clinical abnormalities. Generally, the condition is observed in middle-aged, obese, white males. The symptoms may include, in various combinations, fatigue, headache, weakness, dizziness, pruritus, anxiety, angina, shortness of breath, abdominal pain, paresthesia, and intermittent claudication. Hypertension, myocardial infarction, pulmonary infarction, stroke, hyperuricemia, peptic ulcer, and nephrolithiasis are the most common complications. See also *Vaquez-Osler syndrome (polycythemia vera).*

Gaisböck, F. Die Bedeutung der Blutdruckmessung für die Praxis. *Deut. Arch. Klin. Med.*, 1905, 83:363-409.
Brown, S. M., *et al.* Spurious (relative) polycythemia: A nonexistent disease. *Am. J. Med.*, 1971, 50:200-7.

Gaisböck syndrome. See *Gaisböck disease.*

GAL plus disease. See *mucolipidosis I.*
galactorrhea-amenorrhea syndrome. See *amenorrhea-galactorrhea syndrome.*
galactorrhea-amenorrhea-hyperprolactinemia syndrome. See *amenorrhea-galactorrhea syndrome.*
α-**galactosidase A (GLA) deficiency.** See *Fabry syndrome.*
GALANT, J. S. (German physician)
Hirschsprung-Galant infantilism. See *Hirschsprung syndrome.*
GALEAZZI, RICCARDO (Italian orthopedic surgeon, 1866-1952)
Galeazzi fracture. Synonym: *Galeazzi lesion.*

Fracture of the radial shaft at the junction of the middle distal thirds complicated by a dislocation of the distal radioulnar joint.

Galeazzi, R. Über ein besonderes Syndrom bei Verletzungen im Bereich der Unterarmaknochen. *Arch. Orthop. Unfall. Chir.*, 1934, 35:557-62.

Galeazzi lesion. See *Galeazzi fracture.*

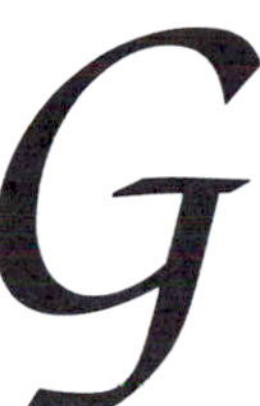

GALLAIS, ALFRED (French physician)
Cooke-Apert-Gallais syndrome. See *Cushing syndrome.*
Cooke-Gallais syndrome. See *Cushing syndrome.*
Gallais syndrome. See *congenital adrenal hyperplasia.*
Gallais syndrome. See *Cushing syndrome.*
gallstone ileus. See *Bouveret syndrome (1).*
gamma chain disease. See *under heavy chain disease.*
GAMMEL, JOHN A. (American physician)
Gammel syndrome. See *erythema gyratum repens.*
GAMSTORP, INGRID (Swedish physician)
Gamstorp syndrome. Synonyms: *adynamia episodica hereditaria, hereditary episodic adynamia, hyperkalemic periodic paralysis, hyperpotassemic periodic paralysis, periodic paralysis.*

Attacks of spontaneously abating paralysis, particularly of the muscles of the extremities and trunk, occurring mainly in children under the age of 10 years. In most patients, the attacks occur during rest after exertion, lasting at most 1 hour. The severity varies from slight weakness of a single extremity to acute states in which the patients becomes immobilized. Mild symptoms involving the muscles innervated by the cranial nerves may be associated. Damp and cold weather seems to exacerbate the attacks. Hyperkalemia without any increase in the excretion of potassium in the urine is a constant feature. Administration of potassium, even in minimal doses, precipitates the attacks of paralysis. The syndrome is transmitted as an autosomal dominant trait.

Gamstorp, I. Adynamia episodica hereditaria. *Acta Paediat., Uppsala,* 1956, 45(Suppl 108):1-126.

Gamstorp-Wohlfart syndrome. A syndrome, transmitted as an autosomal dominant trait, characterized by myokymia, myotonia, muscle wasting, and hyperhidrosis.

Gamstorp, I., & Wohlfart, G. A syndrome characterized by myokymia, myotonia, muscular wasting and increased perspiration. *Acta Psychiat. Neur. Scand.*, 1959, 34:181-94.

gangliocytoma dysplasticum. See *Lhermitte-Duclos disease.*

ganglion geniculi syndrome. See *Melkersson-Rosenthal syndrome.*

ganglioside lipidosis. See *Tay-Sachs syndrome, under Tay, Warren.*

gangliosidosis G_{M1} type I. Synonyms: *Caffey pseudo-Hurler syndrome, Hurler-like syndrome, Landing syndrome, Norman-Landing syndrome, pseudo-Hurler syndrome, generalized gangliosidosis, generalized infantile gangliosidosis with bony involvement, infantile generalized gangliosidosis, neurovisceral lipidosis.*

A ganglioside storage disorder caused by β-galactosidase deficiency and ganglioside G_{M1} storage in neurons and in the hepatic, splenic, and other histiocytes, and in the renal glomerular epithelium. The symptoms become apparent shortly after birth; they include retarded psychomotor development, failure to thrive, startle reaction to sound, feeding difficulty, hepatosplenomegaly, and Hurler (gargoyle-like) facies (coarse facial features, macrocephaly, broad nose, frontal bossing, long philtrum, prominent maxilla, and macroglossia). They are followed by deglutition disorders, sucking difficulty, blindness, deafness, restricted joint movement, gingival hypertrophy, cerebral degeneration, retinitis pigmentosa, kyphoscoliosis, hepatomegaly, splenomegaly, cherry-red spots of the macula, seizures, and terminal decerebrate rigidity. Bronchopneumonia occurs in the second year of life. Bony changes consist of excessive periosteal formation of the long bones, faulty diaphyseal constriction of the short bones, wide ribs, coarse trabeculation, pelvic dysplasia, constriction and irregular formation of the long bones, vertebral defects, bullet-shaped phalanges, and proximally pointed metacarpal bones. Pathological findings include severe cerebral degeneration and accumulation of ganglioside in neurons, renal glomerular epithelium, and hepatic, splenic, and other histiocytes; vacuolated lymphatics; foam cells in the bone marrow; and glomerular ballooning. Mucopolysacchariduria may occur. The syndrome is transmitted as an autosomal recessive trait.

Landing, B. H., *et al.* Familial neurovisceral lipidosis. *Am. J. Dis. Child.*, 1964, 108:503-82. Norman, R. M., *et al.* Tay-Sachs disease with visceral involvement and its relation to gargoylism, *Arch. Dis. Child.*, 1964, 39:634-40. Caffey, J. Gargoylism (Hunter-Hurler disease, dysostosis multiplex, lipochondrodystrophy); prenatal and neonatal bone lesions and their early postnatal evolution. *Bull. Hosp. Joint. Dis.*, 1951, 12:38-66. O'Brien, J. S. The gangliosidoses. In: Stanbury, J. B., Wyngaarden, J. B., & Fredrickson, D. S., eds. *The metabolic basis of inherited disease.* 4th ed. New York, McGraw-Hill, 1978, pp. 841-65.

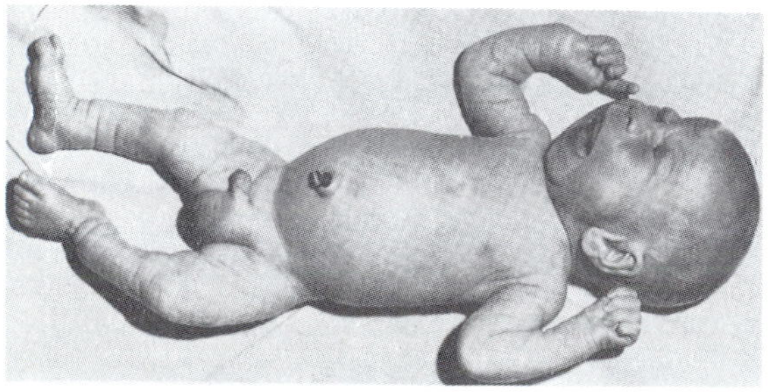

Gangliosidosis G_{M1} type I
Scott, R., et. al: *J.Pediatr.*, 71:357, 1967. St. Louis: C.V. Mosby Co.

gangliosidosis G_{M1} type II. Synonyms: *Derry syndrome, juvenile G_{M1} gangliosidosis.*

A ganglioside storage disorder characterized by deficiency of isozymes B and C of β-galactosidase with resulting accumulation of ganglioside G_{M1} in the brain and excessive amounts of keratosulfatelike mucopolysaccharide in the visceral organs. The affected infants appear normal at birth. Locomotor ataxia, the initial symptom with onset at about one year of life, is followed by strabismus, inability to control hand movements, loss of speech, muscle weakness of the extremities, rapidly progressive psychomotor retardation, dullness of senses, lethargy, seizures, decerebrate rigidity, and terminal bronchopneumonia at the age of 3 to 10 years. Nystagmus, blindness, and mild vertebral, metacarpal, and pelvic defects are often associated. The syndrome is transmitted as an autosomal recessive trait.

Derry, D. M., *et al.* Late infantile systemic lipidosis. Major monosialogangliosidosis. Delineation of two types. *Neurology*, 1968, 18:340-8. O'Brien, J. S. The gangliosidoses. In: Stanbury, J. B., & Wyngaarden, J. B., & Fredrickson, D. S., eds. *The metabolic basis of inherited disease.* 4th ed. New York, McGraw-Hill, 1978, pp. 841-65.

gangliosidosis G_{M2} type 0. See *Sandhoff syndrome.*

gangliosidosis G_{M2} type I. See *Tay-Sachs syndrome, under Tay, Warren.*

gangliosidosis G_{M2} type II. See *Sandhoff syndrome.*

gangliosidosis G_{M2} type III. Synonyms: *Bernheimer-Seitelberger syndrome, Bielschowsky amaurotic idiocy, Bielschowsky syndrome, Dollinger-Bielschowsky syndrome, Jansky-Bielschowsky syndrome, Seitelberger disease, juvenile G_{M2} gangliosidosis, late infantile amaurotic idiocy, late infantile ganglioside lipidosis.*

A rare form of ganglioside storage disorder, transmitted as an autosomal recessive trait, characterized by onset of symptoms between the ages of 2 and 4 years. Most patients die by the age of 4 to 8 years. After a normal or slightly retarded development, first symptoms consist of petit mal or grand mal seizures and myoclonic jerks evoked by sensory stimuli. Next to follow are incoordination, tremor, ataxia, spastic weakness, increased tendon reflexes, Babinski signs, mental deterioration, and dysarthria. Associated symptoms may include mutism, blindness due to retinal degeneration with retinitis pigmentosa, EEG spikes induced by photic stimuli, and occasional microcephaly. Partial deficiency of hexaminidase and abnormal accumulation of ganglioside G_{M2} are the metabolic defects. Pathological findings show the presence of inclusions (translucent vacuoles) in the lymphocytes, azurophilic granules in the neutrophils, neuronal loss in the cerebral and cerebellar cortices, and curvilinear storage particles and osmophilic granules in the neurons.

Bielschowsky, M. Über spätinfantile familiäre amaurotische Idiotie mit Kleinhirnsymptonen. *Deut Zschr. Nervenheilk.*, l914, 50:7-29. Bernheimer, H., & Seitelberger, F. Über das Verhalten der Ganglioside im Gehirn bei 2 Fällen von spätinfantiler amaurotischer Idiotie, *Wien. Klin. Wschr.*, 1968, 80:163-4. O'Brien, J. S. The gangliosidoses. In: Stanbury, J. B., Wyngaarden, J. B., & Fredrickson, D. S., eds. *The metabolic basis of inherited disease.* 4th ed. New York, McGraw-Hill, 1978, pp. 841-65. Dollinger, A. Zur Klinik der infantilen Form der familiären amaurotischen Idiotie (Tay-Sachs). *Zschr. Kin-*

derheilk., 1919, 22:167-94. Goebel, H. H., *et al.* An ultrastructural study of the retina in the Jansky-Bielschowsky type of neuronal ceroidipofuscinosis. *Am. J. Ophth.*, 1977, 83(Ser 3):70-9.

gangliosidosis G_{M2}-hexosaminidase A and B deficiency syndrome. See *Sandhoff syndrome.*

gangliosympathicoblastoma. See *Hutchinson disease, under Hutchinson, Sir Robert Grieve.*

gangrena spontanea chirurgigorum. See *Charcot syndrome (3).*

gangrene of the scrotum. See *Fournier disease.*

GANONG, WILLIAM FRANCIS (American physician, born 1895)

Lown-Ganong-Levine (LGL) syndrome. See *Clerc-Lévy-Cristeco syndrome.*

GANS (granulomatous angiitis of the nervous system) syndrome. Vasculitis of cerebral and spinal cord leptomeningeal and parenchymal small arteries, occurring more often in males than in females. The most frequent symptoms include headache, muscle weakness, confusion, mental disorders, nausea, vomiting, aphasia or dysphasia, seizures, lethargy, memory disorders, loss of consciousness, incoordination, numbness, and stiff neck. Preceding or associated disorders may include hypertension, Hodgkin disease, non-Hodgkin lymphoma, lymphocytic leukemia, renal transplant complications, cancer (of the colon or breast, and tonsils), sarcoidosis, recent upper respiratory infection, ileitis, trauma, and diabetes mellitus. Associated findings include fever, hypertension, maculopapular rash, hemiplegia or single limb paresis, pathologic reflexes of the lower limb, fundus oculi abnormalities, ataxia, tremor, myelopathy, Horner syndrome, and lesions of the cranial nerves. Cerebral angiography shows abnormalities of large, intermediate, and small arteries, such as beading, aneurysms, and eccentric or circumstantial vascular abnormalities. Herpes zoster ophthalmicus with delayed contralateral hemiplegia is sometimes associated. The etiology is unknown.

Craviato, H., & Feigin, I. Noninfectious granulomatous angiitis with predilection for the nervous system. *Neurology*, 1959, 9:599-609. Sigal. L. H. The neurologic presentation of vasculitic and rheumatologic syndromes. *Medicine*, 1987, 66:157-80.

GANSER, SIGBERT JOSEPH MARIA (German psychiatrist, 1853-1931)

Ganser syndrome. Synonyms: *acute hallucinatory mania, approximate answers syndrome, balderdash syndrome, hysterical pseudodementia, nonsense syndrome, pseudodementia syndrome.*

A dissociative disorder, originally described in male prisoners with brain injuries, characterized by peculiar irrelevant verbal responses to questioning, hallucinations, clouded sensorium, somatic conversion, and amnesia.

Ganser. Über einen eigenartigen hysterischen Dämmerzustund. *Arch. Psychiat., Berlin,* 1898, 30:633-40. *Diagnostic and statistical manual of mental disorders.* 3rd ed. Washington, American Psychiatric Association, D. C., 1987, p. 277.

GÄNSSLEN, MAX (German physician, 1895-1969)

Gänsslen disease. Synonyms: *constitutional familial leukopenia, constitutional familial neutropenia, familial neutropenia.*

A familial form of constitutional leukopenia transmitted as an autosomal dominant trait.

Gänsslen, M. Konstitutionelle familiäre Leukopenie (Neutropenie). *Klin. Wschr.*, 1941, 20:922-5.

Gänsslen syndrome. See *Minkowski-Chauffard syndrome.*

Gänsslen-Erb syndrome. See *Minkowski-Chauffard syndrome.*

Minkowski-Chauffard-Gänsslen syndrome. See *Minkowski-Chauffard syndrome.*

GAPO (growth retardation-alopecia-pseudo-anodontia-progreessive optic atrophy) syndrome. A rare syndrome, transmitted as an autosomal recessive trait, characterized by growth retardation, alopecia, pseudo-anodontia, optic atrophy, small face, wide anterior fontanel, flat nasal bridge, frontal bossing, umbilical hernia, mental retardation, mild skin laxity, prominent veins on the scalp, hyperconvex nails, hypoplasia of the breasts, and delayed bone maturation in children.

Tipton, R. E., & Gorlin, R. J. Growth retardation, alopecia, pseudo-anodontia, and optic atrophy-The GAPO syndrome: Report of a patient and review of the literature. *Am. J. Med. Genet.*, 1984, 19:209-16.

GARBE, WILLIAM (Canadian dermatologist, born 1908)

Sulzberger-Garbe syndrome. See *under Sulzberger.*

GARCIA, CARLOS A. (New Orleans physician)

Garcia-Lurie syndrome. Synonyms: *aprosencephaly syndrome, aprosencephaly-atelencephaly syndrome, atelencephalic microcephaly syndrome, XK syndrome, XK-aprosencephaly syndrome.*

A syndrome of agenesis of prosencephalic structures, atelencephaly, and microcephaly with faulty midface development and cyclopia. Associated abnormalities may include craniofacial disproportion with sloping forehead, flat nasal bridge, hypertelorism, thumb hypoplasia, simian creases, oligodactyly with fan-shaped toes, syndactyly, hypogonadism, small penis, hypospadias, dysplasia of the labia majora and clitoris, mobile cecum, adrenal hypoplasia, and ventricular septal defect. In the synonym **XK syndrome,** the letter "X" stands for the unreported name of the patient of Garcia and Duncan, and "K" for the initial of Lurie's patient.

Laziuk, G. I., Lur'e, I. V., & Cherstvoi, E.D. Gennye sindromy mnozhestvennykh vrozhdennykh porokov razvitiia. *Arkh. Pat., Moskva*, 1977, 39(3):3-11. Lurie, I. W., *et al.* Brief clinical reports: Aprosencephaly-atelencephaly and the aprosencephaly (XK) syndrome. *Am. J. Med. Genet.*, 1979, 3(303-9. Garcia, C. A., & Duncan, C. Atelencephalic microcephaly. *Dev. Med. Child. Neurol.*, 1977, 19:227-32.

GARCIN, RAYMOND (French physician, born 1897)

Bertolotti-Garcin syndrome. See *Garcin syndrome.*

Garcin syndrome. Synonyms: *Bertolotti-Garcin syndrome, Garcin-Guillain syndrome, Schmincke tumor-unilateral cranial paralysis syndrome, half-base syndrome, hemipolyneuropathy-cranial paralysis syndrome, unilateral global involvement of cranial nerves.*

A rare syndrome of unilateral involvement of all or nearly all cranial nerves in tumors of the nasopharynx and base of the skull (including Schmincke tumor or lymphoepithelioma) without affecting the brain itself.

*Garcin, R. *Le syndrome paralytique unilatéral global des nerfs crâniens.* Paris, 1927 (Thesis). Guillain, G., Alajuoua-

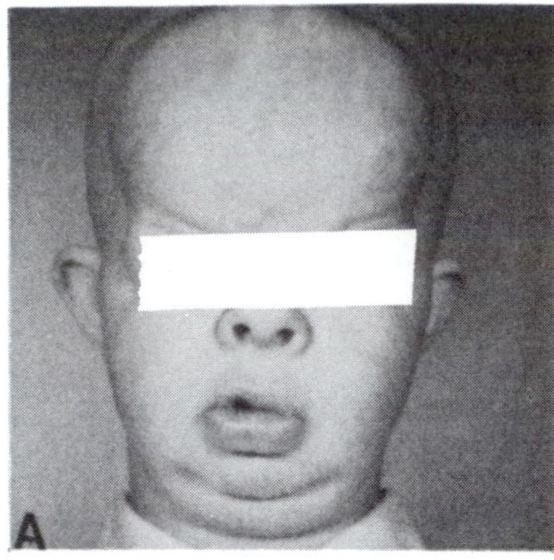

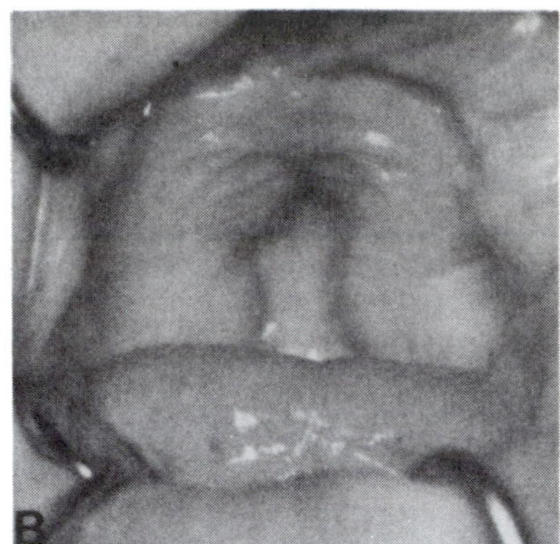

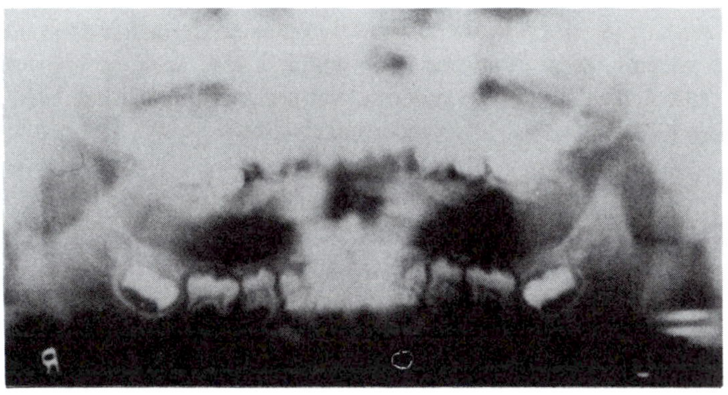

GAPO syndrome
Gorlin, R.J.: "Selected ectodermal dysplasias." In Salinas, C.F., Opitz, J.M., Paul, N.W. (eds): *Recent Advances in Ectodermal Dysplasias.* New York: Alan R. Liss, Inc. for the March of Dimes Birth Defects Foundation BD:OAS 24(2):123-148, 1988, with permission.

nine, R., & Garcin, R. Le syndrome paralytique unilatéral global des nerfs crâniens. *Bull. Soc. Méd. Hôp. Paris*, 1926, 50:456-60.

Garcin-Guillain syndrome. See *Garcin syndrome.*

GARDNER, ELDON JOHN (American physician, born 1909)

Gardner syndrome (GS). Synonyms: *Gardner-Bosch syndrome, hereditary adenomatosis, hereditary polyposis and osteomatosis, intestinal polyposis, osteomatosis-intestinal polyposis syndrome.*

An autosomal dominant syndrome characterized by polyposis of the large intestine, multiple osteomas, epidermoid cysts of the skin, and desmoids or fibromas of the skin. Polyposis involves mainly the colon and rectum (the small intestine being involved infrequently) and has a tendency to undergo malignant changes. The mandible, maxilla, and frontal bones are the primary sites of osteoma, but smaller osteomas may also occur on the long bones. Epidermoid cysts appear on the scalp, face, trunk, or extremities. Fibromas, desmoid tumors, lipomas, and lipofibromas are also found on the skin. Compound odotomas, unerupted teeth, and hypercementosis are present in some cases.

Gardner, E. J. A genetic and clinical study of intestinal polyposis, a predisposing factor for carcinoma of the colon and rectum. *Am. J. Hum. Genet.*, 1951, 3:167-76. Bosch Millares, J., & Bosch Hernandez, J. El sindrome de Gardner-Bosch. *Rev. Españ. Apar. Digest.*, 1963, 22:1017-44.

pre-Gardner syndrome. A complex of clinical conditions resulting from the genetic heterogeneity, variation in penetrance, and expressivity of the Gardner syndrome that, in time, will acquire all the characteristics of the Gardner syndrome.

Helson, L. Pre-Gardner's syndrome, thyroglossal cysts and undifferentiated tumor of neural crest origin. *Anticancer Res.*, 1984, 4:247-50.

GARDNER, FRANK H. (American physician)

Gardner-Diamond syndrome. See *auto-erythrocyte sensitization syndrome.*

GARDNER, HERMAN L. (American physician)

Gardner syndrome. See *Gardner vaginitis.*

Gardner vaginitis. Synonyms: *Gardner syndrome, desquamative inflammatory vaginitis, exudative vaginitis, vaginitis ulcerosa.*

Inflammation of the vaginal structures, especially the posterior fornix and the ectocervix. The affected parts, fiery red areas with well-delineated margins sometimes with serpiginous configurations, are easily traumatized and develop ulcerations and ecchymotic bleeding points and streaks. In some cases, the epithelium presents a grayish pseudomembrane that peels off, exposing inflamed red surfaces.

Gardner, H. L. Desquamative inflammatory vaginitis: A newly defined entity. *Am. J. Obstet. Gynecol.*, 1968, 102:1102-5.

GARDNER, L. I. (American physician)

Gardner-Silengo-Wachtel syndrome. Synonym: *genitopalatocardiac syndrome.*

The concurrence of pseudohermaphroditism, micrognathia, cleft palate, and heart defect. Low-set ears, double-outlet right ventricle, ventricular septal defect, gonadal dysgenesis, cleft lip, transposition of the great vessels, right-sided aortic arch, polycystic kidneys, and hypospadias are the principal abnormalities of this syndrome. The karyotype is either 46,XY or 46,dup. The syndrome appears to be inherited as an autosomal recessive or an X-linked recessive trait. Oral contraceptives are suspected as a probable causative agent.

Gardner, L. I., *et al.* 46,XY female: Anti-androgenic effect of oral contraceptive? *Lancet,* 1970, 2:667-8. Silengo, M., *et al.* A 46,XY infant with uterus, dysgenetic gonads, and multiple anomalies. *Humangenetik,* 1974, 25:65-8. *Wachtel, S. S. *H-Y antigen and the biology of sex determination.* New York, Grune & Stratton, 1983, pp. 224-5.

GARDNER, W. J. (American physician)

Gardner syndrome. Synonyms: *acoustic neurinoma syndrome, neurofibromatosis type NF2.*

A familial disorder, transmitted as an autosomal dominant trait, characterized by usually bilateral neurinomas of the acoustic nerve with progressive hearing loss and neurological complications. Increasing intracranial pressure with papilledema may result in blindness. Encroachment on adjacent cranial nerves, palsies of nerves adjacent to the tumor, cerebellar ataxia, and severe headache are the additional complications.

Gardner, W. J., & Frazier, C. H. Bilateral acoustic neurofibromas. A clinical study and survey of a family of five generations with bilateral deafness in 38 members. *Arch. Neur. Psychiat., Chicago,* 1930, 23:266-302.

GAREIS, FRANK J. (American physician)

Gareis syndrome. Synonym: *mental retardation-clasped thumb syndrome.*

X-linked mental retardation associated with bilateral clasp-thumb anomaly (absent extensor pollicis brevis tendons).

Gareis, F. J., & Mason, J. D. X-linked mental retardation associated with bilateral clasp thumb anomaly. *Am. J. Med. Genet.,* 1984, 17:333-8.

gargoylism. See *mucopolysaccharidosis I-H.*

GARIN

Garin-Bujadoux syndrome. See *Bannwarth syndrome.*

GARLAND

Bruns-Garland syndrome. See *under Bruns.*

GARLAND, HUGH (British physician)

Bland-White-Garland syndrome. See *under Bland.*

Marinesco-Garland syndrome. See *Marinesco-Sjögren syndrome.*

Marinesco-Sjögren-Garland syndrome. See *Marinesco-Sjögren syndrome, under Marinescu, Gheorge.*

GARRE, CARL (Swiss surgeon, 1857-1928)

Garré osteomyelitis. Synonyms: *idiopathic cortical sclerosis, osteomyelitis sicca, sclerosing nonsuppurative osteomyelitis.*

Nonsuppurative sclerosing osteomyelitis marked by increased density and gradual development of a spindle-shaped sclerotic thickening of the cortex. The long bones are most commonly affected, but involvement of the mandible may also occur, characterized by a hard nontender mass of bone overlying the affected jaw. Staphylococci, streptococci, and mixed organisms appear to be the pathogens most frequently associated with the disease.

Garré, C. Über besondere Formen und Folgezustände der akuten infektiösen Osteomyelitis. *Beitr. Klin. Chir.,* 1893, 10:241-98.

GARROD, SIR ARCHIBALD EDWARD (British physician, 1819-1907)

Garrod ablinism. See *albinism I syndrome.*

Garrod pads. Excrescences almost always confined to the dorsal aspects of the proximal interphalangeal joints, and rarely affecting the terminal joints of the fingers. The excresences are usually present on both hands, varying in size from that of a pea to half the size of a hazel nut. Although usually central in position, they may incline to one or the other side of a joint. Sometimes the pads are painless, but more often pain is present, especially when the fingers are flexed.

Garrod, A. E. On an unusual form of nodule upon the joint of the fingers. *St. Batholomew Hosp. Rep., London,* 1893, 29:157-61.

GAS (general adaptation syndrome). See *Selye syndrome.*

gas gangrene of the scrotum. See *Fournier disease.*

GASS

Hruby-Irvine-Gass syndrome. See *Irvine-Gass syndrome.*

Irvine-Gass cystoid macular edema. See *Irvine-Gass syndrome.*

Irvine-Gass syndrome. See *under Irvine.*

GASSER, CONRAD JOHANN (Swiss physician, born 1912)

Gasser syndrome (1). See *hemolytic-uremic syndrome.*

Gasser syndrome (2). Synonyms: *acute benign erythroblastopenia, acute erythroblastopenia, reticulocytopenia.*

A transitory aplastic crisis marked by the disappearance of normoblasts from the bone marrow and reticulocytes from the bone marrow and peripheral blood. Allergic disorders, toxicity, and infections are suspected in the etiology. In the original report, children between the ages of 1 and 12 years were affected.

Gasser, C. Akute Erythroblastopenie. 10 Fälle aplastischer Erythroblastenkrisen mit Riesenproerythroblasten bei allergisch-toxischen Zustandasbildern. *Helvet. Paediat. Acta,* 1949, 4:107-43.

Gasser-Karrer syndrome. Fatal hemolytic anemia, originally described in a premature infant, associated with severe anisocytosis, decaying of the spherocytes, and the presence of remnants of chromatin and Heinz bodies. Monocytosis is observed in the blood and bone marrow, and the number of macrophages in the bone marrow is generally decreased. Autopsy findings show severe hemosiderosis of a hypoplastic liver and spleen and giant cells in the adrenal cortex.

Gasser, C., & Karrer, J. Deletäre hämolytische Anämie mit "Spontan-Innenkörper-Bildung bei Frühgeburt. *Helvet. Paediat. Acta,* 1948, 3:387-403.

Vahlquist-Gasser syndrome. See *under Vahlquist.*

GASTAUT, HENRI JEAN PASCAL (French physician, born 1915)

Gastaut syndrome (1). Synonyms: *self-induced photosensitive epilepsy, sunflower syndrome.*

Photosensitive epilepsy with heliotropism and arm rocking movements, interpreted as an attempt to seek a source of light in self-induced epilepsy. In the report of Ames and Saffer, the mother was sensitive to flicker, but her daughter was insensitive despite frequent heliotropic attacks.

Gastaut, H. L'épilepsie photogénique. *Rev. Prat., Paris,* 1951, 1:105-9. Ames, F. R., & Saffer, D. The sunflower syndrome. A new look at "self-induced" photosensitive epilepsy. *J. Neur. Sc.,* 1983, 59:1-11.

Gastaut syndrome (2). Synonyms: *Lennox-Gastaut syndrome, hemiconvulsion-hemiplegia-epilepsy (HHE) syndrome.*

Unilateral convulsions associated with hemiplegia and epilepsy in young children. Unconsciousness, epigastric, pharyngeal, or abdominal aura, a sensation of fear, and sucking movements are the principal symptoms. Cerebral edema and injuries are the suspected causes.

Gastaut, H., *et al.* Le syndrome "hémiconvulsion-hémiplegie-épilepsie (syndrome H.H.E.) *Rev. Neur., Paris,* 1957, 97:37-52.

Lennox-Gastaut syndrome (LGS). See *Gastaut syndrome (2).*

gastric acid aspiration syndrome. See *Mendelson syndrome.*

gastric hypersecretion-peptic ulceration-pancreatic tumor syndrome. See *Zollinger-Ellison syndrome.*

gastric juice aspiration syndrome (GJA-S). See *Mendelson syndrome.*

gastric outlet syndrome. See *Bouveret syndrome (1).*

gastric remnant syndrome. See *postgastrectomy syndrome.*

gastric sclerosis. See *Brinton disease.*

gastric-lined esophagus. See *Barrett syndrome.*

gastrinoma syndrome. See *Zollinger-Ellison syndrome.*

gastritis hypertrophica gigantea. See *Ménétrier syndrome.*

gastrocardial symptom complex. See *Bergmann syndrome.*

gastrocardial syndrome. See *Roemheld syndrome.*

gastrocnemius muscle syndrome. See *popliteal artery entrapment syndrome.*

gastrocutaneous syndrome. A familial syndrome, transmitted as an autosomal dominant trait with high penetrance and variable expressivity, characterized by peptic ulcer, hiatal hernia, multiple lentigines, café-au-lait spots, apparent hypertelorism, and myopia. Other probable but rarer components include ischemic heart disease, congenital heart disease, and maturity-onset diabetes. Symptoms of peptic ulcer and hiatal hernia usually start in the second or third decade and are associated in some instances with increased acid secretion and abnormal dermatoglyphics.

Halal, F., *et al.* Gastro-cutaneous syndrome: Peptic ulcer/hiatal hernia, multiple lentigines/café-au-lait spots, hypertelorism, and myopia. *Am. J. Med. Genet.,* 1982, 11:161-76.

gastroesophageal laceration syndrome. See *Mallory-Weiss syndrome.*

gastroesophageal laceration-hemorrhage syndrome. See *Mallory-Weiss syndrome.*

gastrosuccorhea. See *Rejchman disease.*

gastroxynsis. See *Rossbach disease.*

GAUCHER, PHILIPPE CHARLES ERNEST (French physician, 1854-1918)

Gaucher disease. Synonyms: *Gaucher syndrome, Gaucher-Schlagenhaufer disease, cerebroside lipidosis, familial splenic anemia, glucosyl ceramide lipidosis.*

A sphingolipid storage disorder characterized mainly by the presence of Gaucher cells (enlarged lipid-laden histiocytes that also stain for carbohydrate when exposed to the periodic acid Schiff reagent), enlarged spleen and liver, and increased serum acid phosphatase activity. The condition is classified into three types, involvement of the brain serving as the basis for the classification: **Type I** (chronic noneuropathic, or adult, Gaucher disease), **Type II** (acute neuropathic Gaucher disease), and **Type III** (subacute neuropathic, or juvenile, Gaucher disease). **Type I** is the most frequent form, occurring in Ashkenazi Jews more often than any other ethnic group. The symptoms consist of bouts of pain, abdominal distention, liver and spleen enlargement, easy bruising, and hemorrhagic episodes. Endarteritis, with resulting osteomyelitis and focal avascular necrosis, causes rarefaction of bone cortices and pathological femur and hip fractures. Pneumonia is the usual cause of death. The term **adult Gaucher disease** appears to be inaccurate, since onset of symptoms may take place from infancy to childhood. **Type II** is marked by protruberant abdomen, enlarged spleen and liver, and central nervous system involvement manifested by motor function disorders and spasticity. Strabismus, muscular hypertonicity, retroflexion of the head, rigidity of the neck, trismus, dysphagia, laryngeal stridor, hyperreflexia, plantar extensor responses, and sometimes seizures are usually present. Death, caused by pulmonary involvement, takes place within 9 months from the onset of symptoms. **Type III** is characterized chiefly by liver and spleen enlargement and neurological disorders, mainly convulsions, EEC abnormalities, muscular hypertonicity, strabismus, and coordination disorders. Children are most frequently affected. When occurring in young adults, the condition may be associated with mental disorders, grand mal epilepsy, tremor, and gait disorders. All three types are genetically transmitted as an autosomal recessive trait.

*Gaucher, P. C. *De l'épitheliome primitif de la rate: hypertrophie idiopathique de la rate sans leucémie.* Paris, 1882 (Thesis). Schlagenhaufer, F. Über meist familiär vorkommende, histologisch charakteristische Splenomegalien (Typ Gaucher). (Eine Systemerkrankung des lymphatisch-hämopoetischen Apparates). *Virchows Arch. Path.,* 1907, 187:125-63.

Gaucher syndrome. See *Gaucher disease.*

Gaucher-Schlagenhauer syndrome. See *Gaucher disease.*

GAULE, JUSTUS (German physician, born 1849)

Gaule spots. A form of corneal degeneration characterized by sharply defined lesions, seen in keratitis of neurological origin.

Gaule, J. Der Einfluss des Trigeminus auf die Hornhaut. *Zbl. Physiol.,* 1891, 5:409-15.

GAULT, FERNAND (French physician, 1873-1936)

Devic-Gault syndrome. See *Devic syndrome.*

GAUTHIER, G. (French physician)

de Morsier-Gauthier syndrome. See *olfactogenital syndrome.*

gay bowel syndrome. A wide spectrum of sexually transmitted diseases in male homosexuals, including intestinal or anorectal diseases caused by bacterial, parasitic, protozoal, and viral infections.

Kazal, H. L., *et al.* The gay bowel syndrome: Clinicopathologic correlation in 260 cases. *Ann. Clin. Lab. Sc.*, 1976, 6:184-92.

gay compromise syndrome. See *acquired immunodeficiency syndrome.*

gay-related immunodeficiency (GRID) syndrome. See *acquired immunodeficiency syndrome.*

GAYET, CHARLES JULES ALPHONSE (French physician, 1833-1904)

Gayet disease. See *Wernicke syndrome.*

Gayet-Wernicke syndrome. See *Wernicke syndrome.*

GB. See *Guillain-Barré syndrome.*

GBS. See *Guillain-Barré syndrome.*

GCPS (Greig cephalopolysyndactyly syndrome). See *Greig syndrome.*

GCS. See *Gianotti-Crosti syndrome.*

GDXY (XY gonadal dysgenesis). See *chromosome XY female syndrome.*

GEE, SAMUEL JONES (British physician, 1839-1911)

Gee disease. See *celiac disease.*

Gee-Herter disease. See *celiac disease.*

Gee-Herter-Heubner disease. See *celiac disease.*

Gee-Thaysen disease. See *celiac disease.*

GEHRIG, HENRY LOUIS (American baseball player, 1903-1941)

Lou Gehrig disease. See *amyotrophic lateral sclerosis.*

geleophysic dwarfism. See *Spranger syndrome (2).*

GELINEAU, JEAN BAPTISTE EDOUARD (French psychiatrist, born 1859)

Gélineau syndrome. Synonyms: *genuine narcolepsy, hypnolepsy, narcolepsy, narcolepsy-catalepsy syndrome, narcoleptic syndrome, paroxysmal sleep, sleep epilepsy.*

An irresistible urge to sleep for brief periods, occurring during any activity and at any time of day. The condition is associated with a tetrad of manifestations: (1) Sleep attacks (occurring suddenly and being often REM sleep attacks), (2) catalepsy (often precipitated by surprise or anger), (3) hypnotic hallucinations, and (4) sleep paralysis (see *Rosenthal disease*, under *Rosenthal, Curt*).

Gélineau, De la narcolepsie. *Gaz. Hôp., Paris*, 1880, 53:626-8; 635-7.

GELLERSTEDT, NILS (Swedish physician, born 1896)

Ceelen-Gellerstedt syndrome. See *under Ceelen.*

GENEE, E.

Genée-Wiedemann syndrome. Synonym: *postaxial acrofacial dysostosis syndrome (POADS).*

A mental retardation-multiple congenital anomalies syndrome, transmitted as an autosomal recessive trait, characterized by acrofacial dysostosis with lower limb involvement, supernumerary vertebrae and other vertebral segmentation and rib defects, atrial and ventricular septal defects, supernumerary nipples, single umbilical artery, cleft palate, malformed ears and eyelids, and absence of the hemidiaphragm. Limb abnormalities vary from mild forms, such as hypoplasia of the fifth toes, to severe types, such as total absence of the fibulae and polydactyly and phocomelia with hypoplastic pectoral girdle (scapulae).

Genée, E. Une forme extensive de dysostose mandibulo-faciale. *J. Génét. Hum., Geneva*, 1969, 17:45-52.
Wiedemann, H. R. Missbildungs-Retardierungs-Syndrom mit Fehlen des 5. Strahls an Händen und Füssen, Gaumenspalte, dysplastischen Ohren und Augenlidern und radioulnarer Synostose. *Klin. Pädiat., Stuttgart*, 1973, 185:181-6. Opitz, J. M., & Stickler, G. B. The Genée-Wiedemann syndrome, an acrofacial dysostosis-further observations. *Am. J. Med. Genet.*, 1987, 27:971-5.

general adaptation syndrome (GAS). See *Selye syndrome.*

general arthritic paralysis. See *Klippel disease.*

general arthritic pseudoparalysis. See *Klippel disease.*

general paralysis. See *Bayle disease.*

general paresis. See *Bayle disease.*

generalized angiomatosis. See *Osler-Rendu-Weber syndrome.*

generalized aphthosis. See *Behçet syndrome.*

generalized capillary and arteriolar thrombosis. See *Moschcowitz syndrome.*

generalized chondromalacia. See *Meyenburg-Altherr-Uehlinger syndrome.*

generalized elastolysis. See *cutis laxa syndrome.*

generalized fibromatosis. See *Meyenburg disease.*

generalized follicle hyperplasia of lymph nodes and spleen. See *Brill-Symmers syndrome.*

generalized gangliosidosis. See *gangliosidosis G_{M1} type I.*

generalized glycogenosis. See *glycogen storage disease II.*

generalized hemopoietic hypoplasia. See *Vaal-Seynhaeve syndrome.*

generalized infantile gangliosidosis with bony involvement. See *gangliosidosis G_{M1} type I.*

generalized lipodystrophy. See *Berardinelli-Seip syndrome.*

generalized muscle rigidity syndrome. See *stiff-man syndrome.*

generalized neurodermatitis. See *Besnier prurigo.*

generalized neuromuscular exhaustion syndrome. See *Nielsen syndrome, under Nielsen, Johannes Mygaard.*

generalized osseous dystrophy syndrome. See *Melnick-Needles syndrome.*

generalized salivary gland virus infection. See *Wyatt disease, under Wyatt, John Poyner.*

generalized spine hyperkeratosis and universal alopecia and deafness. See *KID syndrome.*

generalized subacute thrombophilia. See *Nygaard-Brown syndrome.*

generalized verrucosis. See *Lewandowski-Lutz syndrome.*

generalized xanthonatosis with calcified adrenals. See *Wolman syndrome.*

geniculate syndrome. See *Hunt syndrome (2).*

geniculate ganglion syndrome. See *Hunt syndrome (2).*

geniculate neuralgia. See *Hunt syndrome (2).*

genital dwarfism. See *chromosome XO syndrome.*

genital retraction syndrome. Synonym: *Koro.*

A belief or delusion of retraction of the penis into the abdomen, originally considered to be a Chinese and Indonesian culture-bound syndrome, which recently has been noted to occur in other societies.

Fishbain, D. A., *et al.* "Koro" (genital retraction syndrome): Psychotherapeutic interventions. *Am. J. Psychother.*, 1989, 43:87-91.

genito-anorectal elephantiasis. See *Huguier-Jersild syndrome.*

genito-oral aphthosis with uveitis and hypopyon. See *Behçet syndrome.*

genitodystrophic gerodermia. See *Rummo-Ferranini syndrome, under Rummo, A.*

genitodystrophic xeroderma. See *Rummo-Ferranini syndrome, under Rummo, A.*

genitopalatocardiac syndrome. See *Gardner-Silengo-Wachtel syndrome, under Gardner, L. I.*

genu recurvatum-uterine retroversion-dysmenorrhea syndrome. See *Chapple syndrome (2).*

genuine narcolepsy. See *Gélineau syndrome.*

GERALD, PARK S. (American physician)

Say-Gerald syndrome. See *VATER association.*

GERARD

Gérard-Marchand fracture. Fracture of the radius with an outward dislocation of the lower fragment, pulling of the hand in the varus position, and resulting in a typical deep cutlike depression, reportedly described by Gérard and Marchand.

GERBASI, MICHELE (Italian physician, born 1900)

Gerbasi anemia. Synonyms: *Gerbasi syndrome, pseudo-Biermer anemia, pseudo-pernicious anemia of infants.*

Periniciosiform anemia in breast-fed infants, probably due to deficiency of Castle factor in maternal milk.

Gerbasi, M. Anemia perniciosiforme osservata in bambini ad allattamento materno esclusivo e protratto. *Pediatria, Napoli,* 1940, 48:505-26.

Gerbasi syndrome. See *Gerbasi anemia.*

GERHARDT, CARL ADOLF CHRISTIAN JAKOB (German physician, 1833-1902)

Gerhardt disease. See *Mitchell syndrome (1).*

Gerhardt syndrome. Bilateral abductor paralysis of the larynx.

Gerhardt, C. Studien und Beobachtungen über Stimmbandlähmung. *Arch. Path. Anat., Berlin,* 1863, 27:68-98; 296-321.

GERKEN, H. (German pediatrician)

Appelt-Gerken-Lenz syndrome. See *Roberts syndrome.*

GERLIER, E. FELIX (Swiss physician, 1840-1914)

Gerlier disease. Synonyms: *Gerlier syndrome, endemic paralytic vertigo, kubisagari, paralytic vertigo.*

An endemic disease that is usually restricted to small geographic areas in Switzerland, France, and Japan, and is characterized by the sudden onset of vertigo, together with visual disorders, including diplopia, photopsia, photophobia, and blepharoptosis. Severe headache, pain of the nuchal and spinal muscles, inability to hold the head up, and generalized muscle weakness follow. The disorder is transitory, and patients, usually farm workers exposed to cattle, recover within a few months. The etiology is unknown.

Gerlier. Une épidémie de vertige paralysant. *Rev. Méd. Suisse Rom.,* 1887, 7:5-29.

Gerlier syndrome. See *Gerlier disease.*

GERMAN, J.

German syndrome. See *fetal trimethadione syndrome.*

germinal aplasia syndrome. See *Sertoli cell only syndrome.*

geroderma osteodysplastica hereditaria (GOH). See *geroderma osteodysplastica syndrome.*

geroderma osteodysplastica syndrome. Synonyms: *Bamatter syndrome, Bamatter-Franceschetti-Klein-Sierro syndrome, Walt Disney dwarf, geroderma osteodysplastica hereditaria (GOH).*

A syndrome trasmitted as an X-linked trait with occasional manifestations in females, characterized by growth retardation, hyperlaxity, atrophy, and premature aging of the skin, in association with generalized osteoporosis and predispostion to fractures. Associated disorders include joint muscle hypotonia, hernias, pes planus, hip dislocation, platyspondyly with biconcave vertebrae, thin skin with prominent veins, malocclusion, sunken eyes, and microcorneae.

Bamater, F., Franceschetti, A., Klein, D., & Sierro, A. Gérodermie ostéodysplastique, héréditaire. Un nouveau biotype de la "progeria." *Confin. Neur., Basel,* 1949, 9:397; *Ann. Paediat., Basel,* 1950, 174:12-7.

GEROLD, M.

Baller-Gerold syndrome. See *under Baller.*

GEROTA, DIMITRU (Roumanian anatomist, 1867-1939)

Gerota fascitis. See *Ormond syndrome.*

Gerota syndrome. See *Ormond syndrome.*

GERSTMANN, JOSEF (Austrian physician, 1887-1969)

Gerstmann syndrome (GS) (1). Synonyms: *Gerstmann-Sträussler disease (GSD), Gerstmann-Sträussler syndrome (GSS)), Gerstmann-Sträussler-Scheinker disease (GSSD), cerebral amyloidosis with spongiform encephalopathy, spinocerebellar degeneration-dementia-plaque-like deposits syndrome.*

A familial neurological syndrome transmitted as an autosomal dominant trait. Slowly developing dysarthria and cerebellar ataxia in the fifth decade are the earliest symptoms. They are followed by the absence of reflexes in the legs, bradykinesia, pyramidal signs, and dementia. Nystagmus occurs in some cases. Death follows 2 to 10 years after the onset of symptoms. Pathological findings consist of disseminated amyloid plaques throughout the central nervous system; massive plaques in the cerebral cortex; degeneration of the spinocerebellar and corticospinal tracts, posterior columns of the spinal cord, and gray matter in the Purkinje cells, granule cells, neurons of the cerebral cortex, and caudate nuclei; and spongy changes in the cerebral cortex and caudate nuclei.

Gerstmann, J., Sträussler, E., & Scheinker, I. Über eine eigenartige hereditär-familiäre Erkrankung des Zenetralnervensystems. Zugleich ein Beitrag zur Frage des vorzeitigen lokalen Altern. *Zschr. Ges. Neur. Psychiat.,* 1936, 154:736-62.

Gerstmann syndrome (GS) (2). Synonyms: *Gerstmann-Badal syndrome, angular gyrus syndrome, angularis syndrome, dyscalculia and right-left disorientation, finger agnosia, gyrus angularis syndrome.*

Loss of visual recognition of the finger, confusion of laterality, apractic loss of finger demonstration, agraphia, and dyscalculia in lesions of the anterior portion of the brain in the region of the angular gyrus.

Gerstmann, J. Fingeragnosie: Eine umschriebene Störung der Orientierung am eigenen Körper. *Wien. Klin. Wschr.,* 1924, 37:1010-2. Critchley, M. The enigma of Gerstmann's syndrome. *Brain,* 1966, 89(pt.2):183-98.

Gerstmann-Badal syndrome. See *Gerstmann syndrome (2).*

Gerstmann-Sträussler disease (GSD). See *Gerstmann syndrome (1).*

Gerstmann-Sträussler syndrome (GSS). See *Gerstmann syndrome (1).*

Gerstmann-Sträussler-Scheinker disease (GSSD). See *Gerstmann syndrome (1).*

GESCHICKTER, CHARLES F. (American physician)

Geschickter tumor. Synonyms: *Geschickter-Copeland tumor, paraosteal osteoma, sarcoma osteogenes parostale, sarcoma osteogenes juxtacorticale.*

A bone tumor histologically similar to myositis ossificans, which occurs in both malignant and benign forms (the malignant type being more common), usually at the lower end of the femur or upper humerus. Adults between the ages of 20 and 40 years are most frequently affected. X-ray findings show a mass about 5 to 10 cm in diameter that is densely ossified, circumscribed, and occurring outside the bone, but contiguous with it. A typical tumor is fused with the periosteum and usually encapsulated at its outer margins. The tumor has a firm, dry, striated surface simulating fibrosed cancellous bone. Microscopically, adult bone fibrous tissue predominates but foci of fibrospindle cell sarcoma are found at the periphery in some cases.

Geschickter, C. F., & Copeland, M. M. Parosteal osteoma of bone: A new entity. *Ann. Surg.*, 1951, 133:790-807.

Geschickter-Copeland tumor. See *Geschickter tumor.*

GESCHWIND, N.

Geschwind syndrome. See *disconnection syndrome.*

GHON, ANTON (Prague pathologist, 1866-1936)

Ghon focus. See *Ghon primary lesion.*

Ghon primary lesion. Synonyms: *Ghon focus, Ghon tubercle.*

The primary parenchymal lesion of pulmonary tuberculosis in children.

Ghon, A. *Der primäre Lungenherd bei der Tuberkulose der Kinder.* Berlin, Urbach & Schwarzenberg, 1912.

Ghon tubercle. See *Ghon primary lesion.*

GIACCAI, L. (Physician in Lebanon)

Giaccai syndrome. Synonyms: *neurogenic acro-osteolysis, neurotrophic osseous atrophy.*

Progressive plantar ulceration resulting in mutilation of the feet, associated with sensory disturbances of the extremities. The symptoms become apparent in childhood or early adolescence, usually as slightly painful plantar ulcerations which become purulent and discharge bony spicules. The initial lesions heal spontaneously, but new ulcers appear in a few months or years, accompanied by fever which abates as the discharge commences. In time, the feet become swollen and mutilated and walking becomes difficult. Disorders of pain, heat, and touch sensibility involving all the extremities usually follow. Acro-osteolysis with osteomyelitic changes, bone rarefaction, osteosclerosis, formation of sequestra, and fragmentation of the shafts and distal epiphyses are the principal radiographic findings. Bone changes are of the osteolytic type, the shafts being destroyed while the epiphyses remain as loose bony spicules which undergo reabsorption or are eliminated as sequestra. The syndrome occurs as a familial or sporadic disorder; the sporadic type being often unilateral, usually in association with spinal disorders (syringomyelia, spina bifida, or myelodysplasia) and cogenital foot defects (flatfoot, talipes equinovarus, and the like). Males are more frequently affected than females.

Giaccai, L. Familial and sporadic neurogenic acro-osteolysis. *Acta Radiol., Stockholm,* 1952, 38:17-29.

GIACOBINI, GENARO (Argentine physician, 1889-1954)

Lucherini-Giacobini syndrome. See *under Lucherini.*

GIACOMINI, CARLO (Italian physician, 1841-1898)

Giacomini disease. A rare form of hereditary microcephaly, transmitted as an autosomal recessive trait, usually associated with mental retardation and a wide variety of ocular defects, such as chorioretinal dysplasia, microphthalmia, and embryonic remnants (persistence of the primary vitreous or its minor forms).

Alzial, C., *et al.* Ocular abnormalities of true microcephaly. *Ophthalmologica, Basel,* 1980, 180:333-9. Graux, P., *et al.* Étude génétique de la microcéphalie héréditaire idiopathique (maladie de Giacomini); à propos d'une fratrie comportant 7 microcéphales. *Rev. Neur., Paris,* 1970, 123:423-5.

GIANOTTI, FERDINANDO (Italian physician, born 1920)

Gianotti disease. See *Gianotti-Crosti syndrome.*

Gianotti-Crosti syndrome (GCS). Synonyms: *Gianotti disease, acrodermatitis papulosa eruptiva infantum, acrodermatitis papulosa infantum, eruptive papulous dermatitis of the extremities, infantile acrolocalized papulovesicular syndrome, infantile lichenoid acrodermatitis, infantile papular acrodermatitis (IPA), papular acrodermatitis, papular acrodermatitis of childhood, papulovesical acrolocalized syndrome.*

An exanthematous eruption of the extremities, that appears suddenly in young children and disappears without treatment within 30 to 70 days. The lesions are red, copper, or purple papules with clear limits, ranging in size from that of a pinhead to larger discoid lesions. Purpura, liver disorders, and polyadenopathy are associated. The condition appears to be related to viral infections.

Crosti, A., & Gianotti, F. Dermatose éruptive acrosituée d'origine probablement virosique. *Dermatologica, Basel,* 1957, 115:671-7.

GIANSANTI, JOSEPH S. (American dentist)

Witkop-Weech-Giansanti syndrome. See *tooth-nail syndrome.*

giant condyloma acuminatum of the penis. See *Buschke-Loewenstein tumor.*

giant condyloma of the penis. See *Buschke-Loewenstein tumor.*

giant follicle hyperplasia. See *Brill-Symmers syndrome.*

giant follicle lymphoma. See *Brill-Symmers syndrome.*

giant follicle lymphosarcoma. See *Brill-Symmers syndrome.*

giant follicular lymphadenopathy. See *Brill-Symmers syndrome.*

giant follicular lymphoblastoma. See *Brill-Symmers syndrome.*

giant hypertrophic gastritis. See *Ménétrier syndrome.*

giant hypertrophy of gastric mucosa. See *Ménétrier syndrome.*

giant lymph node hyperplasia (GLNH). See *Castleman disease.*

giant lymphoid hyperplasia of the mediastinum. See *Castleman disease.*

giant platelet syndrome. See *Bernard-Soulier syndrome, under Bernard, Jean.*

giant urticaria. See *Quincke edema.*

giant-cell arteritis. See *Horton disease (1).*

giant-cell chondrodysplasia. See *spondylohumerofemoral hypoplasia syndrome.*

giant-cell granulomatous myocarditis. See *Fiedler myocarditis.*

giant-cell myocarditis. See *Fiedler myocarditis.*

giant-cell pneumonia. See *Hecht pneumonia, under Hecht, Victor.*

giant-cell pseudotuberculous thyroiditis. See *de Quervain disease (2), under Quervain, Fritz, de.*

giant-cell thyroiditis. See *de Quervain disease (2), under Quervain, Fritz, de.*

GIBERT, CAMILLE MELCHIOR (French physician, 1797-1866)

Gibert disease. Synonyms: *Hebra disease, herpes tonsurans maculosus, pityriasis circinata, pityriasis macu-*

lata et circinata, pityriasis rosea, squamous roseola.

An acute, self-limited, inflammatory disease of the skin characterized by oval or circinate macules distributed symmetrically over the trunk and extremities. The individual lesions are usually yellowish, pinkish, or reddish and vary in size from 0.5 to 5.0 cm in diameter. A single large plaque precedes the general eruption by about 1 to 2 weeks. The eruption disappears normally after 4 to 8 weeks, and recurrences are rare.

*Gibert. *Traité pratique des maladies de la peau*. Paris, Plon, 1860, p. 402.

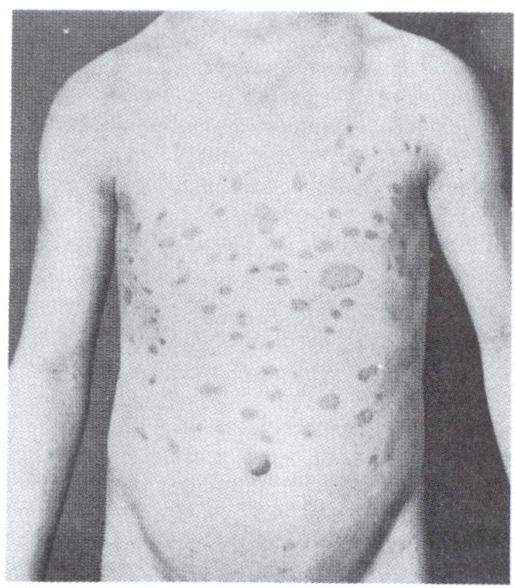

Gibert disease
Nelson, W.E. (eds): *Textbook of Pediatrics*, 8th ed. Philadelphia, W.B. Saunders Co., 1964.

Gibraltar fever. See *brucellosis.*

GIBSON, JOHN LOCKHART (Australian ophthalmologist, 1860-1944)

Gibson glioma. Intraocular glioma of the optic nerve.

Gibson, J. L. Intra-ocular glioma of the optic nerve of each eye. *Brit. J. Ophth.*, 1921, 5:67.

GIBSON, QUENTIN HOWIESON (British physician)

Gibson disease. Synonyms: *Gibson methemoglobinemia, congenital idiopathic methemoglobinemia, idiopathic methemoglobinemia.*

A hereditary hematological disease, transmitted as an autosomal recessive trait, characterized by the presence in the blood of methemoglobin, resulting in the inability of hemoglobin to combine efficiently with oxygen, with secondary persistent slate-gray cyanosis. Fatigability and dyspnea after physical effort are the main complaints. Deficiency of NADH-dependent methemoglobin reductase is the cause. See also *Stokvis-Talma syndrome.*

Gibson, Q. H. The reduction of methemoglobin in red blood cells and studies on the cause of idiopathic methaemoglobinemia. *Biochem. J.*, 1948, 42:13-33. Schwartz, J. M., & Jaffé, E. R. Hereditary methemoglobinemia with deficiency of NADH dehydrogenase. In: Stanbury, J. B., Wyngaarden, J. B., & Fredrickson, D. S., eds. *Metabolic basis of inherited disease*. 4th ed. New York, McGraw-Hill, 1978, pp. 1452-64.

Gibson methemoglobinemia. See *Gibson disease.*

GIEDION, ANDREAS (Swiss physician)

Giedion syndrome. See *trichorhinophalangeal syndrome.*

Langer-Giedion syndrome. See *under Langer.*

Schinzel-Giedion syndrome. See *under Schinzel.*

GIERKE, EDGAR OTTO CONRAD, VON (German physician, 1877-1945)

Fibiger-Debré-von Gierke syndrome. See *congenital adrenal hyperplasia.*

Gierke disease. See *glycogen storage disease I.*

van Creveld-von Gierke syndrome. See *glycogen storage disease I.*

von Gierke disease. See *glycogen storage disease I.*

gigantism. See *Marie syndrome (2), under Marie, Pierre.*

GILBERT, JUDSON BENNETT (American physician, born 1896)

Gilbert syndrome. Synonym: *choriogenic gynecomastia.*

An association of malignant testicular tumors with gynecomastia, high titers of chorionic gonadotropic hormones, and the presence of folliculin.

Gilbert, J. B. Studies in malignant testis tumor. II. Syndrome of choriogenic gynecomastia; report of six cases and review of one hundred and twenty-nine. *J. Urol.*, 1940, 44:345-57.

GILBERT, NICOLAS AUGUSTIN (French physician, 1858-1927)

Gilbert disease. See *Gilbert syndrome.*

Gilbert syndrome (GS). Synonyms: *Gilbert disease, Gilbert-Lereboullet syndrome, Meulengracht icterus, Meulengracht syndrome, benign unconjugated hyperbilirubinemia, cholemia familiaris simplex, chronic intermittent juvenile jaundice, congenital familial cholemia, constitutional hepatic dysfunction, constitutional hyperbilirubinemia, constitutional liver dysfunction, familial cholemia, familial nonhemolytic jaundice, familial nonhemolytic bilirubinemia, hereditary nonhemolytic bilirubinemia, hereditary nonhemolytic jaundice, hyperbilirubinemia I, icterus intermittens juvenilis, idiopathic hyperbilirubinemia, physiologic cholemia, unconjugated benign bilirubinemia, unconjugated hyperbilirubinemia.*

A benign familial disorder, transmitted as an autosomal dominant trait, in which unconjugated hyperbilirubinemia occurs in the absence of structural liver disease and overt hemolysis, with considerable daily fluctuations of the bilirubin level. Jaundice may be detected shortly after birth or later in life. Scleral jaundice is a constant feature. Asthenia, fatigue, anxiety, nausea, and abdominal pain occur in most cases. The symptoms may be precipitated by exertion, alcohol, or infection.

Gilbert, A., Castaigne, J., & Lereboullet, P. De l'ictère familial. Contribution à l'étude de la diathèse biliaire. *Bull. Soc. Méd. Hôp.*, 1900, 17:948-59. Gilbert, A., & Lereboullet, P. La cholémie simple familiale. *Sem. Méd., Paris*, 1901, 21:241-3. Meulengracht, E. Icterus intermittens juvenilis (chronischer intermittierender juveniler Subikterus). *Klin. Wschr.*, 1939, 18:118-21.

Gilbert-Lereboullet syndrome. See *Gilbert syndrome.*

GILBERT, W. (German ophthalmologist)

Gilbert syndrome. See *Behçet syndrome.*

Gilbert-Behçet syndrome. See *Behçet syndrome.*

GILBERT-DREYFUS, SAVOIE (French physician)

Gilbert-Dreyfus syndrome. A familial form of pseudohermaphroditism characterized by male phenotype, hypospadias, gynecomastia, scanty axillary hair, absent beard, and almost normal testes. The patient described by Gilbert-Dreyfus was capable of erection and ejaculation. The estrogen level was below normal and the buccal smear was chromatin-negative.

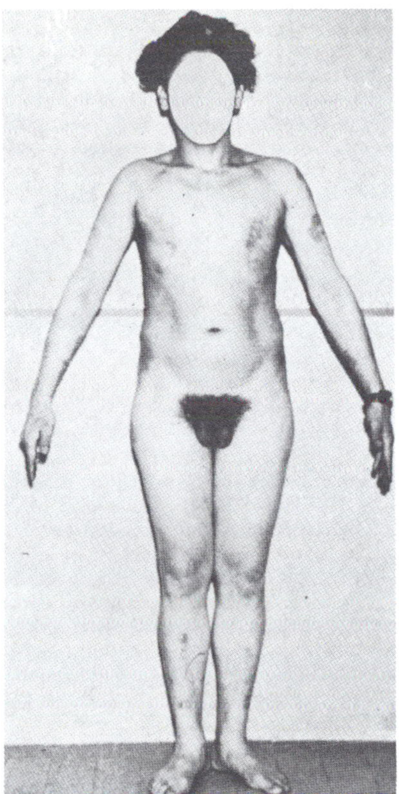

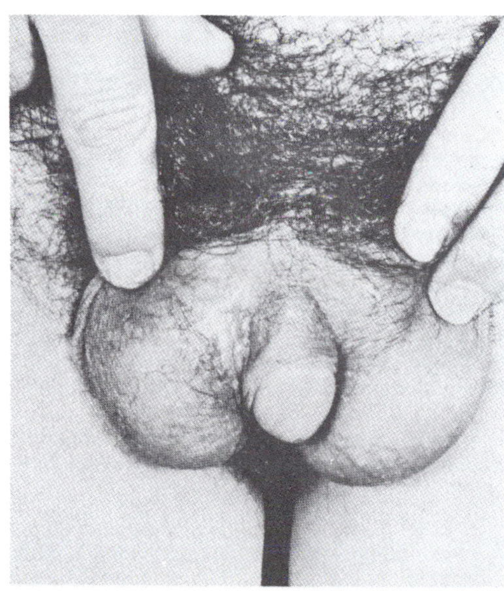

Gilbert-Dreyfus syndrome
Federman, D.D.,: *Abnormal Sexual Development.* Philadelphia, W.B.

Gilbert-Dreyfus, S., *et al*. Étude d'un cas familial d'androgynoïdisme avec hypospadias grave, gynécomastie et hypooestrogénie. *Ann. Endocr., Paris*, 1957, 18:93-101.

GILCHRIST, THOMAS CASPER (American physician)

Gilchrist disease. Synonyms: *Gilchrist mycosis, American blastomycosis, blastomycetic dermatitis, dermatitis blastomycetica, North American blastomycosis, oidiomycosis.*

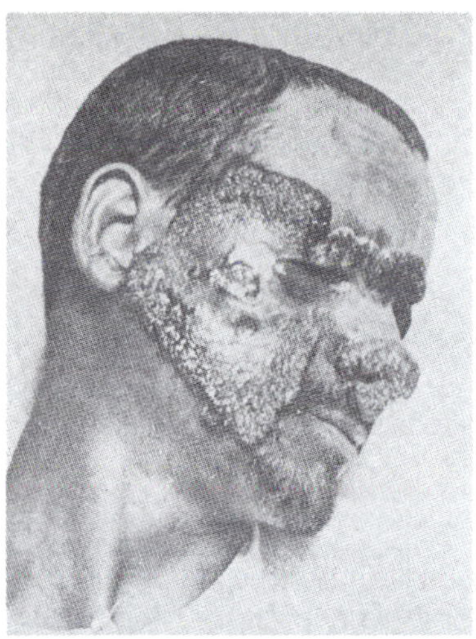

Gilchrist disease
Andrew, G.C. & A.N. Domonkos: *Diseases of the Skin.* 5th ed. Philadelphia: W.B. Saunders Co., 1963.

A chronic progressive, cutaneous, systemic, or combined systemic and cutaneous disease caused by the fungus *Blastomyces dermatitidis*, which occurs almost exclusively in North America. The cutaneous lesions are characterized by papules or papulopustules which develop into crusted, warty eruptions, and oozing sinuses. Areas of the face, particularly the facial orifices, are common sites. Oral lesions are not as prominent as those of the skin, minute ulcers being the most visible features. The oral infection may represent spreading of facial lesions to the nasal, oral, and conjunctival mucous membrane, or it may be primary.

Gilchrist, T. A. A case of blastomycetic dermatitis in man. *Johns Hopkins Hosp. Rep.*, 1896, 1:169-90.

Gilchrist mycosis. See *Gilchrist disease.*

GILFORD, HASTINGS (British physician, 1861-1941)

Gilford syndrome. See *Hutchinson-Gilford syndrome, under Hutchinson, Sir Jonathan.*

Hutchinson-Gilford progeria. See *Hutchinson-Gilford syndrome, under Hutchinson, Sir Jonathan.*

Hutchinson-Gilford progeria syndrome (HGPS). See *Hutchinson-Gilford syndrome, under Hutchinson, Sir Jonathan.*

Hutchinson-Gilford syndrome. See *under Hutchinson, Sir Jonathan.*

GILLES DE LA TOURETTE, GEORGES EDMOUND ALBERT BRUTUS (French physician, 1855-1909)

Gilles de la Tourette syndrome (GTS). Synonyms: *Brissaud disease, Guinon disease, Tourette syndrome (TS), chorea variabilis, compulsive tic, coprolalia-compulsive tic syndrome, habit spasm, mimic spasm, myospasia impulsiva.*

A psychoneurological disorder characterized by chorea, coprolalia, echolalia, and tic. The affected children, usually boys between the ages of 5 and 10 years, develop tics of the hands, arms, or face, spreading to other parts of the body, so that the child has some combination of frequent repetitive facial grimaces, throwing out the arms, contraction of the leg muscles, involuntary kicking, blepharospasms, rubbing of the face, putting the thumbs to the mouth, and hitting or handling other parts of the body. This is followed by compulsive repetitive noises like grunting or hiccuping, which subsequently become frank obscenities. The course of the illness varies. In some patients, the disorders tend to abate, whereas in others they progress to severe disability. The syndrome occurs most frequently in Ashkenazie Jews and persons of Mediterranean extraction, rarely in black children. Transmission as an autosomal dominant trait is suspected.

Gilles de la Tourette. Étude sur une affection nerveuse charactérisée par de l'incoordination motrice accopagnée d'echolalie et de coprolalie (jumping, latah, myriachit). *Arch. Neur., Paris,* 1885, 9:19-42; 158-20 Brissaud, E. La chorée variable de dégenérés. *Rev. Neur., Paris,* 1896, 4:417-31. Guinon, G. Sur la maladie des tics convulsifs. *Rev. Méd., Paris,* 1886, 6:50-80.

Tourette syndrome (TS). See *Gilles de la Tourette syndrome.*

Tourette-like syndrome (TLS). A form of tardive dyskinesia with symptoms of involuntary movements and vocalization, similar to those seen in the Gilles de la Tourette syndrome, believed to be due to chemical denervation hypersensitivity of dopamine receptors following chronic neuroleptic blockage.

Klawans, H. L., *et al.* Gilles de la Tourette syndrome after long term chlorpromazine therapy. *Neurology,* 1978, 28:1064-8.

GILLESPIE, F. D. (American ophthalmologist)

Gillespie syndrome (1). See *oculodentodigital syndrome.*

Gillespie syndrome (2). Synonym: *aniridia-cerebellar ataxia-mental retardation syndrome.*

A rare hereditary syndrome, probably transmitted as an autosomal recessive trait, characterized by partial or complete aniridia, aplasia involving only the pupillary zone of the iris (circumpupillary iris aplasia); congenital nonprogressive cerebellar ataxia with hypotonia; and oligophrenia.

Gillespie, F. D. Aniridia, cerebellar ataxia and oligophrenia in siblings. *Arch. Ophth., Chicago,* 1965, 73:338-41.

GILMOUR

Horton-Gilmour disease. See *Horton disease (1).*

GIMARD, MARTIN JULES LOUIS ALEXANDRE, DE. See MARTIN DE GIMARD, JULES LOUIS ALEXANDRE

gingival fibromatosis-hypertrichosis syndrome. Synonyms: *congenital gingival hyperplasia-hypertrichosis syndrome, congenital macrogingivae-hypertrichosis syndrome, elephantiasis gingivae-hypertrichosis syndrome, fibromatosis gingivae-hypertrichosis syndrome.*

A syndrome of early generalized hypertrichosis and gingival fibromatosis, sometimes associated with epilepsy, mental retardation, and other disorders. Most cases follow a dominant pattern of inheritance, but some are sporadic.

Ruggles, S. D. Primary hypertrophy of the gums. *JAMA,* 1925, 84:20. Witkop, C. J., Jr. Heterogeneity in gingival fibromatosis. *Birth Defects,* 1971, 7(7):210-21.

gingivitis expulsiva. See *Fauchard disease.*

gingivopericementitis. See *Fauchard disease.*

gingivostomatitis syndrome. Synonyms: *atypical gingivostomatitis, idiopathic gingivostomatitis, plasma-cell gingivitis, plasmocytosis of the gingiva.*

An association of cheilitis, glossitis, and gingivitis, believed to be caused by hypersensitivity, associated with cyclic hormonal imbalance. The gingiva appears uniformly inflamed and deeply pink, but remains stippled, with edema of the free and attached gingivae. Histological studies show intense plasma-cell infiltration in the lamina propria.

Kerr, D. A., *et al.* Idiopathic gingivostomatitis. *Oral Surg.,* 1971, 32:402-23.

GIOCONDA. See MONA LISA

GIOVANNINI, SEBASTIANO (Italian physician, 1851-1920)

Giovannini disease. A fungal infection that produces a nodular disease of the hair.

*Giovannini, S. Über die normale Entwicklung und über einige Veränderungen der menschlichen Haare. *Vjschr. Derm. Syph.,* 1887, 14: 1049-75.

GIROUX, JEAN MARIE (Canadian physician)

Giroux-Barbeau syndrome. A neurocutaneous syndrome, transmitted as an autosomal dominant trait, characterized by focal erythematous, hyperkeratotic plaques which are either present at birth or appear shortly thereafter, followed by the development of progressive neurologic disorders in adulthood. The plaques vary in form and intensity and tend to subside during the summer months, most disappearing by the age of 25 years, sometimes to reappear after the age of 40 years. Neurological complications usually consist of decreased tendon reflexes, nystagmus, dysarthria, and severe gait ataxia. The original cases were reported in a family of French Canadian ethnic background.

Giroux, J. M., & Barbeau, A. Erythrodermatodermia with ataxia. *Arch. Derm., Chicago,* 1972, 106:183-8.

GITLIN, D. (American physician)

Bruton-Gitlin syndrome. See *Bruton syndrome.*

GIUFFRIDA-RUGGIERI, VINCENZO (Italian physician, 1872-1922)

Giuffrida-Ruggieri stigma. An abnormally shallow glenoid fossa.

Giuffrida-Ruggieri, V. *Sulla dignità morfologica dei segni detti "degenerativi."* Roma, Laescher, 1879.

GJA-S (gastric juice aspiration syndrome). See *Mendelson syndrome.*

GJESSING, LEIV ROLVSSOEN. (Norwegian physician, born 1918)

Gjessing syndrome. Periodic catatonic stupor and excitement coinciding with nitrogen retention and responding to thyroid therapy.

Gjessing, R. Disturbances of somatic function in catatonia with a periodic course, and their compensation. *J. Ment. Sc.,* 1938, 84:608-21.

GLA (alpha-galactosidase A) deficiency. See *Fabry syndrome.*

glandular fever. See *Filatov disease.*

GLANZMANN, EDUARD (Swiss physician, 1887-1959)

Glanzmann dysporia. See *Andersen triad.*

Glanzmann syndrome. See *Glanzmann thrombasthenia.*

Glanzmann thrombasthenia (GT, GTA). Synonyms: *Glanzmann syndrome, Glanzmann-Naegeli syndrome, Revol syndrome, athrombocytopenic purpura, congenital hemorrhagic thrombocytic dystrophy, diacyclothrombopathy, glycoprotein IIb-III (GP IIb-III) complex deficiency, hemorrhagic thrombasthenia, hereditary thrombasthenia, hereditary thrombocytopenic purpura, plate-*

let fibrinogen receptor deficiency, platelet glycoprotein IIb-III deficiency, thrombocytasthenia, thrombocytopathic purpura.

A hereditary hemorrhagic disorder due to platelet glycoprotein IIb-III deficiency, marked by purpura, prolonged bleeding time, capillary fragility, mild thrombocytopenia, impaired clot retraction, ecchymoses, petechiae, gingival bleeding, epistaxis, menorrhagia, metrorrhagia, gastrointestinal hemorrhage, and excessive postoperative hemorrhage. Defective pseudopod formation and failure of the blood platelets to spread in contact with wettable surfaces are its main features. Low ATP concentrations; faulty glycolysis with or without decreased levels of pyruvate kinase, phosphoglyceraldehyde dehydrogenase, and ATPase; ADP deficiency; and diminished contents of glutathione reductase and glutathione peroxidase in the blood platelets are its principal biochemical defects. The syndrome is generally transmitted as an autosomal recessive trait, but some cases are known to be transmitted as an autosomal dominant trait.

*Glanzmann, E. Hereditäre hämorrhagische Thrombasthenie. Ein Beitrag zur Pathologie der Blutplättchen. *Jb. Kinderh.*, 1918, 88:1-42; 113-41. Revol, L. Nouveau type de dysmorphie thrombocytaire. La diacyclothrombopathie. *Lyon Méd.*, 1950, 183:213-8.

Glanzmann-Naegeli syndrome. See *Glanzmann thrombasthenia.*

Glanzmann-Riniker alymphoplasia. See *severe mixed immunodeficiency syndrome.*

Glanzmann-Riniker syndrome. See *severe mixed immunodeficiency syndrome.*

Glanzmann-Saland syndrome. Severe polyneuritis following diphtheria.

Glanzmann, E., & Saland, S. Seltene postdiphtherische Lähmungen. *Schweiz. Med. Wschr.*, 1935, 16:2-5.

glaucomatocyclitic crises. See *Posner-Schlossman syndrome.*

glazed tongue. See *Möller glossitis.*

GLENARD, FRANTZ (French physician, 1848-1920)

Glénard syndrome. Synonyms: *enteroptosis, splanchnoptosis, visceroptosis.*

A downard displacement of the viscera that may be associated with neurasthenic disorders. The symptoms include muscle tonus disorders, bulging of the abdomen, abdominal pain, a "sinking feeling," backache, vertigo, tachycardia, vasomotor disorders, nausea, vomiting, constipation alternating with diarrhea, headache, fatigability, lethargy, insomnia, anemia, and general nervousness.

Glénard, F. Neurasthénie et entéroptose. *Sem. Méd., Paris*, 1886, 6:211-2.

GLINSKI, LEON KONRAD (Polish physician, 1870-1918)

Glinski-Simmonds syndrome. See *Sheehan syndrome.*

glioma sarcomatodes. See *Cushing medulloblastoma.*

glioma-polyposis syndrome. See *Turcot syndrome.*

GLISSON, FRANCIS (British physician, 1597-1677)

Glisson disease. Synonyms: *English disease, morbus anglicus, morbus anglorum, rachitis, rickets.*

A metabolic disease of infancy and childhood, in which vitamin D deficiency results in failure of calcification of growing bones, associated with bending of bones, hypertrophy of epiphyseal cartilage, widening of the epiphyseal plate (seen on the x-ray as a widened radiolucent zone) with flaring and cupping and irregularity of the epiphyseal-metaphyseal junction, swelling along the costochondral junctions (rachitic rosary), swelling at the ends of the long bones, and delayed closure of the fontanels. The symptoms usually include apathy, listnessness, weakness, hypotonia, growth retardation, misshapen and somewhat soft head with frontal bossing, delayed dentition, hypoplasia of the dental enamel, protruding abdomen, waddling gait, swelling of the joints, and pathological fractures in severe cases. See also Lightwood-Albright syndrome and hypophosphatemic familial rickets.

*Glisson, F. De rachitide, sive morbo puerili qui vulga rickets dictor. London, 1650.

GLNH (giant lymph node hyperplasia). See *Castleman disease.*

global demyelination. See *Schilder disease.*

globoid cell cerebral sclerosis. See *Krabbe disease.*

globoid cell leukodystrophy. See *Krabbe disease.*

globoid cell sclerosis. See *Krabbe disease.*

globozoospermia. See *round-head spermatozoa syndrome.*

glomangioma. See *Barré-Masson syndrome, under Barré, Jean Alexandre.*

glomerulonephritis. See *Klebs disease.*

glomerulonephritis-male pseudohermaphroditism-nephroblastoma syndrome. See *Drash syndrome.*

glomerulonephritis-pulmonary hemorrhage syndrome. See *Goodpasture syndrome.*

glomus tumor. See *Barré-Masson syndrome, under Barré, Jean Alexandre.*

glossitis exfoliativa. See *Möller glossitis.*

glossitis rhombica mediana. See *Brocq-Pautrier syndrome.*

glossitis superficialis chronica. See *Möller glossitis.*

glossodynia exfoliativa. See *Möller glossitis.*

glossolabiolaryngeal paralysis. See *Duchenne paralysis.*

glossolabiopharyngeal paralysis. See *Duchenne paralysis.*

glossolaryngoscapulopharyngeal hemiplegia. See *Collet-Sicard syndrome.*

glossopalatine ankylosis syndrome. Synonyms: *ankyloglossia superior, ankyloglossum superius syndrome.*

Adherence of the tongue to the roof of the mouth, often associated with other abnormalities. The tongue is usually attached to the hard palate, but may also be adherent to the maxillary alveolar ridge or, in some instances, to the lower edge of the nasal septum. Associated anomalies may include high-arched palate, cleft palate, mandibular hypoplasia, hypodontia, temporomandibular joint ankylosis, facial paralysis, and limb malformations, such as syndactyly, digital hypoplasia, lobster claw deformity, and monodactyly involving the hands and feet. The etiology is unknown.

*Kettner. Kongenitaler Zungendefekt. *Deut. Med. Wschr.*, 1907, 33:532. *Kramer, W. Zur Entstehung der angeborenen Gaumenspalte. *Zbl. Chir.*, 1911, 38:385-7.

glossopharyngeal neuralgia syndrome. Synonym: *Weisenburg syndrome.*

A rare condition occurring chiefly in the elderly, which may be precipitated by swallowing, yawning, or caughing, characterized by paroxysms of sharp shooting pain extending from the trigger zone in the posterior pharynx or tonsillar fossa and spreading to the ear, nasopharynx, and posterior part of the tongue.

Occasional severe attacks may be interspersed among numerous mild attacks. The pain is usually followed by homolateral lacrimation and salivation. Tinnitus, partial deafness, and facial tics may occur between attacks of pain. See also *headache syndrome*.

Reichert, F. L. Neuralgias of the glossopharyngeal nerve with particular reference to sensory, gustatory, and secretory functions of the nerves. *Arch., Neur. Psychiat.*, 1934, 32:1032-7. Weisenburg, T. H. Cerebello-pontile tumor diagnosed for six years as tic douloureux.. The symptoms of irritation of the ninth and twelfth cranial nerves. *JAMA*, 1910, 54:1600-4.

glossy tongue. See *Möller glossitis*.

glucagon-secreting carcinoma of pancreas. See *glucagonoma syndrome*.

glucagonoma syndrome. Synonym: *glucagon-secreting carcinoma of pancreas*.

A frequently maligant and metastasizing glucagon-secreting tumor of the pancreas with characteristic skin lesions **(necrolytic migratory erythema, NME)** marked by circinate and gyrate areas of blistering and erosive erythema of the face, lower abdomen, perineum, buttocks, and distal extremities. Glossitis, stomatitis, and angular cheilitis are frequently associated. There are spontaneous periods of remission and exacerbation with residual hyperpigmentation at the sites of healed lesions. Other features include weight loss, normochromic normocytic anemia, increased fasting blood glucose levels, depressed plasma amino acid levels, hypercholesterolemia, elevated plasma ketones in the presence of normal free fatty acids in the blood plasma, and high plasma glucagon levels. The syndrome appears to be transmitted as an autosomal dominant trait. Some cases occur in families with the multiple endocrine neoplasia syndrome I (q.v.).

Becker, S. W., *et al.* Cutaneous manifestations of internal malignant tumors. *Arch. Derm. Syph., Chicago,* 1942, 45:1069. Mac Gavran, M. H., *et al.* A glucagon-secreting carcinoma of pancreas. *N. Engl. J. Med.,* 1966, 274:1408-13.

α-1,4-glucan:alpha-1,4-glucan 6-glucosyl transferase deficiency. See *glycogen storage disease IV*.

glucoadipositas hepatomegalica. See *Debré syndrome (2)*.

glucose-6-phosphatase (G6P) deficiency. See *glycogen storage disease I*.

α-1,4-glucosidase deficiency. See *glycogen storage disease II*.

glucosyl ceramide lipidosis. See *Gaucher disease*.

gluten-induced enteropathy. See *celiac disease*.

gluten-sensitive enteropathy. See *celiac disease*.

glycogen disease (I, II, III. IV, V, VI, VII, VIII). See *glycogen storage disease (I, II, III, IV, V, VI, VII, VIII)*.

glycogen disease of muscle. See *glycogen storage disease VII*.

glycogen heart disease. See *glycogen storage disease II*.

glycogen infiltration. See *Armani-Ebstein nephropathy*.

glycogen nephrosis. See *Armani-Ebstein nephropathy*.

glycogen storage disease I. Synonyms: *Gierke disease, van Creveld-von Gierke syndrome, von Gierke disease, glucose-6-phosphatase (G6P) deficiency, glycogen disease I, glycogenosis I, hepatonephromegalia glycogenica, hepatorenal glycogenosis, liver glycogen disease*.

An inborn error of glycogen metabolism due to glucose-6-phosphatase (G6P) deficiency, involving chiefly the liver and kidneys. The symptoms are usually present at birth or appear shortly thereafter. They include short stature; prominent abdomen due to massive hepatomegaly; adiposity with accumulation of fat in the cheeks, buttocks, and subcutaneous tissues; flabby and poorly developed muscles; nephromegaly; ocular disorders, including corneal clouding and discrete yellow paramacular lesions in the fundi; osteoporosis due to negative calcium balance in chronic acidosis; xanthomas of the extensor surfaces of the extremities; epistaxis and postoperative hemorrhagic complications secondary to impaired platelet function; steatorrhea; hypoglycemia and high blood levels of lactates, pyruvates, triglycerides, phospholipids, cholesterol, and uric acid; ketosis; convulsions; and the Fanconi syndrome (aminoaciduria, glycosuria, and phosphaturia). The syndrome is transmitted as an autosomal recessive trait.

Gierke, E., von. Hepato-nephromegalia glycogenica (Glycogenspeicherkrankheit der Leber und Nieren). *Beitr. Path. Anat.*, 1929, 82:497-513. Creveld, S., van. Chronische hepatogene Hypoglykamie im Kindersalter. *Zschr. Kinderh.*, 1932, 52:299-324.

glycogen storage disease II. Synonyms: *Pompe disease, acid maltase deficiency, α-1,4-glucosidase deficiency, cardiac glycogenosis, cardiomegalia glycogenica diffusa, generalized glycogenosis, glycogen disease II, glycogen heart disease, glycogenosis II, glycogenosis-cardiac syndrome*.

An inborn error of metabolism due to α-1,4-glucosidase deficiency, characterized by deposition of glycogen in various tissues, including muscle, liver, heart, tongue, and central nervous system cells (motor nuclei of the brain stem and anterior horn of the spinal cord). The first (infantile) form is characterized by muscle hypotonia, ECG abnormalities, poor weight gain, dyspnea, circumoral cyanosis, absence of deep tendon reflexes, mental retardation, macroglossia, cardiomegaly, and cardiorespiratory failure. The symptoms appear by the age of 2 months and death follows by the age of 5.5 months. The second type occurs in infants and young children and is marked by a variable involvement of organs and a relatively slow progress. Most patients die by the age of 19 years. The third (adult) type has a mild course and is characterized mainly by muscle weakness without enlargement of the affected organs. The syndrome is transmitted as an autosomal recessive trait.

Pompe, J. C. Over idiopatische hypertrophie van het hart. *Ned. Tschr. Geneesk.*, 1932, 76:304-5.

glycogen storage disease III. Synonyms: *Cori disease, Forbes disease, amylo-1,6-glucosidase deficiency, debrancher deficiency syndrome, glycogen disease III, glycogenosis III, limit dextrinosis*.

An inborn error of metabolism due to amylo-1,6-glucosidase deficiency, characterized by abnormal deposition of glycogen in various tissues, including muscles (leading to progressive myopathy in older patients), heart (causing cardiomegaly), and liver (causing hepatomegaly which, with growth retardation, are the principal early symptoms). The course of this syndrome is similar to that of glycogen storage disease I, except for its mildness, presence of splenomegaly in some cases, and returning of the liver to its normal size at puberty. Associated disorders may include hypoglycemia with convulsions, elevated blood lipid level, and increased blood transaminase content.

Mild hepatitis, cirrhosis, muscle wasting, and fatigability are frequently associated. The syndrome is transmitted as an autosomal recessive trait.

*Cori, G. T. Biochemical aspects of glycogen deposition disease. *Bibl. Paediat., Basel,* 1958, No. 66:344-58. Forbes, G. B. Glycogen storage disease. Report of a case with abnormal glycogen structure in liver and skeletal muscle. *J. Pediat.,* 1953, 42:645-53.

glycogen storage disease IV. Synonyms: *Andersen disease, Najjar-Andersen syndrome, α,4-glucan: α1,4-glucan-6-glucosyl transferase deficiency, amylopectinosis, brancher deficiency, familial cirrhosis with deposition of abnormal glycogen, glycogen disease IV, glycogenosis IV, liver cirrhosis-abnormal glycogen syndrome.*

An inborn error of glycogen metabolism due to α 1,4-glucan:α1,4-glucan-6-glucosyl transferase deficiency. After a normal appearance at birth, the affected infants develop muscle hypotonia, retarded growth, splenomegaly, and progressive hepatomegaly with cirrhosis leading to death in the second year of life. The glycogen is abnormal, having long outer chains similar to those in amylopectin (hence the synonym **amylopectinosis**). The syndrome is transmitted as an autosomal recessive trait.

Andersen D. H. Familial cirrhosis of the liver with storage of abnormal glycogen. *Lab. Invest.,* 1956, 5:11-20.

glycogen storage disease V. Synonyms: *McArdle disease, McArdle-Schmid-Pearson syndrome, glycogen disease V, glycogenosis V, glycolysis myopathy syndrome, glycometabolic myopathy syndrome, muscle phosphorylase deficiency, myophosphorylase deficiency glycogenosis.*

An inborn error of glycogen metabolism due to muscle phosphorylase deficiency. The affected children appear normal early in life, but late in childhood and adolescence they tire easily. During the later stages of adolescence and adulthood, they suffer from severe cramps and myoglobinuria after exercise. About the age of 40 years, cramps and myoglobinuria are less conspicuous but muscle wasting and weakness become progressively worse. Degradation of glycogen to lactate was suggested by McArdle as the cause of this disorder. The syndrome is transmitted as an autosomal recessive trait.

McArdle, B. Myopathy due to a defect in muscle glycogen breakdown. *Clin. Sc., London,* 1951, 10:13-35. Schmid, R., & Hammaker, L. Hereditary absence of muscle phosphorylase (McArdle's syndrome). *N. Engl. J. Med.,* 1961, 264:223-5. Pearson, C. M. A metabolic myopathy due to absence of muscle phosphorylase. *Am. J. Med.,* 1961, 30:502-17.

glycogen storage disease VI. Synonyms: *Hers disease, glycogen disease VI, glycogenosis VI, hepatic phosphorylase deficiency.*

An inborn glycogen metabolism disorder due to hepatic phosphorylase deficiency, characterized by mild to moderate hypoglycemia, mild ketosis, growth retardation, and prominent hepatomegaly due to abnormal glycogen deposition. Deficiency of leukocyte phosphorylase occurs in some cases. The syndrome is believed to be transmitted as an autosomal recessive trait.

Hers, H. G. Études enzymatiques sur fragments hépatiques: Application à la classification des glycogénoses. *Rev. Internat. Hepatol.,* 1959, 9:35-55.

glycogen storage disease VII. Synonyms: *Tarui disease, glycogen disease VII, glycogenosis VII, muscle phosphophosphofructokinase deficiency, phosphofructokinase (PFK) deficiency.*

An inborn error of glycogen metabolism characterized by phosphofructokinase deficiency in the muscles, associated with abnormal deposition of glycogen in muscle tissues. The symptoms are similar to those seen in glycogen storage disease V (muscle cramps and myoglobinuria after extertion). There is an increase in the concentration of glucose-6-phosphate and fructose-6-phosphate in muscles and low muscle fructose-1,6-diphosphate. Autosomal recessive inheritance is suspected.

Tarui, S., *et al.* Phosphofructokinase deficiency in skeletal muscle. A new type of glycogenosis. *Biochem. Biophys. Res. Commun.,* 1965, 19:517-23.

glycogen storage disease VIII. Synonyms: *glycogen disease VIII, glycogenosis VIII, hepatic phosphorylase kinase deficiency.*

An inborn glycogen metabolism disorder characterized by liver phosphorylase kinase deficiency and abnormal glycogen deposition in the liver. Asymptomatic hepatomegaly is the principal symptom. X-linked inheritance is suspected.

Hug, G., *et al.* Deficient activity of diphosphophosphorylase kinase and accumulation of glycogen in the liver. *J. Clin. Invest.,* 1969, 48:704-15.

glycogenosis (I, II, III, IV, V, VI, VII, VIII). See *glycogen storage disease (I, II, III, IV, V, VI, VII, VIII).*

glycogenosis-cardiac syndrome. See *glycogen storage disease II.*

glycolipid lipidosis. See *Fabry syndrome.*

glycolysis myopathy syndrome. See *glycogen storage disease V.*

glycometabolic myopathy syndrome. See *glycogen storage disease V.*

glycoprotein IIb-III (GP IIb-III) complex deficiency. See *Glanzmann thrombasthenia.*

glycoprotein storage disease. Synonym: *Zugibe disease.*

A syndrome, probably transmitted as an autosomal recessive trait, characterized mainly by abnormal glycoprotein storage and splenomegaly. The presence of large eosinophilic granules in reticuloendothelial cells of the spleen and bone marrow and elevated urinary hexosamine levels are the principal biochemical cytological features.

Zugibe, F. T., *et al.* Glycoprotein storage disease. A new entity. *Am. J. Med.,* 1969, 47:135-40.

goat fever. See *brucellosis.*

GODFRIED, EMANUEL GERARD (Dutch physician)

Godfried-Prick-Carol-Prakken syndrome. Synonym: *cardiocutaneous syndrome.*

A familial syndrome consisting of the Recklinghausen syndrome (1), atrophoderma vermiculatum, mongoloid facies, mental retardation, and heart defect, including congenital heart block.

Carol, W. L., Godfried, E. G., Prakken, J. R., & Prick, J. J. v. Recklinghausenschen Neurofibromatosis, Atrophodermia vermiculata und kongenitale Herzanomalie als Hauptkennzeichen eines familiärhereditären Syndroms. *Dermatologica, Basel,* 1940, 81:345-65.

GODTFREDSEN, ERIK (Danish radiologist)

Godtfredsen syndrome. Synonyms: *cavernous sinus-*

nasopharyngeal tumor syndrome, cavernous sinopharyngeal tumor syndrome.

Oculomotor paralysis, trigeminal neuralgia, and hypoglossal paralysis produced by infiltration of nasopharyngeal tumors into the base of the skull and adjacent structures and compression of the hypogossal nerve by enlarged retropharyngeal lymph nodes.

Godtfredsen, E. Ophthalmo-neurological symptoms in connection with malignant nasopharyngeal tumours. *Brit. J. Ophth.*, 1947, 31:78-100. Godtfredsen, E. Ophthalmological and neurological symptoms in malignant nasopharyngeal tumors. A clinical study comprising 454 cases. *Acta Ophth.*, 1944. Suppl. 22.

GODWIN, JOHN T. (American physician)

Godwin tumor. Synonym: *benign lymphoepithelial lesion of the parotid gland.*

A benign, painless lesion of the parotid gland, with xerostomia, characterized by massive infiltration of the lobules of the gland by a proliferative lymphoid tissue with differentiation to germinal centers and atrophy of the glandular acini.

Godwin, J. T. Benign lymphoepithelial lesion of the parotid gland (adenolymphoma, chronic inflammation, lymphoepithelioma, lymmphocytic tumor, Mikulicz disease). Report of eleven cases. *Cancer,* 1952, 5:1089-103.

GOEDEL, A. (German physician)

Epstein-Goedel syndrome. See *Mortensen disease.*

GOEMINNE, LUC (Belgian physician)

Goeminne syndrome. Synonyms: *cervicodermorenogenital dysplasia, torticollis-keloids-cryptorchidism-renal (TKCR) dysplasia syndrome.*

A congenital syndrome of progressive muscular torticollis with facial asymmetry; keloids of the chest and arms, which appear at puberty; cryptorchism; adult seminiferous tubular failure with oligospermia; renal atrophy with pyelonephritis and hypertension; external urethral meatus stenosis; pigmented nevi of the face, neck, and trunk; basocellular epithelioma of the cheek; varicose veins of the leg; gastric hyperacidity; asthmatic bronchitis with emphysema; clinodactyly of the toes; and hyperpigmentation of the eyelids. The syndrome is transmitted as an X-linked trait.

Goeminne, L. A new probably X-linked inherited syndrome; Congenital muscular torticollis, multiple keloids, cryptorchidism and renal dysplasia. *Acta Genet. Med. Gemel.,* 1968, 17:439-67.

GOGH, VINCENT, VAN (Dutch post impressionist painter, 1853-1890)

van Gogh syndrome. See *Munchausen syndrome.*

GOH (**g**eroderma **o**steodyplastica **h**ereditaria). See *geroderma osteodyplastica syndrome.*

goiter-deaf mutism syndrome. See *Pendred syndrome.*

GOLABI, MAHIN (American pediatrician)

Golabi-Rosen syndrome (GRS). Synonym: *mental retardation-overgrowth syndrome.*

An X-linked mental retardation multiple congenital anomalies syndrome characterized by pre- and postnatal overgrowth, coarse facies, supernumerary nipples, intestinal anomalies, supernumerary ribs, defects of the sacrum and tailbone, and digital malformations. Orofacial characteristics include macrostomia, macrocephaly, hypertelorism, short and broad nose, grooved upper lip, tongue and gingiva, submucous clefts, and cleft palate. Finger abnormalities consist of hypoplastic index fingernails, hypoplasia of distal phalanges, syndactyly, and clinodactyly. Hepatomegaly, intestinal obstruction, Meckel diverticulum, inguinal hernia, large cystic kidneys, cryptorchism, and coccygeal skin tags may be associated.

Golabi, M., & Rosen, L. A new X-linked mental retardation-overgrowth syndrome. *Am. J. Med. Genet.*, 1984, 17:345-58. Optiz, J. M. The Golabi-Rosen syndrome-Report of a second family. *Am. J. Med. Genet.*, 1984, 17:359-66.

GOLDBERG, MINNI BERELSON (American physician, born 1900)

Goldberg-Maxwell syndrome. See *testicular feminization syndrome.*

Goldberg-Maxwell-Morris syndrome. See *testicular feminization syndrome.*

Goldberg-Morris syndrome. See *testicular feminization syndrome.*

GOLDBERG, MORTON E. (American physician)

Goldberg syndrome. A syndrome combining clinical features of mucopolysaccharidoses, sphingolipidoses, and mucolipidoses, characterized by dwarfism, gargoylelike facies, mental retardation, seizures, corneal opacity, cherry-red spots of the macula lutea, dysostosis multiplex, and hearing loss. Deficiency of ß-galactosidase is the principal biochemical feature. The syndrome is transmitted as an autosomal recessive trait.

Goldberg, M. F., *et al.* Macular cherry-red spot, corneal clouding, and ß-galactosidase deficiency. *Arch. Intern. Med.,* 1971, 128:387-98.

GOLDBLATT, HARRY (American physician, born 1891)

Goldblatt hypertension. See *Goldblatt syndrome.*

Goldblatt syndrome. Synonyms: *Goldblatt hypertension, renovascular hypertension.*

Severe systolic hypertension due to obstruction of the renal arteries.

Goldblatt, H., *et al.* Studies on experimental hypertension. I. The production of persistent elevation of systolic blood pressure by means of renal ischemia. *J. Exp. Med.*, 1934, 59:347-79.

GOLDBLOOM, RICHARD B. (American physician, born 1924)

Scriver-Goldbloom-Roy syndrome. See *under Scriver.*

GOLDEN, RICHARD L. (American physician)

Golden-Lakin syndrome. A syndrome, originally reported in two brothers, characterized by pterygium colli, pectus excavatum, kyphoscoliosis, fixed flexion of the knee without popliteal webs, atrophy of calf muscles, pes cavus, clubfeet, defective ossification of the lamina of the vertebrae, dolichocephaly, small mandible, bifid uvula, pointed facies, camptodactyly, and stiff distal interphalangeal joints.

Golden, R. L., & Lakin, H. The *forme fruste* in Marfan's syndrome. *N. Engl. J. Med.*, 1959, 260:797-801.

GOLDEN, ROSS (American physician, born 1889)

Golden-Kantor syndrome. Steatorrhea associated with a roentgenological picture of "moulage sign," dilation, and segmentation of the small intestine; dilation and redudancy of the colon; faint filling of the gallbladder; and bone changes, including osteoporosis, deformity, and growth retardation.

Golden, R. The small intestine and diarrhea. *Am. J. Roentgen.*, 1936, 36:892-901. Kantor, J. L. The roentgen diagnosis of idiopathic steatorrhea and allied conditions.

Practical value of the "moulage sign." *Am. J. Roentgen.*, 1939, 41:758-78.

GOLDENHAR, MAURICE (Swiss physician)

Goldenhar syndrome (GS). See *oculo-auriculovertebral dysplasia.*

Goldenhar-Gorlin syndrome. See *oculo-auriculovertebral dysplasia.*

GOLDFARB, ALVIN F. (American physician)

Slotnick-Goldfarb syndrome. See *under Slotnick.*

GOLDFLAM, SAMUEL (Polish neurologist, 1852-1932)

Erb-Goldflam disease. See *Erb-Goldflam syndrome, under Erb, Wilhelm Heinrich.*

Erb-Goldflam syndrome. See *under Erb, Wilhelm Heinrich.*

Erb-Oppenheim-Goldflam syndrome. See *Erb-Goldflam syndrome, under Erb. Wilhelm Heinrich.*

Hoppe-Goldflam syndrome. See *Erb-Goldflam syndrome, under Erb, Wilhelm Heinrich.*

GOLDMAN

Favre-Goldman syndrome. See *under Favre.*

GOLDSCHEIDER, JOHANN KARL AUGUST EUGEN ALFRED (German physician, 1858-1935)

Goldscheider disease. See *epidermolysis bullosa syndrome.*

GOLDSTEIN, HYMAN ISAAC (American physician, 1887-1954)

Goldstein hematemesis. See *Osler-Rendu-Weber syndrome.*

Goldstein heredofamilial angiomatosis. See *Osler-Rendu-Weber syndrome.*

GOLDSTEIN, KURT (German-born American pathologist, 1878-1965)

Goldstein-Reichmann syndrome. A cerebellar syndrome characterized by disorders of equilibrium and movement, and associated with distorted perception of space, time, and weight. The symptoms include unsteady gait with an inability to walk in a straight line and a tendency to fall down, adiachokinesia, a tendency to overestimate the weight of objects, an inability to point, megalographia, clipped speech, hyperflexibility of joints, abnormal reflexes, and intention tremor.

Goldstein, K., & Reichmann, F. Beiträge zur Kauistik und Symptomatologie der Kleinhinerkrankungen (in beson deren zu den Störungen der Bewegungen der Gewichts-, Raum- und Zeitschätzung). *Arch. Psychiat., Berlin*, 1915-16, 56:466-521.

GOLE, L. (French physician)

Touraine-Solente-Golé (TSG) syndrome. See *pachydermoperiostosis syndrome.*

golfer's elbow. See *under overuse syndrome.*

GOLTZ, ROBERT WILLIAM (American dermatologist, born 1923)

Goltz syndrome. Synonyms: *Goltz-Gorlin syndrome, focal dermal hypoplasia (FDH) syndrome.*

A congenital syndrome, probably transmitted as an X-linked dominant trait, that is lethal in males. It consists of atrophy and linear pigmentation of the skin with occasional papillomatosis, keratosis, and focal aplasia distributed chiefly on the trunk and limbs; multiple papillomatoses of the labial, oral, and anal mucosae and leukokeratosis of the oral mucosa; occasional alopecia of the scalp; thin dystrophic nails; hypoplasia of the dental enamel with microdontia and notching of the teeth; thin helix of the ear; coloboma of the iris and choroid with strabismus and microphthalmia; adactyly, syndactyly, or polydactyly; dysplasia of the clavicle; scoliosis; spina bifida; and frequent mental retardation. Moderate short stature, joint hypermobility, congenital heart defects, and other abnormalities may be associated.

Goltz, R. W. Focal dermal hypoplasia. *Arch. Dermatol.*, 1962, 86:708-17. Gorlin, R., *et al.* Focal dermal hypoplasia syndrome. *Acta Derm. Venereol., Stockholm*, 1963, 42:421-40.

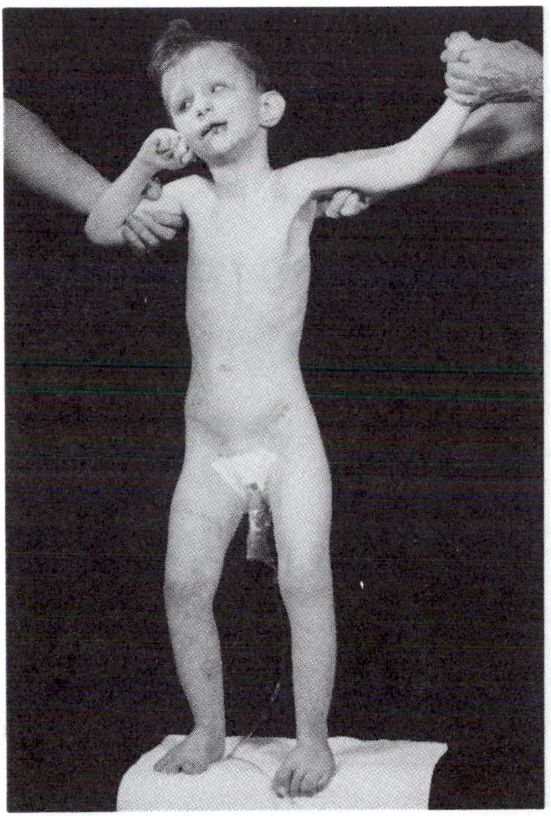

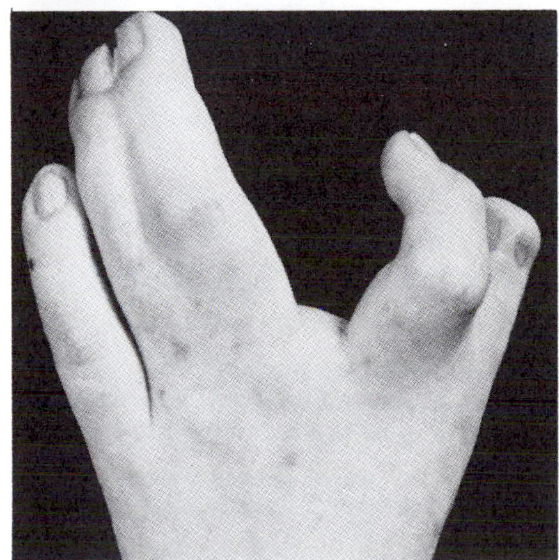

Goltz syndrome
Courtesy Dr. Robert J. Gorlin, Minneapolis, MN.

Goltz-Gorlin syndrome. See *Goltz syndrome.*

Gorlin-Goltz syndrome. See *nevoid basal-cell carcinoma syndrome.*

GOMBAULT, FRANÇOIS ALEXIS ALBERT (French physician, 1844-1904)

Gombault degeneration. See *Déjérine-Sottas syndrome.*

Gombault neuritis. See *Déjérine-Sottas syndrome.*

gonadal agenesis syndrome. See *chromosome XO syndrome.*

gonadal dysgenesis syndrome. See *chromosome XO syndrome.*

gonadal dysgenesis, XX type. See *Perrault syndrome.*

gonadoblastoma. See *Scully tumor.*

goniodysgenesis. See *Rieger syndrome.*

gonococcal arthritis-dermatitis syndrome. See *under arthritis-dermatitis syndrome.*

gonococcal perihepatitis. See *Fitz-Hugh syndrome.*

gonococcal peritonitis of the upper abdomen. See *Fitz-Hugh syndrome.*

GOOD, ROBERT A. (American physician)

Bridges-Good syndrome. See *chronic granulomatous disease of childhood.*

Good syndrome. Synonyms: *hypogammaglobulinemia-thymoma syndrome, thymoma-agammaglobulinemia syndrome, thymoma with immunodefificiency.*

A rare form of primary humoral and cellular immunodeficiency associated with thymoma, complicated by various infections, diarrhea, and blood cell dyscrasias. The complications may also include dermatomyositis, mucocutaneous candidiasis, myasthenia gravis, and other disorders.

Good, R. A. Agammaglobulinemia; a provocative experiment of nature. *Bull. Univ. Minn. Hosp.*, 1954, 26:1-19.

GOODALL, JOHN FRANCIS (British physician)

Goodall disease. See *Spencer disease.*

GOODMAN, RICHARD M.

Goodman camptodactyly. See *Tel Hashomer camptodactyly syndrome.*

Goodman syndrome (1). A syndrome of onychodystrophy, sensorineural deafness, and triphalangeal thumb. Associated abnormalities may include grand mal seizures, dermatoglyphic abnormalities, and hypoplasia of the distal phalanges. The mode of inheritance is not clear.

Goodman, R. M., *et al.* Hereditary congential deafness with onychodystrophy. *Arch. Otolaryng.*, 1969, 90:96-9.

Goodman syndrome (2). See *Tel Hashomer camptodactyly syndrome.*

GOODPASTURE, ERNEST WILLIAM (American physician, 1886-1960)

Goodpasture syndrome (GS, GPS). Synonyms: *glomerulonephritis-pulmonary hemorrhage syndrome, hemorrhagic and interstitial pneumonitis with nephritis, lung purpura with nephritis, pneumorenal syndrome, pulmonary hemosiderosis with glomerulonephritis.*

A progressive, usually fatal illness of young male adults, characterized by severe glomerulonephritis with diffuse pulmonary intra-alveolar hemorrhage. It begins as hemoptysis, anemia, and dyspnea, which are followed by hematuria and proteinuria. Hemoptysis is usually accompanied by the "butterfly-wing" type of pulmonary infiltrates that radiate from each hilar region and are visible on x-rays. Weakness, cough, pallor, low-grade fever, and tachycardia are the additional symptoms. Pathologically, there are changes typical of glomerulonephritis, hemorrhages into the alveolar spaces, deposits of hemosiderin, and thickening of the alveolar septa. Uremia is the usual cause of death.

Goodpasture, E. W. The significance of certain pulmonary lesions in relation to the etiology of influenza. *Am. J. Med. Sc.*, 1919, 158:863-70.

Goodpasture-like syndrome. A syndrome with symptoms similar to those seen in the Goodpasture syndrome, including diffuse intrapulmonary hemorrhage with glomerulonephritis.

Pearl, R. G., & Rosenthal, M. H. Metabolic alkalosis due to plasmapheresis. *Am. J. Med.*, 1985, 79:391-3.

goosey. See *jumping Frenchmen of Maine syndrome.*

GOPALAN, C.

Gopalan syndrome. See *burning feet syndrome.*

GORDAN, GILBERT S. (American physician, born 1916)

Gordan-Overstreet syndrome. Synonym: *androgenicity-gonadal dysgenesis syndrome.*

A variant of the Turner syndrome (see *chromosome XO syndrome*) characterized by ovarian dysgenesis, mild virilization, primary amenorrhea, lack of development of the breasts with widely spaced nipples, growth retardation, and increased excretion of gonadotropins.

Gordan, G. S., Overstreet, W. W., *et al.* A syndrome of gonadal dysgenesis. A variety of ovarian agenesis with androgenic manifestations. *J. Clin. Endocr.*, 1955, 15:1-12.

GORDON, HYMIE (South African physician)

Gordon syndrome. Synonym: *distal arthrogryposis type IIa.*

A syndrome of camptodactyly, cleft palate, and clubfoot, sometimes associated with bifid uvula, nevus flammeus, dermatoglyphic abnormalities, omphalocele, stenosis of the spinal canal, narrowed intervertebral spaces, and cryptorchism. Most affected individuals are short and have short necks. The involvement is more severe in males than in females. The syndrome is transmitted as an autosomal dominant trait with reduced penetrance in variable expressivity.

Gordon, H., *et al.* Camptodactyly, cleft palate, and club foot. A syndrome showing the autosomal-dominant pattern of inheritance. *J. Med. Genet.*, 1969, 6:266-74.

GORDON, RICHARD D. (Australian physician)

Gordon syndrome. A syndrome of hypertension, hyperkalemic acidosis, and low plasma renin and aldosterone.

Gordon, R. D., *et al.* Hypertension and severe hyperkalaemia associated with suppression of renin and aldosterone and completely reversed by dietary sodium restriction. *Aust. Ann. Med.*, 1970, 4:287-94.

GORDON, ROBERT STANTON, JR.

Gordon disease. See *protein-losing gastroenteropathy.*

GORHAM, LEMUEL WHITTINGTON (American physician, 1885-1968)

Breschet-Gorham syndrome. See *Gorham syndrome.*

Gorham syndrome. Synonyms: *Breschet-Gorham syndrome, Gorham-Stout syndrome, acute bone absorption, disappearing bone disease, massive osteolysis syndrome, osteophthisis, phantom bone, phantom clavicle.*

The gradual and often complete unicentric resorption of a bone or group of bones, affecting chiefly children and young adults, males and females about equally. The lesions usually cross the joint and lead to pathologic fractures; ends of the involved bones become tapered. Angiomas, usually hemangiomas, are found in the affected bones or in the surrounding soft tissues. The symptoms include pain, chylous or serosanguineous pleural effusions, and progressive deformity. Involvement of the thoracic cage is usually fatal. The etiology is unknown.

Gorham, L. W., *et al.* Disappearing bones: A rare form of massive osteolysis. Report of two cases, one with autopsy findings. *Am. J. Med.*, 1954, 17:674-82. Gorham, L. W., & Stout, A. P. Massive osteolysis (acute spontaneous absorption of bone, phantom bone, disappearing bone); its relation to hemangiomatosis. *J. Bone Joint Surg.*, 1955, 37(A):985-1004.

Gorham-Stout syndrome. See *Gorham syndrome.*

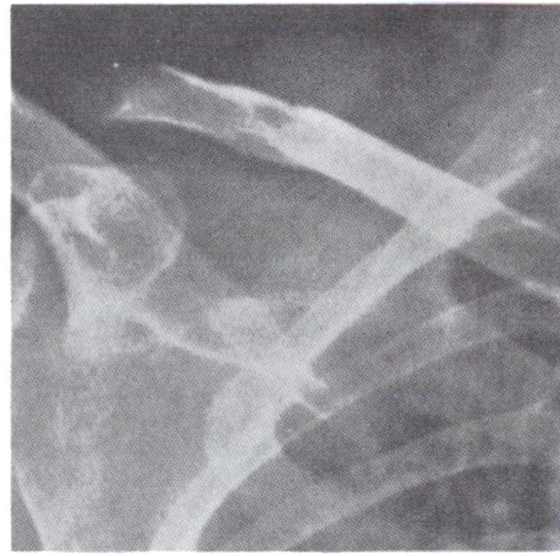

Gorham syndrome
Aegerter, E. & J.A. Kirkpatrick, Jr.: *Orthopedic diseases.* 3rd ed. Philadelphia: W.B. Saunders Co., 1968.

GORLIN, ROBERT JAMES (American oral pathologist and geneticist, born 1923)

Goldenhar-Gorlin syndrome. See *oculo-auriculovertebral dysplasia.*

Goltz-Gorlin syndrome. See *Goltz syndrome.*

Gorlin syndrome (1). See *orofaciodigital syndrome I.*

Gorlin syndrome (2). See *frontometaphyseal dysplasia.*

Gorlin syndrome (3). See *nevoid basal-cell carcinoma syndrome.*

Gorlin syndrome (4). See *megepiphyseal dwarfism.*

Gorlin syndrome (5). See *LEOPARD syndrome.*

Gorlin-Chaudhry-Moss syndrome. A syndrome of craniosynostosis, midfacial hypoplasia, hypertrichosis, and anomalies of the heart, eyes, teeth, and external genitalia. Additional facial defects include antimongoloid palpebral slant, inability to completely open or close the eyes, colobomas of the upper eyelids, microphthalmia, and hyperopia. Oral anomalies include malocclusion, high-arched narrow palate, hypodontia, microdontia, and abnormally shaped teeth. Roentgenographic findings show premature synostosis of the coronal sutures, hypoplasia of the nasal and maxillary bones, brachycephaly, hypertelorism, clival hypoplasia, and elevation of the lesser sphenoid wings. Patent ductus arteriosus, hypoplasia of the labia majora, and umbilical hernia are usually associated. Autosomal recessive transmission is suspected.

Gorlin, R. J., Chaudhry, A. P., & Moss, M. L. Craniofacial dysostosis, patent ductus arteriosus, hypertrichosis, hypoplasia of labia majora, dental and eye anomalies-a new syndrome? *J. Pediat.*, 1960, 56:778-85.

Gorlin-Cohen syndrome. See *frontometaphyseal dysplasia.*

Gorlin-Goltz syndrome. See *nevoid basal-cell carcinoma syndrome.*

Gorlin-Holt syndrome. See *frontometaphyseal dysplasia.*

Gorlin-Pindborg syndrome. See *popliteal pterygium syndrome.*

Gorlin-Psaume syndrome. See *orofaciodigital syndrome I.*

Gorlin-Sedano syndrome. Synonym: *cryptodontic brachymetacarpalia.*

A syndrome of short metacarpal and metatarsal bones, short terminal thumbs, short straight clavicles, and multiple impacted teeth, transmitted as an autosomal dominant trait.

Gorlin, R. J., & Sedano, H. O. Cryptodontic brachymetacarpalia. *Birth Defects*, 1971, 7(7):200-3.

Gorlin-Vickers syndrome. See *mucosal neuromas syndrome.*

GOSSELIN, LEON ATHANASE (French physician, 1815-1887)

Gosselin fracture. A V-shaped fracture of the distal end of the tibia, with extension into the ankle joint.

*Gosselin, L. A. *Des fractures en V et de leurs complications.* Paris, Claye, 1866.

Gotthard tunnel disease. See *Griesinger disease.*

GOTTRON, HEINRICH A. (German physician, 1890-1974)

Arndt-Gottron syndrome. See *under Arndt.*

GOTTRON, HEINRICH ADOLF (German physician, 1890-1974)

Arndt-Gottron scleromyxedema. See *Arndt-Gottron syndrome.*

Gottron syndrome. Synonym: *familial acrogeria.*

A familial form of progeria in which the premature aging of the skin and growth retardation are restricted to the hands and feet. The great majority of cases are consistent with the autosomal recessive mode of transmission, but some authors suggest a dominant mode of inheritance. The symptoms appear early in childhood and include acral atrophy and hyperpigmentation of the skin, presence of prominent blood vessels on the trunk, easy bruising and scar formation, nail abnormalities, elastosis perforans, small stature, and various bone defects. Degeneration of collagen and elastic fibers in the dermis is the principal histopathological feature of this syndrome.

Gottron, H. Familiäre Akrogerie. *Arch. Derm. Syph., Berlin,* 1940-41, 181:571-83.

GOUGEROT, CLAUDE (French physician)

Gougerot syndrome. See *Falta syndrome.*

GOUGEROT, HENRI (French dermatologist, 1881-1955)

Beuermann-Gougerot disease. See *Schenck disease.*

Gougerot disease. Synonyms: *Gougerot trilogy, Gougerot trisymptomatic disease.*

A skin disease characterized by 3 principal symptoms: Erythematous papular lesions, purpuric macules, and dermal or dermohypodermal nodules. The lesions appear chiefly on the legs and thighs, but other parts of the body may be affected. Arthralgia, fever, malaise, and headache may be associated. The lesions appear in crops, each attack lasting from 2 weeks to 2 months, separated by symptom-free periods. Typically, the papules are 2 to 20 mm in diameter and resemble erythema multiforme lesions,. The purpuric nodules are 1 to 5 mm in diameter, and the nodules vary from 2 to 7 mm and are covered by apparently normal skin. Histological findings include increased vascularity and capillaritis, fibroid necrosis of the connective tissue, and leukocytic infiltrates.

Gougerot, H., *et al.* Trisymptome atypique. *Bull. Soc. Fr. Derm. Syph.*, 1951, 58:386.

Gougerot trilogy. See *Gougerot disease.*

Gougerot trisymptomatic disease. See *Gougerot disease.*

Gougerot-Blum syndrome. Synonyms: *dermatitis lichenoides purpurica pigmentosa, pigmented purpuric lichenoid dermatitis.*

A purpuric skin eruption occurring most frequently on the lower limbs and characterized by lichenoid plaques composed of rust-colored papules, some of which may be both purpuric and telangiectatic.

Gougerot, & Blum. Purpura angiosclèreux prurigineaux avec éléments lichenoïdes. (Présentation de malade). *Bull. Soc. Fr. Derm. Syph.*, 1925, 32:161-3.

Gougerot-Carteaud papillomatosis. See *Gougerot-Carteaud syndrome.*

Gougerot-Carteaud syndrome. Synonyms: *Gougerot-Carteaud papillomatosis, confluent and reticulated papillomatosis, cutaneous papillomatosis, papillomatosis confluens et reticularis, papillomatosis cutis, pseudoacanthosis nigricans.*

Progressive papillomatosis appearing in the intermammary and epigastric regions as round, flat-topped, slightly cornified lesions with sharply defined borders. The lesions are about 1 to 2 mm in diameter at the onset, eventually attaining a size of 4 to 5 mm. They evolve in color from bright red to gray and brown. As the epidermis thickens, the lesions increase in size and some may resemble juvenile warts. The eruption typically forms a rhomboid outline, eventually spreading over the breasts and toward the pubis, sacrum, and other areas.

Gougerot, & Carteaud. Papillomatose pigmentée inominée. Cas pour diagnostic *Bull. Soc. Fr. Derm. Syph.*, 1927, 34:719-21.

Gougerot-Hailey-Hailey disease. See *Hailey-Hailey disease, under Hailey, William Howard.*

Gougerot-Houwer-Sjögren syndrome. See *Sjögren syndrome, under Sjögren, Henrik Samuel Conrad.*

Gougerot-Ruiter syndrome. Synonyms: *Ruiter disease, allergic cutaneous arteriolitis, allergic vasculitis (AV), arteriolitis allergica, cutaneous allergic vasculitis, dermatitis nodularis nonnecroticans, leukocytoclastic vasculitis, nodular dermal allergid, vasculitis superficialis.*

An allergic skin disease characterized by erythema, papules, vesicles, pustules, exudation, urticarial edema, cutaneous hemorrhage, telangiectases, and arteriolitis of the cutaneous vessels.

Gougerot, H. Septicémie chronique indéterminée caractérisée par de petits nodules dermiques ("dermatitis nodularis non necroticans"), éléments érythémato-papuleux, purpura. *Bull. Soc. Fr. Derm. Syph.*, 1932, 39:1192-4. Ruiter, M., & Brandsma, C. H. Arteriolitis allergica. *Dermatologica, Basel*, 1948, 97:265-71.

Gougerot-Sjögren syndrome. See *Sjögren syndrome, under Sjögren, Henrik Samuel Conrad.*

reverse Gougerot-Sjögren syndrome. See *Creyx-Lévy syndrome.*

GOUVERNEUR, R. (French physician)

Gouverneur syndrome. Vesicointestinal fistula with suprapubic pain, frequency dysuria, urinary pain, and tenesmus. Pneumaturia, fecaluria, and rectal micturition may be associated.

Gouverneur, R., *et al.* Les fistules colo-vésicales d'origine diverticulaire. *J. Chir., Paris,* 1938, 51:215-31.

GOWERS, SIR WILLIAM RICHARD (British physician, 1845-1915)

Gowers syndrome (1). Synonyms: *distal late hereditary myopathy, hereditary distal myopathy.*

A type of muscular dystrophy that begins as paresis and atrophy of the extensor and small muscles of the distal portions of the extremities and spreads proximally. The symptoms, usually weakness and clumsiness of the hands, become evident during adulthood, but reports that children are also affected suggest that this may be a congenital disorder, probably transmitted as an autosomal dominant trait.

Gowers, W. R. Myopathy of a distal form. *Brit. Med. J.*, 1902, 2:89-92.

Gowers syndrome (2). Irregularity of the pupillary light reflex, seen in tabes dorsalis.

Gowers, W. R. *A manual of disease of the nervous system*. 2nd ed. Philadelphia, Blakiston, 1895. Vol. 1, p. 407.

Gowers syndrome (3). Synonym: *vasoconstriction syncope.*

Attacks of paresthesia, dyspnea, precordial discomfort, depressed pulse, pallor, and cramps occurring chiefly in women with a history of migraine, epilepsy, or mental problems.

Gowers, W. R. *Vagal and vaso-vagal attacks*. London, 1907. Vol. 1, pp. 1551-4.

Gowers-Paton-Kennedy syndrome. See *Kennedy syndrome.*

G6P (glucose-6-phosphatase) deficiency. See *glycogen storage disease I.*

GP IIb-III complex deficiency. See *Glanzmann thrombasthenia.*

GPS. See ***g**ray **p**latelet **s**yndrome.*

GPS. See ***G**ood**p**asture **s**yndrome.*

GRADENIGO, GIUSEPPE (Italian physician, 1859-1926)

Gradenigo syndrome. Synonyms: *Gradenigo triad, Lannois-Gradenigo syndrome, apex of petrous bone syndrome, petrous apicitis.*

Paralysis of the sixth cranial nerve with or without involvement of the ophthalmic branch of the fifth nerve, associated with lesions of the apex of the petrous bone and mastoiditis. Transient involvement of the third and fourth cranial nerves may be present, and facial paralysis may also occur. Severe pain of the area supplied by the ophthalmic branch, photophobia, excessive lacrimation, fever, and reduced corneal sensitivity are the principal symptoms. Inner ear infections, trauma, meningitis, extradural abscess, and hemorrhage are possible causes. The **Gradenigo triad** consists of otitis, abducens paralysis, and deep pain.

Gradenigo, G. Sulla leptomeningite circumscritta e sulla paralisi dell'adducente di origine otitica. *Gior. Accad. Med. Torino*, 1904, 4(10):59-84; 270-367.

Gradenigo triad. See *Gradenigo syndrome.*

Lannois-Gradenigo syndrome. See *Gradenigo syndrome.*

GRAEFE, ALBRECHT FRIEDRICH WILHELM ERNST, VON (German ophthalmologist, 1828-1870)

Graefe-Sjögren syndrome. Synonyms: *Graefe-Lindenov syndrome, Hallgren syndrome, Sjögren syndrome, von Graefe-Lindenov syndrome.*

A hereditary, familial syndrome of retinitis pigmentosa, congenital deafness, and spinocerebellar ataxia, which may be associated with congenital cataracts and mental retardation. The syndrome is transmitted as an autosomal recessive trait. According to Sjögren, the syndrome consists of spinocerebellar ataxia, congenital cataract, and mental retardation; according to Hallgren, it is an association of retinitis pigmentosa, congenital deafmutism, and vestibulocerebellar ataxia with cataract and mental disorders.

Graefe, A., von. Exceptionelles Verhalten des Gesichtsfeldes bei Pigmententartung der Netzhaut. *Arch. Ophth., Berlin*, 1948, 4:250-3. Sjögren, T. Hereditary congenital spinocerebellar ataxia accompanied by congenital cataract and oligophrenia. A genetic and clinical investigation. *Confinia Neur., Basel*, 1950, 10:293-308. Hallgren, B. Retinitis pigmentosa in combination with congenital deafness and vestibulocerebellar ataxia; with psychiatric abnormality in some cases. A clinical and genetic study. *Acta Genet., Basel*, 1958, 8:97-104. Hallgren, B. Retinitis pigmentosa combined with congenital deafness; with vestibulo-cerebellar ataxia, and mental abnormality in a proportion of cases. A clinical and genetico-statistical study. *Acta Psychiat. Scand.*, 1959, 34(Suppl. 138):1-97.

Graefe-Usher syndrome. See *Usher syndrome.*

Graefe syndrome. Synonyms: *chronic progressive ophthalmoplegia, ophthalmoplegia chronica progressiva, ophthalmoplegia externa chronica progressiva internuclearis, primary chronic progressive ophthalmoplegia, ptosis myopathica.*

Progressive oculomotor paralysis that starts with the external muscles before the internal muscles become involved. Bilateral ptosis, diplopia, mydriasis, and pupil rigidity may occur.

Graefe, A. F., von. Demonstration in der Berliner Meizinischen Gesellschaft. *Berlin. Klin. Wschr.*, 1868, 5:127.

von Graefe-Lindenov syndrome. See *Graefe-Sjögren syndrome.*

graft-versus-host disease (GVHD). See *under graft-versus-host syndrome.*

graft-versus-host reaction (GVHR). See *under graft-versus-host syndrome.*

graft-versus-host syndrome. The immunological response to a graft rich in immunologically competent cells against the genetically nonidentical tissues of the recipient. Tissues especially rich in immunologically competent cells capable of inducing a graft-vs-host reaction include the spleen, lymph nodes, thoracic duct lymph, and to a lesser degree the bone marrow and peripheral blood. Cutaneous changes, diarrhea, and liver dysfunction are the principal clinical features. The inflammatory reaction by the donor cells against a specific host organ is termed **graft-versus-host reaction;** the sum of reactions in an individual patient is known as the **graft-versus-host disease** or **syndrome.** The disorder occurs most frequently as a complication of bone marrow transplantation used in the treatment of acute leukemia and some immunodeficiency diseases.

Farmer, E. R., & Hood, A. F. Graft-versus-host disease. In: Fitzpatrick, T. B., Eisen, A. Z., Wolff, K., Freedberg, I. M., & Austen, K. F., eds. *Dermatology in general medicine.* 3rd ed., New York, McGraw-Hill, 1987, pp. 1344-52.

GRAHAM, C. BENJAMIN (American radiologist)

Arkless-Graham syndrome. See *acrodysostosis.*

GRAHAM, EVARTS AMBROSE (American physician, 1883-1957)

Brock-Graham syndrome. See *middle lobe syndrome.*

Graham-Burford-Mayer syndrome. See *middle lobe syndrome.*

GRAHAM LITTLE. See LITTLE, ERNEST GORDON GRAHAM

GRAM, HANS CHRISTIAN JOACHIM (Danish physician, 1853-1938)

Gram syndrome. Synonyms: *adiposalgia arthriticohypertonica, adiposalgia genus medialis, adiposis dolorosa-arthritis genuum-hypertensio arterialis, juxta-articular adiposis dolorosa, pseudogonitis.*

A syndrome of adiposis dolorosa, arthritis deformans of the knee joints, and arterial hypertension occurring in climacteric multiparae.

Gram, H. C. A symptom-triad of the post-climacteric period. (Adiposis dolorosa-arthritis genuum-hypertensio arterialis). *Acta Med. Scand.*, 1930, 73:139-207.

GRANCHER, JACQUES JOSEPH (French physician, 1843-1907)

Grancher disease. Synonym: *splenopneumonia.*

Pneumonia with splenization of the lung.

Grancher. La spléno-pneumonie. *Union Méd., Paris*, 1883, 36:1078-81; 1108-12; 1117-21.

GRANT

Grant syndrome. A familial syndrome in the osteogenesis imperfecta group, transmitted as an autosomal dominant trait, and characterized by persistent wormian bones, blue sclerae, mandibular hypoplasia, shallow glenoid fossae, and campomelia. The syndrome was named after the surname of the affected family.

Maclean, J. R., *et al.* The Grant syndrome. Persistent wormian bones, blue sclerae, mandibular hypoplasia, shallow glenoid fossae and campomelia-an autosomal dominant trait. *Clin. Genet.*, 1986, 29:523-9.

granular cell hypertrophy. See *Lhermitte-Duclos disease.*

granular cell myoblastoma. See *Abrikossov tumor.*

granular conjunctivitis. See *trachoma.*

granular dystrophy of the cornea. See *Groenouw dystrophy (1).*

granule cell hypertrophy of the cerebellum. See *Lhermitte-Duclos disease.*

granulocytic hypoplasia. See *Schultz syndrome.*

granulocytosis. See *Schultz syndrome.*

granuloma fungoides. See *mycosis fungoides.*

granuloma-arteritis-glomerulonephritis syndrome. See *Wegener granulomatosis.*

granulomatosis benigna. See *Besnier-Boeck-Schaumann syndrome.*

granulomatosis disciformis chronica et progressiva. See *Miescher-Leder granulomatosis.*

granulomatosis pseudosclerodermiformis tuberculoidea chronica. See *Miescher-Leder granulomatosis.*

granulomatous angiitis of the nervous system syndrome. See *GANS syndrome.*

granulomatous myocarditis. See *Fiedler myocarditis.*

granulomatous thyroiditis. See *de Quervain disease (2), under Quervain, Fritz, de.*

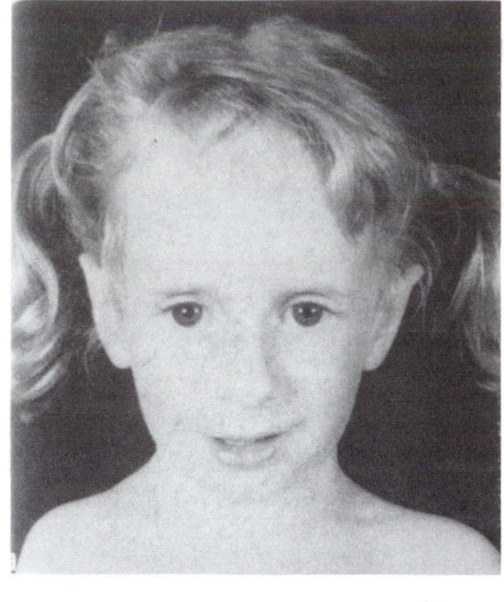
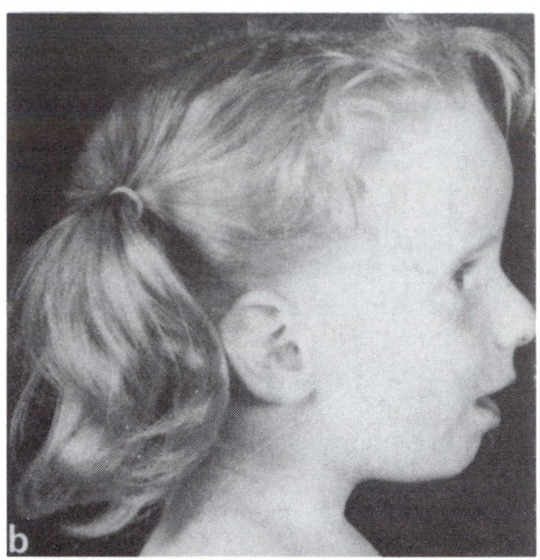
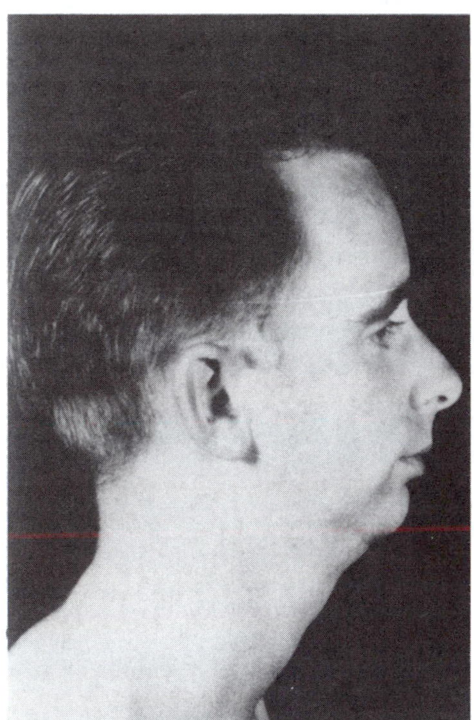
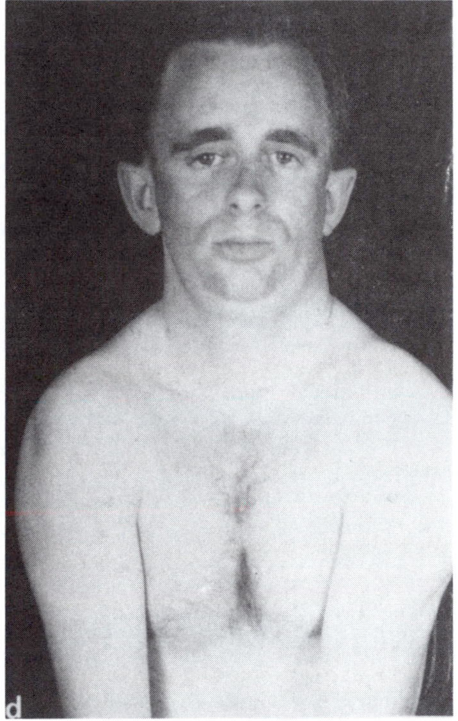

Grant syndrome
Maclean, Robert J., R. Brian Lowry, & Betty J. Wood, *Clinical Genetics* 29:523-529, 1986. Munksgaard International Publishers, Copenhagen, Denmark.

GRÄSBECK, RALPH (Finnish physician, born 1930)

Imerslund-Gräsbeck syndrome. See *under Imerslund.*

Imerslund-Najman-Gräsbeck syndrome. See *Imerslund-Gräsbeck syndrome.*

GRASER, ERNST (German physician, 1860-1929)

Graser diverticulum. Synonym: *sigmoid diverticula.* Multiple diverticula of the sigmoid.

Graser, E. Über multiple falsche Darmdivertikel in der Flexura sigmoidea. *Münch. Med. Wschr.*, 1899, 46:721-3.

GRAUHAM

Grauham syndrome. A syndrome of polydactyly, cleft lip and palate, and urogenital malformations.

Töllner, U., *et al.* Heptacarpo-octatarso-dactyly combined with multiple malformations. *Eur. J. Pediat.*, 1981, 136:207-10.

GRAVES, IRISH JAMES (Irish physician, 1795-1853)

Graves disease. See *Basedow disease.*

GRAWITZ, PAUL ALBERT (German pathologist, 1850-1932)

Grawitz tumor. Synonyms: *hypernephroid tumor, hy-*

pernephroma, struma suprarenalis cystica hemorrhagica.

A malignant tumor of the kidney, most commonly occurring in the fifth or sixth decade of life. A typical lesion is a yellow or orange mass about 5 to 15 cm in diameter, with irregular cystic and hemorrhagic areas. Most tumors are composed of polygonal clear cells in tubules or papillary formations with a high concentration of lipids. Glycogen may be present in some clear cells. Solid cells are also present. Grawitz's original contention that tumors originate from ectopic adrenal tissue is no longer supported.

Grawitz, P. A. Die sogenannten Lipome der Niere. *Arch. Path., Berlin*, 1883, 93:39-63.

gray baby syndrome. Synonym: *grey toddler.*

A potentially fatal chloramphenicol poisoning in newborn infants following maternal administration of the drug during pregnancy. The symptoms include gray skin color, abdominal distention, vomiting, progressive cyanosis, irregular respiration, hypothermia, and shock. Loss of the ability to clear the drug via the placenta at the time of birth is the cause of increased concentration of chloramphenicol in infants.

Burns, L. E., *et al.* Fatal circulatory collapse in premature infants receiving chloramphenicol. *N. Engl. J. Med.*, 1959, 261:1318-21. Sutherland, J. M. Fatal cardiovascular collapse in infants receiving large amounts of chloramphenicol. *Am. J. Dis. Child.*, 1959, 97:761-7.

gray platelet syndrome (GPS). Synonym: *platelet alpha-granule deficiency.*

An inherited disorder, probably transmitted as an autosomal recessive trait, characterized by a marked decrease or absence of α-granules and platelet-specific α-granule proteins in blood platelets. The platelets are large and appear gray in light microscopy.

Raccuglia, G. Gray platelet syndrome: A variety of qualitative platelet disorder. *Am. J. Med.*, 1971, 51:818-28.

greater superficial petrosal neuralgia. See *Sluder neuralgia.*

GREBE, HANS (German physician)

Grebe chondrodysplasia. See *Grebe disease.*

Grebe disease. Synonyms: *achondrogenesis, Brazilian type; achondrogenesis, Grebe type; Grebe chondrodysplasia; Grebe and Quelce-Salgado syndrome.*

A short-limbed dwarfism characterized by hypomelia affecting the lower limbs more severely than the upper ones. The shortening increases in severity from the proximal to the distal segments. The hands are extremely short with toelike fingers, and the feet are in the valgus position. Polydactyly occurs in some cases. The condition is believed to be transmitted as an autosomal recessive trait.

Grebe, H. Die Achondrogenesis: ein eifach rezessives Erbmerkmal. *Fol. Hered. Path.*, 1952, 2:23-9. Quelce-Salgado, A. A new type of dwarfism with various bone aplasias and hypoplasia of the extremities. *Acta Genet., Basel*, 1964, 14:63-6.

Grebe and Quelce-Salgado syndrome. See *Grebe disease.*

green cancer. See *Balfour disease.*

GREENFIELD, JOSEPH GODWIN (British physician, 1884-1958)

Greenfield syndrome. See *metachromatic leukodystrophy.*

Scholz-Greenfield syndrome. See *metachromatic leukodystrophy.*

GREENHOW, EDWARD HEADLAM (British physician, 1814-1888)

Greenhow disease. Synonyms: *parasitic melanoderma, vagabonds' disease, vagrants' disease.*

Discoloration and excoration of the skin in pediculosis, caused by scratching.

Greenhow, E. H. A case of vagabond's discoloration simulating the bronzed skin of Addison's disease. *Tr. Clin. Soc. London*, 1876, 9:44-7.

greeting spasms. See *West syndrome.*

GREGG, NORMAN MCALISTER (Australian ophthalmologist)

Gregg syndrome. See *under congenital rubella syndrome.*

GREGOIRE

Gregoire syndrome. A severe complication of venous thrombosis characterized by obstruction of major veins and spasm of the arteries.

Ermolaev, V. L. Bolezn' Greguara. *Khirurgiia, Moskva*, 1978, No. 8:73-6.

GREIG, DAVID MIDDLETON (Scottish physician, 1864-1936)

Greig cephalopolysyndactyly (GCPS) syndrome. See *Greig syndrome.*

Greig ocular hypertelorism syndrome. Synonyms: *dystopia canthorum, hypertelorism.*

A condition in which there is an abnormal increase in the interorbital distance. It is no longer regarded as a distinct entity, but as a malformation that may occur in a variety of different syndromes.

Greig, D. M. Hypertelorism. A hitherto undifferentiated congenital cranio-facial deformity. *Edinb. Med. J.*, 1924, 31:560-93.

Greig syndrome. Synonyms: *Greig cephalopolysyndactyly (GCPS) syndrome, cephalopolysyndactyly syndrome, cephalosyndactyly syndrome, polysyndactyly-craniofacial anomalies syndrome, polysyndactyly-craniofacial dysmorphism syndrome, polysyndactyly-dyscrania syndrome, frontodigital syndrome.*

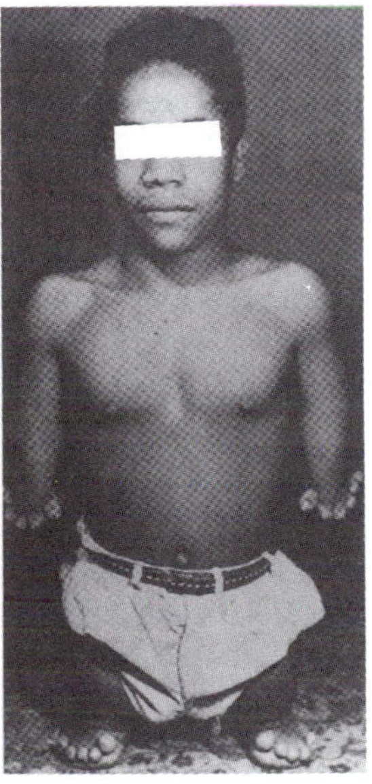

Grebe disease
Quelco-Salgado, A: *Acta-Genet.* 14:63, 1963. New York: Human Genetics.

A syndrome of digital malformations and cranial deformity, consisting of postaxial polydactyly, preaxial polysyndactyly, syndactyly, and peculiar shape of the skull characterized by a large cranial vault with a large forehead, high bregma, and occasional hypertelorism. The syndrome is transmitted as an autosomal dominant trait. The syndrome has been tentatively assigned to chromosome 7 on the basis of its association with balanced translocation involving the short arm of chromosome 7.

Greig, D. M. Oxycephaly. *Edinb. Med. J.*, 1926, 33:189-218; 280-302; 357-76. Marshall, R. E., & Smith, D. W. Frontodigital syndrome: a dominantly inherited disorder with normal intelligence. *J. Pediat.*, 1970, 77:129-33.

GREITHER, ALOYS (German physician)

Greither keratosis. See *Unna-Thost syndrome, under Unna, Paul Gerson.*

Greither syndrome. See *Unna-Thost syndrome, under Unna, Paul Gerson.*

GREPPI, ENRICO (Italian physician, born 1896)

Rietti-Greppi-Micheli syndrome. See *under Rietti.*

grey todler. See *gray baby syndrome.*

GRID (gay-related immunodeficiency) syndrome). See *acquired immunodeficiency syndrome.*

GRIESINGER, WILHELM (German physician, 1817-1868)

Duchenne-Griesinger disease. See *Duchenne muscular dystrophy.*

Duchenne-Griesinger syndrome. See *Duchenne muscular dystrophy.*

Griesinger disease. Synonyms: *Gotthard tunnel disease, ancylostomiasis, Egyptian chlorosis, hookworm disease, miners' anemia, tunnel anemia, uncinariasis.*

A tropical disease caused by infection with the intestinal nematode *Ancylostoma duodenale* and *Necator americanus*, and characterized by severe anemia and cardiac incompetence.

Griesinger, W. Klinische und anatomische Beobachtungen über die Krankheit von Egypten. *Arch. Physiol. Heilk.*, 1854, 13:528-75.

GRIFFITHS, D. LLOYD (British orthopedic surgeon)

Phillips-Griffiths syndrome. See *under Phillips.*

GRIGNOLO, ANTONIO (Italian ophthalmologist)

Grignolo syndrome. A syndrome of ankylopoietic spondylarthritis, hypopyon, iritis, uveitis, polymorphic exudative erythema, and ankylosis, with frequent exacerbations of symptoms.

Grignolo, A. Über einen bisher noch nicht beschriebenen Symptomenkomplex; rezidivierende Hypopyoniritis, polymorphes Erythema exudativum und Spondylarthritis ankylopoetica. *Ophthalmologica, Basel*, 1949, 118:989-97.

GRINDON, JOSEPH (American physician, 1858-1950)

Grindon disease. Synonym: *echolic folliculitis.*

An inflammatory disease of the hair follicles characterized by extrusion of cells from portions of the root sheath, the cells being threaded over the hair and carried up with it in its growth. The process is repeated from time to time until successive masses, bearing a superficial resemblance to nits, are strung along the hair. The disorder is accompanied by a slight redness about the follicular orifice, is chronic in character, and results in reversible alopecia.

Grindon, J. A peculiar affection of the hair follicles. *J. Cutan. Dis.*, 1897, 15:256-9.

GRINSPAN, D. (Argentine physician)

Grinspan syndrome. A syndrome of erosive lichen ruber planus, diabetes mellitus, and hypertension.

Grinspan, d., *et al.* Lichen ruber planus de la muqueuse buccale. Son association à diabète. *Bull. Soc. Fr. Derm. Syph.*, 1966, 73:898-902.

GRISCELLI, CLAUDE (French physician)

Griscelli syndrome. Synonyms: *Chédiak-Higashi-like syndrome, pseudo-Chédiak-Higashi syndrome.*

A syndrome of partial albinism and immunodeficiency associated with frequent pyogenic infections, acute episodes of fever, neutropenia, and thrombocytopenia. The pigmentary dilution is characterized by large clumps of pigment in the hair shafts and accumulation of melanosomes and melanocytes. Melanocytes have few short dendritic expansions and keratinocytes are depigmented. Langerhans cells are absent or almost absent in the skin. The syndrome is transmitted as an autosomal recessive trait.

Griscelli, C., *et al.* A syndrome associating partial albinism and immunodeficienccy. *Am. J. Med.*, 1978, 65:691-702.

GRISEL, P. (French physician)

Grisel syndrome. Synonyms: *atlanto-axial rotary displacement, inflammatory dislocation of the atlanto-axial joint, nasopharyngeal torticollis, nontraumatic dislocation of the atlanto-axial joint, spontaneous dislocation of the atlanto-axial joint, spontaneous hyperemic dislocation of the atlanto-axial joint, torticollis atlanto-epistrophealis.*

Nontraumatic atlanto-axial subluxation, following peripharyngeal inflammation, resulting in torticollis.

Grisel, P. Enucléation de l'atlas et torticolis nasopharyngien. *Presse Méd.*, 1930, 38:50-3.

GROB, MAX (Swiss physician, 1901-1976)

Grob syndrome. A variant of the orofaciodigital syndrome (I), consisting of partial alopecia, epicanthus, cleft lip, cleft palate, multiple ridges in the mucous membranes of the jaws, fissured tongue, brachydactyly, clinodactyly, mental deficiency, and a nose with a broad bridge, flat base, and small orifices.

Grob, M. Dysplasia linguo-facialis (Grob). In his: *Lehrbuch der Kinderchirurgie*, Stuttgart, 1957, pp. 98-100.

GROCCO, PIETRO (Italian physician, 1856-1916)

Grocco-Poncet disease. See *Poncet disease.*

GROENOUW, ARTHUR (German ophthalmologist, 1862-1945)

Groenouw dystrophy (1). Synonyms: *Fleischer dystrophy, Groenouw-Fleischer dystrophy, familial granular dystrophy of the cornea, granular dystrophy of the cornea, nodular corneal dystrophy, noduli corneae.*

Corneal dystrophy, transmitted as an autosomal dominant trait, characterized by hyaline degeneration in the absence of acid mucopolysaccharide deposition. The disorder has a protracted course and is marked by the appearance between the ages of 5 to 10 years of whitish spots between the superficial layers of the stroma, which later aggregate into elevated masses surrounded by an apparently normal cornea. Photophobia, eye irritation, and erosions may occur in later stages. Blindness may develop by the end of the third decade. Sporadic cases are occasionally observed.

Groenouw, A. Knötchenförmige Horhauttrübungen (Noduli corneae). *Arch. Augenh.*, 1889-90; 21:281-9. Fleischer, B. Über familiäre Hornhautentartung. *Arch. Augenh.*, 1905, 53:263-344.

Groenouw dystrophy (2). Synonyms: *Fehr dystrophy, local corneal mucopolysaccharidosis, macular corneal dystrophy, spotted corneal dystrophy.*

Hereditary corneal dystrophy, inherited as an autosomal recessive trait, characterized by the appearance between the ages of 5 and 9 years of discrete gray opacities scattered over the corneal surface, with intervening cloudy spaces. Larger spots of various shapes become evident by the fourth decade. Photophobia, pain, reduced sensitivity, erosion, foreign body sensation, and, eventually, blindness are usually associated. An inborn mucopolysaccharide metabolism disorder is believed to be the cause, and synthesis of corneal sulfate and other glucosaminoglycans may be abnormal.

Groenouw, A. Knötchenförmige Horhauttrubüngen (Noduli corneae). *Arch. Augenh.*, 1890, 21:281-9. Fehr. Über familiäre, fleckige Hornhaut-Entartung. *Zbl. Prakt. Augenh.*, 1904, 28:1-11.

Groenouw-Fleischer dystrophy. See *Groenouw dystrophy (1).*

GROFFITH, JOSEPH (British physician)

Groffith degeneration. Degeneration of undescended testes.

*Groffith, J. The structural changes in the testicle of the dog when it is replaced within the abdominal cavity. *J. Anat. Physiol.*, 1893, 27:483-500.

GROLL, A. (American physician)

Groll-Hirschowitz syndrome. A familial syndrome, transmitted as an autosomal recessive trait, characterized by sensory deafness, mesenteric diverticula of the small bowel, and progressive neuropathy. Gastrointestinal disorders are cachexia, diarrhea, loss of gastric motility, fat malabsorption with steatorrhea, multiple diverticula, jejunal ulceration, and protein-losing enteropathy. Involvement of the vagus nerve with a loss of the carotid sinus reflex, gastric motility disorders, and tachycardia; peripheral sensory neuropathy; absent tendon reflexes; and ophthalmoplegia are the neurological components. Associated disorders may include absent or carious teeth, short fifth finger, pes cavus, dysarthria, and blepharoptosis. The age of onset varies from 3 to 25 years.

Groll, A., & Hirschowitz, B. I. Steatorrhea and familial deafness in two siblings. *Clin. Res.*, 1966, 14:47. Hirschowitz, B. I., Groll, A., & Ceballos, R. Hereditary nerve deafness in 3 sisters with absent gastric motility, small bowel diverticulitis and ulceration and progressive sensory neuropathy. *Birth Defects*, 1972, 8(2):27-41.

GRÖNBLAD, ESTER ELISABETH (Swedish physician, born 1898)

Darier-Grönblad-Strandberg syndrome. See *pseudoxanthoma elasticum.*

Grönblad-Strandberg syndrome. See *pseudoxanthoma elasticum.*

Grönblad-Strandberg-Touraine syndrome. See *pseudoxanthoma elasticum.*

Groote Eylandt syndrome. See *amyotrophic lateral sclerosis-parkinism-dementia complex.*

GROSS, ROBERT EDWARD (American physician, born 1905)

Ladd-Gross syndrome. See *under Ladd.*

GROSS, SAMUEL DAVID (American physician, 1805-1884)

Gross disease. Synonyms: *encysted rectum, sacciform disease of the anus, sacs of the anus.*

A disease of the anus marked by sacculation of the walls with the development of large pouches that may become receptacles of hardened feces and inspissated mucus. The disease is usually observed in elderly patients.

Gross, S. D. *System of surgery; pathological, diagnostic, therapeutic, and operative.* Philadelphia, Blanchard & Lea, 1864, pp. 573-4.

GROSSMAN, HERMAN (American physician)

Winchester-Grossman syndrome. See *carpotarsal osteolysis syndrome (recessive form).*

GROUCHY, JEAN (Dutch-born physician in France, born 1926)

de Grouchy syndrome. See *chromosome 18p deletion syndrome.*

GROVER, R. W. (American physician)

Grover disease. Synonym: *transient acantholytic dermatosis (TAD).*

A pruritic, self-limited acantholytic skin disease characterized by the sudden onset of severe pruritus associated with an eruption of smooth or warty papules, papulovesicles, eczematous plaques, or shiny translucent nodules, which may resemble basal cell carcinoma. Bullous lesions may occur in some cases. The trunk, neck, and proximal parts of the limbs are the most common sites. The disorder may spontaneously remit within weeks or months or may persist and recur over a period of years. Males over the age of 40 years are most frequently affected. The etiology is unknown.

Grover, R. W. Transient acantholytic dermatosis. *Arch. Derm., Chicago,* 1970, 101:426-34.

growth hormone-deficiency-hypogammaglobulinemia syndrome. See *Fleisher syndrome.*

growth retardation-alopecia-pseudoanodontia-progressive optic atrophy syndrome. See *GAPO syndrome.*

growth retardation-pulmonary hypertension-aminoaciduria syndrome. See *Rowley-Rosenberg syndrome.*

GRS. See *Golabi-Rosen syndrome.*

GRUBER, GEORG BENITO OTTO (German pathologist, 1884-1977)

Gruber syndrome. See *Meckel syndrome, under Meckel, Johann Friedrich, Jr.*

Meckel-Gruber syndrome. See *Meckel syndrome, under Meckel, Johann Friedrich, Jr.*

GRUBER, WENZEL LEOPOLD (Anatomist in St. Petersburg, 1814-1890)

Gruber hernia. Synonym: *hernia mesogastrica interna.*

Internal mesogastric hernia with incarceration of the ileum in the omentum.

Gruber, W. L. Über einen Fall nicht incarcerierter, ober mit Incarceration des Ileum durch das Omentum complicierter Hernia interna mesogastrica. *Oesterr. Zschr. Prakt. Heilk.*, 1863, 9:325-30; 341-5.

GRUBY, DAVID (French physician, 1810-1898)

Gruby disease. Synonym: *tinea tonsurans.*

Tinea capitis in children caused by infection with the fungus *Trichophyton tonsurans.*.

Gruby, D. Recherches sur la nature, le siége et le développment du porrigo decalvans ou phytoalopécie. *C. Rend. Acad. Sc., Paris*, 1843, 17:301-3.

GRUDZINSKI, ZYGMUNT (Polish radiologist, 1870-1929)

Grudzinski osteochondropathy. See *Silfverskiöld syndrome.*

GRUMBACH, MELVIN M. (American physician)

Hoyt-Kaplan-Grumbach syndrome. See *septo-optic dysplasia.*

Van Wyk-Grumbach syndrome. See *under van Wyk.*

GRÜTZ, OTTO (German physician, born 1886)

Bürger-Grütz syndrome. See *under Bürger.*

GS. See *Gardner syndrome, under Gardner, Eldon John.*

GS. See *Gerstmann syndrome (1 and 2).*

GS. See *Goodpasture syndrome.*

GS (Goldenhar syndrome). See *oculo-auriculovertebral dysplasia.*

GSD (Gerstmann-Sträussler disease). See *Gerstmann syndrome (1).*

GSELL, OTTO ROBERT (Swiss physician, born 1902)

Gsell-Erdheim syndrome. Synonyms: *medionecrosis aortae idiopathica, medionecrosis idiopathica aortae, medionecrosis idiopathica cystica.*

Necrosis of the medial layer of the aorta without inflammatory changes, often leading to aortic rupture.

Gsell, O. Wandnekrosen der Aorta als selbständige Erkerankung und ihre Beziehung zur Spontanruptur. *Virchows Arch. Path.*, 1928, 270:1-36. Erdheim, J. Medionecrosis aortae idiopathica. *Virchows Arch. Path.*, 1929, 273:454-79.

GSS (Gerstmann-Sträussler syndrome). See *Gerstmann syndrome (1).*

GSSD (Gerstmann-Sträussler-Scheinker disease). See *Gerstmann syndrome (1).*

GT. See *Glanzmann thrombasthenia.*

GTA. See Glanzmann thrombasthenia.

GTS. See Gilles de la Tourette syndrome.

Guadalajara camptodactyly syndrome type I. A familial syndrome of camptodactyly and multiple abnormalities transmitted as an autosomal recessive trait. Maxillofacial defects include frontal and ethmoidal sinus agenesis, abnormal canine teeth, absence of the right upper incisor, crowding of the teeth, and mandibular prognathism. Spinal anomalies consist of cuboid vertebrae, variable dimensions of the transverse apophysis in the lumbar bodies, and spina bifida occulta. Depressed sternal lower half and twelfth rib hypoplasia are the thoracic features. The pelvis is gyneco-anthropoid with hypoplastic iliac bones. Limb abnormalities include fibular hypoplasia, mild metaphyseal broadening, interphalangeal subluxation of the first toe, bilateral hallux valgus, tarsometatarsal luxation of the third and fourth metatarsal bones with metatarsophalangeal subluxation, tubular metacarpal bones, hypoplasia of the second phalanx of the fifth finger, and hypoplasia of the second, third, and fourth metacarpal bones.

Cantú, J. M., *et al.* Guadalajara camptodactyly syndrome. A distinct probably autosomal recessive disorder. *Clin. Genet.*, 1980, 18:153-9.

Guadalajara camptodactyly syndrome type II. A familial syndrome, transmitted as an autosomal recessive trait, characterized by dwarfism, camptodactyly, mental retardation, and multiple abnormalities. Craniofacial defects include microcephaly and occasional blepharoptosis, microphthalmia, low-set ears, and micrognathia or retromicrognathia. Abnormalities of the extremities consist of camptodactyly, ulnar deviation of digits, talipes, prominent talus, overlapping toes, short second toe, aplastic or hypoplastic patella, and, sometimes, syndactyly. Associated anomalies may include scoliosis, pectus excavatum, congenital hip dislocation, hypoplastic pubic region, short neck, and hypogonadism.

Cantú, J. M., *et al.* Guadalajara camptodactyly syndrome type II. *Clin. Genet.*, 1985, 28:54-60.

Guam disease. See *amyotrophic lateral sclerosis-parkinsonism-dementia complex.*

Guam syndrome. See *amyotrophic lateral sclerosis-parkinsonism-dementia complex.*

GUBLER, ADOLPHE MARIE (French physician, 1821-1879)

Gubler hemiplegia. See *Millard-Gubler syndrome.*

Gubler paralysis. See *Millard-Gubler syndrome.*

Gubler tumor. Dorsal tumor of the hand in lead poisoning paralysis.

Gubler, A. De la tumeur dorsale des mains dans la paralysie saturnine des extenseurs des doigts. *Union Méd., Paris*, 1868, 6:2-8; 15-9; 26-30.

Millard-Gubler syndrome. See *under Millard.*

GUERIN, ALPHONSE FRANÇOIS MARIE (French physician, 1816-1895)

Guérin fracture. See *Le Fort fracture I.*

GUERIN, JULES RENE (French physician, 1801-1886)

Guérin-Stern syndrome. See *arthrogryposis multiplex congenita syndrome.*

GUERTIN, ANDRE (French physician)

Guertin syndrome. See *Bergeron disease.*

GUIBAUD, P. (French physician)

Guibaud-Vainsel syndrome. Synonyms: *carbonic anhydrase II deficiency, marble bone disease, osteopetrosis-renal tubular acidosis syndrome.*

A familial syndrome, transmitted as an autosomal recessive trait, characterized by osteopetrosis and renal tubular acidosis. The symptoms include spontaneous fractures, short stature, mental retardation, malocclusion, and optic nerve compression with visual disorders. Calcification of the basal ganglia may develop later. Carbonic anhydrase II deficiency is believed to be the cause of the osteoclast function and abnormal bone resorption.

Guibaud, P., *et al.* Ostéopétrose et acidose rénale tubulaire. Deux cas de cette association dans une fratrie. *Arch. Fr. Pédiat.*, 1972, 29:269-86. Vainsel, M., *et al.* Osteopetrosis associated with proximal and distal tubular acidosis. *Acta Paediat. Scand.*, 1972, 61:429-34.

GUILFORD, SIMEON HAYDEN (American dentist, 1841-1919)

Guilford disease. See *hypohidrotic ectodermal dysplasia syndrome.*

Guilford syndrome. A syndrome of anodontia, inability to smell or taste, hypotrichosis, and anhidrosis.

Guilford, S. H. A dental anomaly. *Dent. Cosmos*, 1883, 25:113-8.

GUILLAIN, GEORGES (French physician, 1876-1961)

Garcin-Guillain syndrome. See *Garcin syndrome.*

Guillain-Barré syndrome. Synonyms: *Guillain-Barré-Strohl syndrome, Landry paralysis, Landry-Guillain-Barré syndrome, Landry-Kussmaul syndrome, acute ascending polyradiculoneuritis, acute idiopathic polyneuritis, acute infective polyneuritis, acute inflammatory demyelinating polyradiculoneuropathy (AIDP), acute plexitis, acute polyneuritis with facial diplegia, acute polyneuronitis, acute polyradiculitis, acute postinfective polyneuropathy, celluloradiculoneuritis, encepha-*

lomyeloradiculoneuritis, febrile polyneuritis, inflammatory polyneuropathy, infectious neuronitis, infectious polyneuronitis, myeloradiculitis, neuritis with albuminocytologic dissociation, neuromyelitis hyperalbumenotica, neuronitis, polyneuritis acuta ascendens, polyneuritis with facial diplegia, polyradiculitis, polyradiculoneuritis, radiculoneuritis, schwannosis.

An acute paralytic disease, most frequently affecting young adults, believed to be a form of an autoimmune disease with a delayed hypersensitivity reaction. Progressive, usually symmetrical, muscle weakness and paralysis and hyporeflexia are the early symptoms. Weakness usually begins in the lower extremities and spreads upwardly (ascending paralysis), eventually involving the upper extremities and face. The paralytic stage begins with pain and paresthesia and is followed by severe weakness. Choked disks, paralysis of facial and cranial nerves, and bulbar paralysis may occur. Additional symptoms may include fever, chills, weight loss, sensory disorders (mainly disorders of vibration sensation and a slight loss of pinprick sensation), and orthostatic hypotension or hypertension. The severity of symptoms varies, ranging from a mild footdrop, as the only symptom in mild cases, to ataxia, ophthalmoplegia, and hyporeflexia **(Fisher syndrome)** in severe cases, to flaccid quadriplegia with disorders of respiration, swallowing, speech, and eye movements in very severe cases. Pathological changes consist mainly of demyelination in the spinal roots, limb girdle plexuses, and proximal nerve trunks, sometimes also involving the distal nerves and autonomic ganglia. Most patients recover complete muscle function, but some severe cases are followed by disability; the mortality rate is about 5 percent. The etiology is unknown, but most affected persons have a history of respiratory infection or gastrointestinal illness about one month before the onset of symptoms. Other predisposing factors include viral infections, including infectious mononucleosis, hepatitis, and Epstein-Barr virus infection; prior surgery, pregnancy; and neoplasms, especially lymphomas. Some patients have been recently vaccinated against rabies and swine influenza.

Guillain, G., Barré, J., & Strohl, A. Sur un syndrome de radiculonévrite avec hyperalbuminose du liquide céphalo-rachidien sans réaction cellulaire. Remarques sur les caractères cliniques et graphiques des réflexes tendineux. *Bull. Soc. Méd. Hôp. Paris*, 1916, 40:1462-70. Landry, O. Note sur la paralysie ascendante aiguë. *Gaz. Hebd. Méd., Paris*, 1859, 6:472-4; 486-8. Kussmaul, A. *Zwei Fälle von Paraplegie mit tödlichem Ausgang ohne anatomisch nachweisbare oder toxische Ursache*. Erlangen, 1859.

Guillain-Barré-Strohl syndrome. See *Guillain-Barré syndrome.*

Landry-Guillain-Barré syndrome. See *Guillain-Barré syndrome.*

GUINON, GEORGES (French physician, 1859-1929)

Guinon disease. See *Gilles de la Tourette syndrome.*

GULIENETTI, R. (Italian physician)

Rosselli-Gulienetti syndrome. See *under Rosselli.*

GULL, SIR WILLIAM WHITEY (British physician, 1816-1890)

Addison-Gull syndrome. See *under Addison.*

Gull syndrome. Synonyms: *adult cretinism, adult myxedema, cachexia strumipriva.*

An adult form of hypothyroidism, usually in women, characterized by intolerance to cold, decreased appetite, gain of weight, dry and cold skin, constipation, puffiness, dry hair, mental dulling, decreased sweating, bradycardia, prolonged reflex time, carotinuria, and excessive and prolonged menses. Congestive heart failure, pernicious anemia, hypothermia, stiffness of joints, depression, and peripheral neuropathies may occasionally occur.

*Gull, W. W. On a cretinoid state supervening in adult life in women. *Tr. Clin. Soc. London*, 1874, 7:180-5.

Gull-Sutton syndrome. Synonym: *arteriocapillary fibrosis.*

Arteriosclerotic fibrosis of the kidney.

Gull, W. W., & Sutton, H. G. On the pathology of the morbid state commonly called chronic Bright's disease with contracted kidney ("arterio-capillary fibrosis". *Med. Chir. Tr., London*, 1872, 37:273-326.

GUNN, ROBERT MARCUS (British ophthalmologist, 1850-1909)

Gunn syndrome. Synonyms: *Marcus Gunn phenomenon, Marcus Gunn ptosis, Marcus Gunn syndrome, Marcus Gunn synkinesis, jaw-winking syndrome, winking-jaw syndrome.*

Unilateral ptosis of the eyelid with exaggerated opening of the eye during mastication or movements of the mandible. The etiology is unknown, but a hereditary pattern of transmission is suspected.

Gunn, R. M. Congenital ptosis with peculiar associated movement of the affected lid. *Tr. Ophth. Soc. U. K.*, 1883, 3:283-7.

inverted Marcus Gunn syndrome. See *Marin Amat syndrome.*

Marcus Gunn phenomenon. See *Gunn syndrome.*

Marcus Gunn ptosis. See *Gunn syndrome.*

Marcus Gunn syndrome. See *Gunn syndrome.*

Marcus Gunn synkinesis. See *Gunn syndrome.*

GÜNTHER, HANS (German physician, 1884-1956)

Günther disease (1). See *congenital erythropoietic porphyria.*

Günther disease (2). See *myoglobinuric myositis.*

gustatory lacrimation syndrome. Synonyms: *Bogorad syndrome, crocodile tears syndrome, gustolacrimal reflex, paroxysmal lacrimation.*

Unilateral paroxysmal lacrimation during the act of eating or drinking. The disorder has followed facial palsy and has also been seen in association with neurosyphilis, acoustic neuroma, vascular diseases, and the Hunt syndrome. Misdirected nerve fiber regeneration is believed to be the cause of this disorder. See also *Frey syndrome.*

*Bogorad, F. A. [A symptom of crocodile tears]. *Vrach. Delo*, 1928, 11:1328-30.

gustatory sweating. See *Frey syndrome.*

gustatory sweating and flushing. See *Frey syndrome.*

gustolacrimal reflex. See *gustatory lacrimation syndrome.*

GUTIERREZ, ROBERT (American physician, born 1895)

Gutierrez syndrome. Synonym: *horseshoe kidney.*

Horseshoe kidney associated with abdominal pain about the epigastric or umbilical region, chronic constipation with or without gastrointestinal disorders, and urinary disorders with early signs of chronic nephritis.

Gutierrez, R. The clinical management of the horseshoe kidney. II. *Am. J. Surg.*, 1932, 15:132-65.

guttate iritis. See *Doyne iritis.*

guttate parapsoriasis. See *Brocq disease (2).*

GUTTMANN, E. (German physician)

Bodechtel-Guttmann disease. See *van Bogaert encephalitis.*

GUY PATIN. See PATIN, GUI

GUYON, FELIX JEAN CASIMIR (French physician, 1831-1920)

Guyon tunnel syndrome. See *ulnar tunnel syndrome.*

loge de Guyon syndrome. See *ulnar tunnel syndrome.*

tunnel of Guyon syndrome. See *ulnar tunnel syndrome.*

GVHD (**g**raft-**v**ersus-**h**ost **d**isease. See *under graft-versus-host syndrome.*

GVHR (**g**raft-**v**ersus-**h**ost **r**eaction). See *under graft-versus-host syndrome.*

gynecomastia-aspermatogenesis syndrome. See *chromosome XXY syndrome.*

gyrate scalp. See *pachydermoperiostosis syndrome.*

gyrus angularis syndrome. See *Gerstmann syndrome (2).*

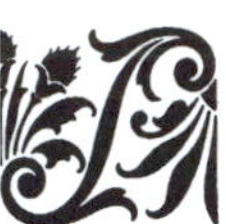

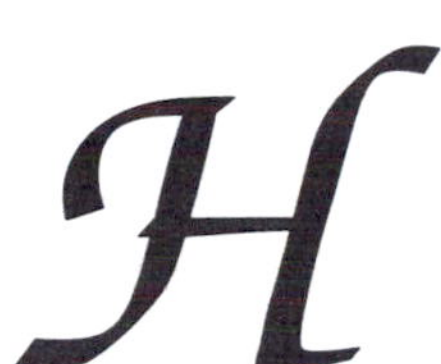

H disease. See *Hartnup disease, and see heavy chain disease.*

4H (hypothalamic hamartoblastoma-hyperphalangeal-hypoendocrine-hypoplastic anus) syndrome. See *Hall syndrome, under Hall, J. G.*

H γ-2 disease. See *heavy chain disease.*

H_3O syndrome. See *Prader-Willi syndrome.*

HA (Hakim-Adams) syndrome. See *Hakim syndrome.*

HAAB, OTTO (Swiss ophthalmologist, 1850-1931)

Biber-Haab-Dimmer syndrome. See *under Biber.*

Haab-Dimmer syndrome. See *Biber-Haab-Dimmer syndrome.*

HAAS

Haas disease. See *Panner disease (2).*

HABER, HENRY (British physician)

Haber syndrome (HS). A form of genodermatosis, transmitted as an autosomal dominant trait, characterized by facial rosacea-like lesions and multiple intraepidermal epitheliomas. The syndrome has a slowly progressive course, beginning in childhood and proceeding with pustular flare-ups. Pigmented keratotic lesions of the trunk, which resemble seborrheic warts, appear during the second decade of life. Xerosis of the lower extremities and a burning sensation of the face may be associated. Sunlight tends to aggravate the facial lesions. A necklace of basaloid cells around the hair and sebaceous follicle is the principal histopathological feature.

Sanderson, K. V. & Wilson, H. T. Haber's syndrome. Familial rosacea-like eruption with intraepidermal epithelioma. *Brit. J. Derm.*, 1965, 77::1-8.

HABERMANN, RUDOLF (German dermatologist, 1884-1941)

Mucha-Habermann syndrome. See *under Mucha.*

habit spasm. See *Gilles de la Tourette syndrome.*

habitus phthisicus. See *Stiller asthenia.*

HADFIELD, GEOFFREY (British physician, born 1889)

Clarke-Hadfield syndrome. See *Andersen triad.*

HADORN, WALTER (Swiss physician, 1898-1948)

Albright-Hadorn syndrome. See *under Albright.*

haematoporphyria congenita. See *congenital erythropoietic porphyria.*

Haemophilus influenzae B laryngitis. See *Kleinschmidt syndrome.*

HAENEL, HEINRICH (HANS) G. (German physician, 1874-1942)

Haenel syndrome. Synonym: *tabetic ocular anesthesia syndrome.*

Absence of pain on pressure applied to the eye in the late stage of neurosyphilis.

Haenel. Ein neues Tabessymptom. *Neurol. Zbl.*, 1909, 28:1199.

HAFERKAMP, OTTO (German physician, born 1929)

Haferkamp syndrome. A variant of the Gorham syndrome characterized by an association of generalized hemangiomatosis and osteolysis that does not cause complete disappearance of the bones. Lipid metabolism disorders; fatty degeneration of the liver, kidney, and tumor tissue; arteriosclerosis of the renal and splenic arteries; blood protein changes; and myelophthisic and leukoerythroblastic anemia usually occur.

Haferkamp, O. Über das Syndrom: Generalisierte maligne Hämangiomatosis und Osteolysis. *Zschr. Krebsforsch.*, 1962, 64:418-26.

Haff disease. Myoglobinuria associated with severe pain in the limbs and a sense of weariness. Epidemics of this condition, first described in fishermen in 1924, 1925, and 1940, were said to be caused by arsine introduced into the Haff waters (a lagoon in East Prussia, connecting with the Baltic Sea) by wastes from cellulose plants.

Assmann, H. *et al.* Beobachtungen und Untersuchungen bei der Haffkrankheit. *Deut. Med. Wschr.*, 1933, 59:122-6.

HAGBERG

Hagberg-Santavuori syndrome. See *Haltia-Santavuori syndrome.*

HAGEMAN, JOHN

Hageman factor deficiency. Synonyms: *Hageman trait, factor XII deficiency.*

A blood coagulation disorder due to factor XII deficiency, transmitted as an autosomal recessive trait and marked by a prolonged coagulation time, usually without hemorrhagic complications, except for some rare instances in which there may may be some mild bleeding. Localization of the Hageman factor locus is believed to be on the short arm of chromosome 7. The disorder was named after John Hageman, the patient in whom factor XII was first detected.

Ratnoff, O. D. *et al.* The demise of John Hageman. *N. Engl. J. Med.*, 1979:260-1.

Hageman trait. See *Hageman factor deficiency.*

HAGLUND, SIMS EMIL PATRIK (Swedish physician, 1870-1937)

Haglund syndrome (1). Tenodynia, tendinitis ossificans, and bursitis in the region of the Achilles tendon, resulting from lesions of the calcaneus at its junction with the Achilles tendon.

Haglund, P. Beitrag zur Klinik der Achillessehne. *Zschr. Orthop. Chir.*, 1927-28, 49:49-58.

Haglund syndrome (2). Fracture of the bony nucleus of the calcaneus at its junction with the Achilles tendon, often without apparent damage to the cartilage or the periosteum, observed in juveniles.

Haglund, P. Über Fraktur des Epiphysenkrens des Calcaneus, nebst allgemeinen Bemerkungen über einige ähnliche juvenile Knochenkeraverletzungen. *Arch. Chir., Berlin,* 1907, 82:922-30.

Haglund-Läwen-Fründ syndrome. See *Büdinger-Ludloff-Läwen syndrome.*

HAGNER, KARL

Hagner syndrome. See *Marie-Bamberger syndrome, under Marie, Pierre.*

HAGNER, WILHELM

Hagner syndrome. See *Marie-Bamberger syndrome, under Marie, Pierre.*

HAILEY, HUGH (American dermatologist, born 1909)

Gougerot-Hailey-Hailey disease. See *Hailey-Hailey disease, under Hailey, William Howard.*

Hailey-Hailey disease. See *under Hailey, William Howard.*

HAILEY, WILLIAM HOWARD (American dermatologist, 1898-1967)

Gougerot-Hailey-Hailey disease. See *Hailey-Hailey disease.*

Hailey disease. See *Hailey-Hailey disease.*

Hailey-Hailey disease. Synonyms: *Gougerot-Hailey-Hailey disease, Hailey disease, chronic recurrent acantholysis, dyskeratoid dermatosis, dyskeratosis bullosa hereditaria, familial benign chronic pemphigus, familial benign pemphigus, familial chronic pemphigus, pemphigus familiaris chronicus, recurrent herpetiform dermatitis repens.*

A skin disease characterized by pemphigus with clusters of small vesicles arising on an erythematous base; these change to rupturing flaccid bullae, leaving eroded areas covered by an amber-colored crust. In their centers, the lesions show healing processes with pigmentation or moist areas. The lesions tend to spread peripherally, involving the neck, axillae, groin, and the genital, perianal, periumbilical, and other regions, being limited to a few sites at one time, and occasionally to a single area. After a period of several months, the eruption heals without scarring. Recurrences usually occur in the same locations. Involvement of the oral mucosa, larynx, esophagus, vulva, and vagina may be observed in some cases. The disorder is transmitted as an autosmal dominant trait.

Hailey, H., & Hailey H. Familial benign chronic pemphipus. *Arch. Derm., Chicago,* 1939, 39:679-85. Gougerot, H. La priorité du pemphigus chronique familial héréditaire benin. *Ann. Derm. Syph., Paris,* 1950, 10:361-3. Gougerot, H., & Allé. Forme de transition entre la dermatite polymorphe douloureuse Brocq-Duhring et le pemphigus congénital familial héréditaire. *Arch. Derm. Syph., Paris,* 1933, 5:255-7.

hair follicle tumor. See *Miescher trichofolliculoma.*

hair strangulation. See *tourniquet syndrome.*

HAIR-AN (hyperadrogenism-insulin resistance-acanthosis nigricans) syndrome. A syndrome of increased androgen production, insulin resistance, and acanthosis nigricans in women. The symptoms include hirsutism, acne, oily skin, occasional obesity, amenorrhea, frequent symptoms of diabetes mellitus (polyuria and polydipsia), and velvety hyperpigmented lesions on the neck, axillae, and under the breasts. Associated symptoms may include skin tags, acral changes suggestive of acromegaly, balding, enlarged clitoris, male habitus, and variable-sized ovaries.

Barbieri, R. L., & Ryan, K. J. Hyperandrogenism, insulin resistance, and acanthosis nigricans syndrome: A common endocrinopathy with distinct pathophysiologic features. *Am. J. Obst. Gyn.*, 1983, 147:90-101.

hair-brain syndrome. Synonyms: *Amish brittle hair syndrome, brittle hair-intellectual impairment-decreased fertility-short stature (BIDS) syndrome, trichothiodystrophy.*

A syndrome transmitted as an autosomal recessive trait, characterized by a short stature, mental deficiency, hair shaft abnormalities with brittle hair, and poor sexual maturation with infertility. Associated disorders may include lack of growth, unusual facies, dental abnormalities, ichthyosis, cataracts, fragility of the nails (trichothyodystrophy). Grooved surfaces and absence of scales on the hair are the main pathological features. Biochemical findings include sulfur deficiency in the hair and nails and low cystine levels. Most reported cases were observed in an Amish kindred. See also *Tay syndrome,* under *Tay, Chong Hai.*

Allen, R. J. Neurocutaneous syndromes in children. *Postgrad. Med. J.*, 1971, 50:83-9. Jackson, C. E., *et al.* "Brittle" hair with short stature, intellectual impairment with decreased fertility; an autosomal recessive syndrome in an Amish kindred. *Pediatrics,* 1974, 54:201-7. Jorizzo, J. L., *et al.* Lamellar ichthyosis, dwarfism, mental retardation, and hair shaft abnormalities. A link *J. Am. Acad. Dermatol.*, 1980, 2:309-17.

hairless pseudofemale. See *testicular feminization syndrome.*

hairless women syndrome. See *testicular feminization syndrome.*

hairy elbows syndrome. Synonym: *familial hypertrichosis cubiti.*

A localized form of familial hypertrichosis involving the elbow regions. The condition was originally observed in several members of an Amish family.

Beighton, P. Familial hypertrichosis cubiti: Hairy elbows syndrome. *J. Med. Genet.*, 1970, 7:158-60.

HAJDU, NICHOLAS (Radiologist in England)

Hajdu syndrome. See *Hajdu-Cheney syndrome.*

Hajdu-Cheney syndrome. Synonyms: *Cheney syndrome, Hajdu syndrome, acro-osteolysis syndrome, arthrodento-osteodysplasia (ADOD).*

A hereditary form of acro-osteolysis associated with short stature, characteristic facies, and slowly progressive skeletal dysplasia which affects the skull, spine, and long bones. Cranial abnormalities include wormian bones, failure of ossification of sutures, absence of the frontal sinus, elongated sella turcica, basilar impression, bathrocephaly, and micromandible. Resorption of the alveolar process and early loss of teeth are the principal dental features. Spinal anomalies consist of biconcave vertebrae and kyphoscoliosis. Short distal digits and nails with acro-osteolysis are the main limb anomalies. Crowded carpal bones and joint laxity are usually associated. The syndrome is transmitted as an autosomal dominant trait; sporadic cases are believed to represent a fresh gene mutation.

Hajdu, N., & Kauntze, R. Cranio-skeletal dysplasia. *Brit. J. Radiol.*, 1948, 21:42-8. Cheney, W. D. Acro-osteolysis, *Am. J. Roentgen.*, 1965, 94:595-607.

HAKIM, S.

Hakim syndrome. Synonyms: *Hakim-Adams (HA) syndrome, normal pressure hydrocephalus, normotensive hydrocephalus, progressive normotensive hydrocephalus in adults.*

A syndrome of dementia, gait apraxia, and urinary incontinence in conjunction with ventricular enlargement in the absence of cerebrospinal fluid pressure disorders.

Hakim, S., & Adams, R. D. The special problem of symptomatic hydrocephalus with normal cerebrospinal fluid pressure. *J. Neur. Sc.*, 1965, 2:307-27.

Hakim-Adams syndrome. See *Hakim syndrome.*

pseudo-Hakim-Adams syndrome. A syndrome with symptoms similar to those in the Hakim syndrome, characterized by dementia with ventricular dilatation, minimal dyscalculia and dyspraxia, increased aphasia, anxiety and depression, and occasional gait and sphincter control disorders.

De Mol, J., *et al.* Pseudo-syndrome de Hakim et Adams. Étude neuropsychologique de 23 cas de faux diagnostic dea syndrome de Hakim et Adams. *Acta Neur. Belg.*, 1982, 82:197-208.

HAKOLA, H. PANU A. (Finnish physician)

Hakola syndrome. Synonym: *lipomembranous polycystic osteodysplasia-dementia syndrome.*

A progressive illness, transmitted as an autosomal recessive trait, characterized by lipomembranous polycystic osteodysplasia and dementia. The early symptoms, having onset in early adult life, consist of skeletal changes, mainly pain, tenderness, and swelling of the ankles and wrists after stress or minor injury. They are followed by frequent fractures, sometimes after only a minor injury. The last to appear are the neuropsychiatric symptoms, including exaggerated deep reflexes, pathological reflexes, abnormal movements, myoclonic twitches, motor aphasia, memory disorders, euphoria, lack of inhibitions, atrophy of the optic disks, impotence or frigidity, EEG disorders, and finally, epileptic seizures, extrapyramidal symptoms, trembling, ataxia, and urinary incontinence. Cystic changes in the humerus, radius, ulna, carpal bones, metacarpal bones, and other bones are the principal radiological findings.

Hakola, H. P. Neuropsychiatric and genetic aspects of a new hereditary disease characterized by progressive dementia and lipomembranous polycystic osteodysplasia. *Acta Psychiat. Scand.*, 1972, Suppl. 232:1-173.

hakuri. See *Sakamoto disease.*

HALASZ, NICHOLAS A. (American physician)

Halasz syndrome. See *scimitar syndrome.*

HALBAN

Halban syndrome. Synonym: *corpus luteum persistens.*

A syndrome seen in young women with benign ovarian tumors, in which there is persistence of the corpus luteum with amenorrhea and symptoms resembling pregnancy.

Aschheim, S., & Varangot, J. Verkannte Schwangershaft. *Arch. Gyn., München,* 1953, 183:275-80.

HALBEISEN, WILLIAM A. (American physician, born 1915)

Stryker-Halbeisen syndrome. See *under Stryker.*

HALBERTSMA, NICOLAAS ADOLF (Dutch physician, born 1889)

van der Hoeve-Halbertsma-Waardenburg syndrome. See *Waardenburg syndrome (2).*

HALBRECHT, J. (American physician)

Halbrecht syndrome. Synonyms: *ABO erythroblastosis, icterus neonatorum precox.*

Jaundice of newborn infants that appears within 24 hours after birth and is related to maternal-fetal ABO incompatibility.

Halbrecht, J. Role of hemagglutinins anti-A and anti-B in pathogenesis of jaundice of the newborn (icterus neonatorum precox). *Am. J. Dis. Child.*, 1944, 68:248-9.

half-base syndrome. See *Garcin syndrome.*

HALL, BRYAN D. (American physician)

Curry-Hall syndrome. See *Weyers syndrome (3).*

HALL, J. G. (American physician)

Hall syndrome. Synonyms: *Pallister-Hall syndrome, congenital hypothalamic hamartoblastoma, hypothalamic hamartoblastoma-hyperphalangeal hypoendocrine-hypoplastic anus (4H) syndrome, hamartopolydactyly syndrome, microphallus-imperforate anus-syndactyly-hamartoblastoma-abnormal lung lobulation-polydactyly (MISHAP) syndrome, renal-anal-lung-polydactyly-hamartoblastoma (RALPH) syndrome.*

A lethal syndrome of hypothalamic hamartoblastoma, postaxial polydactyly, microphalus, and imperforate anus. Some patients also exhibit laryngeal clefts, abnormal lung lobulation, renal agenesis and/or renal dysplasia, short fourth metacarpals, congenital heart defect, and growth retardation. All cases thus far reported have been sporadic, but maternal insecticide and pesticide exposure were reported in some instances.

Hall, J. G., Pallister, P. D., *et al.* Congenital hypothalamic hamartoblastoma, hypopituitarism, imperforate anus, and postaxial polydactyly-A new syndrome? I. Clinical, causal, and pathogenic considerations. *Am. J. Med. Genet.*, 1980, 7:47-74.

Pallister-Hall syndrome. See *Hall syndrome.*

HALL, MARSHALL (British physician, 1790-1857)

Hall syndrome. Synonyms: *hydrocephaloid affection, spurious hydrocephalus.*

Cerebral disorders associated with anemia in children with symptoms simulating those seen in hydrocephalus.

*Hall, M. *An assay on a hydrocephaloid affection in infants arising from exhaustion*. London, Sherwood, 1836.

HALLER, J. ALEX (American physician)

Cantrell-Haller-Ravitch syndrome. See *thoraco-abdominal syndrome.*

HALLERMANN, WILHELM (German ophthalmologist, born 1901)

Hallermann syndrome. See *Hallermann-Streiff syndrome.*

Hallermann-Streiff syndrome (HSS). Synonyms: *François dyscephalia, François dyscephalic syndrome, Hallermann syndrome, Hallermann-Streiff-François syndrome, Ullrich and Fremerey-Dohna syndrome, bird-like facies, dyscephalia mandibulo-oculofacialis, dyscephalia oculomandibulofacialis, dyscephaly-congenital cataract-hypotrichosis syndrome, mandibulofacial dysmorphia, mandibulo-oculofacial dyscephaly, mandibulo-oculofacial dysmorphism, oculomandibulo-*

dyscephaly (OMD), oculomandibulodyscephaly-hypotrichosis syndrome, oculomandibulofacial syndrome.

A syndrome of birdlike facies with hypoplastic mandible, beaked nose, dwarfism, hypotrichosis, microphthalmia, and congenital cataract. Brachycephaly, frontal bossing, open lambdoidal and longitudinal sutures, and delayed closure of fontanels are usually associated. Glaucoma, aphakia, nystagmus, strabismus, and blue sclerae are the additional ocular features. The scalp skin is thin and taut with prominent veins. Hypotrichosis is usually general. Mental retardation occurs in some cases. Osteoporosis, syndactyly, lordosis, scoliosis, spina bifida, and winged scapulae are the skeletal abnormalities. Hypoplasia of the mandible is generally associated with double chin and central cleft or dimple. Dental abnormalities include edentia, persistence of deciduous teeth, malocclusion, malformed teeth, rampant caries, and supernumerary teeth. Most cases are sporadic. See also *Seckel syndrome.*

Hallermann, W. Vogelgesich und Cataracta congenita, *Klin. Mbl. Augenh.*, 1948, 113:315-8. Streiff, E. B. Dysmorphie mandibulo-faciale (tête d'oiseau) et alterations oculaires. *Ophthalmologica, Basel*, 1950, 120:7983. François, J. Un nouveau syndrome: dyscéphalie avec tête d'oiseau et anomalies dentaires, nanisme, hypotrichose, atrophie cutanée, microphthalmie, et cataracte congénitale. *Bull. Soc. Belge Opht.*, 1957, 117:569-97. Ullrich, O., & Fremerey-Dohna, H. Dyskephalie mit Cataracta congenita und Hypotrichose als typischer Merkmalskomplex. *Ophthalmologica, Basel*, 1953, 125:73-90; 144-54.

Hallermann-Streiff-François syndrome. See *Hallermann-Streiff syndrome.*

HALLERVORDEN, JULIUS (German physician, 1882-1965)

Hallervorden-Spatz syndrome (HSS). Synonyms: *pigmentary degeneration syndrome of globus pallidus, progressive pallidal degeneration syndrome.*

A familial syndrome, transmitted as an autosomal recessive trait, characterized by muscle tonus disorders, involuntary movements, and progressive dementia. Early symptoms appear in children or adolescents and consist of muscle rigidity, choreoathetosis, abnormal posture, and torsion spasm. They are followed by cerebellar ataxia, speech disorders, progressive mental deterioration, and death about 10 years later. Accumulation of pigmented materials in the globus pallidus and pars reticulata of the substantia nigra with discoloration, the presence of pigmented iron-containing concretions and granules, loss of nerve fibers, and localized swellings of the axons are the principal pathological findings.

Hallervorden, J., & Spatz, H. Eigenartige Erkrankung im extrapyramidalen System mit besonderer Beteiligung des Globus pallidus und der Substantia nigra: Ein Beitrag zu den Bezhiehungen zwischen diesen beiden Zentren. *Zschr. Neur.*, 1922, 79:254-302.

HALLGREN, BERTIL (Swedish physician)

Alström-Hallgren syndrome. See *Alström syndrome.*

Hallgren syndrome. See *Graefe-Sjögren syndrome.*

HALLIDAY, JOHN (Australian physician)

Halliday hyperostosis. Severe osteosclerotic changes in the skull, maxillary regions, ribs, and clavicles with osteoblastic activity in many bones. The syndrome was described originally in a 3-year-old girl.

Halliday, J. A rare case of bone dystrophy. *Brit. J. Surg.*, 1949-50, 37:52-63.

HALLOPEAU, FRANÇOIS HENRI (French physician, 1842-1919)

epidermolysis bullosa dystrophica Hallopeau-Siemens (EBDH). See *Hallopeau-Siemens syndrome.*

Hallopeau disease (1 and 2). See *Hallopeau syndrome (1 and 2).*

Hallopeau syndrome (1). Synonyms: *Csillag disease, Hallopeau disease, von Zambusch disease, chronic atrophic lichenoid dermatitis, dermatitis lichenoidea chronica, dermatitis lichenoidea chronica atrophicans, lichen albus, lichen planus morphoeicus, lichen planus sclerosus et atrophicus, white spots disease.*

A chronic atrophic skin disease characterized by irregular, firm, mother-of-pearl or ivory-colored flat-topped papules with erythematous halos surrounding the white spots. The papules are round or oval; they have shining smooth surfaces and contain dark, comedolike plugs or minute depressions caused by former plugs. In advanced stages, coalescing papules may form large lesions and atrophy may occur. Bullae, hemorrhage, hyperpigmentation, and exfoliation may be present. The disease is usually observed in women, the upper chest, back, and anogenital area being the common sites.

Hallopeau, H. Lichen plan scléreux. *Ann. Derm. Syph., Paris*, 1889, 20:447-9. Csillag, J. Dermatitis lichenoides chronica atrophicans (Lichen albus v. Zambusch). In: Neisser, A., & Jacobi. E., eds. *Ikonographia dermatologica*. Berlin, 1909, pp. 147-51. Zambusch, L., von. Über Lichen albus, eine bisher unbeschriebene Erkrankung. *Arch. Derm. Syph., Berlin*, 1906, 82:339-50.

Hallopeau syndrome (2). Synonyms: *Hallopeau disease, acrodermatitis continua, acrodermatitis perstans.*

A chronic form of dermatitis usually of the hands, and less frequently the feet. Vesicles, bullae, and pustules, often following an injury or paronychia, develop initially on the palmar surfaces of the fingers and spread to the dorsal areas and palms. Thickening, dystrophy, and furrowing of the nails follow. In the generalized form, patches of various sizes may spread to most parts of the body. The disorder is caused by bacterial infections, usually by *Staphylococcus aureus*. It is considered by some authors to be a variant of Crocker disease.

Ormsby, O. S., & Montgomery, H. *Diseases of the skin*. Philadelphia, Lea & Febiger, 1954, pp. 396-9.

Hallopeau syndrome (3). Synonyms: *Hallopeau-Leredde syndrome, dermatitis pustularis, dermatitis vegetans, pyoderma verrucosum, pyodermatitis vegetans, pyodermia vegetans, vegetative pyoderma.*

A skin disorder, believed to be caused by a staphylococcal superinfection, characterized by miliary pustules surrounded by a hyperemic base on the axillae, scalp, groin, genitalia, lips, and oral mucosa. Coalescing pustules form crust-covered patches with vegetating surfaces beneath. The oral ulcers are caused by ruptured pustules. Histologically, the disorder is similar to pemphigus vulgaris.

*Hallopeau, F. H. Sur une nouvelle forme de dermatite pustuleuse chronique en foyer à progression excentrique. *Cong. Internat. Derm. Syph., Paris*, 1889, p. 544.

Hallopeau-Leredde syndrome. See *Hallopeau syndrome (3).*

Hallopeau-Siemens syndrome. Synonyms: *epidermoly-*

sis bullosa dystrophica Hallopeau-Siemens (EBDH), dystrophia bullosa atrophicans congenita, dystrophia bullosa congenita, dystrophia cutis spinosa congenita, epidermolysis bullosa dystrophica (EBD), epidermolysis bullosa hereditaria dystrophica polydysplastica, epidermolysis bullosa polydystrophica.

A destructive form of epidermolysis bullosa of the hands, feet, elbows, and knees. Mucous surfaces, especially of the conjunctiva and cornea, may be affected. Esophageal stricture and syndactyly occur in severe cases. The dental enamel is usually defective. The condition is inherited as an autosomal recessive trait and may be present at birth or appear early in infancy. Histological findings include collagenolytic changes. Increased capacity to synthesize and secrete collagenase may be observed in cultured fibroblasts.

Hallopeau, F. H. Sur une dermatose bulleuse infantile avec cicatrices indélébiles, kystes epidemiques et manifestations buccales. *Ann. Derm. Syph., Paris,* 1890, 1:414.

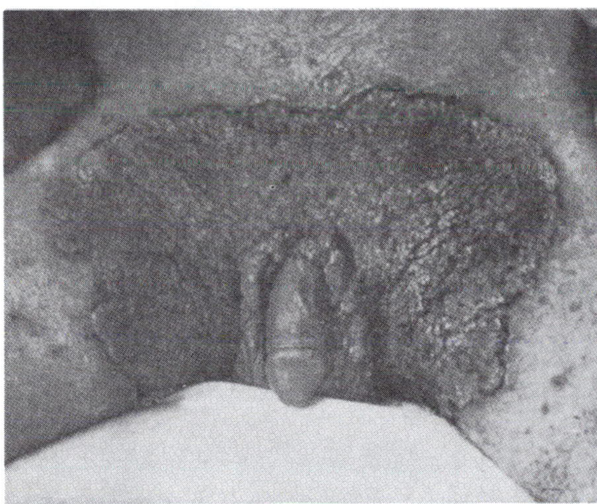

Hallopeau syndrome (3)
Andrew, G.C. & A.N. Domonkos: *Diseases of the Skin,* 5th ed. Philadelphia: W.B. Saunders Co., 1963.

hallucinosis syndrome. See *organic hallucinosis syndrome.*

halo leukoderma. See *Sutton halo nevus, under Sutton, Richard Lighburn.*

HALPERN, L. (Israeli physician)

Halpern syndrome. Synonyms: *acute transient monocular disequilibrium, dysequilibrium syndrome (DES), sensimotor induction in unilateral disequilibrium syndrome, sensorimotor induction syndrome.*

A dysequilibrium syndrome (not to be confused with the *disequilibrium syndrome*), marked by the displacement of vertical and horizontal axes. The condition is induced by looking with the affected eye only, is further aggravated by applying red filters to the eye and is corrected by blue filters. Hagberg defines the syndrome as "a nonprogressive neurologic condition dominated throughout childhood by incapability of or pronounced difficulty in maintaining upright body position and in experiencing the position of the body in space, i.e., a lack of sense of equilibrium." Major features are the postural abnormalities manifested by unilateral displacement and sensory disturbances in the form of altered perception. A wide variety of congenital abnormalities, including mental retardation, cerebral palsy, retarded motor development, and muscle hypotonia may be observed in most cases. The patient usually complains of nausea, occasional vomiting, and dizziness occurring spontaneously or after change in the position of the head. The patient often suffers from a sensation that his eye is "swimming," impaired perception of colors, distorted perception of objects, and unsteady gait. Nonprogressive cerebellar disorders are considered to be the cause. Low serum dopamine-ß-hydrolase activity is the principal metabolic defect. The syndrome is believed to be transmitted as an autosomal recessive trait.

Halpern, L. Das Syndrom des sensorimotorischen Induktion. *Schweiz. Arch. Neur. Psychiat.,* 1969, 103:1-23. Halpern, L. The syndrome of sensimotor induction in disturbed equilibrium. *Arch. Neur. Psychiat.,* 1949, 62:330-54. Bental, E., & Hammond-Tooke, G. D. Vertigo and drop attacks caused by acute transient monocular disequilibrium (Halpern's syndrome). *J, Neur.,* 1979, 222:59-66. Hagbert, B., *et al.* The dysequilibrium syndrome in cerebral palsy. Clinical aspects and treatment. *Acta Paediat. Scand.,* 1972, 61(Suppl. 226):1-63.

HALTIA, M. (Finnish physician)

Haltia-Santavuori neuronal ceroid-lipofuscinosis. See *Haltia-Santavuori syndrome.*

Haltia-Santavuori syndrome. Synonyms: *Hagberg-Santavuori syndrome; Haltia-Santavuori neuronal ceroid lipofuscinosis; Santavuori disease; neuronal ceroid lipofuscinosis, infantile Finnish type.*

An inborn error of metabolism, transmitted as an autosomal recessive trait, characterized by a progressive encephalopathy with onset in the second year of life. The symptoms include mental retardation, muscle hypotonia, ataxia, myoclonic jerks, knitting hyperkinesia, convulsions, microcephaly, blindness due to optic atrophy and hypopigmented retinal dystrophy, and EEG abnormalities. Stellate posterior polar cataracts and retinal degeneration with hyperpigmented "bony spicules" may occur. A decrease in lipid-bound *N*-acetylneuraminic acid is the principal biochemical defect. Histological findings show neuronal destruction accompanied by a massive occurrence of frequently binucleated phagocytes and hypertrophic fibrillary astrocystes in the cerebral cortex. The remaining neurons and glial cells contain autofluorescent granules with the staining properties of lipofuscin and strong acid phosphatase activity.

Santavuori, P., Haltia, M., *et al.* Infantile type of so-called neuronal ceroid-lipofuscinosis. I. A clinical study of 15 patients. *J. Neur. Sc.,* 1973, 18:257-67. Haltia, M., Rapola, J., Santavuori, P., & Keranen, A. Infantile type of so-called neuronal ceroid-lipofuscinosis. II. Morphological and biochemical studies. *J. Neur. Sc.,* 1973, 18:269-85.

HALUSHI BEHÇET. See BEHÇET, HALUSHI

hamartoma of the cerebellum. See *Lhermitte-Duclos disease.*

hamartomatous meningeal melanosis. See *neurocutaneous melanosis.*

hamartopolydactyly syndrome. See *Hall syndrome, under Hall, J. G.*

HAMMAN, LOUIS (American physician, 1877-1946)

Hamman syndrome. Synonym: *subcutaneous emphysema-pneumomediastinum syndrome.*

A syndrome of subcutaneous emphysema and pneumomediastinum associated with pain, subcutaneous and retroperitoneal emphysema, obliteration of the cardiac dullness, crunching sounds over the heart synchronous with the cardiac cycle (Hamman sign), increased mediastinal pressure, dyspnea, cyanosis, engorged veins, circulatory failure, pneumothorax, and roentgenographic evidence of air in the mediastinum.

Hamman, L. Mediastinal emphysema. *JAMA*, 1945, 128:1-6. Reeder, S. R. Subcutaneous emphysema, pneumomediastinum, and pneumothorax in labor and delivery. *Am. J. Obst. Gyn.*, 1986, 154:487-9.

Hamman-Rich syndrome. Synonyms: *Corrigan cirrhosis, diffuse idiopathic interstitial pulmonary fibrosis, diffuse interstitial pulmonary fibrosis, diffuse sclerosing alveolitis, fibroid phthisis, fibrosing lung disease, idiopathic fibrosing alveolitis (IFA), idiopathic pulmonary fibrosis, interstitial fibrosis of the lung, progressive chronic interstitial pulmonary fibrosis, pulmonary fibrosis, usual interstitial pneumonia (UIP).*

An acute or chronic pulmonary disease of unknown etiology, associated with insidious onset which is followed by cough, dyspnea, tachypnea, cyanosis, fatigability, loss of weight, clubbing of the fingers, pulmonary hypertension, cor pulmonale, right cardiac failure, and progressive pulmonary insufficiency due to diffuse interstitial fibrosis and round-cell or plasma-cell infiltration of the interstitial tissue and alveolar structures, which result in capillary block. Radiologically, the disease is manifested by parenchymal and hilar densities, pneumothorax, bronchial and hilar dilatation, and loss of lung volume. The disease may occur at any age but most commonly it is observed in the fifth decade. See also *Fränkel disease*.

Hamman, L., & Rich, A. Acute diffuse interstitial fibrosis of the lungs. *Bull. Johns Hopkins Hosp.*, 1944, 74:177-212. Corrigan, D. J. On cirrhosis of the lung. *Dublin J. Med. Sc.*, 1838, 13:266-86.

hammer finger. See *camptodactyly syndrome*.

HAMMOND, WILLIAM ALEXANDER (American neurologist, 1828-1900)

Hammond syndrome. Synonyms: *athetosis, athetosis duplex.*

An extrapyramidal disorder characterized by dyskinesia with slow, writhing, purposeless movements. The hands and face are usually affected. Lesions of the midbrain, thalamic nuclei, pallidostriatum, and internal capsule of the cerebral cortex are the cause of this disorder. The globus pallidus, nucleus ruber, and corticospinal tracts may also be involved. Sustained contractions at the end of an athetotic movement are called **athetotic dystonia**.

Hammond, W. A. Athetosis. *Med. Times Gaz., London*, 1871, 2:747-8.

HAMSTORN

Hamstorn syndrome. Synonym: *familial intermittent adynamia.*

Paroxysmal myoplegia due to hyperkalemia, reportedly described by Hamstorn.

Il'ina, N. A. O paroksizmal'noi mioplegii. *Zh. Nevropat. Psikhiat.*, 1963, 63:1352-6.

HANAULD

Coote-Hanauld syndrome. See *cervical rib syndrome*.

HAND, ALFRED, JR. (American physician, 1868-1949)

Hand disease. See *Hand-Schüller-Christian syndrome*.

Hand-Rowland disease. See *Hand-Schüller-Christian syndrome*.

Hand-Schüller-Christian (HSC) syndrome. Synonyms: *Christian syndrome, Hand disease, Hand-Rowland disease, Schüller disease, Schüller-Christian disease, chronic disseminated histiocytosis X, craniohypophyseal xanthoma, cholesterol granulomatosis, lipoid granulomatosis, lipoid histiocytosis, xanthomatous granuloma syndrome, xanthomatous reticuloendotheliosis.*

A chronic disseminated form of histiocytosis X, occurring most often in children and young adults, characterized by dissemination of histiocytes and a triad of clinical symptoms: exophthalmos, diabetes insipidus, and osteolytic bone lesions. The histiocytes contain little lipid, hence the disorder has been classified as a **nonlipid reticuloendotheliosis.** Tumorlike masses of cholesterol-loaded histiocytes cause exophthalmos by pushing against the eyeball; they may also compress the pituitary and hypothalamus. The symptoms include eczematous eruption, xanthomata, lymph node enlargement, hepatosplenomegaly, and pulmonary infiltrations. Oral lesions include red, soft gingivae, loose or shedding teeth, and mandibular erosion. Roentgenographically, the affected teeth appear to "float"; bone destruction is marked by radiolucent areas of various shapes and degrees, and rarefaction in the medullary spaces is indicated by poorly outlined lacunae. The skull bones may assume an irregular or serpinginous pattern. The lesions present yellow areas with dark patches of old hemorrhages. Histologically, the lesions are masses of granulation tissue made up mostly of proliferating histiocytes, with some eosinophils present.

Hand, A., Jr. Polyuria and tuberculosis. *Arch. Pediat., N. Y.*, 1893, 10:673-5. Christian, H. Defects in membranous bones, exophthalmos and diabetes insipidus; an unusual syndrome of dyspituitarism. *Med. Clin. N. America*, 1920, 3:849-71. Rowland, R. S. Xanthomatosis and the reticuloendothelial system. Correlation of an unidentified group of cases described as defects in membraneous bones, exophthalmos and diabetes insipidus (Christian's syndrome). *Arch. Int. Med.*, 1928, 42:611-74. Schüller, A. Über eigenartige Schädeldefekte im Jugendalter. *Fortsch. Geb. Röntgen.*, 1915:23:12-8.

hand and foot syndrome. See *under sickle cell anemia*.

hand-arm vibration syndrome. See *vibration syndrome*.

hand-foot-and-mouth disease. See *hand-foot-and-mouth syndrome*.

hand-foot-and-mouth syndrome. Synonyms: *hand-foot-and-mouth disease, stomatitis vesiculosa cum exanthemata.*

A viral disease of children, usually under 10 years of age, caused by coxsackieviruses, especially those of Group A, type 16. The symptoms appear after an incubation period of 2 to 6 days, consisting of superficial vesicles on the borders of the palms and soles and ventral surfaces of the fingers and toes; they first appear as red papules, about 2 to 10 mm in diameter, which change to flaccid gray vesicles that resolve in about 10 days. The oral lesions consist of 5 to 10 painful aphthae, under 2 mm in diameter, involving any part of the mouth and lips; they subside and heal within a week or 10 days. Mild anorexia, fever, malaise, and cervical adenitis may be present.

Robinson, C. R., *et al.* Report on an outbreak of febrile illness with pharyngeal lesions and exanthem. *Canad. Med. Assoc. J.*, 1958, 79:615-21. Cherry, J. D., & John, C.

L. Hand, foot, and mouth syndrome. *Pediatrics*, 1966, 37:637-43.

hand-foot-genital (HFG) syndrome. Synonym: *hand-foot-uterus (HFU) syndrome.*

The principal features of this syndrome consist of small feet with short toes, abnormal thumbs, and duplication of the genitalia in females or hypospadias in males. Stubby thumbs with hypoplastic thenar eminences and incurved little fingers, short thumbs due to shortness of the first metacarpals, and prominent pseudoepiphyses of the distal ends of the first metacarpals are the main hand defects. Most patients also have clinodactyly, brachymesophalangy, and fused trapezium and scaphoid. Short feet are combined with shortening of the calcaneus and fusion of the cuneiform bone, either to the navicular or metatarsal bones. Genital anomalies vary from uterus duplex unicollis to double uterus and cervix with subseptate vagina, or deviation of the vagina to one side. Dermatoglyphic abnormalities and ulnar defects are frequently associated. The syndrome is transmitted as an autosomal dominant trait with variable expressivity.

Stern, A. M., *et al.* The hand-foot-uterus syndrome. A new hereditary disorder characterized by hand and foot dysplasia, dermatoglyphic abnormalities, and partial duplication of the female genital tract. *J. Pediat.*, 1970, 77:109-16.

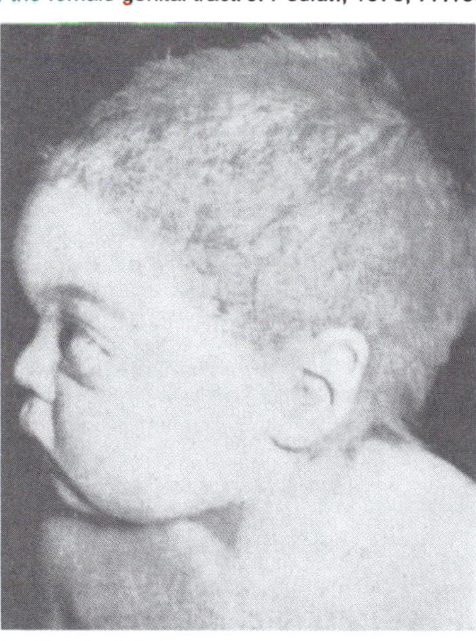

Hand-Schüller-Christian syndrome
Courtesy of Professor Hooft. From Jules Francois: *Heredity in Ophthalmology*. St. Louis: C.V. Mosby Co., 1961.

hand-foot-uterus (HFU) syndrome. See *hand-foot-genital syndrome.*

hand-ipsilateral thorax syndrome. See *Poland syndrome.*

HANE (**h**ereditary **a**ngio**n**eurotic **e**dema). See *under Quincke edema.*

HANHART, ERNST (Swiss physician, 1891-1973)

Hanhart disease. See *Hanhart syndrome (4).*

Hanhart dwarfism. See *Hanhart syndrome (1).*

Hanhart nanism. See *Hanhart syndrome (1).*

Hanhart syndrome (1). Synonyms: *Hanhart dwarfism, Hanhart nanism, ateliotic dwarfism with hypogonadism, idiopathic hypopituitary dwarfism, panhypopituitarism, pituitary dwarfism.*

Hereditary hypopituitarism with proportionate dwarfism and adiposogenital dystrophy, transmitted as an autosomal recessive trait. Growth retardation is usually observed between the ages of 1.5 and 6 years, after a normal infancy and early childhood. Heavy deposits of adipose tissue on the breasts and abdomen, underdevelopment of the secondary sex characteristics, typical facies, and diminished or absent libido are the principal features. Occasionally, brachycephaly and mental retardation may be seen. The syndrome was originally observed in inbred populations in certain areas of Switzerland and on the Island of Veglia in the Adriatic.

Hanhart, E. Über heredodegenerativen Zwergwuchs mit Dystrophia adiposo-genitalis. *Arch. Julius Klaus Stift.*, 1925, 1:181-257.

Hanhart syndrome (2). Synonyms: *aglossia-adactylia syndrome, hypoglossia-hypodactyly syndrome, mandibular dysostosis and peromelia, oro-acral syndrome, oromandibular limb hypoplasia, peromelia-micrognathia syndrome.*

A rare syndrome of combined hypoplasia of the tongue and limbs, the tongue being decreased in size but very seldom completely absent. Orofacial anomalies usually include a narrow face, recessed or hypoplastic mandible, apparent maxillary prognathism, frequent gingival abnormalities, absence of the lower incisors, intraoral bands, fusion of infra-oral structures, and cleft palate. A wide variety of limb defects may be associated, such as a decrease in the number of digits, cleft hand, hemimelia of all four limbs, and syndactyly. Additional findings may include low birth weight and paralysis of the cranial nerves. Mental retardation is rare. The syndrome occurs sporadically, but some apparently hereditary cases transmitted as an autosomal dominant trait have been reported.

Hanhart, E. Über die Kombination von Peromelie mit Mikrognathie, eine neues Syndrom beim Menschen, entsprechend der Akroteriasis congenita von Wriedt und Mohr beim Rinde. *Arch. Julius Klaus Stift.*, 1950, 25:531-44. Kettner. Kongenitaler Zungendefekt. *Deut. Med. Wschr.*, 1907, 33:532. Meyer, M. W. Über das angeborene Fehlen der Zunge und die dadurch bedingte Behinderung des Säuglings. *Jb, Kinderheilk.*, 1849, 13:328-54. Rosenthal, R. Aglossia congenita: Report of a case of the condition combined with other congenital malformations. *Am. J. Dis. Child.*, 1932, 44:383-9.

Hanhart syndrome (3). See *Richner-Hanhart syndrome.*

Hanhart syndrome (4). Synonym: *Hanhart disease.*

Familial spastic paraplegia associated with mental deficiency and transmitted as an autosomal recessive trait.

*Hanhart, E. *Eine Sippe mit einfach-rezessiver Diplegia spastica infantilis (Little-scher) aus einem Schweizeren Inzuchtgebiet*. Erbarzt, 1936.

Richner-Hanhart syndrome. See *under Richner.*

HANN, F., VON (Hungarian physician)

Hann disease. An association of posterior pituitary lesions with diabetes insipidus.

Hann, F., von. Über die Bedeutung der Hypophysenveränderungen bei Diabetes insipidus. *Frankfurt. Zschr. Path.*, 1918, 21:337-65.

HANOT, VICTOR CHARLES (French physician, 1844-1896)

Hanot cirrhosis. Synonyms: *biliary cirrhosis, cholangiolitic biliary cirrhosis, hypertrophic liver cirrhosis, splenomegalic cirrhosis.*

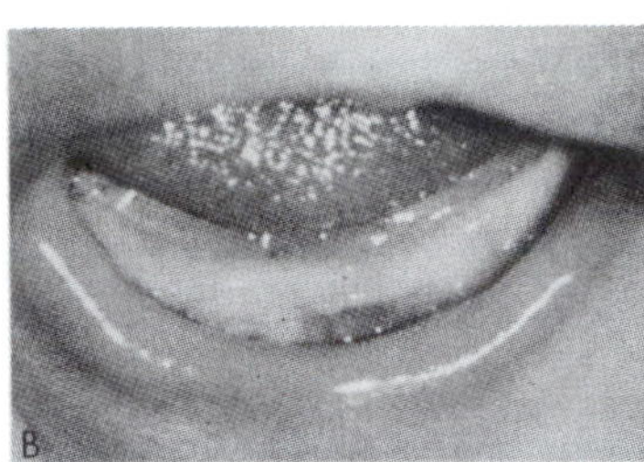
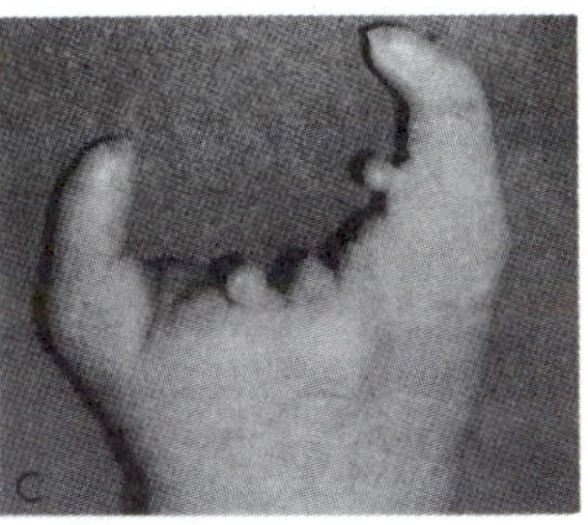

Hanhart syndrome (2)
Hall, B.D.: "Aglossia-adactylia." In Bergsma, D. (ed): Part XI. *Orofacial Structures.* Baltimore: Williams & Wilkins for the National Foundation-March of Dimes BD:OAS VII(7):233-236, 1971, with permission.

Hypertrophic cirrhosis of the liver with infection, fever, inflammation of the portal area, and extrahepatic obstruction of the bile ducts. Hepatomegaly, jaundice, and splenomegaly are the principal symptoms.

*Hanot, V. C. *Étude sur une forme de cirrhose hypertrophique du foi. Cirrhose hypertrophique avec ictère chronique.* Paris, 1875 (Thesis).

Hanot-Chauffard syndrome. See *Troisier-Hanot-Chauffard syndrome.*

Hanot-Kiener syndrome. Synonym: *diffuse mesenchymal hepatitis with nodular lymphomatosis.*

Perilobal cholestasis with hepatitis due to obstruction of the bile ducts by giant peripheral lymphoid follicles that enclose the source of the Hering canals and the terminal portion of the hepatic ducts.

Albot, G., & Lunel, J. L'hépatite mésenchymateuse diffuse avec lymphomatose nodulaire de Hanot et Kiener. *Path. Biol., Paris.*, 1961, 9:1239-50.

Hanot-MacMahon-Thannhauser syndrome. Synonyms: *MacMahon-Thannhauser syndrome, Thannhauser-Magendantz syndrome, pericholangiolitic biliary cirrhosis, xanthomatous biliary cirrhosis.*

An association of xanthomata of the skin of the plain and tuberous variety, hepatomegaly, splenomegaly, chronic obstructive jaundice, extremely high total cholesterol and lecithin in the blood serum, low neutral fats in the blood serum, and transparent blood serum. Histological findings show a nonspecific, chronic inflammatory reaction about the small bile ducts and junction ducts in the portal area, blocking of the finest bile ducts and subsequent intralobular stasis, lack of involvement of the large bile ducts, and absence of foam cells in the liver.

MacMahon, H. E., & Thannhauser, S. J. Xanthomatous biliary cirrhosis (a clinical syndrome). *Ann. Int. Med.*, 1949, 30:121-79. Thannhauser, S. J., & Magendantz, H. The different clinical groups of xanthomatous diseases; a clinical physiological study of 22 cases. *Ann. Int. Med.*, 1938, 11:1662-746.

Hanot-Rössle syndrome. Nonobstructive extrahepatic cholangitis with obstructive intrahepatic cholangitis, and cholestasis due to duodenal dyskinesia and duodenobiliary reflux, occurring in a generalized infection.

Albot, G., & Kopandji, M. La cholangiolite obstructive au cours des cholangites diffuses non oblitératantes ou maladie de Hanot-Rössle. *Sem. Hôp., Paris*, 1962, 38:3213-31.

Troisier-Hanot-Chauffard syndrome. See *under Troisier.*

HANSEN, GERHARD HENRIK ARMAUER (Norwegian physician, 1841-1912)

Hansen disease (HD). Synonyms: *elephantiasis graecorum, leontiasis, lepra, lepra arabum, leprosy, satyriasis.*

A chronic infectious disease caused by *Mycobacterium leprae*, and characterized by granulomatous lesions of the skin, mucous membranes, peripheral nervous system, and bones. Three types are recognized: tuberculoid, lepromatous, and borderline leprosy. **Tuberculoid leprosy** is manifested by sharply demarcated hypopigmented macules which gradually become elevated and circinate or gyrate. The lesions spread, and there is central healing. In time, they become anesthetic, and there is a loss of sweat glands and follicles and enlargement of peripheral nerves, especially the ulnar, peroneal, and greater auricular nerves, leading to severe pain and muscle atrophy. Contractures of the hands and feet usually follow. Involvement of the facial nerve causes logophthalmos, exposure keratitis, corneal ulcers, and blindness. **Lepromatous leprosy** is characterized by macules, nodules, and plaques, which are ill-defined and have indurated and convex centers. The face, wrists, elbows, buttocks, and knees are mainly affected. Gradually, there is a loss of the eyebrows, followed by thickening of the face and forehead (leonine facies) and the earlobes becoming pendulous. In advanced stages, there are nasal complications which include obstruction, septal perforation, and collapse with resulting saddle nose. Other symptoms include hoarseness, laryngitis, keratitis, iridocyclitis, painless lymphadenopathy, scarring of the testes, and gynecomastia. **Borderline leprosy** is characterized by lesions which resemble those of tuberculoid leprosy. They are greater in number than those in the tuberuloid type and are usually poorly defined. Involvement of the nerves is common, but the eyebrows and nasal regions are generally spared, and anesthesia is less severe than in other types of leprosy. Variability of skin lesions, whereby papules and plaques may coexist in the same patient, is characteristic for borderline leprosy, which is sometimes referred to as **dimorphic leprosy.** See also *Danielssen-Boeck disease.*

Hansen, G. H. *Indberetning til det Norske medicinske Selskob i Christiania am en med understottelse of selskabet foretagen reise for at anstille undersogelser angaende spedalskhendens arsager, tidels udforte sommen med forstander* Hartwig. 1874, pp. 1-88. Miller, R. A. Leprosy (Hansen's disease). In: Braunwald, E., Isselbacher, K. J., Petersdorf, R. G., Wilson, J. D., Martin, J. B., & Fauci, A. S., eds. *Harrison's principles of internal medicine.* 11th ed. New York, McGraw-Hill, 1987, pp. 633-7.

happy puppet syndrome. Synonyms: *Angelman syndrome, puppet children, puppetlike syndrome.*

A disorder, transmitted as an autosomal recessive trait, occurring in children who laugh frequently for almost any reason and whose movements are jerky like those of a marionette, or puppet. Associated disorders include mental and motor retardation, epilepsy, ataxic gait or complete inability to walk, muscle hypotonia, EEG abnormalities, and peculiar facies marked by a protruding jaw and tongue, microcephaly, occipital depression, and blue eyes.

Angelman, H. "Puppet children." A report of three cases. *Develop. Med. Child. Neurol.*, 1965, 7:681-8.

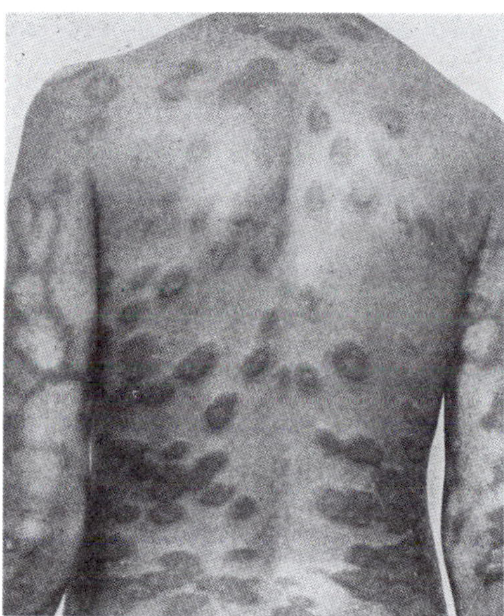

Hansen disease
Andrews, G.C., & A.N. Domonkos: *Diseases of the Skin.* Phildelphia: W.B. Saunders Co., 1963.

HAPSBURG (A German family that has furnished kings to the Holy Roman Empire, Austria, Spain, and other European countries).

disease of Hapsburgs. See *hemophilia A.*

HARADA, E. (Japanese physician)

Harada disease. See *Harada syndrome.*

Harada syndrome. Synonyms: *Harada disease, uveocutaneomeningo-encephalitic syndrome, uveoencephalitis, uveomeningitis syndrome, uveomeningoencephalitis.*

A form of uveomeningoencephalitis observed chiefly in the Far East, possibly of viral etiology, with temporary or permanent loss of hearing and visual acuity, and depigmentation or loss of the hair. Ocular symptoms include uveitis, choroiditis, and retinal detachment. The course lasts from 2 to 8 months. The symptoms overlap those of the Vogt-Kayanagi syndrome.

*Harada, E. [Clinical study of nonsuppurative choroiditis. A report of acute diffuse choroiditis]. *Acta Soc. Ophth. Jpn.*, 1926, 30:356.

Vogt-Koyanagi-Harada (VKH) syndrome. See *Vogt-Koyanagi syndrome, under Vogt, Alfred, and see Harada syndrome.*

HARBITZ, FRANCIS (Norwegian physician, 1867-1950)

Harbitz-Müller disease. Synonyms: *essential familial hypercholesterolemia, essential familial hypercholesterolemic xanthomatosis, familial cholesterolemia, hypercholesterolemia-xanthomatosis syndrome, hyperlipoproteinemia type II.*

A familial form of hyperlipoproteinemia characterized by high blood cholesterol levels (more than 300 mg/dl), associated with high concentrations of low-density lipoproteins (LDL) due to a deficiency of a cell surface receptor that regulates LDL and degradation of cholesterol synthesis. Xanthomas, arcus corneae, and premature arteriosclerotic coronary disease are the principal clinical features; death from myocardial infarction usually takes place before the age of 30 years. Hypercholesterolemia is usually present at birth, but arcus corneae and xanthomas begin to appear later. Xanthomas, presenting orange-yellowish lesions, are usually located in the Achilles and extensor tendons of the hands, tuberous xanthomas are generally found over the elbows, and subperiostesal xanthomas are located below the knee and over the olecranon process. Additional lesions may include palpebral xanthomas (xanthelasmas), elevated plantar xanthomas, elevated xanthomas of the extremities and buttocks, and xanthomas of the interdigital spaces. Histological findings show accumulation of cholesterol within histiocytic foam cells, lipid being present in cytoplasmic drops that are not bound by membranes. The condition is transmitted as an autosomal dominant trait, being more severe in persons inheriting two doses of the gene (i.e.,. homozygotes) than in those inheriting one dose (i.e., heterozygotes). See also *Bürger-Grütz syndrome.*

Müller, C. Xanthomata, hypercholesterolemia, angina pectoris. *Acta Med. Scand.*, 1938, 89(Suppl):75-84. Harbitz, F. Svulster inndeholdende xanthomae. *Norsk. Mg. Laegevid.*, 1925, 86:321-48. Fredrickson, D. S., Goldstein, J. L., & Brown, M. S. The familial hyperlipoproteinemias. In: Stanbury, J. B., Wyngaarden, J. B., & Fredrickson, D. S., eds. *The metabolic basis of inherited disease.* 4th ed. New York, McGraw-Hill, 1978, pp. 604-55.

Raeder-Harbitz syndrome. See *aortic arch syndrome.*

HARBOE

Bickel-Bing-Harboe syndrome. See *Bing-Neel syndrome, under Bing, Jens.*

hard chancre. See *Hunter chancre, under Hunter, John.*

HARD ± E (hydrocephalus-retinal dysplasia-encephalocele) syndrome. See *Walker-Warburg syndrome, under Walker, Arthur Earl.*

HARE, EDWARD SELLECK (British physician, 1812-1838)

Hare syndrome. See *Pancoast syndrome.*

HARGRAVE, ROBERT L. (American physician)

Strasburger-Hawkins-Eldridge-Hargrave-McKusick syndrome. See *symphalangism syndrome.*

HARKAVY, JOSEPH (American physician, born 1890)

Harkavy syndrome. The occurrence in periarteritis nodosa of asthma, recurrent pulmonary infiltrations, eosinophilic polyserositis, pleurisy, pericarditis, and neurological symptoms, probably due to an allergic reaction.

Harkavy, J. Vascular allergy. Pathogenesis of bronchial asthma with recurrent pulmonary infiltrations and eosinophilic polyserositis. *Arch. Int. Med., Chicago*, 1941, 67:709-34.

harlequin fetus. See *ichthyosis congenita syndrome.*

harlequin ichthyosis. See *ichthyosis congenita syndrome.*

HARLEY, GEORGE (British physician, 1829-1896)

Harley disease. See *Dressler syndrome, under Dressler, D. R.*

HARNASCH, HANS MAX EMIL (German physician, born 1907)

Harnasch disease. Acro-osteolysis of the phalangeal diaphyses of the hand and foot, with consecutive involvement of the jaws, acromion, and clavicle, reportedly described by Harnasch.

HARPER, P. S. (British physician)

Young-Harper syndrome. See *under Young, I. D.*

HARPER, RITA G. (American physician)

Harper dwarfism. Synonym: *Harper syndrome.*

A variant of the Seckel syndrome characterized by low birth weight and short length, craniofacial abnormalities (microcephaly, hypoplastic mandibular rami and cheek bones, large eyeballs and orbits in comparison with facial structures, micrognathia, high-arched or cleft palate, prominent nose, low-set lobeless ears), alternating strabismus, hypodontia, enamel hypoplasia, atrophied teeth, hip dislocation, wide separation of the first and second toes with bunching and fusion of the plantar interphalangeal creases, absence of the interphalangeal skin crease of the first digit, hypogonadism, and cryptorchism. Radiological findings include premature closure of sutures, "hammered silver" skull, facial asymmetry, hypertelorism, dislocation of the radius at the elbow, hypoplastic radial head, incurving of distal phalanges, 11 rib-bearing dorsal vertebrae, sacralization of the vertebrae, absence of inferior pubic rami and horizontal ischia, shortening of the fibula with nonformation of the tibiofibular joint, absence of the accessory metacarpal and midphalangeal ossification centers.

Harper, R. G. Bird-headed dwarfs (Seckel's syndrome). A familial pattern of developmental, dental, skeletal, genital, and central nervous system anomalies. *J. Pediat.,* 1967, 70:799-804. Bixler, D., & Antley, R. M. Microcephalic dwarfism in sisters. *Birth Defects,* 1974, 10(7):161-5.

Harper syndrome. See *Harper dwarfism.*

HARRINGTON, ETHEL REGAN (American physician, born 1891)

Helmholz-Harrington syndrome. See *under Helmholz.*

HARRIS, B. T. (British physician)

Harris neuralgia. See *Horton neuralgia.*

HARRIS, SEALE (British physician, 1870-1957)

Harris syndrome. Synonyms: *functional hypoglycemic syndrome, hyperinsulinism syndrome, hypoglycemic syndrome, organic hyperinsulinism.*

Excessive insulin production with hypoglycemia, associated with hunger, jitteriness, tachycardia, and flushing, occurring in conditions such as functional disorders of the pancreas, hyperplasia of the islands of Langerhans, or insulinoma.

Harris, S. Hyperinsulinism and disinsulinism. *JAMA,* 1924, 83:729-33.

HARRISON, CHARLES VICTOR (British pathologist, born 1907)

Harrisons-Vaughan disease. See *Vaughan disease.*

HARRISON, P. (Irish physician)

Harrison-Smyth syndrome. See *subclavian steal syndrome.*

HART, EDWARD WATSON (British physician)

Hart syndrome. See *Hartnup disease.*

HARTMANN, FRITZ (German physician, 1871-1937)

Hartmann apraxia. Synonym: *frontal apraxia.*

Apraxia resulting from tumors of the frontal lobe.

Hartmann, F. Beiträge zur Apraxielehre. *Mschr. Psychiat. Neur.,* 1907, 21:97-118; 248-70.

HARTNUP

Hartnup disease. Synonyms: *Hart syndrome, Hartnup syndrome, H disease, pellagra-cerebellar ataxia-renal aminoaciduria syndrome.*

An inherited metabolic disease, transmitted as an autosomal recessive trait, originally observed in four of eight children whose parents were first cousins. The symptoms consist mainly of a pellagra-like skin rash over the face, neck, hands, and legs; episodic personality changes characterized by emotional lability, uncontrolled temper, confusion, and hallucinations; fully reversible cerebellar ataxia with unsteady gait, intention tremor, and dysarthria; vertigo; syncope; nystagmus; spastic episodes; blapharoptosis; diplopia, severe headache; intermittent muscle pain; and variable EEG disorders. The attacks may be pecipitated by exposure to sunlight, sulfonamides, and psychological stress, when associated with inadequate or irregular diet. Abnormal amino acid transport is the principal metabolic disorder of this syndrome. It consists of excretion of increased amounts of neutral amino acids, indicans (mainly indoxyl sulfate), and nonhydroxylated indole metabolities. The syndrome was designated after the family name (Hartnup) of patients in whom it was first observed.

Baron, D. N., *et al.* Hereditary pellagra-like skin rash with temporary cerebellar ataxia, constant renal amino-aciduria, and other bizarre biochemical features. *Lancet,* 1956, 2:421-8. Jepson, J. B. Hartnup disease. In: Stanbury, J. B., Wyngaarden, J. B., & Fredrickson, D. S., eds. *The metabolic basis of inherited disease.* 4th ed. New York, McGraw-Hill, 1978, pp. 1563-77.

Hartnup syndrome. See *Hartnup disease.*

HASHIMOTO, HAKARU (Japanese pathologist, 1881-1934)

Hashimoto disease. Synonyms: *Hashimoto struma, Hashimoto thyroiditis, lymphocytic thyroiditis, lymphomatoid goiter, struma lymphomatosa.*

A progressive painless enlargement of the thyroid gland with goiter, with or without pressure symptoms, occurring most commonly in menopausal women and believed to be caused by autoimmune processes in the body. It may be associated with other autoimmune conditions, such as rheumatoid arthritis or the Sjögren syndrome. Pathologically, it presents lymphocytic infiltration heavily admixed with plasma cells, leading to atrophy of the parenchyma.

Hashimoto, H. Zur Kenntnis der lymphomatösen Veränderung der Schilddrüse (Struma lymphomatosa). *Arch. Klin. Chir., Berlin,* 1912, 97:219-48.

Hashimoto struma. See *Hashimoto disease.*

Hashimoto thyroiditis. See *Hashimoto disease.*

HASSALL, ARTHUR HILL (British physician, 1817-1894)

Hassall-Henle warts. Small hyaline excrescences in the periphery of the Descemet membrane which contain bonded material, believed to be collagen, in which numerous cracks and fissures are filled with extrusions of the corneal epithelium. The condition is probably associated with the aging processes.

Hogan, M. J., & Zimmerman, L. E. *Ophthalmic pathology. An atlas and textbook.* 2nd ed. Philadelphia, Saunders, 1962, pp. 288-9.

HATT (heparin-associated thrombocytopenia andthrombosis). See *white clot syndrome.*

HAUDEK, MARTIN (Austrian physician, 1880-1931)

Haudek niche. See *Haudek syndrome.*

Haudek syndrome. Synonym: *Hauden niche.*

A budlike prominence seen on roetgenograms of the stomach in peptic ulcer.

Haudek, M. Zur röntgenologischen Diagnose der Ulzserationen in der Pars media des Magens. *Munch. Med. Wschr.*, 1910, 57:1587-91.

HAUPTMANN, A.

Hauptmann-Thannhauser syndrome. Muscle dystrophy, with early contractures and cardiomyopathy, transmitted as an autosomal dominant trait. The clinical picture is characterized by early contractures through muscular shortening, beginning in the first or second decade, and atrophy, mainly affecting the humeral and peroneal muscles with some pelvic girdle involvement, and cardiomyopathy.

*Hauptmann, A., & Thannhauser, S. J. Muscular shortening and dystrophy. A heredofamilial disease. *Arch. Neur. Psychiat.*, 1941, 46:654. Becker, P. E. Dominant autosomal dystrophy with early contractures and cardiomyopathy (Hauptmann-Thannhauser). *Hum. Genet.*, 1986, 74:184.

HAUSER, G.

Rokitansky-Küster-Hauser (RKH) syndrome. See *Mayer-Rokitansky-Küster syndrome.*

von Rokitansky-Hauser syndrome. See *Mayer-Rokitansky-Küster syndrome.*

HAVEN, HALE (American neurologist, born 1902)

Haven syndrome. See *scalenus anticus syndrome.*

HAVLIKOVA, DANA (Czech physician)

Havlikova syndrome. A familial syndrome characterized by congenital hepatosplenomegaly, exocrine pancreatic insufficiency, chronic liver damage, chronic pulmonary disease, failure to thrive, growth retardation, and retarded motor and mental development.

Havlikova, D., *et al.* The syndrome of congenital pancreatic insufficiency, chronic respiratory disease and chronic liver damage. *Acta Paediat. Scand.*, 1967, 56:676-80.

HAWKINS, CAESAR HENRY (British physician, 1798-1884)

Hawkins keloid. See *Alibert disease (1).*

HAWKINS, MARGARET R. (American physician)

Strasburger-Hawkins-Eldridge syndrome. See *symphalangism syndrome.*

Strasburger-Hawkins-Eldridge-Hargrave-McKusick syndrome. See *symphalangism syndrome.*

HAXTHAUSEN, HOLGER (Danish physician, 1892-1959)

Blegvad-Haxthausen syndrome. See *under Blegvad.*

Haxthausen disease. See *Haxthausen panniculitis.*

Haxthausen hyperkeratosis. See *Haxthausen syndrome.*

Haxthausen panniculitis. Synonyms: *Haxthausen disease, adiponecrosis a frigore, adiponecrosis subcutanea neonatorum, cold panniculitis.*

Formation in otherwise normal newborn infants of movable, indurated subepidermal masses (panniculitis), usually on the cheeks and, less commonly, other parts of the body. Exposure to cold appears to be the precipitating factor.

Haxthausen, H. Adiponecrosis a frigore. *Brit. J. Derm.*, 1941, 53:83-9.

Haxthausen syndrome. Synonyms: *Haxthausen hyperkeratosis, climacteric keratosis, climacteric keratosis palmaris et plantaris, hyperkeratosis palmoplantaris climacterica, keratoderma climacterica, keratodermia climacterica.*

Circumscribed hyperkeratosis, mainly of the palms and soles, occurring in climacteric women. Various general signs and symptoms, of which obesity and arterial hypertension are most frequently observed, are associated.

Haxthausen, H. Keratoderma climactericum. *Brit. J. Derm.*, 1934, 46:161-7.

HAY, R. J. (British physician)

Hay-Wells syndrome. See *AEC syndrome.*

hay asthma. See *Bostock catarrh.*

hay fever. See *Bostock catarrh.*

HAYEM, GEORGES (French physician, 1841-1933)

Hayem anemia. See *Hayem-Widal syndrome.*

Hayem icterus. See *Hayem-Widal syndrome.*

Hayem-Faber syndrome. See *Faber syndrome.*

Hayem-Widal syndrome. Synonyms: *Abrami disease, Hayem anemia, Hayem icterus, Widal disease, Widal syndrome, Widal-Abrami syndrome, acholuric hemolytic icterus with splenomegaly, acquired hemolytic anemia, acquired hemolytic jaundice, hemolytic icteroanemia, icteroanemia, icterohemolytic anemia.*

An acquired hemolytic anemia in which the erythrocytes are formed normally but are destroyed prematurely as a result of hemolytic processes. The red cells may be destroyed by the spleen when it is enlarged (hypersplenism), by antibodies or complement as a result of autoimmunization or alloimmunization, and by certain drugs and chemicals, such as arsenic, copper, chloramine, amphotericin, and other substances.

Widal, F., & Abrami, P. Ictère hémolytique non congénitaux avec anémie. Recherches de la résistance globulaire par la procédé de hématies déplasmatisées. *Presse Méd.*, 1907, 15:749. Hayem, G. Sur une variété particulière d'ictère chronique. Ictère infectieux chronique splénomégalique. *Presse Méd.*, 1898, 6:121-6.

Jaksch-Hayem syndrome. See *Jaksch syndrome.*

Jaksch-Hayem-Luzet syndrome. See *Jaksch syndrome.*

late chlorosis of Hayem. See *Faber syndrome.*

HAYGARTH, JOHN (British physician, 1740-1827)

Haygarth nodes. Nodular swelling of the joints in arthritis deformans.

Haygarth, J. A clinical history of the nodosity of the joints. In his: *A clinical history of diseases.* London, 1805. Vol. 2, p. 155.

HAYMAKER, WEBB (American physician)

olivopontocerebellar atrophy (OPCA), Schut-Haymaker type. See *OPCA IV, under olivopontocerebellar atrophy.*

Schut-Haymaker syndrome. See *OPCA IV, under olivopontocerebellar atrophy.*

HAYWARD, JAMES R. (American dentist)

Juberg-Hayward syndrome. See *under Juberg.*

HCE. See ***h**ypoglossal **c**arotid **e**ntrapment syndrome.*

HD. See ***H**odgkin **d**isease.*

HD (Hirschprung disease). See *Hirschprung syndrome.*

HD (Huntington disease). See *Huntington chorea.*

HDL (high-density lipoprotein) deficiency. See *Tangier disease.*

HEAD, HENRY (British physician, 1861-1940)

Head syndrome. See *Head-Holmes syndrome.*

Head-Holmes syndrome. Synonym: *Head syndrome.*

Sensory changes produced by lesions of the cerebral cortex and other parts of the brain.

Head, H., & Holmes, G. Sensory disturbances from cerebral lesions. *Brain*, 1911-12, 34:102-254.

head cold. See *common cold syndrome.*

headache syndrome. Synonym: *cephalgia.*

Any ache, pain, unpleasant sensation, or tenderness in the head. Usually, the term is restricted to conditions affecting the cranial vault, but in an extended sense it is also applied to painful conditions of the entire head, including the face and neck. The terms **headache** and **migraine** (v.i.) are often used interchangeably. The scope of the headache syndrome includes the following conditions: **Alcohol migraine**-due to the breakdown of ethyl alcohol to acetaldehyde. **Allergic migraine**-caused by allergens, usually in food, which trigger the release of serotonin and histamine. **Altitude headache**-occurring at altitudes above 8,000-12,000 feet, which is characterized by a throbbing pain that may be generalized or restricted to the frontal region, and is aggravated by coughing, exertion, or lying down. **Carotidynia**-pain in the carotid region (see *Hilger syndrome*). **Chinese restaurant syndrome**-q.v. **Chocolate migraine**-due to the presence of phenylethylamine in chocolate, which triggers the release of serotonin and causes a reaction to cerebral deficiency of monoamine oxidase. **Circulatory migraine**-due to blood pressure changes (hypotension or hypertension). **Cluster headache**-see *Horton neuralgia.* **Congestion neuralgia**-attributed to congestion or hyperemia. **Dental headache**-associated with toothache, postextraction disorders, and various dental conditions, believed to be a form of referred pain. **Endocrine migraine**-caused by augmented serotonin release precipitated by endocrine factors. **Exertional headache**-short attacks of migraine following an intense physical effort. **Extracranial headache**-due to any extracranial cause. **Geniculate neuralgia**-see *Hunt syndrome (2).* **Glossopharyngeal neuralgia**-see *glossopharyngeal neuralgia syndrome.* **Helmet headache**-marked by pain involving the upper half of the head. **Hemiplegic migraine (ophthalmoplegic migraine)**-associated with hemiplegia that may persist after the headache. **Horton headache (Horton migraine)**-see *Horton neuralgia.* **Hot-dog headache**-bitemporal headache with facial flushing occurring after eating preserved meats containing nitrites. **Hunt syndrome**-q.v. **Ice-cream headache**-midfrontal or retro-auricular migraine after consumption of ice-cream. **Intracranial headache**-due to any intracranial cause. **Menstrual migraine**-occurring before, during, or after menstruation owing to the presence in the blood of abnormal amounts of bradykinin or prostaglandin. **Migraine (blind headache, hemicrania, migraine syndrome)**-a pain syndrome of varying degrees of severity, lasting from a few minutes to several days, often associated with nausea, vomiting, flushing, gastrointestinal disorders, vertigo, and photophobia. The headache is usually unilateral at the beginning, but may spread to other parts of the head. Attacks may be preceded by various prodromal symptoms, such as scotoma, visual field defects, and visual disorders. Painful contractions of the neck and head muscles may occur. **Muscle contraction headache (nervous headache, psychogenic headache, tension headache)**-a steady ache in the temporal, occipital, parietal, or frontal region, associated with a feeling of tightness and cramps of the muscles in the neck and upper back. **Nasociliary neuralgia**-see *Charlin syndrome.* **Ophthalmic headache**-resulting from visual disorders. **Optic migraine**-see *Bárány syndrome.* **Paratrigeminal syndrome**-see *Raeder syndrome.* **Puncture headache (leakage headache, lumbar puncture headache, postspinal headache)**-a dull, usually pulsating headache most often in the occipital area, occurring 12 to 24 hours after lumbar puncture. **Sexual headache**-an attack of headache either preceding or following an orgasm. **Sphenopalatine neuralgia**-see *Sluder neuralgia.* **Spinal migraine**-caused by spinal disorders, such as spinal nerve compression, intervertebral disk subluxation, or whiplash injury. **Styloid syndrome**-see *Eagle syndrome.* **Superior laryngeal neuralgia**-unilateral paroxysms of pain in the ear, throat, and mandible that are precipitated by swallowing, shouting, or head turning, affecting mainly middle-aged males (see also *Arnold neuralgia).* **Tolosa-Hunt syndrome**-q.v. **Traumatic migraine**-secondary to some types of trauma. **Trigeminal neuralgia**-q.v. **Vacuum headache**-due to obstruction of the outlet of the frontal sinus. **Vidian neuralgia**-see *Vail syndrome.* **Yellow cheese migraine**-caused by the presence of tyramine in cheese. **Weather migraine**-headache precipitated by climatic changes. **Hemicrania cerebellaris**-see *Bárány syndrome.* **Painful ophthalmoplegia**-see *Tolosa-Hunt syndrome.*

Sulman, F. G. Migraine and headache due to weather and allied causes and its specific treatment. *Upsala J. Med. Sc.*, 1980, 31(Suppl):41-4. Rose, F. C. The classification of headache. *Neuroepidemiology*, 1985, 4:193-203. Classification of headache. *Arch. Neurol., Chicago*, 1962, 6:173-6.

heart and hand syndrome (1). See *Holt-Oram syndrome.*

heart and hand syndrome (2). Synonym: *Tabatznik syndrome.*

An association of cardiac arrhythmia with brachytelephalangy of the thumbs with shortening and hypoplasia of the fourth and fifth metacarpals in some cases. Additional disorders include sloping shoulders, hypoplasitc deltoid muscles, short arms, flaring of the lower end of the humerus, flaring and obliquity of the lower end of the radius, and absent styloid process of the ulna. The syndrome is transmitted as a dominant trait.

Temtamy, S., & McKusick, V. The genetics of hand malformations. *Birth Defects*, 1978, 14(3):241-4.

heart and hand syndrome (3). A syndrome of intraventricular conduction defects and sick sinus syndrome with brachydactyly C, originally reported in three generations. The syndrome is believed to be transmitted as an autosomal dominant trait.

Ruiz de la Fuente, S., & Prieto, F. Heart-hand syndrome. III. A new syndrome in three generations. *Hum. Genet.*, 1980, 55:43-7.

heart block-retinitis pigmentosa-ophthalmoplegia syndrome. See *Kearns-Sayre syndrome.*

heart-upper limb syndrome. See *Holt-Oram syndrome.*

heavy chain disease. Synonyms: *H disease, Hγ2 disease.*

A disorder of γ-globulin in patients with malignant lymphoma associated with secretion of a monoclonal heavy chain or heavy fragment by the neoplastic cells. **gamma-chain disease (γ-G type** and **Franklin disease)** is characterized by a protein antigenically related to the Fc fragment of the heavy chain of γ-G. Clinical symptoms include lymphadenopathy, splenomegaly, fever, anemia, and occasional hepatomgealy. Leukopenia and thrombocytopenia are usually present. Excessive susceptibility to bacterial infection is common. Oral manifestations include erythema and edema of the soft palate and uvula associated with Waldeyer's ring involvement. The bone marrow and lymph nodes contain atypical immature plasma cells with an admixture of atypical lymphocytes, reticulum cells, and eosinophils. The abnormal serum and urine protein show fast γ and β slow mobility; its molecular weight is about 53,000. It is immunologically related to γ-G globulin and is similar to the fast chain. The level of normal immunoglobulins is usually depressed. **Alpha chain disease (α-A type)** was originally described in a young Arab woman with malignant lymphoma of the intestine. It has been also observed in non-Ashkenazi Jews living in the Middle East and sometimes other ethnic and racial groups. In the original report, the abnormal protein found in serum, urine, and saliva was closely related to γ-A1 and devoid of light chains. Some normal γ-A was present; γ-G and γ-M were abnormally low. Clinical symptoms in the original case included amyloid deposits, bone pain, lymphoproliferative disorders, and carpal-tunnel syndrome, but no eosinophilia, lymphadenopathy, or recurrent infection present in other forms of heavy chain disease. **MU (μ) chain disease** is a rare disorder characterized by secretion into the plasma of free heavy chains. Major complaints include retroperitoneal adenopathy and hepatosplenomegaly. Lymphoplasmacytic cells may occur in the bone marrow. Most patients have large amounts of kappa-L chain in the urine. The monoclonal lymphoid cells of the neoplasm appear to have a defect in the heavy-light chain assembly.

Franklin, E. C., *et al.* Heavy chain disease-A new disorder of serum gamma-globulin. Report of the first case. *Am. J. Med.*, 1964, 37:332-50.

HEBERDEN, WILLIAM, SR. (British physician, 1710-1801)

Heberden asthma. Synonyms: *Elsner asthma, Rougnon de Magny disease, angina pectoris, cardiac asthma, stenocardia.*

A clinical syndrome of chest pain caused by a relative oxygen deficiency in the heart muscle, occurring in the presence of arteriosclerotic coronary artery disease and, less commonly, ventricular hypertrophy, left ventricle outflow obstruction, aortic regurgitation, cardiomyopathy, and other pathological conditions of the heart. The syndrome is characterized by a distinctive radiating precordial pain, often precipitated by physical effort or emotional stress. See also *Prinzmetal angina* and *chest wall syndrome.*

Heberden, W. Some account on a disorder of the breast. *Tr. Roy. Coll. Phys., London*, 1772, 2:59-67.

Heberden nodes. Synonyms: *Bouchard disease, Heberden syndrome, Heberden-Bouchard disease, Rosenbach disease, arthritic nodes.*

Nodes produced by calcific spurs of the articular cartilage at the base of the terminal phalanges in osteoarthritis.

*Heberden, W. De nodis digitorum. In his: *Commentarii de morborum historia et curatione*. London, Payne, 1802. Rosenbach, O. Die Auftreibung der Endophalangen der Finger-eine bisher nocht nicht beschriebene tropische Störung. *Zbl. Nervenh.*, 1890, 13:199-205.

Heberden syndrome. See *Heberden nodes.*

Heberden-Bouchard disease. See *Heberden nodes.*

HEBRA, FERDINAND, VON (Austrian physician, 1816-1880)

Hebra disease (1). See *Gibert disease.*

Hebra disease (2). See *Kaposi disease (2).*

Hebra prurigo. See *Hebra syndrome.*

Hebra syndrome. Synonyms: *Hebra prurigo, von Hebra syndrome, prurigo agria, prurigo ferox, prurigo gravis, prurigo hebrae, prurigo mitis.*

A chronic skin disorder that usually begins during infancy in the form of an urticarial rash followed by millet-sized or slightly larger pruritic papules which eventually become covered by a blood-colored crust. The disorder persists through life.

*Hebra, F., von. *Traite pratique de maladies de la peau*. Paris, 1854.

von Hebra syndrome. See *Hebra syndrome.*

HECHT, FREDERICK (American physician, born 1930)

Beals-Hecht syndrome. See *congenital contractural arachnodactyly syndrome.*

Hecht syndrome. See *trismus-pseudocamptodactyly syndrome.*

Hecht-Beals-Wilson syndrome. See *trismus-pseudocamptodactyly syndrome.*

Hecht-Jarvinen syndrome. See *popliteal pterygium syndrome.*

HECHT, JACQUELINE T. (American physician)

Hecht-Scott syndrome. Synonym: *limb deficiency-heart malformation syndrome.*

A familial syndrome, transmsitted as an autososomal recessive trait, characterized by terminal transverse limb defects associated with congenital heart malformations. Acheiria, apodia, hemimelia, oligosyndactyly, and tibial bowing are the principal abnormalities of the limbs.

Hecht, J. T., & Scott, C. I., Jr. Limb deficiency syndrome in half-sibs. *Clin. Genet.*, 1981, 20:432-7.

HECHT, VICTOR (Austrian physician)

Hecht pneumonia. Synonyms: *Hecht syndrome, giant-cell pneumonia, interstitial giant-cell pneumonia.*

A chronic or subacute form of interstitial pneumonia occurring in infants and young children, and characterized by multinucleate giant-cell inclusion bodies.

Hecht, V. Die Riesenzsellpneumonie im Kindesalter. Eine histologisch-experimentelle studie. *Beitr. Path. Anat.*, 1910, 48:263-310.

Hecht syndrome. See *Hecht pneumonia.*

HECK, JOHN W. (American dentist, born 1923)

Heck disease. Synonym: *focal epithelial hyperplasia.*

Hyperplasia of the buccal, labial, and lingual mucosae, characterized by multiple, soft, sessile papules, with the lower lip seeming to be affected most frequently. First observations were made in a group of American Indian children, and later commonly found among Greenland Eskimos.

Achard, H. O., Heck, W. J., & Stanley, H. R. Focal epithelial hyperplasia found in Indian children. *Oral Surg.*, 1965, 20:201-12. Hettwer, K. J., & Rodgers, M. S. Focal epithelial hyperplasia (Heck's disease) in a Polynesian. *Oral Surg.*, 1966, 22:46-70.

HEDBLOM, CARL ARTHUR (American physician, 1879-1934)

Hedblom syndrome. Synonym: *acute primary diaphragmitis.*

Acute primary myositis of the diaphragm characterized by inspiratory pain, limited chest mobility, and upper abdominal pain. Onset may be sudden, with pain on the affected side over the costal margin and on the shoulder. Radiologically, there is a gradual flattening of the diaphragmatic dome. The disease was named Jaonnides in honor or Dr. Carl A. Hedblom.

Joannides, M. Acute primary diaphragmatitis (Hedblom's syndrome). *Dis. Chest*, 1946, 12:89-110.

HEDDA GABLER. See GABLER, HEDDA

HEDERICH, H.

Piulachs-Hederich syndrome. See *under Piulachs.*

HEDGE, ALICE N. (American physician)

Stanbury-Hedge defect. See *under Stanbury.*

HEDH (hypohidrotic ectodermal dysplasia with hypothyroidism) syndrome. A hypohidrotic form of ectodermal dysplasia associated with hypothyroidism and ciliary dyskinesia, transmitted as an autosomal recessive trait. Associated disorders include urticaria pigmentosa-like skin pigmentation with increased mast cell and melanin deposition in the dermis, ciliary abnormalities of the bronchi associated with recurrent respiratory infections, sparse scalp and eyebrow hair, pigmentation disorders of the mucous membranes, and shriveled nails.

Pabst, H. F., *et al.* Hypohidrotic ectodermal dysplasia with hypothyroidism. *J. Pediat.*, 1981, 98:223-7.

HEDINGER, CHRISTOPH ERNST (Swiss physician, born 1917)

Hedinger syndrome. See *carcinoid syndrome.*

HEERFORDT, CHRISTIAN FREDERIK (Danish ophthalmologist, 1871-1953)

Heerfordt syndrome. Synonyms: *febris uveoparotidea, neuro-uveoparotitis syndrome, uveoparotid fever, uveoparotitic paralysis, uveoparotitis.*

A disorder, sometimes associated with sarcoidosis, consisting chiefly of uveitis, parotid enlargement, mild fever, and facial paralysis. Prodromal symptoms usually include weakness, cough, polyuria, dry mouth, and gastrointestinal disorders. Associated disorders may include vocal cord paralysis, deafness, blepharoptosis, dysphagia, mild cervical lymphadenopathy, and skin rash. Persons in their second or third decade are most commonly affected.

Heerfordt, F. F Über eine "Febris uveo-parotidea subchronica" an der Glandula parotis und an der Uvea des Auges lokalisiert und häufig mit Paresen cerebrospinaler Nerven kompliziert. *Graefes Arch. Ophth.*, 1909, 70:254-73.

HEGGLIN, ROBERT MARQUARD (Swiss physician, born 1907)

Fanconi-Hegglin syndrome. See *under Fanconi.*

Hegglin anomaly. See *May-Hegglin anomaly.*

Hegglin syndrome (HS). Synonym: *energetic-dynamic heart insufficiency.*

Myocardial contraction with the rapid expulsion of blood from the ventricles during systole, so that the second sound is abnormally close to the first sound and the QT space is increased.

Hegglin, R. L'insuffisance cardiaque énergéto-dynamique. *Cardiologia, Basel*, 1949, 65:77.

May-Hegglin anomaly. See *under May, Richard.*

May-Hegglin syndrome. See *May-Hegglin anomaly, under May, Richard.*

HEIDENHAIN, ADOLF (German neurologist, born 1893)

Heidenhain syndrome. Synonyms: *dementia-cortical presenile degeneration syndrome, presenile dementia-cortical blindness syndrome, subacute spongious encephalopathy of the Heindenhain type.*

A type of presenile dementia associated with blindness, ataxia, dysarthria, athetotic movements, and rigidity of all four limbs. Histological findings show neuronal lesions and astrocytic proliferations in the cerebral cortex, and less extensively in the basal ganglia, with status spongiosus. Some writers suggest that this disorder and the Nevin syndrome are analogous and that both are variants of the Jakob-Creutzfeld syndrome.

Heidenhain, A. Klinische und anatomische Untersuchungen über eine eigenartige organische Erkrankung des Zentralnervensystems im Praesenium. *Zschr. Ges. Neur. Psychiat.*, 1929, 118:49-114.

subacute spongious encephalopathy of the Heidenhain type. See *Heidenhain syndrome.*

HEILMEYER, LUDWIG (German physician, 1899-1969)

Heilmeyer-Schöner erythroblastosis. See *Heilmeyer-Schöner syndrome.*

Heilmeyer-Schöner syndrome. Synonym: *Heilmeyer-Schöner erythroblastosis.*

Anemia characterized by severe disintegration of erythrocytes, leading to hematogenous jaundice, associated with rapid bone regeneration. The blood contains a high proportion of reticulocytes, a constantly increasing volume of nucleated erythroblasts, and a large number of megaloblastlike erythrocytes. Biopsy usually shows proliferation of nucleated proerythrocytes, with supression of leukocytes in the bone marrow, liver, and spleen.

Heilmeyer, L., & Schöner, W. Die chronische reine Erythroblastose des Erwachsenen als leukämie-parallel Prozess des erythrocytären Systems. *Deut. Arch. Klin. Med.*, 1940-41, 187:225-48.

HEINE, JACOB, VON (German physician, 1806-1879)

Heine-Medin disease. Synonyms: *anterior poliomyelitis, infantile paralysis, polio, poliomyelitis.*

An acute infectious disease caused by the poliovirus (an RNA virus of the enterovirus group of the picornavirus family). The virus usually enters the body by the oral route and initially replicates in the oropharyngeal and intestinal mucosa, eventually invading the lymph nodes, with Peyer patches being the early manifestations of infection. Clinical characteristics may range from no apparent illness to flaccid paralysis with fatal respiratory failure. In a mild form, the so-called minor illness, there is usually fever, malaise, nausea, vomiting and diarrhea. A mild nervous system involvement may be manifested by only asymptomatic meningitis (**nonparalytic poliomyelitis**). **Paralytic poliomyelitis** is usually preceded by stiff neck, muscle aches and cramps (sometimes with transient fasciculation), headache, and fever. Onset of flaccid paralysis is sudden and its progress is rapid, involving mainly the lower limbs and the lower trunk. The appearance of agitation, a sense of fear, and delirium may indicate involvement of the brain stem. Paralysis is usually associated with a variety of complications, including nystagmus, facial paralysis (usually restricted to one or several muscles), and paralysis of the masticatory, deglutition, and laryngeal muscles. Other associated disorders may include hypertension, tachycardia, pulmonary edema, cardiac arrhythmia, bulbar paralysis, and respiratory failure with terminal sleep apnea.

Heine, J. *Beobachtungen über Lähmungszustände der untern Extremit- äten und deren Behandlung*. Stuttgart, Köhler, 1840. Medin, O. En epidemi af infantil paralysi. *Hygeia, Stockholm*, 1890, 52:657-68.

HEINER, DOUGLAS C. (American physician)

Heiner syndrome. Synonyms: *Heiner-Sears syndrome, milk precipitin syndrome, pulmonary milk allergy syndrome.*

Chronic pulmonary disease, iron-deficiency anemia, recurrent diarrhea, and failure to thrive associated with the presence of precipitating antibodies against cow's milk in the blood serum. Associated symptoms include cough, dyspnea, wheezing, recurrent respiratory infections, retarded growth, gastrointestinal disorders, pulmonary hemosiderosis, and atelectasis.

Heiner, D. C., & Sears, J. W. Chronic respiratory disease associated with mulitple circulating precipitins in cow's milk. *Am. J. Dis. Child.*, 1960, 100:500-2.

Heiner-Sears syndrome. See *Heiner syndrome.*

HELLER, ARNOLD LUDWIG GOTTHILF (German pathologist, 1840-1913)

Heller-Döhle disease. Synonyms: *Heller-Döhle mesoaortitis, luetic aortitis, syphilitic aortitis.*

Aortitis secondary to syphilis, sometimes complicated by aortic valve insufficiency, coronary stenosis, and aortic aneurysm.

*Heller, A. L. Über die syphilitische Aortitis und ihre Bedeutung für die Enstehung von Aneurysmen. *Verh. Deut. Path. Ges.*, 1900, p. 346. *Döhle, K. G. *Ein Fall von eigentümlicher Aortenerkrankung bei einem Syphilitischen*. Kiel, Lipsius & Tischer, 1885.

Heller-Döhle mesoaortitis. See *Heller-Döhle disease.*

HELLER, CARL GEORGE (American physician, born 1913)

Heller-Nelson syndrome. A variant of the Klinefelter syndrome characterized by small atrophic testes, hyalinization of the tunica propria of the seminiferous tubules, clumping of Leydig cells, azospermia, and elevation of urinary gonadotropins. Delayed bone development and various degrees of eunuchoidism, such as gynecomastia, genital infantilism, sparse or absent body hair, high-pitched voice, poor muscle development, poor quality of Leydig cells, and depressed levels of 17-ketosteroids and estrogens may be associated.

Heller, C. G., & Nelson, W. O. Hyalinization of the seminiferous tubules associated with normal or failing Leydig-cell function. Discussion of relationship of eunuchoidism, gynecomastia, elevated gonadotropins, depressed 17-ketosteroids and estrogens. *J. Clin. Endocr.*, 1945, 5:1-12.

HELLER, JULIUS (German physician, 1864-1931)

Heller disease. Synonym: *dystrophia unguium mediana canaliformis.*

Dystrophic, median, canaliform depressions on the fingernails without apparent organic cause. In the original report, only the thumb nails were affected.

Heller, J. Zur Kazuistik seltener Nagelkrankheiten. XVIII. Dystrophia ungium [sic] mediana canaliformis. *Derm. Zschr.*, 1927, 51:416-9.

HELLER, THEODOR O. (Austrian neurologist, born 1869)

Heller dementia. See *Heller syndrome.*

Heller syndrome. Synonyms: *Heller dementia, Heller-Zappert syndrome, Weygandt-Heller syndrome, childhood dementia, childhood psychosis, childhood schizophrenia, dementia infantilis, symbiotic psychosis.*

A developmental disorder characterized by impairment in the development of reciprocal social interaction and imaginative activity, associated with mental retardation and restricted field of interests and activities. Onset is usually observed during early childhood; irritability, tantrums, and other behavior disorders are the early symptoms. Later, the child becomes withdrawn, incontinent, mute, and, in some instances, completely helpless. Pathological examination may reveal lipoid deposits, sclerotic changes, and other brain abnormalities, but there does not seem to be any pattern in structural cerebral changes. The severity and expression of symptoms vary.

Diagnostic and statistical manual of mental disorders. 3rd ed. Washington, D. C., American Psychiatric Association, 1987, pp. 33-7. Heller, T., & Zappert, J. Geistige Schwächezustände bei Kindern. *Zeit. Allg. Wien. Med.*, 1909, p. 209. Zappert, J. Dementia infantilis (Heller). *Mschr. Kinderh.*, 1922, 22:389-97.

Heller-Zappert syndrome. See *Heller syndrome.*

Weygandt-Heller syndrome. See *Heller syndrome.*

HELLERSTRÖM, SVEN CURT ALFRED (Swedish dermatologist, born 1901)

Hellerström disease. Erythema chronicum migrans (Lipschütz erythema) associated with meningitis, following a tick bite.

Hellerström, S. Erythema chronicum migrans Afzelli. *Acta Derm. Vener., Stockholm*, 1930, 11:315-21.

HELLP (hemolysis-elevated liver enzymes-low platelet count) syndrome. A pre-eclamptic or eclamptic disorder with the findings of hemolysis (microangiopathic hemolytic anemia), elevated liver function tests, and thrombocytopenia. Severe hypertension may be associated. Laboratory findings usually show abnormal serum glutamate oxaloacetate transaminase (SGOT) and glutamate pyruvate transaminase (SGPT) levels. Clinical symptoms may include malaise, nausea, epigastric pain, right upper quadrant tenderness, and edema.

Weinstein, L. Syndrome of hemolysis, elevated liver enzymes, and low platelet count: A severe consequence of hypertension in pregnancy. *Am. J. Obst. Gyn.*, 1982, 142:159-67.

helmet headache. See *under headache syndrome.*

HELMHOLZ, HENRY FREDERIC (American physician, 1882-1958)

Helmholz-Harrington syndrome. Synonym: *corneal opacity-cranioskeletal dysostosis syndrome.*

Congenital clouding of the cornea associated with various abnormalities. Restricted motion of the joints, short and thick clawlike hands, feet with limited extension, lumbar kyphosis, scaphocephalic head, and mental retardation were observed in the original four cases.

Helmholz, H. F., & Harrington, E. R. A syndrome characterized by congenital clouding of the cornea and by other anomalies. *Am. J. Dis. Child.*, 1931, 41:793-800.

HELWEG-LARSEN, HANS F. (Danish physician)

Helweg-Larsen syndrome. Synonym: *anhidrosis-neurolabyrinthitis syndrome.*

A familial syndrome, transmitted as an autosomal dominant trait, characterized by congenital anhidrosis and neurolabyrinthitis. There is a marked reduction in the number of sweat glands, and those that are present are hypertrophied.

Helweg-Larsen, H. F., & Ludvigsen, K. Congenital familial anhidrosis and neurolabyrinthitis. *Acta Derm. Vener., Stockholm,* 1946, 26:489-505.

HELWIG, ELSON BOWMAN (American physician, born 1907)

Helwig disease. Synonym: *inverted follicular keratosis.*

A benign epithelial tumor occurring most frequently as a single lesion of the face in older age groups. Histologically, the lesion is characterized by invaginating cup-shaped and fingerlike tumors consisting of peripheral cells that resemble basal cells but are smaller, and squamoid cells in the center, which form numerous structures.

*Helwig, E. B. "Inverted follicular keratosis." Seminar on the skin. *International Congress of Clinical Pathology*. Washington, D. C., 1954. Mehregan, A. H. Inverted follicular keratosis. *Arch. Derm., Chicago*, 1964, 89:229-35.

hemangiectasia hypertrophica. See *Klippel-Trénaunay-Weber syndrome.*

hemangioblastomatosis. See *Hippel-Lindau syndrome.*

hemangioma-consumptive coagulopathy syndrome. See *Kasabach-Merritt syndrome.*

hemangioma-thrombocytopenia syndrome. See *Kasabach-Merritt syndrome.*

hemangioma-thrombopenia syndrome. See *Kasabach-Merritt syndrome.*

hemangiomatosis-intravascular coagulation syndrome. See *Kasabach-Merritt syndrome.*

hematogenic albuminuria. See *Bamberger albuminuria, under Bamberger Heinrich, von.*

hematogenous jaundice. See *Loutit anemia.*

hematomole. See *Breus mole.*

hematomyelia centralis. See *Minor disease.*

hematoporphyria congenita. See *congenital erythropoietic porphyria.*

hematuria-nephropathy-deafness syndrome. See *Alport syndrome.*

hematuric familial nephropathy. See *Alport syndrome.*

hematuric hereditary nephritis. See *Alport syndrome.*

hemi 3 (hemihypertrophy-hemiparesthesia-hemiareflexia) syndrome. A developmental syndrome of hypertrophy involving a half or a quadrant of the body (without affecting the face), areflexia and ipsilateral decreased pain and temperature sense, progressive scoliosis, and foot deformities on the enlarged side. On the larger side, there is hypertrophy of the muscles and increased muscular strength, as well as an increase in diameter, but not in length, of long bones. A defect of the dorsal lip of the neural tube or the neural crest is the suspected cause.

Nudleman, K., *et al.* The hemi 3 syndrome. Hemihypertrophy, hemihypaesthesia [sic], hemiareflexia and scoliosis. *Brain,* 1984, 107(Pt 2):533-46.

hemiacrosomia. See *Curtius syndrome (1).*

hemianalgesia alterna subbulbaris. See *Opalski syndrome.*

hemiasomatognosia. See *Anton-Babinski syndrome.*

hemiatrophia faciei. See *Romberg syndrome (2).*

hemiatrophia faciei progressiva. See *Romberg syndrome (2).*

hemic myeloma. See *Kahler disease.*

hemichondrodysplasia. See *Ollier syndrome.*

hemiconvulsions-hemiplegia-epilepsy (HHE) syndrome. See *Gastaut syndrome (2).*

hemicrania. See *migraine, under headache syndrome.*

hemicrania cerebellaris. See *Bárány syndrome.*

hemifacial hyperplasia-strabismus syndrome. See *Bencze syndrome.*

hemifacial hypertrophy. See *Curtius syndrome (1).*

hemifacial microsomia (HM). See *oculo-auriculovertebral dysplasia.*

hemigigantism. See *Curtius syndrome (1).*

hemignathia and microtia syndrome. See *oculo-auriculovertebral dysplasia.*

hemihypertrophy-intestinal web-preauricular skin tag-congenital corneal opacity syndrome. See *HIPO syndrome.*

hemimacrosomia. See *Curtius syndrome (1).*

hemiparaplegic syndrome. See *Brown-Séquard syndrome.*

hemiplegia abducentofacialis alternans. See *Foville syndrome.*

hemiplegia alternans. See *Millard-Gubler syndrome.*

hemiplegia alternans hypoglossica. See *Jackson-MacKenzie syndrome, under Jackson, John Hughlings.*

hemiplegia alternans inferior. See *Foville syndrome.*

hemiplegia alternans inferior pontina. See *Foville syndrome.*

hemiplegia alternans oculomotorica. See *Leyden paralysis (1).*

hemiplegia alternans superior peduncularis. See *Leyden paralysis (1).*

hemiplegia cruciata abducentis inferior. See *Millard-Gubler syndrome.*

hemiplegia et hemiparaplegia spinalis. See *Brown-Séquard syndrome.*

hemiplegia oculomotorica. See *Leyden paralysis (1).*

hemiplegic migraine. See *under headache syndrome.*

hemipolyneuropathy-cranial paralysis syndrome. See *Garcin syndrome.*

hemochromatosis (HFE). See *Recklinghausen-Applebaum disease.*

hemodialysis disequilibrium. See *disequilibrium syndrome.*

hemogenia. See *Werlhof disease.*

hemogenic syndrome. See *Werlhof disease.*

hemoglobin C thalassemia. See *Zuelzer-Kaplan syndrome (2).*

hemoglobin S disease. See *sickle cell anemia.*

hemoglobinopathy. See *thalassemia syndrome.*

hemolytic anemia-hyperlipemic alcoholic syndrome. See *Zieve syndrome.*

hemolytic crisis. See *Owren syndrome (1).*

hemolytic icteroanemia. See *Hayem-Widal syndrome.*

hemolytic icterus. See *Loutit anemia.*

hemolytic jaundice. See *Loutit anemia.*

hemolytic-uremic syndrome (HUS). Synonyms: *Gasser syndrome, uremic-hemolytic syndrome.*

A disease of infants and children characterized mainly by hemolytic anemia and uremia. Prodromal symptoms consist of a flu-like illness, vomiting, abdominal pain, and diarrhea with or without bloody stools. Major clinical characteristics include gastrointestinal hemorrhage, oliguria or anuria, hematuria, hypertension, coma or stupor, abnormal erythrocytes, thrombocytopenia, uremia, hypocalcemia or hyponatremia, acute abdomen, respiratory disorders, ulcerative colitis, edema, cardiomegaly, congestive heart failure, and neurological complications, usually epileptic seizures, behavioral changes, diplopia, vertigo, hemiparesis, decerebrate state, and ataxia.

Gasser, C., *et al.* Hämolytisch-urämische Syndrome: Bilaterale Nierenrindennekrosen bein akuten erworbenen hämolytischen Anämien. *Schweiz. Med. Wschr.*, 1955, 85:905-9.

hemophagocytic reticulosis. See *Omenn syndrome.*

hemophilia II. See *Christmas disease.*

hemophilia A. Synonyms: *disease of Hapsburgs, bleeder's disease, disease of kings.*

A genetically determined blood coagulation disorder, especially one which is caused by inadequate prothrombin utilization due to a lack of plasma thromboplastin in factor VIII, IX, or XI deficiency. The most common is **classic hemophilia (hemophilia A)**, caused by factor VIII deficiency, and characterized generally by a prolonged coagulation time and a bleeding tendency that may result in hemarthroses and uncontrolled hemorrhage, even after a trivial injury or minor surgical intervention. This type is transmitted as an X-linked recessive trait with parents transmitting the gene to daughters, who in turn transmit it to one-half of their daughters and one-half of their sons. As a rule, only males are affected but some cases have been reported in females. The disorder is usually present at birth, but may go unrecognized for many years. Spontaneous periodic remissions and exacerbations are common. Oozing of blood from many sites in the oral cavity is the most obvious symptom. Tooth extraction and tonsillectomy may produce fatal hemorrhage. Hemophilia was relatively common in inbred European royal families, including the Hapsburgs, hence its synonyms. See also *Willebrand-Jürgens syndrome (pseudohemophilia).*

Hynes, H. E., *et al.* Development of the present concept of hemophilia. *Mayo Clin. Proc.*, 1969, 434:193. Hougie, C. Hemophilia and related conditions-congenital deficiencies of prothrombin (factor II), factor V, and factors VII to XII. In: Williams, W. J., Beutler, E., Erslev, A. J., & Lichtman, M. A., eds. *Hematology,* 3rd ed. New York, McGraw-Hill, 1983, pp. 1381-99.

hemophilia B (HEMPB). See *Christmas disease.*

hemophilia C. See *Rosenthal disease, under Rosenthal, Robert Louis.*

hemophiloid state A. See *Owren syndrome (2).*

hemophiloid state C. See *Christmas disease.*

hemopoietic dysplasia. See *myelodysplastic syndrome.*

hemorrhagic and interstitial pneumonitis with nephritis. See *Goodpasture syndrome.*

hemorrhagic atelectasis. See *adult respiratory distress syndrome.*

hemorrhagic bronchitis. See *Castellani bronchitis.*

hemorrhagic capillary toxicosis. See *Schönlein-Henoch purpura.*

hemorrhagic diathesis-acute progranulocytic leukemia syndrome. See *disseminated intravascular coagulation syndrome.*

hemorrhagic familial nephritis. See *Alport syndrome.*

hemorrhagic fever with renal syndrome (HFRS). Synonyms: *Churilov disease, endemic nephrosonephritis, epidemic hemorrhagic fever (EHF), epidemic mesonephritis, epidemic nephritis (EN), epidemic nephrosonephritis, far eastern hemorrhagic fever, Korean hemorrhagic fever (KHF), Manchurian hemorrhagic fever, nephropathia epidemica (NE), Omsk fever, Songo fever, viral hemorrhagic fever (VHF).*

An acute infectious disease caused by the Hantaan virus (a single-stranded RNA virus of the family Bunyaviridae), occurring in northeastern Asia and parts of eastern and northern Europe. Its main characteristics include fever, prostration, vomiting, proteinuria, hemorrhagic manifestations, shock, and renal failure. Major epidemics occurred in Asia, including the 1951 epidemic among United Nations personnel in Korea. There are two basic forms: A mild form **(nephropathia epidemica)** observed mainly in Scandinavia, and the severe form **(epidemic hemorrhagic fever)** occurring mainly in northeastern Asia. **Nephropathia epidemica** is characterized by initial high fever, backache, headache, and abdominal pain, followed in a few days by hemorrhages (including conjunctival hemorrhage), palatine petechiae, petechial rash, and, finally, oliguria, azotemia, proteinuria, hematuria, leukocyturia, and polyuria. Complete recovery takes place in a few weeks. **Epidemic hemorrhagic fever** is characterized by an incubation period of 10 to 25 days. The febrile or invasive phase is accompanied by vague prodromal symptoms followed by the abrupt onset of chills, fever, headache, backache, abdominal pain, and myalgia. Associated symptoms include constant anorexia, thirst, frequent vomiting and nausea. Additional symptoms include photophobia, pain on movement of the eyes, generalized erythema, dermographism, slight edema of the upper eyelids, conjunctival petechiae, subconjunctival hemorrhage, petechiae of the palate and other parts of the body, enlargement of the lymph nodes, and abdominal and costal tenderness. The hypotensive phase occurs on about the fifth day and sometimes results in shock. The oliguric (hemorrhagic or toxic) phase appears during the eighth day and is associated with return of blood pressure to normal or hypertensive levels, accompanied by weakness, thirst, vomiting, hiccups, hyperkalemia, hyperphosphatemia, and hypocalcemia. With onset of diuresis, there may be neurological complications (disorientation, restlessness, lethargy, paranoid delusions, seizures) and occasional pulmonary infection with edema. This phase is followed by a slow recovery.

Sanford, J. P. Arbovirus infections. In: Braunwald, E., Isselbacher, K. J., Petersdorf, R. G., Wilson, J. D., Martin, J. B., & Fauci, A. S., eds. *Harrison's principles of internal medicine.* 11th ed. New York, McGraw-Hill, 1987, pp. 717-31. Johnson, K. M. Hemorrhagic fever with renal syndrome (HFRS). In: Wyngaarden, J. B., & Smith, L. H., Jr., eds. *Cecil textbook of medicine.* Philadelphia, Saunders, 1985, pp. 1757-8.

hemorrhagic lung syndrome. See *adult respiratory distress syndrome.*

hemorrhagic purpura. See *Werlhof disease.*

hemorrhagic scurvy. See *Möller-Barlow disease.*

hemorrhagic shock-encephalopathy syndrome. See *shock-encephalopathy syndrome.*

hemorrhagic thrombasthenia. See *Glanzmann thrombasthenia.*

hemorrhagic thrombocythemia. See *Mortensen disease.*

hemosiderosis of the lung. See *Ceelen-Gellerstedt syndrome.*

HEMPAS (hereditary erythroblastic multinuclearity with positive acidified serum test) syndrome. Synonym: *congenital dyserythropoietic anemia type II.*

A syndrome of hereditary erythroblastic anemia with megaloblastoid changes and a tendency for multinuclearity among mature red blood cell precursors.

Faruqui, S., *et al.* Normal serum ferritin level in a patient with HEMPAS syndrome and iron overload. *Am. J. Clin. Path.,* 1982, 78:97-101.

HEMPB (hemophilia B). See *Christmas disease.*

HEMRI (hereditary multifocal relapsing inflammation) syndrome. The concurrence of different subgroups of seronegative arthritis, spondylitis, acute anterior uveitis, psoriasis, and inflammatory bowel disease, different HLA-B antigens being associated with a variety of clinical signs.

Moller, P., & Berg, K. Ankylosing spondylitis is part of a multifactorial syndrome: Hereditary multifocal relapsing inflammation (HEMRI). *Clin. Genet.,* 1984, 26:187-97.

HENCH, PHILIP SHOWALTER (American physician, 1896-1965)

Hench-Rosenberg syndrome. Synonym: *palindromic rheumatism.*

A joint disease of adult men and women, characterized by sudden and rapidly developing afebrile attacks of arthritis, periarthritis, and occasional paraarthritis, with pain, swelling, redness, and disability, usually but not always, affecting a single joint. The attacks last a few hours or days and then disappear completely, frequently to recur at irregular intervals. There are no joint deformities or roentgenographic manifestations.

Hench, P. S., & Rosenberg, E. F. Palindromic rheumatism. A "new" recurring disease of joints (arthritis, periarthritis, para-arthritis) apparently producing no articular residues-report of thirty-four cases; its relation to "angioneural arthrosis," "allergic rheumatism" and rheumatoid arthritis. *Arch. Int. Med., Chicago,* 1944, 73:293-321.

HENDERSON, MELVIN STARKEY (American physician, 1883-1954)

Henderson-Jones syndrome. See *Reichel syndrome.*

Reichel-Jones-Henderson syndrome. See *Reichel syndrome.*

HENKIN, R. I. (American physician)

Henkin syndrome. A syndrome characterized by decreased taste acuity, perverted sense of taste, decreased olfactory sense, perverted sense of odors, sensation of foul odors in the nasopharynx, and salty, sweet, sour, bitter, or metallic taste. Associated disorders may include vertigo, hearing loss, decreased libido, and hypertenion. The etiology is unknown.

Henkin, R. I., *et al.* Idiopathic hypogusia with dysgrusia, hyposmia and dysosmia: A new syndrome, *JAMA.* 1971, 11:1328-30.

HENLE, FRIEDRICH GUSTAV JACOB (German anatomist, 1809-1885)

Hassall-Henle warts. See *under Hassall.*

HENNEBERG, RICHARD (German physician, 1868-1962)

Scholz-Bielschowsky-Henneberg syndrome. See *metachromatic leukodystrophy.*

HENNEBERT, CAMILLE (Belgian physician, 1867-1962)

Hennebert syndrome. Synonym: *luetic-otitic-nystagmus syndrome.*

Nystagmus and vertigo on air compression of the auditory meatus, seen in congenital syphilis.

Hennebert, C. Réactions vestibulaires dans les labyrinthites hérédosyphiliques. *Arch. Internat. Laryng., Paris,* 1909, 28:93-6.

HENOCH, EDUARD HEINRICH (German physician, 1820-1910)

Henoch chorea. Synonyms: *chorea electrica, electric chorea, electrolepsy, spasmodic tic.*

Chronic progressive chorea of children, marked by violent and sudden movements. This disorder is similar to Bergeron disease.

*Henoch, E. H. *Beitrage zur Kinderheilkunde.* N. F. Berlin, 1868. p. 113.

Henoch disease. See *Schönlein-Henoch purpura.*

Henoch-Schönlein syndrome (HS, HSS). See *Schönlein-Henoch purpura.*

Schönlein-Henoch disease. See *Schönlein-Henoch purpura.*

Schönlein-Henoch purpura. See *under Schönlein.*

Schönlein-Henoch syndrome. See *Schönlein-Henoch purpura.*

heparin-associated thrombocytopenia and thrombosis (HATT). See *white clot syndrome.*

heparitinuria. See *mucopolysaccharidosis III.*

hepatic coma. See *hepatic encephalopathy syndrome.*

hepatic ductal hypoplasia-multiple malformation syndrome. See *Alagille syndrome.*

hepatic encephalopathy syndrome. Synonyms: *hepatic coma, portal-systemic encephalopathy.*

A syndrome of advanced, decompensated liver disease and/or extensive portal-systemic shunting complicated by neurological disorders. Common precipitating factors contributing to liver failure consist of viral hepatitis, liver cirrhosis, herpes simplex infection, Reye syndrome, hepatic vein occlusion, fatty liver in pregnancy, gastrointestinal hemorrhage, increased intake of protein, axotemia, hypokalemia, constipation, anesthesia in surgery, hypoxia, alkalosis, and toxic reaction to hepatotoxic drugs and chemicals such as acetominophen, halothane, carbon tetrachloride, and yellow phosphorus. Apathy, lack of awareness, euphoria, anxiety, restlessness, and short attention span are the manifestations of the first stage of encephalopathy. They are followed by lethargy, drowsiness, and disorientation in the second stage, deep somnolence in the third stage, and coma in the final stage.

Scharschmidt, B. F. Acute and chronic hepatic failure with encephalopathy. In: Wyngaarden, J. B., & Smith, L. H., Jr., eds. *Cecil textbook of medicine.* 17th ed. Philadelphia, Saunders, 1985, pp. 845-8.

hepatic nephropathy. See *hepatorenal syndrome.*

hepatic phosphorylase deficiency. See *glycogen storage disease VI.*

hepatic phosphorylase kinase deficiency. See *glycogen storage diease VIII.*

hepatic vein thrombosis. See *Budd-Chiari syndrome.*

hepatitis A. See *Botkin disease.*

hepatitis B-associated arthritis-dermatitis syndrome. See *under arthritis-dermatitis syndrome.*

hepatitis epidemica. See *Botkin disease.*

hepatocerebral degeneration. See *Wilson disease, under Wilson, Samuel Alexander Kinnier.*

hepatocerebral dystrophy. See *Wilson disease, under Wilson, Samuel Alexander Kinnier.*

hepatofacioneurocardiovertebral syndrome. See *Alagille syndrome.*

hepatolenticular degeneration. See *Wilson disease, under Wilson, Samuel Alexander Kinnier.*

hepatolienal fibrosis. See *Banti syndrome.*

hepatomegalic glucoadiposity. See *Debré syndrome (2).*

hepatonephritis serosa acuta. See *hepatorenal syndrome.*

hepatonephromegalia glycogenica. See *glycogen storage disease I.*

hepatopancreatic alcoholic syndrome. See *Zieve syndrome.*

hepatorenal glycogenosis. See *glycogen storage disease I.*

hepatorenal syndrome (HRS). Synonyms: *Heyd syndrome, bile nephrosis, cholemic nephrosis, functional renal failure, hepatic nephropathy, liver-kidney disease.*

Impaired renal function in patients with liver diseases. Hepatic disorders in which renal failure may occur include liver cirrhosis, fulminant liver failure, acute viral hepatitis, fatty liver in pregnancy, obstructive jaundice, liver neoplasms, and postoperative complications of liver surgery. Laboratory findings include axotemia, oliguria, low urinary sodium concentration, high urine osmolality, and normal fresh urine sediment. Postmortem examination shows normal or nearly normal kidneys.

Heyd, C. G. The liver and its relation to chronic abdominal infection. *Ann. Surg.*, 1924, 79:55-77. Helvig, F. C., & Schutz, C. B. A liver kidney syndrome. Clinical, pathological and experimental studies. *Surg. Gynec. Obst.*, 1932, 55:570-80.

hepatosplenomegalic lipoidosis. See *Bürger-Grütz syndrome.*

HERBERT, HERBERT (British ophthalmologist, 1865-1942)

Herbert pits. Cavities in the cornea filled by a clear epithelial tissue which remain at the site of resolved trachoma follicles.

Herbert, H. Trachomatous pannus and associated corneal changes. *Tr. Ophth. Soc. U. K.*, 1904, 24:67-77.

hereditary acrolabial telangiectasia syndrome. A familial syndrome, transmitted as an autosomal dominant trait, characterized by bluish discoloration of the vermilion border of the lips, nipples, and nail beds; discrete telangiectasia of the chest, elbows, and dorsa of the hands; varicosities of the lower parts of the legs; and migraine. The presence of extensive, dilated, horizontal subpapillary telangiectases in the tissues of the lips and elbows is the principal histological feature; histochemical examination shows activity of adenosine triphosphatase and leucine aminopeptidase around dilated vessels.

Millns, J. L., & Dicken, C. H. Hereditary acrolabial telangiectasia. A report of familial blue lips, nails, and nipples. *Arch. Derm., Chicago* 1979, 115:474-8.

hereditary acromelalgia. See *restless leg syndrome.*

hereditary adenomatosis. See *Gardner syndrome, under Gardner, Eldon John.*

hereditary amyloid nephropathy. See *Ostertag syndrome.*

hereditary angioedema. See *Quincke edema.*

hereditary angioneurotic edema (HANE). See *Quincke edema.*

hereditary areflexic dystasia. See *Roussy-Lévy syndrome.*

hereditary arthro-ophthalmopathy. See *Stickler syndrome.*

hereditary ataxia. See *Friedreich ataxia, under Friedreich, Nicolaus.*

hereditary benign intraepithelial dyskeratosis. See *Witkop-Von Sallmann syndrome.*

hereditary benign intraepithelial dyskeratosis. See *Witkop-Von Sallmann syndrome.*

hereditary black blood disease. See *Tamura-Takahashi disease.*

hereditary cerebellar ataxia. See *Marie syndrome (1), under Marie, Pierre.*

hereditary cerebellar ataxia with spasticity. See *Marie syndrome (1), under Marie, Pierre.*

hereditary chondrodysplasia. See *mucopolysaccharidosis IV-A.*

hereditary chorea. See *Huntington chorea.*

hereditary cutaneomandibular polyoncosis. See *nevoid basal-cell carcinoma syndrome.*

hereditary dark teeth. See *dentinogensis imperfecta.*

hereditary deforming chondrodysplasia. See *multiple cartilaginous exostoses syndrome.*

hereditary distal myopathy. See *Gowers syndrome (1).*

hereditary dystopic lipoidosis. See *Fabry syndrome.*

hereditary ectodermal polydysplasia. See *hypohidrotic ectodermal dysplasia syndrome.*

hereditary elliptocytosis. See *Dresbach anemia.*

hereditary epiphyseal dysplasia. See *multiple epiphyseal dysplasia I.*

hereditary episodic adynamia. See *Gamstorp syndrome.*

hereditary epistaxis. See *Osler-Rendu-Weber syndrome.*

hereditary epithelial corneal dystrophy. See *Meesmann dystrophy.*

hereditary essential myoclonus. See *Friedreich disease (1), under Friedreich, Nicolaus.*

hereditary factor X deficiency. See *Stuart-Prower factor deficiency.*

hereditary familial angiomatosis. See *Osler-Rendu-Weber syndrome.*

hereditary familial congenital hemorrhagic nephritis. See *Alport syndrome.*

hereditary familial hypogonadism. See *Reifenstein syndrome.*

hereditary giant platelet syndrome. See *Bernard-Soulier syndrome, under Bernard, Jean.*

hereditary gingival fibromatosis. See *Zimmermann-Laband syndrome.*

hereditary goiter-deafness syndrome. See *Pendred syndrome.*

hereditary hemangiomatosis of the central nervous system. See *Hippel-Lindau syndrome.*

hereditary hemorrhagic telangiectasia (HHT). See *Osler-Rendu-Weber syndrome.*

hereditary hemorrhagic thrombasthenia. See *Willebrand-Jürgens syndrome.*

hereditary hyaloretinal degeneration. See *Wagner syndrome, under Wagner, H.*

hereditary hyperphosphatasia. See *hyperphosphatasia-osteoctasia syndrome.*

hereditary hypochondroplasia. See *hypochondroplasia syndrome.*

hereditary hypophosphatemia. See *hypophosphatemic familial rickets.*

hereditary leptocytosis. See *Cooley anemia.*

hereditary lymphedema praecox. See *Meige syndrome (1).*

hereditary lymphedema type I. See *Nonne-Milroy syndrome.*

hereditary lymphedema type II. See *Meige syndrome (1).*

hereditary macrothrombocytopathia-nephritis-deafness syndrome. See *Epstein triad, under Epstein, C. J.*

hereditary malformation of the vertebral bodies. See *spondylothoracic dysplasia.*

hereditary metaphyseal dysostosis, Schmid type. See *Schmid metaphyseal chondrodysplasia syndrome, under Schmid, Franz.*

hereditary motor and sensory neuropathy I (HMSN I). See *Charcot-Marie-Tooth syndrome.*

hereditary mucoepithelial dysplasia. Synonym: *Witkop syndrome.*

A familial syndrome of multiple abnormalities, transmitted as an autosomal dominant trait, affecting oral, nasal, vaginal, urethral, anal, vesical, and conjunctival mucosae. The symptoms include cataract, follicular keratosis, nonscarring alopecia, and terminal lung disease. Severe photophobia, tearing, and nystagmus in infancy are the early signs. They are followed by keratitis, corneal vascularization, and cataracts. Redness of the periorificial mucosa of the oral cavity, nose, anus, and vagina may be observed early. Chronic rhinorrhea and repeated upper respiratory tract infections, often progressing to bilateral pneumonia, are accompanied by the loss of the hair, diarrhea, occasional melena, enuresis, pyuria, and hematuria. Spontaneous pneumothorax is frequent, terminating in fibrocystic lung disease and cor pulmonale. Mucosal epithelial changes (including dyshesion), thinning, dyskeratosis, lack of maturation and cornification, presence of vacuoles and inclusions, lack of keratohyalin granules, paucity of desmosomes, formation of bands and aggregates of filamentous fibers and structures in the cytoplasm resembling desmosomes and gap junctions, and abnormal Pap smear of the vagina are the main histopathological findings.

Witkop, Carl J., Jr. *et al.* Hereditary mucoepithelial dysplasia: A disease apparently of desmosome and gap junction formation. *Am. J. Genet.*, 1979, 31:414-27.

hereditary multicentric osteolysis. See *Torg syndrome.*

hereditary multifocal relapsing inflammation. See *HEMRI syndrome.*

hereditary multiple ankylosing arthropathy. See *symphalangism syndrome.*

hereditary multiple benign cystic epitheliomas. See *Brooke epithelioma.*

hereditary multiple diaphyseal sclerosis. See *Ribbing syndrome.*

hereditary multiple exostoses. See *multiple cartilaginous exostoses syndrome.*

hereditary myotonia. See *Thomsen disease.*

hereditary nephritis. See *Alport syndrome.*

hereditary nephritis-deafness syndrome. See *Alport syndrome.*

hereditary nephropathy-deafness syndrome. See *Alport syndrome.*

hereditary neuropathic amyloidosis. See *amyloid neuropathy type I.*

hereditary nonhemolytic bilirubinemia. See *Gilbert syndrome, under Gilbert, Nicolas Augustin.*

hereditary nonhemolytic jaundice. See *Gilbert syndrome, under Gilbert, Nicolas Augustin.*

hereditary nonpolyposis colorectal cancer (HNPCC) syndrome. A neoplastic disease transmitted as an autosomal recessive trait, comprising the **hereditary site-specific colon cancer (HSSCC, Lynch syndrome I)**, and the **cancer family syndrome (CFS, Lynch syndrome II)**. The first type is characterized by an early-onset proximal colonic carcinoma, and the second by an early-onset proximal colonic carcinoma associated with other extracolonic adenocarcinomas, particularly endometrial carcinoma. The term *cancer family syndrome* is sometimes used in connection with other familial cancers.

Lynch, H. T., *et al.* A family study of adenocarcinoma of the colon and multiple primary cancer. *Surg. Gynec. Obst.*, 1972, 134:781-6. Lynch, H. T., *et al.* Hereditary nonpolyposis colorectal cancer (Lynch syndromes I and II). I. Clinical description and resource. *Cancer*, 1985, 56:934-8.

hereditary nonspherocytic hemolytic anemia (HNSHA). See *Crosby syndrome, under Crosby, William H.*

hereditary oligophrenic cerebrolental degeneration. See *Marinesco-Sjögren syndrome, under Marinescu, Gheorghe.*

hereditary onycho-osteodysplasia (HOOD). See *nail-patella syndrome.*

hereditary onycho-osteodysplasia syndrome (HOODS). See *nail-patella syndrome.*

hereditary opalescent dentin. See *dentinogenesis imperfecta.*

hereditary opalescent teeth. See *dentinogenesis imperfecta.*

hereditary optic atrophy. See *Leber disease.*

hereditary optic neuritis. See *Leber disease.*

hereditary optic neuropathy. See *Leber disease.*

hereditary osteochondrodystrophy. See *mucopolysaccharidosis IV-A.*

hereditary osteolysis with hypertension and nephropathy. See *Thieffry-Shurtleff syndrome.*

hereditary ovalocytosis. See *Dresbach anemia.*

hereditary palmoplantar keratoderma. See *Unna-Thost syndrome, under Unna, Paul Gerson.*

hereditary plasma thromboplastin component (PTC) deficiency. See *Christmas disease.*

hereditary polyposis and osteomatosis. See *Gardner syndrome, under Gardner, Eldon John.*

hereditary polytopic enchondral dysostosis. See *mucopolysaccharidosis IV-A.*

hereditary progressive arthro-ophthalmopathy. See *Stickler syndrome.*

hereditary proximal neurogenic muscular atrophy. See *Wohlfart-Kugelberg-Welander syndrome.*

hereditary proximal spinal muscular atrophy. See *Wohlfart-Kugelberg-Welander syndrome.*

hereditary pseudohemophilia. See *Willebrand-Jürgens syndrome.*

hereditary PTC (plasma thromboplastin component) **deficiency.** See *Christmas disease.*

hereditary recurrent cholestasis with lymphedema. See *Aagenaes syndrome.*

hereditary red cell aplasia. See *Diamond-Blackfan syndrome.*

hereditary renal adysplasia. See *Winter syndrome.*

hereditary renal agenesis. See *Winter syndrome.*

hereditary renal-retinal dysplasia. See *Senior syndrome (1).*

hereditary sensory and autonomic neuropathy IV (HSAN-IV). See *Swanson syndrome.*

hereditary sensory radicular neuropathy. See *Thévenard syndrome.*

hereditary sideroblastic anemia. See *Rundles-Falls syndrome.*

hereditary site-specific colon cancer (HSSCC). See *under hereditary nonpolyposis colorectal cancer syndrome.*

hereditary somatomedin deficiency. See *Laron dwarfism.*

hereditary spherocytosis (HS). See *Minkowski-Chauffard syndrome.*

hereditary spongy dystrophy. See *Canavan syndrome.*

hereditary startle syndrome. Synonyms: *hyperexplexia, stiff baby syndrome.*

A syndrome of young infants, transmitted as an autosomal dominant trait, characterized by exaggerated startle reaction that may cause a generalized hypertonic response and falling. The affected infants tend to assume a fetal position, becoming "frozen" and being unable to execute protective movements when falling down. Injuries, particularly of the face and head may result. The hypertonia lessens or disappears during sleep and with holding the infant. Sitting, walking, and other motor activities are delayed because of hypertonia. The electromyographic activity is usually normal. See also *stiff man syndrome..*

Suhren, O., *et al.* Hyperexplexia. A hereditary startle syndrome. *J. Neur. Sc.*, 1966, 3:577-605.

hereditary symmetrical aplastic nevi of the temples. See *Brauer syndrome, under Brauer, August.*

hereditary thrombasthenia. See *Glanzmann thrombasthenia.*

hereditary thrombocytopathic purpura. See *Glanzmann thrombasthenia.*

hereditary trichodysplasia. See *Unna syndrome, under Unna, Marie.*

hereditary vitelliform macular degeneration. See *Best macular degeneration.*

hereditary vitelliruptive macular degeneration. See *Best macular degeneration.*

hereditary vitreoretinal degeneration. See *Wagner syndrome, under Wagner, H.*

heredoataxia cerebellaris. See *Marie syndrome (1), under Marie, Pierre.*

heredoataxia hemerolopica polyneuritiformis. See *Refsum disease.*

heredofamilial angiomatosis. See *Osler-Rendu-Weber syndrome.*

heredopathia atactica polyneuritiformis. See *Refsum disease.*

HERLITZ, CARL GILLIS (Swedish pediatrician, born 1902)

Herlitz syndrome. See *epidermolysis bullosa syndrome.*

HERMAN, EUFEMIUSZ (Polish physician)

Herman syndrome. A syndrome of livedo racemosa universalis, pyramidal and extrapyramidal disorders, speech disorders, and mental disorders followed by hypertension and convulsions, which occur after closed head injuries.

Herman, E. Niezwykły zespól pourazowy: livedo racemosa universalis u osobnika z objawami piramidowo-pozapiramidowymi i zaburzeniami psychicznymi. *Warsz. Czas. Lek.*, 1937, 14:107-9.

HERMANN, PIERRE (French ophthalmologist)

Hermann syndrome. Synonym: *microphthalmos-retinitis pigmentosa-glaucoma syndrome.*

A familial syndrome, transmitted as an autosomal dominant trait, characterized by microphthalmia, retinitis pigmentosa, and glaucoma, with cataract in some cases.

Hermann, P. Le syndrome microphtalmie-rétinite pigmentaire-glaucome. *Arch. Opht., Paris*, 1958, 18:17-24.

HERMANS, P. E. (American physician)

Hermans syndrome. Late-onset _-globulin deficiency with nodular lymphoid hyperplasia of the ileum. Recurrent infections and diarrhea are the principal symptoms.

Hermans, P. E. Nodular lymphoid hyperplasia of the small intestine and hypogammaglobulinemia: Theoretical and practical considerations. *Fed. Proc.*, 1967, 26:1606-11.

HERMANSKY, F. (Czech physician)

Hermansky-Pudlak syndrome (HPS). Synonyms: *albinism-hemorrhagic diathesis syndrome, oculocutaneous albinism-hemorrhagic diathesis syndrome.*

A hereditary syndrome, transmitted as an autosomal recessive trait, characterized by oculocutaneous albinism, bleeding tendency, (especially after the use of aspirin), storage-pool deficiency in platelets, and accumulation of ceroid-lipofuscin materials in reticuloendothelial and mucosal cells. The affected patients have scant white hair, white-pink skin, translucent irides, minimally pigmented ocular fundi, and nystagmus; those exposed to sunlight have reddish brown hair, pigmented nevi, and freckles. Blood platelets contain low amounts of ADP and ATP.

Hermansky, F., & Pudlak, P. Albinism associated with hemorrhagic diathesis and unusual pigmented reticular cells in the bone marrow: Report of two cases with histochemical studies. *Blood*, 1959, 14:162-9.

hernia inguinoperitonealis incarcerata. See *Krönlein hernia.*

hernia mesogastrica interna. See *Gruber hernia, under Gruber, Wenzel Leopold.*

hernia retroperitonealis. See *Treitz hernia.*

herpangina. See *Zahorsky syndrome (2).*

herpes angina. See *Zahorsky syndrome (2).*

herpes circinatus bullosus. See *Duhring disease.*

herpes tonsurans maculosus. See *Gibert disease.*

herpes zoster auricularis. See *Hunt syndrome (2).*

herpes zoster oticus. See *Hunt syndrome (2).*

herpes zoster syndrome. See *Hunt syndrome (2).*

herpetic keratitis. See *Schmidt keratitis, under Schmidt, Rolf.*

HERRENSCHWAND, FRIEDRICH, VON (German ophthalmologist, born 1881)

Herrenschwand syndrome. Synonym: *sympathetic heterochromia.*

A difference in color of the irides caused by sympathetic lesions, that may be associated with the Bernard-Horner syndrome.

Herrenschwand, F., von. Über verschiedene Arten von Heterochromia iridis. *Klin. Mbl. Augenh.*, 1918, 60:467-94.

HERRICK, JAMES BRYAN (American physician, 1861-1954)

Herrick syndrome. See *sickle cell anemia.*

HERRMANN, CHRISTIAN, JR. (American physician)

Herrmann disease. A familial syndrome, transmitted as an autosomal dominant trait, characterized by photomyoclonus, hearing loss, diabetes mellitus, and nephropathy. Personality changes, depression, seizures, dementia, nystagmus, ataxia, speech disorders, hemiparesis, hemianopsia, hemihypesthesia, and depressed reflex responsiveness may be associated.

Herrmann, C., Jr., *et al.* Hereditary photomyoclonus associated with diabetes mellitus, deafness, nephropathy, and cerebral dysfunction. *Neurology,* 1964, 14:212-21.

HERRMANN, JÜRGEN (German-born physician in the United States, born 1941)

Herrmann syndrome. See *facio-audio-symphalangism syndrome.*

Herrmann-Optiz syndrome. Acrocephalosyndactyly characterized by acrocephaly, peculiar facies, brachysyndactyly of the hands, monodactyly of the feet, and various associated abnormalities. Craniofacial anomalies include hypertelorism, bitemporal flattened head, hypoplastic supraorbital ridges, prominent eyes, shallow orbits, micrognathia, high-arched palate, and small, low-set, posteriorly rotated malformed ears. Strabismus, limitation of movement of the elbow joints, asymmetry of the chest, cryptorchism, rectal prolapse, mental retardation, low birth weight, and reduced stature were associated in the original case reported in a boy whose parents and five sibs were normal.

Herrmann, J., & Optiz, J. M. An unusual form of acroscephalosyndactyly. *Birth Defects,* 1969, 5(3):39-42.

Herrmann-Pallister-Optiz syndrome. A syndrome of craniosynostosis, symmetrical limb abnormalities, and cleft lip and palate. The symptoms usually include microbrachycephaly, synostosis involving chiefly the cranial suture, open sagittal and lambdoid sutures, patent metopic suture, hypertelorism, occipital capillary hemangioma, protruding ears, deviation of the nasal septum, mental retardation, aplasia of the radius, short ulna, and hands in the valgus position. Originally, three metacarpals were missing and the third finger was split. Congenital hip dislocation, dysplasia of the femoral heads and necks, and ankylosis of the knees may be associated. The etiology is unknown.

Herrmann, J., Pallister, P. D., & Opitz, J. M. Craniosynostosis and craniosynostosis syndromes. *Rocky Mt. Med. J.* 1969, 66:45-56.

HERS, G. H. (French biochemist)

Hers disease. See *glycogen storage disease VI.*

HERSMAN, C. F. (American physician)

Hersman disease. Idiopathic progressive enlargement of the hands.

Hersman, C. F. A case of progressive enlargement of the hands. *Internat. Med. Mag., Philadelphia,* 1894, 3:662-5.

HERTER, CHRISTIAN ARCHIBALD (American physician, 1865-1910)

Gee-Herter disease. See *celiac disease.*

Gee-Herter-Heubner disease. See *celiac disease.*

Herter infantilism. See *celiac disease.*

Heubner-Herter disease. See *celiac disease.*

HERTWIG, PAULA (German physician, born 1889)

Hertwig-Weyers syndrome. See *Weyers oligodactyly syndrome.*

HERTWIG, RICHARD (German zoologist, 1850-1937)

Hertwig-Magendie syndrome. Synonym: *skew deviation.*

A dissociation of gaze characterized by a downward and inward rotation of the eyes on the side of a cerebellar lesion and an upward and outward deviation on the contralateral side.

Jaensch, P. A. Bemerkungen zum Hertwig-Magendie Syndrom. *Klin. Mbl. Augenh.,* 1958, 133:866-9.

HERVA, RIITTA (Finnish physician)

Salonen-Herva-Norio syndrome. See *hydrolethalus syndrome.*

HERXHEIMER, KARL (German physician, 1861-1944)

Herxheimer disease. Synonyms: *Pick disease, Pick-Herxheimer syndrome, Taylor disease, acrodermatitis atrophicans chronica, acrodermatitis chronica atrophicans (ACA), atrophia cutis idiopathica progressiva, dermatitis atrophicans diffusa progressiva, dermatitis chronica atrophicans, erythromelia.*

A chronic, progressive skin disease of the extremities. In the early stages, it is characterized by a diffuse or localized erythema of an extremity, spreading along the extensor surfaces, with swelling and doughy consistency of the underlying epidermis. In a few weeks, the inflammatory phase is replaced by atrophy of the skin, causing it to resemble tissue paper (cigarette paper skin), which may be lifted and pushed into folds (Nikolsky sign). Hair loss, decreased sweat and sebum production, and hypopigmentation are usually associated. Additional disorders may include fibrosis, sclerosis, ulnar and tibial bands (dense fibrotic bands over the respective bones, usually with atrophic plaques), fibromas, pseudoscleródermatous patches on the dorsal side of the foot, restricted joint movement, anetoderma, cutaneous and subcutaneous calcification, ulceration, tumor development on atrophic areas (usually squamous cell carcinoma), and lymphocytic infiltration. The condition is usually observed in Europe. The wood tick, *Ixodes ricinus,* is the major vector; antibodies to a tick spirochete similar to that found in Lyme disease can be identified by laboratory tests.

Herxheimer, K., & Hartmann, K. Über Acrodermatitis chronica atrophicans. *Arch. Derm. Syph., Berlin,* 1902, 61:57-76. *Pick, P. J. Erythromelie. *Festschr. Kaposi, Wien,* 1900, p. 915. Burgdorf, W. H. C., & Goltz, R. W. Anetoderma (macular atrophy) and acrodermatitis chronica atrophicans. In: Fitzpatrick, T. B., Eisen, A. Z., Wolff, K., Freedberg, I. M., & Austen, K. F., eds. *Dermatology in general medicine.* 3rd ed. New York, McGraw-Hill, 1987, pp. 1925-30.

Pick-Herxheimer syndrome. See *Herxheimer disease.*

HES. See ***h**yper**e**osinophilic **s**yndrome.*

HESSELBACH, FRANZ CASPAR (German physician, 1759-1816)

Hesselbach hernia. A hernia with diverticula through the cribriform fascia.

Hesselbach, F. C. *Anatomisch-chirurgische Abhandlung über den Ursprung der Leistenbrüche.* Wurzbury, Baumgartner, 1806.

heterochromia cyclica. See *Fuchs heterochromic cyclitis.*

heterochromia iridis. See *Fuchs heterochromic cyclitis.*

heterochromic cyclitis. See *Fuchs heterochromic cyclitis.*

HEUBNER, OTTO JOHANN LEONHARD (German physician, 1843-1926)

Gee-Herter-Heubner disease. See *celiac disease.*

Heubner-Herter disease. See *celiac disease.*

Heubner-Schilder syndrome. See *Schilder disease.*

HEYD, CHARLES GORDON (American physician, born 1884)

Heyd syndrome. See *hepatorenal syndrome.*

HEYDE, E. C. (American physician)

Heyde syndrome. A syndrome of calcific aortic stenosis and gastrointestinal bleeding.

Heyde, E. C. Gastrointestinal bleeding in aortic stenosis. *N. Engl. J. Med.*, 1958, 259:196.

HFE (hemochromatosis). See *Recklinghausen-Applebaum disease.*

HFG. See *hand-foot-genital syndrome.*

HFRS. See *hemorrhagic fever with renal syndrome.*

HFU (**h**and-**f**oot-**u**terus syndrome). See *hand-foot-genital syndrome.*

HGPS (hereditary giant platelets syndrome). See *Bernard-Soulier syndrome.*

HGPS (**H**utchinson-**G**ilford **p**rogeria **s**yndrome). See *Hutchinson-Gilford syndrome, under Hutchinson, Sir Jonathan.*

HHE (**h**emiconvulsion-**h**emiplegia-**e**pilepsy) **syndrome.** See *Gastaut syndrome (2).*

HHH syndrome. See *hyperornithinemia-hyperammonemia-homocitrullinuria syndrome.*

HHHO (**h**ypotonia-**h**ypomentia-**h**ypogonadism-**o**besity) **syndrome.** See *Prader-Willi syndrome.*

HHT (**h**ereditary **h**emorrhagic **t**elangiectasia). See *Osler-Rendu-Weber syndrome.*

HI (**h**ypomelanosis **I**to). See *Ito hypomelanosis.*

hiatus hernia syndrome. See *Bergmann syndrome.*

HICKS, ERIC PERRIN (British physician)

Hicks syndrome. See *Thévenard syndrome.*

hidradenitis suppurativa. See *Verneuil disease.*

hidrocystoma. See *Robinson disease, under Robinson, Andrew Rose.*

hidrotic ectodermal dysplasia. See *Clouston syndrome.*

HIE (**h**yper-Ig**E**) syndrome. See *Job syndrome.*

HIGASHI, OTOKATA (Japanese physician)

Béguez César-Steinbrinck-Chédiak-Higashi syndrome. See *Chédiak-Higashi syndrome.*

Chédiak-Higashi syndrome (CHS). See *under Chédiak.*

Chédiak-Higashi-like syndrome (1). See *pseudo-Chédiak-Higashi syndrome (1), under Chédiak.*

Chédiak-Higashi-like syndrome (2). See *Griscelli syndrome.*

pseudo-Chédiak-Higashi syndrome (1). See *under Chédiak.*

pseudo-Chédiak-Higashi syndrome (2). See *Griscelli syndrome.*

HIGASHI, OTOTAKA (Japanese physician)

Arakawa-Higashi syndrome. See *under Arakawa.*

high altitude disease. See *Monge disease.*

high altitude erythremia. See *Monge disease.*

high T_4 syndrome. Synonym: *euthyroid hyperthyroxinemia.*

A syndrome of transient rise in the serum thyroxine (T_4) concentrations of unknown etiology, associated with fever, tremor, tachycardia, atrial fibrillation, ophthalmopathy, restlessness, nervousness, hyperactivity, and emotional disorders.

Borst, G. G., *et al.* Euthyroid hyperthyroxinemia. *Ann. Intern. Med.*, 1983, 98:366-78. Jackson, I. M. D., & Cobb, W. E.. Disorders of the thyroid. In: Kohler, P. O., & Jordan, R. M., eds. *Clinical endocrinology.* New York, Wiley, 1986, pp. 73-165.

high-density lipoprotein (HDL) deficiency. See *Tangier disease.*

HILDENBRAND, JOHANN VALENTIN ELDER, VON (Austrian physician, 1763-1818)

Hildenbrand disease. Synonyms: *camp fever, epidemic louse-borne fever, jail fever, ship fever, typhus, typhus fever.*

An acute disease caused by *Rickettsia prowazekii* infection, transmitted by the human body louse and characterized by sudden onset of fever, macular rash, and mental disorders (dullness, stupor, and coma). After the incubation period of 8 to 12 days, the early symptoms include malaise and headache, which are followed by fever, weakness, prostration, myalgia, chills, flushing, rash, and mental disorders. Suffused conjunctivae, photophobia, and occasional deafness, tinnitus, vertigo, cough, nausea, vomiting, and diarrhea or constipation are the associated symptoms.

Hildenbrand, J. V. E., von. *Über den ansteckenden Typhus. Nebst einigen Winken zur Beschränkung oder gänzlichen Tilgug der Kriegspest, und mehrerer anderer Menschenseuchen.* Wien, Camesino, 1815.

HILGER, JEROME ANDREW (American physician, born 1912)

Hilger syndrome. Synonyms: *carotid pain, carotidodynia, carotidynia.*

A type of the headache syndrome (q.v.) characterized by pain in the head and neck regions due to vasodilation of the carotid arteries and their branches.

Hilger, J. A. Carotid pain. *Laryngoscope*, 1949, 59:829-38.

HIMELFARB, ALBERT J. (American physician, born 1909)

Weinberg-Himelfarb syndrome. See *under Weinberg.*

HINES, EDGAR ALPHONSO (Born 1906)

Hines-Bannick syndrome. Intermittent attacks of profuse sweating followed by hypothermia, reportedly described by Hines and Bannick.

HINGLAIS, N. (French physician)

Berger-Hinglais syndrome. See *Berger syndrome, under Berger, J.*

HINMAN, FRANK, JR. (American physician)

Hinman syndrome. Synonyms: *achalasia of the urinary tract, detrussor-sphincter dyssynergia, dysfunctional bladder, dysfunctional lazy bladder, nonneurogenic neurogenic bladder (NNNB), nonneurogenic neuromuscular dysfunction, occult neurogenic bladder, pseudoneurogenic bladder, pseudo-obstructed bladder, silent neurogenic bladder, subclinical neurogenic bladder, vesicular-voluntary sphincter dyssynergia.*

A urinary disorder characterized by day and night wetting with futile attempts by the affected child at urinary sphincter control in the face of uncontrollable bladder contractions. Vesicular trabeculation, distortion of ureterovesicular orifices, and dilatation of the upper tract, along with residual urine and consequent bacteriuria are associated. Urodynamic findings show incoordination between detrusor contraction and urethral sphincter relaxation.

Hinman, F., Jr. *Non-neurogenic neurogenic bladder. Annual Meeting of American Urological Asociation, Chicago, May 16-20, 1971. Hinman, F., Jr. Nonneurogenic neurogenic bladder (the Hinman syndrome)-14 years later. J. Urol., Baltimore, 1986, 136:769-77.*

hip synovitis in childhood. See *observation hip syndrome.*

HIPO (hemihypertrophy-intestinal web-preauricular skin tag-congenital corneal opacity) syndrome. A congenital syndrome of hemihypertrophy, intestinal web, preauricular skin tag, and congenital corneal opacity. Associated disorders include upper lid coloboma, epibulbar dermoids, lipodermoids, facial bone dysostosis, micrognathia, low-set malformed ears, malocclusion, tooth abnormalities, and neonatal intestinal obstruction.

Hanley, T. B., & Simon, J. W. Congenital HIPO syndrome. *Ann. Ophth.*, 1984, 16:342-4.

HIPPEL, EUGEN, VON (German ophthalmologist, 1867-1939)

Hippel syndrome. See *Hippel-Lindau syndrome.*

Hippel-Czermak syndrome. See *Hippel-Lindau syndrome.*

Hippel-Lindau disease. See *Hippel-Lindau syndrome.*

Hippel-Lindau syndrome (HLS). Synonyms: *Hippel syndrome, Hippel-Czermak syndrome, Hippel-Lindau disease, Lindau disease, Lindau tumor, von Hippel-Lindau (VHL) syndrome, angiomatosis retinae, angiomatosis retinae cystica, angioreticuloma cerebelli, cerebelloretinal hemangioblastomatosis, cerebroretinal syndrome, hemangioblastomatosis, hereditary hemangiomatosis of the central nervous system, retinal angiomatosis, retinal capillary hamartoma, retinocerebral angiomatosis, viscerocystic retinoangiomatosis syndrome.*

Angiomata of the retina and hemangioblastoma of the cerebellum and walls of the fourth ventricle are the cardinal features of this syndrome. Hemangioma of the spinal cord and pheochromocytoma, sometimes with spinal hypertension, and hypernephromalike renal tumors occur in some patients. Ocular complications include glaucoma, angiomatosis of the iris, vitreous hemorrhage, vascular tortuosity and dilation, retinal hemorrhage and exudates, retinitis proliferans, angiomata of the optic nerve, papilledema, retinal detachment, and macular accumulation of lipid materials. Hemangiomata of the face, adrenals, lungs, and liver, and multiple cysts of the pancreas and kidneys may occur in some cases. The syndrome is transmitted as an autosomal dominant trait with varying expression, the symptoms not being apparent until the third decade of life.

Hippel, E., von. Vorstellung eines Patienten mit einem sehr ungewöhnlichen Aderhautleiden. *Bericht 24 Versammlung der Ophth. Ges.*, 1895, p. 169. Lindau, A. Studien über Kleinhirnzysten. Bau, Pathogenese und Beziehungen zur Angiomatosis retinae. *Acta Path. Microb. Scand.*, 1926, 3(Suppl):1-128. *Czermak. *Verh. Ophth. Ges. Wien*, 1905, p. 184.

von Hippel-Lindau (VHL) syndrome. See *Hippel-Lindau syndrome.*

HIPPOCRATES (Late 5th century B.C. Greek physician)

digital hippocratism. See *Marie-Bamberger syndrome, under Marie, Pierre.*

HIPPOCRATES OF COS (Late 5th century B.C. Greek physician)

hippocratic fingers. See *Marie-Bamberger syndrome, under Marie, Pierre.*

HIRSCH, J. S.

Hirsch syndrome. Osteitis fibrosa generalista (Recklinghausen disease 2) of the ribs, sternum, and metacarpal bones, associated with pachyderma, reportedly described by Hirsch.

HIRSCHFELD, FELIX VICTOR BIRCH (German physician, born 1842)

Hirschfeld disease. An acute form of diabetes mellitus.

*Hirschfeld, F. Vorläufige Mitteilung über eine besondere klinische Form des Diabetes. *Zbl. Med. Wiss* 1890, 18:164-6; 193-5.

HIRSCHHORN, KURT (American physician)

Wolf-Hirschhorn syndrome. See *chromosome 4p deletion syndrome.*

HIRSCHOWITZ, B. I. (American physician)

Groll-Hirschowitz syndrome. See *under Groll.*

HIRSCHSPRUNG, HARALD (Danish pediatrician, 1830-1916)

Hirschsprung disease (HD, HRSD). See *Hirschsprung syndrome.*

Hirschsprung disease-pigmentary anomaly syndrome. See *Shah-Waardenburg syndrome.*

Hirschsprung syndrome. Synonyms: *Hirschsprung disease (HD, HRSD), Hirschsprung-Galant infantilism, aganglionic megacolon, colonic aganglìosis, congenital megacolon, megacolon congenitum.*

Distention of the colon (megacolon) due to congenital absence of intramural neural plexuses (agangliosis) caused by arrested caudal migration of cells from the neural crest cells that develop as intramural plexuses. The aganglionic segment extends from the internal anal sphincter proximally and is located within the rectum and sigmoid colon, being permanently contracted and devoid of peristaltic activity, thus causing the colon to be distended with fecal material and gases. Constipation, intestinal obstruction, and meconium ileus are the most common complications in early infancy; the symptoms become less severe later in life, but constipation and recurrent fecal impaction may persist. Male infants are more commonly affected than females. The condition is sometimes associated with the Down and the Waardenburg syndromes. Its transmission is believed to be polygenetic, but some cases are inherited as an autosomal recessive trait.

*Hirschsprung, H. Stuhlträgheit Neugeborener infolge von Dilatation und Hypertrophie des Colons. *Jahrb. Kinderh.*, 1888, 27:1-7.

Hirschsprung-Galant infantilism. See *Hirschsprung syndrome.*

HIS

His syndrome. Synonym: *formicophilia.*

A form of zoophilia in which arousal and orgasm are produced by crawling or nibbling by small animals and insects such as snails, frogs, or ants.

Dewaraja, R., & Money, J. Transcultural sexology; formicophilia, a newly named paraphilia in a young Buddhist male. *J. Sex. Marital Ther.*, 1986, 12:139-45.

HIS, WILHELM, JR. (German physician, 1863-1934)

Werner-His disease. See *under Werner, Heinrich.*

histamine cephalgia. See *Horton neuralgia.*

histamine headache. See *Horton neuralgia.*

histamine neuralgia. See *Horton neuralgia.*

histiocytic medullary reticulosis (HMR). See *Omenn syndrome.*

histiocytic medullary reticulosis-like (HMR-like) syndrome. A syndrome characterized by symptoms similar to those in histiocytic medullary reticulosis (see *Omenn* *syndrome*), consisting of fever, weight loss, jaundice, lymphadenopathy, hepatosplenomegaly, pancytopenia, and tissue infiltration by atypical histiocytes or macrophages. In one form, the syndrome occurs as a self-limiting condition secondary to viral and other infections, and, in the other, as a preterminal complication of a preexisting malignancy.

Manoharan, A., *et al.* Histiocytic medullary reticulosis complicating chronic lymphocytic leukaemia: Malignant or reactive? *Scand. J. Haemat.*, 1981, 26:5-13.

histoplasmosis. Synonym: *Darling disease.*

A systemic infectious disease caused by the fungus *Histoplasma capsulatum*, which is found in the soil contaminated with chicken, bat, and bird droppings; its spores are inhaled and spread to the blood through the pulmonary lymphatic system. **Primary histoplasmosis**, the most common form, is characterized by flulike symptoms, such as cough, fever, headache, myalgia, stomach cramps, and, in severe cases, dyspnea, cyanosis, chest pain, and pericarditis. Erythema nodosum or multiforme, rash, and arthralgia may be present in some cases. Radiological findings include hilar lymphadenopathy, patchy bronchopneumonia, pleural effusions, granulomas with caseation necrosis, calcification at pulmonary parenchymal and hilar loci (**Ghon complex**), and coin lesions. **Reinfection histoplasmosis** is marked by a short incubation peroid and clinical course, miliary lung nodules, and lack of hilar involvement. **Chronic pulmonary histoplasmosis** occurs most commonly in middle-aged males with preexisting emphysema. The symptoms include emphysematous bleb, cough, fever, malaise, infarctlike necrosis, and fibrous lesions. Thick-walled communicating lung cavities (marching cavities) and bronchogenic spread, resulting in pneumonitis and fibrosis. are the principal pathological features. **Disseminated histoplasmosis**, occurring most often in middle-aged males, follows immunosuppression with arousal of disease from latency. The symptoms include weight loss, fever, weakness, malaise, hepatosplenomegaly, lymphadenopathy, and bone marrow disorders with anemia, leukopenia, and thrombocytosis. Dysphagia and hoarseness due to oropharyngeal, nasopharyngeal, and laryngeal ulcers, are usually present. Other symptoms include gastrointestinal bleeding ulcers, malabsorption, intestinal obstruction or perforation, adrenal insufficiency, respiratory infection, endocarditis, embolism, meningitis, osteomyelitis, and kidney, prostate, and skin lesions.

Darling, S. T. A protozoan general infection producing pseudotubercles in the lungs and focal necrosis in the liver, spleen, and lymph nodes. *JAMA*, 1906, 46:1283-5. Drutz, D. J. Histoplasmosis. In: Wyngaarden, J. B., & Smith, L. H., Jr., eds. *Cecil textbook of medicine.* 17th ed. Philadelphia, Saunders, 1985, pp. 1759-61.

HITZIG, JULIUS EDUARD (German physician, 1838-1907)

Hitzig syndrome. Synkinesis of the orbicularis and other muscles innervated by the seventh cranial nerve, said to be described by Hitzig.

HLHS. See *hypoplastic left heart syndrome.*

HLP (hyperkeratosis lenticularis perstans). See *Flegel disease.*

HLS. See *Hippel-Lindau syndrome.*

HLVS (hypoplastic left ventricle syndrome). See *hypoplastic left heart syndrome.*

HM (hemifacial microsomia). See *oculo-auriculovertebral dysplasia.*

HMC. See *hypertelorism-microtia-clefting syndrome.*

HMD (hyaline membrane disease). See *neonatal respiratory distress syndrome.*

HMR (histiocytic medullary reticulosis). See *Omenn syndrome.*

HMR-like syndrome. See *histiocytic medullary reticulosis-like syndrome.*

HMSN I (hereditary motor and sensory neuropathy I). See *Charcot-Marie-Tooth disease.*

HNPCC. See *hereditary nonpolyposis colorectal cancer syndrome.*

HNSHA (hereditary nonspherocytic hemolytic anemia. See *Crosby syndrome, under Crosby, William H.*

HOCHENEGG, JULIUS, VON (Austrian physician, born 1859-1940)

Hochenegg ulcer. Synonym: *ulcus callosum recti.*

A hard rectal tumor with central ulceration, associated with stenosis, defecation difficulty, blood and mucus in the feces, colic, meteorism, and loss of appetite.

Hochenegg, J. Über Ulcus callosum recti und diesen Behandlung. *Wien. Klin. Wschr.*, 1926, 39:522-4.

HOCKEY, ATHEL (Australian physician)

Hockey syndrome. An X-linked mental retardation syndrome associated with precocious puberty and obesity.

Hockey, A. X-linked intellectual handicap and precocious puberty with obesity in carrier females. *Am. J. Med. Genet.*, 1986, 23:127-37.

HODARA, MANEHEM (Turkish physician, died 1926)

Hodara disease. A form of trichorrhexis of the scalp.

*Hodara, M. Über die Trichorrhexis der Kophaares der Konstantinopoler Frauen. *Mschr. Prakt. Derm.*, 1894, 19:173-88.

HODGE, HAROLD CARPENTER (American dentist, born 1904)

Capdepont-Hodge syndrome. See *dentinogenesis imperfecta.*

HODGKIN, THOMAS (British physician, 1798-1866)

Hodgkin disease (HD). Synonyms: *Bonfils disease, Hodgkin granuloma, Hodgkin syndrome, Hodgkin-Paltauf-Sternberg disease, Paltauf-Sternberg disease, Pel-Ebstein disease, Sternberg disease, fibromyeloid medullary reticulosis, lymphogranuloma, lymphogranulomatosis maligna, lymphomatosis granulomatosa, malignant lymphogranuloma, malignant lymphogranulomatosis, malignant lymphoma.*

A neoplastic disease of unknown etiology, considered to be a form of malignant lymphoma. It usually begins as a painless enlargement of the cervical lymph nodes, followed by splenomegaly, abdominal pain, weakness, anorexia, loss of weight, cough, dyspnea, and occasional itching. The lesions present a wide variety of histological patterns from almost pure lymphocytic infiltrates to histiocytic giant cells. Reed-Sternberg cells (giant tumor cells measuring up to 40 μ in diameter and having abundant cytoplasm, which are irregular in shape and vary in staining reaction from acidophilic to basophilic) are typical of this condition. Cell nuclei are large, sometimes occupying half a cell, some cells having two or more nuclei.

Hodgkin, T. On some morbid appearances of the absorbent glands and spleen. *Med. Chir. Tr., London*, 1832, 17:68-114. Pel, K. P. Zur Symptomatologie der sog.

Pseudo-Leukämie. *Berlin. Klin. Wschr.*, 1885, 22:3-7. Paltauf, R. Lymphosarkom (lymphosarkomatose, Pseudoleukämie, Myelom, Chlorom). *Erg. Allg. Path.*, 1897, 3:652:91. Sternberg, C. Lymphogranulomatose und Reticuloendotheliose. *Erg. Allg. Path.*, 1936, 30:1-76. Ebstein, W. Das chronische Rückfallsfieber, eine neue Infectionskrankheit. *Berlin. Klin Wschr.*, 1887, 24:565-8. *Bonfils, É. A. *Quelques réflexions sur un cas d'hypertrophie ganglionaire générale: avec fistules lymphatiques et avec cachexie, sans leucémie.* Clermont, 1857.

Hodgkin granuloma. See *Hodgkin disease.*

Hodgkin syndrome. See *Hodgkin disease.*

Hodgkin-Paltauf-Sternberg disease. See *Hodgkin disease.*

HODGKIN, W. E.

Rapp-Hodgkin ectodermal dysplasia. See *under Rapp.*

HODGSON, JOSEPH (British physician, 1788-1869)

Hodgson disease. Aneurysmal dilation of the aorta seen in enlargement of the heart.

Hodgson, J. *A treatise on the diseases of the arteries and veins, containing the pathology and treatment of aneurisms and wounded arteries.* London, Underwood, 1815.

HOET, JOSEPH JULES (Belgian physician, born 1925)

Hoet-Abaza syndrome. Postpartum diabetes mellitus and obesity.

Gilbert-Dreyfus, *et al.* A propos du syndrome de Hoet-Abaza. *Gaz. Hôp., Paris*, 1958, 130:447-51.

HOEVE, JAN, VAN DER (Dutch ophthalmologist, born 1878)

van der Hoeve disease. See *osteogenesis imperfecta syndrome (dominant form).*

van der Hoeve-de Kleyn syndrome. See *osteogenesis imperfecta syndrome (dominant form).*

van der Hoeve-Halbertsma-Waardenburg syndrome. See *Waardenburg syndrome (2).*

HOFFA, ALBERT (German physician, 1859-1908)

Hoffa fatty tissue hypertrophy. See *Hoffa-Kastert syndrome.*

Hoffa syndrome. See *Hoffa-Kastert syndrome.*

Hoffa-Kastert syndrome. Synonyms: *Hoffa fatty tissue hypertrophy, Hoffa syndrome.*

Chronic synovitis of the knee joint accompanied by lipomatous degeneration of the corpus adiposum genus, resulting in tumor-like lesions and filamentous adhesions that cause restricted joint movement.

Hoffa, A. Zur Bedeutung des Fettgewebes für die Pathologie des Kniegelenks. *Deut. Med. Wschr.*, 1904, 30:337-8. Kastert, J. Die Verwachsung des Kniegelenkfettkörpers als selbständiges Krankheitsbild. *Chirurg, Berlin*, 1953, 24:390-4.

HOFFMANN, AUGUST (German physician, 1887-1929)

Bouveret-Hoffmann syndrome. See *Bouveret syndrome (2).*

HOFFMANN, ERICH (German physician, 1868-1959)

Hoffmann-Zurhelle syndrome. Synonyms: *lipomatosis cutis superficialis, nevus lipomatodes cutaneus superficialis, nevus lipomatodes superficialis subepidermalis.*

A superficial lipomatous nevus of the gluteal region, characterized by yellowish nodules that may coalesce into large plaques.

Hoffmann, E., & Zuerhelle, E. Über eine Naevus lipomatodes cutaneus superficialis der linken Glutäalgegend. *Arch. Derm. Syph., Berlin*, 1921, 130:327-33.

HOFFMANN, JOHANN (German physician, 1857-1919)

Charcot-Marie-Tooth-Hoffmann syndrome. See *Charcot-Marie-Tooth syndrome.*

Hoffmann atrophy. See *Werdnig-Hoffmann syndrome.*

Hoffmann syndrome. Synonym: *hypothyroid myopathy.*

Myxedema associated with muscle weakness, hypertrophy, and pseudomyotonia. Presence of painful spasms and pseudomyotonia is the major point of difference with the Debré-Semelaigne syndrome.

Hoffmann, J. Weiterer Beitrag zur Lehre von der Tetanie. *Deut. Zschr. Nervenh*, 1897, 9:278-90.

Werdnig-Hoffmann disease (WHD). See *Werdnig-Hoffmann syndrome.*

Werdnig-Hoffmann syndrome. See *under Werdnig.*

HOGAN

Sanders-Hogan syndrome. See *Sanders syndrome.*

HOGAN, G. R. (American physician)

Dreifuss-Emery-Hogan syndrome. See *Emery-Dreifuss syndrome.*

HOGG, GEORGINA R. (Canadian physician)

Birt-Hogg-Dubé syndrome. See *under Birt.*

HOIGNE, ROLF VICTOR (Swiss physician, born 1023)

Hoigné syndrome. Embolism and mental complications following intramuscular injection of procaine penicillin, believed to be caused by penetration of the drug into the blood stream. Neurological disorders include severe agitation, confusion, visual and auditory hallucinations, vertigo, sense of fear and panic, seizures, and psychotic reactions. See also *Nicolau syndrome.*

Hoigné, R., & Krebs, A. Kombinierte anaphylaktische und embolishtoxische Reaktionen durch akzidentelle intravaskuläre Injektion von Procain-Penicillin. *Schweiz. Med. Wschr.*, 1964, 94:610-4. Hoigné, R., & Schoch, K. Anaphylaktischer Schock und akute, nich allergische Reaktionen nach Procain-Penicillin. *Schweiz. Med. Wschr.*, 1959, 89:1350-6.

holiday heart syndrome. Paroxysms of arrhythmia occurring particularly after holiday or weekend bouts of drinking. Persons with a history of alcoholic cardiomyopathy are most frequently affected.

Ettinger, P. O.*et al.* Arrhythmias and the "holiday heart!" Alcohol-associated ventricular paroxysmal tachycardia. *Am. Heart J.*, 1978, 95:555.

HOLLÄNDER, EUGEN (German physician, 1867-1932)

Holländer-Simons syndrome. See *Barraguer-Simons syndrome.*

HOLLISTER, DAVID W. (American physician)

Hollister-Hollister syndrome. Synonym: *long-thumb brachydactyly syndrome.*

A syndrome, transmitted as an autosomal dominant trait, characterized by brachydactyly, clinodactyly, small hands and feet, narrow shoulders with short clavicles, pectus excavatum, apparent cardiomegaly, murmur of pulmonic stenosis, possible heart conduction defects, restriction of movement of the shoulder and metacarpophalangeal joints, and mild shortness of the limbs.

Hollister, D. W., & Hollister, W. G. The "long-thumb" brachydactyly syndrome. *Am. J. Med. Genet.*, 1981, 8:5-16.

Levy-Hollister syndrome. See *lacrimo-auriculodentodigital syndrome.*

HOLLISTER, WILLIAM G. (American physician)

Hollister-Hollister syndrome. See *under Hollister, David W.*

HOLMES, GORDON MORGAN (British neurologist, 1876-1965)

Adie-Holmes syndrome. See *Adie syndrome.*

Head-Holmes syndrome. See *under Head.*

Holmes disease. Synonym: *cerebello-olivary degeneration.*

Degeneration of the cerebellum and olivary nucleus associated with progressive ataxia.

Holmes, G. A form of familial degeneration of the cerebellum. *Brain,* 1907, 30:466-89.

Holmes syndrome. Space perception disorders caused by brain injuries and characterized by an inability to recognize the position, distance, and size of objects in space, in association with impaired fixation, disorders of accommodation and convergence, and absence of the blinking reflex.

Holmes, G. Disturbances of visual orientation. *Brit. J. Ophth.*, 1918, 2:449-68; 506-16.

Stewart-Holmes syndrome. See *under Stewart, T. G.*

HOLMES, LEWIS B. (American physician)

Hootnick-Holmes syndrome. See *under Hootnick.*

Mirhosseini-Holmes-Walton syndrome. See *under Mirhosseini.*

holoprosencephaly anomalad. See *holoprosencephaly syndrome.*

holoprosencephaly syndrome. Synonyms: *Kundrat syndrome, arhinencephaly, holoprosencephaly anomalad, holotelencephaly.*

A congenital syndrome of multiple abnormalities characterized by failure of cleavage of the prosencephalon with faulty midline facial development. Facial defects may include cyclopia, monophthalmia or anophthalmia, synophthalmia, arhinia and other nose abnormalities, micrognathia, ethmocephaly, hypertelorism, cebocephaly, and premaxillary agenesis. Associated abnormalities usually consist of hypotelorism, flat nose, cleft lip and palate, iris coloboma, and other deformities. Alobar or semilobar brain deformity is the usual feature. Holoprosencephaly is not considered an independent entity but a component of several syndromes.

*Kundrat, H. *Arhincephalies als typische Art von Missbildung.* Graz, Leuschner & Lubensky, 1882. DeMyer, W. W., *et al.*, Familial alobar holoprosencephaly (arhinencephaly) with median cleft lip and palate. *Neurology,* 1963, 13:913-8. Gorlin, R. J., Pindborg, J. J., & Cohen, M. M., Jr. *Syndromes of the head and neck.* 2nd ed. New York, McGraw-Hill, 1976.

holotelencephaly. See *holoprosencephaly syndrome.*

HOLT, J. F. (American physician)

Gorlin-Holt syndrome. See *frontometaphyseal dysplasia.*

HOLT, MARY CLAYTON (British physician)

Holt-Oram syndrome. Synonyms: *atriodigital dysplasia, atrio-extremital dysplasia, cardiac-limb syndrome, cardiomelic syndrome, cardio-osseous syndrome, digito-atrial dysplasia, heart and hand syndrome, heart-upper limb syndrome, upper limb-cardiovascular syndrome.*

A syndrome combining upper limb abnormalities and congenital heart diseases. The limb defects are bilateral but not necessarily symmetric and range from minimal changes to phocomelia. Typically, the thumb may be absent or may be triphalangeal or fingerlike. Hypoplasia of the radius and extra carpal bones may occur. Narrow shoulders are common. Cardiovascular defects are varied and may include atrial septal defect, sometimes with arrhythmia, ventricular septal defect, and patent ductus arteriosus. Hypertelorism, pulmonary stenosis, pectus excavatum, small scapulae, and absence of one or more ossification centers in the wrist may be associated. The syndrome is transmitted as an autosomal dominant trait.

Holt, M., & Oram, S. Familial heart disease with skeletal malformations. *Brit. Heart J.*, 1960, 22:236-42.

HOLT, SARAH B. (British physician)

Holt syndrome. A familial syndrome of polydactyly and brachymetapody transmitted as an autosomal dominant trait.

Holt, S. B. Polydactyly and brachymetapody in two English families. *J. Med. Genet.*, 1975, 12:355-66.

HOLTERMÜLLER, K. (German pediatrician)

Holtermüller-Wiedemann syndrome. Synonyms: *cloverleaf skull, Kleeblattschädel, Kleeblattschädel anomald, Kleeblattschädel anomaly, trefoil skull syndrome.*

A congenital form of hydrocephalus resulting from intrauterine craniosynostosis with bulging through the cranial sutures, giving the skull a flattened, cloverleaflike configuration. The degree of severity varies and different sutures may be involved. When the anomaly is severe, the ears are displaced downward, facing the shoulders. Midface hypoplasia with relative mandibular prognathism are usually associated. The nasal bridge is usually depressed, and in some cases the nose may be beaklike. Proptosis, hypertelorism, and antimongoloid palpebral fissures are common. Inability to close the eyelids may lead to corneal ulcers and clouding. Venous distention of the scleras, eyelids, scalp, and periorbital areas are usually visible. Iris coloboma, blindness, nasolacrimal duct obstruction, cardiovascular defects, macrostomia, macroglossia, and other complications may be associated. The syndrome may occur as an isolated anomaly or in association with other syndromes.

Holtermüller, K., & Wiedemann, H. R. Kleeblattschädel-Syndrom. *Med. Mschr.*, 1960, 14:439-46.

HOLZKNECHT, GUIDO (Austrian physician, 1872-1931)

Holzknecht syndrome. A roentgenographic symptom complex of bronchial stenosis in which during inspiration the mediastinum is displaced to the right and the heart disappears from the left chest and reappears on the right side.

Holzknecht, G. Ein neues radioscopisches Symptom bein Bronchialstenose und Methodisches. *Wien. Klin. Rundsch.*, 1899, 13:785-7.

HOMEN, ERNST ALEXANDER (Finnish physician, 1851-1926)

Homen syndrome. Lesions of the lenticular nucleus causing generalized rigidity of the legs, associated with vertigo, amnesia, apraxia, speech disorders, and cerebral and mental deterioration.

Homen, E. A. Eine eigenthümliche Familiienkrankheit, unter der Form Einer progressiven Dementia mit besonderem anatomischen Befund. *Neurol. Zbl.*, 1890, 9:514-8.

homocystinuria syndrome. Synonyms: *Carson-Neill syndrome, cystathionine beta-synthase (CBS) deficiency.*

An inborn error of metabolism characterized by cystathionine synthetase deficiency with accumulation in tissues of homocystine and methionine and deficiency of cystathione and cystine. Ectopia lentis, thromboembolism of medium-sized arteries and veins, malar flushing and livedo reticularis, osteoporosis,

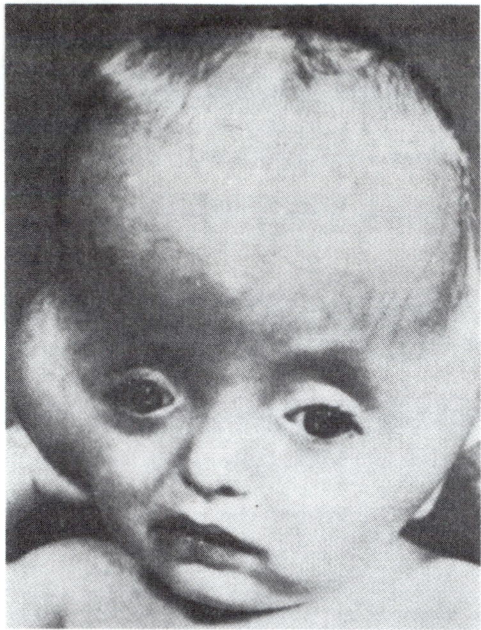

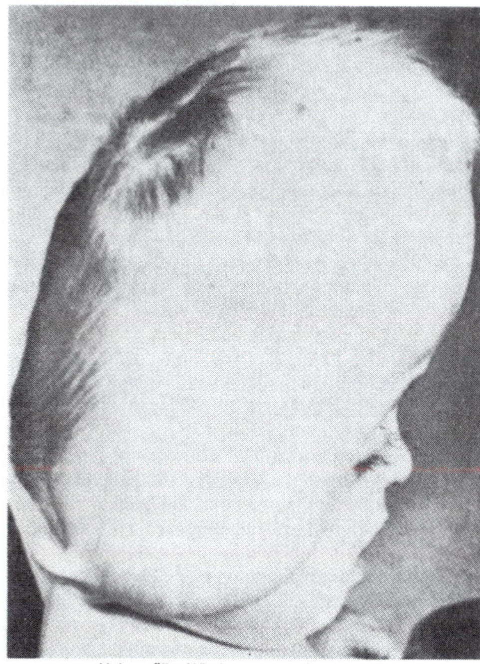

Holtermüller-Wiedemann syndrome
Angle, C.R., M.S. McIntire & R.C. Moore: *Am. J. Dis. Child,* 114:200, 1967.
Chicago: American Medical Assoc.

sparse fine hair, cataract, optic atrophy, cystic degeneration of the retina, retinal detachment, glaucoma, hepatomegaly, and hernia are the major elements of this syndrome. Less common disorders include mental retardation, the Marfan syndrome, dolichostenomelia, pectus carinatum, kyphoscoliosis, and other defects. The syndrome is transmitted as an autosomal recessive trait.

Carson, N. A., & Neill, D. W. Metabolic abnormalities detected in a survey of mentally backward individuals in Northern Ireland. *Arch. Dis. Child.*, 1962, 37:505-13.

Gerritsen, T., *et al.* The identification of homocystine in the urine. *Biochem. Biophys. Res. Commun.*, 1962, 9:493-6.

homozygous beta-thalassemia. See *Cooley anemia.*

homozygous hemoglobin S disease. See *sickle cell anemia.*

honeycomb degeneration of the retina. See *Doyne choroiditis.*

HOOD (hereditary onycho-osteo-dysplasia). See *nail-patella syndrome.*

HOODS (hereditary onycho-osteo-dysplasia syndrome). See *nail-patella syndrome.*

HOOFT, C. (Belgian physician)

Hooft syndrome. Synonyms: *familial hypolipidemia, hypolipidemia S.*

A familial syndrome, transmitted as an autosomal recessive trait, combining a variety of clinical and biochemical abnormalities. Clinical features include growth retardation beginning during the second year of life, erythematosquamous skin lesions on the face and limbs, abnormalities of the hair, nails, and teeth, and occasional tapetoretinal degeneration. Biochemical findings include decreased blood lipid, ATP, and phospholipid levels; increased tubular phosphate reabsorption; abnormal tryptophan metabolism with indoluria and aminoaciduria; and faulty glycolysis.

Hooft, C., *et al.* Familial hypolipidemia and retarded development without steatorrhea. Another inborn error of metabolism? *Helvet. Paediat. Acta*, 1962, 17:1-23.

hookworm disease. See *Griesinger disease.*

HOOTNICK, D. (American physician)

Hootnick-Holmes syndrome. Synonym: *familial polysyndactyly-craniofacial anomalies syndrome.*

A familial syndrome, transmitted as an autosomal dominant trait, characterized by craniofacial anomalies (frontal bossing, scaphocephaly, hypertelorism, downward palpebral slant), hand and foot abnormalities (broad thumbs, preaxial polydactyly, postaxial polydactyly, broad great toes, syndactyly), and nervous system disorders (mental retardation, craniosynostosis, cerebral anomalies, divergent strabismus).

Hootnick, D., & Holmes, L. B. Familial polysyndactyly and craniofacial anomalies. *Clin. Genet.*, 1972, 3:128-34.

HOPF, GUSTAV (German dermatologist, 1900-1979)

Hopf disease. See *Hopf keratosis.*

Hopf keratosis. Synonyms: *Hopf disease, acrodermatitis verruciformis, acrokeratosis verruciformis.*

Localized, symmetrical, flat, wartlike epithelial nevi, usually on the dorsal surfaces of the hands and feet, transmitted as an autosomal dominant trait. The lesions may be present at birth, or they may appear later in infancy as papules or at puberty as ichthyosis. Opaque, brittle, and striated nails are usually associated.

*Hopf, G. Über eine bisher nicht beschriebene disseminierte Keratose (Akrodermatosis verruciformis). *Derm. Zschr.*, 1931, 60:227-50.

HOPKINS, I. J. (Australian physician)

Hopkins syndrome. A poliomyelitislike illness (lower motor neuron paralysis of the arms and legs) associated with acute bronchial asthma and immunodeficiency.

Hopkins, I. J. A new syndrome: Poliomyelitis-like illness associated with acute asthma in childhood. *Austral. Paediat. J.*, 1974, 10:273-6.

HOPMANN, CARL MELCHIOR (German physician, 1844-1925)

Hopmann papilloma. A polyp of the nasal mucosa having the appearance of a papilloma.

Hopmann, C. M. Die papillären Geschwülste der Nosenschleimhaut. *Arch. Path. Anat., Berlin*, 1883, 93:213-58.

HOPPE, HERMANN HENRY (German physician, 1867-1929)

Hoppe-Goldflam syndrome. See *Erb-Goldflam syndrome, under Erb, Wilhelm Heinrich.*

HORAN, M. B. (Australian physician)

Nance-Horan syndrome (NHS). See *under Nance.*

horizontal linear atelectasis. See *Fleischner syndrome.*

horizontal maxillary fracture. See *Le Fort fracture I.*

HÖRLEIN, PHILLIPP HEINRICH (German physician, 1882-1954)

Hörlein-Weber disease. Synonym: *chronic familial methemglobinemia.*

A hematological disorder, characterized by chronic familial methemoglobinemia with cyanosis, transmitted as an autosomal dominant trait. The presence of methemoglobin that differs from other types by its behavior in the red field in spectrum analysis is its main feature.

Hörlein, H., & Weber, G. Über chronische familiäre Hethämoglobinämie und eine neue Modifikation des Methämoglobins. *Deut. Med. Wschr.*, 1948, 73:476-8.

HORNER, JOHANN FRIEDRICH (Swiss ophthalmologist, 1831-1886)

Bernard-Horner syndrome. See *Horner syndrome.*

Claude Bernard-Horner syndrome. See *Horner syndrome.*

Horner sympton complex. See *Horner syndrome.*

Horner syndrome (HS). Synonyms: *Bernard syndrome, Bernard-Horner syndrome, Claude Bernard syndrome, Claude Bernard-Horner syndrome, Horner symptom complex, Horner triad, Mitchell syndrome, cervical sympathetic paralysis syndrome, oculopupillary syndrome, oculosympathetic syndrome.*

A neurological disorder in which interruption of the sympathetic pathways produces ophthalomoplegia, miosis, blepharoptosis, relative ocular hypotonia, apparent enophthalmos and ipsilateral facial cutaneous hyperemia, anhidrosis, and vasodilatation. It may be produced by section of the nerve, trauma, neoplasms, thrombosis, substernal thyroid, and syphilitic aneurysm of the brachiocephalic trunk, situated anywhere along the sympathetic pathways, from the hypothalamus to the sympathetic innervation of the facial sweat glands.

Horner, J. f. Über eine Form von Ptosis. *Klin. Mbl. Augenheilk.*, 1869, 7:193-8. Bernard, C. Des phénomènes oculopupillaires produits par la section du nerf sympathique cervical; il sont indépendants des phénomenes vasculaires colorifique de lat tête. *C. Rend. Acad. Sc., Paris*, 1862, 55:381-8. *Mitchell, S. W., *et al. Gunshot wounds and other injuries on nerves.* Philadelphia, Lippincott, 1864.

Horner syndrome, incomplete. See *Raeder syndrome.*

Horner syndrome, partial. See *Raeder syndrome.*

Horner triad. See *Horner syndrome.*

Horner-Trantas spots. Synonym: *Trantas dots.*

Small chalky concretions seen on the conjunctiva in the later stages of vernal conjunctivitis.

Trantas. Sur le catarrhe printanier. *Arch. Opht., Paris*, 1910, 30:593-621.

reverse Horner syndrome. A disease in which the symtoms are opposite to those in the Horner syndrome, consisting mainly of hyperhidrosis, alopecia, and ipsilateral pupillary dilatation.

Cole, M., *et al.* The reverse Horner syndrome. *J. Thorac. Cardiovasc. Surg.*, 1970, 59:603-6.

HORNOVA, J. (Czech physician)

Hornová-Dluhosová syndrome. A familial syndrome of primary amyloidosis of the gingiva and conjunctiva, congenital cataracts, atrophy of the bulbus oculi, corneal leukoma, and mental retardation.

Hornová, J., & Dluhosová, O. Primary amyloidosis of gingiva and conjunctiva and mental disorder in brother and sister. *Oral Surg.*, 1968, 25:457-64.

horseshoe kindey. See *Gutierrez syndrome.*

HORTON, BAYARD TAYLOR (American physician, born 1895)

Bing-Horton syndrome. See *Horton neuralgia.*

Horton arteritis. See *Horton disease (1).*

Horton disease (1). Synonyms: *Horton arteritis, Horton temporal arteritis, Horton-Gilmour disease, Horton-Magath-Brown syndrome, arteritis cranialis, arteritis temporalis, cranial arteritis, giant-cell arteritis, senile arteritis, temporal arteritis, temporal megacellular arteritis.*

A form of the headache syndrome (q.v.) characterized by inflammation of the temporal and other cranial arteries, usually occurring during the sixth and seventh decades. A pulseless, enlarged superficial artery and a severe throbbing headache are the principal symptoms. Facial edema; visual disorders, including diplopia; hearing disorders; involvement of the third, fourth, and sixth cranial nerves; facial neuralgia; cerebral thrombosis; and mental disorders may occur. The diseased artery is narrowed by granulomatous lesions located at the junction between the media and intima. Histiocytes, lymphocytes, plasma cells, eosinophils, and a large number of giant cells are usually present in the tissue. The disorder normally involves the cranial arteries, but the aorta, coronary artery, and other vessels may also be involved. A bacterial infection is suspected as a probable cause.

Horton, B. T., Magath, T. B., & Brown, G. E. Arteritis of the temporal vessels. A previously undescribed from. *Arch. Int. Med., Chicago*, 1934, 53:400-9.

Horton disease (2). See *Horton neuralgia.*

Horton headache. See *Horton neuralgia.*

Horton migraine. See *Horton neuralgia.*

Horton neuralgia. Synonyms: *Bing erythroprosalgia, Bing syndrome, Bing-Horton syndrome, Harris neuralgia, Horton disease, Horton headache, Horton migraine, ciliary neuralgia, cluster headache, erythromelalgia of the head, erythroprosalgia, facial vagosympathetic algia, histamine cephalgia, histamine neuralgia, histamine headache, periodic migrainous neuralgia.*

Unilateral headaches (see under *headache syndrome*) occurring in clusters, particularly in middle-aged males. Severe pain is centered behind or close to the eye, but may extend to the cheek or the occipital area. Ipsilateral nasal congestion, suffusion of the eye, excessive lacrimation, and facial redness and swelling may accompany or precede the headache. The duration of pain is usually less than 2 hours and commonly less than 30 minutes. The recurrent attacks often appear within a period of 24 hours, sometime during sleep.

Horton, B. T. The use of histamine in the treatment of specific types of headaches. *JAMA,* 1941, 116:377-83. Harris, B. T. *Neuritis and neuralgia.* London, 1926. Bing, R. Über traumatische Erythromelalgie und Erythroprosopalgie. *Nervenarzt,* 1930, 3:506-12.

Horton temporal arteritis. See *Horton disease (1).*

Horton-Gilmour disease. See *Horton disease (1).*

Horton-Magath-Brown syndrome. See *Horton disease (1).*

Hutchinson-Horton syndrome. See *under Hutchinson, Sir Jonathan.*

hospital addiction. See *Munchausen syndrome.*

hospital hobo. See *Munchausen syndrome.*

hospital vagrant. See *Munchausen syndrome.*

hot-dog headache. See *under headache syndrome.*

HOTS (**h**ypercalcemia-**o**steolysis-**T**-cell **s**yndrome). Hypercalcemia and bone resorption associated with T-cell lymphoma. Retrovirus C is suspected as the causative agent.

Grossman, B., *et al.* Hypercalcemia associataed with T-cell lymphoma-leukemia. *Am. J. Clin. Path.,* 1981, 75:149-55. Pierard, G. E., *et al.* Neoplastic proliferation in a case of epidermotropic high-grade malignant lymphoma associated with hypercalcemia. *Dermatologica, Basel,* 1985, 171:278-82.

HOUSSAY, BERNARDO ALBERTO (Argentine physiologist, born 1887)

Houssay phenomenon in man. See *Houssay syndrome.*

Houssay syndrome. Synonyms: *Houssay phenomenon in man, Houssay-Biasotti syndrome, spontaneous remission of diabetes mellitus, vanishing diabetes mellitus.*

Spontaneous remission of diabetes mellitus in patients suffering from destructive diseases of the anterior pituitary gland. This is the clinical counterpart of posthypophysectomy remission of diabetes mellitus in pancreatectomized animals, observed during experiments by Houssay and Biasotti.

*Houssay, B. A., & Biasotti, A. La diabete pancreática de los perros hipofisoprivos. *Rev. Soc. Argent. Biol.,* 1930, 6:251-96.

Houssay-Biasotti syndrome. See *Houssay syndrome.*

HOUSTON, C. STUART (Canadian physician)

Ives-Houston syndrome. See *under Ives.*

HOUWER, A. W. M. (Dutch physician)

Gougerot-Houwer-Sjögren syndrome. See *Sjögren syndrome, under Sjögren, Henrik Samuel Conrad.*

HOWEL-EVANS, W. (British physician)

Howel-Evans syndrome. A familial skin disease, transmitted as an autosomal dominant trait, characterized by diffuse hyperkeratosis palmaris et planaris associated with carcinoma of the esophagus.

Howel-Evans, W., *et al.* Carcinoma of the esophagus with keratosis palmaris et plantaris (tylosis): A study in two families. *Q. J. Med.,* 1958, 27:413.

HOWES

Howes-Pallister-Landor syndrome. See *Landor-Pallister syndrome.*

HOWSHIP, JOHN (British physician, 1781-1841)

Howship-Romberg syndrome. Synonym: *neuralgia obturatoria.*

Neuralgic pain in the leg secondary to obturator hernia.

Howship, J. *Practical remarks on the discrimination and appearance of surgical disease.* London, Churchill, 1840. *Romberg, M. H., von. In: Dieffenbach, ed. *Operativer Chirurgie.* Leipzig, 1848.

HOYT, W. F. (American physician)

Hoyt-Kaplan-Brumbach syndrome. See *septo-optic dysplasia.*

HOZAY, JEAN (French neurologist)

Hozay syndrome. See *van Bogaert-Hozay syndrome.*

van Bogaert-Hozay syndrome. See *under van Bogaert.*

HPS. See ***H**ermansky-**P**udlak **s**yndrome.*

HR (**h**ypophosphatemic **r**ickets). See *hypophosphatasia syndrome, and see hypophosphatemic familial rickets*

HRS. See ***h**epato**r**enal **s**yndrome.*

HRSD (**H**i**r**sch**s**prung **d**isease). See *Hirschsprung syndrome.*

HRUBY

Hruby-Irvine-Gass syndrome. See *Irvine-Gass syndrome.*

HS. See ***H**aber **s**yndrome.*

HS. See ***H**egglin **s**yndrome.*

HS. See ***H**orner **s**yndrome.*

HS. See ***h**ypereosinophilic **s**yndrome.*

HS (**H**enoch-**S**chönlein) syndrome. See *Schönlein-Henoch purpura.*

HS (**h**ereditary **s**pherocytosis). See *Minkowski-Chauffard syndrome.*

HS (**H**urler **s**yndrome). See *mucopolysaccharidosis I-H.*

HSA (**h**yperosmnia-**s**leep **a**pnea) **syndrome.** See *sleep apnea-hypersomnelence syndrome.*

HSAN-IV (**h**ereditary **s**ensory and **a**utonomic **n**europathy-IV). See *Swanson syndrome.*

HSC. See ***H**and-**S**chüller-**C**hristian syndrome.*

HSS. See ***H**allermann-**S**treiff **s**yndrome.*

HSS. See ***H**allervorden-**S**patz **s**yndrome.*

HSS (**H**enoch-**S**chönlein **s**yndrome). See *Schönlein-Henoch purpura.*

HSSCC (**h**ereditary **s**ite-**s**pecific **c**olon **c**ancer). See *under hereditary nonpolyposis colorectal cancer syndrome.*

HÜBNER, OTTO (German physician)

Nierhoff-Hübner syndrome. See *under Nierhoff.*

HUCHARD, HENRI (French physician, 1844-1910)

Huchard ataxia. Hysterical ataxia.

Huchard, H. Caractère, moeurs, état mental des hystériques. *Arch. Neur., Paris,* 1882, 3:187-211.

Huchard disease. Prolonged arterial hypertension, thought to be a cause of arteriosclerosis.

Huchard, H. Principales causes de l'artério-sclérose. *Rev. Gen. Clin. Ther., Paris,* 1909, 23:322-5.

HUCK FINN. See HUCKLEBERRY FINN

HUCKLEBERRY FINN. (The central character in the "Adventures of Huckleberry Finn." by S. L. Clemens (Mark Twain)

Huck Finn syndrome (1 and 2). See *Huckleberry Finn syndrome (1 and 2).*

Huckleberry Finn syndrome (1). Synonyms: *Huck Finn syndrome, persistent truancy, truancy syndrome.*

The condition or act of shirking or neglecting one's duties or obligations, as when staying away from school without permission, arising from parental rejection, feelings of rejection, and superior intelligence.

Rodin, A. E., & Key, J. D.*Encyclopedia of medical eponyms derived from literary characters.* Melbourne, Fl., Robert E. Krieger, 1989. Andriola, J. Truancy syndrome. *Am. J. Orthopsychiat.,* 1946, 16:174-6.

Huckleberry Finn syndrome (2). Synonym: *Huck Finn syndrome.*

Social and psychological maladjustment of normal or bright children of retarded parents.

O'Neill, A. M. Normal and bright children of mentally retarded parents: The Huck Finn syndrome. *Child Psychiat. Hum. Dev.*, 1985, 15:255-68.

HUDSON, ARTHUR CYRIL (British ophthalmologist, 1875-1962)

Hudson line. See *Hudson-Stähli line.*

Hudson-Stähli line. Synonyms: *Hudson line, Stähli line, linea corneae senilis, superficial senile line.*

A greenish, brownish, or yellowish pigmented line occurring in apparently normal eyes in the elderly, as well as in some pathological conditions in both old and young persons. The line may be seen horizontally slightly below the center of the cornea. Hemosiderin is the suspected cause of pigmentation. The line generally corresponds to a tear in the Bowman membrane, although some cases were observed without apparent changes in the membrane of the stroma. Degenerative changes, exposure, and action of the lids are the suspected pathogenic factors in senile cases.

Stähli, J. Über den Fleischerschen Ring beim Keratokonus und eine neue typelpigmentation der normalen Kornea. *Klin. Mbl. Augenh.*, 1918, 60:721-41. *Hudson, A. C. A note on certain peculiar pigmentary markings of the cornea. *Roy. London Ophth. Hosp. Rep.*, 1911, 18:198.

HUET, G. J. (Dutch physician, born 1879)

Pelger-Huët anomaly. See *under Pelger.*

Pelger-Huët phenomenon. See *Pelger-Huët anomaly.*

HUGHES, JOHN PATTERSON (British physician)

Hughes-Stovin syndrome. A combination of thrombosis of the pulmonary arteries and peripheral veins, including the vena cava, veins of the limbs, jugular vein, superior sagittal sinus, and right side of the heart. The symptoms usually include headache, fever, cough, hemoptysis, and papilledema.

Hughes, J. P., & Stovin, P. G. I. Segmental pulmonary artery aneurysm with peripheral venous thrombosis. *Brit. J. Dis. Chest*, 1959, 53:19-27.

HUGHLINGS JACKSON. See JACKSON, JOHN HUGHLINGS

HUGUENIN, GUSTAV (Swiss physician, 1841-1920)

Huguenin edema. Acute brain edema.

Huguenin, G. Über Hirnoedem. *Corresp. Schweiz. Arzte*, 1889, 19:321-30.

HUGUIER, PIERRE CHARLES (French physician, 1804-1873)

Huguier-Jersild syndrome. Synonyms: *Jersild syndrome, anorectogenital elephantiasis, elephantiasis genitoanorectalis, elephantiasis genitorectalis, genitoanorectal elephantiasis.*

Lymphedema of the rectal and external genital regions, frequently with stricture of the anus and introitus vaginae, caused by syphilis, gonorrhea, ulcers, or lymphogranuloma venereum.

Huguier, P. C. Mémoire sur l'esthiomène ou dartre rongeante de la région vulvo-anale. *Mem. Acad. Nat. Méd., Paris*, 1849, 14:501-96. Jersild, O. Elephantiasis genitoanorectalis. *Derm. Wschr.*, 1933, 96:433-8.

humeroperoneal neuromuscular disease. See *scapuloperoneal syndrome.*

humeroscapular periarthrosis. See *Forestier syndrome (1).*

HÜNERMANN, CARL (German physician)

Conradi-Hünermann syndrome. See *under Conradi, Erich.*

Hünermann syndrome. See *Conradi-Hünermann syndrome, under Conradi, Erich.*

HUNNER, GUY LEROY (American physician, 1868-1957)

Hunner ulcer. Synonym: *panmural fibrosis.*

Interstitial cystitis with thickening and ulceration of the bladder, occurring in menopausal women, frequently after pelvic surgery.

Hunner, G. L. Consideration on a new viewpoint on the etiology of renal tuberculosis. *Am. J. Obst. Gyn.*, 1932, 24:703-28.

HUNT, ANDREW DICKSON, JR. (American physician, born 1915)

Hunt epilepsy. Synonym: *pyridoxine-dependent epilepsy.*

Infantile epileptic convulsions caused by pyridoxine-deficient diets.

Hunt, A. D., *et al.* Pyridoxine dependency: Report of a case of intractable convulsions in an infant controlled by pyridoxine. *Pediatrics*, 1954, 14:140-5.

HUNT, JAMES RAMSAY (American neurologist, 1872-1937)

Hunt disease. See *Hunt syndrome (3).*

Hunt paralysis. Synonyms: *Ramsay Hunt paralysis, corpus striatum syndrome, juvenile paralysis agitans, pallidal atrophy, pallidopyramidal disease, paralysis agitans juvenilis.*

A variant of the Parkinson syndrome, caused by degeneration of the globus pallidus, with onset between the ages of 13 and 30 years. The symtoms resemble those of the adult form of parkinsonism. Involvement of the substantia nigra and the pyramidal tracts may occur.

Hunt, J. R. Progressive atrophy of the globus pallidus (primary atrophy of the pallidal system). A system disease of the paralysis agitans type, characterized by atrophy of the motor cells of the corpus striatum. A contribution to the function of the corpus striatum. *Brain*, 1917, 40:58-148.

Hunt syndrome (1). Synonyms: *Ramsay Hunt syndrome (RHS), dentate cerebellar ataxia, dentatorubral atrophy, dyssynergia cerebellaris myoclonica (DCM), dyssynergia cerebellaris progressiva.*

A syndrome in which the most characteristic symptom is intention tremor that generally begins locally in one extremity and spreads gradually, eventually involving the entire voluntary motor system. Unsteady gait, errors in estimating the range, direction, and force of voluntary movements; muscular hypotonia; asthenia; and adiadochokinesia are associated. Convulsions and myoclonic jerks may also occur. Loss of cells in the dentate nuclei, degeneration of the red nuclei, and demyelination of the brachium conjunctivum are the principal pathological findings. The average age of onset is 30 years. When myoclonus epilepsy is associated, the syndrome is referred to as **dyssynergia cerebellaris myoclonica**.

Hunt, J. R. Dyssynergia cerebellaris myoclonica-primary atrophy of the dentate system. A contribution to the pathology and symptomatology of the cerebellum. *Brain*, 1921, 44:490-538.

Hunt syndrome (2). Synonyms: *Ramsay Hunt syndrome (RHS), cephalic zoster syndrome, geniculate ganglion syndrome, geniculate neuralgia, geniculate syndrome, herpes zoster auricularis, herpes zoster oticus, herpes zoster syndrome.*

Herpes zoster infection of the geniculate ganglion with involvement of the external ear and oral mucosa. The symptoms include facial paralysis; severe pain of the external auditory meatus and pinna (geniculate neuralgia); vesicular eruption in the peritonsillar region, oropharynx, and tongue; decreased salivation; hoarseness; loss of sensation in the face; tinnitus; decreased lacrimation; hearing disorder; and vertigo.

Hunt, J. R. On herpetic inflammation of the geniculate ganglion. A new syndrome and its complications. *J. Nerv. Ment. Dis.*, 1907, 34:73-96.

Hunt syndrome (3). Synonyms: *Hunt disease, Ramsay Hunt syndrome (RHS), artisan's palsy, metal turner's paralysis.*

Occupational compression neuritis of the deep palmar branch of the ulnar nerve. See also *overuse syndrome.*

Hunt, J. R. Occupational neuritis of the deep palmar branch of the ulnar nerve. *J. Nerv. Ment. Dis.*, 1908, 35:673-89.

Ramsay Hunt paralysis. See *Hunt paralysis.*

Ramsay Hunt syndrome (RHS) (1, 2, and 3). See *Hunt syndrome (1, 2, and 3).*

HUNT, WILLIAM EDWARD (American physician, born 1921)

Tolosa-Hunt ophthalmoplegia. See *Tolosa-Hunt syndrome.*

Tolosa-Hunt syndrome (THS). See *under Tolosa.*

HUNTER, ALASDAIR G. W. (Canadian physician)

Hunter-Fraser syndrome. A hereditary syndrome, transmitted as an autosomal dominant trait with reduced penetrance, exhibiting mental retardation; characteristic facial appearance with microcephaly, a small oval face, almond-shaped eyes, blepharoptosis, small nose, and small downturned mouth; minor acroskeletal anomalies; and, less commonly, craniosynostosis, heart defects, and limited elbow extension. X-ray findings show cone epiphyses and shortness of the middle, second, and fifth phalanges, shortening of the distal phalanges and thumbs, and hypoplasia of the distal phalanges.

Hunter, A. G. W., McAlpine, P. J., Rudd, N. L., & Fraser, F. C. A "new" syndrome of mental retardation with characteristic facies and brachyphalangy. *J. Med. Genet.*, 1977, 14:430-7.

HUNTER, CHARLES (British physician, 1872-1955)

Hunter syndrome. See *mucopolysaccharidosis II.*

HUNTER, JOHN (British physician, 1728-1793)

Hunter chancre. Synonyms: *hard chancre, hunterian chancre, indurated chancre.*

A firm, elevated papule of the penis, vulva, or cervix in primary syphilis.

*Hunter, J. *A treatise on the venereal disease.* London, 1786.

HUNTER, WILLIAM (British physician, 1861-1937)

Hunter glossitis. Synonyms: *atrophic glossitis, bald tongue of pernicious anemia.*

A condition of the tongue, seen in pernicious anemia, characterized by glossitis, glossodynia, glossopyrosis, and altered sense of taste, which may undergo spontaneous remission but invariably reappears. The pain and burning sensation are usually confined to the tongue, but may also extend to other parts of the oral mucosa. Ultimately, the tongue becomes atrophied and assumes a beefy red color and a smooth shiny appearance, sometimes with small ulcers spreading over its surface.

Hunter, W. Further observations on pernicious anemia (severe cases): A chronic infective disease: Its relation to infection from the mouth and stomach; suggested serum treatment. *Lancet*, 1900, 1:221-4; 296-9; 371-7.

hunterian chancre. See *Hunter chancre, under Hunter, John.*

HUNTINGTON, GEORGE (American physician, 1850-1916)

Huntington chorea. Synonyms: *Huntington disease (HD), Huntington syndrome, Lund-Huntington chorea, chorea chronica progressiva, chorea chronica progressiva hereditaria, degenerative chorea, hereditary chorea, microcellular striatal syndrome, progressive chorea.*

A rare familial neurological disease, usually occurring during the fourth or fifth decade, marked by progressive development of grimacing, gesticulation, ataxic movements, finger twitching, dysarthria, speech disorders, rigidity without involuntary movement, and akinesia. The face, arms, and trunk are initially affected by the choreic movement. Mental symptoms include dullness, indifference, memory lapses, impulsiveness, anxiety, euphoria, depression, and general mental deterioration. The classic choreic form is usually one of abnormal involuntary movements (chorea) accompanied by intellectual impairment and various psychiatric disturbances. The rigid form involves muscular rigidity, slowness of movement, tremor, the bend-forward posture similar to that in Parkinson disease, and mental deterioration. The syndrome is transmitted as an autosomal dominant trait.

Huntington, G. On chorea. *Med. Surg. Reporter, Philadelphia*, 1872, 26:317-21. *Lund, J. C. Chorea Sti Viti i Saetersdalen Uddrag af Distrikslaege J. C. Lunds Meidicinalberetnig for 1860. *Norges officielle statistickk.* 1882. C. No. 4.

Huntington disease (HD). See *Huntington chorea.*

Huntington syndrome. See *Huntington chorea.*

Lund-Huntington chorea. See *Huntington chorea.*

HUNTLEY, CAROLYN COKER (American physician, born 1924)

Wiskott-Aldrich-Huntley syndrome. See *Wiskott-Aldrich syndrome.*

HUPPERT, KARL HUGO (German physiologist, 1832-1904)

Huppert disease. See *Kahler disease.*

HURLER, GERTRUD (German physician, 1889-1965)

Caffey pseudo-Hurler syndrome. See *gangliosidosis G_{M1} type I.*

compound Hurler-Scheie disease. See *mucopolysaccharidosis I-H/S.*

forme fruste of Hurler syndrome. See *mucopolysaccharidosis I-S.*

Hurler disease. See *mucopolysaccharidosis I-H.*

Hurler syndrome (HS). See *mucopolysaccharidosis I-H.*

Hurler-like syndrome. See *gangliosidosis G_{M1} type I.*

Hurler-Scheie syndrome. See *mucopolysaccharidosis I-H/S.*

Pfaundler-Hurler syndrome. See *mucopolysaccharidosis I-H.*

pseudo-Hurler polydystrophy. See *mucolipidosis III.*

pseudo-Hurler syndrome. See *gangliosidosis G_{M1} type I.*

Spät-Hurler syndrome. See *mucopolysaccharidosis I-S.*

HURST, EDWARD WESTON (Australian physician)

Hurst disease. Synonym: *leukoencephalitis acuta hemorrhagica.*

An acute type of hemorrhagic leukoencephalitis occurring in hitherto healthy persons, usually 30 to 40 years of age. A respiratory tract infection may precede the onset, and after a fulminant course the patient becomes comatous and death takes place within a few days. Histologically, the changes are localized in the white matter of the brain, and are characterized by hemorrhages, perivascular leukocyte infiltrations, fibrinoid vascular degeneration, and demyelination.

Hurst, E. W. Acute haemorrhagic leukoencephalitis: Previously undefined entity. *Med. J. Australia*, 1941, 2:1-6.

HUS. See *hemolytic-uremic syndrome.*

husband abuse. See *battered spouse syndrome.*

husband beating. See *battered spouse syndrome.*

HUTCHINSON, JONATHAN, JR. (British ophthalmologist)

Siegrist-Hutchinson syndrome. See *under Siegrist.*

HUTCHINSON, SIR JONATHAN (British physician, 1828-1913)

Hutchinson disease (1). Synonyms: *angioma serpiginosum, infectious angioma, nevus infectiosus, nevus lupus.*

A skin disease characterized by minute vascular ectasias appearing as compressible red or purple punctate lesions, arranged in a serpiginous pattern. The lesions usually occur symmetrically on the extremities. The fundamental lesion is a dilatation of a small vessel of the papillary or subpapillary regions of the skin. Onset, in most instances, is before the age of 16 years, and females are usually affected.

*Hutchinson, J. *A peculiar form of serpiginous and infective naevoid disease*. 1889.

Hutchinson disease (2). Synonyms: *Hutchinson-Tay choroiditis, Tay choroiditis, Tay disease, choroiditis guttata senilis.*

A senile degeneration of the choroid marked by yellow spots around the macula lutea, resulting from atheromatous changes.

*Hutchinson, J. *Illustrations of clinical surgery*. London, Churchill, 1875, Vol. 1, pp. 49-52. *Tay, W. Symmetrical changes in the region of the yellow spot in each eye of an infant. *Tr. Opt. Soc. U.K.*, 1881, 1:55-7.

Hutchinson freckle. Synonyms: *Dubreuilh melanosis, circumscribed precancerous melanosis, dermoepidermal nevus, infectious lentigo, infective senile freckle, intraepidermal malignant melanoma, lentigo maligna, melanosis circumscripta precancerosa, melanotic freckle, precancerous melanosis, senile melanotic freckle, tardive nevus.*

A precancerous condition occurring chiefly during middle and old age. The typical lesion starts on the facial skin as a small dark brown or sepia spot. Among various macules there may be simultaneous expansion and regression, but eventually they coalesce to form irregular pigmented areas, often reaching 10 cm in diameter. Thickening, induration, papules, verrucae, and ulceration signal the onset of malignancy. The average period from onset to development of malignant melanoma is about 10 years.

Hutchinson, J. Senile freckle with deep staining-a superficial epithelioma of the cheek. *Arch. Surg., London*, 1892, 3:159. Dubreuilh, M. W. De la mélanose circonscrite précancéreuse. *Ann. Derm. Syph., Paris*, 1912, 3:129-51; 205-30.

Hutchinson incisor. See *Hutchinson teeth.*

Hutchinson melanotic disease. Synonyms: *melanotic panaritium, melanotic whitlow, subungual melanotic whitlow.*

A melanotic tumor of the nail bed associated with melanotic tissue forming under and around the nail.

Hutchinson, J. Melanotic disease of the great toe following a whitlow of the nail. *Tr. Path. Soc., London*, 1857, 8:404-5.

Hutchinson prurigo. Synonyms: *erythema perstans solare, prurigo estivalis, summer acne, summer prurigo.*

An eruption of nodular and papular, pruritic, urticarialike lesions on parts of the body exposed to the sun, usually beginning in the spring and disappearing spontaneously in the fall, reportedly described by Hutchinson.

Hutchinson teeth. Synonyms: *Hutchinson incisor, screwdriver teeth.*

A tooth abnormality seen in congenital syphilis, characterized by convergence of both lateral margins toward the incisal edge, giving the permanent incisors a screwdriverlike shape, sometimes associated with notching of the incisal edges or depressions in the labial surfaces immediately above the cutting edge.

Hutchinson, J. Report on the effects of infantile syphilis in marring the development of the teeth. *Tr. Path. Soc., London*, 1858, 9:449-55.

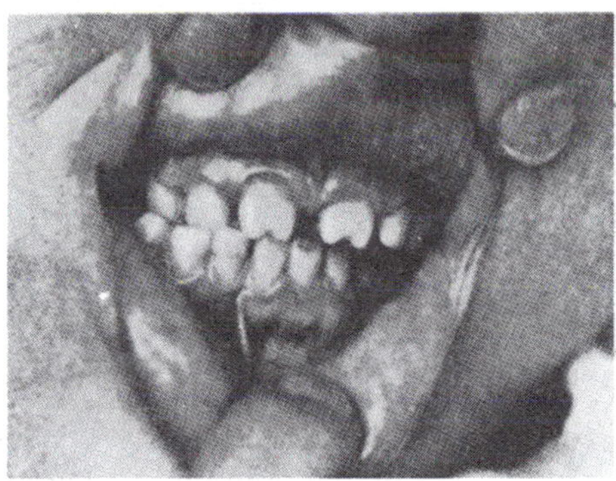

Hutchinson teeth
Nelson, W.E. (ed.): *Textbook of Pediatrics*, 9th ed.
Philadelphia: W.B. Saunders Co., 1969.

Hutchinson triad. Interstitial keratitis, deafness due to lesions of the eighth cranial nerve, and Hutchinson teeth in congenital syphilis.

Hutchinson, J. On the different forms of inflammation of the eye consequent to inherited syphilis. *Ophth. Hosp. Rep.*, 1858, 1:191-203; 226-44; 1859, 2:54-105; 1860, 3:258-83.

Hutchinson-Boeck disease. See *Besnier-Boeck-Schaumann syndrome.*

Hutchinson-Boeck granulomatosis. See *Besnier-Boeck-Schaumann syndrome.*

Hutchinson-Gilford progeria. See *Hutchinson-Gilford syndrome.*

Hutchinson-Gilford progeria syndrome (HGPS). See *Hutchinson-Gilford syndrome.*

Hutchinson-Gilford syndrome. Synonyms: *Gilford syndrome, Hutchinson-Gilford progeria, Hutchinson-Gilford progeria syndrome (HGPS), premature aging syndrome, premature senility syndrome, progeria syndrome, senilism syndrome.*

Pseudosenility characterized mainly by a birdlike, old facial appearance and dwarfism. After an apparently normal development during the first year of life, the face assumes peculiar characteristics, marked by sclerodermalike skin, midfacial cyanosis, subcutaneous lipodystrophy, hydrocephalic appearance (whereby the face becomes disproportionately small with frontal and parietal bossing), midfacial hypoplasia, thin lips, small thin nose, prominent scalp veins, small ears without lobes, and prominent eyes. The eyebrows and lashes are usually lost and scalp hair is replaced by a downy fuzz. Associated defects usually include delayed dentition, flexion of the knees and a "horse-riding" stance, wide-based shuffling gait, coxa valga, acro-osteolysis of the phalanges, delicate and osteoporotic bones, limited extension of the small joints because of periarticular fibrosis, cardiac murmurs, hypertension, atherosclerosis, cerebrovascular accidents, open cranial sutures, persistent frontanels, thin clavicles, and occasional onychodystrophy, high-pitched voice, and decreased sweating. The syndrome is transmitted as a genetic trait but the mode of inheritance is unknown. See also *Werner syndrome,*. under *Werner, Otto,* and *Souques-Charcot geroderma.*

Hutchinson, J. Case of congenital absence of hair with atrophic condition of the skin and its appendages. *Lancet*, 1886, 1:923. Gilford, H. Progeria; a form of senilism. *Practitioner, London*, 1904, 73:188-217.

Hutchinson-Horton syndrome. Horton disease (1), consisting of inflammation of the temporal and other cranial arteries, associated with involvement of the large arteries, including the aorta and its major branches.

Horton, B. T., *et al.* Arteritis of the temporal vessels. A previously undesribed form. *Arch. Intern. Med., Chicago*, 1934, 53:400-9. *Hutchinson, J. Diseases of the arteries. I. On a peculiar form of thrombotic form of thrombotic arteritis of the aged which is sometimes productive of gangrene. *Arch. Surg.*, 1889, 1:323.

Hutchinson-Tay choroiditis. See *Hutchinson disease (2).*

Hutchinson-Weber-Peutz syndrome. See *Peutz-Jeghers syndrome.*

HUTCHINSON, SIR ROBERT GRIEVE (British physician, 1871-1943)

Hutchinson disease. Synonyms: *Abercrombie tumor, Parker syndrome, Pepper disease, Smith syndrome, adrenal medullary neuroblastoma, adrenalin-secreting neuroblastoma, gangliosympathicoblastoma, malignant hypernephroma, neuroblastoma sympathicum embryonale, suprarenal sarcoma, sympathicoma, sympathogonioma, sympathoma embryonale.*

A malignant tumor usually observed in children and adolescents. The adrenal gland is the usual site, but other organs, especially those in the abdominal and thoracic cavities, may be affected. The tumors are gray or purplish-gray, soft, lobular lesions about 80 to 150 gm in weight. Histologically, they are characterized by clusters of small and dark cells without any particular pattern, although rosettes are formed by typical lesions. Metastases to the liver, lungs, and bones are common. Earlier theories that tumors of the right adrenal gland tend to metastasize to the liver **(Pepper syndrome)** and tumors of the left adrenal metastasize to the skull **(Hutchinson disease)** are no longer supported. Elevated levels of epinephrine, norepinephrine, and their metabolites are usually found in the urine.

Hutchinson, R. On suprarenal sarcoma in children with metastases to the skull. *Q. J. Med., Oxford*, 1907, 1:33-8. Smith, J. Case of adrenal neuroblastoma. *Lancet*, 1932, 2:1214-5. Pepper, W. A study of congenital sarcoma of the liver and suprarenal, with a report of a case. *Am. J. Med. Sc.*, 1901, 121:287-99. Abercrombie, J. Multiple sarcomata of the cranial bones. *Tr. Path. Sc. London*, 1880, 31:216-23. Parker, R. W. Diffuse sarcoma of the liver, probably congenital. *Tr. Path. Soc. London*, 1880, 31:290-3.

HUTINEL, VICTOR HENRI (French physician, 1849-1933)

Hutinel cirrhosis. Synonyms: *Hutinel disease, cardiotuberculous cirrhosis of the liver.*

Cirrhosis of the liver associated with tuberculous pericarditis in children.

Hutinel. Cirrhoses cardiaques et cirrhoses tuberculeuses chez l'efant. *Rev. Mens. Mal Enf.*, 1893, 11:529-74; 1894, 12:15-25.

Hutinel disease (1). Synonym: *infectious erythema.*

Erythema due to an infection. See also *Sticker disease.*

Hutinel, V. H. Notes sur quelques erythemes infectieux. *Arch. Gén. Méd., Paris*, 1892, 2:263-91; 385-403.

Hutinel disease (2). See *Hutinel cirrhosis.*

Hutinel-Pick syndrome. See *Pick disease, under Pick, Friedel.*

HVS. See ***h**yper**v**entilation **s**yndrome.*

HVS. See ***h**yper**v**iscosity **s**yndrome.*

hyaline disease of the lungs. See *neonatal respiratory distress syndrome.*

hyaline membrane disease (HMD). See *neonatal respiratory distress syndrome.*

hyalinosis cutis et mucosae. See *Urbach-Wiethe syndrome.*

hydantoin syndrome. See *fetal hydatoin syndrome.*

hydatid fremitus. See *Blatin syndrome.*

HYDE, JAMES NEVIN (American dermatologist, 1840-1910)

Hyde syndrome. Synonyms: *eczema verrucosum callosum, lichen corneus disseminatus, lichen corneus obtusus, lichen ruber obtusus, lichen ruber obtusus corneus, neurodermatitis nodulosa, nodular lichenification, nodular prurigo, prurigo nodularis, tuberosis cutis pruriginosa, urticaria perstans verrucosa.*

A severe, pruritic, nodular and verrucous skin eruption consisting of lesions 3 to 10 mm in diameter, usually found in adult women on the back, extremities, and thighs. Scratching causes furrowing and hemorrhage from the nodules.

Hyde, J. N. *A practical treatise on disease of the skin, for the use of students and practitioners.* 3rd ed. Philadelphia, Lea & Febiger, 1883.

hydroa herpetiformis. See *Duhring disease.*

hydroa pruriginosa. See *Duhring disease.*

hydrocephaloid affection. See *Hall syndrome, under Hall, Marshall.*

hydrocephalus, X-linked. See *Bickers-Adams syndrome.*

hydrocystoma mammae. See *Cheatle disease.*

hydrolethalus syndrome. Synonym: *Salonen-Herva-Norio syndrome.*

A lethal syndrome, transmitted as an autosomal recessive trait, characterized by hydrocephalus, occipital bone defect, small mandible, cleft lip and palate, small anomalous tongue, small and deep-set eyes, anomalous nose, low-set malformed ears, laryngo-

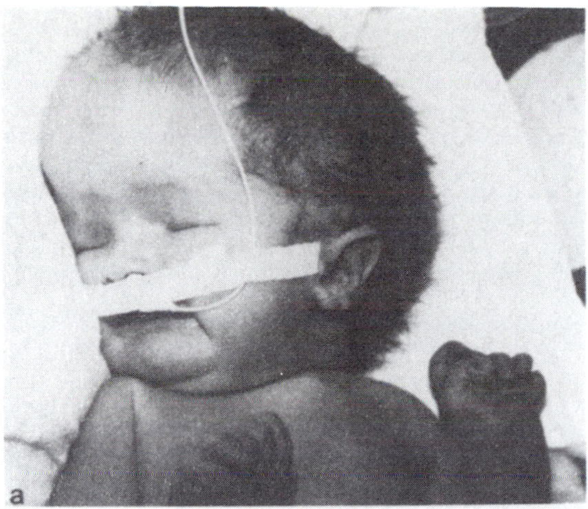

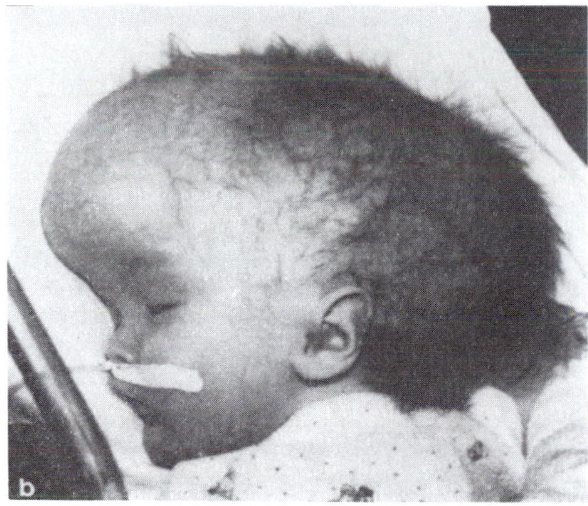

Hydrolethalus syndrome
Aughton, David J. & Suzanne B. Cassidy, *American Journal of Medical Genetics* 27:935-942, 1987. New York: Alan R. Liss, Inc.

tracheo-bronchial abnormalities, defective lung lobation, congenital heart defect, abnormal kidneys, abnormal genitalia (including uterus duplex/bicornis), polydactyly of the fingers and toes, and club foot. Most infants are stillborn, those who are born alive die shortly after birth.

Salonen, R., Herva, R., & Norio, R. The hydrolethalus syndrome: delineation of a "new," lethal malformation syndrome based on 28 patients. *Clin. Genet.*, 1981, 19:321-30.

hydrometrocolpos-polydactyly syndrome. See *McKusick-Kaufman syndrome.*

hydromyelia. See *Morvan disease.*

hydrops congenitus. See *Schridde syndrome.*

17-α-hydroxylase deficiency syndrome (17-OHDS). A syndrome of pseudohermaphroditism in males, amenorrhea with underdeveloped breasts in females, absence of pubic hair, hypertension, and hypokalemia due to 17-α-hydroxylase deficiency.

New, M. I. Male pseudohermaphroditism due to 17-alpha-hydroxylase deficiency. *J. Clin. Invest.*, 1970, 49:1930-41. Scaroni, C., *et al.* Renin-angiotensin-aldosterone system: A long-term follow-up study in 17-alpha-hydroxylase deficiency syndrome (17OHDS). *Clin. Exp. Hypertens. [A]*, 1986, 8:773-80.

hygromatosis lipocalcinogranulomatosa progressiva. See *Teutschländer syndrome.*

hyoid syndrome. See *Eagle syndrome, under Eagle, Watt Weems.*

hyper-IgE (HIE) syndrome. See *Job syndrome.*

hyperabduction syndrome. Synonyms: *Wright syndrome, perabduction syndrome, pectoralis minor syndrome, subcoracoid-pectoralis minor syndrome.*

Compression of the brachial plexus and the axillary artery and vein at the point where the pectoralis minor tendon inserts into the coronoid process of the scapula when the arm is hyperabducted, causing paresthesia and pain in the hand and arm. Sleeping or working with the arm above the head is believed to aggravate this disorder.

Wright, I. S. The neurovascular syndrome produced by perabduction of the arms. The immediate change produced in 150 normal controls, and the effects of some persons of prolonged hyperabduction of the arms, as in sleeping, and in certain occupations. *Am. Heart J.*, 1945, 29:1-19.

hyperactive behavior syndrome. See *attention deficit-hyperactivity disorder.*

hyperactive carotid sinus syndrome. See *carotid sinus syndrome.*

hyperactive child. See *attention deficit-hyperactivity disorder.*

hyperactive child syndrome. See *attention deficit-hyperactivity disorder.*

hyperactive syndrome. See *attention deficit-hyperactivity disorder.*

hyperammonemia (I and II). See *under hyperammonemic syndrome.*

hyperammonemia-hyperornithinemia-homocitrullinuria (HHH) syndrome. An amino acid metabolism disorder, transmitted as an autosomal recessive trait, characterized by simultaneously occurring hyperammonemia, hyperornithinemia, and homocitrullinuria. Seizures and mental retardation are the main clinical features. Diminished ornithine transport into mitochondria with ornithine accumulation in the cytoplasm and diminished ability to clear carbamoyl phosphate and ammonia loads are the basic causative factors.

Shih, V. E., *et al.* Hyperornithinemia, hyperammonemia and homocitrullinuria. A new disorder of amino acid metabolism associated with myoclonic seizures and mental retardation. *Am. J. Dis. Child.*, 1969, 117:83-92.

hyperammonemic syndrome. Elevated blood ammonia levels occurring as the result of disorders of ammonia metabolism in liver diseases, inborn deficiencies of urea cycle enzymes, disorders of ornithine and lysine metabolism, inborn errors of branched-chain amino acid catabolism, and deficiences of dietary proteins in susceptible individuals. Constipation and febrile illness are some of the contributing factors. Neurological disorders, the principal features of ammonia poisoning, include mental deficiency, episodic stupor, cerebral atrophy, brain edema, ventricular dilatation, headache, disruption of neuronal microtubules, changes in Alzheimer type II astrocyte nuclei, decerebrate rigidity with or without seizures, and coma. Alkalosis, fever, hypoxia, hyperglycemia, irritability, muscle hypertonia alternating with hypotonia, and sometimes hepatomegaly are associated. There are several forms of this syndrome, but ornithine transcarbamylase deficiency and carbamyl phosphate synthetase deficiency are considered the principal ones. Ornithine transcarbamylase deficiency (hyperammonemia I, OTC deficiency, ornithine carbamyl transferase deficiency), a hereditary disorder transmitted as an autosomal X-linked trait, is characterized by hyperammonemia, increased blood glutamine concentration, and increased urinary excretion of orotic acid. The affected infants appear normal at birth but shortly become lethargic and develop feeding problems, failure to thrive, rapid respiration, altered muscle tone, convulsions, and sometimes hypothermia. Respiratory distress and death usually follow within the first week of life. **Carbamyl phosphate synthetase (CPS) deficiency syndrome (hyperammonemia II, CPS deficiency syndrome)**, a rapidly fatal hereditary disorder transmitted as an autosomal recessive trait, is characterized by hyperammonemia, increased concentrations of blood alanine and glutamine, and normal orotic acid excretion. Clinical features consist of protein intolerance, vomiting, lethargy, mental retardation, central nervous system disorders, and terminal coma. Some authors classify OTC and CPS deficiencies as hyperammonemia I and II, respectively; others refer to OTC as hyperammonemia II and CPS as hyperammonemia I.

Freeman, J. M., *et al.* Ammonia intoxication due to a congenital defect of urea synthesis. *J. Pediat.*, 1964, 65:1039-40. Russell, A., *et al.* Hyperammonaemia. A new instance of an inborn enzymatic defect of the biosynthesis of urea. *Lancet*, 1962, 2:699-700. Shih, V. E. Urea cycle disorders and other hyperammonemic syndromes. In: Stanbury, J. B., Wyngaarden, J. B., & Fredrickson, D. S., eds. *The metabolic basis of inherited disease.* 4th ed. New York, McGraw-Hill, 1978, pp. 362-86.

hyperandrogenism-insulin resistance-acanthosis nigricans syndrome. See *HAIR-AN syndrome.*

hyperbilirubinemia I. See *Gilbert syndrome, under Gilbert, Nicolas Augustin.*

hyperbilirubinemia II. See *Dubin-Johnson syndrome.*

hypercalcemia-hypocalciuria syndrome. See *familial hypercalcemia-hypocalciuria syndrome.*

hyperchloremic acidosis with nephrocalcinosis. See *Lightwood-Albright syndrome.*

hyperchlorhydria. See *Rossbach disease.*

hypercholesterinemic xanthomatosis. See *Bürger-Grütz syndrome.*

hypercholesterolemia-xanthomatosis syndrome. See *Harbitz-Müller disease.*

hyperchondroplasia. See *Marfan syndrome (1).*

hypercorticism. See *Cushing syndrome.*

hypercortisolism. See *Cushing syndrome.*

hyperdynamic beta-adrenergic circulatory state. See *hyperkinetic heart syndrome.*

hyperemesis hiemis. See *Spencer disease.*

hyperemia of the ovary. See *Taylor syndrome, under Taylor, Howard Canning, Jr.*

hypereosinophilic syndrome (HES, HS). A disorder of unknown cause, characterized by the presence in the blood of more than 1500 eosinophils per cc for longer than 6 months. The disease occurs mainly in males 20 to 50 years of age. Fever, weight loss, anorexia, fatique, malaise, and skin rash are the principal symptoms. Other abnormalities include the following disorders in a descending order of frequency: Löffler endomyocardial fibrosis, cardiovascular complications (arrhythmia, pericarditis, thromboembolic disease in medium to large blood vessels, endocardial thrombi), lymph node enlargement, splenomegaly, ocular complications (retinal and choroidal vascular occlusion, disorders of ocular fixation), excessive sweating, gastrointestinal disorders (diarrhea, malabsorption, enteritis), central nervous system lesions (poor coordination, hemiplegia, Balint syndrome, cerebral thrombosis and embolism, and cranial myeloblastoma), pulmonary involvement (cough, sparse but viscous sputum, susceptibility to infection) muscle pain and weakness due to eosinophilic myositis and perimyositis, renal impairment (proteinuria, hypertension, interstitial fibrosis, tubular atrophy, glomerular lesions), splenic infarction, and joint disease (pain, stiffness, effusions). Pathological findings usually show perineutrophilic infiltrates and a high percentage of nucleated cells in the bone marrow (eosinophils in all stages of maturation).

Griffin, H. Z. Persistent eosinophilia with hyperleukocytosis and splenomegaly. *Am. J. Med. Sc.*, 1919, 158:618-29. Hardy, W. R., & Anderson, R. E. The hypereosinophilic syndromes. *Ann. Intern. Med.*, 1968, 68:1220-9. Spry, C. J. The hypereosinophilic syndrome: Clinical features, laboratory findings and treatment. *Allergy*, 1982, 37:539-51.

hyperexplexia. See *hereditary startle syndrome.*

hyperextension-hyperflexion syndrome. See *whiplash syndrome.*

hypergammaglobulinemic hepatitis. See *Bearn-Kunkel syndrome.*

hyperglobulinemic purpura. See *Waldenström syndrome (2), under Waldenström, Jan Gösta.*

hyperglobulinemic purpura syndrome. See *Waldenström syndrome (2), under Waldenström, Jan Gösta.*

hyperimmunoglobulin E recurrent infection syndrome. See *Job syndrome.*

hyperimmunoglobulinemia E syndrome. See *Job syndrome.*

hyperinsulinism syndrome. See *Harris syndrome, under Harris, Seale.*

hyperkalemic periodic paralysis. See *Gamstorp syndrome.*

hyperkeratosis excentrica. See *Mibelli disease (2).*

hyperkeratosis follicularis et parafollicularis in cutem penetrans. See *Kyrle disease.*

hyperkeratosis follicularis et parafollicularis penetrans. See *Kyrle disease.*

hyperkeratosis lenticularis perstans (HLP). See *Flegel disease.*

hyperkeratosis palmaris et plantaris. See *Unna-Thost syndrome, under Unna, Paul Gerson.*

hyperkeratosis palmoplantaris climacterica. See *Haxthausen syndrome.*

hyperkeratosis palmoplantaris-gingival hyperkeratosis syndrome. A syndrome, transmitted as an autosomal dominant trait, combining keratinization of the attached labial and lingual gingivae and keratosis palmaris et plantaris. Hyperhidrosis may be associated.

Raphael, A. L., *et al.* Hyperkeratosis of gingival and plantar surfaces. *Periodontics*, 1968, 6:118-20.

hyperkeratosis palmoplantaris-periodontoclasia syndrome. See *Papillon-Lefèvre syndrome.*

hyperkeratosis penetrans. See *Kyrle disease.*
hyperkinemia. See *hyperkinetic heart syndrome.*

hyperkinetic syndrome. See *attention deficit disorder-hyperactivity disorder.*

hyperkinetic heart syndrome. Synonyms: *hyperdynamic beta-adrenergic circulatory state, hyperkinemia.*

A syndrome of cardiac overactivity and hypercontractility characterized by an increased rate of ejection of blood with each beat, but not necessarily an increased output of blood per minute, associated with severe anxiety, which is responsive to beta-blockade.

Starr, I., & Jonas, L. Supernormal circulation in resting subjects (hyperkinemia). With a study of the relation of kinemic abnormalities to the basal metabolic rate. *Arch. Intern. Med., Chicago,* 1943, 71:1-22. Gorlin, R. The hyperkinetic heart syndrome. *JAMA,* 1962, 182:823-9.

hyperkinetic-minimal brain dysfunction syndrome. See *attention deficit-hyperactivity disorder.*

hyperlipemia-hemolytic anemia-icterus syndrome. See *Zieve syndrome.*

hyperlipoproteinemia type C-II. See *apolipoprotein C-II deficiency syndrome.*

hyperlipoproteinemia type I. See *Bürger-Grütz syndrome.*

hyperlipoproteinemia type IA. See *Bürger-Grütz syndrome.*

hyperlipoproteinemia type IB. See *apolipoprotein C-II deficiency syndrome.*

hyperlipoproteinemia type II. See *Harbitz-Müller syndrome.*

hyperlucent lung syndrome. See *Swyer-James syndrome.*

hypermetabolic hypoproteinemia. See *protein-losing gastroenteropathy.*

hypernephroid tumor. See *Grawitz tumor.*
hypernephroma. See *Grawitz tumor.*
hyperornithinemia I. See *hyperornithinemia-hyperammonemia-homocitrullinuria syndrome.*

hyperornithinemia-hyperammonemia-homocitrullinuria (HHH) syndrome. Synonym: *hyperornithinemia I.*

An amino acid metabolism disorder, transmitted as an autosomal recessive trait, characterized by hyperammonemia, homocitrullinemia, myoclonic seizures, mental retardation, and protein intolerance. It is due to diminished ornithine transport into mitochondria, with ornithine accumulation in the cytoplasm and faulty carbamoyl clearance and ammonia load. An enzymatic defect is believed to be the cause.

Shih, V. E., *et al.* Hyperornithinemia, hyperammonemia, and homocitrullinemia: A new disorder of amino acid metabolism associated with myoclonic seizures and mental retardation. *Am. J. Dis. Child.,* 1969, 117:83-92. Valle, D., & Simeli, O. The hyperornithinemias. In: Stanbury, J. B., Wyngaarden, J. B., Fredrickson, D. S., eds. *Metabolic basis of inherited disease.* 5th ed. New York, McGraw-Hill, 1983, pp. 382-401.

hyperosteogenesis periosteoenchondralis fetoinfantilis regressiva. See *Caffey-Silverman syndrome.*

hyperostosis corticalis deformans juvenilis. See *hyperphosphatasia-osteoctasia syndrome.*

hyperostosis corticalis generalisata familiaris. See *van Buchem syndrome, under Buchem, Francis Steven Peter, van.*

hyperostosis corticalis infantilis. See *Caffey-Silverman syndrome.*

hyperostosis frontalis interna. See *Morgagni-Stewart-Morel syndrome.*

hyperostosis generalisata with pachydermy syndrome. See *pachydermoperiostosis syndrome.*

hyperostotic dwarfism. See *Lenz-Majewski syndrome.*
hyperphenylalaninemia. See *phenylketonuria.*
hyperphosphatasia tarda. See *van Buchem syndrome, under Buchem, Francis Stevem Peter, van.*

hyperphosphatasia-osteoctasia syndrome. Synonyms: *Bakwin-Eiger syndrome, juvenile Paget disease, chronic hyperphosphatasia, chronic idiopathic hyperphosphatasia, chronic osteopathy-hyperphosphatasia syndrome, familial osteoctasia-macrocranium syndrome, hereditary hyperphosphatasia, hyperostosis corticalis deformans juvenilis, infantile hyperphosphatasia, osteochalasia desmalis familiaris, osteoctasia-hyperphosphatasia syndrome.*

A bone dysplasia associated with elevated serum alkaline and acid phosphatase, uric acid, and aminopeptidase, and urinary peptide-bound hydroxyproline and uric acid. The symptoms appear in late infancy and consist of small stature, hearing loss, angioid streaks of the retina, optic atrophy, hypertension, blue sclerae, dental caries, fusiform swelling and bowing of the tubular bones, and multiple fractures. Radiographic findings include bone demineralization, widening of the short tubular bones, thickening of the calvaria, replacement of cortical structures by strands of longitudinal trabeculae or thinning of the inner cortex of the bowed tubular bones, osteoporosis, prominent frontal and mastoid areas, pectus carinatum, and kyphoscoliosis. The symptoms vary, demineralization and osteoporosis being very severe in some cases and mild in others. The syndrome is transmitted as an autosomal recessive trait with variability of expression.

Bakwin, H., & Eiger, M. S. Fragile bones and macrocranium. *J. Pediat.,* 1956, 49:558-64.

hyperpigmentation-hypohidrosis syndrome. See *Naegeli syndrome, under Naegeli, Oskar.*

hyperplasia fascialis ossificans. See *fibrodysplasia ossificans progressiva.*

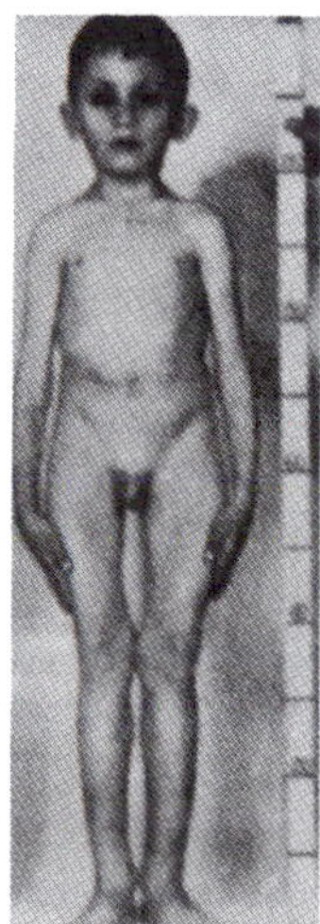
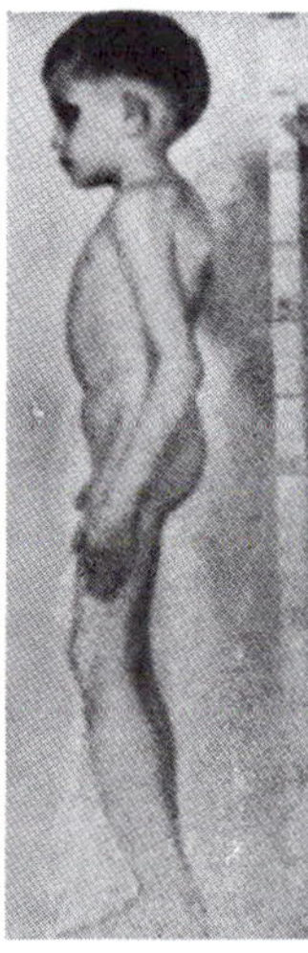

Hyperphosphatasia-osteoctasia syndrome
Andrews, G.C. & A.N. Domonkos: *Diseases of the Skin.* 5th ed. Philadelphia: W.B. Saunders Co., 1963.

hyperplasia fascialis progressiva. See *fibrodysplasia ossificans progressiva.*
hyperplastic achondroplasia. See *metatropic dwarfism syndrome.*
hyperplastic achondroplasia foetalis. See *metatropic dwarfism syndrome.*
hyperplastic osteoarthritis. See *Marie-Bamberger syndrome, under Marie, Pierre.*
hyperplastic periostosis. See *Caffey-Silverman syndrome.*
hyperplastic scleritis. See *Schöbl scleritis.*
hyperpotassemic periodic paralysis. See *Gamstorp syndrome.*
hyperprolactinemia syndrome. The presence in the blood of high levels of prolactin, usually associated with galactorrhea, ovulation and menstrual disorders, sterility, and, less commonly, intractable headache and visual disorders. Common causes of this syndrome include chronic use of psychotropic drugs, anxiolytic agents, tricyclic antidepressants, dopamine antagonists, antihypertensive agents, opiates, steroids, isoniazid, cimetidine, and disorders such as liver cirrhosis, renal failure, hypothyroidism, adrenal hyperplasia, polycystic ovary syndrome, tabes dorsalis, syringomyelia, Parkinson disease, histiocytosis X, sarcoidosis, porphyria, ectopic prolactin-releasing tumors, herpes zoster, postmastectomy complications, postthoracotomy complications, burns and abscesses involving the chest wall, pituitary adenoma, craniopharyngioma, pinealoma, meningioma, astrocytoma, encephalitis, head trauma, pseudotumor cerebri, empty sella syndrome, and neurofibromatosis.

Blackwell, R. E. Diagnosis and treatment of prolactinemic syndromes. *Obstet. Gyn. Annual,* 1985, 14:310-27.

hyperprolactinemia-amenorrhea-galactorrhea syndrome. See *amenorrhea-galactorrhea syndrome.*
hyperprolactinemic chronic anovulation syndrome. See *amenorrhea-galactorrhea syndrome.*
hypersensitive xiphoid syndrome. See *xiphoid syndrome.*
hypersensitivity angiitis. See *Zeek disease.*
hypersensitivity pneumonitis. See *Ramazzini syndrome.*
hypersomnia-bulimia syndrome. See *Kleine-Levin syndrome.*
hypersomnia-megaphagia syndrome. See *Kleine-Levin syndrome.*
hypersomnia-sleep apnea (HSA) syndrome. See *sleep apnea-hypersomnolence syndrome.*
hypertelorism. See *Greig ocular hypertelorism syndrome.*
hypertelorism-hypospadias syndrome (1). See *Elsahy-Waters syndrome.*
hypertelorism-hypospadias syndrome (2). Synonyms: *Opitz syndrome, BBB syndrome, BBG syndrome.*

A syndrome in which males have hypospadias of variable degree and hypertelorism, whereas heterozygous females display only hypertelorism. Associated defects may include mental retardation, cleft lip and palate, multiple lipomata, and cardiovascular disorders. Additional genitourinary anomalies may include cryptorchism, vesicoureteral reflux, and upper urinary tract defects. The syndrome is believed to be genetically transmitted, but the mode of inheritance is unclear. See also *Elsahy-Waters syndrome.* Some authors suggest that this and the hypospadias-dysphagia syndrome (G syndrome) represent the same entity, hence the designation ***BBBG syndrome.***

Opitz, J. M., *et al.* The BBB syndrome. Famalial telecanthus with associated congenital anomalies. *Birth Defects,* 1969, 5(2):86-94. *Christian, J. C., *et al.* Familial telecanthus with associated congeital anomalies. *Birth Defects,* 1969, 5(2):82-5. Verloes, A., *et al.* BBBG syndrome or Opitz syndrome: New family. *Am. J. Med. Genet.,* 1989, 34:313-6.

hypertelorism-microtia-clefting (HMC) syndrome. Synonym: *Bixler syndrome.*

A familial syndrome of hypertelorism, microtia, and clefts of the lip, palate, and nose, associated with psychomotor retardation, atresia of the auditory canals, microcephaly, steep mandibular angles, thenar eminence hypoplasia, kidney ectopy, and cardiovascular defects. The syndrome is believed to be transmitted as an autosomal recessive trait.

Bixler, D., Christian, J. C., & Gorlin, R. J. Hypertelorism, microtia, and facial clefting: A new inherited syndrome. *Birth Defects,* 1969, 5(2):77-81.

hypertensive diencephalic syndrome. See *Page syndrome.*
hypertensive ischemic ulcers of the leg. See *Martorell syndrome (1).*
hyperthecosis of the ovary. See *polycystic ovary syndrome.*
hyperthrombocytic myelosis. See *Mortensen disease.*
hyperthymic syndrome. See *Pende syndrome.*
hypertonic polycythemia. See *Gaisböck disease.*
hypertonic-dyskinetic syndrome. See *Zappert syndrome.*
hypertoxic schizophrenia. See *Bell mania, under Bell, Luther Vos.*
hypertrophic gastritis. See *Brinton disease.*
hypertrophic gastropathy. See *Ménétrier syndrome.*
hypertrophic interstitial neuritis. See *Déjerine-Sottas syndrome.*
hypertrophic interstitial neuropathy. See *Déjerine-Sottas syndrome.*
hypertrophic interstitial polyneuritis. See *Déjerine-Sottas syndrome.*
hypertrophic interstitial radiculoneuropathy. See *Déjerine-Sottas syndrome.*
hypertrophic liver cirrhosis. See *Hanot cirrhosis.*
hypertrophic neuritis. See *Roussy-Cornil syndrome.*
hypertrophic neuritis syndrome. See *Déjerine-Sottas syndrome.*
hypertrophic osteodermopathy. See *pachyderomoperiostosis syndrome.*
hyperventilation syndrome (HVS). Rapid irregular breathing (tachypnea) with intermittent deep sighing respiration, usually precipitated by emotional tension, resulting in low partial pressure of carbon dioxide ($PaCO_2$), low tidal carbon dioxide, and respiratory alkalosis. Associated symptoms include breathlessness, flushing, fear of the inability to breathe, vertigo, fatique, muscle weakness, tinnitus, tetany, cramps, paresthesia, emotional sweating, chest tightness, feeling of suffocation, headache, dry throat, and, sometimes, syncope.

White, P. D., & Hahn, R. G. The symptom of sighing in cardiovascular. diagnosis. With spirographic observations. *Am. J. Med. Sc.,* 1929, 177:179-88. Maytum, C. K. Tetany caused by functional dyspnea with hyperventilation: Report of a case. *Proc. Staff Meet. Mayo Clin.,* 1933, 8:282-4.

hyperviscosaemia. See *hyperviscosity syndrome.*

hyperviscosity syndrome (HVS). Synonyms: *blood hyperviscosity syndrome, hyperviscosaemia.*

A hemorheological disorder, characterized by blood flow resistance due to the presence of the formed elements of the blood, especially the red cells and plasma proteins. Other factors influencing blood viscosity include red cell aggregation, red cell internal viscosity, red cell flexibility, molecular size and shape of blood proteins, interaction of blood proteins and cellular elements, and the properties of the vascular bed. Macroglobulinemia, mainly increased concentrations of IgM monoclonal proteins and IgA M components, is the principal cause of hyperviscosity. The symptoms are related to circulatory disorders due to increased resistance of blood flow. They include changes in the fundus oculi marked by alternating bulges and constrictions in the retinal veins, hemorrhage, and exudates; neurological disorders, including headache, vertigo, somnolence, stupor, coma, pareses, jacksonian or generalized seizures, deafness, cerebral hemorrhage, polyneuropathies, and other conditions resulting from cerebrovascular circulatory insufficiency; myopathies; cardiac failure, especially in the elderly; fatigue; anorexia; weakness; and a variety of other disorders.

Wintrobe, M. M., Lee, G. R., Boggs, D. R., Bithell, T. C., Foerster, J., Athens, J. W., & Lukens, J. N. Hyperviscosity syndrome. In: *Clinical hematology.* 8th ed. Philadelphia, Lea & Febiger, 1981. pp. 1732-3. Dintefass, L. Blood high viscosity syndromes and hyperviscosaemia. In his: *Blood viscosity, hyperviscosity & hyperviscosaemia.* Lancaster, Pennsylvania, MTP Press, 1985, pp. 163-339.

hypervitaminosis hydrocephalus. See *Marie-Sée syndrome, under Marie, Julien.*

hypnolepsy. See *Gélineau syndrome.*

hypo-alpha-lipoproteinemia. See *Vergani syndrome.*

hypo-hyperparathyroidism. See *Costello-Dent syndrome.*

hypo-osmolality in beer drinkers. See *beer drinker syndrome.*

hypoadrenocorticism. See *Addison disease.*

hypoaldosteronism-hyporeninemia syndrome. See *hyporeninemic hypoaldosteronism syndrome.*

hypoandrogenic syndrome with normal spermatogenesis. See *Pasqualini syndrome.*

hypocalcemia-hypocalciuria syndrome. See *familial hypercalcemia-hypocalciuria syndrome.*

hypochondria. See *Cheyne disease, under Cheyne, George.*

hypochondriasis. See *Cheyne disease, under Cheyne, George.*

hypochondroplasia syndrome. Synonyms: *chondrohypoplasia, hereditary hypochondroplasia.*

An autosomal dominant syndrome characterized by micromelic dwarfism, mild joint relaxation, small feet and hands with short tubular bones, rectangular skull, frontal bossing, slight lumbar lordosis, protuberant abdomen, bowlegs, and limited elbow extension. Radiographic findings include shortening of the pedicles, increased dorsal concavity of lumbar vertebrae, short and square tubular bones, short and broad femoral neck, elongated distal ends of the fibula, and bony spinal canal narrowing caudally. Mental retardation and brachycephaly may occur. The symptoms become apparent during childhood.

Ravenna, F. Achondroplasie et chondrohypoplasie. Contribution clinique. *Nouv. Icon. Salpetr.*, 1913, 26:157-84. Léri, A., & Linossier. Hypochondroplesie héréditaire. *Bull. Mem. Soc., Méd. Hôp., Paris*, 1924, 48:1780-7.

hypochromic-achlorhydric anemia. See *Faber syndrome.*

hypodivergent face. See *short face syndrome.*

hypogammaglobulinemia-thymoma syndrome. See *Good syndrome.*

hypogenital dystrophy with diabetic tendency syndrome. See *Prader-Willi syndrome.*

hypoglossal carotid entrapment (HCE) syndrome. Vascular and neurological disorders due to involvement of the external and internal carotid arteries and the hypoglossal nerve in inflammatory diseases of the upper respiratory tract, tonsillitis, and lymph node enlargement. Embolism, focal intimal hyperplasia, and diaphragm formation may result from inflammation of the nasopharynx and tonsils with secondary scar formation and fusion of the carotid arteries and the hypoglossal nerve. A lymph node enlarged by infection or neoplastic changes may cause arterial obstruction or hypoglossal paralysis. Tension on the hypoglossal nerve cuts into the internal carotid artery and causes fracture of the intima, thus precipitating dissection and giving rise to internal carotid artery thrombosis and distal embolism.

Carney, A. L., & Anderson, E. M. Hypoglossal carotid entrapment syndrome. *Adv. Neur.*, 1981, 30:223-47.

hypoglossia-hypodactylia syndrome. See *Hanhart syndrome (2).*

hypoglycemia-mesenchymal tumor syndrome. See *Doege-Potter syndrome.*

hypoglycemic syndrome. See *Harris syndrome, under Harris, Seale.*

hypogonadism-anosmia syndrome. See *olfactogenital syndrome.*

hypogonadism-spermatogenesis syndrome. See *Pasqualini syndrome.*

hypogonadotropic hypogonadism-anosmia syndrome. See *olfactogenital syndrome.*

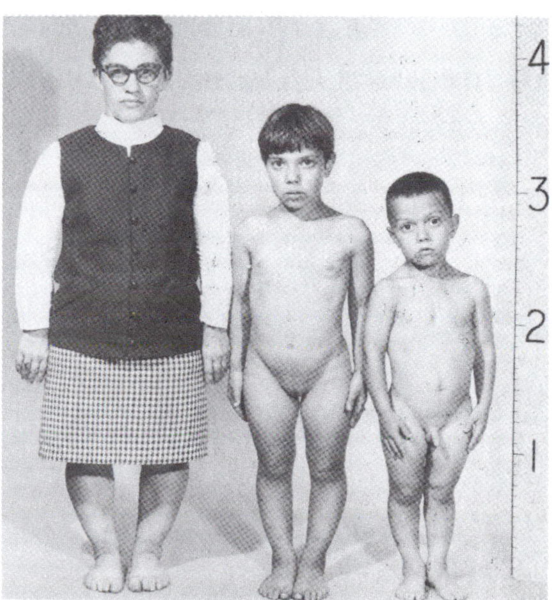

Hypochondroplasia syndrome
Beals, R.K.: *J. Bone Joint Surg. (Am.)*, 51:728, 1969. Boston: Journal of Bone & Joint Surgery. By permission.

hypohidrotic ectodermal dysplasia syndrome. Synonyms: *Christ-Siemens-Touraine syndrome, Christ-Siemens-Weech syndrome, Guilford disease, Jacquet syndrome, Siemens dermatosis, Siemens syndrome, Weech syndrome, anhidrosis hypotrichotica, anhidrosis polydysplastica, anhidrotic ectodermal dysplasia, anhidrotic hereditary ectodermal dysplasia, hereditary ectodermal polydysplasia.*

Ectodermal dysplasia characterized by hipohidrosis, hypotrichosis, and anodontia. The combination of prominent frontal bones, wide, high, and scanty eyebrows, saddle nose, thick lips, hypognathia, and pointed chin gives the affected persons strikingly similar facies. The patients are usually small and delicately proportioned with soft, white, dry skin; feminine appearance; fine stiff, short blond hair; and absent or scanty eyelashes and eyebrows. Intolerance to heat and hyperpyrexia after only mild exertion are caused by absence or decreased number of sweat glands. Hypoplasia of the sebaceous glands causes frequent eczema, especially during childhood. Teeth are few and those that are present are often delayed in eruption. Gonadal anomalies, absence of nipples and mammary glands, cleft palate, mental retardation, finger abnormalities, microphthalmia, and other defects are occasionally associated. The syndrome is usually transmitted as an X-linked trait, the gene being carried by the female and manifested in the male, but some cases have been also reported in females. See also *anhidrotic ectodermal dysplasia, autosomal recessive.*

Christ, J. Über die kongenit. ektodermalen Defekte und inhre Beziehungen zu einander; vikariirendes Pigment für Haartbildung. *Arch. Derm. Syph., Berlin*, 1913, 116:685-703. Siemens, H. W. Studien über Verehung von Hautkrankheiten XII. Anhidrosis hypotrichotica. *Arch. Derm. Syph., Berlin*, 1937, 175:565-77. Jacquet, L. Les rapports de la pelade avec les lésions dentaires. *Presse Méd.*, 1900, 8327-8. Touraine, A. L'"anidrose avec hypotrichose et anodontie." (Polydysplasie ectodermique hereditaire.) *Presse Méd.*, 1936, 44:145-9. Weech, A. A. Hereditary ectodermal dysplasia (congenital ectodermal defect). A report of two cases. *Am. J. Dis. Child.*, 1929, 37:766-90. Guilford, S. Eine Zahnanomalie. *Wien. Med. Wschr.*, 1883, 33:1116.

hypohidrotic ectodermal dysplasia with hypothyroidism. See *HEDH syndrome.*

hypohidrotic onychodental dysplasia syndrome. See *amelo-onychohypohidrotic syndrome.*

hypokalemic alkalosis. See *Bartter syndrome.*

hypokalemic periodic paralysis. See *Westphal syndrome, under Westphal, Karl Friedrich Otto.*

hypolipidemia S. See *Hooft syndrome.*

hypomagnessemia. See *magnesium deficiency syndrome.*

hypomelanosis Ito (HI). See *Ito hypomelanosis.*

hypomelia-hypotrichosis-facial hemangioma syndrome. See *pseudothalidomide syndrome.*

hyponatremia syndrome. See *low salt syndrome.*

hypophosphatasia syndrome. Synonyms: *Rathbun syndrome, hypophosphatemic rickets (HR), osteodysmetamorphosis foetalis, phosphoethanolaminuria.*

An inherited metabolic abnormality, transmitted as an autosomal recessive trait, characterized by a deficiency of serum and tissue alkaline phosphatase and high levels of phosphoethanolamine in the urine. The severity of the syndrome varies, ranging from lethal to mild forms with survival into adult life. The lethal form is characterized by a globular and soft head (caput membranaceum); short, deformed, flaccid extremities; respiratory distress; and death within a few hours or days after birth. Radiological findings show absence of ossification of major parts of the calvaria, base of the skull, and face; absence of ossification of short tubular bones; irregular metaphyseal ossification; poor ossification of the vertebrae; small scapulae; and poorly ossified scapulae and pelvic bones. The mild form (**hypophosphatasia tarda**) is characterized by rachitic bone lesions, such as rosary, bowed legs, painful extremities, and defective gait; craniosynostosis; open cranial sutures; bulging fontanels; prominent scalp veins; failure to thrive; vomiting; anorexia; constipation; fever; convulsions; muscle hypotonia; early shedding of deciduous teeth; anodontia; and multiple fractures. Radiological findings in hypophosphatasia tarda include delayed ossification of the skull, defective ossification of the ribs and long bones, irregular metaphyseal margins, bowing of the extremities, pseudofractures, and ectopic calcification, especially in spinal ligaments and joint cartilage.

Rathbun, J. C. "Hypophosphatasia," new developmental anomaly. *Am. J. Dis. Child.*, 1948, 75:822-31.

hypophosphatasia tarda. See *under hypophosphatasia syndrome.*

hypophosphatemia, X-linked. See *hypophosphatemic familial rickets.*

hypophosphatemic familial rickets. Synonyms: *Albright-Butler-Bloomberg syndrome, familial hypophosphatemia, hereditary hypophosphatemia, hypophosphatemic rickets (HR), phosphate diabetes, primary vitamin D-resistant rickets, vitamin D-resistant rickets, X-linked phosphatemia, X-linked phosphatemic rickets.*

A metabolic syndrome, transmitted as an X-linked trait, characterized by hypophosphatemia, elevated serum alkaline phosphatase, diminished tubular reabsorption of phosphate with resulting hyperphosphaturia, and faulty intestinal absorption of calcium. The symptoms include short-limbed dwarfism affecting the lower extemeties, bowing of the lower limbs, genua vara, occasional genua valga, costochondral beading, enlarged wrists and ankles, enamel hypoplasia, delayed dentition, and premature loss of permanent dentition. Associated disorders include waddling gait, protuberant abdomen and, less commonly, dolichocephaly and craniosynostosis. The affected persons are unresponsive to vitamin D. Radiological manifestations are those of rickets and include osteomalacia, bowing of the tubular bones, Looser zones, increased bone density and coarse trabeculae, bone spurs and ossicles, slipped capital femoral epiphyses, arthritic changes, and spinal cord compression. Onset usually takes place after 6 months of age. See also *Glisson disease* and *Lightwood-Albright syndrome.*

Albright, F., Butler, A. M., & Bloomberg, E. Rickets resistant to vitamin D therapy. *Am. J. Dis. Child.*, 1937, 54:529-47.

hypophosphatemic rickets (HR). See *hypophosphatasia syndrome, and see hypophosphatemic familial rickets*

hypophosphatemic rickets, X-linked. See *hypophosphatemic familial rickets.*

hypophosphatemic rickets-osteomalacia-linear nevus sebaceous syndrome. Synonyms: *Feuerstein-Mims syndrome with resistant rickets, vitamin D-resistant rickets-epidermal nevus syndrome.*

An association of congenital anomalies affecting multiple body systems (especially the skin, skeleton, and central nervous system), epidermal nevus syndrome, rickets, and osteomalacia that is resistant to vitamin D therapy.

Moorjani, R., & Shaw, N. A. Feuerstein and Mims syndrome with resistant rickets. *Pediat. Radiol.*, 1976, 5:120. Carey, D. E., *et al.* Hypophosphatemic rickets/osteomalacia in linear sebaceous nevus syndrome. A variant of tumor induced osteomalacia. *J. Pediat.*, 1986, 109:994-1000.

hypophosphatemic rickets-renal hyperglycinuria-renal glycosuria-glycylprolinuria syndrome. See *Scriver-Goldbloom-Roy syndrome.*

hypophyseal basophilic adenoma. See *Cushing syndrome.*

hypophyseal basophilism. See *Cushing syndrome.*

hypophyseal dwarfism with infantilism. See *Lorain-Levi syndrome.*

hypophyseal infantilism. See *Lorain-Levi syndrome.*

hypophyseal nanism. See *Burnier syndrome.*

hypophyseal syndrome. See *Fröhlich syndrome, under Fröhlich, Alfred.*

hypophyseothalamic syndrome. See *Fröhlich syndrome, undera Fröhlich, Alfred.*

hypopituitarism syndrome. See *Sheehan syndrome.*

hypoplastic anemia of childhood. See *Diamond-Blackfan syndrome.*

hypoplastic left heart complex. See *hypoplastic left heart syndrome.*

hypoplastic left heart syndrome (HLHS). Synonyms: *hypoplastic left heart complex, hypoplastic left ventricle syndrome (HLVS), left ventricular hypoplasia.*

A congenital cardiac anomaly characterized by hypoplasia of the left cardiac chambers, atresia or stenosis of the aortic and/or mitral orifices, and hypoplasia of the aorta. Endocardial fibroelastosis involving the left atrium and ventricle is often associated. Heart failure may occur during the first week of life.

Lev, M. Pathologic anatomy and interrelationship of hypoplasia of the aortic tract complex. *Lab. Invest.*, 1952, 1:61-70. Strong, W. B., *et al.* Hypoplastic left ventricle syndrome. *Am. J. Dis. Child.*, 1970, 120:511-4.

hypoplastic left ventricle syndrome (HLVS). See *hypoplastic left heart syndrome.*

hypoplastic right heart complex. See *hypoplastic right heart syndrome.*

hypoplastic right heart syndrome. Synonyms: *hypoplastic right heart complex, right ventricular hypoplasia.*

A heart anomaly characterized by atresia or stenosis on the right side of the heart associated with hypoplasia of the right ventricle and left ventricular hypertrophy. A right-to-left intracardiac shunt, usually at the atrial level, is associated. Tricuspid atresia and pulmonary atresia or severe pulmonary stenosis with an intact ventricular septum are the cause of this syndrome. Early neonatal congestive heart failure is a frequent complication. See also *Uhl anomaly.*

Medd, W. E., *et al.* Isolated hypoplasia of the right ventricle and tricuspid valve in siblings. *Brit. Heart J.*, 1961, 23:25. Taussig, H. B. Clinical and pathological findings in congenital malformations of heart due to defective development of right ventricle associated with tricuspid atresia or hypopasia. *Bull. Johns Hopkins Hosp.*, 1936, 59:435.

hypoplastic right ventricle. See *Uhl anomaly.*

hypopotassemic periodic paralysis. See *Westphal syndrome, under Westphal, Karl Friedrich Otto.*

hypoprothrombinemia. See *Owren syndrome (2).*

hypopyon recidivans. See *Behçet syndrome.*

hypopyon ulcer. See *Saemisch ulcer.*

hyporeninemic hypoaldosteronism (SHH) syndrome. Synonym: *hypoaldosteronism-hyporeninemia syndrome.*

A metabolic syndrome, usually observed in middle-aged or elderly individuals, characterized by low levels of plasma renin and aldosterone concentrations, in association with chronic renal insufficiency, caused by diabetes mellitus, gout, pyelonephritis, nephrolithiasis, cystic disease, hypertensive nephrosclerosis, or abuse of analgesics. Tubulointerstitial damage is the principal renal feature. Hypertension complicates most cases, but normal blood pressure, even hypotension, may occur in some instances. Restricted sodium intake and diuresis may cause hyperkalemia, hyperchloremic acidosis, hyponatremia, and increased plasma renin activity.

Hudson, J. B., *et al.* Hypoaldosteronism: A clinical study of a patient with an isolated adrenal mineralocorticoid deficiency resulting in hyperkalemia and Stokes-Adams attacks. *N. Engl. J. Med.*, 1957, 257:529-36.

hyposmia-hypogonadotropic hypogonadism syndrome. See *olfactogenital syndrome.*

hypospadias-dysphagia syndrome. Synonyms: *Opitz-Frias syndrome, BBG syndrome, G syndrome.*

A syndrome of characteristic facies, hypospadias, hypertelorism, and esophageal defect with swallowing difficulty. Prominent occipital and parietal eminences, hypertelorism, narrow slitlike palpebral fissures with a slight antimongoloid slant, and epicanthal folds are the principal facial features. Micrognathia, flat nasal bridge, anteverted nostrils, and flat philtrum may be

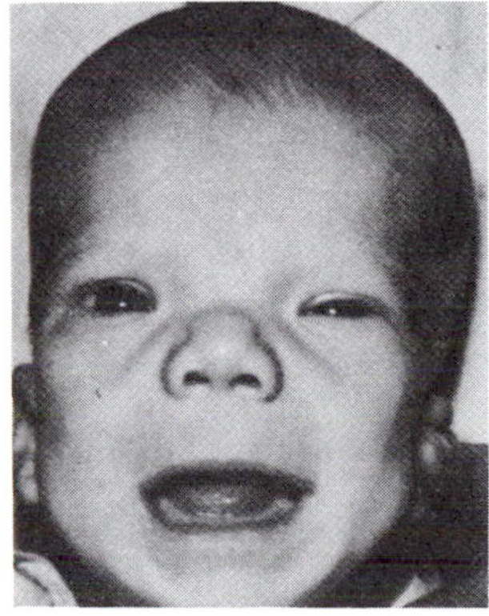

Hypospadias-dysphagia syndrome
Opitz, J.M., J.L. Frias, J.E. Gutenberger, J.R. Pellett: "The G syndrome of multiple congenital anomalies." In Bergsma, D. (ed): Part II, *Malformation Syndromes.* Baltimore: Williams & Wilkins for the National Foundation-March of Dimes BD:OAS V(2):95-101, 1969, with permission.

present. Genitourinary defects consist chiefly of hypospadias, bifid scrotum, and cryptorchism in males; female genitalia being generally normal. High bifurcation of the trachea; hypoplasia of one lung, epiglottis, vocal cords, and larynx; ankyloglossia; bifid uvula; cleft lip and palate; imperfotate anus; and other abnormalities may be associated. The early symptoms include a hoarse cry, stridulous respiration, and difficulty in swallowing, choking, coughing, and cyanosis, sometimes followed by aspiration pneumonia. The syndrome appears to have autosomal dominant inheritance. The designation *G syndrome* stems from the surname of the first reported family. Some authors suggest that this and the hypertelorism-hypospadias syndrome (BBB syndrome) represent the same entity, hence the designation *BBBG syndrome*.

Optiz, J. M., Frías, J. L., Gutenberger, J. E., & Pellett, J. R. The G syndrome of multiple congenital anomalies. *Birth Defects*, 1969, 5(2):95-101. Verloes, A., *et al.* BBBG syndrome or Opitz syndrome: New family. *Am. J. Med. Genet.*, 1989, 34:313-6.

hypothalamic syndrome. Any syndrome caused by dysfunction of the hypothalamus, including diabetes insipidus, body temperature regulation disorders, inappropriate ADH secretion, Fröhlich syndrome, appetite disorders, Cushing ulcer, emotional and behavior disorders, and Kleine-Levin syndrome.

Adams, R. D., & Victor, M. Hypothalamic syndromes. In their: *Principles of neurology.* 3rd ed. New York, McGraw-Hill, 1985, pp. 413-5.

hypothalamic hamartoblastoma-hyperphalangeal-hypoendocrine hypoplastic anus (4H) syndrome. See *Hall syndrome, under Hall, J. G.*

hypothenar hammer syndrome. Synonym: *post-traumatic digital ischemia.*

Digital ischemia caused by compression of the distal ulnar artery against the hook of the hamate, occurring in persons who repeatedly strike the hypothenar eminence when using hammers or similar tools. Arteriography shows irregularity or occlusion of the ulnar artery, occlusion of digital arteries, and intraluminal emboli at the sites of distal obstruction. Clinically, the fingers are cold, pale, and ulcerated with thickening and tenderness in the hypothenar eminence area. The syndrome is considered a form of reversible Raynaud phenomenon.

Barker, N. W., *et al.* Arterial occlusion in the hand and fingers associated with repeated occupational trauma. *Proc. Mayo Clin.*, 1944, 19:345. Conn, J., Jr., *et al.* Recognition of hypothenar hammer syndrome. *Surgery*, 1970, 68:1122.

hypothyroid myopathy. See *Debré-Semelaigne syndrome.*

hypothyroid myopathy. See *Hoffmann syndrome, under Hoffmann, Johann.*

hypothyroid phrynoderma. See *Vilanova-Cañadell syndrome.*

hypothyroidism-large muscle. See *Débre-Semelaigne syndrome.*

hypotonia-hypomentia-hypogonadism-obesity (HHHO) syndrome. See *Prader-Willi syndrome.*

hypotonia-obesity-hypogonadism-mental retardation syndrome. See *Prader-Willi syndrome.*

hypotrichosis congenita hereditaria. See *Unna syndrome, under Unna, Marie.*

hypotrichosis with pili torti. See *Unna syndrome, under Unna, Marie.*

hypothalamic hypoventilation syndrome. A state in which there is a reduced amount of air entering the pulmonary alveoli, usually caused by extrapulmonary disorders, such as lesions of nerves supplying the respiratory muscles, thoracic injuries, airway obstruction, or depression of the respiratory center in the medulla oblongata by drugs, anesthesia, or injury. Hypoventilation is a component of various conditions, including respiratory distress, Ondine, Pickwick, and other syndromes. **Central hypoventilation syndrome (CHS)** is a late-onset type of hypoventilation in children, which is associated with central lesions, mainly of the hypothalamus.

West, J. B. Disturbances of respiratory function. In: Braunwald, E., Isselbacher, K. J., Petersdorf, R. G., Wilson, J. D., Martin, J. B., & Fauci, A. S., eds. *Harrison's principles of internal medicine.* 11th ed. New York, McGraw-Hill, 1987, pp. 1049-56.

hypoxic hyperventilation. See *adult respiratory distress syndrome.*

hysteria. See *Briquet syndrome (1), under Briquet, Pierre.*

hysterical chorea. See *Bergeron disease.*

hysterical dysbasia. See *Blocq syndrome.*

hysterical glossolabial hemispasm. See *Brissaud-Marie syndrome.*

hysterical nongaseous abdominal bloating. See *Alvarez syndrome.*

hysterical pseudodementia. See *Ganser syndrome.*

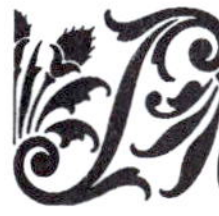

I

I cell disease (ICD, inclusion cell disease). See *mucolipidosis II.*

IADH. See *inappropriate antidiuretic hormone secretion syndrome.*

IADHS. See *inappropriate antidiuretic hormone secretion syndrome.*

IAS. See *infant apnea syndrome.*

IBIDS (ichthyosis-brittle hair-impaired intelligence-decreased ferility-short stature) **syndrome.** See *Tay syndrome, under Tay, Chong Hai.*

IBRAHIM, MURAD JUSSUF BEY (Egyptian physician, 1877-1953)

Beck-Ibrahim syndrome. See *under Beck, Soma Cornelius.*

Ibrahim disease. See *Beck-Ibrahim syndrome, under Beck, Soma Cornelius.*

IBS. See *irritable bowel syndrome.*

ICD (I-cell disease). See *mucolipidosis II.*

ice cream headache. See *under headache syndrome.*

ichthyosiform dermatosis with systemic lipidosis. See *Chanarin-Dorfman syndrome.*

ichthyosis congenita. See *Carini syndrome.*

ichthyosis congenita syndrome. Synonyms: *Riecke syndrome, harlequin fetus, harlequin ichthyosis, ichthyosis fetalis gravis, intrauterine ichthyosis.*

An autosomal recessive form of ichthyosis that is incompatible with extrauterine life. The affected infants are usually of low birth-weight and die within 1 week after birth. The lesions consist of diamond-shaped plaques, up to 4-5 cm on one side, arranged in a pattern similar to that of lamellar ichthyosis. See also *Carini syndrome.*

Thomson, M. S., & Wakeley, C. P. The harlequin foetus. *J. Obstet. Gynaec. Brit. Emp.*, 1921, 28:190-203. Smith, R. W. A case of intrauterine ichthyosis. *Am. J. Obstet. Gyn.*, 1880, 13:458-61. Riecke, E. Über Ichthyosis congenita. *Arch. Derm. Syph., Berlin*, 1900, 54:289-340.

ichthyosis fetalis gravis. See *ichthyosis congenita syndrome.*

ichthyosis linearis circumflexa. See *Rille-Còmel disease.*

ichthyosis palmaris et plantaris. See *Unna-Thost syndrome, under Unna, Paul Gerson.*

ichthyosis palmaris et plantaris corneae. See *Unna-Thost syndrome, under Unna, Paul Gerson.*

ichthyosis sebacea. See *Carini syndrome.*

ichthyosis-brittle hair-impaired-intelligence-decreased fertility-short stature (IBIDS) syndrome. See *Tay syndrome, under Tay, Chong Hai.*

ichthyosis-hypogonadism-mental retardation-epilepsy syndrome. See *Rud syndrome.*

ichthyosis-mental retardation-epilepsy-hypogonadism syndrome. See *Rud syndrome.*

ichthyosis-oligophrenia-epilepsy syndrome. See *Rud syndrome.*

ichthyotic idiocy. See *Sjögren-Larsson syndrome, under Sjögren, Karl Gustaf Torsten.*

ICS (irritable colon syndrome). See *irritable bowel syndrome.*

icteroanemia. See *Hayem-Widal syndrome.*

icterogenic spirochaetosis. See *leptospirosis.*

icterohemolytic anemia. See *Hayem-Widal syndrome.*

icterus intermittens juvenilis. See *Gilbert syndrome, under Gilbert, Nicolas Augustin.*

icterus neonatorum precox. See *Halbrecht syndrome.*

icterus-hepatic pigmentation syndrome. See *Dubin-Johnson syndrome.*

ictus laryngis. See *Charcot vertigo.*

ICU (immunologic contact urticaria). See *under contact urticaria syndrome.*

idiopathic acroparesthesia. See *Wartenberg disease (1).*

idiopathic atrophoderma. See *Pasini-Pierini syndrome.*

idiopathic benign pericarditis. See *Porter syndrome.*

idiopathic carpotarsal osteolysis of François syndrome. See *François syndrome (2).*

idiopathic cortical sclerosis. See *Garré osteomyelitis.*

idiopathic cyclic edema. See *cyclical edema syndrome.*

idiopathic detrussor-sphincter dyssynergia. See *Hinman syndrome.*

idiopathic diffuse esophageal spasm. See *Bársony-Polgár syndrome (2).*

idiopathic eosinophilic lung disease. See *pulmonary infiltration with eosinophilia syndrome.*

idiopathic familial brain calcification. See *Fahr syndrome.*

idiopathic familial cerebrovascular ferrocalcinosis. See *Fahr syndrome.*

idiopathic familial generalized osteophytosis. See *pachydermoperiostosis syndrome.*

idiopathic fibrosing alveolitis (IFA). See *Hamman-Rich syndrome.*

idiopathic flat detachment of the retina. See *Masuda-Kitahara disease.*

idiopathic gangrene of the male genitalia. See *Fournier disease.*

idiopathic gangrene of the scrotum. See *Fournier disease.*

idiopathic gingivostomatitis. See *gingivostomatitis syndrome.*

idiopathic granulomatous myocarditis. See *Fiedler myocarditis.*

idiopathic hemorrhagic sarcoma. See *Kaposi sarcoma.*

idiopathic hyperbilirubinemia. See *Rotor syndrome, and see Gilbert syndrome, under Gilbert, Nicolas Augustin.*

idiopathic hypercalcemia-supravalvular aortic stenosis syndrome. See *Williams syndrome, under Williams, J. C. P.*

idiopathic hyperglobulinemia. See *Waldenström syndrome (2), under Waldenström, Jan Gösta.*

idiopathic hyperlipemia. See *Bürger-Grütz syndrome.*

idiopathic hypertrophic osteoarthropathy. See *pachydermoperiostosis syndrome.*

idiopathic hypochromic anemia. See *Faber syndrome.*

idiopathic hypochronemia. See *Faber syndrome.*

idiopathic hypopituitary dwarfism. See *Hanhart syndrome (1).*

idiopathic hypoproteinemia. See *protein-losing gastroenteropathy.*

idiopathic hypoprothrombinemia. See *Alexander syndrome, under Alexander, Benjamin.*

idiopathic hypothalamic hypogonadism (IHH). See *olfactogenital syndrome.*

idiopathic hypoventilation (syndrome). See *Ondine curse.*

idiopathic leukopenia. See *Schultz syndrome.*

idiopathic lipoidosis. See *Bürger-Grütz syndrome.*

idiopathic megatrachea with tracheomalacia. See *Mounier-Kuhn syndrome.*

idiopathic methemoglobinemia. See *Gibson disease, under Gibson, Quentin Howieson and see Stokvis-Talma syndrome.*

idiopathic multiple hemorrhagic pigmented sarcoma. See *Kaposi sarcoma.*

idiopathic necrosis of femoral head. See *Chandler syndrome, under Chandler, Fremont Augustus.*

idiopathic orthostatic hypotension (IOH). See *Bradbury-Eggleston syndrome.*

idiopathic parenchymatous contracted kidney. See *familial juvenile nephrophthisis.*

idiopathic pulmonary atrophy. See *Burke syndrome.*

idiopathic pulmonary fibrosis. See *Hamman-Rich syndrome.*

idiopathic pulmonary hemosiderosis (IPH). See *Ceelen-Gellerstedt syndrome.*

idiopathic refractory anemia. See *myelodysplastic syndrome.*

idiopathic renal acidosis. See *Lightwood-Albright syndrome.*

idiopathic retroperitoneal fibrosis. See *Ormond syndrome.*

idiopathic sciatica. See *Putti syndrome.*

idiopathic short face. See *short face syndrome.*

idiopathic splenomegaly syndrome. See *tropical splenomegaly syndrome.*

idiopathic steatorrhea. See *see celiac disease, and see Whipple disease.*

idiopathic thrombocytopenic purpura (ITP). See *Werlhof disease.*

idiopathic thrombopenic purpura. See *Werlhof disease.*

idiopathic unilateral hyperlucent lung syndrome. See *Swyer-James syndrome, under Swyer, Paul Robert.*

idiopathic vitamin K deficiency in infancy. See *acquired prothrombin complex deficiency syndrome.*

idiotia phenylketonurica. See *phenylketonuria.*

idiotia xerodermica. See *de Sanctis-Cacchione syndrome.*

IESHIMA, ATSUSHI (Japanese physician)

Ieshima syndrome. A familial syndrome, transmitted as an autosomal recessive trait, characterized by psychomotor retardation, peculiar facies, and multiple abnormalities. Craniofacial anomalies consist of microcephaly, facial asymmetry, arched eyebrows, hypertelorism, blepharoptosis, depressed nasal bridge, small nose, anteverted nostrils, microtia, micrognathia, and cleft palate. Cryptorchism, shawl scrotum, and microphallus are the genital components of the syndrome. Associated defects and disorders include short neck, pulmonary hypertension, patent ductus arteriosus, bone deformities, deafness, muscle hypotonia, brisk tendon reflexes, feeding difficulty, respiratory disorders, and recurrent infections.

Ieshima, A., *et al.* Peculiar face, deafness, cleft palate, male pseudohermaphroditism, and growth and psychomotor retardation; a new autosomal recessive syndrome? *Clin. Genet.*, 1986, 30:136-41.

IFA (idiopathic fibrosing alveolitis). See *Hamman-Rich syndrome.*

IG (irritable gut). See *irritable bowel syndrome.*

IgA disease. See *Berger syndrome, under Berger, J.*

IgA nephropathy. See *Berger syndrome, under Berger, J.*

IgG-IgA nephritis. See *Berger syndrome, under Berger, J.*

IHH (idiopathic hypothalamic hypogonadism). See *olfactogenital syndrome.*

ileal kink. See *Lane kink, under Lane, Sir Willilam Arbuthnot.*

ileal meconium plug. See *meconium plug syndrome.*

iliac horn syndrome. See *nail-patella syndrome.*

iliac vein compression. See *Cockett syndrome.*

iliotibial band friction syndrome. An overuse syndrome (q.v.), observed most commonly in long-distance runners, characterized by pain on the outer aspect of the knee in close relation to the lateral femoral epicondyle. It is caused by friction of the iliotibial band over the lateral epicondylar prominence. The condition is aggravated by long distance running or excessive striding, being more severe when running downhill.

Renne, J. W. The iliotibial band friction syndrome. *J. Bone Joint Surg.*, 1975, 57A:1110-1.

illusion of doubles. See *Capgras syndrome.*

illusion of negative doubles. See *Capgras syndrome.*

imbecillitas phenylpyruvica. See *phenylketonuria.*

IMERSLUND, OLGA (Norwegian physician)

Imerslund anemia. See *Imerslund-Gräsbeck syndrome.*

Imerslund syndrome. See *Imerslund-Gräsbeck syndrome.*

Imerslund-Gräsbeck syndrome. Synonyms: *Imerslund anemia, Imerslund syndrome, Imerslund-Najman-Gräsbeck syndrome, congenital vitamin B_{12} malabsorption syndrome, familial selective malabsorption syndrome, selective vitamin B_{12} malabsorption, selective vitamin B_{12} malabsorption-proteinuria syndrome.*

A familial syndrome, transmitted as an autosomal recessive trait, characterized by juvenile pernicious anemia (due to selective malabsorption of vitamin B_{12})

and proteinuria. Onset takes place between the ages of 5 months and 4 years. Pallor, weakness, irritability, dyspnea, fever, gastrointestinal disorders with diarrhea and vomiting, lack of appetite, glossitis, jaundice, heart murmurs, and proteinuria are the principal symptoms. Transient neurological disorders, pyoderma, hepatomegaly, hemorrhage, edema, and premature graying of the hair may be present. Urinary tract abnormalities (usually different stages of duplication of the kidney, pelvis, and ureters) are sometimes observed. See also *malabsorption syndrome.*

Imerslund, O. Idiopathic chronic megaloblastic anemia in children. *Acta Paediat., Uppsala*, 1960, 49(Suppl. 119):1-115. Gräsbeck, R. Familjar selektiv B12-malabsorption med proteinuri. Ett perniciosaliknande syndrom. *Nord. Med.*, 1960, 63:322-3.

Imerslund-Najman-Gräsbeck syndrome. See *Imerslund-Gräsbeck syndrome.*

imidazole syndrome. See *Bessman-Baldwin syndrome.*

immediate reactivities syndrome (SIR). See *contact urticaria syndrome.*

immune-complex disease. See *serum sickness syndrome.*

immunoglobulin A nephropathy. See *Berger syndrome, under Berger, J.*

immunologic contact urticaria (ICU). See *under contact urticaria syndrome.*

immunosialadenitis. See *Sjögren syndrome, under Sjögren, Henrik Samuel Conrad.*

impending ischemic contracture. See *compartment syndrome.*

impetigo contagiosa streptogenes. See *Fox impetigo, under Fox, William Tilbury.*

impetigo parasitaria. See *Fox impetigo, under Fox, William Tilbury.*

impetigo simplex. See *Fox impetigo, under Fox, William Tilbury.*

impetigo vulgaris. See *Fox impetigo, under Fox, William Tilbury.*

inappropriate ADH syndrome. See *inappropriate antidiuretic hormone secretion syndrome.*

inappropriate antidiuretic hormone secretion syndrome (IADH, IADHS, SIADH). Synonyms: *Schwartz-Bartter syndrome, inappropriate ADH syndrome.*

Hyponatremia with corresponding hypo-osmolality of the serum and extracellular fluid, continued renal excretion of sodium, absence of clinical evidence of fluid volume depletion (i.e., normal skin turgor and blood pressure), osmolality of urine greater than that appropriate for concomitant tonicity of plasma (i.e., urine less than maximally dilute), and normal renal and adrenal function. The syndrome is due to excessive retention of water that persists despite a concomitant reduction in the osmolality of the extracellular fluid. It is found in association with various vasopressin-secreting tumors, with small-cell and oat-cell carcinomas of the lungs being the most frequent cause of this syndrome. Other disorders complicated by SIADH include malignant tumors with autonomous release of vasopressin (carcinoma of the pancreas and duodenum, thymoma, reticulum-cell sarcoma, lymphosarcoma, and Hodgkin disease), lung diseases (tuberculosis, abscesses, pneumonia, empyema, and obstructive diseases), central nervous system disorders (skull fractures, subdural hematoma, subarachnoid hemorrhage, cerebral thrombosis, cerebral atrophy, encephalitis, tuberculous meningitis, purulent meningitis, Guillain-Barré syndrome, lupus erythematosus, and acute intermittent porphyria), adverse reactions to some drugs, hypothyroidism, and positive pressure respiration.

Schwartz, W. B., *et al.* A syndrome of renal sodium loss and hyponatremia probably resulting from inappropriate secretion of antidiuretic hormone. *Am. J. Med.*, 1957, 23:529-42. Bartter, F. C., & Schwartz, W. B. The syndrome of inappropriate secretion of antidiuretic hormone. *Am. J. Med.*, 1967, 42:790-806.

inclusion body encephalitis. See *van Bogaert encephalitis.*

inclusion cell (I cell) disease. See *mucolipidosis II.*

incontinentia pigmenti (IP). See *Bloch-Sulzberger syndrome.*

incontinentia pigmenti achromians (IPA). See *Ito hypomelanosis.*

Indian childhood cirrhosis. See *Sen syndrome (1).*

Indiana type amyloid neuropathy. See *amyloid neuropathy type II.*

indiscretion enteritis. See *rebelaisian syndrome.*

indurated chancre. See *Hunter chancre, under Hunter, John.*

induratio penis plastica. See *Peyronie disease.*

indurative pneumonia. See *Fränkel disease.*

infancy-onset diabetes mellitus with multiple epiphyseal dysplasia syndrome. See *Wolcott-Rallison syndrome.*

infant apnea syndrome (IAS). Synonym: *near miss sudden infant death syndrome.*

An episode in which there is a history of the baby having in the past appeared lifeless, requiring mouth-to-mouth resuscitation. Causes may include gastroesophageal reflux, encephalitis, convulsions, periventricular edema, Arnold-Chiari malformation, and milk allergy. See also *sudden infant death syndrome, neonatal respiratory distress syndrome*, and *Wilson-Mikity syndrome.*

Camfield, P., *et al.* Infant apnea syndrome. A prospective evaluation of etiologies. *Clin. Pediat.*, 1982, 21:684-7.

infant respiratory distress syndrome (IRDS). See *neonatal respiratory distress syndrome.*

infant rumination syndrome. See *rumination syndrome.*

infantile acro-localized papulovesicular syndrome. See *Gianotti-Crosti syndrome.*

infantile amaurotic familial idiocy. See *Tay-Sachs syndrome, under Tay, Warren.*

infantile atrophy. See *marasmus syndrome.*

infantile cortical hyperostosis. See *Caffey-Silverman syndrome.*

infantile eczema. See *Besnier prurigo.*

infantile generalized gangliosidosis. See *gangliosidosis G_{M1} type I.*

infantile genetic agranulocytosis. See *Kostmann syndrome.*

infantile hemorrhagic diathesis. See *Möller-Barlow disease.*

infantile hyperphosphatasia. See *hyperphosphatasia-osteoctasia syndrome.*

infantile lichnoid acrodermatitis. See *Gianotti-Crosti syndrome.*

infantile muscular atrophy. See *Werdnig-Hoffmann syndrome.*

infantile myoclonic encephalopathy. See *Kingsbourne syndrome.*

infantile myxedema. See *Brissaud infantilism.*
infantile myxedema-muscular hypertrophy syndrome. See *Debré-Semelaigne syndrome.*
infantile necrotizing encephalomyelopathy. See *Leigh syndrome.*
infantile obstructive jaundice. See *bile plug syndrome.*
infantile optic atrophy-ataxia syndrome. See *Behr syndrome (2).*
infantile osteochondritis. See *Calvé syndrome.*
infantile osteosclerosis. See *osteopetrosis with precocious manifestations syndrome.*
infantile papular acrodermatitis (IPA). See *Gianotti-Crosti syndrome.*
infantile papulovesicular acrolocalized syndrome. See *Gianotti-Crosti syndrome.*
infantile paralysis. See *Heine-Medin disease.*
infantile partial striatal sclerosis. See *Vogt syndrome, under Vogt, Cécile.*
infantile polymyoclonus. See *Kingsbourne syndrome.*
infantile pseudospondylitis. See *Calvé syndrome.*
infantile pulmonary reticuloendotheliosis. See *Marie syndrome, under Marie, Julien.*
infantile salaam. See *West syndrome.*
infantile scurvy. See *Möller-Barlow disease.*
infantile spasms with mental retardation. See *West syndrome.*
infantile spastic diplegia. See *Little disease, under Little, William John.*
infantile spinal muscular atrophy. See *Werdnig-Hoffmann syndrome.*
infantile spongy degeneration. See *Canavan syndrome.*
infantile thoracic dystrophy. See *Jeune syndrome.*
infantile tremor syndrome. See *Zappert syndrome.*
infantile triploidy syndrome. See *chromosome triploidy syndrome.*
infantile X-linked agammaglobulinemia. See *Bruton syndrome.*

infectious angioma. See *Hutchinson disease (1), under Hutchinson, Sir Jonathan.*
infectious chorea. See *Sydenham chorea.*
infectious edematous polyneuritis. See *Debré-Marie syndrome (1).*
infectious eosinophilia. See *Frugoni disease.*
infectious erythema. See *Huttinel disease (1), and see Sticker disease.*
infectious hepatitis. See *Botkin disease.*
infectious lentigo. See *Hutchinson freckle, under Hutchinson, Sir Jonathan.*
infectious lymphocytosis. See *Smith disease, under Smith, Carl Henry.*
infectious mononucleosis. See *Filatov disease.*
infectious neuronitis. See *Guillain-Barré syndrome.*
infectious polyneuritis. See *Guillain-Barré syndrome.*
infectious reticulosis. See *Letterer-Siwe syndrome.*
infectious spirochetal jaundice. See *leptospirosis.*
infectious spondylitis. See *Bechterew-Strümpell-Marie syndrome, under Bekhterev.*
infectious uroarthritis. See *Reiter syndrome.*
infective hepatitis. See *Botkin disease.*
infective senile freckle. See *Hutchinson freckle, under Hutchinson, Sir Jonathan.*
inferior nucleus ruber syndrome. Synonyms: *Claude syndrome, Claude-Loyez syndrome, rubrospinal cerebellar syndrome, rubrospinal cerebellar peduncle syndrome.*

A neurological disorder in which mesencephalic lesions obstruct branches of the paramedian arteries supplying the inferior nucleus ruber, with ipsilateral paralysis of the oculomotor and trochlear nerves and contralateral hemianesthesia.

Claude, H. Syndrome pédonculaire de la région de noyau rouge. *Rev. Neur., Paris,* 1912, 23:311-3.

inferior protuberance syndrome. See *Millard-Gubler syndrome.*
infiltrative eosinophilia. See *pulmonary infiltration with eosinophilia syndrome.*
inflammatory dislocation of atlanto-axial joint. See *Grisel syndrome.*
inflammatory hereditary degeneration of the macula. See *Sorsby macular degeneration.*
inflammatory polyneuropathy. See *Guillain-Barré syndrome.*
inflammatory rhizomelic rheumatism. See *Forestier syndrome (1).*
influenza bacillus syndrome. See *Kleinschmidt syndrome.*
ingravescent apoplexy. See *Broadbent syndrome.*
inguinoperitoneal hernia. See *Krönlein hernia.*
iniencephaly. See *under Klippel-Feil syndrome.*
inoculation adenitis. See *cat scratch disease.*
inoculation lymphoreticulosis. See *cat scratch disease.*
INSLEY, J. (British physician)
Insley-Astley syndrome. See *Weissenbacher-Zweymüller syndrome.*
inspissated bile syndrome. See *bile plug syndrome.*
insufficientia vertebrae. See *Schanz syndrome.*
insulin resistance-pineal hyperplasia syndrome. See *Rabson-Mendenhall syndrome.*
intercapillary glomerulosclerosis. See *Kimmelstiel-Wilson syndrome.*
interfetal transfusion syndrome. See *twin transfusion syndrome.*
interhemispheric disconnection syndrome. See *under disconnection syndrome.*
intermediate beta-thalassemia. See *Rietti-Greppi-Micheli syndrome.*
intermittent claudication. See *Charcot syndrome (3).*
intermittent hemoglobinuria. See *Dressler syndrome, under Dressler, D. R.*
intermittent hydrarthrosis. See *observation hip syndrome.*
intermittent insufficiency of the basilar arterial system syndrome. See *Millikan-Siekert syndrome.*
intermittent limping syndrome. See *Charcot syndrome (3).*
intermittent myoplegia. See *Westphal syndrome, under Westphal, Karl Friedrich Otto.*
intermittent venous claudication. See *Paget-Schroetter syndrome.*
internal chondromatosis. See *Ollier syndrome.*
internal myxedema. See *Escamilla-Lisser syndrome.*
internuclear ophthalmoplegia. See *Bielschowsky-Lutz-Cogan syndrome, under Bielschowsky, Alfred.*
internuclear paralysis. See *Lhermitte syndrome.*
interpositio hepatodiaphragmatica. See *Chilaiditi syndrome.*
interstitial fibrosis of the lung. See *Hamman-Rich syndrome.*
interstitial giant-cell pneumonia. See *Hecht pneumonia, under Hecht, Victor.*

interstitial ossifying myositis. See *fibrodysplasia ossificans progressiva.*
interstitial pancreatitis. See *Zoepffel edema.*
interstitial pulmonary fibrosis of prematurity. See *Wilson-Mikity syndrome, under Wilson, Miriam Geisendorfer.*

intestinal bacterial overgrowth syndrome. See *bacterial overgrowth syndrome.*
intestinal bypass dermatosis-arthritis syndrome. See *bowel bypass syndrome.*
intestinal carcinoid syndrome. See *carcinoid syndrome.*
intestinal grippe. See *Spencer disease.*
intestinal infantilism. See *celiac disease.*
intestinal lipodystrophy. See *Whipple disease.*
intestinal lipogranulomatosis. See *Whipple disease.*
intestinal polyposis I. See *Peutz-Jeghers syndrome.*
intestinal polyposis II. See *Gardner syndrome, under Gardner, Eldon John.*
intestinal polyposis-cutaneous pigmentation syndrome. See *Peutz-Jeghers syndrome.*
intestinal polyposis-glioma syndrome. See *Turcot syndrome.*
intestinal stasis. See *Lane syndrome, under Lane, Sir William Arbuthnot.*
intestinal stasis syndrome. See *blind loop syndrome.*
intracerebellar atrophy. See *olivopontocerebellar atrophy.*
intracerebral symmetrical centrolobar sclerosis. See *Schilder-Foix disease.*
intracranial exostosis. See *Morgagni-Stewart-Morel syndrome.*
intracranial headache. See *under headache syndrome.*
intraepidermal acanthoma. See *Borst-Jadassohn epithelioma.*
intraepidermal malignant melanoma. See *Hutchinson freckle, under Hutchinson, Sir Jonathan.*
intrahemispheric disconnection syndrome. See *under disconnection syndrome.*
intramuscular hernia. See *Birkett hernia.*
intraparietal hernia. See *Birkett hernia.*
intraphepatic bile duct cysts. See *Caroli syndrome (2).*
intrauterine adhesions (IUA). See *Asherman syndrome.*
intrauterine amputation. See *amniotic band syndrome.*
intrauterine facial necrosis. See *oculo-auriculovertebral dysplasia.*
intrauterine ichthyosis. See *ichthyosis congenita syndrome.*
intrauterine parabiotic syndrome. See *twin transfusion syndrome.*
intrauterine synechiae. See *Asherman syndrome.*
intravascular coagulation syndrome. See *disseminated intravascular coagulation syndrome.*
invasive fibrous thyroiditis. See *Riedel disease.*
inverse Chiari type 2 syndrome. See *primary transtentorial cerebellar displacement syndrome.*
inverted follicular keratosis. See *Helwig disease.*
inverted Marcus Gunn syndrome. See *Marin Amat syndrome.*
inverted Marfan syndrome. See *Weill-Marchesani syndrome, under Weill, Georges.*
IOH (**i**diopathic **o**rthostatic **h**ypotension). See *Bradbury-Eggleston syndrome.*
Iowa-type amyloidosis. See *amyloid neuropathy type III.*
IP (**i**ncontinentia **p**igmenti). See *Bloch-Sulzberger syndrome.*
IPA (**i**ncontinentia **p**igmenti **a**chromians). See *Ito hypomelanosis.*
IPA (**i**nfantile **p**apular **a**crodermatitis). See *Gianotti-Crosti syndrome.*
IPH (**i**diopathic **p**ulmonary **h**emosiderosis). See *Ceelen-Gellerstedt syndrome.*

ipsiphilia compulsiva proctalgenica. See *Socrates syndrome.*
IRDS (**i**nfant **r**espiratory **d**istress **s**yndrome). See *neonatal respiratory distress syndrome.*
IRGANG, S. (French dermatologist)
Kaposi-Irgang disease. See *under Kaposi-Kohn.*
iridocorneal mesodermal dysgenesis. See *Rieger syndrome.*
iridocyclitis heterochromica. See *Fuchs heterochromic cyclitis.*
iridocyclitis recidivans. See *Behçet syndrome.*
iridocyclitis recidivans purulenta. See *Behçet syndrome.*
iridocyclitis septica. See *Behçet syndrome.*
iridocyclitis with hypopyon. See *Behçet syndrome.*
iridodental dysplasia. See *Weyers syndrome (2).*
iridoplegia interna. See *Adie syndrome.*
iritis guttata. See *Doyne iritis.*
iritis septica. See *Behçet syndrome.*
iron overload syndrome. See *Recklinghausen-Applebaum disease.*
iron storage disease. See *Recklinghausen-Applebaum disease.*
irritable bowel syndrome (IBS). Synonyms: *Smith disease, adaptive colitis, colonic neurosis, excitable colon syndrome, irritable colon syndrome, irritable gut (IG), mucoenteritis, mucous colitis, nervous diarrhea, painful irritable bowel, painless diarrhea, painless irritable bowel, spastic bowel syndrome, spastic colon, unstable colon.*

A gastrointestinal motor disorder characterized by altered bowel habits in the absence of inflammatory changes or other forms of recognizable organic pathology. Two forms are recognized: A **painful type** which is associated with either diarrhea or constipation or both, and a **painless type** which is directly related to stressful conditions. Associated symptoms include abdominal pain that may be mild, moderate, or severe and localized or diffuse; abdominal distention with belching and flatus; the presence of mucus in the stools; and abdominal distention associated with belching, dyspepsia, heartburn, pyrosis, and vomiting. Dysmenorrhea occurs in most affected women. The disorder is known to occur in persons who are otherwise normal but are exposed to stressful conditions.

McHardy, G., *et al.* Psychophysiologic gastrointestinal reactions: Therapeutic observations. *Postgrad. Med.*, 1962, 31:346. Schuster, M. M. Irritable bowel syndrome. In: Sleisenger, M. H., & Fordtran, J. S., eds. *Gastrointestinal disease. Pathophysiology, diagnosis, management.* 3rd ed. Philadelphia. Saunders, 1983. p. 880-96.

irritable breast. See *Cooper neuralgia.*
irritable colon syndrome (ICS). See *irritable bowel syndrome.*
irritable gut (IG). See *irritable bowel syndrome.*
irritable heart. See *Da Costa syndrome, under Da Costa, Jacob Mendez.*
irritable hip. See *observation hip syndrome.*

irritation syndrome. See *Reilly syndrome, under Reilly, J.*

IRVINE, S. R. (American ophthalmologist)

Hruby-Irvine-Gass syndrome. See *Irvine-Gass syndrome.*

Irvine-Gass cystoid macular edema. See *Irvine-Gass syndrome.*

Irvine-Gass syndrome. Synonyms: *Hruby-Irvine-Gass syndrome, Irvine-Gass cystoid macular edema.*

Vitreous incarceration in the wound and cystoid edema after cataract surgery. Light sensitivity and visual deterioration are the principal symptoms.

Irvine, S. R. Newly defined vitreous syndrome following cataract surgery. Interpreted according to recent concepts of structure of vitreus. *Am. J. Ophth.*, 1953, 36:599-619.

ISAMBERT, EMILE (French physician, 1828-1876)

Isambert disease. Acute pharyngolaryngeal miliary tuberculosis.

*Isambert, É. *De la tuberculose miliaire aigue pharyngo-laryngée.* Paris, 1871.

ischemic contracture of the heart. See *stone heart syndrome.*

ischemic hepatitis. See *shock liver syndrome.*

ischemic hypertensive leg ulcer. See *Martorell syndrome (1).*

ischias. See *Cotugno syndrome.*

ischiopatellar dysplasia. See *Scott-Taor syndrome, under Scott, J. E.*

ISO, RYOSUKE (Japanese physician)

Iso-Kikuchi syndrome. Synonym: *congenital onychodysplasia of the index finger (COIF) syndrome.*

A hand abnormality characterized by congenital anonychia, micronychia, or polyonychia of the index finger. In the initial report, only the index finger was involved and there were no underlying bone or joint deformities, but later findings indicate a possibility that digits other than the index finger may be involved, and that some cases may show nail or bone abnormalities or both. The characteristic bone abnormalities include terminal bifurcation of the distal phalanges, brachymesophalangia of the fifth fingers, syndactyly, congenital flexion deformity, range of motion abnormalities, and soft tissue thickening. Radiographic findings may show hypoplasia and narrowing of the distal phalanges with terminal enlargement. Other defects may include onychodystrophy, hemionychogryposis, abnormal lanula, nail malalignment, nail thickening, and micronychia. Iso's report specified the nongenetic and nonfamilial nature of this syndrome, but more recent reports indicate a possibility of transmission as an autosomal trait with variable expressivity, X-linked inheritance not being ruled out.

Iso, R. [Congenital defect of the nail of the index finger and its reconstruction]. *Orthop. Surg.*, 1969, 20:1383-4. Iso, R. [Congenital defect of the nail of the index finger and its reconstruction]. *Clin. Orthop. Surg.*, 1969, 4:672-7. Kikuchi, I. Congenital onychodysplasia of the index fingers. *Arch. Derm., Chicago,* 1974, 110:743-6.

isolated granulomatous myocarditis. See *Fiedler myocarditis.*

isolated myocarditis. See *Fiedler myocarditis.*

isotretinoin embryopathy. See *fetal Accutane syndrome.*

ISRAELS, MARTIN CYRIL GORDON (British physician, born 1906)

Israëls-Wilkinson anemia. See *Wilkinson anemia, under Wilkinson, John Frederick.*

itching purpura. See *Casalá-Mosto disease.*

ITO, MINOR (Japanese physician)

Ito hypomelanosis. Synonyms: *Ito syndrome, hypomelanosis of Ito (HI), incontinentia pigmenti achromians (IPA).*

A hereditary neurocutaneous syndrome characterized chiefly by a bizarre, more or less symmetrical leukoderma marked by depigmented streaks, patches, and whorls, sometimes associated with hyperkeratosis follicularis. Neurological features usually consist of cerebral seizures, psychomotor retardation, and macrocephaly. Strabismus, myopia, and changes in the fundus oculi are the common ophthalmological complications. Additional disorders may include coarse facies, hypertelorism, malformed ear auricles, high-arched palate, cleft palate, hamartomas of the incisors, unilateral leg shortness, scoliosis, and hip dysplasia and dislocation. Genetic transmission is suspected, probably as an autosomal dominant trait.

Ito, M. Studies on melanin. XI. Incontinentia pigmenti achromians. A singular case of nevus depigmentosus systematic N. S. bilateralis. *Tohoku J. Exp. Med., Suppl.*, 1952, 55:57-9.

Ito nevus. Synonym: *nevus fuscoceruleus acromiodeltoideus.*

A pigmented nevus of the lateral cervical area, upper thorax, and right shoulder.

Ito, M. Studies on melanin. XXII. Nevus fuscocaeruleus acromiodeltoideus. *Tohoku J. Exp. Med.*, 1954, 60:10.

Ito syndrome. See *Ito hypomelanosis.*

ITP (idiopathic thrombocytopenic purpura). See *Werlhof disease.*

ITSENKO, N. M. (Russian physician)

Itsenko-Cushing syndrome. See *Cushing syndrome.*

IUA (intrauterine adhesions). See *Asherman syndrome.*

IVANOV (IWANOFF), VLADIMIR P. (Russian physician, born 1861)

Blessig-Iwanoff cyst. See *Blessig-Iwanoff disease.*

Blessig-Iwanoff disease. See *under Blessig.*

IVEMARK, BJÖRN ISAAC ISAACSON (Swedish physician, born 1925)

Ivemark syndrome. See *asplenia syndrome.*

IVES, ELIZABETH J. (Canadian physician)

Ives-Houston syndrome. Synonym: *microcephaly-micromelia syndrome.*

A hereditary syndrome, transmitted as an autosomal recessive trait, marked by intrauterine growth retardation, microcephaly, severe limb malformations, and perinatal death. The elbows are fused, forearms are shortened and usually contain only a single bone, and the hands have only two to four malformed digits. Generally, there are two well-developed central digits with a less well-developed index finger and a fifth finger that sometimes arises from the bifid metacarpal bone. The thumb may be absent and the ulna and radius are hypoplastic. The syndrome was first observed in a consanguineous, predominantly Cree Indian community in Saskatchewan, Canada.

Ives, E. J., & Houston, C. S. Autosomal recessive microcephaly and micromelia in Cree Indians. *Am. J. Med. Genet.*, 1980, 7:351-60.

IVIC syndrome. A hereditary syndrome, transmitted as an autosomal dominant trait, marked chiefly by hypoplasia of the radius, hearing disorders, external ophthalmoplegia, thrombocytopenia, and leukocytosis. Mild incomplete right bundle branch block and imperforate anus may occur. There is an early delayed growth in the forearms, clavicles, and skull and permanent growth retardation of the spine. Dermatoglyphic abnormalities are present. Hand anomalies consist of hypoplasia of the thumb or its distal placement, occasional triphalangeal thumbs, hypoplasia of the thenar muscles, some instances of polydactyly and hypoplasia of the carpal bones, and fusion of hypoplastic carpal bones. The syndrome is named for the *Instituto Venezolano de Investigaciones Cientificas (IVIC).*

Arias, S., *et al.* The IVIC syndrome: A new autosomal dominant complex pleiotropic syndrome with radial ray hypoplasia, hearing impairment, external lo ophthalmoplegia, and thrombocytopenia. *Am. J. Med. Genet.,* 1980, 6:25-59.

ivory bones. See *Albers-Schönberg syndrome.*

IWANOFF, VLADIMIR P. See IVANOV, VLADIMIR P.

Page #	Term	Observation

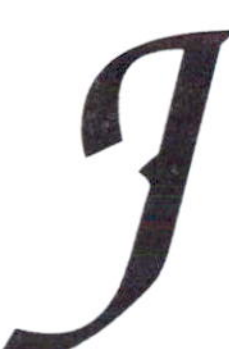

JACCOUD, FRANÇOIS SIGISMOND (French physician, 1830-1913)
Jaccoud arthritis. See *Jaccoud syndrome.*
Jaccoud arthropathy. See *Jaccoud syndrome.*
Jaccoud disease. See *Jaccoud syndrome.*
Jaccoud polyarthritis. See *Jaccoud syndrome.*
Jaccoud syndrome. Synonyms: *Jaccoud arthritis, Jaccoud arthropathy, Jaccoud disease, Jaccoud polyarthritis, chronic postrheumatic arthritis, chronic postrheumatic fever arthropathy.*

A deforming arthropathy of the hands and feet in young adults with a history of recent rheumatic fever or systemic lupus erythematosus. A typical deformity consists mainly of ulnar deviation of the metacarpophalangeal joints, the hand being deviated medially at the wrist. Subluxation of the proximal phalanges may cause a hooklike deformity on the volar aspect of the metacarpal heads. The toes may also be affected, and rheumatic nodules are frequently present. Fibrosis of the periarticular tissues with abnormal synovium is the principal pathologic feature.

Jaccoud, S. *Leçons de clinique médicale faites à l'Hôpital de la Charité.* 2nd ed. Paris, Delahoye, 1869.

Jaccoud-like arthropathy. Resorptive arthropathy with episodes of tendon rupture in patients with systemic lupus erythematosus.

Muniain, M., & Spilberg, I. Opera-glass deformity and tendon rupture in a patient with systemic lupus erythematosus. *Clin. Rheumatol.*, 1985, 4:335-9.

jackknife spasm. See *West syndrome.*

JACKSON, A. D. M.
Jackson-Lawler syndrome. Synonym: *pachyonychia congenita II.*

A variant of the Jadassohn-Lewandowski syndrome, consisting of congenital pachyonychia, hyperhidrosis of palms and soles, hyperkeratosis palmaris et plantaris, and follicular keratosis, but lacking oral leukokeratosis. Additional defects include natal teeth and cutaneous epidermoid cysts, especially of the head, neck, and upper chest. Corneal dystrophy and hoarse voice may be associated. The syndrome is transmitted as an autosomal dominant trait.

Jackson, A. D., & Lawler, S. D. Pachyonychia congenita: A report of six cases in one family. *Ann. Eugen.*, 1951-52, 16:142-6.

JACKSON, HENRY, JR. (American physician)
Parker-Jackson syndrome. See *under Parker, Frederick, Jr.*
JACKSON, JOHN HUGHLINGS (British neurologist, 1835-1911)
Bravais-Jackson epilepsy. See *Jackson epilepsy.*
Hughlings Jackson syndrome. See *Jackson-MacKenzie syndrome.*
Jackson epilepsy. Synonyms: *Bravais-Jackson epilepsy, cortical epilepsy, focal epilepsy, jacksonian epilepsy, partial cortical epilepsy.*

Seizures involving one or several parts of the body on the same side. The attacks may begin as spasms of a single part, usually the angle of the mouth, the index finger, the great toe, or the thumb, and progress to other areas. Consciousness is retained unless the seizures spread to the opposite side of the body. Jacksonian seizures indicate focal lesions on the contralateral side of the brain, usually in the area of the motor cortex.

Jackson, J. H. Unilateral epileptiform seizures, attended by temporary defect of sight. *Med. Times Gaz., London*, 1863, 1:5888. *Bravais, L. F. *Recherches sur les symptômes et le traitement de l'épilepsie hémiplégique.* Paris, 1827 (Thesis).

Jackson syndrome. See *Jackson-MacKenzie syndrome.*
Jackson-MacKenzie syndrome. Synonyms: *Hughlings Jackson syndrome, Jackson syndrome, MacKenzie syndrome, dysphagia-dysphonia syndrome, hemiplegia alternans hypoglossica, vago-accessory-hypoglossal syndrome.*

Unilateral paralysis of the soft palate, pharynx, larynx, sternocleidomastoid muscle, tongue, and trapezius muscle caused by dysfuncion of the tenth, eleventh, and twelfth cranial nerves secondary to cerebral or medullary lesions.

Jackson, J. H. Case of paralysis of the tongue from haemorrhage in the medulla oblongata. *Lancet*, 1872, 2:770-3. *MacKenzie, S. Two cases of associated paralysis of the tongue, soft palate, and vocal cord on the same side. *Tr. Clin. Soc. London*, 1886, 19:317-9.

jacksonian epilepsy. See *Jackson epilepsy.*
JACOB, ARTHUR (Irish physician, 1790-1874)
Jacob ulcer. See *Krompecher tumor.*
JACOB, EUGENE C. (American physician, born 1905)
Jacob syndrome. See *oculo-orogenital syndrome.*
JACOB, OCTAVE (French physician)
Jacob disease. Permanent constriction of the mandible with the inability to open the mouth, reportedly described by Jacob in 1899.

Tarel. Constriction des mâchoires extra-articulaires de'origine osseuse-maladie de Jacob. *J. Stomat. Belg.*, 1965, 7:105-21.

JACOBI, EDUARD (German physician 1862-1915)

Jacobi disease. Synonym: *poikiloderma atrophicans vasculare.*

Poikiloderma that resembles radiodermatiti, which is characterized by extensive telangiectasia, pigmentation, and atrophy of the skin and oral mucosa. Initially, red patches appear on various parts of the body and enlarge gradually, eventually occupying large areas. Individual lesions range in color from red to brown and consist of telangiectases, minute petechial hemorrhages, pigmented areas, and lichenoid papules covered by scales. This disease and Petges-Cléjat syndrome are similar in many respects.

Jacobi, Fall zur Diagnose. (Poikilodermia vascularis atrophicans). *Verh. Deut. Derm. Ges.*, 1906. 9 Cong., pp. 321-3.

JACOBSEN, PETREA (Danish physician)

Jacobsen syndrome. See *chromosome 11q deletion syndrome.*

JACOD, MAURICE (French physician, born 1880)

Jacod syndrome. Synonyms: *Jacod triad, Negri syndrome, Negri-Jacod syndrome, Silvio Negri syndrome, retrosphenoidal syndrome, retrosphenoidal space syndrome.*

A neurological disorder characterized by ophthalmoplegia, optic tract lesions with unilateral amaurosis, and trigeminal neuralgia. It is caused by middle cranial fossa tumors (nasopharyngeal in origin), involving the nerves passing through the foramen ovale, foramen rotundum, and sphenoidal fissure (second, third, fourth, fifth, and sixth cranial nerves).

Jacod, M. Sur la propagation intracrânienne des sarcomes de la trompe d'Eustache, syndrome du carrefour pétro-sphénoidal, paralysie de 2e, 3e, 4e, 5e, et 6e paires crâniennes. *Rev. Neur., Paris,* 1921, 28:33-8. Negri, S. La sindroma di Silvio Negri. Storia d'un tumore della base del cranio. Cenni sulla malatia del Comm. Mons. Bernardo Raineri Reperto necroscopico. *Riv. Otoneurooft., Bologna*, 1935, 12:515-22.

Jacod triad. See *Jacod syndrome.*

Negri-Jacod syndrome. See *Jacod syndrome.*

JACQUET, LEONARD MARIE LUCIEN (French physician, 1860-1914)

Jacquet syndrome. See *hypohidrotic ectodermal dysplasia syndrome.*

JADASSOHN, JOSEF (German dermatologist in Bern, 1863-1936)

Borst-Jadassohn epithelioma. See *under Borst.*

Jadassohn disease (1). Synonyms: *atrophia maculosa cutis, maloculopapular erythrodermia.*

A skin disorder marked by slightly elevated, lentil-shaped, red papules which at first appear in the elbow area and later spread to other parts of the arm and forearm, including the dorsum of the hand. As the disease progresses, the affected area becomes painful and the papules atrophy, gradually forming slight depressions in the skin. Periodically there are new crops of papules, which also atrophy, so that eventually the entire area becomes covered with atrophied depressions and the skin assumes a red, thin, wrinkled, papery appearance. Jadassohn suggested that selective atrophy of elastic fibers is the cause.

Jadassohn. Über eigenartige Form von "Atrophia maculosa cutis." *Verh. Deut. Derm. Ges.*, 1890-91:342-58.

Jadassohn disease (2). See *Jadassohn nevus sebaceus.*

Jadassohn nevus sebaceus. Synonyms: *Jadassohn disease, linear nevus sebaceus anomalad, nevus sebaceus of Jadassohn (SNJ), sebaceus nevus syndrome.*

A type of yellowish to orange or tan plaquelike lesions, usually present at birth, most commonly occurring in the midfacial area, sometimes also affecting the trunk and limbs. Hyperpigmentation, hyperkeratosis, and neurological complications such as seizures and mental deficiency are usually present. Associated disorders may include esotropia, conjunctival lipodermoid lesions, corneal opacity, colobomas of the eyelids and choroid, hydrocephalus, cerebral cortical lesions, alopecia, coarctation of the aorta, ventricular septal defects, tooth enamel hypoplasia, kidney hamartomas, and nephroblastomas. The etiology is unknown.

*Jadassohn, J. Bemerkungen zur Histologie der systematisierten Naevi und über "Talgdrüsen-Naevi." *Arch. Derm. Syph., Berlin*, 1895, 88:355-94.

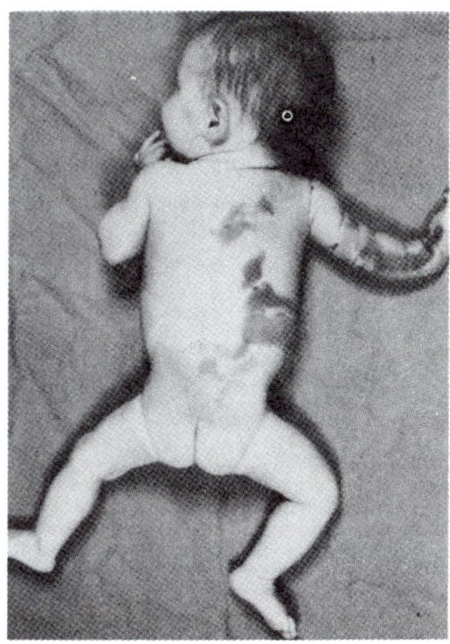

Jadassohn nevus sebaceous
Lansky, L.L., et al.: *Am. J. Dis. Child.* 123:587, 1972. Chicago: American Medical Assocation.

Jadassohn-Lewandowski syndrome. Synonyms: *pachyonychia congenita, pachyonychia ichthyosiforme.*

An association of congenital pachyonychia, hyperhidrosis of the palms and soles, follicular keratosis, hyperkeratosis palmaris et plantaris, and oral leukokeratosis. The nail lesions are usually present at birth or shortly after, but those of the skin become apparent later during infancy or early childhood. Eruption of bullae, which break and become infected and painful, takes place on the plantar surfaces of the toes and heels. Hyperhidrosis of the palms and soles is a constant feature, but other parts of the skin are dry and have a mildly ichthyotic appearance. There may be eruption of follicular papullae on the elbows, knees, buttocks, and popliteal areas, usually in association with verrucous lesions, acanthosis, and parakeratosis, which cause the skin to become thickened. Additional disorders may include alopecia, hoarse voice (because of thickening of the larynx), and mental retardation. The syndrome is transmitted as an autosomal dominant trait. Without leukosis, the condition is known as the *Jackson-Lawler syndrome.*

Jadassohn, J., & Lewandowski, F. Pachyonychia congenita. Keratosis disseminata circumscripta (follicularis),

Tylomata, Leukokeratosis linguae. In: Neisser, A., & Jacobi, E., eds. *Ikonographia dermatologica.*, Berlin, Urbach & Schwarzenberg, 1906, pp. 29-31.

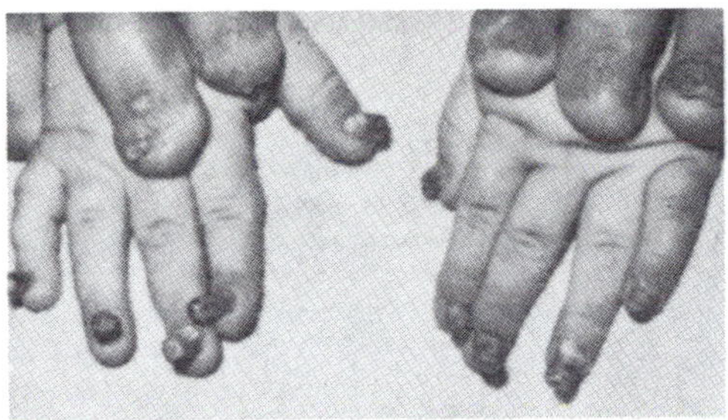

Jadassohn-Lewandowski syndrome
Nelson, W.E. (ed.): *Textbook of Pediatrics*, 8th ed. Phildelphia: W.B. Saunders Co., 1964.

Jadassohn-Tièche nevus. Synonyms: *benign mesenchy mal melanoma, blue neuronevus, blue nevus, chro matophoroma, dermal melanocytoma, melanofi broma.*

A sharply defined, round or oval, slightly elevated, hard, blue to blue-black, benign melanocytic tumor. Individual nevi vary in size from 2 to 15 mm in diameter, and are found most commonly on the face, forearms, hands, buttocks, and occasionally in the oral cavity. Histologically, the lesion consists of mixtures of melanoccytes, fibrillar cells, collangenous fibrous tissue, and nervelike cells. Spindle-shaped, bipolar, dendritic cells grouped in the lower two-thirds of the cutis are the principal features.

*Jadassohn, J. *Dermatologie, Wien,* 1938:429. Tièche, M. Über benigne Melanome ("Chromatophorome") der Haut-"blaue Naevi." *Virchows Arch. Path.*, 1906, 186:212-29.

nevus sebaceus of Jadassohn. See *Jadassohn nevus sebaceus, under Jadassohn, Josef.*

JADASSOHN, W. (Swiss physician)

Franceschetti-Jadassohn syndrome. See *Naegeli syndrome, under Naegeli, Oskar.*

Naegeli-Franceschetti-Jadassohn syndrome. See *Naegeli syndrome, under Naegeli, Oskar.*

JAFFE, HENRY LEWIS (American physician, born 1896)

Jaffe-Lichtenstein dysplasia. See *Jaffe-Lichtenstein syndrome.*

Jaffe-Lichtenstein fibrous dysplasia. See *Jaffe-Lichtenstein syndrome.*

Jaffe-Lichtenstein syndrome. Synonyms: *Jaffe-Lichtenstein dysplasia, Jaffe-Lichtenstein fibrous dysplasia, Jaffe-Lichtenstein-Uehlinger syndrome, fibrocystic disease, fibrous bone dysplasia, fibrous osteoma, localized fibrous dysplasia of bone, localized fibrous lesion, monostotic fibrous dysplasia, nonosteogenic fibroma, ossifying fibroma, osteitis fibrosa cystica, osteitis fibrosa disseminata, osteitis fibrosa juvenilis, osteodystrophia disseminata, osteodystrophia fibrosa universalis, osteofibrosis, osteofibrosis deformans juvenilis, polyostic fibrous dysplasia, skeletal cystofibromatosis.*

A dysplastic bone disease characterized by excessive proliferation of fibrous tissues. The symptoms consist of painful bone deformities associated with pathological fractures, limping, unequal limb length, skull asymmetry, leontiasislike appearance, scoliosis, lordosis, and chest deformity. Radiological findings show predominantly unilateral skull thickening, sclerosis at the base of the skull, cystic lesions of the cranial bones, obliteration of the paranasal sinuses, patchy rarefaction of the shafts of the tubular bones, sclerosis of the spongiosa with internal atrophy of the cortex of the tubular bones, ground-glass appearance and loculation of the lytic lesions, elongation or shortening of the affected bones, and premature epiphyseal closure. Onset usually takes place during the first 2 decades of life with symptoms of the monostotic form sometimes manifested in later adulthood. Heredity does not appear to be a factor. A similar condition with patchy skin pigmentation and sexual precocity is known as the *McCune-Albright syndrome.*

Jaffe, H. L. "Osteid-osteoma," benign osteoblastic tumor composed of osteoid a typical bone. *Arch. Surg.*, 1935, 31:709-28. Lichtenstein, L. Polyostic fibrous dysplasia. *Arch. Surg.*, 1938, 36:874. Jaffe, H. L., & Lichtenstein, L. Non-osteogenic fibroma of bone. *Am. J. Path,* 1942, 18:205-15.

Jaffe-Lichtenstein-Uehlinger syndrome. See *Jaffe-Lichtenstein syndrome.*

JAHNKE

Jahnke syndrome. See *Sturge-Weber syndrome.*

jail fever. See *Hildenbrand disease.*

JAKOB, ALFONS (German physician, 1884-1931)

Creutzfeldt-Jakob disease (CJD). See *Jakob-Creutzfeldt syndrome.*

Jakob pseudosclerosis. See *Jakob-Creutzfeldt syndrome.*

Jakob-Creutzfeldt syndrome. Synonyms: *Creutzfeldt-Jakob disease (CJD), Jakob pseudosclerosis, abiotrophic dementia, corticopallidospinal degeneration, corticostriatal-spinal degeneration, spastic pseudosclerosis.*

A syndrome of motor, sensory, and mental disturbances, including stiffness and weakness of the limbs, progressive dementia, convulsive seizures, and various pyramidal and extrapyramidal symptoms. Pathologically, there is widespread degeneration and atrophy of the cerebral cortex, basal ganglia, and thalamus, with the presence of coarse and fine vacuoles in all cortical layers (status spongiosus). The condition is usually fatal within a few months or years. Middle-aged and elderly persons are usually affected. Some writers consider this syndrome a variant of the Nevin and the Heidenhain syndromes.

Jakob, A. Über eigenartige Erkrankung des Zentralnervensystems mit bemerkenswertem anatomischen Befunde (Spastische Pseudosklerose-Encephalomyelopathie mit disseminierten Degenerationsherden). *Zschr. Ges. Neur. Psychiat.*, 1921, 64:147-228. *Creutzfeldt, H. G. Über eine eigenartige herdförmige Erkrankung des Zentralnervensystems. In: Nissl, F., & Alzheimer, A., eds. *Histologie und Histopathologie.* Jena, 1921, p. 1.

JAKSCH, RUDOLF, RITTER VON WARTENHORST (Austrian physician, 1855-1940)

Jaksch anemia. See *Jaksch syndrome.*

Jaksch syndrome. Synonyms: *Jaksch anemia, Jaksch-Hayem syndrome, Jaksch-Hayem-Luzet syndrome, von Jaksch anemia, von Jaksch-Luzet syndrome, anemia pseudoleukemica, anemia pseudoleukemica infantum, anemia splenica pseudoleukemica infantum, pseudoleukemia infantum.*

A chronic anemic disease of infants and children under the age of 3 years, simulating leukemia and associated with splenomegaly, hepatomegaly, lymph node enlargement, hemoglobin deficiency, anisocytosis, numerous erythroblasts and macroblasts, leukocytosis, and lymphocytosis. The anemia may be associated with a variety of conditions, including rickets, malnutrition, congenital syphilis, gastrointestinal disorders, tuberculosis, iron deficiency, and thalassemia. See also *Bennett disease (leukemia).*

Jaksch, R., von. Über Leukämie und Leukocytose im Kindesalter. *Wien. Klin. Wschr.*, 1889, 2:435-7; 456-8. Hayem, G. *Du sang et de ses altérations pathologiques*. Paris, Masson, 1889, p. 864. Luzet, C. L'anémie infantile pseudoleucémique. *Arch. Gen. Méd., Paris*, 1891, 1:579-92.

Jaksch Wartenhorst syndrome. See *Meyenburg-Altherr-Uehlinger syndrome.*

Jaksch-Hayem syndrome. See *Jaksch syndrome.*

Jaksch-Hayem-Luzet syndrome. See *Jaksch syndrome.*

von Jaksch anemia. See *Jaksch syndrome.*

von Jaksch Wartenhorst syndrome. See *Meyenburg-Altherr-Uehlinger syndrome.*

von Jaksch-Luzet syndrome. See *Jaksch syndrome.*

JAKSCH-WARTENHORST, RUDOLF. See JAKSCH, RUDOLF, RITTER VON WARTENHORST

Jamaican neuropathy. See *Strachan syndrome.*

JAMES, G. C. W. (American physician)

Swyer-James syndrome (SJS). See *under Swyer, Paul Robert.*

Swyer-James-Macleod syndrome. See *Swyer-James syndrome, under Swyer, Paul Robert.*

JAMPEL, ROBERT STEVEN (American physician, born 1926)

Schwartz-Jampel syndrome. See *under Schwartz, Oscar.*

JANBON, MARCEL MARIE JOSEPH (French physician, born 1898)

Janbon syndrome. Synonyms: *antibiotic enteritis, choleriform enteritis, choleriform syndrome.*

A gastrointestinal syndrome resembling cholera, which is produced by oxytetracycline therapy. After administration of the drug, there is a sudden attack of epigastric pain, watery diarrhea, vomiting, fever, dehydration, collapse, peculiar facies, anuria, and azotemia. Fecal analysis usually reveals the disappearance of normal intestinal flora, which is replaced by oxytetracycline-resistant strains of pathogenic staphylococci.

Janbon, M., *et al.* Le syndrome choleriforme de la terramycine. *Montpellier Méd.*, 1952, 41-42:300-11.

JANEWAY, THEODORE CALDWELL (American physician, 1872-1917)

Janeway spots. Nodular hemorrhagic spots of the palms and soles seen in subacute bacterial endocarditis.

*Janeway, T. C. Certain clinical observations upon heart disease. *Med. News*, 1899, 75:257-62.

JANSEN, MURK (Dutch orthopedic surgeon, 1863-1935)

dysostosis metaphysaria, Jansen type. See *Jansen metaphyseal chondrodysplasia syndrome.*

dysostosis metaphysaria, Murk Jansen type. See *Jansen metaphyseal chondrodysplasia syndrome.*

Jansen metaphyseal chondrodysplasia syndrome. Synonyms: *Jansen syndrome; Murk Jansen syndrome; dysostosis metaphysaria, Jansen type; dysostosis metaphysaria, Murk Jansen type; metaphyseal dysostosis, Jansen type; metaphyseal dysostosis, Murk Jansen type; osteochondrodysplasia metaphysaria, Jansen type.*

An autosomal dominant syndrome of dwarfism with extremely short lower extremities and severe anterior bowing with a resulting monkeylike squating stance; small immature facies with prominent eyes, mild supraorbital and frontal hyperplasia, and micrognathia; and prominent joints with restricted mobility and ligament hyperlaxity. Small thoracic cage, hyperostosis of the calvarium, thick cranial base, clubfoot, and occasional deafness may be associated. Hypercalcemia is a constant feature. Major radiographic findings include rachitiform metaphyseal lesions, cortical erosion, increased subperiosteal bone formation, widening and fragmentation of the metaphyses, separation of epiphyseal ossification centers from the metaphyses, and demineralization.

Jansen, M. Über atypische Chondrodystrophie (Achondroplasie) und über eine noch nicht beschriebene angeborene Wachstumsstörung des Knochensystems: metaphysäre Dysostosis. *Zschr. Orthop. Chir.*, 1934, 61:253-86.

Jansen syndrome. See *Jansen metaphyseal chondrodysplasia syndrome.*

metaphyseal dysostosis, Jansen type. See *Jansen metaphyseal chondrodysplasia syndrome.*

metaphyseal dysostosis, Murk Jansen type. See *Jansen metaphyseal chondrodysplasia syndrome.*

Murk Jansen syndrome. See *Jansen metaphyseal chondrodysplasia syndrome.*

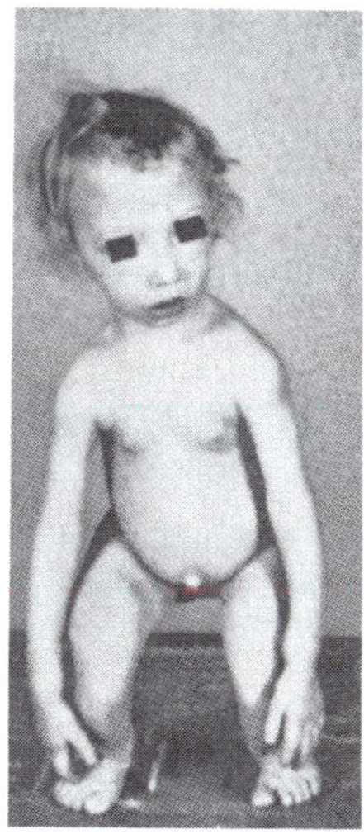
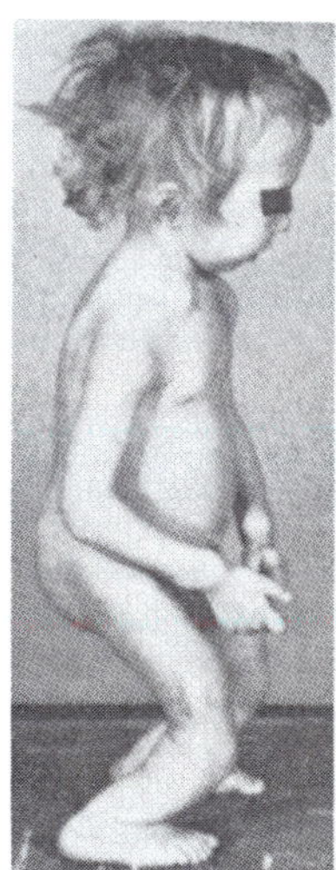

Jansen metaphyseal chondrodysplasia syndrome
Rubin, P.:, *Dynamic Classification of Bone Dysplasias.* Chicago, Year Book Medical Publishers, Inc., 1964.

osteochondrodysplasia metaphysaria, Jansen type. See *Jansen metaphyuseal chondrodysplasia syndrome.*

JANSKY, JAN (Czech physician, 1873-1921)

Jansky-Bielschowsky syndrome. See *gangliosidosis G_{M2} type III.*

JANUS (An ancient Roman god of gates and doorways, having two faces and looking in the opposite directions)

Janus syndrome. See *Swyer-James syndrome.*

Japanese disease. See *Flexner dysentery.*

Japanese multisystem syndrome. See *POEMS syndrome.*

JARCHO, SAUL (American physician, born 1906)

Jarcho syndrome. Synonyms: *carcinoma-disseminated thrombocytopenic purpura syndrome, thrombocytopenic purpura-disseminated carcinoma syndrome.*

Metastatic carcinoma of the bone marrow associated with thrombocytopenic purpura and leukoerythroblastic anemia.

Jarcho, E. Diffusely infiltrative carcinoma. A hitherto undescribed correlation of several varieties of tumor metastasis. *Arch. Pathol.*, 1936, 22:674-96.

Jarcho-Levin syndrome. See *spondylothoracic dysplasia.*

JARVINEN, JUDITH M. (American scientist)

Hecht-Jarvinen syndrome. See *popliteal pterygium syndrome.*

JATZKEWITZ, H. (German biochemist)

Sandhoff-Jatzkewitz syndrome. See *Sandhoff syndrome.*

jaw winking syndrome. See *Gunn syndrome.*

JAYLE, GAETAN E. (French ophthalmologist, born 1904)

Jayle-Ourgaud syndrome. Synonym: *ataxic nystagmus.*

Paralysis of the median rectus muscle in lateral gaze associated with nystagmoid movements of the contralateral eye during the same lateral conjugate movement.

*Hugonnier, R., & Magnard, P. Paralysie internucléaire antérieure. *Bull. Soc. Opht. France*, 1958, 58:265-68. Orowski, W. J., *et al.* Bielschowsky-Lutz-Cogan syndrome. *Am. J. Ophth.*, 1965, 59:416-30.

JBS. See *Johanson-Blizzard syndrome, under Johanson, Ann.*

JEANSELME, ANTOINE EDOUARD (French physician, 1858-1935)

Jeanselme nodules. Synonyms: *Lutz-Jeanselme syndrome, juxta-articular nodosities.*

Subcutaneous fibrous nodules at articulations or under the skin covering the bone, seen in treponemal diseases, such as yaws and syphilis. Preferred sites are the knee and elbow or under the skin covering the tibia, elbow, or, more rarely, the ribs, trochanter, or malleoli. Nodules related to syphilis are known as *syphilitic fibromatous nodules.*

*Lutz, A. *Mh. Prakt. Derm.*, 1892, 14:30. *Jeanselme, E. Nodosites juxtaarticulaires. *Cong. Colonial Paris, Sect. Méd. Hyg. Colon.*, 1904, p. 15.

Lutz-Jeanselme syndrome. See *Jeanselme nodules.*

JEFFERSON, SIR GEOFFREY (British neurologist, born 1886)

Jefferson syndrome. Synonym: *aneurysm of internal carotid artery.*

Aneurysm of the internal carotid artery with involvement of the visual pathways, classified by Jefferson as follows: (1) **Posterior cavernous syndrome**, with involvement of the whole trigeminal nerve, resulting in oculomotor, sometimes only abducens, paralysis. The motor root of the trigeminal nerve may be affected. (2) **Middle cavernous syndrome**, with involvement of only the first and second divisions of the trigeminal nerve, resulting in oculomotor paralysis. (3) **Anterior cavernous syndrome**, with involvement of only the first division of the trigeminal nerve, resulting in paralysis of the muscles supplied by the superior division of the oculomotor nerve, or of all nerves supplying the mobility of the eye.

Jefferson, G. On the saccular aneurysm of the internal carotid artery in cavernous sinus. *Brit. J. Surg.*, 1938-39, 26:267-302.

JEGHERS, HAROLD JOSEPH (American physician, born 1904)

Jeghers syndrome. See *Peutz-Jeghers syndrome.*

Peutz-Jeghers hamartosis. See *Peutz-Jeghers syndrome.*

Peutz-Jeghers syndrome (PJS). See *under Peutz.*

Peutz-Touraine-Jeghers syndrome. See *Peutz-Jeghers syndrome.*

jejunal diverticulosis-macrocytic anemia-steatorrhea syndrome. The concurrence of massive diverticulosis of the jejunum, macrocytic anemia, and steatorrhea.

Badendoch, J., *et al.* Massive diverticulosis of small intestine with steatorrhea and megaloblastic anemia. *Q. J. Med.*, 1955, 24:321. Taybi, H. *Radiology of syndromes.* Chicago, Year Book, 1975, p. 77.

jejunal neoplasm syndrome. See *Dudley-Klingenstein syndrome.*

JENSEN, EDMUND (Danish ophthalmologist, 1861-1950)

Jensen disease. Synonyms: *juxtapapillary choroiditis, juxtapapillary retinopathy, retinochoroiditis juxtapapillaris.*

Circumscribed choroiditis adjacent to the optic disc, characterized by retinal edema with white cotton wool-like patches in the affected area, small lipoid deposits, and occasional exudates and hemorrhage visible under the ophthalmoscope. Decreased central visual acuity and visual field defect are the principal subjective symptoms. Narrowing of the retinal arteriole supplying the involved area usually occurs.

Jensen, E. Retino-choroiditis juxtapapillaris. *Graefes Arch. Ophth.*, 1909, 69:41-8.

jerking stiff-man syndrome. Synonym: *stiff man-myoclonus syndrome.*

An association of muscle rigidity with a peculiar myoclonus. The course is progressive and is characterized by a sustained, predominantly axial rigidity affecting chiefly the paraspinal and abdominal muscles and increased muscle tone in the legs. Repetitive myoclonic jerks may be elicited by touching the perioral region or stretching the muscles of the head and neck. Jaw jerks, downbeat nystagmus, and brisk lower limb reflexes with ankle clonus are associated. Electromyographic findings show normal activity on voluntary movement with absence of activity at rest in the arms and legs but with continuous activity of normal motor units in erector spinae, persisting during attempted relaxation. Pneumoencephalography and computed tomography indicate evidence of brain stem and cerebellar atrophy. See also *stiff man syndrome.*.

Leigh, P. N. *et al.* A patient with reflex myoclonus and muscle rigidity: "Jerking stiff-man syndrome." *J. Neurol. Neurosurg. Psychiat.*, 1980, 43:1125-31.

JERSILD, PETER CHRISTIAN OLAF (Danish physician, 1867-1950)

Huguier-Jersild syndrome. See *under Huguier.*

Jersild syndrome. See *Huguier-Jersild syndrome.*

JERVELL, ANTON (Norwegian physician, born 1901)

Jervell and Lange-Nielsen syndrome. See *under long QT syndrome.*

JESSNER, MAX (American physician)

Jessner disease. See *Jessner-Kanoff disease.*

Jessner-Kanoff disease. Synonym: *Jessner disease.*

Benign lymphocytic infiltration of the skin, affecting primarily the face and occasionally appearing on other parts of the body.

Jessner, M., & Kanoff, N. B Lymphocytic infiltration of the skin. *Arch. Derm. Syph., Chicago,* 1953, 60:447-9.

Sontheimer, R. D., *et al.* Lupus erythematosus. In: Fitzpatrick, T. B., Eisen, A. Z., Wolff, K., Freedberg, I. M., & Austen, K. F., eds. *Dermatology in general medicine.* 3rd ed. New York, McGraw-Hill, 1987, pp. 1816-34.

JEUNE, MATHIS (French pediatrician, born 1910)

Jeune syndrome. Synonyms: *asphyxiating thoracic dysplasia, asphyxiating thoracic dystrophy, infantile thoracic dystrophy, thoracic-pelvic-phalangeal dystrophy (TPPD).*

Congenital polychondrodystrophy in which a narrow and rigid thoracic cage results in asphyxia. The affected infants exhibit short-limb dwarfism, short ribs, small thoracic cage, irregular epiphyses and metaphyses with cone-shaped epiphyses, and early fusion between the epiphyses and metaphyses of the distal and middle phalanges. Occasional defects include polydactyly, lacunar skull, chronic nephritis, and other disorders. The syndrome is believed to represent a spectrum of disorders with a wide variability in clinical and radiological manifestations. Many infants die in infancy because of asphyxia; some survive infancy but die later in childhood of juvenile nephrophthisis. Most cases are transmitted as an autosomal recessive trait. Some authors suggest that, because of their overlapping features, the Ellis-van Creveld syndrome, the Jeune syndrome, and renohepatopancreatic dysplasia form parts of a single disease spectrum, rather than being distinct entities.

Jeune, M., *et al.* Polychondrodystrophie avec blocage thoracique d'évolution fatale. *Pediatrie, Lyon*, 1954, 9:390-2. Brueton, L. A., *et al.* Ellis-van Creveld syndrome, Jeune syndrome, and renal-hepatic-pancreatic dysplasia: Separate entities or disease spectrum? *J. Med. Genet.*, 1990, 27:252-5.

Jeune-Tommasi syndrome. Synonym: *ataxia-deafness-cardiomyopathy syndrome.*

A familial syndrome, transmitted as an autosomal recessive trait, characterized by cerebellar ataxia, progresive sensorineural hearing loss, mental deficiency, lentigines of the skin, and myocardial sclerosis. Intention tremor, hypotonia, scanning speech, pallor of the optic disks, depressed reflexes, muscle atrophy, small incisor teeth, and dental caries are usually present. Autopsy findings include interstitial myocardial fibrosis, portal fibrosis, and degeneration of the spinocerebellar tracts.

Jeune, M., Tommasi, M., *et al.* Syndrome familial associant ataxie, surdité et oligophrénie. Sclérose myocardiaque d'évolution fatale chez l'un des enfants. *Pédiatrie, Paris,* 1963, 18:984-7.

JIRASEK, ARNOLD (Prague surgeon, 1880-1960)

Jirásek-Zuelzer-Wilson syndrome. Synonyms: *Zuelzer-Wilson syndrome, agangliosis of the entire colon, congenital neurogenic ileus, total colonic agangliosis.*

Obstructive ileus in newborn infants in the absence of mechanical causes due to agangliosis of the entire colon. The symptoms, which begin at birth or within the first few days or weeks of life, include abdominal distention, vomiting, severe constipation, and anorexia.

Jirásek, A. Über einige intramurale Ursachen der Krämpfe des Verdauungskanals. *Acta Chir. Scand.*, 1926, 59:91-9. Zuelzer, W. W., & Wilson, J. L. Functional intestinal obstruction on a congenital neurogenic basis in infancy. *Am. J. Dis. Child.*, 1948, 75:40-75.

JOANNY, J.

Léri-Joanny syndrome. See *Léri syndrome (1).*

JOB (In the Old Testament, a man whose faith in God overcame the test of repeated calamities)

Job abscess. See *Job syndrome.*

Job syndrome. Synonyms: *Buckley syndrome, hyper-IgE (HIE) syndrome, hyperimmunoglobulinemia E, hyperimmunoglobulin E recurrent infection syndrome.*

An immunological disorder characterized by recurrent pyogenic infection and cold staphylococcal abscesses **(Job abscesses)**, occurring from birth, originally described in fair-skinned, red-haired females. Its characteristics include recurrent cutaneous, articular, and pulmonary abscesses, growth retardation, coarse facies, chronic dermatitis, immediate hypersensitivity with high serum concentrations of immunoglobulin E and eosinophilia, and an impaired ability of peripheral blood neutrophils and monocytes to kill ingested opsonized bacteria. The syndrome is believed to be transmitted as an autosomal recessive trait. The condition is named after Job, who, according to the Old Testament (Job 2:7), was covered by Satan with boils from the sole of his foot to his crown. See also *chronic granulomatous disease of childhood.*

Davis, S. D. *et al.* Job's syndrome. Recurrent, "cold", staphylococcal abscesses. *Lancet,* 1966, 1:1013-5. Buckley, R. H., *et al.* Extreme hyperimmunoglobulinemia E and undue susceptibility to infection. *Pediatrics,* 1972, 49:59-70.

JOHANSON, ANN (American physician)

Johanson-Blizzard syndrome (JBS). Ectodermal dysplasia with endocrine and exocrine insufficiency and growth and mental deficiency. Craniofacial defects consist of microcephaly, hypoplastic or aplastic alae nasi, midline scalp defects, and oligodontia. Hypothyroidism is the chief endocrine feature, and pancreatic insufficiency with resulting malabsorption is the main exocrine disorder. Associated anomalies include imperforate anus, rectovaginal fistula, double or septate vagina, single urogenital orifice, deafness, muscle hypotonia, and sometimes strabismus, enlarged clitoris, and recurrent urinary infections. The syndrome is transmitted as an autosomal recessive trait.

Johanson, A., & Blizzard, R. A syndrome of congenital aplasia of the alae nasi, deafness, hypothyroidism, dwarfism, absent permanent teeth, and malabsorption. *J. Pediat.*, 1971, 79:982-7.

JOHANSSON, SVEN (Swedish physician, born 1880)

Larsen-Johansson syndrome. See *under Larsen, Christian Magnus Falsen Sinding.*

Sinding Larsen-Johansson syndrome. See *Larsen-Johansson syndrome, under Larsen, Christian Magnus Falsen Sinding.*

JOHNIE MCL

Johnie McL disease. See *mucopolysaccharidosis I-H.*

JOHNSON

Reye-Johnson syndrome. See *Reye syndrome.*

JOHNSON, FRANK B. (American physician, born 1919)

Dubin-Johnson syndrome (DJS). See *under Dubin.*

Dubin-Johnson-Sprinz syndrome. See *Dubin-Johnson syndrome.*

JOHNSON, FRANK CRAIG (American pediatrician, 1894-1934)

Stevens-Johnson syndrome (SJS). See *under Stevens.*

JOHNSON, LORAND VICTOR (American ophthalmologist, born 1905)

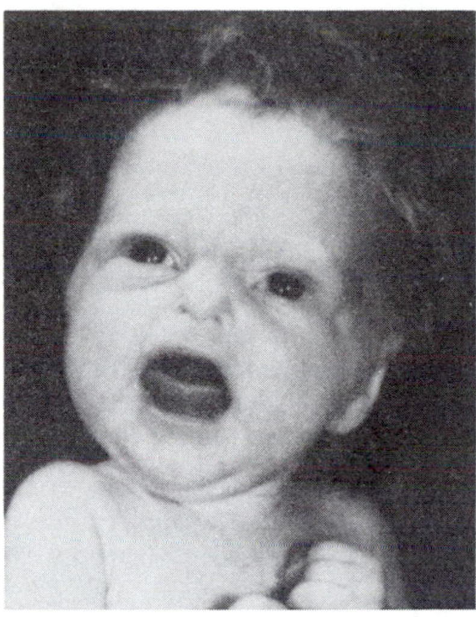

Johanson-Blizzard syndrome
Gorlin, R.J.: "Selected ectodermal dysplasias." In Salinas, C.F., Opitz, J.M., Paul, N.W. (eds): *Recent Advances in Ectodermal Dysplasias*. New York: Alan R. Liss, Inc. for the March of Dimes Birth Defects Foundation BD:OAS 24(2):123-148, 1988, with permission.

Johnson syndrome. Synonyms: *adherence syndrome, adherence syndrome of the lateral or superior rectus muscles, adherent lateral syndrome, pseudoparalysis of the lateral or superior rectus muscles.*

Lateral rectus paralysis caused by adherence of the lateral rectus muscle to the inferior oblique muscle, usually observed in children under 3 years of age.

Johnson, L. V. Adherence syndrome (pseudoparalysis of lateral or superior rectus muscles). *Arch. Ophth., Chicago*, 1950, 44:870-8.

JOHNSON, RONALD C. (American physician)

Opitz-Johnson-McCreadie-Smith syndrome. See *Opitz trigonocephaly syndrome.*

JOHNSTONE, A. S.

Allison-Johnstone anomaly. See *Barrett syndrome.*

joint contractures-dwarfism-normal intelligence syndrome. A familial syndrome, transmitted as an autosomal dominant trait, characterized by dwarfism associated with abnormal joint mobility and flexed distal phalanges, wrists, elbows, feet, and knees, without any apparent skeletal abnormality.

Stoll, C., *et al.* Contracture articulaire avec petite taille et intelligence normale: Un syndrome familial autosomique dominant. *J. Génét. Hum.*, 1980, 28:299-304.

JOLLIFFE, NORMAN HAYHURST (American physician, 1901-1961)

Jolliffe syndrome. See *nicotinic acid deficiency encephalophathy.*

JONES, BENCE. See BENCE JONES, HENRY

JONES, HENRY BENCE. See BENCE JONES, HENRY

JONES, HUGH T. (American physician, born 1892)

Henderson-Jones syndrome. See *Reichel syndrome.*

Reichel-Jones-Henderson syndrome. See *Reichel syndrome.*

JONES, MARILYN C. (American physician)

Jones syndrome. A familial syndrome, transmitted as an autosomal dominant trait, characterized by tetralogy of Fallot associated with low birth weight, characteristic facies (broad forehead, proptotic appearance in infancy, prominent nasal tip, preauricular pits), clinodactyly of the fifth finger (short or incurved fingers), distal transverse palmar creases, thenar crease hypoplasia, and cryptorchism.

Jones, M. C., & Waldman, J. D. An autosomal dominant syndrome of characteristic facial appearance, preauricular pits, fifth finger clinodactyly, and tetralogy of Fallot. *Am. J. Med. Genet.*, 1985, 22:135-41.

JONES, WILLIAM A. (American dentist)

Jones disease. See *cherubism.*

Jones syndrome. See *cherubism.*

JONKERS, GARRIT HENDRIK (Dutch ophthalmologist)

Waardenburg-Jonkers disease. See *under Waardenburg.*

JORGENSON, RONALD J. (American physician)

Jorgenson syndrome. A familial form of ectodermal dysplasia, transmitted either as an X-linked or autosomal dominant trait, characterized by unusual dermatoglyphics, hypotrichosis, hypohidrosis, nail dystrophy, and defective teeth. The hair is usually sparse or normal at birth but is shed by the end of the second decade. Xerophthalmia, sometimes leading to blindness, may be associated. See also *Basan syndrome.*

Jorgenson, R. J. Ectodermal dysplasia with hypotrichosis, hypohidrosis, defective teeth, and unusual dermatoglyphics (Basan syndrome?). *Birth Defects*, 1974, 10(4):323-5.

JOSEPH, ANTONE (Portuguese seaman from the Azores, who settled in California in 1845)

Joseph disease. Synonyms: *Azorean disease, Machado disease, Machado-Joseph disease (MJD), Machado-Joseph Azorean disease (MJAD), Thomas disease, autosomal dominant striatonigral degeneration, nigrospinal-dentatal degeneration with nuclear ophthalmoplegia, striatonigral degeneration.*

A dominantly inherited neurologic disorder reported in two Azorean-Portuguese families in Massachusetts (**Machado disease**), followed by a report in the Thomas family (**Thomas disease**) and in another Portuguese family, the Joseph family in California (**Joseph disease**). **Machado disease** was marked by progressive cerebellar disease with distal extremity atrophy and sensory loss beginning in the fifth decade; segmental demyelination being its chief pathological feature. **Thomas disease** was marked mainly by gait ataxia, external ophthalmoplegia, faciolingual fasciculation, and spasticity and rigidity of the limbs. Its pathological features included neuronal loss of the substantia nigra, dentate nuclei, and the Clarck column of the spinal cord, in association with demyelination in the posterior columns, lateral corticospinal, and spinothalamic tracts of the spinal cord. Clinical characteristics of **Joseph disease** included progressive motor system disease beginning the second of third decades with unsteadiness of gait, stiffness and spasticity of the lower limbs, slow and indistinct speech due to pharyngeal weakness, impaired visual acuity, nystagmus, ophthalmoplegia, prominent eyes, faciolingual fasciculation, and dystonia of the head, face, extremities and trunk in several instances. Urinary incontinence occurred in some cases. Intelligence was normal. Patellar and ankle conus was occasionally observed. Pathological changes included neuronal loss of the striatum, substantia nigra, basis pontis, dentate nucleus, cerebellar cortex, and anterior horns of the spinal cord. Low cerebrospinal fluid homovanillic acid was relative to the loss of dopamine synthesizing cells of the nigrostriatal pathways. Four types of this syndrome are now recognized: **Type I** occurs with pyramidal and extrapyramidal lesions usually in the second or third decades; **Type II** occurs with cerebellar deficits and other motor features; **Type III** occurs with cerebellar deficit and motor and sensory polyneuropathy, having an onset in the fifth to the seventh decades; and **Type IV** occurs with mild cerebellar deficits and a distal motor sensory neuropathy or amyotrophy, in association with parkinsonian features. The syndrome has been traced to Antone Joseph, who settled in California in 1845, and whose two children suffered from this disorder. The disease has also been reported in Japanese, Italian, and other ethnic groups.

Nakano, K. K., *et al.* Machado disease: A hereditary ataxia in Portuguese immigrants to Massachusetts. *Neurology,* 1972, 22:49-55. Woods, B. I., & Schaumburg, H. H. Nigro-spino-dentatal degeneration with nuclear ophthalmoplegia: A unique and partially treatable clinicopathological entity. *J. Neur. Sc.,* 1972, 17:149-66. Rosenberg, R. N., *et al.* Biochemical study of a new genetic disorder. *Neurology,* 1976, 26:703-14.

Machado-Joseph Azorean disease (MJAD). See *Joseph disease.*

Machado-Joseph disease (MJD). See *Joseph disease.*

JOSEPH, R. (French physician)

Joseph syndrome. A syndrome, transmitted as an autosomal recessive trait, characterized by early onset of convulsions, mental retardation, mild elevation of cerebrospinal fluid protein, and aminoaciduria (proline, hydroxyproline, and glycine). Some authors do not consider this syndrome an independent entity.

Joseph, R., *et al.* Maladie familiale associant des convulsions à début tres précoce, une hyperalbuminorachie et une hyperaminoacidurie, *Arch. Fr. Pediat.,* l958, 15:374-87.

JOSEPH, SISTER. See DEMPSEY, MARY JOSEPH, SISTER

JOSEPHS, HUGH WILSON (American pediatrician, born 1892)

Josephs-Diamond-Blackfan anemia. See *Diamond-Blackfan syndrome.*

Josephs-Diamond-Blackfan syndrome. See *Diamond-Blackfan syndrome.*

JOUBERT, MARIE (Canadian physician)

Joubert syndrome. Synonyms: *Joubert-Boltshauser syndrome, Mohr syndrome variant.*

A rare familial syndrome of agenesis of the cerebellum, cerebellar ataxia, mental retardation, episodic hyperpnea with hyperventilation, abnormal eye movements (nystagmus and irregular jerky movements), rhythmic protrusion of the tongne, and colobomata of the retina and choroid. Muscle hypotonia, high insertion of the tentorium, meningocele, hydrocephalus, microcephaly, agenesis of the corpus callosum, and polydactyly occur in some cases. Most patients die in infancy or early childhood. The syndrome is believed to be transmitted as an autosomal recessive trait.

Joubert, M., *et al.* Familial agenesis of the cerebellar vermis. A syndrome of episodic hyperpnea, abnormal eye movements, ataxia, and retardation. *Neurology,* 1969, 19:813-25.

Joubert-Boltshauser syndrome. See *Joubert syndrome.*

JPD (juvenile plantar dermatosis). See *wet and dry foot syndrome.*

JUBERG, RICHARD C. (American physician)

Juberg-Hayward syndrome. Synonym: *orocraniodigital syndrome.*

A familial syndrome of cleft lip, cleft palate, hypoplastic thumbs, and microcephaly, originally observed in five of six children of normal and unrelated parents. The syndrome is transmitted as an autosomal recessive trait.

Juberg, R. C., & Hayward, J. R. A new familial syndrome of oral, cranial, and digital anomalies. *J. Pediat.*, 1969, 74:755-62.

Juberg-Marsidi syndrome. A syndrome of mental retardation, deafness, flat nasal bridge, eye abnormalities (small fissures, exotropia, light retinal pigmentation, and epicanthus), rudimentary scrotum, cryptorchidism, and micropenis, transmitted as an X-linked trait. In the original report, the proband also had onychodystrophy of the fingers and toes.

Juberg, R. C., & Marsidi, I. A new form of X-linked mental retardation with growth retardation, deafness, and microgenitalism. *Am. J. Hum. Genet.*, 1980, 32:714-22..

jugular foramen syndrome. See *Vernet syndrome.*

JUHEL-RENOY, JEAN EDOUARD (French physician, 1855-1894)

Juhel-Rénoy syndrome. Bilateral renal cortical necrosis.

Juhel-Rénoy, E. De l'anurie précoce scarlatineuse. *Arch. Gén. Méd., Paris*, 1886, 17:385-410.

JULES FRANÇOIS. See FRANÇOIS, JULES

JULIEN MARIE. See MARIE, JULIEN

JULIUSBERG, FRITZ (German dermatologist, born 1872)

Kaposi-Juliusberg dermatitis. See *Kaposi varicelliform eruption.*

jumper syndrome. Injuries sustained by persons who have jumped or have fallen from considerable heights, consisting mainly of hemorrhagic shock, spinal shock, intra-abdominal injuries, retroperitoneal injuries and hemorrhage, head injuries, thoracic injuries, multiple fractures, and hollow viscus perforation.

Scalea, T., *et al.* An analysis of 161 falls from a height: The "jumper syndrome." *J. Trauma*, 1986, 26:706-12.

jumping Frenchmen of Maine syndrome. Synonyms: *goosey, jumping syndrome, latah-like reaction.*

An exaggerated startle reflex, consisting of a violent jump, in association with inconsistent echolalia and a tendency to carry out orders in a reflex manner, even when they are dangerous. The original cases were reported in French-Canadians living in Canada and the northern parts of Maine and New Hampshire. The syndrome is believed to be transmitted as an autosomal recessive trait. Some authors consider this disorder to be a psychological rather than neurological condition. See also *latah syndrome.*

Beard, G. M. Remarks upon "jumpers or jumping Frenchmen." *J. Nerv. Ment. Dis.*, 1878, 5:526.

jumping syndrome. See *jumping Frenchmen of Maine syndrome.*

junction scotoma. See *Traquair scotoma.*

JUNET, ROBERT MAURICE (Swiss physician, born 1907)

Troell-Junet syndrome. See *under Troell.*

JÜNGLING, OTTO (German physician, 1884-1944)

Jüngling disease. See *Perthes-Jüngling disease.*

Jüngling polycystic osteitis. See *Perthes-Jüngling disease.*

Perthes-Jüngling disease. See *under Perthes.*

JÜRGENS, RUDOLF (German physician, 1898-1961)
Willebrand-Jürgens syndrome. See *under Willebrand.*
JUSSE (French physician)
Rimbaud-Jusse syndrome. See *Rimbaud-Passouant-Vallat syndrome.*
jute-spinner's melanosis. See *Riehl melanosis.*

JUTRAS, ALBERT (Canadian physician)
Roy-Jutras syndrome. See *pachydermoperiostosis syndrome.*
juvenile amaurotic familial idiocy. See *Stock-Spielmeyer-Vogt syndrome.*
juvenile deforming metatarsophalangeal osteochondritis. See *Köhler disease (2).*
juvenile diabetes-dwarfism-obesity syndrome. See *Mauriac syndrome, under Mauriac, Pierre.*
juvenile epithelial corneal dystrophy. See *Meesmann dystrophy.*
juvenile epithelial degeneration of the cornea. See *Meesmann dystrophy.*
juvenile familial nephropathy-tapetoretinal degeneration syndrome. See *Senior syndrome (1).*
juvenile G_{M1} gangliosidosis. See *gangliosidosis G_{M1} type II.*
juvenile G_{M2} gangliosidosis. See *gangliosidosis G_{M2} type III.*
juvenile ganglioside lipidosis. See *Stock-Spielmeyer-Vogt syndrome.*
juvenile head trauma syndrome. See *traumatic spreading depression syndrome.*
juvenile hereditary disciform macular degeneration. See *Stargardt syndrome.*
juvenile hyperuricemia syndrome. See *Lesch-Nyhan syndrome.*
juvenile idiopathic osteoporosis. See *Dent-Friedman syndrome.*
juvenile kyphosis. See *Scheuermann disease.*
juvenile macular degeneration. See *Stargardt syndrome.*
juvenile malignant nephrosclerosis. See *Ask-Upmark syndrome.*
juvenile melanoma. See *Spitz nevus.*
juvenile muscular dystrophy. See *Erb syndrome (1), under Erb, Wilhelm Heinrich.*
juvenile osteopathia patellae. See *Larsen-Johansson syndrome, under Larsen, Christian Magnus Falsen Sinding.*
juvenile osteoporosis. See *Dent-Friedman syndrome.*
juvenile Paget disease. See *hyperphosphatasia-osteoectasia syndrome.*
juvenile paralysis agitans. See *Hunt paralysis, under Hunt, James Ramsay.*
juvenile plantar dermatosis (JPD). See *wet and dry foot syndrome.*
juvenile progressive spinal muscular atrophy. See *Wohlfart-Kugelberg-Welander syndrome.*
juvenile rheumatoid arthritis. See *Still syndrome.*
juvenile spinal muscular atrophy. See *Wohlfart-Kugelberg-Welander syndrome.*
juvenile tropical pancreatitis syndrome. A disease of undernourished young people on low-protein diets, occurring in some tropical countries, and characterized by abdominal pain, diabetes, steatorrhea, pancreatitis, and pancreatic calcification. It appears to be caused by blockage of the pancreatic ducts by laminated secretions or inspissated mucus which form plugs, most of which eventually calcify. A high-protein diet is believed to restore normal pancreatic juice secretion, resulting in plug dislodgment. Repeated infections and anorexia are the most common complications.

Nwokolo, C., & Oli, J. Pathogenesis of juvenile tropical pancreatitis syndrome. *Lancet,* 1980, 1:456-9.

juvenile-adolescent spondylitis. See *Bechterew-Strümpell-Marie syndrome, under Bekhterev.*
juxta-articular adiposis dolorosa. See *Gram syndrome.*
juxta-articular nodosities. See *Jeanselme nodules.*
juxta-articular nodules. See *Robles disease.*
juxtaglomerular hyperplasia syndrome. See *Bartter syndrome.*
juxtaglomerular hyperplasia-hyperelectrolytemia syndrome. See *Wohlmann-Caglar syndrome.*
juxtapapillary choroiditis. See *Jensen disease.*
juxtapapillary retinopathy. See *Jensen disease.*

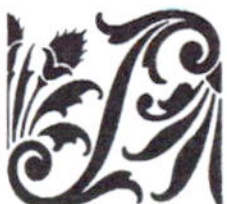

Page #	Term	Observation

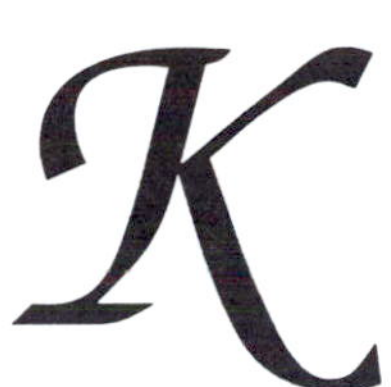

Kabuki make-up syndrome (KMS). Synonym: *Niikawa-Kuroki syndrome.*

A multiple abnormality syndrome, transmitted as an autosomal dominant trait, characterized by unusual facies, postnatal dwarfism, mental retardation, cleft or high-arched palate, scoliosis, short fifth finger, persistence of finger pads, otitis media, and bone defects, especially of the spine, hands, and hip joint. Facial abnormalities consist mostly of long palpebral fissures with eversion of the lateral third of the lower eyelids (hence the term *Kabuki make-up syndrome*), broad and depressed nasal tip, and large protruding ears. The syndrome has been seen almost exclusively in children of Japanese extraction, but some cases have been reported in other racial and ethnic groups.

Kuroki, Y., *et al.* A new malformation syndrome of long palpebral fissures, large ears, depressed nasal tip and skeletal anomalies associated with postnatal dwarfism and mental retardation. *J. Pediat.*, 1981, 99:570-3. Nikawa, N., *et al.* Kabuki make-up syndrome: A syndrome of mental retardation, unusual facies, large and protruding ears, and postnatal growth deficiency. *J. Pediat.*, 1981, 99:565-9.

KAESER, H. E. (Swiss physician)

Kaeser syndrome. See *scapuloperoneal syndrome.*

KAHLER, OTTO (Austrian physician, 1849-1893)

Kahler disease. Synonyms: *Huppert disease, Kahler syndrome, Kahler-Bozzolo disease, Rustitskii disease, Rustitzky disease, von Rustitzky disease, hemic myeloma, lymphocytic myeloma, multiple myeloma, myeloid tumor, myelomatosis, myelomatous pseudoleukemia, plasmocytic myeloma, plasmocytic sarcoma, plasmocytoma.*

A fatal disseminated malignant disease (multiple myeloma) of middle or later life, in which clones of transformed plasma cells proliferate in the bone marrow, causing disturbances of its function. Associated disorders usually include osteolysis, bone pain, spontaneous fractures, hypercalcemia, anemia caused by decreased erythropoiesis and increased hemolysis, Bence Jones protein in the urine, calcium nephropathy, amyloidosis, uremia, occasional oliguria with kidney failure, immunodeficiency with susceptibility to respiratory infection, hyperviscosity syndrome, cryoglobulinemia, hyperlipoproteinemia, hemorrhagic diathesis, high erythrocyte sedimentation rate, and rouleaux formation on blood smear.

Kahler, O. Zur Symptomatologie des multiplen Myeloms. Beobachtung von Albuminurie. *Prag. Med. Wschr.*, 1889, 14:33-5; 45-9. Huppert. Ein Fall von Albumosurie. *Prag. Med. Wschr.*, 1889, 14:35-6. Rustitzky. Multiples Myelom. *Deut. Zschr. Chir.*, 1873, 3:162.

Kahler syndrome. See *Kahler disease.*

Kahler-Bozzolo disease. See *Kahler disease.*

KAJII, TADASHI (Japanese physician)

Sugio-Kajii syndrome. See *trichorhinophalangeal dysplasia type III.*

KALISCHER, SIEGFRIED (German physician, born 1862)

Kalischer syndrome. See *Sturge-Weber syndrome.*

KALLMANN, FRANZ JOSEF (German-born American psychiatrist, 1897-1965)

Kallmann syndrome (KS). See *olfactogenital syndrome.*

Kallmann-des Morsier syndrome. See *olfactogenital syndrome.*

Maestre de San Juan-Kallmann syndrome. See *olfactogenital syndrome.*

Maestre de San Juan-Kallmann-de Morsier syndrome. See *olfactogenital syndrome.*

Maestre-Kallmann-de Morsier syndrome. See *olfactogenital syndrome.*

Kandahar sore. See *Alibert disease (2).*

KANDINSKII, VIKTOR KH. (Russian psychiatrist, 1825-1889)

Kandinskii-Clérambault complex. See *Kandinskii-Clérambault syndrome.*

Kandinskii-Clérambault syndrome. Synonyms: *Kandinskii-Clérambault complex, automatism, S syndrome.*

A condition in which the activities are carried out without conscious knowledge on the part of the subject. Several types are recognized: **Ambulatory automatism** is marked by a rhythmic form of automatic activity; **ambulatory comitial automatism** pertains to automatic acts in epileptic patients; **command automatism** refers to a condition in which the patient obeys a command, without exercising critical judgment; and **primary postictal automatism** is a form of psychomotor epilepsy.

Kandinskii, V. Kh. *O psevdogalliutsinatsiiakh. Kritiko-klinicheskii etud'.* St. Petersburg, 1890. Clérambault, G. G., de. Syndrome mécanique et conception mécaniciste des psychoses hallucinatoires. *Ann. Méd. Psychol., Paris,* 1927, 85:398-413.

kangri cancer. See *Neve cancer.*

KANOFF, NORMAN B. (American physician)
Jessner-Kanoff disease. See *under Jessner.*
KANTOR, JOHN LEONARD (American radiologist, 1890-1947)
Golden-Kantor syndrome. See *under Golden.*
KAPETANAKIS, J.
Doucas-Kapetanakis disease. See *Casalá-Mosto disease.*
KAPLAN, EUGENE (American physician)
Zuelzer-Kaplan syndrome (1). See *Crosby syndrome, under Crosby, William.*
Zuelzer-Kaplan syndrome (2). See *under Zuelzer.*
KAPLAN, HERBERT (American physician, born 1929)
Kaplan-Klatskin syndrome. The concurrence of psoriasis, sarcoidosis, and gout.

Kaplan, H., & Klatskin, G. Sarcoidosis, psoriasis and gout: Syndrome or coincidence? *Yale J. Biol. Med.*, 1960, 32:335-52.

KAPLAN, S. L. (American physician)
Hoyt-Kaplan-Grumbach syndrome. See *septo-optic dysplasia.*
KAPOSI, MORITZ. See KAPOSI-KOHN, MORITZ
KAPOSI-KOHN, MORITZ (Hungarian dermatologist, 1837-1902)
Kaposi angiomatosis. See *Kaposi sarcoma.*
Kaposi dermatitis. See *Kaposi varicelliform eruption.*
Kaposi dermatosis. See *xeroderma pigmentosum syndrome.*
Kaposi disease (1). Synonyms: *Wise-Rein disease, lichen ruber moniliformis, lichen universalis moniliformis, morbus moniliformis lichenoides.*

A skin disease in which numerous whitish punctiform papules and brownish macules are arranged in a necklacelike pattern. Histological findings include an exudative inflammatory reaction in the upper cutis, degeneration of the blood vessels, tissue disintegration, cellular infiltrates, and connective tissue displacement.

*Kaposi, M. Lichen ruber moniliformis. *Vjschr. Derm.*, 1886, 13:571. Wise, F., & Rein, C. R. Lichen ruber moniliformis (morbus moniliformis lichenoides). Report of a case and description of a hitherto to unrecorded histologic structure. *Arch. Derm. Syph., Chicago*, 1936, 34:830-49.

Kaposi disease (2). Synonyms: *Devergie disease, Hebra disease, Tarral-Besnier disease, lichen acuminatus, lichen ruber, lichen ruber acuminatus, pityriasis pilaris, pityriasis rubra pilaris.*

A chronic, mildly inflammatory, exfoliative disease of the skin, characterized by dry, acuminate papules about 1 mm in diameter surrounding hair follicles with horny plugs and scales which dip into the follicle. The papules vary in color from that of normal skin to pink, rose-yellow, or red. Erythematous plaques may be formed by coalescing papules, leaving islands of normal skin. The disease often starts insidiously with scaling of the scalp and forehead or erythema of the face and ears, but it may eventually spread to the entire body. As the disease progresses, there may be heavy mortarlike, dirty scaling of the face with a "plaster cast" appearance, a thick skull cap may be formed by scales and crusts, palmar and plantar keratoderma may develop, and pruritus is common. In the generalized exfoliative stage, chills, fever, malaise, and diarrhea may occur. They are followed by infections and blood disorders.

Kaposi, M. Lichen ruber acuminatus und Lichen ruber planus. *Arch. Derm. Syph., Wien*, 1895, 31:1-32. Devergie, M. G. Pityriasis pilaris, maladie de la peau non décrite par les dermatologistes. *Gaz. Hebd. Méd., Paris*, 1856, 3:197-201. Besnier, E. Observations pour servis a l'histoire clinique de pityriasis rubra pilaris. *Ann. Derm. Syph., Paris*, 1889, 11:253-87; 398-427; 485-544.

Kaposi disease (3). Synonyms: *lichen planus bullosus, lichen ruber pemphigoides.*

A rare variant of lichen planus with extensive bullae, reportedly first described at a meeting of the Vienna Dermatological Society in 1891.

Kaposi disease (4). See *Kaposi sarcoma.*
Kaposi eczema. See *Kaposi varicelliform eruption.*
Kaposi haemangiosarcoma. See *Kaposi sarcoma.*
Kaposi sarcoma. Synonyms: *Kaposi angiomatosis, Kaposi disease, Kaposi haemangiomatosis, Kaposi sarcomatosis, Kaposi syndrome, angioreticulosarcomatosis, angiosarcoma pigmentosum, idiopathic hemorrhagic sarcoma, idiopathic multiple hemorrhagic pigmented sarcoma, multiple idiopathic hemorrhagic sarcoma, sarcoma idiopathicum hemorrhagicum, sarcoma idiopathicum multiplex hemorrhagicum.*

Multiple neoplasms of the skin characterized by bluish red or dark brown nodules and plaques with an ulcerative tendency. Distal parts of the extremities are most frequently affected. However, visceral lesions occur in some instances; the gastrointestinal system, liver, lungs, and retroperitoneal or mesenteric lymph nodes are the most common sites. Histologically, the picture varies with the age of the lesion; younger lesions are angiomatous, whereas fibrosis and deposits of blood pigment are characteristic of older lesions. Generally, the Kaposi sarcoma is most common in older persons, but it is also frequently associated with

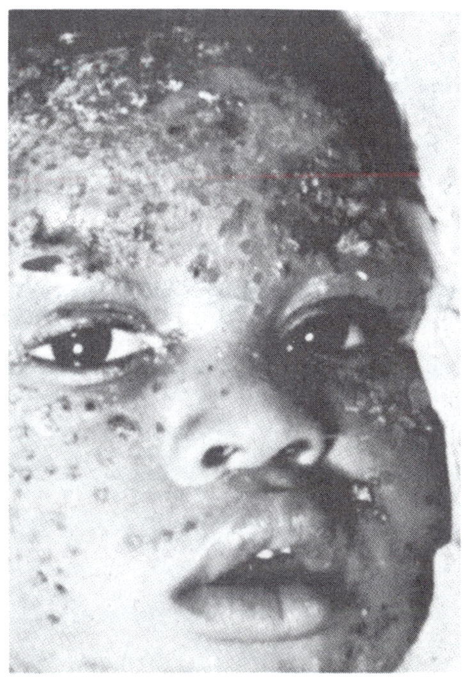

Kaposi varicelliform eruption
Nelson, W.E. (Ed.): *Textbook of Pediatrics*, 9th ed. Philadelphia: W.B. Saunders Co., 1969.

patients of all ages who are suffering from the acquired immunodeficiency syndrome (AIDS).

Kaposi, M. Idiopathisches multiples Pigmentsarkom der Haut. *Arch. Derm. Syph., Berlin*, 1872, 4:265-73.

Kaposi sarcomatosis. See *Kaposi sarcoma.*

Kaposi syndrome. See *Kaposi sarcoma.*

Kaposi varicelliform eruption. Synonyms: *Kaposi dermatitis, Kaposi eczema, Kaposi-Juliusberg dermatitis, eczema herpeticum, eczema herpetiformis, eczema vaccinatum, pustulosis herpetica infantum, pustulosis vacciniformis acuta, pustulosis varioliformis, varioliform pyoderma.*

A diffuse eruption of umbilicated vesicles and pustules resembling varicella, occurring on the skin of the upper trunk, neck, and scalp of patients with active dermatitis, particularly atopic eczema. High fever may accompany the eruption, which may last for several days to a week. Both the vaccinia virus and the herpes simplex virus have been isolated.

*Kaposi, M. *Pathologie und Therapie der Hautkrankheiten.* Berlin, 1887, p. 483. Juliusberg, F. Über Pustulosis acuta varioliformis. *Arch. Derm. Syph., Berlin*, 1898, 46:21-8.

Kaposi-Besnier-Libman-Sacks syndrome. See *Libman-Sacks syndrome.*

Kaposi-Irgang disease. Synonym: *lupus erythematosus profundus.*

A clinical variety of discoid lupus erythematosus in which the cutaneous infiltrate occurs in the deep parts of the corium, with only slight microscopic epidermal changes.

Hebra, F., & Kaposi, M. On disease of the skin, including exanthemata. *New Sydenham Society, London*, 1875, 4:1-247. Irgang, S. Apropos du lupus erythemateux profond. *Ann. Derm. Syph., Paris*, 1954, 81:246-9.

Kaposi-Juliusberg dermatitis. See *Kaposi varicelliform eruption.*

Kaposi-like angiodermatitis. See *Bluefarb-Stewart syndrome.*

Kaposi-like stasis dermatitis. See *Bluefarb-Stewart syndrome.*

Kaposi-Spiegler sarcomatosis. See *Bäfverstedt syndrome.*

pre-Kaposi sarcoma. Abnormal vascular proliferations which evolve into the Kaposi sarcoma in the acquired immunodeficiency syndrome (AIDS). q.v.

Schwartz, J. L., *et al.* Pre-Kaposi's sarcoma. *J. Am. Acad. Derm.*, 1984, 11(2 Pt 2):377-80.

pseudo-Kaposi angiodermatitis. See *Bluefarb-Stewart syndrome.*

pseudo-Kaposi stasis dermatitis. See *Bluefarb-Stewart syndrome.*

KARRER, J. (Swiss physician, born 1919)

Gasser-Karrer syndrome. See *under Gasser.*

KARSCH, JOHANNES (German physician)

Karsch-Neugebauer syndrome. Synonym: *split foot/split hand-congenital nystagmus syndrome.*

A rare syndrome of split foot and hand associated with congenital nystagmus. Strabismus, late cataracts, and pigmentary changes in the retina may be associated. The syndrome is believed to be transmitted as an autosomal recessive trait.

Karsch, J. Erbliche Augenmissbildung in Verbindung mit Spalthand und -Fuss. *Zschr. Augenheilk.*, 1936, 89:274-9. Neugebauer, H. Spalthand und -Fuss mit familiärer Besonderheit. *Zschr. Orthop.*, 1962, 95:500-6.

KARTAGENER, MANES (Swiss physician, 1897-1975)

Kartagener disease. A mild form of pulmonary infiltration occurring in eosinophilia and differing from Loffler disease by its chronic course. See also *Löffler disease, pulmonary infiltration with eosinophilia syndrome, Löhr-Kindberg syndrome,* and *Magrassi-Leonardi syndrome.*.

Kartagener, M. Das chronische Lungeninfiltrat mit Blueteosinophilie. *Schweiz. Med. Wschr.*, 1942, 72:862-4.

Kartagener syndrome (KS). Synonyms: *Kartagener triad, sinusitis-bronchiectasis-situs inversus syndrome.*

A syndrome of paranasal sinusitis, bronchiectasis, and situs inversus. Associated disorders may include frequent bronchitis, colds, bouts of pneumonia, anosmia, cough productive of foul-smelling phlegm, rheumatoid arthritis, renal abnormalities, turricephaly, heart defects, malformations of retinal vessels, anomalous subclavian artery, dextrocardia, and other abnormalities. The syndrome is transmitted as an autosomal recessive trait.

Kartagener, M. Zur Pathogenese der Bronchiektasien. Bronchiektasien bei Situs viscerum inversus. *Beitr. Klin. Tuberk.*, 1933, 83:489-501.

Kartagener triad. See *Kartagener syndrome.*

KASABACH, HAIG H. (American physician, 1898-1943)

Kasabach-Merritt syndrome. Synonyms: *cavernous hemangioma-thrombocytopenia syndrome, hemangioma-consumptive coagulopathy syndrome, hemangioma-thrombocytopenia syndrome, hemangioma-thrombopenia syndrome, thrombopenia-hemangioma syndrome.*

A rare congenital blood disorder characterized by subcutaneous or visceral hemangiomas and thrombocytopenia, frequently associated with microangiopathic hemolytic anemia and disseminated intravascular coagulation syndrome (q.v.). Most capillary and cavernous hemangioms regress spontaneously in time.

Kasabach, H. H., & Merritt, K. K. Capillary hemangioma with extensive purpura. Report of a case. *Am. J. Dis. Child.*, 1940, 59:1063-70.

KASHIN (KASCHIN), NIKOLAI IVANOVICH (Russian physician, 1825-1872)

Kaschin-Beck disease. See *Kashin-Bek disease.*

Kashin-Bek disease. Synonyms: *Bek disease, Kaschin-Beck disease, Aso volcanic disease, endemic polyarthritis, osteo-arthrosis deformans endemica, osteochondritis deformans endemica, osteochondroarthrosis deformans endemica, Tokut-ze disease, Urov disease.*

A slowly progressive, degenerative osteoarthrosis of the spine and joints of the extremities, occurring in children in northern Siberia, northern China, and Northern Korea. The early symptoms are insidious; first, a painless thickening of the joints and gradually an aching muscular weakness, fatigability, and extensive symmetrical enlargement of the wrists and interphalangeal joints. In the second stage, there is paresthesia, stiffness, cramping, a sensation of coldness of the hands and feet, intra-articular loose bodies, and arthralgia. In the third stage, the chief features are osteoarthrosis deformans, limitation of motion which eventually becomes disabling, severe muscular weakness with atrophy, reduction of height as a result of shortening of extremities, and lordosis. In advanced stages, patients assume a characteristic posture with the head is pulled backward and the knees slightly bent. Extra-articular complications may include heart disorders, hypothyroidism, gastric hypoacidity, anemia, and lymphocytosis. Ingestion of cereals infected with the fungus *Sporotrichella* is the suspected etiologic factor.

*Bek, E. V. K voprosu ob obezabrazhivaiushchem endemicheskom osteoartritu (osteoarthritis deformans endemica) v Zabaikal'skoi oblasti. *Russkii Vrach*, 1906, 5:74-5. *Kashin, N. I. *Moskov. Med. Gaz.*, 1861:5-7; 39-51.

KAST, ALFRED (German physician, 1856-1903)
Kast syndrome. See *Maffucci syndrome.*
Maffucci-Kast syndrome. See *Maffucci syndrome.*
KASTERT, JOSEF (German physician, born 1910)
Hoffa-Kastert syndrome. See *under Hoffa.*
Katayama fever. See *Katayama syndrome.*
Katayama syndrome. Synonyms: *Katayama fever, schistosomiasis japonica.*

A parasitic disease caused by *Schistosoma japonicum* infection, named after the district in Japan where the condition is endemic. The schistosome infects humans and domestic animals (cats, dogs, and cattle), snails of the genus *Onchomelania* being the intermediate hosts. The symptoms usually begin a few days after the infection and consist of fever, anorexia, abdominal pain, headache, hepatosplenomegaly, eosinophilia, increased serum immunoglobulin levels, and, less commonly, diarrhea, nausea, and vomiting. Dyspnea indicates the presence of the parasites or their eggs in the lungs, and disorientation, focal jacksonian epilepsy, and generalized encephalitis are symptomatic of invasion of the brain. Pathological features consist mainly of granulomatous lesions in the intestines, liver, lungs, and occasionally brain due to the presence of eggs of the parasites.

Walt, F. The Katayama syndrome. *S. Afr. Med. J.*, 1954, 28:89-93. Mahmoud, A. A. F. Schistosomiasis (bilharziasis). In: Wyngaarden, J. B., & Smith, L. H., Jr., eds. *Cecil textbook of medicine*. 17th ed. Philadelphia, Saunders, 1985, pp. 1809-15.

KATSANTONI, A.
Côté-Katsantoni syndrome. See *under Côté.*
KAUFMAN, H. E. (American opthalmologist)
Franceschetti-Kaufman dystrophy. See *Franceschetti dystrophy.*
Kaufman dystrophy. See *Franceschetti dystrophy.*
KAUFMAN, ROBERT L. (American physician)
Kaufman syndrome (1). See *VATER association.*
Kaufman syndrome (2). See *McKusick-Kaufman syndrome.*
Kaufman syndrome (3). Synonym: *oculocerebrofacial syndrome.*

A familial syndrome, transmitted as an autosomal recessive trait, marked by mental retardation, mongoloid palpebral slant, microcornea, strabismus, myopia, optic atrophy, high-arched palate, preauricular skin tags, and small mandible.

Kaufman, R. L., *et al.* An oculocerebrofacial syndrome. *Birth Defects*, 1971, 7(1):135-8.

McKusick-Dungy-Kaufman syndrome. See *McKusick-Kaufman syndrome.*
McKusick-Kaufman syndrome (MKS). See *under McKusick.*
KAUFMANN, EDUARD (German physician, 1860-1931)
Abderhalden-Kaufmann-Lignac syndrome. See *cystinosis.*
Kaufmann syndrome. See *achondroplasia.*
Parrot-Kaufmann syndrome. See *achondroplasia.*
KAWAKITA, YUKIO (Japanese physician)
Kawakita syndrome. See *moyamoya syndrome.*

KAWASAKI, T. (Japanese physician)
Kawasaki syndrome (KS). Synonyms: *acute febrile infantile mucocutaneous lymph node syndrome, mucocutaneous lymph node syndrome (MCLS, MLNS).*

A disease of the skin and mucous membranes of infants and young children characterized by fever lasting 1 to 2 weeks and not responding to antibiotics; conjunctival congestion associated with dilated blood vessels and occasional uveitis; changes involving the lips and oral cavity, usually reddening of the lips, sometimes with fissuring, swollen and reddened tongue with hypertrophied papillae, white coating of the tongue, reddened pharynx, and occasional bucal mucosal ulceration; changes in the hands and feet, consisting of reddening of the palms and soles early during the course of the disease, followed by swelling of the fingers and toes, often with a bluish tint of the skin, and peeling of the fingertips or toes, sometimes involving the entire sole of the foot; transverse grooving of the toenails or fingernails in advanced stages; polymorphous exanthema; and lymph node enlargement, usually confined to nodes of the neck. Associated disorders may include myocarditis or pericarditis, diarrhea, arthritis or arthralgia, aseptic meningitis, and mild jaundice. Laboratory findings usually show proteinuria, leukocytes in urinary sediment, slight decrease in erythrocyte and hemoglobin levels, increased erythrocyte sedimentation rate, increased C-reactive protein level, increased α-2-globulin, and negative antistreptolysin O test. Normally, the syndrome is not lethal, but some fatalities have been reported. The etiology is unknown.

Kawasaki, T. MCLS-clinical observations of 50 cases. *Jpn. J. Allergy*, 1967, 16:178-98.

KAWASHIMA, H. (Japanese physician)
Kawashima-Tsuji syndrome. A hereditary syndrome, originally reported in a mother and son, characterized by microcephaly, mental retardation, deafness, and dysmorphic face with facial asymmetry, prominent glabella, low-set cup-shaped ears, thick protruding lips, and micrognathia.

Kawashima, H., & Tsuji, N. Syndrome of microcephaly, deafness/malformed ears, mental retardation, and peculiar facies in a mother and son. *Clin. Genet.*, 1987, 31:303-7.

KAYSER, BERNHARD (German ophthalmologist, 1869-1954)
Kayser-Fleischer ring. Synonym: *Fleischer-Strümpell ring.*

A gray-green to red-gold pigmented ring at the outer border of the cornea seen in Wilson disease.

Kayser, B. Über einen Fall von angeborener grünlicher Verfärbung des Cornea. *Klin. Mbl. Augenh.*, 1902, 40(2):22-5. Fleischer, B. Zwei weitere Fälle von grünlicher Verfäubung der Kornea. *Klin. Mbl. Augenh.*, 1903, 41(1):489-91.

KAYSER, HEINRICH (German physician)
Brion-Kayser disease. See *Schottmüller disease.*
KAZNELSON
Kaznelson syndrome. See *Faber syndrome.*

KBG syndrome. A multiple abnormality syndrome, transmitted as an autosomal dominant trait, marked by mental retardation, short stature, speech defects, characteristic facies (biparietal prominence, brachycephaly, round face, telecanthus, wide eyebrows, short alveolar ridges), dental abnormalities (macrodontia, oligodontia, tooth malposition, enamel hypoplasia), skeletal defects (cervical ribs, vertebral anomalies, short femoral neck, short tubular bones of the hands, delayed bone age), and hand defects (syndactyly of the toes, distal axial triradius, and simian creases). The condition has been designated KBG syndrome, using the patient's initials in the first report.

Herrmann, J., *et al.* The KBG syndrome—A syndrome of short stature, characteristic facies, mental retardation, microdontia and skeletal anomalies. *Birth Defects,* 1975, 11(5):7-18.

KCS (keratoconjunctivitis sicca). See *Sjögren syndrome, under Sjögren, Henrik Samuel Conrad.*

KDS (Kocher-Debré-Semelaigne syndrome). See *Debré-Semelaigne syndrome.*

KEARNS, THOMAS P. (American ophthalmologist)

Kearns syndrome. See *Kearns-Sayre syndrome.*

Kearns-Sayre syndrome (KSS). Synonyms: *Barnard-Scholz syndrome, Kearns syndrome, external ophthalmoplegia-retinitis pigmentosa-heart block syndrome, heart block-retinitis pigmentosa-ophthalmoplegia syndrome, oculocraniosomatic disease (OCSD), ophthalmoplegia-pigmentary retinal degeneration-cardiomyopathy syndrome, ophthalmoplegia plus syndrome, ophthalmoplegia-retinal degeneration syndrome, ophthalmoplegic retinal degeneration syndrome.*

A syndrome of myopathy of the external ocular muscles, ophthalmoplegia, retinitis pigmentosa, and heart block. Progressive weakness of muscles of the eyelids and blepharoptosis are the earliest signs. Some cases present progressive paralysis, decreased hearing for high tones, dysphonia, dysphagia ataxia, spasticity, mental deficiency, and congestive heart failure. The syndrome is sometimes classified as the infantile form (with early onset, rapid progress, multisystem involvement, and a severe course), and juvenile and adult forms with onset in the second and third decades respectively, and a generally slower and less severe course. Most cases are sporadic, but autosomal dominant inheritance has been suggested in some instances.

Kearns, T. P., & Sayre, G. P. Retinitis pigmentosa, eaxternal opthalmoplegia and complete heart block. *Arch. Ophth., Chicago,* 1958, 60:280-9. Barnard, R. I., & Scholz, R. O. Ophthalmoplegia and retinal degeneration. *Am. J. Ophth.*, 1944, 27:621-4.

KEHRER, FERDINAND ADALBERT (German physician, 1883-1966)

Kehrer-Adie syndrome. See *Adie syndrome.*

KEIPERT, J. A. (Australian physician)

Keipert syndrome. A familial syndrome, probably transmitted as an autosomal or X-linked recessive trait, marked mainly by abnormal facies and broad terminal phalanges of the fingers and toes. Mental retardation, hydrocephalus, ocular abnormalities, and hearing loss are present in some cases. Facial characteristics consist mainly of a large nose with a high bridge, large rounded columella, prominent alae, and protruding lip with a cupid's bow. Clinodactyly of the short fifth fingers, medial rotation of the toes, and short phalanges are also present.

Keipert, J. A., *et al.* A new syndrome of broad terminal phalanges and facial abnormalities. *Austral. Paediat. J.,* 1973, 9:10-3.

KEITH, N. M. (American physician)

Wagener-Keith syndrome. See *Wagener syndrome.*

KELLY, ADAM BROWN (British physician, 1865-1941)

Kelly syndrome. See *Plummer-Vinson syndrome.*

Paterson-Brown Kelly syndrome. See *Plummer-Vinson syndrome.*

Paterson-Kelly syndrome. See *Plummer-Vinson syndrome.*

keloidal blastomycosis. See *Lobo disease.*

KEMPE, C. H. (American physician)

Caffey-Kempe syndrome. See *battered child syndrome.*

KENNEDY, ROBERT FOSTER (American neurologist, 1884-1952)

Foster Kennedy syndrome (FKS). See *Kennedy syndrome.*

Gowers-Paton-Kennedy syndrome. See *Kennedy syndrome.*

Kennedy syndrome. Synonyms: *Foster Kennedy syndrome (FKS), Gowers-Paton-Kennedy syndrome, basofrontal syndrome.*

An association of ipsilateral optic atrophy and scotoma and contralateral papilledema occurring in tumors or other lesions, such as abscesses or aneurysms, of the frontal lobe or in sphenoid meningioma. Anosmia may occur.

Kennedy, F. Retrobulbar neuritis as an exact diagnostic sign of certain tumors and abscesses in the frontal lobe. *Am. J. Med. Sc.*, 1911, 142:355-68.

KENNY, FREDERIC MARSHAL (American physician, born 1929)

Kenny syndrome. Synonyms: *Kenny-Caffey syndrome, Kenny-Linarelli syndrome, dwarfism-congenital medullary stenosis syndrome, tubular stenosis-hypocalcemia-convulsions-dwarfism syndrome, tubular stenosis-periodic hypocalcemia syndrome.*

A syndrome of dwarfism, inner cortical thickening with stenosis of the medullary cavities of the tubular bones, small face, frontal bossing, episodes of hypocalcemic tetany, convulsions, and hyperphosphatemia. Occasional symptoms may include myopia and hypotrichosis. Autosomal dominant transmission is suspected.

Kenny, F. M., & Linarelli, L. Dwarfism and cortical thickening of tubular bones. *Am. J. Dis. Child.*, 1966, 111:201-7. Caffey, J. Congenital stenosis of medullary spaces in tubular bones and calvaria in two proportionate dwarfs-mother and son; coupled with transitory hypocalcemic tetany. *Am. J. Roentgen.*, 1967, 100:1-11.

Kenny-Caffey syndrome. See *Kenny syndrome.*

Kenny-Linarelli syndrome. See *Kenny syndrome.*

keratitis epithelialis punctata. See *Koeppe disease (1).*

keratitis maculosa. See *Sanders syndrome.*

keratitis nummularis. See *Dimmer keratitis, and see Sanders syndrome.*

keratitis parenchymatosa annularis. See *Vossius keratitis.*

keratitis punctata superficialis. See *Fuchs syndrome (2).*

keratitis subepithelialis. See *Sanders syndrome.*

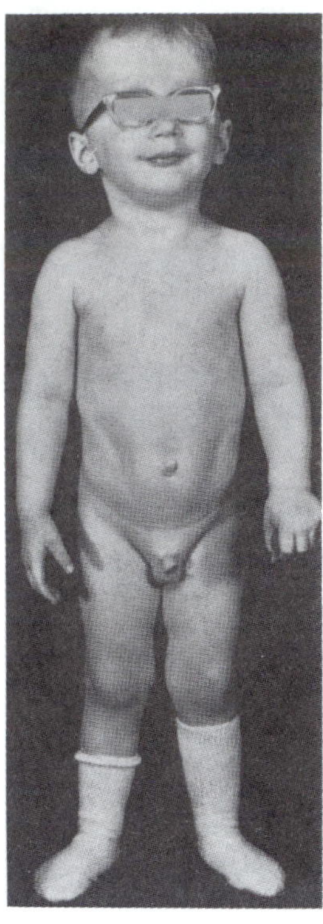

Kenny syndrome
Kenny, F.M. & Linarelli, L.: "Dwarfism and cortical thickening of tubular bones." *Am. J. Dis. Child,* 111:201, 1966. Chicago: American Medical Association.

keratitis superficialis herpetica with striations. See *Schmidt keratitis, under Schmidt, Rolf.*

keratitis superficialis punctata. See *Sanders syndrome.*

keratitis-deafness syndrome. See *Cogan syndrome (1).*

keratitis-ichthyosis-deafness syndrome. See *KID syndrome.*

keratoangioma. See *Mibelli disease (1).*

keratoconjunctivitis epidemica. See *Sanders syndrome.*

keratoconjunctivitis sicca (KCS). See *Sjögren syndrome under Sjögren, Henrik Samuel Conrad.*

keratoderma climacterica. See *Haxthausen syndrome.*

keratoderma hereditarium mutilans (KHM). See *Vohwinkel syndrome.*

keratodermia climacterica. See *Haxthausen syndrome.*

keratoerythrodermia variabilis. See *Mendes Da Costa syndrome.*

keratolysis bullosa congenita. See *epidermolysis bullosa syndrome.*

keratolysis exfoliativa congenita. See *continual skin peeling syndrome.*

keratolysis palmoplantaris with periodontopathy. See *Papillon-Lefèvre syndrome.*

keratoma dissipatum hereditarium palmare et plantare. See *Unna-Thost syndrome, under Unna, Paul Gerson.*

keratoma excentricum. See *Mibelli disease (2).*

keratoma hereditarium mutilans. See *Vohwinkel syndrome.*

keratoma palmare et plantare hereditarium. See *Unna-Thost syndrome, under Unna, Paul Gerson.*

keratosis extremitatum hereditaria progradiens. See *Unna-Thost syndrome, under Unna, Paul Gerson.*

keratosis follicularis. See *Darier disease (1).*

keratosis follicularis acneiformis. See *Morrow-Brooke syndrome.*

keratosis follicularis contagiosa. See *Morrow-Brooke syndrome.*

keratosis follicularis serpiginosa. See *Lutz-Miescher syndrome, under Lutz, Wilhelm.*

keratosis follicularis spinulosa decalvans. See *KID syndrome.*

keratosis follicularis spinulosa decalvans cum ophiasi. See *Siemens syndrome (1).*

keratosis palmaris et plantaris. See *Unna-Thost syndrome, under Unna, Paul Gerson.*

keratosis palmaris et plantaris-corneal dystrophy syndrome. See *Richner-Hanhart syndrome.*

keratosis palmoplantaris transgradiens. See *mal de Meleda.*

keratosis palmoplantaris with periodontopathy. See *Papillon-Lefèvre syndrome.*

keratosis rubra figurata. See *Mendes Da Costa syndrome.*

keratosis vegetans. See *Darier disease (1).*

keratosulfaturia. See *mucopolysaccharidosis IV-A.*

KERSHNER, RICHARD DUDLEY (American physician, born 1923)

Kershner-Adams syndrome. Synonym: *chronic nonspecific suppurative pneumonitis.*

A chronic, nonspecific, suppurative, inflammatory lung disease unrelated to abscesses and bronchiectasis. The main symptoms include productive cough, hemoptysis, and chest pain. Adult and middle-aged women are most commonly affected.

Kershner, R. D., & Adams, W. E. Chronic nonspecific suppurative pneumonitis. *J. Thorac. Surg.*, 1948, 17:495-511.

Keshan disease. A frequently fatal form of endemic cardiomyopathy, believed to be due to selenium deficiency, occurring in children and young women living in a belt extending from northeast to southwest China. The syndrome was originally reported in 1935.

Observations on effect of sodium selenite in prevention of Keshan disease. *Chinese Med. J.*, 1979, 92:471-6. Epidemiologic studies on the etiologic relationship of selenium and Keshan disease. *Chinese Med. J.* 1979, 92:477-82.

keto acid decarboxylase deficiency. See *maple syrup urine disease.*

ketotic hyperglycinemia syndrome. Synonym: *propionic acidemia.*

An inherited metabolic disorder, transmitted as an autosomal recessive trait, characterized by vomiting, lethargy, convulsions, hypertonia, respiratory disorders, growth and psychomotor retardation, and terminal coma in early infancy. Ketotic attacks may be induced by milk protein and casein hydrolysate. Blood analysis shows elevated levels or propionic acid, glycine, butanone, and various fatty acids. The disorder may occur in association with numerous acidurias of infancy, including methylmalonic acidemia, isovaleric acidemia, and lactic acidemia.

Rosenberg, L. E., *et al.* Methylmalonic aciduria: An inborn error leading to metabolic acidosis, long-chain ketonuria and intermittent hyperglycinemia. *N. Engl. J. Med.*, 1968, 278:1319.

KEUTEL, JÜRGEN (German physician)

Keutel syndrome (1). A syndrome, originally described in two siblings from a consanguineous marriage, consisting of peripheral pulmonary stenosis without cardiac lesions, brachytelephalangism, neural hearing loss, and abnormal calcification and/or ossification of the cartilage of the external ear, nose, larynx, trachea, and ribs. The syndrome is transmitted as an autosomal recessive trait.

Keutel, J., *et al.* A new autosomal recessive syndrome; peripheral pulmonary stenoses, brachytelephalangism, neural hearing loss, and abnormal cartilage calcification/ossification. *Birth Defects*, 1972, 8(5):60-8.

Keutel syndrome (2). Humero-radial synostosis, originally described in two brothers from a consanguineous marriage, associated with deformity of the humerus, lack of motion in the elbow, meningocele, flat cervical vertebrae, rib hypoplasia, dysplastic pelvis, hip subluxation, flexion contractures of the knees, high-arched palate, and anorchia. Motor and mental development were subnormal. The syndrome is believed to be transmitted as an autosomal recessive trait.

Keutel, J., *et al.* Eine wahrscheinlich autosomal recessive vererbte Skeletmissbildung mit Humeroradialsynostose. *Humangenetik*, 1970, 9:43-53.

KHAW, KON-T.

Shwachman-Diamond-Oski-Khaw syndrome. See *Shwachman syndrome.*

KHM (**k**eratoderma **h**ereditarium **m**utilans). See *Vohwinkel syndrome.*

KHS. See ***k**inky **h**air **s**yndrome.*

KID (**k**eratitis-**i**chthyosis-**d**eafness) **syndrome.** Synonyms: *corneal leukomas in ichthyosis, generalized spiny hyperkeratosis and universal alopecia and deafness, keratosis follicularis spinulosa decalvans.*

A congenital syndrome of keratitis, ichthyosis, and deafness associated with a variety of other disorders. Ichthyosis appears in the form of erythematous thickened skin that desquamates in the first few weeks of life and is frequently followed by erythematous, sometimes verrucous, plaques. Keratitis usually leads to photophobia, decreased visual acuity, and sometimes blindness. About half of the patients have absent or scanty hair; secondary scalp infection with scarring causing further loss of hair. Leukonychia and onychodystrophy may be noted in some cases. Many patients exhibit areas of decreased or absent sweating. Increased susceptibility to skin infections with purulent draining abscesses and an offensive odor is a common complication. Associated disorders may include vitamin A deficiency, leukoplakia, perioral fissures, fissured tongue, dental caries, delayed dentition, pyoderma, acne, urinary tract infections, and heat intolerance. The syndrome is suspected of being transmitted as an autosomal recessive trait. The synonym *keratosis follicularis spinulosa decalvans* is sometimes used to designate the *Siemens syndrome (1).*

Skinner, B. A., *et al.* The keratitis, ichthyosis, and deafness (KID) syndrome. *Arch. Derm., Chicago,* 1981, 117:285-9.

KIENBÖCK, ROBERT (Austrian physician, 1871-1953)

Kienböck atrophy. See *Sudeck syndrome.*

Kienböck disease. Synonyms: *aseptic necrosis of the lunate bone, lunatomalacia.*

Progressive necrosis of the lunate bone, sometimes leading to fragmentation of the bone, which may be associated with degenerative changes in the wrist. The etiology is unknown, but some cases have been observed in persons using pneumatic tools, others following dislocation of the lunate bone, and still others in patients having the ulna shorter than the radius (the *ulna-minus variant*).

Kienböck, R. Über traumatische Malacie des Mondbeins und ihre Folgezustände: Entartungsformen und Kompressionsfrakturen. *Fortschr. Röntgen.*, 1910-11, 16:77-103.

Kienböck dislocation. Synonym: *Kienböck luxation.*

Isolated dislocation of the semilunar bone.

Kienböck, R. Über Luxationen im Bereiche der

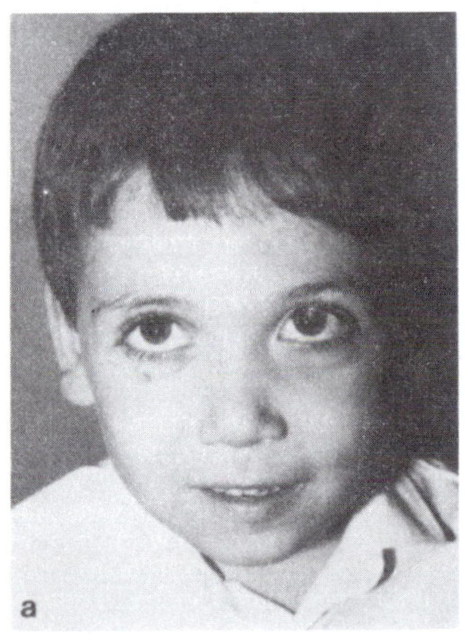

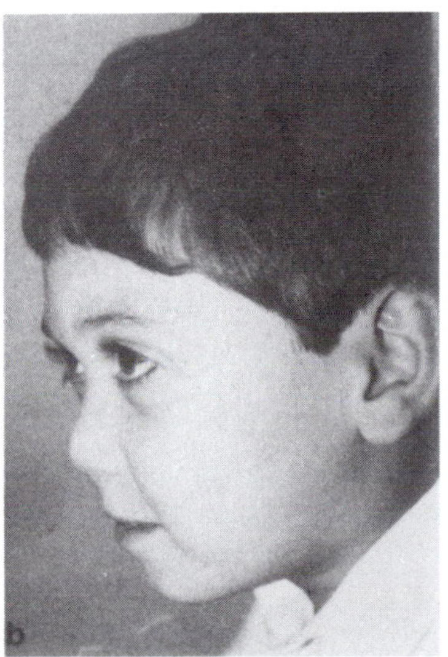

Keutel syndrome (1)
Cormode, Edward J., Malcolm Dawson & R. Brian Lowry, *American Journal of Medical Genetics* 24:289-294 1986. New York: Alan R. Liss, Inc.

Handwurzel. A. Dorsale Luxation der Hand in der perilunären Gelenkslinie und isolierte volare Luxation des Os lunatum. B. Dorsale Luxation der Mittelhand. *Fortschr. Röntgen.*, 1910, 16:103-15.

Kienböck luxation. See *Kienböck dislocation.*

Kienböck syringomyelia. Traumatic syringomyelia.

*Kienböck, R. Kritik der sonenannten "traumatischen Syringomyelie." *Jb. Psychiat.*, 1902, 21:50-210.

KIENER, FRANZ (German neurologist)

Becker-Kiener muscular dystrophy. See *Becker muscular dystrophy, under Becker, Peter Emil.*

Becker-Kiener syndrome. See *Becker muscular dystrophy, under Becker, Peter Emil.*

KIENER, PAUL LOUIS ANDRE (French physician, 1841-1895)

Hanot-Kiener syndrome. See *under Hanot.*

KIESER, WILLIBALD (German physician)

Turner-Kieser syndrome. See *nail-patella syndrome.*

KIHARA, ITARU (Japanene physician)

Robertson-Kihara syndrome. See *under Robertson, under Robertson, P. W.*

KIKKAWA, YUMIO (Japanese physician)

Kikkawa syndrome. See *tubulointerstitial nephritis-uveitis syndrome.*

KIKUCHI, ICHIRO (Japanese physician)

Iso-Kikuchi syndrome. See *under Iso.*

KILIAN, HERMANN FRIEDRICH (German physician, 1800-1863)

Kilian pelvis. Synonyms: *osteomalacic pelvis, pelvis obtecta.*

Pelvic deformity in osteomalacia.

*Kilian, H. F. *De spondylolisthesis gravissimae pelvogustiae caussa nuper detecta commentatio anatomico-obstetrica.* Bonnae, Georgii, 1854.

KILLIAN, WOLFGANG (Austrian physician)

Killian syndrome. See *chromosome 12p tetrasomy syndrome.*

Pallister-Killian syndrome. See *chromosome 12p tetrasomy syndrome.*

Teschler-Nicola and Killian syndrome. See *chromosome 12p tetrasomy syndrome.*

KILOH, LESLIE GORDON (Australian physician)

Kiloh-Nevin syndrome (1). Synonyms: *anterior interosseous nerve syndrome (AINS, AIS), cubital tunnel syndrome.*

Lesions of the anterior interosseous nerve (a motor branch of the median nerve) with paralysis of the long flexor muscle of the thumb, the deep flexor muscle of the index finger, and the quadrate pronator muscle, without sensory disorders. Injuries of the forearm (including supracondylar fractures) are the main cause.

Kiloh, L. G., & Nevin, S. Isolated neuritis of the anterior interosseous nerve. *Brit. Med. J.*, 1952, 1:850-1.

Kiloh-Nevin syndrome (2). Synonyms: *Nevin syndrome, myopathic external ophthalmoplegia, ocular myodystrophy, ocular myopathy, ophthalmoplegia externa progressiva.*

syndrome of retinitis pigmentosa, neurogenic amyotrophy, and external ophthalmoplegia, with or without heart block.

Kiloh, L. G., & Nevin, S. Progressive dystrophy of the external ocular muscles (ocular myopathy). *Brain*, 1951, 74:115-43.

KIMMELSTIEL, PAUL (American physician, 1900-1970)

Kimmelstiel-Wilson syndrome. Synonyms: *diabetes mellitus-hypertension-nephrosis syndrome, diabetes-nephrosis syndrome, diabetic glomerulohyalinosis, diabetic glomerulosclerosis, diabetic nephroangiopathy, intercapillary glomerulosclerosis, renal glomerulohyalinosis-diabetes syndrome.*

A kidney disease characterized by hypertension, proteinuria, renal lesions, edema, and glomerulonephrosis seen in patients with diabetes mellitus of several years duration. Arteriosclerosis of the renal artery is a frequent complication. Pathological findings usually include capillary or intercapillary glomerulosclerosis, eosinophilic nodules, and hyaline degeneration of the renal arterioles.

Kimmelstiel, P., & Wilson, C. Benign and malignant hypertension and nephrosclerosis. A clinical and pathological study. *Am. J. Pathol.*, 1936, 12:45-81.

KIMURA, TETSUJI (Japanese physician)

Kimura disease. Synonyms: *angioblastic lymphoid hyperplasia with eosinophilia, angiolymphoid hyperplasia with eosinophila, eosinophilic lymphofolliculosis of the skin.*

Angiolymphoid hyperplasia with eosinophilia of unknown etiology occurring chiefly in adults 20 to 40 years of age. The principal lesions are flesh-colored solitary or multiple subcutaneous nodules, about 2 cm or more in diameter, usually found on the ears, cheeks, temples, and parotid areas. Associated disoders may include regional lymphadenopathy, lichen amyloidosis, and hyperimmunoglobulinemia E. Histopathological findings consist mainly of poorly defined areas of vascular proliferation with masses of endothelial cells and eosinophilic and focal lymphocytic infiltrations.

Kimura, T., *et al.* On the unusual granulation combined with hyperplastic changes of lymphocytic tissues. *Tr. Soc. Path. Jpn.*, 1948, 37:179-80.

KINDBERG, MICHEL LEON

Löhr-Kindberg syndrome. See *under Löhr.*

Löhr-Léon Kindberg syndrome. See *Löhr-Kindberg syndrome.*

KINDLER, WERNER (German physician, born 1895)

Zange-Kindler syndrome. See *under Zange.*

KING, FREDERICK A. (American scientist)

Zeman-King syndrome. See *under Zeman.*

KING, J. O. (Australian physician)

King syndrome. Synonym: *malignant hyperthermia-myopathy-multiple anomalies syndrome.*

A genetic syndrome exhibiting characteristic facies (down-slanting palpebral fissures, malar hypoplasia, blepharoptosis or blepharophimosis, micrognathia, low-set ears), short stature, delayed motor development, progressive myopathy with muscle weakness, kyphoscoliosis, pectus carinatum, cryptorchism, predisposition to the malignant hyperthermia syndrome (q.v.), and elevated serum creatine phosphokinase levels. The syndrome is transmitted as an autosomal dominant trait.

King, J. O., *et al.* Inheritance of malignant hyperpyrexia. *Lancet*, 1972, 1:365-70.

KINGSBOURNE, M. (British physician)

Kingsbourne syndrome. Synonyms: *ataxia-opsoclonus-myoclonus syndrome, dancing eye syndrome, dancing eye and dancing feet syndrome, dancing eye syndrome with myoclonic ataxia, dancing eyeball syndrome, infantile myoclonic encephalopathy, infantile polymyoclonus, myoclonic encephalopathy syndrome, oculo-*

cerebromyoclonic syndrome, opsoclonic encephalopathy, rapid irregular movement of the eyes and limbs syndrome.

A rare neurological disorder, usually observed in children under the age of 3 years. The symptoms include myoclonus (irregular rapid jerky movements of the limbs and trunk), opsoclonus (irregular jerky movements of the eyes), ataxia, intention tremor, and nystagmus. Occult neuroblastoma may be present in some cases.

Kingsbourne, M. Myoclonic encephalopathy in infants. *J. Neurol. Neurosurg. Psychiat.*, 1962, 25:271-6.

kinky hair syndrome (KHS). Synonyms: *Menkes syndrome, Menkes kinky hair syndrome (MKHS), steely hair syndrome, trichopoliodystrophy.*

An inherited defect of intestinal copper absorption, characterized by sparse, stubby, twisted, and fractured hair (pili torti), mental retardation, growth retardation, and focal cerebral and cerebellar degeneration. The symptoms include failure to thrive, increased muscle tone, severe spasticity, drowsiness, lethargy, hypothermia, convulsions, pudgy pale face, persistent wormian bones, widening of the metaphyses with formation of lateral spurs which fracture, tortuosity of the cerebral vessels, and disintegration of the internal elastic lamina of arteries with thickening of the intima, sometimes leading to obliteration of major arteries. Metabolic features consist of low levels of serum copper, serum copper oxidase (ceruloplasmin), and liver copper. The syndrome is transmitted as an X-linked recessive trait. See also *trichodento-osseous syndrome.*

Menkes, J. H., *et al.* A sex-linked recessive disorder with retardation of growth, peculiar hair and focal cerebral and cerebellar degeneration. *Pediatrics*, 1962, 29:764-79.

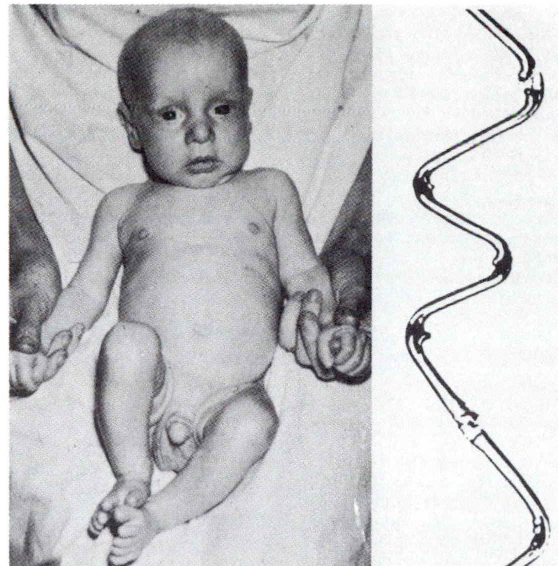

Kinky hair syndrome
Menkes, J.H. et. al: *Pediatrics*, 29:764, 1962, by permission.

KINNIER WILSON. See WILSON SAMUEL ALEXANDER KINNIER

KIRNER, J. (German physician)

Kirner deformity. Synonym: *dystelephalangy.*

Usually symmetric palmar bending involving the shaft of the terminal phalanges of the fifth digit of the hands and often associated with epiphyseal separation. The disorder is transmitted as an autosomal dominant trait, with some sporadic cases also occurring.

Kirner, J. Doppelseitige Verkrümmungen des Kleinfingerendgliedes als selbständiges Krankheitsbild. *Fortschr. Geb. Röntgen.*, 1927, 36:804-6.

kissing osteophytes. See *Baastrup syndrome.*

kissing spine. See *Baastrup syndrome.*

KITAHARA, S. (Japanese ophthalmologist)

Kitahara disease. See *Masuda-Kitahara disease.*

Masuda-Kitahara disease. See *under Masuda.*

KITAMURA, KANEIHIKO (Japanese physician)

Kitamura disease. Synonyms: *acropigmentatio reticularis, reticulate acropigmentation, reticulate acropigmentation of Kitamura (RAPK).*

A pigmentary disorder characterized by a network of sharply demarcated, slightly depressed macules, palmar pits, and breaks in the epidermal rete ridge patterns, appearing on the hands and feet during the first and second decades of life. The lesions darken gradually and extend proximally to involve other parts of the body. Epidermal atrophy, an increased number of basal melanocytes, and the absence of pigmentary incontinence in the upper dermis are the principal histopathological features. The disorder is believed to be transmitted as an autosomal dominant trait.

*Kitamura, K., & Akamatsu, S. *Rinsho-no-Hifu-Hitsmyo.* 1943, 8:201. Kitamura, K., *et al.* Eine besondere Form der Akropigmentation: Acropigmentatio reticularis. *Hautarzt, 1953,* 4:152-6. Griffiths, W. A. Reticulate acropigmentation of Kitamura, *Brit. J. Derm.*, 1976, 95:437-43.

KJELLBERG, S. R.

Waldenström-Kjellberg syndrome. See *Plummer-Vinson syndrome.*

KLATSKIN, GERALD (American physician)

Kaplan-Klatskin syndrome. See *under Kaplan, Herbert.*

KLAUDER, JOSEPH VICTOR (American physician, born 1888)

Klauder disease. See *Rosenbach erysipeloid, under Rosenbach, Anton Julius Friedrich.*

Klauder syndrome. See *Stevens-Johnson syndrome.*

KLEBS, THEODOR ALBRECHT EDWIN (German physician, 1834-1913)

Klebs disease. Synonym: *glomerulonephritis.*

A form of nephritis characterized by inflammatory and/or necrotizing lesions of the kidney glomeruli.

*Klebs, T. A. *Handbuch der pathologische Anatomie.* 1 Abt. Berlin, Hirschwald, 1870, pp. 644-8.

Klebsiella pneumonia. See *Friedländer pneumonia.*

Kleeblattschädel. See *Holtermüller-Wiedemann syndrome.*

Kleeblattschädel anomalad. See *Holtermüller-Wiedemann syndrome.*

Kleeblattschädel anomaly. See *Holtermüller-Wiedemann syndrome.*

KLEIN, DAVID (Swiss physician)

Bamatter-Franceschetti-Klein-Sierro syndrome. See *geroderma osteodysplastica syndrome.*

Champion-Cregan-Klein syndrome. See *popliteal pterygium syndrome.*

Franceschetti-Klein-Wildervanck syndrome. See *Wildervanck syndrome (1).*

Franceschetti-Zwahlen-Klein syndrome. See *mandibulofacial dysostosis.*

Klein syndrome. See *Waardenburg syndrome (2).*

Klein-Waardenburg syndrome. See *Waardenburg syndrome (2).*

Wildervanck-Waardenburg-Francheschetti-Klein syndrome. See *Wildervanck syndrome (1).*

KLEINE, WILLI (German physician)

Kleine-Levin syndrome. Synonyms: *Critchley syndrome, Kleine-Levin-Critchley syndrome, hypersomnia-bulimia syndrome, hypersomnia-megaphagia syndrome, periodic hypersomnia-megaphagia syndrome, periodic somnolence and morbid hunger syndrome.*

A disorder most frequently affecting young males characterized by attacks of somnolence accompanied by excessive food intake, which may occur every 3 to 6 months and last from 2 to 3 days. Confusion, irritability, restlessness, euphoria, hallucinations, delusions, and schizophreniform states often precede, accompany, or follow the attacks of abnormal eating.

Kleine, W. Periodische Schlafsucht. *Mschr. Psychiat.*, 1925, 57:285-320. Levin, M. Periodic somnolence and morbid hunger. A new syndrome. *Brain*, 1936, 59:494-504.

Kleine-Levin-Critchley syndrome. See *Kleine-Levin syndrome.*

KLEINSCHMIDT, HANS (German physician, 1885-1977)

Kleinschmidt syndrome. Synonyms: *cherry-red epiglottitis, Haemophilus influenzae B laryngitis, influenza bacillus syndrome.*

Haemophilus influenzae B influenza which begins as acute phlegmonous epiglottitis and is followed by mediastinitis, pleurisy, pericarditis, and bronchopneumonia. The hematogenous spreading of the pathogen may result in meningitis, subcutaneous abscesses, and empyema of various joints.

Kleinschmidt, H. Ein charakteristisches Syndrom durch Influenzabazilleninfektion. *Kinderarztl. Prax.*, 1939, 10:53-8.

KLEIST, KARL (German physician, born 1879)

Kleist apraxia. See *Mayer-Gross apraxia.*

KLEYN, A., DE (Dutch ophthalmologist)

van der Hoeve-de Kleyn syndrome. See *osteogenesis imperfecta (dominant form).*

KLINEFELTER, HARRY FITCH, JR. (American physician, born 1912)

Klinefelter syndrome (KS). See *chromosome XXY syndrome.*

Klinefelter-Reifenstein-Albright syndrome. See *chromosome XXY syndrome.*

KLINGENSTEIN, PERCY (American physician, born 1896)

Dudley-Klingenstein syndrome. See *under Dudley.*

KLINGER, HEINZ KARL ERNST (German pathologist, born 1907)

Klinger syndrome. See *Wegener granulomatosis.*

Wegener-Churg-Klinger syndrome. See *Wegener granulomatosis.*

KLIONSKY, BERNARD LEON (American physician, born 1925)

Sweeley-Klionsky disease. See *Fabry syndrome.*

KLIPPEL, MAURICE (French neurologist, 1858-1942)

Klippel disease. Synonyms: *general arthritic paralysis, general arthritic pseudoparalysis.*

Generalized arthritic paralysis in erderly persons who have cerebral arteriosclerosis.

Klippel, M. De la pseudoparalysie generale arthritique. *Rev. Méd., Paris*, 1892, 12:280-5.

Klippel-Feil anomalad. See *Klippel-Feil syndrome.*

Klippel-Feil syndrome. Synonyms: *Klippel-Feil anomalad, congenital brevicollis, congenital osseous torticollis syndrome, congenital synostosis of cervicothoracic vertebrae syndrome, congenital webbed neck syndrome.*

A syndrome of shortened neck, low hairline, and a reduced number of cervical vertebrae or multiple hemivertebrae fused into a single osseous mass. Associated anomalies include webbing of the neck, torticollis, spina bifida, meningomyelocele, syringomyelia, occipital bone defects, Sprengel deformity, cervical ribs, hydrocephalus, oxycephaly, scoliosis, lordosis, facial asymmetry, cleft palate, micrognathia, mental retardation, deafness, strabismus, nystagmus, spastic quadriplegia, synkinesis, ataxia, anesthesia, paresthesia, and various muscle abnormalities. Heart defects may occur. A severe form of this syndrome is known as *iniencephaly.* When associated with the Bonnevie-Ullrich syndrome, it is called the *Nielsen disease.* The etiology is unknown.

Klippel, M., & Feil, A. Un cas d'absence des vertèbres cervicales avec cage thoracique remantant jusqu'a la base de crâne (cage thoracique cervicale). *Nouv. Icon. Salpêt.*, 1912, 25:223-50.

Klippel-Feldstein syndrome. Synonym: *simple familial cranial hypertrophy.*

Familial hypertrophy of the cranial vault without any apparent functional disorders.

Klippel, M., & Feldstein, E. L'hypertrophie cranienne simple familiale. *Nouv. Icon. Salpêt.*, 1913, 26:445-51.

Klippel-Trénaunay syndrome. See *Klippel-Trénaunay-Weber syndrome.*

Klippel-Trénaunay-Parkes Weber syndrome. See *Klippel-Trénaunay-Weber syndrome.*

Klippel-Trénaunay-Weber (KTW) syndrome. Synonyms: *Klippel-Trénaunay syndrome, Klippel-Trénaunay-Parkes Weber syndrome, Ollier-Klippel-Trénaunay-Weber syndrome, Parkes Weber syndrome, Weber syndrome, angio-osteohypertrophy syndrome, hemangiectasia hypertrophica, hemangiectatic hypertrophy of Parkes Weber, naevus vasculosus osteohypertrophicus, nevus osteohypertrophicus, nevus varicosus osteohypertrophicus, osteo-angiohypertrophy, phlebarteriectasis. osteohypertrophic varicose syndrome.*

A syndrome of generally unilateral hypertrophy of the soft and bone tissue, hemangiomata, nevus flammeus, and varicose veins usually involving the legs, buttocks, abdomen, and lower trunk. Vascular anomalies may be present at birth or may appear in infancy. Occasional abnormalities may include arteriovenous fistulae, lymphamgiomatous anomalies, macrodactyly, syndactyly, polydactyly, oligodactyly, neonatal and childhood ulcers, cutis marmorata, telangiectasia, asymmetric facial hypertrophy (usually associated with mental retardation, micro- or macrocephaly, and intracranial calcifications), glaucoma, cataracts, heterochromia, aberrant major blood vessels, and growth disorders (tall or short stature). Some writers consider the **Weber syndrome** a separate entity because of proportionate (instead of disproportionate) macroscopic changes, the presence of arteriovenous fistulae, the absence of vascular nevi and lymphangiomas, and deep venous anomalies. Most cases are sporadic but some are familial.

Klippel, M., & Trénaunay, P. Du naevus variqueux ostéohypertrophique. *Arch. Gen. Méd., Paris*, 1900, 3:641-72. Weber, F. P. Angioma-formation in connection with hypertrophy of limbs and hemi-hypertrophy. *Brit. J. Derm.*, 1907, 19:231-5. Konrad, E. A., & Meister, P. F. P. Weber-Syndrom. Definition und differentialdiagnostische Abgrenzung. *Pathologe*, 1981, 2:103-5.

Ollier-Klippel-Trénaunay-Weber syndrome. See *Klippel-Trénaunay-Weber syndrome.*

KLOEPFER, H. W.

Kloepfer syndrome. Complete blindness beginning at about 2 months of age, associated with blistering after exposure to sunlight, arrest of growth at the age of 5 or 6 years, and progressive mental retardation.

*Kloepfer, H. W. Progress report on study of a type of progressive juvenile dementia with oligophrenia and erythremia. *10th Internat. Cong. Genet.*, Montreal, 1958.

KLOSTERMANN, G. F.

Klostermann syndrome. See *Peutz-Jeghers syndrome.*

Peutz-Klostermann syndrome. See *Peutz-Jeghers syndrome.*

KLOTZ, HENRI PIERRE (French physician, born 1910)

Klotz syndrome. A syndrome of primary amenorrhea, genital infantilism, aplasia of the labia minora, small nonovulating ovaries with primordial follicles and progressive sclerosis, male chromosomal sex, slightly mongoloid facies, and occasional hypertrichosis.

Klotz, H. P., *et al.* Aplasie des petites lèvres, infantilisme génital et sclérose ovarienne chez des femmes présentant un sexe génétique mâle. *Ann. Endocr., Paris*, 1958, 19:751-67.

KLUMPKE. See DEJERINE-KLUMPKE, AUGUSTA

KLÜVER, HEINRICH (German-born American neruologist, born 1897)

Klüver-Bucy syndrome (KBS). Synonyms: *Klüver-Bucy-Terzian syndrome, temporal lobectomy behavior syndrome.*

Behavioral changes following temporal lobectomy, originally observed in rhesus monkeys, consisting of a tendency to examine all objects orally; hypermetamorphosis with a tendency to touch everything in sight; increased sexual behavior, including, auto-, hetero-, and homosexual activity; bulimia with the development of an appetite for meat; memory disorders; placidity, flattened affect and petlike compliance with a lack of aggressive affective behavior; and an inability to recognize people. The full syndrome is not common in humal subjects. Etiologic factors include trauma and various brain lesions.

Klüver, H., & Bucy, P. C. "Psychic blindness" and other symptoms following bilateral temporal lobectomy in rhesus monkeys. *Am. J. Physiol.*, 1937, 119:352-3. Terzian, H., & Ore, G. D. Syndrome of Klüver and Bucy. Reproduced in man by bilateral removal of the temporal lobe. *Neurology*, 1955, 5:373-80.

Klüver-Bucy-Terzian syndrome. See *Klüver-Bucy syndrome.*

KMS. See ***k**washiorkor-**m**arasmus **s**yndrome.*

KMS. See ***K**abuki **m**ake-up **s**yndrome.*

KNAPP, HERMAN JAKOB (American ophthalmologist, 1832-1911)

Knapp streaks. Synonym: *angioid streaks.*

Pigmented striae in the retina resembling obliterated blood vessels, frequently seen in pseudoxanthoma elasticum, and usually associated with diseases of the choroidal vessels in which there is rupture of the lamina vitrea and macular hemorrhage.

Knapp, H. On the formation of dark angioid streaks as an unusual metamorphosis of retinal hemorrhage. *Arch. Ophth., Chicago*, 1892, 21:289-92.

knapsack paralysis. See *Rieder paralysis.*

KNIEST, WILHELM (German pediatrician)

Kniest disease. Synonyms: *Kniest dysplasia, Kniest syndrome, metatropic dwarfism type II, Swiss cheese cartilage syndrome.*

An inherited form of bone dysplasia transmitted as an autosomal dominent or X-linked trait. The symptoms consist of peculiar facies with midfacial hypoplasia, depressed nasal bridge and occasional shallow orbits with protruding eyes; short trunk with dorsal kyphosis, lumbar lordosis, and, less frequently, thoracic scoliosis in the later course of the disease; short and broad thorax with sternal protrusion; short extremities with prominent joints and restricted joint mobility; cleft palate; hearing loss; occasional myopia; retinal detachment; and club feet. Some manifestations, such as short stature, prominent knees, cleft palate, and/or club feet, may be present at birth, but the full expression usually occurs by the age of 3 years.

Kniest, W. Zur Abgrenzung der Dysostosis enchondralis von der Chondrodystrophie. *Zschr. Kinderheilk.*, 1952, 70:633-40.

Kniest dysplasia. See *Kniest disease.*

Kniest syndrome. See *Kniest disease.*

KNORR, AUGUST (German physician)

Lichtenstein-Knorr syndrome. See *under Lichtenstein, Heinz.*

knuckle pads syndrome. See *Bart-Pumphrey syndrome, under Bart, Robert S.*

knuckle pads-leukonychia-sensineural deafness syndrome. See *Bart-Pumphrey syndrome, under Bart, Robert S.*

KNUD FABER. See FABER, KNUD HELGE

KÖBBERLING, J. (German physician)

Köbberling-Dunnigan syndrome. Synonyms: *Dunnigan syndrome, familial partial lipodystrophy.*

An X-linked dominant syndrome, lethal in the hemizygous state, characterized by the absence of subcutaneous fat from the limbs and trunk with normal or excessive adipose tissue on the face and neck. Two types are recognized: **Type 1**, in which the loss of subcutaneous fat is confined to the limbs, sparing the face and trunk; and **Type 2**, in which the trunk is also affected, except for the vulva. Insulin-resistant diabetes mellitus, hyperlipoproteinemia, and acanthosis nigricans are present in some but not all patients.

Köbberling, J., *et al.* Lipodystrophy of the extremities. A dominant inherited syndrome associated with lipoatrophic diabetes. *Humangenetik*, 1975, 29:111-20. Dunnigan, M. G., *et al.* Familial lipoatrophic diabetes with dominant transmission. A new syndrome. *Q. J. Med.*, 1974, 169:33-48. Köbberling, J., & Dunnigan, M. G. Familial partial lipodystrophy: two types of an X linked dominant syndrome, lethal in the hemizygous state. *J. Med. Genet.*, 1986, 23:120-7.

KÖBNER, HEINRICH (German dermatologist, 1838-1904)

Köbner syndrome. See *epidermolysis bullosa syndrome.*

KOBY, FREDERIC EDOUARD (French ophthalmologist)

Koby cataract. Synonym: *floriform cataract.*

A familial form of cataract marked by multiple, annular, floriform opacities of different colors and sizes arranged around the sutures of the embryonic nucleus, and probably transmitted as an autosomal domin- ant trait.

Koby, F. E. Cataracte familiale d'un type particulier, se transmettant apparenment suivant le mode dominant. *Arch. Opht., Paris*, 1923, 40:492-503.

KOCHER, EMIL THEODOR (Swiss physician, 1841-1917)

Kocher-Debré-Semelaigne (KDS) syndrome. See *Debré-Semelaigne syndrome.*

KOEBNER, HEINRICH. See KÖBNER, HEINRICH

KOEPPE (KOEPP), LEONHARD (German ophthalmologist, 1884)

Koeppe disease (1). Synonyms: *epithelial punctate keratitis, keratitis epithelialis punctata.*

Fine or coarse, white, punctate, epithelial lesions of the cornea with an areolar or stellate configuration, seen in various viral diseases.

Koeppe, L. Klinische Beobachtungen mit der Nernstspaltlampe und dem Horhautmikroskop. 8. Über zwei weitere bisher nicht beschriebene Hornhautveränderungen im Bilde der Nernstspaltlampe. *Graefes Arch. Ophth.*, 1917, 94:250-66.

Koeppe disease (2). Synonym: *dystrophia hyaliniformis lamellosa corneae.*

A form of corneal dystrophy in which a sharply defined grayish white band on an apparently unchanged cornea is visible to the naked eye. Under the microscope, the band is seen as a diffuse white area covered with spots and having an irregular border with a zig-zag pattern, while the seemingly normal cornea is actually covered with opaque areas. Under the slit lamp, the epithelium in the affected zone appears to be slightly edematous with irregular thickening, and elevations and in the vicinity of the Bowman membrane, there are grayish-blue or grayish-brown hyaline or hyalinoid diffuse granular deposits.

Koeppe, L. Klinische Beobachtungen mit der Nernstspaltlampe und dem Hornhautmikroskop. 8. Über zwei weiter bisher nicht beschriebene Hornhautveränderungen im Bilde der Nornstspaltlampe. *Graefes Arch. Ophth.*, 1917, 94:250-66.

Koeppe nodules. Small white nodules at the pupillary margin of the iris, which are symptomatic of granulomatous uveitis.

Adler, F. H. *Textbook of ophthalmology*. 7th ed. Philadelphia, Saunders, 1962, p. 282.

KOERBER, HERMANN (German ophthalmologist, born 1878)

Koerber-Salus-Elschnig syndrome. Synonyms: *nystagmus retractorius, retraction nystagmus, sylvian aqueduct syndrome, upper sylvian aqueduct syndrome.*

A syndrome in which lesions of the aqueduct of Sylvius produce impaired vertical gaze, vertical nystagmus, retraction nystagmus, convergence nystagmus, pupillary abnormality, convergence spasm, and extraocular palsies. Associated disorders include headache, dizziness, and tremor.

Koerber, H. Über drei Fälle von Retraktionsbewegung des Bulbus (Nystagmus retractorius). *Ophth. Klin., Stuttgart*, 1903, 7:65-7. Salus, R. Über erworbene Retraktionsbewegungen der Augen. *Arch. Augenheilk.*, 1911, 68:61-76. Elschnig, A. Nystagmus retractorius, ein cerebrales Herd-Symptom. *Med. Klin., Berlin*, 1913, 9:8-11.

KOFFERATH, WALTER (German physician)

Kofferath syndrome. Synonym: *obstetric diaphragmatic paralysis.*

Unilateral phrenic paralysis in newborn infants caused by birth injury of the phrenic or cervical nerves, most frequently produced by forceps delivery. It results in diaphragmatic relaxation, dyspnea, cyanosis, unilateral edema of the neck, inspiratory thoracic asymmetry, and frequently, the Duchenne-Erb syndrome.

Kofferath, W. Über einen Fall von recthtsseitiger Erbscher Lähmung und Phrenikuslähmung nach Zangenextraktion. *Mschr. Geburtsch. Gyn.*, 1921, 55:33-8.

KÖHLER, ALBAN (German physician, 1874-1947)

Freiberg-Köhler disease. See *Köhler disease (2).*

Köhler disease (1). Synonyms: *Köhler-Mouchet disease, Panner disease, os naviculare pedis retardatum, osteochondrosis juvenilis, tarsal scaphoiditis.*

Epiphyseal ischemic necrosis of the tarsal navicular bone and, less frequently, the patella.

Köhler, A. Über eine häufige, bisher anscheinend unbekannte Erkrankung einzelner kindlicher Knochen. *Münch. Med. Wschr.*, 1908, 55:1923-5.

Köhler disease (2). Synonyms: *Freiberg infraction, Freiberg-Köhler disease, juvenile deforming metatarsophalangeal osteochondritis.*

An injury of the head of the metatarsal bone, presenting the picture of subchondral cancellous bone necrosis. Osteonecrosis of the metatarsal head from a subchondral bone fatigue fracture is believed to be the cause.

Köhler, A. Eine typische Erkrankung der 2 Metatarsophalangealgelenkes. *Münch. Med. Wschr.*, 1920, 67:1289-90. Freiberg, A. H. The so-called infraction of the second metatarsal bone. *J. Bone Joint Surg.*, 1926, 8:257-61.

Köhler-Mouchet disease. See *Köhler disease (1).*

Köhler-Stieda-Pellegrini syndrome. See *Stieda-Pellegrini syndrome.*

KOHLER, ELAINE (American physician)

Thieffry-Kohler syndrome. See *Thieffry-Shurtleff syndrome.*

KÖHLMEIER, W. (German physician)

Köhlmeier syndrome. See *Degos syndrome.*

Köhlmeier-Degos syndrome. See *Degos syndrome.*

KOHLSCHÜTTER, A.

Kohlschütter syndrome. See *amelocerebrohypohidrosis syndrome.*

KOHN, GERTRUDE (American physician)

Winter-Kohn-Mellman-Wagner syndrome. See *Winter syndrome.*

KOJEWNIKOFF, ALEKSEI IAKOVLEVICH. See KOZHEVNIKOV, ALEKSEI IAKOVLEVICH

KOJEWNIKOFF, ALEXIS J. See KOZHEVNIKOV, ALEKSEI IAKOVLEVICH

KOK, O. (Dutch physician)

Kok disease. A hereditary disease, transmitted as an autosomal dominant trait, characterized by onset at birth with hypertonia in flexion, which disappears during sleep but reappears on awakening; exaggerated startle response to sudden sensory stimuli, sometimes associated with acute diffuse hypertonia and falling down; and strong brainstem reflexes, notably the head-retraction reflex.

Kok, O., & Bruyn, G. W. An unidentified hereditary disease. *Lancet*, 1962, 1:1359.

KOLOPP, P. (French physician)

Woringer-Kolopp syndrome. See *under Woringer, Frederic.*

KÖNIG, FRANZ (German physician, 1832-1910)

König disease (1). Synonyms: *König syndrome, Paget quiet necrosis of bone, arthrolithiasis, loose bodies in the joints, osteochondritis dissecans, osteochondrolysis.*

A disease of the tubular bones in adult males, in which osteochondritis is associated with subchondral inflammatory processes and necrotic dissection of fragments of the cartilage, resulting in loose bodies in the bone and joint cavities.

*König, F. *Lehrbuch der Allgemeinen Chirurgie für Aerzte und Studierende.* Berlin, 1889, p. 751.

König disease (2). See *König syndrome (2).*

König syndrome (1). See *König disease (1).*

König syndrome (2). Synonym: *König disease.*

Cecum mobile and local infection of the cecum and terminal ileum associated with abdominal distention, hyperperistalsis, episodes of constipation or diarrhea, colic simulating intestinal obstruction, and intestinal spasms in the right lower quadrant.

König, F. Die stricturirende Tuberculose des Darmes und ihre Behandlung. *Deut. Zschr. Chir.*, 1892, 34:65-81.

KÖNIGSTEIN, H. (German physician)

Königstein-Lubarsch syndrome. See *Lubarsch-Pick syndrome.*

KONJETZNY, GEORG ERNST (German physician, born 1880)

Konjetzny gastritis. Inflammatory chronic lymphatic gastritis simulating cancer, associated with hypertrophy and ulcer of the gastric mucosa, reportedly described by Konjetzny.

KONOVALOV, N. V. (Russian physician)

Wilson-Konovalov disease. See *Wilson disease, under Wilson, Samuel Alexander Kinnier.*

KOPITS, EUGEN (Hungarian orthopedic surgeon)

Kopits-Matolscy syndrome. See *popliteal pterygium syndrome.*

KOPLIK, HENRY (American physician, 1858-1927)

Koplik spots. Synonym: *Filatov spots.*

Small, irregular, bright red spots on the buccal and lingual mucosae, with minute bluish white specks in the center of each spot, which are pathognomic of beginning measles.

Koplik, H. The diagnosis of the invasion of measles from a study of the exanthema as it appears on the buccal mucous membrane. *Acta Pediat., N. Y.*, 1896, 13:918-22.

Korean hemorrhagic fever (KHF). See *hemorrhagic fever with renal syndrome.*

KORNZWEIG, ABRAHAM LEON (American physician)

Bassen-Kornzweig syndrome. See *under Bassen.*

koro. See *genital retraction syndrome.*

KOROVNIKOV, A. F. (Russian physician)

Korovnikov disease. See *Korovnikov syndrome.*

Korovnikov syndrome. Synonym: *Korovnikov disease.*

Splenomegaly with thrombocytosis and gastrointestinal hemorrhage beginning between the ages of 20 and 40 years, usually in the form of hematemesis and melena, followed by leukopenia, hypochromic anemia, and thrombocytosis.

Korovnikov, A. F. Splenopatii s subtrombotsitozom i gastroenterorragiiami. *Klin. Med., Moskva*, 1936, 14:714-21.

KORSAKOV (KORSAKOFF), SERGEI SERGEEVICH (Russian psychiatrist, 1854-1900)

Korsakoff psychosis (KP). See Korsakoff syndrome.

Korsakoff syndrome (KS). Synonyms: *Korsakoff psychosis (KP), Meynert amentia, amnestic confabulatory psychosis, amnestic psychosis, amnestic syndrome, cerebropathia psychica toxemica, polyneuritic psychosis, psychosis associated with polyneuritis, psychosis polyneuritica.*

A psychiatric disorder characterized mainly by amnesia with a tendency to confabulate, with or without polyneuropathy. Other symptoms may include delirium, anxiety, fear, a sense of panic, depression, confusion, and delusions. It is usually seen in alcoholics **(alcoholic Korsakoff syndrome or AKS)**,but it may also occur in nonalcoholic persons with head injuries, brain tumors, pregnancy toxemias, and toxic or deficiency diseases. When associated with Wernicke disease, the disorder is known as the *Wernicke-Korsakoff syndrome.*

*Korsakov, S. S. Ob alkogol'nom paraliche. *Vestn. Psychiat.*, 1887, vol. 4.

Wernicke-Korsakoff complex. See *Wernicke-Korsakoff syndrome.*

Wernicke-Korsakoff syndrome (WKS). See *under Wernicke.*

KOSCHEWNIKOFF, ALEXEI J. See KOZHEVNIKOV, ALEKSEI IAKOVLEVICH

KOSCHEWNIKOW, ALEKSEI J. See KOZHEVNIKOV, ALEKSEI IAKOVLEVICH

KOSHEVNIKOFF, ALEXIS J. See KOZHEVNIKOV, ALEKSEI IAKOVLEVICH

KOSTMANN, ROLF (Swedish physician, born 1909)

Kostmann agranulocytosis. See *Kostmann syndrome.*

Kostmann syndrome. Synonyms: *Kostmann agranulocytosis, agranulocytosis infantilis hereditaria, congenital agranulocytosis, infantile genetic agranulocytosis.*

A familial form of agranulocytosis, transmitted as an autosomal recessive trait, originally observed in the Parish of Overkalix in northern Sweden. The syndrome is characterized by early onset of symptoms, complete or almost complete lack of granulocytes in the peripheral blood, a skin infection manifested by boils and phlegmons, retarded or blocked maturation of the myelopoietic cells in the bone marrow, and early death due to recurrent infections. In addition, there may be variable monocytosis and hypergammaglobulinemia.

Kostmann, R. Infantile genetic agranulocytosis (agranulocytosis infantilis hereditaria). A new recessive lethal disease in man. *Acta Paediat., Uppsala*, 1956, 45(Suppl. 105):1-78.

KOSZEWSKI, BOHDAN JULIUSZ (Polish physician, born 1918)

Koszewski syndrome. Synonym: *congenital osteosclerosis.*

Congenital diffuse generalized hyperostosis.

Koszewski, B. J. Angeborene diffuse generalisierte Hyperostose. *Schweiz. Zschr. Path. Anat.*, 1949, 12:41-53.

KOUSSEFF, BORIS G. (American physician)

Kousseff syndrome. A familial syndrome, transmitted as an autosomal recessive tait, characterized by sacral meningocele, conotruncal cardiac defects, unilateral renal agenesis, low-set and posteriorly angulated ears, retrognathia, and short neck with a low posterior hairline.

Kousseff, B. G. Sacral meningocele with conotruncal heart defects: A possible autosomal recessive trait. *Pediatrics,* 1984, 74:395-8.

KOYANAGI, YOSHIZO (Japanese physician, born 1880)

Vogt-Koyanagi syndrome. See *under Vogt, Alfred.*

Vogt-Koyanagi-Harada (VKH) syndrome. See *Vogt-Koyanagi syndrome, under Vogt, Alfred, and see Harada syndrome.*

KOZHEVNIKOV (KOSHEWNIKOFF), ALEKSEI IAKOVLEVICH (Russian physician, 1836-1902)

Koshewnikoff syndrome. See *Kozhewnikov syndrome.*

Kozhevnikov epilepsy. See *Kozhevnikov syndrome.*

Kozhevnikov syndrome. Synonyms: *Kojewnikoff syndrome, Koshewnikoff syndrome, Kozhevnikov epilepsy, continuous epilepsy, epilepsia partialis continua, epilepsia partialis continua corticalis, partial epilepsy, polyclonia continua epileptoides.*

Clonic muscular twitching repeated at fairly regular intervals in one part of the body for a period of days or weeks. Each twitch is an abrupt jerk lasting one-fourth of a second, usually involving one muscle group but occasionally including other related muscles on the same side or in the same limb, without relation to consciousness. The muscles involved are chiefly the flexors of the limbs, the lateral flexors of the neck, and facial muscles. Kozhevnikov suspected that the essential lesions were located in the cortex, but subsequent studies indicate that structures other than the cortex also may be involved.

Kozhevnikov, A. I. *Osobyi vid kortikal'noi epilepsii.* Moskva, 1952. Kozhevnikov, A. I. Osobyi vid kortital'noi epilepsii. *Med. Obzor,* 1894, 42:97-118.

KOZLOWSKI, BOGUMIL (Polish ophthalmologist, born 1907)

Kozlowski degeneration. Synonym: *degeneratio hyaloidea granuliformis corneae.*

Yellow granular opacity of the cornea and warty projections on the surface produced by deposition of hyaline material in the lower half of the cornea.

Kozlowski, B. Szczególna postac zwyrodnienia szklistego rogówki. *Klin. Oczna,* 1953, 23:249-53.

KOZLOWSKI, KAZIMIERZ (Polish physician)

chondrodysplasia spondylometaphysia, Kozlowski type. See *Kozlowski spondylometaphyseal dysplasia syndrome.*

dysostosis spondylometaphysaria, Kozlowski type. See *Kozlowski spondylometaphyseal dysplasia syndrome.*

dysplasia spondylometaphysaria, Kozlowski type. See *Kozlowski spondylometaphyseal dysplasia syndrome.*

Kozlowski spondylometaphyseal dysplasia syndrome. Synonyms: *Kozlowski syndrome; Kozlowski-Maroteaux-Spranger syndrome; chondrodysplasia spondylo-metaphysaria, Kozlowski type; dysostosis spondylometaphysaria, Kozlowski type; dysplasia spondylo-metaphysaria, Kozlowski type; spondylometaphyseal dysplasia, Kozlowski type.*

A syndrome of short-trunk dwarfism, waddling gait in early childhood, limited joint mobility, kyphoscoliosis in childhood and adolescence, and occasional hyperopia and genua valga. Radiographic findings show platyspondyly, broad and short basilar parts of the iliac bone, widening sclerosis and irregularity of the metaphyses of the tubular bones and epiphyseal ossification centers, irregular carpal bones, and short hand bones. Onset usually takes place during the second years of life. The syndrome is transmitted as an autosomal dominant trait.

Kozlowski, K., Maroteaux, P., & Spranger, J. La dysostose spondylométaphysaire. *Presse Méd.,* 1967, 75:2769-74.

Kozlowski syndrome. See *Kozlowski spondylometaphyseal dysplasia syndrome.*

Kozlowski-Maroteaux-Spranger syndrome. See *Kozlowski spondylometaphyseal dysplasia syndrome.*

pseudo-achondroplastic spondyloepiphyseal dysplasia, Kozlowski type. See *under pseudo-achondroplastic spondyloepiphyseal dysplasia.*

spondylometaphyseal dysplasia, Kozlowski type. See *Kozlowski spondylometaphyseal dysplasia syndrome.*

KP (Korsakoff psychosis). See *Korsakoff syndrome.*

KRABBE, KNUDD HARALDSEN (Danish physician, 1885-1961)

Christensen-Krabbe disease. See *Alpers syndrome.*

Krabbe disease. Synonyms: *Krabbe leukodystrophy, Krabbe syndrome, diffuse globoid body sclerosis, diffuse globoid cell cerebral sclerosis, familial infantile diffuse brain sclerosis, globoid cell cerebral sclerosis, globoid cell leukodystrophy, globoid cell sclerosis.*

An inborn metabolic disease, transmitted as an autosomal recessive trait, characterized by onset of symptoms before the age of 6 months and death by the end of the first year of life, survival beyond 2 years being very rare. Early manifestations include generalized rigidity, fretfulness, apathy, loss of head control, vomiting, hyperirritability, bouts of crying, and spasticity. They are followed by opisthotonic recurvation of the neck and trunk, adduction of the legs, flexion of the arms, clenching of the fists, Babinski signs, and hyper-

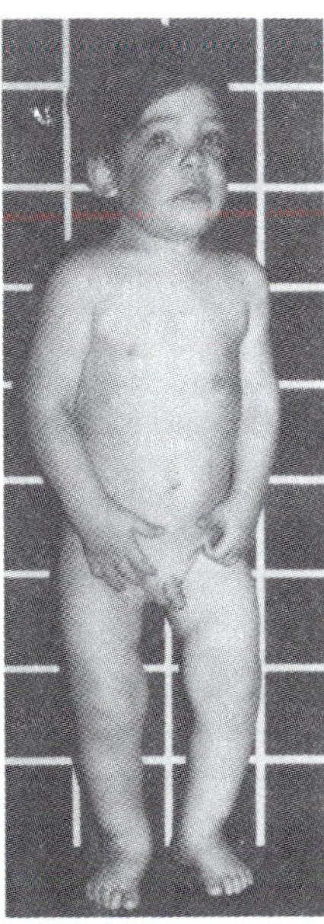

Kozlowski spondylometaphyseal dysplasia syndrome
Riggs, W., Jr. & Summitt, R.L.: *Radiology,* 101:375, 1971. Oak Brook, IL.: Radiological Society of North America, Inc.

reactive reflexes. The advanced stages are marked by blindness, optic atrophy, convulsions, deafness, and cachexia. The metabolic defect is the lack of galactocerebrosidase with resulting accumulation of galactocerebroside, especially in the white matter of the brain. The principal pathologic findings include demyelination and gliosis in the cerebrum, brain stem, spinal cord, and nerves, and the presence of globoid cells (large histiocytes containing accumulated metabolites) and of Schwann cells.

Krabbe, K. H. A new familial infantile form of diffuse brain sclerosis. *Brain,* 1916, 39:74-114.

Krabbe leukodystrophy. See *Krabbe disease.*

Krabbe syndrome. See *Krabbe disease.*

Sturge-Weber-Krabbe syndrome. See *Sturge-Weber syndrome.*

KRAEMER, RICHARD. See KRÄMER, RICHARD

KRAMER, FRANZ (German neurologist, born 1878)

Kramer-Pollnow disease. A neurological disorder characterized by the sudden onset of progressive hyperkinesia between the ages of 1 and 4 years, followed by mental retardation, retrogression of speech efficiency, and anxiety.

Kramer, F., & Pollnow, H. Über eine hyperkinetische Erkrankung im Kindesalter. *Mschr. Psychiat. Neur.*, 1932, 82-83:1-40.

KRÄMER (KRAEMER), RICHARD (German ophthalmologist, born 1878)

Krämer disease. Synonyms: *episcleritis metastatica furunculiformis, pyogenic metastatic scleritis, suppurative scleritis.*

Suppurative scleritis characterized by an abscess that is produced by a bacterial embolus in a scleral vessel. Frequently, there are metastatic deposits in the inner eye. High immunity of the sclera is believed to be the cause of embolization of microorganisms, staphylococci being the most frequently isolated pathogens.

Krämer, R. Episkleritis metastatica furunculiformis. *Klin. Mbl. Augenh.*, 1921, 66:441-50.

KRAUPA, ERNST (German ophthalmologist)

Fuchs-Kraupa syndrome. See *Fuchs dystrophy.*

Kraupa syndrome. See *Fuchs dystrophy.*

kraurosis vulvae. See *Breisky disease.*

KRAUSE, ARLINGTON COLTON (American ophthalmologist, born 1896)

Krause syndrome. Synonyms: *congenital encephalo-ophthalmic dysplasia, encephalo-ophthalmic syndrome.*

A syndrome of retinal and cerebral dysplasia, marked by microphthalmos; retinal choroid and optic nerve malformations; retinal glial membranes, cones, and septa; persistent remains of the hyaloid artery; hypertrophy, hyperplasia or aplasia of the brain and cerebellum; and microcephaly. Mental retardation, hydrocephalus, blindness, enophthalmos, microphthalmos, strabismus, retinal atrophy, gliosis, retinal and vitreous hemorrhages, synechiae, glaucoma, and cataract are the most common clinical features. The disease is most most frequently observed in premature infants and in single infants of multiple births.

Krause, A. C. Congenital encephalo-ophthalmic dysplasia. *Arch. Ophth., Chicago*, 1946, 36:387-444.

KREIBIG, WILHELM (German ophthalmologist)

Kreibig opticomalacia. An acute unilateral disorder of vision with sclerosis of the retinal vessels and optic nerve atrophy, leading to complete blindness. The contralateral eye shows blurring of the papillary margin and slight intrapapillary hemorrhage. Pathologically, there is softening of the optic nerve between the chiasma and the papilla, with sclerosis in the supplying vessels. The disease, which is painless, is usually observed in elderly arteriosclerotic patients.

Hruby, K. Über einige neuere Krankheitsbilder in der Augenheilkunde. *Wien. Klin. Wschr.*, 1949, 61:693-5.

KRETSCHMER, ERNST (German psychiatrist, 1888-1964)

Kretschmer syndrome. See *apallic syndrome.*

KRIDA, ARTHUR (American physician, born 1888)

Bakwin-Krida syndrome. See *metaphyseal dysplasia syndrome.*

KRISHABER, MAURICE (French physician, 1836-1883)

Krishaber disease. Synonym: *cerebrocardiac syndrome.*

A disorder charactererized by tachycardia, vertigo, hyperesthesia, insomnia, and a peculiar feeling that one's head is empty.

Krishaber, M. *De névropathie cérébro-cardiaque*. Paris, Masson, 1873.

KROMPECHER, EDMUND (German physician, 1870-1926)

Krompecher carcinoma. See *Krompecher tumor.*

Krompecher tumor. Synonyms: *Jacob ulcer, Krompecher carcinoma, basal-cell carcinoma, epithelioma basocellulare, rodent ulcer.*

A slow-growing epithelial tumor, usually of the face, derived from basal cells, occurring as a pinhead-to pea-sized pearly nodule with a central depression and a telangiectatic border. Such nodules usually ulcerate and may be locally malignant, but they seldom metastasize. Prolonged exposure to sunlight and wind is believed to be the contributing factor.

Krompecher, E. Des drüsenartige Oberflächenepithelkrebs. Carcinoma epitheliale adenoides. *Beitr. Path. Anat.*, 1900, 28:1-41. *Jacob, A. Observations on ulcers of peculiar character, which attack the eyelids and other parts of the face. *Dublin Hosp. Rep.*, 1827, 4:231-9.

KRÖNLEIN, RUDOLF ULRICH (German physician, 1847-1910)

Krönlein hernia. Synonyms: *hernia inguinoperitonealis incarcerata, inguinoperitoneal hernia.*

A double hernia protruding into the inguinal canal and from the internal inguinal ring into the subperitoneal tissue.

Krönlein, R. U. Hernia inguino-peritonealis incarcerata. *Arch. Klin. Chir., Berlin*, 1876, 19:408-27.

KRÜGER, K. H. (German physician)

Curtius-Krüger syndrome. See *Curtius syndrome (2).*

KRUKENBERG, FRIEDRICH ERNST (German physician, born 1871-1946)

Axenfeld-Krukenberg spindle. See *Krukenberg spindle.*

Krukenberg spindle. Synonyms: *Axenfeld-Krukenberg spindle, bilateral congenital melanosis of the cornea.*

A congenital, vertical, spindle-shaped, symmetrical deposition of brown pigment in the deep layers of the cornea.

Krukenberg, F. Beiderseitige angeborene Melanose der Hornhaut. *Klin. Mbl.*, 1899, 37:254-8.

Krukenberg tumor. Synonym: *fibrosarcoma ovarii mucocellulare carcinomatodes.*

A bilateral ovarian tumor with fibromyxomatous stroma and scattered mucin-secreting signet cells, which is considered to be a metastasis of gastric carcinoma. Typically, the tumor is a large, grayish white, solid lesion.

Krukenberg, F. Über das Fibrosarcoma varii mucocellulare (carcinomatodes). *Arch. Gyn., Berlin*, 1896, 50:287-321.

KRUSE, WALTHER (German bacteriologist, 1864-1943)

Shiga-Kruse disease. See *under Shiga.*

KS. See *Kawasaki syndrome.*

KS. See *Kartagener syndrome.*

KS (Kallmann syndrome). See *olfactogenital syndrome.*

KS (Klinefelter syndrome). See *chromosome XXY syndrome.*

KS-mucopolysaccharidosis. See *mucopolysaccharidosis IV-A.*

KSS. See *Kearns-Sayre syndrome.*

KTW. See *Klippel-Trénaunay-Weber syndrome.*

kubisagari. See *Gerlier disease.*

KUFS, H. (German neurologist, 1871-1955)

Kufs disease. See *Kufs syndrome.*

Kufs syndrome. Synonyms: *Kufs disease, Kufs-Mayer disease, adult ceroid lipofuscinosis, adult amaurotic familial idiocy, adult ganglioside lipidosis, late familial amaurotic idiocy, late ganglioside lipidosis, neuronal ceroid lipofuscinosis (NCL).*

An adult form of amaurotic familial idiocy, transmitted as an autosomal recessive trait (dominant transmission has also been reported), beginning in early adult life. Progressive mental deterioration, faulty memory, apathy, generalized muscular rigidity, cerebellar syndrome, extrapyramidal symptoms, myoclonic jerks, ataxia, tremor, and epileptic seizures are the chief symptoms. Histological findings include extensive storage of ceroid-lipofuscin in the central nervous system, liver, myocardium, and retina (without any ocular manifestations).

Kufs, H. Über eine Spätform der amaurotischen Idiotie und ihre heredofamiliären Grundlagen. *Zschr. Neur. Psychiat.*, 1925, 95:169-88.

Kufs-Mayer disease. See *Kufs syndrome.*

KUGEL, MAURICE ALEXANDER (American physician, 1899-1946)

Kugel-Stoloff syndrome. Synonym: *congenital idiopathic hypertrophy of the heart.*

A childhood disease of unknown etiology, characterized by myocardial fibrosis appearing in the first years of life, an afebrile course, enlargement of the heart, dyspnea, cyanosis, and sudden death.

Kugel, M. A., & Stoloff, E. G. Dilation and hypertrophy of the heart in infants and in young children, with myocardial fibrosis (so called congenital idiopathic hypertrophy). *Am. J. Dis. Child.*, 1933, 45:828-64.

KUGELBERG, ERIC KLAS HENRIK (Swedish physician, born 1913)

Kugelberg-Welander syndrome. See *Wohlfart-Kugelberg-Welander syndrome.*

Wohlfart-Kugelberg-Welander syndrome. See *under Wohlfart.*

KULENKAMPFF, C. (German physician)

Kulenkampff-Tarnow syndrome. See *tardive dyskinesia syndrome.*

KÜMMELL, HERMANN (German physician, 1852-1937)

Kümmell disease. See *Kümmell-Verneuil disease.*

Kümmell kyphosis. See *Kümmell-Verneuil disease.*

Kümmell spondylitis. See *Kümmell-Verneuil disease.*

Kümmell-Verneuil disease. Synonyms: *Kümmell disease, Kümmell kyphosis, Kümmell spondylitis, post-traumatic spondylitis, spondylitis post-traumatica, spondylopathia traumatica.*

Injury (without fracture) of a vertebra, which produces gradual compression and collapse of the vertebral body due to circulatory disorders with resulting rarefying osteitis. Pain, weakness, kyphosis, and a wedge-shaped vertebra are the principal symptoms. Some authors suggest the possibility of a latent fracture during the initial injury.

Kümmel, H. Über die traumatischen Erkrankungen der Wirbelsäuld. *Deut. Med. Wschr.*, 1985, 21:180-1.

KUNDRAT, HANS (Austrian physician, 1845-1893)

Kundrat disease. Synonyms: *lymphoblastoma, lymphocytic reticulosarcoma, lymphocytoma, lymphosarcoma.*

A malignant tumor of the lymphoid tissue composed of lymphocytes and lymphoblasts. A typical tumor forms an invasive mass of soft, gray to pink tissue with areas of necrosis. It may metastasize, but its expansion is usually accomplished by invasive growth, with permeation of the capsule of the involved node by lymphocytes and lymphoblasts and infiltration of the surrounding tissue.

Kundrat. Über Lympho-Sarcomatosis. *Wien. Klin. Wschr.*, 1893, 6:211-3; 234-9.

Kundrat syndrome. See *holoprosencephaly syndrome.*

KUNKEL, HENRY GEORGE (American physician, born 1916)

Bearn-Kunkel syndrome. See *under Bearn.*

Bearn-Kunkel-Slater syndrome. See *Bearn-Kunkel syndrome.*

Kunkel syndrome. See *Bearn-Kunkel syndrome.*

KUROKI, Y. (Japanese physician)

Niikawa-Kuroki syndrome. See *Kabuki make-up syndrome.*

KURZ, JAROMIR (Czech ophthalmologist, born 1895)

Kurz syndrome. Congenital blindness with a high degree of axial hypermetropia (averaging 8 diopters), enophthalmos, pupillary areflexia, and searching eye movements. Mental retardation may appear later in life.

Kurz, J. Syndrom vrozené slepoty. *Cesk. Ofthal.*, 1951, 7:377-87.

Kuskokwim syndrome. Synonym: *arthrogryposis-like syndrome.*

A disorder originally described in an inbred Eskimo population in a limited area surrounding the delta of the Kuskokwin River in Alaska. The most constant features include hypoplasia of the first or second lumbar vertebral body, producing a gibbus in infants; progressive elongation of the pedicle of the fifth lumbar vertebra, producing spondylolisthesis; osteolytic areas in the outer clavicle and proximal humerus in children; and hypoplasia of the patella associated with knee contractures. The familial pattern suggests autosomal recessive inheritance.

Wright, G., & Aase, J. The Kuskokwin syndrome: An inherited form of arthrogryposis in the Alaskan Eskimo. *Birth Defects*, 1969, 5(3):91-4.

KÜSS, GEORGES (French physician, 1877-1967)

Küss disease. Stenosis of the rectum and sigmoid due to inflammatory processes, such as perirectitis and perisigmoiditis, in the surrounding tissue.

Küss, G. Les rétrécissements pseudo-cancéreux péricoliques pelviens. *Bull. Acad. Nat. Méd., Paris*, 1950, 134:377-80.

KUSSMAUL, ADOLF (German physician, 1822-1902)

Kussmaul aphasia. A voluntary refraining from speech in mental disorders.

Kussmaul, A. *Die Störungen der Sprache. Versuch einer Pathologie der Sprache*. Leipzig, Vogel, 1877.

Kussmaul breathing. See *Kussmaul respiration.*

Kussmaul coma. See *under Kussmaul respiration.*

Kussmaul disease. See *Kussmaul-Maier syndrome.*

Kussmaul respiration. Synonym: *Kussmaul breathing.*

Deep, rapid respiration characteristic of the air hunger in diabetic or renal acidosis or coma (**Kussmaul coma**).

Kussmaul, A. Zur Lehre von Diabetes mellitus. Über eine eigenthümliche Todesort bei Diabetischen, über Acetonämie, Glycerin-Behandlung des Diabetes und Einspirtzungen von Diastase in's Blut bei dieser Krankheit. *Deut. Arch. Klin. Med.*, 1874, 14:l-46.

Kussmaul-Maier syndrome. Synonyms: *Kussmaul disease, arteritis nodosa, classic periarteritis nodosa, necrotizing angiitis, panangiitis, panarteritis, periarteritis nodosa, polyarteritis acuta nodosa, polyarteritis nodosa.*

A vascular disease involving the middle-sized and smaller arteries and characterized by visible and palpable nodules along their courses. Arterial bifurcations and branchings are the primary sites of lesions. A typical lesion is marked by edema, fibrous exudations, fibrinoid necrosis, and infiltration of polymorphonuclear neutrophils. The initial lesions are gradually replaced by necrosis, granulation, and scar tissue, which lead to occlusion, thrombosis, infarction, and formation of aneurysms that sometimes rupture. The symptoms are varied and include fever, muscle pain, tachycardia, weight loss, polyneuritis, and myocardial infarction. Renal involvement is usually manifested by glomerulitis and renal polyarteritis. Pain in the umbilical region or the right upper quadrant, anorexia, nausea, and vomiting indicate arterial lesions in the viscera. Hypersensitivity is believed to be the cause, but the pathogenic mechanism is unknown.

Kussmaul, A., & Maier, R. Über eine bisher nicht beschriebene eigentümliche Arterienerkrankung (Periarteritis nodosa), die mit Morbus Brightii und rapid fortschreitender allgemeiner Muskellähmung einhergeht. *Deut. Arch. Klin. Med.*, 1866, 1:484-518.

Landry-Kussmaul syndrome. See *Guillain-Barré syndrome.*

KÜSTER, HERMANN (German gynecologist)

Küster syndrome. See *Mayer-Rokitansky-Küster syndrome.*

Mayer-Rokitansky-Küster (MRK) syndrome. See *under Mayer.*

Rokitansky-Küster-Hauser (RKH) syndrome. See *Mayer-Rokitansky-Küster syndrome.*

kwashiorkor. Synonyms: *kwashiorkor syndrome, malignant malnutrition, nutritional edema syndrome, pluridefìciency syndrome, protein malnutrition.*

A nutritional deficiency syndrome due to inadequate protein intake with a low or normal caloric nutrition, which is seen most frequently in children older than 2 years. The symptoms include pitting edema due to hypoalbuminemia, ascites, stunted growth, apathy, indifference to environment, irritability, fatty liver with protuberant abdomen, skin rash, ulcers, depigmentation, loss of hair, anorexia, diarrhea, decreased heart size, decreased muscle volume, atrophic changes in the pancreas and intestine, slow wound healing, body temperature disorders, and immunologic deficiency. Hematological changes include decreased blood volume and low hematocrit. Kwashiorkor is prevalent in economically depressed areas of Africa, Asia, and South and Central America. The name "kwashiorkor" derives from "the disease the first child gets when the second is on the way" in the Gia dialect in Ghana.

Williams, C. D. Kwashiorkor. *JAMA*, 1953, 153:1280-5.

kwashiorkor syndrome. See *kwashiorkor.*

kwashiorkor-like syndrome. A nutritional-deficiency syndrome occurring in adults with symptoms similar to those of kwashiorkor.

Gofferje, H., *et al.* Mangelernahrung im Alter: Diagnostik und Therapie. *Zschr. Gerontol.*, 1980, 13:52-61. Gofferje, H., *et al.* Untersuchgen zur Mangelernährung in einer medizinischen Klinik. *Zschr. Ernahrungswiss*, 1979, 18:62-70.

kwashiorkor-marasmus syndrome (KMS). Synonyms: *marasmic kwashiorkor, protein-calorie malnutrition (PCM), protein-energy malnutrition (PEM).*

A nutritional deficiency syndrome combining the features of kwashiorkor (a nutritional deficiency syndrome resulting from inadequate protein intake) with a low or normal caloric intake and marasmus (relatively inadequate intake of all nutrients).

Bhattacharyya, A. K. Kwashiorkor-marasmus syndrome (KMS): A suggested nomenclature for protein-energy malnutrition (PEM) and a composite (clinical and anthropometric) classification. *Bull. Calcutta School Trop. Med.*, 1981, 29:125-30. Bhattacharyya, A. K. Protein-energy malnutrition (kwashiorkor-marasmus syndrome): Terminology, classification and evolution. *World Rev. Nutr. Diet.*, 1986, 47:80-133.

KWOK, R. H. M. (American physician)

Kwok quease. See *Chinese restaurant syndrome.*

kyphosis dorsalis adolescentium. See *Scheuermann disease.*

kyphosis dorsalis juvenilis. See *Scheuermann disease.*

kyphosis of adolescence. See *Scheuermann disease.*

KYRLE, JOSEF (Austrian dermatologist, 1880-1926)

Kyrle disease. Synonyms: *hyperkeratosis follicularis et parafollicularis in cutum penetrans, hyperkeratosis follicularis et parafollicularis penetrans, hyperkeratosis penetrans.*

A skin disease characterized by horny papules at or near the follicular orifices, which may affect any site except the palms, soles, and mucous membranes. The eruptions may be generalized or localized. The primary lesions are cone-shaped, slightly elevated, gray, brown or flesh-colored papules with central adherent scales or cornified cones surrounded by an inflammatory halo. Histologically, large masses of keratin are present in or just outside the orifice of the hair follicle. Beneath the plug, the epidermis may be acanthotic or atrophic with flattening of the rete. In some instances, plugs penetrate into the corium.

Kyrle, J. Über einen ungewöhnlichen Fall von universeller follikulärer und parafollikulärer Hyperkeratose. (Hyperkeratosis follicularis et parafollicularis in cutem penetrans). *Arch. Derm. Syph., Berlin*, 1916, 123:466-93.

KZ (Konzentrationslager) syndrome. See *concentration camp survivor syndrome.*

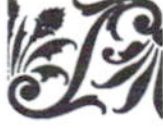

Page #	Term	Observation

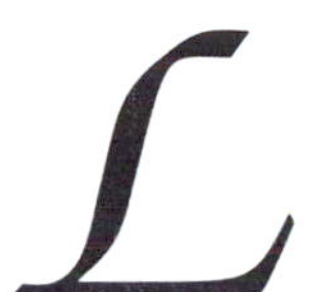

LABAND, PETER F. (Dentist in Trinidad)

Laband syndrome. See *Zimmermann-Laband syndrome.*

Zimmermann-Laband syndrome (ZLS). See *under Zimmermann.*

LABBE, ERNEST MARCEL (French physician, 1870-1939)

Labbé syndrome. Intermittent hypertension associated with adrenal tumors.

Labbé, M. *et al.* Crises solaires et hypertension paroxystique en rapport avec une tumeur surrénale. *Bull. Soc. Méd. Hôp. Paris*, 1922, 46:982-90.

LABHART, A. (Swiss physician)

Prader-Labhart-Willi syndrome (PLW, PLWS). See *Prader-Willi syndrome.*

Prader-Labhart-Willi-Fanconi syndrome. See *Prader-Willi syndrome.*

labile factor deficiency. See *Owren syndrome (2).*

labyrinthine hydrops. See *Ménière syndrome.*

lacerocondylar space syndrome. See *Collet-Sicard syndrome.*

lacrimo-auriculodentodigital (LADD) syndrome. Synonyms: *Levy-Hollister syndrome, lacrimo-auriculo-radiodental (LARD) syndrome.*

A familial syndrome of aplasia or hypoplasia of the lacrimal puncta associated with obstruction of the nasal lacrimal puncta, cup-shaped ears, hearing loss, mild hypodontia, enamel dysplasia, and various finger abnormalities (mainly fifth finger clinodactyly, duplication of the distal phalanges of the thumbs, triphalangeal thumbs, and syndactyly). Individual features of this syndrome may be inherited as an autosomal dominant trait.

Levy, W. J. Mesoectodermal dysplasia. A new combination of anomalies. *Am. J. Ophth.*, 1967, 63:978-82. Hollister, D. W., *et al.* The lacrimo-auriculo-dento-digital syndrome. *J. Pediat.*, 1973, 83:438-44.

lacrimo-auriculoradiodental (LARD) syndrome. See *lacrimo-auriculodentodigital syndrome.*

lactorrhea-amenorrhea syndrome. See *amenorrhea-galactorrhea syndrome.*

lacunar dementia. See *Binswager disease.*

lacunar optic atrophy. See *Schnabel atrophy.*

LADD. See *lacrimo-auriculodentodigital syndrome.*

LADD, WILLIAM EDWARDS (American physician, born 1880)

Ladd syndrome. Congenital obstruction of the duodenum, manifested by severe vomiting taking place shortly after birth or after the first feeding.

Ladd, W. E. Congenital obstruction of the duodenum in children. *N. Engl. J. Med.*, 1932, 206:277-83.

Ladd-Gross syndrome. Icterus neonatorum associated with astresia of the bile ducts.

Ladd, W. E., & Gross, R. E. *Abdominal surgery in infancy and childhood.* Philadelphia, Saunders, 1941, pp. 260-75.

LAENNEC, RENE THEOPHILE HYACINTHE (French physician, 1781-1826)

Laennec cirrhosis. Synonyms: *Morgagni-Laennec syndrome, alcoholic cirrhosis, fatty nutritional cirrhosis, liver cirrhosis with alcohol abuse, portal cirrhosis, septal cirrhosis.*

Cirrhosis of the liver seen in chronic alcoholism and malnutrition. Early liver changes, consisting of hepatomegaly (sometimes reaching extreme proportions) and fatty degeneration due to fatty infiltration of liver cells, are followed by a gradual decrease of fat, coinciding with a progressive increase of fibrous scarring, nodular degeneration, and shrinking of the liver, the surface of which is covered by multiple brown or yellow nodules, separated by a gray fibrous framework.

*Laennec, R. T. *Traité de l'auscultation médicale et des maladies du poumon et du coeur.* Paris, 1819.

Morgagni-Laennec syndrome. See *Laennec cirrhosis.*

LAERE, J., VAN. See VAN LAERE, J.

LAFFER, B. W. (American physician)

Laffer-Ascher syndrome. See *Ascher syndrome.*

LAFORA, GONZALO RODRIGUEZ (Spanish neurologist, born 1887)

Lafora disease. Synonyms: *Lafora-Unverricht disease, Lundborg-Unverricht disease, Unverricht syndrome, Baltic myoclonus, progressive myoclonus epilepsy with Lafora bodies.*

Familial progressive myoclonus epilepsy, transmitted as an autosomal recessive trait, characterized by convulsions, myoclonic jerking, abnormal EEG, and mental deterioration leading to dementia. The age of onset is 10 to 19 years, with progressive deterioration and death 2 to 10 years later. The presence of Lafora bodies (fibrillary elements made of polyglucosan associated with endoplasmic reticulum and ribosomal material) is the principal pathologic feature. Lafora bodies are usually found throughout the central nervous system, being most common in the basal ganglia and the dentate nucleus, and, sometimes, in the liver and myocardium.

Lafora G. R. Über das Vorkommen amyloider Körperchen im Inneren der Ganglienzellen; ein Beitrag zum Studium der amyloiden Substanz im Nervensystem. *Virchows Arch. Path.*, 1911, 205:295-303. Unverricht, H. *Die Myoklonie.* Leipzig, Deutiche, 1891. Lundborg, H. *Die progressive Myoklonusepilepsie.* Upsala, 1903.

Lafora-Unverricht disease. See *Lafora disease.*

Lahore sore. See *Alibert disease (2).*

LAKIN, HAROLD (American physician)

Golden-Lakin syndrome. See *under Golden.*

LAMB (**l**entigines-**a**trial myxoma-**m**ucocutaneous myxomas-**b**lue nevi) **syndrome.** See *cutaneous lentiginosis with atrial myxoma syndrome.*

LAMBERT, EDWARD HOWARD (American physician, born 1915)

Eaton-Lambert myasthenic syndrome. See *Eaton-Lambert syndrome, under Eaton, Lealdes McKendree.*

Eaton-Lambert syndrome (ELS). See *under Eaton, Lealdes McKendree.*

Eaton-Lambert-Rooke syndrome. See *Eaton-Lambert syndrome, under Eaton, Lealdes McKendree.*

Lambert-Eaton myasthenic syndrome (LEMS, LES). See *Eaton-Lambert syndrome, under Eaton, Lealdes McKendree.*

myasthenic syndrome of Eaton and Lambert (MSEL). See *Eaton-Lambert syndrome, under Eaton, Lealdes McKendree.*

LAMBLING, ANDRE (French physician, born 1899)

Lambling syndrome. See *postgastrectomy syndrome.*

lamellar desquamation of the newborn. See *Carini syndrome.*

lamellar exfoliation of the newborn. See *Carini syndrome.*

lamellar ichthyosis. See *Carini syndrome.*

lamelliform atelectatic foci. See *Fleischner syndrome.*

laminar osteochondritis. See *Martin du Pan-Rutishauser disease.*

LAMY, MAURICE EMILE JOSEPH (French physician, born 1985)

Debré-Lamy-Lyell syndrome. See *toxic epidermal necrolysis.*

Lamy-Maroteaux syndrome (1). See *diastrophic dwarfism syndrome.*

Lamy-Maroteaux syndrome (2). Synonyms: *acro-osteolysis without neuropathy, dominant acro-osteolysis.*

A familial form of osteolysis, transmitted as an autosomal dominant trait, characterized by onset between the ages of 8 and 22 years, slow dissolution of bones of the phalanges of the hands and feet, ulcers of the fingers and soles of the feet, disappearance of bone sequestra, and loss of the digits on healing. A similar condition may be produced on exposure to vinyl chloride.

Lamy, M., & Maroteaux, P. Acro-osteolyse dominante. *Arch. Fr. Pediat.*, 1961, 18:693-702. Harris, D. K., & Adams, W. G. Acro-osteolysis occurring in men engaged in the polymerizaticn of vinyl chloride. *Brit. Med. J.*, 1967, 3:712-4.

Maroteaux-Lamy syndrome (1). See *mucopolysaccharidosis VI.*

Maroteaux-Lamy syndrome (2). See *pyknodysostosis.*

Maroteaux-Lamy syndrome (3). See *spondyloepiphyseal dysplasia tarda.*

pseudo-achondroplastic spondyloepiphyseal dysplasia, Maroteaux-Lamytype. See *under pseudo-achondroplastic spondyloepiphyseal dysplasia.*

LANCEREAUX, ETIENNE (French physician, 1829-1910)

Lancereaux diabetes. Diabetes mellitus with severe emaciation.

Lancereaux. Le diabète maigre: ses symptomês, son évolution, son pronostic et son traitement;; ses rapports avec les altérations du pancreas. Étude comparative du diabète maigre et du diabète gras. Coup d'oeil rétrospectif sur les diabètes. *Union Méd., Paris*, 1880, 29:161-7; 205-11.

LANDING, BENJAMIN HARRISON (American physician, born 1920)

Landing syndrome. See *gangliosidosis G_{M1} type I.*

Landing-Oppenheimer syndrome. Synonym: *ceroid storage disease.*

Lipidosis in children, probably transmitted as an autosomal recessive trait, characterized by an increased susceptibility to infection and by ceroid infiltrations of the liver, spleen, and small intestine.

Landing, B. H., & Shirkey, H. S. A syndrome of recurrent infection and infiltration of viscera by pigmented lipid histiocytes. *Pediatrics*, 1957, 20:431-8. Opppenheimer, E. H., & Andrews, E. C., Jr. Ceroid storage disease in childhood. *Pediatrics*, 1959, 23:1091-1102.

Norman-Landing syndrome. See *gangliosidosis G_{M1} type I.*

LANDOR, J. V. (Physician in Malaya)

Howes-Pallister-Landor syndrome. See *Landor-Pallister syndrome.*

Landor-Pallister syndrome. Synonyms: *Howes-Pallister-Landor syndrome, avitaminosis B.*

A nutritional riboflavin deficiency characterized by eczematous eruption of the scrotum and a sore mouth. Associated symptoms include glossitis and white and cracked angles of the lips (perlèche) in early stages, followed by subacute degeneration of the spinal cord and visual deficiency. It was originally observed in the prison population in Singapore and Johore. According to some writers, this and the Strachan syndrome are the same entity.

Landor, J. V., & Pallister, R. A. Avitaminosis B_2. *Tr. Roy. Soc. Trop. Med. Hyg.*, 1935, 29:121-34.

LANDOUZY, LOUIS THEOPHIL JOSEPH (French neurologist, 1845-1917)

Erb-Landouzy-Déjerine syndrome. See *Landouzy-Déjerine syndrome.*

Landouzy disease. See *leptospirosis.*

Landouzy syndrome. Muscular atrophy associated with sciatica.

Landouzy, J. T. De la sciatique et de l'atrophie musculaire qui peut la complique. *Arch. Gén. Méd., Paris*, 1875, 25:303-25; 424-43; 562-78.

Landouzy-Déjerine dystrophy. See *Landouzy-Déjerine syndrome.*

Landouzy-Déjerine syndrome. Synonyms: *Erb-Landouzy-Déjerine syndrome, Landouzy-Déjerine dystrophy, facioscapulohumeral muscular dystrophy (FSHD).*

A hereditary form of progressive muscular dystrophy transmitted as an autosomal dominant trait. Onset usually takes place during childhood and adolescence with atrophic changes in the muscles of the shoulder girdle and face. Inability to raise the arms above the head, myopathic facies, eyelids that remain partly open in sleep, and inability to whistle or to purse the lips (tapir mouth) due to weakness of the facial muscles are the principal clinical features. Deafness and tortuosity of the retinal vessels may be associated.

Landouzy, L., & Déjerine, J. De la myopathie atrophique progressive (myopathie héréditaire, débutant dans l'enfance, par la face, sans altération du système nerveux). *C. Rend. Acad. Sc., Paris*, 1884, 98:53-5. Erb, W. H. Dystrophia musculorum progressiva. *Deut. Zschr. Nervenheilk*, 1891, 1:173.

LANDRY, JEAN BAPTISTE OCTAVE (French physician, 1826-1865)

Landry paralysis. See *Guillain-Barré syndrome.*

Landry-Guillain-Barré syndrome. See *Guillain-Barré syndrome.*

Landry-Kussmaul syndrome. See *Guillain-Barré syndrome.*

LANDSTEINER, KARL (Austrian-born American physician, 1868-1943)

Donath-Landsteiner syndrome. See *under Donath.*

LANE, JOHN EDWARD (American physician, 1872-1933)

Lane disease. Synonyms: *acroerythema symmetricum naeviforme, erythema palmaris hereditaria, erythema palmoplantare, palmar syndrome, palmoplantar erythema, red palms.*

A skin disease, believed to be hereditary, that occurs in both sexes and is characterized by bright red coloration of the palms, without apparent cause. Some cases of erythema appear during pregnancy and disappear after delivery.

Lane, J. E. Erythema palmare hereditarium (red palms). *Arch. Derm., Chicago*, 1929, 20:445-8.

LANE, SIR WILLIAM ARBUTHNOT (British physician, 1856-1943)

Arbuthnot Lane syndrome. See *Lane syndrome.*

Lane bands. Adhesions between tight loops of the terminal ileum which may extend as ligamentous bands to the right fossa.

*Lane, W. A. *The kink of the ileum in chronic intestinal stasis*. London, Nisbet, 1910.

Lane disease. See *Lane syndrome.*

Lane kink. Synonyms: *angulation of the ileum, ileal kink.*

Kinking of an anomalous band of the distal portion of the ileum (Lane bands), resulting in intestinal obstruction.

*Lane, W. A. *The kink of the ileum in chronic intestinal stasis*. London, Nisbet, 1910.

Lane syndrome. Synonyms: *Abruthnot Lane syndrome, Lane disease, colonic inertia-rectal obstruction syndrome, intestinal stasis.*

A syndrome of colonic inertia, contraction and lack of relaxation of the pelvic muscles (mainly of the puborectalis muscle), and rectal obstruction. The syndrome occurs almost exclusively in women and may be associated with galactorrhea, urological defects, abnormal manometric esophageal recordings, the Raynaud phenomenon, edema, orthostatic hypotension, neurological disorders, and abnormalities of the mesenteric plexus of the colon. See also *blind loop syndrome..*

Lane, W. A. The obstruction of the ileum which develops in chronic intestinal stasis. *Lancet*, 1910, 1:1193-4.

LANGDON DOWN. See DOWN, JOHN LANGDON HAYDON

LANGE, CORNELIA, DE (Pediatrician in Amsterdam, 1871-1950)

Brachmann-Cornelia de Lange (BCDL) syndrome. See *de Lange syndrome (1).*

Bruck-de Lange syndrome. See *de Lange syndrome (2).*

Cornelia de Lange syndrome (CLS). See *de Lange syndrome (1 and 2).*

de Lange syndrome (1). Synonyms: *Brachmann-Cornelia de Lange (BCDL) syndrome, Cornelia de Lange syndrome (CLS), Lange syndrome, Amsterdam dwarf, Amsterdam type, status degenerativus amstelodamensis, typus degenerativus amstelodamensis.*

A syndrome of growth deficiency, mental retardation, anomalies of the extremities, and characteristic facies. Low birth weight after full-term pregnancy and a low-pitched growling cry are the early symptoms. Craniofacial features consist mainly of microbrachycephaly, confluent eyebrows (synophrys), low and curly eyelashes, low hairline, thin lips and downturned upper lip (carp mouth), long philtrum, high-arched palate, cleft palate, and micrognathia. Musculoskeletal abnormalities include hypertonicity, small hands and feet with small and tapered digits, syndactyly between the second and third toes, proximal insertion of the thumb, short and curved fifth finger, phocomelia, and oligodactyly. Cutis marmorata, circumoral cyanosis, generalized hypertrichosis, hypoplastic nipples and umbilicus, and simian creases are the principal dermatological features. The majority of those affected have diminished sucking and swallowing capacity, failure to thrive, predisposition to respiratory tract infections, and frequent vomiting with aspiration pneumonia. Mental retardation is usually severe. Most patients die before the age of 6 years. The etiology is unknown.

Lange, C., de. Sur un type nouveau de dégénération (Typus amstelodamensis). *Arch. Méd. Enf., Paris*, 1933, 36:713-9. Brachmann, W. Ein Fall von symmetrischer Monodaktylie durch Ulnadefekt, mit symmetrischer Flughautbildung in den Ellenbeugen, sowie anderen Abnormitäten (Swerghaftigkeit, Halsrippen, Behaarung). *Jb. Kinderheilk.*, 1916, 84:225-235.

de Lange syndrome (2). Synonyms: *Bruck-de Lange syndrome, Cornelia de Lange syndrome (CLS), Lange syndrome, congenital muscular hypertrophy-cerebral syndrome.*

A syndrome of congenital muscular hypertrophy, extrapyramidal disorders, and mental deficiency. A short broad throat and neck, broad shoulders, short and thick extremities, and symmetrical hypertrophy of the muscles give the affected child the appearance of a wrestler. The muscles are hypertophied, hypertonic, and hard. The legs may be extended, the arms may be flexed; the head is usually bent backward, the tongue and ears may be large, there may be asymmetrical skull development, and the hairline may be low. Pathological changes usually include porencephaly, underdevelopment of various parts of the brain, distention of the cerebral ventricles, asymmetry of the brain, large vermis, status spongiosus, destruction of the cerebral cortex, hypertrophy of the fornix, thickening of the esophagus and intestines, and small heart. The affected infants usually die before reaching 2 years of age. There appears to be a familial tendency.

Lange, C., de. Congenital hypertrophy of the muscles, extrapyramidal motor disturbances and mental deficiency. A clinical entity. *Am. J. Dis. Child.*, 1934, 48:243-68. Bruck, F. Über einen Fall von kongenitaler Makroglossie, kombiniert mit allgemeiner wahrer Muskelhypertrophie und Idiotie. *Deut. Med. Wschr.*, 1889, 15:229-32.

Lange syndrome. See *de Lange syndrome (1 and 2).*

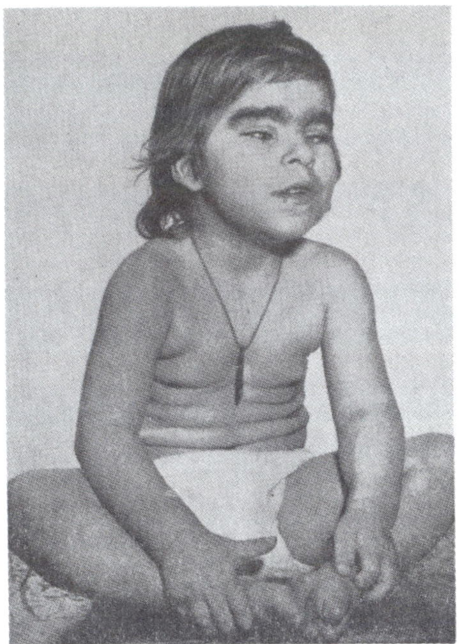

De Lange syndrome (1)
Falek, A., R. Schmidt & G.A. Jervis: *Pediatrics* 37:92, 1966.

LANGE-NIELSEN, FRIEDRIK (FRED) (Norwegian physician)

Jervell and Lange-Nielsen syndrome. See *under long QT syndrome.*

LANGER, LEONARD O., JR. (American physician)

Langer mesomelic dysplasia. See *Langer syndrome.*

Langer syndrome. Synonyms: *Langer mesomelic dysplasia; mesomelic dwarfism of the hypoplastic ulna, fibula and mandible type; mesomelic dwarfism, Langer type.*

A syndrome of short-limbed dwarfism with mesomelic micromelia and hypoplastic mandible. Major radiographic findings show shortening of the long tubular bones, usually involving their middle segments; hypoplasia of the distal portion of the ulna and absence of its ossified distal epiphysis; bowing of the radius and absence of its proximal epiphysis; hypoplasia of the proximal portion of the fibula and absence and poor ossification of its head; and shortening of the tibia and defect of its ossification centers. The symptoms are present at birth. The syndrome is transmitted as an autosomal recessive trait.

Langer, O. Mesomelic dwarfism of the hypoplastic ulna, fibula, mandible type. *Radiology*, 1967, 89:654-60.

Langer-Giedion syndrome. Synonyms: *Alè-Calò syndrome, acrodysplasia-dysostoses syndrome, multiple exostoses-mental retardation (MEMR) syndrome, trichorhino-auriculophalangeal multiple exostoses (TRAMPE) dysplasia, trichorhinophalangeal dysplasia type II (TRP II).*

A syndrome of unknown etiology, characterized by multiple exostoses, peculiar facies, and loose redundant skin. Facial features include a bulbous nose with thickened septum and alae, wide prominent philtrum, thin upper lip, and small mandible. Redundant skin and muscular hypotonia in infants usually regress with age. Cutaneous symptoms also include maculopapular nevi of the scalp, face, neck, trunk, and limbs. Cone-shaped epiphyses usually involve multiple phalanges, metacarpals, and metatarsals. Sparse hair, joint laxity, microcephaly, and mental retardation are included in this syndrome. Occasional deafness, hypochromic anemia, thin hypomineralized bones, clinobrachydactyly, bowed femurs, and hernia may be associated.

Langer, L. O., Jr. The thoracic-pelvic-phalangeal dystrophy. *Birth Defects*, 1969, 5(4):218-9. Hall, B. D., Langer, L. O., Jr., Giedion, A., *et al*. Langer-Giedion syndrome. *Birth Defects*, 1974, 10(12):147-64. Giedion, A. Das tricho-rhino-phalangeale Syndrom. *Helvet. Paediat. Acta*, 1966, 21:475. Alè, G., & Calò, S. Su di un caso di disostosi

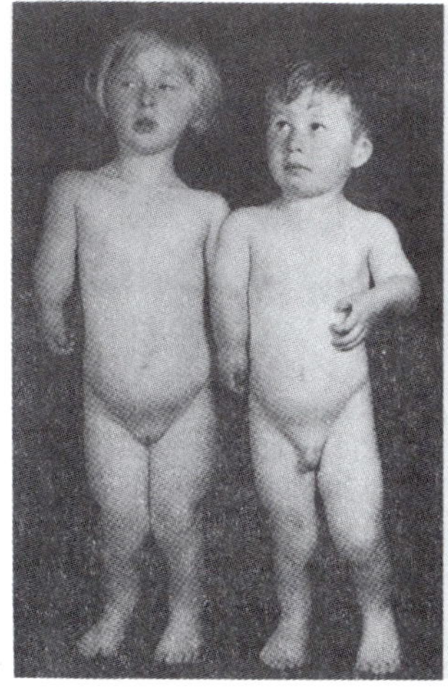

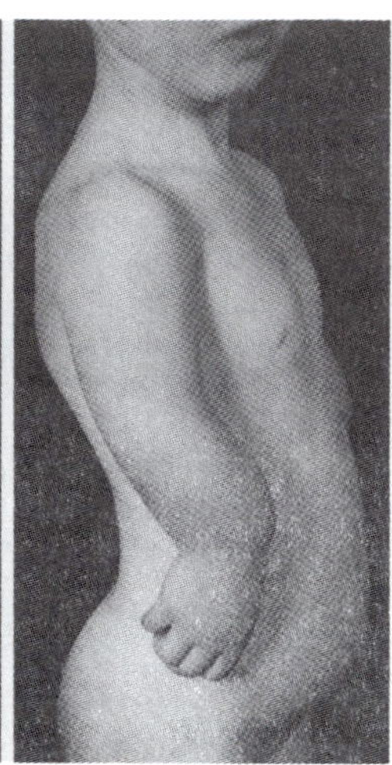

Langer syndrome
Blockley, N.J. & J.H. Lawrie: *J. Bone Joint Surg. (Br.)*, 45:745, 1963. Churchill Livingstone Medical Journals, Edinburgh, Scotland.

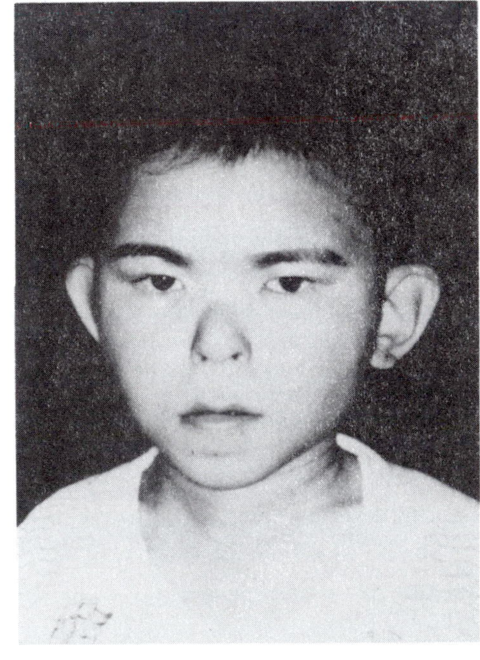

Langer-Giedion syndrome
Okuno, T., A. Inoue, T. Asakura & S. Nakao: *Clinicial Genetics* 32:40-45, 1987. Munksgaard International Publishers, Copenhagen, Denmark.

periferica associata con esostosi osteogeniche multiple ed iposomia disuniforme disarmonica. *Ann. Radiol. Diagn., Bologna*., 1961, 34:376-85.

mesomelic dwarfism, Langer type. See *Langer syndrome.*

LANGMEAD

Fere-Langmead lipomatosis. See *under Fere.*

LANGUEPIN, ANNE (French pediatrician)

Fèvre-Languepin syndrome. See *popliteal pterygium syndrome.*

LANNELONGUE, ODILON MARC (French physician, 1840-1911)

Lannelongue disease. See *Osgood-Schlatter syndrome.*

Lannelongue-Osgood-Schlatter syndrome. See *Osgood-Schlatter syndrome.*

LANNOIS, MAURICE (French physician, born 1856)

Lannois-Gradenigo syndrome. See *Gradenigo syndrome.*

laparotomophilia migrans. See *Munchausen syndrome.*

LARD (lacrimo-auriculoradiodental) syndrome. See *lacrimo-auriculodentodigital syndrome.*

lardaceous disease. See *amyloidosis.*

large atypical mole syndrome. See *dysplastic nevus syndrome.*

large spindle and/or epithelioid nevus. See *Spitz nevus.*

LARON, ZVI (Israeli physician)

Laron dwarfism. Synonyms: *Laron syndrome, Laron-type dwarfism (LTD), hereditary somatomedin deficiency, pituitary dwarfism.*

A familial syndrome, transmitted as an autosomal recessive trait, characterized by dwarfism, an abnormally high plasma concentration of growth hormone, and low somatomedin activity. The symptoms include delayed motor and skeletal maturation, hypoplasia of the base of the skull with small face and mandible, delayed closure of the fontanels, saddle nose, hypotrichosis, delayed dentition, tooth discoloration, crowding of defective teeth, high-pitched voice, acromicria, infantile genitalia, thin and underdeveloped muscle, and osteoporosis. Most early observations of this syndrome were made in children of Jewish and Oriental origins; later cases were reported in other ethnic groups.

Laron, Z., *et al.* Genetic pituitary dwarfism with high serum concentration of growth hormone. A new inborn error of metabolism. *Israel J. Med. Sc.*, 1966, 2:152-5.

Laron syndrome. See *Laron dwarfism.*

Laron-type dwarfism (LTD). See *Laron dwarfism.*

LARSEN, CHRISTIAN MAGNUS FALSEN SINDING (Norwegian physician, 1866-1930)

Larsen-Johansson syndrome. Synonyms: *Sinding Larsen-Johansson syndrome, juvenile osteopathia patellae, osteopathia patellae juvenilis.*

A painful condition of the patella precipitated by overstraining or trauma, usually observed in adolescents. X-ray findings show calcium deposits and signs of periostitis.

Larsen, S. En hittil ukjendt sygdom i patella. *Norsk. Mag. Laegevid.*, 1921, 19:856-8. Johansson, S. En förut icke beskriven sjukdom i patella. *Hygiea*, 1922, 84:161-6.

Sinding Larsen-Johansson syndrome. See *Larsen-Johansson syndrome.*

LARSEN, LOREN JOSEPH (American orthopedic surgeon, born 1914)

Larsen syndrome. Synonym: *multiple congenital dislocation syndrome.*

A syndrome of multiple congenital dislocations associated with characteristic facial features (flat facies with prominent forehead, depressed nasal bridge, and hypertelorism). Dislocations involve the elbows, hips, knees, and other joints, and are accompanied by pes equinovalgus or equinovarus. Hand abnormalities include cylindrical fingers, short metacarpals, and spatulate thumbs. Laxity of the costochondral cartilage, cleft palate, and cleft uvula are common. Both dominant and recessive forms of inheritance have been reported.

Larsen, L. J., *et al.* Multiple congenital dislocations associated with characteristic facial abnormality. *J. Pediat.*, 1950, 37:574-81.

LARSSON, TAGE KONRAD LEOPOLD (Swedish physician, born 1905)

Sjögren-Larsson syndrome (SLS). See *under Sjögren, Karl Gustaf Torsten.*

laryngeal chorea. See *Schroetter chorea.*

laryngeal syncope. See *Charcot vertigo.*

laryngeal vertigo. See *Charcot vertigo.*

laryngitis. See *common cold syndrome.*

LAS. See *laxative abuse syndrome.*

LASLETT, E. E. (British physician)

Laslett syndrome. See *bradycardia-tachycardia syndrome.*

LASSUEUR, AUGUSTE (Swiss physician, 1874-1949)

Graham Little-Lassueur-Feldman syndrome. See *Little syndrome, under Little, Ernest Gordon Graham.*

Lassueur-Graham Little syndrome. See *Little syndrome, under Little, Ernest Gordon Graham.*

Lassueur-Graham Little triad. See *Little syndrome, under Little, Ernest Gordon Graham.*

Lassueur-Little syndrome. See *Little syndrome, under Little, Ernest Gordon Graham.*

Piccardi-Lassueur-Little syndrome. See *Little syndrome, under Little, Ernest Gordon Graham.*

latah. See *latah syndrome.*

latah reaction. See *latah syndrome.*

latah syndrome. Synonyms: *latah, latah reaction.*

A condition of exaggerated startle reaction to a stimulus, consisting of violent jumps, echolalia with yelling out frank obscenities, and a tendency to carry out orders in a reflex manner. The condition is considered a culture-bound syndrome occurring mainly in Malaysia and Indonesia, but has been observed also in other parts of the world (see the *jumping Frenchmen of Maine syndrome*).

Clifford, H. C. Some notes and theories concerning latah. In his: *Studies in brown humanity.* Grant Richards, London, 1898. Simmons, R. C. The resolution of the latah paradox. *J. Nerv. Ment. Dis.*, 1980, 168:195-206.

latah-like reaction. See *jumping Frenchmen of Maine syndrome.*

late cerebromacular degeneration. See *Bessman-Baldwin syndrome.*

late chlorosis of Hayem. See *Faber syndrome.*

late distal hereditary myopathy. See *Welander syndrome.*

late familial amaurotic idiocy. See *Kufs syndrome.*

late ganglioside lipidosis. See *Kufs syndrome.*

late infantile amaurotic idiocy. See *gangliosidosis G_{M2} type III.*

late infantile ganglioside lipidosis. See *gangliosidosis G_{M2} type III.*

late onset lymphedema. See *Meige syndrome (1).*
late osteosclerosis. See *Albers-Schönberg syndrome.*
latent bone cyst. See *Stafne cyst.*
lateral asymmetry. See *Curtius syndrome (1).*
lateral bulbar syndrome. See *Wallenberg syndrome.*
lateral facial dysplasia (LFD). See *oculo-auriculovertebral dysplasia.*
lateral femoral paresthesia. See *Rot-Bernhardt syndrome, under Rot, Vladimir Karlovich.*
lateral medullary infarction syndrome. See *Wallenberg syndrome.*
lateral medullary syndrome. See *Wallenberg syndrome.*
lateral wall of the cavernous sinus syndrome. See *cavernous sinus syndrome.*
laterality anomalad. See *asplenia syndrome, and see polysplenia syndrome.*
LATHAM, A. D. (New Zealand physician)
Latham-Munro syndrome. A familial syndrome, transmitted as an autosomal recessive trait, characterized by congenital deaf-mutism, myoclonus, and grand mal epilepsy. Pscyhotic disorders and harelip or cleft palate are present in some patients.

Latham, A. D., & Munro, T. A. Familial myoclonus epilepsy associated with deaf-mutism in a family showing other psychobiological abnormalities. *Ann. Eugen., London,* 1937, 8:166-75.

lattice corneal dystrophy. See *Biber-Haab-Dimmer syndrome.*
LAUBER, HANS (Swiss-born ophthalmologist in Austria, born 1876)
Lauber disease. Synonyms: *fundus albipunctatus cum hemeralopia, fundus punctatus albescens, retinitis punctata albescens.*

An association of congenital stationary or very slowly progressive hemeralopia with fine whitish spots in the deep layers of the retina.

Lauber, H. Die sogenante Retinitis punctata albescens. *Klin. Mbl. Augenh.,* 1910, 48:133-48.

laughing and weeping syndrome. See *pathologic laughing and weeping syndrome.*
LAUGIER, STANISLAS (French physician, 1799-1872)
Laugier hernia. A femoral hernia perforating the Gimbernat ligament.

Laugier. Note sur une nouvelle espèce de hernie de l'abdomen à travers le ligament de Gimbernat. *Arch. Gén. Méd., Paris,* 1833, 2:27-37.

LAUNOIS, PIERRE EMILE (French physician, 1856-1914)
Launois syndrome. Synonym: *pituitary gigantism.*

Primary gigantism affecting chiefly males, usually beginning before puberty, with rapid growth and closing of the epiphyses. The disease may be associated with subnormal mentalilty, cephalgia, and visual defects. Pituitary hyperplasia and chromophobe adenoma with excessive somatotropin production are considered to be the cause.

Launois, P. E., & Roy, P. *Étude biologique sur les géants,* Paris, Masson, 1904.

Launois-Bensaude syndrome. See *Madelung syndrome.*
Launois-Cléret syndrome. See *Fröhlich syndrome, under Fröhlich, Alfred.*
Madelung-Launois-Bensaude syndrome. See *Madelung syndrome.*
laurel fever. See *Engel syndrome.*
LAURENCE, JOHN ZACHARIAH (British ophthalmologist, 1830-1874)
Laurence-Biedl syndrome. See *Laurence-Moon-Biedl syndrome.*
Laurence-Moon syndrome. See *Laurence-Moon-Biedl syndrome.*
Laurence-Moon-Biedl syndrome. Synonyms: *Bardet-Biedl syndrome, Laurence-Biedl syndrome, Laurence-Moon syndrome, Laurence-Moon-Biedl-Bardet syndrome (LMBB, LMBBS).*

A hereditary syndrome of childhood, transmitted as an autosomal recessive trait, with obesity, retinitis pigmentosa, mental retardation, polydactyly, and hypogonadism as the main features. Other abnormalities, such as ataxia, dwarfism, renal defects (including glomerulonephritis), diabetes insipidus, clinodactyly of the fifth finger, hypospadias, anal atresia, deafness, and heart defects may also occur. Ocular complications usually include coloboma, optic atrophy, scotoma, nyctalopia, strabismus, and nystagmus. Because of the wide variety of clinical symptoms, the syndrome is sometimes classified as complete, incomplete, abortive, atypical, and extensive types. The syndrome occurs more frequently in males than in females, usually in those of consanguineous parents.

Laurence, J. Z. & Moon, R. C. Four case of "retinitis pigmentosa," occurring in the same family, and accompanied by general imperfections of development. *Ophth. Rev., London,* 1866, 2:32-41. *Bardet, G. *Sur un syn-*

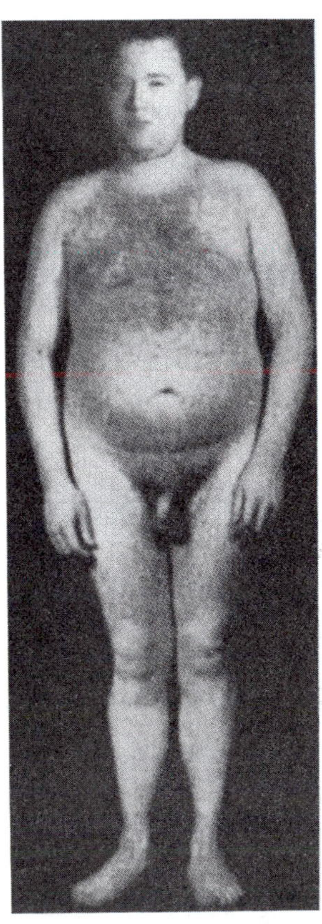

Laurence-Moon-Biedl syndrome
Francois, Jules: *Heredity in ophthalmology.* St. Louis: C.V. Mosby Co., 1961.

drome d'obésité congénitale avec polydactylie et retinite pigmentaire. Paris, 1920. (Thesis). Biedl, A. G. Schwisterpaar mit adiposo-genitaler Dystrophie. *Deut. Med. Wschr.*, 1922, 48:1630.

Laurence-Moon-Biedl-Bardet syndrome (LMBB, LMBBS). See *Laurence-Moon-Biedl syndrome.*

LAVY, NORMAN W. (American physician)

Lavy-Palmer-Merritt syndrome. See *spondylothoracic dysplasia.*

LÄWEN, ARTHUR (German physician, 1876-1958)

Büdinger-Läwen syndrome. See *Büdinger-Ludloff-Läwen syndrome.*

Büdinger-Ludloff-Läwen syndrome. See *under Büdinger.*

Haglund-Läwen-Fründ syndrome. See *Büdinger-Ludloff-Läwen syndrome.*

LAWFORD

Lawford syndrome. See *Sturge-Weber syndrome.*

LAWLER, S. D.

Jackson-Lawler syndrome. See *under Jackson, A. D. M.*

LAWRENCE, ROBERT DANIEL (British physician)

Berardinelli-Seip-Lawrence syndrome. See *Berardinelli-Seip syndrome.*

Lawrence syndrome. See *Berardinelli-Seip syndrome.*

Seip-Lawrence syndrome. See *Berardinelli-Seip syndrome.*

laxative abuse syndrome (LAS). A syndrome caused by chronic abuse of laxatives, mimicking inflammatory bowel disease or malabsorption. It is characterized by a wide range of clinical and metabolic symptoms, including diarrhea alternating with constipation, nausea, weight loss, melanosis coli, cathartic colon, mental problems (including anorexia nervosa), and metabolic disoders, such as acid-base disturbances, metabolic alkalosis, hyperuricemia, sodium and potasium depletion, water-electrolyte balance disorders, calcinosis, and hyperaldosteronism. The condition is considered a variant of the Munchausen syndrome.

Oster, J. R., *et al.* Laxative abuse syndrome. *Am. J. Gastroenterol.*, 1980, 74:451-8. Jimenez, R. A., & Larson, E. B. Case report. Tumoral calcinosis: an unusual complication of the laxative abuse syndrome. *Am. J. Med. Sc.*, 1981, 282:141-7.

LAXOVA, RENATA

Neu-Laxová syndrome. See *under Neu.*

Waisman-Laxová syndrome. See *under Waisman.*

LAZARUS (A brother of Mary and Martha, whom Jesus raised from the dead)

Lazarus complex. Synonym: *Lazarus syndrome.*

A condition observed among survivors of cardiac arrest, characterized by anxiety, depression, recurrent nightmares, and a feeling of alienation. Most affected persons eventually overcome mood disturbancess and adjust to the memory of their traumatic experience.

Druss, R. G., & Kornfeld, D. S. Survivors of cardiac arrest: A psychiatric study. *JAMA*, 1967, 201:291-6. Hackett, T. P. The Lazarus complex revisited. *Ann. Intern. Med.*, 1972, 76:135-7.

Lazarus syndrome. See *Lazarus complex.*

lazy sinus syndrome. See *sick sinus syndrome.*

LAZZARONI-FOSSATI, F. (Italian physician)

Lazzaroni-Fossati syndrome. Synonym: *fibrochondrogenesis.*

A lethal form of dwarfism, transmitted as an autosomal recessive trait, characterized by a round and flat facies with prominent eyes and cleft palate, narrow chest, macromelia, enlarged joints, and proportionate head and trunk. Short ribs with wide and cupped anterior ends, short tubular bones with broad and slightly irregular metaphyses, flat vertebral bodies, small ilia with narrow sacrosciatic notches, short and relatively broad ischia and public bones, and generalized skeletal dysplasia are the principal radiological findings.

Lazzaroni-Fossati, F., *et al.* La fibrochondrogenese. *Arch. Fr. Pediat.*, 1978, 35:1096-104.

LE FORT, LEON CLEMENT (French surgeon, 1829-1893)

Le Fort fracture. Le Fort fracture I (Guérin fracture, horizontal maxillary fracture) is a horizontal segmented fracture of the alveolar process of the maxilla, in which the teeth are usually contained in the detached portion of the bone. **Le Fort fracture II (pyramidal fracture)** is either unilateral or bilateral, in which the body of the maxilla is separated from the facial skeleton, the separated part being pyramidal in shape; the fracture may extend through the body of the maxilla down the midline of the hard palate, through the floor of the orbit, and into the nasal cavity. **Le Fort fracture III (craniofacial dysjunction, transverse facial fracture)** is a type of maxillary fracture in which the entire maxilla and one or more facial bones are completely separated from the craniofacial skeleton; such fractures are almost always accompanied by multiple fractures of the facial bones.

Guérin, A. F. Des fractures des maxillaires supérieurs. Nouveau moyen de les reconnaitre dans les cas fréquents ou elles ne s'accompagnment pas de déplacement. *Arch. Gen. Méd., Paris*, 1866, 2:5-13.

lead colic. See *lead poisoning.*

lead intoxication syndrome. See *lead poisoning.*

lead line. See *under lead poisoning.*

lead poisoning. Synonyms: *Remak paralysis, Remak syndrome, lead intoxication syndrome, neuritis saturnina, plumbism, saturnism.*

In children, poisoning is usually caused by chewing leaded paint. The symptoms include anorexia, apathy, vomiting, vague abdominal pain, clumsiness, and ataxia. As the illness progresses, vomiting becomes more persistent and apathy leads to drowsiness and stupor interspersed with periods of irritability. In severe cases, there is terminal coma with seizures. Pathological findings show acute encephalopathy with swelling and herniation of the temporal lobes and cerebellum, ischemic foci in the cerebrum and cerebellum, and deposition of proteinaceous material and mononuclear inflammatory cells around small blood vessels. In adults, lead intoxication is caused mostly by exposure to lead dust and fumes resulting from burning lead and evaporation of leaded gasoline. The symptoms include colic, anemia, and peripheral neuropathy. **Lead colic** is sometimes precipitated by an intercurrent infection or by alcohol intoxication and is characterized by severe abdominal pain, often with rigidity of abdominal muscles. A black line of lead sulfide **(lead line)** may develop along the gingival margin.

*Remak, E. J. Zur Pathogenese der Bleilahmungen. *Arch. Psychiat., Berlin,* 1876, 4:1. Adams, R. D., & Victor, M. *Principles of neurology.* 3rd ed. New York, McGraw-Hill, 1985, pp. 848-50.

leakage headache. See *puncture headache under headache syndrome.*
lean spastic dwarfism. See *Coffin syndrome (2).*
leather bottle stomach. See *Brinton disease.*
LEBER, THEODOR (German ophthalmologist, 1840-1917)
Leber amaurosis. See *Leber syndrome.*
Leber atrophy. See *Leber disease.*
Leber disease. Synonyms: *Leber atrophy, Leber hereditary optic atrophy, Leber optic neuropathy, hereditary optic atrophy, hereditary optic neuritis, hereditary optic neuropathy.*

A hereditary disease transmitted as an X-linked trait, usually through the mother, occurring predominantly in postadolescent males. The condition is marked by the sudden appearance of bilateral cloudiness of vision, followed by scotoma, rapid deterioration of central vision, and occasional color vision disorders, and is associated with atrophy of the optic nerve fibers and the retina. Multiple aneurysms of small arteries, retinal exudates, macular lesions, and retinal detachment are the principal pathological features.

*Leber, T. Über hereditäre und kongenital-angelegte Sehnervenleiden. *Arch. Ophth., Berlin*, 1871, 17:249-91.

Leber hereditary optic atrophy. See *Leber disease.*
Leber optic neuropathy. See *Leber disease.*
Leber syndrome. Synonyms: *Leber amaurosis, amaurosis congenita, dysgenesis neuroepithelialis retinae, hereditary epithelial aplasia, heredoretinopathia congenitalis, retinal aplasia.*

Total or nearly total blindness present at birth or shortly thereafter, associated with an apparently normal fundus, which is characterized by pendular or searching nystagmus, sunken eyeballs, photophobia, and the digito-ocular sign. Strabismus, keratoconus, retinal changes, pale or atrophic optic disks, changes that resemble those in retinitis pigmentosa, chorioretinitis, and fundal changes appear later. Mental retardation, epileptic seizures, and hearing disorders frequently occur. The disease is transmitted as both autosomal dominant and autosomal recessive traits.

Leber, T. Über Retinitis pigmentosa und angeborene Amaurose. *Arch. Ophth., Berlin*, 1869, 15:1-25.

LEDDERHOSE, GEORG (German physician, 1855-1925)
Ledderhose syndrome. Plantar aponeurositis and fibrous nodules of the flexor tendons resulting in clawfoot.

Ledderhose. Über Zerresungen der Plantarfascie. *Langenbeck Arch. Klin. Chir.*, 1895, 48:853-6.

LEDER, MAX (Swiss dermatologist, born 1912)
Miescher-Leder granulomatosis. See *under Miescher.*
LEDERER, MAX (American physician, 1885-1952)
Lederer anemia. Synonyms: *Lederer disease, Lederer-Brill syndrome, acute febrile hemolytic anemia, acute febrile pleiochromic anemia.*

Acquired hemolytic anemia, usually occurring in children with a recent history of infection. The anemia is associated with fever, lethargy, abdominal pain, nausea, and vomiting. Massive hemolysis is indicated by anemia, jaundice, and hemoglobinuria. Spherocytosis and splenomegaly are frequently associated. Pathological findings include visceral edema and fatty degeneration, hyaline thrombi, enlarged and congested liver, congested spleen, histiocytic proliferation, giant cell formation, and bone marrow hyperplasia.

*Lederer, M. A form of acute hemolytic anemia, probably of infectious origin. *Am. J. Med.*, 1925, 170:500-1.

Lederer disease. See *Lederer anemia.*
Lederer-Brill syndrome. See *Lederer anemia.*
LEE, B. (American physician)
Cooley-Lee syndrome. See *Cooley anemia.*
LEE, ROBERT (British physician, 1793-1877)
Lee polyp. Uterine polyp.

Lee, R. Observations on fibro-calcaerous tumours and polyps of the uterus. *Med. Chir. Tr., London*, 1835, 19:94-133.

LEEDS, NORMAN E. (American physician)
Leeds syndrome. See *moyamoya syndrome.*
LEFEVRE, PAUL (French dermatologist)
Papillon-Lefèvre syndrome (PLS). See *under Papillon, M.*
left renal vein compression syndrome. See *nutcracker syndrome.*
left ventricular hypoplasia. See *hypoplastic left heart syndrome.*
leg jitters. See *restless leg syndrome.*
LEGAL, EMMO (German physician, 1859-1922)
Legal disease. Synonym: *cephalalgia pharyngotympanica.*

A peculiar form of the headache syndrome (q.v.) related to diseases of the pharynx and middle ear and characterized by points douloureux in the regions of the temporal and occipital nerves.

Legal, E. Über eine öftere Ursache des Schläfen und Hinterhaptskopfschmerzes (Cephalalgia pharyngotympanica). *Deut. Klin. Med.*, 1886-87, 40:201-16.

LEGG, ARTHUR THORNTON (American physician, 1874-1939)
Calvé-Legg-Perthes syndrome. See *under Calvé.*
Legg disease. See *Calvé-Legg-Perthes disease.*
Perthes-Calvé-Legg-Waldenström syndrome. See *Calvé-Legg-Perthes syndrome.*
LEHMANN, ORLA (Swedish physician)
Börjeson-Forssman-Lehmann syndrome (BFL, BFLS). See *Börjeson syndrome.*
LEICHTENSTERN (LICHTENSTERN), OTTO MICHAEL LUDWIG (German physician, 1845-1900)
Leichtenstern syndrome. Pernicious anemia associated with tabes dorsalis.

*Leichtenstern, O. Über progressive perniziöze Anämie bei Tabeskranken. *Deut. Med. Wschr.*, 1884, 10:849-50.

Strümpell-Leichtenstern encephalitis. See *under Strümpell.*
LEIGH, ARCHIBALD DENIS (British neurologist, born 1915)
Leigh syndrome. Synonyms: *infantile necrotizing encephalomyelopathy, subacute necrotizing encephalomyelopathy (SNE).*

A hereditary neurological syndrome of infants, transmitted as an autosomal recessive trait and characterized by a wide range of symptoms, which may include muscle hypotonia with weakness of the neck muscles and drooping of the head; mental retardation; motor disturbances, including jerky, choreiform, and ataxic movements and inability to walk; anorexia; vomiting; crying bouts; abnormal respiration, especially episodic hyperventilation, apnea, and gasping; ocular problems, such as external ophthalmoplegia, nystagmus, disorders of gaze similar to those seen in the Wernicke syndrome, and blindness; neurological complications consisting of seizures, myoclonus, areflexia, slowed nerve conduction velocity, and nerve atrophy; somnolence; and other disorders. Pathological findings show bilateral symmetrical foci of necrosis and spongiform degeneration, vascular proliferation, and gliosis in the thalamus, midbrain, medulla oblongata, and spinal cord. Demyelination is present in the peripheral nerves. The affected areas show vascular, microglial, and histiocytic proliferations and a less marked increase in astrocytes. Biochemical abnormalities include the presence in body fluid of adenosine triphosphate phosphoryl transferase (an enzyme that catalyzes the formation of thiamine triphosphate from thiamine pyrophosphate) and pyruvate metabolism.

Leigh, D. Subacute necrotizing encephalomyelopathy in an infant. *J. Neur. Psychiat., London,* 1951, 14:216-21.

LEINER, KARL (Austrian physician, 1871-1930)

Leiner dermatitis. Synonyms: *Leiner disease, Leiner-Moussus disease, dermatitis exfoliativa generalisata, eczema universale seborrheicum, erythrodermia desquamativa in infants, seborrheic diathesis in infants.*

An exfoliative disease of the skin in newborn infants, beginning as seborrheic eczematoid lesions of the scalp and face or the gluteal region, eventually spreading to other areas. The skin lesions, consisting of dry desquamative areas or seborrheic scales, are usually associated with gastrointestinal disorders, including diarrhea. Keratitis and corneal ulcers may occur. Breast-fed infants are most frequently affected.

Leiner, K. Über Erythrodermia desquamativa, eine eigenartige universelle Dermatose der Brustskinder. *Arch. Derm. Syph., Berlin,* 1908, 89:65-76; 163-89.

Leiner disease. See *Leiner dermatitis.*

Leiner-Moussus disease. See *Leiner dermatitis.*

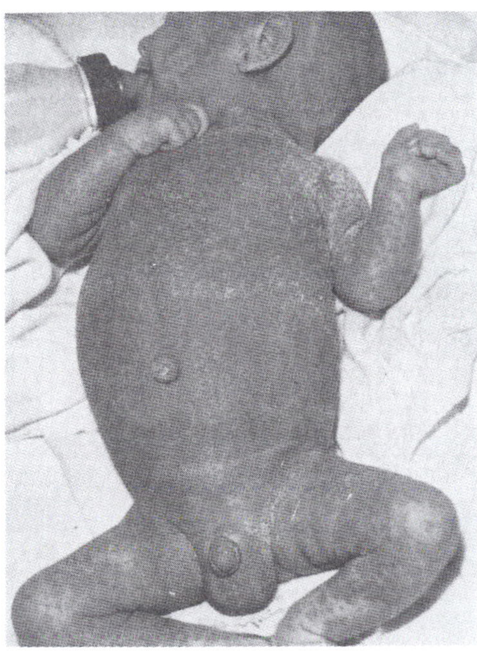

Leiner dermatitis
Nelson, W.E. [ed.: *Textbook of Pediatrics.* 8th ed. Philadelphia: W.B. Saunders Co., 1964.

leishmaniasis tropica. See *Alibert disease (2).*

LEITNER, J. (Swiss physician)

Leitner syndrome. Synonym: *pulmonary tuberculous eosinophilic syndrome.*

Eosinophilic infiltrations of the lungs associated with pulmonary tuberculosis.

Leitner, J., *et al.* Über flüchtige hyperergische Lungeninfiltrate mit Eosinophilie Bei Tuberkulose. *Beitr. Klin. Tuberk.,* 1936, 88:388-420.

LEJEUNE, JEROME JEAN LOUIS MARIE (French pediatrician, born 1926)

Lejeune syndrome. See *chromosome 5p deletion syndrome.*

LEJONNE, N. J. (French physician)

Céstan-LeJonne syndrome. See *Emery-Dreifuss syndrome.*

LELEK, I.

Schwarz-Lélek syndrome. See *under Schwarz, L.*

LELOIR, HENRI CAMILLE (French physician, 1855-1896)

Leloir disease. See *lupus erythematosus.*

LEMIEUX, GUY (Canadian physician)

Lemieux-Neemeh syndrome. A familial syndrome, transmitted as an autosomal dominant trait, combining Charcot-Marie-Tooth disease with progressive deafness. Onset takes place during childhood and consists of progressive distal muscle atrophy, nephritis, proteinuria, and sensorineural hearing loss. Progressive weakness, difficulty in walking and holding objects, claw hand, foot drop, and decreased nerve conduction follow shortly.

Lemieux, G., & Neemeh, J. A. Charcot-Marie-Tooth disease and nephritis. *Canad. Med. Assoc. J.,* 1967, 97:1193-8.

LEMLI, LUC (American physician)

Smith-Lemli-Opitz syndrome (SLO, SLOS) (I and II). See *under Smith, David W.*

LEMS (**L**ambert-**E**aton **m**yasthenic **s**yndrome). See *Eaton-Lambert syndrome, under Eaton, Lealdes McKendree.*

LENNOX, WILLIAM GORDON (American physician, 1884-1960)

Lennox syndrome. Synonyms: *minor epileptic status, petit mal, petit mal epilepsy.*

Epileptic encephalopathy in children characterized electroencephalographically by diffuse slow spike waves, frequently recurring epileptic seizures, and a high incidence of mental retardation. The symptoms consist mainly of head-drop attacks or head-nodding spells and brief tonic seizures, occurring most frequently during sleep. The attacks are frequent but their course may fluctuate widely.

Lennox, W. G. *Epilepsy and related disorders.* Boston, Little Brown, 1960, Vol. 1, pp. 66-173.

Lennox-Gastaut syndrome (LGS). See *Gastaut syndrome (2).*

LENOBLE, E. (French physician)

Lenoble-Aubineau syndrome. Synonyms: *myoclonic nystagmus, nystagmus-myoclonus syndrome.*

Congenital nystagmus, transmitted as an X-linked trait, associated with tremor of the head and arms, fasciculation of the muscles, vasomotor disorders, and overactive reflexes. Cold and mechanical stimuli may precipitate the attacks.

Lenoble, E., & Aubineau, E. Une variété nouvelle de myoclonie congénitale, pouvant être héréditaire et familiale, à nystagmus constant (nystagmus myoclonie). *Rev. Méd., Paris,* 1906, 26:471-515. Van Bogaert, L., & De Savitsch, E. Sur une maladie congénitale et hérédofamiliale comportant un tremblement rythmique de la tête, des globes oculaires et des membres supérieurs. (Ses relations avec le nystagmus-myoclonie et le nystagmus congénital héréditaire). *Encephale*, 1937, 32:113-9.

lentiginopolypose digestive syndrome. See *Peutz-Jeghers syndrome.*

lentiginosis profusa syndrome. See *LEOPARD syndrome.*

lentigo maligna. See *Hutchinson freckle, under Hutchinson, Sir Jonathan and see xeroderma pigmentosum syndrome.*

LENZ, WIDUKIND D. (German physician, born 1919)

Appelt-Gerken-Lenz syndrome. See *Roberts syndrome.*

Lenz dysmorphogenetic syndrome. See *Lenz syndrome (2).*

Lenz microphthalmia syndrome. See *Lenz syndrome (2).*

Lenz syndrome (1). See *Wiedemann syndrome (1).*

Lenz syndrome (2). Synonyms: *Lenz dysmorphogenetic syndrome, Lenz microphthalmia syndrome.*

A syndrome of ocular, skeletal, renal, dental, genital, and other abnormalities. The principal ocular anomaly is unilateral or bilateral microphthalmia ranging to anophthalmia, associated with mongoloid palpebral slant, microcornea, strabismus, nystagmus, and epicanthal folds. Orofacial anomalies include malformed ears, micrognathia, high-arched palate, crooked anterior teeth, and agenesis of the permanent incisors. Musculoskeletal disorders include camptodactyly and clinodactyly of fingers, duplication of the thumb, syndactyly of the toes, gap between first and second toes, flatfoot, calcaneovalgus deformity, talipes varus, short stature, cylindrical thorax, clavicular defects, low scapulae, notching of the vertebrae, cubitus valgus, limited extension of the hip joint, genua valga, and internally rotated knees. Renal agenesis, hydroureters, and hypospadias are the principal genitourinary defects. The patients may be mentally retarded. The syndrome is transmitted as a X-linked trait.

Lenz, W. Recessiv-geschlechtsgebundene Mikrophthalmie mit multiplen Missbildungen. *Zschr. Kinderheilk.*, 1955, 77:384-90.

Lenz-Majewski hyperostotic dwarfism. See *Lenz-Majewski syndrome.*

Lenz-Majewski syndrome. Synonyms: *Lenz-Majewski hyperostotic dwarfism, hyperostotic dwarfism.*

A syndrome of multiple congenital anomalies, mental retardation, and progressive skeletal sclerosis. Clinical characteristics include emaciation, growth retardation, delayed closure of the fontanels, progeria, hypertelorism, choanal atresia, dental enamel hypoplasia, hyperextensibility of the joints, symphalangism, interdigital webbing, cryptorchism, loose and atrophic skin, and prominent superficial veins. Roentgenographic findings show progressive sclerosis of the craniofacial skeleton and vertebrae, broad clavicles and ribs, short middle phalanges, metaphyseal and epiphyseal hyperostosis, delayed bone maturation, defective modeling of the diaphyses, and thickening of bone cortices. The syndrome is believed to be transmitted as an autosomal dominant trait.

Lenz, W. D., & Majewski, F. A generalized disorder of connective tissue with progeria, choanal atresia, symphalangism, hypoplasia of dentine and craniodiaphyseal hyperostosis. *Birth Defects*, 1974, 10(12):133-6. Robinow, M., *et al.* The Lenz-Majewski hyperostotic syndrome. A syndrome of multiple congenital anomalies, mental retardation, and progressive sclerosis. *J. Pediat.*, 1977, 91:417-21.

LEON KINDBERG. See KINDBERG, MICHEL LEON

LEONARDI, GIUSEPPE (Italian physician)

Magrassi-Leonardi pneumonia. See *Magrassi-Leonardi syndrome.*

Magrassi-Leonardi syndrome. See *under Magrassi.*

leontiasis. See *Hansen disease.*

leontiasis ossea. See *McCune-Albright syndrome.*

LEOPARD, leopard syndrome (multiple **l**entigines-**e**lectrocardiographic abnormalities-**o**cular hypertelorism-**p**ulmonary stenosis-**a**bnormalities of genitalia-**r**etardation of growth-sensorineural **d**eafness). Synonyms: *Gorlin syndrome, Moynahan syndrome, cardiocutaneous syndrome, lentiginosis profusa syndrome, multiple lentigines syndrome, progressive cardiomyopathic lentiginosis.*

A syndrome characterized usually by triangular face, with frontal bossing, hypertelorism, blepharoptosis, epicanthus, and low-set ears. Pterygium colli is frequently associated. Multiple lentigines do not occur in all cases; in some patients, they are present at birth, appearing anywhere on the skin. A superiorly oriented mean QRS axis in the frontal plane, generally located between -60º and -120º (S1, S2, S3 pattern) is the characteristic electrocardiographic feature. Pulmonary valvular stenosis is the most common cardiac defect. Complete bundle branch block and complete heart block may be associated. Genitourinary malformations usually consist of hypospadias, cryptorchidism, and late menarche. Growth retardation is the principal

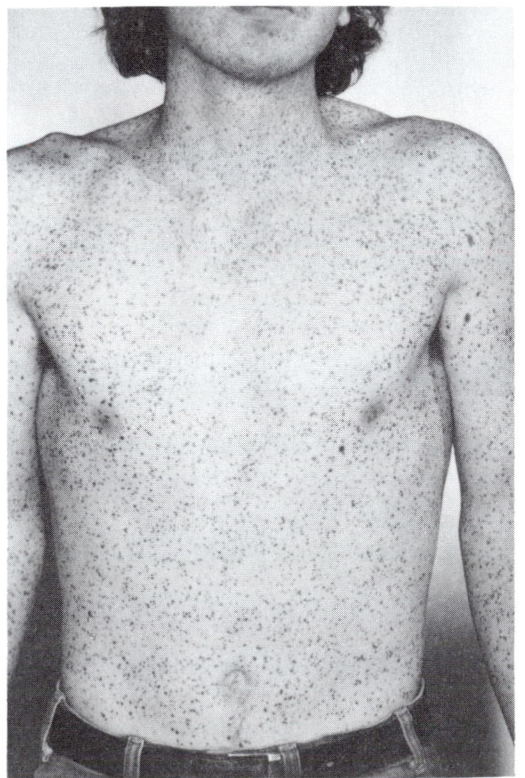

LEOPARD syndrome
Courtesy of Dr. Robert J. Gorlin, Minneapolis, MN.

skeletal component. Pectus carinatum or excavatum, kyphosis, carpal and tarsal fusion, hyperextensibility of the metacarpophalangeal joints, winging of the scapulae, spina bifida occulta, cubitus valgus, and other osteoarticular defects may occur. Neurological features consist mainly of mild mental retardation and sensorineural deafness. The syndrome is transmitted as an autosomal dominant trait with high penetrance and variation in expression. Some authors suggest that this and the Watson syndrome are essentially indistinguishable from the Noonan syndrome.

Gorlin, R. J., *et al.* Multiple lentigines syndrome, complex comprising multiple lentigines, electrocardiographic conduction abnormalities, ocular hypertelorism, pulmonary stenosis, abnormalities of genitalia, retardation of growth, sensorineural deafness and autosomal dominant hereditary pattern. *Am. J. Dis. Child.,* 1969, 117:652-62. Moynahan, E. J. Progressive cardiomyopathic lentiginosis: First report of autopsy findings in a recently recognized inheritable disease (autosomal dominant). *Proc. R. Soc. Med.,* 1970, 63:448-51.

LEOPOLD-LEVY, E. (French physician, 1868-1933)

Léopold-Lévy syndrome. Synonym: *paroxysmal thyroid instability.*

Hyperthyroidism associated with periods of instability.

Léopold-Lévy, E., & Rotschild, H., de. Sur un travail relatif à l'instabilité thyroïdienne et sa forme paroxystique. *Bull. Acad. Méd., Paris,* 1909, 61:586-90.

LEOTTA, NICOLO (Italian physician, born 1878)

Leotta syndrome. Perivisceritis, on the right side in the subhepatic area, of appendicular origin.

Tulia Martini. Las apendiculo-colecistopatias a sindrome seudo-ulceroso. (Interesante secuelas de una apendicitis cronica). *Dia Med., Buenos Aires,* 1941, 13:913-20.

LEPINE, JEAN (French physician)

Lépine-Froin syndrome. See *Froin syndrome.*

lepra. See *Hansen disease.*

lepra alphos. See *Willan lepra.*

lepra arabum. See *Hansen disease.*

lepra Graecorum. See *Willan lepra.*

lepra tuberoanesthetica. See *Danielssen-Boeck disease.*

leprechaunism. See *Donohue syndrome.*

leprosy. See *Hansen disease.*

leptomeningioma. See *Cushing tumor.*

leptospiral jaundice. See *leptospirosis.*

leptospirosis. Synonyms: *Fiedler disease, Landouzy disease, Mathieu disease, Vasilev disease, Weil disease, Weil icterus, Weil syndrome, canicola fever, epidemic spirochetal jaundice, Fort Bragg fever, icterogenic spirochetosis, infectious spirochetal jaundice, leptospiral jaundice, leptospirosis icterohaemorrhagica, peapicker disease, spirochaetosis icterohaemorrhagica, spirochematosis icterohaemorrhagica.*

An enzootic disease caused by *Leptospira interrogans* infection and transmitted to man by animals, including rodents, skunks, foxes, cattle, and dogs. After an incubation period of 1 to 2 weeks, the symptoms may include fever, headache, myalgia, jaundice, widespread hemorrhage with purpura or petechiae, gastrointestinal disorders (nausea, vomiting, abdominal pain), oliguria, cough, renal insufficiency, lymphadenopathy, and conjunctival effusion, occurring in various combinations. Neurological manifestations usually consist of changes in consciousness, hypesthesia, encephalitis, and cranial nerve palsies. Hepatomegaly, bile staining, and enlargement of the heart and kidneys are the main pathological features. The illness lasts from 4 to 9 days. The term **Weil disease (syndrome)** applies to the severe form of leptospirosis.

Weil, A. Über eine eigentümliche, mit Milztumor, Icterus und Nephritis einhergehende, acute Infectionskrankheit. *Deut. Arch. Klin. Med.,* 1886, 39:209-32. Landouzy. Typhus hépatique. *Gaz. Hôp. Paris,* 1883, 56:913-4. Mathieu, A. Typhus hépatique benin; rechute, guérison. *Rev. Méd., Paris,* 1886, 6:633-9. *Vasiliev, N. Infektsionnaia zheltukha. *Ezhened. Klin. Gaz., St. Petersburg,* 1888, 8:429. McClain, J. B. Leptospirosis. In: Wyngaarden, J. B., & Smith, L. H., Jr., eds. *Cecil textbook of medicine.* 17th ed. Philadelphia, Saunders, 1985, pp. 1666-8.

leptospirosis icterohaemorrhagica. See *leptospirosis.*

leptotrichosis of the conjunctiva. See *Parinaud oculoglandular syndrome.*

LEREBOULLET, PIERRE (French physician, 1874-1944)

Gilbert-Lereboullet syndrome. See *Gilbert syndrome, under Gilbert, Nicolas Augustin.*

LEREDDE, EMILE (French dermatologist, born 1866)

Hallopeau-Leredde syndrome. See *Hallopeau syndrome (3).*

LERI, ANDRE (French neurologist, 1875-1930)

Léri disease (1). See *Léri syndrome (1).*

Léri disease (2). Synonym: *lumbarthria.*

Paroxysmal pain precipitated by exposure to cold and high humidity. On bending forward, there is protrusion of the lumbar apophyses and a depression between the first lumbar and the twelfth thoracic vertebrae, giving the spinal column a wavy appearance. On standing erect, the torso is inclined forward. Roentgenographic findings show a characteristic triad: decalcification, "vertèbre en diable" (strangulation of the vertebral body between osteophytes pressing on the superior and inferior surfaces), and "parrot beak".

Chevalier, G. Deux cas de lumbarthrie (maladie de Léri). *Marseille Méd.,* 1933, 70:(pt 2):247-8.

Léri pleonosteosis syndrome. Synonym: *pleonosteosis familiaris.*

A hereditary congenital disease characterized mainly by osseous abnormalities due to precocious and excessive ossification of the bones of cartilaginous origin associated with enlargement of the epiphyses. Osteoarticular defects include contractures and thickening of the joints, especially in the hands and feet; broad thumbs and great toes with short spadelike hands; enlargement of the paranasal sinuses; genu recurvatum; enlargement of neural arches of the cervical vertebrae; and generalized limitation of joint mobility. Cutaneous changes consist mainly of hollow palms with thickened palmar and forearm fasciae, accentuated skin creases between thick palmar pads, and nodules. Mongoloid palpebral slant, laryngeal stenosis, thickening of the eyelids, shuffling gait, and short stature are usually associated. The syndrome is transmitted as an autosomal dominant trait.

Léri, A. Une dystrophie osseuse généralisée congénitale et héréditaire; la pléonosteose familiale. *Presse Méd., Paris,* 1922, 30:13.

Léri syndrome (1). Synonyms: *Léri disease, Léri-Joanny syndrome, flowing hyperostosis, flowing periostitis, melorheostosis, osteopathia hyperostotica, osteopathia* *hyperostotica congenita membri unius, osteosis eburnisans monomelica.*

A bone dysplasia characterized in children by irregular linear areas of increased density along the shafts of the long bones. Less frequently, it affects single bones (the **monostotic form**), whole limb (the **monomelic form**), or multiple bones (the **polystotic form**), seen on the roentgenogram. In adults, x-ray findings show linear densities associated with areas of osteophytic periosteal excrescences resembling melted wax flowing down the side of a candle, hence the synonym **melorheostosis.** Ectopic bone formation, shortening, or occasional lengthing, and abnormal bowing of affected bones may be associated. Clincal features usually include joint contractures of bones and palmar and plantar fasciae, limb inequality, bowing of the affected limbs, increased limb circumference, arthralgia and swelling of the joints, shiny and erythematous skin, subcutaneous edema, muscle atrophy and weakness, and sclerodema of the affected limbs. The symptoms usually appear early in childhood. The etiology is unknown.

Léri, A., & Joanny. Une affection non décrite des os: Hyperostose "en coulée" sur toute la longuer d'un membre ou "mélorhéostose." *Bull. Soc. Méd. Hôp.*, Paris, 1922, 46:1141-5.

Léri syndrome (2). See *Léri-Weill syndrome.*
Léri-Joanny syndrome. See *Léri syndrome (1).*

Léri-Weill syndrome. Synonyms: *dyschondrosteosis, polytopic enchondral dysostosis.*

A skeletal dysplasia combining dorsal subluxation of the distal end of the ulna (Madelung deformity) with mesomelic short stature. Major radiographic features consist of shortness of the radius in relation to the ulna, ulnar and palmar slant of radial articular surface and triangularization of the distal radial epiphysis, dorsal subluxation of the ulna, triangularization of the carpal bones, and shortness of the tibia with prominent medial portion of the proximal tibia. The syndrome is transmitted as an autosomal dominant trait with a somewhat more severe expression in the female.

Léri, A., & Weill, J. Une affection congenitale et symétrique du dévelopement osseux. La dyschondrostéose. *Bull. Soc. Méd. Hôp. Paris*, 1929, 53:1491-4.

Marie-Léri syndrome. See *under Marie, Pierre.*

LERICHE, RENE (French physician, 1879-1955)

Leriche syndrome (LS) (1). Synonyms: *aortic bifurcation occlusion syndrome, chronic aorto-iliac occlusion, terminal aortic thrombosis.*

Thrombotic obliteration above or at the bifurcation of the aorta, usually affecting adult males. Inability to maintain penile erection, extreme fatigability, soft tissue atrophy of the lower limbs, pallor of the legs and feet on standing, slow wound healing, slight hypertension, and absent or very feeble pulse over the aorta and iliac arteries and in the periphery are the usual symptoms.

Leriche, R. De la résection du carrefour aortico-iliaque avec double sympathectomie lombaire pour thrombose artérique de l'aorte. Le syndrome de l'oblitération termino-aortique par artérite. *Presse Méd.*, 1940, 48:33-604.

Leriche syndrome (LS) (2). See *Sudeck syndrome.*
Sudeck-Leriche syndrome. See *Sudeck syndrome.*

LERMOYEZ, J.
Fernand Widal-Lermoyez syndrome. See *Widal-Lermoyez syndrome.*
Widal-Lermoyez syndrome. See *under Widal.*
LERMOYEZ, MARCEL (French physician, 1858-1929)
Lermoyez syndrome. Synonyms: *Lermoyez vertigo, symptomatic Ménière syndrome, tinnitus-deafness-vertigo syndrome.*

A disorder originally attributed to vasospasm of the internal auditory artery, that is characterized by tinnitus and deafness which improve with the onset of vertigo. Vomiting and nausea usually occur. The syndrome is observed most frequently during the third or fourth decade. Allergy is the suspected cause. See also *Ménière syndrome.*

Lermoyez, M. Le vertige qui fait entendre. (Angiospasme labyrinthique). *Ann. Mal. Oreille*, 1929, 48:575-83.

Lermoyez vertigo. See *Lermoyez syndrome.*
LEROY, EMILE (French physician, born 1873)
Fiessinger-Leroy syndrome. See *Reiter syndrome.*
Fiessinger-Leroy-Reiter syndrome. See *Reiter syndrome.*
LEROY, JULES G. (Belgian geneticist)
Leroy syndrome. See *mucolipidosis II.*
LES (Lambert-Eaton myasthenic syndrome). See *Eaton-Lambert syndrome, under Eaton, Lealdes McKendree.*
LESCH, MICHAEL (American pediatrician, born 1939)
Lesch-Nyhan syndrome (LNS). Synonyms: *juvenile hyperuricemia syndrome, primary hyperuricemia syndrome.*

An X-linked purine metabolism disorder affecting only male children, whereby hypoxanthine guanine phosphoribosyltransferase (HGPRT) deficiency results in overproduction of purine and consequently uric acid. Patients are normal at birth but become irritable by 2 months of age and during the second year of life are aggressive and self-destructive, biting the lower lip and, less commonly, the upper lip, cheeks, fingers, and hands, sometimes also using the fingers to mutilate their ears and noses. Associated disorders include mental retardation, spastic cerebral palsy, choreoathetosis, renal uric acid calculi, gouty tophi, and uric acid nodules.

Lesch, M., & Nyhan, W. L. A familial disorder of uric acid metabolism and central nervous system function. *Am. J. Med.*, 1964, 36:561-70.

LESCHKE, ERICH FRIEDRICH WILHELM (German physician, 1887-1933)
Leschke syndrome. Synonyms: *congenital pigmentary dystrophy, dystrophia pigmentosa.*

General asthenia, brown maculae of the skin, and hyperglycemia are the principal elements of this disorder, which may be an early manifestation of hemochromatosis (bronze diabetes) or xanthoma diabeticorum.

*Leschke, E. Über Pigmentierung bei Funktionsstörungen der Niebenniere und des sympathischen Nervensystems bei der Recklinsghausenschen Krankheit. *Berlin Med. Ges.*, 1922. (Abstr. in *Klin. Wschr.*, 1922, 28:1433).

LESNIOWSKI, ANTONI (Polish physician, born 1867)
Crohn-Lesniowski disease. See *Crohn disease.*
lethal catatonia. See *Bell mania, under Bell, Luther Vos.*
lethal faciocardiomelic dysplasia. See *faciocardiomelic dysplasia.*
lethal multiple pterygium syndrome. A lethal syndrome characterized by multiple pterygia, congenital hip contractures, lung hypoplasia, facial abnormalities, and hydrops. Hydranencephaly may be associ-

ated. The syndrome is believed to be transmitted as an autosomal recessive trait. See also *multiple pterygium syndrome* and *popliteal pterygium syndrome.*

Gitlin, M. E., & Pryse-Davis, J. Pterygium syndrome. Case reports. *J. Med. Genet.*, 1976, 13:249-51. Mbakop, A., *et al.* Lethal multiple pterygium syndrome: Report of a new case with hydranencephaly. *Am. J. Med. Genet.*, 1986, 25:575-9.

lethal omphalocele-cleft palate syndrome. A lethal syndrome, transmitted as an autosomal recessive trait, of omphalocele and cleft palate variably associated with uterus bicornis, duplex uvula, and hydrocephalus.

Czeizel, A. A new lethal omphalocele-cleft palate syndrome? *Hum. Genet.*, 1983, 64:99.

lethargic encephalitis. See *van Bogaert encephalitis.*

LETTERER, ERICH (German physician, born 1895)

Abt-Letterer-Siwe syndrome. See *Letterer-Siwe syndrome.*

Letterer reticulosis. See *Letterer-Siwe syndrome.*

Letterer-Siwe disease. See *Letterer-Siwe syndrome.*

Letterer-Siwe syndrome. Synonyms: *Abt-Letterer-Siwe syndrome, Letterer reticulosis, Letterer-Siwe disease, acute disseminated histiocytosis X, aleukemic reticulosis, infectious reticulosis, malignant reticulosis, nonlipid reticuloendotheliosis, subacute disseminated histiocytosis X.*

An acute disease characterized by proliferation of nonlipid histiocytes that have abundant acidophilic cytoplasm and are often vacuolated. Early symptoms include red to brown firm nodules resembling insect bites, followed by maculopapular rash or multiple nodules that sometimes ulcerate and hemorrhage. Other symptoms consist of persistent spiking fever, hepatomegaly with or without jaundice, splenomegaly, enlargement of the lymph nodes, and hyperplasia of the gingiva. Anemia, leukopenia, thrombocytopenia, and hemorrhagic diathesis may occur. The pathological picture is dominated by histiocytic infiltration of the reticuloendothelial system, especially the liver, lymph nodes, spleen, skin, and, in advanced stages, bone. Infants and young children are most frequently affected, but an adult form may occur.

Abt, A. F., & Demenholz, E. J. Letterer-Siwe's disease. Splenohepatomegaly associated with widespread hyperplasia of nonlipoid-storing macrophages; discussion of the so-called reticulo-endothelioses. *Am. J. Dis. Child.*, 1936, 51:499-522. Letterer, E. Aleukämische Retikulose (Ein Beitrag zu den proliferativen Erkrankungen des retikuloendothelialen Apparates). *Frankf. Zschr. Path.*, 1924, 30:377-94. Siwe, S. Die Retikuloendotheliose, ein neues Krankheitsbild unter den Hepatosplenomegalien. *Zschr. Kinderheilk.*, 1933, 55:212-47.

leucinosis. See *maple syrup urine disease.*

leukemia. See *Bennett disease, under Bennett, John Hughes.*

leukocytoclastic vasculitis. See *Gougerot-Ruiter syndrome.*

leukoderma acquisitum centrifugum. See *Sutton halo nevus, under Sutton, Richard Lighburn.*

leukodystrophia cerebri progressiva metachromatica diffusa. See *metachromatic leukodystrophy.*

leukodystrophy, type Scholz. See *metachromatic leukodystrophy.*

leukoencephalitis acuta hemorrhagica. See *Hurst disease.*

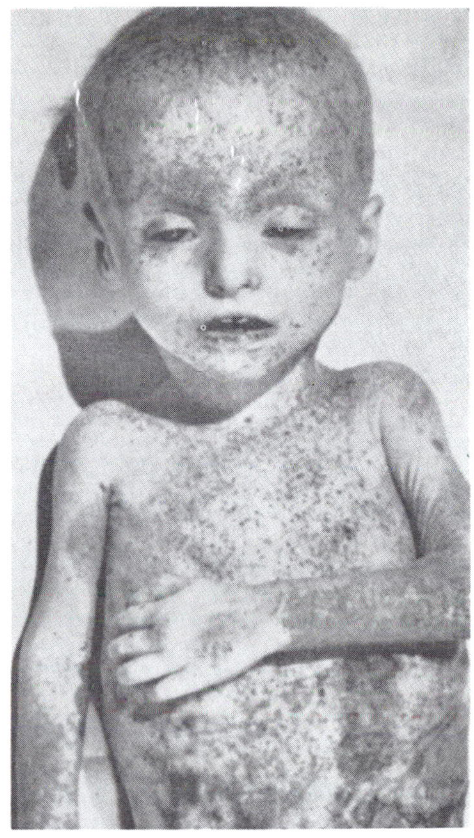

Letterer-Siwe syndrome
Aegerter, E. & J.A. Kirkpatrick, Jr.: *Orthopedic Diseases*, 3rd ed. Philadelphia: W.B. Saunders Co., 1968.

leukoencephalitis periaxialis concentrica. See *Baló syndrome.*

leukoencephalitis subacuta sclerosans. See *van Bogaert encephalitis.*

leukoerythroblastic anemia. See *Vaughan disease.*

leukoerythroblastosis. See *Vaughan disease.*

leukokraurosis. See *Breisky disease.*

leukonychia totalis-multiple sebaceous cysts-renal calculi syndrome. A familial syndrome, transmitted as an autosomal trait, characterized by total leukonychia, sebaceous cysts, and kidney calculi.

Gorlin, R. J., *et al.* Leukonychia totalis, multiple sebaceous cysts and renal calculi: A syndrome. Birth Defects, 1975, 11(5):19-21.

leukopenia. See Schultz syndrome.

levator syndrome. Synonyms: coccygodynia, levator ani syndrome, levator ani spasm syndrome, levator spasm syndrome, proctalgia fugax, proctodynia.

Pain, pressure, and discomfort in the region of the rectum, sacrum, and coccyx, which appear to be aggravated by sitting; gluteal discomfort and high rectal distress are usually associated. Tenderness and muscle spasm affecting the levator ani muscles are the principal symptoms of this disorder. The etiology is unknown. See also Thaysen syndrome.

Simpsom, J. Y. Coccygodynia and diseases and deformities of the coccyx. *Med. Times Gaz.*, 1959, 40:1031. Thiele, G. H. Tonic spasm of the levator ani, coccygeus and pyriformis muscles. *Tr. Am. Proct. Soc.*, 1936, 37:145-55.

levator ani spasm syndrome. See *levator syndrome.*

levator ani syndrome. See *levator syndrome.*

levator spasm syndrome. See *levator syndrome.*

LEVENTHAL, MICHAEL LEO (American gynecologist, born 1901)

Stein-Leventhal syndrome. See *polycystic ovary syndrome.*

LEVER, WALTER FREDERICK (American physician, born 1909)

Lever adenoacanthoma. Synonyms: *adenoacanthoma of sweat glands, adenoid squamous cell carcinoma, squamous cell epithelioma.*

Small, slowly growing tumors of the skin composed of squamous cells which form both solid and glandular proliferations into the dermis. They occur most frequently in aged persons, with the face and, occasionally, the hands and arms being the sites most frequently affected. The tumor is considered to be a squamous cell carcinoma with distinctive adenoid proliferations, dyskeratosis, and acantholytic cells. Senile keratoses are often associated.

Lever, W. F. Adenoacanthoma of sweat glands; carcinoma of sweat glands with glandular and epidermal elements. Report of 4 cases. *Arch. Derm., Chicago*, 1947, 56:157-71.

LEVI, E. (French physician)

Levi syndrome. See *Lorain-Levi syndrome.*

Lorain-Levi syndrome. See *under Lorain.*

LEVIN, L. S. (American physician)

Levin syndrome. See *cranio-ectodermal dysplasia syndrome.*

LEVIN, MAX (American physician, born 1901)

Kleine-Levin syndrome. See *under Kleine.*

Kleine-Levin-Critchley syndrome. See *Kleine-Levin syndrome.*

LEVIN, PAUL M. (American physician)

Jarcho-Levin syndrome. See *spondylothoracic dysplasia.*

LEVINE, IRVING M. (American physician)

Levine-Critchley syndrome. Synonyms: *choreoacanthocytosis, neuroacanthocytosis.*

A hereditary syndrome, transmitted as an autosomal dominant trait, combining acanthocytosis with neurological disorders and apparently normal blood lipoproteins. Tic, grimacing, movement disorders, swallowing difficulty, muscle weakness and cramps, fatigability, poor coordination, hyporeflexia, chorea, seizures, and other neurological complications are usually associated with this syndrome.

Levine, I. M., *et al.* Hereditary neurological disease with acanthocytosis. A new syndrome. *Arch. Neurol., Chicago*, 1968, 19:403-9. Critchley, E. M. R., *et al.* Acanthocytosis, normolipoproteinemia and multiple tics. *Postgrad. Med. J.*, 1970, 46:698-701.

LEVINE, SAMUEL ALBERT (American physician, 1891-1966)

Lown-Ganong-Levine (LGL) syndrome. See *Clerc-Lévy-Cristesco syndrome.*

LEVY, GABRIELLE (French neurologist, 1886-1935)

Roussy-Lévy syndrome (RLS). See *under Roussy.*

LEVY, JACQUES (French physician)

Clerc-Lévy-Cristesco (CLC) syndrome. See *under Clerc.*

LEVY, ROBERT (French physician)

Creyx-Lévy syndrome. See *under Creyx.*

LEVY, WALTER J. (Ophthalmologist in Johannesburg)

Levy-Hollister syndrome. See *lacrimo-auriculodentodigital syndrome.*

LEWANDOWSKI (LEWANDOWSKY), FELIX (German dermatologist, 1879-1921)

Jadassohn-Lewandowski syndrome. See *under Jadassohn, Josef.*

Lewandowski periporitis. Synonym: *furunculus atonicus.*

Mulltiple abscesses in newborn infants. The condition begins as inflammation of the sweat glands and is followed by formation of superficial pustules and abscesses, usually due to a staphylococcal infection. See also *Job syndrome.*

Lewandowsky, F. Zur Pathogenese der multiplen Abszesse im Säuglingsalter. *Arch. Derm. Syph., Berlin*, 1906, 80:179-91.

Lewandowski tuberculid. Synonyms: *rosacea-like tuberculid, rosacea-like tuberculosis.*

Tuberculosis of the skin characterized by lesions which range in size from that of a pinhead to that of a barleycorn, and which are often present in large numbers on the cheeks and forehead, some being flush with the skin and some slightly elevated. They differ from the lesions of rosacea in that they are yellowish or yellow-brown in color and do not disappear entirely on diascopic pressure. The bluish red color of the skin of the face and individual telangiectasia complete the resemblance to rosacea.

Lewandowsky, F., & Lutz, W. Ein Fall einer bisher nicht beschriebenen Hauterkrankung (Epidermodysplasia verruciformis). *Arch. Derm. Syph., Berlin*, 1922, 41:193-202.

Lewandowski-Lutz syndrome. Synonyms: *epidermodysplasia verruciformis, generalized verrucosis, verrucosis generalisata et disseminata.*

A generalized skin disease which most frequently appears in infancy and childhood and is marked by flat, warty, and lichenoid papules that are gray, pink, violet, red, or brown, about 2 to 15 mm in diameter. Pathological findings show a "basket-weave" arrangement of the stratum corneum and vacuolation of the prickle cell layer, especially of the stratum granulosum; the nuclei of the vacuolated cells are shriveled and pyknotic. The disease is considered to be a precancerous form of epithelial nevi.

Lewandowsky, F., & Lutz, W. Ein Fall einer bisher noch nicht beschriebenen Hauterkrankung (Epidermodysplasia verruciformis). *Arch. Derm. Syph., Berlin*, 1922, l41:193-202.

LEWANDOWSKY, FELIX. See LEWANDOWSKI, FELIX

LEWIS, C. S. (American physician)

symphalangism, C. S. Lewis type. Symphalangism involving the first metacarpophalangeal joint in a father and two sons, described by C. S. Lewis in his autobiography.

Lewis, C. S. *Surprised by joy. The shape of my early life.* New York, Harcourt, Brace & World, 1955, p. 12. Temtamy, S. A., & McKusick, V. A. The genetics of hand malformations. *Birth Defects*, 1978, 14(3):500-1.

LEWIS, GEORGE MICHAEL (British physician)

Lewis disease. Familial congenital hepatic glycogenosis due to hepatic glycogen synthetase deficiency, associated with convulsions and hypoglycemia after overnight fasting. Originally, the disease was observed in twins, one mentally retarded and the other with below average intelligence.

Lewis, G. M., *et al.* Infantile hypoglycaemia due to inherited deficiency of glycogen synthetase in liver. *Arch. Dis. Child., London*, 1963, 38:40-8.

LEYDEN, ERNST VICTOR, VON (German physician, 1832-1910)

Leyden ataxia. See *Westphal-Leyden syndrome, under Westphal, Alexander Karl Otto.*

Leyden neuritis. Synonym: *lipomatous neuritis.*

Neuritis complicated by destruction of the nerve fibers and their replacement by fatty tissue.

Leyden, E. Über Poliomyelitis und Neuritis. *Zschr. Klin. Med.*, 1879-80, 1:387-434.

Leyden paralysis (1). Synonyms: *Leyden syndrome, Weber paralysis, Weber symptom, Weber-Leyden syndrome, cerebral peduncle syndrome, hemiplegia alternans oculomotorica, hemiplegia alternans superior peduncularis, hemiplegia oculomotorica.*

Partial or complete oculomotor paralysis and contralateral hemiplegia due to lesions of the nucleus of the third cranial nerve and its ventral fibers crossing the midbrain and the pyramidal tract.

Leyden, E. *Klinik der Rückenmarks-Krankheiten*. Berlin, Hirschwald, 1875, Vol. 2, p. 65. Weber, H. A contribution to the pathology of the crura cerebri. *Med. Chir. Tr., London*, 1863, 46:121-39.

Leyden paralysis (2). A rapidly fatal form of paralysis affecting all four extremities that follows epileptiform seizures, observed in patients with hemorrhage of the pons and medulla oblongata.

Leyden, E. *Klinik der Rückenmarks-Krankheiten*. Berlin, Hirschwald, 1875, Vol. 2, p. 64.

Leyden syndrome. See *Leyden paralysis (1).*

Leyden-Moebius syndrome. Synonyms: *limb-girdle muscular weakness and atrophy; limb-girdle muscular dystrophy (LGMD); limb-girdle syndrome (LGS); muscular dystrophy I; muscular dystrophy, Leyden-Moebius type; myopathic limb-girdle syndrome; pelvofemoral syndrome.*

A muscle dystrophy involving first either the pelvic or, less commonly, the shoulder girdle, with occasional pseudohypertrophy of the calves. The disorder is transmitted as an autosomal recessive trait, the early symptoms usually becoming apparent in children and, less frequently, adult or middle-age persons.

Leyden, E. *Klinik der Rückenmarks-Krankheiten.* Berlin, Hirschwald, 1876, Vol. 2.

muscular dystrophy, Leyden-Moebius type. See *Leyden-Moebius syndrome.*

Weber-Leyden syndrome. See *Leyden paralysis (1).*

Westphal-Leyden syndrome. See *under Westphal, Alexander Karl Otto.*

LFD (lateral facial dysplasia). See *oculo-auriculovertebral dysplasia.*

LGL (Lown-Ganong-Levine) syndrome. See *Clerc-Lévy-Critesco syndrome.*

LGMD (limb-girdle muscular dystrophy). See *Leyden-Moebius syndrome.*

LGS. See *Lennox-Gastaut syndrome.*

LGS (limb-girdle syndrome). See *Leyden-Moebius syndrome.*

LGV (lymphogranuloma venereum). See *Durand-Nicolas-Favre disease, under Durand, J.*

LHERMITTE, JEAN (French physician, 1877-1959)

Lhermitte syndrome. Synonyms: *anterior internuclear ophthalmoplegia, internuclear paralysis, median longitudinal fasciculus syndrome.*

Oculomotor paralysis with nystagmus and paralysis of abduction during attempted lateral deviation of the eye, reportedly described by Lhermitte.

Lhermitte-Cornil-Quesnel syndrome. Synonym: *progressive pyramidopallidal degeneration.*

Slowly progressive, pyramidopallidal degeneration marked by involuntary crying and laughing; hypertonus and rigidity of the locomotor, cervical and facial muscles; dysarthria; aphonia; dysphagia; abduction of the muscles of the extremities, with the hand held in a position characteristic of paralysis agitans, but without the cogwheel phenomenon and with retention of muscle strength. Inflammation of the basal ganglia and subthalamic region with deposits of calcium-iron salts in the anterior globus pallidus and dentate nucleus are found at autopsy.

Lhermitte, J., Cornil, L., & Quesnel. Le syndrome de la dégénération pyramido-pallidale progressive. *Rev. Neur., Paris*, 1920, 27:262-9.

Lhermitte-Duclos disease. Synonyms: *diffuse cerebellar hypertrophy, gangliocytoma dysplasticum, granular-cell hypertrophy, granule cell hypertrophy of the cerebellum, hamartoma of the cerebellum, purkinjoma.*

A rare, progressive disease of the cerebellum characterized chiefly by histopathological changes and varied clinical symptoms, mainly headache, movement disorders and tremor, visual disturbances, enlarged head suggesting hydrocephalus, and abnormal EEG. Pathological findings show hypertrophy of cerebellar folia containing abnormal ganglion cells in circumscribed areas; tough cerebellar tissue that is poorly demarcated; a thick outer layer of nerve fibers in the cortex, an inner layer having abnormal ganglion cells; enlargement of all granule cells, axons, somas, and dendrites, the number of granule cells being reduced; absence of normal Purkinje cells; and intranuclear inclusion bodies in hypertrophied neurons.

*Lhermitte, J., & Duclos, P. Sur un ganglioneurome diffuse du cortex du cervelet. *Bull. Assoc. Fr. Cancer*, 1920, 9:99. Ambler, M., *et al.* Lhermitte-Duclos disease (granule cell hypertrophy of the cerebellum). Pathological analysis of the first familial cases. *J. Neuropath. Exp. Neurol.*, 1969, 28:622-47.

Lhermitte-McAlpine syndrome. Pyramidal and extrapyramidal syndrome in middle-aged and elderly persons. The initial symptoms consist of periods of excitation and depression, which are followed by paresthesia and rigidity of the lower extremities with ataxic gait or inability to walk; abolition of abdominal reflexes; lack of spontaneous movements, mobile spasms, and tremor; dysarthria; mental deterioration with apathy, hallucinations, negativism, delirium, and confusion; and death within a year. Pathologically, the syndrome is characterized by lesions of the frontal and temporal lobes, the corpus striatum, the ventromedian nuclei of the thalamus, bulbar nuclei and anterior cornual cells of the spinal cord, Betz cells and layers of the cerebral cortex, polygonal cells in the striatum, motor cells in the precentral gyrus, and the pyramidal tracts of the spinal cord.

Lhermitte, J., & McAlpine, D. A clinical and pathological résumé of combined disease of the pyramidal and extrapyramidal systems, with special reference to a new syndrome. *Brain*, 1926, 49:157-81.

Lhermitte-Trelles syndrome. Localized lymphoblastic infiltrations of the peripheral nervous system, associated with paresis and amyotrophia, reportedly described by Lhermitte and Trelles.

LIAN, CAMILLE (French physician)

Lian-Siguier-Welti syndrome. The coexistence of diaphragmatic hernia or eventration with venous thrombosis.

Lian, C., Siguier, F., & Welti, J. J. Le syndrome "hernie diaphragmatique ou éventration diaphragmatique et thromboses veineuses." *Presse Méd., Paris*, 1953, 61:145-6.

LIBMAN, EMANUEL (American physician, 1872-1946)

Kaposi-Besnier-Libman-Sacks syndrome. See *Libman-Sacks syndrome.*

Libman endocarditis. See *Libman-Sacks syndrome.*

Libman-Sacks disease. See *Libman-Sacks syndrome.*

Libman-Sacks syndrome. Synonyms: *Kaposi-Besnier-Libman-Sacks syndrome, Libman endocarditis, Libman-Sacks disease, Osler-Libman-Sacks disease, abacterial endocarditis, atypical verrucous endocarditis, nonbacterial verrucous endocarditis, verrucous endocarditis, verrucous noninfective endocarditi.*

Noninfective endocarditis in systemic lupus erythematosus, characterized by the presence on heart valves and/or chordae tendineae of sterile, verrucous lesions composed of fibrin strands. Polymorphonuclear leukocytes, lymphocytes, and histiocytes infiltrate the affected structures. Granular, basophilic clumps of cellular debris similar to LE cells in the bone marrow (the hematoxylin bodies) are the characteristic pathological features of this disease.

Libman, E., & Sacks, B. A hitherto undescribed form of valvular and mural endocarditis. *Tr. Assoc. Am. Physicians*, 1923, 38:46-61.

Osler-Libman-Sacks disease. See *Libman-Sacks syndrome.*

lichen acuminatus. See *Kaposi disease (2).*

lichen albus. See *Hallopeau syndrome (1).*

lichen chronicus circumscriptus. See *Brocq disease (1).*

lichen corneus disseminatus. See *Hyde syndrome.*

lichen corneus obtusus. See *Hyde syndrome.*

lichen myxoedematous. See *Arndt-Gottron syndrome.*

lichen nitidus. See *Pinkus disease, under Pinkus, Felix.*

lichen planus. See *Wilson disease (2), under Wilson, Sir William Erasmus.*

lichen planus bullosus. See *Kaposi disease (3).*

lichen planus et acuminatus atrophicans. See *Little syndrome, under Little, Ernest Gordon Graham.*

lichen planus morphoeicus. See *Hallopeau syndrome (2).*

lichen planus sclerosus et atrophicus. See *Hallopeau syndrome (1).*

lichen psoriasis. See *Wilson disease (2), under Wilson, Sir William Erasmus.*

lichen ruber. See *Kaposi disease (2).*

lichen ruber acuminatus. See *Kaposi disease (2).*

lichen ruber follicularis decalvans. See *Little syndrome, under Little, Ernest Gordon Graham.*

lichen ruber moniformis. See *Kaposi disease (1).*

lichen ruber obtusus. See *Hyde syndrome.*

lichen ruber obtusus corneus. See *Hyde syndrome.*

lichen ruber pemphigoides. See *Kaposi disease (3).*

lichen ruber planus. See *Wilson disease (2), under Wilson, Sir William Erasmus.*

lichen simplex chronicus. See *Brocq disease (1).*

lichen universalis moniliformis. See *Kaposi disease (1).*

lichenification. See *Brocq disease (1).*

LICHTENSTEIN, HEINZ (German physician)

Lichtenstein-Knorr syndrome. A familial syndrome, transmitted as an autosomal recessive trait, characterized by ataxia and progressive sensorineural hearing loss.

Lichtenstein, H., & Knorr, A. Über einige Fälle von fortschreitender Schwerhörigkeit bei hereditärer Ataxie. *Deut. Zschr. Nervenheilk.*, 1930, 114:1-28.

LICHTENSTEIN, JACK R. (American physician)

Lichtenstein syndrome. A familial syndrome, transmitted as an autosomal recessive trait, characterized by immunodeficiency with frequent infections due to neutropenia and immunoglobulin A deficiency; peripheral osteoporosis with frequent fractures; failure of fusion of posterior spinal arches; subluxation at C1-C2 resulting in long-tract signs; metacarpophalangeal camptodactyly with ulnar deviation of the fingers, simian creases; high axial triradius; giant cyst of the lungs;and peculiar facies characterized by carp mouth, synophrys, and anteverted nostrils. The syndrome was originally reported in monozygotic twins.

Lichtenstein, J. R. A "new" syndrome with neutropenia, immunoglobulin deficiency, peculiar facies and bony anomalies. *Birth Defects*, 1972, 8(3):178-90.

LICHTENSTEIN, LOUIS (American physician, born 1906)

Jaffe-Lichtenstein dysplasia. See *Jaffe-Lichtenstein syndrome.*

Jaffe-Lichtenstein fibrous dysplasia. See *Jaffe-Lichtenstein syndrome.*

Jaffe-Lichtenstein syndrome. See *under Jaffe.*

Jaffe-Lichtenstein-Uehlinger syndrome. See *Jaffe-Lichtenstein syndrome.*

LICHTENSTERN, OTTO MICHAEL LUDWIG. See LECHTENSTERN, OTTO MICHAEL LUDWIG

LICHTHEIM, LUDWIG (German physician, 1845-1915)

Lichtheim aphasia. A form of aphasia in which the patient is unable to speak out but can indicate with his fingers the number of syllables in the word of which he is thinking.

Lichteim, O. On aphasia. *Brain*, 1885, 7:433-84.

Lichtheim syndrome. See *Dana syndrome.*

LIEBENBERG, F. (South African orthopedic surgeon)

Liebenberg syndrome. Congenital multiple anomalies of the elbows, wrists, and hands, transmitted as an autosomal dominant trait, characterized by radial deviation of the hands with some flexion deformity, brachydactyly, club-shaped distal phalanges, small nails without grooves, some instances of camptodactyly of the fifth finger, defects of the carpal bones, and fusion of the triquetrum and pisiform bone.

Liebenberg, F. A pedigree with unusual anomalies of the elbows, wrists and hands in five generations. *S. Afr. Med. J.*, 1973, 47:745-8.

LIEBOW, AVERILL ABRAHAM (American physician, born 1911)

Rosen-Castleman-Liebow syndrome. See *under Rosen.*

LIEOU, YONG CHOEN (Chinese physician in France, born 1879)

Barré-Lieou syndrome. See *under Barré.*

LIEPMANN, HUGO KARL (German neurologist, 1863-1925)

Liepmann disease. Synonym: *apraxia.*

Inability to carry out skilled acts, although motor power and mental capacity are preserved.

Liepmann, N. Das Krankheitsbild der Apraxie ("motorischen Asymbolie") auf Grund eines Falles von einseitiger Apraxie. *Mschr. Psychiat. Neur.*, 1900, 8:15-44; 102-32;182-97.

ligamentum latum laceration syndrome. See *Allen-Masters syndrome, under Allen, William Myron.*

light chain disease. See *Bence Jones proteinuria.*

lightning foot. See *burning feet syndrome.*

LIGHTWOOD, REGINALD (British physician)

Butler-Lightwood-Albright syndrome. See *Lightwood-Albright syndrome.*

Lightwood syndrome. See *Lightwood-Albright syndrome.*

Lightwood-Albright syndrome. Synonyms: *Albright syndrome, Butler-Albright syndrome, Butler-Lightwood-Albright syndrome, Lightwood syndrome, calcinosis infantum, congenital hyperchloremic acidosis syndrome, evolutive tubular nephropathy, hyperchloremic acidosis with nephrocalcinosis, idiopathic renal acidosis, nephrocalcinosis infantum, nephrocalcinosis infantum with hyperchloremic acidosis, nephrocalcinosis with rickets and dwarfism, renal tubular acidosis, rickets with renal tubular acidosis.*

A syndrome of metabolic acidosis, hyperchloremia, inability to acidify urine, hypercalciuria, and hypokalemia attributed to excesssive excretion of bicarbonates and an increase in tubular reabsorption of chlorides. In infants, the symptoms include anorexia, constipation, failure to thrive, wasting, muscle hypotonia, nephrocalcinosis, and vomiting; in older children, they may also include rickets, bone deformities, pathological fractures, and growth retardation. See also *Glisson disease* and *hypophosphatemic familial rickets.*

Lightwood, R. Calcium infarction of the kidney in infants. *Arch. Dis. Child., London*, 1935, 10:205-6. Albright, F., *et al.* Metabolic studies and therapy in a case of nephrocalcinosis with rickets and dwarfism. *Bull Johns Hopkins Hosp.*, 1940, 66:7-33. Butler, A., *et al.* Dehydration and acidosis with calcification at renal tubules. *J. Pediat.,*, 1936, 8:489-99.

LIGNAC, GEORGE OTTO EMIL (Dutch pediatrician, 1891-1954)

Abderhalden-Kaufmann-Lignac syndrome. See *cystinosis.*

Lignac disease. See *cystinosis.*

Lignac-Fanconi syndrome. See *cystinosis.*

Lignac-Fanconi-Debré syndrome. See *cystinosis.*

ligneous phlegmon. See *Reclus disease.*

ligneous thyroiditis. See *Riedel disease.*

limb deficiency-heart malformation syndrome. See *Hecht-Scott syndrome, under Hecht, Jacqueline T.*

limb reduction-ichthyosis syndrome. A congenital syndrome of unilateral hypomelia associated with heart defect and ichthyosis. Osseous changes include unilateral shortness of the limbs, sometimes accompanied by absent scapula, rib dysplasia, webbed elbows and knees, and rib abnormalities. Absent septum, valvular defect, and truncus arteriosus are the principal heart anomalies. Most patients die shortly after birth.

Falek, A., *et al.* Unilateral limb and skin deformities with congenital heart disease in twin siblings. A lethal syndrome. *J. Pediat.*, 1968, 73:910.

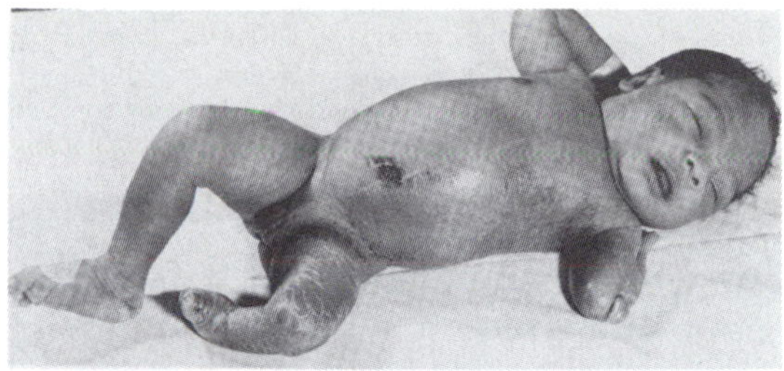

Limb reduction-ichthyosis syndrome
Falek, A., et al.: *J. Pediatr.* 73:910, 1968. St. Louis: C.V. Mosby Co.

limb-girdle dystrophy. See *Erb syndrome (1), under Erb, Wilhelm Heinrich.*

limb-girdle muscular dystrophy (LGMD). See *Leyden-Moebius syndrome.*

limb-girdle muscular weakness and atrophy. See *Leyden-Moebius syndrome.*

limb-girdle syndrome. See *Leyden-Moebius syndrome.*

limit dextrinosis. See *glycogen storage disease III.*

limy bile syndrome. Synonyms: *disappearing limy bile, milk of calcium bile.*

A form of cholelithiasis characterized by precipitation of calcium carabonate in a chronically inflamed gallbladder and bile ducts, causing the bile to become milky and opaque to x-rays. The condition is most common in children, being rare in adults. Abdominal pain, dyspepsia, and vomiting are the principal clinical symptoms.

Churchman, J. W. Acute cholecystitis with large amounts of calcium soap in the gallbladder. *Johns Hopkins Hosp. Bull.*, 1911, 22:223-4.

LINARELLI, LOUIS (American physician)

Kenny-Linarelli syndrome. See *Kenny syndrome.*

LINDAU, ARVID (Swedish physician, 1892-1958)

Hippel-Lindau disease. See *Hippel-Lindau syndrome.*

Hippel-Lindau syndrome (HLS). See *under Hippel.*

Lindau disease. See *Hippel-Lindau syndrome.*

Lindau tumor. See *Hippel-Lindau syndrome.*

von Hippel-Lindau (VHL) syndrome. See *Hippel-Lindau syndrome.*

LINDENOV

von Graefe-Lindenov syndrome. See *Graefe-Sjögren syndrome.*

LINDER, DAVID (American physician)

Taybi-Linder syndrome. See *under Taybi.*

linea corneae senilis. See *Hudson-Ståhli line.*

linear atelectasis. See *Fleischner syndrome.*

linear nevus sebaceus anomalad. See *Jadassohn nevus sebaceus, under Jadassohn, Josef.*

linear nevus sebaceus of Feuerstein and Mims. See *epidermal nevus syndrome.*

linear nevus sebaceus syndrome. See *epidermal nevus syndrome.*

linear verrucous epidermal nevus. See *epidermal nevus syndrome.*

lingual mandibular bone cavity. See *Stafne cyst.*

linitis plastica. See *Brinton disease.*

lioderma essentialis cum melanosis et telangiectasia. See *xeroderma pigmentosum syndrome.*

lip pit-cleft lip or palate syndrome. See *van der Woude syndrome.*

lipalgia. See *Dercum syndrome.*

lipid histiocytosis. See *Niemann-Pick syndrome.*

lipoatrophic diabetes. See *Berardinelli-Seip syndrome.*
lipocalcinogranulomatosis. See *Teutschländer syndrome.*
lipocalcinosis progradiens. See *Teutschländer syndrome.*
lipochalicogranulomatosis. See *Teutschländer syndrome.*
lipochondrodystrophy. See *mucopolysaccharidosis I-H.*
lipodystrophia intestinalis. See *Whipple disease.*
lipodystrophia progressiva seu paradoxa. See *Barraquer-Simons syndrome.*
lipofibrocalcareous myopathy. See *Mattioli-Foggia and Raso syndrome.*
lipoglycoproteinosis. See *Urbach-Wiethe syndrome.*
lipogranulomatosis intramuscularis progressiva. See *Teutschländer syndrome.*
lipogranulomatosis subcutanea. See *Rothmann-Makai syndrome.*
lipoid granulomatosis. See *Hand-Schüller-Christian syndrome.*
lipoid histiocytosis. See *Hand-Schüller-Christian syndrome.*
lipoid nephrosis. See *nephrotic syndrome, and see Munk disease.*
lipoid proteinosis. See *Urbach-Wiethe syndrome.*
lipomata diffusa symmetrica. See *Medelung syndrome.*
lipomatosis cutis superficialis. See *Hoffmann-Zurhelle syndrome, under Hoffman, Erich.*
lipomatosis diffusa symmetrica. See *Medelung syndrome.*
lipomatosis dolorosa. See *Dercum syndrome.*
lipomatous neuritis. See *Leyden neuritis.*
lipomelanotic reticulosis. See *Pautrier-Woringer syndrome.*
lipomembranous polycystic osteodysplasia-dementia syndrome. See *Hakola syndrome.*
lipomucopolysaccharidosis. See *mucolipidosis I.*
lipophagic intestinal granulamatosis. See *Whipple disease.*
lipoprotein lipase deficiency. See *Bürger-Grütz syndrome.*
LIPSCHÜTZ, BENJAMIN (Austrian physician, 1878-1931)
Lipschütz erythema. Synonyms: *Afzelius erythema, erythema chronicum migrans.*

A febrile migrating form of erythema characterized by edematous pinkish red rings that range in diameter from 5 to 7 mm and slowly enlarge, while healing in the center.

Lipschütz, B. Zur Kenntnis der "Erythema chronicum migrans." *Acta Derm. Vener., Stockholm*, 1931, 12:100-2. Afzelius, A. Erythema chronicum migrans. *Acta Derm. Vener., Stockholm*, 1921, 2:120-5.

Lipschütz ulcer. Synonyms: *acute vulvar ulcer, ulcus vulvae acutum.*

A simple acute ulcer of the vulva or the lower vagina, which forms a round shallow lesion without causing serious discomfort. *Bacillus crassus* infection is believed to be the cause.

Lipschütz, B. Über Ulcus vulvae acutum. *Wien. Klin. Wschr.*, 1918, 31:461-4.

LIPSITCH, L. S. (American physician)
Rytand-Lipsitch syndrome. See *under Rytand.*
LIS. See *locked-in syndrome.*
LISON, MICHAEL (Israeli physician)
Lison syndrome. A familial syndrome, transmitted as an autosomal recessive trait, characterized by distinct facies with sharp features, pointed nose and chin and high cheek bones; premature graying of scalp hair, eyebrows, and eyelashes; diffuse vitiligo; hyperpigmentation of exposed areas of the body; lentigines; increased deep tendon reflexes; Babinski reflex; footdrop; spastic gait; spinal deformities consisting of scoliosis, kyphosis, and lordosis; and muscle atrophy of the lower limbs.

Lison, M., *et al.* Progressive spastic paraparesis, vitiligo, premature graying, and distinct facial appearance: A new genetic syndrome in 3 sibs. *Am. J. Med. Genet.*, 1981, 9:351-7.

LISSAUER, HEINRICH (German psychiatrist, 1861-1891)
Lissauer atrophy. See *Lissauer paralysis.*
Lissauer dementia. See *Lissauer paralysis.*
Lissauer paralysis. Synonyms: *Lissauer atrophy, Lissauer dementia.*

Diffuse atrophy of the cerebral cortex associated with dementia paralytica, epileptiform and apoplectiform seizures, hemiplegia, aphasia, transient amblyopia, and facial paralysis.

Storch, E. Über einige Fälle atypischer progressiver Paralyse. Nach einem hinterlassenen Manuskript Dr. H. Lissauer's. *Mschr. Psychiat.*, 1901, 9:401-34.

lissencephaly. See *Norman-Roberts syndrome, and see Miller-Dieker syndrome, under Miller, James Q.*
LISSER, HANS (American physician, born 1888)
Escamilla-Lisser syndrome. See *under Escamilla.*
Escamilla-Lisser-Shepardson syndrome. See *Escamilla-Lisser syndrome.*
LITTLE, ERNEST GORDON GRAHAM (British physician, 1867-1950)
Graham Little syndrome. See *Little syndrome.*
Graham Little-Lassueur-Feldman syndrome. See *Little syndrome.*
Lassueur-Graham Little syndrome. See *Little syndrome.*
Lassueur-Graham Little triad. See *Little syndrome.*
Lassueur-Little syndrome. See *Little syndrome.*
Little syndrome. Synonyms: *Graham Little syndrome, Graham Little-Lassueur-Feldman syndrome, Lassueur-Graham Little triad, Lassueur-Little syndrome, Piccardi-Lassueur-Little syndrome, folliculitis decalvans, folliculitis decalvans et atrophicans, lichen planus et acuminatus atrophicans, lichen ruber follicularis decalvans.*

A progressive form of cicatricial alopecia of the scalp, sometimes also involving the axillae and pubic area, associated with keratosis pilaris which may be widespread. Residual atrophic scars occur only on the scalp.

Little, G. Folliculitis decalvans et atrophicans. *Brit. J. Derm.*, 1915, 27:183-5. Feldman, S. Lichen planus et acuminatus atrophicans. Folliculitis decalvans et lichen spinulosus of Little. *Arch. Derm., Chicago,* 1936, 34:378-97.

Piccardi-Lassueur-Little syndrome. See *Little syndrome.*
LITTLE, WILLIAM JOHN (British physician, 1810-1894)
Little disease. Synonyms: *cerebral diplegia, cerebral spastic paralysis, congenital spastic diplegia, diplegia spastica infantilis, infantile spastic diplegia, spastic diplegia.*

A disease of newborn infants, which results from several disorders, including birth injury, asphyxia neonatorum, prematurity, and maternal illness during pregnancy. The symptoms are caused by central nervous system injury and include various degrees and combinations of palsy, hemiplegia, paraplegia, quadriplegia, spasticity, convulsions, mental deficiency, dyskinetic or ataxic disorders, and ocular disturbances such as optic atrophy, nystagmus, and cataract.

Little, W. J. On the influence of abnormal parturition, difficult labours, premature birth, and asphyxia neonatorum, on the mental and physical conditions of the child, especially in relation to deformities. *Tr. Obst. Soc., London*, 1862, 3:293-344.

LITTRE, ALEXIS (French physician, 1658-1725)

Littre hernia. Synonym: *diverticular hernia.*

Hernial protrusion of an intestinal diverticulum.

Littre. Observation sur une nouvelle éspece de hernie. *Hist. Acad. Roy. Sc., Paris*, 1700, (impr. 1719), pp. 300-10.

livedo reticularis-cerebrovascular syndrome. See *Sneddon syndrome (2).*

liver cirrhosis with alcohol abuse. See *Laennec cirrhosis.*

liver cirrhosis-abnormal glycogen syndrome. See *glycogen storage disease IV.*

liver cirrhosis-polycythemia syndrome. See *Mosse syndrome, under Mosse, Max.*

liver glycogen disease. See *glycogen storage disease I.*

liver-kidney syndrome. See *hepatorenal syndrome.*

LLOYD-THOMAS, HYWEL GEOFFREY LOYD (British physician)

Evans and Lloyd-Thomas syndrome. See *under Evans, William.*

LMBB (Laurence-Moon-Bield-Bardet) syndrome. See *Laurence-Moon-Biedl syndrome.*

LMBBS (Laurence-Moon-Biedl-Bardet syndrome). See *Laurence-Moon-Biedl syndrome.*

LMR (lymphocytic meningoradiculitis). See *Bannwarth syndrome.*

LNS. See *Lesch-Nyhan syndrome.*

lobar atrophy. See *Pick syndrome, under Pick, Arnold.*

LOBO, JORGE (Brazilian physician)

Lobo disease. Synonym: *keloidal blastomycosis.*

Chronic benign blastomycosis caused by infection with *Loboa loboi* and characterized by keloidal tumors of the skin. This disease, predominant in South American countries, is sometimes confused with South American blastomycosis (the Lutz-Splendore-de Almeida syndrome).

*Lobo, J. Um caso de blastomicose produzido por uma specie nova, encontrada em Recife. *Rev. Med., Pernambuco*, 1931, 1:763-5.

LOBSTEIN, JOHANN FRIEDRICH GEORG CHRISTIAN (Strassburg physician, 1777-1835)

Ekman-Lobstein syndrome. See *osteogenesis imperfecta syndrome (dominant form).*

Lobstein syndrome. See *osteogenesis imperfecta syndrome (dominant form).*

lobster-claw defect with ectodermal defects syndrome. See *EEC syndrome.*

local corneal mucopolysaccharidosis. See *Groenouw dystrophy (2).*

localized cicatricial pemphigoid. See *Brunsting disease.*

localized fibrous lesion (of bone). See *Jaffe-Lichtenstein disease.*

localized scleroderma. See *Addison keloid.*

locked-in syndrome (LIS). Synonym: *de-afferented state.*

A tetraplegic, mute but fully alert state which results when the the descending motor pathways are interrupted by infarction of the ventral pons. The patients are fully awake, responsive and sentient, although the repertoire of response is limited to blinking and jaw and eye movements.

Plum, F., & Posner, J. B. *The diagnosis of stupor and coma.* 2nd ed. Philadelphia, Saunders, 1972. Jennett, B., & Plum, B. Peristent vegetative state after brain damage. A syndrome in search of a name. *Lancet*, 1972, 1:734-7.

locomotor ataxia. Synonyms: *Duchenne disease, Duchenne syndrome, posterior spinal sclerosis, tabes dorsalis.*

Degeneration of the posterior roots and posterior column of the spinal cord and the brain stem, marked by attacks of pain; a peculiar gait; progressive ataxia; loss of reflexes; functional disorders of the bladder, gastrointestinal tract, and larynx; and impotence. The disorder develops as a sequel of tertiary syphilis and appears to affect middle-aged males most frequently.

Duchenne. De l'ataxie locomotrice progressive, récherches sur une maladie caracterisée specialement par les troubles généreaux de la coordination de movements. *Arch. Gén. Méd., Paris*, 1858, 12:641-52.

loculation syndrome. See *Froin syndrome.*

LOEFFLER, WILHELM. See LÖFFLER, WILHELM

LOEFGREN, SVEN HALVAR. See LÖFGREN, SVEN HALVAR

LOEHLEIN, MAX HERMANN FRIEDRICH. See LÖHLEIN, MAX HERMANN FRIEDRICH

LOEHR, HANS. See LÖHR, HANS

LOEWENSTEIN, LUDWIG W. (American physician)

Buschke-Loewenstein tumor. See *under Buschke.*

LOEWENTHAL, LEONARD JOSEPH ALPHONSE (British physician)

Loewenthal purpura. See *Casalá-Mosto disease.*

LÖFFLER, WILHELM (Swiss physician, 1887-1972)

Löffler disease. Synonyms: *Löffler eosinophilia, Löffler pneumonia, Löffler syndrome.*

A disorder characterized by eosinophilia and benign, transient, migratory or successive pulmonary infiltrates, showing on the radiograph as irregular opacities. The course is usually mild and is marked by weight loss, fever, and night sweating. Immunologic mechanisms are believed to cause this disorder. Some writers restrict the term to eosinophilic pneumonia due to parasitic infiltration; others consider it a synonym for the *pulmonary infiltration with eosinophilia syndrome.* See also *Kartagener disease, Löhr-Kindberg syndrome,* and *Magrassi-Leonardi syndrome.*

Löffler, W. Flüchtige Lungeninfiltrate mit Eosinophilia. *Klin. Wschr.*, 1935, 14:297-9.

Löffler endocarditis. Synonyms: *Löffler endomyocarditis, constrictive fibrous endocarditis, endocarditis fibroplastica with eosinophilia, endocarditis parietalis fibroplastica, fibroplastic endocarditis, fibroplastic endomyocarditis, fibroplastic parietal endocarditis with eosinophilia, parietal fibroplastic eosinophilic endocarditis.*

A progressive, febrile, refractory heart disease associated with eosinophilia and multiple systemic emboli. The acute form is marked by eosinophilic arteritis of various organs including the heart, leading to cardiac enlargement with fibrotic thickening of the endocardium of all chambers, marked by leathery, grayish-white lesions which extend into the myocardium and papillary muscles and chordae tendineae. The insidious form is characterized by a gradual decrease of tolerance to physical effort and symptoms suggesting constrictive pericarditis. Mitral and tricuspid incompetence and regurgitation, murmurs of mitral stenosis, and electrocardiographic S-T segment and T wave abnormalities are the most common manifestations.

Löffler, W. Endocarditis parietalis fibroplastica mit Bluteosinophilie. Ein eigenartige Krankheitsbild. *Schweiz. Med. Wschr.*, 1936, 66:817-20.

Löffler endomyocarditis. See *Löffler endocarditis.*

Löffler eosinophilia. See *Löffler disease.*

Löffler pneumonia. See *Löffler disease.*

Löffler syndrome. See *Löffler disease.*

LÖFGREN, SVEN HALVAR (Swedish physician)

Löfgren syndrome. Synonyms: *bilateral hilar adenopathy syndrome, bilateral hilar lymphoma syndrome*

Erythema nodosum in combination with bilateral hilar lymphomatous lesions that show a negative or weak tuberculin reaction. Adult women, especially those between the ages of 25 to 29 years, are most commonly affected. A relationship to pregnancy and lactation has been observed in earlier reports, but later findings by Löfgren indicate that this disorder is a manifestation of sarcoidosis.

Löfgren, S. Erythema nodosum. Studies on etiology and pathogenesis in 185 women. *Acta Med. Scand.*, 1946, (Suppl 174):1-197.

loge of Guyon syndrome. See *ulnar tunnel syndrome.*

LÖHLEIN, MAX HERMANN FRIEDRICH (German physician, 1877-1921)

Löhlein nephritis. Synonyms: *acute focal nephritis, embolic bacterial glomerulonephritis, embolic nonsuppurative focal nephritis, focal embolic nephritis, focal glomerulonephritis, focal thrombotic glomerulonephritis, multiple glomerular embolization.*

Nephritis in which only a portion of each nephron is involved. The lesions usually consist of hemorragic glomerulonephritis with epithelial proliferation. Once considered to be caused by bacterial embolization, the condition is now believed to be due to immune mechanisms.

Löhlein, M. H. *Über die entzündlichen Veränderungen der Glomeruli der menschlichen Nieren und ihre Bedeutung für die Nephritis.* Leipzig, Hirzel, 1907.

LÖHR, HANS (German physician, 1891-1949)

Löhr-Kindberg syndrome. Synonyms: *Löhr-Léon Kindberg syndrome, eosinophilic pneumopathy.*

A subacute febrile pulmonary disease associated with marked eosinophilia. The syndrome differs from Löffler disease in its subacute and continuous course and lack of hypersensitivity, whereas the Löffler type has a mild and transient course.

*Löhr, H. Über flüchtige Lungeninfiltrierung mit und ohne Eosinophilie des Blutes. *Zschr. Klin. Med.*, 1940, 137:297. Kindberg, L. M., *et al.* Pneumopathie à éosinophiles. *Presse Méd., Paris*, 1940, 48:277-8.

Löhr-Léon Kindberg syndrome. See *Löhr-Kindberg syndrome.*

LOHUIZEN, CATO H. J., VAN (Dutch physician)

Lohuizen disease. Synonyms: *cutis marmorata teleangiectatica congenita (CMTC), phleboctasia congenita generalisata.*

A congenital skin disease, usually transmitted as an autsosomal recessive trait, characterized by cutis marmorata, phlebectasis, telangiectatic nevi, ulcerations, and steady improvement from birth. Most cases are sporadic.

Lohuizen, C. H., van. Über eine seltene angeborene Hautanomalie (Cutis marmorata teleangiectatica). *Acta Derm. Vener., Stockholm*, 1922, 3:202-11.

LOKEN, AAGOT CHRISTIE (Norwegian physician)

Senior-Loken syndrome. See *Senior syndrome (1).*

LONDE, P.

Fazio-Londe paralysis. See *Duchenne paralysis.*

long QT syndrome (LQTS). Synonyms: *prolonged QT interval syndrome, protracted QT, QT interval prolongation, QT prolongation syndrome.*

Prolongation of Q-T interval on the electrocardiogram, usually in association with syncope, ventricular tachyarrhythmia, and sudden death. The disorder may be sporadic or transmitted as a genetic trait. When associated with deaf-mutism and transmitted as an autosomal recessive trait, it is known as the **Jervell and Lange-Nielsen syndrome**, and when transmitted as an autosomal dominant trait, without deafness, it is referred to as the **Romano-Ward syndrome**.

Jervell, A., & Lange-Nielsen, F. Congenital deaf-mutism, functional heart disease with prolongation of the QT interval and sudden death. *Am. Heart J.*, 1957, 54:59-68. Romano, C., *et al.* Aritmie cardiache rare dell'etá pediatrica. II. Accessi sincopali per fibrillazione ventricolare pyrossistica. Presentazione del primo caso della letteratura pediatrica italiana. *Clin. Pediat., Bologna,* 1963, 45:656-83. Ward, O. C. A new familial cardiac syndrome in children. *J. Irish Med. Assoc.*, 1964, 54:103-6.

long-thumb brachydactyly syndrome. See *Hollister-Hollister syndrome, under Hollister, David W.*

LONGHI, GIOVANNI (Italian physician)

Avellis-Longhi syndrome. See *Avellis syndrome.*

loose bodies in the joints. See *König disease (1).*

LOOSER, EMIL (Swiss physician, 1877-1936)

Looser-Debray-Milkman syndrome. See *Milkman syndrome.*

Milkman-Looser syndrome. See *Milkman syndrome.*

LORAIN, PAUL JOSEPH (French physician, 1827-1875)

Lorain syndrome. See *Lorain-Levi syndrome.*

Lorain-Levi syndrome. Synonyms: *Levi syndrome, Lorain syndrome, ateliosis, hypophyseal dwarfism with infantilism. hypophyseal infantilism, pituitary dwarfism, pituitary hypogonadism, pituitary nanism, prepuberal panhypopituitarism.*

A rare form of dwarfism with normal body proportions, slender extremities, underdeveloped secondary sex characteristics, and thyroid and adrenocortical insufficiency. The syndrome is produced by destructive lesions of the anterior pituitary gland, mainly by tumors, such as craniopharyngioma and intrasellar cysts. Onset usually takes place before puberty, after initial normal development. The initial symptoms include retarded growth, sexual infantilism, and high-pitched voice. They are followed by poor dentition and progeria. See also *Burnier syndrome* and *Fröhlich syndrome.*

*Lorain, P. J. *Du féminisme et de l'infantilisme chez les tuberculeux.* Paris, 1871. (Thesis). Levi, E. Contribution à l'étude de l'infantilisme du type Lorain. *Nouv. Icon. Salpetriére*, 1908, 21:297-324; 421-71.

LORRAIN, MAURICE (French physician, born 1867)

Strümpell-Lorrain disease. See *under Strümpell.*

LORTAT-JACOB, ETIENNE MARIE (French dermatologist, born 1902)

Lortat-Jacob disease. Synonyms: *benign mucosal pemphigoid, cicatricial pemphigoid, dermatite bulleuse muco-synéchiante et atrophiante, mucosynechial dermatitis.*

A chronic bullous disease of elderly persons, involving primarily the conjunctival and oral mucous membranes, with scarring. Associated lesions of the face, neck, scalp, legs, and genitalia are seen in about half of the cases. Entropion with secondary blindness and synechiae of the palpebral and bulbar conjunctivae are common. The bullae of the oral mucosa, most commonly affecting the gingivae and edentulous ridges, develop from vesicles about 3 to 6 mm in diameter, which rupture and coalesce, leaving shallow ulcers, and which eventually cause mild scarring. Histologically, the lesions are similar to those seen in erythema multiforme, with subepithelial bullae and late fibrosis.

Lortat-Jacob, E. Benign mucosal pemphigoid, dermatite bulleuse muco-synéchiante et atrophiante. *Brit. J. Derm.*, 1958, 70:361-7.

LOU GEHRIG. See GEHRIG, HENRY LOUIS

LOUIS

Conn-Louis syndrome. See *Conn syndrome.*

LOUIS-BAR, DENISE (French physician)

Louis-Bar syndrome. Synonyms: *Boder-Sedgwick syndrome, ataxia-telangiectasia (AT), ataxia teleangiectasica, cephalo-oculocutaneous telangiectasis.*

A familial disorder characterized by progressive cerebellar ataxia, oculocutaneous telangiectases, and proneness to sinopulmonary infections. The ataxia becomes apparent when the child begins to walk, and the onset of telangiectasia is usually observed at about 5 years of age. Ocular manifestations consist of strabismus, poor ocular convergence, and nystagmus. Neurological symptoms include intention tremor of upper extremities, hypotonia, and diminished tendon reflexes with choreoathetoid movement. The telangiectasia appears first on the bulbar conjunctivae and later on the ears, transnasal (butterfly) area of the face, palate, sternum, antecubical and popliteal fossae, and dorsa of extremities. Dysarthria, drooling, growth retardation, slow slurred speech, jerky eye movements, rapid spasmodic blinking, café-au-lait spots, and keratosis pilaris are the other symptoms. Neoplasms occur in some cases. Most patients die during adolescence. The syndrome is transmitted as an autosomal recessive trait.

Louis-Bar, D. Sur un syndrome progressif comprenant des télangiectasies capillaires cutanées et conjonctivales symétriques, à disposition naevoïde et des troubles cérébelleux. *Confinia Neur., Basel*, 1941-42, 4:32-42.
Boder, E., & Sedgwick, R. P. Ataxia-telangiectasia. A familial syndrome of progressive cerebellar ataxia, oculocutaneous telangiectasia and frequent pulmonary infection. *Pediatrics*, 1958, 21:526-5; 21:526-54.

LOUTIT, JOHN FREEMAN (British physician, born 1910)

Loutit anemia. Synonyms: *acholuric jaundice, hematogenous jaundice, hemolytic icterus, hemolytic jaundice.*

Jaundice and hemolytic anemia associated with hyperbilirubinemia secondary to an increase in erythrocyte and hemoglobin breakdown rates. Complications may include cholelithiasis and brain damage in infants due to deposition of unconjungated bilirubin in the nerve tissue.

Loutit, F. J., & Mollison, P. L. Hemolytic icterus (acholuric jaundice), congenital and acquired. *J. Path. Bact.*, 1946, 58:711-28.

low blood triiodothyronine syndrome. See *low T_3 syndrome.*

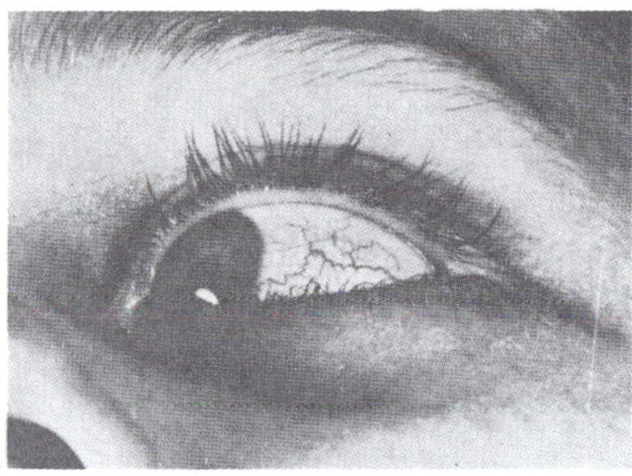

Louis-Bar syndrome
Nelson, W.E. (ed.): *Textbook of Pediatrics,* 9th ed. Philadelphia: W.B. Saunders Co., 1969.

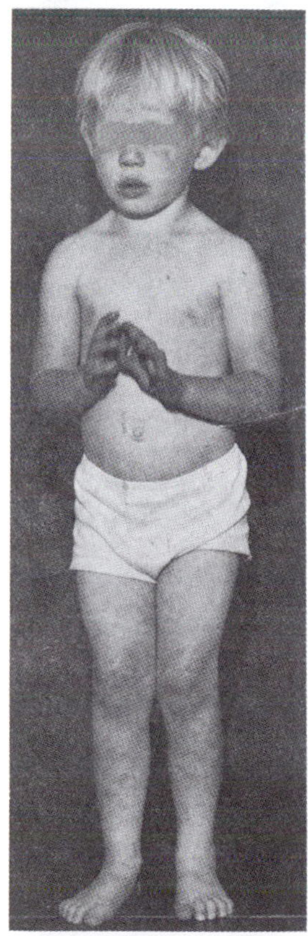

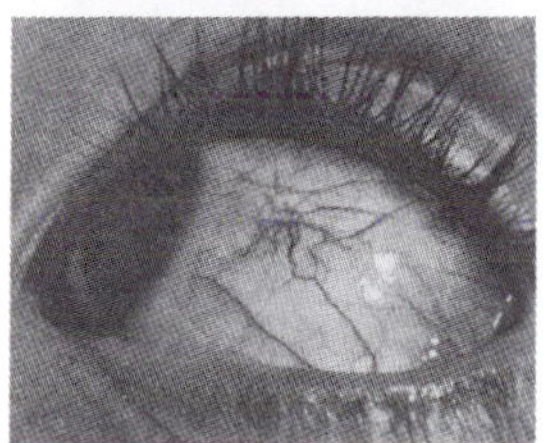

Louis-Bar syndrome
Smith, D.W.: *J. Pediatr.* 70:487. 1967. St. Louis: C.V. Mosby Co.

low conus. See *tethered conus syndrome.*

low salt syndrome. Synonyms: *Schroeder syndrome, hyponatremic syndrome.*

A syndrome of hyponatremia secondary to intensive therapy of congestive heart disease, characterized by rapid physical and mental deterioration, unresponsiveness to mercurial diuretics, a fall in serum chloride levels with azotemia, and renal failure.

*Schroeder, H. A. Renal failure associated with low extracellular chloride: The low salts syndrome. *JAMA,* 1949, 141:117. Vogl, A. The low-salt syndromes in congestive heart failure. *Am. J. Cardiol.,* 1959, 3:192-8.

low T_3 sick syndrome. See *low T_3 syndrome.*

low T_3 syndrome. Synonyms: *euthyroid sick syndrome, low blood triiodothyronine syndrome, low triiodothyronine syndrome, low T_3 sick syndrome, sick euthyroid syndrome.*

A hormonal disorder characterized by reduced conversion of thyroxine (T_4) to triiodothyronine (T_3) due to diminished activity of 5-deiodinase in the liver, kidney, anterior pituitary, and other tissues, in association with a fall in free and serum T_3 levels and marked increase in rT_3 concentrations, T_4 levels remaining normal in most instances. When this phenomenon occurs in the presence of nonthyroidal disorders, the condition is known as the **sick euthyroid syndrome**. Starvation is the main cause, but other conditions associated with impaired conversion of T_4 to T_3 include diabetes mellitus, infections, cancer, liver diseases, renal failure, caloric deprivation (excessive dieting, fasting, and carbohydrate deprivation), surgery, and toxic effects of drugs, such as propylthiouracil, glucocorticoids, proprandrol, and iodine compounds.

Burger, A., *et al.* Reduced active thyroid hormone levels in acute illness. *Lancet,* 1976, 1:653-5. Wartofsky, L., & Burman, K. D. Alterations in thyroid function in patients with systemic illness: The "euthyroid sick syndrome." *Endocr. Rev.,* 1982, 3:164. Jackson, I. M. D., & Cobb, W. E. Disorders of the thyroid. In: Kohler, P. O., & Jordan, R. M., eds. *Clinical endocrinology.* New York, Wiley, 1986, pp. 73-165.

low T_4 syndrome. A condition in euthyroid patients wherein serum thyroxine (T_4), free thyroxine, and thyroxine-binding globulin are reduced.

Jackson, I. M. D., & Cobb, W. E. Disorders of the thyroid. In: Kohler, P. O., & Jordan, R. M., eds. *Clinical endocrinology.* New York, Wiley, 1986, pp. 73-165.

low T_4 and low T_3 syndrome. A condition in euthyroid patients manifested by a low normal to unmeasurable serum thyroxine (T_4) concentrations associated with low triiodothyronine (T_3) levels. Thyroid-stimulating hormone and free T_4 are normal. Sera from sick patients contain inhibitors of T_4 binding which are released from tissues in quantities related directly to the severity of the illness.

Chopra, I. J., *et al.* An inhibitor of the binding of thyroid hormones to serum proteins is present in extrathyroidal tissues. *Science,* 1982, 215:407-9. Jackson, I. M. D., & Cobb, W. E. Disorders of the thyroid. In: Kohler, P. O., & Jordan, R. M., eds. *Clinical endocrinology.* New York, Wiley, 1986, pp. 73-165.

low triiodothyronine syndrome. See *low T_3 syndrome.*

low-angle facial type. See *short face syndrome.*

low-percentage leukemia. See *myelodysplastic syndrome.*

LOWE, CHARLES UPTON (American physician, born 1921)

Lowe syndrome. Synonyms: *Lowe-Terrey-MacLachlan syndrome, oculocerebrorenal (OCR) syndrome.*

Hydrophthalmos, cataracts, mental retardation, vitamin D-resistant rickets, renal tubular dysfunction with aminoaciduria, reduced ammonia production, hypochloremic acidosis, phosphaturia, and hypophosphatemia are the principal features of this syndrome. Associated disorders may include muscle hypotonia, muscle hypoplasia with fatty infiltrations, joint hypermobility, diminished deep tendon reflexes, hyperactivity, episodes of fever, corneal scarring, superficial granulation of the eyes, nystagmus, buphthalmos, glaucoma, growth retardation, hematuria, albuminuria, cryptorchism, seizures, high-pitched cry, pectus excavatum, craniosynostosis, dental cysts, and multiple fractures. Radiological findings show evidence of rickets and osteoporosis. The syndrome is transmitted as an X-linked, incompletely recessive trait, some heterozygote females showing fine lenticular opacities.

Lowe, C. U., Terrey, M., & MacLachlan, E. A. Organic aciduria, decreased renal ammonia productin, hydrophthalmos and mental retardation. A clinical entity. *Am. J. Dis. Child.,* 1952, 83:164-84.

Lowe-Terrey-MacLachlan syndrome. See *Lowe syndrome.*

LÖWENTHAL, ARMAND

Löwenthal sclerosis. A familial syndrome combining generalized muscular sclerosis and blepharoptosis. Its principal features, which are present at birth, are atonic extremities, poorly developed and flaccid muscles (biopsy shows sclerosis of the muscular connective and subcutaneous adipose tissues), rhizomelic contractures, hyperextension of the joints, kyphoscoliosis, fixed position of the head, limitation of movements, wasp waist, spurs of the calcaneum, arched palate, hyperhidrosis, and gradual improvement from birth.

Löwenthal, A. Étude sur les myosites. IV. Sur une forme congénitale et familiale de sclérose musculaire généralisée avec blépharoptose. (Contribution à l'étude des maladies congénitales des muscles et du tissue conjonctif). *Acta Neur. Belg.,* 1952, 52:141-55.

lower brachial plexus palsy. See *Déjerine-Klumpke syndrome.*

lower esophageal ring. See *Schatzki ring.*

lower radicular syndrome. See *Déjerine-Klumpke syndrome.*

lower-face headache. See *Sluder neuralgia.*

lower-half headache. See *Sluder neuralgia.*

LOWN, BERNARD (American physician, born 1921)

Lown-Ganong-Levine (LGL) syndrome. See *Clerc-Lévy-Cristesco syndrome.*

LOWRY, R. BRIAN (Irish physician in Canada)

Coffin-Lowry syndrome (CLS). See *under Coffin.*

Lowry syndrome (1). Synonym: *craniosynostosis-fibular aplasia syndrome.*

A disorder consisting of craniosynostosis involving both coronal and sagittal sutures and symmetric aplasia of the fibulae. Prominent eyes, strabismus, partial cleft palate, high-arched palate, low-set ears, simian creases, cryptorhism, pes equinovarus, short sternum, and pilonidal dimple may be associated. In the original report, two sibs of normal second cousins were affected. Autosomal recessive inheritance is suspected.

Lowry, R. B. Congenital absence of the fibula and craniosynostosis in sibs. *J. Med. Genet.*, 1972, 9:227-9.

Lowry syndrome (2). A syndrome of microcephaly, mental retardation, bilateral cataracts, kyphosis, and limitation of joint movement. Deep-set eyes with narrow palpebral fissures, subluxation of hips, failure to thrive, cryptorchism, microphallus, and sparse hair growth are usually associated. Autosomal recessive transmission is suspected.

Lowry, R. B., *et al.* Cataracts, microcephaly, kyphosis, and limited joint movement in two siblings: A new syndrome. *J. Pediat.*, 1971, 79:282-4.

LOYEZ

Claude-Loyez syndrome. See *inferior nucleus ruber syndrome.*

LQTS. See *long QT syndrome.*

LS. See *Leriche syndrome (1 and 2).*

LTD (Laron-type dwarfism). See *Laron dwarfism.*

LUBARSCH, OTTO (German physician, 1860-1933)

Königstein-Lubarsch syndrome. See *Lubarsch-Pick syndrome.*

Lubarsch syndrome. See *Lubarsch-Pick syndrome.*

Lubarsch-Pick syndrome. Synonyms: *Königstein-Lubarsch syndrome, Lubarsch syndrome, systematized amyloidosis-macroglossia syndrome, systemic amyloidosis syndrome.*

Atypical amyloidosis frequently associated with diffuse enlargement of the tongue (amyloid macroglossia), involvement of the skeletal muscles, and scleroderma. There are extensive deposits of amyoloid substance in the skin, tongue, heart, stomach, intestine, and skeletal muscles, with the liver, kidneys, and adrenals being spared. The presence of Bence Jones protein and atypical plasma cells in the bone marrow suggests a relationship to myeloma.

Lubarsch, O. Zur Kenntnis ungewöhnlicher Amyloidablagerungen. *Virchows Ach. Path.*, 1929, 271:867-89. Pick, L. Über atypische Amyloidalblagerung. *Klin. Wschr.*, 1931, 10:1515. *Königstein, H. Über Amyloidose der Haut. *Arch. Derm. Syph., Berlin*, 1925, p. 330.

LUBS, HERBERT AUGUSTUS, JR. (American physician, born 1929)

Lubs syndrome. A familial form of pseudohermaphroditism. In the original report, the family included five male pseudohermaphrodites, each having an enlarged clitoris, labia with varying scrotal characteristics, and a urogenital sinus containing the urethra. As adults, they had small histologically proven testes in the labioscrotal folds and female breast development and hair distribution. Buccal smears were chromatin-negative.

Lubs, H. A., Jr., *et al.* Familial male pseudohermaphroditism with labial testes and partial feminization. Endocrine studies and genetic aspects. *J. Clin. Endocr.*, 1959, 19:1110-20.

LUCHERINI, TOMMASO (Italian physician, born 1891)

Lucherini syndrome. Synonym: *dystrophic osteoarthropathy.*

Juvenile rheumatoid arthritis associated with iridocyclitis, reportedly described by Lucherini.

Lucherini-Giacobini syndrome. Synonym: *familial endocrine osteochondropathy.*

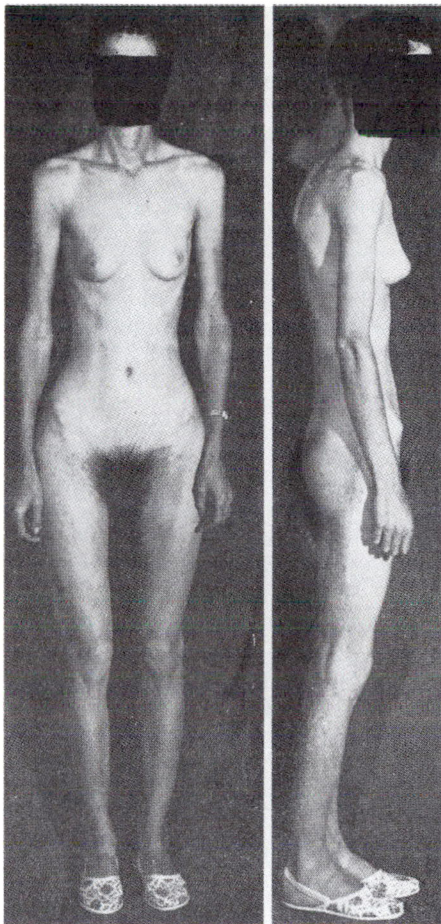

Lubs syndrome
Federman, D.D.: *Abnormal Sexual Development.* Philadelphia: W.B. Saunders Co., 1967.

Precocious macrogenisotomia with multiple epiphyseal disorders, reportedly described by Lucherini and Giacobini.

LUCIANI, LUIGI (Italian physiologist, 1842-1919)

Luciani syndrome. Synonym: *Luciani triad.*

A cerebellar syndrome associated with the triad of asthenia, atonia, and astasia, reportedly described by Luciani.

Luciani triad. See *Luciani syndrome.*

LUDER, JOSEPH (British physician)

Luder-Sheldon syndrome. A form of the renotubular syndrome of Fanconi (adult Fanconi syndrome), transmitted as an autosomal dominant trait, characterized by faulty renal tubular reabsorption of glucose and amino acids, associated with dwarfism due to depletion of some essential amino acids and late rickets. Hypophosphatemia, hypokalemia, acidosis, aminoaciduria, proteinuria, and glycosuria are the usual urinary and hematological findings.

Luder, J., & Sheldon, W. A familiar tubular absorption defect of glucose and amino acids. *Arch. Dis. Child.*, 1955, 30:160-4.

LUDLOFF, KARL (German physician, 1864-1945)

Büdinger-Ludloff-Läwen syndrome. See *under Büdinger.*

LUDWIG, WILHELM FRIEDRICH, VON (German physician, 1790-1865)

Ludwig angina. Synonyms: *angina ludovici, angina ludwigii, phlegmon of the floor of the mouth, submaxillary cellulitis.*

A severe form of cellulitis of the submaxillary space and secondary involvement of the sublingual and submental spaces, usually resulting from an infection of the mandibular molar area or a penetrating injury of the floor of the mouth. The second and third molars are the most common source of infection. From there, the infection perforates the bone, usually the lingual plate, establishes drainage, and thus spreads to other parts. The presenting lesion is a rapidly developing hard swelling of the floor of the mouth, expanding to the parapharyngeal spaces, carotid sheath, pterygopalatine fossa, and neck. Elevation of the tongue, difficulty in eating and swallowing, fever, edema of the glottis, rapid breathing, and moderate leukocytosis are the usual symptoms. Complications may include asphyxia and cavernous sinus thrombosis with subsequent meningitis. Staphylococci are present in nearly all cases, but fusiform bacilli, streptococci, and other bacteria are found in most instances.

*Ludwig, W.F., von. Über eine in neuerer Zeit wiederholt hier vorgekommene Form von Halsentzüng... *Med. Corresp. Württ. Ärztl. Verein.*, 1836, 6:21-5.

luetic aortitis. See *Heller-Döhle disease, under Heller, Arnold Ludwig Gotthilf.*

luetic-otitic-nystagmus syndrome. See *Hennebert syndrome.*

LUETSCHER, JOHN ARTHUR (American physician, born 1913)

Luetscher syndrome. Secondary hyperaldosteronism associated with heart, kidney, and liver diseases.

Lieberman, A. H., & Luetscher, J. A. Clinical implications of excess aldosterone output. *Arch. Klin. Med., Chicago*, 1957, 100:774-9.

lumbar puncture headache. See *puncture headache, under headache syndrome.*

lumbarthria. See *Léri disease (2).*

lumpy jaw. See *Rivalta disease.*

lunatomalacia. See *Kienböck disease.*

LUND, JOHANN CHRISTIAN (Norwegian physician)

Lund-Huntington chorea. See *Huntington chorea.*

LUNDBERG, P. O. (Swedish neurologist)

Lundberg syndrome. A syndrome originally described in three sisters in a sibship of eight, characterized by slowly progressive peripheral paresis of the hands and feet, starting in childhood and leading to moderate incapacitation; absence of tendon reflexes and a reduced motor conduction velocity; moderate mental deliciency; premature menopause at 20-25 years of age; and disproportionate smallness with short arms and legs (acromicria). The syndrome is believed to be transmitted as an autosomal recessive trait.

Lundberg, P. O. Hereditary polyneuropathy, oligophrenia, premature menopause, and acromicria. A new syndrome. *Europ. Neurol.*, 1971, 5:84-98.

LUNDBORG, HERMANN BERNHARD (Swedish physician, 1868-1943)

Lundborg-Unverricht disease. See *Lafora disease.*

lung purpura with nephritis. See *Goodpasture syndrome.*

lupoid hepatitis. See *Beam-Kunkel syndrome, and see Waldenström hepatitis, under Waldenström, Jan Gösta.*

lupus erythematodes. See *lupus erythematosus.*

lupus erythematosus. Synonyms: *Cazenave disease, Leloir disease, lupus erythematodes, lupus sebaceous, seborrhea congestiva, ulerythema centrifugum.*

An autoimmune collagen disease, usually chronic but sometimes acute, which is characterized by erythematous scaling patches of various configurations and sizes on the skin, which cause scarring and atrophy, and by the presence of L.E. cells. Acute disseminated and chronic discoid forms are recognized.

Cazenave, P. L. Des principales formes du lupus et de son traitement. *Gaz. Hôp. Paris,* 1850, 2:393; 1852, 4:114. Leloir. Recherches sur l'histologie pathologique et al nature du lupus érythémateux. *Ann. Der. Syph., Paris,* 1890, 1:708-9.

lupus erythematosus profundus. See *Kaposi-Irgang disease.*

lupus sebaceous. See *lupus erythematosus.*

lupus vulgaris multiplex nonulcerans et nonserpiginosus. See *Mortimer disease.*

LUR'E, I. V. See LURIE, IOSIF V.

LURIE, IOSIF V. (Russian physician)

Garcia-Lurie syndrome. See *under Garcia.*

LUTEMBACHER, RENE (French cardiologist, 1884-1968)

Lutembacher complex. See *Lutembacher syndrome.*

Lutembacher disease. See *Lutembacher syndrome.*

Lutembacher syndrome. Synonyms: *Lutembacher complex, Lutembacher disease, atrial septal defect-mitral stenosis syndrome.*

A combination of atrial septal defect and mitral stenosis.

Lutembacher, R. De la sténose mitrale avec communication interauriculaire. *Arch. Mal. Coeur.*, 1916, 9:237-60.

LUTZ, ADOLFO (Brazilian physician, 1855-1940)

Bielschowsky-Lutz-Cogan syndrome. See *under Bielschowsky, Alfred.*

Lutz disease. See *Lutz-Splendore-de Almeida syndrome.*

Lutz-Jeanselme syndrome. See *Jeanselme nodules.*

Lutz-Splendore-de Almeida syndrome. Synonyms: *de Almeida disease, Lutz disease, Brazilian blastomycosis, paracoccidioidal granuloma, paracoccidioidomycosis.*

A chronic granulomatous disease of the skin, mucous membranes, lymphatic system, and internal organs, caused by the fungus *Paracoccidioides (Blastomyces) brasiliensis*, occurring chiefly in South American farm workers. Picking the teeth with twigs or chewing leaves contaminated with the fungus are the suspected causes. Four principal types are recognized: (1) The **mucocutaneous form,** characterized by papules, chiefly of the oral region, which appear concurrently with lymphatic involvement; (2) the **lymphatic form,** characterized by enlargement of regional lymph nodes; (3) the **visceral form,** involving the spleen, liver, pancreas, intestine, and other internal organs; and (4) the **mixed form,** involving the skin as well as the internal organs and lymphatic system. Initially, the lesion presents a circumscribed ulcer of the gingiva surrounding a tooth, which spreads to other parts of the oral mucosa, producing stomatitis and red-speckled erosions and ulcers. Edema and swelling of the lips, enlargement of the submandibular and cervical lymph nodes, and fistulation usually follow.

Lutz, A. Uma mycose pseudococcidioidica localizada no boca e observada no Brasil. Contribuicao ao conhecimento das hypoblastomycoses americanas. *Impr. Med.,*

Rio, 1908, 16:151-63. Splendore, A. Zimonematosi con localizzazione nella cavita della bocca osservata nel Brasile. *Bull. Soc. Path. Exot., Paris*, 1912, 5:313-9. de Almeida, F. P. Lesoes cutaneas da blastomicose en cabaios experimentalmente infeetados. *An. Fac. Med. S. Paulo*, 1928, 3:59-64.

LUTZ, HENRI CHARLES (French physician)

Lutz-Darier syndrome. See *Darier disease (1).*

LUTZ, WILHELM (Swiss physician, 1888-1958)

Lewandowski-Lutz syndrome. See *under Lewandowski.*

Lutz-Miescher syndrome. Synonyms: *Miescher elastoma, elastoma intrapapillare perforans verruciforme, elastosis perforans serpiginosa (EPS), keratosis follicularis serpiginosa.*

A skin disease, probably genetically transmitted, that affects young males in their twenties more frequently than females. It is characterized by keratotic pale to red papules arranged in an arciform serpiginous pattern and forming a ringed eruption on the posterior or lateral portion of the neck near the hairline. Less frequently, the lesions are located on the extremities. The lesions enlarge by peripheral development of new papules and involute in the center and eventually become atrophic and slightly hypopigmented. Removal of the adherent keratinized caps of the lesions often reveals bleeding craters. The presence of elongated tortuous channels in the epidermis, into which abnormal elastic tissue perforates and is extruded, is the characteristic pathological feature.

Lutz, W. Keratosis follicularis serpiginosa. *Dermatologica, Basel,* 1953, 106:318-20. Miescher, G. Elastoma intrapapillare perforans verruciforme. *Dermatologica, Basel,* 1955, 110:254-66.

LUZET, CHARLES (French physician, born 1863)

Jaksch-Hayem-Luzet syndrome. See *Jaksch syndrome.*

von Jaksch-Luzet syndrome. See *Jaksch syndrome.*

LYELL, ALAN (British dermatologist)

Brocq-Debré-Lyell syndrome. See *toxic epidermal necrolysis.*

Debré-Lamy-Lyell syndrome. See *toxic epidermal necrolysis.*

Lyell syndrome. See *toxic epidermal necrolysis.*

staphylococcal Lyell syndrome. See *staphylococcal scalded skin syndrome.*

staphylogenic Lyell syndrome. See *staphylococcal scalded skin syndrome.*

LYLE, DONALD JOHNSON (American ophthalmologist, born 1895)

Lyle syndrome. Blindness with a normal fundus oculi, due to lesions of the optic radiations and visual cortex or to hysteric disorders.

Lyle, D. J. Diagnosis of visual losses with normal fundus. *Ohio State Med. J.*, 1947, 43:420-1.

Lyme arthritis. See *Lyme disease.*

Lyme borreliosis. See *Lyme disease.*

Lyme disease. Synonyms: *Lyme arthritis, Lyme borreliosis.*

A tickborne spirochetal infectious disease caused by *Borrelia burgdorferi* and characterized mainly by initial erythema, which may be followed by articular, neurological, and cardiac disorders. Erythema chronicum migrans, usually of the thigh, groin, and axilla, is manifested by a red macule or papule at the site of the tick bite, the area of redness expanding until it reaches 3 to 15 cm or more in diameter, usually with a partial central clearing. In a few days there are additional symptoms which occur in descending order of appearance: multiple annular lesions of the skin, lymphadenopathy, pain on neck flexion, malar rash, erythema of the throat, conjunctivitis, tenderness in the right upper quadrant, splenomegaly, hepatomegaly, muscle tenderness, periorbital edema, evanescent skin lesions, abdominal tenderness, and testicular swelling. Other early symptoms may include malaise, headache, fever, chills, stiff neck, arthralgia, myalgias, backache, anorexia, sore throat, nausea, dysesthesia, vomiting, abdominal tenderness, photophobia, stiffness of the hands, dizziness, cough, chest pain, earache, and diarrhea. Some patients develop within several weeks neurologic disorders, which include meningitis, encephalitis, chorea, cranial neuritis, facial palsy, and radiculoneuritis. Cardiac complications may occur in the intermediate stage of disease in a small number of patients, including atrioventricular to complete heart block, myopericarditis, left ventricular dysfunction, and, rarely, cardiomegaly. Arthritis occurs in more than 50% of patients. Violaceous infiltrated plaques or nodules, transverse myelitis, and demyelinating lesions of the central nervous system are the late findings. The condition was first observed in 1977 in a group of children in Lyme, Connecticut, hence its name. See also *Bannwarth syndrome.*

Steere, A. C., *et al.* Lyme arthritis: An epidemic of oligoarticular arthritis in children and adultls in three Connecticut communities. *Arthritis Rheum.*, 1977, 20:7-17. Malawista, S. Lyme disease. In: Wyngaarden, J. B., & Smith, L. H., Jr. eds. Cecil textbook of medicine. 18th ed. Philadelphia, Saunders, 1988, pp. 1726-9.

lymphadenitis nuchalis et cervicalis. See *Piringer-Kuchinka syndrome.*

lymphadenosis benigna cutis. See *Bäfverstedt syndrome.*

lymphedema, early onset type. See *Nonne-Milroy syndrome.*

lymphoblastoma. See *Kundrat disease.*

lymphoblastoma gigantofolliculare. See *Brill-Symmers syndrome.*

lymphocytic meningoradiculitis (MLR). See *Bannwarth syndrome.*

lymphocytic myeloma. See Kahler disease.

lymphocytic radiculomeningitis. See *Bannwarth syndrome.*

lymphocytic reticulosarcoma. See *Kundrat disease.*

lymphocytic thyroiditis. See *Hashimoto disease.*

lymphocytoma. See *Kundrat disease.*

lymphocytoma benignum cutis. See *Bäfverstedt syndrome.*

lymphocytophthisis. See *severe mixed immunodeficiency syndrome.*

lymphogranuloma. See *Hodgkin disease.*

lymphogranuloma inguinale. See *Durand-Nicolas-Favre disease, under Durand, J.*

lymphogranuloma tropicum. See *Durand-Nicolas-Favre disease, under Durand, J.*

lymphogranuloma venereum (LGV). See *Durand-Nicolas-Favre disease, under Durand, J.*

lymphogranulomatosis benigna. See *Besnier-Boeck-Schaumann syndrome.*

lymphogranulomatosis maligna. See *Hodgkin disease.*

lymphoid angiofollicular hyperplasia. See *Castleman disease.*

lymphoma inguinale. See *Durand-Nicolas-Favre disease, under Durand, J.*

lymphomatoid goiter. See *Hashimoto disease.*

lymphomatosis granulomatosa. See *Hodgkin disease.*

lymphomatosis inguinalis suppurativa subacuta. See *Durand-Nicolas-Favre disease, under Durand, J.*

lymphopathia venerea. See *Durand-Nicolas-Favre disease, under Durand, J.*

lymphopenic agammaglobulinemia-short limbed dwarfism syndrome. Synonyms: *ataxia telangiectasia-Swiss type agammaglobulinemia syndrome, Swiss type agammaglobulinemia-achondroplasia syndrome.*

A multiple abnormality syndrome, transmitted as an autosomal recessive trait, characterized by prenatal severe growth deficiency, short and moderately curved limbs with metaphyseal cupping of the radius and ulna, relatively small thorax, short pelvis with large sacrosciatic notch, redundant dyskeratotic and erythematous skin, loss of sparse hair, lymphopenia, agammglobulinemia, and hypoplastic thymus. The symptoms include failure to thrive, repeated episodes of infection, and diarrhea. Bone marrow failure may occur. Most patients die during infancy.

Davis, J. A. A case of Swiss-type agammaglobulinemia and achondroplasia. *Brit. Med. J.,* 1966, 2:1371-4. McKusick, V. A., & Cross, H. E. Ataxia-telangiectasia and Swiss-type agammaglobulinemia. Two genetic disorders of the immune mechanism in related Amish sibships. *JAMA,* 1966, 195:739-45.

lymphoproliferative syndrome, X-linked. See *Wiskott-Aldrich syndrome.*

lymphoreticulosis benigna. See *cat scratch disease.*

lymphosarcoma. See *Kundrat disease.*

LYNCH, HENRY T. (American physician)

Lynch syndrome (I and II). See *under hereditary non-polyposis colorectal cancer syndrome.*

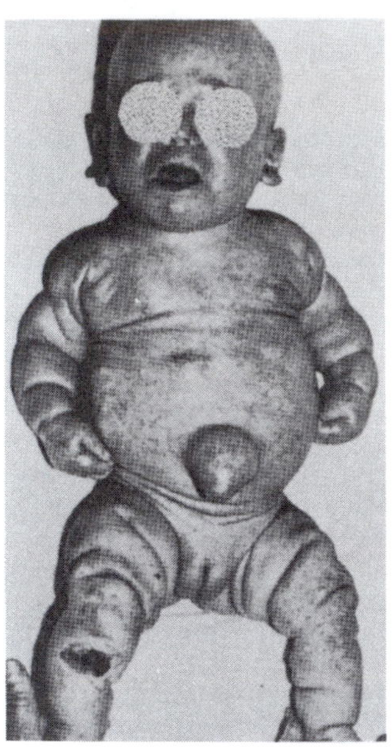

Lymphopenic agammaglobulinemia-short limbed dwarfism syndrome
Gatti, R.A., et al.: *J. Pediatr.* 75:675, 1969. St. Louis: C.V. Mosby Co.

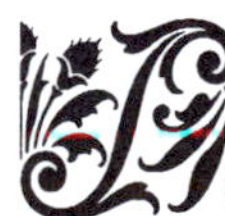

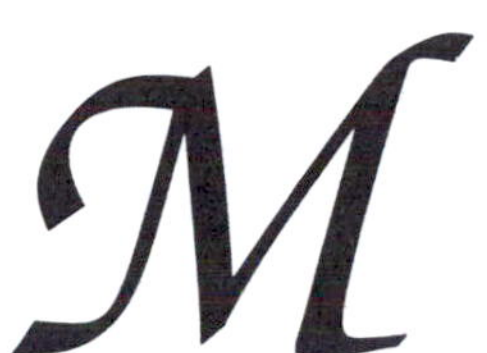

MACH, RENE SIGMUND (Swiss physician, born 1904)

Mach syndrome. Simple adrenal hyperplasia associated with hyperaldosteronism, sodium retention, and edema affecting chiefly the extremities and less frequently the brain, larynx, and eyes.

Mach, R. S., & Müller, A. F. Étude clinique de l'aldostérone. *Schweiz. Med. Wschr.*, 1955, 85:660-1.

MACHACEK

Bloom-Torre-Machacek syndrome. See *Bloom syndrome.*

MACHADO

Machado disease. See *Joseph disease, under Joseph, Antone.*

Machado-Joseph Azorean disease (MJAD). See *Joseph disease, under Joseph, Antone.*

Machado-Joseph disease (MJD). See *Joseph disease, under Joseph, Antone.*

MACKENZIE, SIR STEPHEN (British physician, 1844-1909)

Jackson-MacKenzie syndrome. See *under Jackson, John Hughlings.*

MacKenzie syndrome. See *Jackson-MacKenzie syndrome, under Jackson, John Hughlings.*

MACKLIN, MADGE T. (American physician)

Curth-Macklin syndrome. See *under Ollendorff-Curth, Helene.*

MACLACHLAN, ELSIE A. (American physician)

Lowe-Terrey-MacLachlan syndrome. See *Lowe syndrome.*

MACLENNAN, ALEXANDER (British physician)

MacLennan syndrome. See *Thaysen syndrome.*

MACLEOD, W. M. (British physician)

Macleod syndrome. See *Swyer-James syndrome, under Swyer, Paul Robert.*

Swyer-James-Macleod syndrome. See *Swyer-James syndrome, under Swyer, Paul Robert.*

MACMAHON, H. M. (American physician)

MacMahon-Thannhauser syndrome. See *Hanot-MacMahon-Thannhauser syndrome.*

MACMAHON, HAROLD EDWARD (American physician, born 1901)

Hanot-MacMahon-Thannhauser syndrome. See *under Hanot.*

macrocephaly with feeblemindedness and encephalopathy with peculiar deposits. See *Alexander syndrome, under Alexander, W. Stewart.*

macrocephaly-hamartomas syndrome. See *Bannayan syndrome.*

macrocephaly-pseudopapilledema-hemangiomata syndrome. See *Riley syndrome, under Riley, Harris D., Jr*

macrocytic hemolytic anemia. See *Dyke-Young syndrome.*

macrodactyly-hemihypertrophy-connective tissue nevi syndrome. A congenital syndrome of unknown etiology, characterized by bilateral macrodactyly of the feet, especially of the third, fourth, and fifth toes; asymmetry of the face and arm, one side of the face being overgrown and one forearm and hand being short and stubby; macrocephaly; and systemic pigmented nevi and subcutaneous hemangiomas and lymphangiomas. Associated anomalies include slight facial hemiparesis, unilateral amblyopia with ipsilateral convergent strabismus, and low-set dysplastic ears.

Temtamy, S. A., & Rogers, J. G. Macrodactyly, hemihypertrophy, and connective tissue nevi: Report of a new syndrome and review of the literature. *J. Pediat.*, 1976, 89:924.

macrofollicular lymphoblastoma. See *Brill-Symmers syndrome.*

macrogenitosomia praecox. See *congenital adrenal hyperplasia and see Pellizzi syndrome.*

macroglobulinemia syndrome. See *Waldenström macroglobulinemia, under Waldenström, Jan Gösta.*

macroglobulinemia-neuropsychiatric syndrome. See *Bing-Neel syndrome, under Bing, Jens.*

macroglobulinemic splenomegaly. See *Charmot syndrome.*

macroglossia-omphalocele syndrome. See *Beckwith-Wiedemann syndrome.*

macroglossia-omphalocele-visceromegaly syndrome. See *Beckwith-Wiedemann syndrome.*

macro-orchidism marker X (MOMX) chromosome syndrome. See *chromosome X fragility.*

MACS (medical antishock trousers [MAST]-associated compartment syndrome). See *under compartment syndrome.*

macula halo syndrome. A variant of the Niemann-Pick syndrome characterized by sphingomyelinase deficiency and a ring-form opacity about the foveolas. A secondary hyperlipidemia may also be present. The halos consist of symmetric crystalloid opacities with little or no visual impairment.

Cogan, D. G., *et al.* Macula halo syndrome. Variant of Niemann-Pick disease. *Arch. Ophth.*, 1983, 101:1698-1700.

macular corneal dystrophy. See *Groenouw dystrophy (2).*

macular keratitis. See *Sanders syndrome.*

maculopapular erythrodermia. See *Jadassohn disease (1), under Jadassohn, Josef.*

MADAME FREY. See FREY, LUCIE

MADELUNG, OTTO WILHELM (Surgeon in Strasbourg, 1846-1926)

Madelung deformity. Synonyms: *Madelung subluxation, carpus carvus, manus valga.*

A developmental abnormality of the wrist marked by its displacement by partial fusion of the ulnar side of the radial epiphyses. Onset is usually between 8 and 14 years of age. Disorders associated with this condition include dyschondrosteosis, enchondromatosis, multiple exostoses, Turner syndrome, and susceptibility to trauma.

Madelung. Die spontane Subluxation der Hand nach vorne. *Verh. Deut Ges. Chir.*, 1878, 7:259-76.

Madelung lipoma. See *Madelung syndrome.*

Madelung neck. See *Madelung syndrome.*

Madelung sublaxation. See *Madelung deformity.*

Madelung syndrome. Synonyms: *Buschke disease, Launois-Bensaude syndrome, Madelung lipoma, Madelung neck, Madelung-Launois-Bensaude syndrome, benign symmetrical lipomatosis, cervical lipomatosis, fatty neck, lipomata diffusa symmetrica, lipomatosis diffusa symmetrica, multiple symmetrical lipomatosis, symmetric lipomatosis, symmetric neck lipoma, symmetrical adenolipomatosis.*

Multiple, diffuse, symmetrical lipomata of the neck, sometimes spreading toward the scrotal region and causing vascular compression and tracheal and bronchial obstruction. The disorder may occur as a complication of excessive alcohol consumption.

Madelung, O. Über den Fetthals (diffuses Lipom des Halses). *Arch. Klin. Chir., Berlin*, 1888, 37:106-30. Buschke, A., & Casper, W. Die traumatische Ätiologie und die Begutachtung der symmetrischen Lipomatose. *Klin. Wschr.*, 1929, 8:880-3.

Madelung-Launois-Bensaude syndrome. See *Madelung syndrome.*

Marfan-Madelung symptom complex. See *Marfan-Madelung syndrome.*

Marfan-Madelung syndrome. See *under Marfan.*

madura foot. See *Ballingall disease.*

maduromycosis. See *Ballingall disease.*

MAEDER, G. (Swiss ophthalmologist)

Maeder-Danis dystrophy. Synonyms: *dystrophia filiformis profunda corneae, filiform corneal dystrophy.*

Bilateral corneal dystrophy characterized by corkscrew filaments in the deep layers in front of the Descemet membranes, seen in keratoconus.

Maeder, G., & Danis, P. Sur une nouvelle forme de dystrophie cornéenne (dystrophia filiformis profunda corneae) associée à un kératocône. *Ophthalmologica, Basel*, 1947, 114:246-8.

MAESTRE DE SAN JUAN, A. (Spanish physician)

Maestre de San Juan-Kallmann syndrome. See *olfactogenital syndrome.*

Maestre de San Juan-Kallmann-de Morsier syndrome. See *olfactogenital syndrome.*

Maestre-Kallmann-de Morsier syndrome. See *olfactogenital syndrome.*

MAFFUCCI, ANGELO (Italian pathologist, 1845-1903)

Maffucci syndrome (MS). Synonyms: *Kast syndrome, Maffuci-Kast syndrome, chondrodysplasia-angiomatosis syndrome, chondrodysplasia-hemangioma syndrome, chondrodystrophy with angiomatosis, chondrodystrophy with vascular hamartoma, cutaneous dyschondroplasia-dyschromia syndrome, dyschondroplasia with hemangioma, dyschondroplasia-angiomatosis syndrome, enchondromatosis with hemangiomata.*

An association of vascular lesions (angiomata) with osseous defects (Ollier syndrome or dyschondroplasia), consisting of multiple angiomas, phleboliths, phleboctasia, dyschondroplasia, chondromata, fractures, and other disorders of nonossified cartilage in the metaphyses and diaphyses of the long bones. Most cases are sporadic, but some instances of familial occurrence have been reported.

Maffucci, A. Di un caso encondroma ed angioma multiple *Mov. Med. Chir.*, 1881, 3:399. Kast, & Recklinghausen, Ein fall von Enchondrom mit ungewöhnlicher Multiplikation. *Virchows Arch. Path.*, 1889, 118:1-18.

Maffucci-Kast syndrome. See *Maffucci syndrome.*

MAGATH, THOMAS B. (American physician)

Horton-Magath-Brown syndrome. See *Horton disease (1).*

MAGEE, KENNETH RAYMOND (American physician, born 1926)

Shy-Magee syndrome. See *under Shy.*

MAGENDANTZ, HEINZ (American physician, born 1899)

Thannhauser-Magendantz syndrome. See *Hanot-MacMahon-Thannhauser syndrome.*

MAGENDIE, FRANÇOIS (French physiologist, 1783-1855)

Hertwig-Magendie syndrome. See *under Hertwig, Richard.*

MAGOSS, I. V. (American physician)

Magoss-Walshe syndrome. Synonym: *pre-aortic left renal vein compression syndrome.*

Pre-aortic left renal vein compression by the aorta.

Hu, K. N., Mogoss, I. V., Gerbasi, J. R., Mepani, B. P., & Walshe, J. J. Pre-aortic left renal vein compression syndrome (Magoss and Walshe syndrome). *Internat. Urol. Nephrol.*, 1984, 16:101-7.

MAGRASSI, FLAVIANO (Italian physician, born 1908)

Magrassi-Leonardi pneumonia. See *Magrassi-Leonardi syndrome.*

Magrassi-Leonardi syndrome. Synonyms: *Magrassi-Leonardi pneumonia, eosinophilic-monocytic fever, febris eosinophilica monocytaria.*

Eosinophilic pneumopathy characterized by the presence of monocytic and histiocytic cells in the blood, followed by eosinophilia. The severe form is marked by pleural and pulmonary lesions, cough, and other symptoms suggesting primary atypical pneumonia. In the febrile form, the symptoms include fever, severe malaise, asthenia, myalgia, and cough, which persist for 2 to 3 days. The abortive form is marked by severe symptoms, but there is no fever. A viral etiology was suggested by Magrassi and Leonardi. See also *pulmonary infiltration with eosinophilia syndrome, Löffler disease, Kartagener disease,* and *Löhr-Kindberg syndrome.*

Magrassi, F., & Leonardi, G. Identificazione di una nuova entitá nosologica ad eziologia infettiva; la febbre eosinofilo-monocitaria. Contributo allo studio del problema eziologico della polmonite atipica primaria. *Clinica Nuova*, 1947, 5:177-206.

MAIER, RUDOLF (German physician, 1824-1888)

Kussmaul-Maier syndrome. See *under Kussmaul.*

main en lorgnette. See *Marie-Léri syndrome, under Marie, Pierre.*

MAINZER, FRANK (American radiologist)

Saldino-Mainzer syndrome. See *under Saldino.*

MAIXNER, EMMERICH (Austrian physician, 1847-1920)

Maixner cirrhosis. Synonym: *cirrhosis gastroenterorrhagica seu hemorrhagica.*

A hemorrhagic form of cirrhosis of the liver.

Maixner, E. Über die hämorrhagische Form der Lebercirrhose. *Wien. Med. Wschr.*, 1902, 52:1521-5; passim.

MAJEWSKI, F. (German physician)

Lenz-Majewski hyperostotic dwarfism. See *Lenz-Majewski syndrome.*

Lenz-Majewski syndrome. See *under Lenz.*

Majewski syndrome. Synonyms: *polydactyly with neonatal chondrodystrophy type I; short rib-polydactyly syndrome type I (SRP I); short rib-polydactyly syndrome, Majewski type.*

A lethal form of short-limb dwarfism characterized by a narrow thorax, pre- and/or postaxial polysyndactyly, multiple visceral anomalies, and disproportionately short tibiae. Associated anomalies include protruding abdomen, brachydactyly, peculiar facies (short and flat nose, low-set and malformed ears, and cleft lip and palate), hypoplastic epiglottis, cardiovascular defects (mostly transposition of the great vessels), renal cysts, and genital anomalies. Death takes place shortly after birth. The etiology is unknown.

Majewski, F., *et al.* Polysyndaktylie, verkürzte Gledmassen und Cenitalfehlbildungen: Kennzeichen eines selbstandingen Syndroms? *Zschr. Kinderheilk.*, 1971, 111:118-38.

short rib-polydactyly syndrome, Majewski type. See *Majewski syndrome.*

MAJOCCHI, DOMENICO (Italian physician, 1849-1929)

Majocchi disease. Synonyms: *Majocchi purpura, Majocchi syndrome, purpura annularis, purpura annularis telangiectodes, telangiectasia follicularis annulata.*

A skin disease characterized by purpuric, telangiectatic, and atrophic eruptions that are symmetrical and usually limited to the lower limbs. The initial lesions are annular clusters of capillary dilatations which may thrombose, rupture, and hemorrhage, producing pigmented areas. In the final stage, lesions show central necrosis, scarring, and atrophy with loss of hair. Histological findings include vasculitis in the upper corium, hyalinization of the blood vessels, and inflammatory reactions.

Majocchi, D. Sopra una dermatose telangettode non ancora descritta "purpura annularis," "telangectasia follicularis annulata"; studio clinico. *Gior. Ital. Mal. Vener.*, 1896, 37:242-50.

Majocchi purpura. See *Majocchi disease.*

Majocchi syndrome. See *Majocchi disease.*

MAKAI, ENDRE (Hungarian physician)

Rothmann-Makai panniculitis. See *Rothmann-Makai syndrome.*

Rothmann-Makai syndrome. See *under Rothmann.*

MAKI, Y. (Japanese physician)

Maki syndrome. See *moyamoya syndrome.*

mal de Meleda. Synonym: *keratosis palmoplantaris transgradiens.*

A rare skin disease, transmitted as an autosomal recessive trait, reported in inhabitants of the Adriatic island of Meleda in Yugoslavia, characterized by congenital symmetrical hyperkeratosis palmaris et plantaris and ichthyotic lesions on other parts of the body. The lesions are present at birth or shortly thereafter, and are marked by initial redness followed by hyperkeratosis which spreads to the dorsal surfaces of the hands and feet. Erythematous lesions of the axillary and groin regions are associated. Hyperhidrosis, perioral erythema, and lichnoid plaques may be observed in some cases. See also *Papillon-Lefèvre syndrome.*

Hvorka, O., & Ehlers, E. Mal de Meleda. *Brit. J. Derm.*, 1897, 9:416.

malabsorption syndrome. Faulty absorption of fats, proteins, carbohydrates, minerals, and vitamins by the intestine and loss of essential nutrients in the stools, with resulting wide variety of symptoms. See also *celiac disease*, and see *vitamin E deficiency syndrome.*

Gray, G. M. Maldigestion and malabsorption: Clinical manifestations and specific diagnosis. In: Sleisenger, M. H., & Fordtran, J. S. *Gastrointestinal disease. Pathophysiology, diagnosis, management.* 3rd ed. Philadelphia, Saunders, 1983, pp. 228-56.

malabsorption-pancreatic insuficiency syndrome. See *Shwachman syndrome.*

MALAMUT, GEORGES (French pediatrician)

Maroteaux-Malamut syndrome. See *acrodysostosis.*

MALAN, EDMOND (American physician)

Malan syndrome. A circulatory disorder of the leg and foot due to dilation of the arteriovenous anastomosis in the sole of the foot with shunting of the blood and damage of the contiguous vascular areas.

Malan, E. Vascular syndrome from dilatation of arteriovenous communications of the sole of the foot. *Arch. Surg., Chicago*, 1958, 77:783-95.

MALASSEZ, LOUIS CHARLES (French physician, 1842-1909)

Malassez disease. A testicular cyst.

Malassez, L. C. Note sur un cas de maladie kystique du testicule. *Arch. Physiol., Paris*, 1875, 2:122-35.

male pseudohermaphroditism-nephritis-Wilms tumor syndrome. See *Drash syndrome.*

male Turner syndrome. See *Noonan syndrome.*

male XX syndrome. See *chromosome XX syndrome.*

MALHERBE, ALBERT (French physician, 1845-1915)

Malherbe epithelioma. Synonyms: *Malherbe-Chenantais epithelioma, benign calcifying epithelioma, epithelioma calcificans, pilomatrixoma.*

A disease of the skin, transmitted as an autosomal dominant trait, presenting sharply defined, firm, benign tumors of the face, neck, or arms. A typical lesion is enclosed in a fibrous capsule, is situated deeply in the dermis , and is covered by normal skin, with varying degrees of erythema and discoloration overlying the tumor area. Aggregates of darkly staining cells, foreign body giant-cell reaction, calcification, and occasional ossification of calcified patches are the principal pathological features.

Malherbe, A., & Chenantais, J., fils. Note sur l'épitheliome calcifié des glandes sébacées. *Progr. Méd., Paris*, 1880, 8:826-8.

MALABSORPTION SYNDROME

	PHYSIOLOGIC PATHOLOGY	CLINICAL FEATURES
Diseases of Maldigestion		
Gastic resection with gastrojejunostomy	Decreased pancreatic stimulation because of duodenal bypass. Poor mixing of food, bile, pancreatic enzymes. Decreased intrinsic factor. Bacterial stasis in afferent loop	Weight loss, moderate steatorrhea, anemia (combination of iron, B_{12} malabsorption, folate deficiency)
Pancreatic insufficiency (chronic pancreatitis, pancreatic carcinoma, pancreatic resection, cystic fibrosis)	Reduced intraluminal pancreatic enzyme activity with maldigestion of lipid and protein	History of abdominal pain followed by weight loss. Marked steatorrhea, azotorrhea. Also frequent glucose intolerance (70% in pancreatic insufficiency)
Short gut syndrome. Post-surgical resection or bypass. Crohn's enteritis	Loss of ileal absorbing surface leads to reduced bile salt pool size and reduced vitamin B_{12}	Weight loss, steatorrhea. Abnormal Schilling test, low D-xylose absorption
Bacterial overgrowth syndrome (surgical strictures, blind loops enteric fistulas, multiple jejunal diverticula, scleroderma)	Overgrowth of intraluminal bacteria in jejunum, especially anaerobic organisms, to greater than 10^9/ml, results in deconjugation of bile salts, decreased effective bile pool size; also bacterical unilization of vitamin B_{12}	Weight loss, steatorrhea, Abnormal Schilling test, low D-xylose absorption
Zollinger-Ellison syndrome	Hyperacidity in duodenum inactivates pancreatic enzymes	Ulcer diathesis, steatorrhea
Lactose intolerance	Deficiency of intestinal lactase results in high concentrations of intraluminal lactose with osmotic diarrhea	Affects 70% of U.S. blacks and probably all other noncaucasian races. Varied degrees of diarrhea and cramps after ingestion of lactose-containing foods. Positive lactose tolerance test, decrease intestinal lactase
Diseases of Mucosal Malabsorption		
Celiac disease (glutensensitive enteropathy)	Toxic response to a gluten fraction by surface epithelium results in destruction of absorbing surface	Weight loss, diarrhea, bloating, anemia (low folate, iron), osteomalacia, steatorrhea, azotorrhea, low D-xylose absorption. Flat intestinal biopsy. Responds to gluten restriction
Tropical sprue	Unknown toxic factor results in mucosal inflammation, partial villous atrophy	Weight loss, diarrhea, anemia, (low folate, B_{12}). Steatorrhea. Low D-xylose absorption, abnormal Schilling test. Typical but nonspecific biopsy change
Whipple's disease	Bacterial invasion of intestinal mucosa	Arthritis, hyperpigmentation, lymphadenopathy, serious effusions, fever, weight loss. Steatorrhea, azotorrhea, diagnostic biopsy
Certain parasitic diseases (giardiasis strongyloides, coccidiosis, capillariasis)	Damage to or invasion of surface mucosa	Diarrhea, weight loss, steatorrhea. Organism may be seen on jejunal biopsy or recovered in stool
Immunoglobulinopathy	Decreased local gut defenses, lymphoid hyperplasia, lymphopenia	Frequent association with giardiasis. Hyogammaglobulinemia or isolated IgA deficiency. Diagnostic or typical biopsy changes

From Halsted, C.H., and Halsted, J.A., The Laboratory in Clinical Medicine. 2nd ed. Philadelphia, W.B. Saunders Co., 1981, p. 230.

Malabsorption syndrome
Gray, G.M.: Maldigestion and Malabsorption: Clinical Manifestations and Specific Diagnosis. In Sleisenger, M.H. & J.S. Fordtran: *Gastrointestinal Disease, Pathophysiology, Diagnosis, Management.* 3rd ed. Philadelphia: W.B. Saunders, 1983.

Causes of intestinal bacterial overgrowth (intestinal colonization)

I. Structural abnormalities producing stasis of intestinal contents
  A. Multiple small-bowel diverticula
  B. Strictures
    1. Regional enteritis
    2. Radiation enteritis
    3. Occlusive vascular disease; vasculitis
  C. Billroth II subtotal gastrectomy with afferent loop stasis
  D. Multiple laparotomies resulting in adhesions and partial small-bowel obstruction
II. Fistulas
  A. Gastrocolic, gastroileal, jejunoileal, jejunocolic
III. Motor abnormalities resulting in intestinal hypomotility
  A. Scleroderma
  B. Amyloidosis
  C. Diabetes mellitus
  D. Hypothyroidism
  E. Vagotomy
  F. Intestinal pseudoobstruction
IV. Miscellaneous
  A. Hypogammaglobulinemia
  B. Nodular lymphoid hyperplasia
  C. Pernicious anemia
  D. Pancreatic insufficiency
V. No underlying disorder detected

* *Multiple mechanisms may contribute to malabsorption in these disorders*

Malabsorption syndrome
Braunwald, E., K.J. Isselbacher, R.G. Petersdorf, R.G. Wilson, J.D. Martin, & A.S. Fauci: *Harrison's Principles of Internal Medicine.* 11th ed. New York: McGraw-Hill, 1987.

Malherbe-Chenantais epithelioma. See *Malherbe epithelioma.*
malignant angina. See *Bretonneau disease.*
malignant atrophic papulosis. See *Degos syndrome.*
malignant carcinoid syndrome. See *carcinoid syndrome.*
malignant erythroblastosis. See *Di Guglielmo disease (1).*
malignant fever syndrome. See *malignant hyperpyrexia syndrome.*
malignant granuloma. See *Wegener granulomatosis.*
malignant granulomytous angitis. See *Wegener granulomatosis.*
malignant hypernephroma. See *Hutchinson disease, under Hutchinson, Sir Robert Grieve.*

malignant hyperpyrexia (MH) syndrome. Synonyms: *Ombrédanne syndome, malignant fever syndrome, malignant hyperthermia syndrome, pallor-hyperthermia syndrome, postoperative pallor-hyperthermia syndrome.*

A hypermetabolic, frequently fatal syndrome in susceptible individuals, which is precipitated by depolarizing muscle relaxants (such as succinylcholine), inhalation of anesthetic agents (usually halothane), and various stressing factors. Stiffening of the muscles, rise of body temperature, metabolic acidosis caused by lactic acidemia, and occasional myoglobinuria and renal failure are the principal features of this syndrome. The etiology is unknown, but an inability to control muscle calcium metabolism is suspected as one of the factors. Most cases are sporadic, but inheritance as an autosomal dominant trait occurs in some instances. When associated with multiple abnormalities, the condition is known as the *King syndrome.*

Denborough, M. A., *et al.* Anaesthetic deaths in a family. *Brit. Anaesth.*, 1962, 34:395-6. Ombrédanne, L. De l'influence de l'anesthésique employé dans la genèse des accidents post-opératoires de pâleur-hyperthermie observés chez les nourrissons. *Rev. Méd. Fr.*, 1929, p. 617.

malignant hyperthermia syndrome. See *malignant hyperpyrexia syndrome.*
malignant hyperthermia-myopathy-multiple anomalies syndrome. See *King syndrome.*
malignant lymphogranuloma. See *Hodgkin disease.*
malignant lymphogranulomatosis. See *Hokgkin disease.*
malignant lymphoma. See *Hodgkin disease.*
malignant malnutrition. See *kwashiorkor.*
malignant neuroleptic syndrome. See *neuroleptic malignant syndrome.*
malignant osteosclerosis. See *osteopetrosis with precocious manifestations syndrome.*
malignant papulosis atrophicans. See *Degos syndrome.*
malignant papulosis with atrophy. See *Degos syndrome.*
malignant reticulosis. See *Letterer-Siwe syndrome.*
MALLORY, FRANK BURR (American pathologist, 1862-1941)
Mosse-Marchand-Mallory cirrhosis. See *under Mosse, Alphonse.*
MALLORY, GEORGE KENNETH (American physician, born 1900)
Mallory-Weiss syndrome. Synonyms: *gastroesophageal laceration syndrome, gastroesophageal laceration-hemorrhage syndrome, retching erosion syndrome.*

Massive, painless, and occasionally fatal gastric hemorrhage with hematemesis due to laceration of the gastroesophageal junction, which may develop after severe alcoholic intoxication or as a consequence of malignant tumors, pernicious vomiting of pregnancy, or other diseases. Mallory and Weiss suggested a possible etiologic role of pressure changes in the stomach during the disturbed mechanism of vomiting, together with continuous regurgitation of gastric juice and the local irritant and astringent effects of alcohol, as well as the nature of vascularity of the mucosa.

Mallory, G. K., & Weiss, S. Hemorrhages from lacerations of the cardiac orifice of the stomach due to vomiting. *Am. J. Med. Sc.*, 1929, 178:506-15.

malocclusion-short stature syndrome. A familial syndrome, transmitted as an autosomal recessive trait, characterized mainly by open-bite malocclusion, short stature, and triangular face.

Say, B., *et al.* A familial syndrome of unusual facies with malocclusion and short stature. *Humangenetik*, 1973, 18:279-82.

malpractice stress syndrome. See *battered doctor syndrome.*

Malta fever. See *brucellosis.*

maltreatment syndrome of children. See *battered child syndrome.*

malum cotunnii. See *Cotugno syndrome.*

malum coxae. See *Calvé-Legg-Perthes syndrome.*

malum epiphyseonecroticum vertebrale. See *Scheuermann disease.*

malum rusti. See *Rust disease.*

malum suboccipitale. See *Rust disease.*

malum vertebrale suboccipitale. See *Rust disease.*

mammary Paget disease. See *under Paget.*

MAMOU, HENRI (French physician)

Siegal-Cattan-Mamou disease. See *Reimann periodic disease.*

Manchurian hemorrhagic fever. See *hemorrhagic fever with renal syndrome.*

mandibular dysostosis and peromelia. See *Hanhart syndrome (2).*

mandibulo-acral dysplasia. See *craniomandibular dermatodysostosis.*

mandibulo-oculofacial dyscephaly. See *Hallermann-Streiff syndrome.*

mandibulo-oculofacial dysmorphism. See *Hallermann-Streiff syndrome.*

mandibulofacial dysmorphia. See *Hallermann-Streiff syndrome.*

mandibulofacial dysostosis (MFD). Synonyms: *Berry syndrome, Berry-Treacher Collins syndrome, Franceschetti syndrome, Franceschetti-Zwahlen syndrome, Franceschetti-Zwahlen-Klein syndrome, Thomson complex, Treacher Collins syndrome, Zwahlen syndrome, bilateral facial agenesis, mandibulofacial syndrome.*

A congenital syndrome, transmitted as an autosomal dominant trait with variable expressivity, largely involving structures derived from the first branchial arch, groove, and pouch. Facial characteristics consist of fishlike facies with antimongoloid slant of the palpebral fissures, hypoplasia of the malar bones and mandible, macrostomia, high palate, blind fistulae between the angles of the mouth and ear, low-set small ears, and prolongation of the hairline on the cheek. Deafness, absence or deformities of the external auditory meatus, sclerosis of the middle ear and, less commonly, inner ear, and other ear abnormalities are usually associated. The nasofrontal angle is usually obliterated and the bridge of the nose raised. Mental retardation occurs in some cases.

Collins, E. T. Case with symmetrical congenital notches in the outer part of each lower lid and defective development of the malar bones. *Tr. Ophth. Soc. U. K.*, 1900, 20:190-2. Berry, G. A. Note on a congenital defect (coloboma?) of the lower lid. *Roy. London Ophth. Hosp. Rep.*, 1889, 12:255-7. Franceschetti, A., & Zwahlen. P. Un syndrome nouveau: De la dysostose mandibulofaciale. *Bull. Schweiz. Akad. Wiss.*, 1944, p. 60-6. Franceschetti, A., & Klein, D. The mandibulo-facial dysostosis. A new hereditary syndrome. *Acta Ophth., Copenhagen*, 1949, 27:143-224. *Thomson, A. Notice of several cases of malformation of the external ear, together with experiments on the state of hearing in such persons. *Monthly J. Med. Sc.*, 1846-47, 7:420.

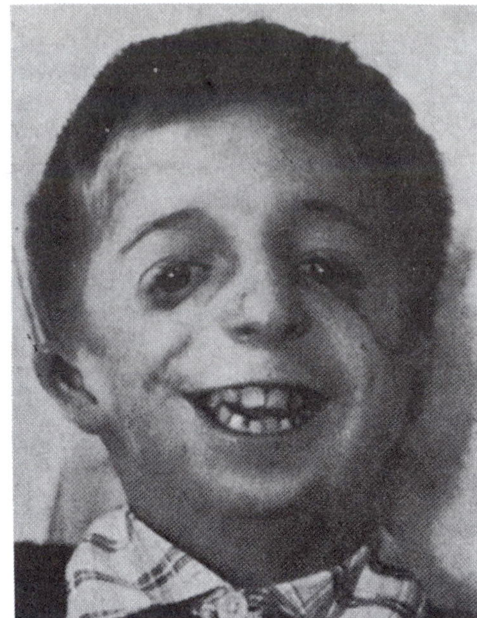

Mandibulofacial dysostosis
Franceschetti, A. & D. Klein, *Acta Ophthalmologica*, 1949, 27 :144. Scriptor Publisher ApS, Copenhagen, Denmark.

mandibulofacial dysostosis with epibulbar dermoids syndrome. See *oculo-auriculovertebral dysplasia.*

mandibulofacial dysostosis with limb malformations syndrome. See *Nager-de Reynier syndrome.*

mandibulofacial syndrome. See *mandibulofacial dysostosis.*

MANKOVSKII (MANKOWSKY), BORIS NIKITICH (Russian physician, 1883-1962)

Mankowsky syndrome. Synonym: *familial dysplastic osteopathy.*

A familial disorder characterized by clubbing of the fingers and toes secondary to various chronic diseases, such as suppurative pulmonary diseases, cardiovascular disorders, and malignant mediastinal tumors. See also *Marie-Bamberger syndrome,* under *Marie, Pierre.*

Mankowsky, B. N., *et al.* Osteopathia dysplastica familiaris (Zur Genese des Syndroms Marie-Bamberger). *Forschr. Geb. Röntgen.*, 1934, 50:542-9.

MANKOWSKY, BORIS NIKITICH. See MANKOVSKII, BORIS NIKITICH

MANN, LUDWIG (German physician, 1866-1936)

Mann syndrome. Contusion of the brain accompanied by generalized coordination disorders characterized by restricted movement of the eye to one side, unsteadiness and swaying of the body toward the damaged side on standing erect with the eyes closed, and difficulty in pointing and in outward turning of the foot on the side of the lesion; increased cerebrospinal fluid pressure; vasomotor hyperexcitability; unilateral diminished corneal and nasal reflexes; deafness; and limpness and hanging of the arm.

Mann, L. Über ein häufig zu beobachtendes Syndrom bei Commotio bzw. Contusio cerebri. *Deut. Med. Wschr.*, 1931, 57:2172-5.

Wernicke-Mann hemiplegia. See *under Wernicke.*

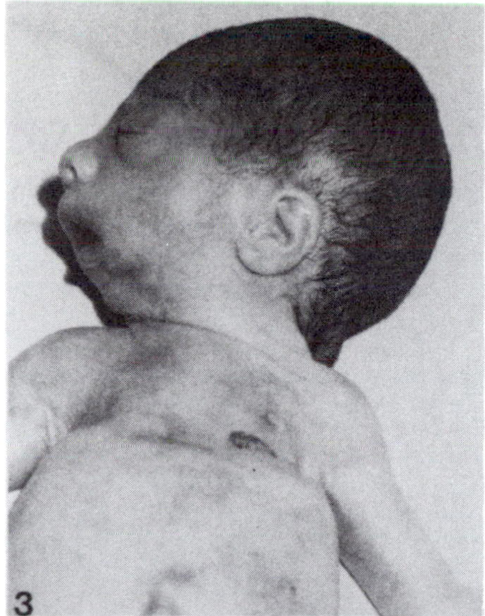

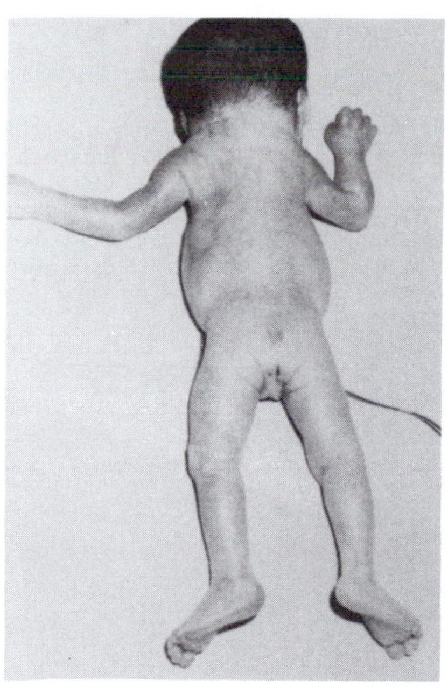

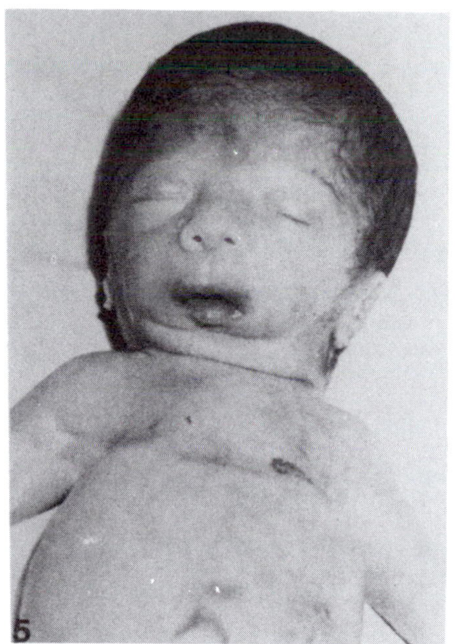

Mandibularfacial dysostosis
Merlob, Paul, Alex Schonfeld, Michael Grunebaum, Naomi Mor & Salomon H. Reisner. *American Journal of Medical Genetics* 26:195- 202, 1987. New York: Alan R. Liss, Inc.

Wernicke-Mann paralysis. See *Wernicke-Mann hemiplegia.*
manus valga. See *Madelung deformity.*
MANZKE, H.
Catel-Manzke syndrome. See *palatodigital syndrome.*
maple syrup urine disease (MSUD). Synonyms: *Menkes disease, branched chain alpha-keto acid dehydrogenase (BCKD) deficiency, branched chain ketoaciduria, keto acid decarboxylase deficiency, leucinosis, maple syrup urine syndrome.*

A hereditary amino acid metabolic disorder, transmitted as an autosomal recessive trait, characterized by deficient activity in the oxidative decarboxylation pathway of leucine, isoleucine, valine, and the corresponding keto acids in body fluids, thus causing the urine to have the odor of maple sypup (hence the name of the disorder). Severe hypotonia, lethargy, feeding difficulty, and hypoglycemia appear in apparently normal infants during the first week of life. Convulsions and decorticate rigidity follow. Most untreated infants die within 1 year.

Menkes, J. H., *et al.* A new syndrome: Progressive familial infantile cerebral dysfunction associated with an unusual urinary substance. *Pediatrics,* 1954, 14:462-6.

maple syrup urine syndrome. See *maple syrup urine disease.*
maplike epithelial dystrophy. See *Cogan dystrophy.*
mar(X) syndrome. See *chromosome X fragility.*

MARAÑON, GREGORIO (Spanish physician, 1887-1960)

Marañón lipomatosis. Synonym: *pseudomuscular hypertrophic lipomatosis.*

Generalized symmetrical lipomas of the muscles, giving the physique of affected persons a wrestlerlike appearance, reportedly described by Marañón.

Marañón syndrome (1). Adiposity, thyrotoxicosis, and fever, often associated with exophthalmos, restlessness, fatigability, and headache, and with leukocytosis and increased erythrocyte sedimentation rate.

Marañón, G. El síndrome adiposidad-Basedow-distermia (A.B.D.). *Med. Españ.*, 1953, 30:509-16.

Marañón syndrome (2). Gynecomastia associated with testicular hypertrophy.

Marañón, G., *et al.* Contribución casuistica al síndrome ambihipergenital (hipertesticulismo con ginecomastia). *Bol. Inst. Pat. Med., Madrid*, 1957, 12:237-40.

Marañón syndrome (3). Ovarian insufficiency associated with severe pain and bone disorders (flatfoot, scoliosis, and other spinal complications).

Marañón, G. Syndrome osteomusculaire douloureux de l'insuffisance ovarique juvénile. *Paris Méd.*, 1930, 1:414-9.

marasmic kwashiorkor. See *kwashiorkor-marasmus syndrome.*

marasmus. See *marasmus syndrome.*

marasmus infantilis. See *marasmus syndrome.*

marasmus lactantium. See *marasmus syndrome.*

marasmus syndrome. Synonyms: *Parrot atrophy, athrepsia, infantile atrophy, marasmus infantilis, marasmus lactantium, pedatrophy, primary infantile atrophy.*

A nutritional deficiency in infants caused by an indadequate food intake, chronic diarrhea, or prolonged negative energy balance. It is characterized by progressive wasting, emaciation, stunted growth, atrophy of muscle and subcutaneous fat, dry skin with decreased turgor, dull appearance, sparse dry hair, and moderate irritability. Edema is usually absent. Pulse, blood pressure, and body temperature may be low. Diarrhea may be associated, but bowel action is generally decreased. When occuring with protein deficiency, the condition is known as the *kwashiorkor-marasmus syndrome.*

Parrot, J. M. *L'athrepsie*, Paris, Masson, 1877.

marble bone disease. See *osteopetrosis with precocious manifestations syndrome.*

marble bone disease. See *Albers-Schönberg syndrome.*

marble bone disease. See *Guibaud-Vainsel syndrome.*

marble disease. See *Albers-Schönberg syndrome.*

march foot. See *Deutschländer disease.*

MARCHAND

Gérard-Marchand fracture. See *under Gérard.*

MARCHAND, FELIX JACOB (German physician, 1846-1928)

Marchand-Waterhouse-Friderichsen syndrome. See *Waterhouse-Friderichsen syndrome.*

Mosse-Marchand-Mallory cirrhosis. See *under Mosse, Alphonse.*

MARCHESANI, OSWALD (German ophthalmologist, 1900-1952)

Marchesani syndrome. See *Weill-Marchesani syndrome, under Weill, Georges.*

Weill-Marchesani syndrome. See *under Weill, Georges.*

MARCHIAFAVA, ETTORE (Italian physician, 1847-1935)

Marchiafava disease. See *Marchiafava-Bignami syndrome.*

Marchiafava hemolytic anemia. See *Marchiafava-Micheli syndrome.*

Marchiafava syndrome. See *Marchiafava-Micheli syndrome.*

Marchiafava-Bignami disease (MBD). See *Marchiafava-Bignami syndrome.*

Marchiafava-Bignami syndrome. Synonyms: *Marchiafava disease, Marchiafava-Bignami disease (MBD), callosal demyelinating encephalopathy, corpus callosum degeneration, primary degeneration of the corpus callosum, progressive alcoholic dementia.*

A neurological disease affecting most frequently adult and middle-aged alcoholic males, also affecting some nonalcoholic subjects. The symptoms vary in severity and type, consisting mainly of nonspecific dementia with manic, paranoid, and delusional states, hallucinosis, delirium, depression, apathy, and disorders similar to those seen in the alcohol withdrawal syndrome (see under *withdrawal syndrome*). Seizures, aphasia, transitory hemiparesis, incontinence, gait abnormalities, and other motor disorders may be associated. Emotional disorders may include acts of violence, moral perversion, and sexual misdemeanors. In its terminal phase, the syndrome is marked by seizures, stupor, and coma. Pathological findings show necrosis of the medial zone of the corpus callosum, with the dorsal and ventral rims being spared. Damage ranges from softening to cavitation and cyst formation. The anterior and posterior commisures, centrum semiovale, subcortical white matter, long association bundles, and middle cerebral peduncles may also be affected. Malnutrition and alcoholism are the suspected causes of this disease, but the pathogenesis is unclear.

Marchiafava, E., & Bignami, A. Sopra un alterazione del corpo calloso osservato da sogetti alcolisti. *Riv. Pat. Nerv.*, 1903, 8:544-9.

Marchiafava-Micheli anemia. See *Marchiafava-Micheli syndrome.*

Marchiafava-Micheli syndrome. Synonyms: *Marchiafava hemolytic anemia, Marchiafava syndrome, Marchiafava-Micheli anemia, Strübing-Marchiafava syndrome, paroxysmal nocturnal hemoglobinuria.*

A rare blood disorder, occurring in both sexes, usually in the third decade of life, marked by chronic hemolytic anemia with attacks of nocturnal paroxysmal hemoglobinuria that may be precipitated by infection, menstruation, blood transfusion, surgery, vaccination, injection of liver extracts, or administration of iron salts. Weakness, abdominal and lumbar pain, jaundice with pallor and yellowish discoloration of the skin and mucous membranes, heart murmurs, splenomegaly, and hemosiderinuria are the principal features. Hemolytic crises also may occur. Pathological findings include systemic venous or portal thrombosis, normoblastic bone marrow hyperplasia, hepatomegaly with necrosis, hemosiderosis, and massive iron deposits in the kidneys.

Marchiafava, E., & Nazari, A. Nuovo contributo allo studio degli itteri cronici emolitici. *Policlinico, Sez. Prat.*, 1911, 18:241-54. Micheli, F. Uno caso di anemia emolitica con emosideriuria perpetua. *Accad. Med. Torino*, 1928, 7:148. Strübing, P. Paroxysmale Hämoglobinurie. *Deut. Med. Wschr.*, 1882, 8:17-21.

Marchiafava-Nazari-Micheli syndrome. See *Marchiafava-Micheli syndrome.*

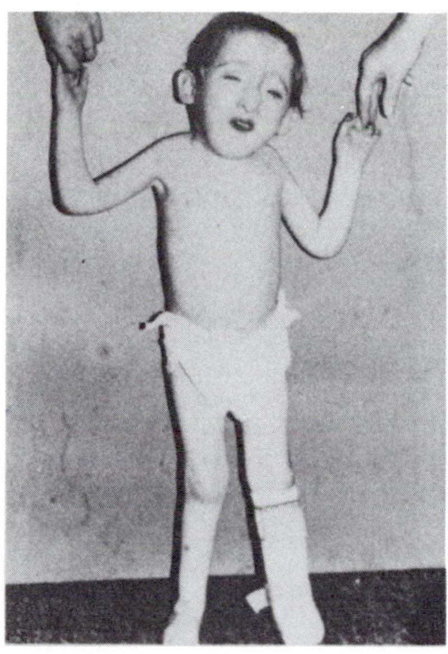

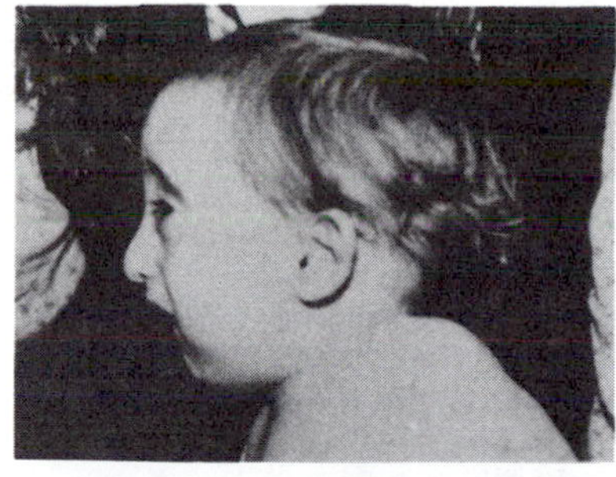

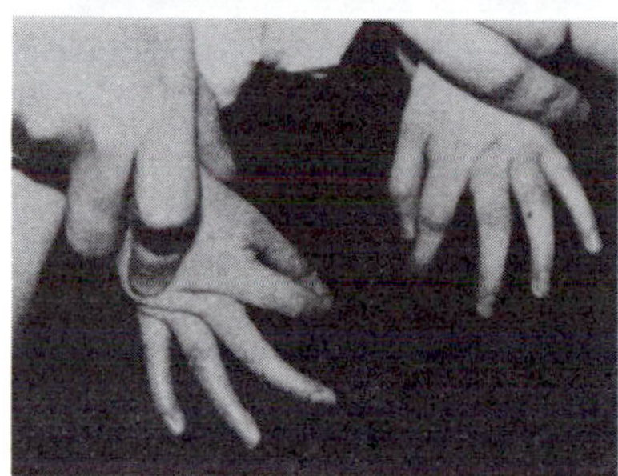

Marden-Walker syndrome
Gossage, David, James M. Perrin & Merlin G. Butler: *American Journal of Medical Genetics* 26:915-919, 1987. New York: Alan R. Liss Inc.

Strübing-Marchiafava syndrome. See *Marchiafava-Micheli syndrome.*

MARCUS GUNN. See GUNN, ROBERT MARCUS

MARDEN, PHILIP M. (American physician)

Marden-Walker syndrome (MWS). A syndrome of multiple abnormalies, transmitted as an autosomal recessive trait, characterized by irreducible joint contractures which disappear during the first year of life, muscular hypotonia, pectus excavatum, arachnodactyly, widely set nipples, and peculiar facies marked by immobile face with sagging cheeks, depressed nasal bridge, pursed lips with eversion of the lower lip, strabismus, blepharophimosis, microstomia, and micrognathia. Other defects include agenesis of the cerebellum and brain stem, decreased deep tendon reflexes, kyphoscoliosis, and myotonia myopathy. Failure to thrive, cleft palate, upward slanting of the palpebral fissures, exotropia, low-set ears, simian creases, abnormal pulmonary return of the heart, and renal microcystic disease may be associated.

Marden, P. M., & Walker, W. A. A new generalized connective tissue syndrome: Association of multiple congenital anomalies. *Am. J. Dis. Child.*, 1966, 112:225-8.

MARFAN, ANTOINE BERNARD JEAN (French pediatrician, 1858-1942)

Dennie-Marfan syndrome. See *under Dennie.*

inverted Marfan syndrome. See *Weill-Marchesani syndrome, under Weill, Georges.*

Marfan abiotrophy. See *Marfan syndrome (1).*

Marfan syndrome (1). Synonyms: *Marfan abiotrophy, acrochondrohyperplasia, arachnodactyly, congenital mesodermal dystrophy, dolichostenomelia, hyperchondroplasia, spider fingers, streblodactyly.*

A connective tissue disorder characterized by a tendency toward tall stature and long, slim limbs, little subcutaneous fat, and muscle hypotonia, associated with arachnodactyly, joint hyperextensibility, lens subluxation, aortic dilatation, and other disorders. Scoliosis, kyphosis, pectus excavatum or carinatum, narrow facies, narrow palate, inguinal or femoral hernias, flatfoot, habitual dislocations, ard arthrogryposis are usually present. Cleft palate or bifid uvula

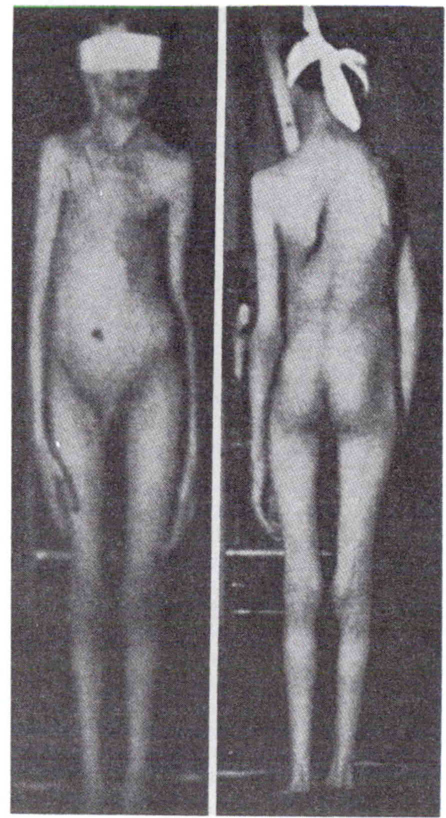

Marfan syndrome (1)
Francois, Jules: *Heredity in Ophthlmology.* St. Louis: C.V. Mosby Co., 1961.

occur in some cases. The teeth may be long and narrow and malocclusion is common. Lens dislocation may be combined with myopia, strabismus, glaucoma, blue sclera, and nystagmus. Cardiovascular defects usually consist of aortic aneurysm, heart enlargement, valvular defects, cystic necrosis of the aorta, and aortic regurgitation. The mean age of survival is 43 years for men and 46 for women. The syndrome is inherited as an autosomal dominant trait.

Marfan, A. B. Un cas de deformation congénitale des quatre membres, plus prononcées aux extrémités, caractérisée par l'allongement des os avec un certain degré d'aminicissement. *Bull. Soc. Méd. Hôp., Paris*, 1896, 13:220-6.

Marfan syndrome (2). See *Dennie-Marfan syndrome.*

Marfan-Achard syndrome. See *Marfan syndrome (1), and see Achard syndrome.*

Marfan-Madelung symptom complex. See *Marfan-Madelung syndrome.*

Marfan-Madelung syndrome. Synonym: *Marfan-Madelung symptom complex.*

A combination of Marfan syndrome (1) and Madelung deformity (q.v.).

Meyer, F. W. Marfan-Madelungscher Symptomkomplex. *Klin. Mbl. Augenh.*, 1957, 130:688-90.

marfanoid hypermobility syndrome. A syndrome of marfanoid habitus with marked hypermobility of joints and hyperextensibity of the skin, but without involvement of the aorta or displacement of the lenses. Floppy mitral valve may be associated. The etiology is unknown.

Walker, B. A., *et al.* The marfanoid hypermobility syndrome. *Ann. Intern. Med.*, 1969, 71:349-52.

MARGHESCU, S. (German physician)

Marghescu and Braun-Falco syndrome. Congenital poikiloderma with bullous eruption transmitted as an autosomal recessive trait. The condition, affecting females more often than males, has its onset during the first weeks of life and is manifested by subepidermal vesicles, followed by erythema that progresses to fully developed poikiloderma by the fourth year of life. The face, extremities, and trunk are most commonly affected. Volar hyperkeratosis may lead to restriction of finger movement. Associated disorders may include proportional dwarfism, tooth anomalies, onychodystrophy, sparse hair, conjunctivitis, blepharitis, corneal opacity, hypogonadism, and gingivitis.

Marghescu, S., & Braun-Falco, O. Über die kongenitalen Poikilodermien; ein analytischer Vers. *Derm. Wschr.*, 1965, 151:9-19.

marginal corneal dystrophy. See *Bietti dystrophy.*

marginal crystalline dystrophy. See *Bietti dystrophy.*

marginal periodontitis. See *Fauchard disease.*

MARGOLIS, EMMANUEL (Israeli physician)

Ziprkowski-Margolis syndrome. See *Woolf syndrome.*

MARIE, JULIEN (French physician, born 1899)

Debré-Julien Marie syndrome (1 and 2). See *Debré-Marie syndrome (1 and 2).*

Debré-Marie syndrome (1 and 2). See *under Debré.*

Foix-Chavany-Marie syndrome (FCMS). See *under Foix.*

Julien Marie syndrome. See *Marie syndrome.*

Julien Marie-Sée syndrome. See *Marie-Sée syndrome.*

Marie syndrome. Synonyms: *Julien Marie syndrome, infantile pulmonary reticuloendotheliosis.*

A cutaneous and pulmonary syndrome of young infants. The skin lesions present small confluent papules covered by brownish crust, and the pulmonary symptoms consist of diffuse roentgenographic opacities and tachypnea. Pathological findings comprise massive, dense, red pulmonary infiltrations with islands of normal tissue; multiple, small, intrapachydermal cavities; and small subpleural emphysematous bullae. Subcutaneous emphysema, mediastinal emphysema, and asphyxia may develop in later stages. There is no fever. Marie considered this syndrome to be a form of reticuloendotheliosis.

Marie, J. *et al.* La réticulose cutanée et pulmonaire apyrétique du nourrisson. Varieté clinique nouvelle de réticuloendothéliose. *Presse. Méd., Paris,* 1941, 49:1146-9.

Marie-Sée syndrome. Synonyms: *Julien Marie-Sée syndrome, acute benign hydrocephalus, acute hydrocephalus in infants, acute hypervitaminosis A syndrome, hypervitaminosis hydrocephalus.*

Acute hydrocephalus in infants receiving large doses of vitamin A. The symptoms, including vomiting, agitation, insomnia, and bulging of the fontanels, appear about 12 hours after the administration of vitamin A and last 24 to 48 hours.

Marie, J., & Sée, G. Hydrocéphalie aiguë bénigne du nourrisson après ingestion d'une dose massive et unique de vitamin A et D. *Arch. Fr. Pediat.*, 1951, 8:563-5.

MARIE, PIERRE (French physician, 1853-1940)

Bamberger-Pierre Marie (BPM) syndrome. See *Marie-Bamberger syndrome, under Marie, Pierre.*

Bechterew-Strümpell-Marie syndrome. See *under Bekhterev.*

Brissaud-Marie syndrome. See *under Brissaud.*

Charcot-Marie syndrome. See *Charcot-Marie-Tooth syndrome.*

Charcot-Marie-Tooth disease (CMTD). See *Charcot-Marie-Tooth syndrome.*

Charcot-Marie-Tooth syndrome (CMTS). See *under Charcot.*

Charcot-Marie-Tooth-Hoffmann syndrome. See *Charcot-Marie-Tooth syndrome.*

Marie anarthria. Synonyms: *Pierre Marie anarthria, accentuated dysarthria.*

Loss of the ability to articulate words in persons with focal cerebral lesions, said to differ from aphasia.

Souques, A. Quelques cas d'anarthrie de Pierre Marie. Aperçu historique sur la localisation du langage. *Rev. Neur., Paris*. 1928, 2:219-68.

Marie ataxia. See *Marie syndrome (1).*

Marie disease. See *Bechterew-Strümpell-Marie syndrome, under Bekhterev.*

Marie syndrome (1). Synonyms: *Marie ataxia, Nonne-Marie syndrome, Nonne-Pierre Marie syndrome, Pierre Marie syndrome, cerebellar hereditary ataxia, congenital cerebellar ataxia, dominant spinopontine atrophy, hereditary cerebellar ataxia, hereditary cerebellar ataxia with spasticity, heredoataxia cerebellaris, spinocerebellar ataxia.*

A hereditary disease of the nervous system, said to be transmitted as an autosomal dominant trait, marked by onset during young adulthood or middle age, spastic ataxic gait, poor coordination, static tremor, exaggerated tendon reflexes, impaired deep sensibility, pain, cramps, paresthesia, and dysarthric speech. Ocular symptoms may include oculomotor paralysis, blindness, and optic atrophy. Mental deterioration and sphincter disorders may occur in advanced stages.

Pathological findings include diminution of the size of the spinal cord and cerebellum; loss of Purkinje cells; gliosis; demyelination of the pyramidal tracts, posterior column, and spinocerebellar tracts; and degeneration of the inferior olive, pontine nuclei, the Clarke column, dentate nucleus, anterior horn cells, and cerebral cortex.

Marie, P. Sur l'hérédo-ataxie cérébelleuse. *Sem. Méd., Paris*. 1893, 13:444-7. Nonne, M. Über eine eigentümliche familiäre Erkrankungsform des Zentralnervensystems. *Arch. Psychiat., Berlin*, 1891, 22:283-316.

Marie syndrome (2). Synonyms: *Pierre Marie disease, acromegaly, pachyacria.*

Hyperfunction of the anterior pituitary gland, usually caused by an adenoma, associated with hypersecretion of growth hormone with secondary overgrowth of the bones, connective tissue, and viscera. Skeletal changes involve mainly the skull and small bones of the hands and feet, resulting in prominent cheek bones; frontal bossing; grossly overdeveloped mandible pressing on the tongue and alveolar processes, with consequent relative mandibular prognathism; and broadening of the hands, fingers, and feet. Enlargement of the soft tissue is usually manifested by large ears and nose; thick lips; enlarged tongue with lobulated margin and papillary hypertrophy, which fills the oral cavity and exerts pressure on the teeth and tips them to the buccal or labial side; coarse facies; fleshy appearance of the hands and feet; widespread splanchnomegaly; and hypertrophy of target organs for anterior pituitary hormones, including the adrenal cortex, thyroid gland, parathyroid glands, and gonads. Sexual disorders, diabetes mellitus, hemianopsia, and increased intracranial pressure may be associated. The term **gigantism** refers to the childhood form of this disease.

Marie, P. Sur deux cas d'acromégalie; hypertrophie singulière non congénitale des extrémités supérieurs, inférieurs et céphalique. *Rev. Méd., Paris*, 1886, 6:297-333.

Marie-Bamberger syndrome. Synonyms: *Bamberger disease, Bamberger-Pierre Marie (BPM) syndrome, Hagner syndrome, Pierre Marie syndrome, Pierre Marie-Bamberger syndrome, acropachia ossea, clubbed finger, digital hippocratism, hippocratic fingers, hyperplastic osteoarthritis, osteoarthropathia hypertrophica, osteopathia hypertrophicans toxica, osteoperiostitis ossificans toxica, osteophytosis, osteopulmonary arthropathy, periostitis hyperplastica, primary hypertrophic osteoarthropathy, pulmonary hypertrophic osteoarthropathy, secondary hypertrophic osteoarthropathy, thoracogenous rheumatic syndrome, toxigenic osteoperiostitis ossificans.*

A syndrome of clubbing of the fingers and toes, periostitis of the distal ends of the long bones, and painful arthritis, occurring in association with pulmonary diseases such as bronchogenic carcinoma, occasional bronchiectasis, or lung abscesses. Periosteal new bone formation involves diaphyses of the tubular bones. The syndrome was first described by Friedreich in brothers Karl and Wilhelm Hagner, hence the synonym **Hagner syndrome**. A familial form of this syndrome is known as the *Mankowsky syndrome* (see under *Mankovskii).*

Marie, P. De l'ostéo-arthropathie hypertrophiante pneumique. *Rev. Méd., Paris*, 1890, 10:1-36. Bamberger, E. Über Knochenveränderungen gei chronischen Lungen- und Herzkrankheiten. *Zschr. Klin. Med.*, 1891, 18:193-217. Friedreich, N. Hyperostose des gesamten Skeletts. *Arch. Path. Anat., Berlin*, 1868, 16:83-7.

Marie-Léri syndrome. Synonyms: *arthritis mutilans, arthropathia mutilans, main en lorgnette, rheumatoid acro-osteolysis, trophopathia myelodysplastica.*

A deformity of the hand caused by osteolysis of the articular surfaces of the fingers and resulting in mobility of the joints in such a way that the fingers may be elongated or shortened like a telescope. The condition is usually seen in some types of rheumatoid arthritis.

Marie, P., & Léri, A. Une varieté de rhumatisme chronique: La main en lorgnette (présentation de pièces et de coupes). *Bull. Soc. Méd. Hôp. Paris*, 1913, 36:104-7.

Marie-Sainton syndrome. See *cleidocranial dysostosis.*

Marie-Strümpell disease. See *Bechterew-Strümpell-Marie syndrome, under Bekhterev.*

Nonne-Marie syndrome. See *Marie syndrome (1).*

Pierre Marie anarthria. See *Marie anarthria.*

Pierre Marie disease. See *Bechterew-Strümpell-Marie syndrome, under Bekhterev.*

Pierre Marie syndrome (1). See *Marie syndrome (1).*

Pierre Marie syndrome (2). See *Marie-Bamberger syndrome.*

Pierre Marie-Bamberger syndrome. See *Marie-Bamberger syndrome.*

Scheuthauer-Marie syndrome. See *cleidocranial dysostosis.*

Scheuthauer-Marie-Sainton syndrome. See *cleidocranial dysostosis.*

MARIE UNNA. See UNNA, MARIE

MARIN AMAT, MANUEL (Spanish ophthalmologist, born 1879)

Marin Amat syndrome. Synonyms: *inverted Marcus Gunn syndrome, reverse jaw-winking syndrome.*

Closure of the eye when the mouth is opened widely or forcibly. Misdirected nerve fiber regeneration is believed to be the most frequent cause.

Marín Amat, M. Contribución al estudio de la curabilidad de las parálisis oculares de origen traumático-substitución funcional del VII por el V par craneal. *Arch. Oft. Hisp. Amer.*, 1918, 18:70-99.

MARINESCO, GEORGE. See MARINESCU, GHEORGHE

MARINESCU (MARINESCO), GHEORGHE (Rumanian physician, 1863-1938)

Marinesco-Garland syndrome. See *Marinesco-Sjögren syndrome.*

Marinesco-Sjögren syndrome (MSS). Synonyms: *Marinesco-Garland syndrome, Marinesco-Sjögren-Garland syndrome, Torsten Sjögren syndrome, cataract-oligophrenia syndrome, hereditary oligophrenic cerebellolental degeneration.*

A rare hereditary syndrome, transmitted as an autosomal recessive trait, and characterized by stationary cerebellar ataxia, often with pyramidal complications, congenital cataract which progresses to blindness, and psychomotor retardation. Bone abnormalities, dwarfism, amd hypogonadism may be associated. Pathological findings may include massive cortical atrophy and enlarged lysosomes containing whorled lamellar or amorphous inclusion bodies, suggesting a lysosomal storage disorder.

Marinesco, G., *et al.* Nouvelle maladie familiale caractérisés par une cataracte congénitale e un arrêt du développement somato-neuro-psychique. *Encéphale,*

1931, 26:97-109. Sjögren, T. Hereditary congenital spinocerebellar ataxia accompanied by congenital cataract and oligophrenia. A genetic and clinical investigation. *Confinia Neur., Basel,* 1950, 10:293-308. Garland, H., & Moorhouse, D. An extremely rare recessive oligophrenia, cataract, and other features. *J. Neur., London,* 1953, 16:110-6.

Marinesco-Sjögren-Garland syndrome. See *Marinesco-Sjögren syndrome.*

MARION, HENRI (French physician)

Marion disease. Synonyms: *bladder neck obstruction, congenital hypertrophy of the bladder neck.*

Hypertrophic obstruction of the bladder neck in children. Congenital excessive development of the prostate in males and of the glands around the bladder neck in females is the cause.

Marion, H. De l'hypertrophie congénitale du col vésical. *J. Urol. Méd. Chir., Paris,* 1927, 23:97-101.

marital violence. See *battered spouse syndrome.*

marker X syndrome. See *chromosome X fragility.*

MARKOE, THOMAS MASTERS (American physician, 1819-1901)

Markoe abscess. Chronic sinuous abscess of the bone.

Markoe, T. M. *A treatise on diseases of the bones.* New York, Appleton, 1872.

MARKUS, C.

Markus syndrome. See *Adie syndrome.*

Markus-Adie syndrome. See *Adie syndrome.*

MAROTEAUX, PIERRE (French pediatrician, born 1926)

Kozlowski-Maroteaux-Spranger syndrome. See *Kozlowski spondylometaphyseal dysplasia syndrome, under Kozlowski, Kazimierz S.*

Lamy-Maroteaux syndrome (1). See *diastrophic dwarfism syndrome.*

Lamy-Maroteaux syndrome (2). See *under Lamy.*

Maroteaux syndrome. See *phalangeal microgeodic syndrome.*

Maroteaux-Lamy syndrome (1). See *mucopolysaccharidosis VI.*

Maroteaux-Lamy syndrome (2). See *pyknodysostosis.*

Maroteaux-Lamy syndrome (3). See *spondyloepiphyseal dysplasia tarda.*

Maroteaux-Malamut syndrome. See *acrodysostosis.*

Maroteaux-Spranger-Wiedemann syndrome. See *metatropic dwarfism syndrome.*

pseudo-achondroplastic spondyloepiphyseal dysplasia, Maroteaux-Lamy type. See *under pseudo-achondroplastic spondyloepiphyseal dysplasia.*

MARSH, SIR HENRY (British physician, 1790-1860)

Marsh disease. See *Basedow disease.*

MARSHALL, DON (American physician)

Marshall syndrome. A syndrome of ectodermal dysplasia, marked by peculiar facies, myopia, and short stature. Facial features include flattened nasal bridge, hypertelorism, anteverted nostrils, thick lips, and hypoplastic mandible. Myopia is associated with congenital or infantile cataracts (spontaneous maturation and absorption of cataracts may occur, causing secondary glaucoma), fluid vitreous body, extra-orbital ocular prominence, and often, alternating esotropia and hypertropia. Female patients are generally short, but the height of the males is about average. The intelligence is slightly subnormal. Sensorineural hearing deficit is common. The skin tends to be soft and dry with little sebaceous secretion and diminished sweating, hence its designation as a form of ectodermal dysplasia. Dental abnormalities consist mainly of hypodontia. The syndrome is transmitted as an autosomal dominant trait.

Marshall, D. Ectodermal dysplasia. Report of kindred with ocular abnormalities and hearing defect. *Am. J. Ophth.,* 1958, 45:143-56.

MARSHALL, RICHARD E. (American physician)

accelerated skeletal maturation, Marshall-Smith type. See *Marshall-Smith syndrome.*

Marshall syndrome. See *Marshall-Smith syndrome.*

Marshall-Smith syndrome (MSS). Synonyms: *Marshall syndrome; accelerated skeletal maturation, Marshall-Smith type.*

A syndrome of accelerated skeletal maturation, failure to thrive, and abnormal facies. Shallow orbits, prominent eyes, antimongoloid palpebral slant, flat nasal bridge, upturned nostrils, microstomia, micrognathia, hypoplastic malar areas, prominent forehead, and flat supraorbital ridges are the principal facial features. Skeletal anomalies include advanced bone age, wide phalanges, prominent calvaria, long cranium, small facial bones, and small ramus of the mandible. Respiratory complications usually consist of choanal atresia or stenosis, abnormal larynx or laryngomalacia, pulmonary hypertension, and atelectasis. Immunodeficiency occurs in some cases. Mental deficiency is the chief neurological feature. The clinical course is marked mainly by pneumonia, stridor, respi-

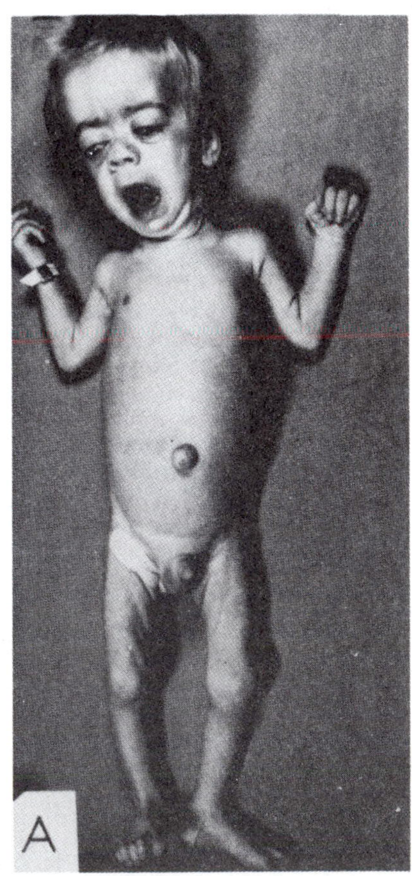

Marshall-Smith syndrome
Marshall, R.E., et al.: *J. Pediatr.* 78:95, 1971.
St. Louis: C.V. Mosby Co.

ratory distress, and death. The etiology is unknown; most cases are sporadic.

Marshall, R. E., Graham, C. B., Scott, C. R., & Smith, D. W. Syndrome of accelerated skeletal maturation and relative failure to thrive: A newly recognized clinical growth disorder. *J. Pediat.*, 1971, 78:95-101.

MARSHALL, WALLACE (American physician)

Marshall-White syndrome. Synonyms: *Bier spots, chronic vasoconstrictor spots.*

Ischemic angiospastic spots on the palms associated with periodic insomnia and tachycardia. The spots are somewhat cooler than the surrounding pinkish skin.

Marshall, W., & White, C. Localized areas of ischemia of the hands. *J. Lab. Clin. Med.*, 1932-33, 18:386-8. Bier, A. Die Entstehung dss Collateralkreislaaufs. II. Der Rückfluss des Blutes aus ischämischen Körpertheilen. *Virchows Arch. Path. Anat.*, 1898, 153:306-34.

MARSIDI, IRENE (American physician)

Juberg-Marsidi syndrome. See *under Juberg.*

MARTIN, A. (German physician)

Bosviel-Martin syndrome. See *Bosviel syndrome.*

Martin syndrome. See *Bosviel syndrome.*

MARTIN, J. PURDON (British physician)

Martin-Bell syndrome (MBS). See *chromosome X fragility.*

Martin-Bell-Renpenning syndrome. See *chromosome X fragility.*

MARTIN DE GIMARD, JULES LOUIS ALEXANDRE (French physician, born 1858)

de Gimard syndrome. See *Martin de Gimard syndrome.*

Gimard syndrome. See *Martin de Gimard syndrome.*

Martin de Gimard syndrome. Synonyms: *de Gimard syndrome, Gimard syndrome, Sheldon necrotic purpura, purpura gangrenosa hemorrhagica, purpura necrotisans.*

A skin disease, usually affecting children, in which purpuric lesions become necrosed and healing is accompanied by separation of the resulting sloughs. It had been suggested that this disorder may be related to the Sanarelli-Shwartzman phenomenon. Except for scarring, there are no sequelae.

*Martin de Gimard. *Purpura hémorrhagique primitif ou purpura infectieux primitif.* Paris, 1884 (Thesis). Sheldon, J. H. Purpura necrotiea. A possible clinical application of the Shwartzman phenomenon. *Arch. Dis. Child.*, 1947, 22:7-13.

MARTIN DU PAN, CHARLES (Swiss physician, 1878-1948)

Martin du Pan-Rutishauser disease. Synonym: *laminar osteochondritis.*

A chronic monoarticular disease occurring chiefly during adolescence and charcterized by pain, progressive ankylosis, and selective destruction of the cartilage due to infiltration of connective tissue between articular cartilage and spongiosa.

Martin du Pan, C., & Rutishauser, E. Un type d'arthrose infantile nouvelle. Ostéochondrite laminaire. *Schweiz. Med. Wschr.*, 1945, 75:955-6.

MARTINELLI, B. (Italian physician)

Campailla-Martinelli syndrome. See *under Campailla.*

MARTORELL, FERNANDO. See MARTORELL OTZET, FERNANDO

MARTORELL OTZET, FERNANDO (Spanish physician, born 1906)

Martorell syndrome (1). Synonyms: *Martorell ulcer, hypertensive ischemic ulcers of the leg, ischemic hypertensive leg ulcer, ulcus cruris hypertonicum.*

Hypertension associated with local gangrene due to obliteration of arteries, with ischemic ulcers of the leg.

*Martorell, F. *Ulcera supramalleolar en los grandes hipertensos.* 1945.

Martorell syndrome (2). See *aortic arch syndrome.*

Martorell ulcer. See *Martorell syndrome (1).*

Martorell-Fabré syndrome. See *aortic arch syndrome.*

Takayasu-Martorell-Fabré syndrome. See *aortic arch syndrome.*

MARTSOLF, J. T.

Martsolf syndrome. See *cataract-mental retardation-hypogonadism syndrome.*

MARY JOSEPH, SISTER. See DEMPSEY, MARY JOSEPH, SISTER

MAS. See ***m**ilk-**a**lkali **s**yndrome.*

MAS. See ***M**cCune-**A**lbright **s**yndrome.*

MAS (Morgagni-Adams-Stokes) syndrome. See *Adams-Stokes syndrome, under Adams, Robert.*

MASA (mental retardation-**a**phasia-**s**huffling gait-**a**bducted thumbs) **syndrome.** A familial syndrome of unknown etiology, consisting of mental retardation, shuffling gait, and adducted thumbs. The syndrome was originally reported in a Mexican-American kindred in which six males and one female were affected in three generations. In addition, the patients showed small body size, exaggerated lumbar lordosis, and hyperactive deep tendon reflexes in the lower limbs.

Bianchine, J. W., & Lewis, R. C., Jr. The MASA syndrome: A new heritable mental retardation syndrome. *Clin. Genet.*, 1974, 5:298-306.

masque ecchymotique. See *Ollivier syndrome.*

MASSHOFF, JOHANN WILHELM (WILLY) (German physician, born 1908)

Masshoff syndrome. Synonym: *mesenteric reticulocytic abscess-forming lymphoadenitis.*

Abscess-forming reticulocytic lymphadenitis of the mesentery. *Pasteurella pseudotuberculosis* is the suspected pathogen.

Masshoff, W. Eine neuartige Form der mesenterialen lymphadenitis. *Deut. Med. Wschr.*, 1953, 78:532-5.

massive osteolysis syndrome. See *Gorham syndrome.*

MASSON, C. B.

Dyke-Davidoff-Masson (DDM) syndrome. See *under Dyke, C. G.*

MASSON, P. (Canadian physician)

Barré-Masson syndrome. See *under Barré, Jean Alexandre.*

Barré-Masson tumor. See *Barré-Masson syndrome, under Barré, Jean Alexandre.*

MASSUMI, RASHID A. (Iranian-born American physician)

Prinzmetal-Massumi syndrome. See *Prinzmetal angina.*

MAST (medical **a**nti**s**hock **t**rousers)-associated compartment syndrome (MACS). See *under compartment syndrome.*

MASTERS, WILLIAM HOWELL (American gynecologist, born 1915)

Allen-Masters syndrome. See *under Allen, William Myron.*

mastitis chronica cystica. See *Cheatle disease.*

mastodynia. See *Cooper neuralgia.*

mastopathia chronica cystica. See *Cheatle disease.*

MASUDA (Japanese ophthalmologist)

Masuda-Kitahara disease. Synonyms: *Kitahara disease, central angiospastic retinopathy, chorioretinitis centralis serosa, idiopathic flat detachment of the retina, preretinal edema, retinitis centralis angioneurotica, retinitis centralis annularis, retinitis centralis capillarospastica, retinitis centralis recidivans, serous central chorioretinitis.*

A circumscribed exudative disorder of the macula lutea, of probable viral origin, seen mainly in Japan and Indonesia.

Kitahara, S. Über klinische Beobachtungen bei der in Japan häufig vorkommenden Chorioretinitis centralis serosa. *Klin. Mbl. Augenh.*, 1936, 97:345-62.

MATHES, PAUL (Austrian physician, 1871-1923)

Mathes mastitis. Synonym: *puerperal mastitis.*

Puerperal inflammation of the breast, apparently restricted to one side. The symptoms include a dark discoloration of the affected area, engorgement and tenderness of the breast, and mild pain. The inflammation usually appears without warning within 2 weeks after delivery and disappears spontaneously in 2 to 3 days.

Mathes, P. Eine typische Form der Brustentzündung im Wochenbett. *Münch. Med. Wschr.*, 1921, I68:15.

MATHIEU, ALBERT (French physician, 1855-1917)

Mathieu disease. See *leptospirosis.*

MATOLCSY, THOMAS (Hungarian physician)

Kopits-Matolscy syndrome. See *popliteal pterygium syndrome.*

MATTIOLI-FOGGIA, CESARE (Italian physician)

Mattioli-Foggia and Raso syndrome. Synonym: *lipofibrocalcareous myopathy.*

A chronic, progressive, recurrent muscular disorder characterized by hard, painless tumors.

Mattioli-Foggia, C. Su un particolare quadro di miopatia lipo-fibro-calcarea. *Riv. Anat. Pat.*, 1948, 1:43-56. Raso, & Mattioli-Faggio. Nuove osservazioni cliniche di miopatia lipo-fibro-calcarea. *Riv. Neur.*, 1949, 19:231-2.

MATZENAUER, RUDOLF (Austrian dermatologist, born 1861)

Matzenauer-Polland syndrome. Synonym: *dermatitis symmetrica dysmenorrhagica.*

A skin disease marked by spontaneous, mostly symmetrical inflammatory lesions followed by chronic fluctuating attacks of erythema and urticarial edema, appearing most frequently in the form of weeping dermatitis, rarely as skin necrosis. Complications usually include vasomotor and mental disorders. Women with dysmenorrhea are most frequently affected.

Metzenauer, R., & Polland, R. Dermatitis symmetrica dysmenorrhoica. Beitrag zur Angioneurosefrage. *Arch. Derm. Syph., Berlin*, 1912, 111:385-54.

MAUGERI, SALVATORE (Italian physician, born 1905)

Maugeri syndrome. Synonyms: *silicotic mediastinitis, silicotic mediastinopathy.*

Asthmatiform dyspnea, laryngotracheal inspiratory turgor, attacks of cough after deep inspiration, and mydriatic anisocoria secondary to mediastinal silicotic lesions.

Maugeri, S. La mediastinite silicotica. *Folia Med.*, 1953, 36:135-43.

MAUNOIR, JEAN PIERRE (French physician, 1768-1861)

Maunoir hydrocele. Synonym: *cervical hydrocele.*

A serous dilation of a persistent cervical cleft or duct or of a deep cervical lymph space.

*Maunoir, J. P. *Mémoires sur les amputations, l'hydrocéle du cou, et l'organisation de l'iris.* Genève, Paschoud, I825. 150 pp.

MAURIAC, CHARLES MARIE TAMARELLE (French physician, 1832-1905)

Mauriac syndrome. Synonym: *erythema nodosum syphiliticum.*

A symmetrical, painful, erythematous nodular eruption on the anterior part of the legs and, less frequently, other parts of the body, which is seen in syphilis.

Mauriac, C. *Pathologie générale de la syphilis tertiaire.* Paris, Capiomont & Renault, 1886, 112 pp.

MAURIAC, LEONARD PIERRE (French physician, born 1882)

Mauriac syndrome. Synonyms: *Pierre Mauriac syndrome, diabetes-dwarfism-obesity syndrome, diabetic dwarfism, secondary diabetic glycogenosis.*

An association of hepatomegaly, dwarfism, and obesity with juvenile diabetes mellitus. Retinopathy is a frequent complication.

Mauriac, P. Hépatomégalie, nanisme, obésite dans le diabète infantile. Pathogénie du syndrome. *Presse Méd.*, 1946, I54:826-7.

Pierre Mauriac syndrome. See *Mauriac syndrome.*

MAXCY, KENNETH FULLER (American bacteriologist, born 1889)

Maxcy disease. A form of typhoid fever endemic in southern United States.

Maxcy, K. F. Clinical observations on endemic typhus (Brill's disease) in southern United States. *U. S. Pub. Health Rep.*, 1926, 41:1213-20.

maxillofacial dysostosis syndrome. Synonym: *dysostosis maxillofacialis.*

A variant of the first and second arch syndrome (q.v.), transmitted as an autosomal dominant trait, characterized by anteroposterior shortening of the maxilla, sometimes associated with relative mandibular prognathism, antimongoloid palpebral slant, ear deformities, and delayed and inarticulate speech.

Villaret, M., & Desoilles, H. L'hypoplasie primitive familiale du maxillaire supérieur. *Ann. Méd., Paris*, 1932, 32:378-81. Peters, A., & Hövels, O. Die Dysostosis maxillofacialis, eine erbliche, typische Fehlbildung des I. Visceralbogens. *Zschr. Menschl. Vererb. Konstitutionsl.*, 1960, 35:434-44.

maxillonasal dysostosis. See *Binder syndrome.*

maxillonasal dysplasia. See *Binder syndrome.*

MAXWELL, ALICE FREELAND (American physician, 1890-1961)

Goldberg-Maxwell syndrome. See *testicular feminization syndrome.*

Goldberg-Maxwell-Morris syndrome. See *testicular feminization syndrome.*

MAY, DUANE L. (American physician)

May-White syndrome. A familial syndrome, transmitted as an autosomal dominant trait with variable penetrance, characterized by myoclonus, cerebellar ataxia, and hearing loss.

May, D. L., & White, H. H. Familial myoclonus, cerebellar ataxia, and deafness. Specific genetically-determined disease. *Arch. Neur., Chicago,* 1968, 19:331-8.

MAY, RICHARD (German physician, 1863-1936)

May-Hegglin anomaly. Synonyms: *Hegglin anomaly, May-Hegglin syndrome.*

A cytoplasmic leukocyte anomaly characterized by Döhle bodies and giant blood platelets, which is inherited as an autosomal dominant trait. Most affected patients are clinically normal, but about one-fourth have a hemorrhagic tendency which is related to thrombocytopenia and abnormal platelet function. The prothrombin consumption test, clot retraction, and other tests may show defective platelet function. Döhle bodies are usually found in the neutrophils, but they may also occur in eosinophils, basophils, monocytes, and lymphocytes.

Hegglin, R. Über eine neue Form einer konstitutionellen Leukozytenanomalie, kombiniert mit Thrombopathie. *Schweiz, Med. Wschr.*, 1945, 75:91-2. May, R. Leukocytenenschlüsse. Kasuistische Mitteilung. *Deut. Arch. Klin. Med.*, 1909, 96:1-6.

May-Hegglin syndrome. See *May-Hegglin anomaly.*

MAYDL, KARL (Austrian physician, 1853-1903)

Maydl disease. See *Calvé-Legg-Perthes syndrome.*

Maydl hernia. Retrograde hernia with strangulation of the intestine in the hernia sac, the loops of the intestine forming a W.

*Maydl, K. *Die Lehre von den Unterleibsbrüchen (Hernien).* Wien, Stefan, 1898.

MAYER (German physician)

Kufs-Mayer disease. See *Kufs syndrome.*

MAYER, AUGUST FRANZ JOSEF KARL (German physician, 1787-1865)

Mayer-Rokitansky syndrome. See *Mayer-Rokitansky-Küster syndrome.*

Mayer-Rokitansky-Küster (MRK) syndrome. Synonyms: *Küster syndrome, Mayer-Rokitansky syndrome, von Rokitansky-Hauser syndrome, Rokitansky-Küster-Hauser (RKH) syndrome, müllerian dysgenesis syndrome, uterus bicornis rudimentarius, uterus bicornis rudimentarius solidus partium excavatum cum vagina solida, uterus bipartitus, uterus bipartitus rudimentarius solidus cum vagina solida.*

A syndrome of aplasia of the mülerian duct, vaginal atresia, variable abnormalities of the uterus (e.g., bicornuate or septate uterus), and other anomalies, including frequent renal agenesis, ectopic kidney, vertebral defect, and skeletal abnormalities.

*Mayer, C. A. J. Über Verdoppelungen des Uterus und ihre Arten nebst Bemerkungen über Hasenscharten und Wolfsrachen. *J. Chir. Augenheilk.*, 1829, 13:525. Rokitansky. Über die sogenannten Verdoppelungen des Uterus. *Med. Jahrb. Öst. Staat.*, 1838, 26:k39-77. Küster, H. Uterus bipartitus solidus rudimentarius cum Vagina solida. *Zschr. Gebur. Gynäk.*, 1910, 67:692-718. Hauser, G. A., & Schreiner, W. E.. Das Mayer-v. Rokitansky-Küster-Syndrom. *Schweiz. Med. Wschr.*, 1961, 91:381-4.

MAYER, JOHN H. (American physician)

Graham-Burford-Mayer syndrome. See *middle lobe syndrome.*

MAYER-GROSS, WILLI (German neurologist, born 1889)

Mayer-Gross apraxia. Synonyms: *Kleist apraxia, constructive apraxia.*

A disturbance in some types of cerebral lesions, which affects formative activities and in which the spatial part of the task is missed, although there is no apraxia of single movements. It results in an inability to draw, to write, or to construct geometric figures with matchsticks.

Mayer-Gross, W. Some observations on apraxia. *Proc. R. Soc. Med.*, 1935, l28:1203-12. *Kleist, K. *Gehirnpathologie.* Leipzig, 1934.

MAYO, WILLIAM JAMES (American physician, 1861-1939)

Mayo anemic spot. An anemic spot visible on the anterior wall of the duodenum at the scar of a duodenal ulcer and corresponding to the area supplied by the supraduodenal artery.

Mayo, W. J. Anemic spot on the duodenum, which may be mistaken for ulcer. *Surg. Obst. Gyn.*, 1908, 6:600-1.

MAYOU, MARMADUKE STEPHEN (British physician, born 1876)

Batten-Mayou syndrome. See *Stock-Spielmeyer-Vogt syndrome.*

maypole deformity. See *apple peel syndrome.*

MAZZA, SALVADOR (Argentine physician, 1886-1946)

Chagas-Mazza disease. See *Chagas disease.*

MBD (Marchiafava-Bignami disease). See *Marchiafava-Bignami syndrome.*

MBD (minimal brain dysfunction). See *attention deficit-hyperactivity disorder.*

MBPA (Munchausen syndrome by proxy and apnea). See *under Munchausen syndrome by proxy.*

MBPS (Munchausen by proxy syndrome). See *Munchausen syndrome by proxy.*

MBS (Martin-Bell syndrome). See *chromosome X fragility.*

MC L., JOHNIE

Johnie McL disease. See *mucopolysaccharidosis I-H.*

MCALPINE, DOUGLAS (British physician, born 1890)

Lhermitte-McAlpine syndrome. See *under Lhermitte.*

MCARDLE, BRIAN (British physician)

McArdle disease. See *glycogen storage disease V.*

McArdle-Schmid-Pearson syndrome. See *glycogen storage disease V.*

MCCORT, JAMES J. (American physician)

Smith-McCort dwarfism. See *Dyggeve-Melchior-Clausen syndrome.*

MCCREADIE, SAMUEL R. (American physician)

Opitz-Johnson-McCreadie-Smith syndrome. See *Opitz trigonocephaly syndrome.*

MCCUNE, DONOVAN JAMES (American physician, born 1902)

Albright-McCune-Sternberg syndrome. See *McCune-Albright syndrome.*

McCune-Albright syndrome. Synonyms: *Albright syndrome, Albright-McCune-Sternberg syndrome, Fuller Albright syndrome, Weil-Albright syndrome, brown spot syndrome, leontiasis ossea, osteitis fibrosa cystica, osteitis fibrosa cystica disseminata, osteitis fibrosa disseminata, osteodystrophia fibrosa.*

A combination of fibrous dysplasia of the bone, brown pigmentation of the skin, and endocrine disorders (chiefly precocious puberty) in females. The long bones are most frequently affected. Other bones involved, in descending order, are the tibia, fibula, pelvis, humerus, radius, and ulna. The femur may become bowed, with shortening of the legs and difficulty in walking because of pain and multiple fractures. Bone lesions may be unilateral. Facial asymmetry occurs in some cases. The skull may be thickened, with obliteration of the foramina and resulting deafness. Pigmentation is of the café-au-lait type. Puberty is usually reached at 5 to 10 years of age. Heredity does not appear to be a factor. A similar condition without skin

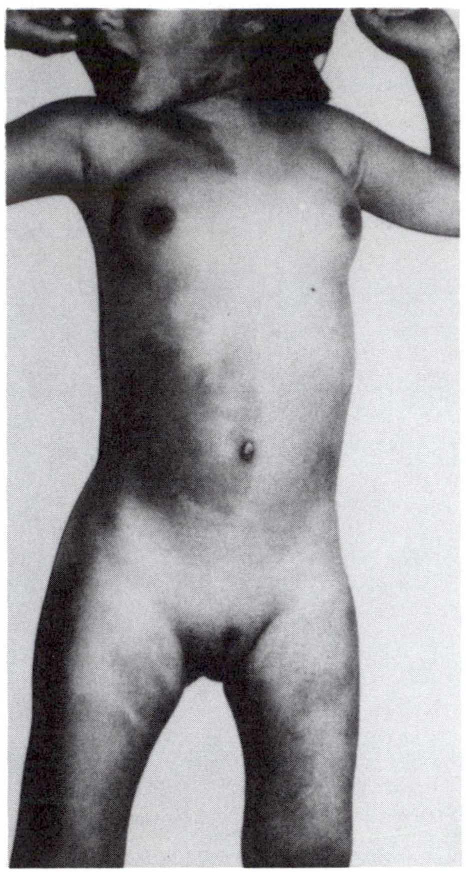

McCune-Albright syndrome
Happle, R.: *Clinical Genetics* 29:321-324, 1986. Munksgaard International Publishers, Copenhagen, Denmark.

pigmentation and precocious puberty is known as the Jaffe-Lichtenstein syndrome.

Albright, F., *et al*. Syndrome characterized by osteitis fibrosa disseminata, areas of pigmentation and endocrine dysfunction, with precocious puberty in females. Report of five cases. *N. Engl. J. Med.*, 1937, 216:727-46. McCune, D., & Bruch, H. Osteodystrophia fibrosa. Report of a case in which the condition was combined with precocious puberty, pathologic pigmentation of the skin and hypertrhyroidism, review of the literature. *Am. J. Dis. Child.*, 1937. 54:806-48. *Weil. [Case presentation of a 9-year-old girl with precocious puberty, fragile bones, and dermal pigmentation] *Klin. Wschr.*, 1922, 1:2114-5.

MCD (minimal cerebral dysfunction). See *attention deficit-hyperactivity disorder.*

MCDONOUGH, KENNETH B.

McDonough syndrome. A multiple congenital anomalies/mental retardation syndrome characterized by mental retardation, congenital heart defect, sternal deformity, kyphosis, craniofacial anomalies (anteverted auricles, upward palpebral slant, and squint), cryptorchism, and other anomalies. The syndrome is believed to be transmitted as an autosomal recessive trait with minor manifestations in heterozygotes. The syndrome was named after Dr. McDonough, who referred to the authors the original family affected with this syndrome.

Neuhauser, G., & Opitz, J. M. Studies of malformation syndromes in man. XXXX. Multiple congenital anomalies/mental retardation syndrome or variant familial developmental pattern: differential diagnosis and description of the McDonough syndrome (with XXY son from XY/XXY father). *Zschr. Kinderheilk.*, 1975, 120:231-42.

MCE. See *multiple cartilaginous exostoses syndrome.*

MCKITTRICK, LELAND STERLING (American physician, born 1892)

McKittrick-Wheelock syndrome. A villous adenoma of the colon and rectum associated with water-electrolyte balance disorders.

McKittrick, L. S., & Wheelock, F. C., Jr. *Carcinoma of the colon*. Springfield, Illinois, Thomas, 1954.

MCKUSICK, VICTOR ALMON (American physician, born 1921)

Cross-McKusick syndrome. See *Troyer syndrome.*

Cross-McKusick-Breen syndrome. See *Cross syndrome.*

Esterly-McKusick syndrome. See *stiff skin syndrome.*

McKusick metaphyseal chondrodysplasia syndrome. Synonyms: *cartilage-hair hypoplasia syndrome; metaphyseal chondrodysplasia, McKusick type.*

A syndrome of short-limb dwarfism, fine sparse hair, eyebrows, and eyelashes, hypoplasia of the cartilage, laxity of the ligaments, and short hands and feet. The skeletal features consist of metaphyseal dysplasia of the long bones, disproportionately long fibulae, moderate flattening of the vertebrae, and normal-sized head. The syndrome was first recognized among the Amish, but has more recently been identified in other groups. It is transmitted as an autosomal recessive trait with reduced penetrance.

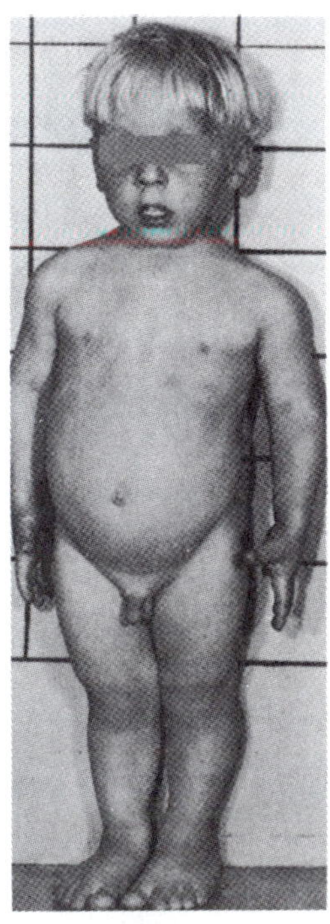

McKusick metaphyseal chondrodysplasia syndrome
McKusick, V.A., et al.: *Bull. Hopkins Hosp.*, 116.285, 1965.

McKusick, V. A., *et al.* Dwarfism in the Amish. II. Cartilage-hair hypoplasia. *Bull. Johns Hopkins Hosp.*, 1965, 116:285-326.

McKusick-Dungy-Kaufman syndrome. See *McKusick-Kaufman syndrome.*

McKusick-Kaufman syndrome (MKS). Synonyms: *Kaufman syndrome, McKusick-Dungy-Kaufman syndrome, hydrometrocolpos-polydactyly syndrome.*

An association of congenital hydrometrocolpos, postaxial polydactyly, and congenital heart defects, two out of three components occurring in many cases. Hydrometrocolpos develops as a result of a transverse vaginal membrane and excessive cervical secretions in response to maternal hormone. Bifid manubrium sterni, urogenital sinus, intestinal malrotation, congenital hip dislocation, polycystic kidney, rectovaginal fistula, imperforate anus, and vaginal duplication may be associated. The syndrome is transmitted as an autosomal recessive trait.

McKusick, V. A., *et al.* Hydrometrocolpos as a simply inherited malformation. *JAMA*, 1964, 189:813-6. Kaufman, R. L., *et al.* Family studies in congenital heart disease. II. A syndrome of hydrometrometrocolpos, postaxial polydactly and congenital heart disease. *Birth Defects*, 1972, 8(5):85-7. Dungy, C. I., *et al.* Hereditary hydometrocolpos with polydactly in infancy. *Pediatrics*, 1971, 47:138-41.

metaphyseal chondrodysplasia, McKusick type. See *McKusick metaphyseal chondrodysplasia syndrome.*

Strasburger-Hawkins-Eldridge-Hargrave-McKusick syndrome. See *symphalangism syndrome.*

MCLEAN, J. M. (American ophthalmologist)

Brown-McLean syndrome. See *under Brown, S. I.*

MCLETCHIE

McLetchie-Aikens syndrome. Synonym: *relapsing myositis.*

Fever followed by oval tumors of the thigh and, after several months, the biceps muscles. Pathologically, the lesions show hyaline necrosis en plaques, necrotic foci, mesenchymal reactions, follicular lesions, and signs of muscular regeneration. The syndrome was reportedly described by McLetchie and Aikens.

MCLS (mucocutaneous lymph node syndrome). See *Kawasaki syndrome.*

MCNS (minimal change nephrotic syndrome). See *nephrotic syndrome.*

MCTD. See *mixed connective tissue disease.*

MD. See *Minamata disease.*

MD (Ménière disease). See *Ménière syndrome.*

MDS. See *Miller-Dieker syndrome, under Miller, James Q.*

MDS. See *myelodysplastic syndrome.*

MEA (multiple endocrine adenomatosis, multiple endocrine adenopathy). See *multiple endocrine neoplasia syndrome.*

MEA I (multiple endocrine adenomatosis I). See *multiple endocrine neoplasia I syndrome.*

MEA-ulcer syndrome. See *multiple endocrine neoplasia I syndrome.*

MEADOW, ROY (British physician)

Meadow syndrome. See *Munchausen syndrome by proxy.*

MEADOW, S. R.

Meadow syndrome. See *fetal hydantoin syndrome.*

MEADOWS, W. R. (American physician)

Meadows syndrome. Synonyms: *postpartum cardiomyopathy, postpartum heart disease.*

A syndrome consisting of dyspnea, precordial pain, congestive heart failure, triple rhythm, tachycardia, embolism, and transient hypertension occurring in the last trimester of pregnancy or in the puerperium.

Meadows, W. R. Idiopathic myocardial failure in the last trimester of pregnancy and the puerperium. *Circulation*, 1957, 15:903-14.

MEANS

Means syndrome. Ophthalmoplegia associated with thyrotoxicosis.

Turut, P., *et al.* Ophtalmoplegie douloureuses recidivantes et syndrome de Means. *Rev. Otoneuropht.*, 1982, 54:47-52.

meat intoxication. See *Aguecheek disease.*

MEB (muscle-eye-brain) disease. See *Santavuori syndrome.*

MECKEL, JOHANN FRIEDRICH, JR. (German physician, 1781-1833)

Meckel diverticulum. Diverticulum of the ileum derived from the unobliterated yolk stalk.

Meckel. Über die Divertikel am Darmkanal. *Arch. Physiol., Halle*, 1809, 9:421-53.

Meckel syndrome (MS). Synonyms: *Gruber syndrome, Meckel-Gruber syndrome, dysencephalia splanchnocystica.*

A congenital syndrome of microcephaly, exencephalocele, microphthalmia, congenital heart defect, polydactyly, cleft lip, cleft palate, and polycystic degeneration of the kidneys, liver, and pancreas. Microcephaly may be associated with holoprosoncephaly, hydrocephalus, occipital encephalocele, and meningoencephalocele. Anencephaly and/or agenesis or hypoplasia of the cerebellum may occur. Polydactyly, the most common skeletal feature, involves all four limbs and presents hexadactyly, heptodactyly, or even a greater number of digits. Talipes equinovarus occurs in some cases. Hypoplastic penis, undescended testes, septate vagina, and bicornuate uterus are the principal genital anomalies. Malrotation of the intestine, cardiovascular defects, and a variety of other defects may be associated. Death usually takes place within the first month of life. The syndrome is transmitted as an autosomal recessive trait, parental consanguinity occurring in some cases.

Meckel, J. F. Beschreibung zweier durch sehr ähnliche Bildungsabweichung entstellter Geschwister, *Deut. Arch. Physiol.*, 1822, 7:99-172. Gruber, G. B. Beiträge zur Frage "gekoppelter" Missbildung (Akrocephalosyndactylie und Dysencephalia splanchnocystica). *Beitr. Path. Anat.*, 1934, 93:459-76.

Meckel-Gruber syndrome. See *Meckel syndrome.*

MECKEL, JOHANN FRIEDRICH, SR. (German anatomist, 1714-1774)

Meckel ganglion neuralgia. See *Sluder neuralgia.*

meconium ileus. See *meconium plug syndrome.*

meconium peritonitis. See *meconium plug syndrome.*

meconium plug syndrome (MPS). Synonyms: *ileal meconium plug, meconium ileus, meconium peritonitis.*

Neonatal intestinal obstruction caused by a plug of inspissated meconium in the large intestine. The symptoms include abdominal distention, vomiting, nausea, and constipation. Hirschprung disease, colonic atresia or stenosis, cystic fibrosis, exocrine pancreatic insufficiency, and neonatal small left colon syndrome are the potential causes.

Clatworthy, H. W., Jr., *et al.* The meconium plug syndrome. *Surgery*, 1956, 39:131-42.

MED I. See *multiple epiphyseal dysplasia I.*

MED II (multiple epiphyseal dysplasia II). See *Conradi-Hünermann syndrome.*

medial gastrocnemius bursitis. See *Baker cyst.*

medial synovial shelf plica syndrome. See *synovial shelf syndrome.*

medial tibial stress syndrome. See *shin splint syndrome.*

medial tibial syndrome. See *compartment syndrome.*

median cleft face syndrome. Synonyms: *DeMyer syndrome, frontonasal dysplasia, frontonasal dysplasia anomalad, median facial dysraphia.*

A defect of midfacial development with cranium bifidum occultum, hypertelorism, and median cleft nose, lip, and palate. Associated anomalies include broad nasal root, abnormal nasal tip, and widow's peak. Secondary telecanthus, epibulbar dermoids, notching of the alae nasi, coronal craniostenosis, and brachycephaly may be associated. Occasional defects may include syndactyly, polydactyly, brachydactyly, umbilical hernia, cryptorchism, and mental retardation. The severity and variety of symptoms vary with individual cases. The median cleft face syndrome and frontofacionasal dysplasia are considered by some writers the same entity.

*Hoppe, I. Eine angeborene Spaltung der Nase. *Preuss. Med. Ztg., Berlin*, 1859, 2:164-5. DeMyer, W. The median cleft face syndrome: Differential diagnosis of cranium bifidum occultum, hypertelorism, and median cleft nose, lip, and palate. *Neurology*, 1967, 17:961-71 Sedano, H. O., *et al.* Frontonasal dysplasia. *J. Pediat.*, 1970, 76:906-13.

median facial dysraphia. See *median cleft face syndrome.*

median facial spasm. See *Meige syndrome (2).*

median longitudinal fasciculus syndrome. See *Lhermitte syndrome.*

median rhomboid glossitis. See *Brocq-Pautrier syndrome.*

medical antishock trousers (MAST)-associated compartment syndrome (MACS). See *under compartment syndrome.*

MEDIN, KARL OSKAR (Swedish physician, 1847-1927)

Heine-Medin disease. See *under Heine.*

medionecrosis aortae idiopathica. See *Gsell-Erdheim syndrome.*

medionecrosis idiopathica aortae. See *Gsell-Erdheim syndrome.*

medionecrosis idiopathica cystica. See *Gsell-Erdheim syndrome.*

Mediterranean anemia. See *Cooley anemia.*

Mediterranean disease. See *Cooley anemia.*

Mediterranean fever. See *brucellosis.*

medullary gonadal dysgenesis. See *chromosome XXY syndrome.*

medullary polycystic kidney. See *Cacchi-Ricci syndrome.*

medullary sponge kidney. See *Cacchi-Ricci syndrome.*

medullary tegmental paralysis. See *Babinski-Nageotte syndrome.*

medullary thyroid carcinoma-pheochromocytoma syndrome. See *multiple endocrine neoplasia II syndrome.*

medulloblastoma cerebelli. See *Cushing medulloblastoma.*

MEEKEREN, JOB, VAN (Amsterdam surgeon, 1611-1666)

Meekeren-Ehlers-Danlos syndrome. See *Ehlers-Danlos syndrome.*

MEESMANN, ALOIS (German ophthalmologist, 1888-1969)

Meesmann dystrophy. Synonyms: *Meesmann-Wilke disease, dystrophia epithelialis corneae, hereditary epithelial corneal dystrophy, juvenile epithelial corneal dystrophy, juvenile epithelial degeneration of the cornea.*

Corneal dystrophy marked by vacuoles loaded with large amounts of glycogen and by cysts containing cellular degeneration products. Onset takes place during the first two years of life as a slight irritation, and is followed by lesions that form multiple punctate opacities of the epithelium and, occasionally, the Bowman membranes, as seen with magnification. It is a familial disorder transmitted as an autosomal dominant trait.

Meesmann, A. Über eine bisher nicht beschriebene, dominant vererbte Dystrophia epithelialis corneae. *Ber. Deut. Ophth. Ges.*, 1938, 52:154-8. Meesmann, A., & Wilke, F. Klinische und anatomische Untersuchungen über eine bisher unbekannte, dominant vererbte Epitheldystrophie der Hornhaut. *Klin. Mbl. Augenh.*, 1939, 103:361-91.

Meesmann-Wilke disease. See *Meesmann dystrophy.*

megacolon congenitum. See *Hirschsprung syndrome.*

megacystis-microcolon-intestinal hyperperistalsis syndrome. Synonym: *Berdon syndrome.*

A familial syndrome of the newborn characterized by intestinal obstruction, microcolon, giant bladder (megacystis), intestinal hypoperistalsis, hydronephrosis, and dilated small bowel. The pathological findings consist of an abundance of ganglion cells in both dilated and narrow areas of the intestine. According to Winter and Knowles, the syndrome is transmitted as an autosomal recessive trait; according to McKusick, it is transmitted as an autosomal dominant trait.

Berdon, W. E., *et al.* Megacystis-microcolon-intestinal hypoperistalsis syndrome: A new case of intestinal obstruction in the newborn: Report of radiologic findings in five newborn girls. *Am. J. Roentgen.*, 1976, 126:957-64. McKusick, V. A. *Mendelian inheritance in man.* 7th ed. Baltimore, Johns Hopkins Univ. Press. 1986, p. 482, No. 15531. Winter, R. M., & Knowles, S. A. S. Megacystis-microcolon-intestinal hypoperistalsis syndrome: Confirmation of autosomal recessive inheritance. *J. Med. Genet.*, 1986, 23:3260-2.

megaencephaly with hyaline panneuropathy. See *Alexander syndrome, under Alexander, W. Stewart.*

megalerythema epidemicum. See *Sticker disease.*

megalerythema infectiosum. See *Sticker disease.*

megalia ossium et cutis. See *pachydermoperiostosis syndrome.*

megaloblastic anemia in infants. See *Zuelzer-Ogden syndrome.*

megatrachea. See *Mounier-Kuhn syndrome.*

megatrachea with tracheomalacia. See *Mounier-Kuhn syndrome.*

megepiphyseal dwarfism. Synonym: *Gorlin syndrome.*

A syndrome of dwarfism, dislocated lenses, staphyloma, glaucoma, mental retardation, depressed nasal

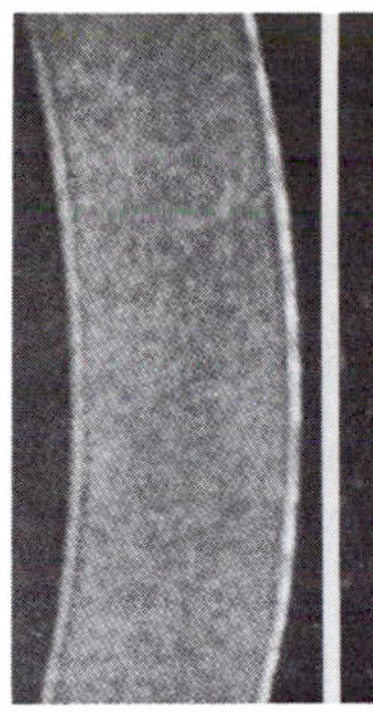
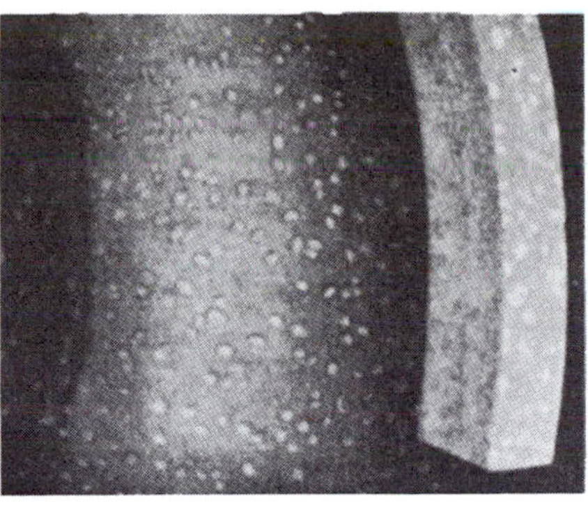
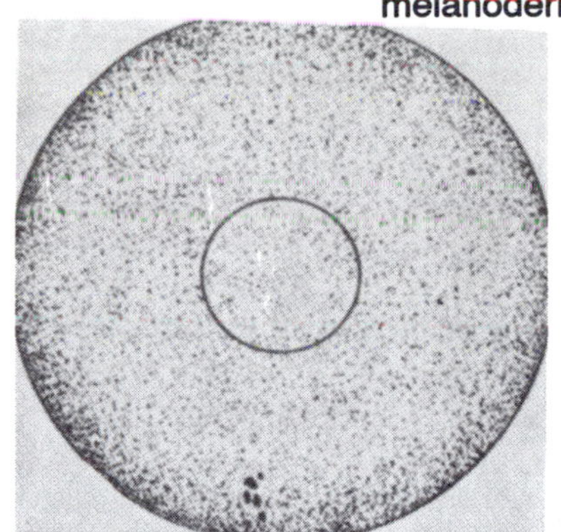

Meesmann dystrophy
Francois, Jules: *Heredity in Ophthalmology.* St. Louis: C.V. Mosby Co., 1961.

bridge, cleft palate, platyspondyly, flared metaphyses, and huge flattened epiphyses widening at the distal ends of the proximal phalanges of the fingers.

Gorlin, R. J., *et al.* Megepiphyseal dwarfism. *J. Pediat.*, 1973, 83:633-5.

MEIBOM (MEIBOMIUS), HEINRICH (German anatomist, 1638-1700)

meibomian cyst. Synonym: *chalazion.*

A small tumor of the eyelid formed by distention of a meibomian gland with secretions.

*Meibomius, H. *De vasis palpebrarum novis epistola.* Halmstäd, Müller, 1666.

MEIGE, HENRY (French physician, 1866-1940)

Brissaud-Meige syndrome. See *Brissaud infantilism.*

Meige syndrome (1). Synonyms: *chronic hereditary trophedema, congenital lymphedema, hereditary lymphedema type II, hereditary lymphedema praecox, late onset lymphedema.*

A familial form of pitting and painless lymphedema of the limbs, with onset in the first or second decade of life, often associated with inflammation and various defects, including distichiasis, extradural cysts, vertebral anomalies, cerebrovascular malformations, yellow nails, and sensorineural hearing loss. It is transmitted as an autosomal dominant trait. **Hereditary lymphedema type I (Nonne-Milroy syndrome)** and **hereditary lymphedema type II (Meige syndrome)** were in the past combined into a single syndrome, the **Nonne-Milroy-Meige syndrome**; they are now divided into two distinct entities.

Meige, H. Le trophoedème chronique héréditaire. *Nouv. Icon. Salpetriere*, 1899, 12:453-80.

Meige syndrome (2). Synonyms: *Brueghel syndrome, blepharospasm-oromandibular dystonia syndrome, median facial spasm.*

A disabling spasm of the facial musculature, most commonly observed in middle-aged or elderly females, although males may be also affected. It consists of primary blepharospasm followed by abnormal facial movement. Squinting may begin unilaterally but soon becomes bilateral. In time, the lower facial muscles becomes involved with yawning, jaw opening, and abnormal tongue movements. Emotional stress and fatigue seem to worsen the abnormal movements. Cervical, laryngeal, pharyngeal, and respiratory muscles may become progressively involved. Torticollis, dystonic writer's cramp, and dystonic posturing of the arms are usually associated. The syndrome is said to have been recognized by Pieter Brueghel, the Elder, who illustrated it in his painting *De Gaper.* The etiology is unknown.

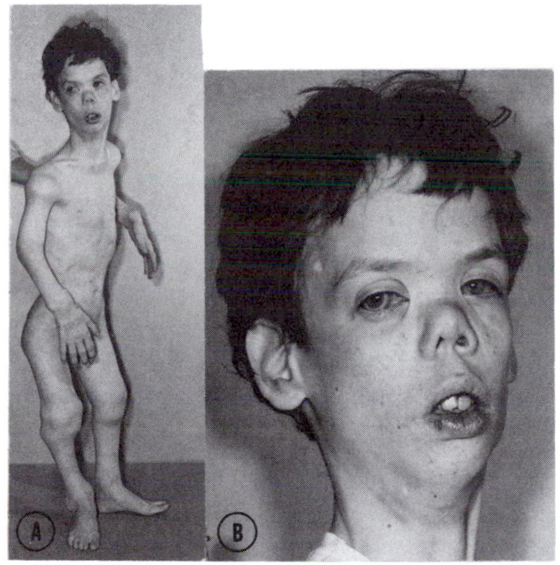

Megepiphyseal dwarfism
Courtesy of Dr. Robert J. Gorlin, Minneapolis, MN.

Meige, H. Les convulsions de la face, une forme clinique de convulsion faciale, bilaterale et mediane. *Rev. Neur., Paris*, 1910, 20:437-43. Marsden, C. D. Blepharospasm-oromandibular dystonia syndrome (Brueghel's syndrome). A variant of adult-onset torsion dystonia? *J. Neurol. Neurosurg. Psychiat.*, 1976, 39:1204-9.

MEIGS, JOE VINCENT (American physician, 1892-1963)

Demons-Meigs syndrome. See *Meigs syndrome.*

Meigs syndrome. Synonyms: *Demons-Meigs syndrome, Meigs-Cass syndrome, ovarian ascites-pleural effusion syndrome.*

A concurrence of ovarian tumors, hydrothorax, and ascites.

Meigs, J. V., & Cass, J. W. Fibroma of the ovary with ascites and hydrothorax with a report of seven cases. *Am. J. Obstet.*, 1937, 33:249-67.

Meigs-Cass syndrome. See *Meigs syndrome.*

melanoblastosis cutis linearis sive systematisata. See *Bloch-Sulzberger syndrome.*

melanocytosis bulbi. See *Ota nevus.*

melanodermatitis toxica. See *Riehl melanosis.*

melanodermic leukodystrophy. See *adrenoleukodystrophy.*

melanofibroma. See *Jadassohn-Tièche nevus, under Jadassohn, Josef.*

melanoplakia-small intestinal polyposis syndrome. See *Peutz-Jeghers syndrome.*

melanosis circumscripta precancerosa. See *Hutchinson freckle, under Hutchinson, Sir Jonathan.*

melanosis corii degenerativa. See *Bloch-Sulzberger syndrome.*

melanosis lenticularis progresiva. See *xeroderma pigmentosum syndrome.*

melanotic freckle. See *Hutchinson freckle, under Hutchinson, Sir Jonathan.*

melanotic panaritium. See *Hutchinson melanotic disease, under Hutchinson, Sir Jonathan.*

melanotic whitlow. See *Hutchinson melanotic disease, under Hutchinson, Sir Jonathan.*

melasma suprarenale. See *Addison disease.*

MELCHIOR, J. C. (Danish physician)

Dyggve-Melchior-Clausen dwarfism. See *Dyggve-Melchior-Clausen syndrome, under Dyggve.*

Dyggve-Melchior-Clausen syndrome (DMC, DMCS). See *under Dyggve.*

melioidosis. See *Whitmore disease.*

melitensis septicemia. See *brucellosis.*

melitococcosis. See *brucellosis.*

MELKERSSON, ERNST GUSTAF (Swedish physician, 1892-1932)

Melkersson-Rosenthal syndrome (MRS). Synonyms: *Melkersson-Rosenthal-Schuermann syndrome, Miescher cheilitis, Miescher syndrome, Rossolimo-Melkersson-Rosenthal syndrome, cheilitis glandularis, cheilitis granulomatosa, essential granulomatous macrocheilitis.*

A disease, usually beginning during childhood or adolescence, consisting of recurrent facial paralysis, facial edema, and fissured tongue. Associated disorders may include acroparesthesia, headache, hyperhidrosis, hypogeusia, xerostomia, blepharospasm, epiphora, and swelling of the hands, chest, and buttocks. The edema usually recurs in the spring and fall, resulting in permanent enlargement of the lips. The etiology is unknown. Some authors divide this disorder into two separate entities: the *Melkersson-Rosenthal syndrome* and *Miescher cheilitis.*

Melkersson, E. Ett fall av recidiverande facialispares i samband med angioneurotisk ödem. *Hygeia,* 1928, 90:737-41. Rosenthal, C. Klinischer biologischer Beitrag zur Konstitutionspathologie. Gemeinsame Auftreten von (rezidivierender familiärer) Facialslähmung angioneurotischem Gesichtsödem und Lingua plicata in Arthritismus-Familien. *Zschr. Ges. Neurol. Psychiat.*, 1931, 475:500. Schuermann, H. H. *Krankheiten der Mundschleimhaut und der Lippen.* 2nd ed. Urbach & Schwarzenberg, Berlin, 1958. Koliadenko, V. G., *et al.* [Rossolimo-Melkersson-Rosenthal syndrome] *Vestn. Dermatol. Venerol.*, 1979, No. 9:22-4. Miescher, G. Über essentielle granulomatöse Makrocheilie (Cheilitis granulomatosa). *Dermatologica*, 1945, 91:57-85.

Melkersson-Rosenthal-Schuermann syndrome. See *Melkersson-Rosenthal syndrome.*

Rossolimo-Melkersson-Rosenthal syndrome. See *Melkersson-Rosenthal syndrome.*

MELLMAN, WILLIAM J. (American physician)

Winter-Kohn-Mellman-Wagner syndrome. See *Winter syndrome.*

MELNICK, JOHN CHARLES (American radiologist, born 1928)

Melnick-Needles syndrome (MNS). Synonyms: *generalized osseous dystrophy syndrome, osteodysplasia, osteodysplasty.*

An autosomal dominant syndrome of craniofacial abnormalities (exophthalmos, puffed cheeks, micrognathia, malocclusion, high and narrow forehead, and large ears), mild bowing of the upper arms and shanks with cubitus valgus and genu valgum, and slight shortening of the distal phalanges, especially the thumbs. The syndrome has its onset in children and is associated with recurrent respiratory and ear infections.

Melnick, J. C., & Needles, C. F. An undiagnosed bone dysplasia. A 2 family study of 4 generations and 3 generations. *Am. J. Roentgen.*, 1966, 97:39-48.

melorheostosis. See *Léri syndrome (1).*

MELTZER, M. (American physician)

Peetoom-Meltzer syndrome. See *arthralgia-purpura-weakness syndrome.*

MEMR (multiple exostoses-mental retardation) syndrome. See *Langer-Giedion syndrome.*

MEN (I, II, IIa, IIb, III). See *multiple endocrine neoplasia syndrome syndrome (I, II, IIa, IIb, III).*

MENDE, IRMGARD (German physician)

Mende syndrome. A congenital familial syndrome combining mongoloid habitus, deaf-mutism, and pigmentation disorders, chiefly partial albinism involving the scalp hair (including white forelock) and pubic and facial hair. Cleft palate, external ear abnormalities, and ocular complications may be present.

Mende, I. Über eine Familie hereditär-degenerativer Taubstummheit mit mongoloidem Einschlag und teilweisen Leukismus der Haut und Haare. *Arch. Kinderh.*, 1926, 79:214-22.

MENDELSON, CURTIS LESTER (American physician, born 1913)

Mendelson syndrome. Synonyms: *acid aspiration syndrome (AAS), acid pulmonary aspiration, aspiration pneumonitis, gastric acid aspiration syndrome, gastric juice aspiration syndrome (GJA-S), peptic aspiration pneumonia, pulmonary acid aspiration.*

Pneumonia with asthmalike symptoms produced by the irritative action of hydrochloric acid in the gastric juice after aspiration of stomach contents during general anesthesia (obstetric anesthesia in the original report). The symptoms include tachypnea, tachycardia, wheezing, rhonchi, crepitant rales, decreased arterial oxygen tension, and, in some severe cases, edema, shock, and death. Abolishment of laryngeal reflexes is believed to be the cause.

Mendelson, C. L. The aspiration of stomach contents into the lungs during obstetric anesthesia. *Am. J. Obst. Gyn.*, 1946, 52:191-205.

MENDENHALL, E. N. (Amearican physician)

Mendenhall syndrome. See *Rabson-Mendenhall syndrome.*

Rabson-Mendenhall syndrome. See *under Rabson.*

MENDES DA COSTA, SAMUEL (Dutch dermatologist, born 1862)

Da Costa syndrome. See *Mendes Da Costa syndrome.*

Mendes Da Costa syndrome. Synonyms: *Da Costa syndrome, erythroderma congenitum symmetricum*

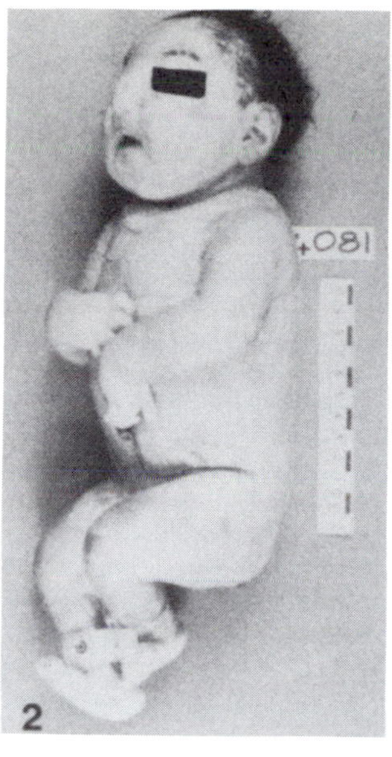
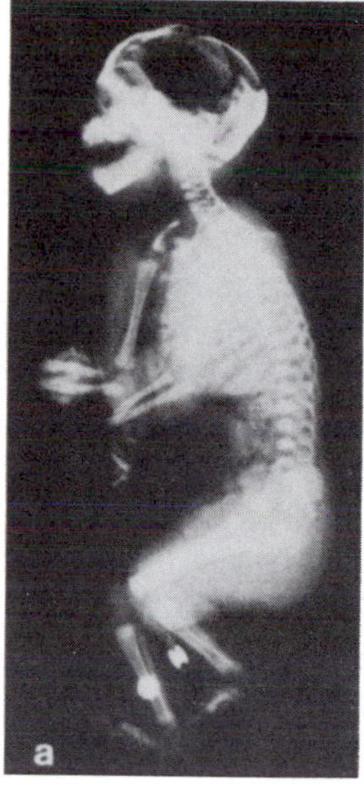
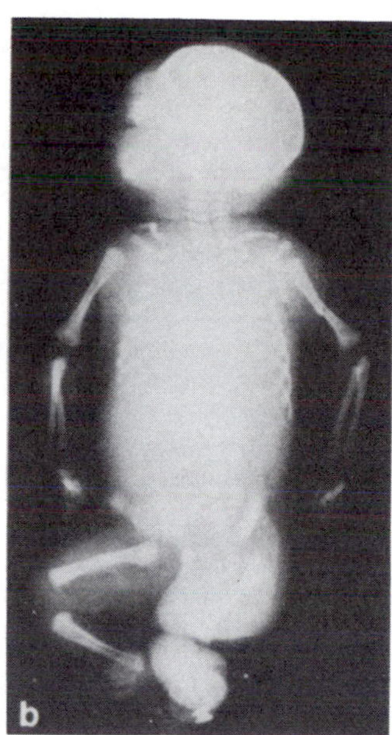

Melnick-Needles syndrome
Donnenfeld, Alan E., Katrina A. Conard, Nancy S. Roberts, Patricia Flint Borns & Elaine H. Zackai: *American Journal of Medical Genetics* 27:159-173 1987. New York: Alan R. Liss, Inc.

progressiva, erythrokeratodermia variabilis (EKV), keratoerythrodermia variabilis, keratosis rubra figurata, variable erythrokeratoderma.

A hereditary skin disease, transmitted as an autosomal dominant trait, characterized by hyperkeratotic plaques with bizarre configurations, associated with sharply outlined independent erythrodermic areas which may assume considerable variations in size, shape, and position from day to day. Onset is in early infancy.

Mendes Da Costa, S. Erythro- et keratodermia variabilis in a mother and daughter. *Acta. Derm. Vener., Stockholm,* 1925, 6:255-61.

MENETRIER, PIERRE EUGENE (French physician, 1859-1935)

Ménétrier syndrome. Synonyms: *chronic hypertrophic gastritis, diffuse gastric polyadenoma, gastritis hypertrophica gigantea, giant hypertrophic gastritis, giant hypertrophy of gastric mucosa, hypertrophic gastropathy, plague-like gastric adenoma, polyadenoma en nappe, villous gastropathy.*

Hypertrophy of the gastric mucosa associated with degenerative changes in the glandular layer, hyperplasia involving the superficial epithelium and remnants of the glandular layer, anacidity or marked hypoacidity, and hypoproteinemia due to leakage of proteins. It is one of the causes of protein-losing gastroenteropathy (q.v.). The symptoms include epigastric pain, edema, ascites, anemia, and frequent eosinophilia.

Ménétrier, P. Des polyadénomes gastriques et de leurs rapports avec le cancer de l'estomac. *Arch. Physiol. Norm. Path.*, 1888, 1:32-55; 236-62.

MENGEL

Mengel bilateral deficiency of abduction. See *Stilling-Türk-Duane syndrome.*

MENIERE, PROSPER (French physician, 1799-1862)

Ménière disease (MD). See *Ménière syndrome.*

Ménière syndrome. Synonyms: *Ménière disease (MD), auditory vertigo, aural vertigo, benign recurrent vertigo syndrome, cochlear hydrops, endolymphatic hydrops, labyrinthine hydrops, oticodynia, recurrent labyrinthine vertigo, vestibular neuronitis.*

Sudden attacks of vertigo, tinnitus, prostration, vomiting, and progressive deafness, associated with distention of the endolymphatic system and degenerative changes of the sensory elements of the internal ear. Onset is usually in the fifth decade, but younger age groups may also be affected. The term *Ménière disease* is sometimes restricted to patients with the triad of vestibular symptoms, auditory symptoms, and aural pressure, in whom the etiologic factor is known; *Ménière syndrome* is used for those whom the cause is unknown. See also *Pedersen syndrome, vestibular syndrome*, and *Lermoyez syndrome.*

Ménière, P. Sur une forme particulière de surdité grave dépendant d'une lésion de l'oreille interne. *Gaz. Méd., Paris*, 1861, 16:29.

symptomatic Ménière syndrome. See *Lermoyez syndrome.*

meningeal angiomatosis with diffuse sclerosis. See *van Bogaert-Divry syndrome.*

meningeal capillary angiomatosis. See *Sturge-Weber syndrome.*

meningeal hydrops. See *pseudotumor cerebri syndrome.*

meningioma. See *Cushing tumor.*

meningitis serosa. See *Schneider disease, under Schneider, Hans.*

meningo-oculofacial angiomatosis. See *Sturge-Weber syndrome.*

meningoblastoma. See *Cushing tumor.*

meningococcic adrenal syndrome. See *Waterhouse-Friderichsen syndrome.*

menisocytosis. See *sickle-cell anemia.*

MENKES, JOHN H. (American physician, born 1928)

Menkes disease. See *maple syrup urine disease.*

Menkes kinky hair syndrome. See *kinky hair syndrome.*

Menkes syndrome. See *kinky hair syndrome.*

menopausal syndrome. See *climacteric syndrome.*

menouria syndrome. See *Youssef syndrome.*

menstrual migraine. See *under headache syndrome.*

menstrual toxic shock syndrome. See *toxic shock syndrome.*

mentagra. See *Alibert disease (3).*

mental deficiency-epilepsy-endocrine disorders syndrome. See *Börjeson syndrome.*

mental retardation, Mietens-Weber type. See *Mietens-Weber syndrome.*

mental retardation, X-linked. See *X-linked mental retardation syndrome.*

mental retardation-aphasia-shuffling gait-adducted thumbs syndrome. See *MASA syndrome.*

mental retardation-clasped thumb syndrome. See *Gareis syndrome.*

mental retardation-overgrowth syndrome. See *Golabi-Rosen syndrome.*

MENZEL, P. (German physician)

Menzel syndrome. See *OPCA I, under olivopontocerebellar atrophy.*

olivopontocerebellar atrophy (OPCA), Menzel type. See *OPCA I, under olivopontocerebellar atrophy.*

meralgia paresthetica. See *Rot-Bernhardt syndrome, under Rot, Vladimir Karlovich.*

MEREDITH, J. M. (American physician)

Coleman-Meredith syndrome. See *Coleman syndrome.*

MERETOJA, J. (Finnish physician)

Meretoja syndrome. See *amyloid neuropathy type IV.*

mermaid syndrome. See *caudal regression syndrome.*

MERRITT, A. DONALD (American physician)

Lavy-Palmer-Merritt syndrome. See *spondylothoracic dysplasia.*

MERRITT, KATHARINE KROM (American physician, born 1886)

Kasabach-Merritt syndrome. See *under Kasabach.*

MERTEN, DAVID F. (American radiologist)

Singleton-Merten syndrome. See *under Singleton.*

MERZBACHER, LUDWIG (German physician, 1875-1942)

Pelizaeus-Merzbacher syndrome. See *under Pelizaeus.*

MES (multiple endocrine syndrome). See *multiple endocrine neoplasia syndrome.*

MESA (myoepithelial sialadenitis). See *Sjögren syndrome, under Sjögren, Henrik Samuel Conrad.*

mesangial IgA/IgG nephropathy. See *Berger syndrome, under Berger, J.*

mesencephalic artery syndrome. Occlusion of a perforating branch of the mesencephalic artery (posterior thalamosubthalamic paramedian artery) associated with akinetic mutism. Disconnection or deafferentiation of thalamic nuclei from ascending midline mesencephalic reticular impulses is believed to be the cause of mutism.

Segarra, J. M. Cerebral vascular disease and behavior. I. The syndrome of mesencephalic artery. *Arch. Neur., Chicago*, 1970, 22:408-18.

mesenchymal hypoglycemic tumor. See *Doege-Potter syndrome.*

mesenteric arteritis syndrome. See *postcoartectomy syndrome.*

mesenteric artery syndrome. See *aortoiliac steal syndrome.*

mesenteric chyladenectasis. See *Whipple disease.*

mesenteric lymphadenitis-upper respiratory tract infection syndrome. See *Brennemann syndrome.*

mesenteric reticulocytic abscess-forming lymphadenitis. See *Massshoff syndrome.*

mesenteric syndrome. See *postcoartectomy syndrome.*

mesoectodermal dysplasia. See *Ellis-van Creveld syndrome.*

mesomelic dwarfism of the hypoplastic ulna, fibula and mandible type. See *Langer syndrome.*

mesomelic dwarfism, Langer type. See *Langer syndrome.*

mesomelic dwarfism, Nievergelt type. See *Nievergelt syndrome.*

metabolic craniopathy. See *Morgagni-Stewart-Morel syndrome.*

metachromatic leukodystrophy (MLD). Synonyms: *Greenfield syndrome; Scholz syndrome; Scholz-Bielschowsky-Henneberg syndrome; Scholz-Greenfield syndrome; van Bogaert-Nijssen syndrome; van Bogaert-Nijssen-Peiffer syndrome; van Bogaert-Nyssen syndrome; van Bogaert-Nyssen-Peiffer syndrome; familial progressive cerebral sclerosis; leukodystrophia cerebri progressiva metachromatica diffusa; leukodystrophy, type Scholz; sulfatide lipidosis.*

A congenital error of metabolism, transmitted as an autosomal recessive trait, consisting of a group of disorders characterized by myelin degeneration with the accumulation of galactosyl sulfatide and other lipids containing a galactosyl-3-sulfate moiety. It is due to arylsulfatase A (cerebroside sulfatase) deficiency and, less commonly, decreased activity of multiple sulfatase. **Late infantile metachromatic leukodystrophy (Greenfield syndrome)**, the most common type, is characterized by normal infancy followed by locomotor disorders between the ages of 12 and 18 months. Associated defects include muscle hypotonia, decreased or absent reflexes (especially of the legs), occasional genu recurvatum, and bilateral plantar responses. Early symptoms are followed by involvement of the arms, slurred speech, deglutition disorders, dementia, optic atrophy, grayish discoloration of the macula lutea, spastic paraplegia or diplegia, increased muscle tone with or without deep tendon reflexes, and ataxia. Eventually, the affected children are bedridden and quadriplegic. There may be decorticate, decerebrate, or dystonic postures with superimposed hypertonic seizures. The children are blind, without speech and volitional movement. **Juvenile metachromatic leukodystrophy** is characterized by onset between the ages of 3 and 21 years of emotional lability, impaired school performance, day dreaming, and gait disorders. Early symptoms are followed by extrapyramidal dysfunction, such as postural abnormalities, increased muscle tone, nystagmus, and intention tremor. **Adult metachromatic leukodystrophy (van Bogaert-Nyssen-Peiffer syndrome)** is marked by onset after the age of 21 years. The symptoms include impaired ability to concentrate, faulty memory, schizophrenialike disorders, emotional lability with episodes of alternating euphoria and depression, spastic movements, and occasional seizures, frequently in association with dementia, slowness and clumsiness of movement, slurred speech, diminished velocity in peripheral nerves, hyperactive deep tendon reflexes, nystagmus, truncal ataxia, intention tremor, flat facial expression, dystonic movements, unilateral pareses and motor impairment, incontinence, inability to speak, and terminal generalized seizures. **Multiple sulfatase deficiency (mucosulfatidosis)** is a rare condition with symptoms similar to those in juvenile metachromatic leukodystrophy. After a slow development, the symptoms may appear during the first year of life. Additional disorders include dry scaly skin, deafness, convexity of the sternum, pectus excavatum, flaring of the ribs, and occasional hepatosplenomegaly. Pathological findings include demyelination of the peripheral nerves, high protein levels in the cerebrospinal fluid, decreased density of the white matter, lesions of the gallbladder, brownish metachromasia in frozen tissue sections stained with acetic cresyl violet, and excess sulfatides in the urine.

Greenfield, J. G. A form of progressive cerebral sclerosis in infants associated with primary degeneration of the interfascicular glia. *J. Neur. Psychopath., London,* 1933, 13:289-302. Bielschowsky, M., & Henneberg, R. Über familiäre diffuse Sklerose (Leukodystrophia cerebri progressiva hereditaria). *J. Psychol., Leipzig,* 1928, 36:131-81. van Bogaert, L. & Nyssen, R. Le type tardif de la leucodystrophie progressive familiale. *Rev. Neur., Paris,* 1936, 65:21-45. Peiffer, J. Über die metachromatischen Leukodystrophien (Typ Scholz). *Arch. Psychother., Berlin,* 1959, 199:386-416. *Scholz, W. Klinische, pathologisch-anatomische und erbbiologische Untersuchungen bei famili- ärer, diffuser Hirnsklerose im Kindersalter (Ein Beitrag zur Lehre von den Heredodegenerationen). *Zschr. Neur.,* 1925, 99:561-717. Dulaney, J. T., & Moser, H. W. Sulfatide lipodosis: metachromatic leukodystrophy. In: Stanbury, J. B., Wyngaarden, J. B., & Fredrickson, D. S., eds. *The metabolic basis of inherited disease.* 4th ed. New York, McGraw-Hill, 1978, pp. 770-809.

metaepiphyseal osteodystrophy of the calcaneum. See *Blencke syndrome.*

metaepiphyseal osteodystrophy of the os calcis. See *Blencke syndrome.*

metaherpetic keratitis. See *Franceschetti dystrophy.*

metal turner paralysis. See *Hunt syndrome (3), under Hunt, James Ramsay.*

metallergic and parallergic reactions. See *excited skin syndrome.*

metameric angiomatosis. See *Cobb syndrome.*

metaphyseal chondrodysplasia, McKusick type. See *McKusick metaphyseal chondrodysplasia syndrome.*

metaphyseal chondrodysplasia, Schmid type. See *Schmid metaphyseal chondrodysplasia syndrome, under Schmid, Franz.*

metaphyseal chondrodysplasia, Wiedemann-Spranger type. See *Wiedemann-Spranger metaphyseal-chondrodysplasia syndrome.*

metaphyseal chondrodysplasia-malabsorption-neutropenia syndrome (MMN). See *Shwachman syndrome.*

metaphyseal dysostosis, Jansen type. See *Jansen metaphyseal chondrodysplasia syndrome.*

metaphyseal dysostosis, Murk Jansen type. See *Jansen metaphyseal chondrodysplasia syndrome.*

metaphyseal dysostosis, Schmid type. See *Schmid metaphyseal chondrodysplasia syndrome, under Schmid, Franz.*

metaphyseal dysostosis-conductive hearing loss-mental retardation syndrome. See *Rimoin syndrome.*

metaphyseal dysostosis-pancreatic insufficiency syndrome. See *Shwachman syndrome.*

metaphyseal dysostosis-pancreatic insufficiency-blood disorder syndrome. See *Shwachman syndrome.*

metaphyseal dysplasia syndrome. Synonyms: *Bakwin-Krida syndrome, Pyle disease, Pyle metaphyseal dysplasia syndrome, Pyle-Cohn syndrome, familial metaphyseal dysplasia.*

A rare congenital syndrome transmitted as an autosomal recessive trait, and characterized by genua valga, occasional joint pain, muscular weakness, mild scoliosis, limited elbow extension, malocclusion, and increased tendency to fractures. Major x-ray findings include hyperostosis of the cranial vault; obtuse mandibular angle; mandibular prognathism; expansion of the ribs, clavicles, and pubic and ischial bones; metaphyseal flare of the tubular bones, extending into the diaphysis; and Erlenmeyer flasklike appearance of the diaphyses in the femur and tibia. The term *Pyle disease* is sometimes also used to designate the *craniometaphyseal dysplasia syndrome.*

Pyle, E. A case of unusual bone development. *J. Bone Joint Surg.,* 1931, 13:874-6. Bakwin, H., & Krida, A. Familial metaphysial dysplasia. *Am. J. Dis. Child.,* 1937, 53:1521-7. Cohn, M. Konstitutionelle Hyperspongiosierung des Skeletts mit partiellen Riesenwuchs. *Fortschr. Röntgen.,* 1933, 47:293.

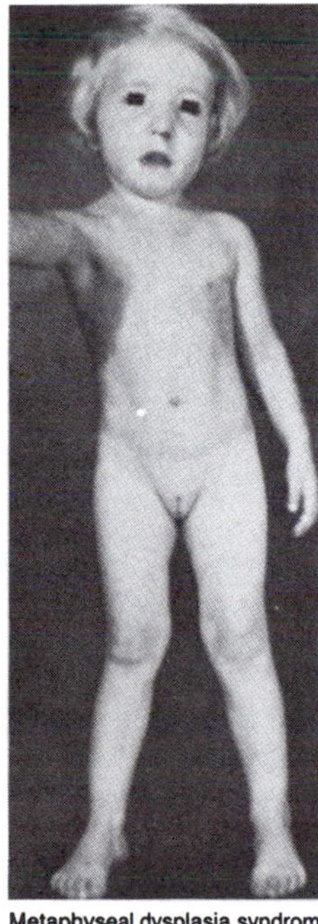
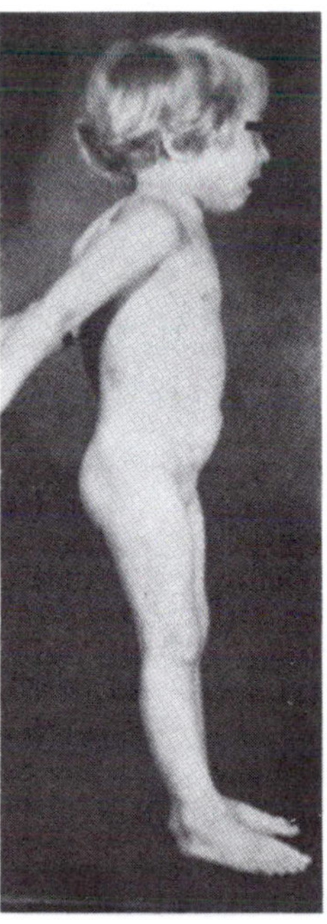

Metaphyseal dysplasia syndrome
Rubin, P., *Dynamic Classification of Bone Dysplasias.* Chicago: Year Book Medical Publishers, 1964.

metastatic carcinoid syndrome. See *carcinoid syndrome.*

metatarsal neuralgia. See *Morton neuralgia, under Morton, Thomas George.*

metatarsal periostitis. See *Busquet disease.*

metatarsalgia anterior. See *Morton neuralgia, under Morton, Thomas George.*

metatarsus atavicus. See *Morton syndrome, under Morton, Dudley J.*

metatarsus primus brevior. See *Morton syndrome, under Morton, Dudley J.*

metatropic dwarfism syndrome. Synonyms: *Maroteaux-Spranger-Wiedemann syndrome, hyperplastic achondroplasia, hyperplastic chondrodystrophia foetalis, metatropic dwarfism type I.*

A syndrome characterized in childhood by dwarfism with normal body length and disproportionately long trunk and short extremities, narrow chest, prominent joints, limited joint movement, and a tail-like appendage overlying the sacrum, and in adults, by short spine, kyphoscoliosis, deformed chest, prominent joints, and frequently a tail-like appendage overlying the sacrum. Radiological findings consist of poor ossification of the vertebral bodies in infancy and platyspondyly and anterior wedging of the vertebral bodies later in life, hypoplasia of the basilar part of the iliac crests and low-set anterosuperior iliac spines, small and deformed capital femoral epiphyses, hyperplasia of the proximal femoral metaphyses, and short tubular bones with metaphyseal flare and epiphyseal dysplasia. Both autosomal recessive and autosomal dominant forms of transmission have been reported.

Maroteaux, P., Spranger, J., & Wiedemann, H. R. Metatropischer Zwerwuchs. *Arch. Kinderheilk.*, 1966, 173:211-26.

metatropic dwarfism type I. See *metatropic dwarfism syndrome.*

metatropic dwarfism type II. See *Kniest disease.*

methionine malabsorption syndrome. Synonyms: *Smith-Strang syndrome, oasthouse syndrome.*

A syndrome of malabsorption of methionine and secondary malabsorption of other amino acids, transmitted as an autosomal recessive trait, in which some of the unabsorbed methionine is converted by colonic bacteria to α-hydroxybutyric acid, giving the urine a characteristic odor similar to that of an oasthouse (a building for drying hops). Mental retardation, diarrhea, convulsions, and polypnea are associated. See also *malabsorption syndrome.*

Smith, A. J., & Strang, J. B. An inhorn error of metabolism with the urinary excretion of alpha-hydroxy-butyric acid and phenylpyruvic acid. *Arch. Dis. Child.*, 1958, 33:109-13. Hooft, C., *et al.* Methionine malabsorption syndrome. *Ann. Paediat., Basel,* 1965, 205:73-104.

MEULENGRACHT, EINAR (Danish physician, 1887)

Meulengracht icterus. See *Gilbert syndrome under Gilbert, Nicolas Augustin.*

Meulengracht syndrome. See *Gilbert syndrome, under Gilbert, Nicolas Augustin.*

Meuse fever. See *Werner-His disease, under Werner, Heinrich.*

MEYENBURG, HANS, VON (Swiss physician, born 1887)

Meyenburg disease. Synonyms: *generalized fibromatosis, fibrosing myositis.*

A rare generalized disease which may affect any muscle or a group of muscles, and which appears within the first 5 years of life. It is characterized by increasing stiffness and absence of pain. At first, the affected muscles become enlarged and indurated; later, they become smaller and contracted, so that eventually the patient becomes completely immobilized. Proliferation of fibroblasts and absence of inflammatory reaction are the main histological features.

Crenshaw, A. H., ed. *Campbell's operative orthopedics.* 4th ed. St. Louis, Mosby, 1963, Vol. 2, p. 1263.

Meyenburg syndrome. See *Meyenburg-Altherr-Uehlinger syndrome.*

Meyenburg-Altherr-Uehlinger syndrome. Synonyms: *Askenazy syndrome, Jaksch Wartenhorst syndrome, Meyenburg syndrome, von Jaksch Wartenhorst syndrome, von Meyenburg syndrome, von Meyenburg-Altherr-Uehlinger syndrome, atrophic polychondritis, chondrolytic perichondritis, chondromalacic arthritis, diffuse perichondritis, familial chronic atrophic polychondritis, generalized chondromalacia, panchondritis, polychondritis chronica atrophicans, polychondritis recidivans et atrophicans, polychondropathy, relapsing polychondritis, rheumatic panchondritis, systemic chondromalacia, systemic panchondritis.*

A disease of the articular and nonarticular cartilages, frequently affecting the nose, throat, ears, epiglottis, larynx, trachea, bronchi, hands, feet, spine, joints, and other organs. The symptoms include painful inflammation of the affected parts with various degrees of severity, and resulting in rhinorrhea, epistaxis, saddle nose, middle and inner ear lesions, deafness, tinnitus, red swollen ears, recurrent laryngitis, dyspnea, cough, hoarseness, fever, and malaise. Ocular manifestations consist of episcleritis, iritis, and cataracts. Anemia, liver function disorders, myocarditis, and aortic valvular insufficiency have been noted in some cases. The illness may become fulminant, with tracheal collapse causing death by airway obstruction. The etiology is unknown.

Meyenburg, von. Über Chondromalacie. *Schweiz. Med. Wschr.,* 1936, 66:1239-40. Altherr, F. Über einen Fall von systematisierter Chondromalacie. *Virchows Arch. Path.,* 1936, 297:445-79. Jaksch-Wartenhorst, R., von. Polychondropathia. *Wien. Arch. Klin. Med.,* 1923, 6:93-100. Harders, H., & Krauspe, C. Über die "systematisierte Chondromalacie" von Meyenburg, Altherr, Uehlinger. *Beitr. Path. Anat.,* 1954, 114:259-70.

von Meyenburg syndrome. See *Meyenburg-Altherr-Uehlinger syndrome.*

von Meyenburg-Altherr-Uehlinger syndrome. See *Meyenhurg-Altherr-Uehlinger syndrome.*

MEYER, HANS WILHELM (Danish physician, 1824-1898)

Meyer disease. Adenoid vegetations of the pharynx.

Meyer, H. W. Om adenoide vegetationer i naesesvoelgrummet. *Hospitalstid. Copenhagen*, 1868, 11:171-81.

MEYER, J.

Meyer dysplasia. See *Meyer syndrome.*

Meyer syndrome. Synonyms: *Meyer dysplasia, dysplasia epiphysealis capitis femoris.*

A syndrome marked by delayed epiphyseal ossification of the femoral heads, diffuse granular pattern of ossification, and aseptic necrosis of the femoral head. In some cases, ossification becomes normal during later childhood.

*Meyer, J. Dysplasia epiphysealis capitis femoris: A clinical-radiological syndrome and its relationship to Legg-Calvé-Perthes disease. *Acta Orthop. Scand*, 1964, 34:183. Taybi, H. *Radiology of syndromes*. Chicago, Year Book, 1975, p. 79.

MEYER, J. E.

Nyssen-van Bogaert-Meyer syndrome. See *under Nyssen.*

MEYER, JULIA (American physician)

Say-Meyer syndrome. See *under Say.*

MEYER-SCHWICKERATH, GERHARD (GERD) (German ophthalmologist, born 1920)

Meyer-Schwickerath and Weyers syndrome. See *oculodentodigital syndrome.*

MEYNERT, THEODOR (Austrian psychiatrist, 1833-1892)

Meynert amentia. See *Korsakoff syndrome, under Korsakov, Sergei Sergeevich.*

MFD. See *mandibulofacial dysostosis.*

MH. See *malignant hyperpyrexia syndrome.*

MIBELLI, VITTORIO (Italian physician, 1860-1910)

Mibelli disease (1). Synonyms: *angiokeratoma, keratoangioma.*

Dark red verrucous lesions, seldom over 3 mm in diameter, that appear on the skin of the fingers and toes, hands, and occasionally knees and elbows. Cavernous capillary dilations are the chief pathological findings.

Mibelli, V. Di una nuova forma di cheratosi "angiocheratoma." *Gior. Ital. Mal. Vener.*, 1889, 30:285-301.

Mibelli disease (2). Synonyms: *Mibelli porokeratosis (MP), porokeratosis of Mibelli (PM), hyperkeratosis excentrica, keratoma excentricum, parakeratosis annularis, parakeratosis paracentrifugata atrophicans, porokeratosis centrifugata atrophicans.*

A rare form of chronic keratoatrophoderma, usually of the bony prominences of the hands and feet, characterized by craterlike keratotic ridges with central atrophy and surrounding grooves. The lesions usually begin as small keratotic papules that spread in a centrifugal pattern. The disease, which usually develops early and persists during life, is inherited as an autosomal dominant trait.

Mibelli, V. Contributo allo studio della ipercheratosi dei canali sudoriferi (porokeratosi). *Gior. Ital. Mal. Vener.*, 1893, 28:313-55.

Mibelli porokeratosis (MP). See *Mibelli disease (2).*

porokeratosis of Mibelli (PM). See *Mibelli disease (2).*

MICHEL

Michel deformity. Complete absence of the inner ear.

Potter, G. D. Inner ear abnormalities in association with congenital atresia of the external auditory canal, including a case of Michel deformity. *Ann. Otol.*, 1969, 78:598-604.

MICHELI, FERNANDO (Italian physician, 1872-1937)

Marchiafava-Micheli anemia. See *Marchiafava-Micheli syndrome.*

Marchiafava-Micheli syndrome. See *under Marchiafava.*

Marchiafava-Nazari-Micheli syndrome. See *Marchiafava-Micheli syndrome.*

Micheli-Rietti syndrome. See *Rietti-Greppi-Micheli syndrome.*

Rietti-Greppi-Micheli syndrome. See *under Rietti.*

Michelin tire baby syndrome. A familial syndrome, transmitted as an autosomal dominant trait, characterized by deep skin folds on the back and around the limbs. The condition is reminescent of that of the mascot of the tire manufacturer, Michelin, hence the name of the syndrome. Nevus lipomatosus under the skin was observed in some patients, others suffered from hemihypertrophy, and one had a deletion of the short arm of chromosome 11 accompanied by mental retardation. There appears to be gradual spontaneous improvement with age.

Ross, C. M. Generalized folded skin with an underlying lipomatous nevus. "The Michelin tire baby." *Arch. Derm., Chicago*, 1969, 100:320-3. Niikawa, N., *et al.* The "Michelin tire baby" syndrome-an autosomal dominant trait. *Am. J. Med. Genet.*, 1985, 22:637-8.

MICHOTTE, L. J. (French physician)

Michotte syndrome. See *Baastrup syndrome.*

microangiopathic hemolytic anemia syndrome. See *disseminated intravascular coagulation syndrome.*

microangiopathic thrombotic hemolytic anemia. See *Moschcowitz syndrome.*

microcellular striatal syndrome. See *Huntington chorea.*

microcephaly-chorioretinopathy syndrome. See *Sabin-Feldman syndrome.*

microcephaly-congenital lymphedema syndrome. A familial syndrome, transmitted as an autosomal dominant trait, characterized by microcephaly and congenital lymphedema.

Leung, A. K. Dominantly inherited syndrome of microcephaly and congenital lymphedema. *Clin. Genet.*, 1985, 27:611-2.

microcephaly-micromelia syndrome. See *Ives-Houston syndrome.*

microcephaly-spastic diplegia syndrome. See *Paine syndrome.*

microcephaly-spastic quadriplegia syndrome. A syndrome of severe microcephaly and spastic quadriplegia transmitted as an autosomal recessive trait.

McKusick, V. V. *Mendelian inheritance in man. Catalogs of autosomal dominant, autosomal recessive, and X-linked phenotypes.* 7th ed. Baltimore, Johns Hopkins Univ., 1986. No. 25128.

microcornea-brachydactyly syndrome. See *Tizzard syndrome.*

microcornea-cataract-coloboma syndrome. A familial syndrome, transmitted as an autosomal dominant trait, characterized by cataract, microcornea, and coloboma.

*Cummings, C., *et al.* Autosomal dominant cataract, coloboma and microphthalmia. *5th Internat. Conf. Birth Defects*, Montreal, 1977.

microcystic dystrophy of the corneal epithelium. See *Cogan dystrophy.*

microdrepanocytic disease. See *Silvestroni-Bianco syndrome.*

microgeodic disease. See *phalangeal microgeodic syndrome.*

micrognathia-glossoptosis syndrome. See *Robin syndrome.*

micrognathia-polydactyly-genital anomalies syndrome. See *Ullrich-Feichtiger syndrome.*

microphallus-imperforate anus-syndactyly-hamartoblastoma-abnormal lung lobulation-polydactyly (MISHAP) syndrome. See *Hall syndrome, under Hall, J. G.*

microphthalmos-microcornea-cataract syndrome. A familial syndrome, transmitted as an autosomal dominant trait, characterized by cataracts associated with microphthalmos and microcornea.

Harman, N. B. Congenital cataract, a pedigree of five generations. *Tr. Ophth. Soc. U. K.*, 1909, 29:101-8.

microphthalmos-retinitis pigmentosa-glaucoma syndrome. See *Hermann syndrome.*

microphthalmos-short stature-multiple joint dislocation syndrome. A familial syndrome, probably transmitted as an autosomal dominant trait, characterized by shortness of stature, mental deficiency, multiple joint dislocations, and eye abnormalities, including microphthalmia, corneal sclerosis, and myopia.

microscopic cystic epithelial dystrophy. See *Cogan dystrophy.*

MIDDELDORPF, K. (German physician)

Middeldorpf tumor. Synonyms: *epidermoid cyst, presacral cyst, presacral dermoid.*

A congenital tumor of the sacral region that contains rudimentary organs.

Middeldorpf, K. Zur Kenntniss der angeborenen Sacralgeschwülste. *Virchows Arch. Path.*, 1885, 101:37-44.

middle alternating hemiplegia. See *Millard-Gubler syndrome.*

middle aortic disease. See *aortic arch syndrome.*

middle aortic syndrome. See *aortic arch syndrome.*

middle cavernous syndrome. See *under Jefferson syndrome.*

middle lobe atelectasis. See *middle lobe syndrome.*

middle lobe syndrome. Synonyms: *Brock syndrome, Brock-Graham syndrome, Graham-Burford-Mayer syndrome, middle lobe atelectasis, right middle lobe syndrome.*

Right lung atelectasis with infection and collapse of the middle lobe due to bronchial compression, usually by enlarged lymph nodes. Cough, wheezing, and recurrent pneumonia are the principal clinical symptoms. Inflammatory diseases with resulting hilar lymphadenopathy bronchiectasis, and carcinoma are the main causes.

Brock, R. C., *et al.* Tuberculous mediastinal lymphadenitis in childhood; secondary effects on the lungs. *Guy's Hosp. Rep.*, 1937, 87:295-317. Graham, E. A., Burford, T. H., & Mayer, J. H. Middle lobe syndrome. *Postgrad. Med.*, 1948, 4:29-34.

midsystolic click-late systolic murmur syndrome. See *mitral valve prolapse syndrome.*

midsystolic click-murmur syndrome. See *mitral valve prolapse syndrome.*

MIEHLKE, ADOLF (German physician, born 1917)

Miehlke-Partsch syndrome. A form of thalidomide-induced embryopathy (the Wiedemann syndrome), that is characterized by ear deformity and abducent paralysis.

Miehlke, A., & Partsch. C. J. Ohrmissbildung Facialis- und Abducenslähmung als Syndrom der Thalidomidschädigung. *Arch. Chir. Ohr. Heilk.*, 1963, 181:154-74.

MIESCHER, GUIDO (Swiss dermatologist, 1877-1961)

Bloch-Miescher syndrome. See *Miescher syndrome (2).*

Lutz-Miescher syndrome. See *under Lutz, Wilhelm.*

Miescher cheilitis. See *Melkersson-Rosenthal syndrome.*

Miescher elastoma. See *Lutz-Miescher syndrome.*

Miescher syndrome (1). See *Melkersson-Rosenthal syndrome.*

Miescher syndrome (2). Synonym: *Bloch-Miescher syndrome.*

A familial syndrome, possibly transmitted as an autosomal recessive trait, characterized by acanthosis nigricans in combination with hypertrichosis, failure to thrive, growth deficiency, lipodystrophylike disorders, insulin-resistant diabetes melliitus, and orofacial deformities with coarse facies. The symptoms appear during early childhood. Acanthosis nigricans involves the neck and axillary, inguinal, and genital regions. Lanugo-type hypertrichosis is observed on the trunk and, occasionally, the extremities. In some cases, there is overabundance of scalp hair. Coarse facies is marked mainly by mandibular prognathism, malocclusion and malformed teeth, and large low-set ears. The body is small and short with a decreased amount of the subcutaneous adipose tissue. Associated disorders may include mental deficiency, high-arched palate, fissured tongue, milky oral mucosa, stubby fingers and toes, and goiter.

Miescher, G. Zwei Fälle von kongenitaler familiärer Akanthosis nigricans, kombiniert mit Diabetes mellitus. *Derm. Zschr.*, 1921, 32-33:276-305.

Miescher syndrome (3). See *Miescher-Leder granulomatosis.*

Miescher trichofolliculoma. Synonyms: *feather hair, hair follicle tumor, trichofolliculoma.*

A benign, organoid, papular tumor of the skin with wooly wisps of immature hair that emerge from a central orifice.

Miescher, G. Trichofolliculoma. *Dermatologica, Basel*, 1944, 89:193.

Miescher-Leder granulomatosis. Synonyms: *Miescher syndrome, granulomatosis disciformis chronica et progressiva, granulomatosis pseudosclerodermiformis tuberculoidea chronica.*

A form of lupoid necrobiosis marked by red to yellowish red flat papular patches of the hands and legs, which show yellowish lupoid spots on pressure. Histologically, there are chronic granulomatous changes in the adventitia, made up of fibroblasts, epithelioid cells, giant cells, aand lymphocytes.

Miescher, G., & Leder, M. Granulomatosis disciformis chronica et progressiva (atypische Tuberkulose). *Dermatologica, Basel*, 1948, 97:25-34.

MIETENS, CARL (German physician)

mental retardation, Mietens-Weber type. See *Mietens-Weber syndrome.*

Mietens syndrome. See *Mietens-Weber syndrome.*

Mietens-Weber syndrome. Synonyms: *Mietens syndrome; mental retardation, Mietens-Weber type.*

A syndrome of mental retardation, corneal opacity, nystagmus, strabismus, small pinched nose, flexion contractures of the elbows, dislocation of the radial head, short ulna and radius, and clinodactyly. In the original report, the parents were second cousins. Autosomal recessive transmission is suspected.

Mietens, C., & Weber, H. A syndrome characterized by conreal opacity, nystagmus, flexion contractures of the elbows, growth failure, and mental retardation. *J. Pediat.*, 1966, 69:624-9.

migraine. See *under headache syndrome.*

migraine syndrome. See *migraine under headache syndrome.*

migratory edema. See *Quincke edema.*

migratory osteolysis of the lower extremities. See *transient osteopenia of the hip syndrome.*

MIKAELIAN, DIRAN O. (Lebanese physician)

Mikaelian syndrome. Synonym: *camptodactyly-ectodermal dysplasia-sensorineural hearing loss syndrome.*

A concurrence of camptodactyly, ectodermal dysplasia, and sensorineural deafness, originally reported in two children of consanguineous marriage. Delayed growth, kyphoscoliosis, dental caries, and coarse and sparse hair are associated. The syndrome is probably transmitted as an autosomal recessive trait.

Mikaelian, D. O., *et al.* Congenital ectodermal dysplasia with hearing loss. *Arch. Otolar.*, 1970, 92:85-9.

MIKITY, VICTOR G. (American radiologist, born 1919)

respiratory distress syndrome of Wilson and Mikity. See *Wilson-Mikity syndrome, under Wilson, Miriam Geisendorfer.*

Wilson-Mikity (WM) syndrome. See *under Wilson, Miriam Geisendorfer.*

MIKULICZ, JOHANN, VON. See MIKULICZ-RADECKI, JAN

MIKULICZ-RADECKI, JAN (Polish surgeon in Germany, 1850-1905)

Mikulicz aphthae. See *Sutton disease, under Sutton, Richards Lighburn, Jr.*

Mikulicz disease. Synonym: *Mikulicz syndrome.*

Bilateral hypertrophy of the lacrimal and salivary glands, associated with xerostomia and decreased or absent lacrimation, which may be caused by tuberculosis, leukemia, lymphosarcoma, poisoning, sarcoidosis, syphilis, or gout. Onset may occur in conjunction with respiratory tract infection, oral infection, or tooth extraction. Some authors consider this disease and the Sjögren syndrome as identical, but others suggest they are separate entities because of the absence rheumatoid arthritis in Mikulicz disease.

Mikulicz, J. Über eine eigenartige symmetrische Erkrankung der Tränenund Mundspeicheldrusen. *Beitr. Chir. Fortschr. Gewidmet Theodor Billroth*. Stuttgart, 1892, pp. 610-30.

Mikulicz syndrome. See *Mikulicz disease.*

mild mountain sickness. See *alpine syndrome.*

MILIAN, GASTON AUGUSTE (French physician, 1871-1945)

Milian erythema. Synonyms: *Milian syndrome, ninth day erythema.*

A toxic disorder characterized by erythema, malaise, headache, fever, and vomiting 7 to 9 days after the first injection of arsphenamine or other drugs.

Milian, G.., & Mansour, M. Erythème polymorphe photobiotrophique avec localisation présternale. *Bull. Soc. Fr. Derm.*, 1932, 39:651-2.

Milian syndrome. See *Milian erythema.*

military posture syndrome. See *costoclavicular compression syndrome.*

milk drinker's syndrome. See *milk-alkali syndrome.*

milk of calcium bile. See *limy bile syndrome.*

milk poisoning. See *milk-alkali syndrome.*

milk precipitin syndrome. See *Heiner syndrome.*

milk-alkali syndrome (MAS). Synonyms: *Burnett syndrome, Cope syndrome, alkalosis syndrome, milk drinker's syndrome, milk poisoning, subacute milk poisoning.*

A disorder associated with excessive intake of milk and absorbable alkali, and characterized by hypercalcemia (without hypercalciuria or hypophosphatemia), normal serum alkaline phosphatase, renal insufficiency, azotemia, alkalosis, calcinosis, and ocular lesions, chiefly band-shaped keratopathy and conjunctivitis with calcification. The symptoms include nausea, vomiting, headache, irritability, vertigo, depression, confusion, weakness, and ataxia. Radiological findings show multiple calcium deposits in soft tissues. Three distinct forms of this condition are recognized: (1) temporary alkalosis and uremia during short intensive treatment with antacids, which disappears when treatment is terminated; (2) a form similar to the first type but accompanied by hypercalcemia **(Cope syndrome)**, and requiring long period for recovery; and (3) and a chronic form characterized by permanent impairment of renal function **(Burnett syndrome)**.

Burnett, C. H., *et al*. Hypercalcemia without hypercalciuria or hypophosphatemia, calcinosis and renal insufficiency. A syndrome following prolonged intake of milk and alkali. *N. Engl. J. Med.*, 1949, 240:787-94. *Cope, C. L. Base changes in the alkalosis produced by the treatment of gastric ulcer with alkalies. *Clin. Sc.*, 1936, 2:287-300.

MILKMAN, LOUIS ARTHUR (American physician, 1895-1951)

Looser-Debray-Milkman syndrome. See *Milkman syndrome.*

Milkman syndrome. Synonyms: *Looser-Debray-Milkman syndrome, Milkman-Looser syndrome, multiple spontaneous idiopathic symmetrical pseudofractures, osteoporosis-osteomalacia syndrome.*

Osteomalacia complicated by multiple, spontaneous, symmetrical fractures, most frequently observed in adult and middle-aged females after severe malnutrition or following pregnancy. The symptoms include severe pain in different parts of the skeleton, fatigability, difficulty in walking, and, in advanced stages, complete disability. Roentgenograms show osteoporosis, demineralization of bone cortex, and poorly healed fractures (pseudo-fractures) and irregular bands of translucency (Looser zones).

Milkman, L. A. Multiple spontaneous idiopathic symmetrical fractures. *Am. J. Roentgen.*, 1934, 32:622-34. Looser. Über pathologische Form von Infraktionen und Callusbildungen bei Rachitis und Osteomalazie und anderen Knochenerkrankungen. *Zbl. Chir.*, 1920, 47:1470-4.

Milkman-Looser syndrome. See *Milkman syndrome.*

MILLARD, AUGUSTE (French physician, 1830-1915)

Millard syndrome. See *Millard-Gubler syndrome.*

Millard-Gubler syndrome. Synonyms: *Gubler hemiplegia, Gubler paralysis, Millard syndrome, abducens-facial hemiplegia alternans, alternate inferior paralysis, hemiplegia alternans, hemiplegia alternans inferior, hemiplegia cruciata abducentis inferior, inferior protuberance syndrome, middle alternating syndrome.*

Unilateral softening of the brain tissue arising from obstruction of the blood vessels of the pons, involving the sixth and seventh cranial nerves and fibers of the corticospinal tract, and associated with paralysis of the abducens and facial nerves and contralateral hemiplegia of the extremities. The muscles of the ipsilateral side of the face are paralysed, and there is paralysis of outward movement of the eye. If, in addition, there is paralysis of inward movement of the other eye in attempting to look toward the side of the lesion, the condition is known as the *Foville syndrome.*

Gubler, A. M. De l'hémiplégie alterne envisagée comme signe de lésion de la protubérance annulaire et comme preuve de la décussation des nerfs faciaux. *Gaz. Hebd. Méd., Paris*, 1856, 3:749-54; 789-92; 811-6.

MILLER, JAMES Q. (American physician)

Miller-Dieker syndrome (MDS). Synonyms: *agyria syndrome, agyria-pachygyria syndrome, lissencephaly syndrome.*

Arrested brain development characterized by smoothness of the surface of the brain, absence of sulci and gyri (agyria), and associated neurological disorders and multiple abnormalities. Brain abnormalities include microcephaly, heterotopias, failure of operculization, hypoplasia of the corpus callosum, and midline calcifications. Neurological disorders consist chiefly of mental retardation, decreased spontaneous activity, early hypotonia followed by hypertonia, feeding difficulty, seizures. and signs of decerebration. Facial features include abnormal irides, tortunous fundal vessels, broad nasal bridge, epicanthus, upturned nares, malpositioned and/or malformed ears, micrognathia, long thin upper lip, delayed dentition, and prominent palatine ridges. High forehead, microcrania, bitemporal hollowing, and prominent occiput are the main cranial defects. Other associated conditions may include failure to thrive, dysphagia, hirsutism, clouding of the corneae, polydactyly, camptodactyly, simian creases, cryptorchism in males and small perineal body in females, and various defects of the heart, kidneys, and gastrointestinal system. Polyhydramnios, decreased fetal movement, neonatal jaundice, infantile spasms, vertical wrinkling of the forehead, and other abnormalities may be present. The syndrome is transmitted as an autosomal recessive trait. Chromosome 17p deletion was reported in some cases. Death usually takes place in early infancy. See also *Norman-Roberts syndrome.*

Miller, J. Q. Lissencephaly in 2 siblings. *Neurology*, 1963, 13:841-50. Dieker, H. The lissencephaly syndrome. *Birth Defects*, 1969, 5(2):53-64. Dobyns, W. B. *et al.* Syndromes of lissencephaly. I. Miller-Dieker and Norman-Roberts syndromes and isolated lissencephaly.*Am. J. Hum. Genet.*, 1984, 18:509-26. Stratton, R. F., *et al.* New chromosomal syndrome: Miller-Dieker syndrome and monosomy 17p13. *Hum. Genet.*, 1984, 67:193-200.

MILLER, JAMES R. (Canadian scientist)

Robinson-Miller-Bensimon syndrome. See *Robinson syndrome, under Robinson, Geoffrey C.*

MILLER, ROBERT W. (American physician)

Miller syndrome. See *aniridia-Wilms tumor syndrome.*

MILLER, S. J. N.

Miller syndrome. See *Sturge-Weber syndrome.*

MILLER, V. (British physician)

Watson-Miller syndrome. See *Alagille syndrome.*

MILLER FISHER. See FISHER, MILLER

MILLIKAN, CLARK HAROLD (American neurologist, born 1915)

Millikan-Siekert syndrome. Synonym: *intermittent insufficiency of the basilar arterial system syndrome.*

Intermittent insufficiency of the basilar artery with symptoms suggesting lesions of the pons, mesencephalon, or occipital lobes, frequently followed by thrombosis of the basilar artery. The symptoms include, in various combinations, loss of consciousness, hemiparesis or hemiplegia, dysarthria, dysphagia, unsteadiness, vertigo, tinnitus, and vomiting. The hemiparesis or hemiplegia may appear on the right side of the body in one attack and on the left side in another.

Millikan, C. H., & Siekert, R. G. Studies on cerebrovascular disease. I. The syndrome of intermittent insufficiency of the basilar arterial system. *Proc. Mayo Clin.*, 1955, 30:61-8.

MILLS, CHARLES KARSNER (American physician, 1845-1931)

Mills disease. Synonyms: *ascending hemiplegia, progressive ascending spinal paralysis.*

A slowly progressive paralysis that initially affects a single lower extremity, then gradually ascends to the upper one on the same side, and eventually involves the extremities on both sides. This disorder is considered to be a form of spinal paralysis, with lesions of the brain being usually present.

Mills, C. K. A case of unilateral progressive ascending paralysis, probably representing a new form of degenerative disease. *J. Nerv. Ment. Dis.*, 1900, 27:195-200.

MILROY, WILLIAM FORSYTH (American physician, 1855-1942)

Milroy disease. See *Nonne-Milroy syndrome.*

Nonne-Milroy syndrome. See under Nonne.

MILTON, JOHN LAWS (British physician, 1820-1898)

Milton disease. See *Quincke edema.*

Milton urticaria. See *Quincke edema.*

mimic spasm. See *Gilles de la Tourette syndrome.*

MIMS, LEROY C. (American physician)

Feuerstein-Mims syndrome. See *epidermal nevus syndrome.*

Feuerstein-Mims syndrome with resistant rickets. See *hypophosphatemic rickets-osteomalacia-linear nevus sebacerous syndrome.*

linear nevus sebaceus of Feuerstein and Mims. See epidermal nevus syndrome.

nevus sebaceus of Feuerstein and Mims. See *epidermal nevus syndrome.*

Schimmelpinning-Feuerstein-Mims syndrome. See *epidermal nevus syndrome.*

Minamata disease (MD). A toxic neurological syndrome caused by ingestion of fish and shellfish contamined by methylmercury, first reported in the mid 50s in fishermen and their families living around Minamata Bay (Kyushu Island) in Japan. Mercury-contaminated effluent from a chemical plant was the original cause of this syndrome. The symptoms include sensory disturbances of distal parts of the extremities followed by ataxia, concentric constriction of the visual field, gait disorders, impaired speech, hearing disorders, muscle weakness, tremor, abnormal eye movement, and occasionally, gustatory changes and mental disorders. Impaired function of the cerebellum and brain stem is the main cause of neurological disturbances.

Kurland, L. H., *et al.* Minamata disease. *World Neurol.*, 1960, 1:370-95. Tamashiro, H. Mortality and survival for Minamata disease. *Internat. J. Epidem.*, 1985, 14:582-8.

miners' anemia. See *Griesinger disease.*

miners' syndrome. See *siderosis-scurvy-osteoporosis syndrome.*

mini-packer. See *under body packer syndrome.*

minimal brain dysfunction (MBD). See *attention deficit-hyperactivity disorder.*

minimal brain dysfunction syndrome. See *attention deficit-hyperactivity disorder.*

minimal cerebral dysfunction (MCD). See *attention deficit-hyperactivity disorder.*

minimal change nephropathy. See *Munk disease.*

minimal change nephrotic syndrome (MCNS). See *nephrotic syndrome.*

MINKOWSKI, OSKAR (German physician, 1858-1931)

Minkowski-Chauffard syndrome. Synonyms: *Gänsslen syndrome, Gänsslen-Erb syndrome, Minkowski-Chauffard-Gänsslen syndrome, acholuric familial jaundice, acholuric jaundice, congenital hemolytic anemia, congenital hemolytic icterus, congenital hemolytic jaundice, congenital microspherocytic hemolytic anemia, constitutional hemolytic jaundice, familial hemolytic jaundice, familial spherocytosis, hereditary spherocytosis (HS), spherocytosis hereditaria (SPH).*

A familial blood disorder characterized by congenital hemolytic anemia with an intrinsic defect in the red blood cells, spherocytosis, splenomegaly, and increased erythrocyte destruction rate. Anemia varies in severity; the spherocytes are usually present at birth, but the symptoms may become evident later in life. Increased osmotic fragility of the erythrocytes, high reticulocyte count, and hemoglobin deficiency in the plasma are the main hematological findings. Associated disorders usually include icterus, gallstones of the pigment type, secondary hyperplasia of the bone marrow and extension of the red marrow into the midshaft of the long bones, presence of urobilinogen in the stools, and occasional extramedullary erythropoiesis with tumorlike paravertebral masses. There may be also a wide variety of complications, such as those involving the skeleton, eyes, and teeth. Roentgenographic findings may show striation and thickening of the frontal and parietal bones and occasional oxycephaly. Persons of northern European origin are affected most frequently, but not exclusively. The syndrome is transmitted as an autosomal dominant trait.

Minkowski, O. Über eine hereditäre, unter dem Bilde eines chronischen Icterus mit Urobilinurie, Splenomegalie und Nierensiderosis verlaufende Affection. *Verh. Deut. Ges. Inn. Med.*, 1900, p. 316-9. Chauffard, M. A. Pathogénie de l'ictére congénital de l'adulte. *Sem. Méd., Paris*, 1907, 27:25-9. Gänsslen, M. Über hämolytischen Ikterus. Nach 25 eigenen Beobachtungen und 10 Milzexstirpationen. *Deut. Arch. Klin. Med.*, 1922, 140:210-26. Jandl, J. H., & Cooper, R. A. Hereditary spherocytosis. In: Stanbury, J. B., Wyngaarden, J. B., & Fredrickson, D. S., eds. *The metabolic basis of inherited disease*. 4th ed. New York, McGraw-Hill, l978, pp. 1396-1409.

Minkowski-Chauffard-Gänsslen syndrome. See *Minkowski-Chauffard syndrome.*

MINOR, LAZAR SALOMONOVICH (Russian physician, 1855-1942)

Minor disease. Synonyms: *Minor-Oppenheim syndrome, central hematomyelia, hematomyelia centralis.*

Paralysis and anesthesia due to extravasation of the blood into or around the spinal cord in injuries not directly involving the spinal cord substance.

Minor, L. Centrale haematomyelie. *Arch. Psychiat., Berlin*, 1892, 24:693-729.

Minor-Oppenheim syndrome. See *Minor disease.*

minor epileptic status. See *Lennox syndrome.*

minor vestibular gland syndrome. A gynecological disorder characterized by introital dyspareunia, erythema around orifices of the minor vestibular glands, and tenderness on palpation over the openings, occurring in young women with a history of candidiasis. Mixed inflammatory infiltrate in the subepithelium and around the glands is the principal pathologic feature. The etiology is unknown.

Marinoff, S. C., & Turner, M. L. Hypersensitivity to vaginal candidiasis or treatment vehicles in the pathogenesis of minor vestibular gland syndrome. *J. Reprod. Med.*, 1986, 31:796-9.

MINOT, FRANCIS (American physician, 1821-1899)

Minot-von Willebrand syndrome. See *Willebrand-Jürgens syndrome.*

MIRHOSSEINI, S. ALI (Physician in the United States)

Mirhosseini-Holmes-Walton syndrome. Synonym: *retinal pigmentaray degeneration-microcephaly-mental retardation syndrome.*

A hereditary syndrome of pigmentary retinal degeneration, cataract, arachnodactyly, hyperextensibility of joints, mental retardation, mild scoliosis, microcephaly, and tall stature, believed to be transmitted as an autosomal recessive trait.

Mirhosseini, S. A., Holmes, L. B., & Walton, D. S. Syndrome of pigmentary retinal degeneration, cataract, microcephaly, and severe mental retardation. *J. Med. Genet.*, 1972, 9:193-6. Mendez H. M. M., *et al.* The syndrome of retinal pigmentary degeneration, microcephaly, and severe mental retardation (Mirhosseini-Holmes-Walton syndrome): Report of two patients. *Am. J. Med. Genet.*, 1985, 22:223-8.

MISHAP (**m**icrophalus-**i**mperforate anus-**s**yndactyly-**h**amartoblatoma-**a**bnormal lung lobulation-**p**olydactyly) **syndrome.** See *Hall syndrome, under Hall, J. G.*

misidentification syndrome. See *Capgras syndrome.*

MITCHELL, SILAS WEIR (American physician, 1829-1914)

Mitchell syndrome (1). Synonyms: *Gerhardt disease, Weir Mitchell disease, acromelalgia, erythromelalgia, erythrothermia, vasomotor paralysis of the extremities.*

A vasomotor disorder marked by sudden onset of pain in the hands and feet, diminution of temperature sense, and occasional glossalgia and feeding difficulty. The fingers and toes usually become red with thickened terminal phalanges and nail beds, and superficial veins are grossly engorged. Although sensitivity to temperature changes is diminished, cold acts as a pain depressor and heat as a stimulator.

*Mitchell, S. W. Clinical lecture on certain painful affections of the feet. *Philadelphia Med. Times*, 1872, 3:81-2; 113-5. Gerhardt, C. Über Erythromelalgie. *Berlin. Klin. Wschr.*, 1892, 29:1125-5.

Mitchell syndrome (2). See *Horner syndrome.*

mitral leaflet prolapse syndrome. See *mitral valve prolapse syndrome.*

mitral systolic click syndrome. See *mitral valve prolapse syndrome.*

mitral valve prolapse (MVP) syndrome. Synonyms: *Barlow syndrome, ballooning mitral cusp syndrome, billowing mitral valve syndrome, click syndrome, click-murmur syndrome, floppy valve syndrome, midsystolic click-late systolic murmur syndrome, midsystolic click-murmur syndrome, mitral leaflet prolapse syndrome, mitral systolic click syndrome, mitral valve prolapse-systolic click (MVP-SC) syndrome, myxomatous mitral valve degeneration, prolapsing mitral leaflet (PML) syndrome, systolic click-late systolic murmur syndrome.*

A relatively common form of cardiac valvular abnormality, occurring in about 5-10 percent of the population, that is characterized by eversion of the mitral valve into the left atrium during ventricular systole. Some cases are asymptomatic, but a pronounced midsystolic click, with or without late systolic murmur, usually indicates the presence of this disorder. Myxomatous changes in the annulus may be associated. The syndrome may occur as a complication of various conditions, including Marfan syndrome, Ehlers-Danlos syndrome, Wolf-Parkinson-White syndrome, Turner syndrome, Noonan syndrome, congenital heart defects, rheumatic endocarditis, coronary diseases, myocarditis, athlete's heart, congestive heart disease, polyarteritis nodosa, relapsing polychondritis, lupus erythematosus, muscular dystrophy, and other disorders.

Barlow, J. B., *et al.* The significance of late systolic murmurs. *Am. Heart J.,* 1963, 66:443-52.

mitral valve prolapse-systolic click syndrome (MVP-SC). See *mitral valve prolapse syndrome.*

MIURA, NOBORU (Japanese dentist)

Cooperman-Miura syndrome. See *under Cooperman.*

mixed chancre. See *Rollet chancre.*

mixed connective tissue disease (MCTD). Synonyms: *Sharp syndrome, mixed connective tissue syndrome.*

A disease characterized by clinical features similar to those of systemic lupus erythematosus, scleroderma, and polymyositis, with serological findings of high titers of speckled pattern fluorescent antinuclear antibody and very high agglutination titers of antibody to an antigen extractable in isotonic buffers from isolated nuclei. The antigen consists of at least two distinct parts: one, sensitive to ribonuclease and trypsin, is a ribonucleoprotein, and the other, resistant to ribonuclease, is identical with the Sm antigen. The antibody to extractable nuclear antigen is directed against the ribonuclease-sensitive ribonucleoprotein antigen and not against the ribonuclease-resistant Sm antigen. Clinically, the disorder is characterized by fever, fatigue, weight loss, dyspnea, synovitis, swelling of the hands, polyarthralgia, dermatomyositis, the Raynaud phenomenon, rheumatoid nodules, high erythrocyte sedimentation rate, anemia, leukopenia, diarrhea, pulmonary insufficiency, esophageal motility disorders, dysphagia, and other symptoms.

Sharp, G. C., *et al.* Mixed connective tissue disease: An apparently distinct rheumatic disease syndrome associated with a specific antibody to an extractable nuclear antigena (ENA). *Am. J. Med.,* 1972, 52:148-59.

mixed connective tissue syndrome. See *mixed connective tissue disease.*

Miyagawanella lymphogranulomatosis. See *Durand-Nicolas-Favre disease, under Durand, J.*

MJAD (**M**achado-**J**oseph **A**zorean **d**isease). See *Joseph disease, under Joseph, Antone.*

MJD. See ***M**seleni **j**oint **d**isease.*

MJD (**M**achado-**J**oseph **d**isease). See *Joseph disease, under Joseph, Antone.*

MKS. See ***M**cKusick-**K**aufman **s**yndrome.*

ML (I, II, III, IV). See ***m**uco**l**ipidosis (I, II, III, IV).*

MLD. See ***m**etachromatic **l**euko**d**ystrophy.*

MLNS (**m**ucocutaneous **l**ymph **n**ode **s**yndrome). See *Kawasaki syndrome.*

MMD (**m**oya**m**oya **d**isease). See *moyamoya syndrome.*

MMM syndrome. Synonyms: *3-M syndrome, 3-M slender-boned dwarfism.*

A familial syndrome, probably transmitted as an autosomal recessive trait, characterized by a low birth weight, proportionate dwarfism, short and broad neck with prominent trapezius muscles, deformed sternum, transverse grooves on the anterior chest, winged scapulae, flat feet with prominent heels, and hatchet-shaped craniofacial configuration with a triangular mouth, wide anteverted nostrils, long philtrum, and full lips. X-ray findings show overtubulated bones, delayed bone maturation, occasional pseudoephiphyses in the second metacarpal bones, narrow medullary space in the metacarpals, slender bones throughout the skeleton, and small pelvis. The syndrome was named after the first letters of the last names of three senior authors of the original report (J. Daniel Miller, Victor A. McKusick, and Paul Malvaux).

Miller, J. D., McKusick, V. A., Malvaux, P., Temtamy, S., & Salinas, C. The 3-M syndrome: A heritable low birthweight dwarfism. *Birth Defects,* 1975, 11(5):39-47.

MMN (**m**etaphyseal chondrodysplasia-**m**alabsorption-**n**eutropenia) **syndrome.** See *Shwachman syndrome.*

MMN (**m**ultiple **m**ucosal **n**euroma) **syndrome.** See *mucosal neuromas disease.*

MMN-pheochromocytoma (**m**ultiple **m**ucosal **n**euromas-pheochromocytoma) **syndrome.** See *mucosal neuromas syndrome.*

MNBCCS (**m**ultiple **n**evoid **b**asal-**c**ell **c**arcinoma **s**yndrome). See *nevoid basal-cell carcinoma syndrome.*

MNS. See ***M**elnick-**N**eedles **s**yndrome.*

MÖBIUS , PAUL JULIUS. See MOEBIUS, PAUL JULIUS

MOEBIUS (MÖBIUS), PAUL JULIUS (German neurologist, 1853-1907)

Leyden-Moebius syndrome. See *under Leyden.*

Moebius anomalad. See *Moebius syndrome (1).*

Moebius syndrome (1). Synonyms: *Möbius syndrome, Moebius anomalad, akinesia algera, congenital abducens-facial paralysis, congenital bulbar paralysis, congenital facial diplegia, congenital facial paralysis, congenital nuclear agenesis, congenital nuclear aplasia, congenital oculofacial paralysis, congenital paralysis of the sixth and seventh nerves.*

Congenital paralysis, usually bilateral, of the external rectus and facial muscles due to aplasia of the nuclei of the abducens and facial nerves, with inability to abduct the eyes beyond the midline, and masklike facies. Other symptoms may include drooling from the corners of the mouth, speech impairment because of difficulty in using the lips, the Bell phenomenon (upward movement of the eyes during attempted closure of the eyelids), and poor eyelid closure, resulting in exposure keratitis. Atrophy of the tongue, paralysis of the masticatory muscles and soft palate, and prominent everted lips are the principal oral disorders. Ear abnormalities, hand defects (including syndactyly), clubfoot, aplasia of the pectoral and sternocleidomastoid muscles, hip dislocation, and other anomalies may be present. The syndrome occurs most commonly as a sporadic disorder, but instances of autosomal dominant inheritance with variable expression have been reported.

Möbius, P. J. Über angeborene doppelseitige Abducens-facialis Lähmung. *Münch. Med. Wschr.,* 1888, 35:91-4; 108-11.

Moebius syndrome (2). Synonyms: *oculomotor recurrent paralysis, ophthalmoplegic migraine, periodic oculomotor paralysis.*

A neurological disorder, characterized by oculomotor paralysis with periodic migraine, which begins as severe vomiting and ophthalmodynia. After an attack, there is a gradual diminishing of symptoms until mydriasis becomes the only sign. Compression of third cranial nerve between the posterior verebral and superior cerebellar arteries is believed to be the cause.

Moebius, P. L. Über periodisch wiederkehrende Oculomotoriuslähmung. *Berlin Klin. Wschr.,* 1884, 21:604-8.

muscular dystrophy, Leyden-Moebius type. See *Leyden-Moebius syndrome.*

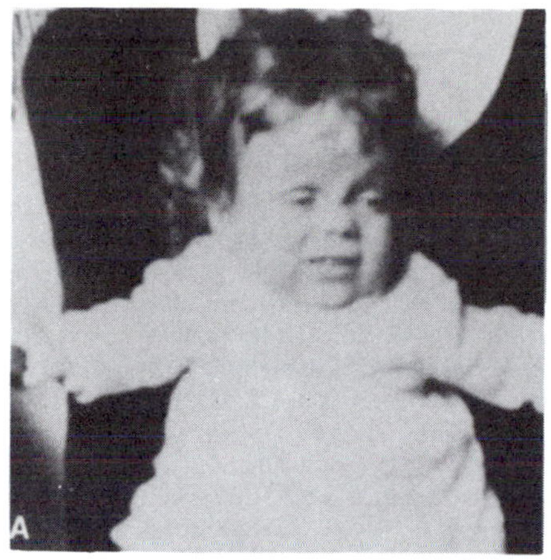
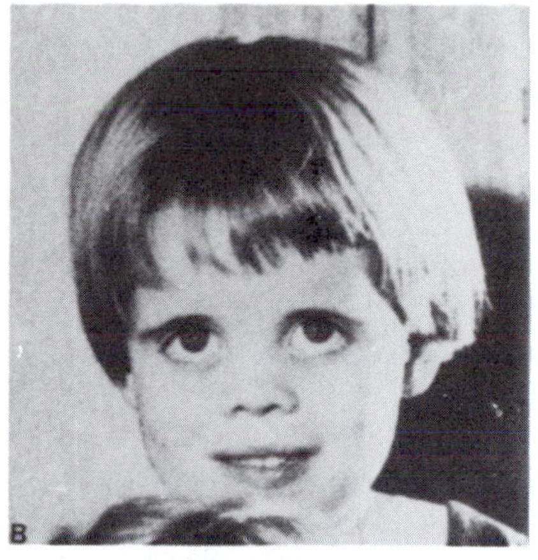
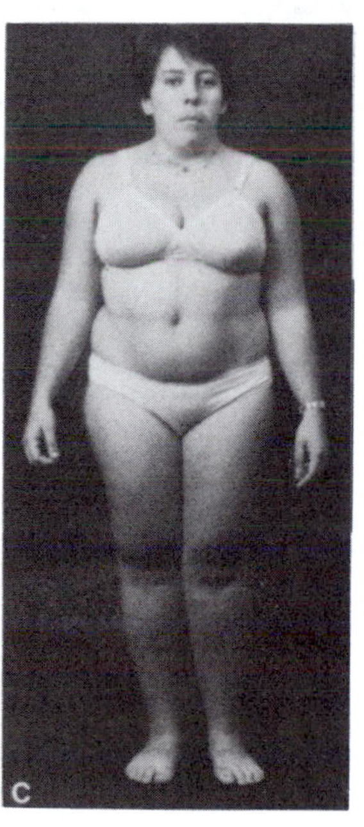
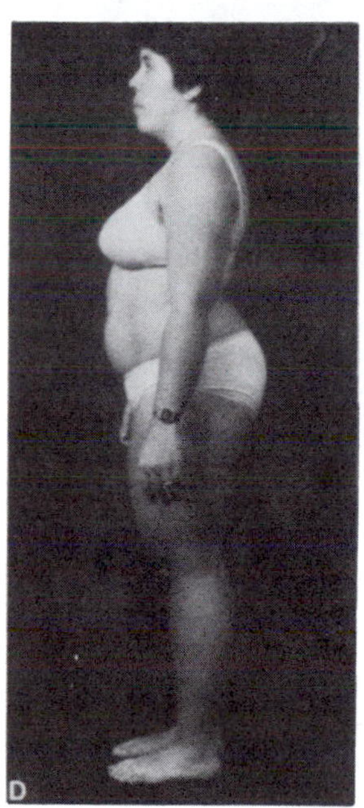

MMM syndrome
Hennekam, Raoul C.M., Jan B. Bijlsma & Jürgen Spranger: *American Journal of Medical Genetics* 28:195-209, 1987. New York: Alan R. Liss Inc.

Poland-Moebius syndrome. See *under Poland.*

MOELLER, JULIUS OTTO LUDWIG. See MÖLLER, JULIUS OTTO LUDWIG

MOELLER-BOECK, CAESAR PETER (Norwegian dermatologist, 1845-1917)

Besnier-Boeck sarcoid. See *Besnier-Boeck-Schaumann syndrome.*

Besnier-Boeck-Schaumann syndrome. See *under Besnier.*

Boeck disease. See *Besnier-Boeck-Schaumann syndrome.*

Boeck lupoid. See *Besnier-Boeck-Schaumann syndrome.*

Boeck miliary lupoid. See *Besnier-Boeck-Schaumann syndrome.*

Boeck sarcoid. See *Besnier-Boeck-Schaumann syndrome.*

Hutchinson-Boeck disease. See *Besnier-Boeck-Schaumann syndrome.*

Hutchinson-Boeck granulomatosis. See *Besnier-Boeck-Schaumann syndrome.*

Moeller-Boeck syndrome. See *Besnier-Boeck-Schaumann syndrome.*

MOENS, E. (Belgian physician)

De Barsy-Moens-Dierckx syndrome. See *under De Barsy.*

MOERSCH, FREDERICK PAUL (American physician, born 1889)

Moersch-Woltman syndrome (MWS). See *stiff man syndrome.*

MOHR, OTTO LOUS (Norwegian geneticist, 1886-1967)

Mohr syndrome I. See *orofaciodigital syndrome II.*

Mohr syndrome II. Synonym: *acrocephalosyndactyly IV (ASC IV).*

A congenital syndrome consisting of sometimes asymmetric acrocephaly and syndactyly that is transmitted as an autosomal dominant trait. Craniofacial features of the disorder consist of a high forehead, thin nose, and ear deformities with open cavum conchae. Soft-tissue syndactyly involves the fourth and fifth

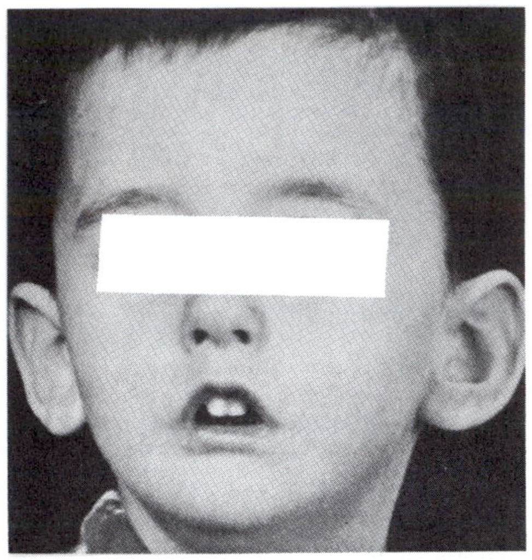

Moebius syndrome (1)
Meyerson, M.D.: The Effect of Syndrome Diagnosis on Speech Remediation. In Shprintzen, R.J., N.W. Paul (eds): *Diagnostic Accuracy: Effect on Treatment Planning.* New York: Alan R. Liss, Inc. for the March of Dimes Birth Defects Foundation BD:OAS 21(2):47-68, 1985, with permission.

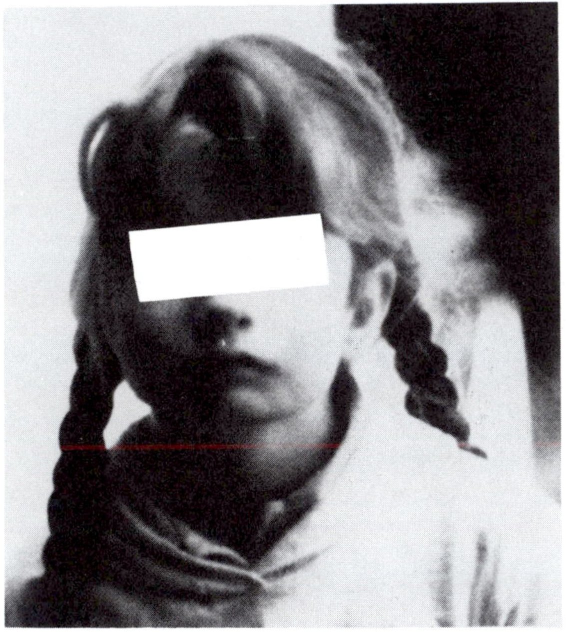

Moebius syndrome (2)
Sogg, R.: *Arch. Ophthalmol.* 65:16, 1961. Chicago: American Medical Association, copyright 1969.

fingers. The syndrome is sometimes identified as acrocephalosyndactyly IV, but it is not included in modern classification schemes of acrocephalosyndactylies.

Mohr. O. L. Dominant acrocephalosyndactyly. *Hereditas,* 1939, 25:193-203.

Mohr syndrome variant. See *Joubert syndrome.*

Mohr-Claussen syndrome. See *orofaciodigital syndrome II.*

Mohr-Wriedt brachydactyly. See *brachdactyly A-2.*

MOLLARET, PIERRE (French neurologist, born 1898)

Debré-Mollaret syndrome. See *cat scratch disease.*

Foshay-Mollaret syndrome. See *cat scratch disease.*

Mollaret meningitis. Synonyms: *benign recurrent aseptic meningitis, benign recurrent endothelial-leukocytic meningitis, recurrent aseptic meningitis.*

Meningitis beginning as sudden attacks of recurrent fever, associated with headache, nausea, vomiting, neck rigidity, malaise, myalgia, and positive Kernig and Brudzinski signs. Mixed pleocytosis, including the endothelial cells, leukocytes, and lymphocytes, accompany the attacks. After three or four days the symptoms disappear, but the attacks recur at regular intervals of several weeks or months.

Mollaret, P. Méningite endothélio-leucocytaire multirécurrente bénigne. Syndrome nouveau ou maladie nouvelle? (Documents cliniques). *Rev. Neur., Paris,* 1944, 76:57-76.

MÖLLER (MOELLER), JULIUS OTTO LUDWIG (German physician, 1819-1887)

Cheadle-Möller-Barlow disease. See *Möller-Barlow disease.*

Möller disease. See *Möller-Barlow disease.*

Möller glossitis. Synonyms: *Moeller glossitis, bald tongue, chronic lingual papillitis, chronic superficial glossitis, glazed tongue, glossitis exfoliativa, glossitis superficialis chronica, glossodynia exfoliativa, glossy tongue, pellagrous tongue, slick tongue, smooth tongue, varnished tongue.*

Superficial excoriation of the tongue, principally of its tip and edges. The lesions are beefy red, well-defined, irregular patches, in which the filiform papillae are thinned or absent and the fungiform papillae are swollen. The surface between the lesions may be smooth, whitish, or opalescent.

Möller. Klinische Bemerkungen über einige weniger bekannte Krankheiten der Zunge. *Deut. Klinik,* 1851, 3:273-5.

Möller-Barlow disease. Synonyms: *Barlow disease, Cheadle disease, Cheadle-Möller-Barlow disease, Möller disease, hemorrhagic scurvy, infantile hemorrhagic diathesis, infantile scurvy.*

A form of scurvy, sometimes observed in artificially fed infants, caused by vitamin C deficiency, and characterized by gingival lesions, hemorrhage, arthralgia, loss of appetite, listlessness, and other symptoms similar to those seen in adult scurvy. Ocular findings may include exophthalmos and conjunctival hemorrhage.

Barlow, T. On cases described as "acute rickets" which are probably a combination of scurvy and rickets, the scurvy being an essential and the rickets a variable element. *Med. Chir. Tr., London,* 1883, 66:159-219. Cheadle, W. B. Scurvy and purpura. *Brit. Med. J.,* 1872, 2:250-2. *Möller, J. O. Über akute Rachitis. *Königsberg Med. Jb.,* 1859, 1:377.

mollities ossium. See *osteogenesis imperfecta syndrome (dominant form).*

moluscum contagiosum. See *Bateman syndrome (1).*

moluscum epitheliale. See *Bateman syndrome (1).*

moluscum sebaceum. See *Bateman syndrome (1).*

MOMX (macroorchidism-marker X) syndrome. See *chromosome X fragility.*

MONA LISA (GIOCONDA), LISA DI ANTON MARIA GHERARDINI (Wife of Francesco del Giocondo, subject of Leonardo da Vinci's portrait, which is known for its subtle smile)

Mona Lisa syndrome. Facial muscle contracture that develops after Bell's palsy when the facial nerve has undergone partial wallerian degeneration and has regenerated, manifested by a Mona Lisa-like smile.

Adour, K. K. Mona Lisa syndrome: Solving the enigma of the Gioconda smile. *Ann. Otol. Rhinol. Laryngol.*, 1989, 98:196-9.

MONAKOW, CONSTANTIN, VON (Swiss physician, 1853-1930)

Monakow syndrome. See *anterior choroidal artery syndrome.*

MÖNCKEBERG, JOHANN GEORG (German pathologist, 1877-1925)

Mönckeberg arteriosclerosis. Synonyms: *Mönckeberg calcification, Mönckeberg degeneration, Mönckeberg sclerosis.*

Calcification of the medial arterial coat, especially in the lower extremities, which forms irregular bands around the affected arteries.

Mönckeberg, J. G. Über die reine Mediaverkalkung der Extremitätenarterien und ihr Verhalten zur Arteriosklerose. *Virchows Arch. Path.*, 1903, 171:141-67.

Mönckeberg calcification. See *Mönckeberg arteriosclerosis.*

Mönckeberg degeneration. See *Mönckeberg arteriosclerosis.*

Mönckeberg sclerosis. See *Mönckeberg arteriosclerosis.*

MONCRIEFF, ALAN AIRD (British physician, born 1901)

Moncrieff syndrome. Synonyms: *Moncrieff-Wilkinson syndrome, sucrosuria-hiatus hernia-mental retardation syndrome.*

A syndrome of sucrosuria, hiatal hernia, and mental retardation transmitted as an autosomal recessive trait. Moncrieff and Wilkinson indicated that the sucrosuria results from a rapid absorption of unsplit disaccharide. In one case, autopsy revealed a congenital defect in the brain.

Moncrieff, A., & Wilkinson, R. H. Sucrosuria with mental defect and hiatus hernia. *Acta Paediat., Stockholm*, 1954, 43(Suppl 100):495-516.

Moncrieff-Wilkinson syndrome. See *Moncrieff syndrome.*

MONDOR, HENRI JEAN JUSTIN (French physician, 1885-1962)

Mondor disease (1). Synonyms: *Mondor phlebitis, Mondor syndrome, cord phlebitis of the chest wall, endophlebitis of the thoraco-epigastric veins, thrombophlebitis of the thoraco-epigastric veins.*

String phlebitis of the subcutaneous veins of the chest and breast extending from the epigastric or hypochondrial region to the axilla. The etiology is unknown, but exertion, infection, and trauma appear to be the contributing factors.

Mondor, H., & Bertrand, I. Thrombo-phlébite et périphlébite de la paroi thoracique antérieure. *Presse Méd., Paris*, 1951, 59:1533-5.

Mondor disease (2). See *Mondor syndrome (2).*

Mondor phlebitis. See *Mondor disease (1).*

Mondor syndrome (1). See *Mondor disease (1).*

Mondor syndrome (2). Synonyms: *Mondor disease, tricolor syndrome.*

Endobacillary septicemia and bacterial shock in septic abortion, caused by *Clostridium perfringens* infection, manifested by red coloration of the skin, red coloration of the urine due to hemoglobinuria, and intense hemolysis with the presence of free hemoglobin.

*Mondor, H. *Les avortements mortels*. Paris, 1936.

MONGE, CARLOS (Peruvian physician, born 1884)

Monge disease. Synonyms: *altitude sickness, Andes disease, chronic mountain sickness, high altitude disease, high altitude erythremia.*

A chronic form of mountain sickness occurring in persons living for long periods at high altitudes, usually at over 14,000 feet, characterized by cyanosis, dyspnea, cough, arrhythmias, headache, dizziness, stupor, muscle and motor disorders, weakness, and pain in the extremities. Depressed respiratory reaction to hypoxia, erythrocytosis with hemoglobin levels reaching 24 gm per deciliter, low minute ventilation with elevated partial pressure of carbon dioxide, and hypoxemia are its principal features.

Monge, C. High altitude disease. *Arch. Intern. Med.*, 1937, 59:32-40.

mongolian spots. See *Brushfield spots.*

mongolism. See *chromosome 21 trisomy syndrome.*

mongoloid idiocy. See *chromosome 21 trisomy syndrome.*

monilethricosis. See *Sabouraud syndrome.*

monilethrix. See *Sabouraud syndrome.*

moniliform hair. See *Sabouraud syndrome.*

monocytic angina. See *Filatov disease.*

monosomy 1pter. See *chromosome 1pter deletion syndrome.*

monosomy 1q. See *chromosome 1q deletion syndrome.*

monosomy 2q. See *chromosome 2q deletion syndrome.*

monosomy 3pter. See *chromosome 3pter deletion syndrome.*

monosomy 3q. See *chromosome 3q deletion syndrome.*

monosomy 4p. See *chromosome 4p deletion syndrome.*

monosomy 4q. See *chromosome 4q deletion syndrome.*

monosomy 5p. See *chromosome 5p deletion syndrome.*

monosomy 5q. See *chromosome 5q deletion syndrome.*

monosomy 6q. See *chromosome 6q deletion syndrome.*

monosomy 7. See *chromosome 7 monosomy syndrome.*

monosomy 7p. See *chromosome 7p deletion syndrome.*

monosomy 7q. See *chromosome 7q deletion syndrome.*

monosomy 8p. See *chromosome 8p deletion syndrome.*

monosomy 8q. See *chromosome 8q deletion syndrome.*

monosomy 9p. See *chromosome 9p deletion syndrome.*

monosomy 10p syndrome. See *chromosome 10p deletion syndrome.*

monosomy 10qter. See *chromosome 10qter deletion syndrome.*

monosomy 11q. See *chromosome 11q deletion syndrome.*

monosomy 12p. See *chromosome 12p deletion syndrome.*

monosomy 13q. See *chromosome 13q deletion syndrome.*

monosomy 14q. See *chromosome 14q deletion syndrome.*

monosomy 16q. See *chromosome 16q deletion syndrome.*

monosomy 17p. See *chromosome 17p deletion syndrome.*

monosomy 18p. See *chromosome 18p deletion syndrome.*

monosomy 18q. See *chromosome 18q deletion syndrome.*

monosomy 20p. See *chromosome 20p deletion syndrome.*

monosomy 20q. See *chromosome 20q deletion syndrome.*

monosomy 21. See *chromosome 21 monosomy syndrome.*
monosomy 21q. See *chromosome 21q deletion syndrome.*
monosomy 22. See *chromosome 22 monosomy syndrome.*
monosomy C. See *chromosome 7 monosomy syndrome.*
monosomy G. See *chromosome 21 monosomy syndrome.*
monostotic fibrous dysplasia. See *Jaffe-Lichtenstein syndrome.*

MONTEGGIA, GIOVANNI BATTISTA (Italian surgeon, 1762-1815)

Monteggia fracture. Fracture of the ulna in the proximal half of the shaft, near the junction of the middle and upper thirds, frequently associated with dislocation of the radial head.

Monteggia, G. B. *Istituzioni chirurgiche*. Milano, Pirotta & Maspero, 1814. Vol. 5.

Montreal platelet syndrome (MPS). See *Bernard-Soulier syndrome.*

MOON, ROBERT C. (American ophthalmologist, 1844-1914)

Laurence-Moon syndrome. See *Laurence-Moon-Biedl syndrome.*
Laurence-Moon-Biedl syndrome. See *under Laurence.*
Laurence-Moon-Biedl-Bardet syndrome (LMBB, LMBBS). See *Laurence-Moon-Biedl syndrome.*

MOORE, EDWARD MOTT (American physician, 1814-1902)

Moore fracture. Fracture of the lower end of the radius with dislocation of the ulna and incarceration of the styloid process under the annular ligament.

*Moore, E. M. *A luxation of the ulna not hitherto described, with a plan of reduction and mode of after-treatment; including the management of Colles' fracture*. Albany, Weed, 1872.

MOORE, MATTHEW THIBAUD (American physician, born 1901)

Moore syndrome. Synonyms: *abdominal epilepsy, paroxysmal abdominal pain syndrome.*

Attacks of paroxysmal abdominal pain symptomatic of epilepsy in children, adolescents, and young adults, occurring in conjunction with electroencephalographic changes and occasional convulsions.

Moore, M. T. Paroxysmal abdominal pain. A form of focal symptomatic epileplsy. *JAMA*, 1944, 124:l561-3.

MOORE, ROBERT A. (American physician)

Dixon-Moore seminoma. See *Dixon-Moore tumor.*
Dixon-Moore tumor. See *under Dixon.*

MOORE, S. (American physician)

Morgagni-Morel-Moore syndrome. See *Morgagni-Steward-Morel syndrome.*

MOORE, W. T. (American physician)

Moore-Federman syndrome. Synonym: *familial dwarfism-stiff joints syndrome.*

A syndrome of dwarfism and limited joint mobility, especially of the elbows, knees, wrists, and fingers. Associated disorders may include thickening of the skin over the affected joints, hyperopia, asthma, hoarse voice, and hepatomegaly. The syndrome is similar to the Léri syndrome and is transmitted as an autosomal dominant trait.

Moore, W. T., & Federman, D. D. Familial dwarfism and "stiff joints." *Arch. Int. Med.*, 1965, 115:398-404.

MOOREN, ALBERT (German ophthalmologist, 1828-1899)

Mooren rodent ulcer. See *Mooren ulcer.*
Mooren ulcer. Synonyms: *Mooren rodent ulcer, chronic serpiginous ulcer, corneal melting syndrome.*

A rare form of corneal ulcer occurring in apparently normal elderly persons. It is marked by a superficial, yellowish gray, infiltrated excavation near the limbus that progresses toward the central cornea with a raised border at the advancing edge.

Mooren, A. *Ophthalmiatrische Beobachtungen*. Berlin, 1867.

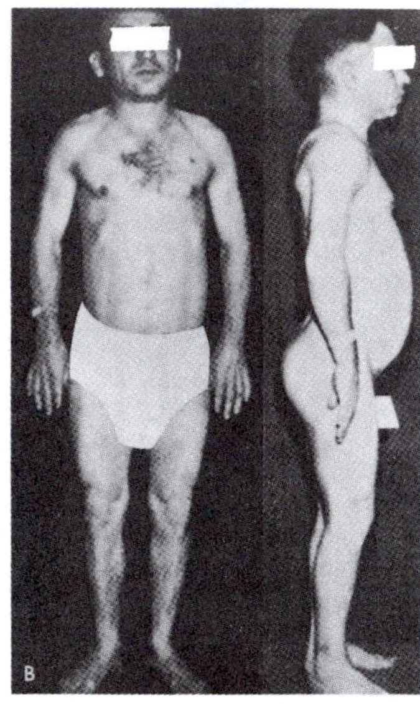

Moore-Federman syndrome
Moore, W.T. & Federman, D.D.: *Arch. Int. Med.* 115:398, 1965. Chicago: American Medical Association.

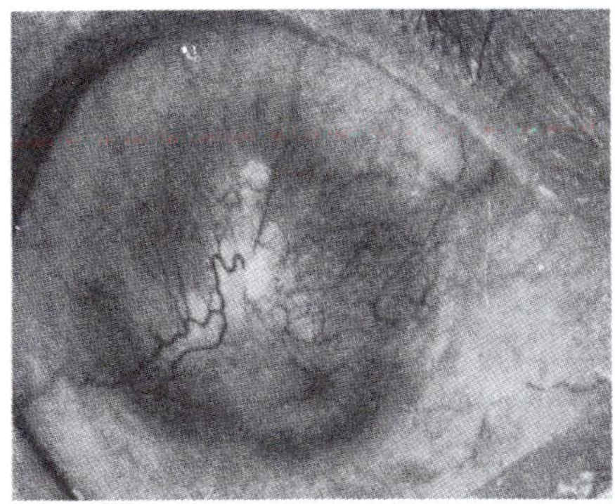

Mooren ulcer
Hansell, Dr. Peter, Dept. of Medical Illustrations, Institute of Ophthalmology, University of London. From S. Duke-Elder & A.G. Leigh: Diseases of the Outer Eye (Part 2). In S. Duke-Elder: *System of Ophthlmology* Vol. VIII. London: Henry Kimpton, 1965.

MORAX, VICTOR (French ophthalmologist, 1866-1935)

Morax-Axenfeld conjunctivitis. Synonyms: *Axenfeld conjunctivitis, diplobacillary conjunctivitis.*

Conjunctivitis caused by *Diplococcus morax-axenfeld* (*Moraxella lacunata*) infection.

*Morax, V. Note sur un diplobacille pathogène pour la

conjonctivite humaine. *Ann Inst. Pasteur*, 1896, 10:337-45. Axenfeld, T. Über die chronische Diplobacillenconjunctivitis. *Zbl. Bakt.*, 1897, 21:1-9.

morbus Addison. See *Addison disease.*

morbus anglicus. See *Glisson disease.*

morbus anglorum. See *Glisson disease.*

morbus asthenicus. See *Stiller asthenia.*

morbus celiacus. See *celiac disease.*

morbus ceruleus. See *Fallot tetralogy.*

morbus coeliacus. See *celiac disease.*

morbus Down. See *chromosome 21 trisomy.*

morbus maculosus hemorrhagicus. See *Werlhof disease.*

morbus maculosus werlhofii. See *Werlhof disease.*

morbus moniliformis lichenoides. See *Kaposi disease (1).*

morbus Ollier. See *Ollier syndrome.*

morbus Petzetakis. See *cat scratch disease.*

MOREL, BENEDICT AUGUSTIN. See MOREL, BENOIT AUGUSTIN

MOREL, BENOIT AUGUSTIN (French alienist, 1809-1873)

Morel disease. Synonyms: *Saunders-Sutton syndrome, alcohol withdrawal delirium, delirium alcoholicum, delirium tremens (DT).*

An acute form of alcohol withdrawal syndrome (see under *withdrawal syndrome*) characterized mainly by cortical and ß-adrenergic hyperexcitability. The symptoms include disorientation, agitation, hallucinations, tremor, seizures, sweating, rapid respiration and pulse rates, hyper- or hypotension, abnormal body temperature, severe muscle cramps, paresthesias, neurological disorders, vomiting, and gastritis. The symptoms usually appear 3 to 5 days after alcohol withdrawal. In untreated cases, disorientation and restlessness may last for several weeks; with adequate treatment, most severe symptoms clear within 10 days. The mortality rate is about 15 per cent.

Morel. B. A. *Traité des maladie mentales.* Paris, 1860, p. 400. Sutton, T. *Tracts on delirium tremens, on some other inflammatory affections, and on the gout.* London, Underwood, 1813. Cutshall, B. J. The Saunders-Sutton syndrome: An analysis of delirium tremens. *Q. J. Stud. Alcohol.*, 1965, 26:423-48.

Morel ear. An ear deformity characterized by maldevelopment of the helix, anthelix, and scaphoid fossa, resulting in obliteration of the folds, the ear being large and smooth, often with a thin edge.

*Morel, B. A. *Traité des dégénerescences physiques, intellectuelles et morales de l'éspéce humaine, etc.* Paris, 1857.

MOREL, FERDINAND (Swiss physician, 1888-1957)

Morel syndrome. See *Morgagni-Stewart-Morel syndrome.*

Morel-Wildi syndrome. Disseminated nodular dysgenesis of the frontal cerebral cortex, manifested as small pearl-like prominences, without any particular clinical manifestations.

Morel, F., & Wildi, E. Dysgénésie nodulaire disséminée de l'écorce frontale. *Rev. Neur., Paris*, 1952, 87:251-70.

Morgagni-Morel-Moore syndrome. See *Morgagni-Stewart-Morel syndrome.*

Morgagni-Stewart-Morel syndrome. See *under Morgagni.*

Stewart-Morel syndrome. See *Morgagni-Stewart-Moral syndrome.*

MOREL-LAVALLEE (French physician)

Morel-Lavallée syndrome. Extravasation of lymph in pockets formed by traumatic separation of the skin from the adjacent soft tissue.

Morel Lavallée. *Traumatismes fermés aux membres inférieurs.* Paris, 1848. (Thesis).

MORGAGNI, GIOVANNI BATTISTA (Italian anatomist and pathologist, 1682-1771)

Morgagni hernia. Anterior diaphragmatic hernia.

Morgagni, G. B. *De sedibus et acusis morborum.* Lib. III, 1761.

Morgagni syndrome. See *Morgagni-Stewart-Morel syndrome.*

Morgagni-Adams-Stokes (MAS) syndrome. See *Adams-Stokes syndrome, under Adams, Robert.*

Morgagni-Laennec syndrome. See *Laennec cirrhosis.*

Morgagni-Morel-Moore syndrome. See *Morgagni-Stewart-Morel syndrome.*

Morgagni-Steward-Morel syndrome. Synonyms: *Morel syndrome, Morgagni syndrome, Morgagni-Morel-Moore syndrome, Stewart-Morel syndrome, calvarial hyperostosis, hyperostosis frontalis interna, intracranial exostosis, metabolic craniopathy.*

A hereditary syndrome of usually symmetrical thickening of the frontal, parietal, or occipital bones due to deposits on the internal aspects of the squama frontalis, occasionally extending to the orbital plate, falx, and squama parietalis. There may be associated menstrual disorders, virilism, hirsutism, mental disorders, fatigue, somnolence, visual disorders, vertigo, tinnitus, obesity, polyphagia, polydipsia, polyuria, loss of sense of smell, decrease in glucose tolerance, convulsions, and involvement of the second, fifth, and seventh cranial nerves with hemiplegia and hemiparesis. Women in the fifth decade of life are most commonly affected. The syndrome is transmitted as an autosomal dominant trait.

Morgagni, G. B. *De sedibus et causis morborum.* Lib. II, 1761. Morel, F. *L'hyperostose frontale interne. Syndrome de l'hyperostose frontale interne avec adipose et troubles cerebraux.* Paris, 1930. Stewart, R. M. Localized cranial hyperostosis in insane. *J. Neur. Psychopath., London,* 1928, 8:321. *Moore, S. *Hyperostosis cranii.* Springfield, Illinoia, Thomas, 1955.

Morgagni-Turner syndrome. See *chromosome XO syndrome.*

Morgagni-Turner-Albright syndrome. See *chromosome XO syndrome.*

sinus of Morgagni syndrome. See *Trotter syndrome.*

MORGAN, A. (British physician)

Zachary-Morgan syndrome. See *under Zachary.*

MORGAN, G. (Australian physician)

Reye-Morgan-Baral syndrome. See *Reye syndrome.*

morphea. See *Addison keloid.*

MORQUIO, LUIS (LOUIS) (Pediatrician in Uruguay, 1867-1935)

Morquio B syndrome. See *mucopolysaccharidosis IV-B.*

Morquio disease. Congenital atrioventricular block associated with a septal defect of the heart.

Jonas, V. *Specialni kardiologie.* Praha, Stat. Zdrav. Makl., 1957. Vol. I, p. 386.

Morquio syndrome. See *mucopolysaccharidosis IV-A.*

Morquio-Brailsford syndrome. See *mucopolysaccharidosis IV-A.*

Morquio-like syndrome. See *mucopolysacchardosis IV-B.*

Morquio-Silfverskiöld syndrome. See *Silfverskiöld syndrome.*

Morquio-Ullrich syndrome. See *mucopolysaccharidosis IV-A.*

MORRIS, JOHN MCLEAN (American physician, born 1914)

Goldberg-Maxwell-Morris syndrome. See *testicular feminization syndrome.*

Goldberg-Morris syndrome. See *testicular feminization syndrome.*

Morris syndrome. See *testicular feminization syndrome.*

MORRISON, ASHTON BYROM (American physician, born 1903)

Verner-Morrison syndrome. See *under Verner.*

MORROW, PRINCE ALBERT (American physician, 1846-1913)

Morrow-Brooke syndrome. Synonyms: *Brooke disease, keratosis follicularis acneiformis, keratosis follicularis contagiosa.*

An apparently infectious skin disease that resembles keratosis follicularis (Darier syndrome). The eruption is usually generalized and symmetrical, involving the nape of the neck, the shoulders, the back, and the extensor surfaces of the extremities. The chief features are keratotic thickening of the skin with deep furrows and comedolike black plugs which later become large brownish papules, which sometimes coalesce. The skin becomes dry and rough. Fissuring of the tongue and leukoplakia are the principal oral manifestations.

Morrow, P. A. Keratosis follicularis associated with fissuring of the tongue and leukoplakia buccalis. *J. Cutan. Dis., N. Y.*, 1886, 4:257-65. *Brooke, H. A. Keratosis follicularis contagiosa. In his: *International atlas of rare skin diseases*. 1892, No. 7, plate 22..**MORSIER, GEORGES, DE** (Swiss physician, born 1894)

de Morsier syndrome (1). See *septo-optic dysplasia.*

de Morsier syndrome (2). See *olfactogenital syndrome.*

de Morsier syndrome (3). Diencephalic lesions associated with a variety of behavioral, psychomotor, and sensory disorders, including impaired memory, mental fatigability, hallucinations, photophobia, perception disturbances, hyperacusia, hyperosmia, difficulty in moving around an axis, and facial and oculomotor spasms. Encephalitis, carbon dioxide poisoning, hypothalamic tumors, and cerebral injuries are the suspected causes.

Morsier, G., de. Pathologie du diencéphale. Le syndrome psychologique et le syndrome sensorio-moteur. *Schweiz. Neur.*, 1944, 54:161-226.

de Morsier-Gauthier syndrome. See *olfactogenital syndrome.*

Kallmann-de Morsier syndrome. See *olfactogenital syndrome.*

Maestre de San Juan-Kallmann-de Morsier syndrome. See *olfactogenital syndrome.*

Maestre-Kallmann-de Morsier syndrome. See *olfactogenital syndrome.*

mort d'amour syndrome. Mort d'amour (death by love) is a condition in men and women with coronary disease in which the excitement and stress during sexual intercourse cause fatal cardiac arrhythmia.

Heggveit, H. A. La mort d'amour. *Am. Heart J.*, 1965, 69:287-94.

mortal catatonia. See *Bell mania, under Bell, Luther Vos.*

MORTENSEN, OLE (Danish physician)

Mortensen disease. Synonyms: *Di Guglielmo disease, Epstein syndrome, Epstein-Goedel syndrome, Revol disease, essential hemorrhagic thrombocythemia, essential thrombocythemia, hemorrhagic thrombocythemia, hyperthrombocytic myelosis, thrombocythemia hemorrhagica, thrombocytic hemorrhage.*

A hematological disorder characterized by prolonged bleeding time in spite of a permanent increase in the blood platelet count, with splenomegaly, an increase in the number of megakaryocytes in the bone marrow, neutrophilic leukocytosis, immature leukocytes in the blood, and occasional eosinophilia. Complications may include thrombosis and gastroduodenitis with hematemesis. The disorder may occur as a complication of leukemia, polycythemia, and splenomegaly.

Mortensen, O. Thrombocythemia hemorrhagica. *Acta Med. Scand.*, 1948, 129:547-59. Revol, L. La myélose hyperthrombocytaire (thrombocytémie hémorrhagique). *Sang*, 1950, 21:409-23. Di Guglielmo, G. Megacariociti e piastrine negli organi emopoietici e nel sangue circolante. *Atti R. Acad. Chir., Napoli*, 1919, 83:19. *Epstein, E., & Goedel, A. Hämorrhagische Thrombocythämie bei vascularer Schrumpfmilz. *Virchows Arch.*, 1934, 292:233-48.

MORTIMER

Mortimer disease. Synonyms: *Mortimer malady, lupus vulgaris multiplex nonulcerans et nonserpiginosus.*

A skin disease characterized by multiple, raised, dusky-red patches that spread slowly in an almost symmetrical pattern. The absence of ulcers and of crust distinguish this entity from lupus vulgaris. The disease was originally described by Hutchinson and named for his patient, Mrs. Mortimer.

Hutchinson, J. Cases of Mortimer's malady (lupus vulgaris multiplex non-ulcerans et non-serpiginosus). *Arch. Surg., London*, 1898, 9:307-14.

Mortimer malady. See *Mortimer disease.*

MORTON, DUDLEY J. (American orthopedic surgeon, 1884-1960)

Morton syndrome. Synonyms: *metatarsus atavicus, metatarsus primus brevior.*

Unusual shortness of the first metatarsal bone associated with tenderness elicited by deep pressure on the sole of the foot at the junction of the second metatarsal and cuneiform bone. Not to be confused with *Morton neuralgia* (under *Morton, Thomas George*).

Morton, D. J. Metatarsus atavicus. The identification of a distinctive type of foot disorder. *J. Bone Joint Surg.*, 1927, 9:531-44.

MORTON, THOMAS GEORGE (American physician, 1835-1903)

Morton disease. See *Morton neuralgia.*

Morton foot. See *Morton neuralgia.*

Morton metatarsalgia. See *Morton neuralgia.*

Morton nerve entrapment syndrome. See *Morton neuralgia.*

Morton neuralgia. Synonyms: *Morton disease, Morton foot, Morton metatarsalgia, Morton nerve entrapment syndrome, Morton neuroma, Morton syndrome, Morton toe, digital neuroma, metatarsal neuralgia, metatarsalgia anterior.*

A disease of the foot occurring spontaneously in middle-aged females and occasionally in males. It is characterized by a sudden cramplike pain in the region of the fourth and, less frequently, the third metatarsophalangeal joint. Compression of the plantar nerve by a tumor, arthritic changes, or bursitis is the common cause. Not to be confused with the *Morton syndrome* (under *Morton, Dudley J.*).

Morton, T. G. A peculiar and painful affection of the fourth metatarsophalangeal articulation. *Am. J. Med. Sc.*, 1876, 71:37-45.

Morton neuroma. See *Morton neuralgia.*

Morton toe. See *Morton neuralgia.*

MORVAN, AUGUSTIN MARIE (French physician, 1819-1897)

Morvan chorea. Synonyms: *Morvan syndrome, chorea fibrillaris, fibrillary chorea, myoclonus multiplex fibrillaris.*

Fibrillary contraction (myoclonus) involving the muscles of the calves, the posterior parts of the thighs, and, less frequently, the trunk.

Morvan. De la chorée fibrillaire. *Gaz. Hebd. Méd., Paris*, 1890, 27:173-6; 186-9; 200-2.

Morvan disease. Synonyms: *Morvan syndrome, analgesic panaris, analgesic paralysis with whitlow, syringomyelia.*

A chronic disease marked by cavities in the spinal cord, usually in the central region and often extending into the medulla (syringobulbia), or inferiorly into the thoracic and lumbar regions of the cord. In some cases, the cavity communicates with the fourth ventricle, when the condition is known as *hydromyelia*. It usually starts insidiously before the age of 30 years and gradually causes muscular weakness, hyperhidrosis, skeletal malformations (chiefly kyphoscoliosis), and analgesia with secondary painless ulcers of the tips of the fingers and the Charcot joint. Dissociation anesthesia, in which the pain and temperature sense are impaired but the sense of touch is retained, and paresthesia are the principal symmptoms. Atrophy of the muscles, fasciculation, and areflexia develop progressively, the upper extremities being chiefly affected. The lower extremities may be involved at the time when the syringomyelic cavity extends into the lateral column of the cord. Warts, bullae, gangrene, contractures, epileptiform seizures, and nocturnal enuresis may occur. This disease is frequently associated with other congenital malformations, such as Arnold-Chiari malformation, Klippel-Feil syndrome and spina bifida.

Morvan. De la parésie analgésique à panaris des extrémités supérieures. *Gaz. Hebd. Méd., Paris*, 1883, 20:580-3; 590-4; 624-6.

Morvan syndrome (1). See *Morvan chorea.*

Morvan syndrome (2). See *Morvan disease.*

mosaic corneal degeneration. See *Vogt degeneration.*

mosaic tetrasomy 12p. See *chromosome 12p tetrasomy syndrome.*

mosaic trisomy 12. See *chromosome 12 trisomy mosaicism.*

MOSCHCOWITZ, ELI (American physician, 1879-1964)

Moschcowitz syndrome. Synonyms: *Baehr-Schiffrin disease, Moschcowitz-Singer-Symmers syndrome, disseminated arteriolar-capillary platelet thrombosis, fulminant thrombotic thrombopenic purpura, generalized capillary and arteriolar thrombosis, microangiopathic thrombotic hemolytic anemia, platelet thrombosis, thrombocytic acroangiothrombosis, thrombohemolytic thrombopenic purpura, thrombotic microangiopathic hemolytic anemia, thrombotic microangiopathy, thrombotic thrombocytopenic purpura (TTP), thrombotic thrombocytic anemia.*

A frequently fatal combination of hemolytic anemia, thrombocytic purpura, neurologic disorders (ischemic complications in the central nervous system), and hyaline thrombosis of the terminal arterioles and capillaries. Jaundice, fever, systemic and retinal hemorrhages, hematuria, confusions, headache, paralysis, paresthesia, convulsions, hemolysis, renal failure, azotemia, and coma are the common manifestations. Pathological findings include disseminated thrombi, chiefly in the brain, adrenals, pancreas, spleen, and gastrointestinal system; gross poikilocytosis; hepatomegaly; and splenomegaly.

Moschcowitz, E. An acute febrile pleiochromic anemia with hyaline thrombosis of the terminal arterioles and capillaries. An undescribed disease. *Arch. Int. Med., Chicago*, 1925, 36:89-93. Baehr, G., Klempferer, P., & Schiffrin, A. Acute febrile anemia and thrombocytopenic purpura with diffuse platelet thromboses of capillaries and arterioles. *Tr. Assoc. Am. Physicians*, 1936, 51:43-58.

Moschcowitz-Singer-Symmers syndrome. See *Moschcowitz syndrome.*

MOSS, MELVIN LIONEL (American physician, born 1923)

Gorlin-Chaudhry-Moss syndrome. See *under Gorlin.*

MOSSE, ALPHONSE (French physician)

Mosse-Marchand-Mallory cirrhosis. A usually fatal form of cirrhosis of the liver complicated by liver atrophy, ascites, and edema that develops after febrile, painful degenerative jaundice. The condition was reportedly described by Mosse in 1879, Marchand in 1895, and Mallory in 1911.

MOSSE, MAX (German physician, born 1873)

Mosse polycythemia. See *Mosse syndrome.*

Mosse syndrome. Synonyms: *Mosse polycythemia, liver cirrhosis-polycythemia syndrome, polycythemia-hepatocirrhosis syndrome.*

An association of liver cirrhosis with polycythemia vera (the Vaquez-Osler syndrome).

Mosse, M. Über Polyzythamie mit Urobilinikterus und Milztumor. *Deut. Med. Wschr.*, 1907, 33:2175-6.

MOSTO, SANTIAGO J. (Argentine physician)

Casalá-Mosto disease. See *under Casalá.*

motion sickness-like syndrome. See *space adaptation syndrome.*

motor aphasia. See *Broca aphasia.*

motor urge incontinence. See *under urge incontinence syndrome.*

mottled enamel. See *Spira disease.*

mottled teeth. See *Spira disease.*

MOUCHET, ALBERT (French physician, born 1869)

Albert Mouchet syndrome. See *Mouchet syndrome.*

Köhler-Mouchet disease. See *Köhler disease (1).*

Mouchet syndrome. Synonym: *Albert Mouchet syndrome.*

Remote paralysis of the cubital nerve after fractures of the external condyle of the humerus.

Mouchet, A. Paralyses tardives du nerf cubital à la suite de fractures du condyle externe de l'humérus. *J. Chir., Paris*, 1914, pp. 437-56.

MOUNIER-KUHN, PIERRE (French physician)

Mounier-Kuhn syndrome. Synonyms: *idiopathic megatrachea with tracheomalacia, megatrachea, megatrachea with tracheomalacia, tracheal diverticu-*

losis, tracheobronchiectasis, tracheobronchiomegaly (TBM), tracheobronchiopathic malacia.

Dilation of the trachea and major bronchi associated with recurrent lower respiratory tract infection. The symptoms include cough, hoarseness, dyspnea, and copious production of sputum. Radiographic findings show emphysema, pulmonary fibrosis, and bullae. Some reported cases have been familial.

Mounier-Kuhn. Dilatation de la trachée, constatation radiographiques et bronchoscopiques. *Lyon Méd.*, 1932, 150:106-19, passim.

MOUNT, LESTER ADRIAN (American physician, born 1910)

Mount syndrome. See *Mount-Reback syndrome.*

Mount-Reback syndrome. Synonyms: *Mount syndrome, familial paroxysmal dystonic choreoathetosis, familial paroxysmal choreoathetosis, paroxysmal dystonic choreoathetosis.*

A hereditary familial disease, transmitted as an autosomal dominant trait, characterized by attacks of choreoathetosis and torsion without loss of consciousness, each episode lasting from a few minutes to several hours. The attacks never occur during sleep and, at their height, are similar to those in Huntington chorea. Alcoholic beverages, coffee, hunger, fatigue, emotional stress, and tobacco are the precipitating factors. The presence of an atypical Kayser-Fleischer ring is the principal ocular feature.

Mount, L. A., & Rebock, S. Familial paroxysmal choreoathetosis. Preliminary report on a hitherto undescribed clinical syndrome. *Arch. Neur., Chicago*, 1940, 44:841-7.

mountain climber's disease. See *D'Acosta disease.*

mountain fever. See *brucellosis.*

mountain sickness. See *D'Acosta disease, and see Monge disease.*

MOUSSUS

Leiner-Moussus disease. See *Leiner dermatitis.*

MOUTOT, HENRI (French physician, born 1880)

Nicolas-Moutot-Charlet syndrome. See *under Nicolas.*

moving toe syndrome. See *restless leg syndrome.*

moyamoya (moya-moya) disease (MMD). See *moyamoya syndrome.*

moyamoya (moya-moya) syndrome. Synonyms: *Kawakita syndrome, Leeds syndrome, Maki syndrome, Taveras syndrome, moyamoya disease (MMD).*

A cerebrovascular disorder marked by progressive obliteration of the intracranial carotid arteries and formation of an extensive vascular network of dilated small branches beyond the stenoses and abundant small collaterals developing from the ascending pharyngeal and meningeal branches of the external carotid artery. The disorder was first reported in Japanese children, and the angiographic appearance of thus formed fine vascular network was described by the Japanese expression "moyamoya," meaning "something hazy, like a puff of smoke drifting in the air," as seen on the radiograph. Acute hemiparesis is the usual initial symptom, but motor disorders, headache, epileptic convulsions, nausea, vomiting, speech disorders, bouts of unconsciousness, visual disorders, involuntary movements, sensory disturbances, intellectual deficit, and subarachnoid hemorrhage may also occur. These symptoms and dysphagia may recur throughout the course of disease. See also *Nishimoto disease.*

Leeds, N. E., & Abbott, K. H. Collateral circulation in cerebrovascular disease in childhood via rete mirabile and perforating branches of anterior choroidal and posterior cerebral arteries. *Radiology*, 1965, 85:628-34. Kawakita, Y., *et al.* Spontaneous thrombosis of the internal carotid artery in children. *Fol. Psychiat. Neur. Jpn.*, 1965, 19:245-55. Taveras, J. M. Multiple progressive intracranial arterial occlusions: A syndrome of children and young adults. *Am. J. Roentgen.*, 1969, 106:235-68. Maki, Y., & Nakata, Y. [Autopsy case of hemangiomatous malformation of bilateral internal carotid artery at the base of the brain] *Brain Nerve, Tokyo*, 1965, 17:764-6.

MOYNAHAN, E. J. (British physician)

Moynahan syndrome (1). A syndrome of multiple symmetrical lentigines, genital hypoplasia, dwarfism, congenital mitral stenosis, and mental deficiency.

Moynahan, E. J. Multiple symmetrical moles, with psychic and somatic infantism and genital hypoplasia. First male case of a new syndrome. *Proc. Roy. Soc. Med.*, 1962, 55:959-60.

Moynahan syndrome (2). Synonyms: *alopecia-epilepsy-oligophrenia syndrome, familial congenital alopecia-epilepsy-mental retardation-unusual EEG syndrome.*

A congenital syndrome, transmitted as an autosomal recessive trait, consisting of alopecia, epilepsy, mental retardation, and abnormal EEG.

Moynahan, E. J. Familial congenital alopecia, epilepsy, mental retardation with unusual electroencephalograms. *Proc. Roy. Soc. Med.*, 1962, 55:411-2.

Moynahan syndrome (3). Synonym: *xeroderma-talipes-enamel (XTE) defect syndrome.*

An ectodermal dysplasia syndrome, transmitted as an autosomal dominant trait, characterized by xeroderma, talipes, and tooth enamel defect. Associated disorders include dry and slow-growing hair, absent eyelashes on the lower lids, scanty hair follicles, small toe nails, and reduced numbers of sweat glands with hypohidrosis.

Moynahan, E. J. XTE syndrome (xeroderma, talipes and enamel defect): A new heredo-familial syndrome: Two cases, homozygous inhritance of a dominant gene. *Proc. R. Soc. Med.*, 1970, 63:447-9.

Moynahan syndrome (4). See *LEOPARD syndrome.*

MOZART, WOLFGANG AMADEUS (Austrian composer, 1756-1791)

Mozart ear. A congenital ear abnormality characterized by fusion of the enlarged portion of the anthelix with the helix, observed in Wolfgang Amadeus Mozart and his father.

García-Cruz, D. A syndrome with mixed deafness, Mozart ear, middle and inner ear dysplasias. *J. Laryng. Otol.*, 1980, 94:773-8. Altmann, F. Malformations of the auricle and the external auditory meatus. *AMA Arch. Otolaryng.*, 1951, 54:115-39.

MP (Mibelli porokeratosis). See *Mibelli disease (2).*

MPS. See *meconium plug syndrome.*

MPS (Montreal pletelet syndrome). See *Bernard-Soulier syndrome.*

MPS (I-H, I-H/S, I-S, II, III, IV-A, IV-B, V, VI, VII). See *mucopolysaccharidosis (I-H, I-H/S, I-S, II, III, IV-A, IV-B, V, VI, VII).*

MRK. See *Mayer-Rokitansky-Küster syndrome.*

MRS. See *Melkersson-Rosenthal syndrome.*

MS. See *Maffucci syndrome.*

MS. See *Munchausen syndrome.*

MS. See *Meckel syndrome.*

MSBP. See *Munchausen syndrome by proxy.*

MSEL (myasthenic syndrome of Eaton and Lambert). See *Eaton-Lambert syndrome, under Eaton, Lealdes McKandree.*

Mseleni disease. See *Mseleni joint disease.*

Mseleni joint disease (MJD). Synonym: *Mseleni disease.*

A chronic, progressively disabling polyarticular disease found in a small area near the Mseleni Mission Station, Ubombo District, Zululand, South Africa. X-ray findings include osteoarthrosis; irregularities in joint spaces, including the hips, knees, and ankles; deformities of the distal ends of the radius, ulna, and carpal bones; brachymetacarpia; and protrusio acetabuli. Etiology is unknown but genetic transmission, manganese deficiency, and mycotoxins are considered as potential causative factors.

Wittman, W., & Fellingham, S. A. Unusual hip disease in remote parts of Zululand. *Lancet*, 1970, 1:842-3.

MSHSC (multiple self-healing squamous carcinoma). See *Ferguson Smith epithelioma, under Smith, John Ferguson.*

MSP. See *Munchausen syndrome by proxy.*

MSS. See *Marshall-Smith syndrome, under Marshall, Richard E.*

MSS. See *Marinesco-Sjögren syndrome, under Marinescu, Gheorghe.*

MSUD. See *maple syrup urine disease.*

MT. See *Muir-Torre syndrome.*

MU chain disease. See *under heavy chain disease.*

MUCHA, VIKTOR (Austrian dermatologist, 1877-1919)

Mucha disease. See *Mucha-Habermann syndrome.*

Mucha-Habermann syndrome. Synonyms: *Mucha disease, Wise disease, acute parapsoriasis varioliformis, pityriasis lichenoides et varioliformis acuta.*

A rare skin disease characterized by the sudden appearance of a polymorphous and polychromatic eruption composed of papules, scaly lesions similar to those in pityriasis rosea, necrotic or hemorrhagic vesicles simulating varicella, and depressed, pigmented, varioliform scars. The cutaneous manifestations are usually unaccompanied by constitutional symptoms and may persist from 1 month to 2 years.

Mucha, V. Über einen der Parakeratosis variegata (Unna) bzw. Pityriasis lichenoides chronica (Neisser-Juliusberg) nahestehenden eigentümlichen Fall. *Arch. Derm. Syph., Berlin*, 1916, 123:586-92. Habermann, R. Über die akut verlaufende, nekrotisierende Unterart der Pityriasis lichenoides (Pityriais lichenoides et varioliformis acuta). *Derm. Zschr.*, 1925, 45:42-8. Wise, F., & Sulzberger, M. B. Pityriasis lichenoides et varioliformis acuta (Habermann). *Med. J. Rec.*, 1930, 132:231.

mucinous alopecia. See *Pinkus disease, under Pinkus, Hermann Karl Benno.*

MUCKLE, THOMAS JAMES (British physician)

Muckle-Wells syndrome. Synonym: *amyloidosis-deafness-urticaria-limb pain syndrome.*

A familial form of amyloidosis, transmitted as an autosomal dominant trait, characterized by nerve deafness, urticaria, limb pain, and nephropathy. Fever, malaise, and arthralgia, appearing in adolescence, are the early symptoms. The nephrotic syndrome (q.v.), leading to fatal uremia, is usually observed in late adult and middle age. Loss of libido, pes cavus, glaucoma, pachyderma, and high erythrocyte sedimentation rate occur in some case. Amyloid deposits in various tissues, small and shriveled kidneys, absence of the organ of Corti, and atrophy of the cochlear nerve are the principal pathological findings.

Muckle, T. J., & Wells, M. Urticaria, deafness and amyloidosis. A new heredo-familial syndrome. *Q. J. Med.*, 1962, 31:235-48.

mucocutaneous candidiasis. See *chronic mucocutaneous candidiasis syndrome.*

mucocutaneous lymph node syndrome (MCLS, MLNS). See *Kawasaki syndrome.*

mucoenteritis. See *irritable bowel syndrome.*

mucolipidosis I (ML I). Synonyms: *GAL plus disease, lipomucopolysaccharidosis.*

An inborn metabolic disorder characterized by the accumulation in tissues of acid mucopolysaccharides and glycolipids. The symptoms include a moderate psychomotor retardation (usually noted in the second year of life), mild Hurler-like (gargoylelike) manifestations appearing after the age of 2 years, hepatosplenomegaly, hernias, muscle wasting, progressive neurologic degeneration, and cherry-red spots of the macula lutea. Associated bony defects include thickening of the calvaria, biconvex vertebral bodies, mild hypoplasia of the basilar part of the ilia, expansion and trabeculation of the ribs, and short tubular bones. High activity of ß-galactosidase and other lysosomal enzymes in the liver tissue is the chief biochemical feature of this syndrome. Pathological findings consist mainly of granulated and vacuolated storage cells in the bone marrow and myelin degeneration. The affected patients may survive into adulthood. The syndrome is transmitted as an autosomal recessive trait.

Spranger, J., *et al.* Lipomucopolysaccharidose. Eine neue Speicherkrankheit. *Zschr. Kinderheilk.*, 1968, 103:285-306.

mucolipidosis II (ML II). Synonyms: *Leroy syndrome, inclusion cell (I cell) disease.*

An inborn error of metabolism, originally described in a girl suspected of having the Hurler syndrome, characterized by unusual cytoplasmic inclusions in cultured fibroblasts (hence the synonyms **I-cell disease** and **inclusion-cell disease**). The syndrome is characterized mainly by Hurler-like facies (gargoylism), low birth weight, growth deficiency, narrow forehead, thin eyebrows, thick and puffy eyelids, inner epicanthic folds, mild corneal opacity, low nasal bridge, anteverted nostrils, long philtrum, and gingival hyperplasia. Early bone defects include mineralization disorders, excessive periosteal new bone formation, diaphyseal expansion of the long bones, short anteroposterior diameter of the vertebrae, anterosuperior hypoplasia of the upper lumbar vertebrae, and pelvic dysplasia, which progressively become more severe later in infancy. Elevated lysosomal hydrolases in body fluids and their partial deficiency in the fibroblasts (enzymes that are required for the catabolism of mucopolysaccharides, glycolipids, and glycoproteins, including α *L*-iduronidase, iduronate sulfatase, ß-glucuronidase, *N*-acetyl-ß-hexosaminidase, arylsulfatase A, ß-galactosidase, α-mannosidase, and ß-*L*-fucosidase) are the principal biochemical features of this syndrome. Death takes place in childhood and is due to heart failure and pneumonia. The syndrome is transmitted as an autosomal recessive trait.

Leroy, J. G., & DeMars, R. I. Mutant enzymatic and cytological phenotypes in cultured human fibroblasts. *Science*, 1967, 157:804-6. Leroy, J. G., *et al.* I-cell disease. A clinical picture. *J. Pediat.*, 1971, 79:360-5.

mucolipidosis III (ML III). Synonyms: *pseudo-Hurler syndrome, pseudopolydystrophy.*

An inborn error of metabolism with features similar to a mild form of the Hurler syndrome. Stiffness and limited mobility, especially in the hands, elbows, shoulders, and knees are the earliest symptoms, usually appearing at the age of 2 to 4 years of life. Associated anomalies include small stature, flat facies with coarse features (gargoyle facies), mild corneal opacity, mild mental retardation, heart defect (usually aortic valve disease with regurgitation), acne, inguinal hernia, and bony anomalies, including mild platyspondyly, wide oar-shaped ribs, skull defects, minor long bone defects, flaring iliac wings, flat femoral epiphyses, pelvic dysplasia, shallow acetabular bones, and coxa valga. The principal biochemical characteristics of this syndrome are elevated levels of lysosomal hydrolases in body fluids and their partial deficiency in the fibroblasts (enzymes that catabolize mucopolysaccharides, glycolipids, and glycoproteins, including α-*L*-iduronidase, iduronate sulfatase, ß-glucuronidase, *N*-acetyl-ß-hexosaminidase, arylsulfatase A, ß-galactosidase, α-mannosidase, and ß-*L*-fucosidase). Most affected patients survive into adulthood. The syndrome is transmitted as an autosomal recessive trait.

Maroteaux, P., & Lamy, M. La pseudo-polydystrophie de Hurler. *Presse Méd.*, 1966, 74:2889-92.

mucolipidosis IV (ML IV). A variant of mucolipidosis in which accumulation of ganglioside and polysaccharide substances occurs most frequently in children of Jewish (Ashkenazi) families. Corneal opacity is present from birth or early infancy. Psychomotor retardation usually does not appear until the end of the first year of life. Retinal degeneration occurs in older children. Conjunctival biopsy shows single-membrane-limited cytoplasmic vacuoles containing fibrillogranular material, membranous lamellae and lamellar and concentric bodies similar to those found in the Tay-Sachs syndrome. Increased levels of lysosomal enzymes are present in fibroblasts and leukocytes. The syndrome is transmitted as an autosomal recessive trait.

Merin, S., *et al.* Mucolipidosis IV: ocular, systemic, and ultrastructural findings. *Invest. Ophth. Vis. Sc.*, 1975, 14:437-48.

mucopolysaccharidosis (MPS). A group of inherited lysosomal storage diseases caused by a deficiency of enzymes involved in degradation of acid mucopolysaccharides (glycosaminoglycans or GAG) and marked by progressive physical and mental deterioration. The number and severity of symptoms vary with each specific form of the disorder, generally consisting of connective tissue thickening due to abnormal deposits of GAG and excessive deposition of pathological materials. A large head, hypertelorism, flat nasal bridge, snub nose, flared nostrils, large lips, prominent tongue, and small or peg-shaped teeth with malocclusion give the face a peculiar coarse appearance. Cardiac lesions may include deposits in the coronary arteries and thickening of the myocardium and cardiac valves. The cornea is usually clear at birth, but shortly thereafter it becomes cloudy with an accumulation of gray punctate opacities. Mental retardation becomes evident during the second year of life. Nasal discharge, noisy breathing, and respiratory infection are frequently associated. Lumbar gibbus, hepatosplenomegaly (due to deposits of GAG) with a prominent abdomen, multiple joint contractures, clawhand, furrowed thick skin, lanugo, extension of the hairline over the cheek, broad stubby fingers, and funnel chest may be present. Neurological complications may include peripheral nerve entrapment syndromes (including the carpal tunnel syndrome), thickening of the meninges that may lead to spinal cord compression, impaired hearing, and hydrocephalus. Changes in the bony skeleton are collectively known as **dysostosis multiplex**; they include: macrocephaly, dyscephaly, J-shaped cella turcica, thick calvaria, wide ribs, wide clavicles, thick scapulae, constricted iliac bodies, dysplasia of the femoral epiphyses, coxa valga, faulty diaphyseal modeling, submetaphyseal constriction, and shortening of the bones and vertebral abnormalities leading to short stature.

McKusick, V. A., Neufeld, E. F., & Kelly, T. E. The mucopolysaccharide storage diseases. In: Stanbury, J. B., Wyngaarden, J. B., & Fredrickson, D. S., eds. *The metabolic basis of inherited disease.* 4th ed. New York, MaGraw-Hill, 1978, pp. 1282-1307.

mucopolysaccharidosis I-H (MPS I-H). Synonyms: *Ellis-Sheldon syndrome, Hurler disease, Hurler syndrome, Johnie McL disease, Pfaundler-Hurler syndrome, Thompson syndrome, dysostotic idiocy, gargoylism, lipochondrodystrophy.*

A metabolic syndrome, transmitted as an autosomal recessive trait, and characterized by faulty degradation of dermatan and heparan sulfate with glycosaminoglycan storage in connective tissues due to α-*L*-iduronidase deficiency. Onset takes place in infants aged 6 to 12 months. Coarse (gargoylelike) facies, rhinorrhea, noisy respiration, corneal opacities, hepatosplenomegaly, cardiac abnormalities, dwarfism, dysostosis multiplex, and mental retardation are the principal symptoms. Most patients die by the age of 5 to 10 years. Johnie Mc L was the patient in whom the syndrome was observed.

Hurler, G. Über einen Typ multipler Abartung, vorwiegend am Skelettsystem. *Zschr. Kinderh.*, 1919, 24:220-34. Pfaundler, M. Demonstrationen über einen Typus kindlicher Dysostose. *Jhrb. Kinderh.*, 1920, 92:420-1. Ellis, R. W., Sheldon, W., & Capon, N. B. Gargoylism (chondro-osteo-dystrophy, corneal opacities, hepato-splenomegaly, and mental deficiency). *Q. J. Med.*, 1936, 5:119-39.

mucopolysaccharidosis I-H/S (MPS I-H/S). Synonyms: *compound Hurler-Scheie disease, Hurler-Scheie syndrome.*

A metabolic syndrome having the characteristics of mucopolysaccharidosis I-H but with a milder and slower progression. It is generally characterized by typical coarse (gargoylelike) facies, corneal opacity, dysostosis multiplex, moderate mental retardation, and dwarfism, most symptoms being half way between those of the Hurler and Scheie syndromes. α-*L*-iduronidase deficiency and faulty degradation of dermatan and heparan sulfate are the principal metabolic features. The affected persons are thought to represent compound heterozygotes inheriting one Hurler and one Scheie gene from each parent.

Hurler, G. Über einen Typ multipler Abartung, vorwiegend

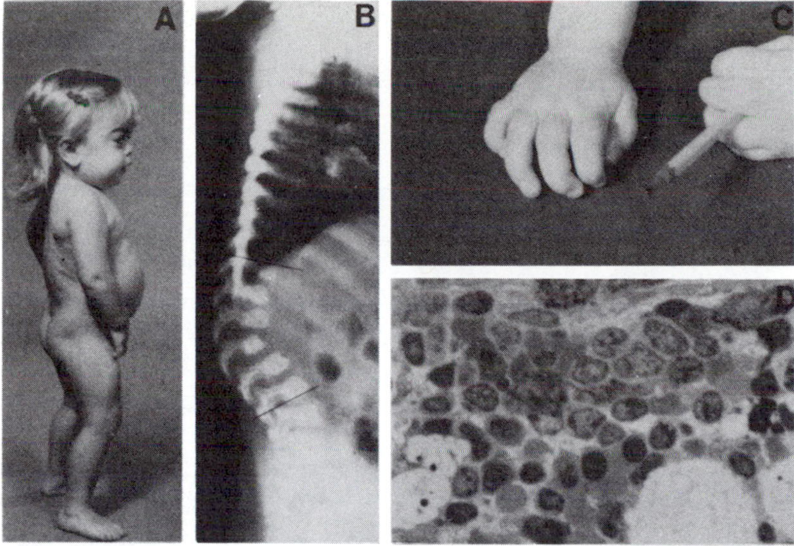

Mucopolysaccharidosis
Whitley, C.B., N.K.C. Ramsay, J.H. Kersey, W. Krivit: Bone Marrow Transplantation for Hurler syndrome: Assessment of Metabolic Correction. In Krivit, W., & N.W. Paul (eds.): *Bone Marrow Transplantation for Treatment of Lysosomal Storage Diseases.* New York: Alan R. Liss, Inc. for the March of Dimes Birth Defects Foundation BD:OAS 22(1):7-24, 1986, with permission.

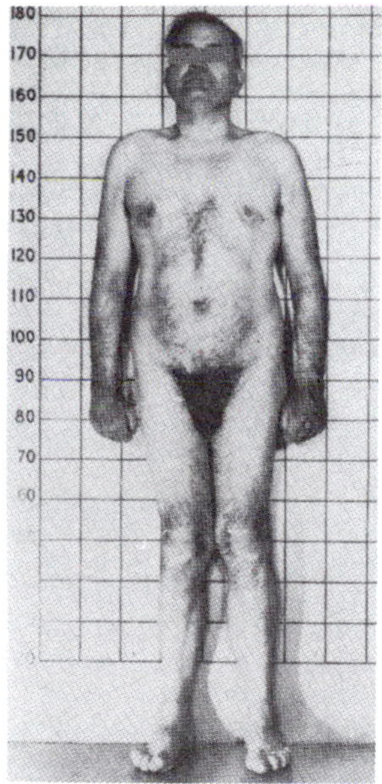

Mucopolysaccharidosis I-S (MPS I-S)
McKusick, V.A.: *Heritable Disorders of Connective Tissue.* St. Louis: C.V. Mosby Co., 1966.

am Skelettsystem. *Zschr. Kinderh.*, 1919, 24:220-34. Scheie, H. G., *et al.* A new recognized forme fruste of Hurler's disease (gargoylism). *Am. J. Ophth.*, 1962, 53:753-69.

mucopolysaccharidosis I-S (MPS I-S). Synonyms: *Scheie syndrome, Spät-Hurler syndrome, Ullrich-Scheie syndrome, forme fruste of Hurler syndrome. Formerly called mucopolysaccharidosis V (MPS V).*

A metabolic syndrome transmitted as an autosomal recessive trait and characterized by faulty degradation of dermatan and heparan sulfate with glycosaminoglycan storage in connective tissues due to α-L-iduronidase deficiency. Onset is at 5 to 15 years of age. Corneal opacity, coarse (gargoyle-like) facies, joint contractures, clawhand, genu valgum, aortic valve lesions, and dysostosis multiplex are the principal features. Normal height and intelligence and long survival distinguishes this disorder from other forms of mucopolysaccharidosis.

Scheie, H. G., *et al.* A new recognized forme fruste of Hurler's disease (gargoylism). Am. J. Ophth., 1962, 53:753-69. Ullrich, O. Die Pfaundler-Hurlersche Krankheit. Erg. Inn. Med. Kinderh., 1943, 63:929-1000. Rampini, R. Der Spät-Hurler (Ullrich-Scheie Syndrom, Mucopolysaccharidose V). Schweiz. Med. Wschr., 1969, 99: 1769-78.

mucopolysaccharidosis II (MPS II). Synonym: *Hunter syndrome.*

A metabolic syndrome transmitted as an X-linked trait affecting only males, which is characterized by faulty dermatan and heparan sulfate degradation with abnormal accumulation of glycosaminoglycan in various cells, including leukocytes, bone marrow, and fibroblasts, due to *L*-sulfoiduronate sulfatase deficiency. The syndrome differs from other forms of MPS by lacking corneal opacity. The severe form is marked by onset at 2 to 4 years, the presence of most symptoms of mucopolysaccharidosis, and death by the age of 10 to 15 years. The symptoms, even in the severe form, are usually milder than those in MPS I-H, except for deafness which is more severe. The mild form is marked by onset in the first decade of life, short stature, joint contractures, dysostosis multiplex, splenomegaly, peripheral nerve entrapment and near-normal intelligence. Life expectancy is about 30 to 60 years, depending on the degree of severity of cardiac lesions.

Hunter, C. A. A rare disease in two brothers. *Proc. Roy. Soc. Med., London*, 1917, 10:104-16.

mucopolysaccharidosis III (MPS III). Synonyms: *Sanfil-*

ippo syndrome, heparitinuria, polydystrophic oligophrenia.

A metabolic syndrome, transmitted as an autosomal recessive trait, characterized by faulty degradation of heparan sulfate and storage of glycosaminoglycan in tissues. Deficiency of heparan sulfate sulfamidase occurs in **MPS III-A**; *N*-acetyl-α-*D*-glucosaminidase in **MPS III-B**; acetyl CoA: α-glucosamide-*N*-acetyltranferase in **MPS III-C**; and *N*-acetyl-α-*D*-glucosaminide-6-sulfatase in **MPS III-D**. Early normal development is usually followed by onset at the age of 2 to 6 years, which includes mental deterioration, hyperactivity and aggressiveness, unsteady gait, muscle atrophy, abundant coarse hair, coarse facies, and dysostosis multiplex, the patient eventually becoming bedridden. Corneal opacity is usually absent, hepatosplenomegaly is mild or absent, and cardiac lesions are rare. Death usually takes place by the time of puberty.

Sanfilippo, S. J., *et al*. Mental retardation associated with mucopolysacchariduria (heparin sulfate type). *J. Pediat.*, 1963, 63:873-8.

mucopolysaccharidosis IV-A (MPS IV-A). Synonyms: *Morquio syndrome, Morquio-Brailsford syndrome, Morquio-Ullrich syndrome, atypical chondrodystrophy, chondrodystrophia tarda, chondro-osteodystrophy, dysostosis enchondralis metaepiphysaria, eccentrochondrodysplasia, eccentro-osteochondrodysplasia, familial osseous dystrophy, hereditary chondrodysplasia, hereditary osteochondrodystrophy, hereditary polytopic enchondral dysostosis, keratosulfaturia, KS mucopolysaccharidosis, osteochondrodystrophia deformans, osteochondrodystrophy, spondylo-epiphyseal dysplasia.*

An inborn error of metabolism, transmitted as an autosomal recessive trait, and marked by faulty degradation of keratan sulfate and chondroitin sulfate, with deposits in tissues of glycosaminoglycans due to *N*-acetylgalactosamine-6-sulfatase deficiency. The syndrome combines peculiar facies, short spine, dwarfism, and skeletal abnormalities. Midface hypoplasia, depressed nasal bridge, flared nostrils, wide mouth, protrusion of the jaws, widely spaced teeth, and enamel hypoplasia are the principal orofacial symptoms. Short-spine dwarfism is followed at the time when the infant begins to walk by vertebra plana, spinal cord compression, instability of short neck, platybasia, enlarged wrists, disproportionately long arms, enlarged knees, genu valgum, flat feet, waddling gait, flaccid muscles, pigeon breast, and prominent abdomen. Fine corneal opacity and impaired hearing are usually associated. Intelligence is usually normal. Death generally takes place in the twenties due to aortic valve diseases.

Morquio, L. Sur une forme de dystrophie osseuse familiale. *Arch. Méd. Enf., Paris*, 1929, 32:129-40. Brailsford, J. F. Chondro-osteo-dystrophy. Roentgenographic & clinical features of a child with dislocation of vertebrae. *Am. J. Surg.*, 1929, 7:404-10. Ullrich, O. Die Pfaundler-Hurlersche Krankheit. Dysostosis multiplex (Hurler)-Dysostotische Idiotie (Hässler)-Familiär-dysostotischer Zwergwuchs; Typ-Pfaundler-Hurler (De Rudder)-Gargoylismus (Ellis-Sheldon und Capon). Ein Beitrag zum Problem pleiotroper Gerwirkung in der Erbpathologie des Menschen. *Erg. Inn. Med. Kinderh.*, 1943, 63:929-1000.

mucopolysaccharidosis IV-B (MPS IV-B). Synonyms: *Morquio B syndrome, Morquio-like syndrome.*

A form of mucopolysaccharidosis with faulty break-

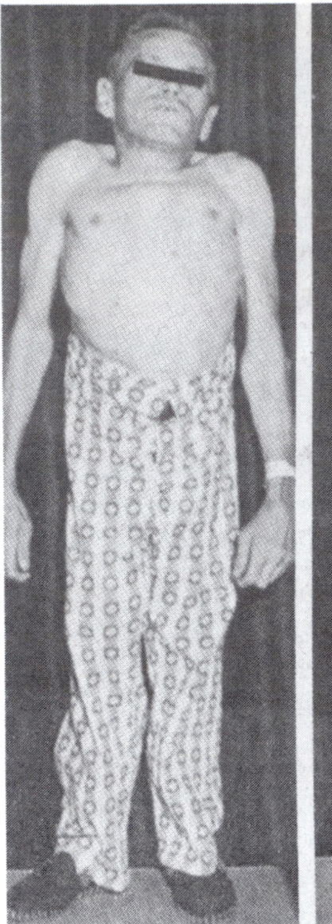
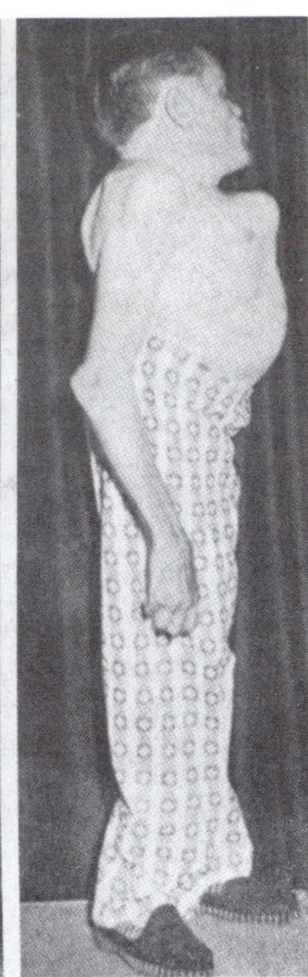

Mucopolysaccharidosis IV-A (MPS IV-A)
Randall, Dr. T.A. From E. Aegerter & J.A. Kirkpatrick, Jr.: *Orthopedic Diseases* 3rd Ed. Philadelphia: W.B. Saunders Co., 1968.

down of keratan sulfate due to ß-galactosidase deficiency. It is marked by short stature, mild pectus carinatum, corneal opacity, odontoid hypoplasia, cervical instability, mild dysostosis multiplex, moderate kyphosis, and mild genu valgum.

Wyngaarden, J. B., & Smith, L. H., Jr., eds. *Cecil textbook of medicine*. 17th ed. Philadelphia, Saunders. 1985, p. 1148. Groebe, H., *et al*. Morquio syndrome (mucopolysaccharidosis IV B) associated with beta-galactosidase deficiency. Report ot two cases. *Am. J. Hum. Genet.*, 1980, 32:258-72.

mucopolysaccharidosis V (MPS V). See *mucopolysaccharidosis I-S.*

mucopolysaccharidosis VI (MPS VI). Synonyms: *Maroteaux-Lamy syndrome, polydystrophic dwarfism.*

A syndrome transmitted as an autosomal recessive trait and marked by faulty degradation of dermatan sulfate with coarse leukocytic granulations and deposits of glycosaminoglycans in tissues due to *N*-acetylgalactosamine-4-sulfatase deficiency. In the severe form, onset at the age of 2 to 4 years is followed by growth retardation, joint contractures, corneal opacity, aortic valve lesions, hip deformity, large head, dysostosis multiplex, and death by the age of 20 years. In the mild form, onset takes place at the age of 5 to 7 years and is followed by growth retardation, dysostosis multiplex, corneal opacities, aortic valve lesions, peripheral nerve entrapment, and longer life expectancy. The intelligence is normal in both types.

Maroteaux, P., & Lamy, M. Hurler's disease, Morquio's disease, and related mucopolysaccharidoses. *J. Pediat.*, 1965, 67:312-23.

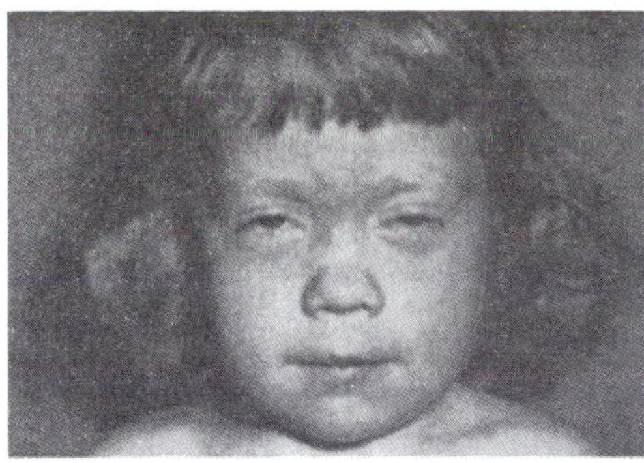

Mucopolysaccharidosis VI (MPS VI)
McKusick, V.A.: *Heritable Disorders of Connective Tissue.* 3rd ed. St. Louis: C.V. Mosby Co., 1966.

mucopolysaccharidosis VII (MPS VII). Synonym: *Sly syndrome.*

A form of mucopolysaccharidosis marked by faulty degradation of heparan, dermatan, and chondroitin sulfate and by leukocytic inclusions caused by ß-glucuronidase deficiency. The onset of symptoms, occurring at the age of 2 years, is followed by dwarfism dysostosis multiplex, pectus carinatum, splenomegaly, heart murmurs, mental retardation, hernias, and respiratory infections. Corneal opacity may be associated.

Sly, W. S. The mucopolysaccharidoses. In: Bondy, P. K., & Rosenberg, L. E., eds. *Metabolic control and disease.* Philadelphia, Saunders, 1980, pp. 545-81. Wyngaarden, J. B., & Smith, L. H., Jr., eds. *Cecil textbook of medicine.* 17th ed. Philadelphia, Saunders, 1985, pp. 1148.

mucosal neuromas syndrome. Synonyms: *Gorlin-Vickers syndrome, Williams-Pollock syndrome, MMN-pheochromocytoma syndrome, multiple mucosal neuroma (MMN) syndrome.*

Multiple endocrine adenomatosis (see under *multiple endocrine neoplasia syndrome*) inherited as an autosomal dominant trait. The syndrome is characterized by multiple mucosal neuromas, primarily involving the lips, anterior tongue, conjunctiva, and nasal and laryngeal mucosa; pheochromocytoma; and medullary carcinoma of the thyroid gland. A marfanoid build and diverticulosis may be associated. Pes cavus, prognathism, and marfanoid appearance of the hand are the principal x-ray findings.

Williams, E. D., & Pollock, D. J. Multiple mucosal neuromata with endocrine tumours: A syndrome allied to von Recklinghausen's disease. *J. Path. Bact.,* 1966, 91:71-80. Gorlin, R. J., Sedano, H. O., Vickers, R. A., & Cervenka, J. Multiple mucosal neuromas, pheochromocytoma and medullary carcinoma of the thyroid: A syndrome. *Cancer,* 1968, 22:293- 9.

mucosal respiratory syndrome. See *Stevens-Johnson syndrome.*

mucoserous dyssecretosis. See *Sjögren syndrome under Sjögren, Henrik Samuel Conrad.*

mucositis necroticans agranulocytica. See *Schultz syndrome.*

mucosulfatidosis. See *metachromatic leukodystrophy.*

mucosynechial dermatitis. See *Lortat-Jacob disease.*

mucous colitis. See *irritable bowel syndrome.*

MUELLER, WALTHER. See MÜLLER, WALTER

MUENCHHAUSEN, BARON, VON. See MUNCHAUSEN, BARON, VON

MUENCHMEYER, ERNST. See MÜNCHMEYER, ERNST

MUIR, E. G. (British physician)

Muir syndrome. See *Muir-Torre syndrome.*

Muir-Torre (MT) syndrome. Synonyms: *Muir syndrome, Torre syndrome, multiple sebaceous neoplasms-visceral carcinoma syndrome.*

An association of sebaceous skin tumors, with or without keratoacanthoma, with visceral malignancies. The skin tumors comprise sebaceous hyperplasia, epitheliomas, and carcinomas, sometimes occurring in various combinations in the same person. Visceral tumors consist mainly of basal and squamous-cell carcinomas occurring with polyps and adenocarcinomas, mainly of the large bowel, small intestine, stomach, and larynx. The syndrome is believed to be transmitted as an autosomal dominant trait with high penetrance and variable expressivity.

Muir, E. G., *et al.* Multiple primary carcinomata of the colon, duodenum, and larynx associated with keratoacanthomata of the face. *Brit, J. Surg.,* 1967, 54:191-5. Torre, D. Multiple sebaceous tumors. *Arch. Derm.,* 1968, 98:549-51.

MULIBREY, mulibrey (muscle-liver-brain-eye) nanism. Synonym: *Perheentupa syndrome.*

A rare syndrome, transmitted as an autosomal recessive trait, characterized by nanism with thin and short limbs and developmental anomalies of the muscles, liver, brain, and eyes. Hypotonia and hepatomegaly are the principal muscular and hepatic components. Cerebral disorders consist of mental retardation and large cerebral ventricles and cisternae. Ocular changes include mild hypertelorism, aggregation and dispersion of pigment in the fundus and characteristic yellowish dots, and hypoplasia of the choroid. Associated craniofacial defects consist mainly of a triangular face with a bulging forehead, low and broad nasal bridge, a mildly hydrocephalic appearance, and prominent veins on the forehead and neck. The voice has a peculiar high-pitched quality. Cardiovascular complications consist of pericardial constriction due to a thickened and adherent pericardium, high venous pressure, cardiomegaly, dilated veins of the neck, and, in some instances, congestive heart failure. The sella turcica is long and shallow. The frontal and sphenoidal sinuses are aplastic or hypoplastic. Some patients exhibit also fibrous dysplasia of the tibia, dental malocclusion, and microglossia.

Perheentupa, J., *et al.* Mulibrey nanism, an autosomal recessive syndrome with pericardial constriction. *Lancet,* 1973, 2:351-5.

MÜLLER, CARL ARNOLDUS (Norwegian physician, born 1886)

Harbitz-Müller disease. See *under Harbitz.*

MULLER, JANS (American physician)

Christian-Andrews-Conneally-Muller syndrome. See *Christian syndrome (1), under Christian, Joe C.*

MÜLLER, WALTHER (German physician, born 1888)

Müller-Ribbing-Clément syndrome. See *multiple epiphyseal dysplasia I.*

Müller-Weiss syndrome. Symmetrical malacia of the os naviculare pedis.

Müller, W. Über eine eigenartige doppelseitige Veränderung des Os naviculare pedis beim Erwachsenen. *Deut. Zschr. Chir.,* 1927, 201:84-7. Weiss, K. Über die

"Malazie" des Os naviculare pedis. *Fortschr. Röntgen.*, 1927, 40:63-7.

Ribbing-Müller syndrome. See *multiple epiphyseal dysplasia I.*

müllerian dysgenesis syndrome. See *Mayer-Rokitansky-Küster syndrome.*

multicentric osteolysis with nephropathy. See *Thieffry-Shurtleff syndrome.*

multicystic kidney. See *Potter syndrome (2), under Potter, Edith Louise.*

multiple basal-cell carcinoma syndrome. See *nevoid basal-cell carcinoma syndrome.*

multiple benign cystic epithelioma. See *Brooke epithelioma.*

multiple benign epithelioma of the scalp. See *Brooke epithelioma.*

multiple benign superficial epithelioma. See *Arning carcinoid.*

multiple cancellous exostoses. See *multiple cartilaginous exostoses syndrome.*

multiple cartilaginous exostoses (MCE) syndrome. Synonyms: *Ehrenfried disease, cancellous exostoses, chondral dysplasia, diaphyseal aclasis, exostosis cartilaginea multiplex, exostotic dysplasia, exostosis multiplex cartilaginea, external chondromatosis syndrome, hereditary deforming chondrodysplasia, hereditary multiple exostoses, multiple cancellous exostoses, multiple cartilaginous exostoses, multiple congenital osteochondromata, multiple exostoses syndrome, multiple osteochondromatosis, multiple osteogenic exostosis, ossified diathesis.*

Bone dysplasia characterized chiefly by exostoses extending from relatively normal diaphyses and irregular expansion of the metaphyses with excrescences projecting from the sides. The principal clinical features consist of multiple bony, sometimes painful, protuberances at the ends of tubular bones, ribs, vertebrae, and iliac crests. Secondary defects include shortening and bowing of the tubular bones, limited joint movement, and ulnar deviation of the hands. Short stature is a variable feature. Major radiographic features include radicular synostoses, tibiofibular synostoses, shortening of the fibula, valgus deformity of the ankle and knee, multiple exotoses of the flat bones, and, less commonly, exostoses of the vertebrae. Onset of symptoms takes place during the first decade of life. The syndrome is transmitted as an autosomal dominant trait with complete penetrance in males and slightly reduced penetrance in females.

Virchow, R. Über multiple Exostosen. *Berl. Klin. Wschr.*, 1891, 82:1082. Krooth, R. S., *et al.* Diaphyseal aclasis (multiple exostoses) on Guam. *Am. J. Hum. Genet.*, 1961, 13:340-7. Solomon, L. Hereditary multiple exostosis. *J. Bone Joint Surg.*, 1963, 45B:292-304. Ehrenfried, A. Multiple cartilaginous exostoses-hereditary deforming chondrodysplasia. A brief report on a little known disease. *JAMA*, 1915, 64:1642-6.

multiple congenital articular rigidity. See *arthrogryposis multiplex congentia syndrome.*

multiple congenital contractures. See *arthrogryposis multiplex congenita syndrome.*

multiple congenital dislocation syndrome. See *Larsen syndrome, under Larsen, Loren Joseph.*

multiple congenital osteochondromata. See *multiple cartilaginous exostoses syndrome.*

multiple cutaneous carcinoid. See *Arning carcinoid.*

multiple enchondromata syndrome. See *Ollier syndrome.*

multiple enchondromatosis. See *Ollier syndrome.*

multiple endocrine adenomas. See *multiple endocrine neoplasia syndrome.*

multiple endocrine adenomatosis (MEA). See *multiple endocrine neoplasia syndrome.*

multiple endocrine adenomatosis I (MEA I). See *multiple endocrine neoplasia I.*

multiple endocrine adenopathy (MEA). See *multiple endocrine neoplasia syndrome.*

multiple endocrine neoplasia (MEN) syndrome. Synonyms: *multiple endocrine adenomas, multiple endocrine adenomatosis (MEA), multiple endocrine adenopathy (MEA), multiple endocrine syndrome (MES).*

A neoplastic syndrome, transmitted as an autosomal dominant trait with complete penetrance and variable expressivity, characterized by the presence of hyperplastic or neoplastic lesions in multiple endocrine systems.

Delellis, R. A., & Wolfe, H. J. Multiple endocrine adenomatosis syndromes. In: Holland, J, F., & Frei, E., III. eds. *Cancer medicine.* 2nd ed, Philadelphia, Lea & Febiger, 1982, pp. 1648-57.

multiple endocrine neoplasia I (MEN I) syndrome. Synonyms: *Wermer syndrome, endocrine adenoma-peptic ulcer syndrome, MEA (multiple endocrine adenomatosis)-ulcer syndrome, multiple endocrine adenomatosis I (MEA I).*

A neoplastic disease, transmitted as an autosomal dominant trait with complete penetrance and variable expressivity, characterized by tumors or hyperplasia of the parathyroid and pituitary glands and the islands of Langerhans with increased incidence of adrenocortical and thyroid disease, the parathyroid gland being most severely affected. Other tumors, including bronchial, gastrointestinal, and mediastinal carcinoids, multiple soft tissue lipomas, and renal cortical neoplasms, are frequently associated. Peptic ulcer with gastric hypersecretion is a common feature of this syndrome. Chromophobic tumors, eosinophilic adenomas with acromegaly, and prolactin-secreting tumor may also occur.

Wermer, P. Genetic aspects of adenomatosis of endocrine glands. *Am. J. Med.*, 1954, 16:363-71.

multiple endocrine neoplasia II (MEN II) syndrome. Synonyms: *Sipple syndrome, medullary thyroid carcinoma-pheochromocytoma syndrome, multiple endocrine neoplasia IIa (MEN IIa) syndrome.*

A neoplastic disease, transmitted as an autosomal dominant trait with complete penetrance and variable expressivity, characterized by a triad of medullary thyroid carcinoma (MTC), pheochromocytoma, and parathyroid hyperplasia or adenoma, in association with elevated calcitonin and catecholamine levels. Other neoplasms found in this syndrome may include glioblastomas and meningiomas.

Sipple, J. H. The association of pheochromocytoma with carcinoma of the thyroid gland. *Am. J. Med.*, 1961, 31:163-6.

multiple endocrine neoplasia IIa (MEN IIa) syndrome. See *multiple endocrine neoplasia II syndrome.*

multiple endocrine neoplasia IIb (MEN IIb) syndrome. See *multiple endocrine neoplasia syndrome III.*

multiple endocrine neoplasia III (MEN III) syndrome. Synonym: *multiple endocrine neoplasia IIb (MEN IIb) syndrome.*

A neoplastic disease, transmitted as an autosomal dominant trait with complete penetrance and variable expressivity, characterized by medullary thyroid carcinoma, pheochromocytoma, mucosal neuromas, and marfanoid habitus. Mucosal neuromas, occurring most often on the lips, are usually present at birth. Additional findings may include hypertrophied corneal nerves and neuromas, neuromatous involvement of the eyelids and conjunctiva, and diffuse gastrointestinal ganglioneurosis, diverticulosis, and megacolon.

Delellis, R. A., & Wolfe, H. J. Multiple endocrine adenomatosis syndromes. In: Holland, J. F., & Frei, E., III., eds. *Cancer medicine.* 2nd ed. Philadelphia, Lea & Febiger, 1982, pp. 1648-57. *Schimke, R. N., *et al.* Syndrome of bilateral pheochromocytoma, medullary thyroid carcinoma and multiple neuromas. *N. Engl. J. Med.,* 1968, 279:1.

multiple endocrine syndrome (MES). See *multiple endocrine neoplasia syndrome.*

multiple epiphyseal dysplasia I (MED I). Synonyms: *Fairbank syndrome, Müller-Ribbing-Clément syndrome, Ribbing disease, Ribbing-Müller disease, dysostosis enchondralis epiphysaria, dysostosis enchondralis polyepiphysaria, dysostosis epiphysealis multiplex, dysplasia epiphysealis multiplex, dystrophia osteochondralis polyepiphysaria, epiphyseal dysplasia, hereditary epiphyseal dysplasia, multiple epiphyseal dysplasia tarda.*

Dysplasia of the epiphyses that results in shortness of stature, and is transmitted as an autosomal dominant trait with complete penetrance and variable expression. Its principal symptoms usually include prominent and painful joints with limited mobility, waddling gait, moderate dwarfism with normal body proportions, thoracic kyphosis, and back pain. The early signs of dysplasia, usually noted after the second year of life, are followed by irregularities of the articular surfaces of the hips, knees, wrists, and hands. Flattening of the vertebral bodies, delayed maturation of the carpal bones, brachydactyly, and other osseous changes may be associated. According to some authors, the term **multiple epiphyseal dysplasia** refers to a single entity; according to others, it includes a group of conditions marked by epiphyseal dysplasia; many restrict the term to the **Conradi-Hünermann syndrome**; and still others differentiate the mild (Ribbing) form, with flat epiphyses and mild involvement of the hands bones, from the severe (Fairbank) form, with small epiphyses, late ossification of irregular carpal bones, and changes of the metacarpal bones and phalanges.

Ribbing, S. Studien über hereditäre, multiple Epiphysenstörungen. *Acta Radiol. Helsingfors,* 1937, Suppl. 34:1-105. Fairbank, T. *An atlas of general affections of the skeleton.* Edinburgh, E. S. Livingstone, 1951, pp. 91-105. *Müller, W. Das Bild der multiplen erblichen Störung der Epiphysenverknocherung. *Zschr. Orthop.,* 1939, 69:257. Fairbank, T. Dysplasia epiphysialis multiplex. *Brit. J. Surg.,* 1947, 34:225-32.

multiple epiphyseal dysplasia II (MED II). See *Conradi-Hünermann syndrome, under Conradi, Erich.*

multiple epiphyseal dysplasia tarda. See *multiple epiphyseal dysplasia I.*

multiple epiphyseal dysplasia with early-onset diabetes mellitus syndrome. See *Wolcott-Rallison syndrome.*

multiple evanescent white dot syndrome. Synonym: *white dot syndrome.*

An eye disease, usually occurring in young persons, characterized by the acute onset of unilateral blindness. Ophthalmoscopic findings consist primarily of small discrete white dots that appear unilaterally at the level of the retinal pigment epithelium or deep retina and a granularity of the fovea. Other clinical signs may include the presence of vitreal cells, retinal vascular sheathing, optic edema, and fluorescein leakage from disk capillaries and late staining of the retinal pigment epithelium. These changes gradually regress for several weeks, and vision returns to normal. Abnormal electroretinographic findings, early receptor potentials, and visual pigment regeneration during the acute phase are followed by almost complete recovery.

Jampol, L. M., *et al.* Multiple evanescent white dot syndrome. Clinical findings. *Arch. Ophth., Chicago,* 1984, 102:671-4. Sieving, P. A., *et al.* Multiple evanescent white dot syndrome. II. Electrophysiology of the the photoreceptors during retinal pigment epithelial disease. *Arch. Ophth., Chicago,* 1984, 102:675-9.

multiple exostoses syndrome. See *multiple cartilaginous exostoses syndrome.*

multiple exostoses-mental retardation (MEMR) syndrome. See *Langer-Giedion syndrome.*

multiple glomerular embolization. See *Löhlein nephritis.*

multiple hamartoma and neoplasia syndrome. See *Cowden syndrome.*

multiple hamartoma syndrome. See *Cowden syndrome.*

multiple hereditary cutaneomandibular polyoncosis. See *nevoid basal-cell carcinoma syndrome.*

multiple hereditary telangiectases with recurrent hemorhage. See *Osler-Rendu-Weber syndrome.*

multiple idiopathic hemorrhagic sarcoma. See *Kaposi sarcoma.*

multiple lentigines syndrome. See *LEOPARD syndrome.*

multiple mucosal neuroma (MMN) syndrome. See *mucosal neuromas syndrome.*

multiple myeloma. See *Kahler disease.*

multiple neurofibromatosis. See *Recklinghausen disease (1).*

multiple nevoid basal-cell carcinoma syndrome (MNBCCS). See *nevoid basal-cell carcinoma syndrome.*

multiple nevoid basal-cell epithelioma-jaw cysts-bifid rib syndrome. See *nevoid basal-cell carcinoma syndrome.*

multiple osteochondromatosis. See *multiple cartilaginous exostoses syndrome.*

multiple osteogenic exostosis. See *multiple cartilaginous exostoses syndrome.*

multiple pterygium syndrome. Synonyms: *Escobar syndrome, familial pterygium syndrome, pterygium syndrome.*

A rare syndrome of short stature, craniofacial anomalies, joint contractures, vertebral fusion anomalies, rocker-bottom feet, and pterygia of the neck, antecubital, digital, popliteal, and intercural areas. Abnormalities of the head usually consist of epicanthal microcephaly, skin folds, long philtrum, antimongoloid palpebral slant, low-set ears, pointed and receding chin, ptosis, down-turned angles of the mouth, cleft lip and palate, and hemangiomas of the forehead. Associated anomalies may include rib defects, scoliosis or lordosis, vertical talus, cryptorchism, hypoplastic labia majora, and mental retardation. Most cases are transmitted as an autosomal recessive trait, some as a dominant trait, and a few are sporadic. See also *lethal multiple pterygium syndrome*, *Bonnevie-Ullrich syndrome*, *arthrogryposis multiplex congenita*, and *popliteal pterygium syndrome*.

Frawley, J. M. Congenital webbing, *Am. J. Dis. Child.*, 1925, 29:799-805. Frias, J. L. *et al.* An autosomal dominant syndrome of multiple pterygium, ptosis, and skeletal abnormalities. *Fourth International Conference on Birth Defects*. Amsterdam, Excerpta Medica, 19. Aarskog. D. Pterygium syndrome. *Birth Defects*, 1971, 7(6):232-4. Escobar, V., *et al.* Multiple pterygium syndrome. *Am. J. Dis. Child.*, 1978, 132:609-11. Scott, C. P. Pterygium syndrome. *Birth Defects*, 1969, 5(2):231-2. Stoll, C., *et al.* Familial pterygium syndrome. *Clin. Genet.*, 1980, 18:317-20.

multiple scleromalacia. See *Paget disease*.

multiple sebaceous neoplasms-visceral carcinoma syndrome. See *Muir-Torre syndrome*.

multiple self-healing squamous carcinoma (MSHSC). See *Ferguson Smith epithelioma, under Smith, John Ferguson*.

multiple spontaneous idiopathic symmetrical pseudofractures. See *Milkman syndrome*.

multiple symmetrical lipomatosis. See *Madelung syndrome*.

multiple synostoses syndrome. Synonyms: *acrocephalo-synankie, polysynostoses syndrome, synostosis multiplex*.

A syndrome of multiple synostoses of various bones and cranial sutures, transmitted as an autosomal dominant trait. Associated defects include hearing disorders, short stature, failure to thrive, mental retardation, and peculiar facies marked by a low frontal hairline, high nasal root with a beaked tip, alar hypoplasia, short philtrum, thin upper lip, and microstomia. Proximal symphalangism is associated with a fusion of other bones, mainly the carpal and tarsal bones. X-ray findings include brachydactyly, absence of distal or middle phalanges with shortening of the fingers of the hands, and dysplastic nails. Cloverleaf skull occurs in some cases.

Maroteaux, P., *et al.* La maladie des synostoses multiples. *Nouv. Presse Méd.*, 1972, 1:3041-7.

multiple synostoses-brachydactyly syndrome. See *facio-audio-symphalangism syndrome*.

multiple synostoses-conductive deafness syndrome. See *symphalangism syndrome*.

multisynostotic osteodysgenesis with fractures. See *Antley-Bixler syndrome*.

multisynostotic osteodysgenesis with long bone fractures. See *Antley-Bixler syndrome*.

MUNCH-PETERSEN, CARL J. (Danish physician, born 1896)

Munch-Petersen encephalomyelitis. See *Redlich encephalitis*.

MUNCHAUSEN, BARON, VON. A teller of exaggerated stories in Raspe's (1737-1794) book, *The Adventures of Baron Munchausen*, based on stories of Baron Karl Friedrich Hieronymus Von Münchhausen, a German soldier and raconteur, whose name was changed in the book by dropping one "h" and an umlaut.

Muenchhausen syndrome. See *Munchausen syndrome*.

Munchausen syndrome (MS). Synonyms: *Ahasuerus syndrome, Muenchhausen syndrome, Münchhausen syndrome, van Gogh syndrome, artifactual illness, chronic factitious disease, chronic factitious disorder with physical symptoms, factitious disease, factitious syndrome, hospital addiction, hospital hobo, hospital vagrant, laparotomophilia migrans, munchausenism,*

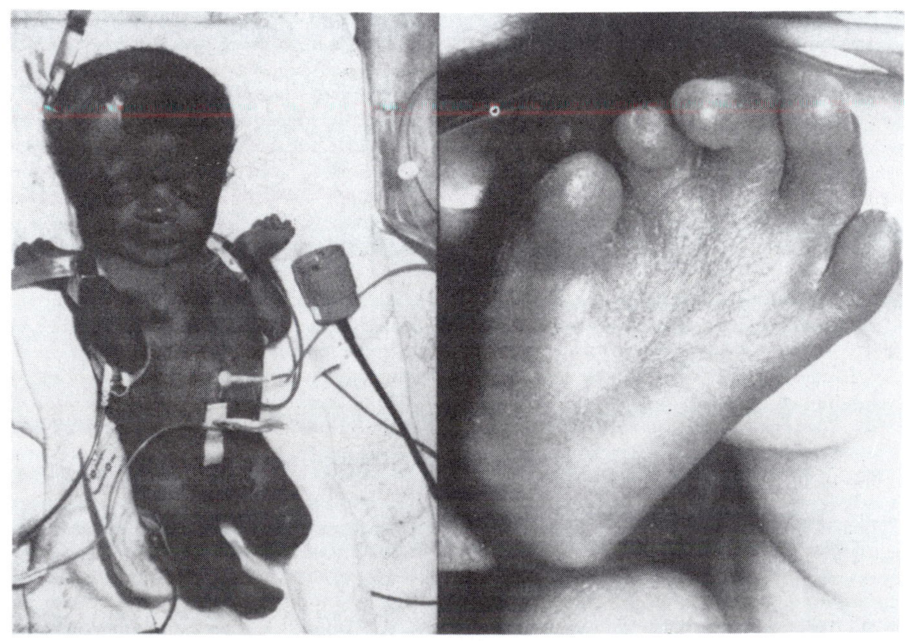

Multiple pterygium syndrome
Robinson, L.K., N.C. O'Brien, M.C. Puckett & M.A. Cox: *Clinical Genetics* 32: 5-9, 1987. Munksgaard International Publishers, Copenhagen, Denmark.

pathomimia, perigrinating problem patient, polysurgical addiction, professional patient, scalpellophilia, SHAFT (sad, hostile, anxious, tenacious) syndrome, surgical mania, tomomania syndrome, toxicomania chirurgica.

A factitious disorder whereby the affected persons wander from hospital to hospital and give dramatic and frequently inconsistent accounts of imaginary severe illnesses. Once admitted to a hospital, they usually create havoc by demanding special attention and quarreling violently with the doctor and nurses and, occasionally, to prove a point, attempt self-mutilation. Physical examination may reveal numerous laparotomy scars, cranial burr holes, or other evidence of previous operations. Substance abuse, particularly of analgesics and sedatives, often medically prescribed, may be the reason for attempts to be hospitalized. Eventually, patients will discharge themselves against advice. Their history may show a long record of previous hospitalizations.

Asher, R. Munchausen's syndrome. *Lancet*, 1951, 1:339-41. Wingate, P. Munchausen's syndrome. *Lancet*, 1951, 1:412-3. Chapman, J. S. Perigrinating problem patients: Munchausen's syndrome. *JAMA*, 1957, 165:927-33. Abram, H. S. The van Gogh syndrome: An unusual case of polysurgical addiction. *Am. J. Psychiat.*, 1966, 123:478-81. Menninger, K. A. Polysurgery and polysurgical addiction. *Psychoanal. Quart.*, 1934, 3:173-99. Rodin, A. E., & Key, J. D. *Encyclopedia of medical eponyms derived from literary characters*. Melbourne, Fl., Krieger, 1988. *Diagnostic and statistical manual of mental disorders*, 3rd. ed. American Psychiatric Association, Washington, D. C., 1980, pp. 288-90.

Munchausen syndrome by proxy (MSBP, MSP). Synonyms: *Meadow syndrome, Munchausen by proxy syndrome (MBPS), Polle syndrome.*

A situation in which one person persistently fabricates symptoms for another, usually a mother inventing symptoms and fabricating signs in relation to her child, and thus causing the child painful and unnecessary physical examinations and treatments. Some children suffer from apnea induced by a parent (**Munchausen syndrome by proxy and apnea** or **MBPA**). The condition was named after Polle, the son of Baron Hieronymus Karl Friedrich von Münchhausen and his second wife, Bernhardine Brun, who was born in 1795 and died 1 year later. The syndrome is considered to be a form of the battered child syndrome (q.v.).

Meadow, R. Munchausen syndrome by proxy: The hinterland of child abuse. *Lancet*, 1977, 2:343-5. Burman, D., & Stevens, D. Munchausen family. *Lancet*, 1977, 2:456.

Münchhausen syndrome. See *Munchausen syndrome.*

munchausenism. See *Munchausen syndrome.*

MÜNCHHAUSEN, BARON VON. See MUNCHAUSEN, BARON VON

MÜNCHMEYER, ERNST (German physician, 1846-1880)

Muenchmeyer syndrome. See *fibrodysplasia ossificans progressiva.*

Münchmeyer syndrome. See *fibrodysplasia ossificans progressiva.*

MUNK, FRITZ (German physician, born 1879)

Munk disease. Synonyms: *epithelial cell disease, lipoid nephrosis, minimal cell disease, minimal change nephropathy.*

A kidney disease characterized by changes in basement membrane permeability to plasma proteins and occurring most commonly in children. The symptoms are similar to those in the nephrotic syndrome (q.v.) but, in some instances, proteinuria may be the only presenting manifestation. The condition may occur alone or in association with Hodgkin disease and other neoplastic diseases in which T-cell function is altered.

Munk, F. Klinische Diagnostik der degenerativen Nierenerkrankungen. *Zschr. Klin. Med.*, 1913, 78:1-52.

MUNRO, T. A. (New Zealand physician)

Latham-Munro syndrome. See *under Latham.*

MÜNZER, FRANZ THEODOR (German neurologist)

Münzer-Rosenthal syndrome. A combination of hallucinations, anxiety, and catalepsy.

Münzer, F. T. Zur Frage der symptomatischen Narkolepsie nach Enzephalitis lethargica. *Mschr. Psychiat. Neurol.*, 1927, 63:97-111. Rosenthal, C. Über das Auftreten von halluzinatorisch-kataleptischen Angstsyndrom Wachanfällen und ählichen Störungen bei Schizophrenen. *Mschr. Psychiat. Neurol.*, 1939-40, 102:11-38.

murderer's thumb. See *brachydactyly D.*

MURK JANSEN. See JANSEN, MURK

MURRAY, JOHN (British physician)

Murray syndrome. Synonyms: *Murray-Puretic-Drescher syndrome, fibromatosis hyalinica multiplex juvenilis.*

Fibromatosis appearing within the first few years of life as hyaline, fibrous, painless lesions of the scalp and other parts of the body, chiefly the gingiva, nail beds, nose, chin, and palmar and digital surfaces. Some lesions progress slowly over a period of several years but others calcify, ulcerate, and gradually disappear. Histologically, the lesions vary; some have abundant connective tissue cells, while others are rich in pseudocartilaginous hyaline matrix. Painful flexion contractures of the elbows, hips, and shoulders, osteolysis of the terminal phalanges, cystic lesions of the long bones, osteoporosis, thoracolumbar scoliosis, reduction of the body weight and height, and delayed sexual maturation are usually associated. The condition is transmitted as an autosomal recessive trait.

Murray, J. On three peculiar cases of molluscum fibrosum in one family. *Med. Chir. Trans., London*, 1873, 56:235-8. Puretic, S., *et al.* A unique form of mesenchymal dysplasia. *Brit. J. Derm.* 1962, 74:8-19. Drescher, E., *et al.* Juvenile fibromatosis siblings (fibromatosis hyalinica multiplex juvenilis). *J. Pediat. Surg.*, 1967, 2:427-36.

Murray-Puretic-Drescher syndrome. See *Murray syndrome.*

muscle compartment syndrome. See *compartment syndrome.*

muscle contraction headache. See *under headache syndrome.*

muscle effort syndrome. See *overuse syndrome.*

muscle pain syndrome. See *fibrositis-fibromyalgia syndrome.*

muscle phosphofructokinase deficiency. See *glycogen storage disease VII.*

muscle phosphorylase deficiency. See *glycogen storage disease V.*

muscle-eye-brain (MEB) disease. See *Santavuori syndrome.*

muscle-tendon syndrome. See *under overuse syndrome.*

muscular dystrophy I. See *Leyden-Moebius syndrome.*

muscular dystrophy, Becker type. See *Becker muscular dystrophy.*

muscular dystrophy, Leyden-Moebius type. See *Leyden-Moebius syndrome.*

muscular rheumatism. See *fibrositis-fibromyalgia syndrome.*
mutational dysostosis. See *cleidocranial dysostosis.*
mutilating keratoderma. See *Vohwinkel syndrome.*
mutilating palmoplantar keratoderma. See *Vohwinkel syndrome.*
MVP. See *mitral valve prolapse syndrome.*
MVP-SC (mitral valve prolapse-systolic click) syndrome. See *mitral valve prolapse syndrome.*
MWS. See *Marden-Walker syndrome.*
MWS (Moersch-Woltman syndrome). See *stiff man syndrome.*
myalgia epidemica. See *Sylvest syndrome.*
myasthenia gravis. See *Erb-Goldflam syndrome, under Erb, Wilhelm Heinrich.*
myasthenia gravis pseudoparalytica. See *Erb-Goldflam syndrome, under Erb, Wilhelm Heinrich.*
myasthenia paroxysmalis angiosclerotica. See *Charcot syndrome (3).*
myasthenic syndrome of Eaton and Lambert (MSEL). See *Eaton-Lambert syndrome, under Eaton Lealdes McKendree.*
myatonia congenita. See *Oppenheim disease, under Oppenheim, Hermann.*
mycetoma. See *Ballingall disease.*
mycosis fungoides. Synonyms: *Alibert-Bazin syndrome, Auspitz dermatosis, Auspitz syndrome, cutaneous T-cell lymphoma, granuloma fungoides, pian fungoides.*

A chronic and usually fatal disease of the reticuloendothelial system. It is a T-cell lymphoma of the skin, frequently also affecting the lymph nodes and viscera. The premycoid or eczematoid stage is characterized by eczematoid eruption, psoriasis, dermatitis exfoliativa, and parapsoriasis. The infiltrative stage is marked by circinate and gyrate elevated plaques of various sizes, usually bluish red, less frequently yellow and brown, often accompanied by pea-sized nodules. The tumor stage is manifested by lesions of various sizes, from that of a pea to that of an orange, usually bluish to brownish red. Extracutaneous dissemination occurs in two-thirds of patients, involving the lymph nodes, lungs, liver, and spleen. The disease seldom occurs before the fifth decade; the survival time is less than 5 years.

*Alibert, J. L. *Description des maladies de la peau.* Bruxelles, Wahlen, 1806, p. 157. *Bazin, A. *Affections cutanees artificielles.* Paris, 1852. *Auspitz, H. Ein Fall von Granuloma fungoides (Mycosis fungoides Alibert). *Wschr. Derm. Syph., Wien,* 1885, 12:123-43.

myelitis necroticans. See *Foix-Alajouanine syndrome.*
myelitis with optic neuritis. See *Devic syndrome.*
myelodysplasia. See *myelodysplastic syndrome.*

myelodysplastic syndrome (MDS). Synonyms: *dyshemopoiesis, dyshemopoietic anemia, dyshemopoietic syndrome, dysmyelopoiesis, dysmyelopoietic syndrome (DMS), hemopoietic dysplasia, idiopathic refractory anemia, low-percentage leukemia, myelodysplasia, preleukemia, preleukemic syndrome, refractory dysmyelopoietic anemia, refractory dysmyelopoietic panmyelopathy, refractory dysmyelopoietic panmyelosis, smoldering leukemia.*

A group of acquired, idiopathic or secondary, progressive cytopenias, usually associated with hyperplastic but ineffective hemopoiesis, involving one or more cell lineages and a risk of transformation to acute

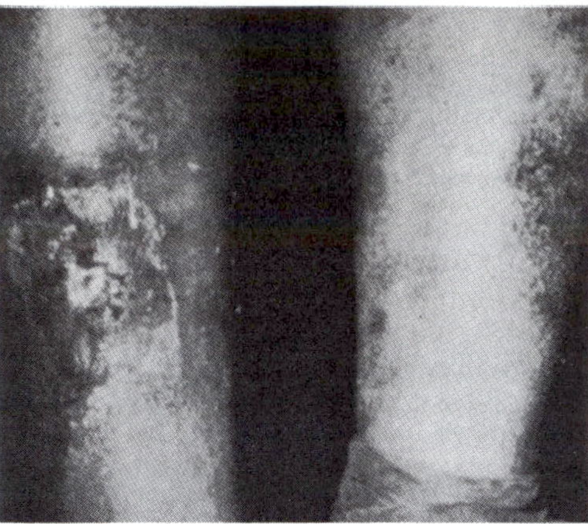

Mycosis fungoides
Glenner, G.G., T.F. Ignaczak & D.L. Page. "The inherited systemic amyloidoses and localized amyloid deposits. In Stanbury, J.B., J.B. Wyngaarden & D.S. Fredrickson, *The Metabolic Basis of Inherited Disease,* 4th ed. New York: McGraw-Hill, 1978, pp 1308-39 (Tables 54-3 and 54-4).

myeloid leukemia. The spectrum of symptoms ranges from relatively stable forms of refractory anemias with functional or morphological abnormalities of the erythroid lineage to acute myeloid leukemia. In the FAB (French-American-British Cooperative Group) classification, MDS includes refractory anemia, acquired idiopathic sideroblastic anemia, refractory anemia with excess of blasts (RAEB), and chronic myelocytic leukemia. It can be also grouped into five broad categories: (1) hereditary conditions, such as the Down and Fanconi syndromes; (2) immune deficiency syndromes; (3) disorders caused by exogenous factors, such as radiations, toxic agents, and infections; (4) primary myelodysplastic syndromes; and (5) other myeloproliferative disorders.

Block, M. *et al.* Preleukemic acute human leukemia. *JAMA,* 1953, 152:1018-28. Ruutu, T. ed. The myelodysplastic syndromes. *Scand. J. Haematol.,* 1986, 36(Suppl. 45):1-139.

myeloid tumor. See *Kahler disease.*
myelomatosis. See *Kahler disease.*
myelomatous pseudoleukemia. See *Kahler disease.*
myelopathia necroticans. See *Foix-Alajouanine syndrome.*
myelopathic albumosuria. See *Bence Jones proteinuria.*
myelopathic muscular atrophy. See *Aran-Duchenne syndrome.*
myelopathic polycythemia. See *Vaquez-Osler syndrome.*
myelophthisic anemia. See *Vaughan disease.*
myeloradiculitis. See *Guillain-Barré syndrome.*
myelosis erythremica. See *Di Guglielmo disease (1).*
MYERS, GARTH G. (American physician)
Smith-Fineman-Myers syndrome. See *under Smith, Richard D.*
MYHRE, S. (American physician)
Ruvalcaba-Myhre-Smith syndrome. See *Ruvalcaba syndrome (2).*
MYHRMAN, GUSTAF CHRISTOFER (Swedish physician, born 1903)
Myhrman-Zetterholm syndrome. Synonym: *nephropathia epidemica.*

A probably infectious disease, occurring predominantly in the northern parts of Scandinavia, marked by the sudden onset of chills, fever, headache, severe abdominal symptoms suggesting appendicitis, malaise, and vomiting, associated with severe proteinuria of short duration, scanty urinary sediment, hyposthenuria, slightly decreased glomerular filtration rate, elevated nonprotein nitrogen level, and low specific gravity of the urine. The course is short and benign.

Myhrman, G. Nephropathia epidemica, a new infectious disease in northern Scandinavia. *Acta Med. Scand.*, 1951, 140:52-6. Zetterholm, S. G. Akuta nefriter simulerande akuta bukfall. *Sven. Läkartidn.*, 1934, 31:425-9.

Myleran toxicity syndrome. See *busulfan toxicity syndrome.*

myo-ossificatio progressiva multiplex. See *fibrodysplasia ossificans progressiva.*

myoblastic myoma. See *Abrikossov tumor.*

myoblastoma granulare. See *Abrikossov tumor.*

myocardial fibrosis. See *Wuhrmann disease.*

myocardial steal. See *coronary steal syndrome.*

myocardosis. See *Wuhrmann disease.*

myoclonic encephalopathy syndrome. See *Kingsbourne syndrome.*

myoclonic nystagmus. See *Lenoble-Aubineau syndrome.*

myoclonus multiplex fibrillaris. See *Morvan chorea.*

myodysplasia fetalis deformans. See *arthrogryposis multiplex congenita syndrome.*

myodysplasia fibrosa multiplex. See *arthrogryposis multiplex congenita syndrome.*

myodystrophia fetalis deformans. See *arthrogryposis multiplex congenita syndrome.*

myoepithelial sialadenitis (MESA). See *Sjögren syndrome, under Sjögren, Henrik Samuel Conrad.*

myofascial pain syndrome. See *fibrositis-fibromyalgia syndrome.*

myofascial trigger point syndrome. Synonym: *trigger point syndrome.*

Myofascial pain elicited by pressure or other stimuli, such as acute or chronic overload of the muscle, on the trigger point. Objective findings include a palpable firm and tense band in the muscle, local twitch response, restricted stretch range-of-motion, and weakness without atrophy. The symptoms consist of stiffness and easy fatigability, spontaneous pain in a distribution predictable for the trigger point, deep tenderness at the trigger point, and referred pain by sustained pressure on the trigger point. See also *fibrositis-fibromyalgia syndrome.*

Simons, D. G. Myofascial trigger points: A need for understanding. *Arch. Phys. Med. Rehabil.*, 1981, 62:97-9. Travell, J. Identification of myofascial trigger point syndromes: A case of atypical fascial neuralgia. *Arch. Phys. Med. Rehabil.*, 1981, 62:100-6. Rubin, D. Myofascial trigger point syndromes: An approach to management. *Arch. Phys. Med. Rehabil.*, 1981, 62:107-10. Reynolds, M. D. Myofascial trigger point syndromes in the practice of rheumatology. *Arch. Phys. Med. Rehabil.*, 1981, 62:111-4. Malzack, R. Myofascial trigger points: Relation to acupuncture and mechanisms of pain. *Arch. Phys. Med. Rehabil.*, 1981, 62:114-7.

myoglobinuric myositis. Synonyms: *Günther disease, myositic myoglobinurica.*

Myositis associated with myoglobinuria. The symptoms include arthralgia, erythema, diarrhea, fever, chills, and fatigability.

Günther, H. Myositis myoglobinurica. *Münch, Med. Wschr.*, 1923, 70:517.

myopathia distalis juvenilis hereditaria. See *Biemond syndrome (5).*

myopathia distalis tarda hereditaria. See *Welander syndrome.*

myopathia osteoplastica. See *fibrodysplasia ossificans progressiva.*

myopathia osteoplastica progressiva. See *Teutschländer syndrome.*

myopathia sclerosans limitans. See *Emery-Dreifuss syndrome.*

myopathic external ophthalmoplegia. See *Kiloh-Nevin syndrome (2).*

myopathic limb-girdle syndrome. See *Leyden-Moebius syndrome.*

myopathy-myxedema syndrome. See *Debré-Semelaigne syndrome.*

myophosphorylase deficiency glycogenosis. See *glycogen storage disease V.*

myorenal syndrome. See *crush syndrome.*

myositis acuta epidemica. See *Sylvest syndrome.*

myositis fibrosa. See *Froriep disease.*

myositis myoglobinurica. See *myoglobinuric myositis.*

myositis ossificans multiplex progressiva. See *fibrodysplasia ossificans progressiva.*

myositis ossificans progressiva. See *fibrodysplasia ossificans progressiva.*

myositis universalis acuta infectiosa. See *Wagner-Unverricht syndrome, under Wagner, Ernst Leberecht.*

myositis with eosinophilia. See *Shulman syndrome, under Shulman, L. E.*

myospasia impulsiva. See *Gilles de la Tourette syndrome.*

myotonia acquisita. See *Talma disease.*

myotonia atrophica. See *myotonic dystrophy syndrome.*

myotonia chondrodystrophica. See *Schwartz-Jampel syndrome, under Schwartz, Oscar.*

myotonia congenita. See *Thomsen disease.*

myotonia congenita intermittens. See *Eulenburg disease.*

myotonia dystrophica. See *myotonic dystrophy syndrome.*

myotonic dystrophy syndrome. Synonyms: *Batten disease, Curschmann-Batten syndrome, Curschmann-Batten-Steinert syndrome, Curschmann-Steinert syndrome, Rossolimo-Curschmann-Batten-Steinert syndrome, Steinert disease, Steinert myopathy, Steinert myotonia, Steinert myotonic dystrophy, congenital myotonic dystrophy, dystrophia myotonica, dystrophia myotonica familiaris, myotonia atrophica, myotonia dystrophica.*

A hereditary familial muscle disease, transmitted as an autosomal dominant trait with complete penetrance and variation in expression, characterized mainly by myotonia, progressive muscle wasting, cataracts, hypogonadism, and mental deterioration. Involvement of the facial and masticatory muscles, especially the temporal muscles, produces a narrow, expressionless, masklike facies and exaggerated forward neck curvature (swan neck). Wasting of the muscles of the extremities progresses distally. Ocular changes include blepharoptosis, dustlike blue-green, red, and yellow opacities in the lens, cataracts, ophthalmoplegia, blepharitis, keratitis sicca, corneal dystrophy, enophthalmos, microphthalmia, choroidal coloboma, dark adaptation disorders, optic atrophy, and other disorders. Heart conduction disorders and arrhythmia are the principal cardiac complications. Respiratory disorders consist mainly of respiratory distress and infections. Testicular atrophy, decreased urinary 17-ketosteroids, increased urinary luteinizing hormone, cryptorchism, amenorrhea, and dysmenorrhea are usually present. Diabetes mellitus, hypothyroidism, and thyroid adenomas may occur in some cases. Dysphagia, nasal regurgitation, gastric bezoars, cholelithiasis, malabsorption, and other gastrointestinal disorders may be associated. Thickening of the calvaria, hyperostosis frontalis interna, small sella turcica, large paranasal sinuses, hypertelorism, kyphoscoliosis, pectus excavatum, and talipes equinovarus are the chief skeletal features of this syndrome.

Steinert, H. Myopathologische Beitrage. I. Über das klinische und anatomische Bild des Muskelschwunds der Myotoniker. *Deut. Zschr. Nervenkeilk.*, 1909, 37:58-104. Curschmann, H. Über familiäre atrophische Myotonie. *Deut. Zschr. Nervenheilk.*, 1912, 45:161-202. Batten, F. E., & Gibbs, H. P. Myotonia atrophica. *Brain*, 1909, 32:187-205. Dzhabarov, D. B. [Vegetative and trophic disorders and the functional status of the sympatho-adrenal system in Rossolimo-Curschmann-Batten-Steinert myotonic dystrophy] *Zh. Nevropat. Psikhiat.*, 1986, 86(3):333-5.

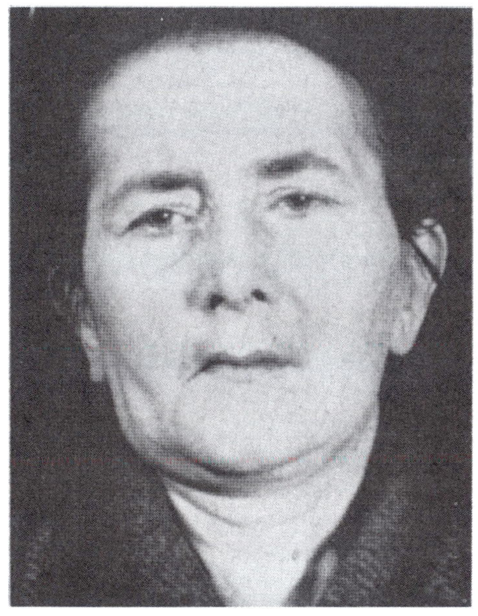

Myotonic dystrophy syndrome
Francois, Jules: *Heredity in Ophthalmology.* St. Louis: C.V. Mosby

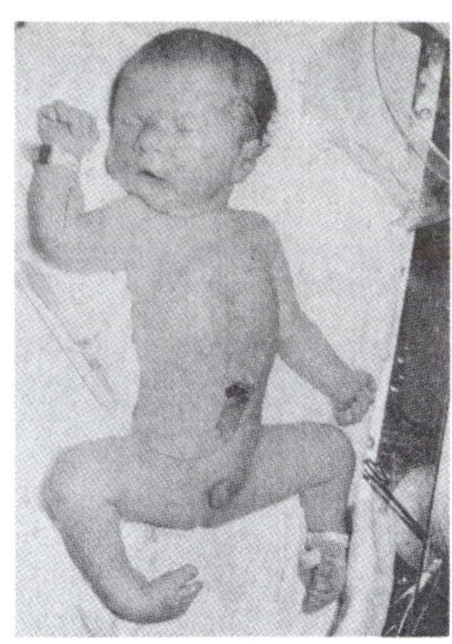

Myotonic dystrophy syndrome
Bell, D.B. & D.W. Smith: *J. Pediatr.* 81:83, 1972. St. Louis: C.V. Mosby Co.

myotonic pupil. See *Adie syndrome.*

myotonic pupillary reaction. See *Adie syndrome.*

myxadenitis labialis. See *Baelz syndrome.*

myxedema heart. See *Zondek syndrome, under Zondek, Hermann.*

myxedema-muscular hypertrophy syndrome. See *Debré-Semelaigne syndrome.*

myxedema-myotonic dystrophy syndrome. See *Debré-Selemaigne syndrome.*

myxomatous mitral valve degeneration. See *mitral valve prolapse syndrome.*

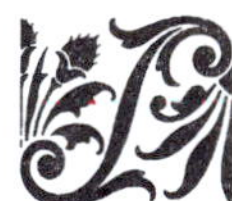

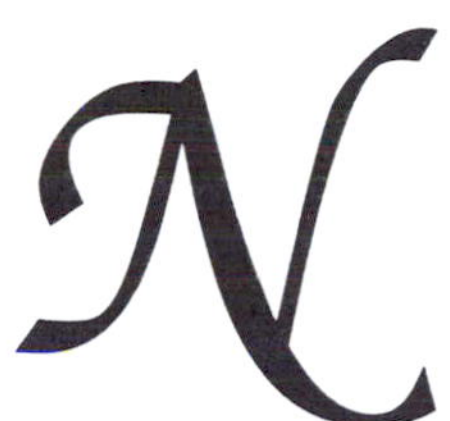

N syndrome. A hereditary syndrome transmitted as either an autosomal recessive or X-linked recessive trait. It combines mental and growth retardation, visual disorders, deafness, dolichocephaly, hypotelorism, scalloped and laterally overlapping upper eyelids, large corneae, abnormal ear auricles, dental dysplasia, generalized skeletal dysplasia (overtubulation of the long bones with the distal bones being relatively shorter than the proximal ones), high fingerprint ridge count, cryptorchidism, hypospadias, and spasticity.

Hess, R. O., *et al.* The N syndrome, a "new" multiple congenital anomaly-mental retardation syndrome. *Clin. Genet.*, 1974, 6:237-46.

NAEGELE, FRANZ KARL. See NÄGELE, FRANZ KARL

NAEGELI, OSKAR (Swiss physician, 1885-1959)

Glanzmann-Naegeli syndrome. See *Glanzmann thrombasthenia.*

Naegeli incontinentia pigmenti. See *Naegeli syndrome.*

Naegeli syndrome. Synonyms: *Franceschetti-Jadassohn syndrome, Naegeli-Franceschetti-Jadassohn syndrome, Naegeli incontinentia pigmenti, chromatophore nevus, hyperpigmentation-hypohidrosis syndrome, reticular pigmented dermatosis.*

A syndrome, transmitted as an autosomal dominant trait, characterized by reticular cutaneous hyperpigmentation, hypohidrosis, hyperkeratosis palmaris et plantaris, and faulty dentition with yellowing of the teeth. Brown, dirty brown, or slate gray pigmentation appears at the age of 2 years, usually involving first the trunk and upper extremities, from where it spreads to other parts.

Naegeli, Familiärer Chromatophorennaevus. *Schweiz. Med. Wschr.*, 1927, 57:48. Franceschetti, A., & Jadassohn, W. A propos de "l'incontinentia pigmenti," délimitation de deux syndromes différents figurant sous le même terme. *Dermatologica, Basel*, 1954, 108:1-28.

Naegeli-Franceschetti-Jadassohn syndrome. See *Naegeli syndrome.*

NAEGELI, OTTO (German physician, 1871-1938)

Naegeli leukemia. Monocytic leukemia in which a moderately large number of cells resemble myeloblasts, or cells of the myeloid series derived from myeloblasts.

Naegeli, O. *Blutkrankheiten und Blutdiagnostik.* 5th ed. Berlin, Springer, 1931.

naevoid basal cell carcinoma syndrome. See *nevoid basal-cell carcinoma syndrome.*

naevus spongiosus albus mucosae. See *white sponge nevus.*

naevus vasculosus osteohypertrophicus. See *Klippel-Trénaunay-Weber syndrome.*

NAFFZIGER, HOWARD CHRISTIAN (American physician, 1884-1961)

Naffziger syndrome. See *scalenus anticus syndrome.*

NÄGELE (NAEGELE), FRANZ KARL (German physician, 1777-1851)

Nägele obliquity. See *Nägele pelvis.*

Nägele pelvis. Synonym: *Nägele obliquity.*

A distorted pelvis in which the conjugate diameter takes an oblique direction.

Nägele, F. K. *Das schräg verengte Becken, nebst einem Anhange über die wichtigsten Fehler des weiblichen Beckens überhaupt.* Mainz, Zabern, 1839, 118 pp.

NAGEOTTE, JEAN (French physician, born 1866)

Babinski-Nageotte syndrome. See *under Babinski.*

NAGER, FELIX ROBERT (Swiss physician, 1877-1959)

Nager acrofacial dysostosis. See *Nager-de Reynier syndrome.*

Nager-de Reynier syndrome. Synonyms: *Nager acrofacial dysostosis, acrofacial dysostosis (AFD), dysostosis mandibularis, mandibulofacial dysostosis with limb malformations syndrome.*

A rare congenital syndrome transmitted as an autosomal recessive trait. It combines the features of mandibulofacial dysostosis with limb abnormalities. Fishlike facies with antimongoloid slant of the palpebral fissures, hypoplasia of the facial bones, macrostomia, underdeveloped mandible, and malformed ears are the main facial features. The hand abnormalities consist mainly of hypoplasia on the preaxial side of the hand, with absent thumbs or radius. In some cases, there are postaxial defects of the hands and polydactyly of the thumbs. Some authors consider any hand malformation with mandibulofacial dysostosis to represent the Nager-de Reynier syndrome, but others restrict its scope to conditions in which there are only preaxial hand deformities.

Nager, F. R., & Reynier, J. P., de. Das Gehörorgan bei den angeborenen Kopfmissbildungen. *Pract. Otorhinolar., Basel*, 1948, 10(Suppl. 2):1-128.

nail dysplasia-hypodontia syndrome. See *tooth-nail syndrome.*

nail dystrophy-deafness syndrome. See *Robinson syndrome, under Robinson, Geoffrey C.*

nail-patella syndrome. Synonyms: *Fong syndrome, Österreicher-Fong syndrome, Trauner-Rieger syndrome, Turner syndrome, Turner-Kieser syndrome, hereditary*

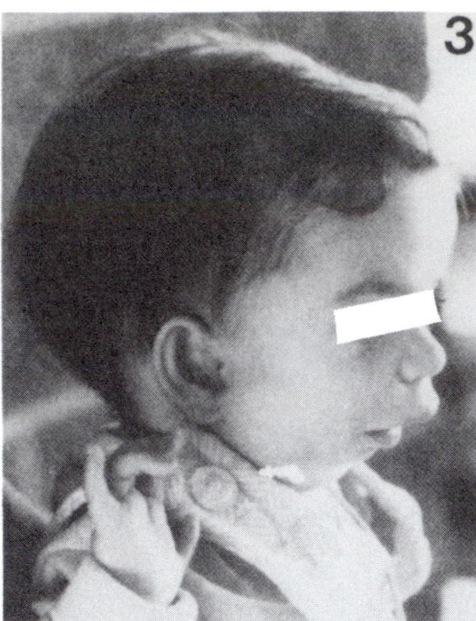

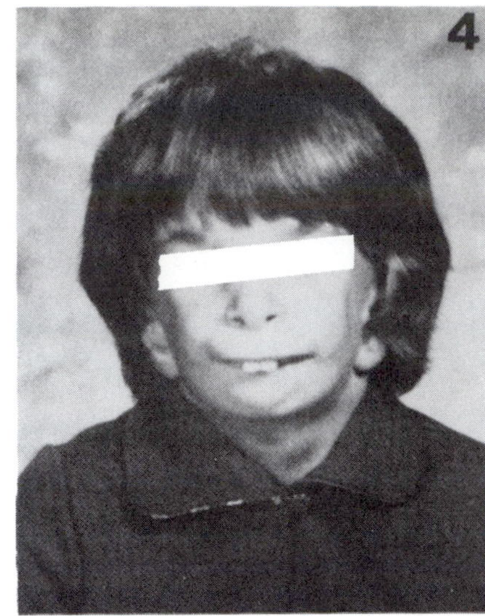

Nager-de Reynier syndrome
Meyerson, M.D.: The Effect of Syndrome Diagnosis on Speech Remediation. In Shprintzen, R.J., & N.W. Paul (eds): *Diagnostic Accuracy: Effect on Treatment Planning.* New York: Alan R. Liss, Inc. for the March of Dimes Birth Defects Foundation BD:OAS 21(2):47-68, 1985, with permission.

onycho-osteodysplasia (HOOD), hereditary onycho-osteodysplasia syndrome (HOODS), iliac horn syndrome, nail-patella-elbow syndrome, onycho-arthrosis, onychomesodysplasia, onycho-osteo-arthrodysplasia, osseous dystrophy-nail dysplasia syndrome, osteo-onychodysostosis, osteo-onychodysplasia, osteo-onychodysplasia-albuminuria.

A hereditary syndrome, transmitted as an autosomal dominant trait, and characterized by anomalies of the patellae, nails, and elbows, in association with iliac horns. The nails of the thumbs are most frequently involved. Abnormalities, usually symmetrical, range from slight longitudinal ridging to complete anonychia. Hypoplasia of the capitellum and radial head results in dislocations and inability to fully extend, pronate, or supinate the elbow. The patellae are often smaller than normal or completely absent. The iliac horns, always bilaterally symmetrical, project from the central area of the external iliac fossa. Clubfoot, hypoplastic scapula, dark cloverleaf pigmentation of the inner margin of the iris, and proteinuria with or without hematuria are frequently present. Associated hand abnormalities may include clinodactyly of the fifth fingers, short middle phalanges, and short third to fifth metacarpals. The syndrome is usually diagnosed during the second or third decade but iliac horns are present from infancy.

Trauner, R., & Rieger, H. Eine Familie mit 6 Fällen von Luxation radii congenita mit übereinstimmenden Anomalien der Finger-und Kniegelenke, sowie der Nagelbildung in 4 Generationen. *Arch. Klin. Chir.*, 1925, 137:659-66. Fong, E. E. "Iliac horns" (symmetrical bilateral central posterior iliac processes). *Radiology*, 1946, 47:517-8. Kieser, W. Die sogenannte Flughaut beim Menschen. Ihre Beziehung zum Status dysraphicus und ihre Erblichkeit. *Zschr. Menschl. Vererb. Konstit.* 1939, 23:594-619. Turner, J. W. A hereditary arthrodysplasia associated with hereditary dystrophy of the nails. *JAMA*, 1933, 100:882-4. Österreicher, W. Nägel- und Skelettanomalien. *Wien. Klin. Wschr.*, 1929, 43:632.

nail-patella-elbow syndrome. See *nail-patella syndrome.*

NAJJAR, VICTOR ASSAD (American physician, born 1914)

Crigler-Najjar syndrome. See *under Crigler.*

Najjar-Andersen syndrome. See *glycogen storage disease IV.*

NAJMAN

Imerslund-Najman-Gräsbeck syndrome. See *Imerslund-Gräsbeck syndrome.*

NAME (nevi-atrial myxoma-**m**yxoid neuro-fibromatosis-**e**phelides) **syndrome.** See *cutaneous lentiginosis with atrial myxomas syndrome.*

NANCE, WALTER E. (American physician)

Nance deafness. See *Nance syndrome.*

Nance dwarfism. See *Nance-Sweeney syndrome.*

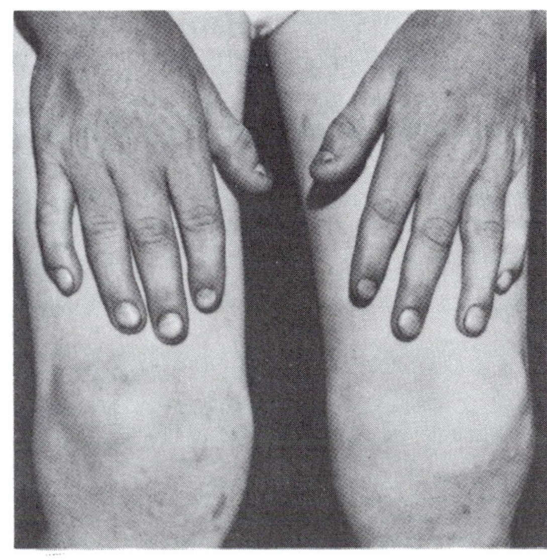

Nail-Patella syndrome
Courtesy of Dr. John Opitz, Helena, MT.

Nance syndrome. Synonyms: *Nance deafness, conductive deafness-stapes fixation syndrome, perilymphatic gusher-deafness syndrome, deafness-perilymphatic gusher syndrome.*

An X-linked otologic disease characterized in males by mixed deafness, vestibular abnormalities, congenital fixation of stapes, and perilymphatic otorrhea on attempted spadectomy. In females, who carry the mutant gene, there are generally subclinical audiologic abnormalities.

Nance, W. E., *et at.* X-linked mixed deafness with congenital fixation of the stapedial footplate and perilymphatic gusher. *Birth Defects,* 1971, 7(4):64-9.

Nance-Horan syndrome (NHS). Synonyms: *brachymetacarpalia-cataract-mesiodens syndrome, X-linked cataract-dental syndrome, X-linked congenital cataracts-microcornea syndrome.*

A congenital syndrome, transmitted as an X-linked trait, characterized by cataracts, impaired vision, extra incisors (mesiodens), incisor diastemas, narrowed incisal edges, anteverted pinnae, and short fourth metacarpals.

Nance, W. E., *et al.* Congenital X-linked cataract, dental anomalies and brachymetacarpalia. *Birth Defects,* 1974, 10(4):285-91. Horan, M. B., & Billson, F. A. X-linked cataract and hutchinsonian teeth. *Austral. Pediat. J.,* 1974, 10:98-102.

Nance-Sweeney syndrome. Synonym: *Nance dwarfism.*

A recessively transmitted chondrodystrophy associated with dwarfism with dispropotionate shortening of the arms and legs; large head with a prominent forehead, saddle nose, prognathia with flattening of the angle of the mandible; malformed calcified external ears; edentia; corneal infiltration; cleft palate; thick and leathery skin (ichthyosis), particularly over the exposed areas of the hands and arms; short fingers; subcutaneous calcification of the hands and fingers; limited movement of the elbows; fusion of the hip joint; and hypoplastic hair. X-ray findings show a champagne glass deformity of the pelvis with calcification of the cartilaginous rim of the ilium; cartilage calcification of the ribs, epiphyseal centers of the scapula, femur, and humerus; S-shaped scoliosis; flattening of the vertebrae; flattening of the base of the skull; and small foramen magnum.

Nance, W. E., & Sweeney, A. A recessively inherited chondrodystrophy. *Birth Defects,* 1970, 6(4):25-7.

nanocephalic dwarfism. See *Seckel syndrome.*

narcolepsy. See *Gélineau syndrome.*

narcolepsy-catalepsy syndrome. See *Gélineau syndrome.*

narcoleptic syndrome. See *Gélineau syndrome.*

nasal leprosy. See *Bergen syndrome.*

nasociliary neuralgia. See *Charlin syndrome.*

nasomaxillary hypoplasia. See *Binder syndrome.*

nasopalpebral lipoma-coloboma syndrome. Synonym: *palpebral coloboma-lipoma syndrome.*

A familial syndrome, transmitted as an autosomal dominant trait, characterized by congenital upper lid and nasopalpebral lipomas, bilateral symmetrical upper and lower palpebral colobomas at the junction of the inner and middle thirds of the lids, telecanthus, and maxillary hypoplasia. The affected individuals have a broad forehead, widow's peak, abnormal patterns of eyebrows and eyelashes, and maldeveloped lacrimal puncta. The interpupillary distance is increased due to divergent strabismus originating from visual interference from inner canthal masses. Persistent epiphora, conjunctival hyperemia, and corneal (and less frequently lens) opacities are secondary to lacrimal puncta defect and the inability to close the eyelids completely.

Penchaszadeh, V. B., *et al.* The nasopalpebral lipoma-coloboma syndrome: A new autosomal dominant congenital nasopalpebral lipomas, eyelid colobomas, telecanthus, and maxillary hypoplasia. *Am. J. Med. Genet.,* 1982, 11:397-410.

nasopharyngeal bursitis. See *Thornwaldt bursitis.*

nasopharyngeal lymphoepithelioma. See *Schmincke tumor.*

nasopharyngeal torticollis. See *Grisel syndrome.*

NAUMOFF, PETER (American physician)

short rib-polydactyly syndrome, Verma-Naumoff type. See *Verma-Naumoff syndrome.*

Verma-Naumoff syndrome. See *under Verma.*

nausea epidemica. See *Spencer disease.*

NAZARI, A. (Italian physician)

Marchiafava-Nazari-Micheli syndrome. See *Marchiafava-Micheli syndrome.*

NBCC. See ***n**evoid **b**asal **c**ell **c**arcinoma syndrome.*

NBCCS. See ***n**evoid **b**asal-**c**ell **c**arcinoma **s**yndrome.*

NBS. See ***n**evoid **b**asal-cell carcinoma **s**yndrome.*

NBS (nursing bottle syndrome). See *baby bottle syndrome.*

NCD (neurocirculatory dystonia). See *Da Costa syndrome, under Da Costa, Jacob Mendez.*

NCL (neuronal ceroid lipofuscinosis). See *Kufs syndrome, and see Stock-Spielmeyer-Vogt syndrome.*

NE (nephropathia epidemica). See *hemorrhagic fever with renal syndrome.*

Neapolitan fever. See *brucellosis.*

near miss sudden infant death syndrome. See *infant apnea syndrome.*

NEBECOURT

Nébecourt syndrome. A syndrome of diabetes mellitus, pituitary dwarfism, and genital infantilism.

Kropf, H. Über Zwergwuchs und Diabetes mellitus. *Ann. Univ. Saraviensis,* 1956, 4:175-92.

NECK, M., VAN. See VAN NECK, M.

neck-face syndrome. See *tardive dyskinesia syndrome.*

neck-tongue syndrome. Synonym: *spinal neck-tongue syndrome.*

Pain in the neck with or without cervical numbness and numbness in the tongue on sudden turning of the head. Compression of the C2 roots in the atlanto-axial space is believed to be the cause, the numbness of the tongue being secondary to compression of proprioceptive fibers from the tongue through the ansa hypoglossi, the cervical plexus, and the C2 roots.

Lance, J. W., & Anthony, M. Neck-tongue syndrome on sudden turning of the head. *J. Neur. Neurosurg. Psychiat.,* 1980, 43:97-101.

necrobiosis lipoidica. See *Oppenheim-Urbach syndrome, under Oppenheim, M.*

necrobiosis lipoidica diabeticorum. See *Oppenheim-Urbach syndrome, under Oppenheim, M.*

necrolytic migratory erythema (NME). See *under glucagonoma syndrome.*

necrotic facial dysplasia. See *oculo-auriculovertebral dysplasia.*

necrotic infectious conjunctivitis. See *Pascheff conjunctivitis.*

necrotizing angiitis. See *Kussmaul-Maier syndrome.*

necrotizing fasciitis of the male genitalia. See *Fournier disease.*
necrotizing granulomatosis. See *Wegener granulomatosis.*
necrotizing infection of the scrotum. See *Fournier disease.*
necrotizing respiratory granulomatosis. See *Wegener granulomatosis.*
necrotizing ulcerative gingivitis. See *Vincent infection.*
NEEDLES, CARL F. (American physician, born 1935)
Melnick-Needles syndrome (MNS). See *under Melnick.*
NEEL, AXEL (Danish physician)
Bing-Neel syndrome. See *under Bing, Jens.*
NEEMEH, JEAN A. (Canadian physician)
Lemieux-Neemeh syndrome. See *under Lemieux.*
NEGRI, SILVIO (Italian physician)
Negri syndrome. See *Jacod syndrome.*
Negri-Jacod syndrome. See *Jacod syndrome.*
Silvio Negri syndrome. See *Jacod syndrome.*
NEILL, CATHERINE A. (British pediatrician)
Neill-Dingwall syndrome. See *Cockayne syndrome.*
NEILL, D. W. (Irish physician)
Carson-Neill syndrome. See *homocystinuria syndrome.*
NELATON, AUGUSTE (French physician, 1807-1873)
Dupuytren-Nélaton disease. See *Nélaton disease.*
Nélaton disease. Synonym: *Dupuytren-Nélaton disease.*

A central tumor of bone.

*Nélaton, A. *Elémens de pathologie chirurgicale*. Paris, 1847-48, Vol. 2, p. 46. *Dupuytren. Des kystes qui se dévelop dans l'épaisseur des os, et de leurs difféntes espéces. In his: *Leçons orales de clinique chirurgicale faites a l'Hôtel-Dieu de Paris*. 1839, pp. 129-48.

Nélaton syndrome. See *Thévenard syndrome.*
Nélaton ulcer. Perforating trophic plantar ulcer.

Nélaton, A. Affection singulière des os du pied. *Gaz. Hôp., Paris*, 1852, 4:13.

NELSON, D. H. (American physician)
Nelson syndrome. Hyperpigmention and pituitary tumors following bilateral adrenalectomy for the Cushing syndrome, associated with elevated levels of circulating adrenocorticotropic hormone (ACTH) and probably melanocyte-stimulating hormone. Progressive visual field defects with bilateral hemianopsia due to a pituitary mass (usually a chromophobe adenoma) and headache are the principal symptoms.

Nelson, D. H., *et al.* ACTH-producing tumor of the pituitary gland. *N. Eng. J. Med.*, 1958, 259:161-4.

NELSON, MATILDA M. (British physician)
Emery-Nelson syndrome. See *under Emery.*
NELSON, WARREN OTTO (American physician, 1906-1964)
Heller-Nelson syndrome. See *under Heller, Carl George.*
nemaline myopathy. See *Shy-Magee syndrome.*
neonatal copper deficiency syndrome. A deficiency syndrome of infants with decreased copper intake in conditions such as prolonged parenteral nutrition, or with poor copper absorption or increased loss associated with protein-losing enteropathy, nephrotic syndrome, cystic fibrosis, and malabsorption syndromes. The symptoms include apathy, failure to thrive, hypotonia, hypothermia, psychomotor retardation, visual disorders, enlarged veins, tortuous arteries, hypopigmentation of the skin and hair, seborrheic dermatitis, and osteoporosis with metaphyseal flaring, cupping, and spurs. Leukopenia, vacuolization, erythroid and myeloid cells in the bone marrow, low serum copper and ceruloplasmin, impaired iron metabolism, and hypochomic anemia that is unresponsive to iron therapy, are the principal laboratory findings.

Sturgeon, P., & Brubaker, C. Copper deficiency in infants. A syndrome characterized by hypocupremia, iron deficiency anemia, and hypoproteinemia. *AMA J. Dis. Child.*, 1956, 92:254-65. Ashkenazi, A., *et al.* The syndrome of neonatal copper deficiency. *Pediatrics*, 1973, 52:525-33.

neonatal hemoglobinuria. See *Winckel-Charrin syndrome.*
neonatal progeroid syndrome. See *Wiedemann-Rautenstrauch syndrome.*
neonatal pseudohydrocephalic progeroid syndrome. See *Wiedemann-Rautenstrauch syndrome.*
neonatal respiratory distress syndrome. Synonyms: *hyaline disease of the lungs, hyaline membrane disease (HMD), infant respiratory distress syndrome (IRDS), perinatal respiratory distress syndrome, pulmonary hyaline membrane disease.*

A life-threatening respiratory disorder of the newborn, occurring most commonly in premature infants, being more frequent in children of diabetic than nondiabetic mothers, especially with delivery by cesarean section. After initial breathing problems are treated, the infants appear to have recovered, but within less than an hour respiration becomes difficult. There is retraction of the lower ribs and sternum on inspiration, and an expiratory grunt becomes audible. Gradually, the breathing rate increases to more than 100 breaths per minute, whereas the actual ventilation efficiency decreases. Rales and cyanosis become apparent. Chest x-ray shows at this stage a ground-glass image. Within 12 to 24 hours, the distress may regress, or there may be worsening of the infant's condition with increased cyonosis, flaccidity, and apnea leading to death. A deficiency of a pulmonary surfactant (lecithin phospholipid) is considered the fundamental defect. See also *Wilson-Mikity syndrome, infant apnea syndrome, sudden infant death syndrome, transient respiratory distress syndrome of the newborn*, and *wet lung syndrome.*

Hochheim, K. Über einige Befunde in den Lungen von Neugeborenen und die Beziehung derselben zur Aspiration von Fruchtwasser. *Zbl. Alg. Pathol.*, 1903, 14:437-8. Johnson, W. C. Pneumonia in newborn infants with lesions resembling pneumonia. *Proc. N. Y. Pathol. Soc.*, 1923, 23:138-42.

neonatal small left colon syndrome. Synonym: *small left colon syndrome.*

A congenital syndrome characterized by a markedly diminished caliber of the colon from the anus to the splenic flexure with a sharp zone of transition at the splenic flexure. The left colon appears to be shortened and lacking the usual tortuosity. The part proximal to the splenic flexure is dilated and distended with a meconium plug causing an obstruction, similar to that seen in the meconium plug syndrome (q.v.).

Davis, W. S., *et al.* Neonatal small left colon syndrome. *Am. J. Roentgen.*, 1974, 120:322-9.

neonatal yusho (PCB-contaminated oil poisoning). See *fetal PCB syndrome.*
neoplastic anorexia-cachexia syndrome. Anorexia with inadequate food intake leading to cachexia in cancer patients.

Krause, R., *et al.* Brain tryptophan and the neoplastic anorexia-cachexia syndrome. *Cancer*, 1979, 44:1003-8.

nephroblastoma. See *Wilms tumor.*

nephrocalcinosis infantum. See *Lightwood-Albright syndrome.*

nephrocalcinosis infantum with hyperchloremic acidosis. See *Lightwood-Albright syndrome.*

nephrocalcinosis with rickets and dwarfism. See *Lightwood-Albright syndrome.*

nephrogenic erythrocytosis. See *Forssell syndrome.*

nephrogenic hepatosplenomegaly. See *Stauffer syndrome.*

nephrogenic polycythemia. See *Forssell syndrome.*

nephropathia epidemica. See *Myhrman-Zetterholm syndrome.*

nephropathia epidemica (NE). See *hemorrhagic fever with renal syndrome.*

nephropathy-male pseudohermaphroditism-Wilms tumor syndrome. See *Drash syndrome.*

nephrophthisis. See *familial juvenile nephrophthisis.*

nephrophthisis-tapetoretinal degeneration syndrome. See *Senior syndrome (1).*

nephrotic syndrome. Synonyms: *Epstein nephrosis, Epstein syndrome, lipoid nephrosis.*

A symptom complex, seen in patients with various forms of glomerular diseases, characterized by an increase in capillary wall permeability to serum protein in association with excretion of large amounts of protein in the urine, hypoalbuminemia, edema, hyperlipidemia, and lipiduria. The complex may be a manifestation of a systemic disease, such as diabetes mellitus, systemic lupus erythematosus, and amyloidosis, but in most adults and some children it is secondary to glomerular diseases, such as minimal change nephrotic syndrome (MCNS), membranous nephropathy, and membranoproliferative glomerulonephritis. The complex also may be associated with occult malignancy. MCNS represents about 75 percent of cases of idiopathic nephrotic syndrome in children and about 20 percent in adults. Nephropathy or glomerulonephropathy with minimal histopathological changes and diffuse epithelial cell effacement or fusion are the only pathological changes that may be observed by electron microscopy. See also *Munk disease.*

Epstein, A. The nephroses. *Bull. N. Y. Acad. Med.,* 1937, 1975, 86:63-71. Watson, G. H., & Miller, V. Arteriohepatic dysplasia. Familial pulmonary arterial stenosis with neonatal liver disease. *Arch. Dis. Child.,* 1973, 48:459-66.

nephrotic-glycosuric dwarfism with hypophosphatemic rickets. See *cystinosis.*

NERI, V. (Italian physician)

Neri-Barré syndrome. See *Barré-Lieou syndrome.*

nerve deafness-distal neurogenic amyotrophy. See *Rosenberg-Chutorian syndrome, under Rosenberg, Roger N.*

nerve deafness-optic nerve atrophy-dementia syndrome. An inherited syndrome, transmitted as an X-linked recessive trait, characterized by sensorineural deafness in infancy, progressive optic atrophy, and dementia beginning in adulthood.

Jensen, P. K. a. Nerve deafness, optic nerve atrophy, and dementia: A new X-linked recessive syndrome? *Am. J. Med. Genet.,* 1981, 9:55-60.

nervous diarrhea. See *irritable bowel syndrome.*

nervous exhaustion. See *Beard syndrome.*

nervous headache. See *muscle contraction headache, under headache syndrome.*

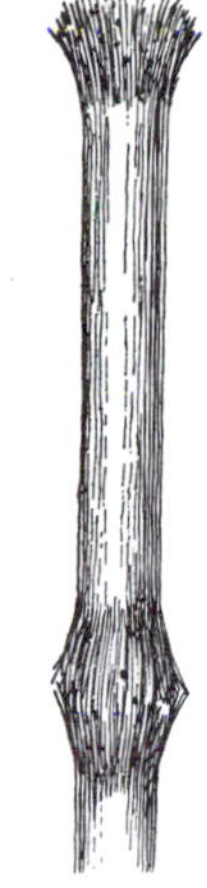

Netherton syndrome
Andrews, G.C. & A.N. Domonkos: *Diseases of the Skin.* 5th ed. Philadelphia: W.B. Saunders, Co., 1963.

nervous heart. See *Da Costa syndrome, under Da Costa, Jacob Mendez.*

NETHERTON, EARL WELDON (American dermatologist, born 1893)

Netherton syndrome. Synonyms: *bamboo hair-erythroderma ichthyosiforme congenitum syndrome, erythroderma ichthyosiforme congenitum-trichorhexis nodosa syndrome.*

A disorder of skin cornification, transmitted as an autosomal recessive trait and marked by ichthyosis linearis circumflexa, that persists from birth with atopic diathesis and nodose swelling of the hair shafts, resembling the joints of bamboo. Ichthyosis linearis circumflexa, a form of generalized hyperkeratosis, in association with desquamation, results in a circinate erythematous base showing a pathognomonic double-edged scale along the margins. Generalized erythroderma of the collodion-baby type may be present at birth. Pruritus, lichenification of flexural surfaces, may occur as a manifestation of atopic dermatitis, affecting chiefly the face, scalp, and eyebrows. Instead of the circinate pattern, some patients exhibit a rash

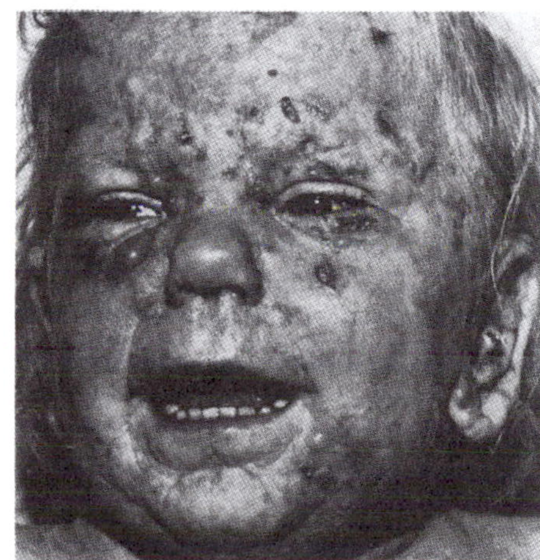

Nettleship syndrome
Nelson, W.E. (ed.): *Textbook of Pediatrics.* 8th ed. Philadelphia: W.B. Saunders Co., 1964.

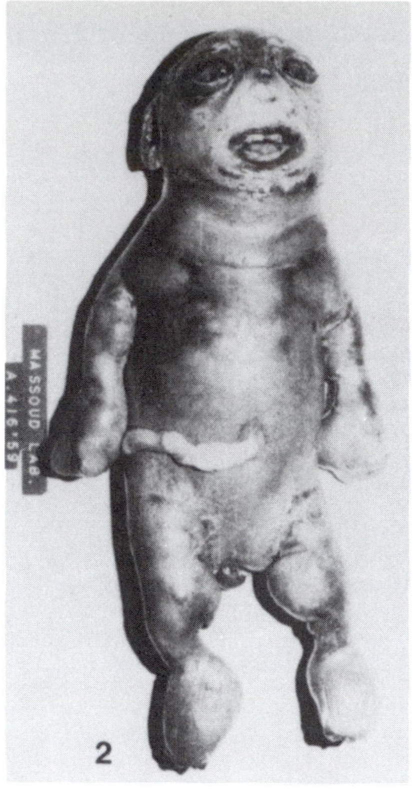

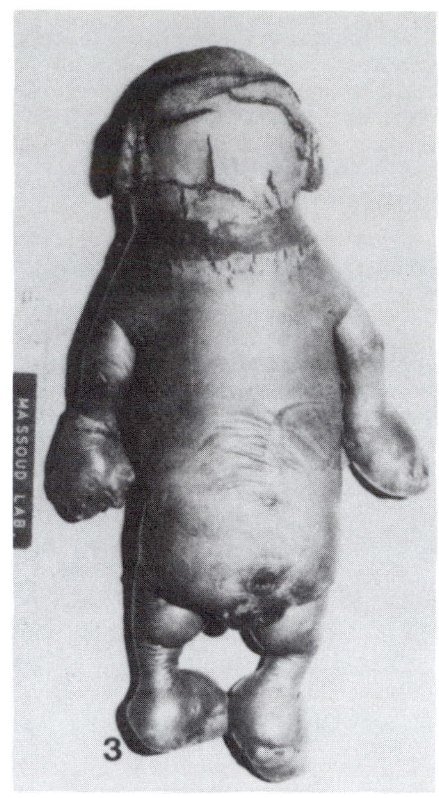

Neu-Laxová syndrome
Karimi-Nejad, Mohammad Haasan, Hooshang Khajavi, Mohammad Jafar Gharavi, & Roxana Karimi-Nejad: *American Journal of Medical Genetics* 28:17-23, 1987. New York: Alan R. Liss, Inc.

resembling lamellar ichthyosis. Additional features may include atopic dermatitis, asthma, anaphylactoid reaction to foods, hypergammaglobulinemia E, aminoaciduria, and impaired cellular immunity.

Netherton, E. A. A unique case of trichorrhexis nodosa-"bamboo hairs." *Arch. Derm., Chicago,* 1958, 78:483-7.

NETTLESHIP, EDWARD (British physician, 1845-1913)

Nettleship syndrome. Synonyms: *urticaria pigmentosa, urticaria xanthelasmoidea.*

A chronic skin disease that usually begins during early childhood, and is characterized by pigmented macules or nodules. The lesions urticate on irritation and contain large numbers of mast cells.

Nettleship, E. Chronic urticaria, leaving brown stains: Nearly two years duration. *Brit. Med. J.*, 1869, 2:435.

NEU, RICHARD L. (American scientist)

Neu syndrome. See *Neu-Laxová syndrome.*

Neu-Laxová syndrome. Synonyms: *Neu syndrome, Neu-Povysilová syndrome.*

A syndrome, believed to be transmitted as an autosomal recessive trait, consisting of microcephaly, lissencephaly, severe subcutaneous edema, atrophic muscles, camptodactyly, syndactyly of toes and fingers, hypoplastic genitalia, and various ocular and cerebral anomalies. Associated defects may include slanted forehead, hypertelorism, a flat nose and nasal bridge, low-set ears, rocker-bottom feet, hypoplastic cerebellum, agenesis of the corpus callosum, intrauterine growth retardation, short neck, ichthyosis, hypoplasia or atelectasis of the lungs, short umbilical cord, hydramnios, and hypoplasia of the placenta.

Neu, R. L., *et al.* A lethal syndrome of microcephaly with multiple congenital anomalies in three siblings. *Pediatrics*, 1971, 47:610-2. Laxová, R., *et al.* A further example of the lethal autosomal recessive condition in sibs. *J. Ment. Defic. Res.*, 1972, 16:139-43. Povysilová, V., *et al.* Letální syndrom mnohocetnych malformaci u trí sourozeňcu. *Cesk. Pediat.*, 1976, 31:190-4.

Neu-Povysilová syndrome. See *Neu-Laxová syndrome.*

NEUGEBAUER, H. (German orthopedic surgeon)

Karsch-Neugebauer syndrome. See *under Karsch.*

NEUHAUSER, EDWARD BLAINE (American physician, born 1908)

Neuhauser-Berenberg syndrome. Synonym: *cardio-esophageal relaxation syndrome.*

Cardio-esophageal relaxation in infants, occurring in nonfunctioning of the cardio-esophageal sphincter, associated with dilation of the esophagus and lack of gastric contractions. Vomiting is the main symptom.

Neuhauser, E. B., & Berenberg, W. Cardioesophageal relaxation as a cause of vomiting in infants. *Radiology*, 1947, 48:480-3.

NEUMANN, ERNST (German physician, 1843-1918)

Neumann syndrome. Synonyms: *congenital epulis, congenital myoblastoma of the newborn, epulis congenita, epulis of the newborn.*

A benign, nonencapsulated, soft, pedunculated tumor of the mucosa of the jaws, usually the maxilla, of newborn infants. It is often found in the incisor region, arising on the crest of the alveolar ridge or process, and is composed of large, closely packed cells showing granular, eosinophilic cytoplasm. The tumor is similar to myoblastoma but is believed to be a separate entity.

*Neumann, E. Ein Fall von congenitaler Epulis. *Arch. Heilk.*, 1871, 12:189.

NEUMANN, ISIDOR ELDER VON HEILWART (Austrian physician, 1837-1906)

Neumann syndrome (1). See *Stevens-Johnson syndrome.*

Neumann syndrome (2). Synonyms: *condylomatosis pemphigoides maligna, erythema bullosum vegetans, pemphigus frambesioides, pemphigus papillaris, pemphigus vegetans.*

A variant of pemphigus vulgaris in which many of the bullous lesions are replaced by malodorous, verrucoid, hypertrophic, vegetative masses, which are usually found on the skin but not on the mucous membranes, except for the vermillion border of the lips. The initial stages are similar to those in pemphigus vulgaris but the denuded ulcerative areas become hypertrophied and are characterized by the presence of vegetative granulation tissue. The lesions may further become dry and verrucous. Secondary bacterial infection is always present.

*Neumann, I. Über Pemphigus vegetans (framboesiodes). *Wien. Med. Bl.*, 1886, 9:46.

neural crest syndrome. See *Brown syndrome, under Brown, Jason W.*

neuralgia mammalis. See *Cooper neuralgia.*

neuralgia nasociliaris. See *Charlin syndrome.*

neuralgia obturatoria. See *Howship-Romberg syndrome.*

neuralgia quinti. See *trigeminal neuralgia.*

neuralgia spasmodica. See *trigeminal neuralgia.*

neuralgic lumbosciatic osteopathy syndrome. See *Camera syndrome.*

neuraoacanthocytosis. See *Levine-Critchley syndrome.*

neurasthenia. See *Beard syndrome, and see fibrositis-fibromyalgia syndrome.*

neurinofibrolipomatosis. See *Recklinghausen disease (1).*

neurinomatosis centralis. See *Bourneville-Pringle syndrome.*

neurinomatosis centralis et peripherica. See *Recklinghausen disease (1).*

neurinomatosis universalis. See *Bourneville-Pringle syndrome.*

neuritis fascians. See *Eichhorst disease.*

neuritis migrans. See *Wartenberg disease (2).*

neuritis multiplex atactica. See *Déjerine syndrome (1).*

neuritis nervi cutanei femoris lateralis. See *Rot-Bernhardt syndrome, under Rot, Vladimir Karlovich.*

neuritis saturnina. See *lead poisoning.*

neuritis with albumino-cytologic dissociation. See *Guillain-Barré syndrome.*

neuro-oculocutaneous angiomatosis. See *Sturge-Weber syndrome.*

neuro-opticomyelitis. See *Devic syndrome.*

neuro-uveoparotitis syndrome. See *Heerfordt syndrome.*

neuroanemic syndrome. See *Dana syndrome.*

neuroangiomatosis encephalofacialis. See *Sturge-Weber syndrome.*

neuroangiosis cruris hemosiderosa. See *Rajka-Szodoray syndrome.*

neuroarthromyodysplasia. See *arthrogryposis multiplex congenita syndrome.*

neuroarthropathy. See *Charcot disease.*

neuroblastoma sympathicum embryonale. See *Hutchinson disease, under Hutchinson, Sir Robert Grieve.*

neurocirculatory asthenia. See *Da Costa syndrome, under Da Costa, Jacob Mendes.*

neurocirculatory dystonia (NCD). See *Da Costa syndrome, under Da Costa, Jacob Mendes.*

neurocutaneous syndrome. See *Sturge-Weber syndrome.*

neurocutaneous melanoblatosis syndrome. See *neurocutaneous melanosis.*

neurocutaneous melanosis. Synonyms: *hamartomatous meningeal melanosis, neurocutaneous melanoblastosis syndrome, neurocutaneous melanosis anomalad.*

A melanocytic form of multiple hamartomas which is present at birth and involves the skin and the central nervous system. Parts of the skin, especially of the lower abdomen, upper thigh, lower runk, thigh, and abdomen, are covered by black, thickened, sometimes hairy pigmented nevi. Thick sheets of melanoblasts cover the pia matter and arachnoid. The symptoms vary from occasional mild central nervous system disorders to frequent seizures and mental retardation. Most affected infants die before the age of two years, but some survive into adult life. The etiology is unknown.

Rokitansky, J. Ein ausgezeichneter Fall von Pigmentmal mit ausgebreiteter Pigmentirung der inneren Hirn- Und Ruckenmarkschäute. *Allg. Wien. Med. Ztg.*, 1861, 6:113.

neurocutaneous melanosis anomalad. See *neurocutaneous melanosis.*

neuroderma*itis circumscripta. See *Brocq disease (1).*

neurodermatitis disseminata. See *Besnier prurigo.*

neurodermatitis nodulosa. See *Hyde syndrome.*

neuroectodermal hamartoma. See *Sturge-Weber syndrome.*

neuroedematous syndrome. See *Debré-Marie syndrome (1).*

neurofaciodigitorenal (NFDR) syndrome. A multiple congenital anomalies/mental retardation syndrome marked by a high and prominent forehead, vertical groove on the tip of the nose, cowlick, malformed ears, acrorenal field defect (incipient unilateral triphalangism, broad halluces with unilateral renal agenesis in one patient), megalencephaly associated with congenital hypotonia, severe mental retardation with high abnormal EEG but without seizures, intrauterine growth retardation, and occasional primordial shortness of stature. The syndrome is transmitted as an autosomal recessive trait.

Freire-Maia, N., *et al.* The neurofaciodigitorenal (NFDR) syndrome. *Am. J. Med. Genet.*, 1982, 11:329-36.

neurofibromatosis. See *Recklinghausen disease (1).*

neurofibromatosis syndrome. See *Recklinghausen disease (1).*

neurofibromatosis type NF2. See *Gardner syndrome, under Gardner, W. J.*

neurofibromatosis-Noonan syndrome. A syndrome combining the characteristics of neurofibromatosis *(see Recklinghausen disease (1))* and the Noonan syndrome, including short stature, blapharoptosis, midface hypoplasia, short neck, and neurofibromatosis. The syndrome is transmitted as an autosomal dominant trait.

Rosenblatt, B., & Kaplan, P. A distinctive facies in neurofibromatosis. *Am. J. Hum. Genet.*, 1983, 35(6):115A.

neurogenic acro-osteolysis. See *Giaccai syndrome.*

neuroglial sclerosis. See *Chaslin syndrome.*

neurohepatic degeneration. See *Wilson disease, under Wilson, Samuel Alexander Kinnier.*

neuroichthyosis-hypogonadism syndrome. See *Rud syndrome.*

neuroleptic malignant syndrome (NMS). Synonym: *malignant neuroleptic syndrome.*

A complication of antipsychotic (neuroleptic) drug therapy, characterized by extrapyramidal symptoms such as parkinsonism, muscle rigidity, dystonia, akinesia, and tremor; autonomic dysfunction, including hyperthermia, tachycardia, diaphoresis, and blood pressure disorders; altered consciousness; leukocytosis; and elevation of creatine phosphokinase levels. Associated disorders may include dehydration, bacterial infection, rhabdomyosis, renal failure, respiratory insufficiency, and dysphagia. Neuroleptic drugs involved in this syndrome may include haloperidol, fluphenazine, chlorpromazine, trifluoroperazine, sulpiride, and thioridazine.

Shalev, A., & Mini, Z. The neuroleptic malignant syndrome. *Acta Psychiat. Scand.*, 1986, 73:337-4. Delay, J., & Deniker. Drug induced extrapyramidal syndrome. In: Vinken, D., & Gruyen, G., eds. *Handbook of clinical neurology.* Vol. 6. New York, Elsevier, 1968, pp. 248-66.

neuroleptic malignant-like syndrome. A neurological withdrawal disorder, similar to the neuroleptic malignant syndrome, characterized by hyperthermia, akinesis, altered consciousness, rigidity, and autonomic dysfunction, occurring after discontinuation of levodopa therapy of parkinsonism.

Friedman, J. H., *et al.* A neuroleptic malignantlike syndrome due to levodopa therapy withdrawal. *JAMA*, 1985, 254:2792-5.

neurolipomatosis. See *Dercum syndrome.*

neurologic-spinal fluid dissociation syndrome. See *Borries syndrome.*

neuromyelitis hyperalbumenotica. See *Guillain-Barré syndrome.*

neuromyelitis optica. See *Devic syndrome.*

neuronal ceroid lipofuscinosis (NCL). See *Kufs syndrome, and see Stock-Spielmeyer-Vogt syndrome.*

neuronal ceroid lipofuscinosis, infantile Finnish type. See *Haltia-Santavuori syndrome.*

neuronitis. See *Guillain-Barré syndrome.*

neuropathic arthritis. See *Charcot disease.*

neuropathic arthropathy. See *Charcot disease.*

neuropathic muscular atrophy. See *Charcot-Marie-Tooth syndrome.*

neuropsychiatric macrohyperglobulinemia syndrome. See *Bing-Neel syndrome, under Bing, Jens.*

neuroptic myelitis. See *Devic syndrome.*

neuroretino-angiomatosis. See *Bonnet-Dechaume-Blanc syndrome, under Bonnet, Paul.*

neurospongioblastoma. See *Cushing medulloblastoma.*

neurospongioblastosis diffusa. See *Bourneville-Pringle syndrome.*

neurospongioma. See *Cushing medulloblastoma.*

neurotabes peripherica. See *Déjerine syndrome (1).*

neurotrophic osseous atrophy. See *Giaccai syndrome.*

neurotrophic trigeminal ulceration. See *trigeminal trophic syndrome.*

neurovertebral dystonia. See *Barré-Lieou syndrome.*

neurovisceral lipidosis. See *gangliodisosis G_{M1} type I.*

neutropenia. See *Schultz syndrome.*

neutropenic hypersplenism-arthritis syndrome. See *Felty syndrome.*

neutrophil dysfunction syndrome. See *chronic granulomatous disease of childhood.*

neutrophilic dermatosis. See *Sweet syndrome.*

NEVE, ERNEST FREDERIC (British physician in Kashmir, 1861-1941)

Neve cancer. Synonym: *Kangri cancer.*

Epithelioma of the skin on the inner sides of the thighs and the anterior surface of the abdomen above and below the umbilicus, caused by the heat and volatile substances produced by the kangri, an earthenware bowl heated by means of charcoal and worn by some Kashmiris against the skin under a single loose garment.

Neve, E. F. Kangri-burn cancer. *Brit. Med. J.*, 1923, 2:1255-6.

nevi epitheliomatosi cystici. See *Brooke epithelioma.*

NEVIN, SAMUEL (British physician, born 1905)

Kiloh-Nevin syndrome (1 and 2). See *under Kiloh.*

Nevin syndrome (1). Synonyms: *presenile spongy encephalopathy, spongiform cerebral atrophy.*

Subacute encephalopathy occurring most commonly between the ages of 50 and 70 years, and characterized by blindness, motor paralysis, speech disorders, cerebellar symptoms, mental disorders, and myoclonus epilepsy. Pathological changes consist of a widespread loss of nerve cells in all layers of the cerebral cortex, especially in the occipital lobe, an associated astroglial reaction in the outer layers, and status spongiosus. Nevin suggested that the disorder is due to a form of vascular dysfunction without gross structural changes in the blood vessels. Some writers consider this and the Heidenhain syndrome to be analogous, both being variants of the Jakob-Creutzfeldt syndrome.

Nevin, S., *et al.* Subacute spongiform encephalopathy-a subacute form of encephalopathy attributable to vascular dysfunction (spongiform cerebral atrophy). *Brain*, 1960, 83:519-64.

Nevin syndrome (2). See *Kiloh-Nevin syndrome (2).*

nevoid amentia. See *Sturge-Weber syndrome.*

nevoid basal-cell carcinoma syndrome (NBCC, NBCCS, NBS). Synonyms: *Gorlin syndrome, Gorlin-Goltz syndrome, basal-cell nevus syndrome, hereditary cutaneomandibular polyoncosis, multiple basal-cell carcinoma syndrome, multiple hereditary cutaneomandibular polyoncosis, multiple nevoid basal-cell carcinoma syndrome (MNBCCS), naevoid basal-cell carcinoma syndrome, nevoid basal-cell epithelioma-jaw cysts-bifid rib syndrome.*

A syndrome of multiple nevoid basal-cell carcinoma, odontogenic keratocyst of the jaw, rib anomalies, and other defects, transmitted as an autosomal dominant trait with high penetrance and variable expressivity. The cutaneous symptoms include multiple nevoid basal-cell carcinomas with calcification, palmoplantar pits, and milia. Multiple jaw cysts and rare instances of fibrosarcoma of the jaws or ameloblastoma are the orofacial manifestations. Abnormalities of the skeletal system consist mainly of frontal and temporoparietal bossing, bridging of the sella, and other bone defects. Bifurcation, sometimes involving several ribs, may be associated with synostosis, pseudarthrosis, and cervical rudimentary ribs. The Sprengel deformity, hooking or dysplasia of the scapulae, and pectus excavatum and carinatum complicate some cases. Neurological features frequently include mental retardation, schizophrenia, congenital hydrocephalus, medulloblastoma, meningioma, nerve deafness, and other disorders. Cardiac fibroma, blindness, hypertelorism, and marfanoid build or unusually great height attained by the affected persons are frequently associated. Some endocrine disorders may occur.

Gorlin, R. J. Nevoid basal-cell carcinoma syndrome. *Medicine,* 1987, 66:98-113. Gorlin, R. J., & Goltz, R. W. Multiple nevoid basal-cell epithelioma, jaw cysts and bifid rib. A syndrome. *N. Engl. J. Med.,* 1960, 262:908-12. Jarisch. Zur Lehre von den Hautgeschwülsten. *Arch. Derm. Syph., Berlin,* 1894, 28:163-222.

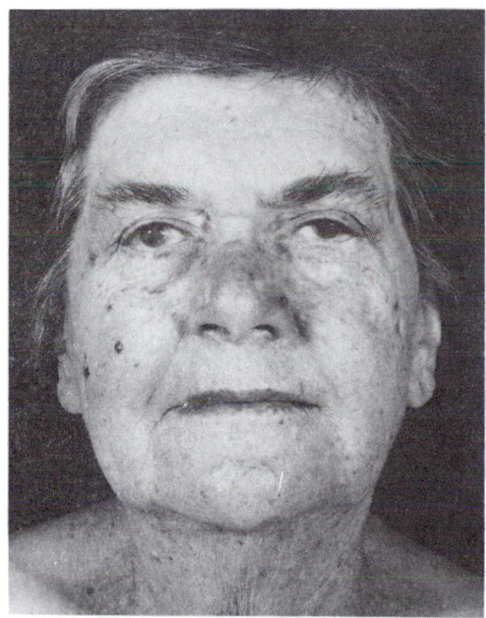

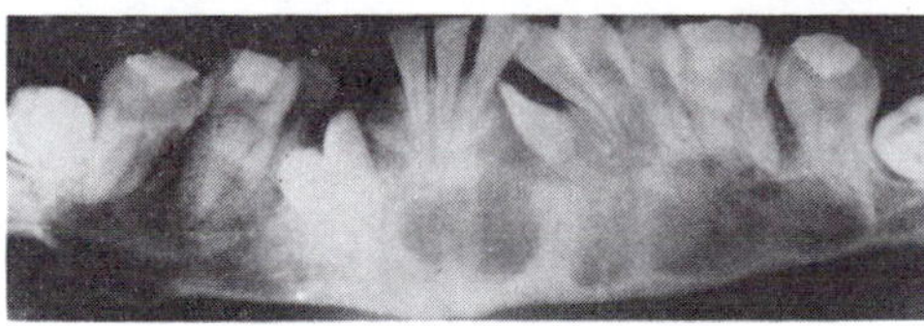

Nevoid basal cell carcinoma syndrome
Courtesy of Dr. Robert J. Gorlin, Minneapolis, MN.

nevoid basal-cell epithelioma-jaw cysts-bifid rib syndrome. See *nevoid basal-cell carcinoma syndrome.*

nevus anemicus. See *Vörner nevus.*

nevus epitheliomatosus sebaceus capitis. See *Wolters nevus.*

nevus follicularis. See *Brooke epithelioma.*

nevus fuscoceruleus. See *Ota nevus.*

nevus fuscoceruleus acromiodeltoideus. See *Ito nevus.*

nevus fuscoceruleus ophthalmomaxillaris. See *Ota nevus.*

nevus infectiosus. See *Hutchinson disease (1), under Hutchinson, Sir Jonathan.*

nevus lipomatodes cutaneus superficialis. See *Hoffmann-Zurhelle syndrome, under Hoffman, Erich.*

nevus lipomatodes superficialis subepidermalis. See *Hoffmann-Zurhelle syndrome, under Hoffman, Erich.*

nevus lupus. See *Hutchinson disease (1), under Hutchinson, Sir Jonathan.*

nevus osteohypertrophicus. See *Klippel-Trénaunay-Weber syndrome.*

nevus pigmentosus systematicus. See *Bloch-Sulzberger syndrome.*

nevus sebaceus linearis. See *epidermal nevus syndrome.*

nevus sebaceus of Feuerstein and Mims. See *epidermal nevus syndrome.*

nevus sebaceus of Jadassohn. See *Jadassohn nevus sebaceus, under Jadassohn, Josef.*

nevus spongiosus albus mucosae. See *white sponge nevus.*

nevus trichoepitheliomatosus adenoides cysticum. See *Brooke epithelioma.*

nevus varicosus osteohypertrophicus. See *Klippel-Trénaunay-Weber syndrome.*

NFDR. See *neurofaciodigitorenal syndrome.*

NHS. See *Nance-Horan syndrome.*

NICOLAS, JOSEPH (French physician, born 1868)

Durand-Nicolas-Favre disease. See *under Durand, J.*

Nicolas-Favre disease. See *Durand-Nicolas-Favre disease, under Durand, J.*

Nicolas-Moutot-Charlet syndrome. Synonym: *epidermolysis bullosa dystrophica ulcerovegetans.*

A familial, congenital, pemphigoid, mucocutaneous disease characterized initially by a single bulla or vesicle, followed by development of ulcerovegetative lesions, and associated with nail dystrophy and laryngeal stenosis due to cicatrization of the mucous membranes.

Nicolas, J., Moutot, H., & Charlet, H. Dermatose congénitale et familiale à lésions trophiques progressives et chroniques ulcéro-végétantes, à début pemphigoïde, avec dystrophies unguéales. Varieté nouvelle de pemphigus congénital de forme dystrophique. *Ann. Derm. Syph., Paris,* 1913, 4:385-414.

NICOLAU, STEFAN GEORGE (Rumanian physician)

Nicolau syndrome. Accidental intra-arterial injection of various drugs (including penicillin) in intended intramuscular injection, resulting in immediate pain at the site of injection, followed by swelling, edema, livid discoloration, and, sometimes, arterial embolism, necrosis, and gangrene. See also *Hoigne syndrome.*

Nicolau, S. Dermite livédoïde et gangréneuse de la fesse consécutive aux injections intra-musculaires dans la syphilis. A propos d'un cas d'embolie artérielle bismuthique. *Ann. Mal. Vener., Paris,* 1925, 20:321-39.

nicotinic acid deficiency encephalopathy. Synonyms: *Jolliffe syndrome, nicotinic acid deficiency syndrome.*

A syndrome of clouding of consciousness followed by coma, cogwheel rigidity of the extremities, and uncontrollable gasping and sucking reflexes due to nicotinic acid deficiency. The syndrome may be associated with nutritional deficiency syndromes, such as Wernicke disease, pellagra, scurvy, and polyneuropathy. There have been no reports of this condition since 1947.

Jolliffe, N., *et al.* Nicotinic acid deficiency encephalopathy. *JAMA,* 1940, 114:307-12.

nicotinic acid deficiency syndrome. See *nicotinic acid deficiency encephalopathy.*

NICU (nonimmunologic contact urticaria). See *under contact urticaria syndrome.*

NIELSEN, HERMAN (Danish physician, 1882-1960)

Nielsen syndrome. Synonyms: *Ullrich-Nielsen syndrome, dystrophia brevicollis congenita.*

A syndrome of short stature, blepharoptosis, cleft palate, abnormal fusion of the vertebrae, pterygium colli, and campodactyly transmitted as an X-linked dominant trait.

Nielsen, H. Dystrofia brevicollis congenita. *Hospitalstidende*, 1934, 77:409-23.

Ullrich-Nielsen syndrome. See *Nielsen syndrome.*

NIELSEN, JOHANNES MYGAARD (Danish-born American neurologist, 1890-1969)

Nielsen syndrome. Synonym: *generalized neuromuscular exhaustion syndrome.*

Weakness with muscular atrophy and fascicular twitching caused by extreme physical exhaustion.

Nielsen, J. M. A subacute generalized neuromuscular exhaustion syndrome. *JAMA*, 1940, 126:801-6.

NIEMANN, ALBERT (German physician, 1880-1921)

Niemann disease. See *Niemann-Pick syndrome.*

Niemann-Pick (NP) syndrome. Synonyms: *Crocker syndrome, Niemann disease, Pick disease, essential lipoid histiocytosis, lipid histiocytosis, phosphatidolipoidosis, phosphatidosis, sphingomyelin lipidosis, sphingomyelinosis, sphingomyelin reticuloendotheliosis.*

An inherited syndrome, transmitted as an autosomal recessive trait, characterized by faulty metabolism of the sphingomyelin-cleaving enzyme, sphingomyelinase, with resulting accumulation of sphingomyelin and cholesterol in foam cells of various organs, including the reticuloendothelial system, liver, spleen, lungs, kidneys, pancreas, and heart. The syndrome occurs primarily in children and is marked by mental and physical retardation, failure to thrive, hepatomegaly, splenomegaly, anemia, cherry red spot of the macula with progressive blindness, Niemann-Pick cells in the bone marrow, widening of the medullary spaces, coarsening of the trabeculae, stippled calcifications in the feet, osteoporosis with spontaneous fractures, coxa valga, pulmonary infiltrations, hepatic and pulmonary calcifications, and calcium deposits in the sacrum and coccyx. About 40% of cases occur in patients of Jewish ancestry. Five clinically distiguishable phenotypes are recognized: **Type A** (the severe infantile form) represents 75 to 80% of all cases, and is characterized by extensive neurological involvement, visceral accumulation of sphingomyelin, and death within the first 3 years of life. **Type B** (the visceral or chronic form) is characterized by. massive visceral involvement with enlargement of various organs but no central nervous system complications; the symptoms appear between 2 and 4 years of life. **Type C** (the subacute or juvenile type) is moderate in course, being similar to Type A but appearing later in life. **Type D** (the Nova Scotia type) has a slow development of symptoms with neurological disorders and appears in early or middle childhood. **Type E** (generally observed in adults) is marked by moderate hepatosplenomegaly and some increase of sphingomyelin in the liver and spleen.

Niemann, A. Ein unbekanntes Krankheitsbild. *Jb. Kinderheilk.*, 1914, 79:1-10. Pick, L. Der Morbus Gaucher und die ihm ähnlichen Krankheiten (die lipoidzellige Splenohepatomegalie Typus Niemann und die diabetische Lipoidzellenhypoplasie der Milz). *Erg. Inn. Med. Kinderh.*, 1926, 29:519-627. Crocker, A. C., & Farber, S. Niemann-Pick disease: A review of eighteen patients. *Medicine, Baltimore*, 1958, 37:1-95.

NIERHOFF, H. (German physician)

Nierhoff-Hübner syndrome. A variant of dysostosis enchondralis characterized by faulty ossification of the skull, vertebrae, ribs, and long bones in newborn infants. Most severely affected is the systemic epiphyseal and metaphyseal ossification of the long bones, a defect that results in shortening of extremities with bowing and thickening of the distal ends. The skull is exceptionally soft. The affected infants die within a few days after birth, usually after an attack of clonic seizures. The syndrome is transmitted as an autosomal dominant trait with incomplete penetration.

Nierhoff, H., & Hübner, O. Familiäre systematisierte enchondrale Dysostose bei 3 Geschwistern. *Zschr. Kinderh.*, 1956, 78:497-521.

NIEVERGELT, KURT (Swiss orthopedic surgeon, born 1913)

mesomelic dwarfism, Nievergelt type. See *Nievergelt syndrome.*

Nievergelt syndrome. Synonyms: *Nievergelt-Erb syndrome; Nievergelt-Pearlman syndrome; mesomelic dwarfism, Nievergelt type.*

A rare bone disease characterized by deformities of the radius, ulna, tibia, and fibula. Shortening and deformity of the lower legs and, occasionally, the forearm and radio-ulnar synostosis are its main features. The tibia and fibula have a characteristic rhomboid form (crura rhomboidei). Synostosis of the tarsal and metatarsal bones, clubfoot, big toe deformities, and dysplasia of the ankle joint may occur. Restricted mobility of the elbows and luxation or subluxation of the radial head are usually present. The disease was originally described in a father and his three sons by different mothers. It is believed to be transmitted as an autosomal dominant trait with variability of expression.

Nievergelt, K. Positiver Vaterschaftnachweis aut Grund erblicher Missbildungen der Extremetaten. *Arch. Julius Klaus Stift.*, 1944, 19:157-60. Pearlman, H. S., *et al.* Familial tarsal and carpal synostosis with radial-head subluxation (Nievergelt's syndrome). *J. Bone Joint Surg.* 1964, 46-A:585-92.

Nievergelt-Erb syndrome. See *Nievergelt syndrome.*

Nievergelt-Pearlman syndrome. See *Nievergelt syndrome.*

night death. See *sudden unexplained death syndrome.*

nigremia. See *Tamura-Takahashi syndrome.*

nigrospinodentatal degeneration with nuclear ophthalmoplegia. See *Joseph disease, under Joseph, Antone.*

NIIKAWA, N. (Japanese physician)

Niikawa-Kuroki syndrome. See *Kabuki make-up syndrome.*

NIJSSEN, RENE. See NYSSEN, RENE

NIKOLSKII (NIKOLSKY), PETR VASILEVICH (Russian physician, 1858-1940)

Nikolskii sign. Synonym: *Nikolsky sign.*

A condition in which the outer layer of the skin is easily removed by a minor injury or rubbing.

Nikolsky sign. See *Nikolskii sign.*

NIKOLSKY, PYOTR VASILYEVICH. See NIKOLSKII, PETR VASILEVICH

ninth day erythema. See *Milian erythema.*
NISBET, WILLIAM (British physician, 1759-1822)
Nisbet chancre. A soft chancre with acute lymphangitis followed by nodular abscesses of the penis.
*Nisbet, W. *First lines on the theory and practice in veneral diseases.* Edinburgh, Elliot, 1787.

NISHIMOTO, A. (Japanese physician)
Nishimoto disease. Synonym: *Nishimoto-Takeuchi syndrome.*
A vascular syndrome, identified mainly by angiographic examination, characterized by bilateral anomalous carotid arteries; stenosis of the intracranial part of the internal carotid artery and/or its main branches, the anterior and middle cerebral arteries; presence of numerous capillarylike vessels at the base of the brain, known as moya-moya (q.v.); a lack of venous drainage from the capillaries, thus contrasting with arteriovenous malformations; and frequent corticodural arterial anastomoses. The condition was once believed to be confined to the Japanese, but it is now known to occur in other ethnic groups.
*Nishimoto, A., & Sugin, R. Hemangiomatous malformations of bilateral internal carotid artery at the base of the brain: Preliminary report. *Ann. Meeting Neuroradiol. Assoc. Japan*, Tokyo, 1964, 5:2-9. *Takeuchi, K. Occlusive diseases of the carotid artery; especially on their surgical treatment. *Shinkei Shimpo,* 1961, 5:511-43. Pecker, J., *et al.* Nishimoto disease: Significance of its angiographic appearance. *Neuroradiology*, 1973, 5:223-30.
Nishimoto-Takeuchi syndrome. See *Nishimoto disease.*
NME (necrolytic migratory erythema). See *under glucagonoma syndrome.*
NMS. See *neuroleptic malignant syndrome.*
NNNB (nonneurogenic neurogenic bladder). See *Hinman syndrome.*
NOACH (neuro-anatomical aberrations-orthoptic anomalies-absence of macular and foveal reflex-congenital nystagmus-hypopigmentation) syndrome. Synonym: *albinism syndrome.*
A hereditary and congenital inborn error of metabolism related to the pigment cell, and resulting in a systemic disorder that is characterized by anomalies of the eyes and hypopigmentation or absence of pigment in the skin, hair, and eyes, and which is associated with neuro-anatomical disorders. See also *albinism.*
Dorp, D. B., van. Albinism, or the NOACH syndrome. (The book of Enoch c.v. 1-20). *Clin. Genet.*, 1987, 31:228-42.

NOACK, M. (German physician)
Noack syndrome. See *Pfeiffer syndrome, under Pfeiffer, Rudolf Arthur.*
nocturnal arm dysesthesia. See *Wartenberg disease (1).*
nocturnal arm paresthesia. See *Wartenberg disease (1).*
nocturnal sleep apnea. See *sleep apnea syndrome.*
nodding spasm. See *West syndrome.*
nodular corneal dystrophy. See *Groenouw dystrophy (1).*
nodular degeneration of the cornea. See *Salzmann dystrophy.*
nodular dermal allergid. See *Gougerot-Ruiter syndrome.*
nodular elastoidosis. See *Favre-Racouchot disease.*
nodular lichenification. See *Hyde syndrome.*
nodular panencephalitis. See *Pette-Döring encephalitis.*
nodular prurigo. See *Hyde syndrome.*
nodular vasculitis. See *Bazin disease.*
noduli corneae. See *Groenouw dystrophy (1).*
nonbacterial regional lymphadenitis. See *cat scratch disease.*
nonbacterial verrucous endocarditis. See *Libman-Sacks syndrome.*
nongonococcal urethritis with conjunctivitis and arthritis. See *Reiter syndrome.*
nonhypoglycemia. See *Yager-Young syndrome.*
nonimmunologic contact urticaria (NICU). See *under contact urticaria syndrome.*
nonlipid reticuloendotheliosis. See *Letterer-Siwe syndrome.*
nonluetic Argyll Robertson pupil. See *Adie syndrome.*
NONNE, MAX (German physician, 1861-1959)
Nonne compression syndrome. See *Froin syndrome.*
Nonne syndrome (1). Cerebellar agenesis.
*Nonne, M. Über das Vorkommen von starker Phase I-Reaktion bei fehlender bei 6 Fällen von Rückenmarkstumor. *Deut. Zschr. Nervenheil.*, 1910, 40:161-7.
Nonne syndrome (2). See *scalenus anticus syndrome.*
Nonne-Froin syndrome. See *Froin syndrome.*
Nonne-Marie syndrome. See *Marie syndrome (1), under Marie, Pierre.*

Nonne-Milroy syndrome. Synonyms: *Milroy disease; congential lymphedema; elephantiasis congenita hereditaria; hereditary lymphedema type I; lymphedema, early onset type.*
A familial form of pitting, painless lymphedema of the limbs, which is present from birth, usually in association with intestinal lymphangiectasia or cholestasis. There is no tendency to ulcerate. The syndrome is transmitted as an autosomal dominant trait with variable expressivity. **Hereditary lymphedema type I (Nonne-Milroy syndrome)** and **type II (Meige syndrome)** were in the past combined into a single syndrome, the **Nonne-Milroy-Meige syndrome;** they are now considered two distinct entities. See also *Quincke edema.*
Nonne, M. Vier Fälle von Elephantiasis congenita hereditaria. *Arch. Path. Anat., Berlin*, 1891, 125:189-96. Milroy, W. F. An undescribed variety of hereditary edema. *N. Y. Med. J.*, 1892, 56:505-8.
Nonne-Pierre Marie syndrome. See *Marie syndrome (1), under Marie, Pierre.*
NONNENBRUCH, WILHELM (German physician, 1887-1955)
Nonnenbruch syndrome. Synonyms: *extrarenal kidney syndrome, extrarenal oliguria.*
Oliguria without renal changes.
Nonnenbruch, W. U. Über das entzündliche Ödem der Niere und das hepatorenale Syndrom. *Deut. Med. Wschr.*, 1937, 63:7-10.
nonneurogenic neurogenic bladder (NNNB). See *Hinman syndrome.*
nonneurogenic neuromuscular dysfunction. See *Hinman syndrome.*
nonobstructive colonic dilatation. See *Ogilvie syndrome.*
nonosteogenic fibroma. See *Jaffe-Lichtenstein disease.*
nonrachitic bowleg in children. See *Erlacher-Blount syndrome.*
nonrecognition misidentification. See *Capgras syndrome.*

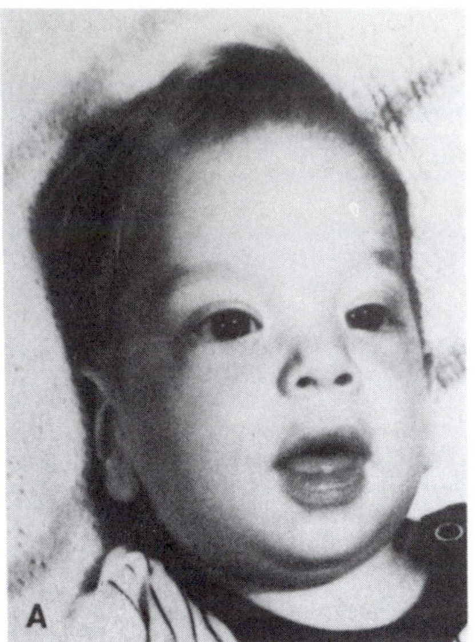

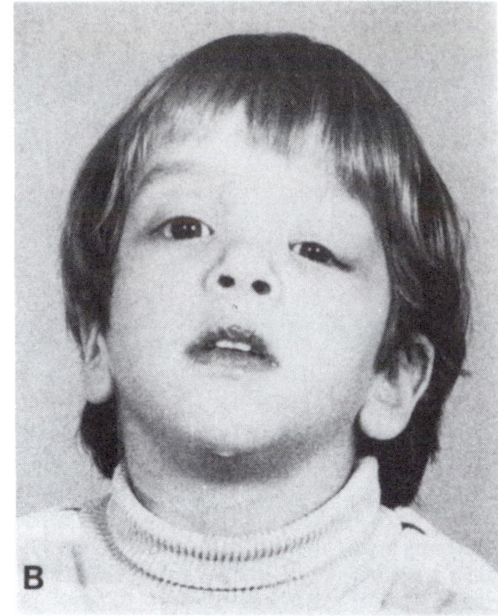

Noonan syndrome
Quattrin, Teresa, Elspeth McPerson & Theodore Putnam, *American Journal of Medical Genetics* 26:645-649, 1987. New York: Alan R. Liss, Inc.

nonsense syndrome. See *Ganser syndrome.*

nonspecific hip synovitis. See *observation hip syndrome.*

nonspecific retroperitoneal inflammation. See *Ormond syndrome.*

nonsyphilitic interstitial keratitis. See *Cogan syndrome (1).*

nontraumatic dislocation of atlanto-axial joint. See *Grisel syndrome.*

nontropical idiopathic splenomegaly. See *Dacie syndrome.*

nontropical sprue. See *Whipple disease.*

nontumorous hypergastrinemic hyperchlorhydria (NTHH) syndrome. See *pseudo-Zollinger-Ellison syndrome, under Zollinger.*

nonuse bone atrophy. See *Allison atrophy.*

NOONAN, JACQUELINE ANNE (American pediatric cardiologist)

neurofibromatosis-Noonan syndrome. See *neurofibromatosis.*

Noonan syndrome. Synonyms: *familial Turner syndrome, female pseudo-Turner syndrome, male Turner syndrome, pseudo-Ullrich-Turner syndrome, Turner-like syndrome, Turner phenotype with normal karyotype, Turner syndrome in female with X chromosome, Ullrich-Noonan syndrome, XX Turner phenotype syndrome, XY Turner phenotype syndrome.*

A congenital syndrome with the Turner phenotype (see *chromosome XO syndrome*) and normal karyotype, marked by growth and mental retardation; seizures; craniofacial abnormalities, consisting of blepharoptosis, antimongoloid slant of palpebral fissures, inner epicanthal folds, hypertelorism, prominent and fleshy low-set abnormal ears, high-arched palate, micrognathia; tooth abnormalities, including malocclusion; neck abnormalities, such as short or webbed neck and low posterior hairline; shield chest with wide-set nipples; cardiovascular defects, including atrial septal defect, pulmonary valvular and supravalvular stenosis, ventricular septal defect, aneurysm of the ventricular septum causing infundibular stenosis, mitral insufficiency, and possible an Ebstein abnormality; and limb defects, mainly cubitus valgus, short stubby hands, and clinodactyly of the fifth fingers. Nerve deafness, kyphoscoliosis, edema of the hands and feet, simian creases, curly hair, skin nevi, keloids, hyperelastic skin, and hypogonadism may be associated. Most cases are sporadic, but an autosomal dominant inheritance has been indicated in some cases. Some writers consider the Noonan and Turner syndromes the same entity, others believe they are separate disorders, and still others consider Watson and LEOPARD syndromes as being indistinguishable from the Noonan syndrome.

Noonan, J. A., & Ehmke, D. A. Associated noncardiac malformations in children with congenital heart disease. *J. Pediat.*, 1963, 63:468-70.

Saldino-Noonan syndrome. See *under Saldino.*

short rib-polydactyly syndrome, Saldino-Noonan type. See *Saldino-Noonan syndrome.*

Turner-Noonan syndrome. See *Noonan syndrome.*

Ullrich-Noonan syndrome. See *Noonan syndrome.*

NORDAU, MAX SIMON (German scientist and social critic, 1849-1923)

Nordau disease. Synonyms: *degeneracy, nordauism.*

Deterioration of the powers of body and mind.

*Nordau, M. S. *Dégénérescence*. Paris, Alcan, 1894.

nordauism. See *Nordau disease.*

NORIO, REIJO (Finnish physician)

Salonen-Herva-Norio syndrome. See *hydrolethalus syndrome.*

normal coronary angina pectoris. See *X syndrome.*

normal pressure hydrocephalus. See *Hakim syndrome.*

NORMAN, MARGARET G. (Canadian physician)

Norman-Roberts syndrome. Synonym: *lissencephaly syndrome.*

A rare congenital syndrome, transmitted as an autosomal recessive trait, characterized by cerebral and craniofacial anomalies and neurological disorders. Brain abnormalities include lissencephaly (widespread agyria), heterotopias, failure of opercularization, enlarged ventricles, and probable hypoplasia of the corpus callosum. Craniofacial abnormalities consist of microcephaly, bitemporal hollowing, prominent occiput, low and sloping forehead, hypertelorism, broad and prominent nasal bridge, and micrognathia. Mental retardation, decreased spontaneous activity, feeding difficult, and seizures are the neurologic manifestations. Low birth weight and clinodactyly are usually associated. See also *Miller-Dieker syndrome.*

Norman, M. G., Roberts, M., *et al.* Lissencephaly, *Canad. J. Neurol. Sc.,* 1976, 3:39-46. Dobyns, W. B., *et al.* Syndromes with lissencephaly. I. Miller-Dieker and Norman-Roberts syndromes and isolated lissencephaly. *Am. J. Med. Genet.,* 1984, 18:509-26.

NORMAN, R. M. (British physician)

Norman-Landing syndrome. See *gangliosidosis G_{M1} type I.*

normotensive hydrocephalus. See *Hakim syndrome.*

NORRIE, GORDON (Danish ophthalmologist, 1855-1941)

Norrie syndrome. Synonyms: *Norrie-Warburg syndrome, atrophia bulborum hereditaria, congenital progressive oculo-acoustico-cerebral degeneration, pseudoglioma congenita.*

A rare X-linked recessive syndrome of retinal malformations, deafness, and mental retardation and/or deterioration. The affected boys present bilateral blindness at birth or during the first month of life, which is associated with pseudoglioma, vitreous opacities, preretinal proliferation, cataracts, corneal opacity, and microphtalmia. Severe progressive mental retardation takes place from 18 months to 5 years. The hearing impairment may appear from childhood to middle life.

Norrie, G. Causes of blindness in children. *Acta Ophth., Copenhagen,* 1927, 5:363-64. Warburg, M. Norrie's disease (atrophia bulborum hereditaria). A report of 11 cases of hereditary bilateral pseudotumor of the retina, complicated by deafness and mental deficiency. *Acta Ophth., Copenhagen,* 1963, 41:134-46.

Norrie-Warburg syndrome. See *Norrie syndrome.*

North American blastomycosis. See *Gilchrist disease.*

Norwegian itch. See *Boeck scabies.*

Norwegian scabies. See *Boeck scabies.*

NOTHNAGEL, CARL WILHELM HERMANN (German physician, 1841-1905)

Nothnagel acroparesthesia. Synonyms: *angiospastic acroparesthesia, vasomotor acroparesthesia.*

Acroparesthesia in adults, secondary to vasomotor disorders, characterized by tingling, numbness, stiffness, cyanosis, blanching, and edema, which may end in recovery or progress on to gangrene. See also *Raynaud syndrome.*

Nothnagel. Zur Lehre von den vasomotorischen Neurosens. *Deut. Arch. Klin. Med.,* 1867, 2:173-91.

Nothnagel syndrome (1). Synonym: *angina pectoris vasomotoria.*

Blanching of the skin, general pallor, and widespread vasoconstriction after exposure to cold. See also *Raynaud syndrome.*

Nothnagel, H. Angina pectoris vasomotoria. *Deut. Arch. Klin. Med.,* 1867, 3:309-22.

Nothnagel syndrome (2). Synonym: *ophthalmoplegia-cerebellar ataxia syndrome.*

Unilateral oculomotor paralysis associated with cerebellar ataxia in lesions of the cerebral peduncles.

Nothnagel, H. *Topische Diagnostik der Gehirnkrankheiten.* Berlin, Hirschwalden, 1879, p. 220.

novobasalioma. See *Arning carcinoid.*

NP. See *Niemann-Pick syndrome.*

NTHH (nontumorous hypergastrinemic hyperchlorhydria) syndrome. See *pseudo-Zollinger-Ellison syndrome, under Zollinger.*

nuchal cyst syndrome. A syndrome consisting of four causally and pathogenetically different entities: (1) nuchal cysts in otherwise normal fetuses; (2) multiple congenital malformations in fetuses with a peculiar appearance; (3) an apparently autosomal recessive syndrome of multiple cysts that extend into deep muscular planes, generalized edema, cleft palate, peculiar skeletal characteristics, acutely angulated ribs producing a bell-shaped cage, and shortened long bones; and (4) multiple inherited abnormalities (multiple pterygium, Roberts syndrome) and chromosomal disorders (trisomy 13, trisomy 21), representing both primary and secondary lesions.

Elejaide, B. R., *et al.* Nuchal cysts syndromes: Etiology, pathogenesis, and prenatal diagnosis. *Am. J. Med. Genet.,* 1985, 21:417-32.

nucleus ambiguus-hypoglossal syndrome. See *Tapia syndrome.*

nummular keratitis. See *Dimmer keratitis.*

nursing bottle syndrome (NBS). See *baby bottle syndrome.*

nursing caries. See *baby bottle syndrome.*

nutcracker phenomenon. See *nutcracker syndrome.*

nutcracker syndrome. Synonyms: *left renal vein compression syndrome, nutcracker phenomenon, renal vein compression syndrome, renal vein entrapment syndrome.*

Compression of the left renal vein between the aorta and superior mesenteric artery, which results in renal vein and left gonadal vein varices. Hematuria and pain are the principal clinical features.

Schepper, A., de. "Nutcracker"-fenomeen van de vena renalis en veneuze pathologie van de linker nier. *J. Belge Radiol.,* 1972, 55:507-11.

nutritional amblyopia. See *Obal syndrome.*

nutritional deficiency syndrome with hypopotassemia. See *Achor-Smith syndrome.*

nutritional dermatosis. See *Stryker-Halbeisen syndrome.*

nutritional edema syndrome. See *kwashiorkor.*

nutritional megaloblastic anemia in India. See *Wills anemia.*

nutritional melalgia. See *burning feet syndrome.*

nutritional sensory neuropathy syndrome. A proprioceptive neuropathy with sensory involvement, including loss of proprioception with resultant pseudoathetosis involving the upper and lower extremities and, occasionally, cranial nerves; motor weakness with absent or decreased reflexes; and fatty deposits about the neurons. A state of nutritional deprivation with or without parenteral hyperalimentation is the cause. The syndrome occurs after gastric stapling for morbid obesity and in association with nutritional disorders or stavation in nonobese patients.

Feit, H., *et al.* Peripheral neuropathy and starvation after gastric partitioning for morbid obesity. *Ann. Intern. Med.,*

1982, 96:453-5. May, W. E.. Nutritional sensory neuropathy. An emerging new syndrome. *Arch. Neur., Chicago,* 1984, 41:559-60.

NYGAARD, KAARE KRISTIAAN (American physician)

Nygaard-Brown syndrome. Synonyms: *essential thrombophilia, generalized subacute thrombophilia.*

An occlusive disease that may involve the arteries of the extremities, brain, kidneys, and heart, preceded by migrating or localized thrombosis. The disease shows a tendency toward relapse, with recurrence of thrombosis. There is associated hypercoagulability of the blood, and gangrene is a frequent complication.

Nygaard, K. K., & Brown, G. E. Essential thrombophilia. Report of five cases. *Arch. Int. Med., Chicago,* 1937, 59:82-106.

NYHAN, WILLIAM LEO (American physician, born 1926)

Lesch-Nyhan syndrome (LNS). See *under Lesch.*

Sakati-Nyhan-Tisdale syndrome. See *under Sakati.*

NYSSEN (NIJSSEN), RENE (Belgian neurologist)

Nyssen-van Bogaert-Meyer syndrome. Synonyms: *atrophia opticocochleodentata, opticocochleodentate degeneration.*

Congenital degeneration of the optic, cochlear, dentate, and medial lemniscal structures, transmitted as an autosomal recessive trait, manifested by optic atrophy with blindness, deafness, defective speech, spasticity, hyperkinetic behavior, contractures, mental deterioration, and death before the age of 10 years. Pathological findings include neuronal loss of the telencephalon with degeneration of corticofugal pathways and gliosis, increasing in severity nucleodistally in the corticonuclear tracts; loss of Purkinje and cerebellar granule cells; possible status marmoratus of the anterior and median thalamus; and degeneration of neurons of the dentate, cochlear, and dorsal medullary nuclei with demyelination and sclerosis of their fiber paths and of the primary optic system.

Nyssen, R., & van Bogaert, L. La dégénérescence systématisée optico-cochléo-dentelée. *Rev. Neur., Paris,* 1934, 2:321-45. Meyer, J. E. Über eine kombinierte Systemerkrankung in Klein, Mittel- und Endhirn. (Dégénérescence systématisée optico-cochléo-dentelée). *Arch. Psychiat. Nervenkr.,* 1949, 182:731-58. Muller, J., & Zeman, W. Dégénérescence systematisée optico-cochléo-dentelée. *Acta Neuropath.,* 1965, 5:26-39.

van Bogaert-Nijssen disease. See *metachromatic leukodystrophy.*

van Bogaert-Nijssen-Peiffer syndrome. See *metachromatic leukodystrophy.*

van Bogaert-Nyssen syndrome. See *metachromatic leukodystrophy.*

van Bogaert-Nyssen-Peiffer syndrome. See *metachromatic leukodystrophy.*

nystagmus retractorius. See Koerber-Salus-Elschnig syndrome.

nystagmus-myoclonus syndrome. See *Lenoble-Aubineau syndrome.*

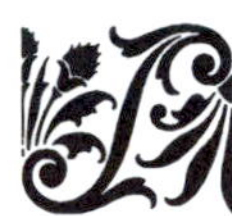

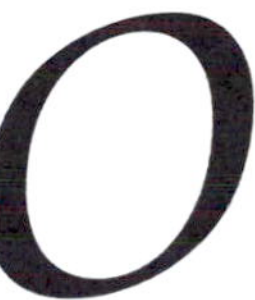

OASD. See *ocular albinism-sensorineural deafness syndrome.*

oasthouse syndrome. See *methionine malabsorption syndrome.*

oat cell carcinoma. See *Barnard carcinoma.*

OAV. See *oculo-auriculovertebral dysplasia.*

OBAL, ADALBERT (American physician)

Obal syndrome. Synonyms: *camp eyes, nutritional amblyopia, polydeficiency-retrobulbar neuritis syndrome.*

Severe malnutrition associated with ocular disorders, including amblyopia, retrobulbar neuritis, scotoma, color vision disturbances, nyctalopia, and photophobia. The symptoms include edema, paresthesia, pruritus, skin eruption, cachexia, diarrhea, polyneuritis, hormonal disorders, impotence, and gynecomastia. The syndrome was observed most frequently among soldiers, prisoners of war, and concentration camp inmates during and after World Wars I and II.

Obal, A. Nutritional amblyopia. *Am. J. Ophth.*, 1951, 34:857-65.

obesity-heart failure syndrome. See *Pickwick syndrome.*

obesity-hypoventilation syndrome (OHS). See *Pickwick syndrome.*

obliteration of supra-aortic branches. See *aortic arch syndrome.*

obliterative brachiocephalic arteritis syndrome. See *aortic arch syndrome.*

O'BRIEN, CECIL STARLING (American physician, born 1889)

O'Brien cataract. Synonyms: *snow-flake cataract, snowstorm cataract.*

A cataract characterized by numerous small grayish flaky opacities, seen most frequently in diabetes mellitus.

O'Brien, C. S., *et al.* Diabetic cataract. Incidence and morphology in 126 diabetic patients. *JAMA*, 1934, 103:892-7.

OBRINSKY, WILLIAM (American physician, born 1913)

Obrinsky syndrome. See *prune belly syndrome.*

observation hip syndrome. Synonyms: *acute transient epiphysitis, coxalgia fugax, coxitis fugax, coxitis serosa seu simplex, hip synovitis in childhood, intermittent hydrathrosis, irritable hip, toxic hip synovitis, transient hip synovitis, nonspecific hip synovitis, phantom hip, transient epiphysitis, transitory coxitis, transitory hip arthritis.*

A transient hip disorder of children and adolescents, characterized by acute pain, limited motion, and limping. Associated disorders may include fever, soft tissue swelling, contracture, increased erythrocyte sedimentation rate, and slight leukocytosis. X-ray findings may show occasional pericapsular inflammation, widening of the joint space, and demineralization; but, in most instances, there are no visible changes. Inflammation due to trauma or infection is believed to be the cause. Complete recovery usually takes place in a few weeks. Children affected by this disorder, often with normal radiograms, are usually admitted to hospitals for observation, hence the designation "observation hip syndrome."

Lovett, R. W., & Morse, J. L. A transient or ephemeral form of hip disease, with a report of a case. *Boston Med. Surg. J.*, 1892, 127:161-3. Butler, R. W. Transitory arthritis of the hip-joint in childhood. An investigation of arthritis of the hip in ninety-seven children. *Brit. Med. J.*, 1933, 1:951-4. Fernandez de Valderrama, J. A. The "observation hip" syndrome and its late sequale. *J. Bone Joint Surg.*, 1963, 45B:462-70.

obstetric diaphragmatic paralysis. See *Kofferath syndrome.*

obstructive azospermia-sinopulmonary infection syndrome. See *Young syndrome, under Young, Donald.*

obstructive lung disease. See *airway obstruction syndrome.*

obstructive pulmonary syndrome. See *airway obstruction syndrome.*

obstructive sleep apnea syndrome (OSAS). See *under sleep apnea syndrome.*

obstructive ventilatory abnormality. See *airway obstruction syndrome.*

obui-himo syndrome. Cyanosis of an upper extremity associated with congenital absence of the cephalic vein in infants carried in the obui-himo (a cloth strap device used in Japan for carrying infants and young children). The symptoms are usually relieved by discontinuing use of the obui-himo.

Osano, M., et al. Cyanosis of the arms associated with anomalies of the veins. Obui-himo syndrome. *Am. J. Dis. Child.*, 1969, 118:473-82.

OCA TY neg (oculocutaneous tyrosinase-negative albinism). See *albinism I syndrome.*

OCA TY pos (oculocutaneous tyrosinase-positive albinism). See *albinism II syndrome.*

occipital-cervical-shoulder girdle syndrome. See *Coleman syndrome.*

occipitofaciocervicothoraco-abdominodigital dysplasia (OFCTAD). See *spondylothoracic dysplasia.*

occlusion of supra-aortic trunk syndrome. See *aortic arch syndrome.*

occult neurogenic bladder. See *Hinman syndrome.*

occupational cervicobrachial disorder. See *shoulder pain syndrome.*

occupational cervicobrachial syndrome. See *overuse syndrome.*

occupational Raynaud disease. See *vibration syndrome.*

occupational stress syndrome. See *burnout syndrome.*

OCR (**o**culo**c**erebro**r**enal) syndrome. See *Lowe syndrome, and see aniridia-Wilms tumor syndrome.*

OCS (**O**ndine **c**urse **s**yndrome). See *Ondine curse.*

OCSD (**o**culo**c**ranio**s**omatic **d**isease). See *Kearns-Sayre syndrome.*

ocular albinism-sensorineural deafness (OASD) syndrome. Synonym: *deafness-ocular albinism syndrome.*

A syndrome of late-onset sensorineural deafness and ocular albinism, transmitted as an X-linked trait.

Winship, I., *et al.* X-linked inheritance of ocular albinism with late-onset sensorineural deafness. *Am. J. Med. Genet.*, 1984, 19:797-803.

ocular and cutaneous melanosis. See *Ota nevus.*

ocular and dermal melanocytosis. See *Ota nevus.*

ocular contusion syndrome. See *Frenkel syndrome.*

ocular myodystrophy. See *Kiloh-Nevin syndrome (2).*

ocular myopathy. See *Kiloh-Nevin syndrome (2).*

ocular retraction syndrome. See *Stilling-Türk-Duane syndrome.*

oculo-auricular vertebral dysplasia. See *oculo-auriculovertebral dysplasia.*

oculo-auriculocutaneous syndrome. See *Burns syndrome.*

oculo-auriculovertebral (OAV) dysplasia. Synonyms: *Goldenhar syndrome (GS), Goldenhar-Gorlin syndrome, branchial arches syndrome, dysplasia oculo-auricularis, facio-auriculovertebral anomalad, first and second branchial arch syndrome, hemifacial microsomia (HM), hemignathia and microtia syndrome, intrauterine facial necrosis, lateral facial dysplasia (LFD), mandibulofacial dysostosis with epibulbar dermoids syndrome, necrotic facial dysplasia, oculo-auriculovertebral syndrome, oculo-auricular vertebral dysplasia, oromandibulo-otic syndrome, otofacial dysostosis, otomandibular syndrome, otomandibular facial dysmorphogenesis.*

An error in the development of the first and second branchial arches, associated with various anomalies. The facies may be striking because of asymmetric hypoplasia of the maxillary, malar, and temporal bones acompanied by hypoplasia of the facial muscles. Some patients show aplasia or hypoplasia of the mandibular ramus and condyle. The mastoid bone may be flattened. One eye may be lower than the other. Vertebral defects usually include occipitalization of the atlas, cuneiform vertebra, synostosis of the cervical vertebrae, supernumerary vertebrae, hemivertebrae, and spina bifida. Ear abnormalities may vary from complete aplasia to distorted and displaced pinna and deafness. Preauricular tags and pits may be associated. Oral abnormalities usually include lateral facial clefts (macrostomia), agenesis of the parotid glands, salivary fistulae, displaced salivary glands, and epibulbar dermoids. Heart defects may consist of ventricular septal defect, patent ductus arteriosus, tetralogy of Fallot, and other abnormalities. A wide variety of other disorders may also occur, including cleft lip or palate, aortic coarctation, strabimus microphthalmia, mental retardation, encephalocele, and other abnormalities. The syndrome is sometimes designated as the **Goldenhar syndrome** (when vertebral defects are present) and **hemifacial microsomia** (when the symptoms are predominantly unilateral). The etiology is unknown.

Goldenhar, M. Associations malformatives de l'oeil et de l'oreille, en particulier le syndrome dermoide epibulbaire-appendices auriculaires-fistula auris congenita et ses relations avec la dysostose mandibulofaciale. *J. Génét. Hum.*, 1952, 1:243-82. Gorlin, R. J., *et al.* Oculoauriculovertebral syndrome. *J. Pediat.*, 1963, 63:991-9.

oculo-auriculovertebral syndrome. See *oculo-auriculovertebral dysplasia.*

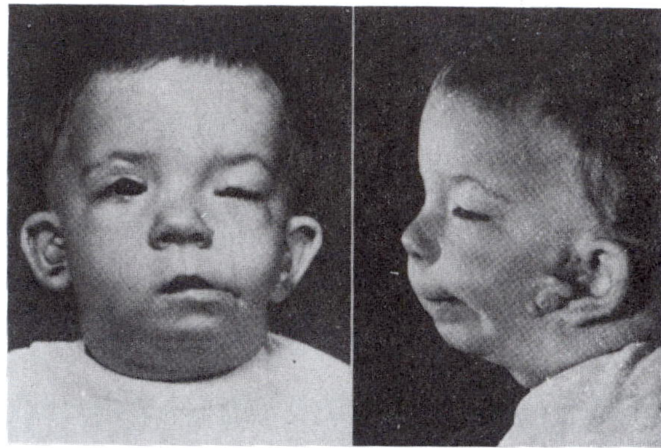

Oculo-auriculovertebral (OAV) dysplasia
Courtesy of Dr. Robert J. Gorlin, Minneapolis, MN.

oculo-orogenital syndrome. Synonyms: *Jacob syndrome, orogenital syndrome.*

A deficiency disease observed in American prisoners of war in Japanese camps during World War II; more than 75% of 8000 Americans were affected after 6 months or more of an inadequate rice diet. It is characterized by exfoliating dermatitis of the scrotum, stomatitis, and conjunctivitis, and is thought to be closely associated with pellagra, but is not pellagra per se. It is probably a result of deficiency of a specific component of the vitamin B complex.

Jacob, E. C. Oculo-oro-genital syndrome: A deficiency disease. *Ann. Int. Ann. Int. Med.*, 1951, 35:1049-54.

oculo-osteocutaneous syndrome. See *Tuomaala syndrome.*

oculo-urethro-articular syndrome. See *Reiter syndrome.*

oculobuccogenital syndrome. See *Behçet syndrome.*

oculocerebral hypopigmentation syndrome. See *Cross syndrome.*

oculocerebrocutaneous syndrome. A syndrome of ocular, cerebral, and cutaneous malformations, transmitted as an autosomal dominant trait, characterized by psychomotor retardation, general asymmetry, orbital cysts, microphthalmia, eyelid coloboma, skull defects, multiple intracranial fluid-filled spaces, accessory facial skin tags and defects, convulsions, skin aplasia or hypoplasia, and punched out defects. Occasional abnormalities may include persistant hyaloid artery, epibulbar dermoid, genital anomalities, rib dysplasia, cleft lip or palate, and agenesis of the corpus callosum.

Delleman, J. W., & Oorthuys, J. W. E. Orbital cysts in addition to congenital cerebral and focal dermal malformations: A new entity? *Clin. Genet.,* 1981, 19:191-8. Delleman, J. W., *et al.* Orbital cyst in addition to congenital cerebral and focal dermal malformations: A new entity. *Clin. Genet.,* 1984, 25:470-2.

oculocerebrofacial syndrome. See *Kaufman syndrome (3), under Kaufman, Robert L.*

oculocerebrofacioskeletal syndrome (COFS). Synonym: *Pena-Shokeir syndrome.*

A familial syndrome, transmitted as an autosomal recessive trait, characterized by microcephaly, ocular abnormalities (cataracts, microphthalmia, narrow palpebral fissures, blepharophimosis), peculiar facies (high nasal bridge, large ears, overhanging upper lip, micrognathia or retrognathia), skeletal defects (kyphosis, arthrogryposis, scoliosis, acetabular dysplasia, coxa valga, camptodactyly, flexion contractures of the knees and elbows, rocker-bottom feet, osteoporosis), widely set nipples, simian creases, longitudinal foot grooves, low birth weight, muscle hypotonia, and failure to thrive.

Pena, S. D. J., & Shokeir, M. H. K. Autosomal recessive cerebro-oculo-facio-skeletal (COFS) syndrome. *Clin. Genet.,* 1974, 5:285-93.

oculocerebromyoclonic syndrome. See *Kingsbourne syndrome.*

oculocerebrorenal (OCR) syndrome. See *Lowe syndrome, and see aniridia-Wilms tumor syndrome.*

oculocraniosomatic disease (OCSD). See *Kearns-Sayre syndrome.*

oculocutaneous albinism with deafness syndrome. See *Woolf syndrome.*

oculocutaneous albinism-hemorrhagic diathesis syndrome. See *Hermansky-Pudlak syndrome.*

oculocutaneous melanocytosis. See *Ota nevus.*

oculocutaneous syndrome. See *Vogt-Koyanagi syndrome, under Vogt, Alfred.*

oculocutaneous tyrosinase-negative albinism (OCA Ty neg). See *albinism I syndrome.*

oculocutaneous tyrosinase-positive albinism (OCA Ty pos). See *albinism II syndrome.*

oculocutaneous tyrosinemia or tyrosinosis. See *Richner-Hanhart syndrome.*

oculodental syndrome. See *Rutherfurd syndrome.*

oculodento-osseous dysplasia (ODOD). See *oculodentodigital syndrome.*

oculodento-osseous syndrome. See *oculodentodigital syndrome.*

oculodentodigital dysplasia (ODD, ODDD). See *oculodentodigital syndrome.*

oculodentodigital syndrome. Synonyms: *Gillespie syndrome, Meyer-Schwickerath and Weyers syndrome, dysplasia oculodentodigitalis, oculodentodigital dysplasia (ODD, ODDD), oculodento-osseous dysplasia (ODOD), oculodento-osseous syndrome.*

A syndrome of ocular abnormalities, such as microcorneas (with or without microphthalmos), fine porous irides, and secondary glaucoma; dental defects, mainly enamel hypoplasia; and digital anomalies, including clinodactyly, camptodactyly, and occasional syndactyly between the fourth and fifth fingers. Associated disorders include thin hypoplastic alae nasi with small nostrils; fine, sparse, slowly growing hair; obtuse mandibular angle and widening of the alveolar ridge of the mandible; widening of the long and short tubular bones; narrow palpebral fissures; and

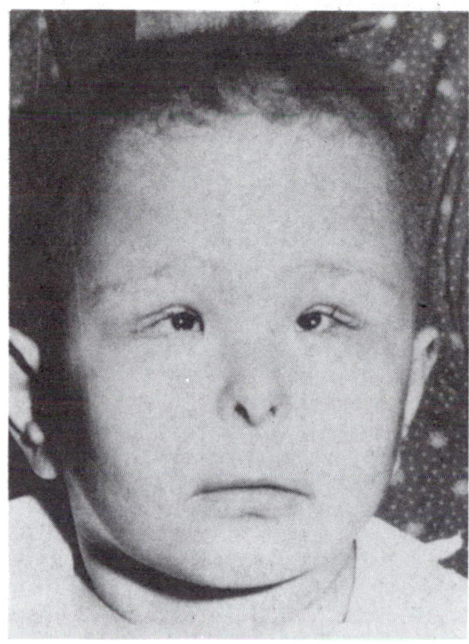

Oculodentodigital syndrome
Traboulsi, Elias I., Bishara M. Faris & Vazken M. Der Kaloustian, *American Journal of Medical Genetics* 24:95-100, 1986. New York: Alan R. Liss, Inc.

epicanthus. Cleft lip and palate, osteoporosis, conductive deafness, cubitus valgus, hip dislocation, and poorly developed teeth may occur. The syndrome is transmitted as an autosomal dominant trait.

Meyer-Schwickerath, G., Grüterich, E., & Weyers, H. Mikrophthalmus-Syndrome. *Klin. Mbl. Augenh.,* 1957, 131:18-30. Gillespie, F. D. A hereditary syndrome: "dysplasia oculodentodigitalis." *Arch. Ophth., Chicago,* 1964, 71:187-92. *Weyers, H., & Meyer-Schwikerath, G. Dysplasia oculo-dento-digitalis, ein neues Ektodermal-Syndrom. *Med. Bilddienst.,* 1959, 2:157-64.

oculodermal melanocytosis. See *Ota nevus.*

oculoglandular syndrome. See *Parinaud oculoglandular syndrome.*

oculomandibulodyscephaly (OMD). See *Hallermann-Streiff syndrome.*

oculomandibulodyscephaly-hypotrichosis syndrome. See *Hallermann-Streiff syndrome.*

oculomandibulofacial syndrome. See *Hallermann-Streiff syndrome.*

oculomotor recurrent paralysis. See *Moebius syndrome (2).*

oculopalatocerebral (OPC) dwarfism. See *oculopalatocerebral syndrome.*

oculopalatocerebral (OPC) syndrome. Synonym: *oculopalatocerebral (OPC) dwarfism.*

A familial syndrome, transmitted as an autosomal recessive trait, characterized by microcephaly, mental retardation, spasticity, connective tissue abnormalities, cleft palate, persistent hypertrophic primary vitreous, and short stature. Associated symptoms include asthma, small hands and feet, large pointed ears, cryptorchism, microphthalmos, deafness, soft skin, visible subcutaneous veins, hypermobility of the joints, limited extension of the elbow, kyphoscoliosis, and hernias.

Frydman, M., *et al.* Oculo-palato-cerebral dwarfism: a new syndrome. *Clin. Genet.,* 1985, 27:414-9.

oculopalatoskeletal syndrome. A syndrome of developmental defects of the anterior chamber of the eye and other anomalies transmitted as an autosomal recessive trait. The symptoms include corneal opacity, the eyelid triad (blepharophimosis, blepharoptosis, and epicanthus inversus), limitation of upward gaze, hypertelorism, cleft lip and palate, mental retardation, deafness, short fifth fingers, spina bifida occulta, closure of the lambdoid suture, abnormal occipital bone, and radioulnar synostosis.

Michels, V. V., *et al.* A clefting syndrome with ocular anterior chamber defect and lid anomalies. *J. Pediat.*, 1978, 93:444-6.

oculopharyngodistal myopathy. See *Satoyoshi syndrome (2).*

oculopupillary syndrome. See *Horner syndrome.*

oculorenal dystrophy. See *Senior syndrome (1).*

oculosympathetic syndrome. See *Horner syndrome.*

oculovertebral dysplasia. See *Weyers-Thier syndrome.*

ODD (oculodentodigital) dysplasia. See *oculodentodigital syndrome.*

ODDD (oculodentodigital dysplasia). See *oculodentodigital syndrome.*

ODELBERG, AXEL AXELSSON (Swedish physician, born 1892)

Odelberg disease. See *Van Neck disease.*

Van Neck-Odelberg syndrome. See *Van Neck disease.*

ODOD (oculodento-osseous dysplasia). See *oculodentodigital syndrome.*

odontogenesis imperfecta. See *dentinogenesis imperfecta.*

odonto-onychodermal dysplasia. Synonyms: *odonto-onychodermal syndrome, tricho-odontodermal dysplasia.*

Ectodermal dysplasia, transmitted as an autosomal recessive trait, characterized by nail dystrophy, malformed teeth (including peg-shaped incisors), erythematous lesions of the face, thickening of the skin, and increased sweating of the palms and soles.

Fadhil, M. Odontoonychodermal dysplasia: A previously apparently undescribed ectodermal dysplasia. *Am. J. Med. Genet.*, 1983, 14:335-46.

odonto-onychodermal syndrome. See *odonto-onychodermal dysplasia.*

odontoma-dysphagia syndrome. An association of multiple odontomas with severe dysphagia transmitted as an autosomal dominant trait.

Schmidseder, R., & Hausamen, J. E. Familiares Auftreten angeborener, multipler Odontome. *Deut. Zahmaerztl. Zschr.*, 1973, 28:626-32.

odontotrichomelic hypohidrotic dysplasia. See *EEC syndrome.*

odontotrichomelic syndrome. See *Freire-Maia syndrome.*

ODYSSEUS. See ULYSSES

OEIS (omphalocele-exstrophy-imperforate anus-spinal defects) complex. Synonyms: *ectopic cloaca, exstrophia splanchnica, extrophy of the cloaca, vesico-intestinal fissure.*

A syndrome combining omphalocele, exstrophy, imperforate anus, and spinal defects. The small bowel, usually ending blindly and often prolapsed into the blind colonic remnant or tailgut, lies just caudal to the bladder. Intestinal malrotation and bowel shortening are common. Abnormalities of the external genitalia are present, with either total absence of any genital structure or various degress of ambiguity. The upper urinary tract is abnormal in many patients. Imperforate anus and abnormalities of the lower spine, such as hemivertebrae or sacral meningocele, are usually associated. Clubfoot and positional deformities of the lower limbs may occur.

Carey, J. C., *et al.* The OEIS complex (omphalocele, exstrophy, imperforate anus, spinal defects). *Birth Defects*, 1978, 14(6B):253-63.

OFCTAD (occipitofaciocervicothoraco-abdomino-digital dysplasia). See *spondylothoracic dysplasia.*

OFD (I, II, III). See *orofaciodigital syndrome (I, II, III).*

OFUJI, SHIGEO (Japanese physician)

Ofuji syndrome. Synonyms: *eosinophilic pustular folliculitis, eosinophilic pustulosis, folliculitis pustulosa eosinophilica.*

A skin disease characterized by recurrent crops of pruritic follicular papulopustules. The lesions, about 1 to 3 cm in diameter, usually begin on the face or upper arm and spread outwardly, fresh eruptions appearing at the periphery of old ones which fade in the centers. The eruptions are arranged in an annular or polycyclic patterns on an erythematous base. Pigmented areas mark the sites of resolved eruptions. Biopsy shows eosinophilic exocytosis of the epidermis with small eosinophilic intraepidermal abscesses, involving the hair follicles and sebaceous glands. Eosinophilia occurs in most cases.

Ofuji, S., *et al.* eosinophilic pustular folliculitis. *Acta. Derm. Vener., Stockholm,* 1970, 50:195-203.

OGDEN, FRANK NEVIN (American physician, born 1895)

Zuelzer-Ogden syndrome. See *under Zuelzer.*

OGILVIE, SIR WILLIAM HENEAGE (British physician)

Ogilvie syndrome. Synonyms: *acute colonic pseudo-obstruction, colonic pseudo-obstruction, false colonic obstruction, nonobstructive colonic dilatation, pseudo-obstruction of the colon, sympathicotonic colonic syndrome.*

A potentially fatal colonic distention in the absence of a mechanical obstruction, usually occurring after surgery or trauma or following a severe pre-existing illness. In the classic Ogilvie syndrome, distention is associated with malignant invasion of the paravertebral ganglia. Rupture of the cecum and peritonitis are the most frequent complications.

Ogilvie, H. Large-intestine colic due to sympathetic deprivation. A new clinical syndrome. *Brit. Med. J.*, 1948, 2:671-3.

OGUCHI, CHUTA (Japanese ophthalmologist, born 1875)

Oguchi disease. Congenital hemerolopia, occurring in Japan, characterized by a golden or grayish white discoloration of the fundus and reduced visual sensitivity after more than 30 minutes in darkness. After a prolonged stay in darkness, the color of fundus reverts to normal and visual sensitivity is restored. The condition is transmitted as an autosomal recessive trait.

Oguchi, C. Über die eigenartige Hemeralopie mit diffuser weissgräulicher Verfärbung des Augenhintergrundes. *Graefes Arch. Ophth.*, 1912, 81:109-17.

OHAHA. See ***o****phthalmoplegia-****h****ypotonia-****a****taxia-****h****ypacusis-****a****thetosis)* **syndrome.**

OHARA, SHOICHIRO (Japanese physician)

Ohara disease. See *Francis disease.*

O'HIGGINS

O'Higgins disease. An anicteric disorder with leukopenia, hypogranulocytosis, blood platelet deficiency with retarded blood coagulation, hypocholesterolemia, hypocalcemia, capillaritis, and equilibrium disorders, usually occurring during the month of May in some areas of Argentina, reportedly described by O'Higgins. Chronic insecticide poisoning is suspected as a possible cause.**OHS (obesity-hypoventilation syndrome).** -See *Pickwick syndrome.*

oidiomycosis. See *Gilchrist disease.*

oil-associated pneumonic paralytic eosinophilic syndrome. See *toxic oil syndrome.*

OKIHIRO, M. M. (Japanese physician)

Okihiro syndrome. Synonym: *Duane-radial ray (DR) syndrome.*

A syndrome of Duane anomaly associated with cervical spine and radial ray abnormalities and deafness, transmitted as an autosomal dominant trait.

Okihiro, M. M., *et al.* Duane syndrome and congenital upper limb anomalies. *Arch. Neur., Chicago,* 1977, 34:174-9.

OLDFIELD, MICHAEL C. (British physician)

Oldfield syndrome. A familial disorder, believed to be transmitted as an autosomal dominant trait, characterized by an association of polyposis of the colon and multiple sebaceous cysts.

Oldfield, M. C. The association of familial polyposis of the colon with multiple sebaceous cysts. *Brit. J. Surg.,* 1954, 41:534-41.

oleogranuloma. See *Rothmann-Makai syndrome.*

olfacto-ethmoidohypothalamic dysplasia. See *olfactogenital syndrome.*

olfacto-ethmoidohypothalamic dysraphia. See *olfactogenital syndrome.*

olfactogenital dysplasia. See *olfactogenital syndrome.*

olfactogenital syndrome. Synonyms: *de Morsier syndrome. de Morsier-Gauthier syndrome, Kallmann syndrome, Kallmann-de Morsier syndrome, Maestre-Kallmann-de Morsier syndrome, Maestre de San Juan-Kallmann syndrome, Maestre de San Juan-Kallmann-de Morsier syndrome, congenital anosmia-hypogonadotropic hypogonadism syndrome, hypogonadism-anosmia syndrome, hypogonadotropic hypogonadism-anosmia syndrome, hyposmia-hypogonadotropic hypogonadism syndrome, idiopathic hypothalamic hypogonadism (IHH), olfacto-ethmoidohypothalamic dysplasia, olfacto-ethmoidohypothalamic dysraphia, olfactogenital dysplasia.*

A disorder of hypothalamic function and reduced pituitary gonadotropic activity with resulting hypogonadism (failure of sexual maturation and retarded primary and secondary sex characteristics), associated with agenesis or hypoplasia of the olfactory bulb with absent or reduced sense of smell. Hypertension, mental retardation, and color blindness may occur. The syndrome is transmitted as an X-linked or autosomal recessive trait.

Kallmann, F. J., & Barrera, S. E. The genetic aspects of primary eunuchoidism. *Am. J. Ment. Defic.,* 1943-44, 48:203-36. Morsier, G., de. Études sur les dysraphies crânioencephaliques. I. Agénesie des lobes olfactifs (télecéphaloschizis latéral) et les commissures calleuse et antérieure (télencéphaloscizis media). La dysplasie olfacto-génitale. *Schweiz. Arch. Neur.,* 1954, 74:309-61. Gauthier, G. La dysplasie olfacto-génitale (agénésie des

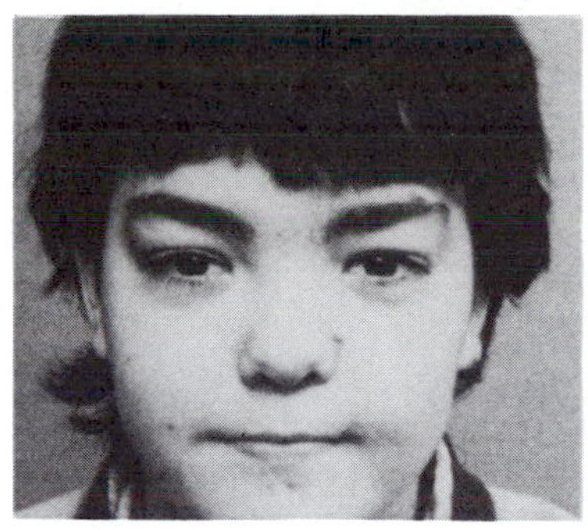

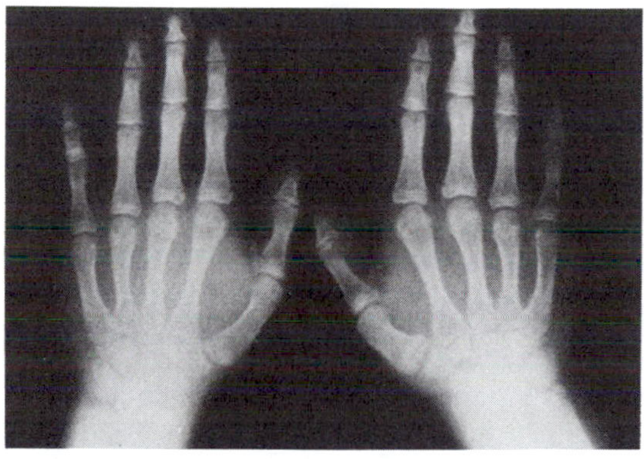

Olfactogenital syndrome
Hunter, Alasdair G.W., William Feldman & Jonathan Miller, *American Journal of Medical Genetics* 24:527-532, 1986. New York: Alan R. Liss, Inc.

lobes olfactifs avec absence de dévelopment gonadique à la puberté). *Acta Neuroveget. Wien,* 1960, 21:345-94. Maestre de San Juan, A. Falta total de los nervios olfactorios con anosmia en un individuo en que existía una atrofia congénita de los testículos y miembro viril. *Siglo Med.,* 1858.

oligodactylia syndrome. See *Weyers oligodactyly syndrome.*

oligohydramnios tetrad. See *Potter syndrome (1), under Potter, Edith Louise.*

oligophrenia-ichthyosis syndrome. See *Sjögren-Larsson syndrome, under Sjögren, Karl Gustaf Torsten.*

OLIVER, C. P. (American physician)

Adams-Oliver syndrome. See *under Adams, Forrest H.*

Oliver syndrome. An association of postaxial polydactyly with mental retardation transmitted as an autosomal recessive trait.

Oliver, C. P. Recessive polydactylism associated with mental deficiency. *J. Hered.,* 1940, 31:365-7.

olivopontocerebellar ataxia. See *olivopontocerebellar atrophy.*

olivopontocerebellar atrophy (OPCA). Synonyms: *Déjerine-Thomas syndrome, cortical cerebellar degeneration, delayed cerebellar ataxic syndrome, delayed cortical cerebellar atrophy, intracerebellar atrophy, olivopontocerebellar ataxia, ponto-olivocerebellar atrophy, presenile cerebellar ataxic syndrome.*

A chronic progressive ataxia which begins in adult or middle life and is characterized by progressive cerebellar atrophy with ataxic disorders of the trunk and limbs, equilibrium and gait disorders, slow voluntary movements, speech disorders, nystagmus, and oscillatory tremor of the head and trunk. Dysarthria, dysphagia, and oculomotor and facial paralysis may be present. Extrapyramidal symptoms include rigidity, immobile facies, and parkinsonian tremor. Knee and ankle jerk reflexes may be absent. Incontinence due to impaired sphincter function is common. Mild dementia may be present in some cases. Pathological findings include shrinkage of the ventral half of the pons, disappearance of the olivary eminence of the ventral surface of the medulla oblongata, and atrophy of the cerebellum. Loss of Purkinje cells, demyelination of the middle cerebellar peduncle and the cerebellar hemispheres, loss of cells in the molecular and granular layers of the pontine nuclei and olives, and degeneration of the posterior columns of the spinocerebellar fibers are often present. The syndrome is sometimes classified as olivopontocerebellar atrophy I, II, III, IV, and V. **OPCA I (Menzel syndrome, olivopontocerebellar atrophy, Menzel type)** is characterized by upper motor neuron and extensor plantar responses. Involuntary choreiform movements may occur. **OPCA II (Fickler-Winkler syndrome; olivopontocerebellar atrophy, Fickler-Winkler type)** is transmitted as an autosomal recessive trait and is marked mainly by the lack of involuntary movements. Albinism may be associated. **OPCA III** is associated with retinal degeneration. **OPCA IV (Schut-Haymaker syndrome; olivopontocerebellar atrophy, Schut-Haymaker type)** has variable symptoms and pathological changes in the inferior olivary nucleus and cerebellum. **OPCA V** occurs with dementia and extrapyramidal signs. Except for OPCA II, all variants of this syndrome are transmitted as an autosomal dominant trait.

Déjérine, J., & Thomas, A. L'atrophie olivo-ponto-cérébelleuse. *Nouv. Icon. Salpetriere,* 1900, 13:330-70. Menzel, P. Beitrag zur Kenntniss der hereditären Ataxie und Kleinhirnatrophie. *Arch. Psychiat. Nervenkr.,* 1890, 22:160-90. Schut, J. W., & Haymaker, W. Hereditary ataxia: Pathologic study of 5 cases of common ancestry. *J. Neuropath. Clin. Neur.,* 1951, 1:183-213. McKusick, V. A. *Mendelian inheritance in man. Catalogs of autosomal dominant, autosomal recessive, and X-linked phenotypes.* 5th ed. Baltimore, Johns Hopkins University Press, 1978, Nos. 16440, 16450, 16460, 16470, 25830. Rowland, L. P. *Merritt's textbook of neurology.* 7th ed. Philadelphia, Lea & Febiger, 1984, pp. 502-3. Fickler, A. Klinische und pathologisch-anatomische Beiträge zu den Erkrankungen des Kleinhirns. *Deut. Zschr. Nervenheilk.,* 1911, 41:306-75. Winkler, C. A case of olivo-pontine cerebellar atrophy and our conceptions of neo- and palaio-cerebellum. *Schweiz. Arch. Neur. Psychiat.,* 1923, 13:684-702.

olivopontocerebellar atrophy (OPCA), Fickler-Winkler type. See *OPCA II, under olivopontocerebellar atrophy.*

olivopontocerebellar atrophy (OPCA), Menzel type. See *OPCA I, under olivopontocerebellar atrophy.*

olivopontocerebellar atrophy (OPCA), Schut-Haymaker type. See *OPCA IV, under olivopontocerebellar atrophy.*

OLLENDORFF, HELENE. See OLLENDORFF-CURTH, HELEN

OLLENDORFF-CURTH, HELEN

Buschke-Ollendorff syndrome. See *under Buschke.*

Curth-Macklin syndrome. A rare form of ichthyosis hystrix, transmitted as an autosomal dominant trait, marked by a wide range of severity, from keratoderma palmaris et plantaris to severe, generalized disorders of cornification. Histopathological findings show binucleate corneocytes and prominent perinuclear shells within granular cells.

Ollendorff-Curth, H., & Macklin. M. T. The genetic basis of various types of ichthyosis in a family group. *Am. J. Hum. Genet.,* 1954, 6:371-82.

OLLIER, LOUIS XAVIER EDOUARD LEOPOLD (French surgeon, 1830-1900)

morbus Ollier. See *Ollier syndrome.*

Ollier disease. See *Ollier syndrome.*

Ollier syndrome. Synonyms: *morbus Ollier, Ollier disease, chondrodysplasia, dyschondroplasia, enchondromatosis, hemichondrodysplasia, internal chondromatosis, multiple enchondromata, multiple enchondromatosis, osteochondromatosis syndrome.*

A disorder of the growing ends of long bones, characterized by local growth deficiency with asymmetric leg shortening, enchondromata that usually appear as multiple swellings of the extremities, and occasional fractures of the affected areas. The lesions are first noted from 1 to 4 years of age with little progression after adolescence. The severity of symptoms varies, ranging from minor changes involving a few bones to extensive lesions in a large number of bones, such as those of the hand, causing deviation of the digits with resulting brachydactyly. Most cases are sporadic but some familial ones have been reported. The term *Ollier syndrome* applies to cases with unilateral involvement; a combination of enchondromatosis with multiple angiomata is known as the *Maffucci syndrome.*

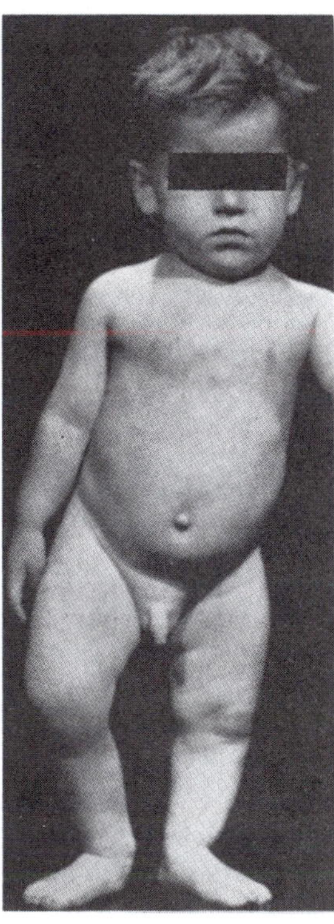

Ollier syndrome
Rubin, P.: *Dynamic Classification of Bone Dysplasias.* Chicago, Year Book Medical Publishers, 1964.

Ollier. De la dyschondroplasie. *Bull. Soc. Chir. Lyon*, 1899-1900, 3:22-7.

Ollier-Klippel-Trénaunay-Weber syndrome. See *Klippel-Trénaunay-Weber syndrome.*

OLLIVIER, D'A. (French physician)

Ollivier syndrome. Synonyms: *masque ecchymotique, traumatic asphyxia syndrome.*

A syndrome of cranial cyanosis, subconjunctival hemorrhage, and vascular engorgement of the head subsequent to crush injury, usually associated with confusion, seizures, loss of consciousness, laceration of the external auditory canal, and various injuries.

Ollivier, d'A. Rélation médicale des evenements survenue au Champs-de-Mars le 14 juin, 1837. *Ann. Hyg., Paris,* 1837, 18:485-9. Landercasper, J., & Cogbill, T. H. Long-term followup after traumatic asphyxia. *J. Trauma,* 1985, 25:838-41.

OLSZEWSKI, JERZY (Polish-born Canadian neurologist, 1913-1966)

Steele-Richardson-Olszewski (SRO) syndrome. See *under Steele.*

ombaja. See *ainhum syndrome.*

OMBREDANNE, LOUIS (French physician, 1871-1956)

Ombrédanne syndrome. See *malignant hyperpyrexia syndrome.*

OMD (**o**culo**m**andibulo**d**yscephaly). See *Hallermann-Streiff syndrome.*

OMENN, G. S. (American physician)

Omenn syndrome (OS). Synonyms: *familial erythrophagocytic lymphohistiocytosis, familial hemophagocytic reticulosis, familial histiocytic reticulosis, familial reticuloendotheliosis with eosinophilia, hemangiophagocytic reticulosis, histiocytic medullary reticulosis, reticuloendotheliosis with eosinophilia.*

A familial disease, transmitted as an autosomal recessive trait, characterized by anemia, eosinophilia, granulocytopenia, and thrombocytopenia. It is caused by phagocytosis of blood cells and replacement of the bone marrow by histiocytic infiltration. The symptoms include failure to thrive, recurrent infections, lymphadenopathy, hepatosplenomegaly, pulmonary infiltration, pancytopenia, and hypergammaglobulinemia. Autopsy findings show massive reticulum cell infiltration of most organs, obliteration of the lymph nodes, and plasmocytosis. Death takes place in infancy or early childhood. See also *histiocytic medullary reticulosis-like syndrome.*

Omenn, G. S. Familial reticuloendotheliosis with eosinophilia. *N. Engl. J. Med.,* 1965, 273:427-32. Farquhar, J. W., & Claireaux, A. E. Familial haemophagocytic reticulosis. *Arch. Dis. Child.,* 1952, 27:519-25.

omentum adhesion syndrome. Synonym: *adherent omentum syndrome.*

Adhesion of the omentum to the parietal peritoneum, usually associated with other adhesions, occurring after abdominal surgery, especially appendectomy. Pain caused by stretching of adhesions is usually aggravated when the patient assumes the erect position and is alleviated in the knee-bent position. About 30% of all cases are asymptomatic.

Knoch, H. G. Über das Netzadhasions-Syndrom. *Zbl. Chir.,* 1963, 88:2017-20.

omoblastoma. See *Ewing sarcoma.*

Omsk fever. See *hemorrhagic fever with renal syndrome.*

onchocerciasis. See *Robles disease.*

onchocercosis. See *Robles disease.*

ONDINE (UNDINE) (A water nymph in an 1814 fairy romance by De La Motte Fouqué and a 1939 play by Jean Giraudous)

Ondine curse. Synonyms: *Ondine curse syndrome (OCS), Ondine syndrome, central alveolar hypoventilation syndrome (CAHS), congenital central aveolar hypoventilation syndrome, congenital central hypoventilation (CCH), congenital hypoventilation syndrome (CHS), failure of respiratory center automaticity, idiopathic hypoventilation, idiopathic hypoventilation syndrome, primary alveolar hypoventilation syndrome, primary central hypoventilation syndrome.*

A syndrome of unknown etiology, characterized by failure of automatic respiratory function with apnea, especially evident during sleep, and retained ability to breathe on command. The term "Ondine curse" is believed to have been coined by Severinghaus, who relates it to the legend of Ondine, who punished her mortal husband for betraying her by depriving him of the ability to breathe automatically. Thus, on falling asleep, he died, not remembering to breathe. Fishman and colleagues have established the criteria for this syndrome: alveolar hypoventilation associated with voracious appetite and transient central diabetes insipidus. The symptoms include lack of energy, somnolence, headache, and some breathlessness on exertion. Cyanosis due to hypoxemia and polycythemia and sensitivity to hypnotics and sedatives are usually present. See also *sleep apnea syndrome.*

Severinghaus, J. W., & Mitchell, R. A. Ondine's curse-failure of respiratory center automaticity while awake. *Clin. Res.,* 1962, 10:122. Fishman, L. S., *et al.* Primary alveolar hypoventilation syndrome (Ondine's curse). Association with manifestations of hypothalamic disease. *Am. J. Dis. Child.,* 1965, 110:155-61.

Ondine curse syndrome (OCS). See *Ondine curse.*

Ondine syndrome. See *Ondine curse.*

ONISHI (Japanese physician)

Takayasu-Onishi syndrome. See *aortic arch syndrome.*

onychia maligna. See *Wardrop disease.*

onycho-mesodysplasia. See *nail-patella syndrome.*

onycho-odontodysplasia-perceptual deafness syndrome. See *Robinson syndrome, under Robinson, Geoffrey C.*

onycho-osteo-arthrodysplasia. See *nail-patella syndrome.*

onychoarthrosis. See *nail-patella syndrome.*

onychodentohypohidrotic syndrome. See *amelo-onychohypohidrotic syndrome.*

onycholysis-hypohidrosis-enamel hypocalcification syndrome. See *amelo-onychohypohidrotic syndrome.*

oophoroma folliculare. See *Brenner tumor.*

OOS (**o**ccupational **o**veruse **s**yndrome). See *overuse syndrome.*

OPALSKI, ADAM (Polish physician, 1897-1963)

Opalski syndrome. Synonyms: *hemianalgesia alterna subbulbaris, partial syndrome of the vertebrospinal artery, subbulbar syndrome.*

A combination of ipsilateral hypoesthesia of pain and temperature in the face, the Bernard-Horner syndrome, and pyramidal paralysis of the extremities, associated with contralateral hypoesthesia of pain and temperature in the trunk and extremities. The suspected cause is a focal lesion of the sub-bulbar region, involving the spinal segment of the trigeminal nerve, the cerebellospinal zone, and the pyramidal tract, resulting from circulatory disorders of the posterior spinal artery. This condition includes all the elements of the Wallenberg syndrome.

Opalski, A. Nowy zespol podopuszkowy. Zespol czesciowy tetnicy kregowo-rezeniowej tylnej. *Pol. Tyg. Lek.*, 1946, 1:397-402.

OPC (oculopalatocerebral) dwarfism or **syndrome.** See *oculopalatocerebral syndrome.*

OPCA (I, II, III, IV, V). See *under olivopontocerebellar atrophy.*

OPD. See *otopalatodigital syndrome.*

ophthalmic crises. See *Pel syndrome.*

ophthalmic headache. See *under headache syndrome.*

ophthalmic-sylvian syndrome. See *Espildora-Luque syndrome.*

ophthalmoencephalomyelopathy. See *Devic syndrome.*

ophthalmomandibulomelic dysplasia. See *Pillay syndrome.*

ophthalmoneuromyelitis. See *Devic syndrome.*

ophthalmoplegia chronica progressiva. See *Graefe syndrome.*

ophthalmoplegia dolorosa. See *Tolosa-Hunt syndrome.*

ophthalmoplegia externa chronica progressiva internuclearis. See *Graefe syndrome.*

ophthalmoplegia externa progressiva. See *Kiloh-Nevin syndrome (2).*

ophthalmoplegia plus syndrome. See *Kearns-Sayre syndrome.*

ophthalmoplegia-ataxia-areflexia syndrome. See *Fisher syndrome, under Fisher, Miller.*

ophthalmoplegia-cerebellar ataxia syndrome. See *Nothnagel syndrome (2).*

ophthalmoplegia-hypotonia-ataxia-hypacusis-athetosis syndrome (OHAHA). A familial syndrome, transmitted as an autosomal recessive trait, characterized by deafness, ophthalmoplegia, ataxia, athetosis, and normal intelligence in all except one of the affected patients in the original report. Inability to speak, strabismus, and a tendency to hold the mouth open give an impression of imbecility.

McKusick, V. A. *Mendelian inheritance in man. Catalogs of autosomal dominant, autosomal recessive, and X-linked phenotypes.* 7th ed. Baltimore, Johns Hopkins Univ. Press, 1986, p. 1173, No. 25812.

ophthalmoplegia-pigmentary retinal degeneration-cardiomyopathy syndrome. See *Kearns-Sayre syndrome.*

ophthalmoplegia-retinal degeneration syndrome. See *Kearns-Sayre syndrome.*

ophthalmoplegic migraine. See *Moebius syndrome (2).*

ophthalmoplegic retinal degeneration syndrome. See *Kearns-Sayre syndrome.*

ophthalmorhinostomatohygrosis. See *Creyx-Lévy syndrome.*

opioid withdrawal syndrome. See *under withdrawal syndrome.*

OPITZ, JOHN MARIUS (American physician, born 1935)

Herrmann-Opitz syndrome. See *under Herrmann.*

Herrmann-Pallister-Opitz syndrome. See *under Herrmann.*

Opitz syndrome. See *hypertelorism-hypospadias syndrome (2).*

Opitz trigonocephaly syndrome. Synonyms: *Opitz-Johnson-McCreadie-Smith syndrome, C syndrome, trigonocephaly syndrome.*

A multiple abnormality syndrome consisting of trigonocephaly, microcephaly, peculiar facies (broad nasal bridge, short nose with a broad root, long philtrum, micrognathia, cowlick, low-set and posteriorly rotated malformed ears, epicanthus, upward slanting palpebral fissures, wide mouth), short neck, attached frenulum, thick anterior alveolar ridges of the palate, polydactyly, syndactyly, bridged palmar creases, short limbs, ulnar deviation of the fingers, varus or equinovarus deformities, joint dislocations and/or contractures, strabismus, cryptorchism, prominent clitoris, neonatal loose skin, hemangiomas, deep sacral dimple, and heart defect. The syndrome is transmited as an autosomal recessive trait. "C" is the first letter of the surname of the affected patients, hence the synonym *C syndrome.*

Opitz, J. M., Johnson, R. C., McCreadie, S. R., & Smith, D. W. The C syndrome of multiple congenital anomalies. *Birth Defects*, 1969, 5(2):161-6.

Opitz-Frias syndrome. See *hypospadias-dysphagia syndrome.*

Opitz-Johnson-McCreadie-Smith syndrome. See *Opitz trigonocephaly syndrome.*

Smith-Lemli-Opitz syndrome (SLO, SLOS) (I and II). See *under Smith, David W.*

OPPENHEIM

Oppenheim syndrome. Synonym: *pituitary pseudotabes.*

Sclerosis of the spinal cord associated with tumor of the pituitary, reportedly described by Oppenheim.

OPPENHEIM, HERMANN (German neurologist, 1858-1919)

Erb-Oppenheim-Goldflam syndrome. See *Erb-Goldflam syndrome, under Erb, Wilhelm Heinrich.*

Minor-Oppenheim syndrome. See *Minor disease.*

Oppenheim disease. Synonyms: *amyatonia congenita, benign congenital hypotonia, congenital atonic pseudoparalysis, myatonia congenita.*

A congenital disorder, transmitted as an autosomal recessive trait, marked by muscular weakness, hypotonicity, and hyperflexibility, observed in floppy infants (excessive mobility of the joints permitting them to assume bizarre postures). Respiratory complications frequently occur. Children who survive more than 18 months after the onset of symptoms may show slow improvement. Some writers consider this syndrome a nonspecific entity.

Oppenheim, H. Über allgemeine und lokalisierte Atonie der Muskulatur (Myotonie) im frühen Kindersalter. Verläufige Mitteillung. *Mschr. Psychiat.*, 1900, 8:232-3.

Schwalbe-Ziehen-Oppenheim syndrome. See *Ziehen-Oppenheim syndrome.*

Ziehen-Oppenheim syndrome. See *under Ziehen.*

OPPENHEIM, MAURICE (Austrian-born American dermatologist, 1876-1949)

Oppenheim-Urbach syndrome. Synonyms: *dermatitis atrophicans maculosa lipoides diabetica, necrobiosis lipoidica, necrobiosis lipoidica diabeticorum.*

A skin disease usually observed in diabetic patients. At onset, the lesions are multiple red or yellowish papules ranging from 1 to 3 mm in diameter, which develop into round or oval sclerodermalike plaques with a cellophanelike surface. The plaques are reddish with yellow depressed centers. The lower limbs are most commonly affected, but the trunk, palms, soles, and forearms may also become involved. Ulceration of the lesions is common. Histologically, there is replacement of collagen fibers by neutral fat. The collagen fibers are pale ,and elastic fibers are absent in zones of necrobiosis. The term **necrobiosis lipoidica**, although often used as a synonym, applies only to cases uncomplicated by diabetes.

Oppenheim, M. Eine noch nicht beschriebene Hauterkrankung bei Diabetes mellitus (Dermatitis atrophicans lipoides diabetica). *Wien. Klin. Wschr.*, 1932, 43:314-5. Urbach, E. Beiträge zu einer physiologischen und pathologischen Chemie der Haut. X. Eine neue diabetische Stoffwechseldermatose: Nekrobiosis lipoidica diabeticorum. *Arch. Derm. Syph., Berlin*, 1932, 166:273-85.

OPPENHEIMER, ELLA H. (American physician)

Landing-Oppenheimer syndrome. See *under Landing.*

opsoclonic encephalopathy. See *Kingsbourne syndrome.*

optic atrophy-ataxia syndrome. See *Behr syndrome (2).*

optic atrophy-polyneuropathy-deafness syndrome. See *Rosenberg-Chutorian syndrome, under Rosenberg, Roger N.*

optic canal syndrome. See *Berlin disease (2).*

optic encephalomyelitis. See *Devic syndrome.*

optic myelitis. See *Devic syndrome.*

optic neuromyelitis. See *Devic syndrome.*

optic neuromyelopathic multiple sclerosis. See *Devic syndrome.*

optic neuromyelopathy. See *Devic syndrome.*

opticocochleodentate degeneration. See *Nyssen-van Bogaert-Meyer syndrome.*

oral epithelial nevus. See *white sponge nevus.*

oral-facial-digital syndrome. See *orofaciodigital syndrome (I, II, III).*

ORAM, SAMUEL (British physician)

Holt-Oram syndrome. See *under Holt.*

ORBELI, DIMITRI J. (Russian physician, died 1971)

Orbeli syndrome. See *chromosome 13q deletion syndrome.*

orbital apex-sphenoidal syndrome. See *Rollet syndrome.*

orbital floor syndrome. Synonym: *Dejean syndrome.*

A neurological disorder characterized by orbital floor lesions associated with exophthalmos, diplopia, superior maxillary pain, and numbness along the trigeminal nerve branches.

Dejean, M. C. Le syndrome du plancher de l'orbite. *Bull. Med. Soc. Fr. Opht.*, 1935, 48:473-85.

orbital inclusion adenoma. See *Warthin tumor.*

orbital periostitis. See *Collier syndrome.*

ORDOÑEZ, J. HERNANDO (Colombian physician)

Ordóñez melanosis. A pigmentation disorder marked by generalized melanoderma, especially of exposed parts of the body; melanosis of the mucous membranes of the mouth, eyes, and vulva; brown pigmentation of the nails; and dark discoloration of the viscera. The disorder is observed mainly in malnourished persons living at high altitudes; pituitary disorders are suspected as contributing factors.

Ordóñez, J. H. Melanosis de causa desconosida. Carencia nutritiva, vida en la altura y trastornos hipofisarios como posible causa. *An. Soc. Biol. Bogotá*, 1946, 2:121-46.

Oregon-type tyrosinemia. See *Richner-Hanhart syndrome.*

organic affective syndrome. A mental disorder due to an organic factor, and characterized by manic- or depressive-like mood disorders. Associated conditions include a mild cognitive impairment, fearfulness, anxiety, irritability, brooding, excessive somatic preoccupation, phobias, panic attacks, tearful and sad appearance, and, frequently, hallucinations and delusions. Delusions of persecution or worthlessness, irritability, and lability of mood occur mainly in the manic type. Poisoning with some substances, such as methyldopa or reserpine, and endocrine disorders, such as hypofunction or hyperfunction of the thyroid gland and adrenal cortex, are the principal etiologic factors.

Diagnostic and statistical manual of mental disorders. 3rd. ed. Washington, D. C., American Psychiatric Association, 1980, p. 137.

organic amnestic syndrome. An organic mental disorder characterized mainly be impairment of memory in the presence of a normal state of consciousness. Associated disorders may include disorientation, confabulation, lack of insight into one's true condition, apathy, lack of initiative, emotional blandness, and shallow affect. Alcoholism with thiamine deficiency and brain lesions, especially damages in the diencephalic and medial temporal structures due to trauma, hypoxia, infarction, and herpes simplex encephalitis are the most common etiologic factors.

Diagnostic and statistical manual of mental disorders. 3rd. ed. Washington, D.C., American Psychiatric Association, 1980, pp. 112-3.

organic brain syndrome. A syndrome of psychological and behavioral changes attributed directly to abnormalities of brain structure or of brain chemistry. Specific conditions included in the scope of this syndrome include delirium syndrome (q.v.), dementia syndrome (q.v.), intoxication, organic affective syndrome (q.v.), organic amnestic syndrome (q.v.), organic delusional syndrome (q.v.), organic hallucinosis syndrome (q.v.), organic personality syndrome (q.v.), and withdrawal syndromes (q.v.).

Diagnostic and statistical manual of mental disorders. 3rd ed. Washington, D. C., American Psychiatric Association, 1980, pp. 103-24. Wells, C. E. Overview of organic mental disorders. In: Kaplan, H. I., & Sadock, B. J., eds. *Comprehensive textbook of psychiatry.* 4th. ed. Baltimore, Williams & Wilkins, 1985, pp. 834-82.

organic delusional syndrome. A mental disorder due to an organic factor, and characterized mainly by the presence of delusions in a normal state of consciousness, persecutory delusions being the most common. Paranoid delusions may occur in amphetamine poisoning, and a delusion that a limb is missing may be present in some brain lesions. Associated disorders may include a mild cognitive impairment, perplexed appearance, disheveled or eccentric dress habits, rambling or incoherent speech, psychomotor disorders, hyperactivity or apathetic immobility, ritualistic and sterotyped behavior, magical thinking, and dysphoria. Intoxication with various substances, such as cannabis, amphetamines, and hallucinogens, temporal lobe epilepsy, and certain brain lesions of the nondominant hemisphere are the principal etiologic factors.

Diagnostic and statistical manual of mental disorders. 3rd ed. Washington, D. C., American Psychiatric Association, 1980, pp. 114-5.

organic hallucinal syndrome. See *organic hallucinosis syndrome.*

organic hallucinatory syndrome. See *organic hallucinosis syndrome.*

organic hallucinosis syndrome. Synonyms: *organic hallucinal syndrome, organic hallucinatory syndrome.*

A mental disorder due to an organic factor, and characterized mainly by persistent or recurrent hallucinations in the presence of a normal state of consciousness. Etiologic factors include prolonged use of alcohol, sensory deprivation (blindness or deafness), and seizures due to brain lesions, especially in the temporal or occipital lobes.

Diagnostic and statistical manual of mental disorders. 3rd. ed. Washington D. C., American Psychiatric Association, 1980, pp. 115-6. Wells, C. E., Overview of organic mental disorders. In: Kaplan, H. I., & Sadock, B. J., eds. *Comprehensive textbook of psychiatry.* 4th ed. Baltimore, Williams & Wilkins, 1985, pp. 834-82.

organic hyperinsulinism. See *Harris syndrome, under Harris, Seale.*

organic personality syndrome. A syndrome of marked changes in personality due to an organic factor. The principal features of this syndrome include emotional lability, lack of impulse control, lack of social judgment, belligerancy and exaggerated aggressiveness, temper outburst with bouts of crying, sexual indiscretions, apathy and indifference to immediate environment, lack of interest in hobbies, humorless verbosity, religiosity, and mild cognitive impairment. Head injuries, vascular brain diseases, brain neoplasms, temporal lobe epilepsy, Huntington chorea, disease of the thyroid gland and adrenal cortex, and ingestion of various substances are the etiologic factors.

Diagnostic and statistical manual of mental disorders. 3rd. ed. Washington, D. C., American Psychiatric Association, 1980, pp. 118-22. Wells, C. E., Overview of organic mental disorders. In: Kaplan, H. I., & Sadock, B. J., eds. *Comprehensive textbook of psychiatry.* 4th ed. Baltimore, Williams & Wilkins, 1985, pp. 834-82.

oriental boil or sore. See *Alibert disease (2).*

ORMOND, JOHN KELSO (American physician, born 1886)

Ormond syndrome. Synonyms: *Gerota fascitis, Gerota syndrome, idiopathic retroperitoneal fibrosis, nonspecific retroperitoneal inflammation, peripyelitis plastica stenosans, perirenal fascitis, periureteral fibrosis, periureteritis fibroplastica, periureteritis plastica et obliterans, sclerosing lipogranuloma, sclerosing retroperitonitis, systemic idiopathic fibrosis.*

Inflammatory retroperitoneal fibrosis of unknown etiology, which may extend into the chest cavity and pelvis, and is usually associated with urinary obstruction. The disease, which occurs twice as often in males as females, usually begins with a loss of appetite and weight, vomiting, radiating backache in the sacral region, constipation, and nausea. Associated symptoms may include anemia, oliguria or anuria, increased erythrocyte sedimentation rate, hypertension, azotemia, and occasional proteinuria or pyuria. Radiological findings may show hydronephritis, ureteral stenosis, vascular narrowing, mediastinal widening, extradural block, esophageal varices, superior vena cava obstruction, intestinal edema, and compression of the gastrointestinal system. Histopathologically, there are fibrous tissues and cellular infiltration within the bounds of the Gerota fascia.

Ormond, J. K. Bilateral ureteral obstruction due to envelopment and compression by an inflammatory retroperitoneal process. *J. Urol.*, 1948, 59:1072-9.

ornithine carbamyl transferase deficiency. See *under hyperammonemic syndrome.*

ornithine transcarbamylase (OTC) deficiency. See *under hyperammonemic syndrome.*

oro-acral syndrome. See *Hanhart syndrome (2).*

orocraniodigital syndrome. See *Juberg-Hayward syndrome.*

orodigitofacial dysostosis. See *orofaciodigital syndrome I.*

orodigitofacial syndrome. See *orofaciodigital syndrome (I, II, III).*

orofaciodigital syndrome I (OFD I). Synonyms: *Gorlin syndrome, Gorlin-Psaume syndrome, Papillion-Léage and Psaume syndrome, dysplasia linguofacialis, orodigitofacial dysostosis, orodigitofacial syndrome.*

A congenital syndrome consisting mainly of orofacial and digital defects, such as hypoplasia of nasal alar cartilages, median pseudocleft of upper lip, asymmetric cleft palate, mental retardation, and various digital malformations. Oral anomalies usually consist of bifid, trifid, or tetrafid tongue, cleft palate, frenulum hyperplasia, and hamartoma of the tongue. The hands generally exhibit brachydactyly, syndactyly, and cystic changes. The feet may show fibular clinodactyly, occasional unilateral polysyndactyly, brachydactyly, and, rarely, supernumerary toes. Sparse hair and transient milia of the ears and face may be associated. The syndrome is inherited as a dominant X-linked trait limited to females and lethal in males.

Papillon-Léage, E. & Psaume, J. Une nouvelle malformation héréditaire de la muqueuse buccale. Brides et freins anormaus. *Rev. Stomat, Paris*, 1954, 55:209-27. Gorlin, R. J., & Psaume. J., Orodigitofacial dysostosis. A new syndrome. A study of 22 cases. *J. Pediat.*, 1962, 61:520-30.

orofaciodigital syndrome II (OFD II). Synonyms: *Mohr syndrome I, Mohr-Claussen syndrome.*

A congenital syndrome occurring in both sexes and consisting mainly of orofacial and digital defects. Oral

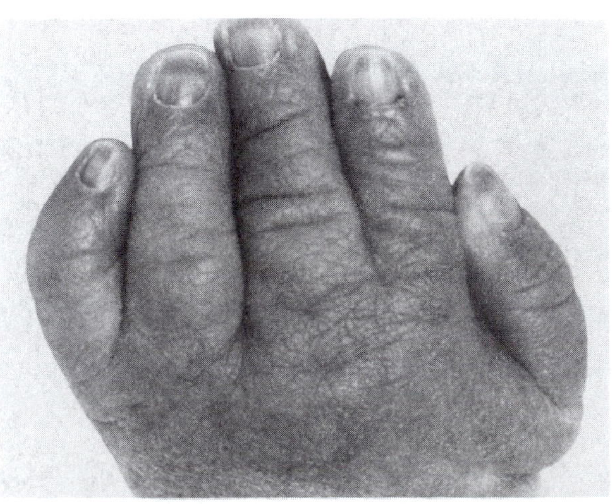

Orofaciodigital syndrome I
Courtesy of Dr. Robert J. Gorlin, Minneapolis, MN.

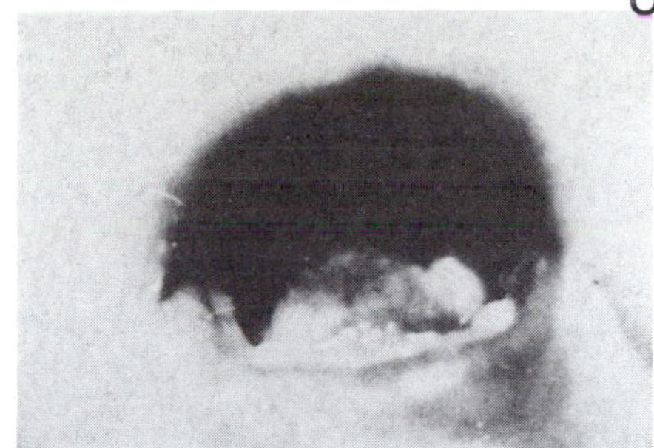

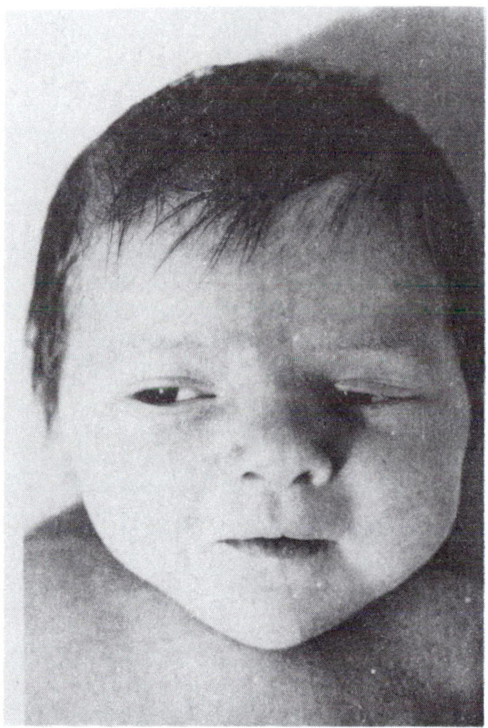

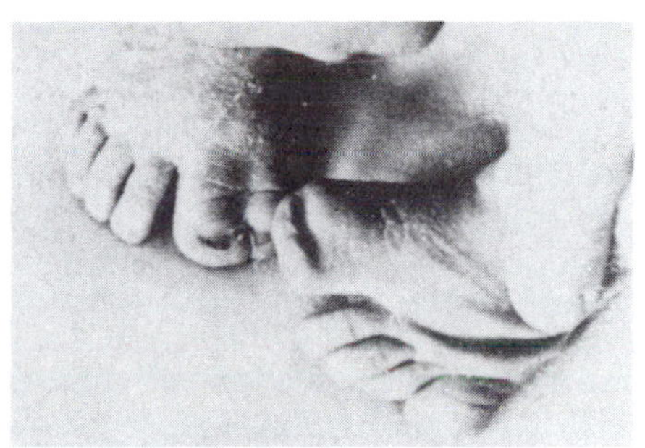

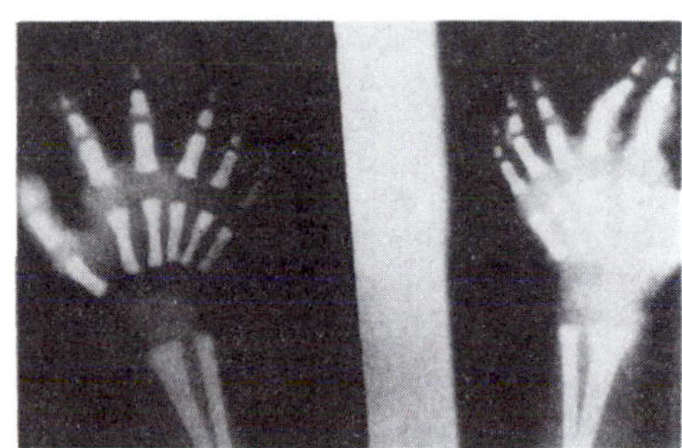

Orofaciodigital syndrome II
Silengo, M.C., G.L. Bell, M. Biagioli & P. Franceschini, *Clinical Genetics* 31:331-336, 1987. Munksgaard International Publishers, Copenhagen, Denmark.

features include lobate tongue, midline clefts of the lips, high-arched palate, hypertrophy of the frenulum, and fatty hamartoma of the tongue. Broad nasal root, broad and bifid nasal tip, dystopia canthorum, hypertelorism, micrognathia, and hypoplasia of the zygomatic arch and maxilla are the principal facial anomalies. Digital abnormalities consist of brachydactyly, syndactyly, clinodactyly, polydactyly, reduplication of the hallux, short and broad navicular bones and first metatarsal bones, and broad and duplicated cuneiform bones. Moderately short stature, metaphyseal irregularities and flaring, and deafness with malformed incus are usually associated. The syndrome is transmitted as an autosomal recessive trait.

Mohr, O. L. A hereditary sublethal syndrome in man. *Skr. Norske Vidensk. Akad.*, 1941, 14:1-18. Claussen, O. Et arvelight syndrom omfattende tungemissdannelse og polydaktyli. *Nord. Med.*, 1946, 30:1147-51.

orofaciodigital syndrome III (OFD III). Synonym: *Sugarman syndrome.*

A syndrome of eye abnormalities, lobulated hamartomatous tongue, dental anomalies in the form of extra small teeth with malocclusion, bifid uvula, postaxial polydactyly of the hands and feet, pectus excavatum, short sternum, kyphosis, motor and mental retardation, lack of response to auditory stimuli, hypotonia hyporeflexia, and abnormal EEG. Antimongoloid narrow palpebral fissures, hypertelorism, bilateral exotropic and ceaseless winking (see-saw winking) blepharospasm are the facial characteristics. The syndrome is believed to be transmitted as an autosomal recessive trait.

Sugarman, G. I., *et al.* See-saw winking in a familial oral-facial-digital syndrome. *Clin. Genet.*, 1971, 2:248-54.

orogenital syndrome. See *oculo-orogenital syndrome.*

orolinguobuccal dyskinesia. See *tardive dyskinesia syndrome.*

oromandibular limb hypoplasia. See *Hanhart syndrome (2).*

oromandibulo-otic syndrome. See *oculo-auriculovertebral dysplasia.*

Oroya fever. See *Carrión disease.*

ORTHMANN, ERNST GOTTLOB (German physician, 1858-1922)

Orthmann tumor. See *Brenner tumor.*

orthostatic hypotensive-dysautonomic-dyskinetic syndrome. See *Shy-Drager syndrome.*

ORTNER, NORBERT (Austrian physician, born 1865)

Ortner syndrome. Synonyms: *cardiomegaly-laryngeal paralysis syndrome, cardiovocal syndrome.*

A heart disease associated with laryngeal paralysis caused by compression of the recurrent laryngeal nerve between the aorta and dilated pulmonary artery, as in pulonary hypertension.

Ortner, N. Reclurrensslähmung bei Mitralstenose. *Wien. Klin. Wschr.*, 1897, 10:753-5.

OS. See *Omenn syndrome.*

os naviculare pedis retardatum. See *Köhler disease (1).*

OSAS (**o**bstructive **s**leep **a**pnea **s**yndrome). See *under sleep apnea syndrome.*

OSEBOLD, WILLIAM R. (American physician)

Osebold-Remondini syndrome. Synonym: *brachydactyly type 6.*

A familial syndrome, transmitted as an autosomal dominant trait, characterized by mesomelic dwarfism, abnormal carpal and tarsal bones, hypoplastic middle phalanges, and bipartite calcanei. The terminal phalanges of the index fingers deviate radially and hamate and capitate bones are joined in the wrist; the bones of the carpus and tarsus coalesce with increasing age.

Osebold, W. R., Remondini, D. J., *et al.* An autosomal dominant syndrome of short stature with mesomelic shortness of limbs, abnormal carpal and tarsal bones, hypoplastic middle phalanges, and bipartite calcanei. *Am. J. Med. Genet.*, 1985, 22:791-809.

OSGOOD, ROBERT BAYLEY (American physician, 1873-1956)

Lannelongue-Osgood-Schlatter syndrome. See *Osgood-Schlatter syndrome.*

Osgood disease. See *Osgood-Schlatter syndrome.*

Osgood-Schlatter syndrome. Synonyms: *Lannelongue disease, Lennelongue-Osgood-Schlatter disease, Osgood disease, Schlatter disease, apophysitis tibialis adolescentium, epiphysitis of the tibial tuberosity, osteochondrosis of the tuberosity of the tibia, periostitis tuberositas tibiae, rugby knee.*

Partial avulsion or strain of the tibial tuberosity resulting from a single injury or, more frequently, repeated flexing of the knee against a tight quadriceps muscle. The injury occurs most frequently in adolescent athletes.

Osgood, R. B. Lesions of the tibial tubercle occurring during adolescence. *Boston Med. Surg. J.*, 1903, 148:114-7. Schlatter, C. Verletzungen des schlnabelförmigen Forsatzes der aberen Tibiaepiphyse. *Beitr. Klin. Chir.*, 1903, 38:874-87.

OSKI, FRANK A. (American physician)

Shwachman-Diamond-Oski-Khaw syndrome. See *Shwachman syndrome.*

OSLER, SIR WILLIAM (Canadian physician, 1849-1919)

Osler disease (1). See *Osler-Rendu-Weber syndrome.*

Osler disease (2). See *Vaquez-Osler syndrome.*

Osler nodes. Cutaneous nodules arising in the course of subacute bacterial endocarditis, often preceded by an aura of burning, throbbing pruritus, or tingling. A typical nodule ranges from a few millimeters to 1.5 cm in diameter. It is reddish purple and may contain a central white opacity. Normally, the lesions are located on the finger pads, the thenar and hypothenar eminences, and the toes; less frequently, on the ears. They generally last for a day or two but may persist for a week, fading without residue.

Osler, W. Chronic infectious endocarditis. *Q, J. Med., Oxford*, 1908-9, 2:219-30.

Osler syndrome. Synonym: *ball-valve gallstone.*

The presence in the diverticulum of Vater of a free-moving gallstone which is larger than the orifice, thus blocking the outflow of bile from the common bile duct in a manner similiar to that of a ball-valve. Jaudice is a common complication.

Osler, W. The ball-valve gall-stone in the common duct. *Lancet*, 1897, 1:1319-23.

Osler-Libman-Sacks disease. See *Libman-Sacks syndrome.*

Osler-Rendu-Weber syndrome. Synonyms: *Babington disease, Goldstein hematemesis, Goldstein heredofamilial angiomatosis, Osler disease, Osler syndrome, Rendu-Osler syndrome, angioma haemorrhagicum hereditaria, familial hemorrhagic telangiectasia, generalized angiomatosis, hereditary epistaxis, hereditary familial angiomatosis, hereditary hemorrhagic telangiectasia, heredofamilial angiomatosis, multiple hereditary telangiectases with recurrent hemorrhage, telangiectasia hereditaria haemorrhagica.*

Pinpoint, spiderlike, and nodular multiple telangiectatic lesions of the face and other parts of the body, giving rise to recurrent epistaxes, melena, hematemesis, genital bleeding, and other hemorrhagic complications with secondary anemia. The skin of the cheeks and nasal orifices is most commonly affected, and the nail beds, the skin of the ears, fingers, toes, and scalp, the nasal mucosa, the bladder, the genitalia, and the pharynx may be involved. The lesions are bright red, violaceous, or purple, blanching under pressure. The syndrome is transmitted as an autosomal dominant trait.

Osler, W. On multiple hereditary telangiectases with recurrent hemorrhage. *Q. J. Med., Oxford*, 1907, 1:53-8. Rendu. Epistaxis répetées chez un sujet porteur de petits angiomes cutanés et muqueux. *Bull. Soc. Méd. Hôp. Paris*, 1896, 13:731-3. Weber P. F. A note on cutaneous telangiectases and their etiology. Comparison with the etiology of haemorrhoids and ordinary varicose veins. *Edinburgh Med. J.*, 1904, 346-9. Goldstein, H. I. Hereditary hemorrhagic telangiectasia with recurring (familial) hereditary epistaxis. *Arch. Int. Med.*, 1921, 27:102-25. Babington, B. G. Hereditary epistaxis. *Lancet*, 1865, 2:362-3.

Rendu-Osler syndrome. See *Osler-Rendu-Weber syndrome.*

Vaquez-Osler erythremia. See *Vaquez-Osler syndrome.*

Vaquez-Osler syndrome. See *under Vaquez.*

OSMED (**o**to**s**pondylo**me**gaepiphyseal **d**ysplasia). See *Weissenbacher-Zweymüller syndrome.*

osseous dystrophy-nail dysplasia syndrome. See *nail-patella syndrome.*

ossified diathesis. See *multiple cartilaginous exostoses syndrome.*

ossifying fibroma. See *Jaffe-Lichtenstein disease.*

ossifying ligamentous spondylitis. See *Bechterew-Strümpell-Marie syndrome, under Bekhterev.*

osteitis condensans ilii. See *Bársony-Polgár syndrome (1).*

osteitis cystica multiplex. See *Perthes-Jüngling disease.*
osteitis cystica multiplex tuberculosa. See *Perthes-Jüngling disease.*
osteitis deformans. See *Paget disease.*
osteitis deformans calcanei. See *Blencke syndrome.*
osteitis fibrosa cystica. See *Jaffee-Lichtenstein syndrome, and see McCune-Albright syndrome.*
osteitis fibrosa cystica disseminata. See *McCune-Albright syndrome.*
osteitis fibrosa disseminata. See *Jaffe-Lichtenstein syndrome.*
osteitis fibrosa generalisata. See *Recklinghausen disease (2).*
osteitis fibrosa juvenilis. See *Jaffe-Lichtenstein syndrome.*
osteitis multiplex cystoides. See *Perthes-Jüngling disease.*
osteo-angiohypertrophy. See *Klippel-Trénaunay-Weber syndrome.*
osteo-arthritis coxae. See *Calvé-Legg-Perthes syndrome.*
osteo-arthropathia hypertrophica. See *Marie-Bamberger syndrome, under Marie, Pierre.*
osteo-arthrosis deformans endemica. See *Kashin-Bek disease.*
osteo-arthrosis interspinalis. See *Baastrup syndrome.*
osteo-onycho-dysostosis. See *nail-patella syndrome.*
osteo-onycho-dysplasia. See *nail-patella syndrome.*
osteo-onycho-dysplasia-albuminuria. See *nail-patella syndrome.*
osteochalasia desmalis familiaris. See *hyperphosphatasia-osteoctasia syndrome.*
osteochondritis deformans endemica. See *Kashin-Bek disease.*
osteochondritis deformans juvenilis. See *Scheuermann disease.*
osteochondritis deformans juvenilis coxae. See *Calvé-Legg-Perthes syndrome.*
osteochondritis deformans tibiae. See *Erlacher-Blount syndrome.*
osteochondritis dissecans. See *König disease (1).*
osteochondritis dissecans of femoral head. See *Chandler syndrome, under Chandler, Fremont Augustus.*
osteochondritis ischiopubica. See *Van Neck disease.*
osteochondritis of the vertebral body. See *Calvé syndrome.*
osteochondritis subepiphysaria. See *Schmid metaphyseal chondrodysplasia syndrome, under Schmid, Franz.*
osteochondritis vertebralis infantilis. See *Calvé syndrome.*
osteochondro-arthrosis deformans endemica. See *Kashin-Bek disease.*
osteochondrodesmodysplasia. See *Rotter-Erb syndrome.*
osteochondrodysplasia metaphysaria, Jansen type. See *Jansen metaphyseal chondrodysplasia syndrome.*

osteochondrodystrophia deformans. See *mucopolysaccharidosis IV-A.*
osteochondrodystrophia foetalis. See *achondroplasia.*
osteochondrodystrophy. See *mucopolysaccharidosis IV-A.*
osteochondrolysis. See *König disease (1).*
osteochondroma of epiphyses. See *Trevor syndrome.*
osteochondromatosis syndrome. See *Ollier syndrome.*
osteochondromuscular dystrophy. See *Schwartz-Jampel syndrome, under Schwartz, Oscar.*
osteochondropathia deformans juvenilis coxae. See *Calvé-Legg-Perthes syndrome.*
osteochondropathia ischiopubica. See *Van Neck disease.*
osteochondrosis calcanei. See *Blencke syndrome.*
osteochondrosis deformans coxae juvenilis. See *Calvé-Legg-Perthes syndrome.*
osteochondrosis juvenilis. See *Köhler disease (1).*
osteochondrosis of the capitellum humeri. See *Panner disease (2).*
osteochondrosis of the capitular epiphysis of the femur. See *Calvé-Legg-Perthes syndrome.*
osteochondrosis of the tuberosity of the tibia. See *Osgood-Schlatter syndrome.*
osteoctasia-hyperphosphatasia syndrome. See *hyperphosphatasia-osteoctasia syndrome.*
osteodental dysplasia. See *cleidocranial dysostosis.*
osteodermopathia hypertrophicans. See *pachydermoperiostosis syndrome.*
osteodermopathic hyperostosis syndrome. See *pachydermoperiostosis syndrome.*
osteodysmetamorphosis foetalis. See *hypophosphatasia syndrome.*
osteodysplasia. See *Melnick-Needles syndrome.*
osteodysplasia endostotica. See *osteopoikilosis syndrome.*
osteodysplasty. See *Melnick-Needles syndrome.*
osteodystrophia chronica deformans. See *Paget disease.*
osteodystrophia chronica deformans hypertrophica. See *Paget disease.*
osteodystrophia deformans. See *Paget disease.*
osteodystrophia disseminata. See *Jaffe-Litchtenstein syndrome.*
osteodystrophia fibrosa. See *McCune-Albright syndrome.*
osteodystrophia fibrosa generalisata. See *Recklinghausen disease (2).*
osteodystrophia fibrosa localisata. See *Paget disease.*
osteodystrophia fibrosa universalis. See *Jaffe-Lichtenstein syndrome.*
osteodystrophia generalisata. See *Recklinghausen disease (2).*
osteodystrophia metaepiphysaria calcanei. See *Blencke syndrome.*
osteofibrosis. See *Jaffe-Lichtenstein syndrome.*
osteofibrosis deformans juvenilis. See *Jaffe-Lichtenstein disease.*
osteogenesis imperfecta congenita-microcephaly-cataract syndrome. See *osteogenesis imperfecta-microcephaly-cataract syndrome.*
osteogenesis imperfecta syndrome (dominant form). Synonyms: *Eddowes syndrome, Ekman syndrome, Ekman-Lobstein syndrome, Lobstsein syndrome, Spurway-Eddowes syndrome, van der Hoeve disease, van der Hoeve-de Kleyn syndrome, brittle bone disease, fragilitas ossium hereditaria, mollities ossium, osteogenesis imperfecta tarda, osteopsathyrosis congenita, osteopsathyrosis idiopathica, osteopsathyrosis idiopathica tarda, thin bone osteogenesis imperfecta.*

A hereditary bone disease, transmitted as an autosomal dominant trait, in which thin bones are abnormally brittle and subject to fractures. Craniofacial defects consist of a small triangular face, craniomalacia, bitemporal bulge, frontal bossing, retarded ossification, wormian bones, and platybasia. The bones show thin cortices, poorly trabeculated spongiosa, thin shafts, multiple poorly united fractures, and translucent, often biconcave vertebral bodies, with dwarfism, callus formation, and thickening of the calvarium. Blue sclerae, peripheral corneal opacities, keratoconus, megalocornea, and hypermetropia are the ocular features. Otosclerosis and deafness are the principal auricular complictions. Dental defects consist mainly of dentinogenesis imperfecta, susceptibility to caries, and yellow or bluish-gray discoloration of the teeth. The syndrome is usually associated with hyperlaxity of the ligaments, genua valga, pes planus, radial dislocation, bleeding tendency due to increased capillary fragility and abnormal thrombocyte function, and thin, translucent skin. Occasional abnormalities may include umbilical hernia, syndactyly, poor muscle development, hypertrophic skin scars, and a host of other defects.

*Lobstein, J. *De la fragilité de os ou l'ostéopsathyrose. Traité de l'anatomie pathologique*. Paris, 1833, Vol 2, pp. 204-12. *Ekman, O. J. *Dissertatio medica. Descriptionem et casus aliquot osteomalaciae sistens*. Uppsala, 1788. Spurway, J. Hereditary tendency to fracture. *Brit. Med. J.*, 1896, 2:844. Eddowes, A. Dark sclerotics and fragilitas ossium. *Brit. Med. J.*, 1900, 2:222. Hoeve, J., van der, & Kleyn, A., de. Blaue Sclera, Knochenbrüchigkeit und Schwerhörigkeit. *Graefes Arch. Ophth.*, 1918, 95:81-93.

osteogenesis imperfecta syndrome (recessive form). Synonyms: *Porak-Durante syndrome, Vrolik disease, Vrolik syndrome, fragilitas ossium, periosteal dysplasia, thick bone osteogenesis imperfecta.*

A congenital bone disease, transmitted as an autosomal recessive trait, in which thick bones are abnormally brittle and subject to fractures. The affected infants frequently are born dead or survive only for a few days; those who survive may live into adulthood with extreme skeletal abnormalities. Short-limb dwarfism, deformed extremities with apparently normal hands and feet, large head, wide fontanels, caput membranaceum, ligament hyperlaxity, muscle hypotonia, proptosis, blue sclerae, small nose with depressed bridge, and inguinal hernia are the principal defects. Hydrocephalus and cerebral hemorrhage may occur. Radiographic findings show multiple fractures of the long bones, which are short, thick, and poorly mineralized; calus formation; multiple wormian bones; generalized osteoporosis; and cystic changes in the long bones of the lower limbs.

Vrolik, W. *Tabulae ad illustrandam embryogenes in hominis et mammalium, tam naturalem quam abnormem*. Lipsiae, Weigel, 1854. Porak, C., & Durante, G. Les micromélies congénitales. Achondroplasie vraie et dystrophie périosteale. *Nouv. Icon. Salpêt.*, 1905, 18:181-538.

osteogenesis imperfecta tarda. See *osteogenesis imperfecta syndrome (dominant form).*

osteogenesis imperfecta-microcephaly-cataract syndrome. Synonym: *osteogenesis imperfecta congenita-microcephaly-cataract syndrome.*

A familial syndrome, transmitted as an autosomal recessive trait, characterized by osteogenesis imperfecta, microcephaly, and cataract. Associated disorders may include prenatal fractures, poorly developed sulci and gyri, short calvaria, hypogonadism, low-set ears, single umbilical artery, hypertelorism, heart defect, shortening and bowing of the lower limbs, and blue sclerae.

Buyse, M., & Bull, M. J. A syndrome of osteogenesis imperfecta, microcephaly, and cataracts. *Birth Defects*, 1978, 14(6B):95-8.

osteoglophonic dwarfism syndrome. A syndrome of rhizomelic dwarfism, flat nasal bridge, craniostenosis, fibrous dysplasia of the mandible, platyspondyly, and metaphyseal defects. The main radiographic findings include metaphyseal lucency, poor modeling of the tubular bones of the hand, conelike epiphyses, small and irregular carpal bones, and poorly developed metaphyses and metacarpals.

Beighton, P., *et al.* Osteoglophonic dwarfism. *Pediat. Radiol.*, 1980, 10:46-50.

osteohypertrophic varicose nevus syndrome. See *Klippel-Trénaunay-Weber syndrome.*

osteoid osteoma. See *Bergstrand disease.*

osteolysis-nephropathy syndrome. See *Thieffry-Shurtleff syndrome.*

osteoma multiplex intramusculare. See *fibrodysplasia ossificans progressiva.*

osteomalacia chronica deformans hypertrophica. See *Paget disease.*

osteomalacic dialysis osteodystrophy. See *aluminum toxicity syndrome.*

osteomalacic pelvis. See *Kilian pelvis.*

osteomatosis-intestinal polyposis syndrome. See *Gardner syndrome, under Gardner, Eldon John.*

osteomyelitis sicca. See *Garré osteomyelitis.*

osteopathia acidotica pseudorachitica. See *Fanconi-Albertini-Zellweger syndrome.*

osteopathia condensans disseminata. See *osteopoikilosis syndrome.*

osteopathia dysplastica familiaris. See *pachydermoperiostosis syndrome.*

osteopathia familiaris neuroendocrina. See *Salvioli syndrome.*

osteopathia fibrosa generalisata. See *Recklinghausen disease (2).*

osteopathia hyperostotica. See *Léri syndrome (1).*

osteopathia hyperostotica congenita membri unis. See *Léri syndrome (1).*

osteopathia hyperostotica scleroticans multiplex infantilis. See *Camurati-Engelmann syndrome.*

osteopathia hypertrophicans toxica. See *Marie-Bamberger syndrome, under Marie, Pierre.*

osteopathia patellae. See *Büdinger-Ludloff-Läwen syndrome.*

osteopathia patellae juvenilis. See *Larsen-Johansson syndrome, under Larsen, Christian Magnus Falsen Sinding.*

osteopathia striata. See *Voorhoeve syndrome.*

osteoperiostitis ossificans toxica. See *Marie-Bamberger syndrome, under Marie, Pierre.*

osteopetrosis with late manifestations. See *Albers-Schönberg syndrome.*

osteopetrosis with precocious manifestations syndrome. Synonyms: *infantile osteosclerosis, ivory bones, malignant osteosclerosis, marble bone disease.*

An early-onset type of bone dysplasia associated with failure to thrive, short stature, anemia, hepatosplenomegaly, macrocephaly, and frequent hydrocephalus, psychomotor retardation, optic atrophy, facial paralysis, delayed dentition, and microdontia. In infants, x-ray findings show increased bone density, lack of corticomedullary differentiation, loss of trabeculae, and metaphyseal undermodeling (club-shaped metaphyses). In adults, the disorder is marked by alternating bands of high- and low-density bone in the tubular bones, arcuate bands in iliac bones, sandwich vertebrae, thickening and sclerosis of the skull, and poor pneumatization of mastoids and paranasal sinuses. Hematological changes include erythroblastosis with anemia, leukocytosis with frequent myeloid reaction, thrombocytopenia, hypocalcemia, and hypo-phosphatemia. The syndrome is transmitted as an autosomal recessive trait.

*Zetterström, R. Osteopetrosis (marble bone disease). Clinical and pathological review. *Mod. Prob. Pediat.*, 1957, 3:488. Spranger, J. W., Langer, L. O., Jr., & Wiedemann, H. R. *Bone dysplasias. An atlas of constitutional disorders of skeletal development*. Philadephia, Saunders, 1974, p. 284.

osteopetrosis-renal tubular acidosis syndrome. See *Guibaud-Vainsel syndrome.*

osteophthisis. See *Gorham syndrome.*

osteophytosis. See *Marie-Bamberger syndrome, under Marie, Pierre.*

osteopoikilia familiaris. See *osteopoikilosis syndrome.*

osteopoikilosis syndrome. Synonyms: *osteodysplasia endostotica, osteopathia condensans disseminata, osteopoikilia familiaris, osteosclerosis disseminata, ostitis condensans generalisata, spotted bone.*

A bone dysplasia characterized mainly by small circumscribed foci of sclerosis, sometimes confluent to form longitudinal bands, affecting chiefly the ends of the tubular bones, including the ossification centers of the epiphyses. Occasional clinical symptoms may include arthralgia, dermatofibrosis lenticularis disseminata, and keloids. The syndrome is transmitted as an autosomal dominant trait.

Green, A. E., *et al.* Melorheostosis and osteopoikilosis. *Am. J. Roentgen.*, 1962, 87:1096-111. Berlin, R. *et al.* Osteopoikilosis-a clinical and genetic study. *Acta Med. Scand.*, 1967, 181:305-14.

osteoporosis acro-osteolytica. See *pyknodysostosis.*

osteoporosis-osteomalacia syndrome. See *Milkman syndrome.*

osteoporosis-pseudoglioma syndrome (OPS). A familial syndrome, transmitted as an autosomal recessive trait, characterized by osteoporosis and pseudoganglioma, frequently in association with laxity of the ligaments and mental retardation. Ocular anomalies may include vitreoretinal dysplasia, phthisis bulbi, blindness, microphthalmia, anterior chamber and lens defects, retrolental mass or falciform fold, and calcifications. Musculoskeletal abnormalities consist of frequent fractures, tubular deformities, wormian bones, kyphosis or kyphoscoliosis, pes planus and/or valgus, hyperextensibility of the joints, limited movement of the forearm, and muscle hypotonia. Short stature, obesity, abnormal EEG, increased deep tendon reflexes, perceptive deafness, facial weakness, hypotrichosis, depressed bridge of the nose, and micrognathia may be present in some cases. Biochemical findings include abnormal blood and urine levels of calcium, phosphorus, alkaline phosphatase, and hydroxyproline.

Pellathy, B. V. Ablatio retinae und Uveitis congenita bei drei Geschwistern. *Zschr. Kinderheilk.*, 1931, 73:249-54. Frontali, M., *et al.* Osteoporosis-pseudoganglioma syndrome. Report of three affected sibs and an overview. *Am. J. Med. Genet.*, 1985, 22:35-47.

osteopsathyrosis congenita. See *osteogenesis imperfecta syndrome (dominant form).*

osteopsathyrosis idiopathica. See *osteogenesis imperfecta syndrome (dominant form).*

osteopsathyrosis idiopathica tarda. See *osteogenesis imperfecta tarda syndrome (dominant form).*

osteopulmonary arthropathy. See *Marie-Bamberger syndrome, under Marie, Pierre.*

osteorhabdotosis. See *Voorhoeve syndrome.*

osteosclerosis disseminata. See *osteopoikilosis syndrome.*

osteosclerosis fragilis generalisata. See *Albers-Schönberg syndrome.*

osteosclerotic anemia. See *Vaughan disease.*

osteosis condensans ilii. See *Bársony-Polgár syndrome (1).*

osteosis eburnisans monomelica. See *Léri syndrome (1).*

ÖSTERREICHER, W.

Österreicher-Fong syndrome. See *nail-patella syndrome.*

OSTERTAG, B.

Ostertag syndrome. Synonyms: *amyloid nephropathy, familial visceral amyloidosis, hereditary amyloid nephropathy.*

A hereditary form of amyloidosis, transmitted as an autosomal dominant trait, characterized by nephropathy, hypertension, hepatomegaly, and splenomegaly. Associated disorders include edema, proteinuria, weakness, and hematuria. The syndrome is familial and is usually fatal within 10 years from its onset. Amyloid deposits in the kidneys, adrenal glands, and liver are the principal pathological findings.

*Ostertag, B. Demonstration einer eigenartigen familiären Paramyloidose. *Zbl. Path.*, 1936, 12:1932, 56:253-4. *Ostertag, B. Familiäre Amyloid-Erkrankung. *Z. Menschl. Vereb. Konstitutionsl.*, 1950, 30:105- 15.

ostitis condensans generalisata. See *osteopoikilosis syndrome.*

OSTRUM, HERMAN WILLIAM (American physician, born 1893)

Furst-Ostrum syndrome. See *under Furst.*

OSUNTOKUN, B. O. (Nigerian physician)

Osuntokun syndrome. Synonym: *congenital pain asymbolia-auditory imperception syndrome.*

A familial syndrome, transmitted as an autosomal recessive trait, characterized by congenital indifference to pain and auditory imperception, wherein the affected children hear speech but are unable to comprehend the symbolic significance of most spoken words.

Osuntokun, B. O., *et al.* Congenital pain asymbolia and auditory imperception. *J. Neurol. Neurosurg. Psychiat.*, 1968, 31:291-6.

OTA, M. T. (Japanese ophthalmologist)

Ota nevus. Synonyms: *aberrant mongolian spot, extrasacral dermal melanosis, melanocytosis bulbi, nevus fuscoceruleus, nevus fuscoceruleus ophthalmomaxillaris, ocular and cutaneous melanosis, ocular and dermal melanocytosis, oculocutaneous melanosis, oculodermal melanocytosis, persistent aberrant mongolian spot, progressive melanosis of the dermis.*

A pigmented nevus of the eyelids, nose, zygomatic and frontal regions, ear lobes, retro-auricular region, and anterior portion of the scalp, usually noted at birth or during the first decade. Commonly, the lesions are unilateral, macular, or slightly raised, and tan-brown,

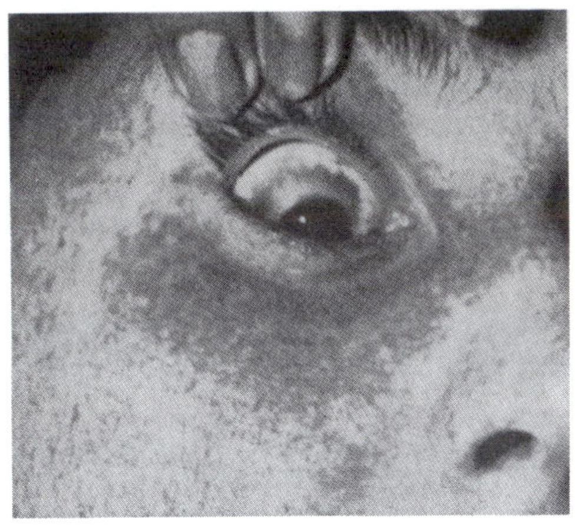

Ota nevus
Kerdel-Vegas, Dr. F. From G.C. Andrews & A.N. Domonkos: *Diseases of the Skin.* 5th ed. Philadelphia: W.B. Saunders Co., 1963.

slate blue, black, or purple. Ipsilateral hyperpigmentation of the cornea, conjunctiva, sclera, uvea, optic papilla, optic nerve, and orbit is frequently associated. There may be pigmentation of the external auditory canal, oral mucosa, gingivae, pharynx, hard palate, nasal mucosa, and leptomeninges. Females of Oriental ancestry and those with a dark skin are most often affected.

*Ota, M. Nevus fusco-coeruleus ophthalmomaxillaris. *Tokyo Med. J.*, 1939, 63:1243-5.

OTC (ornithine transcarbamylase) deficiency. See *under hyperammonemic syndrome.*

otic migraine. See *Bárány syndrome.*

oticodynia. See *Ménière syndrome.*

otitic hydrocephalus. See *pseudotumor cerebri syndrome.*

oto-onychoperoneal syndrome. A familial disorder, transmitted as an autosomal recessive trait, characterized by partial aplasia of the nails, aplasia or hypoplasia of the fibulae, craniofacial abnormalities (dolichocephaly, flaring of the temporal region, flat facies, mongoloid slant of the palpebral fissures, and large dysplastic ears with prominent superior crura and hypoplastic lobules), stubby fingers with immobility of the interphalangeal joints, flattened knuckle creases, pes calcaneovalgus, and contractures of hip, knee, and ankle joint resulting in impaired motor development.

Pfeiffer, R. A. The oto-onycho-peroneal syndrome. *Eur. J. Pediat.,* 1982, 138:317-20.

oto-osteodysplasia syndrome. See *auriculo-osteodysplasia syndrome.*

otocephalia. See *otocephaly syndrome.*

otocephaly syndrome. Synonym: *otocephalia.*

A combination of microstomia, agnathia, and fusion of the external ears in the midline region normally occupied by the mandible (synotia).

Gorlin, R. J., Pindborg, J. J., & Cohen, M. M., Jr. *Syndromes of the head and neck.* 2nd ed., New York, McGraw-Hill, 1976. p. 590-1.

otodental dysplasia. See *otodental syndrome.*

otodental syndrome. Synonym: *otodental dysplasia.*

An autosomal dominant disorder characterized by gigantic globoid teeth and a high-frequency sensorineural deafness.

Levin, L. S., & Jorgenson, E. J. Familial otodentodysplasia: A "new" syndrome. *Am. J. Hum. Genet.*, 1972, 24:61A. Levin, L. S., & Jorgenson, R. J. Otodental dysplasia: A previously undescribed syndrome. *Birth Defects*, 1974, 10(4):310-2.

otofacial dysostosis. See *oculo-auriculovertebral dysplasia.*

otogenic hydrocephalus. See *pseudotumor cerebri syndrome.*

otomandibular dysostosis. See *oculo-auriculovertebral dysplasia.*

otomandibular facial dysmorphogenesis. See *oculo-auriculovertebral dysplasia.*

otopalatodigital (OPD) syndrome. Synonym: *Taybi syndrome.*

A complex of malformations involving chiefly the face, hands, and feet, being more severe in males than females. Facial characteristics include a prominent forehead and supraorbital ridges, broad depressed nasal bridge, hypertelorism, flat midface, and small jaw with a greater than normal mandibular angle, occasional antimongoloid palpebral slant, and a small downturned mouth. Hand and foot anomalies include short spatulate thumbs and hallux, broad second to fourth digital phalanges, mild ulnar clinodactyly of the second and third fingers, mild radial clinodactyly of the fourth and fifth fingers, broad flat feet with spatulate great toes, and wide spaces between the first and second toes. Hip dislocation occurs in some cases. Cleft palate, deafness, short stature, and mental retardation occur only in males. The inheritance pattern is X-linked recessive.

Taybi, H. Generalized skeletal dysplasia with multiple anomalies. A note on Pyle's disease. *Am. J. Roentgen.*, 1962, 88:450-7.

otospondylofacial dysplasia. See *Weissenbacher-Zweymüller syndrome.*

otospondylomegaepiphyseal dysplasia (OSMED). See *Weissenbacher-Zweymüller syndrome.*

OTTO, ADOLF WILHELM (German physician, 1786-1845)

Otto disease. See *Otto-Chrobak syndrome.*

Otto syndrome. See *arthrogryposis multiplex congenita syndrome.*

Otto-Chrobak disease. Synonyms: *Otto disease, arthrokatadysis.*

Osteoarthritic protrusion of the acetabulum, described by Otto in 1816.

Sokolowski, A., & Kopera, Z. Przypadek pierwotnego wglabienia panewki stawu biodrowego (protrusio acetabuli Otto-Chrobak) w wieku mlodocianym. *Post. Reum., Warszawa*, 1957, 3:140-5.

OURGAUD, A. G. (French ophthalmologist)

Jayle-Ourgaud syndrome. See *under Jayle.*

OUS. See *overuse syndrome.*

ovalocytosis. See *Dresbach anemia.*

ovarian ascites-pleural effusion syndrome. See *Meigs syndrome.*

ovarian dwarfism. See *chromosome XO syndrome.*

ovarian dysgenesis-sensorineural deafness syndrome. See *Perrault syndrome.*

ovarian short stature syndrome. See *chromosome XO syndrome.*

OVERSTREET, ERNEST W. (American physician)

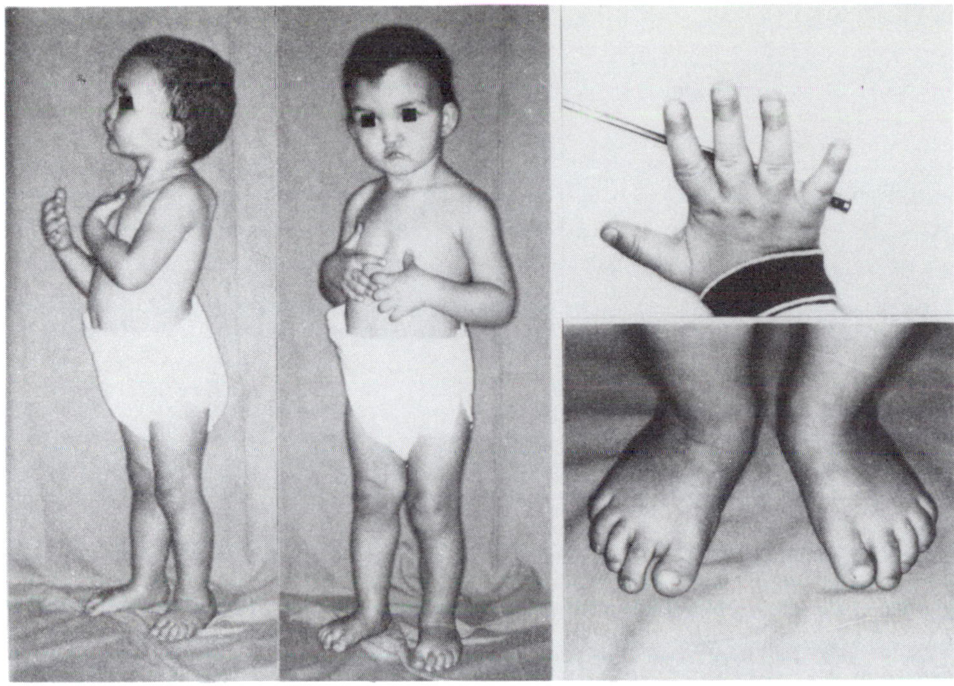

Otopalatodigital syndrome
Pazzaglia, Ugo E. & Giampiero Beluffi: *Clinical Genetics* 30:338-344, 1986. Munksgaard International Publishers, Copenhagen, Denmark.

Gordan-Overstreet syndrome. See *under Gordan.*

overuse syndrome (OUS). Synonyms: *chronic overuse, muscle effort syndrome, occupational cervicobrachial injury, occupational overuse syndrome (OOS), repetition strain injury (RSI), repetitive motion injury, repetitive strain syndrome.*

A group of pathological conditions, usually observed in persons engaged in sports or strenous manual work and in musicians, occurring when a tissue is stressed beyond its anatomical or physiological limits. Included in the group are injuries of the bones, joints, and bursae; musculotendinous lesions; muscle pain and cramps; and nerve entrapment syndromes. Typically, overuse results in microscopic tears of the affected tissue, followed by edema, hemorrhage, inflammatory reaction, and, finally, scar formation. Hypertrophy, stress fractures, vertebral hypertrophy and degenerative changes in the intervertebral disks, bone overgrowth in the joints with spur formation, and resulting limited joint mobility are the principal skeletal overuse injuries. A repeated overload of the musculotendinous system may result in **muscle-tendon syndromes,** including inflammation of the tendon attachment at the lateral or medial epicondyle of the humerus (**tennis** and **golfer elbows**), which are characterized by pain and localized tenderness over the affected tendon or adjacent muscles. Manual workers and musicians often suffer from pain of the wrists, hands, and proximal forearm. Fibrositis is the most common cause of muscle pain, which is sometimes associated with multifocal trigger sites and sleep disorders. Pain in the neck, upper trunk, and lower back may occur after severe strain. Muscle cramps may involve any single muscle or muscle groups; they are usually transient and reversible. **Nerve entrapment syndromes** usually occur at sites where nerves pass between relatively rigid structures, such as bones, tendons, or muscles, or close to the body surface, where they may be compressed externally. Included in this group are the **thoracic outlet syndrome, carpal tunnel syndrome, radial tunnel syndrome, cervical root compression syndrome** (usually involving the sixth, seventh, and eighth cranial nerves), and **pronator syndrome.** The symptoms of nerve compression syndromes consist mainly of pain, paresthesia, and swelling. Occupational palsies are disorders of motor control and involve overused muscles, such as those of the hands and wrists, as in manual workers (especially meat cutters); athletes, writers (**writer cramp**) and computer operators; lips and tongue, as in musicians (see also *Satchmo syndrome*); or muscles of any part of the body engaged in a strenous repetitive activity. Repetitive motions in sign language may cause tendinitis, fasciitis, synovitis, and nerve entrapment of the upper extremities. See also *talar compression syndrome*.

Lederman, R. J., & Calabrese, L. H. Overuse syndromes in instrumentalists. *Med. Probl. Perform. Art.*, 1986, 1:7-11. Howard, N. J. Peritendinitis crepitans; a muscle-effort syndrome. *J. Bone Joint Surg.*, 1937, 19:447-59. Acheson, R. M., *et al.* New Haven survey of joint diseases. XII. Distribution and symptoms of osteoarthritis in the hand with reference to handedness. *Ann. Rheum. Dis.*, 1970, 29:275-86. Cohn, L., *et al.* Overuse syndromes of the upper extremity in interpreters for the deaf. *Orthopedics*, 1990, 13:107-9.

OWENS, R. P. (American physician)

Sensenbrenner-Dorst-Owens syndrome. See *cranioectodermal dysplasia syndrome.*

OWREN, PAUL ARNOR (Norwegian hematologist, born 1905)

Owren crisis. See *Owren syndrome (1).*

Owren syndrome (1). Synonyms: *Owren crisis, aplastic crisis, hemolytic crisis.*

An acute aplastic blood disease marked by hemolytic anemia with complete cessation of erythrocyte production, disappearance of the reticulocytes from the blood, a decrease of normal values of serum bilirubin with urobilinuria, an increase in the level of blood iron, leukopenia, and thrombocytopenia. Spontaneous recovery is a result of a rapid regeneration of the erythropoietic tissue, which causes reticulocytosis, leukocytosis, increase in the thrombocyte count, and a rapid fall in the level of serum iron.

Owren, P. A. Congenital hemolytic jaundice, the pathogenesis of the "hemolytic crisis." *Blood*, 1948, 3:231-48.

Owren syndrome (2). Synonyms: *Ac-globulin deficiency, factor V deficiency, hemophiloid state A, hypoprothrombinemia, labile factor deficiency, parahemophilia A, parahemophilia syndrome, proaccelerin deficiency.*

A congenital blood coagulation disorder, transmitted as an autosomal recessive trait, in which deficiency of factor V (a cofactor in the conversion of prothrombin to thrombin by factor X) results in a hemophilialike syndrome with bleeding that ranges from very mild to fatal. Epistaxis, susceptibility to bruising, hemorrhage after tooth extraction, and bleeding from the gums are the common manifestations. In severe cases, there may be bleeding into the gastrointestinal tract and central nervous system, hematomas, and metrorrhagia. Some patients may show a prolonged bleeding time. Both sexes are affected.

Owren, P. A. Parahaemophilia. Haemorrhagic diathesis due to absence of a previously unknown clotting factor. *Lancet*, 1947, 1:446-8.

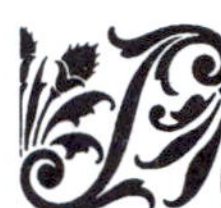

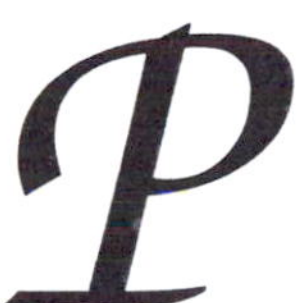

pacemaker syndrome (PS). A complication of ventricular pacing, ranging from occasional mild symptoms to hypotension, congestive heart failure, and neurological disorders. The symptoms may include orthostatic hypotension, tachypnea, neck vein distention, pulmonary rales, edema, regurgitant murmurs, tachycardia, diapheresis, apprehension, lethargy, fatigability, dyspnea, orthopnea, syncope or near-syncope, dizziness, confusion, nocturnal restlessness, right upper quadrant pain, cough, and headache. The syndrome is caused by loss of atrioventricular synchrony, valvular incompetence, asynchronous ventricular contractions, faulty circulatory reflexes, echo beats, or arrhythmias. See also *twidler syndrome.*

Mitsui, T., *et al.* Optimal heart rate in cardiac pacin in coronary sclerosis and nonsclerosis. *Ann. N. Y. Acad. Sc.*, 1969, 167: 745-55.

pacemaker twidler syndrome. See *twidler syndrome.*

pachyacria. See *Marie syndrome (2), under Marie, Pierre.*

pachydermatitis-pachyperiostitis-osteophytosis syndrome. See *pachydermoperiostosis syndrome.*

pachydermia vorticella. See *pachydermoperiostosis syndrome.*

pachydermoperiostosis. See *Brugsch syndrome.*

pachydermoperiostosis syndrome. Synonyms: *Audry syndrome, Friedreich-Erb-Arnold syndrome, Roy syndrome, Roy-Jutras syndome, Touraine-Solente-Golé (TSG) syndrome, Uehlinger syndrome, acromegaloid osteosis, acropachyderma, acropachydermy with pachyperiostosis syndrome, bulldog scalp, cutis verticis gyrata, gyrate scalp, hyperostosis generalisata with pachydermy syndrome, hypertrophic osteodermopathy, idiopathic familial generalized osteophytosis, idiopathic hypertrophic osteoarthropathy, megalia ossium et cutis, osteodermopathia hypertrophicans, osteodermopathic-hyperperiostosis syndrome, osteopathia dysplastica familiaris, pachydermatitis-pachyperiostitis-osteophytosis syndrome, pachydermia orticella, pachyperiosteodermia, pachyhyperiostosis, primary hypertrophic osteoarthropathy, pseudoacromegalic syndrome, washboard scalp.*

An association of clubbing of the digits due to soft tissue hyperplasia; periosteal new bone formation, particularly over the distal endings of the long bones; and coarsening of facial features with furrowing of the face, forehead, and scalp (cutis verticis gyrata). Associated disorders include long extremities, thickening and hyperostosis of the hands and feet, fatigability, blepharitis, and arthralgia. The skin is seborrheic and hyperplastic. Radiological findings consist of cortical thickening and sclerosis of the long bones, expansion of the diaphyses of the long bones in advanced stages, sclerotic rarefaction of the spongiosa with heavy trabeculae along pressure and traction lines, thickening of the calvaria, and enlarged frontal sinuses. The syndrome is transmitted as an autosomal dominant trait with variability of expression, being more severe in males than females. The symptoms appear at the time of puberty. This condition differs from the Brugsch syndrome by the presence of acromegaly.

Touraine, A., Solente, G., & Golé, L. Un syndrome ostéodermopathique. La pachydermie plicaturée avec pachypériostose des extrémités. *Presse Méd.*, 1935, 42:1820-4. Friedreich, N. Hyperostose des gesamten Skeletts. *Arch. Path., Berlin*, 1868, 43:83-7. Uehlinger, E. Hyperostosis generalisata mit Pachydermie. (Idiopatische familiäre generalisierte Osteophytose Friedreich-Erb-Arnold). *Virchows Arch. Path.*, 1942, 308:396-444. Erb, W. Über Akromegalie (krankhaften Riesenwuchs). *Deut. Arch. Klin. Med.*, 1887-88, 42:295-338. Arnold, J. Acromegalie, Pachyacrie oder Ostitis? Ein anatomischer Bericht über den Fall Hagner. *Beitr. Anat.*, 1891, 10:1-80. Roy, J. N. Hypertrophie des tarses palpébraux, des téguments de la face et des extrémités des membres, associée à une osteo-périostose presque généralisée; un syndrome nouveau. *Union Med. Canada*, 1936, 65:517-39. Audry, C. Pachydermie occipitale vorticellée (cutis verticis gyrata). *Ann. Derm. Syph., Paris*, 1909, 10:257-8.

pachyhyperiostosis. See *pachydermoperiostosis syndrome.*

pachyonychia congenita. See *Jackson-Lawler syndrome, under Jackson, A. D. M.* and see *Jadassohn syndrome, under Jadassohn, Josef.*

pachyonychia ichthyosiforme. See *Jadassohn-Lewandowski syndrome, under Jadassohn, Josef.*

pachyperiosteodermia. See *pachydermoperiostosis syndrome.*

PAES. See ***p**opliteal **a**rtery **e**ntrapment **s**yndrome.*

PAGE, IRVINE HEINLY (American physician, born 1901)

Page syndrome. Synonym: *hypertensive diencephalic syndrome.*

A condition usually occurring in association with essential hypertension with irritation of the sympathetic and parasympathetic centers of the diencephalon. The symptoms include vasomotor blushing, perspiration, cyanosis of the fingers, tachycardia, salivation, lacrimation, sensation of choking, labored respiration, and sexual frigidity. The attacks may occur spontaneously but more frequently are precipitated by excitement. The disorder occurs most commonly in young women, but males are occasionally affected.

Page, I. H. A syndrome simulating diencephalic stimulation occurring in patients with essential hypertension. *Am. J. Med. Sc.*, 1935, 190:9-14.

PAGET, SIR JAMES (British physician, 1814-1899)

epithelioma pagetoide. See *Arning carcinoid.*

extramammary Paget disease. A neoplastic disease seen at various sites, most often on the vulva, penis, scrotum, perineum, umbilicus, and axillary regions, which is characterized by an eczematous eruption with weeping and crust formation and the presence of Paget cells. It is a cutaneous manifestation of internal malignancy. Some cases are believed to be familial, transmitted as an autosomal dominant trait.

Armed Forces Institute of Pathology. *Atlas of tumor pathology*. Sect. IX, Fasc. 33, 1960, p. F33(II)-15-27. Helwig, E. B., & Graham, F. N. Anogenital (extramammary Paget's disease). *Cancer*, 1963, 16:387-403. Kuehn, P. G., *et al*. Familial occurrence of extramammary Paget's disease. *Cancer*, 1973, 31:145-8.

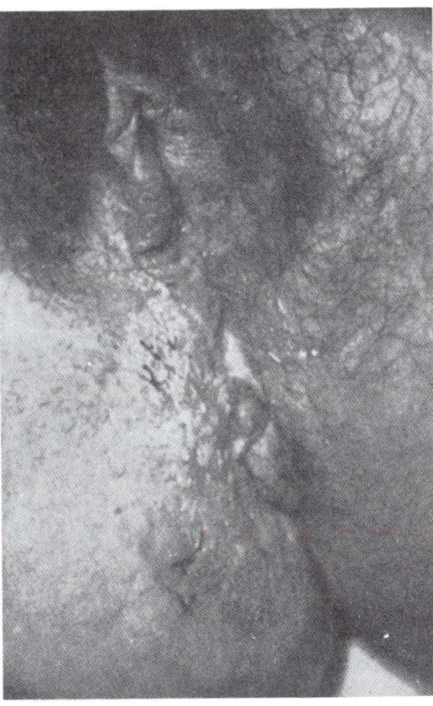

Extramammary Paget disease
Andrews, G.C. & A.N. Domonkos: *Diseases of the Skin.* 5th ed. Philadelphia: W.B. Saunders, Co., 1963.

juvenile Paget disease. See *hyperphosphatasia-osteoctasia syndrome.*

mammary Paget disease. Synonyms: *Paget cancer, Paget carcinoma, Paget nipple, carcinoma simplex of the nipple.*

An eczematoid lesion of the nipple with erosion and exudates, spreading to the areola, and associated with underlying carcinoma of the lactiferous ducts and deeper structures of the breast. The presence of Paget cells is the principal histological feature. Middle-aged women are most frequently affected.

Paget, J. On diseases of the mammary oreola preceding cancer of the mammary gland. *St. Bartholomew Hosp. Rep.*, 1874, 10:87-9.

Paget abscess. Synonym: *residual abscess.*

An abscess that forms about the residue of a former abscess.

Paget, J. On residual abscesses. *St. Bartholomew Hosp. Rep.*, 1869, 5:73-9.

Paget cancer. See *mammary Paget disease.*

Paget carcinoma. See *mammary Paget disease.*

Paget disease. Synonyms: *Paget disease of bone (PDB), Pozzi senile pseudorickets, multiple scleromalacia, osteitis deformans, osteodystrophia chronica deformans hypertrophica, osteodystrophia deformans, osteodystrophia fibrosa localisata, osteomalacia chronica deformans hypertrophica, scleromalacia.*

A slowly progressive bone disease, occurring most frequently in adults over 40 years of age, marked by extensive localized remodeling of one or several bones, including the cranium, clavicles, and long bones, mainly of the lower limbs. Initial changes, consisting of resorption of bone by osteoclasts, are followed by replacement of the bone marrow by vascular fibrous connective tissue and of the bone tissue by coarse, dense, disorganized trabecular structures. Deposition of the new bone causes an increase in irregular cement lines, thus giving the affected bone a characteristic mosaic pattern. Some bones show an increase of density without striations. The remodeling follows the stress exerted by muscle pull and gravity, with resulting bowing of the femur or the tibia and a tendency to deposit the most dense bone on the concave side of the bowed bones. There is enlargement and thickening of the skull. Severe enlargement of the base of the skull may cause basilar impression and compression of the spinal cord, brain stem, cerebellum, and basilar and vertebral arteries, with resulting slurred speech, swallowing difficulty, diplopia, and urinary incontinence. Pathological fractures and bone deformities cause walking problems. Increased skin temperature over the affected bones is due to hypervascularization of the bone beneath and an increase in the blood flow. Associated disorders may include heart enlargement, congestive heart failure, and neoplasms, such as osteosarcoma or giant-cell tumors in the affected bones. Radiographic findings include osteolytic lesions showing as radiolucent areas in the skull, which are known as **osteoporosis circumscripta**, and osteolytic lesions in the long bones with a characteristic sharply

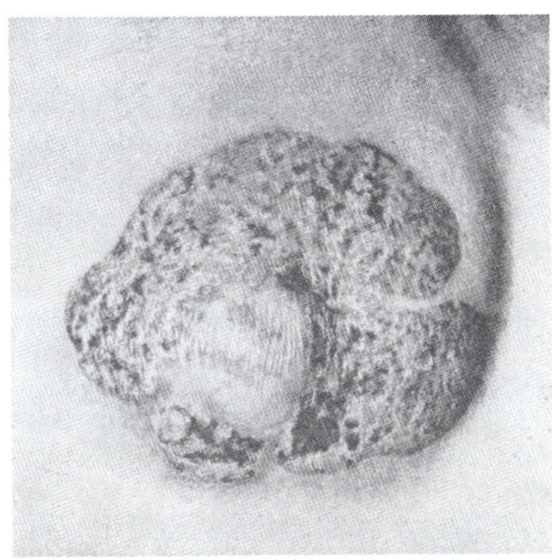

Mammary Paget disease
Andrews, G.C. & A.N. Domonkos: *Diseases of the Skin.* 5th ed. Philadelphia: W.B. Saunders, Co., 1963.

defined V shape, and linear cortical radiolucent areas in the tibia and femur. The etiology is unknown, but some cases are familial; when inherited, the condition is transmitted as an incompletely dominant gene carried on an X-chromosome. When associated with angioid streaks, the condition is known as the *Terry syndrome*.

Paget, J. On a form of chronic inflammation of bones (osteitis deformans). *Med. Chir. Tr., London*, 1877, 60:37-63.

Paget disease of bone. See *Paget disease*.

Paget nipple. See *mammary Paget disease*.

Paget quiet necrosis of bone. See *König disease (1)*.

Paget-Schroetter syndrome. Synonyms: *Paget-von Schroetter syndrome, von Schroetter syndrome, claudicatio venosa intermittens, effort thrombosis, intermittent venous claudication, primary thrombosis of the upper extremity, thrombosis venae axillaris, traumatic thrombosis of the axillary vein.*

Primary thrombosis of the axillary vein with sudden onset of pain, redness, tenderness, increased venous pressure in the affected extremity, and collateral circulation of the arms and shoulders.

Paget, J. *Clinical lectures and assays.* London, Langman, Green, 1875, p. 292. Schroetter, L., von. Erkrankungen der Gefasse. In: *Nothnagels Handbuch der Pathologie und Therapie.* Wien, 1884.

Paget-von Schroetter syndrome. See *Paget-Schroetter syndrome*.

pagetoid epithelioma. See *Arning carcinoid*.

pagetoid reticulosis. See *Woringer-Kolopp syndrome, under Woringer, Frederic.*

pain and spasm syndrome. Throbbing pain or spasm in the chest or parasternal muscles without evidence of myocardial infarction, occurring during intravenous administration of vancomycin.

Gatterer, G. Spasmatic low back pain in a patient receiving intravenous vancomycin during continuous ambulatory peritoneal dialysis. *Clin. Pharm.*, 1984, 3:87-9.

pain asymbolia. See *Schilder-Stengel syndrome*.

PAINE, R. S. (American physician)

Paine syndrome. Synonym: *microcephaly-spastic diplegia syndrome*.

A syndrome, transmitted as an X-linked trait, characterized by microcephaly, arthrogryposis, spastic diplegia, myoclonic convulsions, mental retardation, generalized aminoaciduria, elevated cerebrospinal fluid amino acid level, congenital heart defect, high arched palate, irregular dental arches, and abnormal dermatoglyphics.

Paine, R. S. Evaluation of familial biochemically determined mental retardation in children, with special reference to aminoaciduria. *N. Engl. J. Med.*, 1960, 262:658-65.

painful apicocostovertebral syndrome. See *Pancoast syndrome*.

painful arc syndrome. See *shoulder impingement syndrome*.

painful ecchymotic purpura in women. See *autoerythrocyte sensitization syndrome*.

painful feet syndrome. See *burning feet syndrome*.

painful irritable bowel. See *irritable bowel syndrome*.

painful leg syndrome. See *restless leg syndrome*.

painful lumbar sclerolipoma. See *Copeman-Ackermann syndrome*.

painful ophthalmoplegia. See *Tolosa-Hunt syndrome*.

painless diarrhea. See *irritable bowel syndrome*.

painless irritable bowel. See *irritable bowel syndrome*.

palatodigital syndrome. Synonym: *Catel-Manzke syndrome*.

A syndrome of absence of the hard palate, glossoptosis, and micrognathia (Robin syndrome), occurring in association with an accessory rectangular bone at the base of the proximal phalanx of the index finger, radial deviation and shortening of the finger, and clinodactyly. Heart defect, growth retardation, and talipes equinovarus may occur. The majority of reported cases were in males. The etiology is unknown.

*Catel, W. *Differentialdiagnose von Krankheitsymptomen bei Kindern und Jugendlichen*. 3rd. ed. Stuttgart, Thieme, 1961. Vol.1, p. 218. *Manzke, H. Symmetrische Hyperphalangie des zweiten Fingers durch ein akzessorisches Metacarpale. *Fortschr. Geb. Roentgenstr. Nulklearmed.*, 1966. 105:425.

palatopharyngolaryngeal paralysis. See *Tapia syndrome*.

PALEY, RONALD G. (British physician)

Tunbridge-Paley disease. See *under Tunbridge*.

palindromic rheumatism. See *Hench-Rosenberg syndrome*.

pallidal atrophy. See *Hunt paralysis, under Hunt, James Ramsay*.

pallidopyramidal disease. See *Hunt paralysis, under Hunt, James Ramsay*.

PALLISTER, PHILIP D. (American physician)

Herrmann-Pallister-Opitz syndrome. See *under Herrmann*.

Pallister mosaicism syndrome. See *chromosome 12p tetrasomy syndrome*.

Pallister syndrome (1). Synonym: *W syndrome*.

A multiple congenital anomaly-mental retardation syndrome, transmitted as an X-linked trait, characterized by prematurity, mental retardation, seizures, spasticity, tremor, frontal prominence, anterior cowlick, hypertelorism, antimongoloid slant of the palpebral fissures, alternating internal strabismus, flat and broad bridge and tip of the nose, incomplete median oral cleft, cleft upper lip, absent upper central incisors, medially cleft maxillary arch, anteriorly cleft palate, short and high mandible, cubitus valgus, subluxation of the proximal radioulnar joints, slightly short ulnae, lateral bowing of the radii, camptodactyly, and clinodactyly. The original cases were reported in brothers R. W. and S. W., hence the synonym *W syndrome*.

Pallister, P. D., *et al.* The W syndrome. Studies of malformation syndromes of man XXVIII. *Birth Defects*, 1974, 10(7):51-60.

Pallister syndrome (2). Synonym: *ulnar-mammary syndrome*.

A syndrome of abnormal development of the ulna, forearms, mammary glands, axillary apocrine glands, teeth, palate, vertebrae, and urogenital system, transmitted as an autosomal dominant trait. In the original report, the symptoms included absence of 4th and 5th fingers, metacarpals, triquetrum, hamate and pisiform bones with secondary abnormalities of palmar flexion creases and dermatoglyphics; shortness and malformation of the forearm bones with limitation of pronation and supination and cubitus valgus; cutaneous syndactyly; camptodactyly with subluxation of joints and shortness of fingers; postaxial polydactyly; tapering and hyperextensibility at the proximal interphalangeal joint of the fifth finger; hypoplasia or aplasia of the apocrine glands with absence of body odor, axillary sweating, and acne; hypoplasia or aplasia of the mammary glands and hypoplasia of the areolae and nipples; thoracic scoliosis; increased diameter of maxillary first incisors; absence of the canine teeth; high-arched palate; bifid uvula; kidney malrotation; and imperforate hymen.

Pallister, P. D., *et al.* Studies of malformation syndromes in man XXXXII: A pleiotropic dominant mutation affecting skeletal, sexual and apocrine-mammary development. *Birth Defects*, 1976, 12(5):247-54.

Pallister syndrome (3). See *chromosome 12p tetrasomy syndrome.*

Pallister-Hall syndrome. See *Hall syndrome, see under Hall, J. G.*

Pallister-Killian syndrome. See *chromosome 12p tetrasomy syndrome.*

PALLISTER, R. A. (Physician in Malaya)

Howes-Pallister-Landor syndrome. See *Landor-Pallister syndrome.*

Landor-Pallister syndrome. See *under Landor.*

pallor-hyperthermia syndrome. See *malignant hyperpyrexia syndrome.*

palmar fibromatosis. See *Dupuytren contracture.*

palmar syndrome. See *Lane disease, under Lane, John Edward.*

PALMER, CATHERINE G. (American geneticist)

Lavy-Palmer-Merritt syndrome. See *spondylothoracic dysplasia.*

palmoplantar erythema. See *Lane disease, under Lane, John Edward.*

palmoplantar keratoderma. See *Unna-Thost syndrome, under Unna, Paul Gerson.*

palmus. See *Bamberger disease (1), under Bamberger, Heinrich, von.*

palpebral coloboma-lipoma syndrome. See *nasopalpebral lipoma-coloboma syndrome.*

PALTAUF, RICHARD (Austrian physician, 1858-1924)

Hodgkin-Paltauf-Sternberg disease. See *Hodgkin disease.*

Paltauf-Sternberg disease. See *Hodgkin disease.*

panangiitis. See *Kussmaul-Maier syndrome.*

panarteritis. See *Kussmaul-Maier syndrome.*

panchondritis. See *Meyenburg-Altherr-Uehlinger syndrome.*

PANCOAST, HENRY KHUNRATH (American physician, 1875-1939)

Ciuffini-Pancoast syndrome. See *Pancoast syndrome.*

Pancoast syndrome. Synonyms: *Ciuffini-Pancoast syndrome, Hare syndrome, Pancoast apex syndrome, Pancoast pain syndrome, Pancoast-Tobias syndrome, Tobias syndrome, apicostovertebral syndrome, painful apicocostovertebral syndrome, superior pulmonary sulcus tumor, suprasulcus tumor.*

Destructive lesions of the thoracic inlet with involvement of the brachial and sympathetic plexus or carcinoma of the apex of the lung (**Pancoast tumor**), characterized by pain of the shoulder region radiating toward the axilla and scapula along the ulnar aspect of the arm, sensory and motor disorders and wasting of the muscles of the hand, the Bernard-Horner syndrome, and compression of the blood vessels with edema.

Pancoast, H. K. Superior pulmonary sulcus tumor. Tumor characterized by pain, Horner's syndrome, destruction of bone and atrophy of hand muscles. *JAMA*, 1932, 99:1391-6. Tobías, J. W. Sindrome ápico-costo-vertebral doloroso por tumor apexiano. Su valor diagnóstico en el cáncer primitivo pulmonar. *Rev. Med. Lat. Am.*, 1932, 17:1522-57. Hare, E. S. Tumor involving certain nerves. *London Med. Gaz.*, 98:196-9.

Pancoast apex syndrome. See *Pancoast syndrome.*

Pancoast pain syndrome. See *Pancoast syndrome.*

Pancoast tumor. See *under Pancoast syndrome.*

Pancoast-Tobias syndrome. See *Pancoast syndrome.*

pancreas-blood-bone syndrome. See *Shwachman syndrome.*

pancreatic carcinoma-hypokalemic watery diarrhea syndrome. See *Verner-Morrison syndrome.*

pancreatic cholera. See *Verner-Morrison syndrome.*

pancreatic exocrine insufficiency-metaphyseal dysostosis-dwarfism syndrome. See *Shwachman syndrome.*

pancreatic infantilism. See *Andersen triad.*

pancreatic insufficiency-blood disorder syndrome. See *Shwachman syndrome.*

pancreatic insufficiency-bone marrow dysfunction syndrome. See *Shwachman syndrome.*

pancreatic malignancy syndrome. See *Bard-Pic syndrome, under Bard, Louis.*

pancreaticobiliary syndrome. See *Bard-Pic syndrome, under Bard, Louis.*

pancreaticohepatic syndrome. See *Edelmann syndrome (2).*

pancreaticohepatic syndrome. See *Zieve syndrome.*

pancytopenia-dysmelia syndrome. See *Fanconi anemia.*

pangeria. See *Werner syndrome, under Werner, Otto.*

panhypopituitarism. See *Sheehan syndrome, and see Hanhart syndrome (1).*

panmesenchymal panangitic reaction. See *Slocumb syndrome.*

panmural fibrosis. See *Hunner ulcer.*

PANNER, HANS J. (Danish physician, 1871-1930)

Panner disease (1). See *Köhler disease (1).*

Panner disease (2). Synonyms: *Haas disease, epiphyseal necrosis of the capitellum humeri, osteochondrosis of the capitellum humeri.*

Epiphyseal ischemic necrosis of the capitellum humeri with formation of infarctlike lesions of the epiphyses, which collapse under pressure.

Panner, H. J. An affection of the capitellum humeri resembling Calvé-Perthes disease of the hip. *Acta Radiol., Stockholm*, 1927, 8:617.

panniculitis nodularis febrilis. See *Weber-Christian syndrome, under Weber, Frederick Parkes.*

PAPAS, C. V. (Greek physician)

Bartsocas-Papas syndrome. See *under Bartsocas.*

papillary cystadenolymphoma. See *Warthin tumor.*

papillary cystadenoma. See *Warthin tumor.*

papillary cystadenoma lymphomatosum. See *Warthin tumor.*

papillomatosis confluens et reticularis. See *Gougerot-Carteaud syndrome, under Gougerot, Henri.*

papillomatosis cutis. See *Gougerot-Carteaud syndrome, under Gougerot, Henri.*

PAPILLON, M. (French dermatologist)

Papillon-Lefèvre syndrome (PLS). Synonyms: *hyperkeratosis palmoplantaris-periodontoclasia syndrome, keratosis palmoplantaris with periodontopathy.*

Hyperkeratosis palmaris et plantaris associated with periodontoclasia and premature exfoliation of the teeth. The initial skin lesions usually occur between the ages of 1 and 4 years. Periodontosis becomes evident as soon as the last deciduous tooth has erupted, the teeth being involved in the sequence in which they erupt. Hypotrichosis may be associated. The syndrome is considered a variant of mal de Meleda, and is inherited as an autosomal recessive trait.

*Papillon & Lefèvre. Deux cas de kératodermie palmaire et plantaire symétrique familiale (maladie de Meleda) chez le frère et la soeur. Coexistence dans les deux cas d'alterations dentaires graves. *Bull. Soc. Fr. Derm. Syph.*, 1924, 31:82-7.

PAPILLON-LEAGE, E. (French dentist)

Papillon-Léage and Psaume syndrome. See *orofaciodigital syndrome I.*

PAPP, Z. (Hungarian physician)

Véradi-Papp syndrome. See *under Véradi.*

papular acrodermatitis. See *Gianotti-Crosti syndrome.*

papular acrodermatitis of childhood. See *Gianotti-Crosti syndrome.*

papular and nodular tuberculid. See *Barthélemy disease.*

papular mucinosis. See *Arndt-Gottron syndrome.*

papulosis atrophicans maligna. See *Degos syndrome.*

parabiotic syndrome. See *twin tranfusion syndrome.*

parabiotic twin syndrome. See *twin transfusion syndrome.*

paracoccidioidal granuloma. See *Lutz-Splendore-de Almedica syndrome, under Lutz, Alfredo.*

paracoccidioidomycosis. See *Lutz-Splendore-de Almeida syndrome, under Lutz, Adolfo.*

paradontitis. See *Fauchard disease.*

paraganglioma. See *under pheochromocytoma-islet cell tumor syndrome.*

parahemophilia A. See *Owren syndrome (2).*

parahemophilia syndrome. See *Owren syndrome (2).*

parakeratosis annularis. See *Mibelli disease (2).*

parakeratosis centrifugata atrophicans. See *Mibelli disease.*

parakeratosis psoriasiformis. See *Brocq disease (2).*

paralysis agitans. See *Parkinson syndrome, under Parkinson, James.*

paralysis agitans juvenilis. See *Hunt paralysis, under Hunt, James Ramsay.*

paralysis generalisata progressiva. See *Bayle disease.*

paralysis of the insane. See *Bayle disease.*

paralysis-congenital syphilis syndrome. See *Dennie-Marfan syndrome.*

paralytic dementia. See *Bayle disease.*

paralytic sciatica. See *Putti-Chavany syndrome.*

paralytic vertigo. See *Gerglier disease.*

paramethadione syndrome. See *fetal trimethadione syndrome.*

paramyoclonus multiplex. See *Friedreich disease (1), under Friedreich, Nicolaus.*

paramyotonia congenita. See *Eulenburg syndrome.*

paraneoplastic acrokeratosis. See *Bazex syndrome, under Bazex, A.*

paraneoplastic hypoglycemia-malignant histiocytoma syndrome. See *Doege-Potter syndrome.*

paraneoplastic retinopathy. See *cancer-associated retinopathy syndrome.*

paraneoplastic syndrome (PNS). A symptom complex involving endocrine, metabolic, hematologic, and other disorders that do not appear to be directly related to either the primary local neoplastic lesions or distal metastases of the tumor. The most common are endocrine disorders, which result from the production of hormones or hormonelike substances that are inappropriate to the tissue which produces them, as in the ectopic ACTH production syndrome (q.v.). Paraneoplastic syndromes include the Cushing syndrome due to increased ACTH production in oat-cell bronchogenic carcinoma, malignant thymoma, pancreatic carcinoma, and other neoplasms; hyponatremia due to inappropriate secretion of antidiuretic hormone; hypercalcemia due to cancers with metastases to bone, causing osteolysis and release of calcium into the circulation; hyperthyroidism due to ectopic hormone production in cancers of the hematopoietic system, bronchogenic carcinoma, prostatic carcinoma, and other cancers; hypoglycemia due to mesenchymal sarcoma and, occasionally, carcinoma; polycythemia associated with renal cell carcinoma; elevated serotonin, bradykinin, and histamine eleborated by argentaffinoma in the carcinoid syndrome; and a host of other conditions associated with neoplastic diseases of various organs.

Robbins, S. L., & Cotran, R. S. Paraneoplastic syndromes. In: *Pathologic basis of disease.* 2nd ed. Philadelphia, Saunders, 1979, pp. 190-3.

parangi. See *Charlouis disease.*

paranoia erotica. See *Clérambault syndrome.*

paraosteal osteoma. See *Geschickter tumor.*

parapemphigus. See *Brunsting disease.*

parasitic melanoderma. See *Greenhow disease.*

parastremmatic dwarfism syndrome. Synonyms: *distorted limb dwarfism, parastremmatic dysplasia, twisted limb dwarfism.*

Bone dysplasia characterized by severe dwarfism, a bizarre asymmetric deformity of the legs and arms with genu varum or valgum, bowing of the legs, and twisting of the limbs around their axis. Associated defects usually include brevicollis, kyphoscoliosis, increased anteroposterior diameter of the chest, and joint contractures. Radiographic features include platyspondyly, defective ossification of end plates, radiolucent vertebral bodies, small iliac wings surrounded by irregular ossification, small and poorly ossified femoral heads and necks, short and distorted tubular bones, and irregular ossification of the epiphyses and metaphyses of the tubular bones. Onset takes place in infancy. The syndrome is transmitted as an autosomal dominant or an X-linked dominant trait.

Langer, L. O., Petersen, D., & Spranger, J. An unusual bone dysplasia: Parastsremmatic dwarfism. *Am. J. Roentgen.*, 1970, 110:550-60.

parastremmatic dysplasia. See *parastremmatic dwarfism syndrome.*

paratrigeminal paralysis. See *Raeder syndrome.*

paratrigeminal sympathetic syndrome. See *Raeder syndrome.*

paratrigeminal syndrome. See *Raeder syndrome.*

paratyphoid. See *Schottmüller disease.*

paratyphoid fever. See *Schottmüller disease.*

parchment heart. See *Uhl anomaly.*

parchment right ventricle. See *Uhl anomaly.*

parent abuse. See *battered parent syndrome.*

parent-infant traumatic stress syndrome. See *battered child syndrome.*

PARENTI, GIAN CARLO (Italian physician)

Parenti disease. See *achondrogenesis type I.*

Parenti-Fraccaro syndrome. See *achondrogenesis type I.*

paresthetic meralgia. See *Rot-Bernhardt syndrome, under Rot, Vladimir Karlovich.*

parietal fibroplastic eosinophilic endocarditis. See *Löffler endocarditis.*

parietal hernia. See *Richter hernia.*

parietal syndrome. See *Bianchi syndrome.*

PARINAUD, HENRI (French physician, 1844-1905)

Parinaud conjunctivitis. See *Parinaud oculoglandular syndrome.*

Parinaud conjunctivoadenitis. See *Parinaud oculoglandular syndrome.*

Parinaud oculoglandular syndrome. Synonyms: *Parinaud conjunctivitis, Parinaud conjunctivoadenitis, Parinaud syndrome, cat scratch-oculoglandular syndrome, conjunctivo-glandular syndrome, leptotrichosis of the conjunctiva, oculoglandular syndrome, uniocular granulomatous conjunctivitis with preauricular adenopathy.*

A complication of cat scratch disease (q.v.) manifested by an ocular granuloma or conjunctivitis, with swelling of the parotid area, caused by preauricular lymphadenopathy. See also *Durand-Nicolas-Favre disease*, under *Durand, J.*

Parinaud & Galezowski. Conjoctivite infectieuse transmise par les animaux. *Ann. Ocul., Paris*, 1889, 101:252-3.

Parinaud syndrome. See *Parinaud oculoglandular syndrome.*

PARKER, FREDERICK, JR. (American physician)

Parker-Jackson syndrome. Synonym: *reticulum-cell sarcoma of bone.*

Malignant lymphoma of bone of the undifferentiated or histiocytic type.

Parker, F., Jr., & Jackson, H., Jr. Primary reticulum cell sarcoma of bone. *Surg. Gyn. Obst.*, 1939, 68:45-53.

PARKER, R. W. (British physician)

Parker syndrome. See *Hutchinson disease, under Hutchinson, Sir Robert Grieve.*

PARKES WEBER. See WEBER, FREDERICK PARKES

PARKINSON, JAMES (British physician, 1755-1824)

Parkinson disease (PD). See *Parkinson syndrome.*

Parkinson syndrome. Synonyms: *Parkinson disease (PD), parkinsonism, paralysis agitans, shaking palsy.*

A degenerative disorder of the nervous system, originally defined by Parkinson as "involuntary tremulous motion, with lessened muscular power, in parts not in action and even when supported, with a propensity to bend the trunk forward, and to pass from walking to a running pace, the sense of intellect being unaffected." The syndrome usually occurs in middle or later life and has a progressive, prolonged course. It is characterized by masklike facies with a wide-eyed, unblinking expression, sialorrhea, and greasy skin; dysarthria; stooped posture, cogwheel rigidity; slowness and poverty of movements; alternating tremor; and abnormal gait. Involuntary tremor usually begins in one hand and gradually spreads to both arms and legs; it may disappear momentarily on voluntary movements or during sleep. Pathologically, there is the accumulation of melanin-containing nerve cells in the brain stem, chiefly in the substantia nigra and locus coeruleus, in association with nerve cell loss, reactive gliosis, and eosinophilic inclusions (Lewy bodies). A decrease of dopamine in the caudate nucleus and putamen is the principal biochemical feature of this disorder. Four principal varieties are recognized: **Parkinson disease (paralysis agitans),** which normally occurs during the sixth decade; **encephalitic parkinsonism,** which follows encephalitis and is observed in both children and adults; **arteriosclerotic muscular rigidity,** which is a disease of old age; and **drug-induced parkinsonism,** which is caused by toxic reactions to some medicinal substances and may occur at any age. See also *Hunt paralysis.*

Parkinson, J. *An assay on the shaking palsy.* London, Whittingham & Rowland, 1817.

PARKINSON, SIR JOHN (British physician, born 1885)

Wolff-Parkinson-White syndrome (WPW). See *under Wolff.*

parkinsonism. See *Parkinson syndrome, under Parkinson, James.*

paroxysmal abdominal pain syndrome. See *Moore syndrome, under Moore, Matthew Thibaut.*

paroxysmal atrial tachycardia. See *Bouveret syndrome (2).*

paroxysmal cold hemoglobinuria. See *Donath-Landsteiner syndrome.*

paroxysmal dyspnea. See *Rostan asthma.*

paroxysmal dystonic choreoathetosis. See *Mount-Reback syndrome.*

paroxysmal hematoma of the hand. See *Achenbach syndrome.*

paroxysmal hemoglobinuria. See *Dressler syndrome, under Dressler, D. R.*

paroxysmal hemoglobinuria a frigore. See *Donath-Landsteiner syndrome.*

paroxysmal junctional tachycardia. See *Bouveret syndrome (2).*

paroxysmal lacrimation. See *gustatory lacrimation syndrome.*

paroxysmal nocturnal dyspnea. See *Rostan asthma.*

paroxysmal nocturnal hemoglobinuria. See *Marchiafava-Micheli syndrome.*

paroxysmal paralysis. See *Westphal syndrome, under Westphal, Karl Friedrich Otto.*

paroxysmal polyserositis. See *Reimann periodic disease.*

paroxysmal sleep. See *Gélineau syndrome.*

paroxysmal supraventricular tachycardia (PSVT). See *Bouveret syndrome (2).*

paroxysmal syndrome. See *Reimann periodic disease.*

paroxysmal thyroid instability. See *Léopold-Lévy syndrome.*

paroxysmal ventricular fibrillation. See *torsades de pointes syndrome.*

parricide. See *under battered parent syndrome.*

PARROT, JULES MARIE (French physician, 1839-1883)

Bednar-Parrot disease. See *Parrot syndrome (1).*

Parrot atrophy. See *marasmus syndrome.*

Parrot cicatrix. Whitish cicatrices occurring at the sites of labial fissures, observed in children with congenital syphilis, reportedly described by Parrot.

Parrot disease. See *Parrot syndrome (1).*

Parrot nodes. Syphilitic nodules on the skull, giving it a buttocklike shape, found in infants with congenital syphilis.

Parrot. Lésions du crâne, causées par la syphilis héréditaire. *Progr. Méd., Paris*, 1879, 7:268-9.

Parrot paralysis. See *Parrot syndrome (1).*
Parrot pseudoparalysis. See *Parrot syndrome (1).*

Parrot syndrome (1). Synonyms: *Bednar-Parrot disease, Parrot disease, Parrot paralysis, Parrot pseudoparalysis, Wegner disease, Wegner osteochondritis, syphilitic osteitis of newborn, syphilitic osteochondritis, syphilitic pseudoparalysis.*

Osteochondritis with disabling pain on movement, occurring in infants with congenital syphilis.

Parrot, J. M. Sur une pseudo-paralysie causée par une altération du système osseux chez les nouveau-nées atteints de syphilis héréditaire. *Arch. Physiol., Paris*, 1871-72, 4:319-33. Wegner, G. Über hereditäre Knochensyphilis bei jungen Kindern. *Arch. Path. Anat., Berlin*, 1870, 50:305-22.

Parrot syndrome (2). See *achondroplasia.*
Parrot-Kaumann syndrome. See *achondroplasia.*
PARRY, CALEB HILLIER (British physician, 1755-1822)
Parry syndrome. See *Basedow disease.*
Parry-Romberg syndrome. See *Romberg syndrome (2).*
partial androgen insensitivity syndrome. See *Reifenstein syndrome.*
partial cortical epilspy. See *Jackson epilepsy.*
partial epilepsy. See *Kozhevnikov syndrome.*
partial gigantism. See *Curtius syndrome (1).*
partial lipodystrophy of the cephalothoracic type. See *Barraquer-Simons syndrome.*
partial monosomy 1pter syndrome. See *chromosome 1pter deletion syndrome.*
partial monosomy 1q syndrome. See *chromosome 1q deletion syndrome.*
partial monosomy 2q syndrome. See *chromosome 2q deletion syndrome.*
partial monosomy 3pter syndrome. See *chromosome 3pter deletion syndrome.*
partial monosomy 3q syndrome. See *chromosome 3q deletion syndrome.*
partial monosomy 4p syndrome. See *chromosome 4p deletion syndrome.*
partial monosomy 4q syndrome. See *chromosome 4q deletion syndrome.*
partial monosomy 5p syndrome. See *chromosome 5p deletion syndrome.*
partial monosomy 5q syndrome. See *chromosome 5q deletion syndrome.*
partial monosomy 7p syndrome. See *chromosome 7p deletion syndrome.*
partial monosomy 7q syndrome. See *chromosome 7q deletion syndrome.*
partial monosomy 8p syndrome. See *chromosome 8p deletion syndrome.*
partial monosomy 8q syndrome. See *chromosome 8q deletion syndrome.*
partial monosomy 9p syndrome. See *chromosome 9p deletion syndrome.*
partial monosomy 10p syndrome. See *chromosome 10p deletion syndrome.*
partial monosomy 10qter syndrome. See *chromosome 10qter deletion syndrome.*
partial monosomy 11q syndrome. See *chromosome 11q deletion syndrome.*
partial monosomy 12p syndrome. See *chromosome 12p deletion syndrome.*
partial monosomy 13q syndrome. See *chromosome 13q deletion syndrome.*

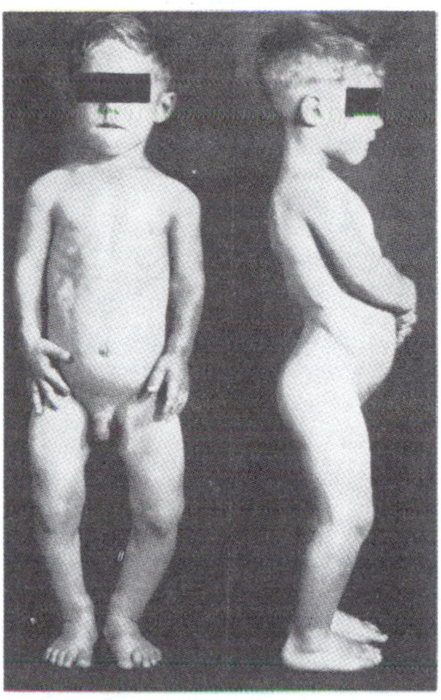

Parrot syndrome (1)
Nelson, W.E., (ed.): *Textbook of Pediatrics.* 8th ed. Philadelphia: W.B. Saunders Co., 1964.

partial monosomy 14q syndrome. See *chromosome 14q deletion syndrome.*
partial monosomy 16q syndrome. See *chromosome 16q deletion syndrome.*
partial monosomy 17p syndrome. See *chromosome 17p deletion syndrome.*
partial monosomy 18p syndrome. See *chromosome 18p deletion syndrome.*
partial monosomy 18q syndrome. See *chromosome 18q deletion syndrome.*
partial monosomy 20p syndrome. See *chromosome 20p deletion syndrome.*
partial monosomy 20q syndrome. See *chromosome 20q deletion syndrome.*
partial monosomy 21q syndrome. See *chromosome 21q deletion syndrome.*
partial syndrome of the vertebrospinal artery. See *Opalski syndrome.*
partial transient osteoporosis. See *transient osteopenia of hip syndrome.*
partial trisomy 1q syndrome. See *chromosome 1q duplication syndrome.*
partial trisomy 2p syndrome. See *chromosome 2p duplication syndrome.*
partial trisomy 2q syndrome. See *chromosome 2q duplication syndrome.*
partial trisomy 3p syndrome. See *chromosome 3p duplication syndrome.*
partial trisomy 3q syndrome. See *chromosome 3q duplication syndrome.*
partial trisomy 4p syndrome. See *chromosome 4p duplication syndrome.*
partial trisomy 4q syndrome. See *chromosome 4q duplication syndrome.*
partial trisomy 5p syndrome. See *chromosome 5p duplication syndrome.*
partial trisomy 5q syndrome. See *chromosome 5q duplication syndrome.*

partial trisomy 6p syndrome. See *chromosome 6p duplication syndrome.*

partial trisomy 6q syndrome. See *chromosome 6q duplication syndrome.*

partial trisomy 7p syndrome. See *chromosome 7p duplication syndrome.*

partial trisomy 7q syndrome. See *chromosome 7q duplication syndrome.*

partial trisomy 8p syndrome. See *chromosome 8p duplication syndrome.*

partial trisomy 8q syndrome. See *chromosome 8q duplication syndrome.*

partial trisomy 10p syndrome. See *chromosome 10p duplication syndrome.*

partial trisomy 10q syndrome. See *chromosome 10q duplication syndrome.*

partial trisomy 11p syndrome. See *chromosome 11p duplication syndrome.*

partial trisomy 11q syndrome. See *chromosome 11q duplication syndrome.*

partial trisomy 12p syndrome. See *chromosome 12p duplication syndrome.*

partial trisomy 12q mosaicism. See *chromosome 12q duplication mosaicism syndrome.*

partial trisomy 12q syndrome. See *chromosome 12q duplication syndrome.*

partial trisomy 13q syndrome. See *chromosome 13q duplication syndrome.*

partial trisomy 14q syndrome. See *chromosome 14q duplication syndrome.*

partial trisomy 15q syndrome. See *chromosome 15q duplication syndrome.*

partial trisomy 16p syndrome. See *chromosome 16p duplication syndrome.*

partial trisomy 16q syndrome. See *chromosome 16q duplication syndrome.*

partial trisomy 17p syndrome. See *chromosome 17p duplication syndrome.*

partial trisomy 17q syndrome. See *chromosome 17q duplication syndrome.*

partial trisomy 18q syndrome. See *chromosome 18q duplication syndrome.*

partial trisomy 19q syndrome. See *chromosome 19q duplication syndrome.*

partial trisomy 20p syndrome. See *chromosome 20p duplication syndrome.*

partial trisomy 20q syndrome. See *chromosome 20q duplication syndrome.*

PARTSCH, C. J. (German physician)

Miehlke-Partsch syndrome. See *under Miehlke.*

PASCHEFF, CONSTANTIN (Bulgarian ophthalmologist, born 1873)

Pascheff conjunctivitis. Synonyms: *conjunctivitis necroticans infectiosa, necrotic infectious conjunctivitis.*

Conjunctivitis with foci of suppurative necrotizing inflammation and swelling in the regional lymph nodes, due to an infection with *Microbacillus polymorphicus necroticans.*

Pascheff, C. Über eine besondere Form von Bindehaut-Entzündung (Conjunctivitis necroticans infectiosa). *Klin. Mbl. Augenh.*, 1916, 57:517-29.

Pascheff folliculoma. Synonym: *trachomatous folliculoma.*

Tumors with lymphoblastic centers formed by masses of confluent trachoma follicles.

Pascheff, C. Researches on the follicular disease of the conjunctiva. Their relation to the laws of true trachoma, its etiology, and unification of conception. *Am. J. Ophth.*, 1932, 15:690-708.

PASCOE, DELMER J. (American physician)

Forney-Robinson-Pascoe syndrome. See *under Forney.*

PASINI, AGOSTINO (Italian dermatologist)

Pasini-Pierini syndrome. Synonyms: *atrophoderma idiopathica progressiva, idiopathic atrophoderma, progressive idiopathic atrophoderma.*

A progressive skin disease, most commonly occurring in young women, characterized by depressed bluish violaceous or brownish-blue lesions with smooth surfaces, varying in size from a few centimeters to large patches. Deep blood vessels are visible beneath the lesions as faint, blurred streaks. The lesions are distributed chiefly on the trunk and back. Edematous changes in the collagen bundles of the deep cutis are the principal pathological features.

Pasini, A. Atrofodermia idiopatica progressiva. (Studio clinico ed istologico). *Gior. Ital. Mal. Vener.*, 1923, 64:785-809. Pierini, L. E., & Vivoli, D. Atrofodermia idiopatica progressiva (Pasini). *Gior. Ital. Derm.*, 1936, 77:403-9.

PASQUALINI, RUDOLFO QUIRINO (Argentine physician, born 1909)

Pasqualini syndrome. Synonyms: *fertile eunuch syndrome, hypogonadism-spermatogenesis syndrome, hypoandrogenic syndrome with normal spermatogenesis.*

Eunuchoidism associated with normal secretion of follicle-stimulating hormone and spermatogenesis.

Pasqualini, R. Q. Sindrome hypoandrogénico con gametogénesis conservada (hypoandrogenic syndrome with normal spermatogenesis). *J. Clin. Endocr.*, 1953, 13:128-9.

PASSARGE, E.

Passarge syndrome. See *anhidrotic ectodermal dysplasia, autosomal recessive.*

PASSOUANT, P. (French physician)

Rimbaud-Passouant-Vallat syndrome. See *under Rimbaud.*

PASSOW, ARNOLD, VON (German ophthalmologist, 1888-1966)

Passow syndrome. An association of Horner syndrome with heterochromia iridis.

Passow, A. Okulare Paresen im Sympathomenbild des "Status dysraphicus," zugleich ein Beitrag zu Aetiologie der Sympathikusparese (Horner-Syndrom und Heterochromia iridis) sowie der Trigeminus Abduzens-und Fazialisparese. *Münch. Med. Wschr.*, 1934, 81:1243-0.

PATAU, KLAUS (German-born physician in America)

Bartholin-Patau syndrome. See *chromosome 13 trisomy syndrome.*

Patau syndrome. See *chromosome 13 trisomy syndrome.*

patellar instability syndrome. See *unstable patella syndrome.*

PATERSON, DONALD ROSE (British physician, 1863-1939)

Paterson-Brown Kelly syndrome. See *Plummer-Vinson syndrome.*

Paterson-Kelly syndrome. See *Plummer-Vinson syndrome.*

pathologic laughing and weeping syndrome. Synonym: *laughing and weeping syndrome.*

Uncontrolled laughing and crying in persons affected with lesions of the forebrain.

Schiffer, R. B., *et al.* Treatment of pathologic laughing and weeping with amitriptyline. *N. Engl. J. Med.*, 1985, 312:1480-2.

pathomimia. See *Munchausen syndrome.*

PATIN, GUI (GUY) (French physician in 17th century)

Guy Patin syndrome. See *fibrodysplasia ossificans progressiva.*

Patin syndrome. See *fibrodysplasia ossificans progressiva.*

PATON, D. (American physician)

Von Sallmann-Paton syndrome. See *Witkop-Von Sallmann syndrome.*

PATON, LESLIE (British physician, born 1872)

Gowers-Paton-Kennedy syndrome. See *Kennedy syndrome.*

PATTERSON, JOSEPH H. (American physician)

Patterson syndrome. Synonym: *pseudoleprechaunism.*

An association of connective tissue and neuroendocrine disorders suggesting leprechaunism because of a somewhat leprechaun-like facies, consisting mainly of bronzed pigmentation of the skin, cutis laxa of the hands and feet, body disproportions, mental retardation, and a variety of bony deformities. Major skeletal anomalies include skeletal dysplasia; kyphoscoliosis; swellings of the distal ends of the long bones with special involvement of the knees, ankles, and wrists; valgus deformities of the ankles; delayed bone maturation; deformities of the ribs, clavicles, and scapulae; thickening of the cranial vault; defects in the occipital bone; thickening of the maxilla and ethmoid bone; malformations of the vertebrae; and deformity and failure of ossification of the pubic bones. Other findings include hirsutism, largely confined to the limbs; grand mal epilepsy, usually occurring in childhood; abnormal dermatoglyphics; precocious puberty; cushingoid features; and excessive production of adrenocortical hormones. The etiology is unknown. See also *Donohue syndrome (leprehaunism).*

Patterson, J. H. Presentation of a patient with leprechaunism. *Birth Defects,* 1969, 5(4):117-21.

paucity of interlobular bile ducts (PILBD). See *Alagille syndrome.*

PAUTRIER, LUCIEN MARIUS ADOLPHE (French physician, 1876-1959)

Brocq-Pautrier glossitis. See *Brocq-Pautrier syndrome.*

Brocq-Pautrier syndrome. See *under Brocq.*

Pautrier abscess. Synonym: *Pautrier microabscess.*

An eosinophil-rich pleomorphic intradermal cellular infiltration with focal collections of reticular cells, observed in mycosis fungoides.

Moore, C. V. Mycosis fungoides. In: Beeson, P. B., & McDermott, W., eds. *Cecil-Loeb textbook of medicine.* 12th ed. Philadelphia, Saunders, 1967, p. 1093.

Pautrier microabscess. See *Pautrier abscess.*

Pautrier-Woringer syndrome. Synonyms: *dermatopathic lymphadenopathy, lipomelanotic reticulosis.*

Lipomelanotic deposits in enlarged lymph nodes occurring in association with a variety of skin diseases. Pruritus may or may not be present.

Pautrier, L. M., & Woringer, F. Note préliminaire sur un tableau histologique particulier de lésions ganglionnaires accompagnant des éruptions dermatologiques généralisées, prurigineuses, de types cliniques différentes. *Bull. Soc. Fr. Derm. Syph.*, 1932, 39:947-55.

PAUZAT, JEAN EUGENE (French physician)

Pauzat disease. Osteoplastic periostitis of the metatarsal bones precipitated by fatigue, especially after prolonged walking.

Pauzat, J. E. De la périostite ostéoplasique des métatarsiens à la suite des marches. *Arch. Méd. Pharm. Mil., Paris*, 1887, 10:337-53.

PAVY, FREDERICK WILLIAM (British physician, 1829-1911)

Pavy disease. Synonyms: *cyclic albuminuria, recurrent physiologic albuminuria.*

Albuminuria in adolescents and young adults, occurring without any appparent cause, and marked by the diurnal appearance of small amounts of albumin in the urine. Pavy described it as follows: "In the early morning the urine is free from albumen. Albumen then shows itself; it may be at 9, 10, or 11 A.M. or not till the early part of the afternoon. After reaching its maximum it declines, and often by the evening it has disappeared by bedtime. The condition noticed may go on not only for weeks and months, but even for years. It is not accompanied by any impairment in health."

Pavy, F. W. Cyclic albuminuria (albuminuria in the apparently healthy). *Lancet*, 1885, 2:706-8.

PAXSON, NEWLIN F. (American physician)

Young-Paxson syndrome. See *under Young, James.*

PAXTON, FRANCIS VALENTINE (British physician, died 1924)

Paxton disease. See *Beigel disease.*

PAYR, ERWIN (German physician, 1871-1946)

Payr syndrome. See *splenic flexure syndrome.*

PBC. See *primary biliary cirrhosis syndrome.*

PBS. See *prune belly syndrome.*

PCB (polychlorinated biphenyl)-induced fetopathy. See *fetal PCB syndrome.*

PCM (protein-calorie malnutrition). See *kwashiorkor-marasmus syndrome.*

PCOD (polycystic ovarian disease). See *polycystic ovary syndrome.*

PCS. See *postcholecystectomy syndrome.*

PCS. See *postconcussive syndrome.*

PCS (postcardiotomy syndrome). See *postpericardiotomy syndrome.*

PCT. See *porphyria cutanea tarda syndrome.*

PD (Parkinson disease). See *Parkinson syndrome, under Parkinson, James.*

PD-AR. See *photosensitivity and actinic reticuloid syndrome.*

PDB (Paget disease of bone). See *Paget disease.*

PDE (progressive dialysis encephalopathy). See *dialysis encephalopathy syndrome.*

peapicker disease. See *leptospirosis.*

PEARLMAN, HUBERT S. (American orthopedic surgeon)

Nievergelt-Pearlman syndrome. See *Nievergelt syndrome.*

PEARSON, CARL M. (American physician)

McArdle-Schmid-Pearson syndrome. See *glycogen storage disease V.*

pectoral aplasia-dysdactylia syndrome. See *Poland syndrome.*

pectoral muscle absence and syndactyly syndrome. See *Poland syndrome.*

pectoralis minor syndrome. See *hyperabduction syndrome.*

pedatrophy. See *marasmus syndrome.*

PEDERSEN, EJNAR (Danish physician)

Pedersen syndrome. Synonyms: *epidemic neurolabyrinthitis, epidemic vertigo, vestibular neuronitis.*

Sudden and protracted vertigo, gradually becoming paroxysmal, usually in association with asthenic symptoms and occasional depression and anxiety. The disease occurs in conjunction with encephalitis. One form is characterized by gastrointestinal complications, and the other by upper respiratory tract infection. The symptoms may include gastroenteritis, fever, nausea, vomiting, abdominal pain, sore throat, dehydration, impaired hearing, nystagmus, and mild hemiplegia. See also *Ménière syndrome*, and *vestibular syndrome*.

Pedersen, E. Epidemic vertigo. Clinical picture, epidemiology and relation to encephalitis. *Brain*, 1959, 82:566-80.

pedionalgia epidemica. See *acrodynia.*

peduncular syndrome. See *Foville syndrome.*

peeling skin syndrome. See *continual skin peeling syndrome.*

PEETOOM, F. (Dutch physician)

Peetoom-Meltzer syndrome. See *arthralgia-purpura-weakness syndrome.*

PEGOT

Pégot-Cruveilhier-Baumgarten syndrome. See *Cruveilhier-Baumgarten syndrome.*

PEIFFER, JÜRGEN (German physician, born 1922)

van Bogaert-Nijssen-Peiffer syndrome. See *metachromatic leukodystrophy.*

van Bogaert-Nyssen-Peiffer syndrome. See *metachromatic leukodystrophy.*

PEL, PIETER KLASSES (Dutch physician, 1852-1919)

Pel crises. See *Pel syndrome.*

Pel-Ebstein disease. See *Hodgkin disease.*

Pel syndrome. Synonyms: *Pel crises, ophthalmic crises, tabetic ciliary neuralgia.*

Ocular crises, particularly paroxysms of ciliary neuralgia and corneal hyperesthesia, associated with tabes dorsalis. Systemic neuralgias, glaucoma, lacrimation, and photophobia may also occur.

Pel, P. K. Augenkrisen bei Tabes dorsalis (Crises ophthalmiques). *Berlin Klin. Wschr.*, 1898, 35:25-7.

pelade. See *Cazenave vitiligo.*

PELGER, KAREL (Dutch physician, 1885-1931)

Pelger anomaly. See *Pelger-Huët anomaly.*

Pelger nuclear anomaly. See *Pelger-Huët anomaly.*

Pelger-Huët anomaly. Synonyms: *Pelger anomaly, Pelger nuclear anomaly, Pelger-Huët phenomenon, false shift to the left.*

A hereditary abnormality of leukocyte maturation, transmitted as an autosomal dominant trait, characterized by decreased segmentation of the nuclei of granulocytes, giving the nuclei a rodlike or dumbbell shape and a coarse lumpy structure; condensation of nuclear chromatin in granulocytes, lymphocytes, and monocytes; and normal cytoplasmic maturation. Döhle bodies may be present. Usually, there are no associated systemic abnormalities.

Pelger, K. Demonstratie van een paar zeldzaam voorkomende typen van bloedlichaampjes en besprecking der patienten. *Ned. Tschr. Geneesk.*, 1928, 72:1178. Huët, G. J. Over eeen familiaire anomalie der leucocyten. *Mschr. Kindergeneesk.*, 1932, 1:173-81.

Pelger-Huët phenomenon. See *Pelger-Huët anomaly.*

peliosis rheumatica. See *Schönlein-Henoch purpura.*

peliosis werlhofii. See *Werlhof disease.*

PELIZAEUS, FRIEDRICH (German physician, born 1850)

Pelizaeus-Merzbacher syndrome. Synonyms: *aplasia axialis extracorticalis congenita, chronic infantile cerebral sclerosis, extracortical axial aplasia, familial centrolobar sclerosis, familial chronic infantile diffuse sclerosis, sudanophilic leukodystrophy.*

An inherited disease of the nervous system, which includes several closely related pathological entities, some being transmitted as an autosomal recessive and others as an X-linked trait. In the first type, onset may take place early in life, and the symptoms include nystagmus, shaking movements of the head (as in spasmus nutans), ataxia, intention tremor, choreiform or athetotic movements of the arms, and retarded psychomotor development with inability to stand up, sit down, or walk. Seizures may be present. The second type is marked by late onset and survival into the second or third decades. The symptoms include pendular nystagmus, choreoathetosis, corticospinal dysarthria, cerebellar ataxia, and mental deficiency. The third type is similar to the Cockayne syndrome and is marked by photosensitivity of the skin, dwarfism, cerebellar ataxia, corticospinal signs, cataracts, retinitis pigmentosa, and deafness. Islands of preserved myelin give a tigroid pattern of degeneration and intact myelin in the cerebrum.

Pelizaeus, F. Über eine eigentümliche Form spastischer Lähmung mit Cerebralerscheinungen auf hereditärer Grundlage (multiple Sklerose). *Arch. Psychiat., Berlin,* 1885, 16:698-710. Merzbacher, L. Weitere Mitteilungen über eine einzigartige hereditär-familiäre Erkrankung des Zentralnervensystems. *Med. Klin., Berlin,* 1908, 4:1952-5. Adams, R. D., & Victor, M. *Principles of neurology.* 3rd ed. New York, McGraw-Hill, 1985, p. 728.

pellagra-cerebellar ataxia-renal aminoaciduria syndrome. See *Hartnup disease.*

pellagrous tongue. See *Möller glossitis.*

PELLEGRINI, AUGUSTO (Italian physician, born 1877)

Köhler-Stieda-Pellegrini syndrome. See *Stieda-Pellegrini syndrome.*

Stieda-Pellegrini syndrome. See *under Stieda.*

PELLIZZI, G. B. (Italian physician)

Pellizzi syndrome. Synonyms: *epiphyseal syndrome, macrogenitosomia praecox, pineal syndrome, quadrigeminal plate syndrome.*

A syndrome of precocious puberty in boys and amenorrhea in postpuberal girls caused by pineal tumors. Similar conditions may be observed in hypothalamic lesions. Destruction of the pineal parenchyma or interruption of thalamopineal connections are believed to be the cause.

Pellizzi, G. B. La sindrome epifisaria "macrogenitosomia precoce." *Riv. Ital. Neuropat.*, 1910, 3:193-207.

pelvic congestion syndrome. See *Taylor syndrome, under Taylor, Howard Canning, Jr.*

pelvic sympathetic syndrome. See *Taylor syndrome, under Taylor, Howard Canning, Jr.*

pelvicocleidocranial dysostosis. See *cleidocranial dysostosis.*

pelvipathia vegetans. See *Taylor syndrome, under Taylor, Howard Canning, Jr.*

pelvis obtecta. See *Kilian pelvis.*

pelvofemoral muscular dystrophy. See *Leyden-Moebius syndrome.*

pelvospondondylitis ossificans. See *Bechterew-Strümpell-Marie syndrome, under Bekhterev.*

PEM (protein-energy malnutrition). See *kwashiorkor-marasmus syndrome.*

pemphigus circinatus. See *Duhring disease.*

pemphigus erythematodes (erythematosus). See *Senear-Usher syndrome.*

pemphigus familiaris chronicus. See *Hailey-Hailey disease, under Hailey, William Howard.*

pemphigus foliaceus. Synonym: *Cazenave disease.*

A chronic form of symmetrical pemphigus in adults, in which flaccid bullae characterize the early phases and generalized exfoliation predominates in the later stages. The bullae are slightly elevated and rupture readily, discharging malodorous fluid and revealing a reddish or purplish moist surface beneath. The lesions spread slowly and symmetrically, and within a few months the entire body is covered with exfoliative lesions. The Nikolsky sign and acantholysis are always present.

Cazenave, P. L. Pemphigus chronique, général; forme rare de pemphigus foliacé; mort; autopsie; altération du foi. *Ann. Mal. Peau,* 1884, 1:208-10.

pemphigus frambesioides. See *Neumann syndrome (2), under Neumann, Isidor Elder von Heilwart.*

pemphigus hereditarius. See *epidermolysis bullosa syndrome.*

pemphigus papillaris. See *Neumann syndrome (2), under Neumann, Isidor Elder von Heilwart.*

pemphigus vegetans. See *Neumann syndrome (2), under Neumann, Isidor Elder von Heilwart.*

PENA, SERGIO D. J. (physician in Canada)

Pena-Shokeir syndrome (1). Synonym: *camptodactyly-ankyloses-facial anomalies-pulmonary hypoplasia syndrome.*

A lethal syndrome, probably transmitted as an autosomal recessive trait, consisting of polyhydramnios, intrauterine growth retardation, short umbilical cord, peculiar facies, limb abnormalities, and pulmonary hypoplasia. Facial characteristics include hypertelorism, low-set deformed ears, depressed tip of the nose, micrognathia, microstomia, and high-arched palate. Limb abnormalities consist of camptodactyly, hypoplastic dermal ridges and creases, clubfeet, rocker-bottom feet, multiple ankyloses and contractures (arthrogryposis), subluxation of the finger joints, and slender bones. Cryprotorchism is the principal genital defect.

Pena, S. D. J., & Shokeir, M. H. K. Syndrome of camptodactyly, multiple ankyloses, facial anomalies, and pulmonary hypoplasia: A lethal condition. *J. Pediat.*, 1974, 85:373-5.

Pena-Shokeir syndrome (2). See *cerebro-oculofacioskeletal syndrome.*

PENDE, NICOLA (Italian physician, born 1880)

Pende syndrome. Synonyms: *hyperthymic syndrome, thymic hypertrophy.*

Thymic hyperfunction associated with adiposity, genital dystrophy, and retarded mental and physical development.

Gualco, S. La sindrome ipertimico di Pende. Modificazioni del quadro ematico e del metabolismo basale mediante roentgenoterapia sul timo. *Riforma Med.*, 1939, 55:1659-62.

PENDRED, VAUGHAN (British physician, 1869-1946)

Pendred syndrome. Synonyms: *deafness-goiter syndrome, goiter-deaf mutism syndrome, hereditary goiter-deafness syndrome.*

A hereditary syndrome, transmitted as an autosomal recessive trait, characterized by congenital perceptive hearing loss and goiter. Abnormal peroxidase activity and perchlorate test are the principal biochemical features.

Pendred, V. Deaf-mutism and goitre. *Lancet,* 1896, 2:532.

PENFIELD, WILDER GRAVES (Canadian physician, born 1891)

Penfield syndrome. Synonym: *autonomic diencephalic epilepsy.*

Attacks of epileptic seizures caused by a tumor pressing on the hypothalamus and accompanied by dilation of the peripheral blood vessels, diaphoresis, sialorrhea, lacrimation, nystagmus, exophthalmos, hypertension, piloerection, hypothermia, tachycardia, and slowing of respiration.

Penfield, W. Diencephalic autonomic epilepsy. *Arch. Neur. Psychiat., Chicago*, 1929, 22:358-74.

penis tourniquet syndrome. Synonym: *annular constriction of the penis.*

Complications following placing on the penis a constricting band, characterized by bluish discoloration of the penis, ecchymosis of the penis and scrotum, dysuria, hematuria, and potential gangrene.

Farah, R., & Cerny, J. C. The penis tourniquet syndrome and penile amputation. *Urology*, 1973, 2:310-1.

penta-X syndrome. See *chromosome XXXXX syndrome.*

pentasomy X syndrome. See *chromosome XXXXX syndrome.*

PEP (pigmentation-edema-plasma cell) dyscrasia syndrome. See *POEMS syndrome.*

PEPPER, WILLIAM (American physician, 1874-1947)

Pepper disease. See *Hutchinson disease, under Hutchinson, Sir Robert Grieve.*

peptic aspiration pneumonia. See *Mendelson syndrome.*

perabduction syndrome. See *hyperabduction syndrome.*

PERHEENTUPA, JAAKKO (Finnish physician)

Perheentupa syndrome. See *MULIBREY nanism.*

periadenitis mucosae necrotica recurrens. See *Sutton disease, under Sutton, Richard Lighburn, Jr.*

periarteritis nodosa. See *Kussmaul-Maier syndrome.*

periarthritis humeroscapularis. See *Duplay bursitis.*

periarthritis of the shoulder. See *Duplay bursitis.*

pericardial pseudocirrhosis of the liver. See *Pick disease, under Pick, Friedel.*

pericholangiolitic biliary cirrhosis. See *Hanot-MacMahon-Thannhauser syndrome.*

peridigital dermatosis. See *wet and dry foot syndrome.*

periextra-articular rheumatism. See *Forestier syndrome (1).*

perigrinating problem patient. See *Munchausen syndrome.*

periluteal phase dysphoric disorder. See *premenstrual syndrome.*

perilymphatic gusher-deafness syndrome. See *Nance syndrome.*

perinatal respiratory distress syndrome. See *neonatal respiratory distress syndrome.*

perineal necrotizing fasciitis. See *Fournier disease.*

periodic abdominalgia. See *Reimann periodic disease.*

periodic allergic conjunctivitis. See *Angelucci syndrome.*

periodic fever. See *Reimann periodic disease.*

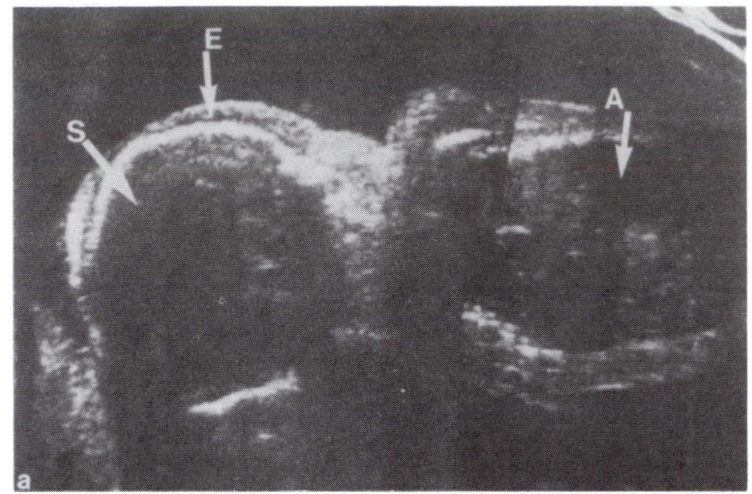

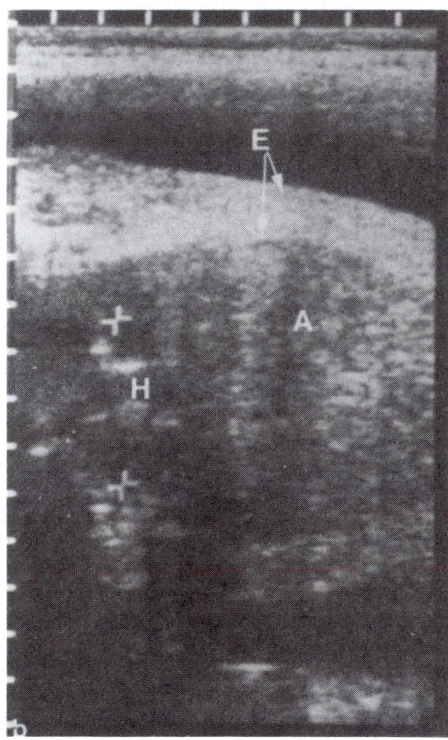

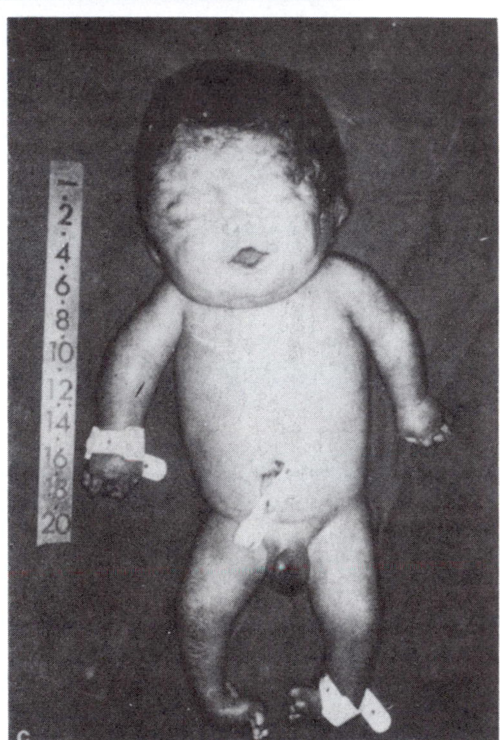

Pena-Shokeir syndrome I
Muller, Linnie M., & Greetje de Jong, *American Journal of Medical Genetics*

periodic hemoglobinuria. See *Dressler syndrome, under Dressler, D. R.*

periodic hypersomnia-megaphagia syndrome. See *Kleine-Levin syndrome.*

periodic leg movement (PLM). See *restless leg syndrome.*

periodic migrainous neuralgia. See *Horton neuralgia.*

periodic oculomotor paralysis. See *Moebius syndrome (2).*

periodic paralysis I. See *Westphal syndrome, under Westphal, Karl Friedrich Otto.*

periodic paralysis II. See *Gamstorp syndrome.*

periodic peritonitis. See *Reimann periodic disease.*

periodic somnolence and morbid hunger syndrome. See *Kleine-Levin syndrome.*

periodontitis simplex. See *Fauchard disease.*

periosteal dysplasia. See *osteogenesis imperfecta syndrome (recessive form).*

periostitis deformans. See *Soriano syndrome.*

periostitis hyperplastica. See *Camurati-Englemann syndrome.*

periostitis hyperplastica. See *Marie-Bamberger syndrome, under Marie, Pierre.*

periostitis tuberositas tibiae. See *Osgood-Schlatter syndrome.*

peripheral cystoid degeneration of the retina. See *Blessig-Iwanoff disease.*

peripheral dysostosis-nasal hypoplasia-mental retardation (PNM) syndrome. See *acrodysostosis.*
peripheral resistance to thyroid hormone. See *Refetoff syndrome.*
periphlebitis retinae. See *Eales syndrome.*
peripyelitis plastica stenosans. See *Ormond syndrome.*
perirenal apoplexy. See *Wunderlich syndrome.*
perirenal fascitis. See *Ormond syndrome.*
perirenal hematoma. See *Wunderlich syndrome.*
perirenal hemorrhage. See *Wunderlich syndrome.*
peritendinitis crepitans. See *under overuse syndrome.*
peritendinitis of the shoulder. See *Duplay bursitis.*
peritendinits calcarea. See *Duplay bursitis.*
periureteral fibrosis. See *Ormond syndrome.*
periureteritis fibroplastica. See *Ormond syndrome.*
periureteritis plastica et obliterens. See *Ormond syndrome.*

PERKINS
Barry-Perkins-Young syndrome. See *Young syndrome, under Young, Donald.*
PERLMAN, M. (Israeli physician)
Perlman familial nephroblastomatosis syndrome. See *Perlman syndrome.*
Perlman syndrome. Synonyms: *Perlman nephroblastomatosis syndrome, fetal gigantism-renal hamartomas-nephroblastomatosis syndrome.*

A familial syndrome, believed to be transmitted as an autosomal recessive trait, consisting of renal dysplasia, Wilms tumor, hyperplasia of the islands of Langerhans with hyperinsulinism, unusual facies, and other congenital defects, including hydramnios, high birth weight, enophthalmos, low-set ears, everted upper lip, sternal defect, capillary hemangiomas of the skin, polycythemia, hypoglycemia, hepatomegaly, and renal disorders which consist of persistent nephrogenesis, hamartomas, nephroblastomatosis, and horseshoe kidney. Most patients die in infancy.

Perlman, M., *et al.* Syndrome of fetal gigantism, renal hamartomas, and nephroblastomatomatosis with Wilms' tumor. *Cancer,* 1975, 35:1212-7.

pernicious anemia. See *Addison-Biermer anemia.*
pernicious anemia of pregnancy. See *Wills anemia.*
pernicious catatonia. See *Bell mania, under Bell, Luther Vos.*
peromelia-micrognathia syndrome. See *Hanhart syndrome (2).*
peroneal muscle atrophy. See *Charcot-Marie-Tooth syndrome.*
PEROUTKA, L. A. (American physician)
Peroutka sneeze. See *ACHOO syndrome.*
PEROUTKA, S. J. (American physician)
Peroutka sneeze. See *ACHOO syndrome.*
PERRAULT, M. (French physician)
Perrault syndrome. Synonyms: *gonadal dysgenesis, XX type; ovarian dysgenesis-sensorineural deafness syndrome.*

A familial syndrome, transmitted as an autosomal recessive trait, characterized by ovarian dysgenesis in female homozygotes and facultative deafness in male and female homozygotes. Right bundle branch block and mental retardation may be associated.

Perrault, M., *et al.* Deux cas de syndrome de Turner avec surdi-mutité dans une meme fratrie. *Bull. Mém Soc. Méd. Hôp. Paris,* 1951, 16:79-84.

PERRY, H. O. (American physician)
Brunsting-Perry syndrome. See *Brunsting disease.*
persistent aberrant mongolian spot. See *Ota nevus.*
persistent galactorrhea-amenorrhea syndrome (PGAS). See *amenorrhea-galactorrhea syndrome.*
persistent truancy. See *Huckleberry Finn syndrome (1).*
PERTHES, GEORG CLEMENS (German physician, 1869-1927)
Calvé-Legg-Perthes syndrome. See *under Calvé.*
Calvé-Perthes disease. See *Calvé-Legg-Perthes syndrome.*
Perthes disease. See *Calvé-Legg-Perthes disease.*
Perthes-Calvé-Legg-Waldenström syndrome. See *Calvé-Legg-Perthes syndrome.*
Perthes-Jüngling disease. Synonyms: *Jüngling disease, Jüngling polycystic osteitis, osteitis cystica multiplex, osteitis multiplex tuberculosa, osteitis multiplex cystoides.*

A slowly progressive form of polycystic osteitis that also involves the surrounding soft tissue, originally observed in the fingers, toes, and nasal bone. Infection with strains of *Mycobacterium tuberculosis* are believed to be responsible.

Jüngling, O. Ostitis tuberculosa multiplex cystica (eine eigenartige Form der Knochentuberkulose). *Forschr. Röntgen.,* 1919-21, 27:375-83.

Peruvian wart. See *Carrión disease.*
PETERS, ALBERT (German ophthalmologist, 1862-1938)
Peters anomaly. Synonyms: *Peters syndrome, congenital central corneal leukoma, dysgenesis mesodermalis corneae.*

A familial developmental defect of the Descemet membrane and deep stromal layers of the cornea. In the mildest expression, a central posterior corneal defect is the only anomaly; in the most pronounced form, the central corneal defect is associated with corneal leukoma, iris and lens adhesions, and microphthalmia. A single congenital anomaly is a frequent occurrence, mental deficiency, craniofacial dysplasia, and urogenital dysgenesis being the most common associated disorders in Peters anomaly. The syndrome is sometimes a component of various systemic disorders.

Peter, A. Über angeborene Defektbildung der Descemet' Membran. *Klin. Mbl. Augenh.,* 1906, 44:27-40; 105-9.

Peters syndrome. See *Peters anomaly.*
Peters-plus syndrome. Peters anomaly (q.v.) associated with short stature, brachymorphy, mental retardation, malformed ears, and cheilo(gnatho)palatoschisis. The condition is relatively mild, but may be lethal in the fetal period.

Schooneveld, M. J., van., *et al.* Peters'-plus: a new syndrome. *Ophth. Paediat. Genet.,* 1984, 4:141-6.

PETGES, GABRIEL (French physician, born 1872)
Petges-Cléjat syndrome. Synonym: *poikilodermatomyositis.*

Poikiloderma characterized by extensive telangiectasia, pigmentation, atrophy of the skin and muscles, and myositis. It is similar to Jacobi disease, except for the presence of myositis and muscular atrophy.

Petges, G., & Cléjat, C. Sclérose atrophique de la peau et myosite généralisée. *Ann. Derm. Syph., Paris,* 1906, 7:550-68.

PETIT, FRANÇOIS POURFOUR, DU (French physician, 1664-1741)
du Petit syndrome. See *Petit syndrome.*
Petit syndrome. Synonyms: *du Petit syndrome, Pourfour du Petit syndrome.*

An oculopupillary disease caused by sympathetic irritation and consisting of mydriasis, exophthalmos, widening of the rima palpebrarum, high intraocular pressure, and changes in the connective tissue of the bulbus oculi and retinal vessels.

Petit. Mémoire dans lequel it est démontré que les nerfs intercostaux fournissent des rameaux qui portent des esprits dans les yeux. Hist. Acad. Sc., Paris, 1727, pp. 1-18.

Pourfour du Petit syndrome. See *Petit syndrome.*

PETIT, JEAN LOUIS (French physician, 1674-1750)

Petit hernia. A lumbar hernia in the Petit triangle (a small triangle between the inferolateral margin of the latissimus dorsi muscle and the external oblique muscle of the abdomen).

*Petit, J. L. *Traité des maladies chirurgicales, et des opérations qui leur conviennent*. Paris, Didot, 1774. Vol. 2, pp. 256-8.

petit mal. See *Lennox syndrome.*

petit mal epilepsy. See *Lennox syndrome.*

petrous apicitis. See *Gradenigo syndrome.*

PETTE, HEINRICH WILHELM (German neurologist, born 1887)

Pette-Döring encephalitis. Synonym: *nodular panencephalitis.*

Encephalitis marked by severe headache, vertigo, bouts of unconsciousness, movement disorders, and delirium. The movement disorders usually include tremor, myoclonus, and chorea, in which the extremities may assume bizarre positions. Anarthria and trismus are frequently present. The fever usually follows an unpredictable curve. Pathological changes are found in most areas of the central nervous system, including the meninges, cerebral cortex, and spinal cord, but the nucleus ruber, substantia nigra, and corpus pallidum are spared. Inflammatory infiltrates are present in the meninges and blood vessels; lymphocytes and plasma cell infiltrates are found in various parts of the brain, and there is usually a severe nodular proliferation in the neuroglia. This disease and van Bogaert encephalitis are considered to be variants of the same entity.

Pette, H., & Döring, G. Über einheimische Panencephalomyelitis vom Character der Encephalitis japonica. *Deut. Zschr. Nervenh.*, 1939, 149:17-44.

PETZETAKIS, M. (Greek physician)

morbus Petzetakis. See *cat scratch disease.*

Petzetakis disease. See *cat scratch disease.*

Petzetakis-Takos syndrome. Synonym: *trophopenic superficial keratitis.*

Superficial keratitis, edema of the eyelids and bulbar conjunctiva, hypoesthesia of the cornea, diminished reflexes of the iris, xerophthalmia, and lesions of the corneal and precorneal layers, observed in severe malnutrition.

Petzetakis, M. Les troubles oculaires pendant la trophopénie (maladie oedémateuse) et l'épidémie de la pellagre (1941-1944). La kératite superficielle trophopénique (kératopathie épithéliale). *Presse Méd., Paris*, 1950, 58:1082-4.

PEUTZ, J. L. A. (Dutch physician)

Hutchinson-Weber-Peutz syndrome. See *Peutz-Jeghers syndrome.*

Peutz syndrome. See *Peutz-Jeghers syndrome.*

Peutz-Jeghers hamartosis. See *Peutz-Jeghers syndrome.*

Peutz-Jeghers syndrome (PJS). Synonyms: *Hutchinson-Weber-Peutz syndrome, Jeghers syndrome, Klostermann syndrome, Peutz syndrome, Peutz-Jeghers hamartosis, Peutz-Klostermann syndrome, Peutz-Touraine syndrome, Peutz-Touraine-Jeghers syndrome, intestinal polyposis, intestinal polyposis-cutaneous pigmentation syndrome, lentiginopolypose digestive syndrome, melanoplakia-small intestinal polyposis syndrome.*

A hereditary syndrome, transmitted as an autosomal dominant trait, characterized by gastrointestinal polyposis, usually benign adenomatous (hamartous) tumors 0.5 to 7.0 cm in diameter, and mucocutaneous pigmentation consisting of discrete brown to bluish-black macules about the lips, oral mucosa, and other facial orifices. Occasional pigmentation may involve the umbilicus, axilla, and shoulders, and polyps are found in the uterus, bladder, and ureters. The pigmentary spots appear from infancy and tend to disappear in the adult. In most instances, polyps appear by the age of 20 years. Cases of malignant degeneration of the polyps have been reported. Abdominal pain, intussusception, and gastrointestinal bleeding with resulting iron-defficiency anemia are the most common symptoms of gastrointestinal involvement. Associated disorders include occasional ovarian cysts and tumors, clubbing of the fingers, and precocious puberty.

Peutz, J. L. Over een zeer merkvaardige, gecombinerde familiaire polyposis van de slijmvliezen, van den tractus intestinalis met die van de neuskeelholte en gepaard met eigenaardige pigmentaties van huiden slijmvliezen. *Ned. Mschr. Genesk.*, 1921, 10:134-46. Jeghers, H., *et al.* Generalized intestinal polyposis and melanin spots on the oral mucosa, lips and digits. A syndrome of diagnostic significance. *N. Engl. J. Med.*, 1949, 241:993-1005. Hutchinson, J. Pigmentation of lip and mouth. *Arch. Surg., London*, 1896, 7:290. Weber, F. P. Patches of deep pigmentation of the oral mucous membrane not connected with Addison's disease. *Q. J. Med., Oxford*, 1919, 12:204-8. Touraine, H., & Couder, F. Syndrome de Peutz (lentigo-polypose digestive). *Ann. Derm. Syph., Paris*, 1945, 5:313. Klostermann, G. F. *Pigmentflecken-polypose. Klinische, histologische and erbbiologische Studien am sogenannten Peutz-Syndrom*. Thieme, Stuttgart, 1960.

Peutz-Klostermann syndrome. See *Peutz-Jeghers syndrome.*

Peutz-Touraine syndrome. See *Peutz-Jeghers syndrome.*

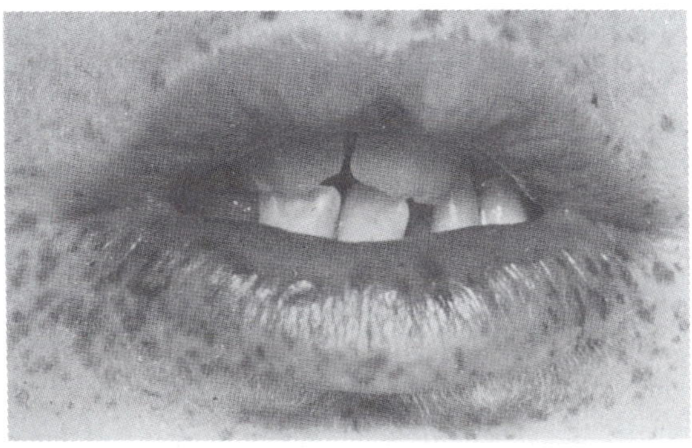

Peutz-Jeghers syndrome
Sheward, J.D.: *Brit. Med. J.* 1:921, 1962. British Medical Association, London, England.

Peutz-Touraine-Jeghers syndrome. See *Peutz-Jeghers syndrome.*

PEYRONIE, FRANÇOIS, DE LA (French physician, 1678-1747)

Peyronie disease. Synonyms: *Van Buren disease, cavernitis fibrosa, fibrous cavernitis, fibrous sclerosis of the penis, induratio penis plastica, penile induration, penis plasticus, plastic induration of the penis, primary indurative cavernositis of the penis, sclerosis fibrosa penis, strabismus of the penis.*

Fibrous thickening of the shaft of the penis associated with pain and curving of the penis toward the affected side during the erection. The process apparently starts as vasculitis in the areolar connective tissue sleeve beneath the tunica albuginea and extends to the adjacent structures. The inflammation is followed by fibrosis, leading to formation of a perivascular fibrous collar and ossification.

*Peyronie, F., de la. Sur quelques obstactles, qui s'opposent à l'éjaculation naturelle de la semence. *Mém. Acad. Chir., Paris*, 1743, 1:425. Van Buren, W. H., & Keyes. E. L. *A practical treatise on the surgical disease of the genito-urinary organs, including syphilis*. 2nd ed. New York, Appleton, 1881, pp. 81-3.

PFAUNDLER, MEINHARD, VON (German pediatrician, 1872-1947)

Pfaundler-Hurler syndrome. See *mucopolysaccharidosis I-H.*

PFEIFER, VICTOR (German physician)

Pfeifer-Weber-Christian disease. See *Weber-Christian syndrome, under Weber, Frederick Parkes.*

PFEIFFER, EMIL (German physician, 1846-1921)

Pfeiffer disease. See *Filatov disease.*

PFEIFFER, RICHARD FRIEDRICH JOHANNES (German bacteriologist, 1858-1945)

Pfeiffer meningitis. Meningitis caused by the Pfeiffer bacillus (*Haemophilus influenzae*).

Pfeiffer, R. F. J. Vorläufige Mitteilungen über die Erreger der Influenza. *Deut. Med. Wschr.*, 1892, 18:28.

PFEIFFER, RUDOLF ARTHUR (German physician, born 1931)

Pfeiffer syndrome. Synonyms: *Noack syndrome, acrocephalosyndactyly IV (ACS IV), acrocephalosyndacyly V (ASC V), acrocephalosyndactyly VI (ACS VI).*

A congenital syndrome, transmitted as an autosomal dominant trait, characterized by acrocephalosyndactyly with craniosynostosis in mild acrocephaly, broad thumbs and great toes, partial soft-tissue syndactyly of the hands and feet, and occasional duplication of the first toes. High forehead, hypertelorism, antimongoloid slant of the palpebral fissures, small nose, narrow maxilla, and high-arched palate are the principal characteristics. The syndrome is variously classified as **acrocephalosyndactyly IV** (Spranger, Langer, and Wiedemann), **acrocephalosyndactyly V** (McKusick), and, occasionally, acrocephalosyndactyly VI.

Pfeiffer, R. A. Dominant erbliche Akrocephalosyndaktylie. *Zschr. Kinderheilk.*, 1964, 90:301-20. McKusick, V. A. *Mendelian inheritance in man*. 5th ed. Baltimore, The Johns Hopkins University Press, 1978, p. 8, No. 10160. Spranger, J. W., Langer, L. O., & Wiedemann, H. R. *Bone dysplasias*. Philadelphia, Saunders, 1974, p. 261. Noack, M. Ein Beitrag zum Krakheitsbid der Akrocephalosyndaktylia. *Arch. Kinderheilk.*, 1959, 160:168-71.

Reinhardt-Pfeiffer syndrome. See *under Reinhardt, K.*

ulnofibular dysplasia, Reinhardt-Pfeiffer type. See *Reinhardt-Pfeiffer syndrome, under Reinhardt, K.*

PFFD (proximal focal femoral deficiency). See *femur-fibula-ulna syndrome.*

PFK deficiency. See *glycogen storage disease VII.*

PFS (primary fibromyalgia syndrome). See *fibrositis-fibromyalgia syndrome.*

PGA (I, II, III). See *polyglandular autoimmune syndrome (I, II, III).*

PGAS (persistent galactorrhea-amenorrhea syndrome). See *amenorrhea-galactorrhea syndrome.*

phacomatosis. See *Bourneville-Pringle syndrome.*

phagodenic gingivitis. See *Vincent infection.*

phalangeal avascular necrosis. See *Thiemann syndrome.*

phalangeal microgeodic syndrome. Synonyms: *Maroteaux syndrome, microgeodic disease.*

A chillblainlike disease of the fingers and occasionally the toes observed during the winter months in infants and children. It is characterized mainly by swelling, redness, heat, and minimal pain. Radiographic findings show small punched out lacunae in the middle and distal phalanges and widening of the involved phalanges. Some cases also show sclerosis in the diaphyses and rarefaction in the metaphyses with occasional spontaneous fractures. There is a spontaneous regression within several months.

Maroteaux, P. Cinq observations d'une affection microgeodique des phalanges du nourrisson d'etiologie inconnue. *Ann. Radiol., Paris*, 1970, 13:229-36.

phantom bone. See *Gorham syndrome.* and see *carpotarsal osteolysis syndrome (dominant and sporadic forms).*

phantom clavicle. See *Gorham syndrome.*

phantom double syndrome. See *Capgras syndrome.*

phantom hip. See *observation hip syndrome.*

pharyngeal bursitis. See *Thornwaldt bursitis.*

pharyngeal pouch syndrome. See *DiGeorge syndrome.*

pharyngitis. See *common cold syndrome.*

pharyngitis vesicularis. See *Zahorsky syndrome (2).*

pharyngolaryngeal paralysis syndrome. See *Collet-Sicard syndrome.*

PHC (premolar hypodontia-**h**yperhidrosis-**c**anities prematura) **syndrome.** See *Böök syndrome.*

phenylalanine hydroxylase deficiency syndrome. See *phenylketonuria.*

phenylketonuria (PKU). Synonyms: *Følling syndrome, hyperphenylalaninemia, idiotia phenylketonurica, imbecillitas phenylpyruvica, phenylalanine hydroxylase deficiency syndrome, phenylpyruvic oligophrenia, phenyluria.*

An inborn error of metabolism, transmitted as an autosomal recessive trait, attributed to a deficiency or defect of phenylalanine hydrolase (the enzyme which catalyzes conversion of phenylalanine to tyrosine), resulting in accumulation of phenylalanine and its metabolic products in body tissues and fluids. The syndrome occurs more commonly in northern Europeans than in the Ashkenazi Jews, Italians, Blacks, and persons of the Mediterranean ancestry. Several varieties are recognized: **Classic phenylketonuria (phenylketonuria I, PKU I, Følling syndrome, hyperphenylalanemia I)** is characterized by an apparently normal appearance at birth, followed in a year or so by

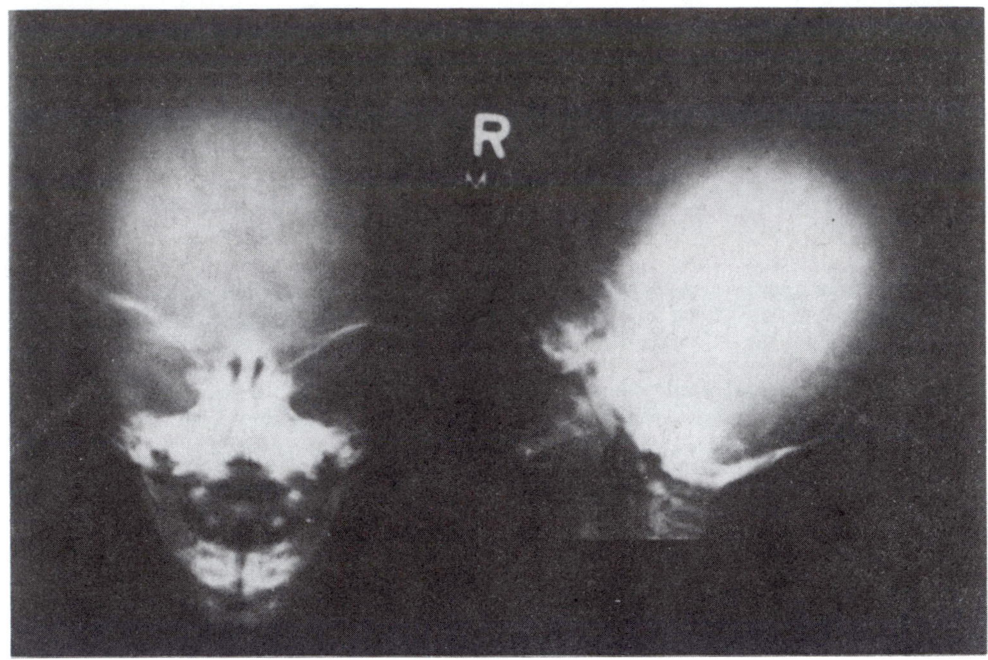

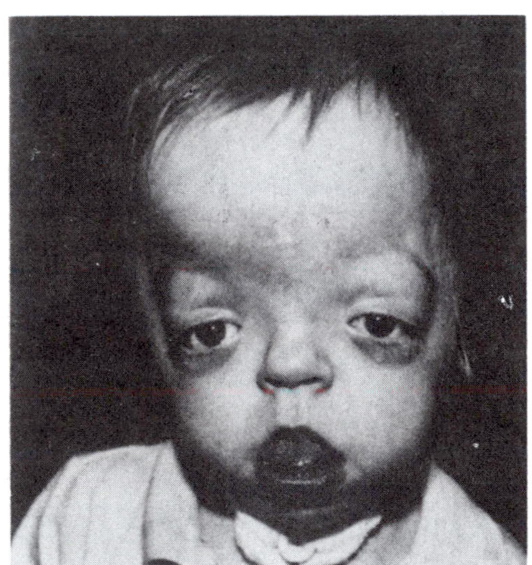

Pfeiffer syndrome
Rasmussen, Sonja A. & Jaime L. Frias, *Clinical Genetics* 33:5-10, 1988. Munksgaard International Publishers, Copenhagen, Denmark.

mental retardation, neurologic manifestations (hyperkinesia, delayed psychomotor development, aggressive behavior, seizures, and microcephaly), light pigmentation, eczema, and a mousy odor, unless treated with diets low in phenylalanine. The affected patients, who are usually blond and blue-eyed, may show poor coordination, tremor, dystonia, athetoid movements, and inability to walk or talk. Their head circumference averages nearly 2 cm less than normal. Prominent maxillae, wide interdental spaces, and enamel hypoplasia may occur. **Phenylketonuria II (PKU II, dihydropteridine reductase deficiency)** is characterized mainly by lack of responsiveness to low phenylalanine diets, feeding difficulty, choking, growth retardation, seizures, abnormal EEG, and disappearance by the age of 18 months of all voluntary movements and social awareness. Dihydropteridine reductase deficiency is said to be the cause of this type. **Phenylketonuria, Tourian and Sidbury type (hyperphenylalaninemia VI)** is also marked by the lack of responsiveness to low phenylalanine dietary therapy, normal phenylalanine hydroxylase, dihydropteridine reductase, and phenylalanine-hydroxylase-stimulating protein. DOPA therapy results in progressive disappearance of myoclonus, uncontrolled movements, tetraplegia, greasy skin, sialorrhea, and hyperthermia.

Følling , A. Über Ausscheidung von Phenylbrenztarubensäure in dem Harn als Stoffwechselanomalie in Verbindung mit Imbezillität. *Hoppe Seyler Zschr. Physiol. Chem.*, 1934, 227:169-76. Bartholome, K., & Byrd, D. J. Tetrahydrobiopterin treatment of variant form of phenylketonuria. *Lancet*, 1975, 2:1042. Tourian, A. Y., & Sidbury, J. Phenylketonuria. In: Stanbury, J. B., Wyngaarden, J. B., & Fredrickson, D. S., eds. *Metabolic basis of inherited disease*. 4th ed. New York, McGraw-Hill, 1978, pp. 240-55.

phenylketonuria, Tourian and Sidbury type. See *under phenylketonuria.*

phenylpyruvic oligophrenia. See *phenylketonuria.*

phenyluria. See *phenylketonuria.*

pheochromocytoma-islet cell tumor syndrome. Tumor producing, storing, and secreting chatecholamines, which are usually benign, and are derived from the adrenal medulla, although some may arise from the chromaffin cells in or about the sympathetic ganglia, when they are known as either **pheochromocytomas** or **paragangliomas.** Hypertension is the most important clinical sign. **Islet-cell tumor**, an insulin-secreting tumor of the islands of Langerhans, produces recurrent fasting hypoglycemia and neurological complications, including headache, visual disorders, confusion, weakness, sweating, palpitations, convulsions, and coma. The presence of these tumors may be associated with various endocrine or nonendocrine familial disorders. Some authors incorporate the syndrome with multiple endocrine neoplasia I and II, while others identify them as being the autosomal dominant endocrine adenomatosis distinct from MEA I, II, and III.

Carney, J. A., *et al.* Familial pheochromoocytoma of the pancreas and islet cell tumor of the pancreas. *Am. J. Med.*, 1980, 68:515-21.

PHILLIPS, C. I. (British ophthalmologist)

Phillips-Griffiths syndrome. A syndrome of bilateral macular coloboma, cleft palate, and digital abnormalities. Long middle phalanges with spindling at proximal interphalangeal joints, hyperextensible middle fingers, flexion deformity of the interphalangeal joints of the middle fingers, hallux valgus, and metatarsals are the principal digital defects. Mental retardation, sloping forehead, platybasia, and various skeletal abnormalities occur in some cases. The syndrome is believed to be transmitted as an autosomal recessive trait.

Phillips, C. I., & Griffiths, D. L. Macular coloboma and skeletal abnormality. *Brit. J. Ophth.*, 1969, 53:346-9.

phlebarteriectasis. See *Klippel-Trénaunay-Weber syndrome.*

phlebectasia of the scrotum. See *Fordyce lesion.*

phlegmon of the floor of the mouth. See *Ludwig angina.*

phobic anxiety-depersonalization syndrome. See *Roth syndrome, under Roth, Martin.*

PHOCAS, B. GERASIME (French physician, 1861-1937)

Tillaux-Phocas disease. See *Cheatle disease.*

phocomelic diabetic embryopathy. See *caudal regression syndrome.*

phosphate diabetes. See *hypophosphatemic familial rickets.*

phosphatidolipoidosis. See *Niemann-Pick syndrome.*

phosphatidosis. See *Niemann-Pick syndrome.*

phosphoethanolaminuria. See *hypophosphatasia syndrome.*

phosphofructokinase deficiency. See *glycogen storage disease VII.*

photic sneeze reflex. See *ACHOO syndrome.*

photodermatitis pigmentaria. See *Freund dermatitis under Freund, Emanuel.*

photosensitivity dermatitis and actinic reticuloid (PD-AR) syndrome. Contact allergic dermatitis in persons suffering from lymphoma-like erythroderma with thickening and ridging of the exposed skin. Sensitivity to oleoresin extracts from Compositae plants is the most common cause.

Ive, F. A. "Actinic reticuloid"; a chronic dermatosis associated with severe photosensitivity and the histological resemblance to lymphoma. *Brit. J. Derm.*, 1969, 81:469-85.

photosensitivity-ichthyosis-brittle hair-intellectual impairment-decreased fertility-short stature (PIBIDS, PIB(D)S) syndrome. See *Tay syndrome, under Tay, Chong Hai.*

PHP (pseudohypoparathyroidism). See *Albright syndrome (1).*

PHPT (pseudohypoparathyroidism). See *Albright syndrome (1).*

physiologic cholemia. See *Gilbert syndrome, under Gilbert, Nicolas Augustin.*

phytanic acid storage disease. See *Refsum disease.*

pian. See *Charlouis disease.*

pian fungoide. See *mycosis fungoides.*

PIAVA (polydactyly-imperforate anus-vertebral anomalies) **syndrome.** See *VATER association.*

PIBIDS, PIBI(D)S (photosensitivity-ichthyosis-brittlehair-intellectual impairment-decreased syndrome fertility-**short stature**) syndrome. See *Tay syndrome, under Tay, Chong Hai.*

PIC, ADRIEN (French physician, born 1863)

Bard-Pic syndrome. See *under Bard, Louis.*

Pic syndrome. See *Bard-Pic syndrome, under Bard, Louis.*

PICCARDI, GEROLAMO (Italian physician)

Piccardi-Lassueur-Little syndrome. See *Little syndrome, under Little, Ernest Gordon Graham.*

PICFS (postinfective chronic fatigue syndrome). See *chronic fatigue syndrome.*

PICK, ARNOLD (Neurologist in Prague, 1851-1924)

Pick atrophy. See *Pick syndrome.*

Pick disease. See *Pick syndrome.*

Pick presenile dementia. See *Pick syndrome.*

Pick syndrome. Synonyms: *Pick atrophy, Pick disease, Pick presenile dementia, lobar atrophy.*

A rare fatal degenerative disease of the nervous system, occurring mostly in middle-aged women. Most cases are transmitted as an autosomal dominant trait. It is characterized by signs of severe frontal or temporal lobe dysfunction, including loss of memory, disorientation, apathy, reduced initiative, lack of insight, and, in later stages, speech disorders, prominent grasp and sucking reflexes, and terminal decerebrate rigidity, dystonia, and tremor. Death takes place about 7 years after the onset of symptoms. Severe atrophy of the anterior parts of the frontal and temporal lobes with a sharp line of demarcation between atrophied and normal tissues is the principal pathologic feature of this syndrome. There may be atrophic changes in the subcortical parts, most notably in the caudate nucleus, putamen, thalamus, and substantia nigra, and in the descending frontopontine structures. Histological examination shows fibrillary intracytoplasmic deposits, consisting of masses of straight fibrils, and densely packed spherical aggregates in some neurons (Pick bodies); otherwise, the findings are similar to those seen in Alzheimer's disease.

Pick. Über die Bezhiehungen der senilen Hirnatrophie zur Aphasie. *Prag. Med. Wschr.*, 1892, 17:165-7.

PICK, FRIEDEL (German physician, 1867-1926)

Hutinel-Pick syndrome. See *Pick disease.*

Pick cirrhosis. See *Pick disease.*

Pick disease. Synonyms: *Hutinel-Pick syndrome, Pick cirrhosis, pericardial pseudocirrhosis of the liver.*

Constrictive pericaditis associated with ascites, cirrhosis of the liver, and fibrosis, with little or no edema and without jaundice.

Pick, F. Über chronische, unter dem Bilde der Lebercirrhose verlaufende Pericarditis (pericarditische Pseudolebercirrhose) nebst Bemerkungen; über die Zuckerausgussleber (Curschmann). *Zschr. Klin. Med.*, 1896, 29:385-410.

PICK, LUDWIG (German physician, 1868-1925)

Lubarsch-Pick syndrome. See *under Lubarsch.*

Niemann-Pick (NP) syndrome. See *under Niemann.*

Pick disease. See *Niemann-Pick syndrome.*

Pick retinitis. Synonyms: *cachexic retinitis, retinitis cachectica et carcinoma ventriculi, retinitis cachecticorum.*

Retinitis with lesions in the vicinity of the papilla, characterized by grayish white spots that originate from vascular anastomoses and spread to other parts of the retina as ill-defined, diffuse areas, sometimes associated with hemorrhage. The disorder usually occurs in cachexic patients with anemia secondary to cancer of the stomach or to gastrointestinal hemorrhage.

Pick, L. Netzhautveränderungen bei chronischen Anämien. *Klin. Mbl. Augenh.*, 1901, 39:177-92.

PICK, PHILIPP JOSEPH (Physician in Prague, 1834-1910)

Pick disease. See *Herxheimer disease.*

Pick-Herxheimer syndrome. See *Herxheimer disease.*

PICKWICK, SAMUEL (The central character in *The Pickwick Papers* by Charles Dickens)

Pickwick (pickwickian) syndrome. Synonyms: *cardiopulmonary obesity syndrome, cardiorespiratory-obesity syndrome, fat Joe's folly, obesity-heart failure syndrome, obesity-hypoventilation syndrome (OHS), respiratory insufficiency of obesity.*

A disorder, named after the fat, red-faced boy in Dickens' *The Pickwick Papers*, characterized by obesity associated with a rapid, shallow breathing pattern that causes a relative increase in dead space ventilation and a reduction in the proportion of each breath available for gas exchange. Alveolar hypoventilation, somnolence and drowsiness, intermittent cyanosis, secondary polycythemia, myoclonic twitching, and finally, right ventricular hypertrophy with failure are usually associated. See also *airway obstruction syndrome.*

Platter, F. *Observationum, in hominis affectibus plerisque corpori et animo, functionum laesione, dolore, aliave molestia et vitio incommodantibus.* Libri tres, Basel, Koenig, 1914, pp. 5-6. Burwell, C. S., *et al.* Extreme obesity associated with alveolar hypoventilation hypoventilation-a pickwickian syndrome. *Am. J. Med.*, 1962, 1956, 21:811-8.

PIE. See *pulmonary infiltration with eosinophilia syndrome.*

piedra. See *Beigel disease.*

PIERINI, LUIGI E. (Italian physician)

Pasini-Pierini syndrome. See *under Pasini.*

PIERRE MARIE. See MARIE, PIERRE

PIERRE MAURIAC. See MAURIAC, LEONARD PIERRE

PIERRE ROBIN. See ROBIN, PIERRE

PIERROU

Friess-Pierrou syndrome. See *under Friess.*

PIETRANTONI, LUIGI (Italian physician)

Pietrantoni syndrome. Mucosal and cutaneous zones of anesthesia and neuralgia of the face and oral cavity, observed in paranasal tumors.

Pietrantoni, L. Zone nevralgiche e zone di anestesia della regione faciale et della cavità orale come sintomi precoci di alcune forme di tumori maligni della cavità paranasali. *Arch. Ital. Otol.*, 1948, 59:105-8..

pig-backed kidney. See *Formad kidney.*

pigeon breeder disease. See *pigeon breeder syndrome.*

pigeon breeder lung. See *pigeon breeder syndrome.*

pigeon breeder syndrome. Synonyms: *bird fancier lung, bird fancier lung syndrome, pigeon breeder disease, pigeon breeder lung.*

Interstitial and alveolar pulmonary disease occurring in persons exposed to pigeons. Chills, fever, dyspnea, and cough are the principal symptoms, which occur a few hours after the exposure. Immunologic examination shows skin reactivity and antibodies to pigeon antigens.

Barboriak, J. J., *et al.* Serological studies in pigeon breeder's disease. *J. Lab. Clin. Med.*, 1965, 65:600-4.

pigmentary cirrhosis. See *Recklinghausen-Applebaum disease.*

pigmentary degeneration syndrome of globus pallidus. See *Hallervorden-Spatz syndrome.*

pigmentary retinal lipoid neuronal heredodegeneration. See *Stock-Spielmeyer-Vogt syndrome.*

pigmentation-edema-plasma cell (PEP) dyscrasia syndrome. See *POEMS syndrome.*

pigmented cosmetic dermatitis. See *Riehl syndrome.*

pigmented epitheliomatosis. See *xeroderma pigmentosum syndrome.*

pigmented hair (hairy) epidermal nevus. See *Becker nevus, under Becker, Samuel William.*

pigmented purpuric lichenoid dermatitis. See *Gougerot-Blum syndrome, under Gougerot, Henri.*

PILBD (paucity of interlobular bile ducts). See *Alagille syndrome.*

pili annulati. See *Sabouraud syndrome.*

pili canaliculi. See *uncombable hair syndrome.*

pili moniliformsis. See *Sabouraud syndrome.*

pili torti-deafness syndrome. See *Björnstad syndrome.*

pili trianguli et canaliculi. See *uncombable hair syndrome.*

PILLAT, ARNOLD (Austrian ophthalmologist, born 1891)

Pillat dystrophy. Familial parenchymatous corneal dystrophy characterized by punctate opacities, chiefly of the deep and middle layers.

Pillat, A. Zur Frage der familiärer Hornhautentartung. Über eine eigenartige tiefe schollige und periphere gitterförmige familiäre Hornhautdystrophie. *Klin. Mbl. Augenh.*, 1940, 104:571-88.

PILLAY, V. K. (Orthopedic surgeon in Singapore)

Pillay syndrome. Synonym: *ophthalmomandibulomelic dysplasia.*

A syndrome of eye abnormalities (corneal opacity and blindness), mandibular defects (temporomandibular fusion, absent coronoid process, and obtuse mandibular angle), and symmetric limb dysplasia (short forearms due to radiohumeral and proximal radioulnar dislocations aplasia of lateral humeral condyle, head of radius, lower third of ulna, and short and bowed radius articulating solely with the lunate bone). The syndrome was first reported in a father and his son and daughter. It is transmitted as an autosomal dominant trait.

Pillay, V. K. Ophthalmo-mandibulo-melic dyspalsia. *J. Bone Joint Surg.*, 1964, 46(A):858-62.

pilodento-ungular dysplasia-microcephaly syndrome. A multiple congenital anomalies/mental retardation syndrome characterized by microcephaly, hypotrichosis, dental anomalies, onychodystrophy, mental retardation, precocious puberty, scoliosis, spasticity, advanced bone age, retrognathia, blue sclerae, strabismus, high-arched palate, clinodactyly, and bilateral transpalmar creases. The syndrome is suspected of being transmitted as an autosomal recessive trait.

Tajara, E. H., *et al.* Pilodentougular dysplasia with microcephaly: A new ectodermal dysplasia/malformation syndrome. *Am. J. Med. Genet.*, 1987, 26:153-6.

pilomatrixoma. See *Malherbe epithelioma.*

PINDBORG, JENS J. (Danish oral pathologist)

Gorlin-Pindborg syndrome. See *popliteal pterygium syndrome.*

pineal syndrome. See *Pellizzi syndrome.*

pineal-neurologic-ophthalmic syndrome. See *Frankl-Hochwart syndrome (2).*

pink disease. See *acrodynia.*

PINKUS, FELIX (German physician, born 1868)

Pinkus disease. Synonym: *lichen nitidus.*

Small, glistening, flesh-colored to reddish-yellow papules or macules that occur in groups (without coalescing) on various parts of the body, with special predilection for the genital area, elbows, axillae, palms of the hands, abdomen, and, occasionally, the oral mucosa and tongue. A typical lesion is located beneath the epidermis and is composed of lymphocytes, histiocytes, and giant cells. The course is slowly progressive.

Pinkus, F. Über eine neue knötchenförmige Hauteruption: Lichen nitidus. *Arch. Derm. Syph., Berlin*, 1907, 85:11-36.

PINKUS, HERMANN KARL BENNO (German-born American dermatologist, born 1905)

Pinkus disease. Synonyms: *alopecia mucinosa, follicular mucinosis, mucinous alopecia.*

An inflammatory skin disease with papular infiltrations and alopecia. Histologically, it is characterized by the accumulation of mucin in the root sheaths of hair follicles and in the secretory epithelium of the sebaceous glands.

Pinkus, H. Alopecia mucinosa. Inflammatory plaques with alopecia characterized by root-sheath mucinosis. *Arch. Derm., Chicago*, 1957, l76:419-26.

Pinkus epithelioma. Synonyms: *Pinkus fibroepithelioma, premalignant fibroepithelioma.*

A variant of basal cell epithelioma, characterized by a slow development, predilection for the lower back, clinical similarity to fibroma or papilloma, and histological resemblance to intracanalilcular fibroadenoma of the breast or reticulated verruca senilis.

Pinkus, H. Premalignant fibroepithelial tumors of skin. *Arch. Derm., Chicago*, 1953, 67:598-615.

Pinkus fibroepithelioma. See *Pinkus epithelioma.*

Pinkus tumor. Synonym: *eccrine poroma.*

A benign tumor originating in the porous epithelium of the epidermal sweat duct unit and clinically resembling papilloma or granuloma. The cells retain the morphological and histochemical characteristicss of the ductal lining cells. The histologic structure of the tumor resembles that of seborrheic verruca and basal cell epithelioma, but it retains the features of the epidermal eccrine sweat duct unit. The nonhairy surfaces of the hands and feet are the usual sites, but some cases have been observed on hair-bearing skin. It appears most commonly in older persons.

Pinkus, H., *et al.* Eccrine poroma. Tumors exhibiting features of the epidermal sweat duct unit. *Arch. Derm., Chicago*, 1956, 74:511-21.

PIÑOL AGUADE, JOAQUIN (Spanish physician, born 1917)

Vilanova-Piñol Aguadé syndrome. See *under Vilanova.*

PIRIE, GEORGE R. (British physician)

Pirie syndrome. See *congenital adrenal hyperplasia.*

PIRINGER, ALEXANDRA. See PIRINGER-KUCHINKA, ALEXANDRA

PIRINGER-KUCHINKA, ALEXANDRA (Austrian physician, born 1912)

Piringer lymphadenitis. See *Piringer-Kuchinka syndrome.*

Piringer-Kuchinka syndrome. Synonyms: *Piringer lymphadenitis, lymphadenitis nuchalis et cervicalis.*

Benign cervical lymphadenitis marked by the presence of epithelioid reticulum cells in the lymph nodes. Toxoplasmosis has been identified as a possible etiologic factor.

Piringer-Kuchinka, A. Eigenartiger mikroskopischer Befund am exzidierten Lymphknoten. *Verh. Deut. Ges. Path.*, 1952, 36:352-62.

Pisa syndrome. A postural disorder characterized by tonic flexion of the trunk to one side, accompanied by its slight rotation, occurring as a side effect after the use of the butyrophenone group of neuroleptic drugs.

Ekbom, K., *et al.* New dystonic syndrome associated with butyrophenone therapy. *Neurology*, 1972, 202:94-103.

PITT, D. B. (Australian physician)

Pitt syndrome. Synonym: *Pitt-Rogers-Danks syndrome.*

A familial syndrome, transmitted as an autosomal recessive trait, characterized by mental and growth retardation and peculiar facies. Craniofacial abnormalities include a wide mouth, short upper lip, flat philltrum, beaked nose, prominent eyes, telecanthus, slanting palpebral fissures, maxillary hypoplasia, low-set ears, highly-arched palate, and microcephaly. Epilepsy and hyperactivity are the additional neurological symptoms. Associated disorders include small hands, unusual palmar creases, talipes, hyperextensible fingers, radioulnar synostosis, and myopia.

Pitt, D. B., Rogers, J. G., & Danks, D. M. Mental retardation, unusual face, and intrauterine growth retardation. A new recessive syndrome? *Am. J. Med. Genet.*, 1984, 19:307-13.

Pitt-Rogers-Danks syndrome. See *Pitt syndrome.*

pituitary basophilism. See *Cushing syndrome.*

pituitary cachexia. See *Sheehan syndrome.*

pituitary dwarfism (1). See *Lorain-Levi syndrome.*

pituitary dwarfism (2). See *Laron dwarfism.*

pituitary dwarfism (3). See *Hanhart syndrome (1).*

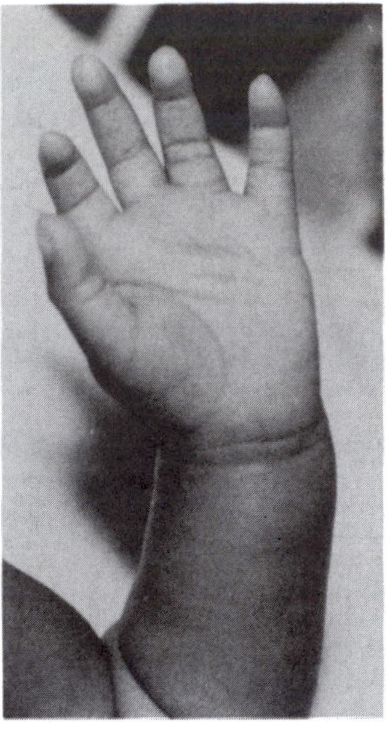
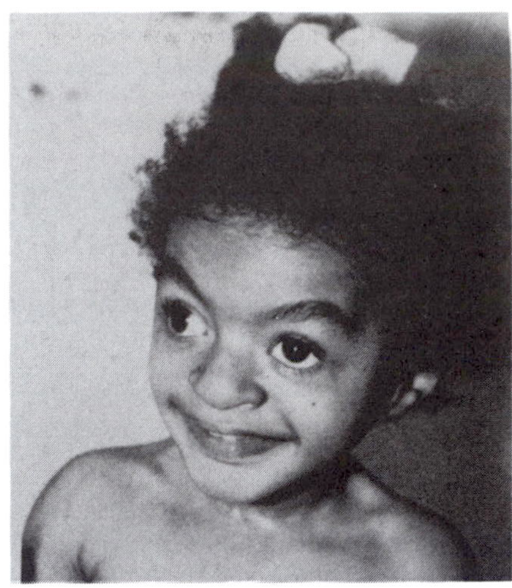

Pitt syndrome
Donnai, Dian: *American Journal of Medical Genetics* 24:29-32 1986. New York: Alan R. Liss, Inc.

pituitary gigantism. See *Launois syndrome.*
pituitary hypogonadism. See *Lorain-Levi syndrome.*
pituitary nanism. See *Lorain-Levi syndrome.*
pituitary pseudotabes. See *Oppenheim syndrome.*
pityriasis circinata. See *Gibert disease, and see Toyama disease.*
pityriasis lichenoides chronica. See *Brocq disease (2).*
pityriasis lichenoides et varioliformis acuta. See *Mucha-Habermann syndrome.*
pityriasis maculata et circinata. See *Gibert disease.*
pityriasis pilaris. See *Kaposi disease (2).*
pityriasis rosea. See *Gibert disease.*
pityriasis rotunda. See *Toyama disease.*
pityriasis rubra pilaris. See *Kaposi disease (2).*
PIULACHS, OLIVA PEDRO (Spanish physician)
Piulachs-Hederich syndrome. Synonym: *tympanites in dolichomegacolon.*

Dolichomegacolon complicated by the sudden appearance of acute paralytic occlusion of the colon with severe gas distention, without any apparent mechanical factor or volvulus.

Piulachs, P., & Hederich, H. La "dilatación aguda de colon," complicación del dolicomegacolon. *Acta Med. Hisp.*, 1947, 5:131-5.

PIV (polydactyly-imperforate anus-vertebral anomalies) syndrome. See *VATER association.*
PJS. See *Peutz-Jeghers syndrome.*
PKU. See *phenylketonuria.*
placental dysfunction syndrome. See *Ballantyne-Runge syndrome.*
plague of Athens. See *Thucydides syndrome.*
plaque-like gastric adenoma. See *Ménétrier syndrome.*
plasma thromboplastin antecedent (PTA) deficiency. See *Rosenthal disease, under Rosenthal, Robert Louis.*
plasma thromboplastin component (PTC) deficiency. See *Christmas disease.*
plasma thromboplastin factor-B (PTF-B) deficiency. See *Christmas disease.*
plasma-cell balanitis. See *Zoon erythroplasia.*
plasma-cell dyscrasia-polyneuropathy-organomegaly-endocrinopathy-M-protein-skin changes syndrome. See *POEMS syndrome.*
plasma-cell gingivitis. See *gingivostomatitis syndrome.*
plasma-cell hepatitis. See *Bearn-Kunkel syndrome, and Waldenström hepatitis, under Jan Gösta.*
plasmacytosis of the gingiva. See *gingivostomatitis syndrome.*
plasmocytic myeloma. See *Kahler disease.*
plasmocytic sarcoma. See *Kahler disease.*
plasmocytoma. See *Kahler disease.*
plaster cast syndrome. See *cast syndrome.*
plastic induration of the penis. See *Peyronie disease.*
platelet alpha-granule deficiency. See *gray platelet syndrome.*
platelet fibrinogen receptor deficiency. See *Glanzmann thrombasthenia.*
platelet glycoprotein Ib deficiency. See *Bernard-Soulier syndrome, under Bernard, Jean.*
platelet glycoprotein IIb-III deficiency. See *Glanzmann thrombasthenia.*
platelet thrombosis. See *Moschcowitz syndrome.*
platelike atelectasis. See *Fleischner syndrome.*
platybasia-cervical synostosis-Sprengel deformity syndrome. See *Furst-Ostrum syndrome.*
platyspondylia. See *Calvé syndrome.*
platyspondylia generalisata. See *Dreyfus syndrome.*
platyspondylia vera generalisata. See *Dreyfus syndrome.*

PLAUT, HUGO CARL (German physician, 1858-1928)
Plaut ulcer. See *Vincent infection.*
Plaut-Vincent infection. See *Vincent infection.*
Plaut-Vincent ulcer. See *Vincent infection.*
pleomorphic-cell sarcoma. See *Abrikossov tumor.*

pleomorphic granular-cell sarcoma. See *Abrikossov tumor.*

pleonosteosis familiaris. See *Léri pleonosteosis syndrome.*

pleuropneumonia-like organism pneumonia. See *Eaton pneumonia, under Eaton, Monroe Davis.*

PLM (periodic leg movement). See *restless leg syndrome.*

PLS. See *Papillon-Lefèvre syndrome.*

PLUMBE, SAMUEL (British dermatologist)

Willan-Plumbe syndrome. See *Willan lepra.*

plumbism. See *lead poisoning.*

PLUMMER, HENRY STANLEY (American physician, 1874-1937)

Plummer adenoma. See *Plummer disease.*

Plummer disease. Hyperthyroidism due to toxic adenoma of the thyroid gland (Plummer adenoma).

Plummer, H. S. The clinical and pathological relationship of simple and exophthalmic goiter. *Am. J. Med. Sc.,* 1913, 146:790-5.

Plummer-Vinson syndrome (PVS). Synonyms: *Kelly syndrome, Paterson-Brown Kelly syndrome, Paterson-Kelly syndrome, Waldenström-Kjellberg syndrome, sideropenic dysphagia.*

A syndrome occurring chiefly in middle-aged women suffering from vitamin B deficiency with iron-deficiency anemia. The principal symptoms include cracks or fissures at the corners of the mouth (perlèche), painful tongue which has a shiny smooth appearance, atrophy of the filiform and later the fungiform papillae, and dysphagia resulting from stenosis or webs of the esophageal mucosa. Lemon-tinted pallor of the skin; spoon-shaped and brittle nails; atrophy and lack of normal keratinization of the mucous membrane of the mouth, esophagus, and upper respiratory tract; and other symptoms of iron deficiency anemia are usually present. Ocular changes may include fissures at the corners of the eyes, blepharoconjunctivitis, keratitis, and hemeralopia. Other findings may include dry and burning eyes, burning and itching of the vulva, atrophy of the vulvar and anal mucosa, and splenomegaly. Cancer of the tongue and upper alimentary tract occurs in some cases. The etiology is unknown.

Plummer, H. S. Diffuse dilatation of the esophagus without anatomic stenosis (cardiospasm). A report of ninety-one cases. *JAMA,* 1912, 58:2013-5. Vinson, P. P. A case of cardiospasm with dilatation and angulation of the esophagus. *Med. Clin, N. America,* 1919, 3:623-7. Paterson, D. R. A clinical type of dysphagia. *J. Laryng. Otol., London,* 1919, 34:285-91. Waldenström, J., & Kjellberg, D. R. The roentgenological diagnosis of sideropnic dysphagia (Plummer-Vinson's syndrome). *Acta Radiol., Stockholm,* 1939, 20:618.

PLUNKETT, EARL R. (Canadian physician)

Carr-Barr-Plunkett syndrome. See *chromosome XXXX syndrome.*

plurideficiency syndrome. See *kwashiorkor.*

pluriglandular insufficiency syndrome. See *Falta syndrome.*

plurisystematic degeneration of the neuraxis. See *Steele-Richardson-Olszewski syndrome.*

PLUTARCH (First century Greek biographer and historian)

Appian-Plutarch syndrome. See *under Appian of Alexandria.*

PLW (Prader-Labhart-Willi) syndrome. See *Prader-Willi syndrome.*

PLWS (Prader-Labhart-Willi syndrome). See *Prader-Willi syndrome.*

PM (porokeratosis of Mibelli). See *Mibelli disease (2).*

PMIS. See *postmyocardial infarction syndrome.*

PML (prolapsing mitral leaflet) **syndrome.** See *mitral valve prolapse syndrome.*

PMR (polymyalgia rheumatica). See *Forestier syndrome (1).*

PMS. See *premenstrual syndrome.*

PMT (premenstrual tension). See *premenstrual syndrome.*

pneumorenal syndrome. See *Goodpasture syndrome.*

PNM (peripheral dysostosis-nasal hypoplasia-mental retardation) **syndrome.** See *acrodysostosis.*

PNS. See *paraneoplastic syndrome.*

POADS (postaxial acrofacial dysostosis syndrome). See *Genée-Wiedemann syndrome.*

POEMS (plasma cell dyscrasia-polyneuropathy-organomegaly-endocrinopathy-M-protein-skin changes) **syndrome.** Synonyms: *Crow-Fukase syndrome, Takatsuki syndrome, Japanese multisystem syndrome, pigmentation-edema-plasma (PEP) cell dyscrasia syndrome.*

A multisystem syndrome characterized by polyneuropathy, organomegaly, endocrinopathy, production of M-protein, skin changes, and other disorders. Neurological symptoms include peripheral neuropathy, papilledema, and increased cerebrospinal fluid proteins. Hepatomegaly, splenomegaly, and lymphadenopathy are the chief forms of organomegaly. Endocrine disorders consist of gynecomastia, hypogonadism, impotence, amenorrhea, glucose intolerance, adrenal insufficiency, and hypothyroidism. IgG and IgA are the immunoglobulins characteristic of this syndrome. Dermatological features are hyperpigmentation, pachyderma, hirsutism, anasarca, white nails, angiomas, and hyperhidrosis. Associated disorders include peripheral edema, ascites, pleural effusion, clubbing of the fingers, and fever. Most, but not all, cases of this syndrome have been reported in Japan.

Crow, R. S. Peripheral neuritis in myelomatosis. *Brit. Med. J.,* 1956, 2:802-4. Takatsuki, K., *et al.* Plasma dyscrasia with polyneuropathy and endocrine disorder: Review of 32 patients. Internat. Cong. Series No. 415. Topics in Hematology. *Proc. 16th Internat. Cong. Hematol.,* Kyoto, Sept. 1976, p. 454. Shimpo, S., *et al.* [Solitary plasmacytoma with polyneuritis and endocrine disturbances] *Nippons Rinsho,* 1968, I26:2444-56 (clinicopathological conference conducted by Masaichi Fukase). Nakanishi, T., *et al.* The Crow-Fukase syndrome: A study of 102 cases in Japan. *Neurology,* 1984, 34:712-21.

Pohvant Valley plague. See *Francis disease.*

poikiloderma atrophicans-cataract syndrome. See *Rothmund-Thomson syndrome.*

poikiloderma atrophicans vasculare. See *Jacobi disease.*

poikiloderma congenita. See *Rothmund-Thomson syndrome.*

poikilodermatomyositis. See *Petges-Cléjat syndrome.*

poikiloscleroderma. See *Rothmund-Thomson syndrome.*

poker back. See *Bechterew-Strümpell-Marie syndrome, under Bekhterev.*

pokkuri. See *sudden unexplained death syndrome.*

POLAND, ALFRED (British physician, 1820-1872)

Poland anomalad. See *Poland syndrome.*

Poland anomaly. See *Poland syndrome.*

Poland complex. See *Poland syndrome.*

Poland syndactyly. See *Poland syndrome.*

Poland syndrome. Synonyms: *Poland anomalad, Poland anomaly, Poland complex, Poland syndactyly, hand and ipsilateral thorax syndrome, pectoral aplasia-dysdactylia syndrome, pectoral muscle absence and syndactyly syndrome.*

Absence of the pectoralis major muscle or its sternal portion associated with ipsilateral shortening of the phalanges with syndactyly (symbrachydactyly). Associated anomalies may include absence of the nipples and areolae, rib defects, and hypoplasia of the hand or the whole arm on the affected side. Most reported cases are sporadic, but some authors suggest genetic inheritance, possibly as an autosomal dominant trait.

Poland, A. Deficiency of the pectoralis muscle. *Guy's Hosp. Rev., London*, 1841, 6:191-3.

Poland-Moebius syndrome. The Poland syndrome (absence of the pectoralis major muscle or its sternal portion associated with ipsilateral shortening of the phalanges with syndactyly) combined with the Moebius syndrome (1) (congenital paralysis of the external rectus and facial muscles due to aplasia of the nuclei of the abducens and facial nerves with inability to abduct the eyes beyond the midline and masklike facies). The syndrome is probably transmitted as a genetic trait.

Parker, D. L., *et al.* Poland-Moebius syndrome. *J. Med. Genet.*, 1981, 18:317-20. Poland, A. Deficiency of the pectoralis muscle. *Guy's Hosp. Rep., London,* 1841, 6:191-3. Moebius, P. J. Über angeborene doppelseitige Abducens-facialis Lähmung. *Münch. Med. Wschr.*, 1888, 35:91-4; 108-11.

POLGAR, FRANZ (Hungarian radiologist)

Bársony-Polgár syndrome (1 and 2). See *under Bársony.*

Brailsford-Bársony-Polgár syndrome. See *Bársony-Polgár syndrome (1).*

polio. See *Heine-Medin disease.*

poliodysplasia cerebri. See *Alpers syndrome.*

poliodystrophia cerebri progressiva. See *Alpers syndrome.*

poliodystrophia cerebri progressiva infantilis. See *Alpers syndrome.*

polioencephalitis hemorrhagica superioris. See *Wernicke syndrome.*

poliomyelitis. See *Heine-Medin disease.*

POLLAND, RUDOLF (Austrian dermatologist, born 1876)

Matzenauer-Polland syndrome. See *under Matzenauer.*

POLLE (A son of Baron Hieronymus Karl Friedrich von Münchhausen)

Polle syndrome. See *Munchausen syndrome by proxy.*

pollenosis. See *Bostock catarrh.*

POLLNOW, HANS (German physician)

Kramer-Pollnow disease. See *under Kramer.*

POLLOCK, D. J. (British physician)

Williams-Pollock syndrome. See *mucosal neuromas syndrome.*

polyadenoma en nappe. See *Ménétrier syndrome.*

polyarteritis acuta nodosa. See *Kusssmaul-Maier syndrome.*

polyarteritis nodosa. See *Kussmaul-Maier syndrome.*

polyarthritis enterica. See *Reiter syndrome.*

polyatresia congenita. See *Weyers syndrome (1).*

polychondritis chronica atrophicans. See *Meyenburg-Altherr-Uehlinger syndrome.*

polychondritis recidivans et atrophicans. See *Meyenburg-Altherr-Uehlinger syndrome.*

polychondropathy. See *Meyenburg-Altherr-Uehlinger syndrome.*

polyclonia. See *Friedreich disease (1).*

polyclonia continua epileptoides. See *Kozhevnikov syndrome.*

polycoric hepatomegaly. See *Debré syndrome (2).*

polycoric hypertrophy. See *Debré syndrome (2).*

polycystic kidney. See *Potter syndrome (2), under Potter, Edith Louise.*

polycystic ovarian disease (PCOD). See *polycystic ovary syndrome.*

polycystic ovary syndrome. Synonyms: *Stein syndrome, Stein-Leventhal syndrome, bilateral polycystic ovarian syndrome, hyperthecosis of the ovary, polycystic ovarian disease (PCOD), sclerocystic ovary syndrome.*

A syndrome of multiple cysts of the ovaries associated with amenorrhea, sterility, frequent hirsutism and obesity, menstrual disorders, and elevated levels of luteinizing and follicle-stimulating hormones. It is usually observed in women in their second or third decade of life. The ovaries are usually enlarged and have thickened capsules and numerous small follicular cysts beneath the capsule. Polycystic ovaries also occur in syndromes of abnormal bleeding with hypermenorrhea and virilism.

Stein, I. F., & Leventhal, M. L. Amenorrhea associated with bilateral polycystic ovaries. *Am. J. Obst. Gyn.*, 1935, 29:181-91.

polycythemia hypertonica. See *Gaisböck disease.*

polycythemia rubra. See *Vaquez-Osler syndrome.*

polycythemia rubra hypertonica. See *Gaisböck disease.*

polycythemia rubra vera. See *Vaquez-Osler syndrome.*

polycythemia vera. See *Vaquez-Osler syndrome.*

polycythemia with chronic cyanosis. See *Vaquez-Osler syndrome.*

polycythemia-hepatocirrhosis syndrome. See *Mosse syndrome, under Mosse, Max.*

polydactyly with neonatal chondrodystrophy type I. See *Majewski syndrome.*

polydactyly with neonatal chondrodystrophy type II. See *Saldino-Noonan syndrome.*

polydactyly with neonatal chondrodystrophy type III. See *Verma-Naumoff syndrome.*

polydactyly-chondrodystrophy syndrome. See *Ellis-van Creveld syndrome.*

polydactyly-imperforate anus-vertebral anomalies (PIV, PIAVA) syndrome. See *VATER association.*

polydeficiency-retrobulbar neuritis syndrome. See *Obal syndrome.*

polydystrophic dwarfism. See *mucopolysaccharidosis VI.*

polydystrophic oligophrenia. See *mucopolysaccharidosis III.*

polyglandular autoimmune (PGA) syndrome. Synonyms: *autoimmune endocrine syndrome, autoimmune polyendocrine syndrome, autoimmune polyglandular syndrome.*

Dysfunction of multiple endocrine glands associated with the presence of circulating organ-specific antibodies directed against the involved glands. The underlying abnormality is probably a defect in T suppressor cell function, but aberrant expression of HLA

DR antigens is also suspected as a pathogenic factor. **Polyglandular autoimmune syndrome type I (PGA I)** occurs in patients who have at least two of the triad of Addison disease, hypoparathyroidism, and chronic mucocutaneous candidiasis. Associated disorders may include gonadal failure, autoimmune thyroid disease and occasional hypopituitarism, insulin-dependent diabetes mellitus, diabetes insipidus, pernicious anemia, vitiligo, alopecia, malabsorption syndrome, and chronic hepatitis. **Polyglandular autoimmune syndrome type II**, or **PGA II**, (synonyms: **Schmidt syndrome, thyroid-adrenocortical insufficiency syndrome)** represents an association of primary adrenal insufficiency with autoimmune thyroid disease and/or insulin-dependent diabetes mellitus. Co-occurring disorders may include gonadal failure, diabetes insipidus, vitiligo, alopecia, pernicious anemia, myasthenia gravis, immune thrombocytopenic purpura, the Sjögren syndrome, and rheumatoid arthritis. **Polyglandular autoimmune syndrome type III (PGA III)** is marked by a thyroid disease and another autoimmune dysfunction, but without the symptoms of the Addison syndrome.

Schmidt, M. B. Eine biglandulare Erkrankung (Nebenniere und Schilddruse) bei Morbus Addisonii. *Verh. Deut. Path. Ges.*, 1926, 21:212-21. Butler, M. G., *et al.* Linkage analysis in a large kindred with autosomal dominant transmission of polyglandular autoimmune disease Type II (Schmidt syndrome). *Am. J. Med. Genet.*, 1984, 18:61-5.

polymorphic macular degeneration of Braley. See *Best macular degeneration.*
polymorphic vitelline macular degeneration. See *Best macular degeneration.*
polymorphous posterior corneal dystrophy (PPCD). See *Schlichting dystrophy.*
polymorphous prurigo syndrome. See *Sulzberger-Garbe syndrome.*
polymorphous ventricular tachycardia. See *torsades de pointes syndrome.*
polymyalgia rheumatica (PMR). See *Forestier syndrome (1).*
polymyositis gregarina. See *Wagner-Unverricht syndrome, under Wagner, Ernst Leberecht.*
polyneuritic psychosis. See *Korsakoff syndrome, under Korsakov.*
polyneuritis acuta ascendens. See *Guillain-Barré syndrome.*
polyneuritis cerebralis menieriformis. See *Frankl-Hochwart syndrome (1).*
polyneuritis cranialis menieriformis. See *Frankl-Hochwart syndrome (1).*
polyneuritis with facial diplegia. See *Guillain-Barré syndrome.*
polyossificatio congenita progressiva. See *fibrodysplasia ossificans progressiva.*
polyosteopathia deformans connatalis regressiva. See *Caffey-Silverman syndrome.*
polyostic fibrous dysplasia. See *Jaffe-lichtenstein syndrome.*
polyostotic infantilia. See *Camurati-Engelmann syndrome.*
polypapilloma tropicum. See *Charlouis disease.*
polyposis-skin pigmentation-alopecia-fingernail changes. See *Cronkhite-Canada syndrome.*
polyradiculitis. See *Guillain-Barré syndrome.*
polyradiculoneuritis. See *Guillain-Barré syndrome.*
polysplenia syndrome. Synonyms: *cardiovascular anomaly-left isomerism syndrome, laterality anomalad, situs ambiguus with left isomerism, situs ambiguus-polysplenia (SAP) syndrome.*

The presence of two or more splenic masses in association with complex heart defects, malposition and maldevelopment of the visceral organs, and abnormal lobation of the lungs. Bilateral bilobed lungs with hyparterial bronchi occur in most cases. Isomerism of the liver is present in some instances; in the remainder, the major lobe may be found on the left rather than the right side, and the gallbladder is usually associated with the major lobe. The stomach is located on the right side in the majority of cases, but it may be found on the same side as the major lobe of the liver. Malrotation of the jejunum and ileum occurs in most patients. Bilateral superior venae cavae are present in some cases. A solitary superior vena cava is usually found on the right side. The hepatic segment of the inferior vena cava is often absent, the vena cava draining by way of the azygos veins. Juxtaposition of the inferior vena cava and abdominal aorta may occur. The pulmonary veins may enter the atria normally, or they may empty into one or the other atrium in its sinus venosus portion; in some cases, the right pulmonary veins enter the right atrium and the left ones the left atrium. Transposition of the great arteries occurs only in a small number of instances. The heart apex is located on the left side in most cases, but the right-sided apex may also occur. A normal heart may be observed in some cases. Somewhat more than a half of the affected infants die within the first year of life. See also *asplenia syndrome.*

Moller, J. H., *et al.* Congenital cardiac disease associated with polysplenia: A development complex of bilateral "left-sidedness." *Circulation*, 1967, 36:789.

polysurgical addiction. See *Munchausen syndrome.*
polysyndactyly-craniofacial anomalies syndrome. See *Greig syndrome.*
polysyndactyly-craniofacial dysmorphism syndrome. See *Greig syndrome.*
polysyndactyly-dyscrania syndrome. See *Greig syndrome.*
polysynostoses syndrome. See *multiple synostoses syndrome.*
polytopic enchondral dysostosis. See *Léri-Weill syndrome, under Léri, André.*
POMPE, JOANN CASSIANUIS (Dutch physician)
Pompe disease. See *glycogen storage disease II.*
POMPEN, ARNOLD WILLEM MARIA (Dutch dermatologist)
Ruiter-Pompen syndrome. See *Fabry syndrome.*
Ruiter-Pompen-Wyers syndrome. See *Fabry syndrome.*

PONCET, ANTONIN (French physician, 1849-1913)
Poncet disease. Synonyms: *Grocco-Poncet disease, Poncet rheumatoid syndrome.*

A form of tuberculous polyarthritis.

Poncet, A. Polyarthrite tuberculeuse simulant les lésions chroniques déformantes. *Gaz. Hôp. Paris.*, 1879, 70:1219.

Poncet rheumatoid syndrome. See *Poncet disease.*
pontine tegmentum syndrome. See *Foville syndrome.*
pontobulbar palsy with deafness. See *Brown-Vialetto-van Laere syndrome, under Brown, C. H.*

pontobulbar palsy with neurosensory deafness. See *Brown-Vialetto-van Laere syndrome, under Brown, C. H.*

ponto-olivocerebellar atrophy. See *olivopontocerebellar atrophy.*

popliteal artery compression syndrome. See *popliteal artery entrapment syndrome.*

popliteal artery entrapment syndrome (PAES). Synonyms: *anomalous position of the popliteal artery syndrome, gastrocnemius muscle syndrome, popliteal artery compression syndrome, trapped popliteal artery syndrome.*

Compression of the popliteal artery, ultimately leading to thrombosis, due to an abnormal anatomical relationship between vessels and muscles within the popliteal fossa, abnormality of the medial head of the gastrocnemius muscle being the principal cause. The disorder occurs most commonly in young male adults. Intermittent unilateral claudication, absence of dorsalis pedis pulse, and weakness of the posterior tibial pulse are the principal symptoms.

Stuart, T. P. Note on a variation in the course of popliteal artery. *J. Anat.,* 1879, 13:162. Servello, M. Clinical syndrome of anomalous position of the popliteal artery. Differentiation from juvenile arteriopathy. *Circulation,* 1962, 26:885-90.

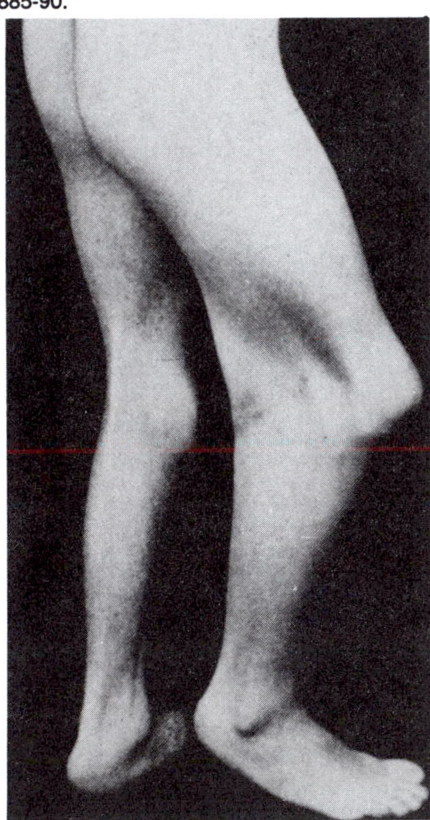

Popliteal artery entrapment syndrome (PAES)
Courtesy Dr. Robert J. Gorlin, Minneapolis, MN.

popliteal bursitis. See *Baker cyst.*

popliteal cyst. See *Baker cyst.*

popliteal pterygium syndrome (PPS). Synonyms: *Champion-Cregan-Klein syndrome, Fèvre-Languepin syndrome, Gorlin-Pindborg syndrome, Hecht-Jarvinen syndrome, Kopits-Matolscy syndrome, Trèlat syndrome, faciogenitopopliteal syndrome, popliteal web syndrome.*

A syndrome of orofacial, genital, and musculoskeletal abnormalities, sometimes associated with mental retardation. The orofacial defects consist of ankyloblepharon filiforme, cleft lip or palate, lower lip pits, ankyloglossia, syngnathia, micrognathia, epicanthal folds, and hypoplastic ear lobes. The cutaneous and musculoskeletal abnormalities include popliteal pterygium, spina bifida occulta, scoliosis, lordosis, hypoplastic or absent digits, finger and toe syndactyly, bipartite or absent patella, pes varus or valgus, pyramidal skin bridges over the great toes, hypoplastic toe nails, brachydactyly of the toes, metatarsal fusion, hypoplastic or supernumerary nipples, oligohydramnios, and arthrogryposis. Genitourinary anomalies are cryptorchidism, small penis, hypoplastic or absent labia minora, clitoromegaly, and absent, hypoplastic, or ectopic scrotum. Inguinal hernia and intercrural pterygium may occur. Autosomal dominant inheritance with variable expressivity and incomplete penetrance is suspected. See also *lethal multiple pterygium syndrome* and *multiple pterygium syndrome.*

Kopits, E. Die als "Flughaut" bezeichneten Missbildungen und deren operative Behandlung. (Musculo-dysplasia congenita.) *Arch. Orthop. Unfallchir.,* 1936-37, 37:539-49. *Trélat, U. Sur un vice conformation très rare de la lèvre-inferieure. *J. Méd. Chir. Prat.,* 1869, 40:860-3. Gorlin, R. J., & Pindborg, J. J. *Syndromes of the head and neck.* McGraw-Hill, New York, 1964, p. 38. Klein, D. Un curieux syndrome héréditaire: chéilo-palatoschizis avec fistules de la lévre inferieure associée à une syndactylie, une onychodysplasie particulière, un ptérygion poplité unilatéral et des pieds varus équins. *J. Génét. Hum.,* 1962, 11:65-71. Champion, R., & Cregan, J. C. F. Congenital popliteal webbing in siblings. *J. Bone Joint Surg.,* 1959, 41-B:355-7. Matolcsy, T. Über die chirurgische Behandlung der angeborenen Flughaut. *Arch. Klin. Chir., Berlin,* 1936, 185:675-81. Hecht, F., & Jarvinen, J. M. Heritable dysmorphic syndrome with normal intelligence. *J. Pediat.,* 1967, 70:927-35. Fèvre, M., & Languepin, A. Les brides cruro-jambieres contenant le nerf sciatique. The syndrome brides poplitées et malformations multiples (division palatine, fistules de la lèvre inferieure, syndactylie des orteils). *Press Méd.,* 1962, 70:615-8. Escobar, V., & Weaver, D. D. The facio-genito-popliteal syndrome. *Birth Defects,* 1978, 14(6B):185-93.

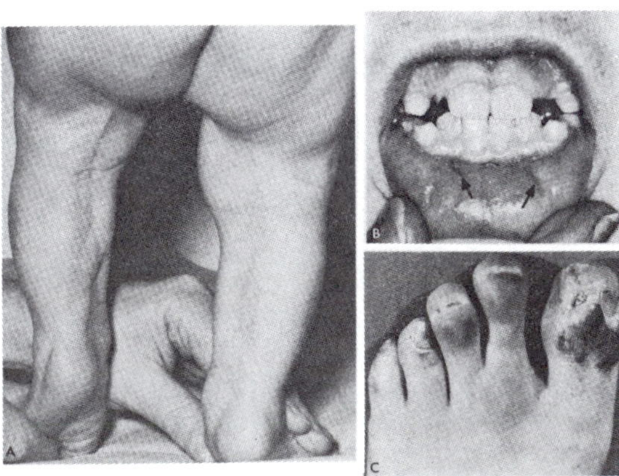

Popliteal pterygium syndrome
Hecht, F., & Jarvinen, J.M.: *J. Pediatr.* 70:927, 1967: St. Louis: C.V. Mosby Co.

popliteal web syndrome. See *popliteal pterygium syndrome.*

poradenitis inguinalis. See *Durand-Nicolas-Favre disease, under Durand, J.*

poradenitis nostras. See *Durand-Nicolas-Favre disease, under Durand, J.*

PORAK, CHARLES (French physician, 1845-1921)

Porak-Durante syndrome. See *osteogenesis imperfecta syndrome (recessive form).*

porokeratosis centrifugata atrophicans. See *Mibelli disease (2).*

porokeratosis of Mibelli (PM). See *Mibelli disease (2).*

porphyria cutanea tarda (PCT) syndrome. Synonyms: *acquired hepatic porphyria, chemical porphyria, symptomatic porphyria.*

A common form of porphyria, transmitted as an autosomal dominant trait, seen most commonly in alcoholics. The symptoms usually occur during the third or fourth decade, rarely before puberty. They include photosensitivity; vesicular, bullous, and ulcerative lesions, chiefly on parts of the skin that are exposed to the sunlight; excessive skin sensitivity to injuries; hyperpigmentation; sclerodermoid plaques; cicatricial alopecia; milia of the fingers and hands; hypertrichosis; and violaceous periorbital suffusion. Associated disorders may include diabetes mellitus, liver tumors, increased liver iron storage, and elevated serum iron levels. The precipitating agents, in addition to ethyl alcohol, may include estrogens (such as those used in oral contraceptives and in the treatment of prostatic carcinoma), hexachlorobenzene, chlorinated phenols, iron, tetrachlorobenzo-*p*-dioxin, and polychlorinated biphenyls. Excessive synthesis of uroporphyrin I due to inhibition of uroporphyrinogen III cosynthetase by ferrous compounds is the principal biochemical feature.

Waldenström, J. Studien über Porphyrie. *Acta Med. Scand,* 1937, Suppl. 82.

porphyria erythropoetica. See *congenital erythropoietic porphyria.*

porphyria hepatica. See *acute intermittent porphyria.*

porphyria intermittens acuta. See *acute intermittent porphyria.*

porrigo. See *Fox impetigo, under Fox, William Tilbury.*

porrigo decalvans. See *Cazenave vitiligo.*

portal cirrhosis. See *Laennec cirrhosis.*

portal-systemic encephalopathy. See *hepatic encephalopathy syndrome.*

PORTER, WILLIAM BRANCH (American physician, born 1888)

Porter syndrome. Synonym: *idiopathic benign pericarditis.*

A type of benign pericarditis that does not belong to the rheumatic, bacterial, or uremic group.

Porter, W. B., *et al.* Nonspecific pericarditis. *JAMA,* 1950, 144:749-53.

Portsmouth syndrome. A hematological disorder characterized by a prolonged bleeding time, reduced platelet adhesiveness, and abnormal or absent collagen-induced platelet aggregation, in the presence of normal exogenous ADP-induced platelet aggregation. The original research on this condition was done in Portsmouth, England, hence its name.

O'Brien, J. R. Platelets: A Portsmouth syndrome? *Lancet,* 1967, 2:258.

Portuguese neuropathic amyloid syndrome. See *amyloid neuropathy type I.*

POSNER, ADOLF (American ophthalmologist, born 1906)

Posner-Schlossman syndrome. Synonyms: *Terrien-Veil syndrome, acute glaucomatocyclitic crises, benign paroxysmal ocular hypertension, cyclic glaucoma, glaucomatocyclitic crises.*

Recurrent episodes of glaucoma with cyclitis that are limited to one, always the same, eye. The symptoms include heterochromia, anisocoria, colored halos or blurring of vision, white color of the eye, and congestion of the sclera or edema of the corneal epithelium. Simultaneous with, or a day or so after, the appearance of hypertension, there are cellular components in the aqueous humor. Within 24 hours, pigmented precipitates on the posterior surface of the cornea are noted. These disappear but, if hypertension persists, fresh ones may appear. Episodes occur with varying frequency and without any apparent cause, lasting for a few hours to 1 month, but rarely over 2 weeks.

Posner, A., & Schlossman, A. Syndrome of unilateral recurrent attacks of glaucoma with cyclitic symptoms. *Arch. Ophth., Chicago,* 1948, 39:517-35. Terrien, F., & Veil, P. De certains glaucomes soi-disant primitifs. *Bull. Soc. Fr. Opht.,* 1929, 42:349-68.

POSPISCHILL

Pospischill-Feyrter aphthoid. See *Pospischill-Feyrter disease.*

Pospischill-Feyrter disease. Synonym: *Pospischill-Feyrter aphthoid.*

A sometimes fatal form of primary herpetic gingivostomatitis affecting chiefly infants and young children who are in poor physical condition. The disease extends to organs other than the mouth and involves the perioral areas, esophagus, genitalia, fingers, and other parts. The primary lesion presents as a vesicle with central invagination and a thick surface, eventually evolving into necrotic plaques, ulcers, and erosions. Painful lymphadenopathy is usually present. The disorder was reportedly first described by Pospischill and Feyrter.

post head trauma syndrome. See *postconcussive syndrome.*

post-sino-cibal syndrome. See *Chinese restaurant syndrome.*

post-transfusion mononucleosis. See *postperfusion syndrome.*

post-transfusion pulmonary syndrome. See *postperfusion lung syndrome.*

post-transfusion purpura. See *Shulman syndrome, under Shulman, N. Raphael.*

post-traumatic apallic syndrome. See *apallic syndrome.*

post-traumatic atelectasis. See *adult respiratory distress syndrome.*

post-traumatic digital ischemia. See *hypothenar hammer syndrome.*

post-traumatic fat embolism syndrome. See *fat embolism syndrome.*

post-traumatic lung failure. See *adult respiratory distress syndrome.*

post-traumatic nevus flammeus. See *Fegeler syndrome.*

post-traumatic occipital-cervical shoulder girdle syndrome. See *Coleman syndrome.*

post-traumatic painful osteoporosis. See *Sudeck syndrome.*

post-traumatic pulmonary insufficiency. See *adult respiratory distress syndrome.*

post-traumatic spondylitis. See *Kümmell-Verneuil disease.*

post-traumatic spreading neuralgia. See *Sudeck syndrome.*

post-traumatic stress disorder (PTSD). See *post-traumatic stress syndrome.*

post-traumatic stress syndrome. Synonyms: *combat fatigue, DaNang syndrome, poststress syndrome, post-traumatic stress disorder (PTSD), stress response syndrome, Vietnam syndrome, war neurosis.*

A syndrome occurring as a reaction to overwhelmingly distressful physical or mental situations, such as wartime experiences, chronic illness, interpersonal conflicts, starvation, threat of harm, imprisonment, rape, natural disasters, torture, trauma, severe pain, and the like. The resulting disorders may include persistently re-experiencing the traumatic event, recurrent dreams of the event, illusions and hallucinations related to the experience, distress on exposure to situations similar to the traumatic experience, avoidance of situations that may bring back the recollection of the event, psychogenic amnesia, disinterest in the immediate environment and family, disinterest in the future, insomnia, irritability, difficulty in concentrating and decreased attention span, hypervigilance, exaggerated startle response, changes in thinking and feeling, impairment of short-term memory, tendency to view minor problems as major, racing thoughts, negative approach to problem solving, rigid thinking, feeling of being victimized, loss of sense of humor, demanding behavior, and escapism. See also *rape trauma syndrome* and *concentration camp survivor syndrome.*

Pavlov, I. P. *Lectures on conditional reflexes.* Translated and edited by W. H. Gant. New York, International Publishing Co., 1941. *Diagnostic and statistical manual of mental disorders.* 3rd ed. Washington, D. C., American Psychiatric Association, 1987, pp. 247-51.

post-tubal ligation syndrome. See *tubal ligation syndrome.*

postaxial acrofacial dysostosis syndrome (POADS). See *Genée-Wiedemann syndrome.*

postcardiotomy syndrome (PCS). See *postpericardiotomy syndrome.*

postcesarean monouria. See *Youssef syndrome.*

postcesarean vesicouterine fistula. See *Youssef syndrome.*

postcholecystectomy sump syndrome. See *sump syndrome.*

postcholecystectomy syndrome (PCS). Synonyms: *Walter-Bohmann syndrome, recurrent biliary tract syndrome.*

Persistence of abdominal symptoms after cholecystectomy, including pain, nausea, or jaundice, due to retained calculi in the common bile duct, stricture of the common bile duct, stenosis of the sphincter of Oddi, or other disorders which were not diagnosed prior to surgery. Postcholecystectomy syndrome with tachycardia, hypopothermia, polypnea, pallor, and cold sweat is referred to as the *Walter-Bohmann syndrome.* See also *sump syndrome.*

Dreiling, D. A. The postcholecystectomy syndrome. The functional aspect of biliary colic persistent after cholecystectomy. *Am. J. Digest Dis.*, 1962, 7:603-12. Akel, S. Kolesistektomiden sonra görülen bir Walter-Bohmann syndromu. *Türk Tip Cem. Mec.*, 1955, 21:225-6.

postcoartectomy syndrome. Synonyms: *mesenteric syndrome, mesenteric arteritis syndrome.*

Complications following surgery of coarctation of the aorta involving the mesenteric artery. It usually occurrs on the third postoperative day and is characterized by abdominal pain and tenderness, ileus, vomiting, fever, melena, leukocytosis, and paradoxical hypertension, followed by bowel necrosis. See also *aortoiliac steal syndrome.*

Clagett, O. T., & Jampolis, R. W. Coartctation of the aorta. A study of seventy cases in which surgical exploration was performed. *Arch. Surg.*, 1951, 63:337-48. Mays, E. T., & Sargeant, C. K. Postocarctectomy syndrome. *Arch. Surg.*, I965, 63:337-48.

postcommissurotomy syndrome. See *postpericardiotomy syndrome.*

postconcussion seizure syndrome. See *traumatic spreading depression syndrome.*

postconcussive syndrome (PCS). Synonym: *posthead trauma syndrome.*

A symptom complex following brain injury, characterized by headache, irritability, dizziness, difficulty with concentration, apprehension, general lack of interest in the surroundings, mild memory impairment, intolerance to alcohol, insomnia, loss of libido, and a feeling of weakness or lightheadedness on turning the head. Potential whiplash injury, damage of neck innervation, and other neurological complications of injury are considered as probable contributing factors, but the etiology and pathogenesis are not understood. See also *traumatic spreading depression syndrome.*

Becker, D. P. Injury of the head and spine. In: Wyngaarden, J. B., & Smith, L. H., Jr., eds. *Cecil textbook of medicine.* 17th ed. Philadelphia, Saunders, 1986, pp. 2170-7.

postdormital paralysis. See *Rosenthal disease, under Rosenthal, Curt.*

postdysenteric rheumatoid. See *Reiter syndrome.*

postdysenteric syndrome. See *Reiter syndrome.*

postenteric rheumatoid. See *Reiter syndrome.*

postepileptic paralysis. See *Todd paralysis, under Todd, Robert Bentley.*

posterior cavernous syndrome. See *under Jefferson syndrome.*

posterior cervical sympathetic syndrome. See *Barré-Lieou syndrome.*

posterior column ataxia. See Biemond syndrome (4).

posterior hernia of the knee. See Baker cyst.

posterior inferior cerebellar artery syndrome. See *Wallenberg syndrome.*

posterior interosseous tunnel syndrome. See *radial tunnel syndrome.*

posterior laterocondylar space syndrome. See *Collet-Sicard syndrome.*

posterior retroparotid space syndrome. See Villaret syndrome.

posterior spinal sclerosis. See locomotor ataxia.

posterior thalamic syndrome. See *Déjerine-Roussy syndrome.*

posterior triangular glossitis. See *Chevallier glossitis.*

posterior uveal bleeding syndrome. Loss of vision secondary to multiple recurrent hemorrhages or serous fluid beneath the retinal pigment epithelium and neurosecretory retina in the posterior fundus.

Kleiner, R. C., *et al.* The posterior uveal bleeding syndrome. *Retina*, 1990, 10:9-17.

posterolateral sclerosis. See *Dana syndrome.*

postgastrectomy syndrome. Synonyms: *Lambling syndrome, afferent loop syndrome, alkaline reflux gastritis, bilious vomiting syndrome, dumping syndrome, gastric remnant syndrome, postgastrectomy malabsorption syndrome, postgastrectomy pseudodeficiency syndrome, postgastric resection syndrome, reflux syndrome, reflux gastritis syndrome, small stomach.*

Complications of gastric resection, consisting of early and late postcibal disorders. The early disorders include: (1) The **early dumping syndrome**, which consists of vasomotor disorders (flushing, arrhythmias, diaphoresis, lightheadedness, tachycardia, and postural hypotension) and affective symptoms (lassitude, desire to lie down, and diminished attention span). The alimentary symptoms, occurring with or without vasomotor and affective symptoms, include a feeling of satiety, nausea, vomiting, abdominal pain, and diarrhea. (2) The **small stomach syndrome** is usually marked by a feeling of early postcibal satiety, often followed by vomiting. This syndrome may also occur after nonresective surgery, such as vagotomy with drainage. Similar symptoms may also occur in congenital microgastria and after surgery for morbid obesity. (3) The **afferent loop syndrome** is characterized by upper abdominal pain due to afferent loop obstruction leading to its distention with resulting feeling of satiety and vomiting. In some cases, there may be vomiting of small amounts of food but, more often, the vomitus contains only a bile-stained liquid (the **bilious vomiting syndrome**). (4) The **alkaline (bile) reflux syndrome** is marked by gastritis associated with reflux of the duodenal contents into the stomach, sometimes triggering abnormal gastrointestinal motor activity and vomiting of bile. Late postcibal symptoms consist mainly of diaphoresis, arrhythmias, lassitude, and loss of consciousness 90 to 180 minutes after a meal (the **late dumping syndrome**). (5) **Postgastrectomy malabsorption (Lambling) syndrome** is characterized by extreme thinness, anemia, hypoproteinemia, edema, and diarrhea due to malabsorption in gastrectomized patients. Hypoglycemia, steatorrhea, weight loss, maldigestion, anemia, bone diseases (osteoporosis, pseudomalacia, and pseudofractures), elevated serum alkaline phosphatase, hypocalcemia, metabolic neuropathies, bezoars, stomal stenosis, intussusception, volvulus, and other disorders may be also associated with postgastrectomy syndromes.

Lambling, A. *et al.* Syndrome carential complexe chez des gastrectomisés. Étude biologique. *Bull. Soc. Méd. Hôp. Paris*, 1949, 65-161-4. Meyer, J. H. Chronic morbidity after ulcer surgery. In: Sleisenger, M. H., & Fordtran, J. S., eds. *Gastrointestinal disease. Pathophysiology, diagnosis, management.* 3rd ed. Philadelphia, Saunders, 1983, pp. 757-79.

postgastrectomy malabsorption syndrome. See *postgastrectomy syndrome.*

postgastrectomy pseudodeficiency syndrome. See *postgastrectomy syndrome.*

postgastric resection syndrome. See *postgastrectomy syndrome.*

posthemiplegic reflex sympathetic dystrophy. See *Sudeck syndrome.*

postinfarction syndrome. See *postmyocardial infarction syndrome.*

postinfarctional sclerodactylia. See *shoulder-hand syndrome.*

postinfection purpura. See *Seidlmayer disease.*

postinfective chronic fatigue syndrome (PICFS). See *chronic fatigue syndrome.*

postmastectomy angiosarcoma. See *Stewart-Treves syndrome, under Stewart, Fred Waldorf.*

postmastectomy lymphangiosarcoma. See *Stewart-Treves syndrome, under Stewart, Fred Waldorf.*

postmastectomy lymphedema. See *Stewart-Treves syndrome, under Stewart, Fred Waldorf.*

postmaturity syndrome. See *Ballantyne-Runge syndrome.*

postmyocardial infarction syndrome (PMIS). Synonyms: *Dressler syndrome, postinfarction syndrome.*

A complication occurring a few weeks or months after myocardial infarction, characterized by protracted or recurrent fever, chest pain, pericardial rub, left pleural effusion, and pericardial effusion. Cardiac tamponade is rare. Most cases also have had earlier postmyocardial pericarditis. Autoimmune mechanisms, viral infection, and pericardial bleeding caused by anticoagulant therapy have been proposed as probable etiologic factors. The syndrome is similar to the postpericardiotomy syndrome (q.v.). See also *shoulder-hand syndrome.*

Dressler, W. Idiopathic recurrent pericarditis. Comparison with the postcommissurotomy syndrome; considerations of etiology and treatment. *Am. J. Med.*, 1955, 18:591-601.

postoperative pallor-hyperthermia syndrome. See *malignant hyperpyrexia syndrome.*

postopertive residual ovary syndrome. See *residual ovary syndrome.*

postpartum cardiomyopathy. See *Meadows syndrome.*

postpartum heart disease. See *Meadows syndrome.*

postpartum hypophyseogenic myxedema. See *Sheehan syndrome.*

postpartum hypopituitarism. See *Sheehan syndrome.*

postpartum necrosis. See *Sheehan syndrome.*

postpartum panhypopituitary syndrome. See *Sheehan syndrome.*

postpartum pituitary cachexia. See *Sheehan syndrome.*

postpartum pituitary insufficiency. See *Sheehan syndrome.*

postpartum pituitary necrosis. See *Sheehan syndrome.*

postperfusion syndrome. Synonym: *post-transfusion mononucleosis.*

A complication appearing in some patients 3 to 7 weeks following heart surgery with extracorporeal profusion, charactertzed by fever, splenomegaly, lymphadenopathy, a macular papular rash, atypical lymphocytes, and a negative heterophil agglutination reaction. The disorder resembles infectious mononucleosis or infectious hepatitis and is believed to be due to the Ebstein-Barr virus or the cytomegalovirus from transfused blood.

Reyman, T. A. Postperfusion syndrome. *Am. Heart J.*, 1966, 72:116-23.

postperfusion lung syndrome. Synonyms: *postperfusion pulmonary syndrome, postperfusion pulmonary vasculitis, post-transfusion pulmonary syndrome, pump lung.*

A frequently fatal respiratory complication (adult respiratory distress syndrome) occurring within the first few hours after heart surgery with extracorporeal perfusion. Its principal features include generalized weakness, anorexia, fever, respiratory insufficiency, hypoventilation, dyspnea, and, sometimes, cyanosis. Auscultation shows coarse rales and rhonchi. Diffuse pulmonary mottling is shown on x-rays. Pulmonary function disorders are demonstrated by impaired blood gas diffusion, hypercapnia, and hypoxemia. Pulmonary arteriovenous shunting past atelectatic alveoli is believed to be the cause. Extensive and diffuse atelectasis with hyperemia and focal hemorrhages, edema, vascular stasis, and frequent congestion with perivascular and intra-alveolar hemorrhages are the main pathologic features of this syndrome. The etiology is unknown but mechanical factors related to the operation, pathological variations in patient population, and factors related to the type of oxygenator used are the suspected causes.

Kolff, W. J., *et al.* Pulmonary complications of open heart operations. Their pathogenesis and avoidance. *Clev. Clin. Q.*, 1958, 25:65-83. Neville, W. E., *et al.* Postperfusion pulmonary vasculitis. *Arch, Surg.*, 1963, 86:126-37.

postperfusion pulmonary syndrome. See *postperfusion lung syndrome.*

postperfusion pulmonary vasculitis. See *postperfusion lung syndrome.*

postpericardiotomy syndrome (PPS). Synonyms: *postcardiotomy syndrome (PCS), postcommissurotomy syndrome.*

A complication of open-heart surgery characterized by fever, chest pain, malaise, arthralgia, and pericardial and pleural effusion occurring 1 to 12 weeks after intracardiac operations. Pericardial friction rub, ST-T changes on ECG, cardiomegaly, and parenchymal infiltrates on chest X-ray are constant features of this syndrome. Cardiac tamponade occurs in some cases. Hematological changes include leukocytosis and elevated erythrocyte sedimentation rate. Reactivation of rheumatic fever, hypersensitivity reaction to blood in the pericardial sac, a poor nutritional status, an autoimmune response, viral infections triggering the autoimmune reaction, and reactivation of a latent viral infection are the suspected etiologic factors. The syndrome was first recognized after mitral valvulotomy, hence the synonym **postcommissurotomy syndrome.** The syndrome is similar in many respects to the postmyocardial infarction syndrome.

Janton, O. H., *et al.* Results of the surgical treatment of mitral stenosis. *Circulation*, 1952, 6:321-33. Soloff, L. A., *et al.* Reactivation of rheumatic fever following mitral commissurotomy. *Circulation*, 1953, 8:481-93.

postprandial cardiogastric syndrome. See *Roemheld syndrome.*

postradiotherapy somnolence syndrome. See *somnolence syndrome.*

postrubella syndrome. See *congenital rubella syndrome.*

postspinal headache. See *puncture headache, under headache syndrome.*

poststress syndrome. See *post-traumatic stress syndrome.*

postural changes-brain tumor syndrome. See *Bruns syndrome.*

postviral asthenia. See *chronic fatigue syndrome.*

postviral fatigue syndrome. See *chronic fatigue syndrome.*

postviral syndrome. See *chronic fatigue syndrome.*

potassium-losing nephritis. See *Conn syndrome.*

POTH, D. O. (American physician)

Poth keratosis. Self-healing multiple keratoses of the skin similar to squamous cell carcinoma, originally observed on the sunburned skin of fishermen in the Gulf of Mexico.

Poth, D. O. Tumor-like keratoses: Report of a case. *Arch. Derm., Chicago*, 1939, 39:228-38.

POTT, SIR PERCIVALL (British physician, 1714-1788)

Pott aneurysm. Synonym: *aneurysmal varix.*

Arteriovenous aneurysm in which blood flows from an artery directly into a a vein without going through a connecting sac, reportedly described by Pott.

Pott caries. See *Pott disease.*

Pott curvature. See *Pott disease.*

Pott disease. Synonyms: *David disease, Pott caries, Pott curvature, tuberculous spondylitis.*

Tuberculosis, usually beginning as osteomyelitis of one or more vertebrae, which involves the adjacent tissue and is frequently complicated by kyphosis (**Pott curvature**), paraplegia, and cold abscesses.

*Pott, P. *Remarks on that kind of palsy of the lower limbs which is frequently found to accompany a curvature of the spine and is supposed to be caused by it, together with its methods of cure.* London, Johnson, 1779. *David, J. P. *Dissertation sur les effets du mouvement et de repos dans les maladies chirurgicales.* Paris, 1779.

Pott fracture. Synonym: *Dupuytren fracture.*

Abduction fracture of the lower segment of the fibula and malleolus of the tibia with rupture of the internal lateral ligament of the ankle, caused by outward displacement of the leg while the foot is fixed.

*Pott, P. *Some few general remarks on fractures and dislocations.* London, Howes, 1769, pp. 57-64. *Dupuytren, G. Sur la fracture des l'extrémité inferieure du peroné, les luxations et les accidents qui en sont la suite. *Ann. Mém. Chir. Hôp., Paris*, 1819, I:1-212.

Pott gangrene. Synonym: *senile gangrene.*

Gangrene in the aged, usually of the extremities, caused by arterial occlusion.

*Pott, P. *Chirurgical observations relative to the cataract, the polypus of the nose, the cancer of the scrotum, the different kinds of ruptures, and the mortification of the toes and feet.* London, Howes, 1775.

Pott paralysis. See *Pott paraplegia.*

Pott paraplegia. Synonym: *Pott paralysis.*

Paraplegia due to spinal cord compression and abscesses in tuberculous spondylitis (Pott disease).

*Pott, P. *Remarks on that kind of palsy of the lower limbs which is frequently found to accompany a curvature of the spine and is supposed to be caused by it, together with its methods of cure.* London, Johnson, 1779.

Pott puffy tumor. Circumscribed edema of the scalp associated with osteomyelitis of the skull.

*Pott, P. *Observations on the nature of consequences of wounds and contusions of the head, fracturess of the skull, concussions of the brain.* London, Hitch & Lowes, 1760.

POTTER, EDITH LOUISE (American physician, born 1901)

Potter facies. See *under Potter syndrome (1).*

Potter syndrome (1). Synonyms: *bilateral renal agenesis (BRA) syndrome, dysplasia renofacialis, oligohydramnios tetrad, renofacial dysplasia, renofacial syndrome.*

A rare syndrome, transmitted as an autosomal recessive trait, characterized by facial abnormalities, renal agenesis (sometimes bilateral) or hypoplasia, and other defects. Facial features, known as the **Potter facies**, consist of flattened palpebral fissures, prominent epicanthus, flattened nasal bridge, mandibular micrognathia, and low-set malformed ears. Pulmonary hypoplasia, oligohydramnios, amnion nodosum, and skeletomuscular abnormalities (such as clubbing of the hands and feet and contractures), frequently occur. Males are more commonly affected than females. The affected infants are usually stillborn or die shortly after birth.

Potter, E. L. Facial characteristics of infants with bilateral renal agenesis. *Am. J. Obst. Gyn.*, 1946, 51:885-8.

Potter syndrome (2). Synonyms: *congenital polycystic disease, fetal polycystic disease, multicystic kidneys, polycystic kidney.*

A group of renal cystic diseases classified by Potter as follows: (1) **Infantile polycystic kidneys**, characterized by hyperplasia of the interstitial portions of the collecting tubules; (2) **multicystic kidney (multilocular cysts, aplastic kidneys)**, characterized by inhibition of the ampullary activity with a reduction in the number of generations of collecting ducts derived from the ureteral bud, the inadequately branched collecting ducts terminating with cysts, with diminution or absence of nephrons; (3) **adult type polycystic kidney (cysts in trisomy, cysts in tuberous sclerosis, medullary sponge kidney)**, characterized by multiple abnormalities of kidney development; and (4) **renal cysts in infants with posterior urethral valves** characterized by injury to ampullae from pressure due to urethral obstruction.

Potter, L. E. *Pathology of the fetus and the newborn.* Year Book, 1952, p. 336. Osathanondh, V., & Potter, E. L. Pathogenesis of polycystic kidneys. *Arch. Path.*, 1964, 77:459-65; 510-2. Elkin, M. Renal cystic disease-an overview. *Semin. Roentgen.*, 1975, 10:99-102.

POTTER, ROY PILLING (American radiologist, born 1879)

Doege-Potter syndrome. See *under Doege.*

potter's thumb. See *brachydactyly D.*

POURFOUR DU PETIT. See PETIT, FRANÇOIS POURFOUR, DU

POUTEAU, CLAUDE (French physician, 1725-1775)

Pouteau fracture. Fracture of the distal end of the radius, a variant of the Colles fracture.

*Poteau, C. *Oeuvres posthumes de M. Poteau.* Paris, Pierres, 1783, Vol. 2. p. 251.

POVYSILOVA, V. (Physician in Czechoslovakia)

Neu-Povysilová syndrome. See *Neu-Laxová syndrome.*

POZZI, SAMUEL JEAN, DE (French physician, 1846-1918)

Pozzi senile pseudorickets. See *Paget disease.*

PPCD (polymorphous posterior corneal dystrophy). See *Schlichting dystrophy.*

PPHP (pseudopseudohypoparathyroidism). See *Albright syndrome (1).*

PPS. See *popliteal pterygium syndrome.*

PPS. See *postpericardiotomy syndrome.*

PRADER, ANDREA (Swiss pediatrician, born 1919)

Fanconi-Prader syndrome. See *adrenoleukodystrophy.*

Prader-Labhart-Willi syndrome (PLW, PLWS). See *Prader-Willi syndrome.*

Prader-Labhart-Willi-Fanconi syndrome. See *Prader-Willi syndrome.*

Prader-Willi syndrome (PWS). Synonyms: *Prader-Labhart-Willi syndrome (PLW, PLWS), Prader-Labhart-Willi-Fanconi syndrome, cardiorespiratory syndrome of obesity in child, H_3O syndrome, hypogenital dystrophy with diabetic tendency syndrome, hypotonia-hypogonadism-obesity (HHHO) syndrome, hypotonia-obesity-hypogonadism-mental retardation syndrome.*

A childhood disease characterized at birth by the lack of spontaneous movements and protective reflexes, thus giving an appearance of severe brain damage. Sucking and swallowing reflexes are absent or decreased. Deficient thermoregulation, amyotonia, hypogonadism (hypoplasia of the scrotum and penis and cryptorchism) are generally associated. After a few weeks or months, the affected children become more responsive and more alert. Areflexia disappears gradually but hypotonia may persist longer. Feeding difficulty also disappears gradually. This phase is marked mainly by mental subnormality, delayed growth and motor development, speech defect, lack of emotional control, hyperphagia or bulimia leading to obesity, hypotonia, hyperlaxity, delayed bone maturation, dental

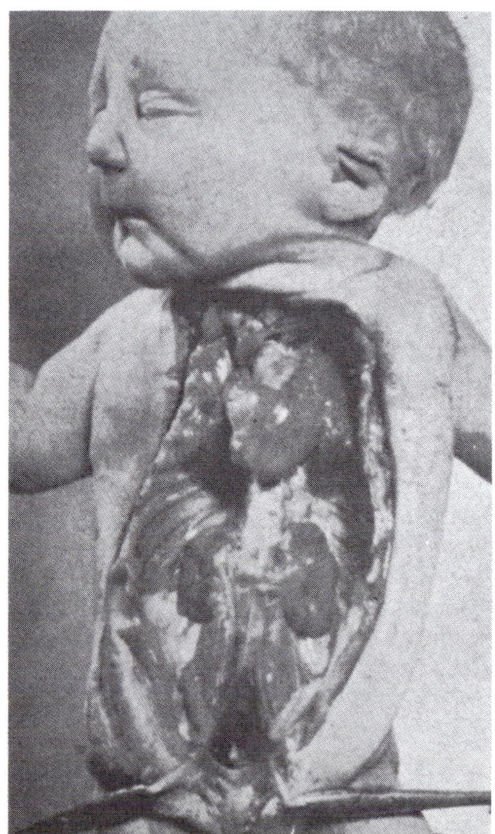

Potter syndrome (1)
Potter, E.L., *Am. J. Obst. & Gynec.* 51 887, 1946. St. Louis: C.V. Mosby Co.

caries, and dental enamel defect. Associated anomalies may include hypertelorism, epicanthus, strabismus, low-set ears, overlapping helix, high-arched palate, micrognathia, acromicria, clinodactyly, mesobrachyphalangy, syndactyly, and other disorders. There is a tendency to develop diabetes mellitus in some patients. Deletions of the long arm of chromosome 15 (15q11-q13) and unbalanced translocation occur in some cases, but most patients have a normal karyotype.

Prader, A. Labhart, A., & Willi, H. Ein Syndrom von Adipositas, Kleinwuchs, Kryptorchismus und Oligophrenie nach myatonieartigem Zustand im Neugeborenenalter. *Schweiz. Med. Wschr.*, 1956, 86:1260-1. *Prader, A., Labhart, A., Willi, H., & Fanconi, G. Ein Syndrom von Adipositas, Kleinwuchs, Kryptorchismus und Idiotie bei Kindern und Erwachsenen, Die als Neugeborene ein myatonieartiges Bild geboten haben. *VIII Internat. Cong. of Paediatrics*, Copenhagen, 1956.

PRAKKEN, JAN ROELOF (Dutch physician, born 1897)

Godfried-Prick-Carol-Prakken syndrome. See *under Godfried.*

PRASAD, ANANDA S. (Iranian physician)

Prasad syndrome. See *zinc deficiency syndrome.*

PRATESI, F. (Spanish physician)

Pratesi syndrome. Synonym: *femoral arteriovenous hyperostomia.*

Intermittent claudication of the lower extremities with cold feet, usually occurring in middle-aged males.

Monserrat, J. Un caso de hiperstomia arteriovenosa femoral. *Angiologia, Barcelona*, 1965, 17:32-4.

pre-aortic left renal vein compression syndrome. See *Magoss-Walshe syndrome.*

pre-Cushing syndrome. See *under Cushing.*

pre-excitation syndrome. A congenital disorder characterized by bypassing a part of the normal heart conduction system by an accessory pathway. Two mechanisms are suspected: (1) an early premature atrial depolarization which traverses the bypass tract and captures the ventricle during its vulnerable period, and (2) ultrarapid tachycardia as a result of atrial fibrillation and the antegrade conduction of the impulse down the anomalous pathway. The rapid ventricular rate may cause inadequate coronary flow with resulting myocardial ischemia. Paroxysmal atrial tachycardia (AV junctional tachycardia) and atrial fibrillation associated with a rapid ventricular response, sometimes resulting in ventricular fibrillation, are the complications. Syndromes of Wolff-Parkinson-White and Lown-Ganong-Levine are the principal forms of the pre-excitation syndrome.

Lown, B. Preexcitation syndromes (Wolff-Parkinson-White and Lown-Ganong-Levine). In: Braunwald, E., ed. *Heart disease. A textbook of cardiovascular medicine.* Philadelphia, Saunders, 1980, p. 788.

pre-Gardner syndrome. See *under Gardner, Eldon John.*

pre-Kaposi sarcoma. See *under Kaposi-Kohn, Moritz.*

pre-Sézary syndrome. See *under Sézary.*

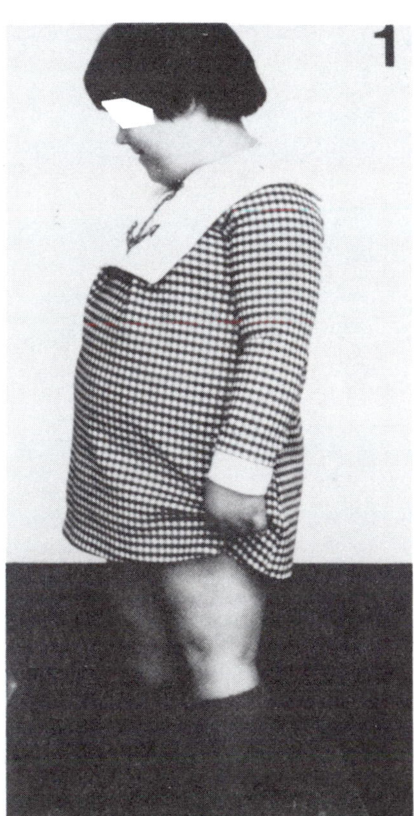

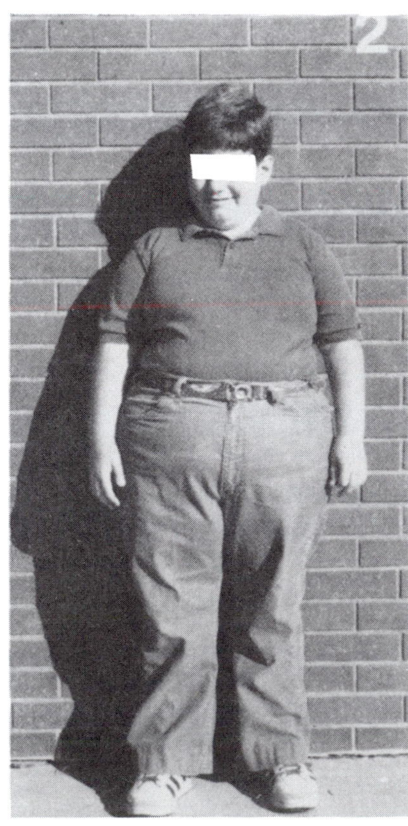

Prader-Willi syndrome
Meyerson, M.D.: The Effect of Syndrome Diagnosis on Speech Remediation. In Shprintzen,R.J., & N.W. Paul(eds): *Diagnostic Accuracy: Effect on Treatment Planning.* New York: Alan R. Liss, Inc. for the March of Dimes Birth Defects Foundation BD:OAS 21(2):47-68, 1985, with permission.

precalyceal tubular ectasia. See *Cacchi-Ricci syndrome.*

precancerous dermatosis. See *Bowen disease, under Bowen, John Templeton.*

precancerous melanosis. See *Hutchinson freckle, under Hutchinson, Sir Jonathan.*

precordial catch syndrome. An anterior chest wall disease occurring usually in apparently healthy young adults and characterized by brief, sharp, severe precordial pain of short duration, taking place at rest, during mild activity, or with bending or slouching. Shallow breathing eases the pain and forced inspiration or asumming a proper posture relieves it.

Sparrow, M. J., & Bird, E. L. "Precordial catch": A benign syndrome of chest pain in young persons. *N. Z. Med. J.*, 1978, 88:325-6.

PREISER, GEORG KARL FELIX (German physician, 1879-1913)

Preiser disease. Progresive necrosis of the scaphoid bone after spraining of the wrist, presumably caused by a vascular disorder.

Preiser, G. Zur Frage der typischen traumatischen Ernährungstörungen der kurzen Hand- und Fusswerzelknochen. *Fortschr. Geb. Röntgen.*, 1911, 17:360-2.

preleukemia. See *myelodysplastic syndrome.*

preleukemic syndrome. See *myelodysplastic syndrome.*

premalignant fibroepithelioma. See *Pinkus epithelioma, under Pinkus, Hermann Karl Benno.*

premature aging syndrome. See *Hutchinson-Gilford syndrome, under Hutchinson, Sir Jonathan.*

premature senility syndrome. See *Hutchinson-Gilford syndrome, under Hutchinson, Sir Jonathan.*

premenstrual syndrome (PMS). Synonyms: *periluteal phase dysphoric disorder, premenstrual phase dysphoric syndrome, premenstrual tension (PMT), premenstrual tension syndrome.*

A cyclic disorder occurring between the last week of the luteal phase and the beginning of the follicular phase of the menstrual cycle, or about one week before and one day after the onset of menstruation. The symptoms are variable, ranging from a mild, almost imperceptible, feeling of discomfort to severe, sometimes incapacitating, physical and emotional disorders. Physical symptoms may include headache, breast swelling (see also *Racine syndrome*) and tenderness, abdominal bloating, weight gain, nausea, vomiting, constipation or diarrhea, increased thirst and appetite, craving for sweet or salty foods, visual disorders, low back pain, pain in the legs, genital pruritus, asthmatic attacks, acneiform eruption, periocular pigmentation, rhinorrhea, epistaxis, vertigo, conjunctivitis, uveitis, hoarseness, sore throat, cystitis, urethritis, and other disorders. Emotional and behavioral changes may include affective lability (sadness, irritability, anger, bouts of crying), anxiety, tension, depression, feeling of hopelessness, decreased interest in work, hobbies, and friends, fatigability, difficulty in concentrating, and hypersomnia or insomnia.

Frank, F. T. Hormonal causes of premenstrual tension. *Arch. Neur. Psychiat.*, 1931, 26:1053-7. *Diagnostic and statistical manual of mental disorders.* 3rd ed. Washington, D. C., American Psychiatric Association, 1987, pp. 367-9.

premenstrual phase dysphoric syndrome. See *premenstrual syndrome.*

premenstrual salivary syndrome. See *Racine syndrome.*

premenstrual tension (PMT). See *premenstrual syndrome.*

premenstrual tension syndrome. See *premenstrual syndrome.*

premolar aplasia-hyperhidrosis-canities syndrome. See *Böök syndrome.*

prenatal dystrophy syndrome. See *Ballantyne-Runge syndrome.*

prepuberal panhypopituitarism. See *Lorain-Levi syndrome.*

prepulseless arteritis. See *aortic arch syndrome.*

preretinal edema. See *Masuda-Kitahara disease.*

presacral cyst. See *Middeldorpf tumor.*

presacral dermoid. See *Middeldorpf tumor.*

presbyophrenia. See *Wernicke dementia.*

presenile cerebellar ataxic syndrome. See *olivopontocerebellar atrophy.*

presenile dementia. See *Alzheimer disease, and see Binswager disease.*

presenile dementia-cortical blindness syndrome. See *Heidenhain syndrome.*

presenile gangrene. See *Buerger syndrome.*

presenile spongy encephalopathy. See *Nevin syndrome (1).*

PRICK, JOSEPH JULES GUILLAUME (Dutch physician, born 1909)

Godfried-Prick-Carol-Prakken syndrome. See *under Godfried.*

PRIEST, W. M. (British physician)

Priest-Alexander syndrome. See *Verner-Morrison syndrome.*

PRIEUR, MAURICE (French physician, born 1885)

Prieur-Trénel syndrome. An association of the Sabouraud syndrome (monilethrix) and cataract.

Prieur, M., & Trénel, M. Monilethrix et cataracte précoce. *Bull. Soc. Opht., Paris*, 1930, 42:794-9.

primary acrodystrophic neuropathy. See *Thévenard sydrome.*

primary aldosteronism. See *Conn syndrome.*

primary alveolar hypoventilation syndrome. See *Ondine curse.*

primary anemia. See *Addison-Biemer anemia.*

primary autonomic insufficiency. See *Bradbury-Eggleston syndrome.*

primary biliary cirrhosis (PBC) syndrome. Synonym: *chronic nonsuppurative destructive cholangitis (CNDC).*

A chronic progressive liver disease manifested by a disturbance in bile secretion and by segmental inflammatory destruction of intrahepatic bile ducts, resulting in a progressive loss of these bile ducts associated with periportal hepatitis and, eventually, liver cirrhosis.

Rubin, E., *et al.* Localization of the basic injury in primary abiliary cirrhosis. *JAMA*, 1963, 183:331-4. Ludwig, J., *et al.* Staging of chronic nonsuppurative destructive cholangitis (syndrome of primary biliary cirrhosis). *Virchows Arch. A Path. Anat. Histol.*, 1978, 379:103-12.

primary central hypoventilation syndrome. See *Ondine curse.*

primary chronic progressive ophthalmoplegia. See *Graefe syndrome.*

primary degeneration of the corpus callosum. See *Marchiafava-Bignami syndrome.*

primary elastolysis. See *cutis laxa syndrome.*

primary erythroblastic anemia. See *Cooley anemia.*

primary familial xanthomatosis. See *Wolman syndrome.*
primary fibromyalgia syndrome (PFS). See *fibrositis-fibromyalgia syndrome.*
primary hyperaldosteronism. See *Conn syndrome.*
primary hypersplenic pancytopenia. See *Dacie syndrome.*
primary hypersplenism. See *Dacie syndrome.*
primary hypertrophic osteoarthropathy. See *pachydermoperiostosis syndrome.*
primary hypertrophic osteoarthropathy. See *Marie-Bamberger syndrome, under Marie, Pierre.*
primary hyperuricemia syndrome. See *Lesch-Nyhan syndrome.*
primary hypoglycemic mesenchymal tumor. See *Doege-Potter syndrome.*
primary idiopathic nontraumatic necrosis of femoral head. See *Chandler syndrome, under Chandler, Fremont Augustus.*
primary indurative cavernositis of the penis. See *Peyronie disease.*
primary infantile atrophy. See *marasmus syndrome.*
primary macroglobulinemia. See *Waldenström macroglobulinemia, under Waldenström, Jan Gösta.*
primary microorchidism. See *chromosome XXY syndrome.*
primary ovarian insufficiency. See *chromosome XO syndrome.*
primary periodontitis. See *Fauchard disease.*
primary postictal automatism. See *Kandinskii-Clérambault syndrome.*
primary red cell aplasia. See *Diamond-Blackfan syndrome.*
primary splenic neutropenia. See *Wiseman-Doan syndrome.*
primary splenic neutropenia with arthritis syndrome. See *Felty syndrome.*
primary splenic thrombocytopenia. See *Werlhof disease.*
primary thrombocytopenia. See *Werlhof disease.*
primary thrombocytopenic purpura. See *Werlhof disease.*
primary thrombosis of the upper extremity. See *Paget-Schroetter syndrome.*
primary transtentorial cerebellar displacement syndrome. Synonym: *inverse Chiari type 2 syndrome.*

Upward displacement of the lobuli quadrangulares and upper brain stem into the supratentorial space through an enlarged tentorial notch. The tentorium cerebelli is hypoplastic and shows a low insertion, thus causing narrowing of the infratentorial space. The displaced structures are impressed between the mediobasal parts of the forebrain, leaving a bowl-shaped excavation after removal of the brain stem and the cerebellum. The basal cisternae may be obstructed by reactively augmented connective tissue, probably causing a further deterioration of spinal fluid circulation, thereby exaggerating the hydrocephalus.

Schmitt, H. P. Syndrome of primary transtentorial cerebellar displacement-"inverse Chiari type II syndrome." *Neuropaediatrie*, 1978, 9:268-76.

primary vitamin-D-resistant rickets. See *hypophosphatemic familial rickets.*
PRINGLE, JOHN JAMES (British physician, 1855-1922)
Bourneville-Pringle syndrome. See *under Bourneville.*
Pringle disease. See *Bourneville-Pringle syndrome.*
PRINZMETAL, MYRON (American physician, born 1908)
Prinzmetal angina. Synonyms: *Prinzmetal syndrome, Prinzmetal variant angina, Prinzmetal-Massumi syndrome, anterior chest wall syndrome, anterior thoracic wall syndrome.*

A variant of angina pectoris (see *Heberden asthma*) due to coronary artery spasm, characterized by chest pain at rest in association with S-T segment deviation. The condition occurs without preceding changes in heart rate and blood pressure. Most patients have underlying coronary artery disease, but some have normal arteries. A prolonged bout of coronary arterial spasm may lead to ventricular arrhythmia, myocardial infarction, heart block, and sudden death. See also *chest wall syndrome.*

Prinzmetal, M., & Massumi, R. A. The anterior chest wall syndrome-chest pain resembling pain of cardiac origin. *JAMA*, 1955, 159:177-84.

Prinzmetal syndrome. See *Prinzmetal angina.*
Prinzmetal variant angina. See *Prinzmetal angina.*
Prinzmetal-Massumi syndrome. See *Prinzmetal angina.*
privet cough. See *Engel syndrome.*
proaccelerin deficiency. See *Owren syndrome (2).*
proctalgia fugax. See *levator syndrome, and see Thaysen syndrome.*
proctodynia. See *levator syndrome.*
professional patient. See *Munchausen syndrome.*
professional stress syndrome. See *burnout syndrome.*
PROFICHET, GEORGES CHARLES (French physician, born 1873)
Profichet disease. Synonym: *calcinosis circumscripta.*

The gradual development of subcutaneous, stonelike, calcareous nodules about the large joints, sometimes involving the tendons and lungs. Complications may include ulceration, atrophy, pain, stiffness, and movement disorders.

*Profichet, G. C. *Sur une variété de concrétion phosphatiques suscutanée (pierre de la peau).* Paris, 1890.

progeria adultorum. See *Werner syndrome, under Werner, Otto.*
progeria-like syndrome. See *Cockayne syndrome.*
progeria syndrome. See *Hutchinson-Gilford syndrome, under Hutchinson, Sir Jonathan.*
progeroid nanism. See *Cockayne syndrome.*
progressive alcoholic dementia. See *Marchiafava-Bignami syndrome.*
progressive ascending spinal paralysis. See *Mills disease.*
progressive bulbar paralysis. See *Duchenne paralysis.*
progressive cardiomyopathic lentiginosis. See *LEOPARD syndrome.*
progressive cerebral degeneration in infancy. See *Alpers syndrome.*
progressive chorea. See *Huntington chorea.*
progressive chronic interstitial pulmonary fibrosis. See *Hamman-Rich syndrome.*
progressive dialysis encephalopathy (PDE). See *dialysis encephalopathy syndrome.*
progressive diaphyseal dysplasia. See *Camurati-Engelmann syndrome.*
progressive dystonia with diurnal fluctuations. See *Segawa syndrome.*
progressive facial hemiatrophy. See *Romberg syndrome (2).*

progressive fibrosing myositis. See *Meyenburg disease.*
progressive hemifacial atrophy. See *Romberg syndrome (2).*
progressive hereditary nephritis. See *Alport syndrome.*
progressive hypertrophic interstitial neuritis. See *Déjerine-Sottas syndrome.*
progressive hypertrophic neuritis. See *Roussy-Cornil syndrome.*
progressive idiopathic atrophoderma. See *Pasini-Pierini syndrome.*
progressive infantile poliodystrophy. See *Alpers syndrome.*
progressive intrahepatic cholestasis. See *Byler disease.*
progressive lenticular degeneration. See *Wilson disease, under Wilson, Samuel Alexander Kinnier.*
progressive lethal granulomatous ulceration of the nose. See *Stewart syndrome, under Stewart, J. P.*
progressive lipodystropohy. See *Barraquer-Simons syndrome.*
progressive melanosis of the dermis. See *Ota nevus.*
progressive muscle tautness syndrome. See *stiff man syndrome.*
progressive muscular atrophy. See *amyotrophic lateral sclerosis.*
progressive muscular dystrophy with fibrillary twitching. See *Wohlfart-Kugelberg-Welander syndrome.*
progressive muscular dystrophy, Duchenne type. See *Duchenne muscular dystrophy.*
progressive myelopathic muscular atrophy. See *Wohlfart-Kugelberg-Welander syndrome.*
progressive myoclonus epilepsy with Lafora bodies. See *Lafora disease.*
progressive normotensive hydrocephalus in adults. See *Hakim syndrome.*
progressive pallidal degeneration syndrome. See *Hallervorden-Spatz syndrome.*
progressive paralysis. See *Bayle disease.*
progressive partial lipodystrophy. See *Barraquer-Simons syndrome.*
progressive pernicious anemia. See *Runeberg anemia.*
progressive pigmentary dermatosis. See *Schamberg disease.*
progressive pigmentary disease. See *Schamberg disease.*
progressive poliodystrophy. See *Alpers syndrome.*
progressive pulmonary dystrophy. See *Burke syndrome.*
progressive pyramidopallidal degeneration. See *Lhermitte-Cornil-Quesnel syndrome.*
progressive recurrent dermatofibroma. See *Darier-Ferrand dermatofibrosarcoma.*
progressive respiratory distress. See *adult respiratory distress syndrome.*
progressive spinal muscular atrophy. See *Werdnig-Hoffmann syndrome* and *Wohlfart-Kugelberg-Welander syndrome.*
progressive spinal muscular atrophy of infants. See *Werdnig-Hoffman syndrome.*
progressive spleno-adenomegalic polyarthritis. See *Still syndrome.*
progressive subcortical arteriosclerotic encephalopathy. See *Binswager disease.*
progressive subcortical encephalitis. See *Binswager disease.*
progressive subcortical encephalitis. See *Binswager disease.*
progressive supranuclear ophthalmoplegia. See *Steele-Richardson-Olszewski syndrome.*
progressive supranuclear palsy. See *Steele-Richardson-Olszewski syndrome.*
progressive tardive muscular dystrophy. See *Becker muscular dystrophy.*
progressive torsion spasm. See *Ziehen-Oppenheim syndrome.*
prolapsing mitral leaflet (PML) syndrome. See *mitral valve prolapse syndrome.*
prolonged gestation syndrome. See *Ballantyne-Runge syndrome.*
prolonged QT interval syndrome. See *long QT syndrome.*
pronator syndrome. See *Seyffarth syndrome.*
pronator teres syndrome. See *Seyffarth syndrome.*
propionic acidemia. See *ketotic hyperglycinemia syndrome.*
prosopagnosia. See *bald soprano syndrome.*
prosopalgia. See *trigeminal neuralgia.*
proteiform syndrome. See *Proteus syndrome.*
protein-calories malnutrition (PCM). See *kwashiorkor-marasmus syndrome.*
protein-energy malnutrition (PEM). See *kwashiorkor-marasmus syndrome.*
protein-losing enteropathy. See *protein-losing gastroenteropathy.*
protein-losing gastroenteropathy. Synonyms: *Gordon disease, essential hypoproteinemia, exudative enteropathy, hypermetabolic hypoproteinemia, idiopathic hypoproteinemia, protein-losing enteropathy, protein-losing syndrome.*

A group of disorders having in common hypoproteinemia due to leakage and intestinal malabsorption of proteins, mainly albumin, associated with diseases of the gastrointestinal mucosa, lymphatic obstruction, and food sensitivity. Ménétrier disease is one of the causes, resulting in the gastric loss of proteins, and intestinal lymphangiectasis produces leakage of proteins in the small intestine. See also *malabsorption syndrome* and *Ménétrier syndrome.*

Gordon, R. S., Jr. Exudative enteropathy. Abnormal permeability of the gastrointestinal tract demonstrable with labeled polyvinylphrrolidone. *Lancet,* 1959, 1:325-6.

protein-losing syndrome. See *protein-losing gastroenteropathy.*
protein malnutrition. See *kwashiorkor.*
proteinosis lipoidea. See *Urbach-Wiethe syndrome.*
PROTEUS (Greek sea god known for his ability to assume different forms)
Proteus syndrome (PS). Synonyms: *Wiedemann syndrome, proteiform syndrome.*

A congenital syndrome, transmitted as an autosomal dominant trait, characterized by a wide spectrum of abnormalities, including usually symmetrical partial gigantism of the hands and/or feet with digital overgrowth and thickening of the palms and soles, pigmented nevi with variable intensity and distribution, hemihypertrophy of various parts (face, ear, shoulder girdle, thorax, arms, or the entire side of the body), subcutaneous hamartomas, skull anomalies (macrocephaly, exostoses, asymmetry, and parieto-occipital protuberances), accelerated growth during early years, and cystiform pulmonary abnormalities.

Associated abnormalities may include macroorchidism, failure of breast development, and goiter.

Wiedemann, H. R., *et al.* The Proteus syndrome. Partial gigantism the the hands and/or feet, nevi, hemihypertrophy, subcutaneous tumors, macrocephaly or other skull anomalies and possible accelerated growth and visceral affections. *Eur. J. Pediat.*, 1983, 140:5-12.

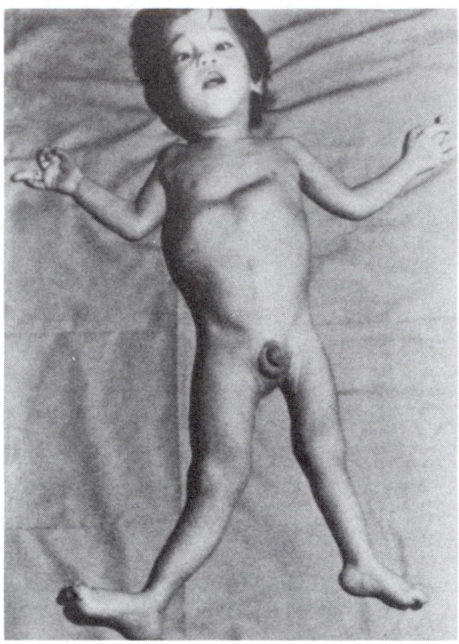

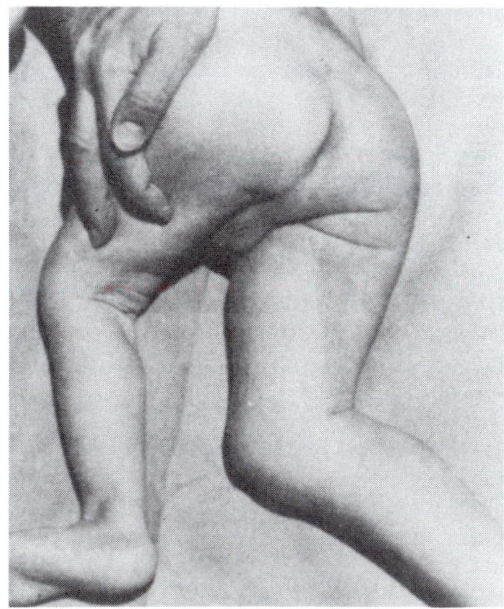

Proteus syndrome
Malamitsi-Puchner, Ariadne, Sophia Kitsiou, & Christos S. Bartsocas, *American Journal of Medical Genetics* 27:119-125, 1987. New York: Alan R. Liss, Inc.

protozoan cell disease. See *Wyatt disease, under Wyatt, John Poyner.*

protracted QT. See *long QT syndrome.*

PROWER

Prower defect. See *Stuart-Prower factor deficiency, under Stuart.*

Prower factor deficiency. See *Stuart-Prower factor deficiency, under Stuart.*

Stuart-Prower factor deficiency. See *under Stuart.*

proximal diabetic neuropathy. See *Bruns-Garland syndrome.*

proximal focal femoral deficiency (PFFD). See *femur-fibula-ulna syndrome.*

proximal spinal muscular atrophy. See *Wohlfart-Kugelberg-Welander syndrome.*

proximal symphalangism syndrome. See *symphalangism syndrome.*

PRS (Pierre Robin syndrome). See *Robin syndrome.*

prune belly syndrome (PBS). Synonyms: *Eagle-Barrett syndrome, Fröhlich syndrome, Obrinsky syndrome, abdominal muscle deficiency anomalad, abdominal muscle deficiency syndrome, abdominal musculature aplasia syndrome, abdominal wall aplasia syndrome, absence of abdominal muscle syndrome, aplastic abdominal muscle syndrome, defective abdominal wall syndrome.*

A syndrome of hypoplasia or aplasia of the abdominal muscle, presenting a thin, loose, wrinkled, and shriveled (prunelike) abdominal wall; persistent furrowlike umbilicus; urinary tract dysplasia; cryptorchism; and other anomalies, including malrotation of the bowel, pigeon breast, hip dislocation, polydactyly, and heart defects. The etiology is unknown.

Obrinsky, W. Agenesis of abdominal muscle with associated malformations of the genitourinary tract. A clinical syndrome. *Am. J. Dis. Child.*, 1949, 77:362-73. *Fröhlich, F. *Der Mangel der Muskeln, Insbesondere der Seitenbauchmuskeln*. Würzburg, 1839. (Thesis). Eagle, J. F., Jr., *et al.* Congenital deficiency of abdominal musculature with associated genito-urinary abnormalities. A syndrome. *Pediatrics*. 1950, 6:721.

prurigo agria. See *Hebra syndrome.*

prurigo-asthma syndrome. See *Besnier prurigo.*

prurigo eczematodes allergicum. See *Besnier prurigo.*

prurigo estivalis. See *Hutchinson prurigo, under Hutchinson, Sir Jonathan.*

prurigo ferox. See *Hebra syndrome.*

prurigo gravis. See *Hebra syndrome.*

prurigo hebrae. See *Hebra syndrome.*

prurigo mitis. See *Hebra syndrome.*

prurigo nodularis. See *Hyde syndrome.*

pruritus hiemalis. See *Duhring pruritus.*

pruritus with lichenification. See *Brocq disease (1).*

PS. See ***p**acemaker **s**yndrome, and see **P**roteus **s**yndrome.*

Ps-ZES. See *pseudo-Zollinger-Ellison syndrome, under Zollinger.*

PSAUME, JEAN (French dentist)

Gorlin-Psaume syndrome. See *orofaciodigital syndrome I.*

Papillon-Léage and Psaume syndrome. See *orofaciodigital syndrome I.*

pseudo-acanthosis nigricans. See *Gougerot-Carteaud syndrome, under Gougerot, Henri.*

pseudo-achondroplasia. See *pseudo-achondroplastic spondyloepiphyseal dysplasia.*

pseudo-achondroplastic spondyloepiphyseal dysplasia. Synonyms: *pseudo-achondroplasia, pseudo-achondroplastic spondyloepiphyseal dysplasia syndrome.*

An inherited skeletal dysplasia in which dwarfism is a major feature. The syndrome is usually recognized in early childhood, abnormal gait and knee joint deformity being the first noticeable symptoms. Major features of this syndrome include disproportionately long trunk with lumbar lordosis and moderate scoliosis, hypermobility of all joints except the elbows, limitation of extension of the elbow joints and genu varum or genu valgum. The facies, intelligence, and life expectancy are normal. Radiographic characteristics include shortness of hands and feet, shortness of the tubular bones typical of micromelia, irregular metaphyses and epiphyses, faulty ossification of the vertebrae, biconvex vertebral bodies, and spatulate ribs. The syndrome is classified as **Type I (Kozlowski type)**, transmitted as an autosomal dominant trait; **Type II (Kozlowski type)**, transmitted as an autosomal recessive trait; **Type III (Maroteaux-Lamy type)**, transmitted as an autosomal dominant trait; and **Type IV (Maroteaux-Lamy type)**, transmitted as autosomal recessive trait.

Maroteaux, P., & Lamy, M. Les formes pseudo-achondroplasiques des dysplasies spondylo-epiphysaires. *Presse Méd.*, 1959, 67:383-6. Ford, N., Silverman, F. N., & Kozlowski, K. Spondylo-epiphyseal dysplasia (pseudoachondroplastic type). *Am. J. Roentgen.*, 1961, 86:462-72.

pseudo-achondroplastic spondyloepiphyseal dysplasia syndrome. See *pseudo-achondroplastic spondyloepiphyseal dysplasia.*

pseudo-achondroplastic spondyloepiphyseal dysplasia, Kozlowski type. See *under pseudo-achondroplastic spondyloepiphyseal dysplasia.*

pseudo-achondroplastic spondyloepiphyseal dysplasia,Maroteaux-Lamy type. See *under pseudo-achondroplastic spondyloepiphyseal dysplasia.*

pseudo-acromegalic syndrome. See *pachydermoperiostosis syndrome.*

pseudo-acromegaly. See *Brugsch syndrome.*

pseudo-actinomycosis. See *Ballingall disease.*

pseudo-Addison syndrome. See *renal salt losing syndrome.*

pseudo-Argyll Robertson syndrome. See *Adie disease.*

pseudo-Bartter syndrome. See *factitious Bartter syndrome, under Bartter.*

pseudo-Biermer anemia. See *Gerbasi anemia.*

pseudo-Chédiak-Higashi syndrome (1). See *under Chédiak.*

pseudo-Chédiak-Higashi syndrome (2). See *Griscelli syndrome.*

pseudo-Cushing syndrome. See *alcohol-induced pseudo-Cushing syndrome.*

pseudo-Hakim-Adams syndrome. See *under Hakim.*

pseudo-Hurler polydystrophy. See *mucolipidosis III.*

pseudo-Hurler syndrome. See *gangliosidosis G_{M1} type I.*

pseudo-infectious anemia of infants. See *Gerbasi anemia.*

pseudo-Kaposi angiodermatitis. See *Bluefarb-Stewart syndrome.*

pseudo-Kaposi stasis dermatitis. See *Bluefarb-Stewart syndrome.*

pseudo-Mangelrachitis. See *pseudo-vitamin D-deficiency rickets syndrome.*

pseudo-obstructed bladder. See *Hinman syndrome.*

pseudo-obstruction of the colon. See *Ogilvie syndrome.*

pseudo-ophthalmoplegia syndrome. See *Rot-Bielschowsky syndrome.*

pseudo-Sjögren syndrome. See *sicca-like syndrome.*

pseudo-Tay-Sachs syndrome. See *Sandhoff syndrome.*

pseudo-Ullrich-Turner syndrome. See *Noonan syndrome.*

pseudo-vitamin D-deficiency rickets syndrome. Synonyms: *pseudo-Mangelrachitis, vitamin D-dependent rickets.*

Rickets responding to large but not small doses of vitamin D. Growth deficiency, muscle hypotonia, tetany, fractures, large fontanels, tooth enamel hypoplasia, and metabolic changes (such as hypocalcemia, elevated serum alkaline phosphatase, mild hypophosphatemia, aminoaciduria, and mild renal tubular acidosis)are associated. The syndrome is transmitted as an autosomal recessive trait, but there is a possibility of autosomal dominant inheritance in some families.

Dent, C. E., *et al.* Hereditary pseudo-vitamin D deficiency rickets ("pseudo-Mangelrachitis"). *J. Bone Joint Surg.*, 1968, 50B:708-19. Prader, A., *et al.* Eine besondere Form der primären Vitamin-D-resisten Rachitis mit Hypocalcämie und autosomal-dominant Erbgang: die hereditäre pseudo-Mangel-Rachitis. *Helvet. Paediat. Acta.*, 1961, 16:452-68.

pseudo-Volkmann syndrome. See *under Volkmann.*

pseudo-Zollinger-Ellison syndrome (Ps-ZES). See *under Zollinger.*

pseudobattered child syndrome. Synonym: *cao gio.*

Multiple ecchymoses produced by abrasive rubbing of a coin over the skin in an attempt to free the body of "bad winds" which, according to Vietnamese folk medicine, are responsible for various physical ailments, including fever, headache, and convulsions. See also *battered child syndrome.*

Primosch, R. E., & Young, S. K. Pseudobattering of Vietnamese children (cao gio). *JADA*, 1980, 101:47-8.

pseudobulbar palsy. See *amyotrophic lateral sclerosis.*

pseudocholera infantum. See *Sakamoto disease.*

pseudocolloid of the lips. See *Fordyce disease.*

pseudocoxalgia. See *Calvé-Legg-Perthes syndrome.*

pseudodementia syndrome. See *Ganser syndrome.*

pseudodiastrophic dwarfism, Burgio type. See *Burgio pseudodiastrophic dwarfism syndrome.*

pseudodiastrophic dysplasia, Burgio type. See *Burgio pseudodiastrophic dwarfism syndrome.*

pseudodiphtheria. See *Epstein syndrome, under Epstein, Alois.*

pseudoencephalitis acuta hemorrhagica superior. See *Wernicke syndrome.*

pseudoencephalitis hemorrhagica superior. See *Wernicke syndrome.*

pseudoglioma congenita. See *Norrie syndrome.*

pseudogonitis. See *Gram syndrome.*

pseudogout syndrome. Synonyms: *articular chondrocalcinosis, calcium gout, calcium pyrophosphate dihydrate deposition (CPPD) syndrome, chondrocalcinosis articularis hereditaria, chondrocalcinosis idiopathica, chondrocalciosynovitis syndrome, crystal synovitis, pseudogout-chondrocalcinosis syndrome.*

A goutlike disease marked by recurrent attacks of pain with soft tissue swelling and joint effusion due to precipitation of calcium pyrophosphate crystals in the synovial fluid and membranes, as well as fibrocartilage and hyaline cartilage of the articular surface. Elbows, wrists, metacarpophalangeal joints, ankles, and knees are most commonly affected. In some cases, the hips, shoulders, and symphysis pubis are also involved. The condition has been reported in cases of chronic renal failure. Radiological findings include subchondral rarefaction, chondrocalcinosis, and calcification of the tendon, bursal, and para-articular structures.

McCarty, D. J., Jr., *et al.* The significance of calcium phosphate crystals in the synovial fluid of arthritic patients. The "pseudogout syndrome." *Ann. Intern. Med.*, 1962, 56:211-45.

pseudogout-chondrocalcinosis syndrome. See *pseudogout syndrome.*

pseudohemophilia. See *Willebrand-Jürgens syndrome.*

pseudohermaphroditism-glomerulopathy-Wilms tumor syndrome. See *Drash syndrome.*

pseudohypertrophic muscular dystrophy. See *Duchenne muscular dystrophy.*

pseudohypertrophic progressive muscular dystrophy, Duchenne type. See *Duchenne muscular dystrophy.*

pseudohypoglycemia syndrome. See *Yager-Young syndrome.*

pseudohypoparathyroidism (PHP, PHPT). See *Albright syndrome (1).*

pseudohypoparathyroidism syndrome. See *Albright syndrome (1).*

pseudoichthyose acuise en taches circulaires. See *Toyama disease.*

pseudoileus. See *Alvarez syndrome.*

pseudoinflammatory fundus dystrophy. See *Sorsby disease.*

pseudoleprechaunism. See *Patterson syndrome.*

pseudoleukemia infantum. See *Jaksch syndrome.*

pseudomeningitis. See *Dupré syndrome.*

pseudomuscular hypertrophic lipomatosis. See *Marañón lipomatosis.*

pseudomyopathic spinal muscular atrophy. See *Wohlfart-Kugelberg-Welander syndrome.*

pseudoneurogenic bladder. See *Hinman syndrome.*

pseudonuchal infantilism. See *chromosome XO syndrome.*

pseudoparalysis of lateral or superior rectus muscles. See *Johnson syndrome, under Johnson, Lorand Victor.*

pseudopolycythemia. See *Gaisböck disease.*

pseudopolydystrophy. See *mucolipidosis III.*

pseudopseudohypoparathyroidism (PPHP). See *Albright syndrome (1).*

pseudorheumatoid arthritis. See *carpotarsal osteolysis syndrome (recessive form).*

pseudorubella. See *Zahorsky syndrome (1).*

pseudosepsis allergica. See *Wissler syndrome.*

pseudosepsis allergica erythemato-arthralgica recidivans. See *Wissler syndrome.*

pseudosepsis allergogenes. See *Wissler syndrome.*

pseudosepticemia syndrome. See *Wissler syndrome.*

pseudosexual precocity. See *congenital adrenal hyperplasia.*

pseudotabes. See *Adie syndrome.*

pseudotabes pupillotonica. See *Adie syndrome.*

pseudothalidomide syndrome. Synonyms: *hypomelia-hypotrichosis-facial hemangioma syndrome, SC syndrome, SC phocomelia syndrome.*

A syndrome resembling thalidomide embryopathy (see *Wiedemann syndrome I*). It is characterized by symmetric reduction deformity of the limbs (upper extremities being more severely affected than the lower ones), flexion contractures of the joints, scanty silvery-blond hair, hypoplastic cartilage of the nose and ears, micrognathia, corneal opacity, blue sclera, growth retardation, and capillary hemangioma of the face, forehead, and ears. Microbrachycephalic skull with wormian bones in the occipital region and mental retardation may be associated. Hand abnormalities include absence of the thumb, shortening of the first metacarpal bone, hypoplasia of the fifth digit, fusion of the fourth and fifth metacarpals, clinodactyly of the second and fifth digits, and hypoplasia of the middle phlanges. The syndrome is believed to be transmitted as an autosomal recessive trait. "S" and "C" are the first letters of surnames of the two patients in whom the syndrome was first reported, hence the synonyms *SC syndrome* and *SC phocomelia syndrome.* Some authors consider this syndrome a variant of the Roberts syndrome.

Hermann, J., *et al.* A familial dysmorphogenetic syndrome of limb deformities, characteristic facial appearance and associated anomalies: The "pseudothalidomide" or "SC-syndrome." *Birth Defects*, 1969, 5(3):81-9.

pseudotoxoplasmosis. See *Sabin-Feldman syndrome.*

pseudotrichinosis. See *Wagner-Unverricht syndrome, under Wagner, Ernst Leberecht.*

pseudotuberculoma silicoticum. See *Shattock disease.*

pseudotuberculosis of lungs with eosinophilia syndrome. See *tropical eosinophilia syndrome.*

pseudotuberculous thyroiditis. See *de Quervain disease (2), under Quervain, Fritz, de.*

pseudotumor cerebri (PTC) syndrome. Synonyms: *Quincke meningitis, Symonds syndrome, benign intracranial hypertension, meningeal hydrops, otitic hydrocephalus, otogenic hydrocephalus, serous meningitis, toxic hydrocephalus.*

A neurological disorder marked by intracranial hypertension associated with papilledema, headache, and paralysis of the sixth cranial nerve. Vomiting, giddiness, blurring of vision, diplopia, and transient convulsions are the principal symptoms. It occurs most commonly in adult women and is believed to be caused by faulty production and absorption of the cerebrospinal fluid, dural sinus thrombosis, inflammatory diseases, endocrine disorders, trauma, immune reactions, and toxicity. The designation "hydrocephalus" appears to be a misnomer.

Quincke, H. Die Lumbopunction des Hydrocephalus. *Berlin. Klin. Wschr.*, 1891, 28:929-38. Symonds, C. P. Otitic hydrocephalus. *Brain*, 1931, 54:55-71.

pseudotumor of the penis. See *Buschke-Loewenstein tumor.*

pseudoxanthoma elasticum (PXE). Synonyms: *Darier-Grönblad-Strandberg syndrome, Grönblad-Strandberg syndrome, Grönblad-Strandberg-Touraine syndrome, angioid streaks-pseudoxanthoma elasticum syndrome, elastica disease, elastorrhexis generalisata, elastosis dystrophica, systemic elastodystrophy.*

A hereditary disease occurring in autosomal dominant and recessive forms. It is due to calcification of elastic fibers and is characterized by raised, yellowish flat papules, especially around the mouth, neck, axillae, elbows, groin, and periumbilical areas, sometimes involving most parts of the skin. The skin becomes inelastic, thickened, and grooved, having an appearance of orange skin (peau d'orange) or a coarse-grained leather. Ocular features usually include angioid streaks, retinal hemorrhage, loss of visual acuity, and, sometimes, macular degeneration and chorioretinitis. Cardiovascular complications generally consist of absence of the pulse in the arms and legs, intermittent claudication, hypertension, angina pectoris, peripheral periarterial calcification, and stenosis of the celiac artery. Epistaxis, hematemesis, subarachnoid hemorrhage, and bleeding from the gastrointestinal organs, kidney, and uterus may occur.

Grönblad, E. Angioid Streaks-Pseudoxanthoma elasticum: Vorläufige Mittelung. *Acta Ophth., Copenhagen*, 1929, 7:329. Strandberg. Pseudoxanthoma elasticum. *Zbl. Haut.*, 1929-30, 31:689. Darrier, J. F. Pseudoxanthoma elasticum. *Mschr. Prakt. Derm.*, 1896, 23:609-17. Van Balen, A. T., & Houtsmuller, A. J. Syndrome of Grönblad-Strandberg-Touraine. *Ophthalmologica*, Basel, 1965, 149:246-7.

psora. See *Willan lepra.*

psoriasiform acrokeratotic dermatosis. See *Bazex syndrome, under Bazex, A.*

psoriasis vulgaris. See *Willan lepra.*

psorospermosis. See *Darier disease (1).*

PSVT (paroxysmal supraventricular tachycardia). See *Bouveret syndrome (2).*

psychic paralysis of visual fixation. See *Bálint syndrome.*

psychogenic headache. See *muscle contraction headache, under headache syndrome.*

psychogenic pupura. See *auto-erythrocyte sensitization syndrome.*

psychose passionelle. See *Clérambault syndrome.*

psychosis associated with polyneuritis. See *Korsakoff syndrome, under Korsakov, Sergei Sergeevich.*

psychosis polyneuritica. See *Korsakoff syndrome, under Korsakov, Sergei Sergeevich.*

PTA (plasma thromboplastin-antecedent) deficiency. See *Rosenthal disease, under Rosenthal, Robert Louis.*

PTC. See *pseudotumor cerebri syndrome.*

PTC (plasma thromboplastin component) deficiency. See *Christmas disease.*

pterygium colli syndrome. See *Bonnevie-Ullrich syndrome.*

pterygium syndrome. See *multiple pterygium syndrome.*

pterygium universalis. See *arthrogryposis multiplex congenita syndrome.*

pterygo-arthromyodysplasia congenita. See *arthrogryposis multiplex congenita syndrome.*

pterygolymphangiectasia syndrome. See *Bonnevie-Ullrich syndrome.*

pterygonuchal infantilism. See *chromosome XO syndrome.*

pterygopalatine neuralgia. See *Sluder neuralgia.*

PTF-B (plasma thromboplastin factor-B) deficiency. See *Christmas disease.*

ptosis adiposa. See *Sichel disease.*

ptosis-epicanthus syndrome. See *Waardenburg syndrome (2).*

ptosis myopathica. See *Graefe syndrome.*

PTSD (post-traumatic stress disorder). See *post-traumatic stress syndrome.*

puberal seminiferous tubule failure. See *chromosome XXY syndrome.*

PUDLAK, P. (Czech physician)

Hermansky-Pudlak syndrome (HPS). See *under Hermansky.*

puerperal mastitis. See *Mathes mastitis.*

pug nose-peripheral dysostosis syndrome. See *acrodysostosis.*

pulmonary acid aspiration. See *Mendelson syndrome.*

pulmonary alveolar proteinosis. See *Rosen-Castleman-Liebow syndrome.*

pulmonary anectasis. See *Wilson-Mikity syndrome, under Wilson, Miriam Geisendorfer.*

pulmonary artery steal syndrome. Synonym: *pulmonary steal syndrome.*

Diversion of blood from the pulmonary circulation by vascular abnormalities, such as pulmonary arteriovenous fistula or vascularization of the right pulmonary lobe by an aberrant coronary artery.

Fried, R., *et al.* congenital pulmonary arteriovenous fistula producing pulmonary arterial steal syndrome. *Pediat. Cardiol.*, 1982, 2:313-8. Briançon, S. *et al.* Vascularisation anormale du lobe pulmonaire inférieur droit par une artère coronaire aberrante. A propos de 2 observations exceptionnelles. *Arch. Mal. Coeur*, 1981, 74:481-6.

pulmonary dysmaturity syndrome. See *Wilson-Mikity syndrome, under Wilson, Miriam Geisendorfer.*

pulmonary emphysema with unilateral transradiancy of one lung. See *Swyer-James syndrome, under Swyer, Paul Robert.*

pulmonary eosinophilia. See *pulmonary infiltration with eosinophilia syndrome.*

pulmonary eosinophilic infiltration. See *pulmonary infiltration with eosinophilia syndrome.*

pulmonary fibrosis. See *Hamman-Rich syndrome.*

pulmonary hemosiderosis with glomerulonephritis. See *Goodpasture syndrome.*

pulmonary hyaline membrane syndrome. See *neonatal respiratory distress syndrome.*

pulmonary hypertrophic osteoarthropathy. See *Marie-Bamberger syndrome, under Marie, Pierre.*

pulmonary infiltration with eosinophilia (PIE) syndrome. Synonyms: *chronic eosinophilic pneumonia (CEP), eosinophilic lung, eosinophilic pneumonia, eosinophilic pneumonitis, eosinophilic pneumopathy, eosinophilic pulmonary infiltrate, eosinophilic pulmonary syndrome, idiopathic eosinophilic lung disease, infiltrative eosinophilia, pulmonary eosinophilic infiltration.*

A disease characterized mainly by pulmonary infiltration and usually, but not always, by peripheral eosinophilia. Clinical manifestations vary and may include cough, asthmatic symptoms, fever, weight loss, and night sweating. Radiographic features consist of irregular opacities about 0.5 to 5.0 cm in diameter. The syndrome includes the following disorders:

I. Eosinophilic pneumonia due to parasitic infestation (**Löffler disease**, q.v.).
II. Chemically-induced pulmonary eosinophilia.
III. Eosinophilic pneumonia associated with the asthmatic syndrome.
  A. Bronchial asthma
  B. Mucoid impaction of the bronchi
  C. Bronchopulmonary aspergillosis
IV. Eosinophilic pneumonia in association with hypersensitivity disorders and systemic angiitis.
  A. Periarterial angiitis
  B. Allergic angiitis and granulomatosis (**Churg-Strauss disease**, q.v.).
V. Eosinophilic pneumonia of unknown etiology

See also *Kartagener disease* and *Magrassi-Leonardi syndrome.*

Mayock, R. L., & Saldana, M. J. Eosinophilic pneumonia. In: Fishman, A. P., ed. *Pulmonary diseases and disorders.* Vol. 1. New York, McGraw Hill, 1980, pp. 926-39. Reeder, W. H., & Goodrich, B. E. Pulmonary infiltration with eosinophilia (P.I.E. syndrome). *Ann. Intern. Med.*, 1952, 36:1217-40.

pulmonary milk allergy syndrome. See *Heiner syndrome.*

pulmonary proteinosis. See *Rosen-Castleman-Liebow syndrome.*

pulmonary steal syndrome. See *pulmonary artery steal syndrome.*

pulmonary valve agenesis syndrome. See *absent pulmonary valve syndrome.*

pulseless arteritis. See *aortic arch syndrome.*

pulseless disease. See *aortic arch syndrome.*

pump lung. See *postperfusion lung-syndrome.*

PUMPHREY, ROBERT E. (American physician, born 1933)

Bart-Pumphrey syndrome. See *under Bart, Robert S.*

punctate epiphyseal dysplasia. See *Conradi-Hünermann syndrome, under Conradi, Erich.*

puncture headache. See *under headache syndrome.*

pupillotonia. See *Adie syndrome.*

puppet children. See *happy puppet syndrome.*

puppet-like syndrome. See *happy puppet syndrome.*

pure alexia. See *alexia without agraphia syndrome.*

pure red cell anemia. See *Diamond-Blackfan syndrome.*

PURETIC, S. (Yugoslav physician)

Murray-Puretic-Drescher syndrome. See *Murray syndrome.*

purkinjoma. See *Lhermitte-Duclos disease.*

purpura abdominalis. See *Schönlein-Henoch purpura.*

purpura anaphylactica. See *Schönlein-Henoch purpura.*

purpura annularis. See *Majocchi disease.*

purpura annularis telangiectodes. See *Majocchi disease.*

purpura feminarum typica. See *David disease, under David W. Walter.*

purpura gangrenosa hemorrhagica. See *Martin de Gimard syndrome.*

purpura hemorrhagica. See *Werlhof disease.*

purpura hyperglobulinemica. See *Waldenström syndrome (2), under Waldenström, Jan Gösta.*

purpura infectiosa acuta. See *Schönlein-Henoch purpura.*

purpura necrotisans. See *Martin de Gimard syndrome.*

purpura pigmentaria progressiva. See *Schamberg disease.*

purpura postinfectiva. See *Seidlmayer disease.*

purpura rheumatica. See *Schönlein-Henoch purpura.*

purpura senilis. See *Bateman purpura.*

purpura thrombopenica. See *Werlhof disease.*

purpura with arthralgia. See *Schönlein-Henoch purpura.*

purpura with visceral manifestations. See *Schönlein-Henoch syndrome.*

PURTSCHER, OTMAR (German ophthalmologist, 1852-1927)

Purtscher disease. Synonyms: *Purtscher retinopathy, angiopathic retinopathy, angiopathia retinae trumatica, traumatic regional angiopathy.*

Traumatic retinopathy marked by edema, exudates, and hemorrhage that appears throughout the retina several days after an injury, which is thought to be caused by posterior retinal microembolization. A fat or air embolism of the retinal vessels and lipemia retinalis with the presence of lymph may also occur.

Purtscher, O. Angiopathia retinae traumatica. Lymphorrhagien des Augengrundes. *Graefes Arch. Ophth.*, 1912, 82:347-71.

Purtscher retinopathy. See *Purtscher disease.*

pustular bacterid. See *Andrews bacterid, under Andrews, George Clinton.*

pustular psoriasis of extremities. See *Barber dermatosis, under Barber, Harold Wordsworth.*

pustulosis herpetica infantum. See *Kaposi varicelliform eruption.*

pustulosis vacciniformis acuta. See *Kaposi varicelliform eruption.*

pustulosis varioliformis. See *Kaposi varicelliform eruption.*

PUTNAM, JAMES JACKSON (American physician, 1846-1918)

Putnam acroparesthesia. See *Wartenberg disease (1).*

Putnam disease. See *Dana syndrome.*

Putnam syndrome. See *Wartenberg disease (1).*

Putnam-Dana syndrome. See *Dana syndrome.*

putrid sore mouth. See *Vincent infection.*

putrid stomatitis. See *Vincent infection.*

PUTTI, VITTORIO (Italian physician, 1880-1940)

Putti syndrome. Synonyms: *idiopathic sciatica, rheumatic sciatica, vertebral sciatica, vertebral syndrome.*

Pain radiating from the back into the buttock and into the lower extremity due to arthrosis of posterior vertebral joints causing irritation of the sciatic nerve. See also *Cotugno syndrome.*

Putti, V. On new conceptions in the pathogenesis of sciatic pain. *Lancet*, 1927, 2:53-60.

Putti-Chavany syndrome. Synonym: *paralytic sciatica.*

Unilateral sciatica with violent attacks of pain radiating from the back into the buttocks and lower extremities, followed by the simultaneous occurrence of foot paralysis, abatement of pain, abolishment of the Achilles reflex, and onset of sensory disorders of the foot.

Putti, V. *Lomboartrite e sciatica vertebrale.* Bologna, 1936. Chavany, J. A. Petite histoire de la sciatique paralysante. *Progr. Méd., Paris*, 1958, 86:427-35.

PVS. See ***P**lummer-**V**inson **s**yndrome.*

PWS. See ***P**rader-**W**illi **s**yndrome.*

PXE. See ***p**seudo**x**anthoma **e**lasticum.*

pyknodysostosis. Synonyms: *Maroteaux-Lamy syndrome, Toulouse-Lautrec disease, osteoporosis acro-osteolytica.*

A congenital syndrome of short-limbed dwarfism, craniofacial abnormalities, increased bone fragility, and dental anomalies. Abnormalities of the skull and face generally consist of disproportionately large calvarium, frontal and occipital bossing, open fontanels, small face, hypoplasia of the angle of the mandible, parrotlike nose, mild exophthalmos, and receding chin. Bone defects may include genu valgum, kyphosis, scoliosis, lumbar lordosis, hypoplasia of the clavicle, pectus excavatum, and short and wide digits. The nails may be thin and hypoplastic. Premature tooth eruption, persistence of primary teeth, malocclusion, and enamel hypoplasia are the principal dental defects. The syndrome is transmitted as an autosomal recessive trait. Parental consanguinity has been noted in some cases. Toulouse-Lautrec is said to have been afflicted with this syndrome.

Maroteaux, P., & Lamy M. La pycnodysostose. *Presse Méd.*, 1962, 70:999-1002. Maroteaux, P., & Lamy, M. The malady of Toulouse-Lautrec. *JAMA*, 1965, 191:715-7.

pyknolepsy. See *Friedmann syndrome (2), under Friedmann, Max.*

PYLE, EDWIN (American physician, born 1892)

Pyle disease. See *metaphyseal dysplasia syndrome.*

Pyle metaphyseal dysplasia syndrome. See *metaphyseal dysplasia syndrome.*

Pyle-Cohn syndrome. See *metaphyseal dysplasia syndrome.*

pylephlebostenosis splenica. See *Wallgren disease.*

pyoderma verrucosum. See *Hallopeau syndrome (3).*

pyodermatitis vegetans. See *Hallopeau syndrome (3).*

pyodermia vegetans. See *Hallopeau syndrome (3).*

pyodermitis chronica vegetans. See *De Azua pseudoepithelioma.*

pyogenic metastatic scleritis. See *Krämer disease.*

pyorrhea. See *Fauchard disease.*

pyorrhea alveolaris. See *Fauchard disease.*

pyramid-hypoglossal syndrome. See *Déjerine syndrome (2).*

pyramidal fracture. See *Le Fort fracture II.*

pyridoxine-dependent epilepsy. See *Hunt epilepsy, under Hunt, Andrew Dickson, Jr.*

pyridoxine responsive anemia. See *Rundles-Falls syndrome.*

pyrroloporphyria. See *acute intermittent porphyria.*

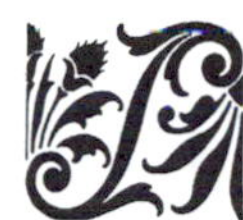

Page #	Term	Observation

QT interval prolongation. See *long QT syndrome.*
QT prolongation syndrome. See *long QT syndrome.*
quadrigeminal plate syndrome. See *Pellizzi syndrome.*
QUARELLI, GUSTAVO (Italian physician)
Quarelli syndrome. Striatopallidal syndrome with parkinsonian tremor, seen in carbon disulfide poisoning.

Quarelli, G. Del tremore parkinsonsimile dell'intossicazione cronico da solfuro di carbonio. *Med. Lavoro*, 1930, 21:58-64.

QUASIMODO (Hunchback of Notre Dame in Victor Hugo's *Notre Dame de Paris*)
Quasimodo syndrome. Severe kyphoscoliosis with respiratory disorders due to thoracic deformity, including obstructive apnea and hypopnea during sleep.

Guilleminault, C., *et al.* Severe kyphoscoliosis, breathing, and sleep. The "Quasimodo" syndrome during sleep. *Chest*, 1981, 79:626-30.

QUELCE-SALGADO, A. (Brazilian physician)
Grebe and Quelce-Salgado syndrome. See *Grebe disease.*
QUERVAIN, FRITZ, DE (Swiss physician, 1868-1940)
de Quervain disease (1). Synonyms: *de Quervain stenosing tendovaginitis, de Quervain syndrome, de Quervain tendinitis, stenosing tendinitis of the abductor longus.*

Tenosynovitis due to relative narrowness of the tendon sheath of the abductor pollicis longus and the extensor pollicis brevis. The disease causes pain, swelling, and tenderness. X-ray findings show a lateral bulge of the skin near the radial styloid. Accumulation of synovial fluid within the tendon sheath enlarges the sheath and deviates the subcutaneous tissue.

*Quervain, F., de. Über eine Form von chronischer Tendovaginitis. *Cor. Bl. Schweiz. Arzte, Basel*, 1895, 25:389-94.

de Quervain disease (2). Synonyms: *de Quervain thyroiditis, giant-cell pseudotuberculous thyroiditis, giant-cell thyroiditis. granulomatous thyroiditis, pseudotuberculous thyroiditis, sclerosing thyroiditis, struma granulomatosa, subacute granulomatous thyroiditis, subacute thyroiditis, thyreoiditis nonpurulenta subacuta.*

A form of subacute thyroiditis that frequently follows a viral infection by several weeks and is most common in males in their third to fifth decades of life. It is characterized by painful enlargement of the thyroid gland in association with fever, chills, malaise, dysphagia, and, sometimes, tachycardia. Follicular cell destruction, lymphocytic and polymorphonuclear leukocyte infiltration, and the presence of multinucleate cells in the thyroid gland are the principal pathological features. Fibrosis may appear in later stages.

Quervain, F., de. Über acute nichteitrige Thyreoiditis. *Arch. Klin. Chir., Berlin*, 1902, 67:706-14.

de Quervain stenosing tendovaginitis. See *de Quervain disease (1).*
de Quervain syndrome (1). See *de Quervain disease (1).*
de Quervain syndrome (2). See *testicular feminization syndrome.*
de Quervain tendinitis. See *de Quervain disease (1).*
de Quervain thyroiditis. See *de Quervain disease (2).*
QUESNEL, MAURICE (French physician)
Lhermitte-Cornil-Quesnel syndrome. See *under Lhermitte.*

QUEYRAT, AUGUSTE (French physician, born 1872)
Queyrat erythroplasia. Synonyms: *erythroplakia, ulcero-membranous balanitis.*

A chronic precancerous condition of the mucous membrane, characterized by painless, but slightly sensitive, red plaques, accompanied by superficial infiltration of the mucosa, and having a tendency to degenerate to epithelioma. The lesions are moist and shiny and usually occur on the glans penis, but they may also affect the female genitalia, lips, and oral mucosa. Occasionally, erythroplasia may exist side by side with leukoplakia. A soft variety found on the oral mucosa, with an irregular outline and a granular or finely nodular surface speckled with small white plaques, is sometimes referred to as **speckled leukoplakia** or **speckled erythroplakia**. Queyrat erythroplasia and Bowen disease are considered as variants of carcinoma in situ.

Queyrat. Erythroplasie du gland. *Bull. Soc. Fr. Derm.*, 1911, 22:378-82.

QUIE, PAUL G. (American physician)
Quie syndrome. See *chronic granulomatous disease of childhood.*
QUINCKE, HEINRICH IRENAEUS (German physician, 1842-1922)
Quincke disease. See *Quincke edema.*
Quincke edema. Synonyms: *Bannister disaese, Milton disease, Milton urticaria, Quincke disease, acute circumscribed edema, acute essential edema, angioneurotic edema, cutaneous angioneurosis, edema cutis circum-*

scriptum, giant urticaria, migratory edema, urticaria edematosa, urticaria gigantea, wandering edema.

A disorder of the skin and subcutaneous and submucosal tissues, characterized by increased vascular permeability and the sudden appearance of painless, circumscribed, nonpitting swellings of the face (around the eyes, chin, and lips), tongue, feet, genitalia, and trunk, which persist from a few hours to 2 or 3 days and then fade, although the attacks may recur often at the same sites. Edema appears in two forms: (1) the hereditary form (**hereditary angioneurotic edema** or **HANE**), which is transmitted as an autosomal dominant trait, involves the larynx and viscera, is marked by abdominal pain, and has occasional severe and fatal respiratory complications; and (2) the sporadic form, which may be caused by allergy, infection, or emotional stress. C1 esterase inhibitor deficiency is believed to be involved in the hereditary form. See also *Nonne-Milroy syndrome*.

Quincke, H. I. Über akutes umbeschriebenes Hautödem. *Mhefte Prakt. Derm.*, 1882, 1:129-31. Milton, J. L. On giant urticaria. *Edinburgh Med. J.*, 1876, 22:513-26. Bannister, H. M. Acute angioneurotic oedema. *J. Nerv. Ment. Dis.*, 1894, 21:627-31.

Quincke meningitis. See *pseudotumor cerebri syndrome.*

QUINQUAUD, CHARLES EUGENE (French physician, 1843-1894)

Quinquaud disease. Synonyms: *acne decalvans, folliculitis decalvans.*

An eruption of purulent pustules or miliary abscesses that involve the hair follicles, produce alopecia, and leave atrophic cicatricial lesions of the scalp.

Quinquaud, C. E. Folliculite destructive des régions velues. *Bull. Soc. Méd. Hôp. Paris*, 1888, 5:395-8.

quintan fever. See *Werner-His disease, under Werner, Heinrich.*

quintuple-X syndrome. See *chromosome XXXXX syndrome.*

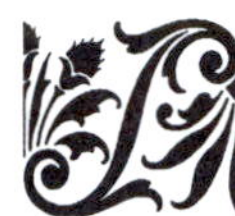

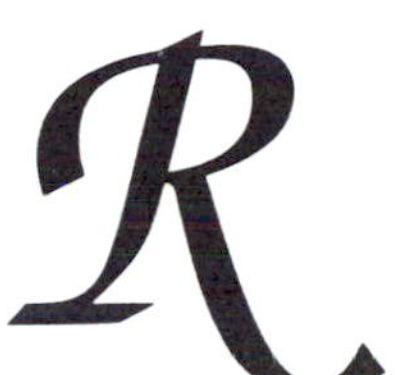

r(2) syndrome. See *chromosome 2 ring syndrome.*
r(6) syndrome. See *chromosome 6 ring syndrome.*
r(7) syndrome. See *chromosome 7 ring syndrome.*
r(9) syndrome. See *chromosome 9 ring syndrome.*
r(10) syndrome. See *chromosome 10 ring syndrome.*
r(11) syndrome. See *chromosome 11 ring syndrome.*
r(12) syndrome. See *chromosome 12 ring syndrome.*
r(13) syndrome. See *chromosome 13 ring syndrome.*
r(14) syndrome. See *chromosome 14 ring syndrome.*
r(15) syndrome. See *chromosome 15 ring syndrome.*
r(17) syndrome. See *chromosome 17 ring syndrome.*
r(18) syndrome. See *chromosome 18 ring syndrome.*
r(21) syndrome. See *chromosome 21 ring syndrome.*
r(22) syndrome. See *chromosome 22 ring syndrome.*
rabbit fever. See *Francis disease.*

rabbit syndrome. A subcategory of the extrapyramidal toxic reactions characterized by perioral muscular movements resembling the rapid, chewing-like movements of the rabbit mouth. Neuroleptic drugs are the principal cause of this illness. Middle-aged and elderly persons are most commonly affected.

Villeneuve, A. The rabbit syndrome. A peculiar extrapyramidal reaction. *Canad. Psychiat. Assoc. J.*, 1972, 17(Suppl. 2):69-72.

RABE, FRITZ (German physician, born 1884)

Rabe-Salomon syndrome. Synonyms: *congenital afibrinogenemia, congenital hypofibrinogenemia, constitutional afibrinogenemia.*

A blood-clotting disorder caused by a lack or deficiency of fibrinogen in the blood, resulting in bleeding from the umbilical cord at birth, ecchymoses, hematomas, spontaneous gingival bleeding, and hemorrhage after tooth extraction. It is a familial condition, occurring in both sexes, transmitted as an autosomal recessive trait.

Rabe, F., & Salomon, E. Über Faserstoffmangel im Blute bei einem Falle von Hämophilie. *Deut. Arch. Klin. Med.*, 1920, 132:240-4.

Rabenhorst syndrome. See *cardio-acrofascial syndrome.*

RABSON, S. M. (American physician)

Rabson-Mendenhall syndrome. Synonyms: *Mendenhall syndrome, insulin resistance-pineal hyperplasia syndrome.*

Insulin-resistant diabetes mellitus, with a decrease in the number of insulin receptors, associated with multiple abnormalities and hypertrophy of the pineal body and adrenal cortex. The symptoms include enlarged genitalia, dental abnormalities (dysplastic teeth, premature tooth eruption), protruding abdomen, peculiar facies (bulging forehead, hypertrichosis), skin disorders (dry skin, acanthosis nigricans), thin limbs, narrow or thickened nails, draining abscesses, recurrent infections, and ketoacidosis. The syndrome is familial and is transmitted as an autosomal recessive trait.

Rabson, S. M., & Mendenhall, E. N. Familial hypertrophy of the pineal body, hyperplasia of adrenal cortex, and diabetes mellitus. *Am. J. Clin. Pathol.*, 1956, 26:283-90
*Mendenhall, E. N. Tumor of the pineal body with high insulin resistance. *J. Indiana Med.*, 1950, 43:32-6.

rachitis. See *Glisson disease.*

RACINE, WILLY (Swiss physician, 1898-1946)

Racine syndrome. Synonym: *premenstrual salivary syndrome.*

Swelling of the salivary glands and breasts occurring 4 or 5 days before menstruation and subsiding with the onset of flow.

Racine, W. Le syndrome salivaire prémenstruel. *Schweiz. Med. Wschr.*, 1939, 69:1204-7.

RACOUCHOT, JEAN (French physician, born 1908)

Favre-Racouchot disease. See *under Favre.*

RADEMACHER

Rademacher disease. Diminished immunity resulting in frequent infections, associated with hypogammaglobulinemia, and complicated by generalized lymphadenopathy. The disease was named after the person in whom it was first observed.

Rademacher's disease. Diminished immunity of an unusual form complicated by lymphadenopathy. *Am. J. Med.*, 1962, 32:80-905.

radial nerve compression. See *radial tunnel syndrome.*
radial nerve entrapment. See *radial tunnel syndrome.*

radial tunnel syndrome. Synonyms: *posterior interosseous tunnel syndrome, radial nerve compression, radial nerve entrapment.*

A syndrome of radial paresthesia and paresis, a popping sensation, and pain in the area of the forearm overlying the radial tunnel, causing painful or restricted motion of the elbow. Compression or entrapment of the nerve in the radial tunnel (the structures surrounding the radial nerve from the furrow between the brachioradialis and radialis in the distal arm to the distal edge of the supinator in the proximal forearm) is caused by trauma; overuse, as in tennis elbow (see under *overuse syndrome*); ganglia; rheumatoid sinovitis; space-occupying lesions; and other conditions. The compression usually occurs at the fibrous tethering bands, the fibrous origin of the extensor carpi radialis brevis, the recurrent radial fan of vessels, and the arcade of Frohse. A condition characterized by entrapment of the radial nerve at two levels is known as the *double-entrapment radial tunnel syndrome.*

Roles, N. C., & Maudsley, R. H. Radial tunnel syndrome. *J. Bone Joint Surg.*, 1972, 54(B):499-508. Moss, S. H., *et al.* Radial tunnel syndrome: A spectrum of clinical presentations. *J. Hand Surg.*, 1983, 8:414-20.

radiculoneuritis. See *Guillain-Barré syndrome.*

RADS. See *reactive airways dysfunction syndrome.*

RADULESCU, A. (Rumanian physician)

Radulescu syndrome. Hypertrophy of the lower limb associated with vascular nevi, osteosclerosis, and acrocyanosis.

Brucar, M., & Gotescu, I. Hipertrofie totala al unuia din membrele inferioare insotita de osteoscleroza in benzi, nev plan vascular si acrocianoza. *Rev. Chir., Bucuresti,* 1976, 25:203-10.

RAEDER, JOHAN GEORG (Norwegian physician, 1889-1956)

Raeder syndrome. Synonyms: *incomplete Horner syndrome, partial Horner syndrome, paratrigeminal paralysis, paratrigeminal syndrome, paratrigeminal sympathetic syndrome.*

A neurological disease, resembling the Horner syndrome, most commonly affecting males in their fifth decade of life. It is due to disruption of the sympathetic pathways by a neoplasm of the middle cranial fossa or a primary tumor of the gasserian ganglion. Blepharoptosis and miosis associated with severe unilateral headache, usually around the eye, or pain in the area of trigeminal distribution are the principal clinical characteristics of this disorder.

Raeder, J. G. "Paratrigeminal" paralysis of the oculopupillary sympathetic. *Brain*, 1924, 47:149-58.

Raeder-Harbitz syndrome. See *aortic arch syndrome.*

RAGHIB, GUNAY (Physician in Indianapolis)

Raghib syndrome. A cardiovascular developmental anomaly consisting of termination of the persistent superior vena cava in the left atrium, atrial septal defect, and absence of the coronary sinus.

Raghib, G., *et al.* Termination of the left superior vena cava in left atrium, atrial septal defect, and absence of coronary sinus. A developmental complex. *Circulation,* 1965, 31:906-18.

RAJKA (Hungarian physician)

Rajka-Szodoray syndrome. Synonym: *neuroangiosis cruris hemosiderosa.*

A vascular disorder of the lower limbs, characterized by capillary bundles, whorls, and subepidermal glomi, leading to diapedesis with microscopic hemorrhage and eventual hemosiderosis.

Szodoray, L., & Sóvári, É. Contribution à l'étude de l'histologie de la neuroangiosis cruris haemosiderosa. *Acta Med. Acad. Sc. Hung.*, 1954, 6:107-15.

RALLISON, M. L. (American physician)

Wolcott-Rallison syndrome. See *under Wolcott.*

RALPH (renal-anal-lung-polydactyly-hamarto-blastoma) syndrome. See *Hall syndrome under Hall, J. G.*

RAMAZZINI, BERNARDINO (Italian physician, 1633-1714)

Ramazzini syndrome. Synonyms: *extrinsic allergic alveolitis, farmer's lung.*

Hypersensitivity pneumonitis in agricultural workers caused by exposure to certain soil microorganisms, including *Micropolyspora faeni, Thermoactinomyces vulgaris, T. sacchari, T. candidus,* and *T. viridis.* In the acute form, the condition is characterized by cough, dyspnea, chills, fever, myalgia, malaise, tachycardia, tachypnea, and rales. The symptoms appear suddenly 4 to 8 hours after the exposure and disappear several hours later. Laboratory findings include leukocytosis, elevated immunoglobulin levels (except for IgE), and rheumatoid factor in some cases. The chronic form, occurring in persons exposed to low levels of antigens over long periods of time, is marked by progressive dyspnea, cough, malaise, weakness, weight loss, and irreversible lung damage.

Ramazzini, B. *De morbus artificium diatriba.* Mutinae, Capponi, 1700. 360 pp.

RAMON, F. (French physician)

Chauffard-Ramon syndrome. See *Still syndrome.*

RAMON, YOCHANAN (Israeli dentist)

Ramon syndrome. Synonym: *cherubism-gingival fibromatosis-epilepsy-mental deficiency syndrome.*

A familial syndrome, transmitted as an autosomal recessive trait, characterized by gingival fibromatosis, fibrous dysplasia of the maxillae, narrow palate, buried teeth, cherubic face with wide and persistent anterior fontanelle, partial epilepsy with secondary generalization, mild mental retardation, growth retardation, hypertrichosis, and juvenile rheumatoid arthritis. See also *cherubism.*

Ramon, Y., *et al.* Gingival fibromatosis combined with cherubism. *Oral Surg.*, 1967, 24:435-48. Pina-Neto, J. M., *et al.* Cherubism, gingival fibromatosis, epilepsy, and mental deficiency (Ramon syndrome) with juvenile rheumatoid arthritis. *Am. J. Med. Genet.*, 1986, 25:433-41.

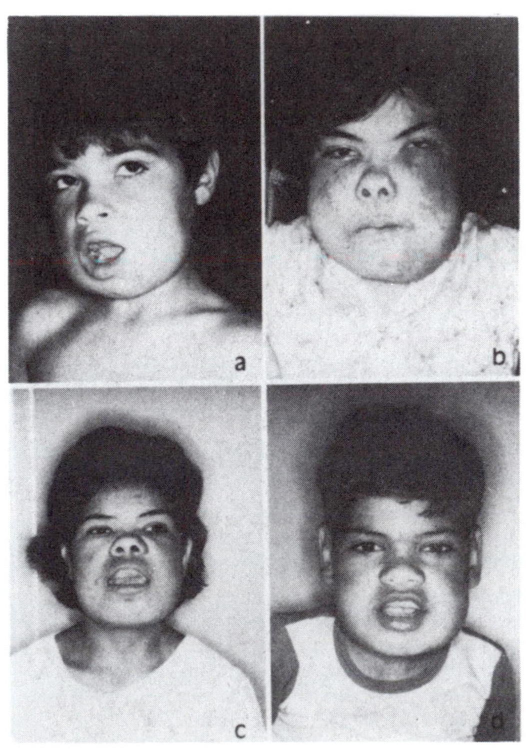

Ramon syndrome
Pina-Neto, Joao M., Aparecida Fatima C. Moreno, Luis Roberto Silva, Maria Angeles S.L. Velludo, Eucia Beatriz L. Petean, Maria Valeriana M. Ribeiro, Luis Athayde-Junior & Julio Cesar Voltarelli, *American Journal of Medical Genetics* 25:433- 441, 1986. New York: Alan R. Liss, Inc.

RAMSAY HUNT. See HUNT, JAMES RAMSAY

rape trauma syndrome. A state occurring after an individual experiences a forced, violent sexual assault, with vaginal, anal, or oral penetration, against the will. The acute phase includes various disorders, especially vaginal and/or anal lacerations, gastrointestinal irritability, muscle tension, sleep disturbances, and emotional changes, such as nightmares and phobias. Long-term effects include changes in lifestyle, social and family relationships, and eating and sleeping patterns; fear of men and of being alone on the street; aversion to sex; and altered personalility. See also *post-traumatic stress syndrome*.

Burgess, A. W., & Homstrom, L. L. Rape trauma syndrome. *Am. J. Psychiat.*, 1974, 1131:981-6. Homstrom, L. L., & Burgess, L. L. Assessing trauma in the rape victim. *Am. J. Nurs.*, 1975, 75:1288-91.

rapid irregular movement of the eyes and limbs syndrome. See *Kingsbourne syndrome.*

RAPK (**r**eticulate **a**cro**p**igmentation of **K**itamura). See *Kitamura disease.*

RAPP, R. S.

Rapp-Hodgkin syndrome. A hereditary syndrome, transmitted as an autosomal dominant trait, characterized by hypohidrosis, cleft lip, cleft palate, narrow dysplastic nails with soft tissue tufting, hypotrichosis (stiff and sparse steel wool hair, sparse eyebrows and lashes, no axillary and pubic hair), hypospadias, and variable short stature. Associated defects may include low nasal bridge, narrow nose, hypodontia, conical teeth, maxillary hypoplasia, absent uvula with functional short palate, epiphora, absent lacrimal puncta, corneal opacity, photophobia, stenosis of the auditory canals, syndactyly, and hypoplastic dermatoglyphics. Childhood hypothermia, purulent conjunctivitis, and otitis media may be associated.

*Rapp, R. S., & Hodgkin, W. E. Anhidrotic ectodermal dysplasia: Autosomal dominant inheritance with palate and lip anomalies. *J. Med. Genet.*, 1968, 5:269-72.

RAPUNZEL (A character in the tale of the brothers Jacob and Wilhelm Grimm [1812] about a young maiden with long hair tresses, who lowered them to the ground to allow her lover to climb up to her window)

Rapunzel syndrome. Trichobezoar in the stomach with a tail-like extension made by long strands of twisted hair, reaching the ileocecal valve.

Vaughan, E. D., *et al.* The Rapunzel syndrome: An unusual complication of intestinal bezoar. *Surgery,* 1968, 63:339-43. Rodin, A., & Key, J. D. *Encyclopedia of medical eponyms derived from literary characters.* Melbourne, Fl., Krieger, 1989.

RASMUSSEN, FRITZ WALDEMAR (Danish physician, 1834-1877)

Rasmussen aneurysm. Dilation of a terminal artery in a tuberculous cavity that may lead to rupture and hemorrhage.

Rasmussen, V. Om haemoptyse, novnlig den lethale, i anatomisk og klinisk henseende. *Hospitalstidende*, 1868, 11:33-6; 45-6; 49-52.

RASO, MARIO (Italian physician, born 1906)

Mattioli-Foggia and Raso syndrome. See *under Mattioli-Foggia.*

rastafarianism syndrome. See *vegans syndrome.*

RATHBUN, JOHN CAMPBELL (American physician, born 1915)

Rathbun disease. See *hypophosphatasia syndrome.*

RAUSCHKOLB, J. E. (American physician)

Cole-Rauschkolb-Toomey syndrome. See *Zinsser-Engmann-Cole syndrome.*

RAUTENSTRAUCH, T. (German physician)

Wiedemann-Rautenstrauch syndrome (WRS). See *under Wiedemann.*

RAVITCH, MARK M. (American physician)

Cantrell-Haller-Ravitch syndrome. See *thoraco-abdominal syndrome.*

RAWLINGS, MAURICE S. (American physician)

Rawlings syndrome. See *straight back syndrome.*

RAY, ISAAC (American psychiatrist, 1807-1881)

Ray mania. Mental derangement with impairment of the moral sense.

Ray, I. *A treatise on the medical jurisprudence of insanity.* London, Henderson, 1837.

RAYER, PIERRE FRANÇOIS OLIVE (French physician, 1793-1867)

Rayer disease. See *Addison-Gull syndrome.*

RAYMOND, FULGENCE (French physician, 1844-1910)

Raymond-Céstan syndrome. A tumor of the cerebral peduncles involving the red nucleus, in association with speech disorders, paralysis of lateral conjugate gaze, ipsilateral abducens palsy, contralateral hemiplegia, and ipsilateral anesthesia of the face, extremities, and trunk.

Raymond, F., & Céstan, R. Sur un cas d'endothéliome épithéliale du noyau rouge. *Rev. Neur., Paris.*, 1902, 10:463-4.

RAYNAUD, A. G. MAURICE

occupational Raynaud disease. See *vibration syndrome.*

Raynaud disease. See *Raynaud syndrome.*

Raynaud gangrene. See *Raynaud syndrome.*

Raynaud phenomenon (RP). See *Raynaud syndrome.*

Raynaud phenomenon-esophageal motor dysfunction-sclerodactyly-telangiectasia syndrome. See *REST syndrome.*

Raynaud syndrome (RS). Synonyms: *Raynaud disease, symmetric asphyxia.*

A peripheral vascular disorder of unknown etiology in which bilateral paroxysmal spasms, usually precipitated by cold or emotional factors, produce cyanosis and pallor of the digits associated with paresthesia, numbness, tingling, and burning. Ulcers and gangrene (**symmetrical gangrene of extremities** or **Raynaud gangrene**) may follow. The syndrome has a special predilection for adult women, usually under the age of 40 years. The term **Raynaud phenomenon** or **RP (acrocyanosis, Crocq disease, Crocq-Cassirer syndrome,** or **acroasphyxia chronica hypertrophica)** applies to a vasomotor disorder characterized by pallor and cyanosis resulting from constriction of the small arteries of the extremities; it is frequently associated with the Raynaud syndrome but may occur independently or with other diseases. See also *Nothnagel syndrome (1).*

Raynaud, A. G. *De l'asphyxie locale et la gangrene symetrique des extremites.* Paris, 1862. (Thesis). Crocq, J. B. De l'"acrocyanose." *Sem. Méd.*, 1896, 16:298. Cassirer, R. *Die vasomotorisch-tropischen Neurosen.* Berlin, Karger, 1901.

RD (**R**eiter **d**isease). See *Reiter syndrome.*

RD syndrome. See *Rolland-Desbuquois syndrome.*

RDS (**r**espiratory **d**istress **s**yndrome). See *adult respiratory distress syndrome, and see neonatal respiratory distress syndrome.*

reactive airways dysfunction syndrome (RADS). An airway obstruction syndrome with asthma-like symptoms due to an exposure to high levels of an irritating aerosol, vapor, fume, or smoke.

Brooks, S. M., *et al.* Reactive airways dysfunction syndrome. Case reports of persistent airways hyperreactivity following high-level irritant exposure. *J. Occup. Med.*, 1985, 27:473-6.

reactive hypoglycemia syndrome. Functional hypoglycemia occurring after eating or following ingestion of sugar, without any evidence of gastric disorders.

Harris, S. Hyperinsulinism and dysinsulism. *JAMA*, 1924, 83:1193-208. Lefèbre, P. J., *et al.* Le syndrome d'hypoglycémie réactionnelle. Mythe ou réalité. *Journ. Annuel. Diabet. Hôtel Dieu*, 1983, p. 111-8.

REAS. See *retained, excluded antrum syndrome.*

REBACK, S. (American physician)

Mount-Reback syndrome. See *under Mount.*

REBELAIS, FRANÇOIS (French writer and physician who described bizarre gustatory habits)

rebelaisian syndrome. Small bowel disease after bizarre massive gustatory insults.

Robin, E. D., *et al.* Indiscretion enteritis. A rebelaisian syndrome. *Am. J. Med.*, 1986, 81:1108-12.

recalcitrant pustular eruption. See *Andrews bacterid, under Andrews, George Clinton.*

receptive aphasia. See *Wernicke aphasia.*

recessive carpotarsal osteolysis. See *Torg syndrome.*

recessive hereditary sensory neuropathy. See *congenital sensory neuropathy syndrome.*

RECKLINGHAUSEN, FRIEDRICH DANIEL, VON (German pathologist, 1833-1910)

Engel-von Recklinghausen syndrome. See *Recklinghausen disease (2).*

Recklinghausen disease (1). Synonyms: *Recklinghausen neurofibromatosis, Recklinghausen syndrome, von Recklinghausen disease, von Recklinghausen neuropathy, multiple neurofibromatoses, neurinofibrolipomatosis, neurinomatosis centralis et peripherica, neurinomatosis universalis, neurofibromatosis, neurofibromatosis syndrome.*

A hereditary syndrome, transmitted as an autosomal dominant trait (about 50% of the cases represent new mutations), and characterized by multiple neurofibromas and skin pigmentation associated with cutaneous, cerebral, cranial, spinal, sympathetic nervous system, skeletal, and other disorders. The syndrome may develop slowly, some manifestations being present at birth and others evolving by the second year of life. The first clinical stigmata are usually café-au-lait spots which increase in size and number. The neurofibromas, varying in size from that of a small pea to a giant pendulous tumor, may appear on any part of the body and there may be malignant degeneration. Schwannomas, fibromas, and other types of neoplasms are also known to occur. Mental retardation, seizures, hydrocephalus, and other neurological complications are frequent. Eye involvement may result in proptosis, muscle palsies, phakoma, glaucoma, corneal opacity, and other ocular complications. Bony anomalies may include kyphoscoliosis, erosion, cystic lesions, lordosis, overgrowth of cranial bones, asymmetry of facial bones, elevation of the scapula, absence of ribs, pseudarthrosis, and other skeletal defects. Macrodactyly, acromegaly, and sexual precocity may also occur.

Recklinghausen, F. D., von. *Über die multiplen Fibrome der Haut und ihre Beziehungen zu den Neuromen.* Berlin, A. Hirschwald, 1882.

Recklinghausen disease (2). Synonyms: *Engel-von Recklinghausen disease, von Recklinghausen disease, osteitis fibrosa cystica, osteitis fibrosa generalisata, osteodystrophia fibrosa generalisata, osteodystrophia generalisata, osteopathia fibrosa generalisata.*

A generalized rarefying bone disorder, seen in advanced hyperparathyroidism, characterized by cysts or brown tumors in the form of deeply pigmented foci consisting of fibrous scarring of the bone with pseudocysts, hemorrhages, and collection of osteoclasts. Bone destruction is often associated with gross deformities, osteomalacia, fractures, tissue resorption, and replacement of destroyed bone with fibrous tissue. The pathogenesis is attributed to excessive production of parathyroid hormone with secondary calcium and phosphorus metabolism disorders and stimulation of osteoclastic bone resorption. Metastatic calcification, especially of the kidneys, and renal failure may occur.

Engel, G. *Über einen Fall cystoider Entartung des gesamten Skeletts.* Giessen, 1864. *Recklinghausen, F. D., von. Die fibröse oder deformierende Ostitis, die Osteomalazie und die osteoplastische Carcinose in ihren gegenseitigen Beziehungen. *Fortschr. R. Virchow*, Berlin, 1891.

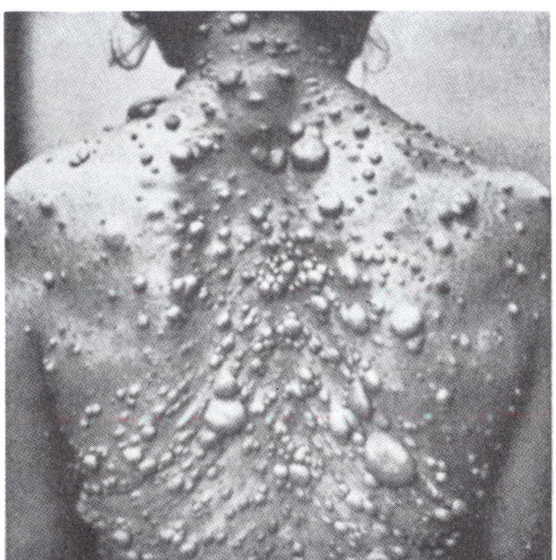

Recklinghausen disease (1)
Andrews, G.C. & A.N. Domonkos: *Diseases of the Skin.* 5th ed. Philadelphia: W.B. Saunders Co., 1963.

Recklinghausen neurofibromatosis. See *Recklinghausen disease (1).*

Recklinghausen syndrome. See *Recklinghausen disease (1).*

Recklinghausen-Applebaum syndrome. Synonyms: *bronze diabetes, bronzed diabetes, hemochromatosis (HFE), iron overload syndrome, iron storage disease, pigmentary cirrhosis.*

A disorder of iron metabolism characterized by a triad of hemosiderosis, liver cirrhosis, and diabetes mellitus. It is caused by massive iron deposits in parenchymal cells that may develop after a prolonged increase of iron absorption. The hereditary type is transmitted as an autosomal recessive trait. Masssive blood transfusions and overmedication with iron compounds with resulting iron overload are the principal causes of the exogenous type, which is most commonly observed in persons over the age of 40 years, and is characterized by bronze-tan discoloration, chiefly of the face, arms, genitalia, and skin folds, in association with iron deposits in the pancreas, liver, endocrine glands, skin, spleen, lymph nodes, and reticuloendothelial cells. Hepatomegaly, weakness, malaise, chronic abdominal pain, loss of libido, loss of weight, portal hypertension, osseous and articular changes, and nonspecific neurological disorders are the most common clinical features. Associated disorders may include esophageal varices, splenomegaly, cardiac arrhythmias, congestive heart failure, arthritis or osteoarthritis (usually involving the metacarpophalangeal, knee, hip, and shoulder joints), synovitis and pseudogout of the knees, testicular atrophy, scanty body hair, hypogonadism, and lethargy. The gene for hemochromatosis is located on the short arm of chromosome 6 and is linked to the HLA locus. Secondary iron overload may occur in hemosiderosis/hemochromatosis due to hemolytic anemia, intermedullary hemolysis, and alcoholic cirrhosis with excess iron deposited in various tissues.

*Recklinghausen, F. D. Über Hämochromatose. *Tagebl. Versam. Natur. Arzte, Heidelberg*, 1889, 62:324. Motulsky, A. G. Hemochromatosis (iron storage disease). In: Wyngaarden, J. B., & Smith, L. H., Jr., eds. *Cecil textbook of medicine*. 17th ed. Philadelphia, Saunders, 1985, pp. 1160-3. Pollycove, M. Hemochromatosis. In: Stanbury, J. B., Wyngaarden, J. B., & Fredrickson, D. S., eds. *The metabolic basis of inherited disease*. 4th ed. New York, McGraw-Hill, 1978, pp. 1127-64. Polly, M. Iron overload syndromes. *Clin. Physiol. Biochem.*, 1986, 4:61-77. Weir, M. P., *et al.* Haemosiderin and tissue damage. *Cell Biochem. Funct.*, 1984, 2:186-94.

von Recklinghausen disease (1 and 2). See *Recklinghausen disease (1 and 2).*

von Recklinghausen neuropathy. See *Recklinghausen disease (1).*

RECLUS, PAUL (French physician, 1847-1914)

Reclus disease. Synonyms: *Cooper disease, ligneous phlegmon.*

Induration of the subcutaneous connective tissue of the neck, with fever, pain, and suppuration.

Reclus, P. Phlégmon ligneux de cou. *Rev. Chir., Paris*, 1896, 16:522-31.

Reclus syndrome. See *Cheatle disease.*

Reclus-Schimmelbusch disease. See *Cheatle disease.*

recrudescent typhus. See *Brill disease.*

rectal crisis. See *Thaysen syndrome.*

rectal shelf. See *Blumer syndrome.*

rectus abdominis muscle syndrome. Synonym: *rectus muscle syndrome.*

A disorder of unknown etiology that produces rupture or tear of the epigastric artery and stretches the rectus cutaneous medialis nerve, producing severe pain.

Jones, T. W., & Merendino, K. A. The deep epigastric artery: Rectus abdominis syndrome. *Am. J. Surg.*, 1962, 103:159-69.

rectus muscle syndrome. See *rectus abdominis muscle syndrome.*

recurrent algetic ophthalmoplegia. See *Tolosa-Hunt syndrome.*

recurrent aseptic meningitis. See *Mollaret meningitis.*

recurrent biliary tract syndrome. See *postcholecystectomy syndrome.*

recurrent febrile nodular panniculitis. See *Weber-Christian syndrome, under Weber, Frederick Parkes.*

recurrent granulomatous dermatitis with eosinophilia. See *Wells syndrome, under Wells, G. C.*

recurrent herpetiform dermatitis repens. See *Hailey-Hailey disease, under Hailey, William Howard.*

recurrent juvenile eczema of the hands and feet. See *wet and dry foot syndrome.*

recurrent labyrinthine vertigo. See *Ménière syndrome.*

recurrent laryngeal neuralgia. See *Arnold neuralgia.*

recurrent ophthalmoplegia dolorosa. See *Tolosa-Hunt syndrome.*

recurrent patellar dislocation. See *unstable patella syndrome.*

recurrent patellar subluxation. See *unstable patella syndrome.*

recurrent physiologic albuminuria. See *Pavy disease.*

recurrent polyserositis. See *Reimann periodic disease.*

recurring scarring aphthae. See *Sutton disease, under Sutton, Richard Lighburn.*

red cell fragmentation syndrome. Fragmentation of the erythrocytes, which may result in hemolytic anemia, due to trauma caused by turbulence of the bloodstream. Abnormalities of the heart valves, malformations of the blood vessels, aortofemoral bypass, vascular grafts, and indwelling hemodialysis catheters are the principal causes.

Nand, S., *et al.* Red cell fragmentation syndrome with the use of subclavian hemodialysis catheters. *Arch. Intern. Med.*, 1985, 145:1421-3.

red diaper syndrome. A condition characterized by red discoloration of diapers, simulating hematuria, due to chromobacterial (*Serratia marcescens*) colonization of the gastrointestinal tract in infants. The bacteria are passed to the diapers, where they cause discoloration after incubation for more than 24 hours at less than body temperature.

Koff, S. A. A practical approach to hematuria in children. *Am. Fam. Physician*, 1981, 23:159-64.

red eye syndrome. See *red-eyed shunt syndrome.*

red-eyed shunt syndrome. Synonym: *red eye syndrome.*

A syndrome of a low-flow carotid-cavernous fistula associated with ocular disorders consisting mainly of dilated and tortuous episcleral veins, an increase in intraocular pressure, the presence of blood in the Schlemm canals, and red eyes. Exophthalmos is common and motility restriction occurs in some patients. Vision is rarely impaired.

Phelps, C. D., *et al.* The diagnosis and prognosis of atypical carotid-cavernous fistula (red-eyed shunt syndrome). *Am. J. Ophth.*, 1982, 93:423-36.

red goggle syndrome. A syndrome named after the red goggles that were used for dark adaptation in the prevideo era of radiology, referring to the use of outdated or inappropriate diagnostic procedures.

Palmer, P. E. S., & Cockshott, W. P. The appropriate use of diagnostic imaging. Avoidance of the red goggle syndrome. *JAMA*, 1984, 252:2753-4.

red man syndrome (RMS). See *red neck syndrome.*

red neck syndrome. Synonym: *red man syndrome (RMS).*

Acute urticarial flushing of the upper torso, arms,

and neck, sometimes extending to the hands, frequently associated with pruritus, caused by intravenous vancomycin. The condition is mediated in part by histamine release.

Garrelts, J. C., & Peterie, J. D. Vancomycin and the "red man's syndrome." *N. Engl. J. Med.*, 1985, 312:245.

red palms. See *Lane disease, under Lane, John Edward.*

red suya syndrome. Hemolytic anemia and jaundice occurring after eating suya (barbecued steak served in fast-food stands in Nigeria). A food-coloring agent, orange-RN (monosodium salt of 1-phenylazo-2-naphthol-6-sulfonic acid), is believed to be the cause.

Akinyanju, O. O., & Odusote, K. A. Red suya syndrome. *Lancet*, 1983, 1:935. Akinyanju, O. O., & Odusote, K. A. Cause of red suya syndrome is food dye orange-RN. *Lancet*, 1983, 2:1314.

REDLICH, EMIL (German physician, 1866-1930)

Redlich encephalitis. Synonyms: *Munch-Petersen encephalomyelitis, Redlich-Flatau syndrome, abortive disseminated encephalomyelitis, disseminated epidemic cerebrospinal meningitis, encephalomyelitis funicularis infectiosa, funicular spinal syndrome.*

A poorly defined form of abortive disseminated encephalomyelitis with lesions distributed throughout the brain and the spinal cord. The symptoms are usually very mild, but the course is protracted. The most common symptoms include tendon reflex disorders, paresthesia, and inflammatory reactions. Redlich suspected that this disorder and Economo disease are variants of the same entity.

Redlich, E. Über abotive Formen der Encephalomyelitis disseminata. *Deut. Med. Wschr.*, 1929, 55:562-3. *Flatau, E. *Warsz. Czas. Lek.*, 1931, p. 49-51. Munch-Petersen, C. J. Encephalo-myelitis disseminata (Redlich) og encephalo-myelitis funicularis infectiosa. *Bibl. Laeger*, 1934, 126:97-132; 138-73.

Redlich-Flatau syndrome. See *Redlich encephalitis.*

redundant lumbar nerve root syndrome. See *redundant nerve root syndrome.*

redundant nerve root syndrome. Synonym: *redundant lumbar nerve root syndrome.*

A neurological disease characterized by large, elongated, tortuous, coiled, and serpiginous nerve roots or roots of the cauda equina. L-3 to S-1 roots are most commonly involved. The symptoms usually include pain in the legs, paraspinal spasm, and a positive Lasègue test. Sphincter disorders and impotence may occur in patients in advanced stages who are nearly paraplegic. X-ray findings usually show lumbar spondylosis with narrowing of the spinal canal. Myelographic examination shows a block with serpiginous filling defects indicating an arteriovenous malformation. Middle-aged males are most frequently affected.

De Lange, S. A. Eine Anomalie der Cauda equina bei einer achondroplastichen Frau. *Acta Neurochir., Wien*, 1967, 16:114-21.

REEDS (**r**etention of tears-**e**ctrodactyly-**e**ctodermal **d**ysplasia-**s**trange hair, skin, and teeth) **syndrome.** A multiple abnormality syndrome, probably inherited as an autosomal dominant trait with reduced penetrance and variable expressivity, characterized by a lobster hand deformity (ectrodactyly) of the hands and feet, nasolacrimal obstruction, and cleft lip and palate. Additional symptoms may include high-arched palate, tearing, keratoconjunctivitis, alopecia, pili torti, graying of the scalp, soft tissue syndactyly, lacrimal duct obstruction, brown atrophic maculae on the extensor surfaces, sparse eyebrows, absence of pigment in the hair shafts, fragmentation of the elastic fibers in the dermis, and, less frequently, microcephaly, mental retardation, inguinal hernia, ureteral malformations, and dental anomalies (anodontia, oligodontia, absence of the central incisors).

Reed, W. B., *et al.* The REEDS syndrome. *Birth Defects*, 1974, 10(5):61-73.

REESE, ALGERON BEVERLY (American ophthalmologist, born 1896)

Cogan-Reese syndrome. See *under Cogan.*

Reese dysplasia. See *Reese syndrome.*

Reese retinal dysplasia. See *Reese syndrome.*

Reese syndrome. Synonyms: *Reese dysplasia, Reese retinal dysplasia, Reese-Blodi syndrome, retinal dysplasia syndrome.*

A syndrome, transmitted as an autosomal recessive trait, characterized mainly by malformation of the retina and persistence of the primary vitreous. Clinically it is a congenital, always bilateral, retinal dysplasia in the form of rosettes, usually associated with microphthalmos, cerebral agenesis, and other abnormalities. The anterior chamber is shallow and synechiae, a persistent pupillary membrane, a white vascularized retrolental membrane, elongated ciliary processes, corneal opacity, and cataracts may be present. Associated abnormalities may include cleft lip, cleft palate, encephalocele, meningocele, pulmonary abnormalities, congenital heart defect, urogenital abnormalities, and skeletal deformities. The characteristic ocular changes in this syndrome are similar to those of the Patau syndrome.

Reese, A. B., & Blodi, F. C. Retinal dysplasia. *Am. J. Ophth.*, 1950, 33:23-32.

Reese-Blodi syndrome. See *Reese syndrome.*

refeeding syndrome. Cardiopulmonary decompensation associated with hypophosphatemia and other metabolic disorders occurring after aggressive total parenteral nutrition in severely malnourished patients.

Weinsier, R. L., & Krumdieck, C. L. Death resulting from overzealous total parenteral nutrition: The refeeding syndrome revisited. *Am. J. Clin. Nutrit.*, 1981, 34:393-9.

REFETOFF, SAMUEL (American physician)

Refetoff syndrome. Synonyms: *Refetoff-DeWind-DeGroot syndrome, deafmutism-goiter-euthyroidism syndrome, peripheral resistance to thyroid hormone, resistance to thyroid hormone, thyroid hormone unresponsiveness.*

An inherited syndrome of peripheral resistance to thyroid hormone, transmitted as an autosomal recessive trait, characterized by increased serum concentrations of thyroxine (T_4) and triiodothyronine (T_3), increased thyroid hormone binding ratio, increased serum T_4 and T_3, and normal to slightly increased thyroid-stimulating hormone (TSH) and TSH response to thyrotropin-releasing hormone. The affected persons are euthyroid to slightly hypothyroid. The symptoms include deaf-mutism, delayed bone maturation, stippled epiphyses, small goiter, nystagmus, elevated serum carotene, low urine hydroxyproline, metachromasia in cultured skin fibroblasts, and high serum protein-bound iodine (PBI). Elevation of serum PBI levels is due to the presence of circulating thyroxine and triiodothyronine in the form of the *L*-isomer, the hormones being normally transferred from blood to tissue and metabolized in excessive amounts, whereby triiodothyronine is converted to thyroxine. The absence of hypermetabolism and the presence of possible hypothyroidism indicate the existence of partial resistance to the peripheral action of thyroid hormone.

Refetoff, S., DeWind, L. T., & DeGroot, L. J. Familial syndrome combining deaf-mutism, stippled epiphyses, goiter and abnormally high PBI: Possible target organ refractoriness to thyroid hormone. *J. Clin. Endrocr. Metab.*, 1967, 27:279-94. Refetoff, S., Degroot, L. J., & Barsano, C. P. Defective thyroid hormone feedback regulation in the syndrome of peripheral resistance to thyroid hormone. *J. Clin. Endocr. Metab.*, 1980, 51:41-5.

Refetoff-DeWind-DeGroot syndrome. See *Refetoff syndrome.*

reflex atelectasis. See *Fleischner syndrome.*

reflex bone atrophy. See *Sudeck syndrome.*

reflex dystrophy of the upper extremity. See *shoulder-hand syndrome.*

reflex iridoplegia. See *Robertson syndrome, under Robertson, Douglas Moray Cooper Lamb Argyll.*

reflex sympathetic dystrophy syndrome (RSD, RSDS). A neurological disorder characterized by pain, hyperalgesia, hyperesthesia, and autonomic dysfunction following injury of an extremity involving a peripheral nerve (especially the sciatic or median nerve). When the injury is characterized by burning pain, the condition is known as **causalgia.** Painful injuries not involving a peripheral nerve occur in post-traumatic painful osteoporosis, shoulder-hand syndrome, Sudeck syndrome, spreading neuralgia, and reflex dystrophy.

Les ouvres d'Ambroise Paré. Paris, Chez G. Buon, 1575. Mitchell, S. W. Morehouse, G. R., & Keene, W. W. *Gunshot wounds and other injuries of nerves.* Philadelphia, Lippincott, 1864. Posner, J. B. Disorders of sensation, In: Wyngaarden, J. B., & Smith, L. H., Jr., eds. *Cecil textbook of medicine.* 17th ed. Philadelphia, Saunders, 1985. pp. 2063-4.

reflux gastritis syndrome. See *postgastrectomy syndrome.*

reflux syndrome. See *postgastrectomy syndrome.*

refractory anemia. See *Davidson anemia.*

refractory dysmyelopoietic anemia. See *myelodysplastic syndrome.*

refractory dysmyelopoietic panmyelopathy. See *myelodysplastic syndrome.*

refractory dysmyelopoietic panmyelosis. See *myelodysplastic syndrome.*

refractory rickets. See *hypophosphatemic familial rickets.*

refrigeration palsy. See *Bell palsy, under Bell, Sir Charles.*

REFSUM, SIGVALD BERNHARD (Norwegian physician, born 1907)

Refsum disease. Synonyms: *Refsum syndrome, Refsum-Thiébaut disease, ataxia hereditaria hemeralopica polyneuritiformis, heredoataxia hemerolopica polyneuritiformis, heredopathia atactica polyneuritiformis, phytanic acid storage disease.*

A rare inherited lipid metabolism disorder, transmitted as an autosomal recessive trait, characterized by phytanic acid accumulation in the blood and tissues. The symptoms consist of retinitis pigmentosa, night blindness, progressive constriction of visual fields, lenticular opacity, peripheral polyneuropathy, absent or diminished deep tendon reflexes, cerebellar ataxia, unsteady gait, Romberg sign, intention tremor, nystagmus, ECG changes, ichthyosis, hyperkeratosis palmaris et plantaris, epiphyseal dysplasia, short metatarsal bones, syndactyly, hammer toe, pes cavus, and osteochondritis.

Refsum, S. Heredoataxia hemerolopica polyneuritiformis-et tidligere ikke beskrevet familiar syndrome? En forelobig moddelelse. *Nord. Med.*, 1945, 28:2682-5. Thiébaut, F., *et al.* Deux syndromes oto-neuro-oculistique d'origine congénitale. Leur rapport avec la phocomatose de van der Hoeve et autres dysplasies neuro-éctodermiques. *Rev. Neur., Paris,* 1939-40, 72:71-5.

Refsum syndrome. See *Refsum disease.*

Refsum-Thiébaut disease. See *Refsum disease.*

REGALA, ARSENIO C. (American physician)

Stransky-Regala syndrome. See *under Stransky.*

regional enteritis. See *Crohn disease.*

regional ileitis. See *Crohn disease.*

regressive periosteal enchondral hyperosteogenesis. See *Caffey-Silverman syndrome.*

REICHEL, PAUL FRIEDRICH (German physician, 1858-1934)

Reichel syndrome. Synonyms: *Henderson-Jones syndrome, Reichel-Jones-Henderson syndrome, synovial osteochondromatosis.*

A condition seen in chondromatosis, characterized by the presence of bodies which contain either cartilage or bone or both. At first, the bodies are attached to the synovial membrane by pedicles, but later they become detached and wander about in the joints, bursae, and tendon sheaths.

Reichel, P. Chondromatose der Kniegelenkskapsel. *Arch. Klin. Chir., Berlin,* 1900, 61:717-24. Jones, H. T. Loose body formation in synovial osteochondromatosis with special reference to the etiology and pathology. *J. Bone Joint Surg.*, 1924, 6:407-58. *Henderson, M. S. Osteocartilaginous joint bodies. *Railway Surg. J.*, 1918, 25:49-53.

Reichel-Jones-Henderson syndrome. See *Reichel syndrome.*

REICHERT, A. (American physician)

Ruvalcaba-Reichert-Smith syndrome. See *Ruvalcaba syndrome (1).*

REICHERT, FREDERICK LEET (American physician)

Reichert syndrome. Synonyms: *cruciate geniculate ganglion neuralgia, tic douloureux of the glossopharyngeal nerve, tic douloureux of Jacobson nerve, tympanic plexus neuralgia.*

Neuralgia of the glossopharyngeal nerve. In the complete form, paroxysms of pain, which start in the tonsillar fossa or base of the tongue, radiate deeply into the ear. Symptoms are associated with salivation, and are precipitated by movements of the tongue or throat. In the partial form, the tympanic plexus is involved and the paroxysms of pain in the vicinity of the external auditory canal occur without any movement of the tongue or pharynx.

Reichert, F. L. Tympanic plexus neuralgia. True tic douloureux of the ear or so-called cruciate geniculate ganglion neuralgia: Cure affected by intracranial section of the glossopharyngeal nerve. *JAMA,* 1933, 100:1744-6.

REICHMANN, FRIEDA (German physician)

Goldstein-Reichmann syndrome. See *under Goldstein.*

REICHMANN, NICOLAS. See REJCHMAN, MIKOLAJ

REIFENSTEIN, EDWARD CONRAD, JR. (American physician, born 1908)

Klinefelter-Reifenstein-Albright syndrome. See *chromosome XXY syndrome.*

Reifenstein syndrome. Synonyms: *hereditary familial hypogonadism, partial androgen insensitivity syndrome.*

A syndrome of male pseudohermaphroditism with partial deficiency of androgen receptors, hypospadias, hypogonadism, gynecomastia, and normal XY karyotype. The affected males are sterile, but germ cells with mitotic activity are present in the testes; there are no spermatozoa. Associated disorders include delayed puberty, absence of the beard, short stature, and abnormally high excretion of follicle-stimulating hormone. The size of the phallus and libido are normal. The syndrome is familial and its transmission is consistent with X-linked recessive inheritance.

Reifenstein, E. C., Jr. Hereditary familial hypogonadism. *Proc. Am. Fed. Clin. Res.*, 1947, 3:86.

REILLY, J. (French physician)

Reilly syndrome. Synonyms: *irritation syndrome, splanchnic vasoplegia, sympathetic irritation syndrome.*

A microcirculatory disorder of various organs, due to irritation of the autonomic nervous system by allergens, bacterial toxins, and physical irritants, marked by vasomotor disorders, increased capillary permeability, edema, and lesions of the reticuloendothelial system.

Reilly, J., *et al.* Hémorragie, lésion vasculaire et lymphatique du tube digéstif détérminées par l'injection périsplanchnique de substances diverses. *C. Rend. Soc. Biol.*, 1934, 116:24-6.

REILLY, WILLIAM ANTHONY (American physician, born 1901)

Alder-Reilly anomaly. See *under Alder.*

REIN, CHARLES R. (American physician)

Wise-Rein disease. See *Kaposi disease (1).*

REINHARDT, K. (German physician)

Reinhardt-Pfeiffer syndrome. Synonyms: *ulnofibular dysplasia, Reinhardt-Pfeiffer type.*

A syndrome of dwarfism with mesomelic brachymelia, radial bowing of the forearm with ulnar deviation of the hand, restricted movement of the forearm, and lateral bowing of the fibula with a cutaneous dimple at the apex of the angulation. Radiographic findings show a shortened ulna with defective ossification of its distal epiphysis and hyperplasia of the interosseous shaft; radial bowing; radiovolar angulation of the articular surface and dislocation of the head; shortening of the fibula and angulation of the shaft; and short and plump tibia with hypoplasia of its distal epiphysis, lateral angulation of the distal articular suface, and fibular deviation of the talus. The syndrome is transmitted as an autosomal dominant trait.

*Reinhardt, K., & Pfeiffer, R. A. Ulno-fibulare Dysplasie. Eine autosomal-dominant vererbte mikromesomelie ähnlich dem Nievergelt Syndrom. *Fortschr. Geb. Roentgen.*, 1967, 107:379-91.

ulnofibular dysplasia, Reinhardt-Pfeiffer type. See *Reinhardt-Pfeiffer syndrome.*

REINKE, FRIEDRICH (German physician)

Reinke edema. Subepithelial edema of the vocal cords produced by drugs, sometimes associated with malignant degeneration.

Reinke, F. Untersuchungen über das menschliche Stimmband. *Fortsch. Med.*, 1895, 13:469-78.

REIS, HEINRICH MARIA WILHELM (German ophthalmologist, born 1872)

Reis-Bücklers syndrome. Synonyms: *Bücklers dystrophy, annular corneal dystrophy, ring-like corneal dystrophy.*

A familial form of corneal dystrophy, transmitted as an autosomal dominant trait, characterized by annular grayish lesions of the Bowman membrane with secondary involvement of the epithelium and superficial part of the stroma. The lesions, after merging, give the impression of a geographic area when viewed under the slit lamp. Ulcers and absence of sensitivity may result. Pathological findings may show complete loss of the Bowman membrane with deposition of eosinophilic PAS-positive subepithelial material or its thickening and degeneration.

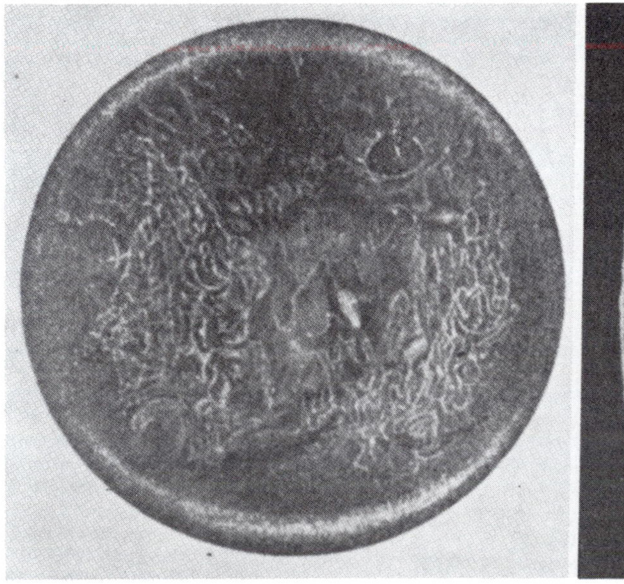

Reis-Bücklers syndrome
Bücklers, M., *Klin. Monats. Augenh.* 114:386, 1949. Stuttgart, W. Germany.

Reis, W. Familiäre, fleckige Hornhautentartung. *Deut. Med. Wschr.*, 1917, 43:575. Bücklers, M. Über eine weitere familiäre Hornhautdystrophie (Reis). *Klin. Mbl. Augenh.*, 1949, 114:386-97.

REITER, HANS CONRAD (German physician, 1881-1969)

Fiessinger-Leroy-Reiter syndrome. See *Reiter syndrome.*

Reiter disease (RD). See *Reiter syndrome.*

Reiter syndrome (RS). Synonyms: *Fiessinger-Leroy syndrome, Fiessinger-Leroy-Reiter syndrome, Reiter disease (RD), Reiter triad, Waelsch urethritis, arthritic spirochetosis, blenorrhagic balantiform keratoderma with oral involvement, conjunctivo-urethrosynovial syndrome, infectious uroarthritis, nongonococcal urethritis with conjunctivitis and arthritis, oculo-urethro-articular syndrome, polyarthritis enterica, postdysenteric rheumatoid, postdysenteric syndrome, Ruhr rheumatism, postenteric rheumatoid, spirochaetosis arthritica, urethral arthritis, urethral rheumatism, urethro-oculosynovial syndrome, uroarthritis.*

A triad of arthritis, conjunctivitis, and urethritis, occurring predominantly in young males, although it has been seen in some females. Urethral involvement consists of itching and burning sensation, reddening of the meatus, and discharge. Cystitis, dysuria, pyuria, and hematuria may be associated. Polyarthritis, usually affecting the weight-bearing joints of the lower limbs, and also involving the shoulder, fingers, and sacrum, is the main feature of this disorder. There may be bone atrophy, decalcification, and a change of color in the skin covering the affected joints. Ocular disorders usually include conjunctivitis with photophobia, epiphora, and mucopurulent discharge. Skin lesions, usually observed on the palms and soles and occasionally on the trunk and extremities, resemble keratosis blennorrhagica and pustular psoriasis. Slightly elevated areas sometimes surrounded by whitish circinate lines are the principal lesions of the buccal mucosa, lips, and gingiva. The palate and tongue may be also involved. The etiology is unclear, but pleuropneumonialike organisms and *Chlamydia* are suspected as possible etiologic factors.

Reiter, H. Über eine bisher unerkannte Spirochäten-Infecktion (Spirochaetosis arthritica). *Deut. Med. Wschr.*, 1916, 42:1535-6. Fiessinger, N., & Leroy, E. Contribution à l'étude d'une épidémie de dysenterie dans la Somme (juliett-octobre, 1916). *Bull. Soc. Méd. Hôp., Paris*, 1916, 40:2030-69. Waelsch, L. Über chronische nicht gonorrhoische Urethritis. *Arch. Derm. Syph., Berlin*, 1916, 123:1089-105.

Reiter triad. See *Reiter syndrome.*

REJCHMAN (REICHMANN), MIKOLAJ (NICOLAS) (Polish physician, 1851-1918)

Reichmann disease. See *Rejchman disease.*

Rejchman disease. Synonyms: *Reichmann disease, gastrosuccorrhea.*

Excessive continuous secretion of gastric juice. See also *Rossbach disease.*

Rejchman, M. Przypadek chorobowo wzmozonego wydzielania soku zoladkowego. *Gaz. Lek., Warszawa*, 1882, 2:516-22.

rejection encephalopathy syndrome. Encephalopathy associated with convulsions, headache, confusion, disorientation, irritability, and papilledema, occurring during rejection crises after kidney transplantation.

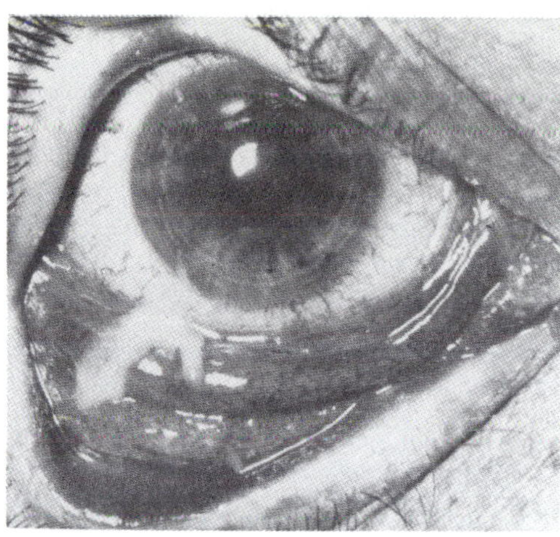

Reiter syndrome
Duke-Elder, S.: *System of Ophthalmology.* Vol. VIII, Part I, Diseases of the outer eye. London: Henry Kimpton, 1965.

Gross, M. L. P., *et al.* Rejection encephalopathy. An acute neurological syndrome complicating renal transplantations. *J. Neur. Sc.*, 1982, 56:23-34.

relapsing myositis. See *McLetchie-Aikens syndrome.*

relapsing nodular panniculitis. See *Weber-Christian syndrome, under Weber, Frederick Parkes.*

relapsing nonsuppurative nodular panniculitis. See *Weber-Christian syndrome, under Weber, Frederick Parkes.*

relapsing polychondritis. See *Meyenburg-Altherr-Uehlinger syndrome.*

relative polycythemia. See *Gaisböck disease.*

REM syndrome. See *reticular erythematous mucinosis syndrome.*

REMAK, ERNST JULIUS (German physician, 1849-1911)

Remak paralysis. See *lead poisoning.*

Remak syndrome. See *lead poisoning.*

remitting seronegative symmetrical synovitis with pitting edema. See *RS3PE syndrome.*

REMONDINI, DAVID J. (American physician)

Osebold-Remondini syndrome. See *under Osebold.*

renal compression syndrome. Perirenal compression of normal kidney parenchyma producing renin-mediated hypertension. Subcapsular hematoma, perirenal fibrosis following surgery or trauma, and congenital lesions are the potential etiologic factors.

Krane, R. J., *et al.* The renal compression syndrome. *Am. J. Surg.*, 1976, 132:396-9.

renal cystine disease. See *cystinosis.*

renal glomerulohyalinosis-diabetes syndrome. See *Kimmelstiel-Wilson syndrome.*

renal salt losing syndrome. Synonyms: *pseudo-Addison syndrome, Thorn syndrome, salt losing nephritis, salt losing nephropathy, salt wasting renal disease, sodium losing nephropathy.*

A disorder simulating Addison disease, characterized by excessive urinary excretion of salt due to faulty renal reabsorption in the absence of adrenocortical dysfunction. A failure to conserve sodium is usually a complication of diseases in which medullary damage is prominent, e.g., analgesic nephropathy, obstructive nephropathy, pyelonephritis, nephronophthisis, and polycystic disease. There may be decreased blood sodium and increased potassium levels. The most prominent symptoms are weakness, fatigue, fainting, giddiness, muscular cramps, anorexia, nausea, vomiting, and, later, hypotension and coma. See also *cerebral salt wasting syndrome.*

Thorn, G. W., *et al.* Renal failure simulating adrenocortical insufficiency. *N. Engl. J. Med.*, 1944, 231:76-85.

renal tubular acidosis. See *Lightwood-Albright syndrome.*

renal tubular acidosis-nerve deafness syndrome. A syndrome, transmitted as an autosomal recessive trait, characterized by renal tubular acidosis, progressive nerve deafness, and carbonic anhydrase B deficiency.

Nance, W. E., & Sweeney, A. Evidence for autosomal recessive inheritance of the syndrome of renal tubular acidosis with deafness. *Birth Defects*, 1971, 7(4):70-72.

renal vein compression syndrome. See *nutcracker syndrome.*

renal vein entrapment syndrome. See *nutcracker syndrome.*

renal-anal-lung-polydactyly-hamartoblastoma (RALPH) syndrome. See *Hall syndrome, under Hall, J. G.*

renal-ocular syndrome. Acute interstitial nephritis with acute iritis in otherwise healthy persons. See also *Senior syndrome (1).*

Steinman, T. I., Silva, P. Acute interstitial nephritis and iritis. Renal-ocular syndrome. *Am. J. Med.*, 1984, 77:189-91.

renal-retinal dysplasia syndrome. See *Senior syndrome (1).*

renal-retinal dystrophy. See *Senior syndrome (1).*

renal-splanchnic steal. See *Alfidi syndrome.*

RENAULT, P. (French physician)

Touraine-Renault syndrome. See *under Touraine, A.*

RENDU, HENRI JULES LOUIS MARIE (French physician, 1844-1902)

Fiessinger-Rendu syndrome. See *Stevens-Johnson syndrome.*

Osler-Rendu-Weber syndrome. See *under Osler.*

Rendu-Osler syndrome. See *Osler-Rendu-Weber syndrome.*

renofacial dysplasia. See *Potter syndrome (1), under Potter, Edith Louise.*

renofacial syndrome. See *Potter syndrome (1), under Potter, Edith Louise.*

RENON, LOUIS (French physician, 1863-1922)

Rénon-Delille syndrome. Synonyms: *acromegaly-thyro-ovarian insufficiency syndrome, thyro-ovarian insufficiency-acromegaly syndrome.*

Thyroid and ovarian insufficiency associated with hypophyseal hyperfunction and acromegaly. Hypotension, tachycardia, hyperhidrosis, oliguria, insomnia, and intolerance to heat may be associated.

Rénon, L., & Delille, A. Insuffisance thyro-ovarienne et hyperactivité hypophysaire (troubles acromégalique). Amélioration par l'opothérapie thyro-ovarienne; augmentation de l'acromégalie par la médication hypophysaire. *Bull. Soc. Méd. Hôp. Paris*, 1908, 25:973-9.

renovascular hypertension. See *Goldblatt syndrome.*

RENPENNING, H. (Canadian physician)

Martin-Bell-Renpenning syndrome. See *chromosome X fragility.*

Renpenning syndrome. See *chromosome X fragility.*

reperfusion syndrome. Tissue edema with capillary swelling taking place immediately after re-establishment of circulation following a period of ischemia. The disorder is frequently observed in the kidneys, myocardium, and brain, and is characterized by exudative edema and microhemorrhage that lead to increased vascular resistance and decreased blood flow. Reperfusion after revascularization of ischemic lower extremities may cause the development of compartment syndrome, myoglobinuria, renal failure, rethrombosis, limb loss, myocardial depression, and death (*revascularization syndrome*).

Shah, D. M., *et al.* Defects in peripheral oxygen utilization following trauma and shock. *Arch. Surg.*, 1981, 116:1277-81. Buchbinder, D., *et al.* Hyperatonic mannitol. Its use in the prevention of revascularization syndrome after acute arterial ischemia. *Arch. Surg.*, 1981, 116:414-21.

repetition strain injury (RSI). See *overuse syndrome.*

repetitive motion injury. See *overuse syndrome.*

repetitive paroxysmal tachycardia. See *torsades de pointes syndrome.*

repetitive strain syndrome. See *overuse syndrome.*

residual abscess. See *Paget abscess.*

residual ovary syndrome. Synonym: *postoperative residual ovary syndrome.*

Pelvic mass, pain, and dyspareunia, singly or in various combinations, seen in patients who have undergone hysterectomy with the preservation of one or both ovaries. The disorder is associated with the presence of adhesions which prevent free access to the peritoneal cavity, thus resulting in an accumulation of follicular products accompanied by the formation of a mass with cystic and solid components.

Grogan, R. H. Residual ovaries. *Obstet. Gynecol.*, 1958, 12:329-32.

resistance to thyroid hormone. See *Refetoff syndrome.*

resistant ovary syndrome. Synonym: *Savage syndrome.*

A syndrome characterized by primary amenorrhea or secondary amenorrhea before the age of 30 years, chromosomal complement 46/XX with normally developed secondary sexual characteristics, increased endogenous production of follicle-stimulating and luteinizing hormones, the presence of morphologically normal ovarian follicles, and resistance to the administration of human gonadotropins.

Jones, G. S., & De Moraes-Ruehsen, M. A new syndrome of amenorrhea in association with hypergonadotropism and apparently normal ovarian follicular apparatus. *Am. J. Obst. Gyn.*, 1969, 104:597-600.

respirator lung syndrome. Synonyms: *Banerjee syndrome, bronchopulmonary dysplasia (BPD).*

A respiratory disorder in newborn infants treated for respiratory distress syndrome with the use of a respirator and 80-100 % oxygen. The symptoms include persistence of the respiratory distress syndrome, radiopacity of the lungs, cystic pulmonary lesions, focal emphysema, and right congestive heart failure.

Banerjee, C. K., *et al.* Pulmonary fibroplasia in newborn babies treated with oxygen and artificial ventilation. *Arch. Dis. Child., Chicago*, 1972, 47:509. Taybi, H. *Radiology of syndromes*, Chicago, Year Book Medical Publishers, 1975, p. 38.

respiratory distress syndrome (RDS). See *adult respiratory distress syndrome, and see neonatal respiratory distress syndrome.*

respiratory distress syndrome of Wilson and Mikity. See *Wilson-Mikity syndrome under Wilson, Miriam Geisendorfer.*

respiratory insufficiency of obesity. See *Pickwick syndrome.*

REST (Raynaud phenomenon-esophageal motor dysfunction-sclerodactyly-telangiectasia) syndrome. A variant of the CREST syndrome characterized by the Raynaud phenomenon, esophageal motor dysfunction, sclerodactyly, and telangiectasia. Complications may include anemia due to gastric hemorrhage.

Allende, H. D., *et al.* Bleeding gastric telangiectasia. Complication of Raynaud's phenomenon, esophageal motor dysfunction, sclerodactyly and telangiectasia (REST) syndrome. *Am. J. Gastroenterol.*, 1981, 75:374-6.

restless leg syndrome (RLS). Synonyms: *Ekbom syndrome, Wittmaack-Ekbom syndrome, anxietas tibiarum, asthenia crurum dolorosa, athenia crurum paresthetica, hereditary acromelalgia, leg jitters, moving toe syndrome, painful leg syndrome, periodic leg movement (PLM).*

A sensory motor disorder characterized by fidgeting and an irrestible urge to move the legs, especially when sitting or lying down. Nonpainful discomfort in the gastrocnemius muscle is the principal feature. In many instances there is paresthesia with creeping crawling, pricking, and itchy sensations that may or may not be associated with pain. Weakness in the legs and a feeling of cold in the feet are sometimes associated. Many patients experience myoclonic jerks. The condition may lead to insomnia. The symptoms usually disappear in the morning. The disorder frequently occurs as a familial condition transmitted as an autosomal dominant trait. Sudden body jerks on falling asleep may be observed also in otherwise normal persons.

Ekbom, K. A. Restless legs. A clinical study of a hitherto overlooked disease in the legs characterized by peculiar paresthesia ("anxietas tibiarum"), pain and weakness and occurring in two main forms, asthenia crurum paraesthetica and asthenia crurum dolorosa. A short review of paresthesias in general. *Acta Med. Scand.*, 1945, Suppl. 158:1-123. *Wittmaack, T. *Pathologie und Therapie der Sensibilitätsneurosen.* Leipzig, 1861. Huizinga, J. Hereditary acromalalgia (or "restless legs"). *Acta Genet. Statist. Med.*, 1957, 7:121-3. Oswald, I. Sudden bodily jerks on falling asleep. *Brain*, 1959, 82:92-103.

retained, excluded antrum syndrome (REAS). Gastrojejunal stomal ulceration after partial gastrectomy with gastrojejunostomy, when the antrum has been retained but excluded from contact with acid secretion or food.

Korman, M. G., *et al.* Hypergastrinaemia due to an excluded gastric antrum. A proposed method for differentiation from the Zollinger-Ellison syndrome. *Aust. NZ J. Med.*, 1972, 2;266-71. Friesen, S. R., & Tomita, T. Further experience with pseudo-Zollinger-Ellison syndrome: Its place in the management of neuroendocrine duodenal ulceration. *World J. Surg.*, 1984, 8:552-60.

retching erosion syndrome. See *Mallory-Weiss syndrome.*

retention hyperlipemia. See *Bürger-Grütz syndrome.*

RETHORE, MARIE ODILE (French physician)

Rethoré syndrome. See *chromosome 9p duplication syndrome.*

reticular dysgenesia. See *Vaal-Seynhaeve syndrome.*

reticular dysgenesis-congenital aleukia syndrome. See *Vaal-Seynhaeve syndrome.*

reticular erythematous mucinosis (REM) syndrome. Synonyms: *Steigleder syndrome, reticulated erythema with mucinosis.*

Reticular erythematosis characterized by a reddish or bluish, sometimes infiltrated, pruritic eruption of the trunk and neck. The lesions are ill defined and frequently irregular in shape. Pathological examination shows perivascular lymphocytic infiltrates. Exposure to sunlight exacerbates the eruption.

Steigleder, G. K., *et al.* Syndrome retikuläre erythematöse Mucinosis (Rundzellenerythematosis). *Zschr. Haut. Geschlkr.*, 1974, 49:235-8.

reticular pigmented anomaly of the flexures. See *Dowling-Degos disease.*

reticular pigmented dermatosis. See *Naegeli syndrome, under Naegeli, Oskar.*

reticulate acropigmentation. See *Kitamura disease.*

reticulate acropigmentation of Kitamura (RAPK). See *Kitamura disease.*

reticulated erythema with mucinosis. See *reticular erythematous mucinosis syndrome.*

reticulated pigmented poikiloderma. See *Riehl melanosis.*

reticulocytopenia. See *Gasser syndrome (2).*

reticuloendotheliosis with eosinophilia. See *Omenn syndrome.*

reticulohistiocytosis cutanea hyperplastica benigna cum melanodermia. See *Sézary syndrome.*

reticulum-cell sarcoma of bone. See *Parker-Jackson syndrome, under Parker, Frederick, Jr.*

retinal angiomatosis. See *Hippel-Lindau syndrome.*

retinal capillary hamartoma. See *Hippel-Lindau syndrome.*

retinal disinsertion syndrome. Retinal disinsertion asociated with subluxation of the lens, microphthalmos, and keratoconus. Mental retardation may be present.

Shammas, H. J., & McGaughey, A. S. Retinal disinsertion syndrome: Report of a case. *J. Pediat. Ophth. Strabismus*, 1979, 16:284-6.

retinal dysplasia syndrome. See *Reese syndrome.*

retinal pigmentary degeneration-microcephaly-mental retardation syndrome. See *Mirhosseini-Holmes-Walton syndrome.*

retinal telangiectasia. See *Coats syndrome.*

retinitis cachectica et carcinoma ventriculi. See *Pick retinitis, under Pick, Ludwig.*

retinitis cachecticorum. See *Pick retinitis, under Pick, Ludwig.*

retinitis centralis angioneurotica. See *Masuda-Kitahara disease.*

retinitis centralis annularis. See *Masuda-Kitahara disease.*

retinitis centralis capillarospastica. See *Masuda-Kitahara disease.*

retinitis centralis recidivans. See *Masuda-Kitahara disease.*

retinitis hemorrhagica externa. See *Coats syndrome.*

retinitis pigmentosa-congenital deafness syndrome. See *Usher syndrome.*

retinitis proliferans. See *Eales syndrome.*

retinitis punctata albescens. See *Lauber disease.*

retino-otodiabetic syndrome. See *Alström syndrome.*
retinocerebral angiomatosis. See *Hippel-Lindau syndrome.*
retinochoroiditis juxtapapillaris. See *Jensen disease.*
retinohepato-endocrinologic (RHE) syndrome. A familial syndrome, transmitted as an autososmal recessive trait, characterized by total color blindness due to progressive cone dystrophy, liver degeneration with elevated transaminase levels and fatty infiltration, and endocrine dysfunction (hypothyroidism, maturity-onset diabetes mellitus, protracted thyrotropic-releasing hormone test response indicating a hypothalamic disorder, defective ACTH reserve, recurrent abortions, and infertility). Hypertension, progressive hearing loss, enlarged sella turcica, and the empty sella syndrome occur in some cases.

Froyshov Larsen, I., *et al.* Familial syndrome of progressive cone dystrophy, degenerative liver disease and endocrine dysfunction. II. Clinical and metabolic studies. *Clin. Genet.*, 1978, 13:176-89.

retinopathy of prematurity. See *retrolental fibroplasia.*
retinoschisis with early hemerolopia. See *Favre-Goldman syndrome.*
retractio bulbi. See *Stilling-Türk-Duane syndrome.*
retraction nystagmus. See *Koerber-Salus-Elschnig syndrome.*
retraction syndrome. See *Stilling-Türk-Duane syndrome.*
retrocalcaneal bursitis. See *Sever syndrome.*
retrocecal hernia. See *Rieux hernia.*
retrolental fibroplasia (RLF). Synonyms: *Terry syndrome, retinopathy of prematurity.*

A disease of premature infants exposed to high oxygen concentrations, in which the chief manifestation is a grayish white, opaque membrane behind each crystalline lens. Other symptoms include dilation and tortuosity of the retinal vessels, hemorrhage, neovascularization of the iris, anterior and posterior synechiae, pallor of the optic disk, retinal folds, retrolental mass, retinal pigmentation changes, leukokoria, myopia, cataract, and retinal detachment. The condition may also occur in infants with immature retinal vessels who have not been exposed to high oxygen concentrations.

Terry, T. L. Extreme prematurity and fibroblastic overgrowth of peristent vascular sheath behind each crystalline lens. I. Preliminary report. *Am. J. Ophth.*, 1942, 25:203-4.

retrolenticular syndrome. See *Déjerine-Roussy syndrome.*
retroparotid space syndrome. See *Villaret syndrome.*
retroperitoneal fibrosis-scleroderma syndrome. Retroperitoneal fibrosis associated with systemic sclerosis in patients positive for the HLA-B27 antigen.

Mansell, M. A., & Watts, R. W. E. Retroperitoneal fibrosis and scleroderma. *Postgrad. Med. J.*, 1980, 56:730-3.

retroperitoneal hernia. See *Treitz hernia.*
retrosphenoidal space syndrome. See *Jacod syndrome.*
retrosphenoidal syndrome. See *Jacod syndrome.*
RETT, ANDREAS (Austrian physician)
Rett syndrome (RS). A mental retardation syndrome, occurring exclusively in females, characterized by acquired microcephaly, severe dementia, autism, loss of purposeful use of the hands, characteristic hand-wringing stereotypy, and jerky ataxia of the trunk. The affected children are born clinically normal, but their psychomotor development stagnates and deteriorates between the ages of 6 months and 2.5 years. After the appearance of initial symptoms there is a period of relative stability, followed by additional symptoms, including epileptic seizures, spastic paraparesis, and vasomotor disorders in the lower limbs. The syndrome is believed to be transmitted as an X-linked dominant trait with lethality in the hemizygous males.

Rett, A. Über eine eigenartiges hirnatrophisches Syndrom bei Hyperammonämie in Kindesalter. *Wien. Klin. Wschr.*, 1966, 116:723-38. Opitz, J. M., Reynolds, J. F., Spano, L. M., & Moser, H. W., eds. The Rett syndrome. *Am. J. Med. Genet.*, 1986, 24(Suppl. 1):1-415.

revascularization syndrome. See *reperfusion syndrome.*
reverse Colles fracture. See *Smith fracture, under Smith, Robert William.*
reverse Gougerot-Sjögren syndrome. See *Creyx-Lévy syndrome.*
reverse Horner syndrome. See *under Horner.*
reverse jaw-winking syndrome. See *Marin Amat syndrome.*
reverse Sjögren syndrome. See *Creyx-Lévy syndrome.*
reverse urea syndrome. See *under disequilibrium syndrome.*
reversed coarctation of aorta. See *aortic arch syndrome.*
REVOL, L. (French hematologist)
Revol disease. See *Mortensen disease.*
Revol syndrome. See *Glanzmann thrombasthenia.*
REYE, E. (German physician)
Reye-Sheehan syndrome. See *Sheehan syndrome.*

REYE, R. D. K. (Australian physician)
Reye syndrome (RS). Synonyms: *Reye-Johnson syndrome, Reye-Morgan-Baral syndrome, fatty liver-encephalopathy syndrome, white liver disease.*

An acute disease of children under the age of 15 years, characterized by fatty degeneration of the liver and encephalopathy. The symptoms, usually appearing after an respiratory tract infection (such as chickenpox or influenza), consist mainly of vomiting and progressive central nervous system disorders manifested by stupor, convulsions, and coma. Laboratory findings show hypoglycemia, metabolic acidosis, increased serum aminotransferases, and high prothrombin time. Pathological changes include fatty vacuolization of the liver and renal tubules, cerebral edema, neuronal degeneration of the brain, astrocytic swelling, and intracranial hypertension. The etiology is unknown but viruses and toxic agents are suspected. Some cases occur after febrile conditions in children who have received aspirin, but others have been observed in the absence of exposure to salicylates.

Reye, R. D., Morgan, G., & Baral, J. Encephalopathy and fatty degeneration of the viscera. *Lancet*, 1963, 2:749-52.

Reye-Johnson syndrome. See *Reye syndrome.*
Reye-like syndrome. A syndrome of vomiting, drowsiness, metabolic acidosis, and encephalopathy, which simulates the Reye syndrome. Medium chain acyl-CoA dehydrogenase deficiency of mitochondrial beta-oxidation frequently masquarades as the Reye syndrome. Reye-like symptoms may be also produced by margosa oil poisoning.

Sinniah, D., & Baskaran, G. Margosa oil poisoning-as a cause of Reye's syndrome. *Lancet*, 1981, I:487-9. Roe, C. R., *et al.* Recognition of medium-chain acyl-CoA dehydrogenase deficiency in asymptomatic siblings of children dying of sudden infant death or Reye-like syndromes. J. Pediat., 1986, 108:13-8.

Reye-Morgan-Baral syndrome. See *Reye syndrome.*

REYNIER, JEAN PIERRE, DE (French physician, born 1914)

Nager-de Reynier syndrome. See under Nager.

REYNOLDS, TELFER B. (American physician)

Reynolds syndrome. A syndrome of chronic liver disease (primary biliary cirrhosis, jaundice, elevated alkaline phosphatase activity), scleroderma, the Raynaud phenomenon, calcinosis cutis, telangiectasia, pruritus, and a positive test for serum mitochondrial activity.

Reynolds, T. B., *et al.* Primary biliary cirrhosis with scleroderma, Raynaud phenomenon and telangiectasia. A new syndrome. *Am. J. Med.*, 1971, 50:302-12.

REYS, L. (French physician)

Weill-Reys syndrome. See *Adie syndrome.*

Weill-Reys-Adie syndrome. See *Adie syndrome.*

rhabdomyosis. See *compartment syndrome.*

RHE. See *retinohepato-endocrinologic syndrome.*

RHEINHARD

Rheinhard myocarditis. Fiedler myocarditis associated with extensive eosinophilic infiltrations.

Larcon, A. A. A propos des gros coeurs dits primitifs. *Gaz. Méd. Hôp. Paris,* 1958, 130:897-907.

rheumapyra. See *Bouillaud syndrome.*

rheumarthritis. See *Bouillaud disease.*

rheumatic brachio-cephalic arteritis. See *aortic arch syndrome.*

rheumatic chorea. See *Sydenham chorea.*

rheumatic fever. See *Bouillaud disease.*

rheumatic pain modulation disorder (RPMD). See *fibrositis-fibromyalgia syndrome.*

rheumatic panchondritis. See *Meyenburg-Altherr-Uehlinger syndrome.*

rheumatic sciatica. See *Putti syndrome.*

rheumatic sialosis. See *Sjögren syndrome, under Sjögren, Henrik Samuel Conrad.*

rheumatism of hypercorticism. See *Slocumb syndrome.*

rheumatismal ossifying pelvispondylitis. See *Bechterew-Strümpell-Marie syndrome, under Bekhterev.*

rheumatismus cordis. See *Bouillaud syndrome.*

rheumatoid acro-steolysis. See *Marie-Léri syndrome, under Marie, Pierre.*

rheumatoid arthritis-hypersplenism syndrome. See *Felty syndrome.*

rheumatoid arthritis-pneumoconiosis syndrome. See *Caplan syndrome.*

rheumatoid arthritis-splenomegaly-leukopenia syndrome. See *Felty syndrome.*

rheumatoid lung silicosis. See *Caplan syndrome.*

rheumatoid pneumoconiosis. See *Caplan syndrome.*

rheumatoid pneumoconiosis syndrome. See *Caplan syndrome.*

rheumatoid spondylitis. See *Bechterew-Strümpell-Marie syndrome, under Bekhterev.*

rheumatopyra. See *Bouillaud disease.*

rhinogenic polyarteritis. See *Wegener granulomatosis.*

rhizomelic syndrome. A familial syndrome, transmitted as an autosomal recessive trait, characterized by rhizomelia of the arms, short stature, hip dislocation, digitalization of the thumb with bifid distal phalanx, microcephaly, large anterior fontanel, micrognathia, and pulmonary stenosis.

Urbach, I. D., *et al.* A new skeletal dysplasia syndrome with rhizomelia of the humeri and other malformations. *Clin. Genet.*, 1986, 29:83-7.

rhizomelic chondrodysplasia punctata syndrome. See *Spranger syndrome (1).*

rhizomelic pseudopolyarthritis. See *Forestier syndrome (1).*

rhizomelic spondylosis. See *Bechterew-Strümpell-Marie syndrome, under Bekhterev.*

RHOADS, C. P. (British physician)

Bomford-Rhoads anemia. See *Davidson anemia.*

RHS (Ramsay Hunt syndrome). See *Hunt syndrome (1, 2, and 3).*

rib gap defects with micrognathia. See *cerebrocostomandibular syndrome.*

rib syndrome. See *slipping rib syndrome.*

rib-tip syndrome. See *slipping rib syndrome.*

RIBBING, SEVED (Swedish radiologist, born 1902)

Müller-Ribbing-Clément syndrome. See *multiple epiphyseal dysplasia I.*

Ribbing disease. See *multiple epiphyseal dysplasia I.*

Ribbing syndrome. Synonym: *hereditary multiple diaphyseal sclerosis.*

A familial syndrome, transmitted as an autosomal dominant trait, characterized by diaphyseal osteosclerosis and hyperostosis affecting one to four long bones.

Ribbing, S. Hereditary, multiple, diaphyseal sclerosis. *Acta Radiol., Stockholm,* 1949, 31:522-36.

Ribbing-Müller disease. See *multiple epiphyseal dysplasia I.*

RICCI, VINCENZO (Italian physician)

Cacchi-Ricci syndrome. See *under Cacchi.*

rice millers' syndrome. A disease due to an exposure to rice husk dust, characterized by irritation of the eyes, skin, and upper respiratory tract and allergic responses such as nasal catarrh, tightness of the chest, asthma, and eosinophilia. Pulmonary opacities, probably representing early stages of silicosis, and extrinsic allergic alveolitis are the principal radiographic findings.

Lim, H. H., *et al.* Rice millers' syndrome: A preliminary report. *Brit. J. Indust. Med.*, 1984, 41:445-9.

RICH, ARNOLD RICE (American physician, born 1893)

Hamman-Rich syndrome. See *under Hamman.*

RICHARDS, B. W. (British physician)

Richards-Rundle syndrome (RRS). Synonym: *familial ataxia-hypogonadism syndrome.*

A familial syndrome of hearing loss, mental retardation, ataxia, hypogonadism, peripheral muscle wasting, and ketoaciduria. The symptoms progress from childhood, eventually becoming static. The syndrome is transmitted as an autosomal recessive trait.

Richards, B. W., & Rundle, A. T. A familial hormonal disorder associated with mental deficiency, deaf-mutism, and ataxia. *J. Ment. Defic.*, 1959, 3:33-55.

RICHARDSON, JOHN CLIFFORD (Canadian neurologist, born 1909)

Steele-Richardson-Olszewski (SRO) syndrome. See *under Steele.*

RICHET, DIDIER DOMINIQUE ALFRED (French physician, 1816-1981)

Demarquay-Richet syndrome. See *van der Woude syndrome.*

RICHNER, HERMANN (Swiss physician, born 1908)

Richner syndrome. See *Richner-Hanhart syndrome.*

Richner-Hanhart syndrome. Synonyms: *Hanhart syndrome, Richner syndrome, keratosis palmaris et plantaris-corneal dystrophy syndrome, oculocutaneous tyrosinemia, oculocutaneous tyrosinosis, Oregon-type tyrosinemia, tyrosine aminotransferase deficiency, tyrosine transaminase deficiency, tyrosinemia type II, tyrosinosis II.*

An inborn error of amino acid metabolism, transmitted as an autosomal recessive trait, typically characterized by keratosis palmaris et plantaris, persistent dendritic lesions of the cornea with unaffected corneal sensitivity, photophobia, tearing, and mental retardation. A deficiency of hepatic tyrosine aminotransferase causes elevated tyrosine levels in the blood. Tyrosine metabolites found in high concentrations in the urine include *p*-hydroxyphenylpyruvic acid, *p*-hydroxyphenylacetic acid, and *N*-acetyltyrosine, as well as unmodified tyrosine. See also *tyrosinosis.*

Richner, H. Hornhautaffektion bei Keratoma palmare et plantare hereditarium. *Klin. Mbl. Augenh.*, 1938, 100:580-8. Hanhart, E. Neue Sonderformen von Keratosis palmoplantaris, u. a. eine regelmässig-dominante mit systematisierten Lipomen, ferner 2 einfach-rezessive mit Schwachsinn und z. T. mit Hornhautveränderungen des Auges (Ektodermalsyndrome). *Dermatologica, Basel,* 1947, 94:286-308.

RICHTER, AUGUSTUS (AUGUST) GOTTLIEB (German surgeon, 1742-1812)

Richter hernia. Synonym: *parietal hernia.*

Strangulated hernia in which only a part of the circumference of the gut is involved.

Richter, A. G. *Abhandlung von den Brüchen.* Göttingen, Dietrich, 1785. Ch. 24, pp. 596-7.

RICHTER, INA M. (American hematologist)

Clough-Richter syndrome. See *cryopathic hemolytic syndrome.*

RICHTER, MAURICE N. (American physician)

Richter syndrome. An association of chronic lymphocytic leukemia with reticulosarcoma.

Richter, M. N. Generalized reticular cell sarcoma of the lymph nodes associated with lymphatic leukemia. *Am. J. Pathol.*, 1928, 4:285-92.

ricin syndrome. See *fetal ricin syndrome.*

rickets. See *Glisson disease.*

rickets with renal tubular acidosis. See *Lightwood-Albright syndrome.*

RIDDOCH, GEORGE (British physician, 1888-1947)

Riddoch syndrome. Synonym: *visual disorientation syndrome.*

Visual disorientation in homonymous half-field without loss of stereoscopic vision, resulting from unilateral lesions of the parietal lobe.

Riddoch, G. Visual disorientation in homonymous half-fields. *Brain,* 1935, 58:376-82.

RIDELL, A. R. (American physician)

Shaver-Ridell syndrome. See *Shaver syndrome.*

RIECKE, E. (German physician)

Riecke syndrome. See *ichthyosis congenita syndrome.*

RIEDEL, BERHHARD MORITZ KARL LUDWIG (Surgeon in Jena, 1846-1916)

Riedel disease. Synonyms: *Riedel struma, Riedel thyroiditis, invasive fibrous thyroiditis, ligneous thyroiditis, strumitis fibrosa, woody thyroid.*

A form of thyroiditis, observed most commonly in middle-aged females, that develops insidiously and is manifested by compression of the surrounding structures. Attacks of suffocation due to compression of the trachea is the usual presenting symptom. The disease gives the thyroid a hard, focal or diffuse nodular appearance. Pathologically, there is a loss of the lobular structure and its replacement by collagen; the presence of the fibrous tissue of muscle fibers derived from the overlying musculature; infiltration of lymphocytes, plasma cells, neutrophils, and eosinophils in the fibrous tissue; and adenomatoid areas in the affected tissue.

Riedel, B. M. Die chronische, zur Bildung eisenharter Tumoren führende Entzündung der Schilddrüse. *Verh. Deut. Ges. Chir.*, 1986, 25:101-5.

RIEDEL, BERNHARD MORITZ KARL LUDWIG (Surgeon in Jena, 1846-1916)

Riedel struma. See *Riedel disease.*

Riedel thyroiditis. See *Riedel disease.*

RIEDER, HERMANN (German physician, 1858-1932)

Rieder paralysis. Synonyms: *knapsack paralysis, stone-carrier paralysis.*

Brachial plexus paralysis due to injury by a knapsack or a hod, as occurs in mortar and brick carriers.

Rieder, H. Die "Steinträger-Lähmung." Eine Form der combinierten Armnerven- oder Brachialplexus-Lähmung. *Münch. Med. Wschr.*, 1893, 40:121-3.

RIEGER, HERWIGH (Austrian physician)

Axenfeld-Rieger syndrome. See *Axenfeld syndrome, and see Rieger syndrome.*

Rieger anomaly. See *Rieger syndrome.*

Rieger malformation. See *Rieger syndrome.*

Rieger syndrome. Synonyms: *Rieger anomaly, Rieger malformation, dysgenesis mesodermalis corneae et iridis, dysgenesis mesostromalis anterior, dysplasia marginalis posterior, goniodysgenesis, iridocorneal mesodermal dysgenesis.*

A syndrome of malformations of the anterior chamber of the eye and the teeth, combining features of the Axenfeld syndrome with oligodontia. Eye anomalies consist of posterior embryotoxon, a prominent Schwalbe ring, iris adhesion to the Schwalbe line, hypoplasia of the anterior stroma of the iris, and occasional glaucoma. Tooth anomalies include anodontia vera, microdontia, and abnormally shaped implanted teeth. Associated symptoms may consist of broad flat nasal root, prominent supraorbital ridges, relative prognathism, and mild telecanthus with or without hypertelorism. A wide spectrum of other defects, such as short stature, myotonic dystrophy, mental deficiency, brachydactyly, clinodactyly, arachnodactyly, and polydactyly, may also occur. The condition is transmitted as an autosomal dominant trait. The Axenfeld and Rieger syndromes are suspected of being expressions of the same gene. When occurring without dental and skeletal defects, the disorder is known as the *Axenfeld syndrome*; when associated with growth retardation, it is called the *SHORT syndrome.*

Rieger, H. Dysgenesis mesodermalis corneae et iridis. *Zschr. Eugenheilk.*, 1935, 86:333. Rieger, H. Beiträge zur Kenntnis seltener Missbildungen der Iris. II. Über Hypoplasie des Irisvorderblattes mit Verlagerung und Entrundung der Papille. *Graefes Arch. Ophth.*, 1935, 133:602-35.

Trauner-Rieger syndrome. See *nail-patella syndrome.*

RIEHL, GUSTAV (Austrian physician, 1855-1943)

Riehl melanosis (RM). Synonyms: *Riehl syndrome, female facial melanosis, jute-spinner's melanosis, melanoder-*

matitis toxica, pigmented cosmetic dermatitis, reticulated pigmented poikiloderma, tar melanosis, war melanosis.

A skin disease marked by brown-violet to black reticular pigmentation of the face, forehead, neck, and occasionally of other parts unprotected by clothing, such as the hands and forearms. An increase of melanophages in the upper dermis and multiplication of the basal lamina are the characteristic histological features of this disorder. The condition was a common occupational disease in Germany during World War I. Photosensitization after exposure to tar, jute, and aniline-containing chemicals were suspected as causative factors. Benzyl salicylate or citral in cosmetics, when applied to the skin of susceptible persons, may cause the same reaction.

Riehl, G. Über eine eigenartige Melanose. *Wien. Klin. Wschr.,* 1917, 30:780-1.

Riehl syndrome. See *Riehl melanosis.*

RIETTI, FERNANDO (Italian physician, born 1929)

Micheli-Rietti syndrome. See *Rietti-Greppi-Micheli syndrome.*

Rietti disease. See *Rietti-Greppi-Micheli syndrome.*

Rietti-Greppi-Micheli syndrome. Synonyms: *Micheli-Rietti syndrome, Rietti disease, constitutional microcythemic anemia, intermediate beta-thalassemia.*

An intermediate form of thalassemia characterized by microcythemia, hemolytic jaundice, hepatomegaly, and splenomegaly.

Greppi, E. Ittero emolitico familiare con aumento della resistanza dei globuli. *Minerva Med.,* 1928, 8(pt 2):1-11. *Rietti, F. Sugli itteri emolitici primitivi. *Atti Accad. Med. Ferrara,* 1924-25, 2:14. *Micheli, F. La splenomegalie emolitiche. *35 Cong. Soc. Ital. Med. Int.,* 1929.

RIEUX, LEON (French physician)

Rieux hernia. Synonym: *retrocecal hernia.*

Retrocecal protrusion of the intestine.

*Rieux, L. *Considérations sur l'étranglement de l'intestin dans la cavité abdominale et sur une mode d'étranglement non décrit par les auteurs.* Paris, 1853. (Thesis).

RIGA, ANTONIO (Italian physician, 1832-1919)

Riga aphthae. See *Riga-Fede disease.*

Riga papilloma. See *Riga-Fede disease.*

Riga-Fede disease. Synonyms: *Cardarelli aphthae, Cardarelli disease, Fede disease, Riga aphthae, Riga papilloma, cachetic aphthae, diphtheroid subglossitis, sublingual fibrogranuloma, sublingual fibroma.*

A small sublingual ulceration in infants with natal or neonatal teeth, caused by rubbing against the lower incisors, most frequently observed in whooping cough.

*Riga, A. *Di una malattia della prima infanzia, probabilmente non trattata, di movimenti patologici.* Napoli, 1881. *Fede, F. Della produzione sottolinguale o malattia di Riga. *I. Cong. Pediat. Ital.,* Napoli, 1891, pp. 251-60.

RIGGS, JOHN M. (American dentist, 1811-1885)

Riggs disease. See *Fauchard disease.*

right hemisphere syndrome. A group of disorders occurring following lesions of the right cerebral hemisphere, including visual and spatial dysfunction, disturbances of body schema (anosognosia or asomatognosia), attention disorders (unilateral spatial neglect, motor impersistence, confusion), emotional changes (aprosodia, indifference to environment), conjugate eye deviation to the right or right grasp reaction, and writing disorders (hypergraphia).

Yamadori, A., *et al.* Hypergraphia: A right hemisphere syndrome. *J. Neur. Neurosurg. Psychiat.,* 1986, 49:1160-4.

right middle lobe syndrome (RMLS). See *middle lobe syndrome.*

right ovarian vein syndrome. Congenital malposition of the right ovarian vein, causing compression of the right ureter and external iliac artery.

*Clark, J. C. The right ovarian vein syndrome. In: Emmet, J. L., ed. *Clinical urography.* Philadelphia, Saunders, vol. 2, 1964, p. 1227.

right pneumonectomy syndrome. A condition characterized by delayed complications of right pneumonectomy, occurring mainly in children and adolescents. Dyspnea and recurrent pulmonary infections in the left lung are the principal clinical symptoms. Radiographic findings include right and posterior deviation of the mediastinum, counterclockwise rotation of the heart and great vessels, herniation of the left lung, and softening of the airways. Computed tomography may show compression of the trachea and left main bronchus between the aorta and pulmonary artery.

Shepard, J. A., *et al.* Right pneumonectomy syndrome: Radiologic findings and CT correlation. *Radiology,* 1986, 161:661-4.

right ventricle obstruction-failure. See *Bernheim syndrome.*

right ventricular hypoplasia. See *hypoplastic right heart syndrome.*

right-sided-aortic arch-mental deficiency-facial dysmorphism syndrome. See *Strong syndrome.*

rigid spinal column syndrome. See *rigid spine syndrome.*

rigid spine syndrome. Synonyms: *Dubowitz syndrome, rigid spinal column syndrome.*

A syndrome, usually occurring in male children, characterized by a slowly progressive muscle weakness and atrophy, limitation of neck and trunk flexion, scoliosis, joint contractures, increased serum creatinine phosphokinase levels, and abnormal electromyographic patterns. The syndrome is believed to be transmitted as an X-linked trait and may be related to the Emery-Dreifuss syndrome.

Dubowitz, V. "Pseudo" muscular dystrophy. *Proc. 3rd Symposium. Research Committee of the Muscular Dystrophy Group of Great Britain,* 1965, pp. 57-73. Dubowitz, V. Rigid spine syndrome in search of a name. *Proc. Roy. Soc. Med.,* 1973, 66:219-20.

RILEY, CONRAD MILTON (American physician, born 1913)

Riley-Day syndrome. Synonyms: *congenital autonomic dysfunction syndrome, familial dysautonomia I, functional dysautonomia.*

A congenital disorder of the autonomic nervous system, transmitted as an autosomal recessive trait, occurring primarily in Ashkenazi Jewish children. It is characterized by the lack of tears, blotching of the skin, hyperhidrosis, postural hypotension, stress hypertension, indifference to pain, emotional instability, corneal ulcers, taste deficiency, decreased fungiform and circumvalate papillae, unexplained bouts of fever, urinary frequency, and absent deep tendon reflexes. The development of Charcot joint, poor coordination, scoliosis, episodic vomiting, growth retardation, dysphagia, and slurred nasal speech appear later in life. Occasional abnormalities may include microcephaly, hydrocephalus, heart defects, mental retardation, and other disorders. Absence of flare skin response to cutaneous histamine and exaggerated response to norepinephrine are constant. Few patients survive beyond adolescence.

Riley, C. M., & Day, R. L., *et al*. Central autonomic dysfunction with defective lacrimation. *Pediatrics*, 1949, 3:468-78.

Riley-Schwachman syndrome. A combination of osseous changes and hyperreflexia, originally described in two children. The symptoms include a peculiar gait characterized by stiff legs, a wide base, calcaneal limp, ankle clonus, and hyperreflexia; symmetric areas of diminished density of long bones and increased density at the base of the skull seen on roentgenograms; concentration of organic matrix and minimal bone resorption; anorexia; emaciation; and excessive fatigability.

Riley, C. M., & Schwachman, H. Unusual osseous disease with neurologic changes; report of two cases. *Am. J. Dis. Child.*, 1943, 66:150-4.

RILEY, HARRIS D., JR. (American physician)

Riley syndrome. Synonyms: *Riley-Smith syndrome, macrocephaly-pseudopapilledema-hemangiomata syndrome.*

A familial syndrome, transmitted an an autosomal dominant trait, combining macrocephaly, pseudopapilledema, and hemangiomata.

Riley, H. D., Jr., & Smith, W. R. Macrocephaly, pseudopapilledema and multiple hemangiomata. A previously undescribed heredofamilial syndrome. *Pediatrics*, 1960, 26:293-300.

Riley-Smith syndrome. See *Riley syndrome.*

RILLE, JOHANN HEINRICH (Austrian physician)

Rille-Comèl disease. Synonyms: *ichthyosis linearis circumflexa, keratosis rubra figurata.*

A rare form of ichthyosis characterized by raised reddish to dark brown lesions arranged in linear serpiginous patterns. The first crops appear shortly after birth, usually on the buttocks, spreading to other parts of the body. After healing of the initial lesions, new ones appear shortly. Associated symptoms include profuse sweating of the palms and soles and hair disorders (trichorrehexis nodosa or invaginata, pili torti or moniliformi, and occasional leukodystrophy of the hair shafts). Acanthopapillomatosis may occur in some cases.

Rille, J. H. Demonstration 87. Vers. Dtsch. Naturforscher und Ärzte. *Derm. Wschr.*, 1922, 75:1204. Comèl, M. Ichtyosis linearis circumflexa. *Dermatologia, Basel*, 1949, 98:133-6.

RIMBAUD, LOUIS (French physician, born 1877)

Rimbaud-Jusse syndrome. See *Rimbaud-Passouant-Vallat syndrome.*

Rimbaud-Passouant-Vallat syndrome. Synonyms: *Rimbaud-Jusse syndrome, comatous encephalitis.*

Febrile encephalitis associated with coma, convulsions, hemiplegia, headache, vertigo, Cheyne-Stokes respiration, and deglutition disorders. Pathological findings include massive demyelination of the peripheral nerves and brain edema. Hypoglycemia, high leukocyte count, and hyperazotemia are found on blood analysis.

Rimbaud, L., Passouant, P., & Vallat, G. Les encéphalites comateuses. *Presse Méd.*, 1951, 59:605-6.

RIMOIN, DAVID L. (Canadian-born physician in the United States)

Rimoin syndrome. Synonym: *metaphyseal dysostosis-conductive hearing loss-mental retardation syndrome.*

A familial syndrome, inherited as an autosomal recessive trait, characterized by short-linbed dwarfism, metaphyseal dysostosis, conductive deafness, and mild mental retardation.

Rimoin, D. L., & McAlister, W. H. Metaphyseal dysostosis, conductive hearing loss and mental retardation: A recessively inherited syndrome. *Birth Defects*, 1971, 7(4):116-22.

ring chromosome 2 syndrome. See *chromosome 2 ring syndrome.*

ring chromosome 6 syndrome. See *chromosome 6 ring syndrome.*

ring chromosome 7 syndrome. See *chromosome 7 ring syndrome.*

ring chromosome 9 syndrome. See *chromosome 9 ring syndrome.*

ring chromosome 10 syndrome. See *chromosome 10 ring syndrome.*

ring chromosome 11 syndrome. See *chromosome 11 ring syndrome.*

ring chromosome 12 syndrome. See *chromosome 12 ring syndrome.*

ring chromosome 13 syndrome. See *chromosome 13 ring syndrome.*

ring chromosome 14 syndrome. See *chromosome 14 ring syndrome.*

ring chromosome 15 syndrome. See *chromosome 15 ring syndrome.*

ring chromosome 17 syndrome. See *chromosome 17 ring syndrome.*

ring chromosome 18 syndrome. See *chromosome 18 ring syndrome.*

ring chromosome 21 syndrome. See *chromosome 21 ring syndrome.*

ring chromosome 22 syndrome. See *chromosome 22 ring syndrome.*

ring constriction syndrome. See *amniotic band syndrome.*

ring dermoid syndrome. A familial disease, transmitted as an autosomal dominant trait, characterized by ocular dermoids. The choristoma involves the limbus and extends anteriorly into the cornea and posteriorly within the conjunctiva. Additional findings include conjunctival plaques of keratinization, hairs, and corneal lipids deposits. An irregular corneal astigmatism, amblyopia, and concomitant strabismus are the secondary features.

Mattos, J., *et al.* Ring dermoid syndrome. A new syndrome of autosomal dominantly inherited, bilateral, annular limbal dermoids with corneal and conjunctival extension. *Arch. Ophth., Chicago*, 1980, 98:1059-61.

ring-like corneal dystrophy. See *Reis-Bücklers syndrome.*

RINIKER, PAUL (Swiss physician)

Glanzmann-Riniker alymphoplasia. See *severe mixed immunodeficiency syndrome.*

Glanzmann-Riniker syndrome. See *severe mixed immunodeficiency syndrome.*

RIOPELLE, JOSEPH LUC (Canadian physician)

Riopelle tumor. A rare renal tumor made of true hypernephroma, sarcoma, and angiomyolipoma, reportedly described in 1945 by Riopelle.

Lagache, G., *et al.* Un nouveau cas de tumeur de Riopelle. *Chirurgie,* 1975, 101:597-604.

RIP VAN WINKLE (A character in Washington Irving's story, who fell into an irresistible sleep for twenty years)

Rip Van Winkle syndrome. A syndrome of irresistible somnolence and confusion. In one report, the affected child, whose father also suffered from hypersomnia, slept 22-23 hours per day and awakened with hallucinations and regressive behavior. In another case, an elderly patient suffered from confusion and somnolence after stroke.

Prendes, J. L., & Rosenberg, S. J. Rip Van Winkle syndrome. Confusion and irresistible somnolence after stroke. *South. Med. J.,* 1986, l79:1162-4. Cutler, E. A., & Marshall, J. R. Rip Van Winkle syndrome in childhood: Familial long-term hypersomnia. *Birth Defects,* 1978, 14(6B):367-8. Rodin, A. E., & Key, J. D. *Encyclopedia of medical eponyms derived from literary characters.* Melbourne, FL, Krieger, 1989.

RITTER, GOTTFRIED. See RITTER VON RITTERSHAIN, GOTTFRIED

RITTER VON JAKSCH, RUDOLF. See JAKSCH, RUDOLF, VON

RITTER VON RITTERSHAIN, GOTTFRIED (Austrian physician, 1820-1883)

Ritter dermatitis. See *staphylococcal scalded skin syndrome.*

Ritter disease. See *staphylococcal scalded skin syndrome.*

Ritter syndrome. See *staphylococcal scalded skin syndrome.*

RIVALTA, SEBASTIANO (Italian veterinarian, 1852-1893)

Rivalta disease. Synonyms: *actinomycosis, big jaw, clams, clyers, lumpy jaw, wooden tongue.*

Any infection with actinomycetes, particularly a chronic disease of cattle caused by *Actinomyces bovis* or of man caused by *A. israelii.* The human type is characterized by multiple indurated abscesses about the face, neck, chest, and abdomen, which discharge through numerous sinuses. Cervicofacial actinomycosis is the most common form, the organisms having gained entrance through soft tissue wounds, through the pulp of a broken-down tooth, or through ducts of the salivary glands. The lesion presents a dark-red discoloration of the skin, slate-blue elevations, multiple nodules with ridges and furrows in the creases of the skin of the neck, distinct boardlike indurations, and multiple sinuses with both macroscopic and microscopic granules in the purulent discharge. The tongue is occasionally the primary site; the lesion is a deep-seated, slow-growing, painless nodule that eventually breaks through the mucosa, discharging a yellowish, purulent material. Gingival lesions are similar to those of the tongue. See also *Ballingall disease (pseudoactinomycosis).*

Rivalta, S. Del cosi detto facino o moccio dei bovini e della cosi detta tuberculosi o mal del rospo (trutta) della lingua dei medisimi animali. *Gior. Anat. Fisiol. Pat. Animali,* 1875, l7:198-217.

RKH (Rokitansky-Küster-Hauser) syndrome. See *Mayer-Rokitansky-Küster syndrome.*

RLF. See *retrolental fibroplasia.*

RLS. See *restless legg syndrome.*

RLS. See *Roussy-Lévy syndrome.*

RM. See *Riehl melanosis.*

RMLS (right middle lobe syndrome). See *middle lobe syndrome.*

RMS (red man syndrome). See *red neck syndrome.*

ROBB-SMITH, A. H. T. (British physician)

Scott and Robb-Smith syndrome. See *under Scott, R. Bodley.*

ROBERT, HEINRICH (German physician)

Robert pelvis. A symmetrical transversely contracted pelvis due to absence of the sacral alae.

*Robert, H. *Beschreibung eines im hachsten Grade querverengtes.* Becken, Karlsrube, 1842.

ROBERTS, JOHN B. (American surgeon)

Roberts syndrome (RS). Synonyms: *Appelt-Gerken-Lenz syndrome, tetraphocomelia-cleft lip-palate syndrome.*

A syndrome of low birth weight, tetraphocomelia, cleft lip and palate, failure to thrive, vitium cordis, and short life expectancy. There are bone defects of all four extremities marked by shortening of the long bones, the middle segments of the limbs being most severely affected; shortening of the thumb and fifth fingers; three-digit hands, which may be attached directly to the shoulder; and osseous syndactyly of the fourth and fifth fingers. Orofacial features consist of hypertelorism, proptosis, and bilateral cleft lip with or without cleft palate. Enlarged phallus, cryptorchism, enlarged clitoris, enlarged or cleft labia minora, and septate vagina are the principal genital anomalies. Ocular disorders may include cataracts, corneal opacity, and colobomas of the eyelids. The pinnae of the ears may be deformed. The syndrome follows an autosomal recessive mode of transmission. Parental consanguinity and occurrence in sibs have been observed in some cases. Some patients have an abnormality of the constitutive heterochromatin (the RS effect), which has been described as a premature separation of the paracentromeric and nucleolar organizing of the Y chromosome. See also *tetraphocomelia-cleft palate syndrome.*

Roberts, J. B. A child with double cleft lip and palate, protrusion of the intermaxillary portion of the upper jaw and imperfect development of the bones of the four extremities. *Ann. Surg.*, 1919, 70:252-61. Appelt, H., Gerken, H., & Lenz, W. Tetraphokomelie mit Lippen-Kiefer-Gaumenspalte und Clitorishypertrophie-ein Syndrom. *Pädiatr. Pädol.*, 1966, 2:119-24. Burns, M. A., & Tomkins, D. J. Hypersensitivity to mitomycin C cell-killing in Roberts syndrome fibroblasts with, but not without, the heterochromatin abnormality. *Mutat. Res.,* 1989, 216:243-9.

ROBERTS, MAUREEN (Canadian physician)

Norman-Roberts syndrome,. See *under Norman.*

ROBERTSON, DOUGLAS MORAY COOPER LAMB ARGYLL (British physician, 1837-1909)

Argyll Robertson pupil. See *Robertson syndrome.*

Argyll Robertson syndrome. See *Robertson syndrome.*

nonluetic Argyll Robertson pupil. See *Adie syndrome.*

pseudo-Argyll Robertson syndrome. See *Adie syndrome.*

Robertson syndrome. Synonyms: *Argyll Robertson pupil, Argyll Robertson syndrome, reflex iridoplegia.*

A frequent symptom of neurosyphilis, especially tabes dorsalis, and other diseases of the central nervous system, in which the pupil is small and responds slowly or not at all to light, but contracts normally on accommodation and convergence.

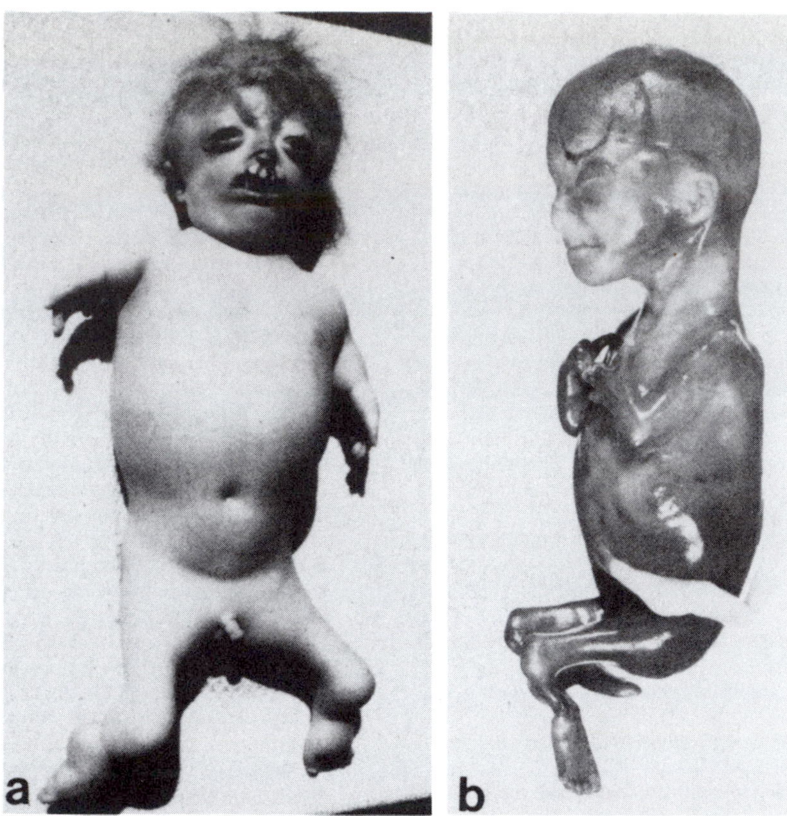

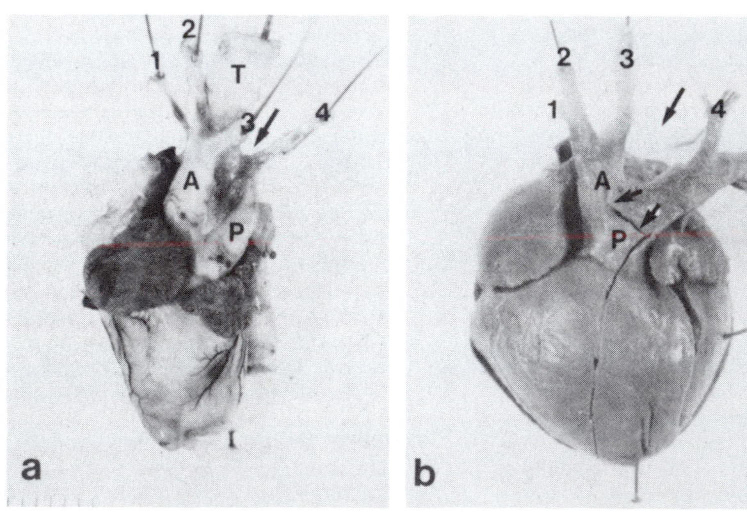

Roberts syndrome
Rehder, H., M.Weber, K. Heyne & M. Lituania: Fetal Pathology - Nonchromosomal. In Gilbert, E.F., J.M. Opitz (eds.): *Genetic Aspects of Development Pathology.* New York: Alan R. Liss, Inc., for the March of Dimes Birth Defects Foundation BD-OAS 23(1) : 131-151, 1987, with permission.

Robertson, A. On an interesting series of eye-symptoms in a case of spinal disease, with remarks on the action of belladonna on the iris, etc. *Edinburgh Med. J.,* 1868, 14:696-708.

ROBERTSON, P. W. (British physician)

Robertson-Kihara syndrome. A syndrome of renal juxtaglomerular cell tumor associated with hypertension, hyperreninemia, and secondary aldosteronism.

Robertson, P. W., *et al.* Hypertension due to a renin-secreting renal tumour. *Am. J. Med.,* 1967, 43:963-76. Kihara, I., *et al.* A hitherto unreported vascular tumor of the kidney: A proposal of "juxtaglomerular cell tumor." *Acta Path. Jpn.,* 1968, 18:197-206. Conn, J. W., *et al.* The syndrome of hypertension, hyperreninemia and secondary aldosteronism associated with renal juxtaglomerular cell tumor (primary renism). *J. Urol.,* 1973, 109:349-55.

ROBIN, PIERRE (French dentist, 1867-1950)

Pierre Robin syndrome. See *Robin syndrome.*

Robin anomalad. See *Robin syndrome.*

Robin anomaly. See *Robin syndrome.*

Robin syndrome. Synonyms: *Pierre Robin syndrome (PRS), Robin anomalad, Robin anomaly, micrognathia-glossoptosis syndrome.*

An abnormality syndrome of brachygnathia and cleft palate, often associated with glossoptosis, backward and upward displacement of the larynx, angulation of the manubrium sterni, and pressure marks on the chest caused by the rami of the mandible. Cleft palate makes sucking and swallowing difficult and permits easy access of fluids to the larynx. Periodic inspiratory distress, exacerbated by feeding or lying the child on its back, is frequent and is initiated by choking. The condition may proceed to stridor, cyanosis, and rib retraction, and is often accompanied by vomiting. The syndrome occasionally occurs without associated abnormalities, but is more likely to be accompanied by various teratogenic syndromes or hereditary conditions, its mode of transmission being that of the syndrome with which it is associated.

*Robin, P. *La glossoptose, un grave danger pour nos enfants.* Paris, 1927.

ROBINOW, MEINHARD (American physician)

Robinow dwarfism. See *Robinow syndrome.*

Robinow syndrome. Synonyms: *Robinow dwarfism, Robinow-Silverman-Smith syndrome, fetal face syndrome.*

A syndrome of peculiar (fetal) facies, mesomelic dwarfism, hemivertebrae, hypoplastic genitalia, and brachydactyly. Craniofacial features consist of macrocephaly, large anterior fontanel, frontal bossing, hypertelorism, small upturned nose, long philtrum, small mouth, micrognathia, hyperplastic alveolar ridges, and crowded teeth. Cryptorchism and small penis, clitoris, and labia majora are the genital features. Occasional abnormalities include nevus flammeus, epicanthus, posterior rotation of the ears, macroglossia, high-arched palate, absent or bifid uvula, broad thumbs and toes, clinodactyly, hyperextensibility of the fingers, short metacarpals, a Madelung-like anomaly of the forearm, and hip dislocation. Transmission as an autosomal dominant trait was suspected in the original report, but some other cases have been sporadic.

Robinow, M., *et al.*. A newly recognized dwarfing syndrome. *Am. J. Dis. Child.*, 1969, 117:645-51.

Robinow-Silverman-Smith syndrome. See *Robinow syndrome.*

ROBINSON, ANDREW ROSE (American physician, 1845-1924)

Robinson disease. Synonym: *hidrocystoma.*

A retention cyst of a sweat gland caused by obstruction of the duct and seen as a discrete, deeply seated, noninflammatory vesicle, about 1 to 5 mm in diameter. It occurs most commonly on the faces of middle-aged women exposed to excessive heat and humidity.

Robinson, A. R. Hidrocystoma. *J. Cutan. Dis.,* 1893, 11:293-303.

ROBINSON, GEOFFREY C. (Canadian physician)

ectodermal dysplasia, Robinson type. See *Robinson syndrome.*

Robinson syndrome. Synonyms: *Robinson-Miller-Bensimon syndrome; ectodermal dysplasia, Robinson type; nail dystrophy-deafness syndrome; onycho-odontodysplasia-perceptual deafness syndrome.*

A syndrome of familial ectodermal dysplasia, transmitted as an autosomal dominant trait, marked by nail hypoplasia and dystrophy, sensorineural deafness, hypodontia, and peg-shaped teeth. Associated defects may include syndactyly, polydactyly, and sweat electrolyte disorders.

Robinson, G. C., Miller, J. R., & Bensimon, J. R. Familial ectodermal dysplasia and sensorineural deafness and other anomalies. *Pediatrics*, 1962, 30:797-802.

Robinson-Miller-Bensimon syndrome. See *Robinson syndrome.*

ROBINSON, SAUL J. (American physician)

Forney-Robinson-Pascoe syndrome. See *under Forney.*

ROBLES, RUDOLFO (South American physician)

Robles disease. Synonyms: *blinding filariasis, coastal erysipelas, craw-craw, juxta-articular nodules, onchocerciasis, onchocercosis.*

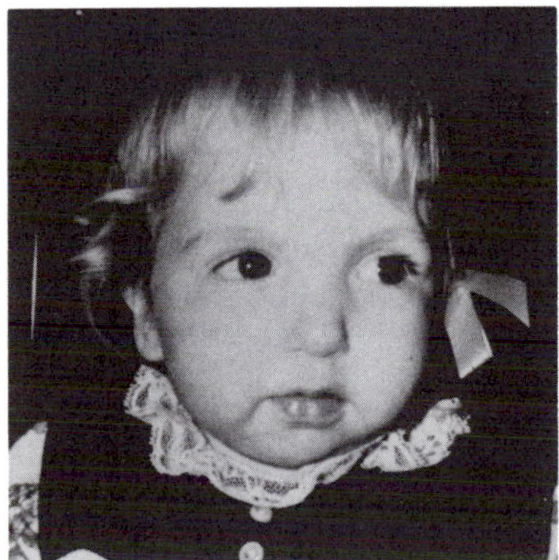

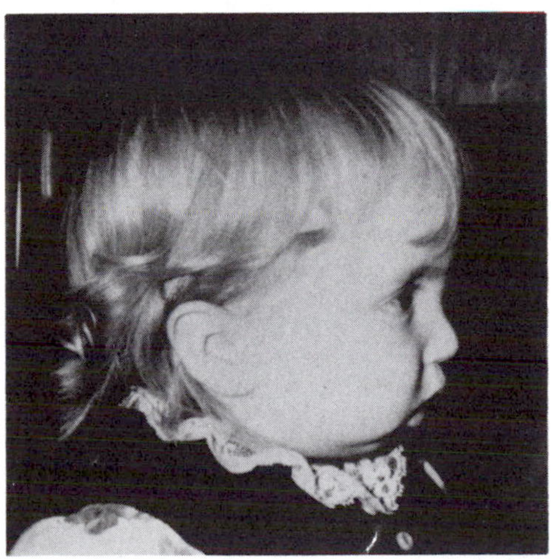

Robin syndrome

Dignan, P. St. J., L.W. Martin & E.J. Zenni, Jr.: *Clinical Genetics* 29-168-173, 1986. Munksgaard International Publishers, Copenhagen, Denmark. 25:119-129, 1986. New York: Alan R. Liss, Inc.

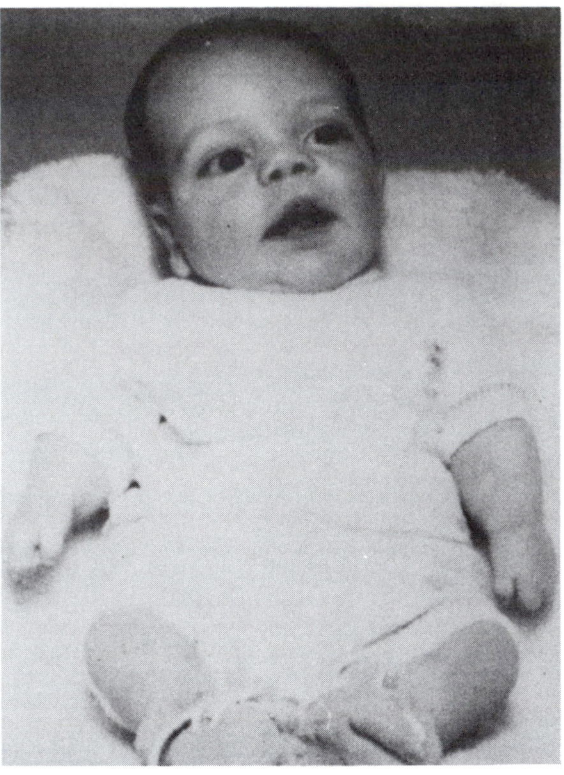
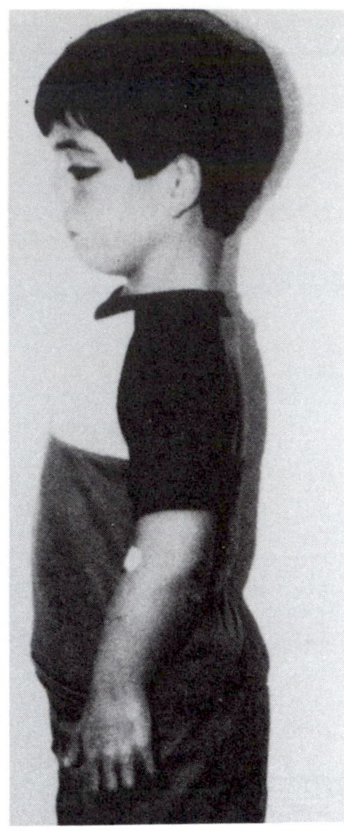

Robinow syndrome
Butler, Merlin G. & William B. Wadlington: *Clinical Genetics* 31:77-85, 1987. Munksgaard International Publishers, Copenhagen, Denmark.

Onchocerca volvulus infection transmitted to man by the black gnats of the genus *Simulium*. The disease occurs mainly in Africa and the Western Hemisphere, where it is confined to certain areas of Guatemala, Mexico, and Venezuela. Two forms of infection are recognized: the **benign type**, produced by adult worms, involves the junctions of the lymphatic vessels in the subcutaneous tissue, with encapsulation of the worms; and the **severe type**, in which microfilaria, after being discharged by adult females into the fibrous tissue, circulates through the subcutaneous lymphatic system, often invading the eyes. In the latter type, the presence of maturing or adult worms provokes a local tissue reaction and the development of tumors about 2 to 10 mm in diameter. Polymorphonuclear leukocytes, plasma cells, eosinophils, and giant cells may be found in the vicinity. Bacterial superinfection, allergic pigmented dermatitis, pruritus, and macular rash may result, and elephantiasis, keratitis, lens atrophy, and blindness may develop after ocular invasion. The condition was described by Robles in 1915, but his report was never published.

ROCH

Roch lipomatosis. A familial form of congenital lipomatosis characterized by hard, painless, movable fatty tumors in the skin, varying in number from 10 to 100 and in size from that of a lentil to that of an orange.

Bernard, H., *et al.* Lipomatose de Roch chez deux soeurs jumelles univitellines. *Presse Méd.*, 1954, 62:579.

ROCHER, HENRI GASTON LOUIS (French physician, born 1876)

Rocher-Sheldon syndrome. See *arthrogryposis multiplex congenita syndrome.*

rock fever. See *brucellosis.*

rod myopathy. See *Shy-Magee syndrome.*

rodent ulcer. See *Krompecher tumor.*

ROEMHELD, LUDWIG (German physician, 1871-1938)

Roemheld syndrome. Synonyms: *Tecklenburg-Roemheld syndrome, gastrocardial syndrome, postprandial cardiogastric syndrome, tympanismus hystericus.*

An association of cardiac and gastrointestinal symptoms, usually observed in excitable individuals, which is characterized by the occurrence of tachycardia immediately after meals. Chest pain, palpitations, cor mobile, and tympanites with gastric dyspepsia are the principal symptoms. See also *Bergmann syndrome.*

Roemheld, L. Der gastro-kardiale Symptomenkomplex, eine besondere Form sogenannter Herzneurose. *Zschr. Phys. Diät. Ther.*, 1912, 16:339-49.

Tecklenburg-Roemheld syndrome. See *Roemheld syndrome.*

ROGER, HENRI LOUIS (French physician, 1809-1891)

Roger disease. A congenital defect of the interventricular septum of the heart.

Roger, H. Recherches cliniques sur la communication congénitale de deux coeurs, par inocclusion du septum interventriculaire. *Bull. Acad. Méd., Paris,* 1879, 8:1074-94; 1189-191.

Roger murmur. A murmur caused by a congenital interventricular septal defect of the heart.

Roger, H. Recherches cliniques sur la communication congénitale de deux coeurs, par inocclusion du septum interventriculaire. *Bull. Acad. Méd., Paris,* 1879, 8:1074-94; 1189-191.

ROGERS, J. G. (Australian physician)

Pitt-Rogers-Danks syndrome. See *Pitt syndrome.*

rogue positive reactions. See *excited skin syndrome.*

ROHR, KARL (German physician)

Rohr agranulocytosis. Agranulocytosis associated with myelogranulocytic hyperplasia.

Rohr, K. Agranulozytosen und blutbildende Organe einschliesslich des lymphatischen und reticulo-histiozytären Systems. In: Jürgens, R., & Waldenström, J., eds. *Nebenwirkungen von Arzneimitteln auf Blut und Knochenmark.* Stuttgart, Schattauer, 1957, pp. 114-28.

ROKITANSKY, KARL FREIHERR, VON (Austrian physician, 1804-1878)

Mayer-Rokitansky syndrome. See *Mayer-Rokitansky-Küster syndrome.*

Mayer-Rokitansky-Küster (MRK) syndrome. See *under Mayer.*

Rokitansky disease. See *Budd-Chiari syndrome.*

Rokitansky-Cushing ulcer. Peptic ulcer secondary to cerebral lesions.

Rokitansky, C. *Handbuch der pathologischen Anatomie.* vol. 3, Wien, Braumüller & Seidel, 1842. Cushing, H. Peptic ulcer and the interbrain. *Surg. Obst.*, 1932, 55:1-34.

Rokitansky-Küster-Hauser (RKH) syndrome. See *Mayer-Rokitansky-Küster syndrome.*

von Rokitansky disease. See *Budd-Chiari syndrome.*

von Rokitansky-Hauser syndrome. See *Mayer-Rokitansky-Küster syndrome.*

ROLLAND, J. C. (French physician)

Rolland-Desbuquois (RD) syndrome. Synonyms: *anisospondylitic camptomicromelic dwarfism; dyssegmental dwarfism (DD), Rolland-Desbuquois type; dyssegmental dysplasia (DD), Rolland-Desbuquois type.*

A lethal syndrome of multiple abnormalities, transmitted as an autosomal recessive trait, characterized by micromelia, cleft palate, and variable limited mobility of the elbow, wrist, knee, and ankle joints. Occasional occipital encephalocele, inguinal hernia, hydronephrosis, hydrocephalus, and patent ductus arteriosus may be associated. Radiographic findings consist of a small cranial vault, moderately narrow chest with short ribs, small scapulae, severe defects in ossification of the vertebral bodies with vertical clefts and faulty segmentation, horizontal acetabular roofs, rounded iliac wings with short diameters, extremely short limbs with a dumbbell-like shape, flaring and irregular metaphyses with slanted ends, absent epiphyses, and short and wide tubular bones with lateral angulation.

Rolland, J. C., Laugier, J., Grenier, B., & Desbuquois, G. Nanisme chondrodystrophique et division palatine chez un nouveau-né. *Ann. Pediat., Paris,* 1972, 19:139-43. Handmaaker, S. H., *et al.* Dyssegmental dwarfism: A new syndrome of lethal dwarfism. *Birth Defects,* 1977, 8(3D):79-90.

ROLLET, J. (French physician)

Rollet syndrome. Synonym: *orbital apex-sphenoidal syndrome.*

A syndrome in which lesions of the apex of the orbit produce sensorimotor ophthalmoplegia and optic atrophy through involvement of the third, fourth, and sixth cranial nerves, with ptosis; diplopia; vasomotor disorders; hyperesthesia or anesthesias of the forehead, upper eyelid, and cornea; retrobulbar neuralgia radiating to the forehead, top of the head, and temples; and visual field defects. Exophthalmos, optic neuritis, and papilledema may occur.

Rollet, & Colrat. Syndrome de l'apex orbitaire (ophthalmoplegie sensorio-sensitivo-motrice d'origine traumatique). *Bull. Soc. Opht. Lyon,* 1926-27, 16:13-4.

ROLLET, JOSEPH PIERRE MARTIN (French physician, 1824-1894)

Rollet chancre. Synonym: *mixed chancre.*

A chancre produced by mixed syphilitic and chancroid infections.

*Rollet, J. P. Coincidence du chancre syphilitique primitif avec la gale, la blénorrhagie, la chancre simple et la vaccina. *Gaz. Méd., Lyon,* 1866, 18:160-3.

ROMANO, C. (Italian physician)

Romano-Ward syndrome. See *under long QT syndrome.*

ROMBERG, MORITZ HEINRICH, VON (German neurologist, 1795-1873)

Cavaré-Romberg syndrome. See *Westphal syndrome, under Westphal, Karl Friedrich Otto.*

Cavaré-Romberg-Westphal syndrome. See *Westphal syndrome, under Westphal, Karl Friedrich Otto.*

Howship-Romberg syndrome. See *under Howship.*

Parry-Romberg syndrome. See *Romberg syndrome (2).*

Romberg disease. See *Romberg syndrome (2).*

Romberg syndrome (1). See *Westphal syndrome, under Westphal, Karl Friedrich Otto.*

Romberg syndrome (2). Synonyms: *Parry-Romberg syndrome, Romberg disease, facial hemiatrophy, facial trophoneurosis, hemiatrophia faciei, hemiatrophia faciei progressiva, progressive facial hemiatrophy, progressive hemifacial atrophy, trophoneurosis.*

A disorder, usually appearing during the first decade of life, characterized by progressive atrophy of some or all tissues on one side of the face, occasionally extending to other parts of the body. It involves the tongue, gingiva, soft palate, the cartilages of the nose, ear, larynx, and palpebral tarsus. Frequent pigmentation disorders, such as heterochromia iridis, vitiligo, and pigmented facial nevi; trigeminal neuralgia; ocular disorders, including strabismus, enophthalmos, blepharoptosis, miosis, uveitis, and optic atrophy; jacksonian epilepsy; and ataxia are associated. Occasional complications may consist of the Horner syndrome, lagophthalmos, and migraine. This condition is believed to be related to scleroderma.

Romberg, M. H., von. Trophoneurosen. In his: *Klinische Ergebnise.* Berlin, Förstner, 1846, pp. 75-81. Parry, C. H. *Collections from the unpublished medical writings.* London, Underwood, 1825.

ROMBO

Rombo syndrome. A familial cutaneous syndrome, believed to be transmitted as an autosomal dominant trait, characterized by vermiculate atrophoderma, milia, hypotrichosis, trichoepitheliomas, basal cell carcinomas, peripheral vasodilation, and cyanosis. The lesions become apparent in late childhood and are most pronounced on the face. Histological findings include irregularly distributed atrophic hair follicles, milia, dilated dermal vessels, and lack of elastin or its clumping. On exposure to cold, there are marked changes in skin temperature. The syndrome was named after the oldest member of the affected family.

Michaëlsson, G., *et al.* The Rombo syndrome: A familial disorder with vermiculate atrophoderma, milia, hypotrichosis, trichoepitheliomas, basal cell carcinomas and peripheral vasodilation with cyanosis. *Acta Derm. Vener., Stockholm,* 1981, 61:497-503.

RONCHESE, F. (American physician)

Ronchese syndrome. A syndrome, transmitted as an autosomal recessive trait, characterized by pili torti of the scalp and eyebrows and dental enamel hypoplasia.

Ronchese, F. Twisted hairs (pili torti). *Arch. Derm. Syph., Chicago,* 1932, 26:98-109.

ROOKE, E. D. (American physician)

Eaton-Lambert-Rooke syndrome. See *Eaton-Lambert syndrome, under Eaton, Lealdes McKendree.*

root puller fracture. See *Schmitt syndrome.*

ROQUES, R. (French physician)

Roques syndrome. Parallel sclerosis of the heart and lungs in chronic cor pulmonale in aged patients.

Roques, R. *et al.* Les scléroses parallèles du coeur et du poumon. *Sem. Hôp. Paris,* 1949, 25:721-4.

rosacea-like tuberculid. See *Lewandowski tuberculid.*

rosacea-like tuberculosis. See *Lewandowski tuberculid.*

ROSAI, JUAN (American physician)

Destombes-Rosai-Dorfman syndrome. See *Rosai-Dorfman syndrome.*

Rosai-Dorfman syndrome. Synonyms: *Destombes-Rosai-Dorfman syndrome, sinus histiocytosis with massive lymphadenopathy (SHML).*

Sinus histiocytosis associated with massive, painless, often bilateral cervical lymphadenopathy. Extranodal involvement may include the orbits, eyelids, upper respitory tract, salivary glands, skin, bones, testes, and occasionally the epidural space and the vertebral canal. Fever, leukocytosis with neutrophilia, elevated erythrocyte sedimentation rate, and hypergammaglobulinemia are the common symptoms. The involved lymph nodes show pericapsular fibrosis, dilation of sinuses, numerous sometimes foamy or atypical intrasinusal histiocytes with abundant clear cytoplasm, and a large collections of plasma cells. Lymphocytes and hematopoietic cells are usually present in the sinus histiocytes. The condition is benign and there is spontaneous regression of symptoms with complete recovery.

Rosai, J., & Dorfman, R. F. Sinus histiocytosis with massive lymphadenopathy. A newly recognized benign clinicopathological entity. *Arch. Path., Chicago,* 1969, 87:63-70.

rose rash in infants. See *Zahorsky syndrome (1).*

ROSEN, LINDA (American pediatrician)

Golabi-Rosen syndrome (GRS). See *under Golabi.*

ROSEN, SAMUEL HARRY (American physician, born 1903)

Rosen neuralgia. Synonym: *tic douloureux of the chorda tympani.*

Neuralgia of the chorda tympani, in which the pain resembles that of tic douloureux.

Rosen, S. Tic douloureux of the chorda tympani. *Arch. Neur. Psychiat., Chicago,* 1953, 69:275-8.

Rosen syndrome. See *Rosen-Castleman-Liebow syndrome.*

Rosen-Castleman-Liebow syndrome. Synonyms: *Rosen syndrome, pulmonary alveolar proteinosis, pulmonary proteinosis.*

A lung disease in which the alveoli are filled with a PAS-positive proteinaceous material rich in lipid. This material appears to be produced by the lining cells, which slough into the lumen, ultimately become necrotic, and yield granules and laminated bodies to the alveolar content. The symptoms include dyspnea, especially on exertion, productive cough, fever, weakness, weight loss, aching, chest pain, and occasional cardiovascular failure.

Rosen, S. H., Castleman, B., & Liebow, A. A. Pulmonary alveolar proteinosis. *N. Engl. J. Med.,* 1958, 258:1123-42.

ROSENBACH, ANTON JULIUS FRIEDRICH (German physician, 1842-1923)

Rosenbach disease. See *Rosenbach erysipeloid.*

Rosenbach erysipeloid. Synonyms: *Klauder disease, Rosenbach disease, crab dermatitis, erysipeloid, swine erysipelas in man.*

A rare disease of traumatized skin caused by *Erysipelothrix rhusopathiae* infection, most commonly affecting kitchen workers, butchers, fishermen, and other persons coming in contact with contaminated meat, animal products, or dead animals. The incubation period ranges from 2 to 7 days. In its mild forms, erythema, burning and itching sensations, and pain at the site of the initial contact, usually involving the hands and finges, are the early symptoms. The subsequent lesions are tender and warm red or purplish eruptions with well-defined raised margins, which spread peripherally. Low-grade fever and malaise are the common systemic manifestations. Regional lymphadenopathy, occasional endocarditis, arthralgia, bronchitis due to inhalation of bacteria, and bacteremia may occur. In the bacteremic form, there may be purpuric and hematomalike lesions and distinctive linear lesions of the creases of the palms and fingers. The term **Rosenbach disease** is frequently used in connection with the mild type, and **Klauder disease** with the diffuse and septicemic type.

*Klauder, J. V., *et al.* A distinctive form of erysipeloid among fish handlers. *Arch. Derm. Syph., Chicago,* 1926, 14:622.

ROSENBACH, OTTOMAR (German physician, 1851-1907)

Rosenbach disease (1). An association of paroxysmal tachycardia with cardiac, respiratory, and gastric disorders.

Rosenbach, O. Beitrag zur Lehre von den Krankheiten des Verdauunbsapparates. *Deut. Med. Wschr.,* 1879, 5:535-8; 555-7.

Rosenbach disease (2). See *Heberden nodes.*

ROSENBERG, ALAN L. (American physician)

Rosenberg-Bergstrom syndrome. A familial syndrome, transmitted as an autosomal recessive trait, characterized by hyperuricemia, renal insufficiency, ataxia, and deafness.

Rosenberg, A. L., Bergstrom, L., *et al.* Hyperuricemia and neurologic deficit. A family study. *N. Engl. J. Med.,* 1970, 282:992-7.

ROSENBERG, EDWARD FRANK (American physician, born 1908)

Hench-Rosenberg syndrome. See *under Hench.*

ROSENBERG, LEON EMANUEL (American physician, born 1933)

Rowley-Rosenberg syndrome. See *under Rowley.*

ROSENBERG, ROGER N. (American physician)

Rosenberg-Chutorian syndrome. Synonyms: *nerve deafness-distal neurogenic amyotrophy syndrome, optic atrophy-polyneuropathy-deafness syndrome.*

A hereditary syndrome of progressive neural hearing loss, polyneuropathy, and optic atrophy. Associated disorders may include speech disorders, muscle weakness, hyporeflexia, unsteady gait, depressed sensory reflexes, and nerve conduction disorders.

Rosenberg, R. N., & Chutorian, A. Familial opticoacoustic nerve degeneration and polyneuropathy. *Neurology*, 1967, 17:827-32.

ROSENBLOOM, ARLAN L. (American physician)

Rosenbloom syndrome. See *Rosenbloom-Frias syndrome.*

Rosenbloom-Frias syndrome. Synonyms: *Rosenbloom syndrome, diabetic stiff joint syndrome.*

A congenital syndrome of small stature, joint rigidity, finger contractures, and diabetes mellitus. Cardiac complications and decreased vital capacity may occur.

Rosenbloom, A. L., & Frías, J. L. Diabetes mellitus, short stature and joint stiffness-a new syndrome. *Clin. Res.*, 1974, 22:92A.

ROSENTHAL, CURT (German physician)

Melkersson-Rosenthal syndrome (MRS). See *under Melkersson.*

Melkersson-Rosenthal-Schuermann syndrome. See *Melkersson-Rosenthal syndrome.*

Münzer-Rosenthal syndrome. See *under Münzer.*

Rosenthal disease. Synonyms: *catalepsy on awakening, delayed psychomotor awakening, postdormital paralysis, sleep paralysis.*

Paralysis on awakening in which the patient, although fully conscious, is unable to move, even though he may be able to move his eyes and speak. The duration of paralysis varies from a few seconds to several minutes. Anxiety and fear of death are usually associated.

Rosenthal, C. Über das verzögerte psychomotorische Erwachen, seine Entstehung und seine nosologische Bedeutung. *Arch. Psychiat., Berlin*, 1827, 81:159-71.

Rossolimo-Melkersson-Rosenthal syndrome. See *Melkersson-Rosenthal syndrome.*

ROSENTHAL, NATHAN (American physician)

Brill-Baehr-Rosenthal disease. See *Brill-Symmers syndrome.*

ROSENTHAL, ROBERT LOUIS (American hematologist, born 1923)

Rosenthal disease. Synonyms: *factor XI deficiency, hemophilia C, plasma thromboplastin-antecedent (PTA) deficiency.*

Hereditary deficiency of factor XI, transmitted as an autosomal recessive trait, characterized mainly by mild bruising, epistaxes, menorrhagia, infrequent hemarthroses, and intramuscular hemorrhage. There may be persistent bleeding after tooth extraction, tonsillectomy, and other surgical operations. Most patients suffering from this condition are of Jewish ancestry.

Rosenthal, R. L., *et al.* New hemophilia-like disease caused by deficiency of a third plasma thromboplastin factor. *Proc. Soc. Exper. Biol. Med.*, 1953, 82:171-4.

roseola infantilis (infantum). See *Zahorsky syndrome (1).*

ROSKE, GEORG (German physician)

Roske-De Toni-Caffey-Silverman syndrome. See *Caffey-Silverman syndrome.*

Roske-De Toni-Caffey-Smyth syndrome. See *Caffey-Silverman syndrome.*

ROSS, ALEXANDER T. (American physician)

Ross syndrome. Synonym: *tonic pupil plus.*

Tonic pupil (pupillary hyporeflexia) whereby the affected pupil does not respond or responds sluggishly to light and is larger than the unaffected pupil in lighted surroundings and smaller in unlighted surroundings. Symptoms occur in association with loss of muscle stretch reflexes in the limbs and hemifacial flushing and loss of sweating. Other symptoms may include emotional disorders and orthostatic hypotension. See also *Adie syndrome.*

Ross, A. T. Progressive selective sudomotor denervation. A case with coexisting Adie's syndrome. *Neurology*, 1958, 8:809-17.

ROSSBACH, MICHAEL JOSEF (German physician, 1842-1894)

Rossbach disease. Synonyms: *gastroxynsis, hyperchlorhydria.*

Excessive secretion of hydrochloric acid by the stomach. See also *Rejchman disease.*

Rossbach, M. J. Nervöse Gastroxynsis, als eine eigene, genau charakterisirbare Form der nervösen Dyspepsie. *Deut. Arch. Klin. Med.*, 1884, 35:383-401.

ROSSELLI, D. (Italian physician)

Rosselli-Gulienetti syndrome. A hereditary syndrome, transmitted as an autosomal recessive trait, marked by hypohidrosis, hair abnormalities (hypotrichosis, brittle and wooly hair, albinoid hypopigmentation), nail disorders (hyperkeratosis, onychoclasis, striae), peculiar facies (mongoloid palpebral slant, epicanthus, marked nasogenial slant, absence of the eyelashes and eyebrows), dermatological changes (dystrophic skin, pityriasis, eczema, seborrhea of the scalp, skin desquamation), limb deformities (syndactyly, hypoplasia of the thumbs), urogenital defects (hypogonadism, renal hypoplasia), cleft lip and/or palate, microdontia, and popliteal and perineal pteryria.

Rosselli, D., & Gulienetti, R. Ectodermal dysplasia. *Brit. J. Plast. Surg.*, 1961, 14:190-204.

ROSSI, ETTORE (Swiss physician)

Rossi syndrome. See *arthrogryposis multiplex congenita syndrome.*

RÖSSLE, R. (German physician, 1876-1956)

Rössle-Urbach-Wiethe syndrome. See *Urbach-Wiethe syndrome.*

RÖSSLE, ROBERT (German physician, 1844-1896)

Hanot-Rössle syndrome. See *under Hanot.*

ROSSOLIMO

Rossolimo-Curschmann-Batten-Steinert syndrome. See *myotonic dystrophy syndrome.*

Rossolimo-Melkersson-Rosenthal syndrome. See *Melkersson-Rosenthal syndrome.*

ROSTAN, LEON LOUIS (French physician, 1790-1866)

Rostan asthma. Synonyms: *cardiac asthma, paroxysmal dyspnea, paroxysmal nocturnal dyspnea.*

Attacks of dyspnea, usually occurring at night in patients with congestive heart failure, associated with fluid accumulation in the interstitial space of the lungs. The congested lung becomes stiffer, resulting in rapid and shallow respiration. Slowing of the airflow, prolonged expiration, wheezing, and hyperinflation of the chest are the main clinical features.

Rostan, L. L. Mémoire sur cette question, l'asthme de vieillards est-il une affection nerveuse? *Nouv. J. Méd. Chir. Pharm.*, 1818, 3:3-30.

ROT (ROTH), VLADIMIR KARLOVICH (Russian neurologist, 1848-1916)

Rot meralgia. See *Rot-Bernhardt syndrome.*

Rot-Bernhardt syndrome. Synonyms: *Bernhardt disease, Bernhardt paralysis, Rot meralgia, Roth meralgia, Roth-Bernhardt syndrome, lateral femoral paresthesia, meralgia paresthetica, neuritis nervi cutanei femoris lateralis, paresthetic meralgia.*

A sensory disorder and paresthesia in the area supplied by the external cutaneous nerve of the thigh, marked by numbness, pain, tingling, formication, burning, heaviness, itching, cramps, and heat sensation on the anterolateral surface of the thigh after prolonged walking or standing. Compression caused by belts and girdles, obesity, shoulder girdle syndrome, postoperative complications, diabetes, and other conditions are suspected as possible causes.

*Roth, W. K. *Meralgia paresthetica*. Berlin, Karger, 1895. Bernhardt, M. Über isoliert im Gebiete des N. cutaneus femoris externus vorkommende Paraesthesien. *Neurol. Zbl.*, 1895, 14:242-4.

Rot-Bielschowsky syndrome. Synonyms: *Roth-Bielschowsky syndrome, pseudo-opthalomplegia syndrome.*

A supranuclear lesion in the temporal lobe associated with paralysis of conjugate gaze in one direction and retention of the slow phase in the absence of vestibular nystagmus.

Roth, W. Pseudobulbärparalyse. *Neurol. Zbl.*, 1909, 28:1126-7. Bielschowsky, A. Das klinische Bild der assozierten Blicklähmung und seine Bedeutung für die topische Diagnostik. *Münch. Med. Wschr.*, 1903, 50:1666-70.

Roth meralgia. See *Rot-Bernhardt syndrome.*

Roth-Bernhardt syndrome. See *Rot-Bernhardt syndrome.*

Roth-Bielschowsky syndrome. See *Rot-Bielschowsky syndrome.*

rotavirus syndrome. An epidemic disease of children caused by rotavirus infection, and characterized by gastroenteritis, diarrhea, vomiting, dehydration, fever, respiratory infection, and otitis media.

Bishop, R. F., *et al.* Detection of a new virus by electron microscopy of faecal extracts from children with acute gastroeneritis. *Lancet*, 1974, 1:149-51. Lewis, H. M., *et al.* A year's experience of the rotavirus syndrome and its association with respiratory illness. *Arch. Dis. Child.*, 1979, 54:339-46.

ROTES-QUEROL, J. (French physician)

Forestier and Rotés-Querol syndrome. See *Forestier syndrome (2).*

ROTH, MARTIN (British physician)

Roth syndrome. Synonyms: *calamity syndrome, phobic anxiety-depersonalization syndrome.*

A form of neurotic illness consisting of a combination of depersonalization and phobic anxiety, some cases having features reminescent of disturbances of temporal lobe function such as *déjà vu* phenomena, metamorphopsia and panoramic memory. In a higher proportion, more variable obsessional, hysterical, and depressive features and vasomotor disturbances occur.

Roth, M. The phobic anxiety-depersonalization syndrome. *Proc. Roy. Soc. Med., London*, 1959, 52:587-95.

ROTH, MORITZ, VON (German physician, 1839-1914)

Roth spot. A small white hemorrhagic spot in the retina sometimes observed in bacterial endocarditis, pernicious anemia, and leukemia.

Roth, M., von. Über Netzhautaffectionen bei Wundfiebern. I. Die embolische Panophthalmitis. *Deut. Zschr. Chir.*, 1872, 1:471-84.

ROTH, WLADIMIR KARLOWICZ. See ROT, VLADIMIR KARLOVICH

ROTHMANN, MAX (German physician, 1868-1915)

Rothmann-Makai panniculitis. See *Rothmann-Makai syndrome.*

Rothmann-Makai syndrome. Synonyms: *Rothmann-Makai panniculitis, lipogranulomatosis subcutanea, oleogranuloma, spontaneous lipogranulomatosis, spontaneous panniculitis.*

Circumscribed panniculitis of the trunk and extremities, most commonly occurring in children, which is characterized by subcutaneous nodules that undergo spontaneous involution without having any systemic manifestations. Some writers question this condition as a distinct entity.

Rothmann, M. Über Entzündung und Atrophie des subcutanen Fettgewebes. *Arch. Path., Berlin*, 1894, 136:159-69. Makai, E. Über Lipogranulomatosis subcutanea. *Klin. Wschr.*, 1928, 7:2343-6.

ROTHMUND, AUGUST, JR., VON (German ophthalmologist, 1830-1906)

Rothmund dystrophy. See *Rothmund-Thomson syndrome.*

Rothmund syndrome. See *Rothmund-Thomson syndrome.*

Rothmund-Thomson syndrome (RTS). Synonyms: *Bloch-Stauffer dyshormonal dermatosis, Rothmund dystrophy, Rothmund syndrome, congenital cutaneous dystrophy, congenital poikiloderma atrophicans vasculare, congenital poikiloderma-juvenile cataracts syndrome, poikiloderma atrophicans-cataract syndrome, poikiloderma congenita, poikiloscleroderma, telangiectasis-pigmentation-cataract syndrome.*

An autosomal recessive syndrome of atrophy, pigmentation, telangiectasia, and a peculiar marmorization of the skin in association with juvenile cataracts, abnormalities of the skeleton, loss of hair, defects of the nails and teeth, and disturbances of sexual development. Associated defects may include macrocephaly with frontal bossing and a broad depressed nasal bridge. The skin is generally normal at birth, but becomes red and swollen about the third to sixth month of life. The exposed surfaces are usually most severely affected; sensitivity to sunlight and blister formation occurring in many cases. Warty hyperkeratosis with late development of squamous cell carcinoma and hyperkeratosis palmaris et plantaris are sometimes present. Scalp, pubic, and axillary hypotrichosis and complete absence of eyebrows and eyelashes are common. Onychodystrophy has been noted in some instances. Short stature occurs in over half the patients. The most common hand findings include absence or hypoplasia of the thumb, resorption of the phalangeal tufts, soft tissue calcification, fusion of the fourth and fifth metacarpals, syndactyly, and brachydactyly. Osteosclerosis, lucency of various bones, and hypoplasia or aplasia of the radius and ulna may be present. Cataract, the principal ocular defect, may be associated with blindness, keratopathy, microcornea, and strabismus. Oral manifestations may include microdontia, crown malformations, delayed or ectopic eruption, missing teeth, and bifid uvula.

Rothmund, A. Über Cataracten in Verbindung mit einer eigentümlichen Hautdegeneration. *Graefes Arch. Klin.*

Ophth., 1868, 14:159-82. Thomson, M. S. Poikiloderma congenitale. *Brit. J. Derm.*, 1936, 48:221-34. Block, B., & Stauffer, H. Skin disease of endocrine origin (dysmormonal dermatosis). *Arch. Derm. Syph., Chicago*, 1929, 19:22-34.

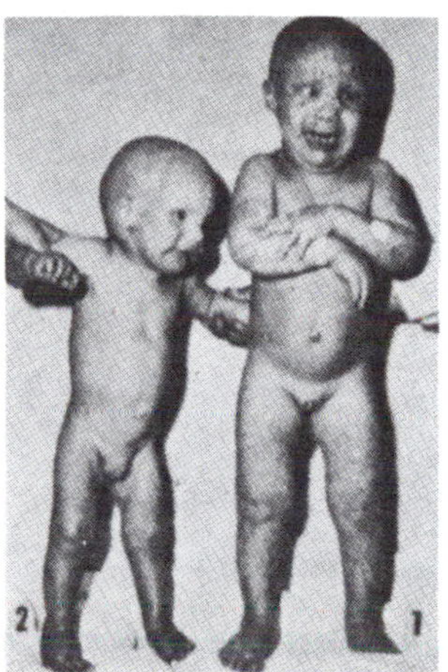

Rothmund-Thomson syndrome
Silver, H.K.: *AM. J. Dis. Child.* 111:183, 1966. Chicago: American Medical Association.

ROTOR, ARTURO B. (Physician in Manila)

Rotor syndrome (RS). Synonyms: *chronic idiopathic jaundice, idiopathic hyperbilirubinemia.*

An idiopathic form of hyperbilirubinemia, transmitted as an autosomal recessive trait, characterized by nonhemolytic jaundice, abdominal pain, epigastric discomfort, and fever. Pathological findings include low-grade pigment deposition, dissociation of liver cells, occasional necrotic foci, and fibrin precipitation. This and the Dubin-Johnson syndrome are similar, except that the Rotor syndrome exhibits increased total urinary coproporphyrin excretion and delayed plasma sulfobromophthalein clearance.

Rotor, A. B., *et al.* Familial non-hemolytic jaundice with direct van den Bergh reaction. *Acta Med. Philip.*, 1948, 5(2):37-49.

ROTTER, WOLFGANG (German physician, born 1910)

Rotter-Erb syndrome. Synonym: *osteochondrodesmodysplasia.*

A combination of deformities of the bones, joints, and tendons, marked by dwarfism, brachycephaly, brachymetapody, multiple metaphyseal lesions, loose joints, multiple dislocations, bilateral clubfoot, pterygium colli, vertebral deformities, including kyphoscoliosis and clefting of the vertebral arches, and cleft palate. Some writers consider this a doubtful entity.

Rotter, W., & Erb, W. Über eine Systemerkrankung des Mesenchyms mit multiplen Luxationen aus angeborener Gelenkschlaffheit und uber Wirbelbogenspalten. *Virchows Arch. Path.*, 1948-49, 316:233-63.

ROUBICEK, M. M.

Zanler-Roubicek syndrome. See *under Zanier.*

ROUGNON DE MAGNY, NICOLAS FRANÇOIS (French physician, 1727-1799)

Rougnon de Magny disease. See *Heberden asthma.*

round-cell sarcoma. See *Ewing sarcoma.*

round-head spermatozoa syndrome. Synonym: *globozoospermia.*

The presence of abnormal round-headed spermatozoa in the ejaculate of infertile males. Some authors suggest transmission as an autosomal dominant trait; others suspect recessive transmission.

Kullander S., & Rausing, A. On round-headed human spermatozoa. *Int. J. Fertil.*, 1975, 20:33-40. Syms, A. J., *et al.* Studies on human spermatozoa with round head syndrome. *Fertil. Steril.*, 1984, 42:431-5.

ROUSSY, GUSTAVE (French physician, 1874-1948)

Darier-Roussy sarcoid. See *under Darier.*

Déjerine-Roussy syndrome. See *under Déjerine.*

Roussy-Cornil syndrome. Synonyms: *hypertrophic neuritis, progressive hypertrophic neuritis.*

A disease of the nervous system, beginning in the fifth decade, characterized by degeneration of the muscles innervated by the affected nerves, particularly amyotrophy of the upper extremities, fibrillation, ataxia, positive Romberg sign, intention tremor, sensory disorders of the hand, and absent or depressed reflexes of the Achilles tendon and foot. Biopsy shows myelin degeneration, nuclear proliferation of the Schwann sheath, axonal changes, and mild hyperplasia of the connective tissue.

Roussy, G., & Cornil, L. Névrite hypertrophique progressive non familiale de l'adulte. *Ann. Méd., Paris*, 1919, 6:296-305.

Roussy-Lévy syndrome (RLS). Synonyms: *abortive type of Friedreich disease, familial claw foot with absent tendon jerks, hereditary areflexic dystasia.*

A familial disease of the nervous system, transmitted as an autosomal dominant trait, characterized by sensory ataxia, pes cavus, and areflexia, affecting at first the lower parts of the legs and progressing slowly to involve the hands. Onset is during infancy or childhood. The symptoms include clumsy gait, equilibrium disorders, awkwardness, weakness and slight atrophy of the muscles of the hands and legs, coldness and cyanosis of the legs, heart anomalies, disorders of the extensor palmar reflexes, loss of sensation (mainly of vibratory and position sense), decreased faradic and galvanic excitability of the muscles, and atypical tremor of the hands marked by tensing of the muscles, which is intensified during movements and absent at rest. Kyphoscoliosis may occur in some cases.

Roussy, G., & Lévy, G. Sept cas d'une maladie familiale particulaire: Troubles de la marche, pieds bots et aréflexie tendineuse généralisée, avec accessoirement, légère maladresse des mains. *Rev. Neur., Paris,* 1926, 1:427-50.

Roux-en-Y syndrome. Postoperative complication after a Roux-en-Y anastomosis (a surgical procedure performed to divert the pancreaticobiliary juices from the gastric pouch), consisting of abdominal pain, nausea, and vomiting, especially after eating.

Mathias, J. R., *et al.* Nausea, vomiting, and abdominal pain after Roux-en-Y anastomosis: motility of the jejunal limb. Gastroenerology, 1985, 88(1 Pt 1):101-7.

ROWELL, NEVILLE R.

Rowell syndrome. A syndrome of erythema multiforme-like lesions associated with discoid lupus erythematosus.

Rowell, N. R., et al. Lupus erythematosus and erythema multiforme-like lesions. A syndrome with characteristic immunological abnormalities. Arch. Derm., Chicago, 1963, 88:176-80.

ROWLAND, RUSSELL STURGIS (American physician, 1874-1938)

Hand-Rowland disease. See *Hand-Schüller-Christian syndrome.*

ROWLEY, PETER TEMPLETON (American physician, born 1929)

Rowley syndrome (1). See *Rowley-Rosenberg syndrome.*

Rowley syndrome (2). A familial syndrome, transmitted as an autosomal dominant trait with variable expressivity and incomplete penetrance, characterized by branchial fistulae and congenital hearing loss with both conductive and sensorineural components. Associated disorders may include low ears with flopped or malformed preauricular appendages, mandibular hypoplasia, and facial paralysis.

Rowley, P. T. Familial hearing loss associated with branchial fistulas. *Pediatrics,* 1969, 44:978-85.

Rowley-Rosenberg syndrome. Synonyms: *Busby syndrome, Rowley syndrome, growth retardation-pulmonary hypertension-aminoaciduria syndrome.*

A familial syndrome, transmitted as an autosomal recessive trait, characterized by retarded growth with muscle hypoplasia, scanty adipose tissue, renal aminoaciduria without elevation of blood amino acid levels and increased plasma unesterified fatty acid concentration, cor pulmonale, recurrent pulmonary infections, alveolar hypoventilation, atelectasis, pulmonary hypertension, and low basal respiratory quotient. Busby is the surname of the affected family in the original report.

Rowley, P. T., *et al.* Familial growth retardation, renal aminoaciduria and cor pulmonale. I. Description of a new syndrome with case reports. *Am. J. Med.,* 1961, 31:187-204. Rosenberg, L. E., *et al.* A new syndrome: Familial growth retardation, renal aminoaciduria and cor pulmonale. II. Investigation of renal function, amino acid metabolism and genetic transmission. *Am. J. Med.,* 1961, 31:205-15.

ROY, CLAUDE CHARLES (American physician, born 1928)

Scriver-Goldbloom-Roy syndrome. See *under Scriver.*

ROY, J. N. (Canadian physician)

Roy syndrome. See *pachydermoperiostosis syndrome.*

Roy-Jutras syndrome. See *pachydermoperiostosis syndrome.*

ROY, JAMES EVANS (American psychiatrist, born 1914)

Friedman-Roy syndrome. See *under Friedman, Arnold Phineas.*

ROYER, PIERRE (French physician)

Royer syndrome. An association of diabetes mellitus with the Prader-Willi syndrome.

Royer, P. Le diabète sucré dans le syndrome de Willi-Prader. *Journ. Ann. Diabét. Hôtel Dieu,* 1963, 4:91-9.

ROZIN, SAMUEL (Israeli physician)

Zondek-Bromberg-Rozin syndrome. See *Zondek syndrome, under Zondek, Bernhard.*

RP (Raynaud phenomenon). See *Raynaud syndrome.*

RPMD (rheumatic pain modulation disorder). See *fibrositis-fibromyalgia syndrome.*

RRS. See *Richards-Rundle syndrome.*

RS. See *Reiter syndrome.*

RS. See *Rett syndrome.*

RS. See *Reye syndrome.*

RS. See *Roberts syndrome.*

RS. See *Rotor syndrome.*

RS3PE (remitting seronegative symmetrical synovitis with pitting edema) syndrome. Symmetrical polysynovitis, involving most appendicular joints and flexor digitorum tendons, associated with pitting edema of the dorsum of the hands and feet. It is usually observed in elderly persons.

McCarty, D. J., *et al.* Remitting seronegative symmetrical synovitis with pitting edema. RS3PE syndrome. *JAMA,* 1985, 254:2763-7.

RSD. See *reflex sympathetic dystrophy syndrome.*

RSDS. See *reflex sympathetic dystrophy syndrome.*

RSH syndrome. See *Smith-Lemli-Opitz syndrome I, under Smith, David W.*

RSI (repetition strain injury). See *overuse syndrome.*

RSS. See *Russell-Silver syndrome.*

RTS. See *Rothmund-Thomson syndrome.*

RTS. See *Rubinstein-Taybi syndrome.*

rubella embryopathy. See *congenital rubella syndrome.*

rubella retinopathy. See *under congenital rubella syndrome.*

rubella syndrome. See *congenital rubella syndrome.*

rubeola syndrome. See *congenital rubella syndrome.*

rubeolar embryopathy. See *congenital rubella syndrome.*

RUBINSTEIN, JACK HERBERT (American pediatrician, born 1925)

Rubinstein syndrome. See *Rubinstein-Taybi syndrome.*

Rubinstein-Taybi syndrome (RTS). Synonyms: *Rubinstein syndrome, broad thumb-mental retardation syndrome.*

A syndrome of short broad terminal phalanges of the thumbs and great toes (brachydactyly D); short stature; mental retardation; motor retardation; facial deformities, including high-arched palate and straight or beaked nose; eye abnormalities, including various combinations of antimongoloid slant, epicanthus, strabismus, cataract, refractive error, high-arched eyebrows, and long lashes; skeletal maturation and head circumference that are below average for the age; and cryptorchism. There is also susceptibility to respiratory infections. Occasionally, there are other skeletal abnormalities, especially of the sternum, ribs, fingers, vertebrae, and toes; deformity of the urinary tract; simian crease; capillary hemangioma; and abnormal electroencephalographic findings. The etiology is unknown; almost all cases have been sporadic.

Rubinstein, J. H., & Taybi, H. Broad thumbs and toes and facial abnormalities. A possible mental retardation syndrome. *Am. J. Dis. Child.,* 1963, 105:588-608.

rubrospinal cerebellar syndrome. See *inferior nucleus ruber syndrome.*

rubrospinal cerebellar peduncle syndrome. See *inferior nucleus ruber syndrome.*

ruby spots. See *De Morgan spots.*

RUD, EINAR (Danish physician, born 1892)

Rud syndrome. Synonyms: *dwarfism-ichthyosiform erythroderma-mental deficiency syndrome, ichthyosis-hypogonadism-mental retardation-epilepsy syndrome, ichthyosis-mental retardation-epilepsy-hypogonadism syndrome, ichthyosis-oligophrenia-epilepsy syndrome, neuroichthyosis-hypogonadism syndrome.*

A syndrome, probably transmitted as an autosomal recessive or X-linked trait, characterized by ichthyosis (usually present from early infancy), psychomotor retardation, epileptic seizures, hypogonadism with eunuchoid apperance, and occasional short stature, retinitis pigmentosa, and polyneuropathy. Some writers consider this and the Sjögren-Larsson syndrome the same entity.

Rud, E. Et tilfaelde al infantislismus med tetani, epilepsy, polyneuritis, ichthiosis og anaemi of pernicios type. *Hospitalstidende*, 1927, 70:525-38.

RUDER, H. J. (American physician)

Ruder syndrome. Adrenal hyperfunction due to micronodular hyperplasia, which is associated with severe osteoporosis, but is unaccompanied by stigmata characteristic of the Cushing syndrome.

Ruder, H. J., *et al.* Severe osteopenia in young adults associated with Cushing's syndrome due to micronodular adrenal disease. *J. Clin. Endocr. Metab.*, 1974, 39:1138-47.

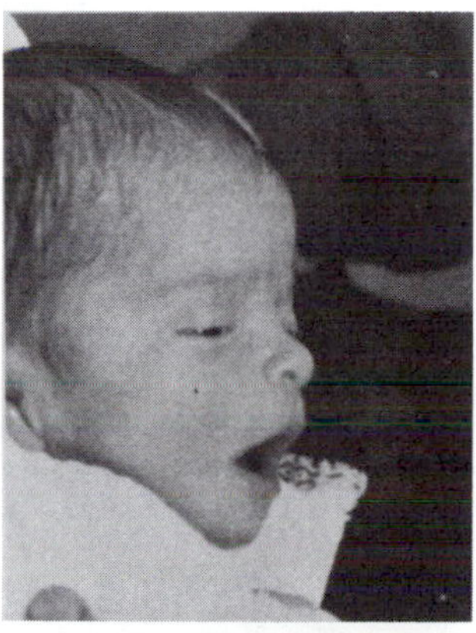

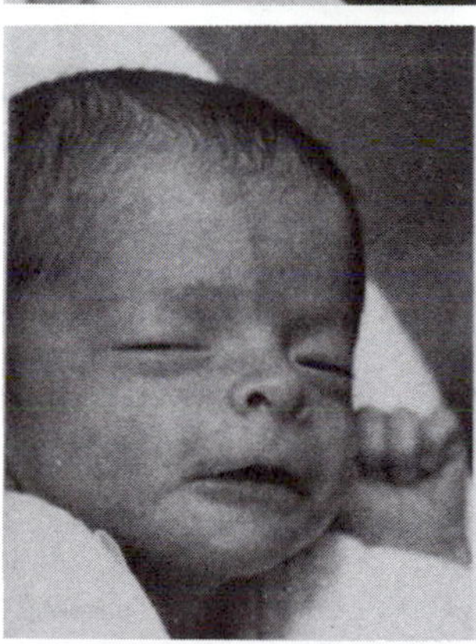

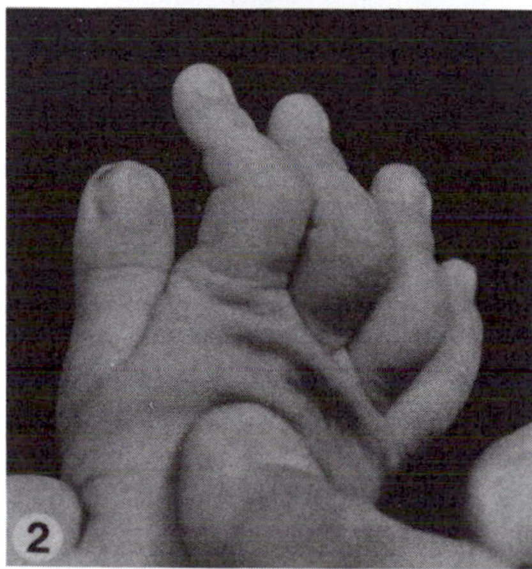

Rubinstein-Taybi syndrome
Cotsirilos, Patricia, JoEllyn C. Taylor, & Reuben Matalon: *American Journal of Medical Genetics* 26:85-93, 1987. New York: Alan R. Liss, Inc.

RÜDIGER, ROSWITHA A. (German physician)

Rüdiger syndrome (1). See *EEC syndrome.*

Rüdiger syndrome (2). A syndrome of shortened extremities, coarse facies, abnormal thickened palms and soles, abnormal dermatoglyphic pattern, abnormal cartilage development in the ears, cleft soft palate, hydronephrosis due to ureteral stenosis, inguinal hernia, and a bicornuate uterus. Originally, the syndrome was reported in two siblings who died in infancy. Autosomal recessive transmission is suspected.

Rüdiger, R. A., *et al.* Severe developmental failure with coarse facial features, distal limb hypoplasia, thickened palmar creases, bifid uvula, and ureteral stenosis. A previously unidentified familial disorder with lethal outcome. *J. Pediat.*, 1971, 79:977-81.

rudimentary testes syndrome. A congenital syndrome characterized by exceedingly small rudimentary testes without any abnormality of male sex differentiation. The testes are composed of scanty, small testicular tubules containing pre-Sertoli cells and some spermatogonia.

Bergada, C., *et al.* Variants of embryonic testicular dysgenesis: Bilateral anorchia and the syndrome of rudimentary testes. *Acta Endocr., Copenhagen,* 1962, 40:521-36.

rugby knee. See *Osgood-Schlatter syndrome.*

Ruhr rheumatism. See *Reiter syndrome.*

RUITER, M. (Dutch physician)

Gougerot-Ruiter syndrome. See *under Gougerot.*

Ruiter disease. See *Gougerot-Ruiter syndrome.*

Ruiter-Pompen syndrome. See *Fabry syndrome.*

Ruiter-Pompen-Wyers syndrome. See *Fabry syndrome.*

RUKAVINA, JOHN G. (American physician)

Rukavina syndrome. See *amyloid neuropathy type II.*

RULF

Rulf convulsions. A familial disorder of children and adolescents characterized by convulsions precipitated by the first purposeful movement following a period of rest, reportedly described by Rulf in 1913.

Davidenkova, E. F. O klinike i patofiziologii intensionnoi sudorogi Riul'fa. *Zh. Nevropat. Psikhiat.*, 1963, 63:1308-12.

rumination syndrome. Synonym: *infant rumination syndrome.*

Regurgitation of previously swallowed food and its rechewing and reswallowing. In infants, the process results in incomplete ingestion of food with secondary inanition, water-electrolyte balance disorders, and, potentially, loss of life.

Cameron, H. C. Some forms of habitual vomiting in infancy. *Brit. Med. J.*, 1925, 1:872-6.

RUMMO, A. (Italian physician)

Rummo-Ferranini syndrome. Synonyms: *genitodystrophic gerodermia, genitodystrophic xeroderma.*

A progeroid syndrome with lax skin, abnormal hair growth, and genital dystrophy with normal or acromegalic appearance.

*Rummo, A., & Ferranini, A. Xeroderma genitodystrofico, nuova entite clinica. *Riforma Med., Napoli,* 1897, 1:340.

RUMMO, GAETANO (Italian physician, 1853-1917)

Rummo disease. Synonym: *cardioptosis.*

Downward displacement of the heart.

Rummo, G. Sulla cardioptosis: Prima abbozzo anatomo-clinico. *Arch. Med. Int., Palermo,* 1898, 1:161-83.

RUNDLE, A. T. (British physician)

Richards-Rundle syndrome (RRS). See *under Richards.*

RUNDLES, RALPH WAYNE (American physician, born 1911)

Rundles-Falls syndrome. Synonyms: *hereditary sideroblastic anemia, pyridoxine-responsive anemia.*

A hereditary form of familial sideroblastic anemia, occurring in males, and characterized by red cell abnormalities, enlargement of the spleen, and responsiveness to pyridoxine. The condition is transmitted by females-many of whom have enlarged spleens and erythrocyte abnormalities without anemia in a manner compatible with sex-linked inheritance in which the abnormality is recessive, or incompletely recessive, in females.

Rundles, R. W., & Falls, H. F. Hereditary (?sex-linked) anemia. *Am. J. Med. Sc.,* 1946, 211:641-58.

RUNEBERG, JOHAN WILHELM (Finnish physician, 1843-1918)

Runeberg anemia. Synonym: *progressive pernicious anemia.*

A progressive form of pernicious anemia characterized by recurrent attacks of symptoms. After the first attack there appears to be a complete regression of the symptoms, followed by a succession of attacks, each being more severe than the preceding one.

Runeberg, J. W. Zur Kenntniss der sogenannten progressiven perniciösen Anämie. *Deut. Arch. Klin. Med.,* 1880-81, 28:499-520.

RUNGE, HANS (German physician, 1892-1964)

Ballantyne-Runge syndrome. See *under Ballantyne.*

Runge syndrome. See *Ballantyne-Runge syndrome.*

RUSSELL (RUSSEL), ALEXANDER (British physician)

Russell dwarf. See *under Russell-Silver syndrome.*

Russell nanism. See *Russell-Silver syndrome.*

Russell syndrome (1). See *Russell-Silver syndrome.*

Russell syndrome (2). See *diencephalic syndrome.*

Russell-Silver syndrome (RSS). Synonyms: *Russell dwarf, Russell nanism, Russell syndrome, Silver syndrome.*

A congenital syndrome of unknown etiology, characterized by prenatal growth deficiency, immature bone development in infancy and early childhood, late closure of the anterior fontanel, small triangular face with down-turned mouth and a prominent sometimes bossed forehead, small mandible and maxilla, developmental asymmetry, brachydactyly, clinodactyly, café-au-lait spots, excessive sweating, hypoglycemia, elevated gonadotropic hormone, hip and elbow dislocation, the Kirner deformity, hypoplasia of the sacral and coccygeal bones, and abnormal sexual development, including hypospadias, cryptorchism, and enlarged clitoris. Renal and/or ureteral defects and mental retardation may occur in some cases. Some authors separate the Russell and Silver syndromes as independent entities. An affected individual is known as the *Russell dwarf.*

Russell, A. A syndrome of "intra-uterine" dwarfism recognizable at birth with cranio-facial dysostosis, disproportionately short arm, and other anomalies (5 examples). *Proc. Roy. Sac. Med., London,* 1954, 47:1040-4. Silver, H. K., *et al.* Syndrome of congenital hemihypertrophy, shortness of stature, and elevated urinary gonadotropins. *Pediatrics,* 1953, 12:368-76.

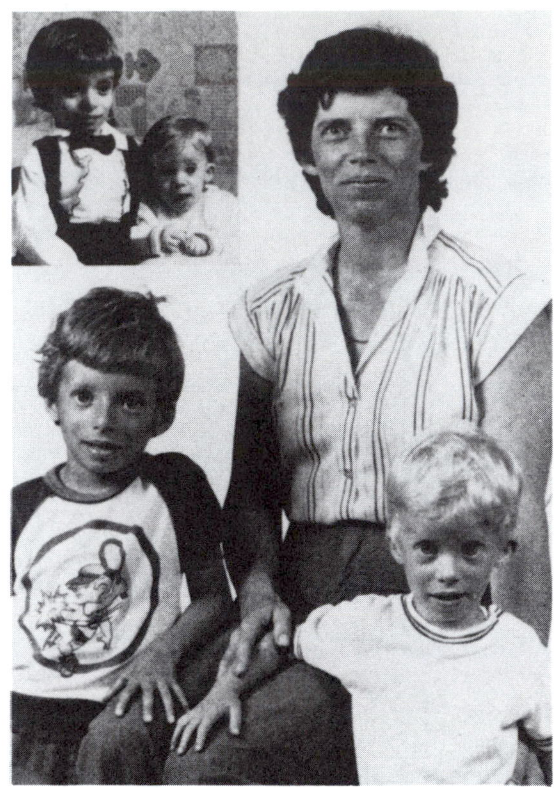

Russell-Silver syndrome
Partington, M.W., *Clinical Genetics* 29:151-156, 1986. Munksgaard International Publishers, Copenhagen, Denmark.

RUST, JOHANN NEPOMUK (Austrian physician, 1775-1840)

Rust disease. Synonyms: *malum rusti, malum suboccipitale, malum vertebrale suboccipitale, suboccipital vertebral disease.*

Lesions of the atlanto-occipital region secondary to tuberculosis, syphilis, neoplasms, fractures, or rheumatism. The symptoms include suboccipital pain and swelling, drooping of the head, trigeminal neuralgia, hypoglossal paralysis, tongue atrophy, and vagus nerve paralysis with cardiac arrhythmia.

Rust, J. N. *Aufsätze und Abhandlungen aus dem Gebiebe der Medizin, Chirurgie und Staatsarzneikunde.* Berlin, Enslin, 1834, Vol. 1, p. 196.

RUSTITSKII (RUSTITZKY, VON RUSTITZKY) (Russian physician)

Rustitskii disease. See *Kahler disease.*

Rustitzky disease. See *Kahler disease.*

Rustitzky syndrome. See *Kahler disease.*

von Rustitzky disease. See *Kahler disease.*

RUSTITZKY, VON. See RUSTITSKII

RUTHERFURD, MARGARET ELIZABETH (British dentist, 1910-1964)

Rutherfurd syndrome. Synonym: *oculodental syndrome.*

A relatively mild form of gingival hypertrophy associated with failure of tooth eruption and a dense curtainlike corneal opacity involving the upper part of each cornea, with root resorption occurring in the primary teeth in the unerupted teeth. The condition is transmitted as an autosomal dominant trait.

Rutherfurd, M. E. Three generations of inherited dental defect. *Brit. Med. J.*, 1931, 2:9-11.

RUTISHAUSER, E. (Swiss physician)

Martin du Pan-Rutishauser disease. See *under Martin du Pan.*

RUVALCABA, R. H. A. (American physician)

Ruvalcaba syndrome (1). Synonym: *Ruvalcaba-Reichert-Smith syndrome.*

A syndrome of mental retardation, short stature, microcephaly, peculiar facies, narrow thoracic cage with pectus carinatum, hypoplastic genitalia, hypoplastic skin lesions, and skeletal deformities. Orofacial features include antimongoloid slant of the palpebral fissures, small narrow nose, and narrow maxilla with crowded teeth. Kyphoscoliosis, osteochondritis of the spine, limitation of elbow movement, shortening of the third to fifth metacarpals with broadening of the distal ends of the fingers, and early fusion of the epiphyses are the principal skeletal features. Inguinal hernia is usually associated. Autosomal recessive transmission is suspected, with X-linked inheritance also being considered. See also *trichorhinophalangeal dysplasia type III.*

Ruvalcaba, R. H. A., Reichert, A., & Smith, D. W. A new familial syndrome with osseous dysplasia and mental deficiency. *J. Pediat.*, 1971, 79:450-5.

Ruvalcaba syndrome (2). Synonym: *Ruvalcaba-Myhre-Smith syndrome.*

A syndrome combining the principal elements of the Sotos syndrome with intestinal polyposis and pigmented lesions (café-au-lait spots) on the penis.

Ruvalcaba, R. H. A., Myhre, S., & Smith, D. W. Sotos syndrome with intestinal polyposis and pigmentary changes of the genitals. *Clin. Genet.*, 1980, 18:413-6.

Ruvalcaba-Myhre-Smith syndrome. See *Ruvalcaba syndrome (2).*

Ruvalcaba-Reichert-Smith syndrome. See *Ruvalcaba syndrome (1).*

RYTAND, D. A. (American physician)

Rytand-Lipsitch syndrome. Total arteriovenous block resulting from destruction of the central area of the conducting system of the heart due to extension of calcification from the fibrous ring of the mitral valve.

Paulsen, S., & Vetner, M. Rytand-Lipsitch syndrome. *Arch. Path., Chicago,* 1975, 99:246-8.

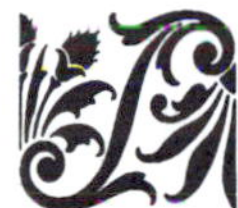

Page #	Term	Observation

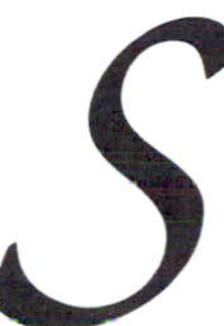

S syndrome. See *Kandinskii-Clérambault syndrome.*

SA. See *sleep apnea* ***syndrome.***

SA (Stokes-Adams) syndrome. See *Adams-Stokes syndrome.*

SABIN, ALBERT BRUCE (American physician, born 1906)

Sabin-Feldman syndrome. Synonyms: *microcephaly-chorioretinopathy syndrome, pseudotoxoplasmosis, seronegative toxoplasmosis.*

A syndrome of toxoplasmosislike symptoms and extensive destruction of brain tissue, hydrocephalus, diffuse cerebral calcification, chorioretinopathy, microcephaly, mental retardation, and bizarre degenerative changes in the small blood vessels. The syndrome has been reported in inbred groups as a hereditary condition transmitted as an autosomal recessive trait.

Sabin, A. B., & Feldman, H. A. Chorioretinopathy associated with other evidence of cerebral damage in childhood. A syndrome of unknown etiology separable from congenital toxoplasmosis. *J. Pediat.,* 1949, 35:296-309. McKusick, V. A., *et al.* Chorioretinopathy with hereditary microcephaly. *Arch. Ophth., Chicago,* 1966, 75:597-600.

Sabinas brittle hair syndrome. See *Sabinas syndrome.*

Sabinas syndrome. Synonyms: *brittle hair-mental deficit syndrome, Sabinas brittle hair syndrome.*

A familial syndrome of brittle hair, mild mental deficiency, and nail dysplasia, originally observed in infants in Sabinas, a small community in northern Mexico. Additional symptoms may include alopecia or hypotrichosis, trichorrhexis nodosa, anodontia, amelogenesis imperfecta, hypohidrosis, cleft lip, webbed knees, deafness, and endocrine disorders. Reduced hair cystine levels, increased copper/zinc ratio, and the presence of arginosuccinic acid in the blood and urine are the principal biochemical features. The syndrome is transmitted as an autosomal recessive trait.

Arbisser, A. I., *et al.* A syndrome manifested by brittle hair, with morphologic and biochemical abnormalities, developlmental delay and normal stature. *Birth Defects,* 1976, 12(5):219-28.

SABOURAUD, RAYMOND JACQUES ADRIAN (French physician, 1864-1938)

Sabouraud syndrome. Synonyms: *beaded hairs, monilethricosis, monilethrix, moniliform hair, pili annulati, pili moniliformis.*

A congenital disease in which the hairs exhibit beadlike or fusiform enlargements and become brittle, being a component of some hereditary syndromes.

Sabouraud, R. Sur les cheveux moniformes. (Trichorrhexies et monilethrix). *Arch. Derm. Syph., Paris,* 1892, 3:781-93.

sacciform disease of the anus. See *Gross disease, under Gross, Samuel David.*

SACHS, BERNARD (American physician, 1858-1944)

pseudo-Tay-Sachs syndrome. See *Sandhoff syndrome.*

Sachs disease. See *Tay-Sachs syndrome, under Tay, Warren.*

Tay-Sachs disease (TSD). See *Tay-Sachs syndrome, under Tay, Warren.*

Tay-Sachs syndrome. See *under Tay, Warren.*

SACK, GEORG (German physician)

Sack syndrome. See *Ehlers-Danlos syndrome.*

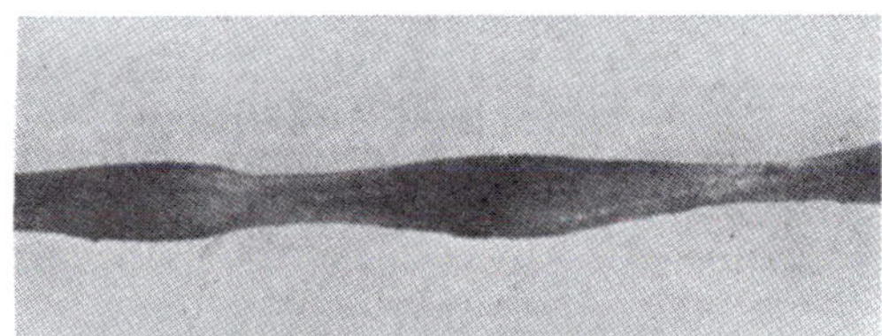

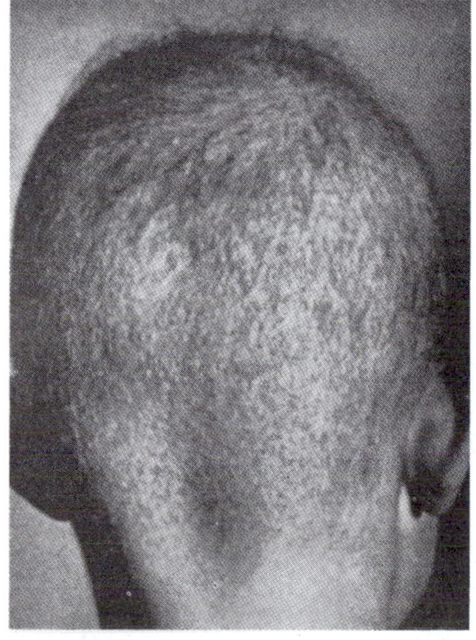

Sabouraud syndrome
Andrews, G.C. & A.N. Domonkos: *Diseases of the Skin.* 5th ed. Philadelphia: W.B. Saunders Co., 1963.

Sack-Barabas syndrome. See *Ehlers-Danlos syndrome.*

SACKS, BENJAMIN (American physician)

Kaposi-Besnier-Libman-Sacks syndrome. See *Libman-Sacks syndrome.*

Libman-Sacks disease. See *Libman-Sacks syndrome.*

Libman-Sacks syndrome. See *under Libman.*

Osler-Libman-Sacks disease. See *Libman-Sacks syndrome.*

sacral agenesis syndrome. See *caudal regression syndrome.*

sacral dysplasia syndrome. See *caudal regression syndrome.*

sacrococcygeal agenesis syndrome. See *caudal regression syndrome.*

sacs of the anus. See *Gross disease, under Gross, Samuel David.*

SAEMISCH, EDWIN THEODOR (German ophthalmologist, 1833-1909)

Saemisch ulcer. Synonyms: *hypopyon ulcer, ulcus corneae serpens.*

Serpiginous ulcer of the cornea characterized by destructive grayish white or yellow discoid lesions that may be associated with keratitis, iridocyclitis, hypopyon, and posterior abscesses of the cornea. Pneumococcal infection following a minor abrasion is the usual cause.

*Saemisch, E. T. *Das Ulcus corneae serpens und seine Therapie; eine klinische Studie.* Bonn, Cohen, 1870.

SAENGER, ALFRED (German physician, 1860-1921)

Saenger syndrome. See *Adie syndrome.*

SAETHRE, HAAKON (Norwegian psychiatrist)

Saethre-Chotzen syndrome. Synonyms: *Chotzen syndrome, Chotzen-Saethre syndrome, acrocephalosyndactyly II (ACS II), acrocephalosyndactyly III (ACS III), dysostosis craniofacialis with hypertelorism.*

A relatively mild form of acrocephalosyndactyly characterized by hypertelorism, cranial synostosis, asymmetry of the skull and orbits (plagiocephaly), low frontal hairline, beaked nose, deviated nasal septum, absent frontonasal angle, blepharoptosis, tear duct stenosis, dermatoglyphic changes, and brachydactyly. Bifid phalanges, absence of first metatarsal bones, cleft palate, strabismus, hydrophthalmos, knee and elbow contractures, and cardiac malformations may be associated. The syndrome is transmitted as an autosomal dominant trait. According to some authorities (McKusick), the syndrome is classified as acrocephalosyndactyly III; according to others (Spranger, Langer, and Wiedemann), as acrocephalosyndactyly II.

Saethre, H. Ein Beitrag zum Turmschädelproblem (Pathogenese, Erblichkeit und Symptomatologie). *Deut. Zschr. Nervenheilk.*, 1931, 117:533-5. Chotzen, F. Eine eigenartige familiäre Entwicklungsstörüng (Akrozephalosyndaktylie, Dysostosis craniofacialis und Hypertlorismus). *Mschr. Kinderheilk.*, 1932, 55:97-122. McKusick, V. A. *Mendelian heritance in man.* 5th ed. Baltimore, The Johns Hopkins University Press, 1978, p. 8 (No. 10140). Spranger, J. W., Langer, L. O., Wiedemann, H. R. *Bone dysplasias*, Philadelphia, Saunders, 1974, p. 261.

safety belt syndrome. See *seat belt syndrome.*

SAHS. See ***s**leep **a**pnea-**h**yper**s**omnolence syndrome.*

SAID (sexually **a**cquired **i**mmuno**d**eficiency) **syndrome.** See *acquired immunodeficiency syndrome.*

SAINT

Saint syndrome. See *Saint triad.*

Saint triad. Synonym: *Saint syndrome.*

A combination of hiatus hernia, diverticulosis, and gallbladder calculi.

Palmer, E. D. Saint's triad (hiatus hernia, gall stones and diverticulosis coli): the problem of properly directing surgical therapy. *Am. J. Digest. Dis.*, 1955, 22:314-5.

SAINTON, RAYMOND (French physician)

Marie-Sainton syndrome. See *cleidocranial dysostosis.*

Scheuthauer-Marie-Sainton syndrome. See *cleidocranial dysostosis.*

SAKAMOTO, A. (Japanese physician)

Sakamoto disease. Synonyms: *alimentary toxicosis, cholera infantum, hakuri, pseudocholera infantum.*

Infantile diarrhea characterized by milky white stools, explosive vomiting, and mild respiratory symptoms, occurring annually and epidemiologically throughout Japan.

*Sakamoto, A. On the pathogenesis of so-called pseudocholera infantum. *Ann. Rep. Coop. Res. (Med.) Minist. Educ.*, 1961, 353-60.

SAKATI, NADIA (American pediatrician)

Sakati syndrome. See *Sakati-Nyhan-Tisdale syndrome.*

Sakati-Nyhan-Tisdale syndrome. Synonyms: *Sakati syndrome, acrocephalopolysyndactyly (ACPS).*

A syndrome of multiple abnormalities involving the head, limbs, heart, ears, and skin. Craniofacial defects consist of a small face, shallow orbits, prominent eyes, acrocephaly, craniosynostosis, dysplastic low-set ears, high-arched palate, maxillary hypoplasia, and crowding of the upper teeth. Patches of alopecia with atrophic skin above the ears, low hairline, and linear cleft like submental scars are usually present. Limb abnormalities include brachydactyly, polydactyly of the fingers and toes, syndactyly of the toes, bowed femora, hypoplastic tibiae, posterior displacement of the fibulae, short hands, cubitus valgus, abduction of the feet, and coxa valga. Congenital heart defect, widely spaced nipples, cryptorchidism, microphallus, and inguinal hernia may be associated. The reported cases are usually sporadic.

Sakati, N., Nyhan, W. L., & Tisdale, W. K. A new case with acrocephalopolysydactyly, cardiac disease, and distinctive defect of the ear, skin, and lower limbs. *J. Pediat.*, 1971, 79:104-9.

salaam convulsions. See *West syndrome.*

SALAMON, T.

Salamon syndrome (1). A syndrome, probably transmitted as a genetic trait, characterized by pili torti, tooth dystrophy, onychodystrophy, verrucae, and conjunctivitis.

Salamon, T., *et al.* The hairs in the syndrome of Netherton and in a peculiar form of ectodermal dysplasia. *Derm. Mschr.*, 1974, 160:362-77.

Salamon syndrome (2). An inherited familial syndrome, transmitted as an autosomal recessive trait, characterized by wooly hair, hypotrichosis, everted lower lip, and large protruding ears.

Salamon, T. Über eine Familie mit recessiver Kraushaarigkeit, Hypotrichose und anderen Anomalien. *Hautarzt*, 1963, 14:540-4.

SALAND, S. (Swiss physician)

Glanzmann-Saland syndrome. See *under Glanzmann.*

SALDINO, RONALD M. (American radiologist)

Saldino syndrome. See *achondrogenesis type II.*

Saldino-Mainzer syndrome. A familial disorder of unknown etiology, characterized by juvenile nephrophthisis, retinitis pigmentosa, cerebellar ataxia, cone-shaped epiphyses of the fingers and toes, and short irregularly ossified femoral heads and necks.

Saldino, R. M., & Mainzer, F. Cone-shaped epiphyses (CSE) in siblings with hereditary renal disease and retinitis pigmentosa. *Radiology*, 1971, 98:39-45.

Saldino-Noonan syndrome. Synonyms: *polydactyly with neonatal chondrodystrophy type II; short rib-polydactyly syndrome type II (SRP II); short rib-polydactyly syndrome, Saldino-Noonan type.*

A congenital syndrome of short limb dwarfism, hydropic appearance with a narrow thorax, very short flipperlike limbs, and postaxial polydactyly. Brachydactyly, prominent abdomen, multiple cardiovascular defects (mostly transposition of the great vessels), hypoplastic lungs, anal atresia, and genital abnormalities are associated. Occasional defects include polycystic kidneys, unossified phalanges, metaphyseal dysplasia, and premature ossification of the epiphyses. Death occurs in utero or shortly after birth. The syndrome is transmitted as an autosomal recessive trait.

Saldino, R. M., & Nooman, C. C. Severe thoracic dystrophy with striking micromelia, abnormal osseous development, including the spine, and multiple visceral anomalies. *Am.J. Roentgen.*, 1972, 114:257-53.

short rib-polydactyly syndrome, Saldino-Noonan type. See *Saldino-Noonan syndrome.*

salivary gland virus disease. See *Wyatt disease, under Wyatt, John Poyner.*

salivary gland virus inclusion disease. See *Wyatt disease, under Wyatt, John Poyner.*

SALLIS, J. G. (Physician in South Africa)

Sallis-Beighton syndrome. See *digitotalar dysmorphism syndrome.*

SALLMANN, LUDWIG, VON. See VON SALLMANN, LUDWIG

SALLY

Sally syndrome. See *Chapple syndrome (2).*

SALOMON, EUGEN (German physician)

Rabe-Salomon syndrome. See *under Rabe.*

SALONEN, RIITA (Finnish physician)

Salonen-Herva-Norio syndrome. See *hydrolethalus syndrome.*

salt losing nephritis. See *renal salt losing syndrome.*

salt losing nephropathy. See *renal salt losing syndrome.*

salt losing syndrome (1). See *cerebral salt wasting syndrome.*

salt losing syndrome (2). See *congenital adrenal hyperplasia.*

salt losing syndrome (3). See *renal salt losing syndrome.*

salt wasting renal disease. See *renal salt losing syndrome.*

saltatory spasms. See *Bamberger disease (1), under Bamberger, Heinrich, von.*

SALUS, ROBERT (Austrian ophthalmologist, born 1877)

Koerber-Salus-Elschnig syndrome. See *under Koerber.*

SALVIOLI, GAETANO (Italian physician, born 1894)

Salvioli syndrome. Synonym: *osteopathia familiaris neuroendocrina.*

A familial syndrome involving the bones, autonomic nervous system, endocrine glands, and phosphorus metabolism. The symptoms include fragilitas ossium, hypophosphatemia, tremor, athetotic chorea, masklike facies, mental deficiency, gynecomastia, hypogenitalism, secondary muscle atrophy, and mild pain. Extensive areas of decalcification and multiple fractures are seen on x-rays.

Salvioli, G. Über eine neue Knochenerkrankung: Osteopathia familiaris neuroendocrina. *Mschr. Kinderh.*, 1954, 102:330-1.

SALZMANN, MAXIMILIAN (German ophthalmologist, 1862-1954)

Salzmann dystrophy. Synonym: *nodular degeneration of the cornea.*

Nodular dystrophy of the cornea characterized by progressive hypertrophic degeneration of the epithelial layer, the Bowman membrane, and the outer portion of the cornea; it is a complication of phlyctenular keratitis or trachoma.

*Salzmann, M. Über eine eigentümliche Form von Hornhautentzündung. *Mitt. Verein. Aerzte Steiermark,* 1916, 53:194-8.

SAMMAN, P. D. (British physician)

Samman-White syndrome. See *yellow nail syndrome.*

SAMPSON, JOHN ALBERTSON (American physician, 1873-1946)

Sampson cyst. Synonyms: *chocolate cyst, endometrial cyst.*

A cyst with chocolatelike contents made of a collection and hemosiderin, with occurrs after local hemorrhage, such as that following mastectomy, or in the ovary in ovarian endometriosis.

Sampson, J. A. Perforating hemorrhagic (chocolate) cysts of the ovary. Their importance and especially their relation to pelvic adenomas or endometrial type ("adenomyoma" of the uterus, rectovaginal septum, sigmoid, etc.). *Arch. Surg., Chicago,* 1921, 3:245-323.

SAMTER, MAX (American physician)

Samter syndrome. Synonym: *aspirin insensitivity.*

Intolerance to aspirin associated with vasomotor rhinitis, with or without nasal polyps, and bronchial asthma. Associated features include eosinophilia, urticaria, and/or angioedema in the absence of significant atopic allergy.

Samter, M., & Beers, R. F., Jr. Concerning the nature of intolerance to aspirin. *J. Allergy,* 1967,40:281-93 Zeitz, H. J., & Jarmoszuk, I. Nasal polyps, bronchial asthma, and aspirin insensitivity: The Samter syndrome. *Compr. Ther.,* 1985, 11(6)21-6.

SANDER, WILHELM (German physician, 1838-1922)

Sander disease. A form of paranoia.

Sander, W. Über eine specielle Form der primären Verrücktheit. *Acta Psychiat., Berlin,* 1868-69, 1:387-419.

SANDERS, MURRAY (American physician, born 1910)

Sanders syndrome. Synonyms: *Sanders-Hogan syndrome, epidemic keratoconjunctivitis, keratitis maculosa, keratitis nummularis, keratitis subepithelialis, keratitis superficialis punctata, keratoconjunctivitis epidemica, macular keratitis, shipyard conjunctivitis.*

An epidemic form of keratoconjunctivitis caused by strains of adenovirus and characterized by acute follicular or pseudomembranous conjunctivitis complicated by subepithelial corneal infiltrates. See also *Dimmer keratitis.*

Sanders, M. Epidemic keratoconjunctivitis ("shipyard conjunctivitis"). I. Isolation of a virus. *Arch. Ophth., Chicago,* 1942, 28:581-6.

Sanders-Hogan syndrome. See *Sanders syndrome.*

SANDHOFF, K. (German biochemist)

Sandhoff disease. See *Sandhoff syndrome.*

Sandhoff syndrome. Synonyms: *pseudo-Tay-Sachs syndrome, Sandhoff disease, Sandhoff-Jatzkewitz syndrome, gangliosidosis G_{M2} type II, gangliosidosis G_{M2} type 0, gangliosidosis G_{M2}-hexosaminidase A and B deficiency syndrome.*

A ganglioside storage disorder characterized by deficiency of both hexosaminidases A and B with resulting accumulation of ganglioside G_{M2}, lipidosis being most prominent in the cortical, cerebellar, spinal, and autonomic nervous system tissues. The syndrome is similar in most respects to the Tay-Sachs syndrome but has no special predilection for any ethnic or racial group. It is characterized chiefly by motor weakness, which may be noted within the first 6 months of life, followed by startle reaction to sharp sound, blindness, psychomotor retardation, doll-like facies, cherry-red spots of the retina, and fatal pneumonia by the age of 3 years. Macroglossia, macrocephaly, hepatosplenomegaly, lumbar gibbus, and mucopolysacchariduria are usually associated. Pathological findings may include foamy histiocytes in the bone marrow and vacuolated histiocytes in the lungs, spleen, lymph nodes, and bone marrow. The syndrome is transmitted as an autosomal recessive trait.

Sandhoff, K., Andreae, U., & Jatzkewitz, H. Deficient hexosaminidase activity in an exceptional case of Tay-Sachs disease. *J. Neurochem.*, 1971, 18:2469-89. O'Brien, J. S. The gangliosidoses. In: Stanbury, J. B., Wyngaarden, J. B., & Fredrickson, D. S., eds. *The metabolic basis of inherited disease.* 4th ed. New York, McGraw-Hill, 1978, pp. 841-65.

Sandhoff-Jatzkewitz syndrome. See *Sandhoff syndrome.*

SANDIFER, PAUL (British radiologist)

Sandifer syndrome. A syndrome characterized by abnormal body posturing and contortions of the neck (torticollis), associated with gastro-esophageal reflux, with or without a hiatus hernia. Paul Sandifer is said to have been the first to recognize this disorder.

Kinsbourne, M. Hiatus hernia with contortions of the neck. *Lancet,* 1964, 1:1058-62. Sutcliffe, J. Torsion spasms and abnormal postures in children with hiatus hernia: Sandifer's syndrome. *Progr. Pediat. Radiol.*, 1969, 2;190-7.

SANDROW, RICHARD E. (American physician)

Sandrow syndrome. A syndrome of polydactyly of the hands and feet, duplication of the carpal and tarsal bones, talipes equinovarus, dislocated knees, colobomas of the nasal alae, and peculiar facies mainly due to partial fusion of the external nares with obstruction of the nasal passages, snorting respiration, and superficial hemangiomata over the temporozygomatic region of the face. The syndrome is believed to be transmitted as a genetic trait.

Sandrow, R. E., *et al.* Hereditary ulnar and fibular dimelia with peculiar facies. A case report. *J. Bone Joint Surg.*, 1979, 52(A):367-80.

SANDWITH, FLEMING MANT (British physician, 1853-1918)

Sandwith bald tongue. An extremely clean tongue sometimes seen in the late stages of pellagra, reportedly described by Sandwith.

SANFILIPPO, SYLVESTER J. (American physician)

Sanfilippo syndrome. See *mucopolysaccharidosis III.*

SANTAVUORI, PIRKKO (Finnish physician)

Hagberg-Santavuori syndrome. See *Haltia-Santavuori syndrome.*

Haltia-Santavuori neuronal ceroid lipofuscinosis. See *Haltia-Santavuori syndrome.*

Haltia-Santavuori syndrome. See *under Haltia.*

Santavuori disease. See *Haltia-Santavuori syndrome.*

Santavuori syndrome. Synonym: *muscle-eye-brain (MEB) disease.*

A congenital syndrome of muscle, brain, and eye disorders, transmitted as an autosomal recessive trait. Ocular manifestations include congenital or infantile glaucoma, persistent hyperplastic primary vitreous, cataract, choroid and retinal hypoplasia, optic atrophy, colobomas of the choroid and retina, and myopia. Congenital muscular dystrophy, characterized by muscular hypotonia and weakness, usually with joint contractures, is the principal muscular component of this syndrome. Neurological defects consist of dilation of the ventricles and exterior liquor spaces, the Dandy-Walker malformation, hypodensity of the white matter, agyria, pachygyria, or microgyria of the cerebral cortex, absence of cortical lamination, cytological abnormalities, frontal adhesions of the hemispheres, pial thickening, stenosis of the aqueduct of Sylvius, micropolygyria of the cerebellum, hypoplasia of the pyramidal tracts, and heterotopias of the brain stem and basal meninges.

*Santavuori, P., *et al.* Muscle, eye and brain disease. A new syndrome. *Neuropädiatrie,* 1977, 8:550. Raitta, C., *et al.* Ophthalmological findings in an new syndrome with muscle, eye and brain involvement. *Acta Ophth., Copenhagen,* 1978, 56:465-72.

SAP (situs ambiguus-polysplenia) syndrome. See *polysplenia syndrome.*

sarcoma idiopathicum hemorrhagicum. See *Kaposi sarcoma.*

sarcoma idiopathicum multiplex hemorrhagicum. See *Kaposi sarcoma.*

sarcoma osteogenes juxtacorticale. See *Geschickter tumor.*

sarcoma osteogenes parostale. See *Geschickter tumor.*

sarcomatosis cutis. See *Bäfverstedt syndrome.*

SARROUY (SARROY), C. (Algerian physician)

Sarrouy disease. Synonym: *Sarroy disease.*

Anemia associated with retarded growth, pallor, hepatosplenomegaly, hepatosplenic hematopoiesis, signs of rickets, bone marrow hypoplasia, and usually terminal marasmus. The disease was originally described in Algerian infants.

Sarrouy, C., *et al.* L'anémie subaigue curable due nourrison avec hypoplasie médullaire et hématopoïesie hépatosplénique. *Algerie Méd.*, 1954, 58:419-25.

SARROY, C. See SARROUY, C.

SAS. See *supravalvular aortic stenosis syndrome.*

SASPP. See *absence of septum pellucidum with porencephalia syndrome.*

Sassoon hospital syndrome. An epidemic disease with symptoms of severe polyuria, thirst, anorexia, weakness, and fatigue caused by a strain of the fungus *Rhizopus nigricans* found on the staple millet grains. The condition was observed in the Sassoon General Hospitals, Poona, Maharashtra, India.

Narasimhan, M. J., Jr., *et al.* Epidemic polyuria in man caused by a phycomycetous fungus (the Sassoon hospital syndrome). *Lancet,* 1967, 1:760-1.

SATCHMO. See ARMSTRONG (SATCHMO), LOUIS DANIEL

SATOYOSHI, EJIRO (Japanese physician)

Satoyoshi syndrome (1). A syndrome of multiple metaphyseal lesions, progressive painful muscle cramps, alopecia, and stunted growth. Radiological findings consist of abnormal ossification of the femur, radius, ulna, and phalanges of the hand. Most cases of this syndrome have been observed in Japan.

Satoyoshi, E., & Yamada, K. Recurrent muscle spasms of central origin. A report of two cases. *Arch. Neur., Chicago,* 1967, 16:254-64.

Satoyoshi syndrome (2). Synonym: *oculopharyngodistal myopathy.*

Oculopharyngeal myopathy, transmitted as an autosomal dominant trait, consisting of slowly progressive blepharoptosis and extraocular palsy associated with weakness of the masseter, facial, and bulbar muscles and distal involvement of the limbs. Retinitis pigmentosa, optic atrophy, endocrine complications, dementia, ataxia, pyramidal disorders, and deafness may occur in some cases. Onset usually takes place in the fifth decade of life.

Satoyoshi, E., & Kinoshita, M. Oculopharyngodistal myopathy. *Arch. Neur., Chicago,* 1977, 34:89-92.

SATTLER, C. HUBERT (Austrian ophthalmologist)

Sattler veil. Corneal edema with blurring of vision, halos, and development of vesiculation due to oxygen deficiency that may result from wearing contact lenses.

Sattler, C. H. Erfahrungen über den Ausgleich von Brechungsfehlern des Auges durch Haftgläser. *Deut. Med. Wschr.,* 1931, 57:312-4.

saturnism. See *lead poisoning.*

satyriasis. See *Hansen disease.*

SAUNDERS, WILLIAM (Scottish physician, 1783-1817)

Saunders-Sutton syndrome. See *Morel disease, under Morel, Benedict Augustin.*

SAUVINEAU, CHARLES (French ophthalmologist, born 1862)

Sauvineau ophthalmoplegia. Oculomotor paralysis associated with horizontal movements of the eyes.

Sauvineau, C. Un nouveau type de paralysie associée des mouvements horizontaux des yeux. *Ann. Ocul., Paris,* 1895, 113:363-4.

SAVAGE

Savage syndrome. See *resistant ovary syndrome.*

SAVILL, THOMAS DIXON (British physician, 1856-1910)

Savill disease. Synonym: *epidemic exfoliative dermatitis.*

An epidemic form of an inflammatory skin disease with more or less generalized erythema and scaling, originally observed during the summer and autumn of 1891 in London asylums and workhouses. The condition may have been associated with either an infectious agent or a drug.

Savill, T. D. On an epidemic skin disease. *Brit. Med. J.,* 1891, 2:1197-202.

SAY, BURHAN (American physician)

Say syndrome (1). See *VATER association.*

Say syndrome (2). A familial syndrome, probably transmitted as an autosomal recessive or X-linked trait, characterized by multiple abnormalities, a chemotactic defect, and transient hypogammaglobulinemia. The anomalies include retarded growth, flexion contractures, neurological development delay, craniofacial defects (microcephaly, craniosynostosis, slopping forehead, beaked and prominent nose with high nasal bridge, carp-shaped mouth, micrognathia), stenosis of the anus, dislocated hip, hypoplastic patellae, scoliosis, small penis and testes, eczematous eruption, and decreased subcutaneous fatty tissue.

Say, B., *et al.* Microcephaly, short stature, and developmental delay with a chemotactic defect and hypogammaglobulinaemia in two brothers. *J. Med. Genet.,* 1986, 23:355-9.

Say-Gerald syndrome. See *VATER association.*

Say-Meyer syndrome. A familial syndrome of trigonocephaly, short stature, and retarded psychomotor development. The pattern of inheritance appears to be X-linked recessive, but the possibility of autosomal dominant inheritance with low expressivity in women could not be excluded. In the original report, additional symptoms included closed posterior fontanel, small anterior fontanel, frontal vertical ridge, narrow forehead, and hypertelorism.

Say, B., & Meyer, J. Familial trigonocephaly associated with short stature and developmental delay. *Am. J. Dis. Child.,* 1981, 135:711-2.

SAYRE, GEORGE P. (American physician)

Kearns-Sayre syndrome (KSS). See *under Kearns.*

SBS. See *short bowel syndrome.*

SBS (shaken baby syndrome). See *battered child syndrome.*

SC syndrome. See *pseudothalidomide syndrome.*

SC phocomelia syndrome. See *pseudothalidomide syndrome.*

scabies crustosa norvegica. See *Boeck scabies.*

scabies norvegica boeckii. See *Boeck scabies.*

SCAGLIETTI, OSCAR (Italian physician)

Scaglietti-Dagnani syndrome. See *Erdheim syndrome.*

scalded skin syndrome. See *staphylococcal scalded skin syndrome, and toxic epidermal necrolysis*

scalenus anticus syndrome. Synonyms: *Cooper syndrome, Haven syndrome, Naffziger syndrome, Nonne syndrome, scalenus neurocirculatory compression syndrome.*

Compression of the brachial plexus and the subclavian artery between a cervical rib and the scalenus anticus muscle or, in the absence of rib abnormality, by large scalene muscle. See also *thoracic outlet syndrome* and *cervical rib syndrome.*

Naffziger, H. C. The scalenus syndrome. *Surg. Gyn. Obst.,* 1937, 64:119-20. Haven, H. Neurocirculatory scalenus anticus syndrome in the presence of developmental defects of the first rib. *Yale J. Biol. Med.,* 1938-39, 11:443-58.

scalenus neurocirculatory compression syndrome. See *scalenus anticus syndrome.*

scalpellophilia. See *Munchausen syndrome.*

scapula congenita elevata. See *Sprengel deformity.*

scapula elevata. See *Sprengel deformity.*

scapulocostal syndrome. Pain of the back and/or shoulder, sometimes referring to the anterior chest wall, or radiating into the forearm, hand, and fingers, often in association with numbness and tingling in the fourth or fifth finger. Some authors believe that changes in the relationship between the scapula and the thoracic wall are the cause; others suspect that the condition may be secondary to long-standing postural habit with round-shoulder deformity causing disturbances in the tissue beneath the scapula or in the muscles of the scapular group.

Michele, A. A., *et al.* Scapulocostal syndrome (fatigue-postural paradox). *NY State J. Med.*, 1950, 50:1353-6. Cohen, C. A. Scapulocostal syndrome: Diagnosis and treatment. *South. Med. J.*, 1980, 73:433-4; 437.

scapulohumeral periarthritis. See *Duplay bursitis.*

scapulohumero-distal muscular dystrophy. See *Emery-Dreifuss syndrome.*

scapuloperoneal amyotrophy. See *scapuloperoneal syndrome.*

scapuloperoneal syndrome (SPS). Synonyms: *Davidenkov syndrome, Kaeser syndrome, humeroperoneal neuromuscular disease, scapuloperoneal amyotrophy.*

A familial neurological disorder, transmitted as either an autosomal dominant or X-linked trait, involving mainly the scapular and peroneal muscles. The syndrome may begin in the shoulder girdle or in the leg muscles, weakness and wasting in scapular and anterolateral leg muscles being its principal features. It may affect the arm, neck, cranial, and trunk muscles, producing deformities of the spine and feet (foot drop and talipes equinovarus) and weakness and contractures of the muscles of the neck and arms. Associated disorders may include heart defect and short heel cord. Autopsy shows muscular atrophy and involvement of caudal cranial nuclei.

Kaeser, H. E. Die familiäre scapuloperoneale Muskelatrophie. *Deut. Zschr. Nervenheilk.*, 1964, 186:379-94. Sulaiman, A. R., *et al.* Scapuloperoneal syndrome. Report of two families with neurogenic muscular atrophy. *J. Neurol. Sc.*, 1981, 52:305-25. Davidenkow, S. Scapuloperoneal amyotrophy. *Arch. Neur. Psychiat., Chicago*, 1939, 41:694-701.

SCARF (skeletal abnormalities-cutis laxa-craniostenosis-psychomotor retardation-facial abnormalities) syndrome. A familial syndrome of cutis laxa, joint hyperextensibility, umbilical and inguinal hernias, craniosynostosis, pectus carinatum, abnormally shaped vertebrae, hypocalcified teeth with hypoplastic enamel, facial abnormalities, wide webbed neck, ambiguous genitalia, nodular liver tumors, and mild psychomotor retardation. The occurrence in two male children related through their mother suggests X-linked recessive inheritance.

Koppe, R., *et al.* Ambiguous genitalia associated with skeletal abnormalities, cutis laxa, craniostenosis, psychomotor retardation, and facial abnormalities (SCARF syndrome). *Am. J. Med. Genet.*, 1989, 34:305-12.

scarlatina anginosa. See *Fothergill disease, under Fothergill, John.*

scarlatinosis. See *Sticker disease.*

SCBG (symmetrical calcification of basal cerebral cerebral ganglia). See *Fahr syndrome.*

SCD (sickle cell disease). See *sickle cell anemia.*

SCE (split hand-cleft lip/palate and ectodermal dysplasia). See *EEC syndrome.*

SCHACHENMANN, GERTRUD (Swiss physician)

Smith-Theiler-Schachenmann syndrome. See *cerebrocostomandibular syndrome.*

SCHÄFER, ERICH (German physician)

Schäfer syndrome. A syndrome of keratosis palmaris et plantaris, hyperhidrosis, leukokeratosis of the oral mucosa, congenital cataract, circumscribed alopecia, pachyonychia, mental deficiency, small stature, and hypogonadism.

Schäfer, E. Zur Lehre von den congenitalen Dyskertosen. *Arch. Derm. Syph., Berlin*, 1925, 148:425-32.

SCHAMBERG, JAY FRANK (American physician, 1870-1934)

Schamberg dermatosis. See *Schamberg disease.*

Schamberg disease. Synonyms: *Schamberg dermatosis, progressive pigmentary dermatosis, progressive pigmentary disease, purpura pigmentaria progressiva.*

A purpuric eruption, usually in males, affecting chiefly the lower extremities and rarely the upper ones. The lesions are flat puncta that spread and blend to form brownish patches. Inflammation of the capillaries of the upper dermis, deposits of hemosiderin, dilation of the blood vessels, and the presence of melanin are the principal pathological features.

Schamberg, J. F. A peculiar progressive pigmentary disease of the skin. *Brit. J. Dermatol.*, 1901, 13:1-5.

SCHANZ, ALFRED (German physician, 1868-1931)

Schanz disease. Traumatic inflammation of the Achilles tendon.

Schanz, A. Eine typische Erkrankung der Achillessehne *Zbl. Chir.*, 1905, 32:1289-91.

Schanz syndrome. Synonyms: *insufficientia vertebrae, spinal insufficiency, vertebral insufficiency.*

A spinal disorder with a feeling of fatigue and pain on pressure or when lying prone.

Schanz, A. Eine typische Erkrankung der Wirbelsäule (Insufficientia vertebrae). *Berlin. Klin. Wschr.*, 1907, 44:986-92.

SCHATZKI, RICHARD (American radiologist, born 1901)

Schatzki ring. Synonym: *lower esophageal ring.*

Annular stricture of the lower esophagus resulting in dysphagia.

Schatzki, R., & Gary, J. E. Dysphagia due to a diaphragm-like localized narrowings in the lower esophagus (lower esophageal ring). *Am. J. Roentgen.*, 1956, 70:911-22.

SCHAUMANN, JÖRGEN (Swedish dermatologist, 1879-1953)

Besnier-Boeck-Schaumann syndrome. See *under Besnier.*

Schaumann disease. See *Besnier-Boeck-Schaumann syndrome.*

SCHEIE, HAROLD GLENDON (American ophthalmologist, born 1909)

compound Hurler-Scheie disease. See *mucopolysaccharidosis I-H/S.*

Hurler-Scheie syndrome. See *mucopolysaccharidosis I-H/S.*

Scheie syndrome. See *mucopolysaccharidosis I-S.*

Ullrich-Scheie syndrome. See *mucopolysaccharidosis I-S.*

SCHEINKER, I. (Austrian physician)

Gerstmann-Sträussler-Scheinker disease (GSSD). See *Gerstmann syndrome (1).*

SCHEINKER, I. MARK (American physician)

Scheinker subependymoma. See *Scheinker tumor.*

Scheinker tumor. Synonym: *Scheinker subependymoma.*

A brain tumor composed predominantly of ectodermal elements derived from the subependymal glia.

Scheinker, I. M. Subepependymoma: A newly recognized tumor of subependymal derivation. *J. Neurosurg.*, 1945, 2:232-40.

SCHENCK, BENJAMIN ROBINSON (American physician, 1873-1920)

Schenck disease. Synonyms: *Beuermann disease, Beuermann-Gougerot disease, sporotrichosis.*

A chronic disease caused by the fungus *Sporothrix schenckii.* The cutaneous lymphatic type is characterized by papules or nodules at the site of implantation of the fungus in a minor injury, usually on the dorsum of the hand, followed by lymphatic spread and development of a chain of ulcerating subcutaneous nodules. The pulmonary type is marked mainly by pneumonia. In the disseminated type, the muscles, bones, joints, eyes, gastrointestinal system, and nervous system usually become involved.

Schenck, B. R. On refractory subcutaneous abscesses caused by the fungus possibly related to the *Sporotricha. Johns Hopkins Hosp. Bull.*, 1898, 9:286-90. Beuermann, de, & Gougerot. *Les sporotrichoses.* Paris, 1912.

SCHEPENS, C. L. (American ophthalmologist)

Criswick-Schepens syndrome. See *under Criswick.*

SCHERER, HANS JOACHIM (Austrian physician, born 1906)

van Bogaert-Scherer-Epstein syndrome. See *under van Bogaert.*

SCHEUERMANN, HOLGER WERFEL (Danish physician, 1877-1960)

Scheuermann disease. Synonyms: *Scheuermann kyphosis, adolescent kyphosis, juvenile kyphosis, kyphosis of adolescence, kyphosis dorsalis adolescentium, kyphosis dorsalis juvenilis, malum epiphyseonecroticum vertebrale, osteochondritis deformans juvenilis, spinal epiphysitis, spinal osteochondritis, vertebral epiphysitis, vertebral osteochondritis.*

Epiphyseal ischemic necrosis seen in late adolescence, usually involving the seventh and tenth thoracic vertebrae, and resulting in osteochondrosis of the vertebral bodies and kyphosis. Some cases are familial and are transmitted as an autosomal dominant trait.

Scheuermann, H. W. Kyfosis dorsalis juvenilis. *Ugeskr. Laeger.*, 1920, 82:385-93.

Scheuermann kyphosis. See *Scheuermann disease.*

SCHEUTHAUER, GUSTAV (German physician, 1832-1894)

Scheuthauer-Marie syndrome. See *cleidocranial dysostosis.*

Scheuthauer-Marie-Sainton syndrome. See *cleidocranial dysostosis.*

SCHIFFRIN, ARTHUR (American pathologist, born 1904)

Baehr-Schiffrin disease. See *Moschcowitz syndrome.*

SCHILDER, PAUL FERDINAND (German-born American physician, 1886-1940)

Addison-Schilder syndrome. See *adrenoleukodystrophy.*

Heubner-Schilder syndrome. See *Schilder disease.*

Schilder disease. Synonyms: *Heubner-Schilder syndrome, encephalitis periaxialis diffusa, global demyelination, progressive subcortical encephalitis, subchronic leukoencephalitis.*

A neurological disease of children and young adults characterized by extensive areas of asymmetrical myelin destruction, often involving the entire lobe or central hemispheres with extensions across the corpus callosum and involving the opposite hemisphere. The optic nerves, brainstem, and spinal cord often show discrete but well-defined lesions of multiple sclerosis. The symptoms usually include dementia, homonymous hemianopia, cortical blindness and deafness, hemiplegia, quadriplegia, and pseudobulbar palsy. Most patients die within a few months after onset; very few survive longer. In the older literature, the scope included some neurological disorders which are now excluded from this group, including familial neuropathies with widespread symmetric destruction and gliosis of the white matter, subacute encephalitis, vascular encephalopathies, and the like.

Schilder, P. Zur Kenntnis der sogenannten diffusen Sklerose (über Encephalitis periaxialis diffusa). *Zschr. Neur.*, 1912, 10:1-60.

Schilder-Foix disease. Synonym: *intracerebral symmetrical centrolobar sclerosis.*

A disease of the central nervous system characterized by nonprogressive sclerotic lesions of the white matter of the cerebral hemispheres, secondary to perinatal anoxic encephalopathy or arteriosclerotic ischemia of the brain.

*Foix, C., & Marie, J. La sclerose cerebrale centrolobaire a tendence symetrique; ses rapports avec l'encephalite periaxiale diffuse. *Encephale,* 1927, 22:81. Schilder, P. Zur frage der Enzephalitis periaxialis diffusa (sogenannte diffuse Sklerose). *Zschr. Ges. Neur.*, 1913, 15:359.

Schilder-Stengel syndrome. Synonyms: *asymbolia for pain, pain asymbolia.*

A condition wherein the affected person, although capable of distinguishing the different types of pain stimuli, does not make any verbal, motor, or emotional responses to noxious irritation.

Schilder, P., & Stengel, E. Das Krankheitsbild der Schmerzasymbolie. *Zschr. Ges. Neur. Psychiat.*, 1930, 129:250-79.

SCHILLING, VICTOR THEODOR ADOLF GEORG (German hematologist, 1883-1960)

Schilling leukemia. Monocytic leukemia characterized by the presence in the blood of large cells derived from the endothelial system, with lacy chromatin, bizarre nuclei, and irregular borders.

Watkins, C. H., & Hall, B. E. Monocytic leukemia of the Naegeli and Schilling types. *Am. J. Clin. Path.*, 1940, 10:387-96.

SCHIMKE, R. NEIL (American physician)

Schimke syndrome. Synonym: *choreoathetosis-mental retardation syndrome.*

A familial syndrome, transmitted as an X-linked trait, characterized by childhood-onset choreoathetosis with later spasticity, postnatal microcephaly, growth and mental retardation, apparent external ophthalmoplegia, and varying degrees of deafness.

Schimke, R. N., *et al.* A new X-linked syndrome comprising progressive basal ganglion dysfunction, mental and growth retardation, external ophthalmoplegia, postnatal microcephaly and deafness. *Am. J. Med. Genet.*, 1984, 17:323-32.

SCHIMMELBUSCH, CURT (German physician, 1860-1895)

Reclus-Schimmelbusch disease. See *Cheatle disease.*

Schimmelbusch disease. See *Cheatle disease.*

SCHIMMELPENNING, G. W. (German phyisician)

Schimmelpenning-Feuerstein-Mims syndrome. See *epidermal nevus syndrome.*

SCHINZEL, A. (Swiss physician)

Schinzel syndrome (1). Synonym: *acrocallosal syndrome (ACS).*

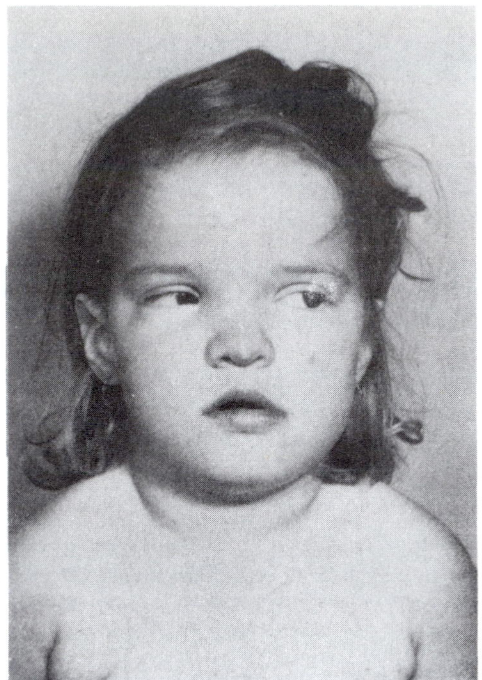
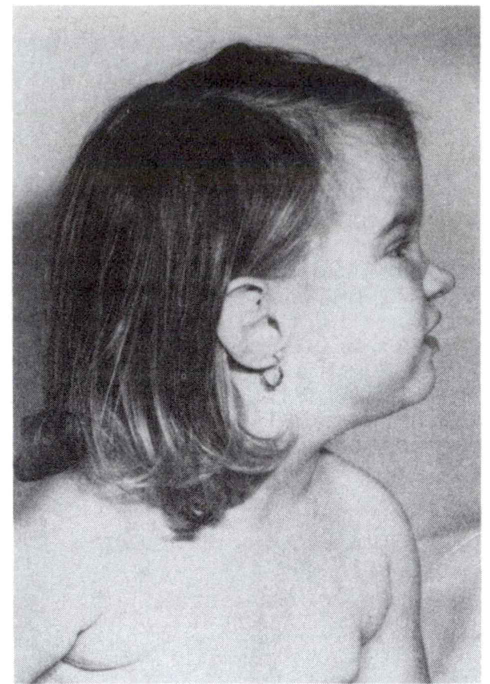
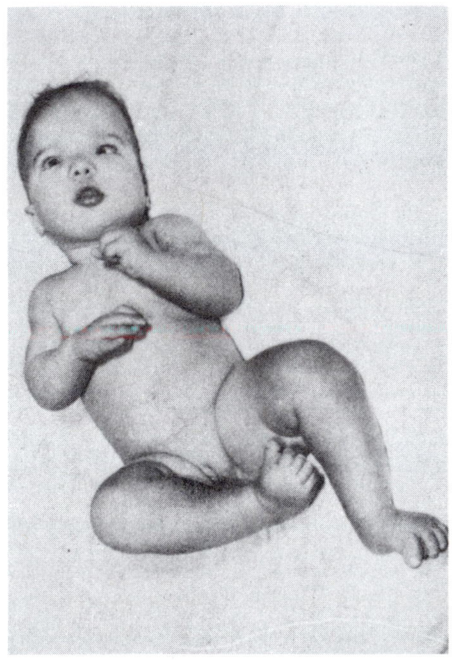
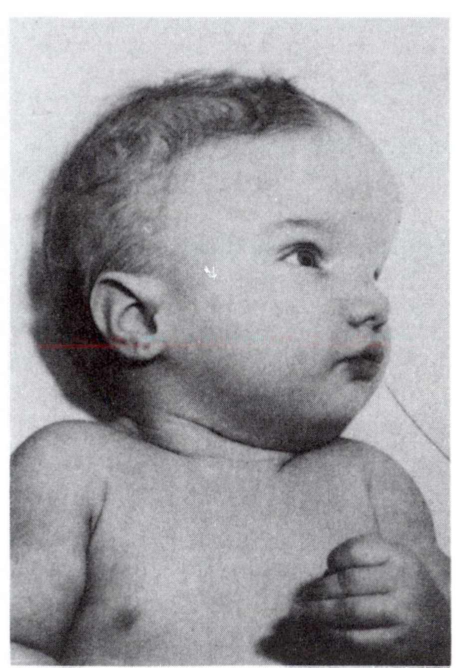

Schinzel syndrome (1)
Schinzel, Albert & Ulrich Kaufmann: *Clinical Genetics* 30: 399- 405, 1986. Munksgaard International Publishers, Copenhagen, Denmark.

A syndrome of peculiar facies, mental retardation, absence of the corpus callosum, and polydactyly. Orofacial features consist of antimongoloid palpebral fissures, macrocephaly, prominent eyes, epicanthal folds, bulging forehead, short nose, and short upper lip. Clinodactyly of the fifth fingers may occur. The affected children are generally hyperreflexic and hypotonic.

Schinzel, A. Postaxial polydactyly, hallux duplication, absence of the corpus callosum, macroencephaly and severe mental retardation. A new syndrome. *Helv. Paediat. Acta*, 1979, 34:141-6.

Schinzel syndrome (2). A familiar syndrome of ulnar ray defects, hand abnormalities, microgenitalism, delayed puberty, obesity, and anal atresia. Hand malformations vary from a stiff fifth finger to hypoplasia of distal phalanges or complete absence of the fourth and fifth fingers and their metacarpals. Genital abnormalities consist of cryptorchism, microphallus, and small scrotum. The syndrome is transmitted as an autosomal dominant trait.

Temtamy, S. A., & McKusick, V. A. The genetics of hand malformations. *Birth Defects*, 1978, 14(3):156-7.

Schinzel-Giedion syndrome. A syndrome of congenital hydronephrosis, skeletal dysplasia, and severe developmental retardation. The principal symptoms are coarse facies characterized by midface hypoplasia, frontal bossing, facial hemangiomas, short nose with anteverted nostrils, malformed ears, protruding large tongue, and hypertelorism; skeletal defects include open cranial sutures, steep short skull, wide occipital synchondrosis, multiple wormian bones, hypoplastic ribs, and broad ribs; limb defects consist of postaxial polydactyly, talipes, mesomelic brachymelia, and hypoplasia of distal phalanges. Choanal stenosis, redundant neck skin, hypoplastic nipples, atrial septal defects, hypoplastic dermal ridges, simian creases, hyperconvex nails, hypospadias, microphallus, hypertrichosis, and seizures are frequently associated. The affected patients usually die in infancy. The syndrome is said to be a single gene autosomal recessive disorder.

Schinzel, A., & Giedion, A. A syndrome of severe midface retraction, multiple skull anomalies, clubfeet, and cardiac and renal malformations in sibs. *Am. J. Med. Genet.*, 1978, 1:361-75.

SCHIRMER, RUDOLF (German ophthalmologist, 1831-1896)

Schirmer syndrome. See *Sturge-Weber syndrome.*

schistosomiasis japonica. See *Katayama syndrome.*

SCHLAGENHAUFER, FRIEDRICH (German physician)

Gaucher-Schlagenhauer syndrome. See *Gaucher disease.*

SCHLATTER, CARL (Swiss physician, 1864-1934)

Lannelongue-Osgood-Schlatter syndrome. See *Osgood-Schlatter syndrome.*

Osgood-Schlatter syndrome. See *under Osgood.*

Schlatter disease. See *Osgood-Schlatter syndrome.*

SCHLESINGER, P.

Fanconi-Schlesinger syndrome. See *Williams syndrome, under Williams, J. C. P.*

SCHLICHTING, HANS (German ophthalmologist)

Schlichting dystrophy. Synonyms: *dystrophia cornealis posterior polymorpha, polymorphous posterior corneal dystrophy (PPCD).*

A familial form of corneal dystrophy, transmitted as an autosomal dominant trait, characterized by polymorphous opacities, vesicles, and depressions in the Descemet membrane, frequently in association with opacities in the deep layers.

Schlichting, H. Blasen- und dellenförmige Endotheldystrophie der Hornhaut. *Klin. Mbl. Augenh.*, 1941, 107:425-35.

SCHLOFFER, HERMANN (German physician, 1868-1937)

Schloffer tumor. An inflammatory tumor of the abdominal wall surrounded by small foreign-body abscesses or granulomas and suppuration.

*Schloffer, H. Chronisch entzündliche Bouchdeckengeschwülst nach Bruchoperationen. *Zbl. Chir.*, 1908, 35:113-5.

SCHLOSSMAN, ABRAHAM (American ophthalmologist, born 1918)

Posner-Schlossman syndrome. See *under Posner.*

SCHMID, FRANZ (German physician)

dysostosis enchondralis, Schmid type. See *Schmid metaphyseal chondrodysplasia syndrome.*

hereditary metaphyseal dysostosis, Schmid type. See *Schmid metaphyseal chondrodysplasia syndrome.*

metaphyseal chondrodysplasia, Schmid type. See *Schmid metaphyseal chondrodysplasia syndrome.*

metaphyseal dysostosis, Schmid type. See *Schmid metaphyseal chondrodysplasia syndrome.*

Schmid metaphyseal chondrodysplasia syndrome. Synonyms: *Schmid syndrome; dysostosis enchondralis, Schmid type; hereditary metaphyseal dysostosis, Schmid type; metaphyseal chondrodysplasia, Schmid type; metaphyseal dysostosis, Schmid type; osteochondritis subepiphysaria.*

An autosomal dominant syndrome of short-limb dwarfism, bowed legs, and waddling gait. Splaying of broad irregular metaphyses, coxa vara, genu varum, limitation of finger extension, and short tubular bones are the principal defects. The initial symptoms (short stature and bowed legs) become apparent during the second year of life.

Schmid, F. Beitrag zur Dysostosis enchondralis metaepiphysaria. *Mschr. Kinderheilk.*, 1963, 97:393-7.

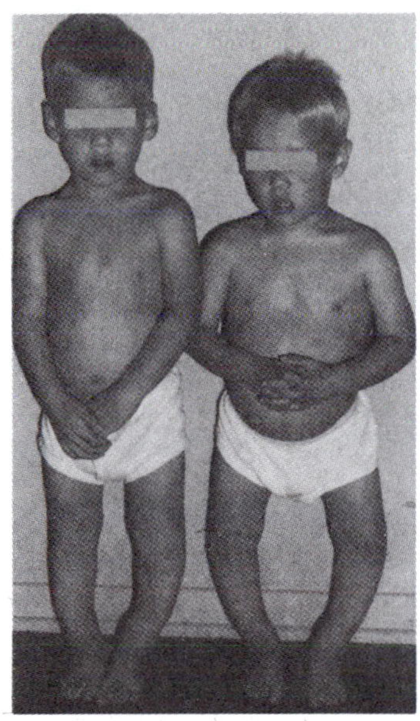

Schmid metaphyseal chondrodysplasia syndrome
Rosenbloom, A.L. & D.W. Smith: *J. Pediatr.* 66:857, 1965. St. Louis: C.V. Mosby Co.

Schmid syndrome. See *Schmid metaphyseal chondrodysplasia syndrome.*

SCHMID, RUDI (Swiss-born American physician, born 1922)

McArdle-Schmid-Pearson syndrome. See *glycogen storage disease V.*

SCHMID, W.

Schmid-Fraccaro syndrome. See *cat eye syndrome.*

SCHMIDT, ADOLF (German physician, 1865-1918)

Schmidt syndrome. Synonym: *vago-accessory syndrome.*

A variant of the Jackson-MacKenzie syndrome, in which unilateral dysfunction of the tenth and eleven cranial nerves produces ipsilateral paralysis of the soft palate, vocal cords, and sternocleidomastoid and trapezius muscles.

Schmidt, A. Casuistische Beiträge zur Nervenpathologie. II. Doppelseitige Accessoriusähmung bei Syringomyelie. *Deut. Med. Wschr.*, 1892, 18:606-8.

SCHMIDT, MARTIN BENNO (German physician, 1863-1949)

Schmidt syndrome. See *under polyglandular autoimmune syndrome.*

SCHMIDT, ROLF (German ophthalmologist, born 1906)

Schmidt keratitis. Synonyms: *herpetic keratitis, keratitis superficialis herpetica with striations.*

Herpetic keratitis with striations on the corneal epithelium.

Schmidt, R. Über die streifenförmige Keratitis superficialis herpetica. *Klin. Mbl. Augenh.*, 1933, 91:47-58.

SCHMIEDEN, V. (German physician)

Schmieden disease. Prolapse of the gastric mucosa into the duodenum.

Schmieden, V. Die Differentialdiagnose zwischen Magengeschwür und Magenkrebs; die pathologische Anatomie dieser Erkrankungen in Beziehung zu ihrer Darstellung in Röntgenbilde. *Arch. Klin. Chir., Berlin*, 1911, 96:253-344.

SCHMINCKE, ALEXANDER (German physician, 1877-1953)

Schmincke tumor. Synonym: *nasopharyngeal lymphoepithelioma.*

A tumor variously considered to be a reticulum cell sarcoma or anaplastic carcinoma with hemolytic infiltration. It originates in the nasopharynx and metastasizes to the lymph nodes.

Schmincke, A. Über lymphoepitheliale Geschwülste. *Beitr. Path. Anat.*, 1921, 68:161-70.

Schmincke tumor-unilateral cranial paralysis syndrome. See *Garcin syndrome.*

SCHMITT, H. G. (German physician)

Schmitt disease. See *Schmitt syndrome.*

Schmitt fracture. See *Schmitt syndrome.*

Schmitt syndrome. Synonyms: *Schmitt disease, Schmitt fracture, Schmitt-Wisser disease, Clay Schveller syndrome [sic], clay shoveler disease, clay shoveler fracture, root puller fracture, stress fracture of the spinous process.*

A variant of the overuse syndrome (q.v.) characterized by fractures of one or more spinous processes of the lower cervical or upper thoracic vertebrae caused by overstraining, as in workers digging through clay (hence the synonym **clay shoveler fracture** or **disease**), metal dippers, and football players. Pain in or adjacent to the midline of the lower neck or between the shoulder blades while lifting or other strenuous activities is the principal clinical symptom. The name is sometimes misspelled in non-English language literature as *Clay Schveller's syndrome.*

Schmitt, H. G., & Wisser, P. Die Schipperkrankheit bei Jugendlichen. *Arch. Klin. Chir., Berlin* 1951, 268:333-40.

Schmitt-Wisser disease. See *Schmitt syndrome.*

SCHMORL, CHRISTIAN GEORG (German physician, 1861-1932)

Schmorl disease. Synonym: *Schmorl hernia.*

Prolapse of the nucleus pulposus.

Schmorl, C. G. Die pathologische Anatomie der Wirbelsäule. *Verh. Deut. Orthop. Ges.*, 1926, 21:3-41.

Schmorl hernia. See *Schmorl disease.*

Schmorl nodes. Usually asymptomatic intervertebral disk protrusions, beginning as a defect in the cortex or end plate of a vertebra, followed by fissures and protrusion of the nucleus pulposus.

Schmorl, G. Über Knorpelknötchen on den Wirbelbandscheiben. *Fortsch. Geb. Roentgen.*, 1928, 38:265-79.

schmutz pyorrhea. See *Fauchard disease.*

SCHNABEL, ISIDOR (Austrian physician, 1842-1908)

Schnabel atrophy. Synonyms: *Schnabel caverns, cavernous optic atrophy, lacunal optic atrophy.*

Cavernous mucoid degeneration of the glia with disappearance of optic nerve fibers and formation of clear pools of mucoid material associated with glaucoma.

Hogan, M. J., & Zimmerman, L. E. *Ophthalmic pathology. An atlas and textbook.* 2nd ed. Philadelphia, Saunders, 1962, p. 627.

Schnabel caverns. See *Schnabel atrophy.*

SCHNEIDER, HANS (Austrian physician)

Schneider disease. Synonym: *meningitis serosa.*

A viral infection occurring during the spring and fall, characterized by the sudden appearance of high fever, chills, nasopharyngitis, arthralgia, malaise, vomiting, and headache. The initial phase lasts about 4 days and, in most instances, is followed by a symptomless period. The second phase varies in severity; in the mildest form it includes involvement of the central nervous system leading to serous meningitis, with severe headache extending to the neck, high fever, nausea, vomiting, and occasional diarrhea. This phase lasts about 3 to 5 days and is followed by complete recovery. A more severe form is meningoencephalitis characterized by sensory disorders, hyperkinesia, tic, and convulsions. The symptoms persist for about 7 to 10 days, and are followed by usually complete recovery. Pakinsonism complicates a small number of cases. The most severe form is marked by meningoencephalitis with symptoms similar to those in poliomyelitis. Paralysis of the muscles of the shouldler girdle appears 5 to 10 days after subsidence of fever.

Schneider, H. Über epidemische akute "Meningitis serosa." *Wien. Klin. Wschr.*, 1831, 44:350-2.

SCHNEIDER, RICHARD C. (American physician)

Schneider syndrome. Synonym: *acute central cervical spinal cord injury syndrome.*

A syndrome of cervical spinal cord injury characterized by motor impairment of the extremities (being more severe in the upper than in the lower limbs), bladder dysfunction (usually urinary retention), and various degrees of sensory deficit below the level of injury. In cases caused by central cord destruction and associated with bleeding and hematomyelia, there may be caudal or cephalad extension of the lesion with further progression of symptoms, sometimes culminating in complete tetraplegia and death. In cases caused by concussion or contusion associated with an edematous central cord involvement, there may be in time a gradual return of normal functions. The lower extremities tend to recover motor activity first, bladder function returns next, and the restoration of strength in the upper limbs is the last phase of recovery.

Schneider, R. C., *et al.* The syndrome of acute central cervical spinal cord injury. *J. Neur. Neurosurg. Psychiat.*, 1958, 21:216-27.

SCHNYDER, WALTER (Swiss ophthalmologist)

Schnyder dystrophy. Synonyms: *crystalline corneal degeneration, degeneratio cristallinea corneae hereditaria.*

A familial form of crystalline corneal degeneration transmitted as an autosomal dominant trait and characterized by symmetrical, grayish, discoid clouding of the central or paracentral parts of the cornea, extending to the limbus, and by the presence of cholesterol crystals. The lesions may be present at birth but, more frequently, appear during infancy or childhood.

Schnyder, W. Mitteilung über einen neuen Typus von familiäre Hornhauterkrankung. *Schweiz. Med. Wschr.*, 1929, 59:559.

SCHÖBL, JOSEF (Ophthalmologist in Prague, 1837-1902)

Schöbl scleritis. Synonym: *hyperplastic scleritis.*

Inflammation of the sclera, in which there is excessive proliferation of fibrous tissue.

Schöbl, J. Über hyperplastische Entzündungen der Augenhäute. *Arch. Augenh.*, 1889, 20:98-122.

SCHOENLEIN, JOHANN LUKAS. See SCHÖNLEIN, JOHANN LUKAS

SCHOLTE, A. J. (Austrian physician)

Cassidy-Scholte syndrome. See *carcinoid syndrome.*

Scholte syndrome. See *carcinoid syndrome.*

SCHOLZ, R. O.

Barnard-Scholz syndrome. See *Kearns-Sayre syndrome.*

SCHOLZ, WILLIBALD OSCAR (German physician, born 1889)

leukodystrophy, type Scholz. See *metachromatic leukodystrophy.*

Scholz syndrome. See *metachromatic leukodystrophy.*

Scholz-Bielschowsky-Henneberg syndrome. See *metachromatic leukodystrophy.*

Scholz-Greenfield syndrome. See *metachromatic leukodystrophy.*

SCHÖNENBERG, HANS (Swiss physician)

Schönenberg syndrome. A syndrome of proportionate dwarfism, congenital blepharoptosis, congenital heart defect, and mental retardation. In the original report, one of the two patients also presented with anomalous arches, retarded bone development, hypospadias, cryptorchism, abnormal EEG, and heart abnormalities, including aortic stenosis and atrial septal defect.

Schönenberg, H. Über ein neues Kombinationsbild multipler abartungen. (Minderwuchs, Vitium cordis, beiderseitige congenitale Ptose). *Ann. Paediat., Basel*, 1954, 182:229-40.

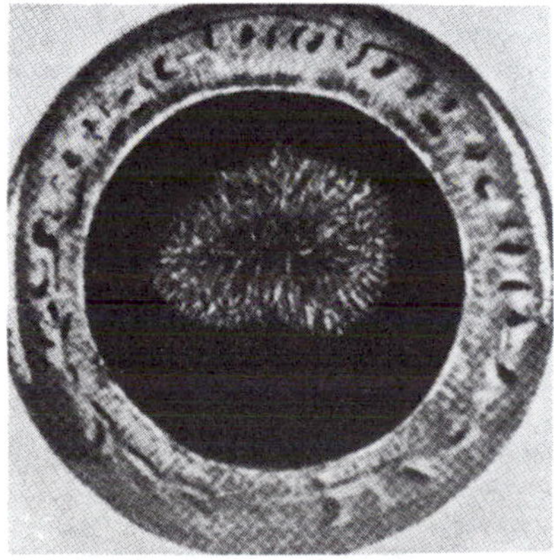

Schnyder dystrophy
Forni, S., *Arch. Ophthalmol.* 11:541,1951. Chicago: American Medical Association.

SCHÖNER, W. (German physician)

Heilmeyer-Schöner erythroblastosis. See *Heilmeyer-Schöner syndrome.*

Heilmeyer-Schöner syndrome. See *under Heilmeyer.*

SCHÖNLEIN, JOHANN LUKAS (German physician, 1792-1864)

Henoch-Schönlein syndrome (HS, HSS). See *Schönlein-Henoch purpura.*

Schönlein purpura. See *Schönlein-Henoch purpura.*

Schönlein-Henoch disease. See *Schönlein-Henoch purpura.*

Schönlein-Henoch purpura. Synonyms: *Henoch disease, Henoch-Schönlein syndrome (HS, HSS), Schönlein purpura, Schönlein-Henoch disease, Schönlein-Henoch syndrome, allergic nonthrombocytopenic purpura, allergic purpura, allergic purpura-arthralgia-gastrointestinal symptoms, anaphylactoid purpura, capillarotoxic purpura, essential athrombopenic purpura, hemorrhagic capillary toxicosis, peliosis rheumatica, purpura abdominalis, purpura anaphylactica, purpura infectiosa acuta, purpura rheumatica, purpura with arthralgia, purpura with visceral manifestations.*

Nonthrombocytic purpura with skin rash, edema, joint pain, and gastrointestinal complications. It is primarily a disease of children, having its greatest frequency in the early spring and fall and occurring more commonly in males than females. In adults, there is no special predilection for either sex. Prodromal symptoms include respiratory infections. Onset is sudden, having anaphylaxis-like characteristics. Malaise, headache, fever, rash, and abdominal and joint pain are the early symptoms. Initial urticarial lesions gradually recede and the skin turns pinkish and red, eventually becoming hemorrhagic. Arthralgia involves chiefly the ankles, knees, hips, wrists, elbows, and fingers. Joint effusion may occur. Edema of the hands, feet, or scalp may be observed in some cases. Colicky abdominal pain is usually associated with melena and guaiac-positive stools. Other symptoms may include hematemesis, intussusception, intestinal perforation, pancreatitis, transient paresis, convulsions, paralysis of some cranial nerves, hematuria, hypertension, transient renal failure with nitrogen retention and oliguria, and intestinal hemorrhage and torsion. Aseptic vasculitis is the principal pathological feature. Radiological findings consist of mucosal edema of the bowel, mucosal intestinal hemorrhage, and signs of bowel perforation and appendicitis.

Henoch, H. Über den Zusammenhang von Purpura und Intestinalstörungen. *Berlin. Klin. Wschr.*, 1868, 5:517-9. Schönlein, J. L. *Allgemeine und spezielle Pathologie und Therapie.* Würzburg, Etlinger, 1832.

Schönlein-Henoch syndrome. See *Schönlein-Henoch purpura.*

SCHOTTMÜLLER, HUGO (German physician, 1867-1936)

Schottmüller disease. Synonyms: *Brion-Kayser disease, enteric fever, paratyphoid, paratyphoid fever.*

An infectious disease caused by any species of *Salmonella* except *S. typhosa.*

Schottmüller. Über eine das Bild des Typhus bietende Erkrankung hervorgerufen durch Typhus ähnliche Bacillen. *Deut. Med. Wschr.*, 1900, 26:511-2. Brion, A., & Kayser, H. Über eine Erkrankung mit dem Befund eines typhus-ähnlichen Bacteriums im Blute (Paratyphus). *Münch. Med. Wschr.*, 1902, 49:611-5.

SCHRIDDE, HERRMANN AUGUST (German physician, born 1875)

Schridde syndrome. Synonyms: *congenital generalized dropsy, fetoplacental anasarca, hydrops congenitus.*

A disease of the prenatal and neonatal periods characterized by hydramnios, edematous swelling of the placenta, umbilical cord, and fetus, most typically manifested by giant swelling of the maternal abdomen. The thickened scalp of the newborn infant overhangs the face and nose and is made up of yellowish gelatin-like subcutaneous fatty tissue with white stripes. Infants usually die within a few days or weeks after birth. Splenomegaly, cardiac hypertrophy, and hemosiderosis of the liver and spleen are found at autopsy. Blood examination shows severe anemia with the presence of erythroblasts, megalocytes, myeloblasts, and myelocytes.

Schridde, H. Die angeborene allgemeine Wassersucht. *Münch. Med. Wschr.*, 1910, 57:397-8.

SCHRÖDER, C. H. (German physician)

Schröder syndrome. A familial disorder of multiple luxations and external ear deformities due to defective differentiation of the embryonal anlage of the articular cartilage. The reported cases have been transmitted as autosomal recessive, dominant, and irregularly dominant traits.

Schröder, C. H. Familiäre kongenitale Luxationen. *Zschr. Orthop. Chir.*, 1932, 57:580-96.

SCHROEDER, HENRY ALFRED (American physician, born 1906)

Schroeder syndrome (1). Synonym: *endocrine hypertensive syndrome.*

A syndrome of obesity occurring at menarche, menopause after multiple pregnancies or gynecologic operations, pale striae on thighs and sometimes upper arms, menstrual irregularities, and abnormally low concentrations of sodium and chloride in the sweat. Additional symptoms include aversion to salty foods, high fluid intake, oliguria, glycosuria, a diabetic type of glucose tolerance curve, a tendency to easy bruising and ecchymoses, and sensitivity of the blood pressure to injected desoxycorticosterone acetate or glucoside..

Schroeder, H. A., *et al.* A syndrome of hypertension, obesity, menstrual irregularities, and evidence of adrenal cortical hyperfunction. *J. Lab. Clin. Med.*, 1949, 34:1745. Schroeder, H. A., *et al.* Studies on "essential" hypertension. V. An endocrine hypertensive syndrome. *Ann. Intern. Med.*, 1954, 40:516-39.

Schroeder syndrome (2). See *low salt syndrome.*

SCHROETTER (SCHRÖTTER), KRISTELLI LEOPOLD, VON (Austrian physician, 1837-1908)

Paget-Schroetter syndrome. See *under Paget.*

Paget-von Schroetter syndrome. See *Paget-Schroetter syndrome.*

Schroetter chorea. Synonyms: *chorea laryngis, diaphragmatic chorea, laryngeal chorea.*

The utterance of a peculiar cry in cases of painless tic.

Schroetter, L., von. Über "Chorea laryngis." *Allg. Wien. Med. Ztg.*, 1879, 24:67-8.

von Schroetter syndrome. See *Paget-Schroetter syndrome.*

SCHRÖTTER, KRISTELLI LEOPOLD, VON. See SCHROETTER, KRISTELLI LEOPOLD, VON

SCHUERMANN, H.

Melkersson-Rosenthal-Schuermann syndrome. See *Melkersson-Rosenthal syndrome.*

SCHÜLLER, ARTHUR (Austrian physician, born 1874)

Hand-Schüller-Christian (HSC) syndrome. See *under Hand.*

Schüller disease. See *Hand-Schüller-Christian syndrome.*

Schüller-Christian disease. See *Hand-Schüller-Christian syndrome.*

SCHULMAN, IRVING (American physician)

Schulman syndrome. See *Schulman-Upshaw syndrome.*

Schulman-Upshaw syndrome. Synonyms: *Schulman syndrome, Upshaw factor deficiency, congenital microangiopathic hemolytic anemia.*

A congenital hematological disease, transmitted as an autosomal recessive trait, characterized by thrombocytopenia with microangiopathic hemolytic anemia caused by a deficiency of the Upshaw factor (a factor in normal plasma that assists in platelet and red cell survival).

Schulman, I., *et al.* Studies on thrombopoiesis. I. A factor in normal human plasma required for platelet production; chronic thrombocytopenia due to its deficiency. *Blood*, 1960, 16:943-57. Upshaw, J. D., Jr. Congenital deficiency of a factor in normal plasma that reverses microangiopathic hemolysis and thrombocytopenia. *N. Engl. J. Med.*, 1978,298:1350-2.

SCHULTZ, WERNER (German physician, 1878-1947)

Schultz angina. See *Schultz syndrome.*

Schultz syndrome. Synonyms: *Schultz angina, agranulocytic angina, agranulocytosis, aneutrocytosis, aneutrophilia, angina agranulocytica, granulocytic hypoplasia, idiopathic leukopenia, leukopenia, mucositis necroticans agranulocytica, neutropenia.*

A hematological disorder marked by a reduced neutrophil count, occurring as an isolated condition or in association with a decrease in other circulating elements of the blood, such as pancytopenia. Decreased production of leukocytes or their excessive destruction are the two basic etiological factors. The causes include idiopathic factors, such as aplastic anemia; bone marrow replacement in leukemia, tumors, fibrosis, or granulomatosis; nutritional deficiencies, such as cobalamin or folic acid deficit; hypersplenism; ionizing radiations; and cytotoxic and other drugs, such as nitrogen mustards or other alkylating agents. Isolated neutropenia may occur as a complication of overwhelming infection and, in some instances, as a secondary disorder in immunologically mediated granulocyte destruction. Clinical characteristics vary from very mild or subclinical to severe forms, in which the symptoms may include prostration, chills, and ulceration of the oral mucosa.

Schultz, W. Über eigenartige Halserkrankungen (a) Monozytenangina, (b) gangränisieriende Prozesse und Defekte des Granulozytensystems. *Deut. Med. Wschr.*, 1922, 48:1495-6.

SCHULTZE, FRIEDRICH (German physician, 1848-1934)

Schultze acroparesthesia. See *Wartenberg disease (1).*

Schultze syndrome. See *Wartenberg disease (1).*

SCHÜRENBERG, E. (German physician)

Axenfeld-Schürenberg syndrome. See *under Axenfeld.*

SCHUT, JOHN W. (American physician)

olivopontocerebellar atrophy (OPCA), Schut-Haymaker type. See *OPCA IV, under olivopontocerebellar atrophy.*

Schut-Haymaker syndrome. See *OPCA IV, under olivopontocerebellar atrophy.*

SCHVELLER, CLAY (A misspelling of "clay shoveler," occasionally seen in the literature)

Clay Schveller syndrome. See *Schmitt syndrome.*

SCHWACHMAN, HARRY (American physician)

Riley-Schwachman syndrome. See *under Riley.*

Schwachman syndrome. A syndrome, probably transmitted as an autosomal recessive trait, characterized by the lack of the exocrine pancreas (which is replaced by adipose tissue), leukopenia, mild skeletal abnormalities (metaphyseal chondrodysplasia, faulty mineralization in the epiphyses, and narrow sacroiliac notch), and deficiency of pancreatic trypsin, lipase, and amylase. Anemia, thrombocytopenia, eczema, immunoglobulin deficiency, cystic fibrosis of the pancreas, and leukemia may be observed in some cases. The symptoms having their onset in infancy, include failure to thrive, diarrhea, steatorrhea, and frequent infections.

Schwachman, H., *et al.* Pancreatic insufficiency and bone marrow dysfunction. A new clinical entity. *J. Pediat.*, 1963, 63:835-7.

SCHWALBE

Schwalbe-Ziehen-Oppenheim syndrome. See *Ziehen-Oppenheim syndrome.*

schwannosis. See *Guillain-Barré syndrome.*

SCHWARTZ, ARIAH (American ophthalmologist)

Schwartz syndrome. A combination of uveitis, high intraocular pressure, and retinal detachment with peripheral tears.

Schwartz, A. Chronic open-angle glaucoma secondary to rhegmatogenous retinal detachment. *Am. J. Ophth.*, 1973, 75:205-11.

SCHWARTZ, OSCAR (American physician, born 1919)

Schwartz syndrome. See *Schwartz-Jampel syndrome.*

Schwartz-Jampel syndrome. Synonyms: *Aberfeld syndrome, Schwartz syndrome, chondrodystropia myotonica, chondrodystrophic myotonia, myotonia chondrodystrophica, osteochondromuscular dystrophy, spondylo-epimetaphyseal dysplasia with myotonia.*

A syndrome, probably transmitted as an autosomal recessive trait, characterized by growth retardation, peculiar facies, skeletal anomalies, and myotonia. The face has a normal appearance at birth but develops into a masklike facies with puckered lips, blepharophimosis, and ptosis of the eyelids because of tonic contractions of the facial muscles. Skeletal and articular disorders consist chiefly of limitation of motion of the hips, wrist, toes, and spine, short vertebrae with brevicollis, fragmentation and flattening of femoral epiphyses, pectus carinatum, acetabular dysplasia, and coxa vara. Because of stiff hips, the gait becomes waddling and progressively difficult. Associated defects include a high-pitched voice, choking on cold liquids, long eyelashes, low hairline, low-set small ears, small testes, high-arched palate, and occasional pes equinovarus.

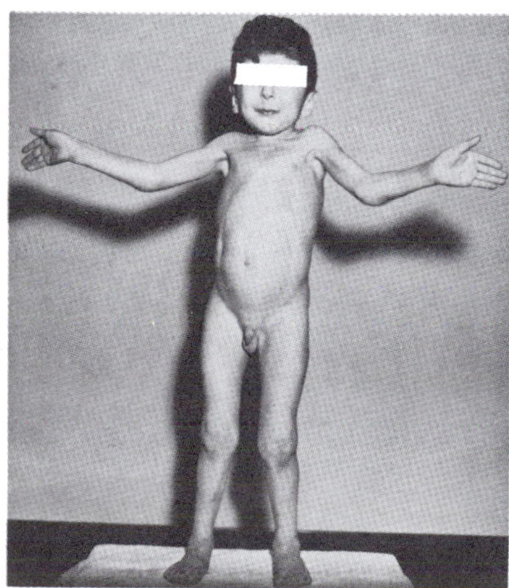

Schwartz-Jampel syndrome
Schwartz, O., & R.S. Jampel: *Arch. Ophthalmol.* 68:62. 1962. Chicago: American Medical Association.

Schwartz, O., & Jampel, R. Congenital blepharophimosis associated with a unique generalized myopathy. *Arch. Ophth., Chicago*, 1962, 68:52-7. Aberfeld, D. C., *et al.* Myotonia, dwarfism, diffuse bone disease and unusual ocular and facial abnormalities (a new syndrome). *Brain*, 1965, 88:313-22.

SCHWARTZ, WILLIAM BENJAMIN (American physician, born 1922)

Schwartz-Bartter syndrome. See *inappropriate antidiuretic hormone secretion syndrome.*

SCHWARZ, L.

Schwarz-Lélek syndrome. Clinical manifestations of this syndrome consist of head enlargement, frontal bossing, thick mandible, and genu valgum. Roentgenographic findings show hyperostosis and sclerosis of the skull, particularly in the frontal and occipital regions, obliteration of the paranasal sinuses, bowing of the humerus and femur, and widening of long bones. Serum alkaline phosphatase is usually elevated.

Lélek, L Camurati-Engelmannsche Erkrankung. *Forschur. Röntgen.*, 1961, 94:702-2. Schwarz, E. Craniometaphyseal dysplasia, *Am. J. Roentgen.*, 1960, 94:466-6.

sciatica. See *Cotugno syndrome.*

SCID (severe combined immunodeficiency) syndrome. See *severe mixed immunodeficiency syndrome.*

scimitar syndrome. Synonyms: *Halasz syndrome, anomalous pulmonary venous connection (APVC), anomalous pulmonary venous return, scimitar vein syndrome, Turkish sabre syndrome.*

A syndrome of hypoplasia of the right lung with dextroposition of the heart, systemic arterial supply to the right lung, and anomalous right pulmonary venous drainage to the inferior vena cava. The principal radiological sign is an arc-ike shadow, resembling the blade of a Turkish sword or scimitar, produced by the anomalous vein which courses downward parallel to the right atrium to its connection with the inferior vena cava. Hypoplasia of the right upper lung segment is the most constant feature of this syndrome. Congenital heart defects, especially atrial septal defect, occur in fewer than a half of all cases. Diaphragmatic anomalies with eventration may occur. Most cases are sporadic but some are transmitted as an autosomal dominant trait.

Halasz, N. A., *et al.* Bronchial and arterial anomalies with drainage of the right lung into the inferior vena cava. Circulation, l956, 14:826-46. Neill, C. A., et al. The familial occurrence of hypoplastic right lung with systemic arterial supply and venous drainage: "Scimitar syndrome." *Bull.*

Johns Hopkins Hosp., 1960, 107:1-21. Cooper, G. Case of malformation of the thoracic viscera: Consisting of imperfect development of right lung and transposition of the heart. London Med. Gaz., 1836, 18:600-2.

scimitar vein syndrome. See *scimitar syndrome.*

sclerema adiposum. See *Underwood syndrome.*

sclerema neonatorum. See *Underwood disease.*

sclerocystic ovary (SCO) syndrome. See *polycystic ovary syndrome.*

scleroderma adultorum. See *Buschke disease (1).*

scleroderma-silicosis syndrome. See *Erasmus syndrome.*

scleromalacia. See *Paget disease.*

sclerosing lipogranuloma. See *Ormond syndrome.*

sclerosing nonsuppurative osteomyelitis. See *Garré osteomyelitis.*

sclerosing retroperitonitis. See *Ormond syndrome.*

sclerosing thyroiditis. See *de Quervain disease (2), under Quervain, Fritz, de.*

sclerosing tubular degeneration. See *chromosome XXY syndrome.*

sclerosis fibrosa penis. See *Peyronie disease.*

sclerosis tuberosa. See *Bourneville-Pringle syndrome.*

sclerosteosis syndrome. Synonym: *cortical hyperostosis with syndactyly.*

A bone dysplasia of infants and children characterized by hyperostosis of the calvaria, base of the skull, and mandible, lack of diaphyseal constriction of the tubular bones, cortical sclerosis and hyperostosis of the tubular bones, syndactyly, radial deviation of the second and third fingers, and onychodysplasia. A broad and flat nasal bridge, hypertelorism, and a prominent mandible are the typical facial characteristics. The syndrome is transmitted as an autosomal recessive trait.

Hansen, H. G. Sklerosteose. In: Opitz, H., & Schmid, F., eds. *Handbuch der Kinderheilkunde*. vol. VI. Berlin, Springer, 1967, pp. 351-5.

sclerotic pedicle syndrome. See *Wilkinson syndrome, under Wilkinson, Robert M.*

SCLS (capillary systemic leak syndrome). See *capillary leak syndrome.*

SCO (sclerocystic ovary) syndrome. See *polycystic ovary syndrome.*

scombroid fish poisoning syndrome. Intoxication with spoiled scombroid fish (members of the suborder *Scombroidei*, family *Scombroidae*, including tuna, mackarel, skipjack, bonito, and wahoo), associated with a histaminelike reaction consisting of facial flushing, burning sensation in the mouth, lightheadedness, headache, nausea, and palpitations. Physical examination shows intense hyperemia of the face, upper chest, back, and proximal third of the arms. A high content of free histidine in the flesh, which when acted on by certain bacteria, particularly *Proteus morgagni*, is decarboxylated to histamine, causes a toxic reaction when unrefrigerated fish is consumed.

Dickinson, G. Scombroida fish poisoning syndrome. *Ann. Emerg. Med.*, 1982, 11:487-9.

SCOTT, C. RONALD (American physician)

Scott syndrome. A hereditary syndrome, transmitted as an X-linked recessive trait, characterized by growth retardation, mental retardation, hirsutism, craniofacial abnormalities (brachycephaly, small mandible, small pointed nose, prominent eyebrows, long dark eyelashes, startled expression), and hand and foot anomalies (soft tissue syndactyly and dermatoglyphic abnormalities).

Scott, C. R., *et al.* A new craniodigital syndrome with mental retardation. *J. Pediat.*, 1971, 78:658-63.

SCOTT, CHARLES I., JR. (American pediatrician)

Aarskog-Scott syndrome (ASS). See *Aarskog syndrome.*

Hecht-Scott syndrome. See *under Hecht, Jacqueline T.*

SCOTT, HENRY HARALD (American physician, born 1874)

Strachan-Scott syndrome. See *Strachan syndrome.*

SCOTT, J. E. (American physician)

Scott-Taor syndrome. Synonyms: *ischiopatellar dysplasia, small patella syndrome.*

A familial syndrome of an aplastic or hypoplastic patella associated with a deformed pelvis at the junction between the ischium and the pubic bone, wherein the synostosis may be absent or replaced by a massive bone formation. A hollow depression in the ilium caudal to the acetabulum occurs in all cases.

*Scott, J. E., & Taor, W. S. The "small patella" syndrome. *J. Bone Joint Surg.*, 1979, 61(A):172.

SCOTT, R. BODLEY (British physician)

Scott and Robb-Smith syndrome. Progressive histiocytic medullary reticulosis.

Scott, R. B., & Robb-Smith, A. H. T. The progressive hyperplasias of the reticulo-endothelial system. *St. Bartholomew Hosp. Rep.*, 1936, 64:143-75.

screwdriver teeth. See *Hutchinson teeth, under Hutchinson, Sir Jonathan.*

SCRIVER, CHARLES ROBERT (American physician, born 1930)

Scriver-Goldbloom-Roy syndrome. Synonym: *hypophosphatemic rickets-renal hyperglycinuria-renal glycosuria-glycylprolinuria syndrome.*

A disorder of amino acid metabolism characterized by hypophosphatemia, rickets, renal hyperglycinuria, renal glycosuria, and glycyl-prolinuria, originally described in an adolescent boy. The primary factor is believed to be a disturbance of renal tubular transport affecting phosphorus, glycine, and glucose, rickets and osteomalacia being secondary to the impaired conservation of phosphorus.

Scriver, C. R., Goldbloom, R. B., & Roy, C. C. Hypophosphatemic rickets with renal hyperglycinuria, renal glucosuria, and glycyl-prolinuria. A syndrome with evidence of renal tubular secretion of phosphorus. *Pediatrics*, 1964, 34:357-71.

scrofulous ulcers of the legs. See *Bazin disease.*

SCULLY, ROBERT EDWARD (American pathologist, born 1921)

Scully tumor. Synonym: *gonadoblastoma.*

An androgen-producing tumor of the ovary, which contains cells of sex cord mesenchyme origin as well as cells of the germ-cell type.

Scully, R. E. Gonadoblastoma. A gonadal tumor related to the dysgerminoma (seminoma) and capable of sex-hormone production. *Cancer*, 1953, 6:455-63.

SD (somatization disorder). See *Briquet syndrome (1), under Briquet, Pierre.*

SD (Still disease). See *Still syndrome.*

SDAT (senile dementia of the Alzheimer type). See *Alzheimer disease.*

SDS. See *Shy-Drager syndrome.*

sea-blue histiocyte disease. Synonym: *sea-blue histiocytosis.*

The presence in the bone marrow and spleen of

histiocytes with blue or blue-green staining cytoplasms, associated with splenomegaly, mild purpura secondary to thrombocytopenia, and, occasionally, liver cirrhosis. The symptoms usually include macular abnormalities, skin pigmentation, neurologic complications, and pulmonary infiltrates. Lipids containing cerebroside and carbohydrate are usually found in the histiocytes. Increased urinary excretion of mucopolysaccharides occurs in some cases. The course is usually benign,but involvement of the bones, lungs, and liver with hepatic failure and gastrointestinal hemorrhage leading to death may occur. Sea-blue histiocytes may also be present in patients with idiopathic thrombocytopenia, chronic myelocytic leukemia, hyperlipoproteinemia, Niemann-Pick syndrome, and other conditions. The syndrome is believed to be transmitted as an autosomal recessive trait.

Silverstein, M. N., *et al.* The syndrome of the sea-blue histiocyte. *N. Engl. J. Med.*, 1970, 282:1-4. Wewalka, F. G. Syndrome of sea-blue histiocyte. *Lancet*, 1970, 2:1248. Zlotnick, A., & Fried, K. Sea-blue histiocyte syndrome, *Lancet*, 1970, 2:776.

sea-blue histiocytosis. See *sea-blue histiocyte syndrome.*

Seabright Bantam syndrome. See *Albright syndrome (1).*

seal finger syndrome. Synonym: *blubber finger.*

A finger infection, caused by some unknown agent, that occurs in persons engaged in slaughtering and skinning seals. Severe pain and swelling are the main symptoms.

Candolin, Y. Seal finger (spekkfinger) and its occurrence in the gulfs of the Baltic Sea. *Acta Chir. Scand.*, 1953, Suppl. 177:7-51.

SEARS, J. W. (American physician)

Heiner-Sears syndrome. See *Heiner syndrome.*

seat-belt syndrome. Synonym: *safety belt syndrome.*

Injuries resulting from wearing an automobile seat belt during traffic accidents, including damages of the abdominal organs (bowel rupture, abdominal wall injuries, liver rupture, and vascular trauma), thoracic trauma (sternal fracture and myocardial contusion), and flexion fractures of the spine.

Garrett, J. W., & Braunstein, P. W. The seat belt syndrome. *J. Trauma*, 1962, 2:220-38.

sebaceous nevus syndrome. See *Jadassohn nevus sebaceus, under Jadassohn, Josef.*

seborrhea congestiva. See *lupus erythematosus.*

seborrheic dermatitis. See *Unna disease, under Unna, Paul Gerson.*

seborrheic diathesis in infants. See *Leiner dermatitis.*

seborrheic eczema. See *Unna disease, under Unna, Paul Gerson.*

seborrheic pemphigus. See *Senear-Usher syndrome.*

SECKEL, HELMUT PAUL GEORGE (American physician, born 1900)

Seckel bird head syndrome. See *Seckel syndrome.*

Seckel nanism. See *Seckel syndrome.*

Seckel syndrome. Synonyms: *Seckel bird head syndrome, Seckel nanism, Virchow-Seckel syndrome, bird-headed dwarfism, birdlike face syndrome, nanocephalic dwarfism.*

A syndrome of intrauterine proportionate dwarfism and birdlike facies with prominent sometimes beaked nose, micrognathia, high-arched palate, cleft palate, low-set lobeless ears, prominent eyes, antimongoloid palpebral fissures, and epicanthus. A small simplified

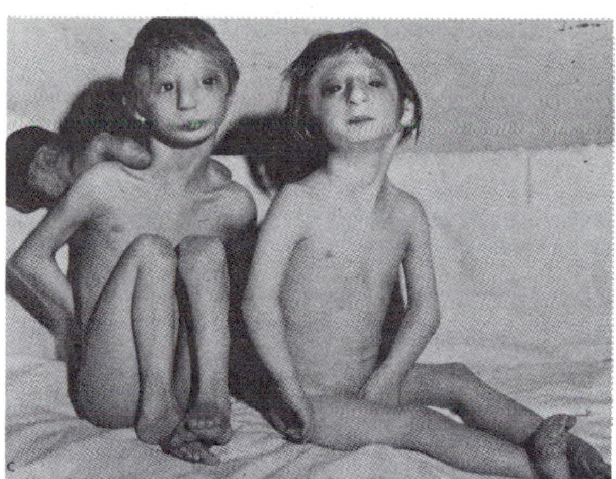

Seckel syndrome
Harper, R.G., et al: *J. Pediatr.* 70:799, 1967. St. Louis: C.V. Mosby Co.

cerebrum resembles the chimpanzee brain (pongidoid micrencephaly). Bone disorders include multiple dislocations, mainly congenital hip dislocation, kyphoscoliosis, sternal defects, absence of the patella, and disorders of bone maturation. Clinodactyly, simian creases, increased distance between the first and second toes, cryptorchism, pancytopenia, mental retardation, abnormalities of pigmentation, hypertrichosis, hypertelorism, chorioretinopathy, strabismus, defects of the epiglottis, hypodontia, malocclusion, and other disorders may occur. Autosomal recessive transmission is suspected. See also *Hallermann-Streiff syndrome.*

Seckel, H. P. *Bird-headed dwarfs; studies in developmental anthropology including human proportions.* Basel, Karger, 1960. Virchow, R. Zwergenkind. *Zschr. Ethnol.*, 1882, 14:215.

Virchow-Seckel syndrome. See *Seckel syndrome.*

second injury syndrome. A non-contact injury in athletes due to poor muscle coordination secondary to inadequate training, poor warm-up, or excessive tiredness.

King, J. Second injury syndrome. *Brit. J. Sports Med.*, 1983, 17:59-60.

secondary degeneration. See *wallerian degeneration, under Waller, Augustus Volney.*

secondary diabetic glycogenosis. See *Mauriac syndrome, under Mauriac, Leonard Pierre.*

secondary hypertrophic osteoarthropathy. See *Marie-Bamberger syndrome, under Marie, Pierre.*

SECRETAN, HENRI FRANÇOIS (Swiss physician, 1856-1916)

Secrétan disease. Post-traumatic hard edema of the dorsum of the hand or foot, resulting in formation of fibrous tisssue and restriction of digital flexion, except of the thumb or great toe.

Secrétan, H. Oedéme dur et hyperplasie traumatique du métacarpe dorsal. *Rev. Méd. Suisse Rom.*, 1901, 21:409-16.

secretoinhibitor syndrome. See *Sjögren syndrome, under Sjögren, Henrik Samuel Conrad.*

SEDAGHATIAN, M. R. (Iranian physician)

Sedaghatian chondrodysplasia. See *Sedaghatian syndrome.*

Sedaghatian syndrome. Synonym: *Sedaghatian chondrodysplasia.*

A familial lethal epimetaphyseal chondrodysplasia, transmitted as an autosomal recessive trait, characterized by rhizomelic dwarfism, platyspondyly, metaphyseal dysplasia, microphthalmia, asymmetric ears, depressed nasal bridge, broad nose, short neck, and prominent sternum. Structural and functional disorders of cartilage and bony tissues affecting the area of the epiphyses and metaphyses, manifested chiefly by irregular ossification and variably constituted bone with persisting cartilage and chondrocytes in the beginning portion of the spongiosa are the principal histological findings.

Sedaghatian, M. R. Congenital lethal metaphyseal chondrodysplasia: A newly recognized complex autosomal recessive disorder. *Am. J. Med. Genet.*, 1980, 6:269-74.
Opitz, J. M., *et al.* Brief clinical report: Sedaghatian congenital lethal metaphyseal chondrodysplasia-observations in a second Iranian family and histopathological study. *Am. J. Med. Genet.*, 1987, 26:583-90.

SEDANO, HEDDIE O. (Argentine oral pathologtst in the United States)

Gorlin-Sedano syndrome. See *under Gorlin.*

SEDGWICK, ROBERT P. (American physician)

Boder-Sedgwick syndrome. See *Louis-Bar syndrome.*

SEDILLOT

Sedillot syndrome. Changes in the genitalia and psychoneurotic disorders of an irritable character developing into true neurosis, believed by Sedillot to be caused by such practices as contraception and masturbation.

Ramirez Prado, C. Sindrome de Sedillot. *Cir. Cirujan.*, 1953, 21:361-70.

SEDLACKOVA, E. (Czech physician)

Sedlácková syndrome. A syndrome of congenital shortening of the velum palatinum, deficient velopalatine closure, speech disorders (mainly hyperrhinophony or palatolaly), and characteristic facies (narrow palpebral fissures, narrow nostrils, wide base of the nose, hypoplastic philtrum, and, less frequently, facial asymmetry, inability to close the eyes, and malformed ears).

Sedlácková, E. Insuficience patrohla tnového záveru vyvojová porucha. *Cas. Lék. Cesk.*, 1955, 94:47-9.
Sedlácková, E. The syndrome of the congenitally shortened velum the dual innervation of the soft palate. *Fol. Phoniat.*, 1967, 19:441-50.

SEE, GEORGES (French physician, born 1904)

Julien Marie-Sée syndrome. See *Marie-Sée syndrome, under Marie, Julien.*

Marie-Sée syndrome. See *under Marie, Julien.*

SEELIGMANN, E. (German physician)

Seeligmann syndrome. See *Carini syndrome.*

SEEMENOVA, EVA (Physician in Ostrava)

Seemenová syndrome. A familial syndrome, transmitted as an autosomal recessive trait, characterized by birdlike facies, microcephaly with normal intelligence, receding mandible, immunodeficiency due to decreased immunoglobulin levels, and risk of lymphoreticular malignant tumors originating in the mediastinum.

Seemenová, E., *et al.* Familial microcephaly with normal intelligence, immunodeficiency, and risk for lymphoreticular malignancies: A new autosomal recessive disorder. *Am. J. Med. Genet.*, 1985, 20:639-48.

SEGAWA, M. (Japanese physician)

Segawa syndrome. Synonym: *progressive dystonia with diurnal fluctuations.*

A familial dystonic syndrome, transmitted as an autosomal dominant trait, characterized by progressive postural and motor disorders with diurnal fluctuations, which appear between the ages of 1 to 9 years and involve all the extremities within 5 years from onset. The symptoms are alleviated by sleep and low doses of L-DOPA.

Segawa, M., *et al.* Hereditary progressive dystonia with marked diurnal fluctuation. *Adv. Neur.*, 1976, 14:215-33.

segmental enteritis. See *Crohn disease.*

segmental ileitis. See *Crohn disease.*

segmental saccular dilatation of the intrahepatic bile ducts. See *Caroli syndrome (2).*

segmental skin hemangioma-spinal meninges hemangioma syndrome. See *Cobb syndrome.*

segmental spasm of esophagus. See *Bársony-Polgár syndrome (2).*

SEIDLMAYER, HUBERT (German physician, 1910-1965)

Seidlmayer disease. Synonyms: *postinfection purpura, purpura postinfectiva.*

Postinfectious purpura of infancy and childhood, characterized by coinlike elevated lesions.

Seidlmayer, H. Die früchtinfantile, postinfektiöse Kokarden-Purpura. *Zschr. Kinderheilk.*, 1940, 61:217-55.

SEIP, MARTIN FREDRIK (Norwegian physician, born 1921)

Berardinelli-Seip syndrome. See *under Berardinelli.*

Berardinelli-Seip-Lawrence syndrome. See *Berardinelli-Seip syndrome.*

Seip syndrome. See *Berardinelli-Seip syndrome.*

Seip-Lawrence syndrome. See *Berardinelli-Seip syndrome.*

SEITELBERGER, FRANZ (Austrian physician)

Bernheimer-Seitelberger syndrome. See *gangliosidosis G_{M2} type III.*

Seitelberger disease (1). See *gangliosidosis G_{M2} type III.*

Seitelberger disease (2). A familial form of demyelinating disease with early onset and absence of stainable myelin. It is a variant of the Pelizaeus-Merzbacher syndrome.

Seitelberger, F. Die Pelizaeus-Merzbachersche Krankheit Klinisch-anatomische Untersuchung zum Problem ihrer Stellung unter dendiffusen Sklerosen. *Wien. Zschr. Nervenh.*, 1954, 9:228-89.

selective vitamin B_{12} malabsorption. See *Imerslund-Gräsbeck syndrome.*

selective vitamin B_{12} malabsorption-proteinuria syndrome. See *Imerslund-Gräsbeck syndrome.*

self-induced photosensitive epilepsy. See *Gastaut syndrome (1).*

self-induced water intoxication and schizophrenic disorders (SIWIS) syndrome. Self-induced water intoxication complicated by schizophrenia. Inappropriate affect, auditory hallucinations, paranoid delusions, and looseness of associations characteristic of schizophrenia are the principal symptoms. Complications include recurrent seizures and coma secondary to hyponatremia, gastrointestinal dilation and hypotonicity, bladder dilation and hypotonicity, and hydronephrosis due to consumption of large quantities of water. Edema, hypotension, and hypovolemia may be present.

Vieweg, W. V. R., *et al.* Evaluation of patients with self-induced water intoxication and schizophrenic disorders (SIWIS). *J. Nerv. Ment. Dis.*, 1984, 172:552-5.

SELTER, PAUL (German pediatrician, born 1866)
Selter disease. See *acrodynia.*
Selter-Swift-Feer syndrome. See *acrodynia.*
SELYE, HANS (Hungarian-born Canadian physician, born 1907)
Selye syndrome. Synonyms: *adaptation syndrome, general adaptation syndrome (GAS), stress syndrome.*

The sum of reactions to prolonged exposure to stress, including enlargement of the adrenal cortex with increased production of corticoid hormones, involution of the thymus and other lymphatic organs, gastrointestinal ulcer, metabolic changes, and variations in the resistance of the organism. The first stage is the **alarm reaction,** consisting of a shock phase and then a countershock phase, followed by the **adaptation stage,** in which the resistance to the original stressor is greater, but the resistance to other stressors is decreased. If the stressor is not removed, the **exhaustion stage** and death will follow. See also *post-traumatic stress syndrome,* and *stress ulcer syndrome.*

Selye, H. *The physiology and pathology of exposure to stress; a treatise based on the concepts of the general-adaptation-syndrome and the diseases of adaptation.* Montreal, 1950.

SEMDJL. See *spondylo-epimetaphyseal dysplasia with joint laxity syndrome.*
SEMELAIGNE, GEORGES (French physician)
Debré-Semelaigne syndrome. See *under Debré.*
Kocher-Debré-Semelaigne (KDS) syndrome. See *Debré-Semelaigne syndrome.*
semimembranosus bursitis. See *Baker cyst.*
seminiferous tubule dysgenesis. See *chromosome XXY syndrome.*
seminoma. See *Chevassu tumor.*
SEN, PRAFULLA KUMAR (Indian physician, born 1915)
Sen syndrome. Synonym: *Indian childhood cirrhosis.*

Infantile cirrhosis of the liver. The condition has its onset in infancy, occurring more commonly in males than in females. It is transmitted as an autosomal recessive trait, familial cases being frequent.

Chaudhuri, A., & Chaudhuri, K. C. The karyotype in Sen's syndrome (infantile cirrhosis of the liver). *Indian J. Pediat.,* 1964, 31(201):309-11.

SENATOR, HERMANN (German physician, 1834-1911)
Banti-Senator disease. See *Banti syndrome.*
Senator angina. An acute and rapidly fatal form of pharyngolaryngeal infection described by Senator in 1888.

Hicquet. Un cas d'angine de Senator? *Ann. Otolar., Paris,* 1951, 68:851-2.

Senator syndrome. See *Banti syndrome.*

SENEAR, FRANCIS EUGENE (American physician, 1889-1958)
Senear-Usher syndrome. Synonyms: *pemphigus erythematodes, pemphigus erythematosus, seborrheic pemphigus.*

An eruption of bullous crusted lesions, usually on the face and chest. On the face, they may occur in the "butterfly" distribution similar to that seen in seborrheic dermatitis and lupus erythematosus. Histologically, the condition is classified with the pemphigus group because of the presence of acantholysis.

Senear, F. E., & Usher, B. An unusual type of pemphigus, combining features of lupus erythematosus. *Arch. Derm., Chicago,* 1926, 3:761-81.

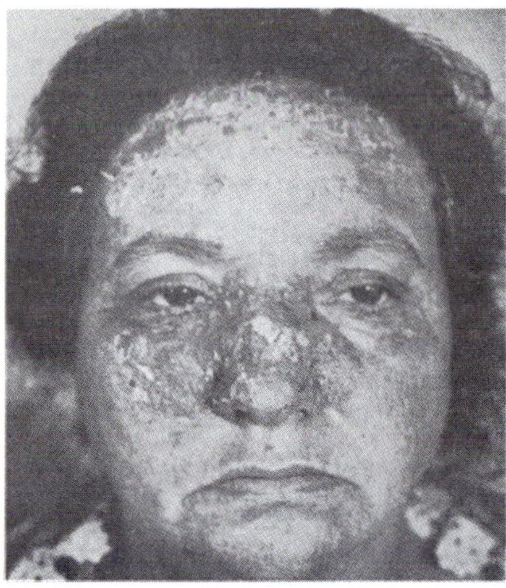

Senear-Usher syndrome
Andrews, G.C. & A.N. Domonkos: *Diseases of the Skin.* 5th ed. Philadelphia: W.B. Saunders Co., 1963.

senile angiomas. See *De Morgan spots.*
senile ankylosing hyperostosis of the spine. See *Forestier syndrome (2).*
senile arteritis. See *Horton disease (1).*
senile cardiac calcification syndrome. Calcific deposits in the heart of elderly individuals, most commonly found in the epicardial coronary arteries, the mitral annular area, the aortic valve cusps, and the left ventricular papillary muscles.

Roberts, W. C. The senile cardiac calcification syndrome. *Am. J. Card.,* 1986, 58:572-4.

senile dementia. See *Alzheimer disease.*
senile dementia of the Alzheimer type (SDAT). See *Alzheimer disease.*
senile gangrene. See *Pott gangrene.*
senile gout. See *Forestier syndrome (1).*
senile melanotic freckle. See *Hutchinson freckle, under Hutchinson, Sir Jonathan.*
senile parenchymatous hypertrophy of the breast. See *Cheatle disease.*
senile rheumatic gout. See *Forestier syndrome (1).*
senilism syndrome. See *Hutchinson-Gilford syndrome, under Hutchinson, Sir Jonathan.*
SENIOR, BORIS (American physician)
Senior syndrome (1). Synonyms: *Senior-Biochi syndrome, Senior-Loken syndrome, hereditary renal-retinal dysplasia, juvenile familial nephropathy-tapetoretinal degeneration syndrome, nephrophthisis-tepetoretinal degeneration syndrome, oculorenal dystrophy, renal-retinal dysplasia syndrome, renal-retinal dystrophy, tubulo-interstitial nephropathy-tapetoretinal degeneration syndrome.*

A congenital disorder combining nephrophthisis and tapetoretinal degeration. In the juvenile type, there is blindness and death from renal failure before the age of 10. The adult type is marked by a later onset and a milder course. Renal involvement consists mainly of polyuria and polydipsia due to impaired urinary concentrating ability of the kidneys. Proteinuria and leukocyturia may be associated. Progressive development of chronic renal failure usually leads to hypertension, anemia, hypocalcemia, and hyperphosphatemia. Aminoaciduria may also occur. **Tapetoretinal degeneration** comprises a group of disorders, including Leber congenital amaurosis and pigmentatary retinal degeneration. The syndrome is believed to be transmitted as an autosomal recessive trait with variable expression. See also *renal-ocular syndrome*.

Senior, B., *et al.* Juvenile familial nephropathy with tapetoretinal degeneration. A new oculorenal dystrophy. *Am. J. Ophth.*, 1961, 52:625-33, Loken, A. C., *et al.* Hereditary renal dysplasia and blindness. *Acta Paediat., Stockholm*, 1961, 50:177-84.

Senior syndrome (2). A congenital syndrome of short stature, minute nails on the small toes bilaterally, mild intellectual retardation, broad nose, wide mouth, shortness of the middle phalanges of the fifth fingers, and fusion of the middle and distal phalanges of the fifth toes.

Senior, B. Impaired growth and onychodysplasia. Short children with tiny toenails. *Am. J. Dis. Child.*, 1971, 122:7-9.

Senior-Biochi syndrome. See *Senior syndrome (1).*

Senior-Loken syndrome. See *Senior syndrome (1).*

SENSENBRENNER, JUDITH A. (American physician)

Sensenbrenner syndrome. See *cranio-ectodermal dysplasia syndrome.*

Sensenbrenner-Dorst-Owens syndrome. See *cranio-ectodermal dysplasia syndrome.*

sensimotor induction in unilateral disequilibrium syndrome. See *Halpern syndrome.*

sensorimotor induction syndrome. See *Halpern syndrome.*

sensory neuropathy syndrome. A disease of the peripheral nervous system in which the primary neuropathological changes involve the nerve cell, characterized by profound sensory ataxia, areflexia, slowed or absent sensory conduction, and widespread sensory loss, primarily of large fiber modalities (proprioceptive sensibility). There is no muscle weakness and muscle and motor conduction is normal. The lesions are most likely confined to the dorsal root and gasserian ganglia. The disease is monophasic, progresses rapidly to a severe, mainly proprioceptive sensory deficit. Little improvement occurs, and the patient remains severely disabled. The condition may be produced by toxins, mercury, adriamycin, some vitamins, or infections, or it can be found in association with neoplasms.

Sterman, A. B., *et al.* The acute sensory neuropathy syndrome: A distinct entity. *Ann. Neurol.*, 1980, 7:354-8.

sensory radicular neuropathy. See *Thévenard syndrome.*

sensory urge incontinence. See *under urge incontinence syndrome.*

sepsis acutissima hyperergica fulminans. See *Waterhouse-Friderichsen syndrome.*

sepsis allergenica. See *Wissler syndrome.*

sepsis hyperergica. See *Wissler syndrome.*

septal cirrhosis. See *Laennec cirrhosis.*

septo-optic dysplasia (SOD). Synonyms: *de Morsier syndrome, Hoyt-Kaplan-Grumbach syndrome, dwarfism-septo-optic dysplasia syndrome, septo-optic dysplasia anomalad, septo-optic dysplasia and pituitary dwarfism syndrome, septo-optic-pituitary dysplasia syndrome.*

A syndrome of growth retardation due to congenital hypopituitarism, associated with hypoplasia of the optic disk, absence of the septum pellucidum and/or corpus callosum, and midline fusion or absence of the basal ganglia, with bitemporal hemianopia, nystagmus, and poor vision. Laboratory findings may show growth hormone, ACTH, and thyroid-stimulating hormone deficiencies.

Morsier, G., de. Études sur les dysraphies, crânio-encéphaliques. III. Agénésie du septum lucidum avec malformation du tractus optique. La dysplasie septo-optique. *Schweiz. Arch. Neur. Neurhochir.*, 1956, 77:267. Hoyt, W. F., Kaplan, S. L., Grumbach, M. M., & Glaser, J. S. Septo-optic dysplasia and pituitary dwarfism. *Lancet*, 1970, 1:893. Kaplan, S. L., *et al.* A syndrome of hypopituitary dwarfism, hypoplasia of the optic nerves, and malformations of the prosencephalon: Report of six patients. *Pediat. Res.*, 1970, 4:480-1.

septo-optic dysplasia and pituitary dwarfism syndrome. See *septo-optic dysplasia.*

septo-optic dysplasia anomalad. See *septo-optic dysplasia.*

septo-optic-pituitary dysplasia syndrome. See *septo-optic dysplasia.*

seronegative toxoplasmosis. See *Sabin-Feldman syndrome.*

seropositive nonsyphilitic pneumopathy. See *Fanconi-Hegglin syndrome.*

serous central chorioretinitis. See *Masuda-Kitahara disease.*

serous meningitis. See *Dupré syndrome, and see pseudotumor cerebri syndrome.*

Sertoli cell only syndrome. Synonyms: *Del Castillo syndrome, germinal aplasia syndrome, testicular dysgenesis syndrome.*

A syndrome, transmitted as an X-linked trait, characterized by seminiferous tubules lined with Sertoli cells, little or no tubular fibrosis, and absent germinal cells, associated with small testes, sterility with azospermia, increased plasma FSH level, normal LH level, and an exaggerated response of LH to GnRH. Exposure to radiations and reaction to some drugs, including cytotoxic agents, are said to be the contributing factors.

Del Castillo, E. B., *et al.* Syndrome produced by the absence of the germinal epithelium without impairment of the Sertoli or Leydig cells. *J. Endocr.*, 1947, 7:493-502.

serum disease. See *serum sickness syndrome.*

serum intoxication. See *serum sickness syndrome.*

serum prothrombin conversion accelerator (SPCA) deficiency. See *Alexander syndrome, under Alexander, Benjamin.*

serum sickness syndrome. Synonyms: *immune-complex disease, serum disease, serum intoxication.*

Hypersensitivity reaction following the administation of a foreign serum or other antigens or certain drugs (the **serum-sickness-like syndrome**), and marked by urticaria, edema, arthralgia, high fever, lymphadenopathy, and prostration. The acute reaction is attributable to the formation of antibodies against the foreign serum, antigen, or drug, which are usually present in excess at initial antibody production. Soluble antigen-antibody complexes that mediate immunologic injury are deposited in tissues. Penicillin, sulfonamides, penicilamine, thiouracil, and other chemotherapeutic agents are the most common causes of this disorder in modern medical practice.

Amos, H. E. Allergic drug reactions. In: Lachmann, P. J., & Peters, D. K., eds. *Clinical aspects of immunology.* vol. 1, 4th ed. London, Blackwell, 1982. pp. 724-44.

serum sickness-like syndrome. See *under serum sickness syndrome.*

SERVELLE, M. (French physician)

Servelle syndrome. A form of osteohypoplastic angiomatosis of the extremities.

Servelle, M. Stase veineuse et croissance osseuse. *Bull. Acad. Nat. Méd., Paris,* 1948, 132:471-4.

SETLEIS, HOWARD (American physician)

Setleis syndrome. A familial syndrome, probably transmitted as an autosomal recessive trait, characterized by an aged, leonine facial appearance; absent eyelashes from either eyelid, or multiple rows of eyelashes on the upper lids with absence of the lashes on the lower eyelids; upward and lateral slanting of the eyebrows; scarlike defects on the temples erroneously attributed to obstetrical forceps; aging-like puckering of the skin around the eyes; scarlike median ridge of the chin; and rubbery appearance of the nose and chin on palpation.

Setleis, H., *et al.* Congenital ectodermal dysplasia of the face. *Pediatrics,* 1963, 32:540-8.

seven point syndrome. Deformities of the head, thorax, pelvis, and contractures of the neck, hip, and feet associated with scoliosis in children. A long C-type lateral curvature of the spine, with a slight rib bump on the convex side and flattening of the concave side of the thorax, is complicated by asymmetrical flattening of the dorsal aspect of the skull (plagiocephaly) and unilateral flattening of the pelvis, occurring almost always on the same side as the concavity of the spinal curvature. Other deformities include calcaneus deformities of the feet and later a rotated posture of the head suggesting torticollis, limitation of abduction of the hip (sometimes associated with dysplasia of the acetabulum), and occasional fixed dorsolumbar kyphosis. Associated disorders are caused by pressure deformation of the skeleton on one side and unilateral contractures of the soft tissue on the contralateral side.

Mau, H. The changing concept of infantile scoliosis. *Internat. Orthop.,* 1981, 5:131-7. Mau, H. Begleiterscheinungen und Verlauf der. sog. Säuglingsskoliose. *Verh. Deut. Orthop. Gesselsch.,* 1963, 97:464-6.

SEVER, JAMES WARREN (American physician, born 1878)

Sever syndrome. Synonym: *retrocalcaneal bursitis.*

Posterior heel pain in otherwise normal and active children, caused by post-traumatic inflammation of the soft tissue of the posterior heel. The loss of the lucent retrocalcaneal recess is the principal radiographic finding.

Sever, J. W. Apophysitis of the os calcis. *N. Y. Med. J.,* 1912, 95:1027-9. Heneghan, M. A., & Wallace, T. Heel pain due to retrocalcaneal bursitis-radiographic diagnosis (with a historical footnote on Sever's disease). *Pediat. Radiol.,* 1985, 15:119-22.

severe combined immunodeficiency (SCID) syndrome. See *severe mixed immunodeficiency syndrome.*

severe combined immunodeficiency with leukopenia. See *Vaal-Seynhaeve syndrome.*

severe mixed immunodeficiency syndrome. Synonyms: *Glanzmann-Riniker alymphoplasia, Glanzmann-Riniker syndrome, alymphocytosis, essential lymphocytophthisis, severe combined immunodeficiency (SCID) syndrome, lymphocytophthisis, Swiss-type agammaglobulinemia, thymic alymphoplasia.*

A hereditary syndrome, transmitted as either an autosomal recessive or X-linked trait, characterized by the lack of delayed hypersensitivity, thymus atrophy, lymphocytopenia, unresponsiveness to the administration of gamma-globulin, and susceptibility to bacterial, fungal, and viral infections. Some infants with the autosomal recessive type have a deficiency of adenosine deaminase, but otherwise the two genetic forms are clinically similar. Watery diarrhea with *Salmonella* and *Escherichia coli* in the stools, lung abscesses caused by *Pseudomonas aeruginosa, Pneumocystis carinii* pneumonia, moniliasis involving the oral and perianal areas, generalized chickenpox, Hecht giant cell pneumonia, cytomegalus or adenovirus and other infections, and death within the first 2 years of life are the major features of this syndrome. Hematological findings include leukopenia, variable lymphocytopenia, and frequent eosinophilia. See also *bare lymphocyte syndrome.*

Glanzmann, E., & Riniker, P. Essentielle Lymphocytophthie. Ein neues Krankheitsbild aus der Säuglingspathologie. *Ann. Paediat., Basel,* 1950, 175:1-32.

sex reversal syndrome. See *chromosome XX syndrome.*

sexual asphyxia syndrome. Synonym: *adolescent sexual asphyxia syndrome.*

Self-hanging while masturbating, in order to achieve maximum sexual gratification.

Rosenblum, S., & Faber, M. M. The adolescent sexual asphyxia syndrome. *J. Am. Acad. Child. Psychiat.,* 1979, 18:546-58.

sexual aversion syndrome. Unwillingness to participate in sexual activity, with avoidance of any touching or communication that might lead to sexual involvement.

Crenshaw, T. L. The sexual aversion syndrome. *J. Sex. Marital. Ther.,* 1985, 11:285-92.

sexual headache. See *under headache syndrome.*

sexually acquired immunodeficiency (SAID) syndrome. See *acquired immunodeficiency syndrome.*

SEYFFARTH, HENRIK (Norwegian physician)

Seyffarth syndrome. Synonyms: *pronator syndrome, pronator teres syndrome.*

An overuse syndrome (q.v.) characterized by lesions of the median nerve secondary to myosis of the pronator teres. The symptoms include a tender and hard pronator teres muscle, being most severe at a point above the median nerve; a tender spot in the thenar eminence; aching pain in the wrist and forearam; and paresthesia in the radial fingers. Excessive straining at work or exercise is believed to be the cause.

Seyffarth, H. Primary myoses in the m. pronator teres as cause of lesion in the n. medianus (the pronator syndrome). *Acta Psych. Neur. Scand.,* 1950, Suppl. 74:251-6.

SEYNHAEVE, VICTORIEN (Dutch physician)

de Vaal-Seynhaeve syndrome. See *Vaal-Seynhaeve syndrome.*

Vaal-Seynhaeve syndrome. See *under Vaal.*

SEZARY, ALBERT (French physician, 1880-1956)

pre-Sézary syndrome. Chronic erythroderma with clinical features similar to those seen in the Sézary syndrome, characterized by intractable erythroderma, an immunologic and histologic picture of chronic exfoliative dermatitis, and less than 1,000 circulating atypical lymphocytes (Sézary cells) per cubic millimeter. The condition usually evolves into the Sézary syndrome.

Winkelmann, R. K., & Caro, W. A. Current problems in mycosis fungoides and Sézary syndrome. *Annu. Rev. Med.*, 1977, 28:251-69.

Sézary reticulosis. See *Sézary syndrome.*

Sézary syndrome (SS). Synonyms: *Sézary reticulosis, Sézary-Baccaredda syndrome, Sézary-Bouvrain syndrome, reticulohistiocytosis cutanea hyperplastica benigna cum melanodermia.*

A syndrome of severe pruritic erythroderma, lymphomatous skin infiltration, and circulating large mononuclear activated T-cells with convoluted nuclei (Sézary cells). Facial infiltration may produce facies leonina. Some patients also have alopecia and nail dystrophy. The Sézary syndrome and mycosis fungoides are considered by some authors the same entity, and by others as two separate forms of the cutaneous T-cell lymphoma (CTCL).

Sézary, A., & Bouvrain, Érythrodermie avec présence de cellules monstreuses dans la derme et le sang circulant. *Bull. Soc. Fr. Derm. Syph.*, 1938, 45:254-60. Baccaredda, A. Reticulohistiocytosis cutanea hyperplastica benigna cum melanodermia. Beitrag zum Studium der peripheren Reticulohistiocytosen. *Arch. Derm. Syph., Berlin,* 1939, 179:209-56.

Sézary-Baccaredda syndrome. See *Sézary syndrome.*

Sézary-Bouvrain syndrome. See *Sézary syndrome.*

SFD (silo filler disease). See *silo unloader syndrome.*

SFORZINI, PAOLO (Italian physician)

Sforzini syndrome. Synonym: *exophthalmia normometabolica hereditaria.*

A hereditary form of exophthalmos associated with gigantism, proportionately long extremities, small head, visceroptosis, emotional excitability, stuttering, and occasional autonomic gastrointestinal dystonia, in the absence of any metabolic or endocrine disorder.

Sforzini, P. Esoftalmia normometabolica ereditaria. (Studio genetico-clinico di una nuova sindrome). *Gazz. Internaz. Med.*, 1955, 59:401-10.

SHÄFER

Shäfer syndrome. Synonym: *congenital dyskeratosis.*

A congenital syndrome of hyperkeratosis palmaris et plantaris, leukokeratosis of the oral mucosa, thick nails, testicular hypoplasia, cataract, corneal dystrophy, mental retardation, and growth retardation, reportedly described by Shäfer.

SHAFT (sad, hostile, anxious, frustrating, tenacious) syndrome. See *Munchausen syndrome.*

SHAH, KRISHNAKUMAR N. (Indian physician)

Shah-Waardenburg syndrome. Synonym: *Hirschsprung disease-pigmentary anomaly syndrome.*

A variant of the Waardenburg syndrome associated with white forelock, white eyebrows and eyelashes, iridochromia iridis, and intestinal obstruction caused by a long-segment Hirschsprung disease. The syndrome is transmitted as an autosomal recessive trait.

Shah, K. N., *et al.* White forelock, pigmentary disorder of irides, and long segment Hirschsprung disease: Possible variant of Waardenburg syndrome. *J. Pediat.*, 1981, 99:432-5.

shaken baby syndrome (SBS). See *battered child syndrome.*

shaken child syndrome. See *battered child syndrome.*

shaking palsy. See *Parkinson syndrome, under Parkinson, James.*

SHAPIRO, WILLIAM R. (American physician)

Shapiro syndrome. Synonym: *spontaneous periodic hypothermia.*

A syndrome of agenesis of the corpus callosum associated with recurrent attacks of hypothermia with chills and sweating, lasting from a few minutes to several weeks, and behavioral retardation. Polydipsia, polyuria, and hyponatremia may be associated. Craniofacial and midline defects are frequent features of this syndrome. Occasional attacks may be triggered by emotional stress or a particular odor.

Shapiro, W. R., *et al.* Spontaneous recurrent hypothermia accompanying agenesis of the corpus callosum. *Brain,* 1969, 92:423-36.

SHARP, GORDON C. (American physician)

Sharp syndrome. See *mixed connective tissue disease.*

SHATTOCK, SAMUEL GEORGE (British physician, 1852-1924)

Shattock disease. Synonyms: *pseudotuberculoma silicoticum, silicotic granuloma.*

Granuloma caused by foreign-body reaction to implanted silica particles.

Shattock, S. G. Pseudotuberculoma of the lip. *Proc. Roy. Soc. Med.*, 1916-17, 10(Sect. Path.):6-17.

SHAVER, CECIL GORDON (Canadian physician)

Shaver syndrome. Synonyms: *Shaver-Ridell syndrome, aluminosis, bauxite workers' disease.*

Interstitial pulmonary fibrosis accompanied by emphysema and pneumothorax, seen in bauxite workers. Histological findings include fibrous changes in the alveolar septa with hyalinization and replacement of the alveolar structures, pigment deposits in fibrosed areas, thickening of the arterial walls, presence of giant cells and cholesterol crystals, inflammatory changes and pigment deposits in the lymph nodes, alveolar pneumonitis, and severe emphysematous alterations.

Shaver, C. G., & Ridell, A. R. Lung changes associated with manufacture of alumina abrasives. *J. Indust. Hyg.*, 1947, l29:145-57.

Shaver-Ridell syndrome. See *Shaver syndrome.*

shawl scrotum syndrome. See *Aarskog syndrome.*

SHEA, M. COYLE, JR. (American physician)

Coyle Shea syndrome. See *Shea syndrome.*

Coyle syndrome. Synonym: *Coyle Shea syndrome.*

Postinflammatory osteogenic fixation of the stapes.

Shea, M. C., Jr. Postinflammatory osteogenic fixation of the stapes. *Laryngoscope,* 1977, 87:2056-65.

SHEEHAN, HAROLD LEEMING (British physician)

Reye-Sheehan syndrome. See *Sheehan syndrome.*

Sheehan syndrome. Synonyms: *Glinski-Simmonds syndrome, Reye-Sheehan syndrome, Simmonds cachexia, Simmonds syndrome, hypopituitarism syndrome, panhypopituitarism, pituitary cachexia, postpartum hypophyseogenic myxedema, postpartum hypopituitarism, postpartum pituitary insufficiency, postpartum necrosis, postpartum panhypopituitary syndrome, postpartum pituitary cachexia, postpartum pituitary necrosis.*

Necrosis of the pituitary gland with complete or partial functional failure of the adenohypophysis and secondary atrophy of the gonads, adrenal cortex, and thyroid gland. Anorexia, atrophy of the genitalia and breasts, bradycardia, hypotension, transient diabetes insipidus, hypoglycemia, amenorrhea, weight loss, loss of body hair, absence of libido, fatigability, depression, hypopituitary coma, hypothyroidism, adrenal insufficiency, gonadal insufficiency, and cachexia may ensue. Vascular disorders resulting in thrombosis and infarction of the pituitary gland were once considered to be the cause, but it is now believed that anoxia secondary to disorders such as excessive hemorrhage and eversion of the uterus is the cause. The term **Sheehan syndrome** applies to necrosis of the pituitary during the postpartum period; **Simmonds syndrome** refers to a similar condition which may occur in both sexes and is unrelated to postpartum complications.

Simmonds, M. Über Hypophysissschwund mit tödlichem Ausgang. *Deut. Med. Wschr.*, 1914, 40:322-3, Glinski, L. K. Z kazuistyki zmian anatomopatologicznych w pszysadce mozgowej. *Przegl. Lek.*, 1913, 52:13-4. Sheehan, H. L. Post-partum necrosis of the anterior pituitary. *J. Path. Bact., London*, 1937, 45:189-214. *Reye, E. Die ersten klinischen Symptome bei Schwund des Hypophysenworderlappens (Simmondsche Krankheit) und ihre erforlgreiche Behandlung. *Deut. Med. Wschr.*, 1928, 54:696.

SHEEHY

Sheehy syndrome. A syndrome reportedly described by Sheehy as a rapidly advancing sensorineural hearing loss in the younger age group.

SHELDON, JOSEPH HAROLD (British physician, 1920-1964)

Freeman-Sheldon syndrome (FSS). See *under Freeman.*

Sheldon necrotic purpura. See *Martin de Gimard syndrome.*

SHELDON, SIR WILFRID (British pediatrician, born 1901)

Ellis-Sheldom syndrome. See *mucopolysaccharidosis I-H.*

Luder-Sheldon syndrome. See *under Luder.*

Rocher-Sheldon syndrome. See *arthrogryposis multiplex congenita syndrome.*

shelf syndrome. See *synovial shelf syndrome.*

shelf syndrome of the knee. See *synovial shelf syndrome.*

shell nail syndrome. A syndrome of atrophy of the nail beds, clubbing, periostitis, and bronchiectasis.

Cornelius, C. E., III, & Shelley, W. B. Shell nail syndrome associated with bronchiectasis. *Arch. Derm., Chicago*, 1967, 96:694-5.

SHEPARDSON, H. C. (American physician)

Escamilla-Lisser-Shepardson syndrome. See *Escamilla-Lisser syndrome.*

SHEPHERD, FRANCIS JOHN (Canadian physician, 1851-1929)

Shepherd fracture. Fracture of the astragalus with detachment of the outer protecting edge.

Shepherd, F. J. A hitherto undescribed fracture of the stragalus. *J. Anat. Physiol., London*, 1882, 17:79-81.

SHERESHEVSKII, N. A. (Russian physician)

Shereshevskii-Turner syndrome. See *chromosome XO syndrome.*

SHH. See ***hyporeninemic hypoaldosteronism syndrome.***

SHIGA, KIYOSHI (Japanese physician, 1870-1957)

Shiga-Kruse disease. Synonyms: *bacillary dysentery, shigellosis.*

An acute infectious disease caused by strains of *Shigella dysenteriae* and marked by abdominal pain, malaise, fever, diarrhea, and tenesmus, mucus, pus, and blood in the stools.

Shiga, K. Über den Dysenteriebazillus (*Bacillus dysenteriae*). *Zbl. Bakt.*, 1898, 14(Part 1):817-28. Kruse, W. Über die Ruhr als Volkskrankheit und ihren Erreger. *Deut. Med. Wschr.*, 1900, 26;637-9.

Shigella dysentery. See *Flexner dysentery.*

shigellosis. See *Shiga-Kruse disease.*

SHIMODA, M. (Japanese physician)

Shimoda immobilithymia. A behavioral disorder characterized by a rigid, excitable, and stubborn personality with depressive tendencies.

Shimoda, M [Preclinical personality of depression] *Psychiat. Neur. Japon.*, 1941, 45:101-2.

shin bone fever. See *Werner-His disease, under Werner, Heinrich.*

shin splint syndrome. Synonyms: *medial tibial stress syndrome, soleus syndrome, tibial stress syndrome.*

A term referring to several pathological conditions, usually caused by athletic injuries, which include: (1) Strains of the tibialis anterior or the tibialis posterior muscles. (2) Tearing of the interosseous membrane between the tibia and the fibula. (3) Irritation of the periosteum due to muscles pulling away from it. (4) Inflammation of the tendons of the dorsiflexors of the foot. (5) Lesions of the soleus muscle. The disorder is characterized by a dull ache to intense pain in the leg and tenderness of the posterior medial border of the tibia. Pain is induced by exercise and is relieved by rest. Tendinitis, myositis, stress fractures, and compartment syndromes are the contributing factors.

Lilletvedt, J., *et al.* Analysis of selected alignment of the lower extremity related to the shin splint syndrome. *J. Am. Podiat. Assoc.*, 1979, 69:211-7. Mubarak, S. J., *et al.* The medial tibial stress syndrome (a cause of shin splints). *Am. J. Sports Med.*, 1982, 10:201-5. Michael, R. H., & Holder, L. E. The soleus syndrome. A cause of medial tibial stress (shin splints). *Am. J. Sports Med.*, 1985, 13:87-94.

ship fever. See *Hildenbrand disease.*

shipyard conjunctivitis. See *Sanders syndrome.*

SHML (**s**inus **h**istiocytosis with **m**assive **l**ymphadenopathy). See *Rosai-Dorfman syndrome.*

shock. See *shock syndrome.*

shock syndrome. Synonyms: *acute circulatory failure, shock.*

A condition of acute peripheral circulatory failure due to derangement of circulatory control or loss of circulating fluid, leading to cellular membrane dysfunction, abnormal cellular metabolism, and eventually cellular death. The causative factors include: (1) Decreased intravascular volume due to acute hemorrhage, excessive fluid loss in diarrhea, dehydration by excessive sweating, polyuria (in diabetes, after diuretic drugs, and/or acute renal failure), peritonitis, pancreatitis, slanchnic ischemia, intestinal obstruction, gangrene, burns, muscle injury, and vasodilatation caused by some drugs, nervous system injuries, gram-negative endotoxins, gram-positive bacteria, acute adrenal insufficiency, and anaphylaxis. (2) Heart disease. (3) Microcirculatory endothelial injury and aggregation of corpuscles in anaphylactic reaction, disseminated intravascular coagulation, burns, trauma, and sepsis. (4) Cellular membrane injury in sepsis, anaphylaxis, ischemia, hypoxia, pancreatitis, and tissue injury.

Abboud, F. M. Shock. In: Wyngaarden, J. B., & Smith, L. H., Jr., eds. *Cecil textbook of medicine.* 17th ed. Philadelphia, Saunders, 1985, pp. 211-25.

shock liver syndrome. Synonym: *ischemic hepatitis.*

Acute liver disease characterized by centrilobular necrosis and a sudden massive increase in transaminase levels (SGOT and SGPT) to more than 20 times the upper limit of normal levels, in response to cellular anoxia and in the absence of viral infections or drug toxicity. The acute phase is followed by complete remission and healing of necrosis within 7 to 10 days.

Birgens, H. S., *et al.* The shock liver: Clinical and biomedical findings in patients with centrilobular liver necrosis following cardiogenic shock. *Acta Med. Scand.*, 1978, 204:417-21. Bynum, T. E., *et al.* Ischemic hepatitis. *Dig. Dis. Sc.*, 1979, 24:129-35.

shock lung. See *adult respiratory distress syndrome.*

shock-encephalopathy syndrome. Synonym: *hemorrhagic shock-encephalopathy syndrome.*

A syndrome in which previously healthy infants suddenly develop severe shock, encephalopathy, hyperthermia, and the disseminated intravascular coagulation syndrome (q.v.), associated with liver enzyme elevation, acidosis, and kidney function disorders. Severe neurological complications and death are frequent.

Bacon, C., *et al.* Heatstroke in well-wrapped infants. *Lancet*, 1979, 1:422-5. Whittington, L. K., *et al.* Hemorrhagic shock and encephalopathy: Further description of a new syndrome. *J. Pediat.*, 1985, 106:599-602.

SHOKEIR, M. H. K. (physician in Canada)

Pena-Shokeir syndrome (1). See *under Pena.*

Pena-Shokeir syndrome (2). See *cerebro-oculofacioskeletal syndrome.*

Shokeir syndrome. A familial syndrome, transmitted as an autosomal dominant trait, characterized by congenital and permanent alopecia, including absence of scalp hair, eyebrows, eyelashes, and axillary hair. Mental subnormalilty and psychomotor epilepsy occur in some cases. Periodontosis is a constant feature.

Shokeir, M. H. K. Universal permanent alopecia, psychomotor epilepsy, pyorrhea and mental subnormality. *Clin. Genet.*, 1977, 11:13-7.

SHONE, JOHN D. (American physician)

Shone syndrome. Coexistence of the parachute mitral valve (one having two leaflets and commissures but the chordae, instead of diverging to insert into two papillary muscles, converge to insert into one major papillary muscle); supravalvular ring of the left atrium (representing a circumferential ridge of connective tissue that arises at the base of the atrial surface of the mitral leaflet and protrudes into the inlet of the mitral valve and, when fully developed, acts as a stenosing perforated diaphragm); subaortic stenosis; and coarctation of the aorta.

Shone, J. D., *et al.* The developmental complex of "parachute mitral valve," supravalvular ring of left atrium, subaortic stenosis, and coaractation of aorta. *Am. J. Cardiol.*, 1963, 11:714-25.

SHORT, D. S.

Short syndrome. See *bradycardia-tachycardia syndrome.*

SHORT (short stature-hyperextensibility of joints or hernia [inguinal] or both-ocular depression Rieger anomaly-teething delay) syndrome. A syndrome of multiple abnormalities, transmitted as an autosomal recessive trait, characterized by lipoatrophy involving mainly the upper limbs and face, slow weight gain, and frequent illness during infancy. The symptoms include a triangular face, telecanthus, growth retardation, deeply set eyes, Rieger anomaly, wide nasal bridge, hypoplastic alae of the nose, micrognathia, anteverted ears, clinodactyly, delayed dentition, lack of subcutaneous fat, hyperextensibility of the joints, deafness, heart murmur, inguinal hernia, delayed bone age, delayed speech, and normal intellect.

Gorlin, R. J., *et al.* Rieger anomaly and growth retardation (the S-H-O-R-T syndrome). *Birth Defects*, 1975, 11(2):46-8. Sensebrenner, J. A., *et al.* A low birthweight syndrome, ?Rieger syndrome. *Birth Defects*, 1975, 11(2):423-6.

short bowel syndrome (SBS). Synonyms: *short gut syndrome, short intestine syndrome, small bowel syndrome.*

A postoperative complication following extensive intestinal resection or jeunoileal bypass for morbid obesity. The severity of resulting malabsorption and the type of symptoms are related to the extent and the level of resection and the amount of absorptive and digestive surfaces of the intestine remaining intact; symptoms may include diarrhea, steatorrhea, weight loss, fatigue, lassitude, weakness, tetany, osteomalacia, osteoporosis, spontaneous fractures, purpura, generalized bleeding, peripheral neuropathy, hypoalbuminemia, ascites, and peripheral edema.

Trier, J. S. The short bowel syndrome. In: Sleisenger, M. H., Fordtran, J. S., Almy, T. P., eds. *Gastrointestinal disease. Pathology, diagnosis, management.* 3rd ed. Philadelphia, Saunders, 1983, pp. 873-9.

short colon-imperforate anus syndrome. See *Zachary-Morgan syndrome.*

short face syndrome. Synonyms: *hypodivergent face, idiopathic short face, low-angle facial type, skeletal type deep bite, vertical maxillary deficiency.*

A dentofacial deformity due to a deficiency in the vertical maxillary growth, presenting a short, square-shaped face, with the maxillary incisors hidden behind the upper lip when the jaw is at rest; a downward curving of the corners of the mouth below the midline; distinct skin folds lateral to the oral commissures when the mandible is in centric occlusion; apparent or actual macrostomia, and an edentulouslike appearance. The upper third of the face tends to be within normal limits, but the middle third usually shows broad nasal bases and large nostrils, the posterior part appearing wide because of prominent mandibular angles due to attachment of the masseter muscles to the laterally flared gonial processes. The maxillary arch is broad and the palatal vault is typically flat. Decreased vertical maxillary height, large freeway space, and low mandibular plane are the chief cephalometric findings. Malocclusion with deep overbite is common. Maxillary buccal cross-bites with interdental spacing are frequently associated.

Bell, W. H. Correction of the short-face syndrome-vertical maxillary deficiency: A preliminary report. *J. Oral Surg.*, 1977, 35:110-9.

short gut syndrome. See *short bowel syndrome.*

short intestine syndrome. See *short bowel syndrome.*

short leg syndrome. Asymmetry of length in the lower extremities. The structural forms are due to trauma or congenital growth inequality; functional (apparent) short legs usually result from soft tissue contractures or foot function disorders.

Vogel, F., Jr. Short-leg syndrome. *Clin. Podiat.*, 1984, 1:581-99.

short PR-normal QRS syndrome. See *Clerc-Lévy-Cristesco syndrome.*

short rib-polydactyly syndrome type I (SRP I). See *Majewski syndrome.*

short rib-polydactyly syndrome type II (SRP II). See *Saldino-Noonan syndrome.*

short rib-polydactyly syndrome type III (SPR III). See *Verma-Naumoff syndrome.*

short rib-polydactyly syndrome, Beemer type. See *Beemer syndrome.*

short rib-polydactyly syndrome, Majewski type. See *Majewski syndrome.*

short rib-polydactyly syndrome, Saldino-Noonan type. See *Saldino-Noonan syndrome.*

short rib-polydactyly syndrome, Verma-Naumoff type. See *Verma-Naumoff syndrome.*

short rib syndrome, Beemer type. See *short rib-polydactyly syndrome, Beemer type, under Beemer.*

shoulder syndrome. A complication of radical neck dissection due to denervation of the trapezius muscle by division of the spinal accessory nerve. The symptoms include trapezius paralysis with a dropped shoulder, a right angle appearance of the shoulder due to atrophy of muscle substance, inability to abduct more than 90 degrees, limitation of forward flexion, abnormal rotation of the scapula, and aching pain.

Szunyogh, B. Shoulder disability following radical neck dissection. *Am. Surgeon,* 1959, 25:194-8. Nahum, A. M., & Marmor, L. A syndrome resulting from radical neck dissection. *Arch. Otolar., Chicago,* 1961, 74:424-8.

shoulder impingement syndrome. Synonyms: *painful arc syndrome, subacromial impingement syndrome.*

Compression of the rotator cuff tendons and subacromial bursa between the humeral head and structures that make up the coracoacromial arch and the humeral tuberosities. The condition is associated with subacromial bursitis and rotator cuff (largely supraspinatus) and bicipital tendon inflammation, with or without degenerative changes in the tendons. Pain that is most severe when the arm is abducted in an arc between 40 and 120 degrees, sometimes associated with tears in the rotator cuff, is the chief symptom. Radiographic findings include the presence of a subacromial spur, degenerative changes in both the humeral tuberosities and acromioclavicular joint, and narrowing of the acromiohumeral distance.

Hardy, D. C., *et al.* The shoulder impingement syndrome: Prevalence of radiographic findings and correlation with response to therapy. *AJR,* 1986, 147:557-61.

shoulder pain syndrome. Synonym: *occupational cervicobrachial disorder.*

An occupational disorder characterized by painful shoulder due to overstraining. Rotator cuff tendinitis is the principal cause. The hypovascularity of the supraspinatus tendon is then likely to be accentuated by intramuscular pressure that reduces the blood flow through the muscle. The strain on the supraspinatus muscle is a factor in producing shoulder pain and disability. See also *overuse syndrome.*

Herberts, P., *et al.* Shoulder pain and heavy manual labor. *Clin. Orthop.,* 1984, No. 191:166-78.

shoulder-hand syndrome. Synonyms: *Steinbrocker syndrome, postinfarctional sclerodactylia, reflex dystrophy of the upper extremity.*

A form of the reflex sympathetic dystrophy syndrome (q.v.) characterized by painful incapacitating disorder of the shoulder in association with ipsilateral pain, stiffness, swelling, and vasomotor changes in the hands, wrists, and arms, resulting in atrophy of the subcutaneous tissue and muscles of the hands, thickening of the skin , and edema, and occasional adhesive capsulitis and sclerodactyly. The syndrome usually occurs in persons over 50 years of age after myocardial infarction, brain neoplasms, cerebrovascular accidents, and trauma to the distal upper extremity. When following hemiplegia, the syndrome develops on the side contralateral to the brain lesion. See also *postmyocardial infarction syndrome..*

Steinbrocker, O. Painful homolateral disability of shoulder and hand with swelling and atrophy of hand. *Ann. Rheum. Dis.,* 1947, 6:80-4.

shrinking lung syndrome. Dyspnea associated with small stiff lungs, which is demonstrable on chest radiographs of patients with systemic lupus erythematosus. Pathological findings include pulmonary and diaphragmatic fibrosis.

Hoffbrand, B. I., & Beck, E. R. "Unexplained" dyspnoea and shrinking lungs in SLE. *Brit. Med. J.,* 1965, 1:1273-7.

shrinking man syndrome. Loss of height in hyperparathyroidism with vertebral involvement and normal hand radiographs. Blood calcium levels are low or normal.

Memmos, D. E., *et al.* The "shrinking man" syndrome. *Nephron,* 1982, 30:106-9.

SHULMAN, L. E. (American physician)

Shulman syndrome. Synonyms: *diffuse fasciitis with eosinophilia, eosinophilic fasciitis, eosinophilic myositis, fasciitis with eosinophilia, myositis with eosinophilia.*

A syndrome characterized by acute onset of erythema, swelling, and induration of the extremities, associated with peripheral eosinophilia, increased erythrocyte sedimentation rate, and hypergammaglobulinemia. Histological findings include deep fascia inflammation, sometimes extending to the muscle and subcutaneous tissue, with the inflammatory cell infiltrate consisting of lymphocytes, plasma cells, and occasional eosinophils.

Shulman, L. E. Diffuse fasciitis with hyperglobulinemia and eosinophilia: A new syndrome? *J. Rheum.,* 1974, 1(Suppl):46. Pincus, S. H. Cutaneous eosinophilic diseases. In: Fitzpatrick, T. B., Eisen, A. Z., Wolff, K., Freedberg, I. M., & Austen, K. F., eds. *Dermatology in general medicine.* 3rd ed., New York, McGraw-Hill, 1987, pp. 1336-44.

SHULMAN, N. RAPHAEL

Shulman syndrome. Synonym: *post-transfusion purpura.*

Development of purpura after blood transfusion due to a mismatched platelet antigen.

Shulman, N. R., *et al.* Immunoreactions involving platelets. V. Post-transfusion purpura due a complement-fixing antibody against genetically controlled platelet antigen. A proposed mechanism for thrombocytopenia and its relevance in "autoimmunity." *J. Clin. Invest.*, 1961, 40:1597-620.

shunt nephritis syndrome. A postoperative syndrome after shunt operation for hydrocephalus, consisting of glomerulonephritis, cryoglobulinemia, and bacteremia. Cutaneous findings of urticaria and vasculitis may be associated. An infected ventriculoatrial shunt is the cause.

Black, J. A., *et al.* Nephrotic syndrome associated with bacteraemia after shunt opertions for hydrocephalus. *Lancet*, 1965, 2:921-6.

shunt syndrome. See *electrical leak syndrome.*

SHURTLEFF, DAVID B. (American physician)

Thieffry-Shurtleff syndrome. See *under Thieffry.*

SHWACHMAN, HARRY (American pediatrician, born 1910)

Shwachman syndrome. Synonyms: *Shwachman-Bodian syndrome, Shwachman-Diamond syndrome, Shwachman-Diamond-Oski-Khaw syndrome, congenital lipomatosis of pancreas-malabsorption-pancreatic insufficiency syndrome, metaphyseal chondrodysplasia-malabsorption-neutropenia (MMN) syndrome, metaphyseal dysostosis-pancreatic insufficiency syndrome, metaphyseal dysostosis-pancreatic insufficiency-blood disorder syndrome, pancreas-blood-bone syndrome, pancreatic exocrine insufficiency-metaphyseal dysostosis-dwarfism syndrome, pancreatic insufficiency-bone marrow dysfunction syndrome.*

An autosomal recessive syndrome of short-limbed dwarfism, malabsorption due to pancreatic insufficiency, loose stools with steatorrhea, recurrent infections, and variable leukopenia, neutropenia, anemia, eczema, and galactosuria. Diminished excretion of pancreatic exocrine enzymes and bicarbonate is a constant feature. Radiological findings show metaphyseal chondrodysplasia, especially of the hip and knee, ossification disorders of the costochondral junctions, coxa vara, clinodactyly, and delayed maturation of the carpal bones. Early symptoms (usually, failure to thrive and recurrent respiratory infections) occur in infancy. If left untreated, death occurs during the first 5 years of life.

Shwachman, H., Diamond, L. K., Oski, F. A., & Khaw, K. T. The syndrome of pancreatic insufficiency and bone marrow dysfunction. *J. Pediat.*, 1964, 65:645-63. Bodian, M., *et al.* Congenital hypoplasia of exocrine pancreas. *Acta Paediat., Stockholm*, 1964, 53:282-93.

Shwachman-Bodian syndrome. See *Shwachman syndrome.*

Shwachman-Diamond syndrome. See *Shwachman syndrome.*

Shwachman-Diamond-Oski-Khaw syndrome. See *Shwachman syndrome.*

SHY, GEORGE MILTON (American physician, 1919-1967)

Shy-Drager syndrome (SDS). Synonym: *orthostatic hypotensive-dysautonomic-dyskinetic syndrome.*

A progressive degenerative disorder of the nervous system in which orthostatic hypotension is associated with urinary and fecal incontinence, bladdder atony, postural dizziness and syncope, decreased sweating, impotence, iris atrophy, external ocular paralysis, tremor, loss of coordination, generalized muscle weakness and neuropathic wasting, and fasciculation. Pathologically, there is a loss of neurons in the central regions of the autonomic nervous system, particularly in the cells of the intermediolateral column of the thoracic spinal cord; cell loss in the peripheral autonomic ganglia, brainstem and basal ganglia; symmetrical neuronal degeneration of the caudate nucleus, substantia nigra, locus coeruleus, olivary nuclei, dorsal vagal nuclei, and the cerebellum; gliosis associated with cell loss; and the presence of Lewy bodies characteristic of the Parkinson syndrome. Onset usually takes place in the sixth or seventh decades, most persons becoming disabled within 5 to 7 years. More males than females are affected. The etiology is unknown.

Shy, G. M., & Drager, G. A. A neurological syndrome associated with orthostatic hypotension. A clinical-pathological study. *Arch. Neur., Chicago*, 1960, 2:511-27.

Shy-Magee syndrome. Synonyms: *central core disease, centronuclear myopathy, nemaline myopathy, rod myopathy.*

A progressive muscle disease characterized by rodlike structures throughout the entire length of the muscle, formed by a core of tightly packed myofibrils in the centers of muscle fibers. The structures have a wormlike appearance, thus the synonym nemaline myopathy. The pathologic fibrillar material is similar to and continuous with the substance that constitutes the Z-bands. The affected infants have the appearance of floppy infants who attain motor development at a slow rate and subsequently develop nonprogressive muscle weakness. The syndrome is probably transmitted as an autosomal dominant trait with wide variability in severity, but some authors suggest the existence of both dominant and recessive forms.

Shy, G. M., & Magee, K. R. A new congenital nonprogressive myopathy. *Brain*, 1956, 79:610-21.

SIADH. See *inappropriate antidiuretic hormone secretion syndrome.*

sialidosis I. See *cherry red spot-myoclonus syndrome.*

SICARD, JEAN ANASTHASE (French physician, 1872-1929)

Brissaud-Sicard syndrome. See *under Brissaud.*

Collet-Sicard syndrome. See *under Collet.*

Sicard syndrome. See *Collet-Sicard syndrome.*

sicca syndrome. See *Sjögren syndrome under Sjögren, Henrik Samuel Conrad.*

sicca-like syndrome. Synonyms: *pseudo-Sjögren syndrome, Sjögren-like syndrome.*

A syndrome with symptoms similar to those seen in the Sjögren syndrome. In one form, it is characterized primarily by parotid enlargement attributed to fatty infiltration of the glands in hyperlipoproteinemia, but without ocular or oral sicca symptoms. In the second form, the syndrome is marked by toxic epidermal necrolysis, xerostomia or keratoconjunctivitis sicca or both, or lymphocytic infiltration of the salivary glands.

Reinertsen, J. L., *et al.* Sicca-like syndrome in type V hyperlipoproteinemia. *Arthritis Rheum.*, 1980, 23:114-8. Roujeau, J. C. Sjögren-like syndrome after drug-induced toxic epidermal necrolysis. *Lancet*, 1985, 1:609-11.

SICHEL, JULES (French ophthalmologist, 1802-1868)

Sichel disease. Synonyms: *Sichel ptosis, ptosis adiposa.*

A form of pseudoptosis in which folds of skin hang from the upper lid margins. Relaxation of the fascial bands that attach the levator of the skin, rather than an accumulation of fat, as previously suspected, is the cause.

Walsh, F. B. *Clinical neuro-ophthalmology. 2nd ed. Baltimore, Williams & Wilkins, 1957, p. 199.*

Sichel ptosis. See *Sichel disease.*

sick building syndrome. Synonyms: *building illness syndrome (BIS), tight building syndrome.*

A sensation of dry mucous membranes and skin, erythema, lethargy, mental fatigue, headaches, high frequency of airway infections, mucosal irritation, cough, hoarseness, wheezing, itching, nausea, dizziness, and unspecified hypersensitivity in persons occupying poorly ventilated school and office buildings which are heavily populated, use needle-felt carpets, are so constructed as to cause dust accumulation and microbial pollution, and have inadequate cleaning services.

Gravesen, S., *et al.* Demonstration of microorganisms and dust in schools and offices. An observational study of non-industrial buildings. *Allergy*, 1986, 41:520-5.

sick cell syndrome. Essential hyponatremia, due to cell osmolality disorders, occurring in a variety of chronic diseases, such as pulmonary tuberculosis, congestive heart failure, liver cirrhosis, and other conditions.

*Elkinton, J. R. Hyponatremia: Clinical state or biochemical sign? *Circulation*, 1956, 14:1027. Flear, C. T. G., & Singh, C. M. Hyponatraemia and sick cells. *Brit. J. Anaesth.*, 1973, 45:976-94.

sick euthyroid syndrome. See *low T_3 syndrome.*

sick headache. See *migraine under headache syndrome.*

sick sinus syndrome (SSS). Synonyms: *lazy sinus syndrome, sinus node dysfunction, sinus node syndrome, sluggish sinus syndrome.*

A cardiac disorder characterized by inability of the sinus node to perform its pacemaking function with resulting heart rate abnormality, which includes the bradycardia-tachycardia syndrome (q.v.). Hypertension or arteriosclerosis is often the cause. The symptoms include severe bradycardia, cessation of sinus rhythm (sinus pause or sinus arrest) with or without the appearance of an ectopic escape rhythm, episodes of sinoatrial exit block, chronic atrial fibrillation with slow ventricular responses in nondigitalized patients, and inability of the heart to resume sinus rhythm following DC cardioversion of atrial fibrillation.

Wenckenbach, K. V. Beitrage zur Kenntnis der menschlichen Herztatigkeit. *Arch. Anat. Physiol.*, 1906, 297:297. Eyster, J, A., & Evans, J. S. Sino-auricular heart block: With report of a case in man. *Arch. Intern. Med.*, 1915, 10:832. Ferrer, M. I. The sick sinus syndrome in atrial disease. *JAMA*, 1968, 206:645-6. Kerr, C. R., *et al.* Sinus node dysfunction. *Cardiol. Clin.*, 1983, 1:187-107.

sickle cell anemia. Synonyms: *Herrick syndrome, African anemia, drepanocytic anemia, hemoglobin S disease, homozygous hemoglobin S disease, menisocytosis, sickle cell disease (SCD), sickle cell syndrome, sicklemia, SS disease.*

Hemolytic anemia, occurring almost exclusively in persons of Negro ancestry, and affecting women more often than men. Crystallization of sickle-cell hemoglobin in the presence of low oxygen tension and reduced pH in the blood are responsible for the sickling phenomenon, resulting in the appearance of sickle-shaped erythrocytes in the blood and increased viscosity of capillary blood. Onset takes place early in life after normal hemoglobin is replaced with sickle-cell hemoglobin, and is marked by arthralgia and abdominal cramps. Greenish-yellow sclerae, blindness, nystagmus, pale mucosae, weakness, fatigability, sinus arrhythmia, prominent pulsation in the neck area, moderate hepatomegaly, hematuria, leg ulcers, kyphosis, scoliosis, oxycephaly, hemiplegia, epistaxis, coma, aphasia, stupor, cranial nerve palsies, headache, and convulsions are the other symptoms. Osteoporosis of the jaws, showing trabecular changes in the alveolar bones and large, irregular spaces on x-rays are the usual oral findings. Another feature is the hand and foot syndrome (dactylitis) in children, characterized by soft tissue swelling, bone resorption in infected or infarcted areas, periosteal elevation, and subperiosteal new bone formation. Sickle-cell anemia is due to the substitution of thymine for adenine in the glutamic acid DNA codon (GAG to GTG), which results in substitution of ß-6-valine for glutamic acid.

Herrick, J. B. Peculiar elongated and sickle-shaped red blood corpuscles in a case of severe anemia. *Arch. Int. Med.*, 1910, 6:517-21. Beutler, E. The sickle cell diseases and related disorders. In: Williams, W. J., Beutler, E., Erslev, A. J., & Lichtman, M. A., eds. *Hematology*, 3rd ed. New York, McGraw-Hill, 1983, pp. 583-609.

sickle cell disease (SCD). See *sickle cell anemia.*

sickle cell syndrome. See *sickle cell anemia.*

sickle/ß+-thalassemia syndrome. A sickling disorder of varying severity, which results from compound heterozygosity for sickle cell trait and ß-thalassemia trait.

Atweh, G. F., & Forget, B. G. Clinical and molecular correlations in the sickle/beta+-thalassemia syndrome. *Am. J. Hemat.*, 1987, 24:31-6.

sicklemia. See *sickle cell anemia.*

SIDBURY, JAMES B. (American physician)

phenylketonuria, Tourian and Sidbury type. See *under phenylketonuria.*

sideropenic dysphagia. See *Plummer-Vinson syndrome.*

siderosis-scurvy-osteoporosis syndrome. Synonym: *miners' syndrome.*

A syndrome of steoporosis, scurvy, and siderosis, occurring almost exclusively among Bantu males, particularly those who live in compounds in South Africa. The fundamental cause appears to be iron overload, resulting from consumption of alcoholic brews containing high concentrations of iron, the excess of iron affecting the metabolism of ascorbic acid, accompanied by a dietary ascorbic acid deficiency. The woody induration of of the legs and scorbutic pseudoscleroderma are manifestations of hemorrhage into the skin and are caused by ascorbic acid deficiency, osteoporosis being a complication of scurvy.

Grusin, H., & Kincaid-Smith, P. S. Scurvy in adult Africans. A clinical, haematological, and pathological study. *Am. J. Clin. Nutrit.*, 1954, 2:323-35. Cosnett, J. E. Miners' syndrome. *South Afr. Med. J.*, 1974, 48:2011.

SIDLER-HUGUENIN, ERNST (Swiss physician, 1869-1922)

Sidler-Huguenin endothelioma. Endothelioma of the optic nerve.

Sidler-Huguenin, E. Ein Endotheliom om Sehnervenkopf. *Graefes Arch. Ophth.*, 1920, 101:113-22.

SIDS. See *sudden infant death syndrome.*

SIEGAL, SHEPPARD (American physician, born 1909)

Siegal-Cattan-Mamou disease. See *Reimann periodic disease.*

SIEGRIST, AUGUST (Swiss ophthalmologist, born 1865)

Siegrist spots. Synonym: *Siegrist streaks.*

A string of pigmented spots along a white sclerosed choroidal vessel.

*Siegrist, A. *9th Internat. Cong. Ophth.*, 1899, p. 131.

Siegrist streaks. See *Siegrist spots.*

Siegrist syndrome. See *Siegrist-Hutchinson syndrome.*

Siegrist-Hutchinson syndrome. Synonyms: *Siegrist syndrome, chorioretinopathia post-traumatica.*

Post-traumatic chorioretinopathy marked by mydriasis, yellowish lesions with pigmented foci, macular disorders, choroid rupture, and atrophy of the optic nerve. Rupture of the ciliary artery and choroid ischemia secondary to subchoroidal hemorrhage are the probable causes.

Hutchinson, J., Jr. Diseases of the choroid. *Tr. Ophth. Soc. U. K.*, 1889, 9:116-25. Siegrist, A Ophthalmologische Studien. *Mittel. Klin. Med. Inst. Schweiz.*, 1895, 3:545-82.

SIEKERT, ROBERT GEORGE (American neurologist, born 1924)

Millikan-Siekert syndrome. See *under Millikan.*

SIEMENS, HERMANN WERNER (German physician, 1891-1969)

Bloch-Siemens syndrome. See *Bloch-Sulzberger syndrome.*

Christ-Siemens-Touraine (CST) syndrome. See *hypohidrotic ectodermal dysplasia syndrome.*

Christ-Siemens-Weech syndrome. See *hypohidrotic ectodermal dysplasia syndrome.*

epidermolysis bullosa dystrophica Hallopeau-Siemens (EBDH). See *Hallopeau-Siemens syndrome.*

Hallopeau-Siemens syndrome. See *under Hallopeau.*

Siemens dermatosis. See *hypohidrotic ectodermal dysplasia syndrome.*

Siemens syndrome (1). Synonyms: *keratosis follicularis spinulosa decalvans, keratosis follicularis spinulosa decalvans cum ophiasi.*

A familial form of keratosis involving the face, neck, forearms, ears, palms and soles, and backs of the hands, associated with loss of the eyebrows, eyelashes, and beard, thickening of the eyelids, blepharitis, ectropion, and corneal changes. Photophobia and lacrimation, the early symptoms, are followed by the skin lesions, which are typically characterized by cornification on the tops of noninflammatory papules, seen as dark shiny thornlike formations. The disorder is transmitted as an X-linked trait, but autosomal dominant inheritance has been also reported. The term *keratosis follicularis spinulosa decalvans* is used also to designate the KID syndrome.

Siemens. Keratosis follicularis spinulosa decalvans. *Arch. Derm. Syph., Berlin*, 1926, 151:384-6.

Siemens syndrome (2). See *hypohidrotic ectodermal dysplasia syndrome.*

Siemens-Bloch pigmented dermatosis. See *Bloch-Sulzberger syndrome.*

SIEMERLING, ERNST (German physician)

Siemerling-Creutzfeldt syndrome. See *adrenoleukodystropophy.*

SIERRO, A.

Bamatter-Franceschetti-Klein-Sierro syndrome. See *geroderma osteodysplastica syndrome.*

sigmoid diverticula. See *Graser diverticulum.*

SIGUIER, FRED (French physician, born 1909)

Lian-Siguier-Welti syndrome. See *under Lian.*

SILENGO, MARGHERITA (Italian physician)

Gardner-Silengo-Wachtel syndrome. See *under Gardner, L. I.*

silent neurogenic bladder. See *Hinman syndrome.*

SILFVERSKIÖLD, NILS OTTO (Swedish physician, born 1888)

Morquio-Silfverskiöld syndrome. See *Silfverskiöld syndrome.*

Silfverskiöld syndrome. Synonyms: *Gruzinski osteochondropathy, Morquio-Silfverskiöld syndrome, achondroplasia atypica, extremity osteochondrodystrophy syndrome.*

A peculiar form of chondrodystrophy, in which development of the forearms and hands is normal. Silfverskiöld described a case in an 11-year-old boy in whom the symptoms included disproportionate dwarfism with short legs, large head, and flattened nose; broad chest; large trochanters; lordosis due to flexion contractures of the hips; genu valgum; coxa vara; loose joints; and powerful musculature. Roentgenological findings showed disorders of enchondral ossification, especially of the lower extremities; irregular lines of ossification, notably of the femoral epiphyses; disturbed periosteal and endosteal ossification; increased epiphyseal and metaphyseal width of the femur and, to a lesser degree, other bones of the arms and legs; small radial and carpal nuclei; small, angular tarsal nuclei; extra metacarpal and metatarsal epiphyses; and decreased density of various bones. The etiology is unknown.

Silfverskiöld, N. A "forme fruste" of chondrodystrophia with changes simulating several of the known "local malacias." *Acta Radiol., Stockholm*, 1925, 4:44-57. Grudzinski, Z. Über eien neue mit Achondroplasie (Chondrodystrophie) verwandté Krankheitsform. (Osteochondropathia multiplex Grudzinski, Achondroplasia atypica Silfverskiöld, Dystrophie spongieuse epiphysaire systematisée Ghimus). *Fortschr. Roentgen.*, 1928, 38:873-82.

silicoarthritis. See *Caplan syndrome.*

silicotic granuloma. See *Shattock disease.*

silicotic mediastinitis. See *Maugeri syndrome.*

silicotic mediastinopathy. See *Maugeri syndrome.*

silo filler disease (SFD). See *silo unloader syndrome.*

silo unloader syndrome. Synonym: *silo filler disease (SFD).*

A potentially fatal condition in farm workers who enter a silo which has been filled within the preceding 7 days. It is characterized by cough, chills, fever, weakness, myalgia, headache, anorexia, and fatigue. Pulmonary function tests and chest x-rays are usually normal. Blood tests show mild alkalosis. The disease occurs when workers inhale the toxic oxides of nitrogen.

Lowry, T. "Silo-filler's disease." A newly recognized syndrome. *Univ. Minn. Med. Bull.*, 1956, 27:203. Pratt, D. S., & May, J. J. Feed-associated respiratory illness in farmers. *Arch. Environment. Health*, 1984, 39:43-8.

SILVER, HENRY K. (American physician, born 1918)

Russell-Silver syndrome (RSS). See *under Russell.*

Silver syndrome. See *Russell-Silver syndrome.*

SILVERMAN, FREDERIC N. (American physician)

Robinow-Silverman-Smith syndrome. See *Robinow syndrome.*

Silverman disease. An abnormality of the sternum

characterized by premature obliteration of its sutures and pigeon breast.

Currarino, G., & Silverman, F. N. Premature obliteration of the sternal sutures and pigeon-breast deformity. *Radiology,* 1958, 70:532-40.

Silverman syndrome (1). See *battered child syndrome.*

Silverman syndrome (2). Synonyms: *dyssegmental dwarfism (DD), Silverman type; dyssegmental dysplasia (DD), Silverman type.*

A lethal bone dysplasia characterized by markedly short stature, short limbs with limited joint mobility, unusual facies, pes equinovarus, bow legs, and hirsutism. Additional anomalies may include hydrocephalus, occipital encephalocele, cleft palate, hydroureters, and other urinary tract abnormalities. Radiographic examination shows faulty segmentation characterized by delayed ossification of the vertebral bodies, lumbosacral kyphosis, small and round iliac bones, wide femoral ends of the femoral and small acetabular bones, narrow chest with broad short ribs and slight anterior cupping, small scapulae with hypoplastic glenoid processes and large humeral processes, short long bones with broad clublike ends, inward bowing of the ulnae, hypoplastic first metacarpal and slightly short and wide remaining metacarpal bones in the hands, and foot anomalies similar to those of the hands.

Fasanelli, S., *et al.* Dyssegmental dysplasia. (Report of two cases with a review of the literature). *Skelet. Radiol.,* 1985, 14:173-7.

SILVERMAN, WILLIAM A. (American physician)

Caffey-Silverman syndrome. See *under Caffey.*

De Toni-Caffey-Silverman syndrome. See *Caffey-Silverman syndrome.*

Roske-De Toni-Caffey-Silverman syndrome. See *Caffey-Silverman syndrome.*

SILVESTRINI, R. (Italian physician)

Silvestrini-Corda syndrome. Synonym: *endocrine deficiency-hepatic cirrhosis syndrome.*

A syndrome of liver cirrhosis associated with impotence, menorrhagia, amenorrhea, postmenopausal bleeding, gynecomastia, testicular atrophy, loss of axillary hair, ascites, and other disorders.

Silvestrini, R. La reviviscenza mammaria nell'uomo affeto da cirrosi del Laennec. *Riforma Med.,* 1926, 42:701-4. Corda, L., & Sulla, C. D. Revivistenza della mammella maschile nella cirrosi epatica. *Minerva Med.,* 1925, 5:1067-9.

SILVESTRONI, E. (Italian physician)

Silvestroni-Bianco syndrome. Synonyms: *constitutional microcytic anemia, microdrepanocytic disease.*

A blood disorder having the characteristics of both sickle cell anemia and Mediterranean anemia.

Silvestroni, E., & Bianco, I. Richerche cliniche, genetiche ed ematologiche sui malati di anemia microcitica costituzionale e di morbo di Cooley. *Haematologica, Pavia,* 1948, 31:135-90. Silvestroni, E., & Bianco, I. Genetic aspects fo sickle-cell anemia and microdrepanocytic disease. *Blood,* 1952, 7:429-35.

SILVIO NEGRI. See NEGRI, SILVIO

SIMENON, GEORGES (French novelist and mystery writer)

Simenon syndrome. See *Clérambault syndrome.*

SIMMONDS, MORRIS (German physician, 1855-1925)

Glinski-Simmonds syndrome. See *Sheehan syndrome.*

Simmonds cachexia. See *Sheehan syndrome.*

Simmonds syndrome. See *Sheehan syndrome.*

SIMONS (SIMON), ARTHUR (German neurologist, born 1879)

Barraquer-Simons syndrome. See *under Barraquer.*

Höllander-Simons syndrome. See *Barraguer-Simons syndrome.*

Simons syndrome. See *Barraquer-Simons syndrome.*

simple achlorhydric acid anemia. See *Faber syndrome.*

simple familial cranial hypertrophy. See *Klippel-Feldstein syndrome.*

simple periodontitis. See *Fauchard disease.*

simple splenic hyperplasia. See *Dacie syndrome.*

SIMPSON, J. L. (American physician)

Simpson dysmorphia syndrome. See *Simpson syndrome.*

Simpson dysplasia syndrome. See *Simpson syndrome.*

Simpson syndrome. Synonyms: *Simpson dysmorphia syndrome, Simpson dysplasia syndrome, bulldog syndrome.*

A familial syndrome, transmitted as an X-linked trait, characterized by bulldog-like facies and multiple abnormalities. The symptoms include above normal birth weight and length, postnatal overgrowth, large head with coarse facies, short nose with wide bridge and upturned tip, widely open mouth, thick lips, midline depression of the lower lip, enlarged tongue with short frenulum, high-arched palate, malocclusion, prognathism, large ears, husky voice, short and broad neck, stocky constitution, pectus excavatum, bundle-branch or AV block, hepatosplenomegaly, and occasional iris coloboma, umbilical or inguinal hernia, cryptorchidism, broad and short hands and feet, hexadactyly, nail dysplasia, abnormal dermatoglyphics, and mental retardation.

Simpson, J. L., *et al.* A previously unrecognized X-linked syndrome of dysmorphia. *Birth Defects,* 1975, 11(2):18-24. Behmel, A., *et al.* A new X-linked dysplasia gigantism syndrome: Identical with the Simpson dysplasia syndrome? *Hum. Genet.,* 1984, 67:409-13.

SIMPSON, SAMUEL LEONARD (American physician)

Simpson syndrome. Synonyms: *adipose gynandrism, adipose gynism.*

A syndrome affecting both sexes. In males, it is marked by accelerated growth; adiposity, often from birth; delayed puberty; feminine appearance, including smooth face, feminine pattern of pubic hair, sparsity of body hair, and feminine pattern of behavior, waddling gait; and red or purple striae distensae. In females, the symptoms include above normal height, adiposity, delayed puberty, red or purple striae distensae which may become white or disappear, and hirsutism. The syndrome may appear after measles or scarlet fever, suggesting hypothalamic mechanisms. Simpson hypothesized an insulotropic action of the pituitary as a possible pathogenic factor.

Simpson, S. L. Acromegaly and gigantism. Including a new syndrome in childhood. *Postgrad. Med. J.,* 1950, 26:201-14.

sin-cib-syn. See *Chinese restaurant syndrome.*

SINDING LARSEN. See LARSEN, CHRISTIAN MAGNUS FALSEN SINDING

SINGER, H. D. (American physician)

Moschcowitz-Singer-Symmers syndrome. See *Moschcowitz syndrome.*

SINGLETON, EDWARD B. (American radiologist)

Singleton-Merten syndrome. A syndrome of calcification of the aortic arch with heart enlargement; osteoporosis involving the cranial vault, long and hand bones with widening of the metacarpals, carpals, and phalanges; and hypoplasia of the tooth buds with hypodontia and occasional failed tooth eruption. Muscle weakness and poor development are usually associated. The syndrome is believed to be transmitted as an autosomal dominant trait.

Singleton, E. B., & Merten, D. F. An unusual syndrome of widened medullary cavities of the metacarpals and phalanges, aortic calcification, and abnormal dentition. *Pediat. Radiol.*, 1973, 1:2-7.

sinobronchial syndrome. Chronic sinus infections in patients with pulmonary diseases, such as asthma, bronchiectasis, recurrent pneumonia, or chronic bronchitis.

McBride, J. T., & Brooks, J. G. Sinobronchial syndrome. *Ear Nose Throat J.*, 1984, 63:177-9.

sinus histiocytosis with massive lymphadenopathy (SHML). See *Rosai-Dorfman syndrome.*

sinus node dysfunction. See *sick sinus syndrome.*

sinus node syndrome. See *sick sinus syndrome.*

sinus of Morgagni syndrome. See *Trotter syndrome.*

sinus tarsi syndrome (STS). See *tarsal sinus syndrome.*

sinusitis-bronchiectasis-situs inversus syndrome. See *Kartagener syndrome.*

SIPPLE, JOHN H. (American physician)

Sipple syndrome. See *multiple endocrine neoplasia II syndrome.*

SIR (**s**yndrome of **i**mmediate **r**eactivities). See *contact urticaria syndrome.*

sirenomelia. See *caudal regression syndrome.*

SIRIS, EVELYN (American physician)

Coffin-Siris syndrome. See *under Coffin.*

Coffin-Siris-Weglenka syndrome. See *Coffin-Lowry syndrome.*

SISTER JOSEPH. See DEMPSEY, MARY JOSEPH, SISTER

SISTER MARY JOSEPH. See DEMPSEY, SISTER MARY JOSEPH

SISYPHUS. (A mythological character, son of Aeoulus and ruler of Corinth, noted for his trickery, who was condemned to roll a stone to the top of a slope, the stone always escaping him near the top)

Sisyphus complex. See *Danaïd syndrome, under Danaïds.*

situs ambiguus with left isomerism. See *polysplenia syndrome.*

situs ambiguus-polysplenia (SAP) syndrome. See *polysplenia syndrome.*

SIWE, STURE AUGUST (Swedish pediatrician, born 1897)

Abt-Letterer-Siwe syndrome. See *Letterer-Siwe syndrome.*

Letterer-Siwe disease. See *Letterer-Siwe syndrome.*

Letterer-Siwe syndrome. See *under Letterer.*

SIWIS. See ***s****elf-****i****nduced* ***w****ater* ***i****ntoxication* ***s****chizophrenic disorder syndrome.*

sixth disease. See *Zahorsky syndrome (1).*

SJAASTAD, OTTAR (Norwegian physician)

Sjaastad syndrome. Synonym: *chronic paroxysmal hemicrania.*

A form of the headache syndrome (q.v.) characterized by frequent attacks of pain of short duration. The pain is severe and unilateral, always occurring on the same side, and is accompanied by nasal congestion and lacrimation on the painful side, but not by visual disorders and nausea or vomiting. The pain is most acute in the temporal region but during some severe attacks may involve the entire half of the head, as well as the neck, shoulder, and arm on the homolateral side.

Sjaastad, O., & Dale, I. A new (?) clinical headache entity "chronic paroxysmal hemicrania." 2. *Acta Neur. Scand.*, 1976, 54:140-59.

SJÖGREN, HENRIK SAMUEL CONRAD (Swedish ophthalmologist, born 1899)

Gougerot-Houwer-Sjögren syndrome. See *Sjögren syndrome.*

Gougerot-Sjögren syndrome. See *Sjögren syndrome.*

pseudo-Sjögren syndrome. See *sicca-like syndrome.*

reverse Gougerot-Sjögren syndrome. See *Creyx-Lévy syndrome.*

reverse Sjögren syndrome. See *Creyx-Lévy syndrome.*

Sjögren syndrome (SS). Synonyms: *Gougerot-Houwer-Sjögren syndrome, Gougerot-Sjögren syndrome, arthro-oculosalivary syndrome, dacryosialadenopathia atrophicans, dacryosialoadenopathy, dacryosialocheilopathy, dry syndrome, immunosialadenitis, keratoconjunctivitis sicca (KCS), mucoserous dyssecretosis, myoepithelial sialadenitis (MESA), rheumatic sialosis, secretoinibitor syndrome, sicca syndrome.*

The concurrence of xerostomia, pharyngolaryngitis sicca, rhinitis sicca, enlarged salivary glands, polyarthritis, and keratoconjunctivitis sicca, observed chiefly in postmenopausal women or younger women after artificial menopause. The face is characterized by enlarged parotid glands. Typical ocular changes consist of dryness, burning sensation, and photophobia due to failure of the lacrimal and conjunctival glands. Dryness of other mucous membranes occurs in the pharynx, larynx and the nasal passages with resulting atrophic rhinitis and reduced sense of smell. Rheumatoid arthritis is the most common articular complication. Xerostomia is often associated with dysphonia, dysphagia, and masticatory problems. The symptoms may include weakness, fatigability, loss of weight, dryness of the skin, purpura, recurrent respiratory infections, the Raynaud phenomenon, and other disturbances. Some authors consider the Sjögren and sicca syndromes as being the same entity; others define the **sicca syndrome** as keratoconjunctivitis sicca and xerostomia with or without salivary gland enlargement, but not with rheumatoid arthritis or other connective tissue disease. Also, some consider the **Mikulicz syndrome** to be identical with the Sjögren's syndrome; according to others, the former does not include rheumatoid arthritis and, therefore, is a separate entity. Polymyositis may be substituted for rheumatoid arthritis as a component of this syndrome.

Sjögren, H. S. Zur Kenntnis der Keratoconjunctivitis sicca (Keratitis filiformis bei Hypofunktion der Tränendrüsen). *Acta Ophth., Copenhagen,* 1933, Suppl. 2:1-151. Gougerot. Insuffisance progressive et atrophie des glandes salivaires et muqueuses de la bouche, des conjonctives (et parfois de muqueuses, nasale, laryngeé, vulvaire). "Serecheresse" de la bouche, des conjonctives, etc. *Bull. Soc. Fr. Derm. Syph.*, 1925, 32:376-9. Houwer, A. W. Corneal infection and joint affections. *Ned. T. Geneesk.*, 1927, 1:2299-2301.

Sjögren-like syndrome. See *sicca-like syndrome.*

SJÖGREN, KARL GUSTAF TORSTEN (Swedish physician, born 1896)

Graefe-Sjögren syndrome. See *under Graefe.*

Marinesco-Sjögren syndrome (MSS). See *under Marinescu, Gheorge.*

Marinesco-Sjögren-Garland syndrome. See *Marinesco-Sjögren syndrome, under Marinescu, Gheorge.*

Sjögren syndrome. See *Graefe-Sjögren syndrome.*

Sjögren-Larsson syndrome (SLS). Synonyms: *ichthyotic idiocy, oligophrenia-ichthyosis syndrome.*

A syndrome of congenital ichthyosis or ichthyosiform erythroderma, spastic paralysis, and mental retardation. Sparse and brittle hair, short stature, pigmentary retinal degeneration, seizures, hypohidrosis, tooth enamel hypoplasia, kyphosis, hypertelorism, and metaphyseal dysplasia with small irregular epiphyses may be associated. The syndrome is transmitted as an autosomal recessive trait. Some writers consider this and the Rud syndrome the same entity.

Sjögren, T., & Larsson, T. Oligophrenia in combination with congenital ichthyosis and spastic disorders. A clinical and genetic study. *Acta Neur. Scand.*, 1957, Suppl. 113:1-112.

Torsten Sjögren syndrome. See *Marinesco-Sjögren syndrome, under Marinescu, Gheorghe.*

SJS. See *Swyer-James syndrome, under Swyer, Paul Robert.*

SJS. See *Sjögren syndrome, under Sjögren Henrik Samuel Conrad.*

skeletal abnormalities-cutis laxa-craniostenosis-psychomotor retardation-facial abnormalities syndrome. See *SCARF syndrome.*

skeletal cystofibromatosis. See *Jaffe-Lichtenstein syndrome.*

skeletal dysplasia-abnormal palmar creases syndrome. See *Tel Hashomer comptodactyly syndrome.*

skeletal dysplasia-blindness-deafness syndrome. A familial syndrome, transmitted as an autosomal dominant trait, characterized by multiple epiphyseal dysplasia, myopia, and conductive deafness. Associated abnormalities include short stature, peculiar facies (round and flat face, small mouth, and snub nose), stubby fingers, short nails, mild valgus deformity of the knees, cataract, and asteroid hyalosis.

Beighton, P., *et al.* Dominant inheritance of multiple epiphyseal dysplasia, myopia and deafness. *Clin. Genet.*, 1978, 14:173-7.

skeletal dysplasia-joint laxity-mental retardation syndrome. A congenital syndrome of mental retardation, skeletal dysplasia, joint laxity, and craniofacial abnormalities. A narrow face, antimongoloid slant of the palpebral fissures, large ears, high-arched palate, and micrognathia are the principal craniofacial defects. Associated anomalies include blue sclerae, pectus carinatum, thoracolumbar scoliosis, joint abnormalities, long hands, simian creases, abnormal toes, and tarsal and metatarsal anomalies.

Katsantoni, A., & Côté, G. B. A syndrome of skeletal dysplasia, joint laxity, and mental retardation. *Prog. Clin. Biol. Res.*, 1982, 104:155-6.

skeletal-type deep bite. See *short face syndrome.*

skew deviation. See *Hertwig-Magendie syndrome, under Hertwig, Richard.*

ski boot compression syndrome. Compression by a ski boot at the ankle causing neuritis of the deep peroneal nerve and synovitis of the extensor tendons.

Lindenbaum, B. L. Ski boot compression syndrome. *Clin. Orthop.*, 1979, No. 140:109-10.

skin fatigue. See *excited skin syndrome.*

skin shedding. See *continual skin peeling syndrome.*

skin-eye-brain-heart syndrome. See *epidermal nevus syndrome.*

SKL (superior limbic keratoconjunctivitis). See *Theodore syndrome.*

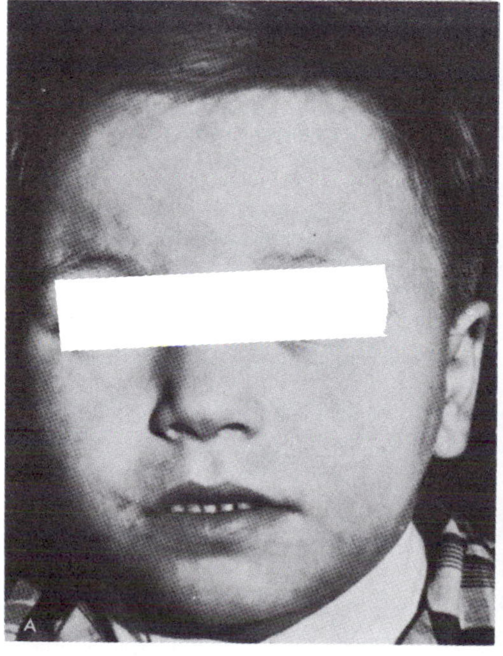

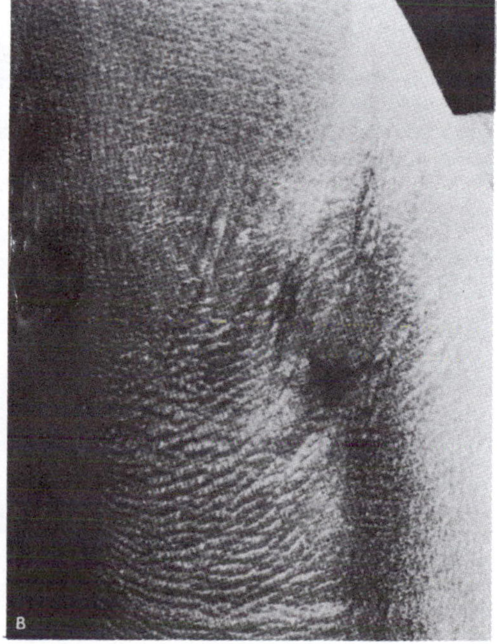

Sjögren-Larsson syndrome
Selmanowitz, V.J. & M.J. Porter: *Am. J. Med.* 42:412, 1967. New York: Yorke Medical Group.

slapped cheek syndrome. See *Sticker disease.*

SLATER, ROBERT JAMES (American physician, born 1923)

Bearn-Kunkel-Slater syndrome. See *Bearn-Kunkel syndrome.*

sleep apnea (SA) syndrome. Synonym: *nocturnal sleep apnea.*

Cessation of respiratory activity at the nostrils and mouth for at least 30 apneic episodes of 10 seconds or longer in both rapid eye movement (REM) and non-rapid eye movement (NREM) sleep during the period of 7 hours of nocturnal sleep. **Obstructive sleep apnea syndrome (OSAS)** is caused by airway obstruction due to backward movement of the tongue, thus narrowing of the upper airway in obese persons, failure of the genioglossus muscle with resulting pharyngeal wall collapse, or enlarged tonsils or adenoids. Complications include hypoxia, cardiac arrhythmias, and pulmonary and systemic hypertension. Snoring, sleep deprivation, somnolence, fatigue, morning headache, behavior changes, and depression are the principal symptoms. **Central sleep apnea syndrome,** marked by cessation of both airflow and respiratory movements, is due to damage of the respiratory centers in the brain, as in bulbar poliomyelitis, brain stem infarct, bilateral cordotomy, the Shy-Drager syndrome, poisoning, or congenital brain defects. The symptoms and complications are similar to those in the obstructive sleep apnea syndrome. See also *airway obstruction syndrome, Pickwick syndrome.* and *Ondine curse.*

Guilleminault, C., & Dement, W. C., eds. *Sleep apnea syndromes.* New York, Liss, 1978, 372 p.

sleep apnea-hypersomnolence (SAHS) syndrome. Synonym: *hypersomnia-sleep apnea (HSA) syndrome.*

Sleep apnea associated with hypersomnolence and loss of upper airway patency.

Sanders, M. H., & Moore, S. H. Inspiratory and expiratory partitioning of airway resistance during sleep in patients with sleep apnea. *Am. Rev. Resp. Dis.,* 1983, 127:554-8.

sleep epilepsy. See *Gélineau syndrome.*

sleep paralysis. See *Rosenthal disease, under Rosenthal, Curt.*

sleep shoulder syndrome. A complaint, usually observed in young to middle-aged persons, characterized by frequent episodes of awakening with pain in the arm and points of tenderness over the ventral belly of the deltoid and the shaft of the humerus. The affected persons sleep on either side or on the abdomen with an arm extended and placed against the side of the head, with the pinna and the temporal area of the skull impinged against the anteromedial inferior aspect of the deltoid area of the forearm. On awakening, there is pain with all movements of the shoulder (especially anteromedial rotation), except external rotation. Pain gradually disappears, to recur the following day. The cause is a traumatic insult of the ventral component of the deltoid and shaft of the humerus, owing to their being compressed by the head. See also *Wartenberg disease (1).*

Wehby, C. T., & Wehby, J. H. Sleep shoulder syndrome. *Ohio State Med. J.,* 1980, 76:691-2.

sleep tetany. See *Wartenberg disease (1).*

sleeping sickness. See *Economo disease.*

slick tongue. See *Möller glossitis.*

slim disease. See *acquired immunodeficiency syndrome.*

slipping patella. See *unstable patella syndrome.*

slipping rib. See *slipping rib syndrome.*

slipping rib cartilage. See *slipping rib syndrome.*

slipping rib syndrome. Synonyms: *Cyriax syndrome, Davies-Colley syndrome, clicking rib syndrome, rib syndrome, rib-tip syndrome, slipping rib cartilage.*

Lesions of the costal cartilage, usually of the 8th, 9th and 10th ribs, causing pain, autonomic symptoms, and a sensation of a slipping movement of the ribs, which is frequently confused with angina pectoris and intra-abdominal disorders. The main symptom, pain radiating to the shoulder joint and arm, is caused by moving and assuming certain postures and is precipitated by a pressure at one or more points on the costal margin. Slipping rib syndrome involving the twelfth rib is known as the *twelfth rib syndrome.*

Cyriax, E. F. On various conditions that may simulate the referred pains of visceral disease, and a consideration of these from the point of view of cause and effect. *Practitioner, London,* 1919, 102:314-22. Rawlings, M. S. The "rib syndrome." *Dis. Chest,* 1962, 41:432-41. Davies-Colley, R. Slipping rib. *Brit. Med. J.,* 1922, 1:432.

slit-ventricle syndrome (SVS). Synonym: *chronic overdrainage syndrome.*

A condition seen in hydrocephalic children with anti-siphon devices connected to the shunts, characterized by overdrainage in the upright patient and the suction-induced collapse of the ventricular wall around the draining catheter, causing an intermittent and ultimately irreversible obstruction of the shunt system, and resulting in an elevated intracranial pressure.

Epstein, F. J., *et al.* Subtemporal craniectomy for recurrent shunt obstruction secondary to small ventricles. *J. Neurosurg.,* 1974, 41:29-31. Gruber, R., *et al.* Experiences with anti-siphon device (ASD) in shunt therapy of pediatric hydrocephalus. *J. Neurosurg.,* 1984, 61:156-62.

SLO. See ***S**mith-**L**emli-**O**pitz syndrome under Smith, David W.*

SLOCUMB, CHARLES HENRY (American physician, born 1905)

Slocumb syndrome. Synonyms: *chronic hypercorticism of rheumatoid arthritis, panmesenchymal panangitic reaction, rheumatism of hypercorticism, steroid pseudorheumatism.*

Hypercorticism resulting from prolonged therapy of rheumatoid arthritis with corticoid steroids. It is characterized by diurnal cycles of tiredness, aching and tightness of the muscles and joints, changes in mood, emotional instability, and difficulty in making voluntary movements. The symptoms are relieved by a short sleep. See also *steroid withdrawal syndrome.*

Slocumb, C. H. Rheumatic complaints during chronic hypercortisonism and syndromes during withdrawal of cortisone in rheumatic patients. *Proc. Mayo Clin.,* 1953, 28:655-7.

SLOS. See ***S**mith-**L**emli-**O**pitz **s**yndrome, under Smith, David W.*

SLOTNICK, EDWARDS A. (American physician)

Slotnick-Goldfarb syndrome. Synonyms: *streaked ovary syndrome, unilateral streaked ovary syndrome.*

Oligomenorrhea progressing into secondary amenorrhea in a normal phenotypic female who has a streaked ovary on one side and a hypoplastic ovary on the opposite side.

Slotnick, E. A., & Goldfarb, A. F. Unilateral streaked ovary syndrome. *Obstet. Gyn.*, 1972, 39:269-73.

slow-channel syndrome. A syndrome, transmitted as an autosomal dominant trait with high penetrance and variable expressivity, characterized by weakness, fatigability, and atrophy of muscles of the neck, shoulder girdle, and forearms, with variable involvement of extraocular, cranial, and limb muscles. Abnormally slow closure of the acetylcholine receptor ion channel is the cause.

Engel, A. G. Myasthenia gravis and other disorders of neuromuscular transmission. In: Braunwald, E., Isselbacher, K. J., Petersdorf, R. G., Wilson, J. D., Martin, J. B., & Fauci, A. S., eds. *Harrison's principles of internal medicine.* 11th ed., New York, McGraw-Hill, 1987, pp. 2079-82.

SLS. See *Sjögren-Larsson syndrome, under Sjögren, Karl Gustaf Torsten.*

SLS (stagnant loop syndrome). See *blind loop syndrome.*

SLUDER, GREENFIELD (American otorhinolaryngologist, 1865-1925)

Sluder disease. See *Sluder neuralgia.*

Sluder headache. See *Sluder neuralgia.*

Sluder neuralgia. Synonyms: *Meckel ganglion neuralgia, Sluder disease, Sluder headache, Sluder syndrome, atypical facial headache, autonomic faciocephalalgia, buccal neuralgia, facial sympathalgia, greater superficial petrosal neuralgia, lower-face headache, lower-half headache, pterygopalatine neuralgia, sphenopalatine ganglion neurosis, sphenopalatine neuralgia.*

A headache syndrome (q.v.) characterized by neuralgia which is often preceded by ethmoidal or sphenoidal sinusitis, occurring most commonly in females after the age of 30 years. The pain is usually unilateral, involving the maxilla, teeth, ear, mastoid, periocular area, the base of the nose, and the area beneath the zygoma, usually in association with itching in the palate, peculiar sense of taste, sneezing, and nasal congestion. The occipital area, neck, shoulder, axilla, breast, arm, and hand are involved in some cases. There may be rhinorrhea, ocular hyperemia, lacrimation, and paresthesia of the skin of the lower face. Vasodilation of the internal maxillary artery, especially the portion supplying the sphenopalatine ganglion, is suspected as the etiologic factor. Some writers dispute the concept of this syndrome.

Sluder, G. The role of the sphenopalatine (or Meckel's) ganglion in nasal headaches. *N. Y. Med. J.*, 1908, 87:989-90.

Sluder syndrome. See *Sluder neuralgia.*

sluggish sinus syndrome. See *sick sinus syndrome.*

SLY, WILLIAM S. (American physician)

Sly syndrome. See *mucopolysaccharidosis VII.*

SMA. See *superior mesenteric artery syndrome.*

SMA I (spinal muscular atrophy I). See *Werdnig-Hoffman syndrome.*

SMA III (spinal muscular atrophy III). See *Wohlfart-Kugelberg-Welander syndrome.*

SMALL, ROBERT G. (American physician)

Small disease. A syndrome, transmitted as an autosomal recessive trait, characterized by retinal changes ranging from tortuous vessels to exudative retinitis, hearing loss, muscle weakness, and mental retardation. Myopathic facies and spinal curvature disorders are associated.

Small, R. G. Coats' disease and muscular dystrophy. *Tr. Am. Acad. Ophth. Otolar.*, 1968, 72:225-31.

small artery syndrome. See *small blood vessel syndrome.*

small blood vessel syndrome. Synonyms: *constitutional arterial narrowing, small artery syndrome.*

Constitutional arterial narrowing, occurring mostly in short females who have mild truncal obesity. It may be normal for a given person but predisposes her to symptomatic generative disease at an early age. It is frequently associated with high bifurcation of the common femoral artery, diminutive ankle pulse, and a tendency for spasm secondary to direct trauma by needle or catheter.

Johnson, T. E. Small blood vessel syndrome. Constitutional arterial narrowing. *Minnesota Med.*, 1969, 52:1903-5.

small bowel syndrome. See *short bowel syndrome.*

small bowel bacterial overgrowth. See *bacterial overgrowth syndrome.*

small intestinal bacterial overgrowth syndrome. See *bacterial overgrowth syndrome.*

small left colon syndrome. See *neonatal small left colon syndrome.*

small patella syndrome. See *Scott-Taor syndrome, under Scott, J. E.*

small stomach syndrome. See *postgastrectomy syndrome.*

SMAS. See *superior mesenteric artery syndrome.*

SMITH, ALLAN J. (British physician)

Smith-Strang syndrome. See *methionine malabsorption syndrome.*

SMITH, CARL HENRY (American physician)

Canale-Smith syndrome. See *under Canale.*

Carl Smith disease. See *Smith disease.*

Smith disease. Synonyms: *Carl Smith disease, acute infectious lymphocytosis, infectious lymphocytosis.*

A benign condition usually characterized by pronounced lymphocytosis and variable clinical manifestations, including fever, respiratory infection, gastrointestinal disorders, and meningoencephalitis, or there may be a complete lack of symptoms. The leukocyte count ranges from 20,000 to 120,000 per cubic millimeter. The majority of affected patients have been children. Infectious mononucleosis, whooping cough, German measles, and other diseases are believed to be the cause.

Smith, C. H. Infectious lymphocytosis. *Am. J. Dis. Child.*, 1941, 62:231-61.

SMITH, DAVID W. (American physician, 1926-1981)

Aase-Smith syndrome. See *under Aase.*

accelerated skeletal maturation, Marshall-Smith type. See *Marshall-Smith syndrome, under Marshall, Richard E.*

Marshall-Smith syndrome (MSS). See *under Marshall, Richard E.*

Opitz-Johnson-McCreadie-Smith syndrome. See *Opitz trigonocephaly syndrome.*

Ruvalcaba-Myhre-Smith syndrome. See *Ruvalcaba syndrome (2).*

Ruvalcaba-Reichert-Smith syndrome. See *Ruvalcaba syndrome (1).*

Smith syndrome. See *Smith-Lemli-Opitz syndrome I.*

Smith-Lemli-Opitz syndrome I (SLO I, SLOS I). Synonyms: *Smith syndrome, RSH syndrome.*

A syndrome of physical and mental retardation, microcephaly, and unusual facies characterized by blepharoptosis, anteverted nostrils, low-set pinnae, and micrognathia. Other abnormalities include syndactyly, genital abnormalities (hypospadias, cleft srcotum, cryptorchism), broad alveolar ridges, and sometimes whitish-blond hair, cataract, cleft palate, and pyloric stenosis. The designation **RSH syndrome** includes initials of the surnames of the first three patients in whom the syndrome was reported. The condition is inherited as an autosomal recessive trait.

Smith, D. W., Lemli, L., & Opitz, J. M. A newly recognized syndrome of multiple congenital anomalies. *J, Pediat.*, 1964, 64:210-7.

Smith-Lemli-Opitz syndrome II (SLO II, SLOS II). A syndrome similar to the Smith-Lemli-Opitz syndrome I (growth and mental retardation, microcephaly, unusual facies, syndactyly, hypospadias, cleft scrotum, cryptorchism, broad alveolar ridges, whitish-blond hair, cataracts, cleft palate, and pyloric stenosis), which, in addition, is characterized by pseudohermaphroditism and frequent early death. Hirschsprung syndrome, unilobated lungs, hexadactyly, congenital heart defect, enlarged adrenals, and Langerhans cell hyperplasia may be associated.

Curry, C. J. R., *et al.* Smith-Lemli-Opitz syndrome-Type II. Multiple congenital anomalies with male pseudohermaphroditism and frequent early lethality. *Am. J. Med. Genet.*, 1987, 26:45-57.

Smith-Theiler-Schachenmann syndrome. See *cerebrocostomandibular syndrome.*

Weaver-Smith syndrome. See *under Weaver, David, D.*

SMITH, E. M. (American physician)

Smith-Thévenard syndrome. See *Thévenard syndrome.*

SMITH, EUSTACE (British physician, 1835-1914)

Smith disease. See *irritable bowel syndrome.*

SMITH, HUGO D. (American physician)

Robinow-Silverman-Smith syndrome. See *Robinow syndrome.*

SMITH, JEAN (British physician)

Smith syndrome. See *Hutchinson disease, under Hutchinson, Sir Robert Grieve.*

SMITH, JOHN FERGUSON (British physician, 1888-1978)

Ferguson Smith epithelioma. Synonyms: *Ferguson Smith keratoacanthoma, multiple self-healing squamous carcinoma (MSHSC).*

A skin neoplasm characterized by a succession of lesions on the apparently normal skin, which are acnelike eruptions with central horny plugs, gradually increasing in size and forming ulcerations. Histologically, the lesions resemble squamous cell carcinoma with epithelial pearls and downgrowths or strands of epidermal cells showing variations in cellular size and staining properties. After a period of several months, the lesions heal spontaneously, leaving scars. The condition is transmitted as an autosomal dominant trait.

Smith, J. F. A case of multiple primary squamous-celled

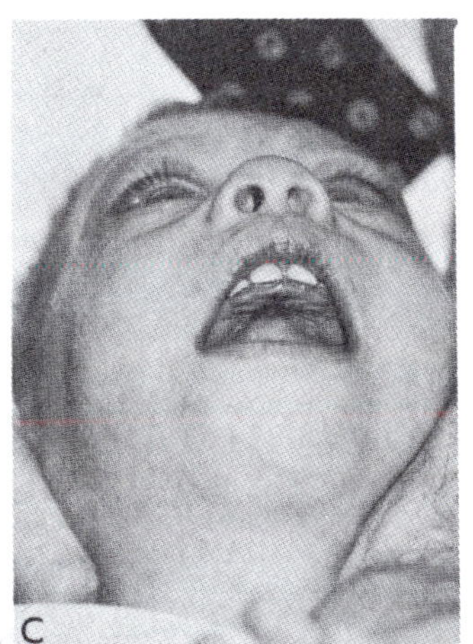

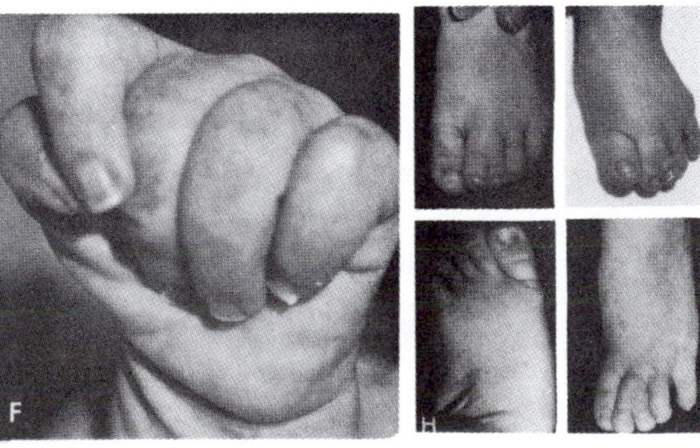

Smith-Lemli-Opitz syndrome (I)
Smith, D.W., et al: *J. Pediatr.* 64:210, 1964. St. Louis: C.V. Mosby Co.

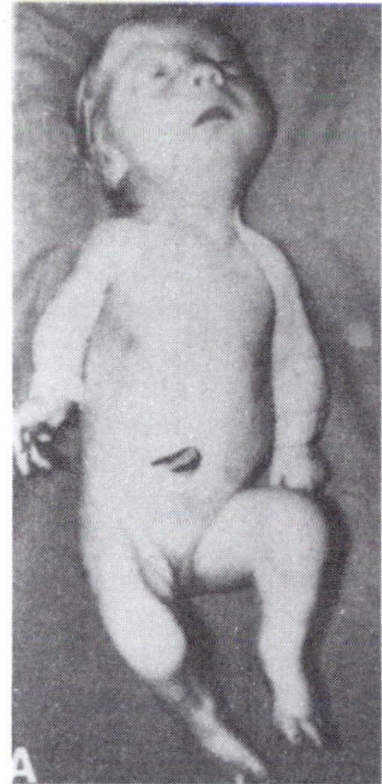
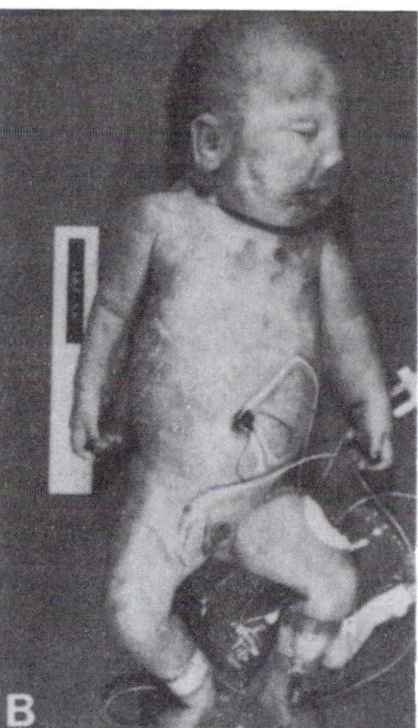
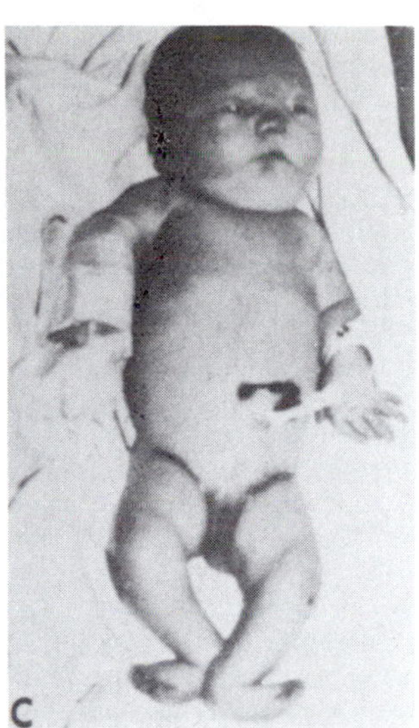

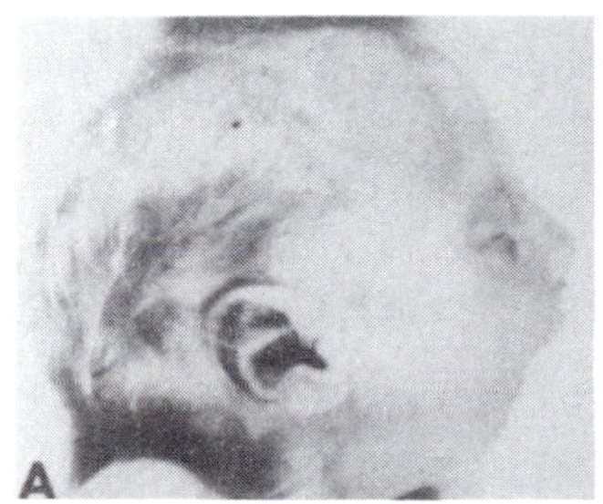
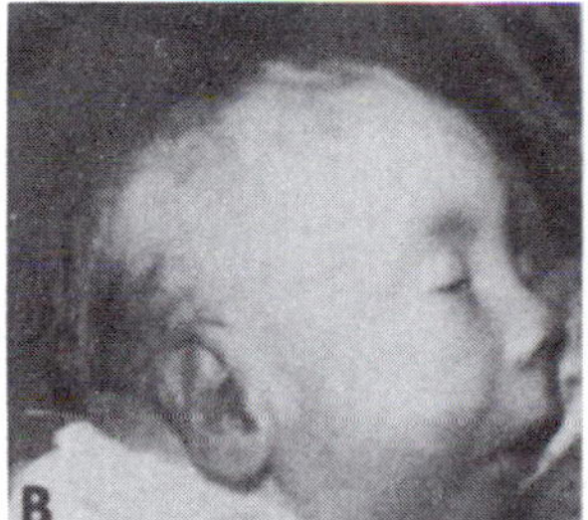
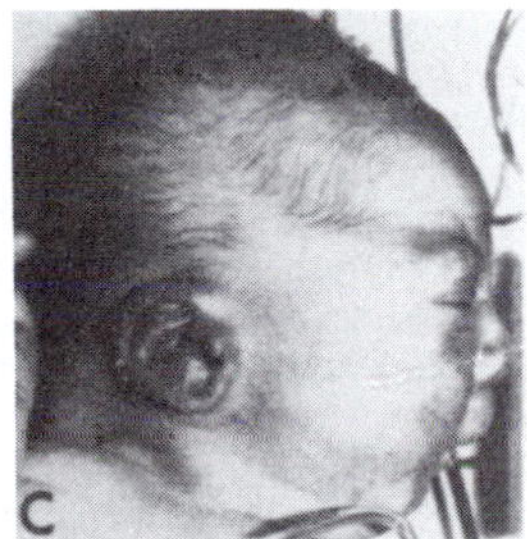

Smith-Lemli-Opitz syndrome II
Curry, Cynthia J.R., John C. Carey, Julie S. Holland, Devinder Chopra, Robert Fineman, Mahin Golabi, Sanford Sherman, Roberta A. Pagon, Judith Allanson, Sally Shulman, Mason Barr, Vicent McGravey, Cyrus Dabiri, Neil Schimke, Elizabeth Ives & Bryan D. Hall: *American Journal of Medical Genetics,* 26:45-57, 1987. New York: Alan R. Liss, Inc.

carcinomata of the skin in a young man, with spontaneous healing. *Brit. J. Derm.,* 1934, 46:267-72.

Ferguson Smith keratoacanthoma. See *Ferguson Smith epithelioma.*

SMITH, LUCIAN S. (American physician, born 1910)

Achor-Smith syndrome. See *under Achor.*

SMITH, RICHARD D. (American physician)

Smith-Fineman-Myers syndrome. A rare hereditary syndrome of mental and growth retardation associated with multiple craniofacial and musculoskeletal abnormalities. Craniofacial defects include microcephaly, dolichocephaly with narrow face, short upslanting palpebral fissures, strabismus, hyperopia, optic nerve hypoplasia, decreased frontonasal angle and nasolabial folds, flat philtrum, prominent upper central incisors, patulous lower lip, bifid uvula, and micrognathia with maxillary prognathism. Other anomalies consist of thin habitus, chest deformity, bridged palmar creases, foot deformities, muscle hypertonia, hyperreflexia, hyperpigmentation, and seizures. The syndrome is transmitted as an X-linked trait.

Smith, R. D., Fineman, R. M., & Myers, G. G. Short stature, psychomotor retardation, and unusual facial appearance in two brothers. *Am. J. Med. Genet.,* 1980, 7:5-9.

SMITH, ROBERT WILLIAM (Irish physician, 1807-1873)

Smith fracture. Synonym: *reverse Colles fracture.*

A flexion and compression fracture of the lower end of the radius with forward displacement of the lower fragment.

Smith, R. W. Fractures of the bones of the fore-arm, in the vicinity of the wrist-joint. In his: *A treatise on fracture in the vicinity of joints, and on certain forms of accidental and congenital dislocations.* Dublin, Hodges & Smith, 1847, pp. 129-75.

SMITH, ROY (American physician)

Smith-McCort dwarfism. See *Dyggve-Melchior-Clausen syndrome.*

SMITH, WILLIAM R. (American physician)

Riley-Smith syndrome. See *Riley syndrome, under Riley, Harris D., Jr.*

smoking stools syndrome. Yellow phosphorus poisoning characterized mainly by a garlic odor of the breath, expelling smoking stools, and cardiovascular collapse. The symptoms of acute yellow phosphorus poisoning may be divided into three phases: the initial symptoms include painful cutaneous burns, oral burning, thirst, vomiting, diarrhea, and severe abdominal pain. Acute cardiovascular collapse may occur at this stage. A symptom-free period, sometimes persisting for as long as several weeks, is followed by the final stage, in which the symptoms are related to systemic toxic effects on the heart, liver, kidneys, and central nervous system. Accidental ingestion of phosphorus-containing rodenticides is the most common cause.

Simon, F. A., & Pickering, L. K. Acute yellow phosphorus poisoning. "Smoking stool syndrome." *JAMA*, 1976, 235:1343-4. Hussey, H. H. Phosphorus poisoning in children. *JAMA*, 1976, 235:1366.

smoldering leukemia. See *myelodysplastic syndrome.*

SMON. See ***s**ubacute **m**yelo-**o**ptico **n**europathy syndrome.*

smooth tongue. See *Möller glossitis.*

SMYTH, A. W. (American physician)

Harrison-Smyth syndrome. See *subclavian steal syndrome.*

SMYTH, F. S. (American physician)

Caffey-Smyth syndrome. See *Caffey-Silverman syndrome.*

Roske-De Toni-Caffey-Smyth syndrome. See *Caffey-Silverman syndrome.*

snapping hip syndrome. Hip pain associated with an audible snapping of the hip during exercise, typically seen in young athletic individuals. The condition traditionally has been associated with a thickened posterior border of the iliotibial band or anterior border of the gluteus maximum slipping over the greater trochanter. Bursography shows subluxation of the iliopsoas tendon to be an apparent cause.

Binnie, J. F. Snapping hip (hanche a ressort, schnellend Hefte). *Ann. Surg.*, 1913, 58:59-66.

snapping scapula syndrome. A disorder of the scapulocostal mechanism characterized by a distinct thump or snapping sound as the scapula is moved across the chest. Chronic, repetitive, forceful action of the shoulder mechanism, producing microtears along the medial border of the scapula and, eventually, causing the development of a spur at the avulsed muscle attachment on the scapula was initially believed to be the cause. Other writers suspect a weakening of the levator scapulae muscle by chronic trauma or, in a patient who has had only one episode of injury, by a major avulsion of its insertion. Poorly coordinated or unbalanced throwing motion in athletes that results in lifting of the periosteal membrane with subperiosteal hemorrhage and subperiosteal ossificatiaon are the suspected etiologic factors. The grating of the ossified mass at the superomedial angle of the scapula on the costal surface produces the audible snapping or thumping sound.

Bateman, J. E. Shoulder injuries in the throwing sports. In: *The American Academy or Orthopedic Surgeons. Symposium on sports medicine.* St. Louis, Mosby, 1969. p. 94. Strizak, A. M., & Cowen, M. H. The snapping scapula syndrome. A case report. *J. Bone Joint Surg.*, 1982, 64A:941-2.

SNE (subacute necrotizing encephalomyelopathy). See *Leigh syndrome.*

SNEDDON, IAN BRUCE (British dermatologist, born 1915)

Duhring-Sneddon-Wilkinson syndrome. See *Sneddon-Wilkinson syndrome.*

Sneddon syndrome (1). See *Sneddon-Wilkinson syndrome.*

Sneddon syndrome (2). Synonyms: *Sneddon-Champion syndrome, livedo reticularis-cerebrovascular syndrome.*

A syndrome of livedo reticularis and cerebrovascular lesions transmitted as an autosomal dominant trait. Livedo involves all the extremities and the trunk, worsening in cold weather and during the acute phase of neurological complications. Chronic ischemia of the extremities is present in all cases; it is associated with acroerythrocyanosis, coldness of the hands and feet, an impaired or absent pulse in posterior tibial and dorsalis pedis arteries, and the Raynaud phenomenon. Adventitial fibrosis, thrombosis, and changes in the media are the principal pathological changes in the digital arteries. Neurological manifestations consist of stroke, transient ischemic attacks, epileptic seizures, and dementia. Angiographic findings show segmental narrowing and dilatation in the palmar digital arteries, together with multiple obstructions and reduced vascular caliber; stenosis in the distal or basal branches of the intracranial arteries; collateral circulation in the brain, including transdural anastomoses and anastomoses between intracranial arteries; and the moyamoya syndrome (q.v.).

Sneddon, I. B. Cerebrovascular lesions and livedo reticularis. *Brit. J. Derm.*, 1965, 77:80-5. Champion, R. H., & Allison, J. R. Livedo reticularis: A review. *Brit. J. Derm.*, 1965, 77:167-79. Rebollo, M., *et al.* Livedo reticularis and cerebrovascular lesions (Sneddon's syndrome). Clinical, radiological and pathological features in eight cases. *Brain*, 1983, 106:965-79.

Sneddon-Champion syndrome. See *Sneddon syndrome (2).*

Sneddon-Wilkinson syndrome. Synonyms: *Duhring-Sneddon-Wilkinson syndrome, Sneddon syndrome, dermatitis pustulosa subcornealis, dermatosis pustulosa subcornealis, subcorneal pustular dermatosis.*

A chronic, recurrent pustular eruption, usually involving the axillae, groins, abdomen, submammary areas, the flexor aspects of the limbs, and, less commonly, the palms and soles. Some itching and burning may be present. Vesicles which rapidly evolve into pustules or small, discrete, flaccid pustules, are the initial lesions. They usually arise in crops and become erythematous within a few hours. There is some pus in the lower parts of the pustules, which tend to coalesce, sometimes forming annular, circinate, or serpiginous patterns. After a few days, they rupture and dry up to form superficial scales and crust. Peripheral spreading and central healing produce numerous erythematous areas in which pustules in the central parts disappear, whereas new crops appear on the peripheries. The eruption may regress and become quiescent for a few days or weeks, to be followed by new eruptions. The condition occurs most frequently in middle-aged women.

Sneddon, I. B., & Wilkinson, D. S. Subcorneal pustular dermatosis. *Brit. J. Derm.*, 1956, 68:385-94.

sneezing from light exposure. See *ACHOO syndrome.*

SNELLEN, HERMAN ADRIANUS (Dutch cardiologist, born 1905)

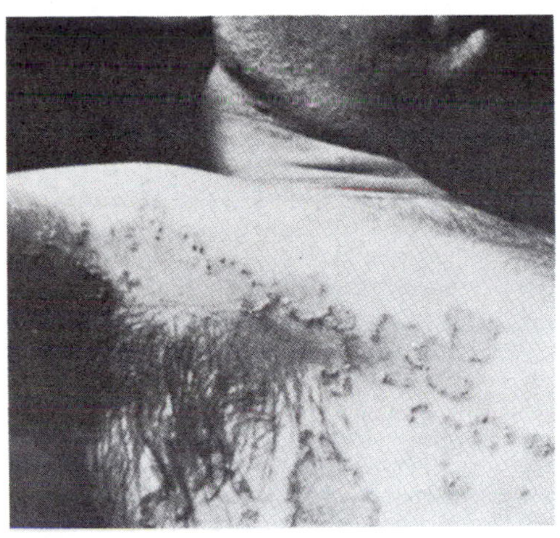

Sneddon-Wilkinson syndrome
Andrews, G.C. & A.N. Domonkos: *Diseases of the Skin.* 5th ed. Philadelphia: W.B. Saunders Co., 1963.

Taussig-Snellen-Albers syndrome. See *under Taussig.*

SNJ (nevus sebaceous of Jadassohn). See *Jadassohn nevus sebaceous.*

snow-flake cataract. See *O'Brien cataract.*

snow-storm cataract. See *O'Brien cataract.*

snowball opacities of the vitreous. See *Benson disease.*

SOCRATES (Athenian philosopher, c.469-c.399 B.C)

Socrates syndrome. Synonym: *ipsiphilia compulsiva proctalgenica.*

A condition generally observed among unfulfilled artists, writers, and scientists, usually those who consider themselves as having been deprived of their rightful recognition and rewards. They imagine themselves as living in a socratic setting, their adoring family and associates sitting respectfully at their feet while they dispense wisdom to the world. They will never tolerate any hint of criticism or any attempt to discuss their views, considering themselves the sole and absolute custodians of the truth.

Stanley, J. Personal communication.

SOD. See *septo-optic dysplasia.*

sodium losing nephropathy. See *renal salt losing syndrome.*

soft chancre. See *Ducrey disease.*

soft hand syndrome. See *Coffin-Lowry syndrome.*

soft tissue overuse syndrome. See *overuse syndrome.*

Sogo fever. See *hemorrhagic fever with renal syndrome.*

SOKOLSKII (SOKOLSKY), GRIGORII IVANOVICH (Russian physician, 1807-1886)

Sokolskii-Bouillaud disease. See *Bouillaud disease.*

Sokolsky-Bouillaud disease. See *Bouillaud disease.*

SOKOLSKY, GRIGORII IVANOVICH. See SOKOLSKII, GRIGORII IVANOVICH

soldier's heart. See *Da Costa syndrome, under Da Costa, Jacob Mendez.*

SOLENTE, G. (French physician)

Touraine-Solente-Golé (TSG) syndrome. See *pachydermoperiostosis syndrome.*

soleus syndrome. See *shin splint syndrome.*

solitary lobar atrophy. See *Burke syndrome.*

solitary rectal ulcer syndrome (SRU, SRUS). Synonym: *solitary ulcer syndrome.*

An uncommon condition usually occurring as a persistent, nonhealing ulcer on the anterior aspect of the rectum. There can also be multiple ulcers or a localized proctitis without ulceration. The exact etiology is unknown, but the condition is often associated with rectal prolapse or a history of straining at stool. Electromyographic findings often show pelvic muscle discoordination during defecation with persistent contraction of the puborectalis muscle. The syndrome occurs in both sexes, usually in persons under the age of 40 years, but older individuals may occasionally be affected.

Levine, M. S., *et al.* Solitary rectal ulcer syndrome: A radiologic diagnosis. *Gastrointest. Radiol.,* 1986, 11:187-93.

solitary ulcer syndrome. See *solitary rectal ulcer syndrome.*

SOLOMON, L. L.

Solomon syndrome. See *epidermal nevus syndrome.*

Solomon-Fretzin-Dewald syndrome. See *epidermal nevus syndrome.*

somatization disorder (SD). See *Briquet syndrome (1), under Briquet, Pierre.*

somatostatinoma syndrome. A somatostatin-producing tumor of the pancreas associated with dyspepsia, steatorrhea, mild diabetes mellitus, and cholelithiasis. The symptoms are believed to be due to somatostatin inhibitory action on the secretion of gastrin, secretin, insulin, and cholecystokinin.

Unger, R. H. Somatostatinoma. *N. Engl. J. Med.,* 1977, 296:998-1000.

somnolence syndrome. Synonym: *postradiotherapy somnolence syndrome.*

Transient cerebral disturbances characterized by somnolence after prophylactic cranial irradiation in children with acute lymphocytic leukemia. The symptoms vary from mild drowsiness to prolonged periods of sleep. Somnolence is often preceded and followed by anorexia and irritability. Some children may develop fever with symptoms of upper respiratory infection, nausea, and vomiting.

Freeman, J. E., *et al.* Somnolence after prophylactic cranial irradiation in children with acute lymphoblastic leukemia. *Brit. Med. J.,* 1973, 4:523-5.

SONNE, CARL OLAF (Danish bacteriologist, 1882-1948)

Sonne disease. See *Sonne dysentery.*

Sonne dysentery. Synonym: *Sonne disease.*

Bacillary dysentery (shigellosis) caused by the Sonne bacillus (*Shigella sonnei*). It is an acute, self-limiting disease of the intestinal tract of humans, which is characterized by diarrhea, fever, and abdominal pain.

Sonne, C. O. Über die Bakteriologie der giftarmen Dysenteriebacillen (Paradysenteriebacillen). *Zbl. Bakt.,* 1915, 75:408-56.

sopite syndrome. A symptom complex centering around drowsiness in motion sickness. The symptoms include yawning, drowsiness, disinclination to work, and lack of participation in group activities.

Graybiel, A., & Knepton, J. Sopite syndrome: A sometimes sole manifestation of motion sickness. *Aviat. Space Environ. Med.,* 1976, 47:873-82.

sorcerer's apprentice syndrome. A compulsive disorder wherein an activity may be preceded by procrastination but, once it is started, it cannot be stopped, as in anorexia-once a diet or a binge is started, it usually continues because the affected person has difficulty stopping it. See also *bulimia syndrome*.

Solyom, L., *et al.* A comparative psychometric study of anorexia nervosa and obsessive aneurosis. *Canad. J. Psychiat.*, 1982, 27:282-6.

sorcery syndrome. An aboriginal behavioral disorder, occurring in cultural situations in which sorcery is an important component of belief systems. It is characterized by severe anxiety and agitation, a breakdown of normal social behavior, and a paranoid preoccupation with personal, physical, and social security.

Reser, J. P., & Eastwell, H. D. Labeling and cultural expectations & the shaping of a sorcery syndrome in aboriginal Australia. *J. Nerv. Ment. Dis.*, 1981, 169:303-10.

SORENSEN, S. STAMPE (Danish physician)

Sorensen syndrome. Mild müllerian anomalies and eugonadotropic oligomenorrhea with demonstrable ovulation in infertile or low-fertility women.

Sorensen, S. S. Minor müllerian anomalies and oligomenorrhea in infertile women. A new syndrome. *Am. J. Obst. Gynec.*, 1981, 140:636-44.

SORIANO, A. (Spanish physician)

Soriano syndrome. Synonym: *periostitis deformans.*

A bone disease characterized by hyperplastic, osteogenic, recurrent osteoperiostitis of the polyostotic type with development of bone tumorlike lesions at the site of osteogenic periostitis. After 2 to 12 months, the lesions regress, often with total involution of the tumors. The attacks may recur at any time during the lifespan, each attack being less intense than the previous one. Anorexia and wasting may occur in severe episodes.

Soriano, M. Periostitis deformans. *Ann. Rheum. Dis.*, 1952, 11:154-61.

SORRELL-DEJERINE, J. (French physician)

Thieffry and Sorrell-Déjerine syndrome. See *Thieffry-Shurtleff syndrome.*

SORSBY, ARNOLD (British ophthalmologist)

Sorsby disease. Synonyms: *dominant generalized fundus dystrophy, pseudoinflammatory fundus dystrophy.*

Dystrophy of the fundus oculi beginning in the fifth decade as unilateral blurring of the central vision followed by a similar disorder in the other eye. Objectively, there is edema, hemorrhage, and exudation in the central area with scar formation and pigment proliferation, which develop into generalized choroidal atrophy. The final stage is characterized by the disappearance of the choroidal vessels, which exposes the sclerotic irregularities, followed by total blindness. The disorder is familial, being transmitted as an autosomal dominant trait.

Sorsby, A., *et al.* A fundus dystrophy with unusual features. (Late onset and dominant inheritance of a central retinal lesion showing oedema, haemorrhage and exudates developing into generalized choroidal atrophy with massive pigment proliferation). *Brit. J. Ophth.*, 1949, 33:67-100.

Sorsby macular degeneration. Synonym: *inflammatory hereditary degeneration of the macula.*

A familial, invariably bilateral and symmetrical form of exudative (or hemorrhagic exudative) macular degeneration which occurs during the third or fourth decade, and eventually develops into chorioretinal atrophy. Generally, this disorder is believed to be transmitted as an autosomal dominant trait, although in a few cases there is evidence of recessive transmission.

Sorsby, A. The dystrophies of the macula. *Brit. J. Ophth.*, 1940, 24:469-529.

Sorsby syndrome. Synonym: *apical dystrophy with macular coloboma syndrome.*

A familial form of brachydactyly B associated with macular coloboma. The syndrome is believed to be transmitted as an autosomal dominant trait.

Sorsby, A. Congenital coloboma of the macula: together with an account of the familial occurrence of bilateral macular coloboma in association with apical dystrophy of hands and feet. *Brit. J. Ophth.*, 1935, 19:64-90.

SOTOS, JUAN F. (American physician)

Sotos syndrome (SS). Synonym: *cerebral gigantism.*

A syndrome of excessive growth, acromegalic features, and a nonprogressive cerebral disorder with mental retardation. Dolichocephaly, macrocrania, hypertelorism, antimongoloid palpebral slant, high-arched palate, frontal bossing, mandibular

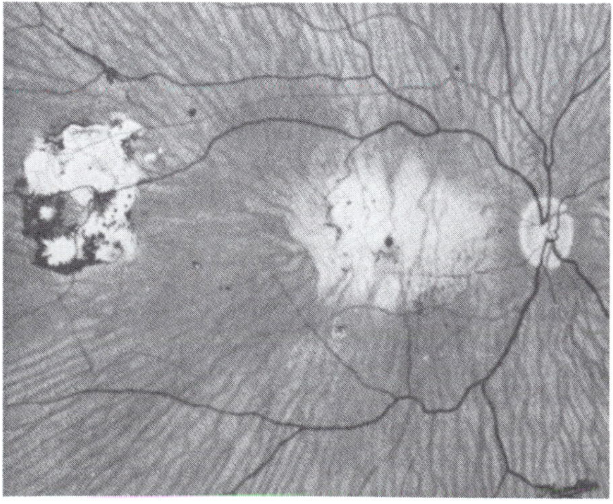

Sorsby macular degeneration
Francois, Jules: *Heredity in Ophthlmology.* St. Louis: C.V. Mosby Co., 1961.

prognathism, and precocious dentition are the principal features. Accelerated skeletal maturation in the absence of obvious endocrine dysfunction is usually associated. Levels of 17-ketosteroids and gonadotropins have been elevated in some cases. Kyphoscoliosis may occur. Pneumoencephalography reveals dilated cerebral ventricles without an obstructive lesion. Convulsions occur but electroencephalographic findings show only some nonspecific abnormalities. Most cases are sporadic but some are transmitted as an autosomal dominant trait.

Sotos, J. F., *et al.* Cerebral gigantism in childhood. A syndrome of excessively rapid growth with acromegalic features and nonprogressive neurologic disorder. *N. Engl. J. Med.*, 1964, 271:109-16.

SOTTAS, JULES (French physician, born 1866)

Déjerine-Sottas syndrome. See *under Déjerine.*

SOULIER, JEAN PIERRE (French physician, born 1915)

Bernard-Soulier syndrome (BSS). See *under Bernard, Jean.*

Soulier-Boffa syndrome. Repeated spontaneous abortions in women with circulating antithromboplastin anticoagulant and thrombosis.

Soulier, J. P., & Boffa, M. C. Avertements à répétition, thrombose et anticoagulants circulants antithromboplastines. *Nouv. Presse Méd.*, 1980, 9:859-64.

SOUQUES, ALEXANDRE ACHILLE (French physician, 1860-1944)

Souques-Charcot geroderma. Synonym: *gerodermia infantilis.*

A variant of the Hutchinson-Gilford syndrome, consisting of loose, shiny, dry skin, subcutaneous atrophy, eunuchoid habitus, and intellectual deficiency, reportedly described by Souques and Charcot.

South American blastomycosis. See *Lutz-Splendore-de Almeida syndrome.*

South American trypanosomiasis. See *Chagas disease.*

SOUTHWORTH, HAMILTON (American physician, born 1907)

Southworth symptom complex. Hematuria, abdominal pain, and nitrogen retention following the administration of sulfapyridine.

Southworth, H., & Cooke, C. Hematuria, abdominal pain and nitrogen retention associated with fulflapyridine. *JAMA*, 1939, 112:1820-1.

space adaptation syndrome. Synonyms: *motion sickness-like syndrome, space motion sickness.*

A disorder, similar in many respects to motion sickness, characterized by a feeling of "fullness" in the head, headache, vomiting, and malaise, occurring after 1 or more days of space flight. The syndrome appears to be associated with a combination of factors, including weightlessness, head movements, and visual-spatial disorientation.

Homick, J. L. Space motion sickness. *Acta Astronaut.*, 1979, 6:1259-72.

space motion sickness. See *space adaptation syndrome.*

Spanish oil syndrome. See *toxic oil syndrome.*

Spanish toxic oil syndrome. See *toxic oil syndrome.*

Spanish toxic syndrome. See *toxic oil syndrome.*

Spanish toxic-allergic syndrome. See *toxic oil syndrome.*

SPANLANG, HERBERT (Austrian physician)

Spanlang-Tappeiner syndrome. Synonyms: *alopecia-hyperhidrosis-corneal dystrophy syndrome, keratosis palmaris et plantaris-corneal dystrophy syndrome.*

A syndrome of congenital zonular corneal opacity with hyperkeratosis palmaris et plantaris, frequently accompanied by cataract, hyperhidrosis, and alopecia. The syndrome is transmitted as an autosomal recessive trait.

Spanlang, H. Beiträge zur Klinik und Pathologie seltener Hornhauterkrankungen. (Dystrophia adiposa corneae, Dyskeratosis corneae congenita). *Zschr. Augenh.*, 1927, 62:21-41. Tappeiner, S. Zur Klinik der idiopathischen diffusen palmoplantaren Keratodermien. *Arch. Derm., Berlin,* 1937, 175:453-66.

spasmodic tic. See *Henoch chorea.*

spasmotic bronchitis-leukocytosis-eosinophilia syndrome. See *tropical eosinophilia syndrome.*

spastic bowel syndrome. See *irritable bowel syndrome.*

spastic colon. See *irritable bowel syndrome.*

spastic diplegia. See *Little disease, under Little, William John.*

spastic paraplegia. See *Erb-Charcot syndrome, under Erb, Wilhelm Ernst.*

spastic pelvic floor syndrome. A functional disorder whereby the pelvic floor muscles contract instead of relaxing during straining, thus causing rectal outlet obstruction and inhibiting defecation with resulting constipation.

Kuijpers, H. C., & Bleijenberg, G. The spastic pelvic floor syndrome: A cause of constipation. *Dis. Colon Rectum,* 1895, 28:669-72.

spastic pseudosclerosis. See *Jakob-Creutzfeldt syndrome.*

spastic spinal paralysis. See *Erb-Charcot syndrome, under Erb, Wilhelm Ernst.*

spastic striated external sphincter syndrome. A variant of the urethral syndrome in women, characterized by incoordination during micturition between a normally sustained detrusor contraction and a spastic striated external sphincter.

Tanagho, E. A., *et al.* Spastic striated external sphincter and urinary tract infection in girls. *J. Urol.*, 1971, 43:69-82.

spastic tabes dorsalis. See *Erb-Charcot syndrome, under Erb, Wilhelm Heinrich.*

SPÄT

Spät-Hurler syndrome. See *mucopolysaccharidosis I-S.*

SPATZ, HUGO (German physician)

Hallervorden-Spatz syndrome (HSS). See *under Hallervorden.*

SPCA (serum prothrombin conversion accelerator) deficiency. See *Alexander syndrome, under Alexander, Benjamin.*

speaking stomach syndrome. Persistent audible gurgling sounds in the gastric region, which occur synchronously with respiration, the respiratory movements causing a displacement of gastric contents. An abnormal pattern of respiration with activity of the abdominal muscles and involvement of the diaphragm are the etiologic factors.

Edwards, D. A. W. The "speaking stomach" syndrome. *Gut*, 1968, 9:732.

specific giant-cell myocarditis. See *Fiedler myocarditis.*

specific productive myocarditis. See *Fiedler myocarditis.*

speckled corneal dystrophy. See *François dystrophy (2).*

speckled erythroplakia. See *under Queyrat erythroplasia.*
speckled leukoplakia. See *under Queyrat erythroplasia.*
SPENCER, WALTER
Spencer disease. Synonyms: *Bradley disease, Goodall disease, epidemic vomiting, hyperemesis hiemis, intestinal grippe, nausea epidemica, winter vomiting disease.*

An epidemic disease, usually occurring during the winter months, characterized by nausea, vomiting, anorexia, abdominal pain, diarrhea and, less frequently, constipation, pale stools, headache, generalized aching, and fever. A viral etiology is suspected.

*Bradley, W. H. Epidemic nausea and vomiting. *Brit. Med. J.*, 1943, 1:309-12. Goodall, J. F. The winter vomiting disease. A report from general practice. *Brit. Med. J.*, 1954, 1:197-8.

SPENS, THOMAS (British physician, 1764-1842)
Spens syndrome. See *Adams-Stokes syndrome, under Adams, Robert.*
SPH (spherocytosis hereditaria). See *Minkowski-Chauffard syndrome.*
sphenopalatine ganglion neurosis. See *Sluder neuralgia.*
sphenopalatine neuralgia. See *Sluder neuralgia.*
spherocytosis hereditaria (SPH). See *Minkowski-Chauffard syndrome.*
spherophakia-brachymorphism syndrome. See *Weill-Marchesani syndrome, under Weill, Georges.*
sphingomyelin lipidosis. See *Niemann-Pick syndrome.*
sphingomyelin reticuloendotheliosis. See *Niemann-Pick syndrome.*
sphingomyelinosis. See *Niemann-Pick syndrome.*
spider fingers. See *Marfan syndrome (1).*
SPIEGHEL (SPIGELIUS), ADRIAAN, VAN DER (Flemish anatomist, 1587-1625)
spigelian hernia. Abdominal hernia through the linea semilunaris, above the epigastric artery.
SPIEGLER, EDUARD (Austrian physician, 1860-1903)
Ancell-Spiegler cylindroma. See *Brooke epithelioma.*
Brooke-Spiegler syndrome. See Brooke epithelioma.
Kaposi-Spiegler sarcomatosis. See *Bäfverstedt syndrome.*
Spiegler-Fendt sarcoid. See *Bäfverstedt syndrome.*
Spiegler-Fendt sarcomatosis. See *Bäfverstedt syndrome.*
SPIELMEYER, WALTER (German physician, 1879-1935)
Stock-Spielmeyer-Vogt syndrome. See *under Stock.*
Vogt-Spielmeyer syndrome. See *Stock-Spielmeyer-Vogt syndrome.*
spigelian hernia. See *under Spieghel, Adriaan, van der.*
SPIGELIUS. See SPIEGHEL, ADRIAAN, VAN DER
SPILLER, WILLIAM GIBSON (American physician, 1864-1940)
Spiller syndrome. Synonym: *epidural ascending spinal paralysis.*

Thrombophlebitis of the meningorachidian veins with subacute and chronic pachymeningitis, causing spinal cord compression and pain, sensory disorders, weakness, ascending paralysis with atrophy of various muscle groups, and transverse myelitis.

Spiller, W. G. Epidural ascending spinal paralysis. *Rev. Neur. Psychiat.*, 1911, 9:494-8.

spillover. See *excited skin syndrome.*
spinal block syndrome. See *Froin syndrome.*
spinal cholesterolosis. See *van Bogaert-Scherer-Epstein syndrome.*
spinal epiphysitis. See *Scheuermann disease.*
spinal hemiparaplegia. See *Brown-Séquard syndrome.*
spinal hereditary ataxia. See *Friedreich ataxia.*
spinal insufficiency. See *Schanz syndrome.*
spinal muscular atrophy I (SMA I). See *Werdnig-Hoffmann syndrome.*
spinal muscular atrophy III (SMA III). See *Wohlfart-Kugelberg-Welander syndrome.*
spinal neck-tongue syndrome. See *neck-tongue syndrome.*
spinal osteochondritis. See *Scheuermann disease.*
spinal traction syndrome. See *cast syndrome.*
spindle cell nevus. See *Spitz nevus.*
spine migraine. See *under headache syndrome.*
spinocerebellar ataxia. See *Marie syndrome (1), under Marie, Pierre.*
spinocerebellar degeneration-dementia-plaque-like deposits syndrome. See *Gerstmann syndrome (1).*
spinocerebellar heredoataxia. See *Friedreich ataxia, under Friedreich, Nicolaus.*
spinophthalmic tract-nucleus ambiguous syndrome. See *Avellis syndrome.*

SPIRA, LEO
Spira disease. Synonyms: *dentes de Chiaie, fluorosis, mottled enamel, mottled teeth.*

A chronic form of hypoplasia of the dental enamel caused by drinking water with a high fluorine content during the time of tooth formation, and characterized by defective calcification that gives a white chalky appearance to the enamel, which will gradually undergo brown discoloration.

*Spira, L. *Franco Brit. Med. Rev.*, 1928, 5:61.

spirochaetosis arthritica. See *Reiter syndrome.*
spirochaetosis icterohaemorrhagica. See *leptospirosis.*
spirochematosis icterohaemorrhagica. See *leptospirosis.*
SPITZ, SOPHIE (American physician)

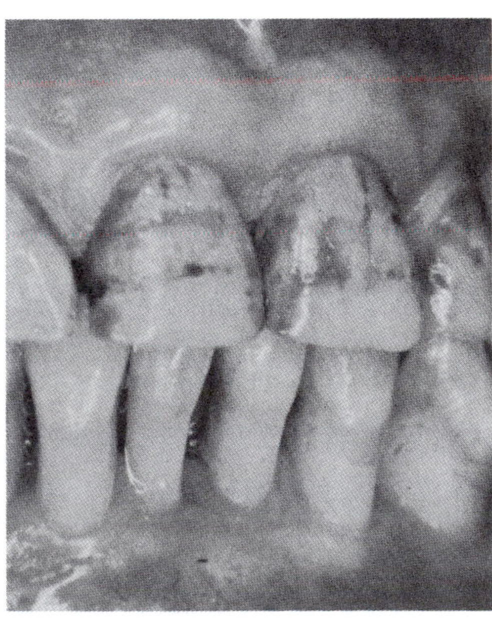

Spira disease
Robbins, S.L.: *Pathology.* 3rd ed. Philadelphia: W.B. Saunders Co., 1967.

Spitz nevus. Synonyms: *benign juvenile melanoma, epithelioid cell nevus, juvenile melanoma, large spindle and/or epithelioid nevus, spindle cell nevus.*

A benign nevus presenting asymptomatic, dome-shaped, smooth, usually pink or tan but sometimes brown or black papules. The lesions may be verrucous but rarely ulcerate; they are relatively superficial and there is generally abrupt transition between the acantholytic loose junctional cells and the still intact adjacent epidermis. There are sharply separated nests of spindle and/or epithelioid cells in the epithelium. Giant nevus cells, when present, have 4 to 5 nuclei. Atypical mitoses are absent. Edema and telangiectasia are present in the subepidermal tissue, and a lymphohistiocytic infiltrate may be seen around the blood vessels in the dermal part of the nevus. Heavy melanization may occur in some cases but, in most instances, pigmentation is scanty.

Spitz, S. Melanomas of childhood. *Am. J. Path.*, 1948, 24:591-602. Bovenmyer, D. A. Spitz's nevus in a black child. *Cutis*, 1981, 28:186-9; 209.

SPITZER, ADRIAN (American physician)

Spitzer-Weinstein syndrome. A syndrome of hyperkalemia, acidosis, and short stature associated with defective renal potassium excretion and decreased hydrogen ion secretion by the distal tubule.

Spitzer, A., *et al.* Short stature, hyperkalemia and acidosis: A defect of renal transport of potassium. *Kidney Internat.*, 1973, 3:251-7. Weinstein, S. F., *et al.* Hyperkalemia, acidosis, and short stature associated with a defect of renal potassium excretion. *J. Pediat.*, 1974, 85:355-8.

splanchnic vasoplegia. See *Reilly syndrome, under Reilly, J.*

splanchnoptosis. See *Glénard syndrome.*

spleen-liver syndrome. See *Banti syndrome.*

SPLENDORE, ALPHONSO (Brazilian physician)

Lutz-Splendore-de Almeida syndrome. See *under Lutz, Adolfo.*

splenic agenesis syndrome. See *asplenia syndrome.*

splenic anemia. See *Banti syndrome.*

splenic flexure syndrome. Synonyms: *Payr syndrome, flexura lienalis syndrome.*

Interposition of the splenic flexure of the colon between the diaphragm, stomach, and spleen, associated with abdominal pain, tenderness of the left abdomen, and abdominal distention.

Payr, E. Über eine eigentümliche, durch abnorm starke Knikungen und Adhäsionen bedingte gutartige Stenose der Flexura lienalis und hepatica coli. *Verh. Deut. Kong Innn. Med.*, 1910, 27:276-305.

splenic neutropenia syndrome. See *Wiseman-Doan syndrome.*

splenic syndrome. Acute splenic sequestration or infarction. The disorder may occur in persons with sickle cell trait who are exposed to high altitudes. Nonblack persons with the trait are suspected of being more susceptible than black persons with the trait.

Rotter, R., *et al.* Splenic infarction in sicklemia during airplane flight: Pathogenesis, hemoglobin analysis, and clinical features in six cases. *Ann. Intern. Med.*, 1956, 44:257-70. Lane, P. A., & Githens, J. H. Splenic syndrome at mountain altitudes in sickle cell trait. Its occurrence in nonblack persons. *JAMA*, 1985, 253:2251-4.

splenic thrombocytopenic purpura. See *Werlhof disease.*

splenogonadal fusion-ectromelia syndrome. See *splenogonadal fusion-peromelia syndrome.*

splenogonadal fusion-peromelia syndrome. Synonym: *splenogonadal fusion-ectromelia syndrome.*

A congenital abnormality characterized by fusion of the testes to the spleen in association with defects of the extremities, including amelia, hemimelia, and phocomelia. Micrognathia may be associated in some cases. Cardiac lesions, including multiple right ventricular diverticula, tricuspid atresia, mitral to semilunar valve discontinuity, and absent muscular outflow tract septum may also occur.

Pommer, G. Verwachsung des linken kryptorchischen Hodens und Nebenhodens mit der Milz in einer Missgeburt mit zahlreichen Bildungsdefecten. *Berl, Naturw. Med. Verh. Innsbruck*, 1887-89, pp. 17-19; 144-8. Putschar, W. G., & Manion, W. C. Splenic-gonadal fusion. *Am. J. Pathol.*, 1956, 32:15-33. Loomis, K. F., *et al.* Unusual cardiac malformations in splenogonadal fusion-peromelia syndrome: relationship to normal development. *Teratology*, 1982, 25:1-9.

splenomegalic cirrhosis. See *Hanot cirrhosis.*

splenomegalic polycythemia. See *Vaquez-Osler syndrome.*

splenopneumonia. See *Grancher disease.*

split foot/split hand-congenital nystagmus syndrome. See *Karsch-Neugebauer syndrome.*

split hand-cleft lip/palate and ectodermal (SCE) dysplasia. See *EEC syndrome.*

split notochord syndrome. A syndrome of combined anterior and posterior spina bifida involving primarily the lumbosacral spine. Associated abnormalities may include meningocele or myelomeningocele, aplasia of the penis, agenesis of the colon, intestinal malrotation, anomalous mesenteric arteries, malformed kidney, bicornuate uterus, and bifurcation of the spinal cord.

Bentley, J. F. R., & Smith, J. R. Developmental posterior enteric remnants and spinal malformations. The split notochord syndrome. *Arch. Dis. Child., London*, 1960, 35:76-86.

spondylitis adolescens. See *Bechterew-Strümpell-Marie syndrome, under Bekhterev.*

spondylitis ankyloarthrica. See *Bechterew-Strümpell-Marie syndrome, under Bekhterev.*

spondylitis atrophica ligamentosa. See *Bechterew-Strümpell-Marie syndrome, under Bekhterev.*

spondylitis deformans. See *Bechterew-Strümpell-Marie syndrome, under Bekhterev.*

spondylitis ossificans ligamentosa. See *Bechterew-Strümpell-Marie syndrome, under Bekhterev.*

spondylitis traumatica. See *Kümmell-Verneuil disease.*

spondylo-arthritis ankylopoietica. See *Bechterew-Strümpell-Marie syndrome, under Bekhterev.*

spondylo-epimetaphyseal dysplasia with joint laxity (SEMDJL) syndrome. A familial syndrome, transmitted as an autosomal recessive trait, characterized by severe dwarfism, articular hypermobility, progressive spinal malalignment, thoracic asymmetry, bilateral dislocation of the radial heads, and bilateral talipes equinovarus. Characteristic but variable features include an oval face, long upper lip, protuberant eyes, blue sclerae, soft and doughy skin with some hyperelasticity, spatulate terminal phalanges (especially of the thumbs), and joint laxity of the hands permitting abnormal positioning. Inconsistent features consist of cleft palate, high-arched palate, heart defect, genu valgum, and congenital hip dislocation. Mental retardation, myopia, ocular lens dislocation, Hirschsprung disease, and unilateral megaureter may occur in some patients. The syndrome was originally reported in several Afrikans families in South Africa.

Beighton, P., & Kozlowski, K. Spondylo-epi-metaphyseal dysplasia with joint laxity and severe, progressive kyphoscoliosis. *Skelet. Radiol.*, 1980, 5:205-12.

spondylo-epimetaphyseal dysplasia with myotonia. See *Schwartz-Jampel syndrome, under Schwartz, Oscar.*

spondylo-epiphyseal dysplasia. See *mucopolysaccharidosis IV-A.*

spondylo-epiphyseal dysplasia congenita. Synonyms: *Spranger-Wiedemann syndrome, dysplasia spondyloepiphysaria congenita.*

A syndrome of dysproportionate dwarfism, short spine, brevicollis, barrel chest, pectus carinatum, genu valgum, flat face, myopia, malar hypoplasia, kyphoscoliosis, and limited joint mobility, especially of the elbows, knees, and hips. Associated defects may include genu varum, hypertelorism, retinal detachment, clubfeet, and cleft palate. Major radiological findings include ovoid or pear-shaped vertebral bodies, poorly ossified flat vertebrae in childhood and flattening of vertebral bodies in adulthood, hypoplasia of the odontoid process, retarded pubic bone ossification, flared broad iliac wings, rhizomelic brachymelia, poorly ossified metaphyses and epiphyses, poor ossification of the femoral head and neck, deformed femoral capital epiphyses, and high greater trochanter in adults. The syndrome is transmitted as an autosomal dominant trait with variability of expression.

Spranger, J. W., & Wiedemann, H. R. Dysplasia spondyloepiphysaria congenita. *Lancet*, 1966, 2:642. Spranger, J. W., & Langer, L. O., Jr. Spondyloepiphyseal dysplasia congenita. *Radiology*, 1970, 94:313-22.

spondylo-epiphyseal dysplasia syndrome, X-linked. See *spondylo-epiphyseal dysplasia tarda.*

spondylo-epiphyseal dysplasia tarda. Synonyms: *Maroteaux-Lamy-syndrome; dysplasia spondyloepiphysaria tarda; spondylo-epiphyseal dysplasia, late type; X-linked spondylo-epiphyseal dysplasia.*

A familial type of bone dysplasia transmitted as an X-linked recessive trait, having onset between the ages of 5 and 10 years. The principal symptoms include short-trunk dwarfism, back pain, pain in the hips, and limitation of joint movement. Associated anomalies consist of platyvertebrae with central humps, epiphyseal irregularities with flat femoral heads, small iliac wings, short femoral neck, brevicollis, kyphoscoliosis, wide and deep chest diameters, small bony pelvis, coxa vara, and osteoarthritic changes in adult life, leading to complete disability by the age of 60 years.

Jacobsen, A. W. Hereditary osteochondrodystrophia deformans. A family with twenty members affected in five generations. *JAMA*, 1939, 113-121-4. Maroteaux, P., Lamy, M., & Bernard, J. La dysplasie spondylo-epiphysaire tardive. *Presse Méd.*, 1957, 65:1205-8.

spondylo-epiphyseal dysplasia, late type. See *spondylo-epiphyseal dysplasia tarda.*

spondylo-epiphyseal dysplasia-diabetes mellitus syndrome. See *Wolcott-Rallison syndrome.*

spondylocostal dysostosis. See *spondylothoracic dysplasia.*

spondylocostal dysplasia. See *spondylothoracic dysplasia.*

spondylohumerofemoral hypoplasia syndrome. Synonyms: *atelosteogenesis, giant-cell chondrodysplasia.*

A syndrome of lethal short-limb skeletal dysplasia with absent or hypoplastic humeri, absent fibulae, hypoplastic vertebrae, and ossification in only the distal phalanges of the hands. Morphologic findings show hypocellular areas of growth plate cartilage containing occasional multinucleated giant cells. Associated disorders include premature birth polyhydramnios, short for gestational age, pointed proximal femur, square distal femur and short ribs. All cases were sporadic in the original report.

Sillence, D, O., *et al.* Spondylohumerofemoral hypoplasia (giant cell chondrodysplasia): A neonatally lethal short-limb skeletal dysplasia. *Am. J. Med. Genet.*, 1982, 13:7-14.

spondylometaphyseal dysplasia, Kozlowski type. See *Kozlowski spondylometaphyseal dysplasia syndrome, under Kozlowski, Kazimierz S.*

spondylopanniculitis. See *Weber-Christian syndrome, under Weber, Frederick Parkes.*

spondylopathia traumatica. See *Kümmell-Verneuil disease.*

spondylorheostosis. See *Forestier syndrome (2).*

spondylosis hyperostotica. See *Forestier syndrome (2).*

spondylothoracic dysplasia. Synonyms: *Jarcho-Levin syndrome, Lavy-Palmer-Merritt syndrome, bizarre vertebral anomalies syndrome, costovertebral dysplasia, costovertebral segmentation anomalies syndrome, costovertebral syndrome, dysplasia spondylothoracica, hereditary malformation of the vertebral bodies, occipitofaciocervicothoraco-abdominodigital dysplasia (OFCTAD), spondylocostal dysostosis, spondylocostal dysplasia.*

A hereditary syndrome involving the spinal column and thoracic cage. Two types are recognized: **Type I** is transmitted as an autosomal recessive trait, and occurs most commonly in children of Puerto Rican ancestry. It is usually fatal in infancy because of pneumonia, respiratory problems, and cardiac failure. Clinical features include short neck, shortness of the of the posterior aspect of the chest, prominent abdomen, long thin limbs with tapering digits, hemivertebrae, block vertetrae, open neural arches, missing vertebral bodies, and fanlike ribs with their posterior convergence. Short-trunk dwarfism, prominent occiput, peculiar facies, low posterior hairline, hernias, and hammer toes may be associated. **Type II**, consisting of hemivertebrae, vertebral fusion, missing ribs, rib fusion, short-trunk dwarfism, and other anomalies, is transmitted as an autosomal dominant trait, and occurs mainly in white children, usually with nearly normal longevity.

Jarcho, S., & Levin, P. M. Hereditary malformation of the vertebral bodies. *Bull. Johns Hopkins Hosp.*, 1938, 62:216-29. Lavy, N. W., Palmer, C. G., & Merritt, A. D. A syndrome of bizarre vertebral anomalies. *J. Pediat.*, 1966, 69:1121-5. Pérez-Comas, A., & García-Castro, J. M. Occipito-facial-cervico-thoracic-abdomino-digital dysplasia: Jarcho-Levin syndrome of vertebral anomalies. *J. Pediat.*, 1974, 85:388-91. Heilbronner, D. M., & Reinshaw, T. S. Spondylothoracic dysplasia. A case report. *J. Bone Joint Surg.*, 1984, 66(A):302-3.

sponge kidney. See *Cacchi-Ricci syndrome.*

spongiform cerebral atrophy. See *Nevin syndrome (1).*

spongioblastosis circumscripta. See *Bourneville-Pringle syndrome.*

spongy degeneration of the nervous system. See *Canavan syndrome.*

spongy degeneration of the white matter. See *Canavan syndrome.*

spontaneous dislocation of atlanto-axial joint. See *Grisel syndrome.*

spontaneous fulminating gangrene of the scrotum. See *Fournier disease.*

spontaneous hyperemic dislocation of the atlanto-axial joint. See *Grisel syndrome.*

spontaneous lipogranulomatosis. See *Rothmann-Makai syndrome.*

spontaneous panniculitis. See *Rothmann-Makai syndrome.*

spontaneous periodic hypothermia. See *Shapiro syndrome.*

spontaneous remission of diabetes mellitus. See *Houssay syndrome.*

spontaneous rupture of the esophagus. See *Boerhave syndrome.*

spontaneous thyrotoxic crisis. See *Waldenström disease, under Waldenström, Jan Gösta.*

SPOONER, WILLIAM ARCHIBALD (Dean of New College, Oxford, 1844-1930)

Spooner syndrome. Synonym: *spoonerism.*

A neurological disorder characterized by an intermediate state between simple absent-mindness and gross brain damage with dysphasia, dysgraphia, and dyspraxia, associated with albinism. The condition is believed to have been the cause of Dr. Spooner's habit of transposing words or sounds (spoonerisms), as in "kinquering congs."

Potter, J. M. Dr. Spooner and his dysgraphia. *Proc. Roy. Soc. Med.,* 1976, 69:639-48. Vaisrub, S. Spooner syndrome. *JAMA,* 1977, 237:677.

spoonerism. See *Spooner syndrome.*

sporadic acropathia ulceromutilans. See *Bureau-Barrrière syndrome.*

sporadic hemophilia. See *Bernuth syndrome.*

sporadic ulcerating and mutilating acropathy (SUMA). See *Bureau-Barrière syndrome.*

sporotrichosis. See *Schenck disease.*

spotted bone. See *osteopoikilosis syndrome.*

spotted corneal dystrophy. See *Groenouw dystrophy (2).*

spousal abuse. See *battered spouse syndrome.*

spouse beating. See *battered spouse syndrome.*

SPRANGER, JÜRGEN W. (German physician)

Kozlowski-Maroteaux-Spranger syndrome. See *Kozlowski spondylometaphyseal dysplasia syndrome, under Kozlowski, Kazimierz S.*

Maroteaux-Spranger-Wiedemann syndrome. See *metatropic dwarfism syndrome.*

metaphyseal chondrodysplasia, Wiedemann-Spranger type. See *Wiedemann-Spranger metaphyseal chondrodysplasia syndrome.*

Spranger syndrome (1). Synonyms: *chondrodysplasia punctata, recessive type; chondrodysplasia punctata, rhizomelic type; rhizomelic chondrodysplasia punctata syndrome.*

A syndrome of disproportionate shortness of stature with short proximal parts of the extremities, flat face with mongoloid features, cataract, ichthyosiform skin changes, and multiple joint contractures. The affected infants fail to thrive and are severely retarded, and usually die in infancy from repeated infections. Only a few infants are known to have survived their first year of life. The syndrome is transmitted as an autosomal recessive trait.

Spranger, J., *et al.* Heterogeneity of chondrodysplasia punctata. *Humangenetik,* 1971, 11:190-212.

Spranger syndrome (2). Synonym: *geleophysic dwarfism.*

A syndrome of small stature, a peculiar but pleasant and even happy natured facial appearance (hence the synonym *geleophysic dwarfism*), dysostosis multiplex-like bone dysplasia affecting predominantly the hands and feet, and an apparently focal accumulation of acid mucopolysaccharides in the liver and possibly cardiovascular tissues. Small hands and feet are noted at birth, psychomotor development is slightly retarded, progressive growth failure and recurrent respiratory infections are observed after the first year of life. Possible soft-tissue infiltration by storage substances is indicated by the full face, especially of the upper lip, which is thick and long, and a flat philtrum. The nose is short with a depressed bridge and anteverted nostrils. Other facial features include hypertelorism, slight mongoloid slanting of the palpebral fissures, a thick nasolabial fold, and micrognathia. There is a disproportionate shortness of stature, particularly affecting the hands and feet. Multiple contractures of the finger joints are present. Hepatomegaly and cardiomegaly occurs in some cases. Cardiac deformities include thickening of the pulmonary and mitral valves and stenosis of the mitral valve. Radiographic findings consist of an elongated sella, ovoid or slightly hook-shaped vertebrae at the thoracolumbar junction, bone shortening of the arms and legs, and shortening and widening or the tubular bones of the hands and feet.

Spranger, J. W., *et al.* Geleophysic dwarfism—A "focal" mucopolysaccharidosis? *Lancet,* 1971, 2:97-8.

Spranger-Wiedemann syndrome. See *spondyloepiphyseal dysplasia congenita.*

Wiedemann-Spranger metaphyseal chondrodysplasia syndrome. See *under Wiedemann.*

SPRENGEL, OTTO GERHARD KARL (German physician, 1852-1915)

Sprengel anomaly. See *Sprengel deformity.*

Sprengel deformity. Synonyms: *Sprengel anomaly, Sprengel shoulder, congenital high scapula, high scapula, scapula congenita elevata, scapula elevata, undescended scapula.*

Congenital elevation of the scapula with rotation of its lower angle toward the spine and scoliosis, sometime with an accessory bone between the scapula and the cervical spine. The arm on the affected side cannot be raised above the right angle. The Klippel-Feil syndrome, syringomyelia, and a cervical rib are often associated. A familial form of the Sprengel deformity is known as *Corno disease.*

Sprengel. Die angeborene Verschiebung des Schulterblattes nach oben. *Arch. Klin. Chir., Berlin,* 1891, 42:545-9.

Sprengel shoulder. See *Sprengel deformity.*

spring catarrh. See *Angelucci syndrome.*

spring conjunctivitis. See *Angelucci syndrome.*

SPRINZ, HELMUTH (German-born American pathologist, born 1911)

Sprinz

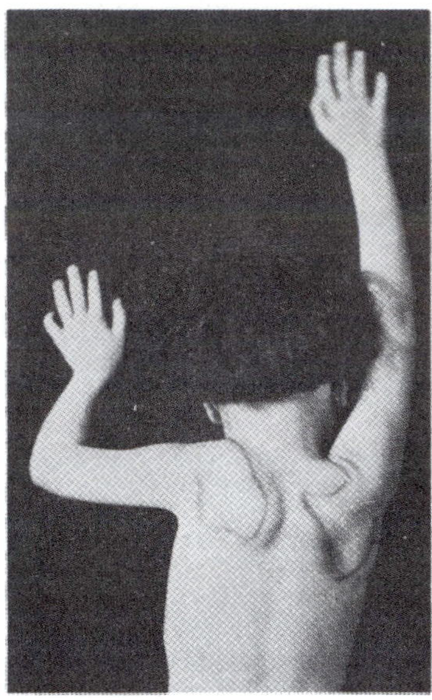

Sprengel deformity
Nelson, W.E. (ed.): *Textbook of Pediatrics.* 9th ed. Philadelphia: W.B. Saunders Co., 1969.

Dubin-Johnson-Sprinz syndrome. See *Dubin-Johnson syndrome.*

Dubin-Sprinz syndrome. See *Dubin-Johnson syndrome.*

SPS. See ***s**capulo**p**eroneal **s**yndrome.*

spun glass hair syndrome. See *uncombable hair syndrome.*

spurious hydrocephalus. See *Hall syndrome, under Hall, Marshall.*

spurious meningocele. See *Billroth disease (1).*

spurious polycythemia. See *Gaisböck disease.*

SPURWAY, JOHN (British physician)

Spurway-Eddowes syndrome. See *osteogenesis imperfecta syndrome (dominant form).*

squamous cell epithelioma. See *Lever adenoacanthoma.*

squamous roseola. See *Gibert disease.*

squint syndrome. See *blind spot syndrome.*

SRB, J.

Srb syndrome. Aplasia and synostosis of the first two ribs with a hornlike bony protrusion of the manubrium and displacement of the synchondrosis, frequently complicated by compression of the nerves and blood vessels.

*Srb, J. Über Missbildung en der ersten Rippe. *Med. Jahr. Kais. Kön. Ges. Arzte, Wien,* 1862-65, 5:75. Wenz, W. Geipert, G. Röntgenologie und Klinik der Srbschen Rippen-Sternum-Anomalie. *Radiologie, Berlin,* 1967, 7:53-8.

SRO. See ***S**teele-**R**ichardson-**O**lszewski syndrome.*

SRP I (short rib-polydactyly syndrome type I). See *Majewski syndrome.*

SRP II (short rib-polydactyly syndrome type II). See *Saldino-Noonan syndrome.*

SRP III (short rib-polydactyly syndrome type III). See *Verma-Naumoff syndrome.*

SRPS (short rib-polydactyly syndrome). See *Majewski syndrome, Saldino-Noonan syndrome, Verma-Naumoff syndrome.*

SRU. See ***s**olitary **r**ectal **u**lcer syndrome.*

SRUS. See ***s**olitary **r**ectal **u**lcer **s**yndrome.*

SS. See ***S**ézary **s**yndrome.*

SS (sickle cell) disease. See *sickle cell anemia.*

SS. See ***S**jögren **s**yndrome, under Sjögren Henrik Samuel Conrad.*

SS. See ***S**otos **s**yndrome.*

SS. See ***S**weet **s**yndrome.*

SSPE (subacute sclerosing panencephalitis). See *van Bogaert encephalitis.*

SSS. See ***s**ick **s**inus **s**yndrome.*

SSSS. See ***s**taphylococcal **s**calded **s**kin **s**yndrome.*

St. Helena familial genu valgum. A familial disorder, transmitted as an autosomal dominant trait, characterized by genu valgum and variable lesser malalignment at the elbows and wrists, occurring as the consequence of hypoplasia of the corresponding bony condyles, with subsequent progressive degenerative osteoarthropathy. The condition occurs in inhabitants of the mid-Atlantic island of St. Helena.

Beighton, P., *et al.* St. Helena familial genu valgum. *Clin. Genet.,* 1986, 30:309-14.

ST. VITUS (Third century Christian child martyr)

chorea St. Viti. See *Sydenham chorea.*

St. Vitus dance. See *Sydenham chorea.*

staccato syndrome. A disorder characterized by abrupt staccato behavior and a disconnected and discontinuous affect, observed in connection with teen-age drug abuse .The symptoms resemble schizophrenia, except that relationships with peers are maintained.

Tec, L. The staccato syndrome: A new clinical entity in search of recognition. *Am. J. Psychiat.,* 1971, 128:647-8.

STAFNE, EDWARD CHRISTIAN (American dentist, born 1894)

Stafne cyst. Synonyms: *Stafne mandibular defect, latent bone cyst, lingual mandibular bone cavity, static bone cavity, static bone cyst.*

A developmental bone inclusion of salivary glandular tissue within or, more commonly, adjacent to the lingual surface of the body of the mandible, forming a deep, circumscribed depression. It is sometimes bilateral, and is believed to be congenital, although it is rarely observed in children, occurring more commonly in males than in females. On the radiograph, it appears as an ovoid radiolucency situated between the mandibular canal and the inferior border of the mandible, just anterior to the angle.

Stafne, E. C. Bone cavities situated near the angle of the mandible. *JADA.,* 1942, 29:1969-72.

Stafne mandibular defect. See *Stafne cyst.*

stagnant loop syndrome (SLS). See *blind loop syndrome.*

STAHL, FRIEDRICH KARL (German physician, 1811-1873)

Stahl ear. A deformed ear in which the helix is broad and coalesces with the anthelix, the fossa ovalis and fossa scaphoidea being almost invisible and the lower part of the helix being obliterated; or one in which there are three instead of two crura anthelicis.

Stahl, F. K. Einige Skizzen über Missgestaltungen des äusseren Ohres. *Allg. Psychiat., Berlin,* 1859, 16:479-90.

STÄHLI, JEAN (Swiss ophthalmologist, born 1890)

Hudson-Stähli line. See *under Hudson.*

Stähli line. See *Hudson-Stähli line.*

STAINTON, C. W. (American dentist)

Sprinz syndrome. See *dentinogenesis imperfecta.*

Stainton-Capdepont syndrome. See *dentinogenesis imperfecta.*

STANBURY, JOHN BRUTON (American physician, born 1915)

Stanbury-Hedge defect. Congenital defective binding of iodine by the thyroid gland in goitrous cretins.

Stanbury, J. B., & Hedge, A. N. A study of a family of goitrous cretins. *J. Clin. Endocr.*, 1950, 10:1471-84.

STANESCO, V. (Rumanian physician)

autosomal dominant osteosclerosis, Stanesco type. See *Stanesco syndrome.*

Stanesco dysostosis syndrome. See *Stenesco syndrome.*

Stanesco dysplasia. See *Stanesco syndrome.*

Stanesco syndrome. Synonyms: *Stanesco dysostosis syndrome; Stanesco dysplasia; autosomal dominant osteosclerosis, Stanesco type; craniofacial dysostosis with diaphyseal hyperplasia.*

A congenital syndrome, transmitted as an autosomal dominant trait, characterized by craniofacial dysostosis, brachycephalic skull, depressions over the frontoparietal and occipitoparietal sutures, poor pneumatization of the frontal and sphenoid bones, short-arm dwarfism, underdeveloped mandible, narrow maxilla, crowded teeth, enamel hypoplasia, small hands with brachydactyly, and thickening of the long bones.

Stanesco, V., *et al.* Syndrome héréditaire dominant, réunissant une dysostose cranio-faciale de type particulier, une insuffisance de croissance d'aspect chondrodystrophique et un épaississement massif de la corticale des os longs. *Rev. Fr. Endocrin. Clin.*, 1963, 4:219-31.

STANLEY, J.

Stanley syndrome (1). Synonym: *proctalgia syndromica terminalis.*

Severe proctalgic pain in conjunction with fatigue, myopia, and scotoma, seen in middle-aged and elderly individuals afflicted with chronic lexicomania. The condition appears to be aggravated by remaining in the sedentary position for long periods of time, and is incurable.

Stanley, J. Personal communication.

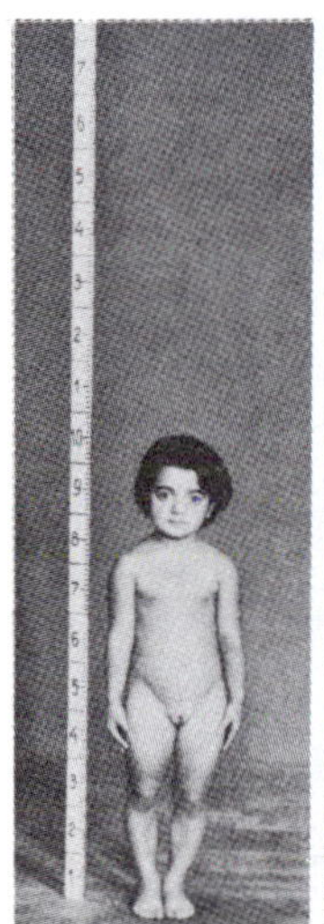
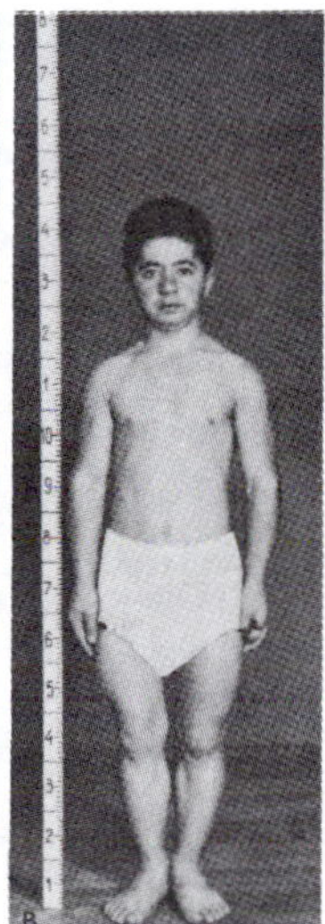
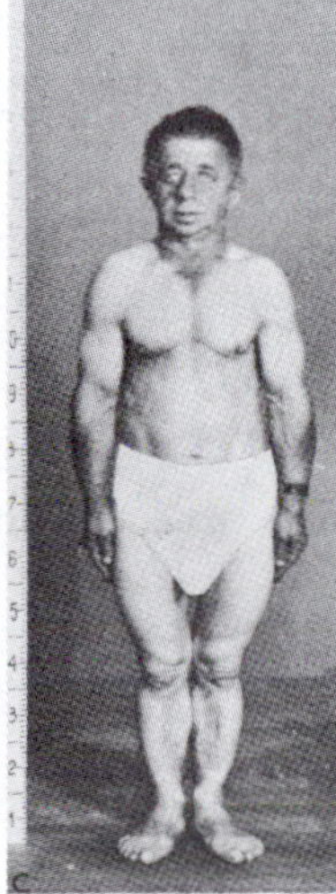

Stanesco syndrome
Stanesco, V., et al.: *Rev. Fr. Endocrinol. Clin.* 4:219, 1963. Editions de Medicine Pratique, Asnieres, France.

Stanley syndrome (2). See *Danaid syndrome, under Danaids.*

staphylococcal Lyell syndrome. See *staphylococcal scalded skin syndrome.*

staphylococcal scalded skin syndrome (SSSS). Synonyms: *Ritter disease, Ritter syndrome, dermatitis erysipelatosa, dermatitis exfoliativa infantum, dermatitis exfoliativa neonatorum (DEN), exfoliative dermatitis of the newborn, staphylococcal Lyell syndrome, staphylogenic Lyell syndrome.*

A form of exfoliative dermatitis caused by an exotoxin (exfoliatin) produced by strains of the bacterium *Staphylococcus aureus*, group 2, phage type 71. Two main types are recognized: The generalized form **(type I**, or **Ritter disease)** and the localized one **(type II)**. **Type I**, usually occuring in children under the age of 5 years (including newborn infants), begins as a localized cutaneous infection with purulent conjunctivitis, otitis media, or occult nasopharyngeal infection, and is characterized by scarlatiniform rash of the perioral area, spreading over the trunk and extremities, and cutaneous tenderness. Friction applied to the skin causes the epidermis to wrinkle and separate (Nikolsky sign). The lesions are initially faint, yellow-orange-amber eruptions. Within 24 to 48 hours there is spontaneous wrinkling of the epidermis, followed by formation of large, flaccid bullae, which spread over all parts of the body but spare the mucous membrane. The bullae burst, exposing red, denuded skin, giving it a burnlike appearance. **Type II** also occurs in children, although adult cases have been reported, and is characterized by bullae filled with cloudy fluid surrounded by an erythematous rim, usually on the exposed parts of the body and around orifices. Skin tenderness is usually absent. In some cases, localized forms progress to the generalized form. The *staphylococcal scalded skin syndrome* and *toxic epidermal necrolysis* were considered in the past the same entity; now they are recognized as separate diseases with different etiologies.

Ritter von Rittershain, G. Dermatitis erysipelatosa. Gangraena. Enkephalitis. *Österr. Jb. Pediat.*, 1870, 1:23-4.

Lyell, A. Toxic epidermal necrolysis, an eruption resembling scalding of the skin. *Brit. J. Derm.*, 1956, 68:355.

staphylococcal toxic shock syndrome. See *toxic shock syndrome.*

staphylogenic Lyell syndrome. See *staphylogoccal scalded skin syndrome.*

staphylohematoma. See *Bosviel syndrome.*

starch granuloma syndrome. Granulomas in the peritoneal cavity caused by starch glove powder introduced into the cavity during surgery. The principal manifestations include metastatic carcinoma-like miliary seedlings in the peritoneal cavity, peritonitis, and granulomatous masses which occur within the abdomen, in surgical incisions, and other parts of the body.

Vellar, I. D. The starch granuloma syndrome. *Med. J. Australia*, 1975, 1:60-2.

STARGARDT, KARL BRUNO (German ophthalmologist, 1875-1927)

Stargardt syndrome. Synonyms: *familial juvenile macular degeneration, juvenile hereditary disciform macular degeneration, juvenile macular degeneration.*

Bilateral, symmetric, slowly progressive macular degeneration transmitted as an autosomal recessive trait. It begins insidiously with gradual deterioration of vision and ends in total blindness. Abnormal pigmentation of the macular region is the early symptom, and this is followed by dark yellow spots that eventually coalesce and by irregular pigmentation of the entire area. Gradually, the foveal and macular reflexes disappear. Grayish spots surrounded by pigmented halos then appear in the centers of the lesions and eventually form well-defined oval areas with visible dirty yellowish retinal vessels. The disorder is congenital, but the first symptoms appear later in childhood.

Stargardt, K. Über familiäre, progressiver Degeneration in der Maculagegend des Auges. *Graefes Arch. Ophth.*, 1909, 71:534-50.

stasibasiphobia. See *Blocq syndrome.*

static bone cavity. See *Stafne cyst.*

static bone cyst. See *Stafne cyst.*

status degenerativus amstelodamensis. See *de Lange syndrome (1), under Lange, Cornelia, de.*

status degenerativus typus rostockiensis. See *Ullrich-Feichtiger syndrome.*

status eczematicus. See *excited skin syndrome.*

status marmoratus. See *Vogt syndrome, under Vogt, Cécille.*

STAUFFER, H.

Bloch-Stauffer dyshormonal dermatosis. See *Rothmund-Thomson syndrome.*

STAUFFER, MAURICE H. (American physician)

Stauffer syndrome. Synonym: *nephrogenic hepatosplenomegaly.*

A rare syndrome of splenomegaly and disturbed liver function with hepatomegaly, occurring in patients with renal neoplasms.

Stauffer, M. H. Nephrogenic hepatosplenomegaly. *Gastroenterology*, 1961, 40:694.

stave of the thumb. See *Bennett fracture, under Bennett, Edward Hallaran.*

steal syndrome. See *aorto-iliac steal syndrome, carotid steal syndrome, coronary steal syndrome, coronary-subclavian steal syndrome, pulmonary artery steal syndrome, subclavian steal syndrome, thyroid steal syndrome.*

STEARNS, GENEVIEVE (American physician)

Boyd-Stearns syndrome. See *under Boyd.*

steatorrhea arthropericarditica. See *Whipple disease.*

STEELE, JOHN C. (Canadian physician)

Steele-Richardson-Olszewski (SRO) syndrome. Synonyms: *plurisystematic degeneration of the neuraxis, progressive supranuclear ophthalmoplegia, progressive supranuclear palsy.*

A neurological syndrome, usually occurring during the sixth decade, characterized by initial impairment of vertical-saccadic movement and a loss of the fast component of optokinetic nystagmus. Ophthalmoplegia, particularly paralysis of the downward gaze and limitation of the upper gaze with preserved lateral gaze, is the cardinal symptom. Associated disorders include pseudobulbar palsy, dysarthria, mild dementia, memory loss, disturbances of balance and gait, masklike facies, weak voice, extreme flexion or extension dystonia of the neck, and axial rigidity, mainly involving the neck and trunk. Pathologically, there is a loss of neurons and gliosis in the tectum and tegmentum of the midbrain, the subthalamic nuclei of Luys, the vestibular nuclei, and the ocular nuclei. Microscopic findings show intracytoplasmic filamentous material in the form of tangled masses (Alzheimer neurofibrillary tangles), composed of straight rather than paired helical filamaents. A slow virus is suspected as the cause.

Steele, J. C., Richardson, J. C., & Olszewski, J. Progressive supranuclear palsy. A heterogenous degeneration involving the brain stem, basal ganglia and cerebellum with vertical gaze and pseudobulbar palsy, nuchal dystonia and dementia. *Arch. Neur., Chicago*, 1964, 10:333- 59.

steely hair syndrome. See *kinky hair syndrome.*

STEIGLEDER, G. K. (German physician)

Steigleder syndrome. See *reticular erythematous mucinosis syndrome.*

STEIN, IRVING FREILER, SR. (American gynecologist, born 1887)

Stein syndrome. See *polycystic ovary syndrome.*

Stein-Leventhal syndrome. See *polycystic ovary syndrome.*

STEINBRINCK, W. (German physician)

Béguez César-Steinbrinck-Chédiak-Higashi syndrome. See *Chédiak-Higashi syndrome.*

Chédiak-Steinbrinck syndrome. See *Chédiak-Higashi syndrome.*

Steinbrinck anomaly. See *Chédiak-Higashi syndrome.*

STEINBROCKER, OTTO (American physician)

Steinbrocker syndrome. See *shoulder-hand syndrome.*

STEINDLER, ARTHUR (American physician, born 1878-1959)

Steindler posterior syndrome. Low back pain.

Steindler, A., & Luck, J. V. Differential diagnosis of pain low in the back; allocation of the source of pain by the procaine hydrochloride method. *JAMA*, 1938, 110:106-13.

STEINER, GABRIEL (German physician, born 1883)

Steiner syndrome. See *Curtius syndrome (1).*

STEINER, L. (German physician)

Steiner-Voerner syndrome. See *carcinoid syndrome.*

STEINERT, HANS (German physician)

Curschmann-Batten-Steinert syndrome. See *myotonic dystrophy syndrome.*

Curschmann-Steinert syndrome. See *myotonic dystrophy syndrome.*

Rossolimo-Curschmann-Batten-Steinert syndrome. See *myotonic dystrophy syndrome.*

Steinert disease. See *myotonic dystrophy syndrome.*

Steinert myopathy. See *myotonic dystrophy syndrome.*

Steinert myotonia. See *myotonic dystrophy syndrome.*

Steinert myotonic dystrophy. See *myotonic dystrophy syndrome.*

STELLWAG, CARL VON CARION (Austrian ophthalmologist, 1823-1904)

Stellwag brawny edema. Gelatinous thickening of the conjunctiva due to generalized infiltration of merged florid blebs, seen in trachoma.

Duke-Elder, S. *Systems of ophthalmology.* London, Kimpton, 1965, Vol. 8, p. 285.

STENGEL, E. (German physician)

Schilder-Stengel syndrome. See *under Schilder.*

stenocardia. See *Heberden asthma.*

stenosing aortitis. See *aortic arch syndrome.*

stenosing tendinitis of the abductor longus. See *de Quervain disease (1), under Quervain, Fritz, de.*

STEPHENS, JAMES (American physician)

Stephens syndrome. A familial syndrome combining the features of Friedreich ataxia and Charcot-Marie-

Tooth disease in association with chronic progressive external ophthalmoplegia.

Stephens, J., *et al.* On familial ataxia, neural amyotrophy, and their association with progressive external ophthalmoplegia. *Brain,* 1958, 81:556-66.

STERN, WALTER G. (American physician)

Guérin-Stern syndrome. See *arthrogryposis multiplex congenita syndrome.*

STERNBERG, CARL, VON (German physician, 1872-1935)

Albright-McCune-Sternberg syndrome. See *McCune-Albright syndrome.*

Hodgkin-Paltauf-Sternberg disease. See *Hodgkin disease.*

Paltauf-Sternberg disease. See *Hodgkin disease.*

Sternberg disease. See *Hodgkin disease.*

sternocostoclavicular hyperostosis syndrome. A bone disease characterized mainly by radiographic signs of enlargement and increased density of the clavicles, sternum, and first ribs, associated with ossification of the sternoclavicular and sternocostal joints. Hyperostosis without osteoclast inclusion is the principal histological characteristic. Subclavian vein occlusion may occur. The etiology is unknown.

Köhler, H., *et al.* Sterno-kosto-klavikuläre Hyperostose. Ein bisher nicht beschriebenes Krankheitsbild. *Deut. Med. Wschr.,* 1975, 100:1519-23.

steroid pseudorheumatism. See *Slocumb syndrome.*

steroid withdrawal syndrome. A group of disorders which follow interruption of corticoid therapy, ranging from nonspecific complaints in the presence of normal adrenal function tests to cardiovascular collapse in patients with severe compromised adrenal function. The disorders associated with glucocorticoid withdrawal include a flaring of the underlying disease as dosage is reduced below that required for its suppression, adrenal insufficiency, and limited pituitary reserve. The symptoms of adrenal insufficiency consist of anorexia, nausea, vomiting, abdominal pain, headache, weight loss, weakness, fatigability, myalgias, lethargy, apathy, confusion, mental disorders, hypotension, impaired response to catecholamines, fever, arthralgia, pericarditis, fasting hypoglycemia, hyponatremia, hypercalcemia, and impaired tolerance to stress. Prolonged symptoms after withdrawal may include arthralgias, malaise, and anorexia. Some patients may develop psychological withdrawal symptoms. See also *Slocumb syndrome.*

Sullivan, J. N. Steroid withdrawal syndromes. *South Med. J.,* 1982, 75:726-33.

STEVENS, ALBERT MASON (American physician, 1884-1945)

Stevens-Johnson syndrome (SJS). Synonyms: *Baader dermatostomatitis, Baader syndrome, Fiessinger-Rendu syndrome, Fuchs syndrome, Klauder syndrome, Neumann syndrome, acute mucocutaneous-ocular syndrome, aphthosis generalisata, bullous malignant erythema multiforme, conjunctivitis et cheilostomatitis pseudomembranacea exanthematodes, conjunctivitis et stomatitis pseudopseudomembranacea, cutaneomucooculoepithelial syndrome, dermatostomatitis, ectodermosis erosiva pluriorificialis, erythema multiforme syndrome, erythema multiforme exudativum, fever-stomatitis-ophthalmia syndrome, mucosal-respiratory syndrome.*

A disease affecting chiefly young adult males, usually during the spring and fall. Upper respiratory tract infections, headache, malaise, nausea, arthritis, and fever are the earliest symptoms. They are followed in a few days by skin lesions consisting of vesiculobullous eruptions, usually on the dorsa of the hands and feet, often also involving other parts of the body. The ocular lesions are also variable, generally involving the conjunctiva. Keratitis, iritis, uveitis, panophthalmia, and blindness are frequently present. The lesions of the penis and vulva are the most common forms of mucous involvement, often leading to balanitis, urethritis, and vulvovaginitis. Mucous lesions may spread to the respiratory tract, causing bronchopneumonia and gastrointestinal disorders with ulceration, proctitis, colitis, and nephritis. Sialorrhea, dysphagia, enlarged cervical lymph nodes, and halitosis are the result of involvement of the oral mucosa. The syndrome is sometimes classified as **erythema multiforme exudativum minor** (a mild form characterized primarily by cutaneous and oromucosal lesions) and **erythema multiforme exudativum major** (a severe form characterized by fever, and ocular, genital, cutaneous, and oral mucosal lesions). Etiologic factors include herpes simplex, allergy, bacterial infections, *Mycoplasma pneumoniae* infection, and adverse reactions to drugs, such as some antibiotics and sulfonamides. The degree of severity and symptoms may vary in the same patient during different attacks.

Stevens, A. M., & Johnson, F. C. A new eruptive fever associated with stomatitis and ophthalmia. Report of two cases in children. *Am. J. Dis. Child.,* 1922, 24:526-33. Baader, E. Dermatostomatitis, *Arch. Derm. Syph., Berlin,* 1925, 149:261-8. Klauder, J. V. Ectodermosis pluriorificialis. Its resemblance to the human form of foot and mouth disease and its relation to erythema multiforme. *Arch. Derm. Syph., Chicago,* 1937, 36:1067-77. Fiessinger, N., & Rendu, R. Sur un syndrome caractérisé par l'inflammation simultaneé de toutes les muqueuses externes coexistant avec une éruption vésiculeuse des quatre membres, non douloureuse et non recidivante. *Paris Méd.,* 1917, 25:54-8. Rendu, R. Sur un syndrome caractérisé par l'inflammation simultanée de toutes les muqueuses externes (conjunctivale, nasale, linguale, buccopharyngée, orale et balanopréputiale) coexistant avec une éruption variceliforme puis purpurique des quatre membres. *Rev. Gen. Clin. Ther.,* 1916, 30:351-8. Fuchs, E. Herpes oris conjunctivae. *Klin. Mbl. Augenh.,* 1876, 14:333-51.

STEWART, DOUGLAS HUNT (American physician, 1860-1930)

Morgagni-Stewart-Morel syndrome. See *under Morgagni.*

Stewart-Morel syndrome. See *Morgagni-Stewart-Morel syndrome.*

STEWART, FRED WALDORF (American physician, born 1894)

Stewart-Treves syndrome (STS). Synonyms: *postmastectomy angiosarcoma, postmastectomy lymphangiosarcoma, postmastectomy lymphedema.*

A tumor in lymphadenomatous extremities following lymph node excision. The incidence appears to be higher in females owing to the higher rate of postoperative lymphedema as a result of mastectomy in breast cancer, but males are also affected. Tumors are identified by some writers as lymphangiosarcoma, but they

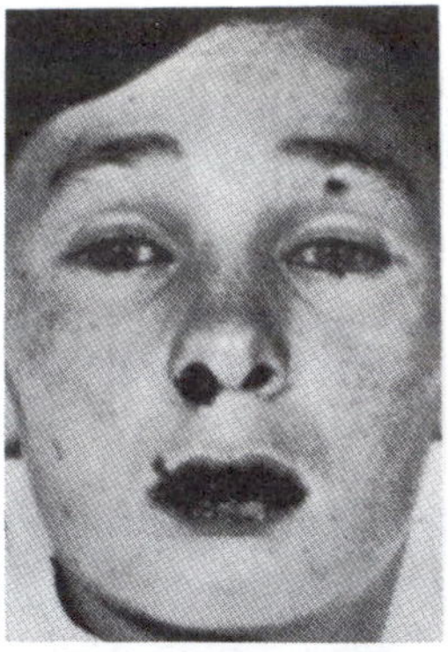

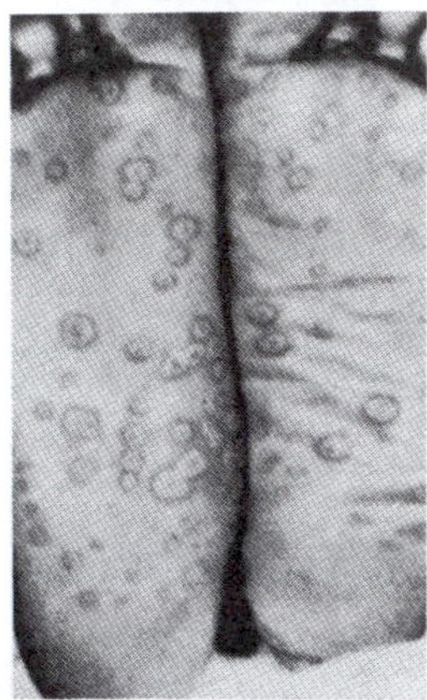

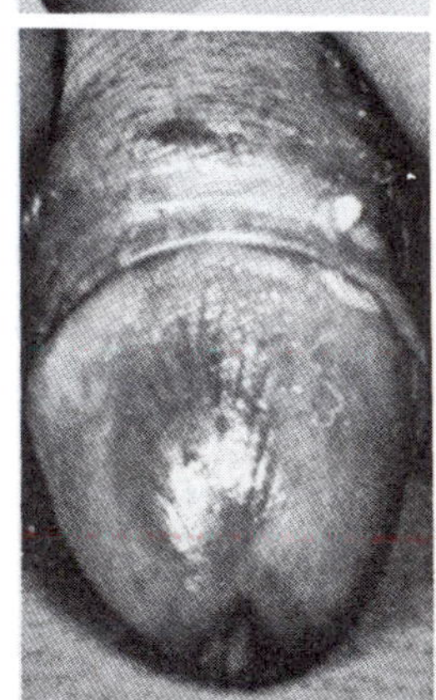

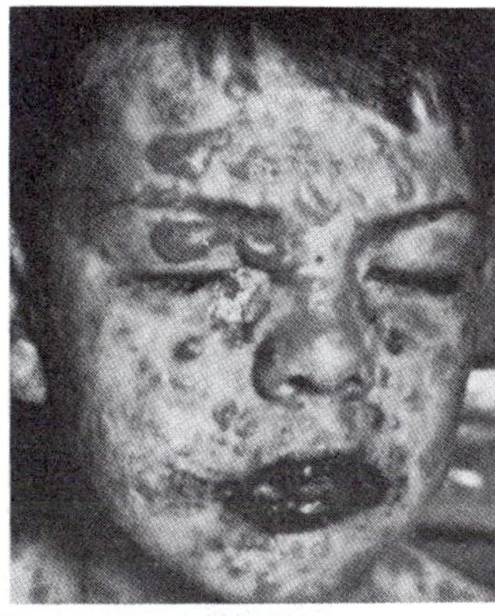

Stevens-Johnson syndrome
Pillsbury, D.M., W.B. Shelley & A.M. Kligman: *Dermatology.* Philadelphia: W.B. Saunders Co., 1956.

are more often classified under the broader group of angiosarcoma.

Stewart, F. W., & Treves, N. Lymphangiosarcoma in postmastectomy lymphedema. A report of 6 cases in elephantiasis chirurgica. *Cancer,* 1948, 1:64-81.

STEWART, J. P. (British physician)

Stewart granuloma. See *Stewart syndrome.*

Stewart syndrome. Synonyms: *Stewart granuloma, progressive granulomatous ulceration of the nose.*

A lethal condition, occurring most frequently in adult males, characterized by progressive destruction of the face, nose, and pharynx by a granulomatous ulcerative lesion of the midline of the face. Bouts of fever and severe hemorrhage are usually associated. Most patients die within 2 years from the onset of symptoms. See also *Wegener granulomatosis.*

Stewart, J. P. Progressive lethal granulomatous ulceration of the nose. *J. Laryng. Otol., London,* 1933, 48:657-701.

STEWART, JANET M. (American physician)

Stewart-Bergstrom syndrome. Synonyms: *arthrogryposis-like anomaly-sensorineural deafness syndrome, camptodactyly-sensorineural hearing loss syndrome.*

An association of camptodactyly and sensorineural hearing loss, originally reported in a family in which 12 persons in five generations were affected. Abnormal dermatoglyphics and wasting of the thenar, hypothenar, and interosseous muscles are associated. The syndrome is transmitted as an autosomal dominant trait.

Stewart, J. M., & Bergstrom, L. Familial hand abnormality and sensori-neural deafness. A new syndrome. *J. Pediat.,* 1971, 78:102-10.

STEWART, T. G. (British physician)

Stewart-Holmes syndrome. Cerebellar lesions associated with epileptic fits, usually manifested by jerking movements of one arm, sometimes also affecting the other arm.

*Stewart, T. C., & Holmes, G. Symptomatology of cerebellar tumors: A study of forty cases. *Brain,* 1904, 27:522-91.

STEWART, W. M.

Bluefarb-Stewart syndrome. See *under Bluefarb.*

STICKER, GEORG (German physician, 1860-1960)

Sticker disease. Synonyms: *erythema infectiosum, fifth eruptive disease, infectious erythema, megalerythema epidemicum, megalerythema infectiosum, scarlatinosis, slapped cheek syndrome.*

An infectious skin disease characterized by an erythematous rash over the malar prominence, which spreads over the arms, thighs, and buttocks, and occasionally over the trunk. The disease is epidemic and occurs most frequently in children. The course varies from 2 to 24 days. See also *Hutinel disease (1)..*

Sticker, G. Die neue Kinderseuche in der Umgebung von Giessen (Erythema infectiosum). *Zschr. Prakt. Arzte,* 1899, 8:353-8.

STICKLER, GUNNAR B. (American pediatrician)

Stickler syndrome. Synonyms: *arthro-ophthalmopathy (AO), hereditary arthro-ophthalmopathy, hereditary progressive arthro-ophthalmopathy.*

A connective tissue dysplasia with pleiotropic manifestations characterized by degenerative articular changes, prominence and hyperextensibility of large joints, flat facies, cleft palate, bifid uvula, myo-

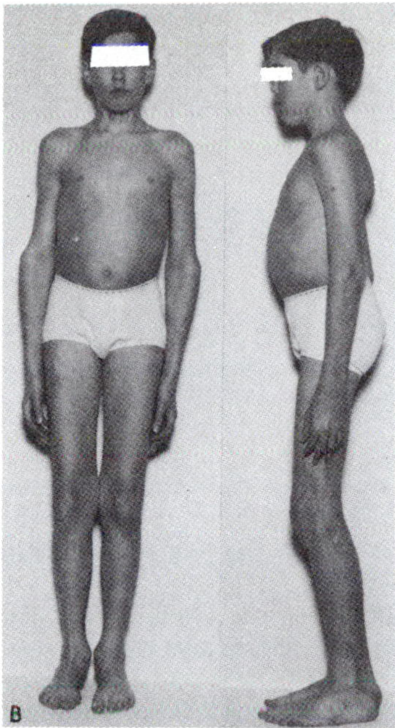

Stickler syndrome
Stickler, G.B., D.G. Pugh: Hereditary Progressive Arthroophthalmopathy. II. Additional Observations on Vertebral Abnormalities, a Hearing Defect, and a Report of a Similar Case. *Mayo Clin. Proc.* 42:495-500, 1967. By permission.

pia, spontaneous retinal detachment, cataracts, and a roentgenographic picture of mild epiphyseal dysplasia and overtubulation of long bones. The face presents slight micrognathia, slight hypertelorism, and epicanthal folds. Hearing loss may occur. The syndrome is transmitted as an autosomal dominant trait with variable expressivity and incomplete penetrance.

Stickler, G. B., *et al.* Hereditary progressive arthro-ophthalmopathy. *Mayo Clin. Proc.*, 1965, 40:433-55.

STIEDA, ALFRED (German physician, 1869-1945)

Köhler-Stieda-Pellegrini syndrome. See *Stieda-Pellegrini syndrome.*

Stieda disease. See *Stieda-Pellegrini syndrome.*

Stieda fracture. See *Stieda-Pellegrini syndrome.*

Stieda-Pellegrini syndrome. Synonyms: *Köhler-Stieda-Pellegrini syndrome, Pellegrini disease, Stieda disease, Stieda fracture.*

Traumatic calcification of the collateral tibial ligament, sometimes occurring as a complication of athletic injuries.

Stieda, A. Über eine typische Verletzung am unteren Femurende. *Arch. Klin. Chir., Berlin,* 1908, 85:815-26. *Pellegrini, A. Ossificazione traumatica del ligamento collaterale tibiale dell'articolazione del ginocchio sinistro. *Clin. Moderna,* 1905, 11:283-8. *Köhler, A. *Die normale und pathologische Anatomie des Hüftgelenkes und Oberschenkels in röntgenograpischer Darstallung.* Hamburg, 1905, p. 140.

stiff baby syndrome. See *hereditary startle syndrome.*

stiff man syndrome. Synonyms: *Moersch-Woltman syndrome (MWS), generalized muscle rigidity syndrome, stiff person syndrome.*

A syndrome, affecting both males and females and characterized by prodromal intermittent aching and tightness of the axial muscles, which progresses to generalized, usually symmetrical stiffness involving the extremities, neck, and trunk. Physical and emotional stimuli precipitate the attacks of paroxysms of painful muscle spasms, which usually last several minutes and may cause fractures. Electromyographic findings show the tonic contraction in a constant firing of impulses, which continues even at rest and is unaffected by attempts of relaxation. Profuse sweating and tachycardia are usually associated. Muscle histology is normal. The hereditary form of the syndrome is transmitted as an autosomal dominant trait, and is characterized by attacks of stiffness precipitated by surprise or minor physical contact, difficulty in sudden movements, the presence of the electromyographic counterpart of the stiffness, continuous activity at rest with normal action potentials, and disappearance of the continuous electrical activity after the administration of diazepam. Onset takes place in infancy with gradual amelioration during the life span. See also *hereditary startle syndrome* and *jerking stiff man syndrome.*

Moersch, F. P., & Woltman, H. W. Progressive fluctuating muscular rigidity and spasm (stiff-man syndrome): Report of a case and some observations in 13 other cases. *Proc. Staff. Meet. Mayo Clin.,* 1956, 31: 421-7. Klein, R., *et al.* Familial congenital disorder resembling stiff-man syndrome. *Am. J. Dis. Child.,* 1972, 124:730-31.

stiff man-myoclonus syndrome. See *jerking stiff-man syndrome.*

stiff person syndrome. See *stiff man syndrome.*

stiff skin syndrome. Synonyms: *Esterly-McKusick syndrome, congenital fascial dystrophy syndrome.*

Flexion contracture of the fingers and toes, limited motion of other joints (including the vertebral column), and sclerodermatoid changes of the skin, giving it stonelike hardness in localized areas, are the principal features of this syndrome. Biopsy of the affected skin shows abnormal amounts of hyaluronidase-digestible acid mucopolysaccharide in the dermis. The occurrence of this disorder in a mother and two children in the original report suggests an autosomal dominant mode of inheritance.

Pichler, E. Hereditäre Kontrakturen mit sklerodermieartigen Hautverahderungen. *Zschr. Kinderheilk.,* 1968, 104:349-61. Esterly, N. B., & McKusick, V. A. Stiff skin syndrome. *Pediatrics,* 1971, 47:360-9.

STILL, SIR GEORGE FREDERICK (British physician, 1868-1941)

Chauffard-Still syndrome. See *Still syndrome.*

Still arthritis. See *Still syndrome.*

Still disease (SD). See *Still syndrome.*

Still syndrome. Synonyms: *Chauffard-Ramon syndrome, Chauffard-Still syndrome, Dreier syndrome, Still arthritis, Still disease (SD), Still-Chauffard-Felty syndrome, arthritis deformans juvenilis, juvenile rheumatoid arthritis, progressive spleno-adenomegalic polyarthritis, systemic onset juvenile rheumatoid arthritis.*

Juvenile rheumatoid arthritis of unknown etiology, beginning in childhood or early adolescence, and characterized by intense arthralgias, swelling and edema of the joints, limitation of movement, anemia, spiking fever, erythematous macular or maculopapular rash, lymph node enlargement, hepatosplenomegaly, sore throat, leukocytosis, weakness, weight loss, and ocular complications, including decreased tear formation, uveitis, scleromalacia perforans, macular edema, choroiditis, papillitis, and keratopathy. Associated disorders may include pneumonia, pericarditis, leukocytosis, increased erythrocyte sedimentation rate, and increased serum glycoproteins and plasma fibrinogen.

Still, G. F. On a form of chronic joint disease in children. *Med. Chir. Tr. Roy. Med. Chir. Soc. London*, 1897, 80:47-59. Chauffard, A. & Ramon, F. Des adénopathies dans le rheumatisme chronic infectieux. *Rev. Méd., Paris*, 1896, 16:345-59.

Still-Chauffard-Felty syndrome. See *Still syndrome, and see Felty syndrome.*

STILLER, BERTHOLD (Hungarian physician, 1837-1922)

Stiller asthenia. Synonyms: *Stiller disease, Stiller habitus, asthenia universalis, habitus asthenicus, morbus asthenicus.*

A condition usually observed in tall and slender individuals, which is characterized by constitutional visceroptosis, neurasthenic tendency, vasomotor weakness, and gastrointestinal atonia.

Stiller, B. *Die asthenische Konstitutionskrankheit (Asthenia universalis congenita, Morbus asthenicus).* Stuttgart, Enke, 1907.

Stiller disease. See *Stiller asthenia.*

Stiller habitus. See *Stiller asthenia.*

STILLING, JAKOB (German ophthalmologist, 1842-1915)

Stilling syndrome. See *Stilling-Türk-Duane syndrome.*

Stilling-Türk-Duane syndrome. Synonyms: *Duane radial dysplasia syndrome, Duane retraction syndrome, Duane syndrome, Mengel bilateral deficiency of abduction, Stilling syndrome, Türk syndrome, Türk-Stilling syndrome, bulbus retractus syndrome, congenital abduction deficiency (CAD), ocular retraction syndrome, retractio bulbi, retraction syndrome.*

A congenital syndrome of ocular and systemic abnormalities that affects females more frequently than males. The affected eye shows complete or, less often, partial absence of abduction and partial or, rarely, complete absence of adduction. On abduction, the affected eye retracts into the orbit, moves in a sharply oblique manner either up and in or down and in, and shows pseudoptosis. There is also paresis or marked deficiency of convergence, the affected eye remaining fixed in the primary position while the unaffected eye is converging. Radiological findings are similar to those seen in the Holt-Oram syndrome and may include triphalangeal or fingerlike thumbs, extra carpal bones, and thumb hypoplasia. The Klippel-Feil deformity, meningocele, scoliosis, and radio-ulnar synostosis may be associated. Supranuclear lesions and aplasia of the abducens nerve with substitute innervation of the lateral rectus muscle were suggested as possible etiologic factors. Autosomal dominant inheritance is suspected. This condition, when associated with cervical spine and radial ray abnormalities and deafness, is known as the *Okihiro syndrome.*

Stilling, J. *Untersuchungen über die Entstehung der Kurzsichtigkeit.* Wiesbaden, Bergmann, 1887. Türk, S. Über Retraktionsbewegungen der Augen. *Deut., Med. Wschr.*, 1896, 22:199. Duane, A. Congenital deficiency of abduction, associated with impairment of adduction, retraction movements, contraction of the palpebral fissure and oblique movements of the eye. *Arch. Ophth., Chicago*, 1905, 34:133-59.

Türk-Stilling syndrome. See *Stilling-Türk-Duane syndrome.*

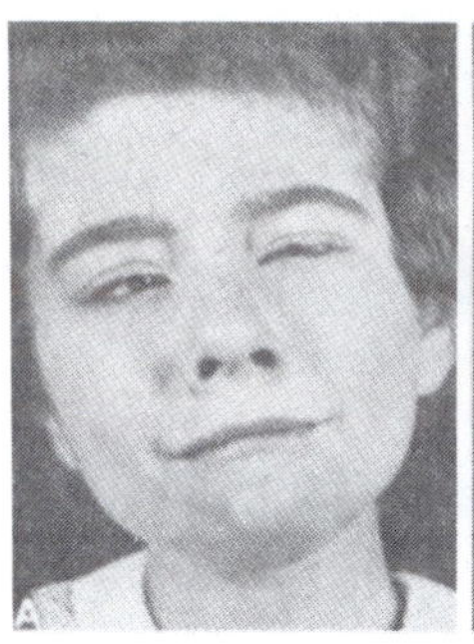

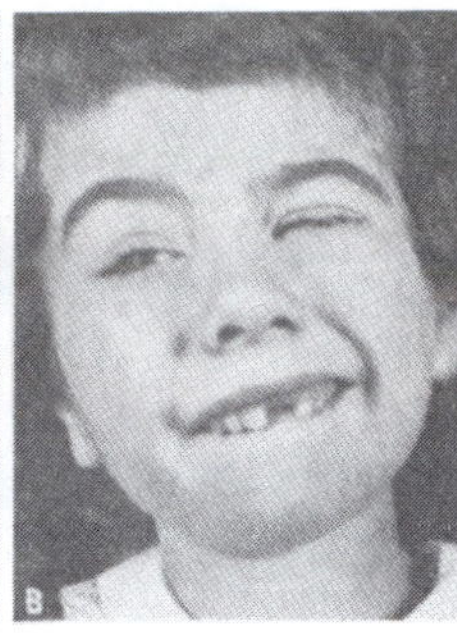

Stilling-Türk-Duane syndrome
Nelson, W.E. (ed.): *Textbook of Pediatrics* 8th ed. Philadelphia: W.B. Saunders Co., 1964.

stippled epiphyses. See *Conradi-Hünermann syndrome, under Conradi, Erich.*

STOCK, WOLFGANG (German physician, born 1876)

Stock-Spielmeyer-Vogt syndrome. Synonyms: *Batten disease, Batten-Mayou syndrome, Vogt-Spielmeyer syndrome, cerebromacular degeneration, cerebromacular dystrophy, juvenile amaurotic familial idiocy, juvenile ganglioside lipidosis, neuronal ceroid lipofuscinosis (NCL), pigmentary retinal neuronal heredodegeneration.*

A juvenile form of amaurotic familial idiocy characterized by cerebroretinal degeneration beginning between the ages of 5 and 6 years. Progressive blindness results from the ocular lesions, which include pathological changes in the retinal rods and cones in addition to ganglion cells, optic atrophy, pigmentary degeneration of the retina, loss of the foveal reflex, gray-brown discoloration of the macula, and threadlike retinal vessels. Diffuse cerebral lesions are manifested by mental deterioration, behavior changes, emotional problems, speech disorders, lack of attention, uncontrolled laughter or weeping, poor memory, restlessness, convulsions, muscle wasting, and rigidity. Death takes place within 10 to 15 years after onset. Brain and rectal biopsies show nerve cells which are heavily laden with lipid and accumulation of lipofuscin in the neuronal perikaryon. The syndrome is transmitted as an autosomal recessive trait.

Vogt, H. Über familiäre amaurotische Idiotie und verwandte Krankheitsbilder. *Mschr. Psychiat.*, 1905, 18:161-71; 310-57. *Spielmeyer, W. Klinische und anatomische Untersuchungen über einen besonderen Fall von amaurotischer Idiotie. *Nissls Beitr. Nerv. Geistes Krkh., Berlin*, 1908. Batten, F. E. Cerebral degeneration with symmetrical changes in the maculae in two members of a family. *Tr. Ophth. Soc. U. K.*, 1903, 23:386-90. Mayou, M. S. Cerebral degeneration with symmetrical changes in the maculae, in three members of a family. *Tr. Ophth. Soc. U. K.*, 1904, 24:142-5. Stock, W. Über eine bis jetzt noch nicht beschriebene Form der familiär auftretenden Netzhautdegeneration bei bleichzeitiger Verblödung und über Pigmentdegeneration der Netzhaut. *Klin. Mbl. Augenh.*, 1908, 5:225-44.

STOCKER, F. W. (Swiss physician)

Stocker line. A brownish or yellowish pigmented line occurring ahead of the advancing edge of a pterygium, attributed to a tear in the Bowman membrane and hemosiderin deposits.

Stocker, F. Eine pigmentierte Hornhautline bei Pterygium. *Schweiz. Med. Wschr.*, 1939, 69:19.

Stockholm syndrome. The positive feelings of the captives toward their captors that are accompanied by negative feeling toward the police. The syndrome was first described in a group of young men and women taken hostages by a bank robber in Stockholm.

Strentz, T. The Stockholm syndrome: Law enforcement policy and ego defenses of the hostage. *Ann. N. Y. Acad. Sc.*, 1980, 347:137-50.

STOJANO, C. (Argentine physician)

Stojano subcostal syndrome. See *Fitz-Hugh syndrome.*

STOKES, WILLIAM (Irish physician, 1804-1878)

Adams-Stokes (AS) syndrome. See *under Adams, Robert.*

Adams-Stokes disease. See *Adams-Stokes syndrome, under Adams, Robert.*

Adams-Stokes syncope. See *Adams-Stokes syndrome, under Adams-Robert.*

Cheyne-Stokes respiration (CSR). See *under Cheyne, John.*

Morgagni-Adams-Stokes (MAS) syndrome. See *Adams-Stokes syndrome, under Adams, Robert.*

Stokes syndrome. See *Adams-Stokes syndrome, under Adams, Robert.*

Stokes-Adams (SA) syndrome. See *Adams-Stokes syndrome.*

STOKVIS, BAREND J. (Dutch physician, 1834-1902)

Stokvis-Talma syndrome. Synonyms: *van den Bergh disease, autotoxic cyanosis, enterogenic cyanosis, idiopathic methemoglobinemia, sulfhemoglobinemia.*

An association of cyanosis, enteritis, and clubbing of the fingers due to methemoglobinemia, occurring in the presence of sulfhemoglobin produced by substances entering the body through the gastrointestinal tract. A congenital variant is known as the *Gibson syndrome.*

Stokvis, B. J. Bijdrage tot de casuistiek der autotoxische enterogene cyanosen (methaemoglobinaemia?) et enteritis parasitaria. *Ned. Tschr. Geneesk.*, 1902, 38:678-93. Talma, S. Intraglobuläre Methämoglobinämie beim Menschen. *Berlin. Klin. Wschr.*, 1902, 39:865-7. Bergh, A. A. H., van den. Enterogene Cyanose. *Deut. Arch. Klin. Med.*, 1905, 83:86-106.

STOLOFF, E. GORDON (American physician)

Kugel-Stoloff syndrome. See *under Kugel.*

stomatitis herpetica. See *Zahorsky syndrome (2).*

stomatitis vesiculosa cum exanthemata. See *hand-foot-and-mouth syndrome.*

stone heart syndrome. Synonym: *ischemic contracture of the heart.*

Irreversible cardiac failure due to ischemic myocardial contracture wherein the heart becomes small and frozen in systole.

Cooley, D. A., *et al.* Ischemic contraction of the heart: "Stone heart." *Am. J. Cardiol.*, 1972, 29:575-7.

stone-carrier paralysis. See *Rieder paralysis.*

STOUT, A. P. (American physician)

Gorham-Stout syndrome. See *Gorham syndrome.*

STOVIN, PETER GEORGE INGLE (British physician)

Hughes-Stovin syndrome. See *under Hughes.*

strabismus of the penis. See *Peyronie disease.*

STRACHAN, WILLIAM HENRY (British physician, 1857-1921)

Strachan syndrome. Synonyms: *Strachan-Scott syndrome, amblyopia-pain neuropathy-orogenital dermatitis syndrome, camp dizziness, Jamaican neuropathy.*

A neurologic disorder of the peripheral and optic nerves, characterized mainly by paresthesia, painful hyperesthesia of the feet, loss of deep and superficial sensations, and ataxia. Associated symptoms may include blindness and pallor of the optic discs, deafness, vertigo, hyporeflexia, angular stomatitis (perlèche), glossitis, scrotal dermatitis, loss of pain and temperature sensation, and less often, drop foot and muscle weakness and atrophy. Pathological findings include damage to the papillomacular bundle of the optic nerve and demyelination of the fibers of the posterior column of the spinal cord. The disorder is due to a nutritional deficiency, the specific agent missing in the food being undetermined. The Jamaican poor were the first individuals in whom this condition was observed. It was later reported in the besieged population of Madrid during the Spanish Civil War, among prisoners of war during World II, and in undernourished populations of Africa and Asia. According to some writers, this and the Landor-Pallister syndrome are the same entity.

Strachan, H. On a form of multiple neuritis prevalent in the West Indies. *Practitioner, London,* 1897, 59:477-84. Scott, H. H. An investigation into an acute outbreak of "central neuritis." *Ann. Trop. Med., Liverpool,* 1918-19, 12:109-96.

Strachan-Scott syndrome. See *Strachan syndrome.*

straight back syndrome. Synonyms: *Rawlings syndrome, flat chest syndrome.*

A syndrome of abnormal curvature of the upper dorsal spine with a narrow anteroposterior diameter of the chest and apparent compression and displacement to the left of the heart, in association with a systolic murmur of the base of the heart, originally believed to be due to torsion of the great vessels. X-ray findings show heart enlargement. Straight back is sometimes associated with the mitral valve prolapse syndrome in which systolic clicks and murmur arise from a floppy mitral valve.

Rawlings, M. S. The "straight back" syndrome. A new cause of pseudoheart disease. *Am. J. Cardiol.*, 1960, 5:333-8. Straight back syndrome. *Lancet,* 1981, 1:540 (Editorial).

STRANDBERG, JAMES VICTOR (Norwegian physician, born 1883)

Darier-Grönblad-Strandberg syndrome. See *pseudoxanthoma elasticum.*

Grönblad-Strandberg syndrome. See *pseudoxanthoma elasticum.*

Grönblad-Strandberg-Touraine syndrome. See *pseudoxanthoma elasticum.*

STRANG, LEONARD B. (British physician)

Smith-Strang syndrome. See *methionine malabsorption syndrome.*

STRANSKY, EUGENE (Austrian-born American physician)

Stransky-Regala syndrome. Chronic familial hemolytic anemnia characterized by extreme erythroblastosis of the bone marrow with a preponderance of immature erythroblasts. After splenectomy, the anemia changes in character, becoming macrocytic and hyperchromic. Initially, the disease was observed among the Filipinos.

Stransky, E.., & Regala, A. C. A new type of familial

congenital chronic hemolytic anemia. *Am. J. Dis. Child.*, 1946, 71:492-505.

STRASBURGER, ARTHUR K. (American physician)

Strasburger-Hawkins-Eldridge syndrome. See *symphalangism syndrome.*

Strasburger-Hawkins-Eldridge-Hargrave-McKusick syndrome. See *symphalangism syndrome.*

STRAUSS, ALFRED A. (American psychiatrist)

Strauss syndrome. A form of cerebral dysfunction in children, manifested by hyperactivity, attentional aberrations (ranging from short attention span to perseveration), impulsivity, emotional lability, easy distractibility, and easy frustration. Lying, fire setting, and cruelty to animals are seen in some cases.

Strauss, A. A., & Lehtinen, L. E. *Psychopathology and education of the brain-injured child.* Grune & Stratton, New York, 1947.

STRAUSS, LOTTE (American physician)

Churg-Strauss syndrome (CSS). See *under Churg.*

Churg-Strauss vasculitis. See *Churg-Strauss syndrome.*

Strauss-Churg-Zak syndrome. See *Churg-Strauss syndrome.*

STRÄUSSLER, E. (Austrian physician)

Gerstmann-Sträussler disease (GSD). See *Gerstmann syndrome (1).*

Gerstmann-Sträussler syndrome (GSS). See *Gerstmann syndrome (1).*

Gerstmann-Sträussler-Scheinker disease (GSSD). See *Gerstmann syndrome (1).*

streaked ovary syndrome. See *Slotnick-Goldfarb syndrome.*

streblodactyly. See *Marfan syndrome (1).*

streblomicrodactyly. See *camptodactyly syndrome.*

STREETER, GEORGE LINIUS (American embryologist, 1873-1948)

Streeter bands. See *amniotic band syndrome.*

Streeter dysplasia. See *amniotic band syndrome.*

STREIFF, ENRICO BERNARD (Swiss ophthalmologist, born 1908)

Hallermann-Streiff syndrome (HSS). See *under Hallermann.*

Hallermann-Streiff-François syndrome. See *Hallermann-Streiff syndrome.*

streptococcal gangrene. See *Fournier disease.*

stress syndrome. See *Selye syndrome.*

stress erythrocytosis. See *Gaisböck disease.*

stress fracture of the spinous process. See *Schmitt syndrome.*

stress gastric bleeding. See *stress ulcer syndrome.*

stress polycythemia. See *Gaisböck disease.*

stress response syndrome. See *post-traumatic stress syndrome.*

stress ulcer syndrome. A syndrome of multiple, punctate, superficial erosions, confined initially to the proximal gastric mucosa, with gastric bleeding, developing in association with some types of central nervous system injury, respiratory insufficiency, acute renal failure, and, especially, sepsis. Active bleeding is usually preceded by an increase in the volume and acidity of aspirated gastric contents, which is also bile stained. Blood coagulation disorders are frequently present.

Lucas, C. E., *et al.* Natural history of surgical dilema of "stress" gastric bleeding. *Arch. Surg.*, 1971, 102:266. Lucas, C. E.. Stress ulceration: The cllinical problem. *World J. Surg.*, 1981, 5:139-51.

striatonigral degeneration. See *Joseph disease, under Joseph, Antone.*

STROHL, ANDRE (French physician, born 1887)

Guillain-Barré-Strohl syndrome. See *Guillain-Barré syndrome.*

STROM, ROAR (Norwegian physician)

Strom-Zollinger-Ellison syndrome. See *Zollinger-Ellison syndrome.*

STRONG, WILLIAM B. (American physician)

Strong syndrome. Synonym: *right-sided aortic archmental retardation-facial dysmorphism syndrome.*

A triad of mental retardation, right-sided aorta, and craniofacial defects, transmitted as an autosomal dominant trait. Right-sided aorta is associated with posterior vascular indentation on the esophagus, heart murmur, abnormal ECG, abnormal x-ray picture of the heart, and unequal blood pressure in the arms. Craniofacial dysmorphism consists of peculiar facies marked by hypoplasia of the maxilla, beaklike nose, antimongoloid palpebral slant, posteriorly rotated large ears, microcephaly, broad forehead, small mouth with down-turned corners, facial asymmetry, long upper lip, and nasal septum deviation.

Strong, W. Familial syndrome of right-sided aortic arch, mental deficiency, and facial dysmorphism. J. Pediat., 1968, 73:882-8.

STRÜBING, PAUL (German physician, born 1852)

Strübing-Marchiafava syndrome. See *Marchiafava-Micheli syndrome.*

struma granulomatosa. See de Quervain disease (2), under Quervain, Fritz, de.

struma lymphomatosa. See *Hashimoto disease.*

struma suprarenalis cystica hemorrhagica. See *Grawitz tumor.*

strumitis fibrosa. See *Riedel disease.*

STRÜMPELL, ERNST ADOLF GUSTAV GOTTFRIED, VON (German physician, 1853-1925)

Bechterew-Strümpell-Marie syndrome. See *under Bekhterev.*

Fleischer-Strümpell ring. See *Kayser-Fleischer ring, under Kayser, Bernhard.*

Marie-Strümpell disease. See *Bechterew-Strümpell-Marie syndrome, under Bekhterev.*

Strümpell disease (1). Synonyms: *acute polioencephalitis, cerebral infantile paralysis.*

The cerebral form of poliomyelitis.

Strümpell, A. Über die acute Encephalitis der Kinder (Polioencephalitis acuta, cerebrale Kinderlähmung). *Jahrb. Kinderh.*, 1884-85, 22:173-8.

Strümpell disease (2). See *Erb-Charcot syndrome, under Erb, Wilhelm Ernst.*

Strümpell-Lichtenstern encephalitis. Synonym: *acute primary hemorrhagic encephalitis.*

Acute hemorrhagic encephalitis characterized by necrosis, hemorrhage, and demyelination of the white matter. The symptoms include fever, headache, cough, stupor, confusion, disorientation, hallucinations, hemihypesthesia, hemiparesis, quadriplegia, facial paralysis, nuchal rigidity, diplopia, papilledema, and dysphasia.

Strümpell, A. Über primäre acute Encephalitis. *Deut. Arch. Klin. Med.*, 1890, 47:53-74. Lichtenstern. Über primäre acute haemorrhagische Encephalitis. *Deut. Med. Wschr.*, 1892, 18:39-40.

Strümpell-Lorrain disease. Synonym: *familial spastic paraplegia.*

A familial form of paraplegia of young adults, in which spasticity is limited mainly to the lower extremities. Degeneration of the pyramidal tract of the spinal cord and of the columns of Goll is the principal histological feature. Ocular complications may include strabismus, pupillary defects, macular degeneration, and optic atrophy. The disorder is transmitted as an autosomal dominant or recessive trait.

Strümpell, A. Beiträge zur Pathologie des Rückenmarks. *Arch. Psychiat., Berlin*, 1880, 10:676-717. *Lorrain, M. *Contribution a l'étude de la paraplégie splasmodique familiale.* Paris, 1898. (Thesis).

Westphal-Strümpell syndrome. See *Wilson disease, under Wilson, Samuel Alexander Kinnier.*

STRYKER, GAROLD V. (American physician, born 1896)

Stryker-Halbeisen syndrome. Synonyms: *deficiency dermatosis, erythroderma-macrocytic anemia syndrome, nutritional dermatosis.*

An association of macrocytic anemia with vitamin B complex deficiency dermatosis, marked by erythroderma of the neck, face, shoulders, chest, and periaxillary areas, that is evanescent, patchy, or diffuse, superficial, pruritic, scaly and dry, or vesicular. In advanced stages, the patches lose their evanescent character and become confluent and the vesiculation tends to disappear. The skin then becomes edematous and slightly thickened.

Stryker, G. V., & Halbeisen, W. A. Determination of macrocytic anemia as an aid in diagnosis of certain deficiency dermatoses. *Arch. Derm. Syph., Chicago*, 1945, 51:116-23.

STS. See *Stewart-Treves syndrome, under Stewart, Fred W.*

STS (sinus tarsi syndrome). See *tarsal sinus syndrome.*

STUART

Stuart defect. See *Stuart-Prower factor deficiency.*

Stuart factor deficiency. See *Stuart-Prower factor deficiency.*

Stuart-Prower factor deficiency. Synonyms: *Prower defect, Prower factor deficiency, Stuart defect, Stuart factor deficiency, factor X deficiency, hereditary factor X deficiency.*

A genetically determined blood coagulation disorder characterized by a deficiency of factor X (known as the Stuart or Prower factor after Mr. Stuart and Miss Prower in whom the factor was first discovered), which occurs in both males and females, and is transmitted as an autosomal recessive trait. The manifestations depend on the degree of depression of factor X and may include moderate to severe bleeding following injury, with rare spontaneous epistaxis, hemarthroses, and gingival hemorrhage.

Telfer, T. P., *et al.* A "new" coagulation defect. *Brit. J. Haemat.*, 1956, 2:308. Hougie, C., & Graham, J. B. The blood clotting role and mode of inheritance of the Stuart factor. A new clotting factor distinct from SPCA. *Bibl. Haemat.*, 1956, Fasc. 7:80. Hougie, C. Hemophilia and related conditions-congenital deficiencies of prothrombin (factor II), factor V, and factors VII to XII. In: Williams, W. J., Beutler, E., Erslev, A.. J., & Lichtman, M. A., eds. *Hematology.* 3rd ed. New York, McGraw-Hill, 1983 , pp.1381-99.

STUART, KENNETH LAMONT (British physician)

Stuart-Bras disease. Synonym: *veno-occlusive disease of the liver.*

A liver disease occurring in the West Indies. The acute stage is characterized by the sudden development of hepatomegaly and ascites, usually in children between 1 and 6 years of age. The primary lesion is a widespread occlusion of the smaller- and medium-sized branches of the hepatic veins, with sinusoidal congestion and pressure necrosis of the parenchymal cells around the central veins. Cirrhosis around the central veins may follow. In the subacute stage, there is persistent, often symptomless, hepatomegaly. The chronic stage may be almost indistinguishable from cirrhosis due to other causes. The etiology is unknown, but plant toxins, especially of "bush tea," *Senecio*, and *Crotalaria retusa*, are suspected.

Stuart, K. L., & Bras, G. Veno-occlusive disease of the liver. *Q. J. Med.*, 1957, 26:291-315.

stub thumb. See *brachydactyly D.*

STUHL, I. (French physician)

Weismann-Netter and Stuhl syndrome. See *Weismann-Netter syndrome.*

STURGE, WILLIAM ALLEN (British physician, 1850-1919)

Sturge disease. See *Sturge-Weber syndrome.*

Sturge syndrome. See *Sturge-Weber syndrome.*

Sturge-Weber anomalad. See *Sturge-Weber syndrome.*

Sturge-Weber syndrome (SWS). Synonyms: *Jahnke syndrome, Kalischer syndrome, Lawford syndrome, Miller syndrome, Parkes Weber syndrome, Parkes Weber-Dimitri syndrome, Schirmer syndrome, Sturge disease, Sturge syndrome, Sturge-Weber anomalad, Sturge-Weber-Dimitri syndrome, Sturge-Weber-Krabbe syndrome, Sturge-Weber-Thoma syndrome, Weber syndrome, Weber-Dimitri syndrome, angioma capillare et venosum calcificans, angiomatosis encephalofacialis, cerebrocutaneous angiomatosis, angiomatosis meningo-ulofacialis, congenital neuroectodermal dysplasia, cutaneocerebral angioma, cutaneocerebral angioma, ectoneurodermal hamartoma, encephalofacial angiomatosis, encephalofacial neuroangiomatosis, encephalotrigeminal angiomatosis, encephalotrigeminal syndrome, meningeal capillary angiomatosis, meningo-oculofacial angiomatosis, neuroangiomatosis encephalofacialis, neurocutaneous syndrome, neuroectodermal hamartoma, neuro-oculocutaneous angiomatosis, nevoid amentia, trigemino-encephalo-angiomatosis.*

A congenital syndrome of venous angiomatosis of the leptomeninges, ipsilateral facial angiomatosis and gyriform calcifications of the cerebral cortex, seizures, mental deficiency, hemiplegia, and ocular involvement, including choroid lesions with secondary glaucoma and buphthalmos. Intraoral angiomata usually affect the buccal mucosa, lips (causing macrocheilia), and, occasionally, the palate, tongue (with hemihypertrophy), and gingivae. Most cases are sporadic.

*Sturge, W. A. Case of partial epilepsy apparently due to lesions of one of vasomotor centers of the brain. *Tr. Clin. Soc. London*, 1879, 12:162-7. Weber, F. P. Right-sided hemihypotrophy resulting from right-sided congenital spastic hemiplegia, with morbid condition of left side of brain, revealed by radiograms. *J. Neur. Psychopath.*, 1922, 3:134-9. Brushfield, T., & Wyatt, W. Sturge-Weber disease. *Br. J. Child. Dis.*, 1927, 24:98-106; 1928, 25:96-101. Dimitri, V. Tumor cerebral congénito (angioma cavernosum). *Rev. Asoc. Med. Argentina*, 1923, 36:1029. Krabbe, K. H. Facial and meningeal angiomatosis associated with calcifications of the brain cortex, a clinical and an anatomopathologic contribution. *Arch. Neur. Psychiat.*, 1934, 32:737-55. Kalischer, S. Ein Fall von Telangiektasie (Angiom) des Gesichts und der weichen Hirnhäute. *Arch. Psychiat., Berlin*, 1901, 34:171-80. Miller, S. J. Ophthalmic aspects of the Sturge-Weber syndrome. *Proc. Roy. Soc. Med.*, 1965, 56:419-21. Schirmer, R. Ein Fall von Telangiektasie. *Albrecht von Graefes Arch. Ophth.*, 1860, 7:119-21. Thoma, K. H. Sturge-Kalischer-Weber syndrome with pregnancy tumors. *Oral Surg.*, 1952, 5:1124-31.

Sturge-Weber-Dimitri syndrome. See *Sturge-Weber syndrome.*

Sturge-Weber-Krabbe syndrome. See *Sturge-Weber syndrome.*

Sturge-Weber-Thoma syndrome. See *Sturge-Weber syndrome.*

stylet injury syndrome. Failure to properly use the stylet when withdrawing a spinal puncture needle, causing aspiration of the lumbar nerve root and adjacent arachnoid, thereby fixing the nerve in the epidural space with resulting painful complications.

Trupp, M. Stylet injury syndrome. *JAMA*, 1977, 237:2524.

stylohyoid syndrome. See *Eagle syndrome, under Eagle, Watt Weems.*

styloid syndrome. See *Eagle syndrome, under Eagle, Watt Weems.*

styloid elongation syndrome. See *Eagle syndrome, under Eagle, Watt Weems.*

styloid process syndrome. See *Eagle syndrome, under Eagle, Watt Weems.*

styloid process-carotid artery syndrome. See *Eagle syndrome, under Eagle, Watt Weems.*

styloid-stylohyoid syndrome. See *Eagle syndrome, under Eagle, Watt Weems.*

Styx syndrome. A psychological condition in patients who have recovered from shock after intramuscular penicillin therapy (Hoigné syndrome), characterized by a feeling that they have returned to life after being at the gate of death, or on the banks of the river Styx.

Vacek, J., & Calková, M. Psychopathologische Reaktionen nach Depot-Penicillin. "Hoigné-Syndrom." *Psychiat. Neur. Med. Psychol., Leipzig*, 1982, 10:602-9.

subacromial bursitis. See *Duplay bursitis.*

subacromial impingement syndrome. See *shoulder impingement syndrome.*

subacute combined degeneration of the spinal cord. See *Dana syndrome.*

subacute combined sclerosis. See *Dana syndrome.*

subacute disseminated histiocytosis X. See *Letterer-Siwe syndrome.*

subacute granulomatous thyroiditis. See *de Quervain disease (2), under Quervain, Fritz, de.*

subacute milk poisoning. See *milk-alkali syndrome.*

subacute myelo-optico neuropathy (SMON) syndrome. A neurotoxic reaction to clioquinol, characterized by subacute myelopathy, optic neuropathy, and peripheral neuropthy occurring in various combinations. Persistent symmetrical dysenthesia usually affecting the legs and trunk is a common feature. Motor involvement is less common, and consists mainly of spastic ataxic paraparesis or, rarely, hypotonic weakness in the lower limbs. Bilateral visual impairment, sometimes resulting in blindness, occurs is some cases. Additional symptoms may include abdominal disorders (pain and diarrhea), consciousness disorders, convulsions, pyramidal signs, hyperreflexia of the lower limbs, the Babinski sign, sphincter disorders of the rectum and bladder, and green tongue. Pathological findings include degenerative changes of the visual pathways, the lateral corticospinal tracts of the lower spinal cord, and the rostral portion of the gracile fasciculi. The condition was reported in various parts of the world but the Japanese appear to be most susceptible to clioquinol toxicity.

Tsubaki, T., *et al.* Subacute myelo-optic neuropthy following abdominal symptoms. A clinical pathological study. *Jpn. J. Med.*, 1965, 4:181. Proceedings from the 1983 Swedish neurotoxicology symposium. Copenhagen, Denmark, April 14-16, 1983. *Acta Neur. Scand.*, 1984, 70(Suppl. 100):1-225.

subacute necrotizing encephalomyelopathy (SNE). See *Leigh syndrome.*

subacute necrotizing myelitis. See *Foix-Alajouanine syndrome.*

subacute panniculitis nodosa migrans. See *Vilanova-Piñol Aguadé syndrome.*

subacute proximal diabetic neuropathy. See *Bruns-Garland syndrome.*

subacute sclerosing encephalopathy. See *van Bogaert encephalitis.*

subacute sclerosing leukoencephalitis. See *van Bogaert encephalitis.*

subacute sclerosing panencephalitis (SSPE). See *van Bogaert encephalitis.*

subacute spongious encephalopathy of the Heidenhain type. See *Heidenhain syndrome.*

subacute thyroiditis. See *de Quervain disease (2), under Quervain, Fritz, de.*

subarachnoid hemorrhage with vitreous hemorrhage. See *Terson syndrome.*

subbulbar syndrome. See *Opalski syndrome.*

subchorial hematoma mole. See *Breus mole.*

subchorial thrombohematoma. See *Breus mole.*

subchronic leukoencephalitis. See *Schilder disease.*

subclavian steal phenomenon. See *subclavian steal syndrome.*

subclavian steal syndrome. Synonyms: *Harrison-Smyth syndrome, subclavian steal phenomenon.*

Diversion of blood flow from the basilar artery to the subclavian artery due to occlusion of its proximal segment, resulting in cerebral ischemia. The symptoms include vertigo and/or presyncope following upper extremity exercise on the side of the occlusion. Absence of the pulse on the affected side, pain and numbness of the arm and hand, headache, and hypotension are the additional symptoms. Arteriosclerosis, thrombosis, vascular anomalies, injuries, tumors, and surgery are the principal causes.

A new vascular syndrome: "The subclavian steal." (Editorial). *N. Engl. J. Med.*, 1961, 265:912. Harrison, P. *The surgical anatomy of the arteries of the human body.* Dublin, Hodges & Smith, 1829. *Smyth, A. W. Successful operation in a case of subclavian aneurysm. *N. Orleans Med. Rec.*, 1866, 1:4.

subclinical neurogenic bladder. See *Hinman syndrome.*

subcoracoid-pectoralis minor syndrome. See *hyperabduction syndrome.*

subcorneal pustular dermatosis. See *Sneddon-Wilkinson syndrome.*

subcortical arteriosclerotic encephalopathy. See *Binswager disease.*

subcortical paraplegia. See *Binswager disease.*
subcortical vascular encephalopathy. See *Binswager disease.*
subcostal syndrome. See *Fitz-Hugh syndrome.*
subcutaneous emphysema-pneumomediastinum syndrome. See *Hamman syndrome.*
subcutaneous nodular sarcoidosis. See *Darier-Roussy sarcoid.*
subcutaneous sarcoidosis. See *Darier-Roussy sarcoid.*
subdeltoid bursitis. See *Duplay bursitis.*
subepiphyseal osteochondropathy. See *Erlacher-Blount syndrome.*
subinvolution and congestion of the ovary. See *Taylor syndrome, under Taylor, Howard Canning, Jr.*
subisthmic coarctation of aorta. See *aortic arch syndrome.*
subjective doubles syndrome. See *Capgras syndrome.*
sublingual fibrogranuloma. See *Riga-Fede disease.*
sublingual fibroma. See *Riga-Fede disease.*
submaxillary cellulitis. See *Ludwig angina.*
suboccipital vertebral disease. See *Rust disease.*
subperiosteal cortical hyperostosis. See *Caffey-Silverman syndrome.*
subphrenic displacement of the colon. See *Chilaiditi syndrome.*
subphrenic interposition syndrome. See *Chilaiditi syndrome.*
subsepsis allergica. See *Wissler syndrome.*
subsepsis hyperergica. See *Wissler syndrome.*
substance withdrawal. See *withdrawal syndrome.*
subungual melanotic whitlow. See *Hutchinson melanotic disease, under Hutchinson, Sir Jonathan.*

SUCKOW, E. E. (American physician)
Brock-Suckow polyposis. See *under Brock.*
sucrosuria-hiatus hernia-mental retardation syndrome. See *Moncrieff syndrome.*
sudanophilic leukodystrophy. See *Pelizaeus-Merzbacher syndrome.*
sudden cardiac death syndrome. Synonym: *sudden death.*

The sudden cessation of cardiac contractions resulting in death. It is most often associated with coronary artery disease, cardiomyopathies, left ventricular hypertrophy, valvular heart disease, and accessory pathways, but it may be due to other causes. Lethal ventricular arrhythmia may occur without associated cardiac pathology, sometimes as a complicataion of severe metabolic disorders.

Willerson, J. T. Sudden cardiac death. In: Wyngaarden, J. B., & Smith, L. H., Jr., eds. *Cecil textbook of medicine.* 17th ed. Philadelphia, Saunders, 1985, pp. 296-7.

sudden death. See *sudden cardiac death syndrome.*
sudden infant death syndrome (SIDS). Synonyms: *cot death, crib death.*

The sudden and unexpected death of an apparently well or almost well infant, which remains unexplained after autopsy. Sudden infant deaths occur almost entirely in the second through the fifth month of life, most infants dying at night. An otherwise normal infant suddenly turns blue, stops breathing, and becomes limp, without crying or struggling. Certain apparently trivial symptoms, such as a mild respiratory infection, are believed to be the contributing factors. See also *infant apnea syndrome, Wilson-Mikity syndrome,* and *neonatal respiratory distress syndrome.*

Bergman, A. B., Beckwith, J. B., & Ray, C. G., eds. *Proceedings of the Second International Conference on Causes of Sudden Death in Infants.* Seattle, Univ. of Washington Press, 1970. 248 pp. Valdes-Dapena, M. Sudden unexpected death in infancy (sudden infant death syndrome ([SIDS]). In: Vaughan, V. C., III, McKay, R. J., & Behrman, R. E., eds. *Nelson textbook of pediatrics.* Philadelphia, Saunders, 1979, pp. 1980-1.

sudden unexplained death syndrome (SUDS). Synonyms: *bangungot, night death, pokkuri, sudden unexplained nocturnal death syndrome.*

The death of an otherwise healthy southeast Asian male, for whom a postmortem examination does not reveal the underlying cause. The victim appears to have been subjected to a violent, terrifying dream from which he cannot be awaked; maligant ventricular arrhythmia is the cause of death. In recent years, cases of sudden unexplained death have been reported in Asian refugees in the United States.

Mendoza de Guazon, M. P. Algunas notas sobre "bangungot." *Rev. Filip. Med. Farm.,* 1917, 8:437-42. Vang Pao, *et al.* Sudden unexpected, nocturnal deaths among Southeast Asian refugees. *MMWR,* 1981, 30:581-4. Parrish, G., & Downes, D. Surveillance for sudden unexplained death syndrome. *JAMA,* 1986, 255:2893.

sudden unexplained nocturnal death syndrome. See *sudden unexplained death syndrome.*

SUDECK, PAUL HERMANN MARTIN (German physician, 1866-1945)
Sudeck atrophy. See *Sudeck syndrome.*
Sudeck porosis. See *Sudeck syndrome.*
Sudeck post-traumatic syndrome. See *Sudeck syndrome.*
Sudeck syndrome. Synonyms: *Kienböck atrophy, Leriche syndrome, Sudeck atrophy, Sudeck porosis, Sudeck post-traumatic syndrome, Sudeck-Leriche syndrome, posthemiplegic reflex sympathetic dystrophy, post-traumatic painful osteoporosis, post-traumatic spreading neuralgia, reflex bone atrophy.*

A variant of the reflex sympathetic dystrophy syndrome (q.v.) caused by injury of an extremity, and characterized by a burning pain that is exacerbated by emotional stress. Initial localized hyperalgesia causes movements of the affected limb or touching the affected site to become excruciatingly painful, gradually spreading to involve the entire extremity. Early vasodilation, whereby the affected extremity becomes warm and dry, changes to vasocontriction with the resulting production of edema, cyanosis, and cool skin. Hyperhidrosis or hypohidrosis, trophic skin disorders, and osteoporosis usually follow, eventually leading to muscle atrophy, ankylosis, and osteoporosis. The terms *Sudeck syndrome* and *reflex sympathetic dystrophy syndrome* are sometimes used synonymously.

Sudeck, P. Über die akute entzündliche Knochenatrophie. *Arch. Klin. Chir., Berlin,* 1900, 62:147-56. Kienböck, R. Über akute Knochenatrophie bei Entzündungsprozessen an den Extremitäten (fälschlich sogenannte Inaktivitätsatrophie des Knochens) und ihre Diagnose nach dem Röntgenbilde. *Wien, Med. Wschr.,* 1901, 51:1346-8; 1389-92; 1427-30; 1462-6; 1508-11; 1591-5. Leriche, R. *The surgery of pain.* (Translated by A. Young). Baltimore, Williams & Wilkins, 1939. Posner, J. B. Disorders of sensation. In: Wyngaarden, J. B., & Smith, L. H., Jr., eds. *Cecil textbook of medicine.* Philadelphia, Saunders, 1985, pp. 2063-4.

Sudeck-Leriche syndrome. See *Sudeck syndrome.*
SUDS. See ***s**udden **u**nexplained **d**eath **s**yndrome.*
SUGARMAN, GERALD I. (American pediatrician)
Sugarman brachydactyly. Brachdactyly with a nonarticulating great toe, which is set dorsal and proximal to the usual position, associated with duplication of the toes. The disorder is probably transmitted as an autosomal recessive trait.

Sugarman, G. I., *et al.* A new syndrome of brachydactyly of the hands and feet with duplication of the first toes. *Birth Defects*, 1974, l0(5):1-8.

Sugarman syndrome. See *orofaciodigital syudrome III.*
SUGIO, YOSHITSUGU (Japanese physician)
Sugio-Kajii syndrome. See *trichorhinophalangeal dysplasia type III.*
sukha pakla. See *ainhum syndrome.*
sulfatide lipidosis. See *metachromatic leukodystrophy.*
sulfhemoglobinemia. See *Stokvis-Talma syndrome.*
sulfone syndrome. Hypersensitivity to sulfones characterized by fever, malaise, weakness, morbilliform eruption, exfoliative dermatitis, jaundice, hepatic dysfunction, lymphadenopathy, and hemolytic anemia.

Tomecki, K. J., & Catalano, C. J. Dapsone hypersensitivity. The sulfone syndrome revisited. *Arch. Derm., Chicago,* 1981, 117:38-9.

SULZBERGER, MARION BALDUR (American physician, born 1895)
Bloch-Sulzberger melanoblastosis. See *Bloch-Sulzberger syndrome.*
Bloch-Sulzberger syndrome. See *under Bloch.*
Sulzberger-Garbe syndrome. Synonyms: *exudative discoid and lichenoid dermatosis, polymorphous prurigo syndrome.*

Chronic exudative discoid and lichenoid dermatosis characterized by sharply demarcated oval or discoid plaques showing rapid variations in consistency and appearance, being at times flat and scaly, at times elevated and edematous, and at times oozing and crusting. Pruritus is the constant feature. The symptoms include crusting plaques on the penis, scaly lesions on the scrotum, cutis anserina, chills, pain, and a burning sensation. Onset is usually sudden, although the generalized eruption is sometimes preceded by a circumscribed dermatitis. In the original report, all patients were of Jewish extraction and in the fourth or fifth decade of life.

Sulzberger, M. B., & Garbe, W. Nine cases of a distinctive exudative discoid and lichenoid chronic dermatosis. *Arch. Derm., Chicago,* 1937, 36:247-78.

SUMA (sporadic ulcerating and mutilating acropathy). See *Bureau-Barrière syndrome.*
summer acne. See *Hutchinson prurigo, under Hutchinson, Sir Jonathan.*
summer prurigo. See *Hutchinson prurigo, under Hutchinson, Sir Jonathan.*
SUMMERSKILL, WILLIAM J. (American physician)
Summerskill-Walshe syndrome. Synonyms: *benign recurrent cholestasis, benign recurrent intrahepatic cholestasis (BRIC).*

A benign liver disease characterized by recurrent episodes of jaundice and cholestasis in association with choluria and pruritus. Conjugated bilirubinemia, increased alkaline phosphatase and transaminase levels in the blood, high leukocyte count, and elevated sedimentation rate are usually observed during the icteric episodes; there are no apparent abnormalities in the interim period.

Summerskill, W. H. J., & Walshe, J. M. Benign recurrent intrahepatic "obstructive" jaundice. *Lancet,* 1959, 2:686-90.

SUMMITT, ROBERT L. (American physician, born 1932)
Summitt syndrome. Synonyms: *acrocephalosyndactyly V, craniosynostosis-syndactyly-obesity syndrome.*

Acrocephalosyndactyly characterized by mild acrocephaly, obesity, variable syndactyly, and minor anomalies of the face. Moderate gynecomastia, scaphocephaly, epicanthal folds, strabismus, high-arched palate, and delayed dental eruption are the principal features of this syndrome. Anomalies of the hands and feet vary from severe to mild syndactyly and clinodactyly. The syndrome is transmitted as an autosomal recessive trait.

Summitt, R. L. Recessive acrocephalosyndactyly with normal intelligence, *Birth Defects*, 1969, 5(3):35-8.

sump syndrome. Synonyms: *choledocho-cholecystoenterostomy sump syndrome, postcholecystectomy sump syndrome.*

A complication of side-to-side choledochoduodenostomy and choledochojejunostomy, whereby a sump (a pit or well) is formed in the distal nonfunctioning limb of the common bile duct where lithogenic bile, gastrointestinal contents, and debris accumulate, resulting in obstruction of the enterostomy stoma and producing cholangitis, pancreatitis, pain, and/or cholestasis. See also *postcholecystectomy syndrome.*

Siegel, J. H. Endoscopic management of the choledochocholecystoenterostomy sump syndrome: Definitive therapy for recurrent cholangitis. *Gastrointest. Endosc.*, 1980, 26:77.

Sunday syndrome. Once-a-week induction with amphetamines of an altered state of consciousness in football players, characterized by analgesia, anger, and violent inclinations.

Golding, L. A., & Barnard, J. R. The effects of *d*-amphetamine sulfate on physical performance. *J. Sports Med.*, 1963, 3:221-4. Mandell, A. J. The Sunday syndrome: A unique pattern of amphetamine abuse indigenous to American professsional football. *Clin. Tox.*, 1979, 15:225-32. Mandell, A. J., *et al.* The Sunday syndrome: From kinetics to altered consciousness. *Fed. Proc.*, 1981, 40:2693-704.

sundown syndrome. A condition observed in institutionalized elderly persons, characterized by agitation, restlessness, and confusion, sometimes associated with wandering about and screaming, most commonly accurring at sunset. Most affected persons suffer from dementia.

Evans, L. K. Sundown syndrome in institutionalized elderly. *J. Am. Geriat. Soc.*, 1987, 35:101-8.

sunflower syndrome. See *Gastaut syndrome (1).*
sunrise syndrome. Superior subluxation of the posterior chamber intraocular lens with resulting progressive loss of vision.

Smith, S. G., & Lindstrom, R. L. Report and management of the sunrise syndrome. *Am. Intra-Ocul. Impl. Soc. J.*, 1984, 10:218-20.

super female. See *chromosome XXX syndrome.*
super male. See *chromosome XYY syndrome.*
superficial epitheliomatosis. See *Arning carcinoid.*
superficial gyrate erythema. See *erythema annulare centrifugum.*

superficial marginal keratitis. See *Fuchs keratitis.*

superficial punctate keratitis. See *Fuchs syndrome (2), and see Thygeson keratitis.*

superficial pustular perifolliculitis. See *Bockhart impetigo.*

superficial senile line. See *Hudson-Stähli line.*

superior facet syndrome. Lumbar nerve root compression by lesions of the superior facets, causing low back pain and sciatica. Degenerative arthritis of the posterior facets (apophyseal arthrosis) is usually the primary cause, with congenital vertebral anomalies, spondylosis, and stenosis of the spinal canal being the contributory factors.

Ghormley, R. K. Low back pain with special reference to the articular facets, with presentation of an operative procedure. *JAMA*, 1933, 101:1773-7. Epstein, J. A., *et al.* Lumbar nerve root compression at the intervertebral foramina caused by arthritis of the posterior facets. *J. Neurosurg.*, 1973, 39:362-9.

superior hemorrhagic polioencephalitis. See *Wernicke syndrome.*

superior laryngeal nerve syndrome. See *Avellis syndrome.*

superior laryngeal neuralgia. See *Arnold neuralgia, and see under headache syndrome.*

superior limbic keratoconjunctivitis (SLK). See *Theodore syndrome.*

superior mediastinal syndrome. Mediastinal tumor causing compression of the trachea and major blood vessels, associated with respiratory and circulatory complications.

Sato, M. [Superior mediastinal syndrome] *Kyobu Geka*, 1985, 38:312-5.

superior mesenteric artery syndrome (SMA, SMAS). Synonyms: *Wilkie disease, Wilkie syndrome, arterial mesenteric duodenal ileus, arteriomesenteric duodenal compression syndrome, arteriomesenteric duodenal ileus, arteriomesenteric occlusion syndrome, duodenal atresia syndrome, duodenal vascular compression syndrome.*

Obstruction of the duodenum between the superior mesenteric artery and retroperitoneal structures, leading to dilation of the proximal duodenum and stomach. The symptoms include epigastric pain, abdominal cramps, bloating, nausea, and bilious vomiting after meals. The syndrome occurs most commonly in persons who have lost a considerable amount of weight, in anorexia nervosa, after prolonged bedrest, after abdominal surgery, or in conjunction with lordosis, pancreatitis, peptic ulcer, and various abdominal inflammatory disorders. An acute angle between the aorta and the superior mesenteric artery is a common angiographic feature.

Wilkie, D. P. The blood supply of the duodenum. With special reference to the supraduodenal artery. *Surg. Gyn. Obst.*, 1911, 13:399-405.

superior oblique tendon sheath syndrome. See *Brown syndrome, under Brown, H. W.*

superior orbital fissure syndrome. An association of ophthalmoplegia, anesthesia of the upper eyelid and forehead, blepharoptosis, exophthalmos, and dilation and fixation of the pupil. The condition may be a complication of facial fractures, or be caused by retrobulbar neoplasms; retrobulbar infections; infections of the meninges, cavernus sinus, and central nervous system; and cavernous sinus hematomas.

Hirschfeld, L. Épanchement de sang dans le sinus caverneux du côté gauche diagnostiqué pendant la vie. *C. Rend. Soc. Biol., Paris*, 1858, 5(2nd series):138-40. Bowerman, J. E. The superior orbital fissure syndrome complicating fractures of the facial skeleton. *Brit. J. Oral Surg.*, 1969, 7:1-6. Zachariades, N. The superior orbital fissure syndrome. Review of the literature and report of a case. *Oral Surg.*, 1982, 53:237-40.

superior pulmonary sulcus syndrome. See *Pancoast syndrome.*

superior pulmonary sulcus tumor. See *Pancoast sydrome.*

superior sulcus tumor. See *Pancoast syndrome.*

superior vena cava syndrome (SVC, SVCS). A partial or complete obstruction of the superior vena cava by neoplasms, lymphadenopathy, fibrosis, thrombosis, aortic aneurysms, mediastinal emphysema, peritonitis, mediastinitis, postoperative complications, and other disorders. The symptoms include swelling of the neck and head, distention and tortuosity of the veins of the neck, thorax, and arms; orbital edema; congestion of the vessels of the oral mucosa; headache; vertigo; somnolence; hoarseness; respiratory problems; cynanosis of the face, neck, arms, and upper trunk; proptosis; syncope; and convulsions. The presence and severity of symptoms depend on the degree of obstruction and collateral circulation.

Hunter, W. History of aneurysms of aorta with some remarks on aneurysms in general. *Med. Observ. Inquiries*, 1747, 1:323. Soloff, L. A. Syndrome of superior vena caval obstruction. *Am. Heart. J.*, 1939, 18:318-28.

supernumerary isochromosome 18 syndrome. See *chromosome +18pi syndrome.*

supine hypotensive syndrome. Hypotension in pregnant women on assuming the supine position due to

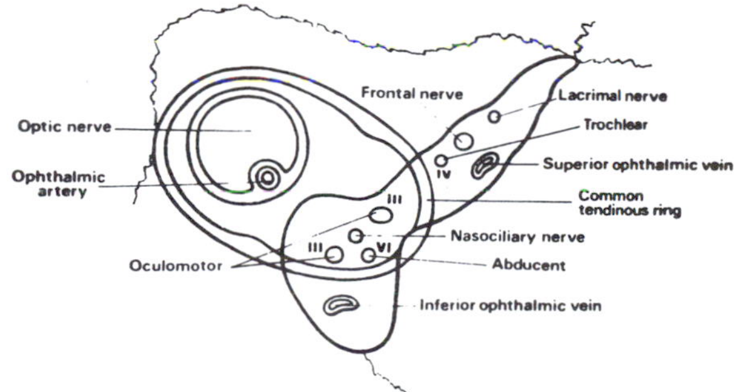

Superior orbital fissure syndrome
Bowerman, John E.: *British Journal of Oral Surgery*. Churchill Livingstone Medical Journals, Edinburgh, Scotland.

reduction of maternal cardiac output and mechanical occlusion of the vena cava by the gravid uterus.

McRoberts, W. A. Postural shock in pregnancy. *Am. J. Obst. Gyn.*, 1951, 62:627. Howard, B. K., *et al.* Supine hypotensive syndrome in late pregnancy. *Obst. Gyn.*, 1953, 1:371.

suppurative inguinal adenitis. See *Durand-Nicolas-Favre disease, under Durand, J.*

suppurative scleritis. See *Krämer disease.*

supraorbital neuralgia. See *Charlin syndrome.*

suprarenal apoplexy. See *Waterhouse-Friderichsen syndrome.*

suprarenal genital syndrome. See *congenital adrenal hyperplasia.*

suprarenal melasma. See *Addison disease.*

suprarenal pseudohermaphroditism-virilism-hirsutism syndrome. See *congenital adrenal hyperplasia.*

suprarenal sarcoma. See *Hutchinson disease, under Hutchinson, Sir Robert Grieve.*

suprascapular entrapment syndrome. See *suprascapular nerve entrapment syndrome.*

suprascapular nerve compression syndrome. See *suprascapular nerve entrapment syndrome.*

suprascapular nerve entrapment syndrome. Synonyms: *suprascapular entrapment neuropathy, suprascapular nerve syndrome, suprascapular nerve compression syndrome.*

Wasting of the supraspinatus and infraspinatus muscles associated with weakness of external rotation and of abduction of the shoulder due to entrapment or compression of the suprascapular nerve. The suprascapular notch is the most frequent site of entrapment; abnormal configuration of the notch, fractures of the scapula, traction, and neoplasms being the most frequent causes.

Clein, L. J. Suprascapular entrapment neuropathy. *J. Neurosurg.*, 1975, 43:337-42. Edeland, H. G., *et al.* Block of the suprascapular nerve in reduction of acute anterior shoulder injury. *Acta Anesth. Scand.*, 1973, 17:46-9.

suprascapular nerve syndrome. See *suprascapular nerve entrapment syndrome.*

suprasulcus tumor. See *Pancoast syndrome.*

supravalvular aortic stenosis (SAS) syndrome. A localized or diffuse narrowing of the ascending aorta beginning at the superior margin of the sinus of Valsalva and varying in severity from slight to severe concentric constrictions to hypoplasia of the entire aorta. The condition may occur as an uncomplicated sporadic entity in otherwise normal patients, as a familial disorder transmitted as an autosomal dominant trait with variable expression, or as a complication of severe idiopathic hypercalcemia.

Mencarelli, L. Stenosi sopravalvolare aortica ad anello. *Arch. Ital. Anat. Path.*, 1930, 1:829-41. Morrow, A. G., *et al.* Supravalvular aortic stenosis; clinical, hemodynamic and pathologic observations. *Circulation*, 1959, 20:1003-10.

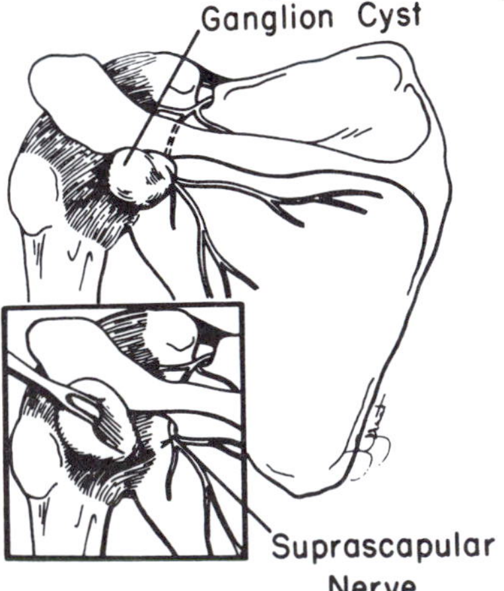

Suprascapular nerve entrapment syndrome
Ganzhorn, Richard W., John T. Hocker, Marshall Horowitz, & Hugh E. Switzer: *J. Bone Joint Surg.* [Am], 63A:494, 1981. Boston: Journal of Bone & Joint Surgery.

surdocardiac syndrome. See *long QT syndrome.*

surgical abdomen. See *acute abdominal syndrome.*

surgical mania. See *Munchausen syndrome.*

survivor syndrome. See *concentration camp survivor syndrome.*

suspended heart syndrome. See *Evans and Lloyd-Thomas syndrome, under Evans, William.*

SUTTON, HENRY GAWEN (British physician, 1837-1891)

Gull-Sutton syndrome. See *under Gull.*

SUTTON, RICHARD LIGHBURN (American dermatologist, 1878-1952)

Sutton disease. Synonyms: *Mikulicz aphthae, chronic necrotic stomatitis, periadenitis mucosae necrotica recurrens, recurring scarring aphthae.*

A recurrent disease of the mucous membranes of unknown etiology, generally considered to be a severe form of recurrent aphthous stomatitis. It is characterized by deep crateriform ulcers with inflamed borders, which leave scars after healing, thus differing from herpes simplex and ordinary recurrent aphthous stomatitis in which there is no scarring. The mucosae of the lips, cheeks, tongue, palate, and anterior tonsillar pillars are most commonly involved, and the pharynx, larynx, and genitalia also are affected in some cases. The gingivae are seldom if ever involved. The recurrent episodes of disease are spaced over a period of several years.

Sutton, R. L., Jr. Recurrent scarring painful aphthae. Amelioration with sulfathiazole in two cases. *JAMA*, 1941, 117:175-6.

Sutton halo nevus. Synonyms: *halo leukoderma, leukoderma acquisitum centrifugum.*

A skin disorder, considered by Sutton to be a form of vitiligo, occurring in the first or second decade of life, and characterized by a nevus in the process of destruction, surrounded by a sharply defined depigmented area. Some nevi undergo active changes and become erythematous, raised, and crusted. Histological examination shows nevus cells and infiltrates of cells of the lymphocyte and monocyte types.

Sutton, R. L. An unusual variety of vitiligo (leucoderma acquisitum centrifugum). *J. Cutan. Dis.*, 1916, 34:797-800.

SUTTON, THOMAS (British physician, 1767-1835)

Saunders-Sutton syndrome. See *Morel disease, under Morel, Benedict Augustin.*

suture barb giant papillary conjunctivitis syndrome. A postoperative complication consisting of a mucoid ocular discharge with blurred vision, a foreign body sensation, upper lid edema, and blepharoptosis concomitant with giant papillae of the upper palpebral conjunctiva caused by a cut exposed suture end that abrades the upper palpebral conjunctiva.

Jolson, A. S., & Jolson, S. C. Suture barb giant papillary conjunctivitis. *Ophth. Surg.*, 1984, 15:139-40.

SVC. See *superior vena cava syndrome.*

SVCS. See *superior vena cava syndrome.*

SVS. See *slit ventricle syndrome.*

swallowing syncope syndrome. Synonyms: *cardiac syncope after swallowing, cardiac syncope after vomiting, vagovagal syncope after swallowing.*

A decrease in cardiac output in response to swallowing with a loss of consciousness. It is believed to be caused by cerebral hypoperfusion due to bradycardia and heart block, which are thought to be mediated by a vagovagal reflex.

Weiss, S., & Ferris, E. B., Jr. Adams-Stokes syndrome with transient complete heart block of vagovagal reflex origin: Mechanism and treatment. *Arch. Intern. Med.*, 1934, 54:931. Shapira, J., & Versano, N. Cardiac syncope associated with vomiting. *Lancet*, 1958, 1:392.

SWAMI, R. K. (Indian physician)

Wadia-Swami syndrome. See *under Wadia.*

SWAN, KENNETH CARL (American ophthalmologist, born 1912)

Swan syndrome. See *blind spot syndrome.*

SWANSON, AUGUST G. (American physician)

Swanson syndrome. Synonyms: *congenital insensitivity to pain with anhidrosis, congenital sensory neuropathy with anhidrosis, familial dysautonomia II, hereditary sensory and autonomic neuropathy IV (HSAN-IV).*

A familial syndrome, transmitted as an autosomal recessive trait, characterized by congenital insensitivity to pain and complete inability to sweat.

Swanson, A. G. Congenital insensitivity to pain with anhidrosis. A unique syndrome in two male siblings. *Arch. Neur., Chicago,* 1963, 8:299-306.

Swedish porphyria. See *acute intermittent porphyria.*

SWEELEY, CHARLES CRAWFORD (American biochemist, born 1930)

Sweeley-Klionsky disease. See *Fabry syndrome.*

SWEENEY, ANNE (American scientist)

Nance-Sweeney syndrome. See *under Nance.*

SWEET, ROBERT DOUGLAS (British dermatologist)

Sweet syndrome (SS). Synonyms: *acute febrile neutrophilic dermatosis, acute neutrophilic dermatosis, febrile neutrophilic dermatosis, neutrophilic dermatosis.*

A skin disease characterized by the abrupt onset of red or bluish, tender papules or nodules on the face, extremities, and upper trunk, accompanied by fever, malaise, and neutrophilic leukocytosis. The lesions show a tendency to coalesce and form irregular, sharply defined plaques, which are often painful and tend to enlarge, eventually resolving without scarring. Some patients experience recurrences. Additional symptoms may include headache, arthralgia, conjunctivitis, and episcleritis. Febrile upper respiratory tract infection, tonsillitis, or influenzalike illness often precede the appearance of skin lesions. Edema of the papillary body and a dense infiltrate of leukocytes in the lower dermis are the principal pathological features. The etiology is unknown.

Sweet, R. D. An acute febrile neutrophilic dermatosis. *Brit. J. Derm.*, 1964, 76:349-56.

SWIFT, H. (Australian physician)

Selter-Swift-Feer syndrome. See *acrodynia.*

Swift disease. See *acrodynia.*

Swift-Feer syndrome. See *acrodynia.*

swine erysipelas in man. See *Rosenbach erysipeloid, under Rosenbach, Anton Julius Friedrich.*

Swiss cheese cartilage syndrome. See *Kniest disease.*

Swiss type agammaglobulinemia. See *severe mixed immunodeficiency syndrome.*

Swiss type agammaglobulinemia-achondroplasia syndrome. See *lymphopenic agammaglobulinemia-short limbed dwarfism syndrome.*

SWS. See *Sturge-Weber syndrome.*

SWYER, G. I. M. (British physician)

Swyer syndrome. See *chromosome XY female syndrome.*

SWYER, PAUL ROBERT (Canadian physician, born 1921)

Swyer-James syndrome (SJS). Synonyms: *Bret syndrome, Janus syndrome, Macleod syndrome, Swyer-James-Macleod syndrome, abnormal transradiancy of one lung, chronic obstructive pseudoemphysema, hyperlucent lung syndrome, idiopathic unilateral hyperlucent lung syndrome, pulmomary emphysema with unilateral transradiancy of one lung, unilateral clear lung, unilateral hyperlucent lung, unilateral hyperlucent lung syndrome, unilateral nonfunctioning lung, unilobar hyperlucency of the lung.*

Hyperlucency of one lung, as seen on x-rays of persons with a history of recurrent pulmonary infections in childhood. Cough, frequent respiratory infections, decreased tolerance to physical effort, hemoptysis, and arterial blood desaturation are the principal clinical symptoms. Additional symptoms include poor air exchange and differences in lung density during expiratory and inspiratory phases, hypoplastic pulmonary vessels, and bronchial dilation. The condition may be observed during the radiographic examination of Fallot tetralogy, with atresia of a branch of the pulmonary artery, or of the truncus arteriosus with a solitary pulmonary artery. See also *Burke syndrome.*

Swyer, P. R., & James, G. C. A case of unilateral pulmonary emphysema. *Thorax,* 1953, 8:133-6. Macleod, W. M. Abnormal transradiancy of one lung. *Thorax,* 1954, 9:147-53. Bret, J. Le syndrome de Janus. *Arch. Mal.Coeur,* 1956, 49:468-72. Hamilton, C. R., Jr., *et al.* The unilateral hyperlucent lung syndrome. *Johns Hopkins Med. J.,* 1968, 123:222-8.

Swyer-James-Macleod syndrome. See *Swyer-James syndrome.*

sycosis barbae. See *Alibert disease (3).*

sycosis simplex. See *Alibert disease (3).*

sycosis staphylogenes. See *Alibert disease (3).*

SYDENHAM, THOMAS (British physician, 1624-1689)

Sydenham chorea. Synonyms: *chorea St. Viti, St. Vitus dance, chorea infectiosa, chorea minor, chorea rheumatica, infectious chorea, rheumatic chorea.*

A disease of the central nervous system associated with distinctive involuntary, purposeless, or seemingly purposeless movements which are intensified by voluntary efforts or by excitement and which disappear during sleep. It is most common between 5 and 15 years of age, but it may occur later in life or be associated with pregnancy (**chorea gravidarum**). In most instances, the involuntary movements are generalized but, in some cases, they flow from site to site (**hemichorea**). Fidgety behavior, dysarthria, clumsiness, impaired gait, speech difficulty, mild muscle weakness, and emotional lability are usually associated. Recovery takes place in 2 to 6 months, but some patients experience the recurrence of symptoms. Scattered vascular lesions in the cerebral cortex, basal ganglia, cerebellum, and brain stem are the principal pathological features. Laboratory findings may reveal a lingering streptococcal infection. Some patients have residual heart valve defects, and behavioral and psychological problems.

*Sydenham, T. *Schedula monitoria de novae febris ingressu.* London, Kettilby, 1686.

SYLVEST, EJNAR OLUF SORENSEN (Danish physician, 1880-1931)

Sylvest syndrome. Synonyms: *Bornholm disease, Bornholm syndrome, Dabney grippe, bamble disease, devil's clutch, devil's grip, endemic myalgia, epidemic myalgia, epidemic pleurodynia, myalgia epidemica, myositis acuta epidemica.*

An acute infectious disease caused by Coxsackie B viral infection. After an incubation period of 2 to 4 days, there is the sudden onset of fever and severe paroxysmal pain in the muscles of the lower chest or abdomen. The epidemic pattern is similar to that of acute poliomyelitis, outbreaks usually occurring during the summer and fall.

Sylvest, E. En Bornholmsk epidemi-Myositis epidemica. *Ugeskr. Laeger,* 1930, 92:798-801. Dabney, W. C. Account of an epidemic resembling dengue which occurred in and around Charlottsville and the University of Virginia in June, 1888. *Am. J. Med. Sc.,* 1888, 96:488-95.

SYLVESTER, PETER E. (British physician)

Sylvester disease. A familial neurological syndrome, transmitted as an autosomal dominant trait, characterized by progressive optic atrophy, progressive deafness, ataxia, and weakness, especially of the shoulder girdle and hands. Associated disorders may include mental deficiency, nystagmus, unsteady gait, fibrillation, postural abnormalities (kyphosis, lordosis, scoliosis), pes cavus, and claw hand.

Sylvester, P. E. Some unusual findings in a family with Friedreich's ataxia. *Arch. Dis. Child.,* 1958, 33:217-21.

sylvian aqueduct syndrome. See *Koerber-Salus-Elschnig syndrome.*

symbiotic psychosis. See *Heller syndrome, under Heller, Theodor O.*

symmelia. See *caudal regression syndrome.*

SYMMERS, DOUGLAS (American physician, 1879-1952)

Brill-Symmers syndrome. See *under Brill.*

Brown-Symmers disease. See *under Brown, Charles Leonard.*

Moschcowitz-Singer-Symmers syndrome. See *Moschcowitz syndrome.*

Symmers syndrome. See *Brill-Symmers syndrome.*

symmetric asphyxia. See *Raynaud syndrome.*

symmetric keratodermia of the extremities. See *Unna-Thost syndrome, under Unna, Paul Gerson.*

symmetric lipomatosis. See *Madelung syndrome.*

symmetric neck lipoma. See *Madelung syndrome.*

symmetrical adenolipomatosis. See *Madelung syndrome.*

symmetrical calcification of basal cerebral ganglia (SCBG). See *Fahr syndrome.*

symmetrical gangrene of extremities. See *Raynaud syndrome.*

SYMONDS, SIR CHARLES PUTNAM (British physician)

Symonds syndrome. See *pseudotumor cerebri syndrome.*

sympathetic heterochromia. See *Herrenschwand syndrome.*

sympathetic irritation syndrome. See *Reilly syndrome, under Reilly, J.*

sympathicoblastoma. See *Hutchinson disease, under Hutchinson, Sir Robert Grieve.*

sympathicotonic colonic syndrome. See *Ogilvie syndrome.*

sympathogonioma. See *Hutchinson disease, under Hutchinson, Sir Robert Grieve.*

sympathoma embryonale. See *Hutchinson disease, under Hutchinson, Sir Robert Grieve.*

symphalangism syndrome. Synonyms: *Cushing symphalangism, Strasburger-Hawkins-Eldridge syndrome, Strasburger-Hawkins-Eldridge-Hargrave-McKusick syndrome, Vesell syndrome, deafness-strabismus-symphalangism syndrome, hereditary multiple ankylosing arthropathy, multiple synostoses-conductive deafness syndrome, proximal symphalangism syndrome, symphalangism-brachydactyly-conductive deafness syndrome, symphalangism-stapes fixation syndrome, symphalangism-strabismus-hearing loss syndrome, symphalangism-surdity syndrome.*

A hereditary syndrome of symphalangism with fusion of the midphalangeal joints; absence of the normal articular folds; fusion of the elbow and carpal and tarsal bones; limitation of motion of the elbow, wrist, and ankle joints; abnormal gait; brachydactyly; cutaneous syndactyly; fusion of the ossicles of the middle ear, leading to conductive deafness; peculiar facies marked by hypoplasia of the alae nasi, long and narrow face, thin upper lip, and broad nasal bridge; and occasional strabismus. The syndrome is transmitted as an autosomal dominant trait with variance in expression. See also the *facio-audio-symphalangism syndrome.*

Cushing, H. Hereditary anchylosis of the proximal phalangeal joints (symphalangism). *Genetics,* 1916, 1:90-106. Vesell, E. S. Symphalangism, strabismus and hearing loss in mother and daughter. *N. Engl. J. Med.,* 1960, 263:839-42. Strasburger, A. K., Hawkins, M. R., Eldridge, R., Hargrave, R. L., & McKusick, V. A. Symphalangism: Genetic and clinical aspects. *Bull. Johns Hopkins Hosp.,* 1965, 117:108-27.

symphalangism, C. S. Lewis type. See *under Lewis, C. S.*

symphalangism-brachydactyly syndrome. See *facio-audio-symphalangism syndrome.*

symphalangism-brachydactyly-conductive deafness syndrome. See *symphalangism syndrome.*

symphalangism-stapes fixation syndrome. See *symphalangism syndrome.*

symphalangism-strabismus-hearing loss syndrome. See *symphalangism syndrome.*

symphalangism-surdity syndrome. See *symphalangism syndrome.*

sympodia. See *caudal regression syndrome.*

symptomatic Ménière syndrome. See *Lermoyez syndrome.*

symptomatic porphyria. See *porphyria cutanea tarda syndrome.*

syndactylic oxycephaly syndrome. See *Apert syndrome.*

syndesmitis ossificans. See *Bechterew-Strümpell-Marie syndrome, under Bekhterev.*

syndrome of immediate reactivities (SIR). See *contact urticaria syndrome.*
synostosis multiplex. See *multiple synostoses syndrome.*
synovial cyst of the politeal space. See *Baker cyst.*
synovial osteochondromatosis. See *Reichel syndrome.*
synovial plica syndrome. See *synovial shelf syndrome.*
synovial shelf syndrome. Synonyms: *medial synovial shelf plica syndrome, shelf syndrome, shelf syndrome of th knee, synovial plica syndrome.*

An intra-articular disease of the knee characterized by thickening and inflammation of the synovial plica, with resulting friction and erosion of the medial femoral condyle, formation of shelflike structures, chondromalacic painful changes within the joint, and snapping, buckling, and catching sensations. Associated findings may include patellar instability and tendinitis, ligamentous instability, and a torn lateral and/or medial meniscus. The disorder is usually caused by strain in athletes and trauma in nonathletes.

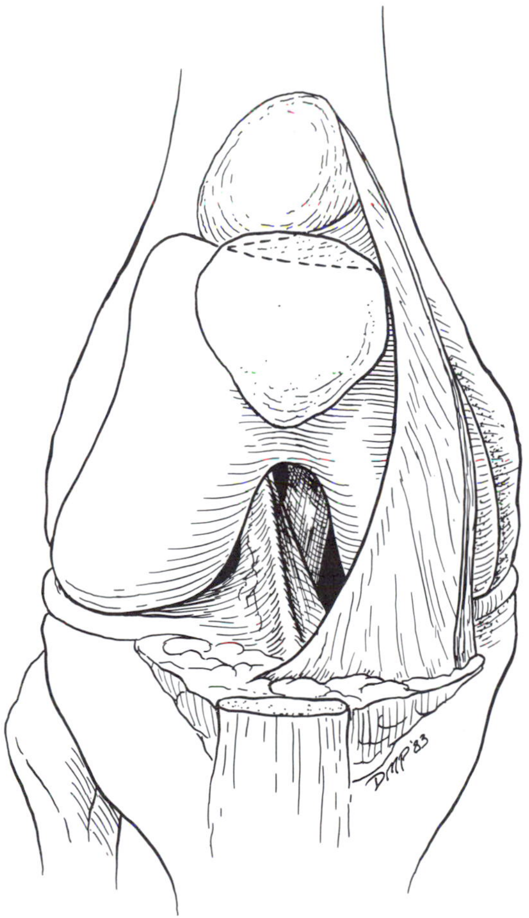

Synovial shelf syndrome
Rovere, George D., M.D. & Daniel M. Adair, .M.D: *American Journal of Sports Medicine* Vol.13 No. 6, 1985. American Orthopaedic Society for Sports Medicine, 0363-5465/85/1306-0382802.00/0.

Hughston, J. C., *et al.* The role of the suprapatellar plica in internal derangement of the knee. *Am. J. Orthop.*, 1963, 5:25-7. *Allen, R. F. *The shelf syndrome. Course on operative arthroscopy.* Center for Health Sciences. UCLA, 1973. *Mizumachi, S., *et al.* So-called synovial shelf in the knee joint. *J. Jpn. Orthop. Assoc.*, 1948, 22:1.

syphilitic aortitis. See *Heller-Döhle disease, under Heller, Arnold Ludwig Gotthilf.*
syphilitic-cardiovascular syndrome. See *Babinski syndrome.*
syphilitic fibromatous nodules. See *Jeanselme nodules.*
syphilitic osteitis of newborn. See *Parrot syndrome (1).*
syphilitic osteochondritis. See *Parrot syndrome (1).*
syphilitic poliomyelitis. See *Erb-Charcot syndrome, under Erb, Wilhelm Ernst.*
syphilitic pseudoparalysis. See *Parrot syndrome (1).*
syringobulbia. See *Morvan disease.*
syringomyelia. See *Morvan disease.*
systematized amyloidosis-macroglossia syndrome. See *Lubarsch-Pick syndrome.*
systemic amyloidosis syndrome. See *Lubarsch-Pick syndrome.*
systemic capillary leak syndrome (SCLS). See *capillary leak syndrome.*
systemic chondromalacia. See *Meyenburg-Altherr-Uehlinger syndrome.*
systemic elastodystrophy. See *pseudoxanthoma elasticum.*
systemic elastorrhexia. See *Touraine syndrome, under Touraine, M. A.*
systemic idiopathic fibrosis. See *Ormond syndrome.*
systemic onset juvenile rheumatoid arthritis. See *Still syndrome.*
systemic panchondritis. See *Meyenburg-Altherr-Uehlinger syndrome.*
systolic click-late systolic murmur syndrome. See *mitral valve prolapse syndrome.*
SZODORAY, L. (Hungarian physician)
Rajka-Szodoray syndrome. See *under Rajka.*

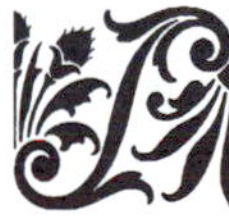

Page #	Term	Observation

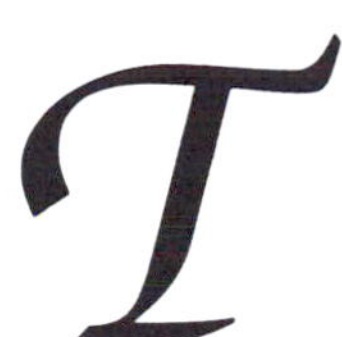

TA (Takayasu arteritis). See *aortic arch syndrome.*

TA-AIDS (transfusion-associated acquired immunodeficiency syndrome). See *under acquired immunodeficiency syndrome.*

TABATZNIK, B. (South African physician)

Berk-Tabatznik syndrome. See *under Berk.*

TABATZNIK, R. (South African physician)

Tabatznik syndrome. See *heart and hand syndrome (2).*

tabes dorsalis. See *locomotor ataxia.*

tabetic ciliary neuralgia. See *Pel syndrome.*

tabetic ocular anesthesia syndrome. See *Haenel syndrome.*

tabetic osteoarthropathy. See *Charcot disease.*

tachybradycardia syndrome. See *bradycardia-tachycardia syndrome.*

tachycardia-bradycardia syndrome. See *bradycardia-tachycardia syndrome.*

TAD (transient acantholytic dermatosis). See *Grover disease.*

TAENZER, PAUL RUDOLF (German physician, 1858-1919)

Taenzer disease. Synonyms: *Unna-Taenzer disease, ulerythema ophryogenes.*

A skin disease characterized by follicular red papules beginning in the eyebrows, spreading to neighboring areas of the face and scalp. Some hairs become finer than normal, some may be broken at the follicles, and some are atrophied. The resulting alopecia is usually permanent.

Taenzer, P. R. Über das Ulerythema ophryogenes, eine noch nicht beschriebene Hautkrankheit. *Mschr. Prakt. Derm.*, 1889, 8:197-208. Unna, P. G. *The histopathology of the diseases of the skin.* New York, Clay, 1896, pp. 1086-9.

Unna-Taenzer disease. See *Taenzer disease.*

TAKAHARA, SHIGEO (Japanese physician)

Takahara syndrome. Synonyms: *acatalasia, acatalasemia, anenzymia catalasea, catalase deficiency.*

A rare syndrome of catalase deficiency, transmitted as an autosomal recessive trait, originally described in Japanese and Korean patients and, more recently, in other racial and ethnic groups. Malignant alveolar pyorrhea and gangrene are the principal symptoms of this syndrome, but only about half of the persons homozygous for acatalasemia have any clinical manifestations; gangrene seldom occurs after puberty. A small painful ulcer in the crevices around the neck of a tooth or, less frequently, the tonsillar lacuna is the initial symptom. In the mild form, painful crateriform ulcers of the free gingiva, which apppear in children as early as 2 to 3 years of age, heal spontaneously. In the moderate form, there may be involvement of the entire gingiva, associated with gangrene and recession and bone loss, resulting in loosening and exfoliation of teeth. In the severe form, the mandible or maxilla is affected, with gangrene, bony sequestration, and invasion of the nasal antrum.

Takahara, S. Progressive oral gangrene probably due to lack of catalase in the blood (acatalasaemia). Report of nine cases. *Lancet*, 1952, 2:1101-4. Aebi, H. E., & Wyss, S. R. Acatalasemia. In: Stanbury, J. B., Wyngaarden, J. B., & Fredrickson, D. S., eds. *The metabolic basis of inherited disease.* 4th ed. New York, McGraw-Hill, 1978, pp. 1792-807.

TAKAHASHI, MATARO (Japanese physician)

Tamura-Takahashi disease. See *under Tamura.*

TAKATSUKI, K. (Japanese physician)

Takatsuki syndrome. See *POEMS syndrome.*

TAKAYASU, MICHISHIGE (Japanese physician, born, 1872)

Takayasu arteritis (TA). See *aortic arch syndrome.*

Takayasu disease. See *aortic arch syndrome.*

Takayasu syndrome. See *aortic arch syndrome.*

Takayasu-Martorell-Fabré syndrome. See *aortic arch syndrome.*

Takayasu-Onishi syndrome. See *aortic arch syndrome.*

TAKEUCHI, K. (Japanese physician)

Nishimoto-Takeuchi syndrome. See *Nishimoto disease.*

TAKOS (Greek physician)

Petzetakis-Takos syndrome. See *under Petzetakis.*

talar compression syndrome. Pain and tenderness usually localized at the posterolateral aspect of the ankle behind the peroneal tendons, caused by impingement of the os trigonum or the Stieda process between the calcaneus and the posterior edge of the tibia. The condition occurs most often in ballet dancers who frequently stand on the tips of their toes, resulting in compression of the posterior structures of the ankle during repeated plantar flexion of the foot. See also *overuse syndrome.*

Quirk, R. Talar compression syndrome in dancers. *Foot Ankle*, 1982, 3:65-8.

TALMA, SAPE (Dutch physician, 1847-1918)

Stokvis-Talma syndrome. See *under Stokvis.*

Talma disease. Synonym: *myotonia acquisita.*

Increased muscular rigidity and spasm of muscles when movements are initiated and a decrease in the degree of relaxation even when the muscle is at rest, associated with normal mechanical and electrical excitability of the motor nerves but with abnormally heightened mechanical and electrical excitability of muscle. In contrast to Thomsen disease, which is congenital, Talma disease usually develops in adult life after trauma, acute infection, or intoxication.

Talma, S. Over myotonia acquisita. *Ned. Tschr. Geneesk.*, 1892, 28:321-8.

TAMURA, AKIRA (Japanese physician)

Tamura-Takahashi disease. Synonyms: *hereditary black blood disease, nigremia.*

A familial disease, transmitted as an autosomal dominant trait, manifested by the dark appearance of the mucous membranes, and probably caused by abnormal absorption layers in heme.

Tamura, A., & Takahashi, M. Study on the hereditary black blood disease (Tamura and Takahashi's disease). *Tohoku J. Exp. Med.*, 1951, 54:209-13.

Tangier disease. Synonyms: *analphalipoproteinemia, familial high-density lipoprotein (HDL) deficiency, high-density lipoprotein (HDL) deficiency.*

Severe deficiency or absence of normal high-density lipoprotein (HDL), transmitted as an autosomal recessive trait, characterized mainly by large orange tonsils and corneal opacity. Additional clinical symptoms may include enlarged lymph nodes, hepatomegaly, splenomegaly, abnormal rectal mucosa, and neuropathy. Neurological abnormalities consist mainly of sensory, motor, or mixed disorders associated with weakness, paresthesias, dysesthesias, sweating, diminished or absent deep tendon reflexes, abnormal proprioception, and loss of pain and temperature sensibilities. Diplopia, blepharoptosis, and oculomotor palsies are the ocular features. Cardiovascular manifestations may include angina pectoris, heart murmur, right bundle branch block, and other disorders. Hypocholesterolemia and reduced HDL levels are the principal laboratory findings. Histological examination shows the thymus and reticuloendothelial cells loaded with a lipid (which consists of cholesterol esters) and intestinal lipid storage. The condition was originally observed among inhabitants of Tangier Island in the Chesapeake Bay, most of whom are descendants of the first settlers. Other affected families have been located in Missouri, Kentucky, and Great Britain.

Frederickson, D. S., *et al.* Tangier disease. *Ann. Intern. Med.*, 1961, 55:1016-31. Herbert, P. N., *et al.* Familial lipoprotein deficiency (abetalipoproteinemia, hypobetalipoproteinemia, and Tangier disease). In: Stanbury, J. B., Wyngaarden, J. B., & Frederickson, D. S., eds. *The metabolic basis of inherited disease.* 4th ed. New York, McGraw-Hill, 1978, pp. 544-88.

TAOR, W. S. (American physician)

Scott-Taor syndrome. See *under Scott, J. E.*

TAPIA, ANTONIO GARCIA (Spanish neurologist, born 1875)

Tapia syndrome. Synonyms: *nucleus ambiguus-hypoglossal syndrome, palatopharyngolaryngeal paralysis, vagohypoglossal syndrome.*

A variant of the Jackson-MacKenzie syndrome, wherein unilateral dysfunction of the tenth and twelfth cranial nerves produces paralysis of the tongue and vocal cords.

Tapia, A. G. Un caso de parálisis del lado derecho de la laringe y de la lengua, con parálisis del esterno-cleido-mastoide y trapecio de mismo lado; acompañado de hemiplejia total temporal del lado izquierdo del cuerpo. *Siglo Med., Madrid*, 1905, 52:211-3.

TAPPEINER, JOSEF (Austrian physician)

Spanlang-Tappeiner syndrome. See *under Spanlang.*

TAR. See *thrombocytopenia-absent radius syndrome.*

tar melanosis. See *Riehl melanosis.*

TARDIEU, AMBROISE (French physician, 1818-1879)

Ambroise Tardieu syndrome. See *battered child syndrome.*

tardive dyskinesia (TD) syndrome. Synonyms: *Kulenkampff-Tarnow syndrome, buccolinguomasticatory syndrome, cervicolinguomasticatory syndrome, faciobuccolinguomasticatory dyskinesia, neck-face syndrome, orolinguobuccal dyskinesia.*

A toxic syndrome of abnormal involuntary movements and motor restlessness due to the use of certain antipsychotic drugs, such as phenothiazines, butyrophenones, or chlorpromazine. The symptoms consist of a combination of spasmodic tension of the muscles of the neck, tongue, floor of the mouth, and pharynx; respiratory disorders; speech disorders; tachycardia; and hypertension. Typically, there are repetitive (stereotypic) rapid movements, most often involving the lower part of the face and muscles of the trunk and extremities. The orolinguobuccal type is marked by movements similar to those in chewing, with the tongue intermittently darting in and out of the mouth. Movements of the trunk may cause repetitive flexion and extension, and constant alternative flexion and extension movements of the limbs give an impression of piano-playing fingers and toes. When standing up, there are repetitive movements of the legs, as if the patient were marching in place. The gait appears to be unaffected by the swinging of the arms.

Sigvald, J., *et al.* Quatre cas de dyskinesie facio-bucco-linguomasticatrice a evolution prolongée secondaire a un traitement par les néuroleptiques. *Rev. Neur., Paris*, 1959, 100:751-5. Fahn, S. Tardive dyskinesia. In: Rowland, L. P., ed. *Merrit's textbook of neurology.* 7th ed. Philadelphia, Lea & Febiger, 1984, pp. 539-41. Kulenkampff, C., & Tarnow, G. Ein eigentümliches Syndrom im oralen Bereich Megaphenapplikation. *Nervenarzt*, 1956, 27:178-80.

tardive muscular dystrophy. See *Emery-Dreifuss syndrome.*

tardive nevus. See *Hutchinson freckle, under Hutchinson, Sir Jonathan.*

target cell anemia. See *Cooley anemia.*

target oval cell syndrome. See *Cooley anemia.*

TARLOV, I. M. (American physician)

Tarlov cyst. A perineural cyst arising from the posterior sacral nerve roots; it can cause sciatica.

Tarlov, I. M. Cysts (perineural) of the sacral roots. Another cause (removable) of sciatic pain. *JAMA*, 1948, 138:740-4.

TARNOW, G. (German physician)

Kulenkampff-Tarnow syndrome. See *tardive dyskinesia syndrome.*

TARRAL, CLAUDIUS (French physician)

Tarral-Besnier disease. See *Kaposi disease (2).*

tarsal kink syndrome. Congenital kinking of the tarsus causing entropion and corneal ulceration.

Bosniak, S., *et al.* Re-examining the tarsal kink syndrome: Considerations of its etiology and treatment. *Ophth. Surg.*, 1985, 16:437-40.

tarsal scaphoiditis. See *Köhler disease (1).*

tarsal sinus syndrome. Synonym: *sinus tarsi syndrome (STS).*

Chronic pain over the lateral ankle with a feeling of hindfoot instability, occurring after ankle sprain. Excessive post-traumatic scarring of the superficial ligamentous floor of the tarsal sinus was believed to be the cause in the original report. Some authors suggest that the pain may develop as a result of hypertrophy, strangulation, pinching, or herniation of the synovial membrane within the sinus tarsi. Other conditions implicated in the etiology include inflammatory conditions in rheumatoid arthritis, ankylosing spondylitis, and gouty arthritis.

O'Connor, D. Sinus tarsi syndrome. *J. Bone Joint Surg.*, 1958, 40(A):720.

tarsal tunnel syndrome. Entrapment of the posterior tibial nerve beneath the flexor retinaculum and deep fascia along the medial border of the foot. The symptoms vary with the degree of nerve compression, and may include tingling, burning, pain, hyperesthesia or hypoesthesia, intrinsic muscle weakness, and vasomotor disorders. Hypertrophic laciniate ligament, hypertrophic abductor hallucis muscle or fascia, pronated forefoot with either a valgus or varus heel, bony changes after fractures, edema with flexor tenoyinovitis, ganglion cysts, flexor tendon cysts, perineural fibrosis, neurilemmoma, varices and thrombi of the posterior tibial vein, and fat within the tarsal tunnel are the main etiologic factors. A compression of the posterior tibial nerve and its branches may occur distal to the laciniate ligament under the fibrous border of the abductor muscles secondary to swelling or hypertrophy of the muscle in runners.

Pollock, L. J., & Davis, L. *Peripheral nerve injuries.* New York, Hoeber, 1933, pp. 32; 484-93. O'Malley, G. M., *et al.* Tarsal tunnel syndrome. A case report and review of the literature. *Orthopedics,* 1985, 8:758-60.

tarso-epiphyseal aclasis. See *Trevor syndrome.*

tarsocarpal acro-osteolysis with or without nephropathy. See *carpotarsal osteolysis syndrome (dominant and sporadic forms).*

tarsomegaly. See *Trevor syndrome.*

TARUI, SEIICHIRO (Japanese physician)

Tarui disease. See *glycogen storage disease VII.*

TAS. See *thoraco-abdominal syndrome.*

TAS (traumatic apallic syndrome). See *apallic syndrome.*

TAUSSIG, HELEN BROOKE (American cardiologist, born 1898)

Taussig-Bing anomaly. See *Taussig-Bing syndrome.*

Taussig-Bing complex. See *Taussig-Bing syndrome.*

Taussig-Bing heart. See *Taussig-Bing syndrome.*

Taussig-Bing malformation. See *Taussig-Bing syndrome.*

Taussig-Bing syndrome. Synonyms: *Taussig-Bing anomaly, Taussig-Bing complex, Taussig-Bing heart, Taussig-Bing malformation, complete dextroposition of the aorta, complete transposition of the aorta and levoposition of the pulmonary artery.*

A double-outlet right ventricle associated with complete transposition of the aorta and incomplete transposition of the pulmonary artery, which overrides the ventricular septum, in association with a large ventricular septal defect located above the septal limb of the crista supraventricularis and below the pulmonary valve. Cardiomegaly and right ventricular hypertrophy are usually present. The syndrome is manifested by pulmonary hypertension, cyanosis, dyspnea on exertion, systolic murmur, loud second pulmonary sound, and polycythemia.

Taussig, H. B., & Bing, R. J. Complete transposition of the aorta and levoposition of the pulmonary artery. Clinical, physiological, and pathological findings. *Am. Heart J.*, 1949, 37:551-9.

Taussig-Snellen-Albers syndrome. Anomalous drainage of the pulmonary vein into the inferior vena cava or into the left innominate vein, associated with septal defect. Situs inversus and pulmonary stenosis may be present. Most patients with partial abnormal drainage enjoy good health until an advanced age.

*Taussig, H. B. *Congenital malformations of the heart.* New York, 1947. Snellen, H. A., & Albers, F. H. The clinical diagnosis of anomalous pulmonary venous drainage. *Circulation,* 1952, 6:801-16.

TAVERAS, JUAN M. (Physician in St. Louis)

Taveras syndrome. See *moyamoya syndrome.*

TAY, CHONG HAI (Singapore physician)

Tay syndrome. Synonyms: *IBIDS (**i**chthyosis-**b**rittle hair-**i**mpaired intelligence-**d**ecreased fertility-**s**hort stature) syndrome; PIBIDS, PIBI(D)S (**p**hotosensitivity-**i**chthyosis-**b**rittle hair-**i**ntellectual impairment-**d**ecreased fertility-**s**hort stature) syndrome.*

A syndrome of congenital ichthyosis with a peculiar anomaly of hair growth (trichothyodystrophy), progerialike facies, and physical and mental retardation. When photosensitivity is present, the syndrome is known an the **PIBIDS** or **PIBI(D)S** syndrome; without photosensitivity, it is referred to as the **IBIDS** syndrome. Ichthyosiform erythroderma occurs during the first week of life with the skin being covered by a smooth, shiny membrane, giving the infant the appearance of a collodion baby. Scales develop within 1 month. Trichothyodystrophy (sulfur-deficient brittle hair) is present early in life but tends to improve during adolescence and adulthood. Lack of subcutaneous fatty tissue causes the cheeks to become sunken, thus giving the affected children a progeroid appearance. Other facial characteristics include beaked nose, receding chin, large protruding ears, and occasional epicanthus. Growth and mental retardation are constant. Dysplastic nails, microcephaly, brain calcification, mild deafness, spasticity, tremor, ataxia, hypogonadism, cataracts, osteosclerosis, hoarse and raspy or high-pitched voice, susceptibility to infections, and other disorders may be associated. Autosomomal recessive transmission is suspected. See also *hair-brain syndrome.*

Tay, C. H. Ichthyosiform erythroderma, hair shaft abnormalities, and mental and growth retardation. A new recessive disorder. *Arch. Derm.*, 1971, 104:4-13. Crovato, F., & Rebora, A PIBI(D)S syndrome: An entity with defect of deoxyribonucleic acid excision repair system. *J. Am. Acad. Derm.*, 1985 13,363-6. Jorizzo, J, L., *et al.* Ichtyosis, brittle hair, impaired intelligence, decreased fertility and short stature (IBIDS) syndrome. *Brit. J. Derm.*, 1982, 106:705-10.

TAY, WARREN (British physician, 1843-1927)

Hutchinson-Tay choroiditis. See *Hutchinson disease (2), under Hutchinson, Sir Jonathan.*

pseudo-Tay-Sachs syndrome. See *Sandhoff syndrome.*

Tay choroiditis. See *Hutchinson disease (2), under Hutchinson, Sir Jonathan.*

Tay disease. See *Hutchinson disease (2), under Hutchinson, Sir Jonathan.*

Tay-Sachs disease (TSD). See *Tay-Sachs syndrome.*

Tay-Sachs syndrome. Synonyms: *Sachs disease, Tay-Sachs disease (TSD), amaurotic familial idiocy, ganglioside lipidosis, gangliosidosis G_{M2} type I, infantile amaurotic idiocy.*

A ganglioside storage disorder occurring predominantly, but not exclusively , in children of Jewish (Ashkenazi) families. Early symptoms become apparent within the first 3 to 6 months of life and include muscle weakness and startle reaction to sharp sounds. The affected infants may learn to crawl or sit unaided but are seldom capable of walking. The initial symptoms are followed by blindness, psychomotor retardation, feeding difficulty (due to deglutition disorders), poor muscle tone, and generalized paralysis. At about 18 months there are convulsions, progressive deafness, blindness, seizures, spasticity, and, ultimately, decerebrate rigidity. Anomalies of the face and head include doll-like facies, macrocephaly, translucent skin, long eyelashes, fine hair, and pale-pink coloration. Cherry-red spots of the maculae are present in some cases. An almost total absence of the enzyme hexosaminidase (while hexosaminidase B activity is increased in the brain) is the most prominent biochemical feature of this syndrome. Pathological changes include storage of sphingolipids (ganglioside G_{M2}) in nerve cells, resulting in their destruction. Neuronal lipidosis of cortical, autonomic, and rectal neurons, with ballooning of the cytoplasm and displacement of the nucleus, is associated. Central demyelination follows axonal degeneration and cortical gliosis. Most affected children die from bronchopneumonia before the age of 3 years. The syndrome is transmitted as an autosomal recessive trait.

Tay, W. Symmetrical changes in the region of the yellow spot in each eye of an infant. *Tr. Ophth. Soc. U. K.*, 1881, 1:57-7. Sachs, B. On arrested cerebral development, with special reference to its cortical pathology. *J. Nerv. Ment. Dis.*, 1887, 14:541-53. O'Brien, J. S. The gangliosidoses. In: Stanbury, J. B., Wyngaarden, J. B., & Fredrickson, D. S., eds. *The metabolic basis of inherited disease.* 4th ed. New York, McGraw-Hill, 1978, pp. 841-65.

TAYBI, HOOSHANG (American radiologist, born 1919)

Rubinstein-Taybi syndrome (RTS). See *under Rubinstein.*

Taybi syndrome. See *oto-palato-digital syndrome.*

Taybi-Linder syndrome. A congenital syndrome, probably transmitted as an autosomal recessive trait, characterized by dwarfism, low birth weight, cerebral dysgenesis, and bone dysplasia. Skeletal manifestations are marked by microcrania, deep intervertebral spaces, decreased vertical vertebral body diameter, irregular metaphyseal borders of the long bones, concave margins of the chondro-osseous junctions of the short tubular bones, shortening of the bones (chiefly the first metacarpal bones, some with triangular configuration, and middle phalanges of the fifth fingers), delayed ossification of the spine, and defective ossification of the pelvic bones.

Taybi, H., & Linder, D. Congenital familial dwarfism with cephaloskeletal dysplasia. *Radiology*, 1967, 89:275-81.

TAYLOR, HOWARD CANNING, JR. (American physician, born 1900)

Taylor syndrome. Synonyms: *congestion-fibrosis syndrome, congestive dysmenorrhea syndrome, hyperemia of the ovary, pelvic congestion syndrome, pelvic sympathetic syndrome. pelvipathia vegetativa, subinvolution and congestion of the uterus.*

A combination of disorders of vascular function of the female genitalia, characterized by arterial dilatation, venous engorgement, and local increase in extravascular fluid retention, and resulting in congestion and fibrosis of the genital system. In the congestive stage, there is uterine and parametrial congestion, cervical hypersecretion, endocervicitis, cervical erosion, peritoneal edema and ascites, ovarian congestion, premenstrual breast engorgement, and mastodynia. In the fibrous stage, there is diffuse hypertrophy of the uterus and cervix, chronic inflammation of the posterior parametrium, inflammation of the Douglas pouch, ovarian fibrocystitis, and chronic fibrous mastitis. Emotional problems, radiating neuralgic pains, palpitations, and indigestion are usually associated. The etiology is unknown, but stress and psychogenic disorders are suspected as the contributing factors.

Taylor, H. C., Jr. Vascular congestion and hyperemia. Their effects on structure and function in the female reproductive system. *Am. J. Obst.*, 1949, 57:211-30; 637-53; 654-68.

TAYLOR, ROBERT WILLIAM (American physician, 1842-1908)

Taylor disease. See *Herxheimer disease.*

TBM (tracheobronchiomegaly). See *Mounier-Kuhn syndrome.*

TCS (tethered cord syndrome). See *tethered conus syndrome.*

TD. See *tardive dyskinesia syndrome.*

TDO. See *trichodento-osseous syndrome.*

TEC. See *transient erythroblastopenia of childhood syndrome.*

TECKLENBURG, F. (German physician)

Tecklenburg-Roemheld syndrome. See *Roemheld syndrome.*

TEDESCI

Tedesci syndrome. Multicentric lipomatosis of unknown etiology, characterized by lipomas of subcutaneous and internal organs containing undifferentiated mesenchymal cells.

Prusov, A. L., *et al.* [Lipomatoz podvzdoshnoi kishki (sindrom Tedesci)] *Khirurgiia, Moskva,* 1986, No. 9:120-1.

tegmental syndrome. See *Benedikt syndrome.*

tegmental mesencephalic paralysis. See *Benedikt syndrome.*

Tel Hashomer camptodactyly syndrome. Synonyms: *Goodman camptodactyly, Goodman syndrome, camptodactyly-muscular hypoplasia syndrome, skeletal dysplasia-abnormal palmar creases syndrome.*

A syndrome of camptodactyly, distinct facies, muscular hypoplasia, skeletal dysplasia, and abnormal palmar creases, occurring in Jewish families of Moroccan and Arab Bedouin origin. The principal features of this syndrome include short stature, brachycephaly, prominent forehead and maxilla, broad mandible, asymmetric facies, hypertelorism, small mouth, high-arched palate, long philtrum, dental crowding, thoracic scoliosis, winging of scapulae, spindle-shaped fingers, club feet, syndactyly, and hypoplasia of the muscles of the chest, pelvis, and limbs. Autosomal recessive inheritance is suspected. The name derives from Tel Hashomer Hospital near Tel

Aviv in Israel, where the first cases were observed.

Goodman, R. M., *et al*, Camptodactyly: occurence in two new genetic syndromes and its relationship to other syndromes. *J. Med. Genet.*, 1972, 9:203-12.

telangiectasia follicularis annulata. See *Majocchi disease.*

telangiectasia hereditaria haemorrhagica. See *Osler-Rendu-Weber syndrome.*

telangiectasia-alopecia syndrome. Synonym: *Bazex syndrome.*

A congenital syndrome of generalized telangiectasia and alopecia associated with systemic abnormalities, including ocular defects, malformed teeth, saddle nose, midfacial hypoplasia, subcutaneous calcifications, brachydctyly with short metatarsal and metacarpal bones, and retarded growth and mental development.

Bazex, J., *et al.* Télangiectasies généralisées, alopécie, syndrome malformatif. *Ann. Derm. Vener., Paris,* 1979, 106:795-800.

telangiectasis-pigmentation-cataract syndrome. See *Rothmund-Thomson syndrome.*

TELFER, M. A. (American physician)

Telfer syndrome. A familial syndrome, transmitted as an autosomal dominant trait, characterized by piebaldism (white forelock and leukoderma), deafness, cerebellar ataxia, impaired motor coordination, and mental retardation.

Telfer, M. A., *et al.* Dominant piebald trait (white forelock and leukoderma) with neurological impairment. *Am. J. Hum. Genet.*, 1971, 23:383-9.

telodiencephalic ischemia. An ischemic disorder of the common pathway of the internal carotid and middle cerebral arteries. The symptoms include contralateral brachiofacial hemiparesis, sometimes with hemianopia and/or aphasia, and ipsilateral thermoregulatory hemihypohidrosis with an ipsilateral central Horner syndrome. It is caused by lesions of the crossed pathways descending from the cerebrum and the uncrossed hypothalamo-spinal sympathetic pathways descending through the subthalamic regions.

Schiffter, R., & Reinhart, K. The telodiencephalic ischemic syndrome. *J. Neur., Berlin,* 1980, 222:265-74.

temporal arteritis. See *Horton disease (1).*

temporal lobe agenesis syndrome. Agenesis or hypogenesis of the temporal lobe, occurring as the primary defect or as a malformation of the brain secondary to congenital or acquired cyst. The condition is characterized by expansion of the body boundaries of the middle cranial fossa or the temporal lobe that is occupied by the cerebrospinal fluid. The symptoms include headache and a hard, nontender bulging of the temporal area of the skull. The affected children usually have normal mentality and neurological signs are frequently absent.

Robinson, R. G. The temporal lobe agenesis syndrome. *Brain,* 1964, 87:87-111.

temporal lobectomy behavior syndrome. See *Klüver-Bucy syndrome.*

temporal megacellular arteritis. See *Horton disease (1).*

temporomandibular syndrome. See *temporomandibular joint syndrome.*

temporomandibular arthrosis. See *temporomandibular joint syndrome.*

temporomandibular dysfunction syndrome. See *temporomandibular joint syndrome.*

temporomandibular joint (TMJ) syndrome. Synonyms: *Costen syndrome, temporomandibular arthrosis, temporomandibular dysfunction syndrome, temporomandibular joint and muscle pain syndrome, temporomandibular joint pain dysfunction syndrome, temporomandibular neuralgia, temporomandibular pain and dysfunction syndrome (TMPDS), temporomandibular syndrome, TMJ dysfunction syndrome, TMJ pain dysfunction syndrome.*

A symptom complex originally described by Costen as consisting of partial deafness, stuffy sensation in the ears (especially during eating), tinnitus, clicking and snapping of the temporomandibular joint, dizziness, headache, and burning pain in the ears, throat, and nose. Later investigators disproved Costen's anatomical and clinical conclusions. According to later studies, the syndrome consists mainly of temporomandibular crepitation, decreased temporomandibular mobility, preauricular and auricular pain, pain on movement, headache, tenderness of the jaws on palpation, and, sometimes, head and nasopharyngeal symptoms. Ear symptoms are very rare.

Costen, J. B. A syndrome of ear and sinus symptoms dependent upon disturbed function of the temporomandibular joint. *Ann. Otol. Rhinol.*, 1934, 43:1-15. Gorlin, R. J., Pindborg, J. J., & Cohen, M. M., Jr. *Syndromes of the head and neck.* 2nd ed. New York, McGraw-Hill, 1976, p. 691-3.

temporomandibular joint and muscle pain syndrome. See *temporomandibular joint syndrome.*

temporomandibular joint pain dysfunction syndrome. See *temporomandibular joint syndrome.*

temporomandibular neuralgia. See *temporomandibular joint syndrome.*

temporomandibular pain and dysfunction syndrome (TMPDS). See *temporomandibular joint syndrome.*

TEMTAMY (EL-TEMTAMY), SAMIA ALI (Egyptian physician)

Temtamy brachydactyly. See *brachydactyly A-4.*

TEN. See *toxic epidermal necrolysis.*

tendon sheath adherence syndrome. See *Brown syndrome, under Brown, H. W.*

TENNESSON, HENRI (Franch physician, 1836-1913)

Besnier-Tennesson syndrome. See *Besnier-Boeck-Schaumann syndrome.*

tennis elbow. See *under overuse syndrome, and see under radial tunnel syndrome.*

tension headache. See *muscle contraction headache, under headache syndrome.*

terminal aortic thrombosis. See *Leriche syndrome (1).*

terminal ileitis. See *Crohn disease.*

TERREY, MARY (American physician)

Lowe-Terrey-MacLachlan syndrome. See *Lowe syndrome.*

TERRIEN, FELIX (French ophthalmologist, 1872-1940)

Terrien-Veil syndrome. See *Posner-Schlossman syndrome.*

TERRIER, LOUIS FELIX (French physician, 1837-1908)

Courvoisier-Terrier syndrome. See *Bard-Pic syndrome, under Bard, Louis.*

TERRY, THEODORE LASATER (American ophthalmologist, 1899-1946)

Terry syndrome (1). Angioid streaks of the retina associated with osteitis deformans (Paget disease).

Terry, T. L. Angioid-streaks and osteitis deformans. *Tr. Am. Ophth. Soc.*, 1934, 32:555-73.

Terry syndrome (2). See *retrolental fibroplasia.*

TERSON, ALBERT (French ophthalmologist, 1867-1935)

Terson syndrome. Synonyms: *subarachnoid hemorrhage with vitreous hemorrhage, vitreous hemorrhage-ruptured cerebral aneurysm syndrome.*

Vitreous hemorrhage associated with a sudden increase in intracranial venous pressure that ruptures the epi- and peri-papillary capillaries and causes subarachnoid hemorrhage.

Terson, A. Hémorragie dans le corps vitré ou cours d'une hémorragie cérébrale. *Ann. Oculist.*, 1912, 147:410-7.

TERZIAN, H. (American neurologist)

Klüver-Bucy-Terzian syndrome. See *Klüver-Bucy syndrome.*

TES (toxic epidemic syndrome). See *toxic oil syndrome.*

TESCHENDORF, WERNER (German radiologist)

Bársony-Teschendorf syndrome. See *Bársony-Polgár syndrome (2).*

TESCHLER-NICOLA, M.

Teschler-Nicola and Killian syndrome. See *chromosome 12p tetrasomy syndrome.*

testicular dysgenesis syndrome. See *Sertoli cell only syndrome.*

testicular feminization (TF, TFM). See *testicular feminization syndrome.*

testicular feminization syndrome (TFS). Synonyms: *de Quervain syndrome, Goldberg-Maxwell syndrome, Goldberg-Maxwell-Morris syndrome, Goldberg-Morris syndrome, Morris syndrome, androgen-insensitivity syndrome (AIS), androgen receptor deficiency, androgen-resistance syndrome, dihydrotestosterone receptor (DHTR) deficiency, hairless pseudofemale, hairless women syndrome, testicular feminization (TF, TFM).*

A familial form of male pseudohermaphroditism which can be transmitted as either an X-linked recessive trait or a sex-linked autosomal trait. The syndrome of complete testicular feminization include: female habitus and breast development, scanty or absent axillary and pubic hair, female external genitalia with underdeveloped labia and a blind-ending vagina, absence of internal genitalia except for rudimentary anlage and gonads that may be intra-abdominal, histological picture of the gonads suggesting cryptorchism, resistance to the androgenic and anabolic effects of testosterone, elevated gonadotropin levels, and production of testostosterone and estrogens at levels that are equal or higher than in males. Genetic study shows male sex chromatin and 46,XY karyotype.

*de Quervain, F. Ein Fall von Pseudohermaphrodismus masculinus. *Schweiz. Med. Wschr.*, 1923, 53:563. Goldberg, M. B., & Maxwell, A. F. Male pseudohermaphroditism proved by surgical exploration and microscopic examination. A case report with speculations concerning pathogenesis. *J. Clin. Endocr.*, 1948, 8:367-79. Morris, J. M. The syndrome of testicular feminization in male pseudohermaphrodites. *Am. J. Obst.*, 1953, 65:1192-211. Leinzinger, E. "Hairless woman," der männliche Scheinzwitter mit testiculärer Feminisierung. *Wien. Med. Wschr.*, 1974, 124:443-8. Wilson, J. D., & Macdonald, P. C. Male pseudohermaphroditism due to androgen resistance: testicular feminization and related syndromes. In: Stanbury, J. B., Wyngaarden, J. B., & Fredrickson, D. S., eds. *The metabolic basis of inherited disease*. 4th ed. New York, McGraw-Hill, 1978, pp. 894-913.

tethered conus syndrome. Synonyms: *cord contraction syndrome, cord traction syndrome, filum terminale syndrome, low conus, tethered cord syndrome (TCS), tethered spinal cord syndrome.*

A developmental anomaly of the lumbosacral spinal cord caused by lipomeningocele, thickened filum terminale, diastematomyelia, and arachnoiditis. Tethering prevents free movements of the cord within the spinal canal, leading to undue traction on the distal cord and potential ischemic damage of the cord and spinal roots. Complications may include gait disturbances, foot deformities, scoliosis, and bladder and bowel dysfunctions. Usually associated are progressive neurological symptoms, consisting of paralysis, muscle atrophy, sensory loss of the lower limbs, and low back pain, sometimes radiating to the lower limbs. Other findings include spinal dysraphia, intradural lipoma, hypertrichosis, pigmented nevi, dimples and dermal sinuses in the lumbar area, and limb length asymmetry. The syndrome is usually diagnosed in children, but is also found in adults.

Garceau, G. J. The filum terminale syndrome (the cord contraction syndrome). *J. Bone Joint Surg.*, 1953, 35A:711.

tethered cord syndrome (TCS). See *tethered conus syndrome.*

tethered spinal cord syndrome. See *tethered conus syndrome.*

tetralogy of Fallot (TF). See *Fallot tetralogy.*

tetraphocomelia-cleft lip-palate syndrome. See *Roberts syndrome.*

tetraphocomelia-cleft palate syndrome. A familial syndrome, originally reported in identical twins, characterized by severe, symmetrical phocomelia with short stature, cleft palate, identical facies, and 11 ribs. Arm deformities include humeral hypoplasia, a severe radial clubbed hand deformity, radius hypoplasia or aplasia, and a reduction in the first ray of the hands. One twin had a small cutaneous appendage instead of the left thumb. Femoral aplasia, the feet in equinovarus position, and severe adduction of the forefoot are the principal defects of the lower limbs. Craniofacial appearance consists mainly of a round face and a long upper lip with a deep philtrum. See also *Roberts syndrome.*

Fryns, H., *et al.* The tetraphocomelia-cleft palate syndrome in identical twins. *Hum. Genet.*, 1980, 53:279-81.

tetraploidy. See *chromosome tetraploidy syndrome.*

tetrasomy 9p. See *chromosome 9p tetrasomy syndrome.*

tetrasomy 12. See *chromosome 12p tetrasomy syndrome.*

tetrasomy 12p. See *chromosome 12p tetrasomy syndrome.*

tetrasomy 18p. See *chromosome 18p tetrasomy syndrome.*

tetrasomy Y. See *chromososme XYYYY syndrome.*

TEUTSCHLÄNDER, OTTO (German physician, 1874-1950)

Teutschländer syndrome. Synonyms: *calcifying collagenolysis, calcinosis interstitialis universalis, calcinosis lipogranulomatosa progradiens, calcinosis multiplex lipogranulomatosa, dystrophic metalipoid calcinosis, hygromatosis lipocalcinogranulomatosa progressiva, lipocalcinogranulomatosis, lipocalcinosis progradiens, lipochalicogranulomatosis, lipogranulomatosis intramuscularis progressiva, myopathia osteoplastica progressiva, tumoral calcinosis.*

Painless, calcified masses, ranging in size from a few millimeters to several centimeters in diameter, located over the extensor surface of the joints; the hip, elbow, ankle, wrist, shoulder, and foot being most commonly affected. There is tissue necrosis, especially of the fatty tissue, with granuloma formation in the later stages. Limited joint movement is usually associated. The disease generally occurs before the age of 20 years.

Teutschländer. Über progressive lipogranulomatose der Muskulatur. Zugleich ein Beitrag zur Pathogenese der Myopathia osteoplastica progressiva. *Klin. Wschr.*, 1935, 14:451-3.

TF. See *testicular feminization syndrome.*

TF (tetralogy of Fallot). See *Fallot tetralogy.*

TFM. See *testicular feminization syndrome.*

TFS. See *testicular feminization syndrome.*

thalamic hyperesthetic anesthesia. See *Déjerine-Roussy syndrome.*

thalamic pain syndrome. See *Déjerine-Roussy syndrome.*

thalamic syndrome. See *Déjerine-Roussy syndrome.*

thalassemia syndrome. A group of inherited hematological disorders, transmitted as an autosomal recessive trait, characterized by a reduced rate of synthesis of one or more of the globin chains of hemoglobin, usually in association with imbalanced globin chain production with precipitation of excess chain, inclusion body formation, faulty erythropoiesis, and shortened red cell survival. According to early classifications, the severe homozygous form was named **thalassemia major,** and the heterozygous forms were designated according to their severeity as **thalassemia minor** or **thalassemia minima.** According to more recent classsifications, two basic types are recognized: the first group consists of hemoglobinopathies, such as sickle-cell anemia, which are caused by structural changes in one of the globin chains; and the second consists of hemoglobinopathies which are caused by structural changes in the rate of synthesis of one or more of the globin chains. Thalassemias are now classified according globin chains which are synthesized at a reduced rate; the main subtypes have been defined alpha-, beta-, gamma-, and delta-thalassemias; the Greek letters being the designations for the specific globin chains. Beta-thalassemia causes Cooley anemia (q.v.).

Cooley, T. B., & Lee, P. A series of cases of splenomegaly in children with anemia and peculiar bone changes. *Tr. Am. Pediat. Soc.*, 1925, 37:29. Weatherall, D. J. The thalassemias. In: Williams, W. J., Beutler, E., Erslev, A. J., & Lichtman, M. A., eds. *Hematology*, 3rd ed. New York, McGraw-Hill, 1983, pp. 493-521.

thalassemia major. See *Cooley anemia.*

thalassemia-hemoglobin C disease. See *Zuelzer-Kaplan syndrome (2).*

thalassemic syndrome. See *Cooley anemia.*

thalidomide syndrome. See *Wiedemann syndrome (1).*

thalidomide embryopathy. See *Wiedemann syndrome (1).*

thalidomide phocomelia. See *Wiedemann syndrome (1).*

thanatophoric dwarfism syndrome. A lethal form of achondroplasia of the newborn, characterized chiefly by disproportionate dwarfism with very short extremities and relatively normal trunk, narrow thorax, and disproportionately large head with depressed nasal bridge and protruding ears. Death takes place in infancy. Associated defects include frontal bossing, cloverleaf skull, bulging eyes, bowed limbs, redundant skin folds, short ribs, flattening of the vertebrae, and other disorders.

Maroteau, P., *et al.* Le nanisme thanatophore. *Presse Méd.*, 1967, 75:2519-24.

THANNHAUSER, SIEGFRIED JOSEF (German-born American physician, born 1885)

Hanot-MacMahon-Thannhauser syndrome. See *under Hanot.*

Hauptmann-Thannhauser syndrome. See *under Hauptmann.*

MacMahon-Thannhauser syndrome. See *Hanot-MacMahon-Thannhauser syndrome.*

Thannhauser-Magendantz syndrome. See *Hanot-MacMahon-Thannhauser syndrome.*

THAYSEN, THORNWALD EJNAR HESS (Danish physician, 1883-1936)

Gee-Thaysen disease. See *celiac disease.*

Thaysen syndrome. Synonyms: *MacLennan syndrome, proctalgia fugax, rectal crisis.*

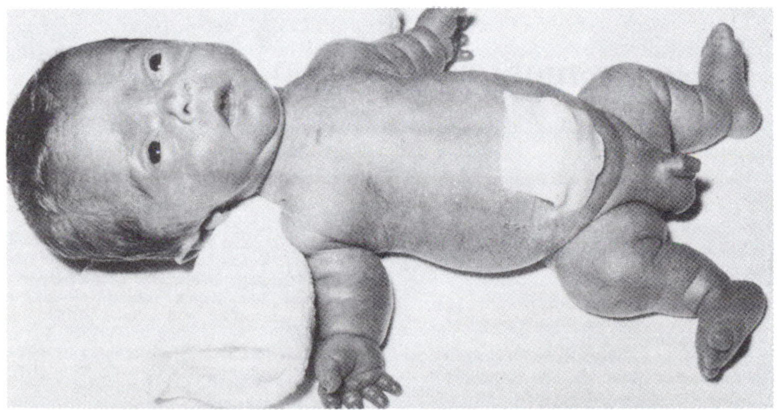

Thanatophoric dwarfism syndrome
Giedion, A.: Thanatophoric Dwarfism. *Helv. Paediat. Acta* 23, 175-183, 1968.

Intermittent attacks of intense pain of short duration occurring in the region of the anorectal ring and the internal anal sphincter. The syndrome may be associated with precordial pressure, pallor, perspiration, and syncope. See also the *levator syndrome.*.

MacLennan, A. A short note on rectal crises of nontabetic origin. *Glasgow Med. J.*, 1917, 88:129-31. Thaysen, T. E. Proctalgia fugax. A little known form of pain in the rectum. *Lancet*, 1935, 2:243-6.

THEILER, KARL (Swiss physician)

Smith-Theiler-Schachenmann syndrome. See *cerebrocostomandibular syndrome.*

THEODORE, FREDERICK H. (American ophthalmologist)

Theodore syndrome. Synonym: *superior limbic keratoconjunctivitis (SLK).*

A recurrent eye disease characterized by inflammation of the tarsal conjunctiva of the upper eyelid, inflammation of the upper bulbar conjunctiva, fine punctate fluorescein or rose bengal staining of the cornea at the upper limbus and the adjacent conjunctiva above the limbus, superior limbic proliferation, and the occurrence of filaments situated at the superior limbus or in the upper part of the cornea in about one-third of all cases.

Theodore, F. H. Further observations on superior limbic keratoconjunctivitis. *Tr. Am. Acad. Ophth. Otolar.*, 1967, 71:341-51.

thermic stress syndrome. A group of pharmacogenetic disorders precipitated by physical, thermic, and anesthetic stress, which include heat stroke, malignant hyperpyrexia, sudden death syndrome in athletes, recurrent rhabdomyolysis with myoglobinuria, and exercise myoglobinuria.

Meyers, E. F. Thermic stress syndrome. *Prev. Med.*, 1979, 8:5202.

thesaurismosis hereditaria. See *Fabry syndrome.*

thesaurismosis hereditaria lipoidica. See *Fabry syndrome.*

thesaurismosis lipoidica. See *Fabry syndrome.*

THEVENARD, ANDRE (French physician)

Smith-Thévenard syndrome. See *Thévenard syndrome.*

Thévenard syndrome. Synonyms: *Denny-Brown syndrome, Hicks syndrome, Nélaton syndrome, Smith-Thévenard syndrome, acrodystrophic neuropathy, acropathia ulceromiliaris, familial acropathia ulceromutilans, familial neurovascular dystrophy, familial perforating ulcer of the foot, hereditary sensory radicular neuropathy, primary acrodystrophic neuropathy, sensory radicular neuropathy, ulcerative mutilating acropathy.*

A rare hereditary syndrome characterized by sensory disorders of the lower extremities, leading to perforating ulceration of the feet and destruction of the underlying bones. Primary degeneration of the posterior root ganglia is the chief pathological feature, and ulceration of the pressure points of the feet is the earliest symptom. Bone lesions usually include acroosteolysis, destruction of the metatarsophalangeal joints, Charcot arthropathy of the lower limbs, hemarthrosis, osteoporosis, fractures, and dislocations. Elephant foot, vasomotor disorders, and hypertrichosis are usually associated. Shooting pain and progressive deafness with atrophy of the cochlear and vestibular ganglia are the common features. Optic atrophy was observed in Thévenard's but no other cases. The syndrome is usually transmitted as an autosomal dominant trait but recessive and sporadic cases have been reported.

Thévenard, A. L'acropathie ulcéro-mutilante familiale. *Rev. Neur., Paris*, 1942, 74:193-212. Smith, E. M. Familial neurotrophic osseous atrophy: A familial neurotrophic condition of the feet with anesthesia and loss of bone. *JAMA*, 1934, 102:593-5. Hicks, E. P. Hereditary perforating ulcer of the foot. *Lancet*, 1922, 1:319-21. Nélaton. Affection singuliere des os du pied. *Gaz. Hôp, Paris*, 1852, 4:13-20. Denny-Brown, D. Hereditary sensory radicular neuropathy. *J. Neur. Neurosurg. Psychiat., London*, 1948, 14:237-52.

thiamine-responsive anemia syndrome. Anemia associated with diabetes mellitus and deafness, that responds only to therapeutic doses of thiamine.

Rogers, L. E., *et al.* Thiamine-responsive megaloblastic anemia. *J. Pediat.*, 1969, 74:494-504.

THIBIERGE, GEORGES (French physician)

Thibierge-Weissenbach syndrome. Synonym: *calcinosis cutis-scleroderma syndrome.*

Generalized calcinosis of the skin with scleroderma. Esophageal disorders, gastrointestinal complications, pulmonary hypofunction with or without pulmonary fibrosis, and intervertebral calcifications may be associated. The term Thibierge-Weissenbach syndrome is sometimes used in the literature as a synonym for the CRST syndrome.

Thibierge, G., & Weissenbach, R. J. Concrétions calcaires sous-cutanées et sclérodermia. *Ann. Derm. Syph., Paris*, 1911, 2:129-55.

thick bone osteogenesis imperfecta. See *osteogenesis imperfecta syndrome (recessive form).*

thick skull syndrome. Synonym: *dik kop disease.*

A hereditary bone disorder, transmitted as an autosomal recessive trait, characterized by overgrowth of the skull with entrapment of the cranial nerves. The disorder is a complication of osteoporosis, which includes bone fragility and osteomyelitis, particularly of the jaw. It was first observed in South African patients who had a variety of other defects, including craniometaphyseal dysplasia, pycnodysostosis, van Buchem disease, and osteosclerosis.

Beighton, P. Dik kop disease: a variety of osteoporosis. *J. Bone Joint Surg.*, 1975, 57B:260.

THIEBAUT, F. (French physician)

Refsum-Thiébaut disease. See *Refsum disease.*

THIEBAUT, M. F. (French physician)

Thiébaut syndrome. See *van Bogaert-Scherer-Epstein syndrome.*

THIEFFRY, STEPHANE (French physician)

Thieffry and Sorrell-Déjerine syndrome. See *Thieffry-Shurtleff syndrome.*

Thieffry-Kohler syndrome. See *Tieffry-Shurtleff syndrome.*

Thieffry-Shurtleff syndrome. Synonyms: *Thieffry-Kohler syndrome, Thieffry and Sorrell-Déjerine syndrome, hereditary osteolysis with hypertension and nephropathy, multicentric osteolysis with nephropaphy, osteolysis-nephropathy syndrome.*

Idiopathic hereditary osteolysis, transmitted as an autosomal dominant trait with variable expressivity, characterized by arthritic symptoms in early childhood with swelling of the joints and surrounding soft tissues, followed by osteolysis of the carpal and tarsal joints and leading to complete disappearance of the involved bones. Vascular nephropathy and hypertension occur in some patients. Associated disorders include marfanoid habitus, frontal bossing, micrognathia, pes cavus, plantar cysts, and occasional scoliosis, and elbow involvement. Elevated alkaline phosphatase, high normal excretion of peptide-bound hydroxyproline, and engorgement of polymorphonuclear leukocytes with metachromatic materials during the inflammatory stages are usually present.

Thieffry, S., & Sorrell-Déjerine, J. Forme spéciale d'ostéolyse essentielle héréditaire et familiale à stabilisation spontanée, survenant dans l'enfance. *Presse Méd.*, 1958, 66:1858-61. Shurtleff, D. B., *et al.* Hereditary osteolysis with hypertension and nephropathy. *JAMA*, 1964, 188:363-8. Kohler, E., *et al.* Hereditary osteolysis. A clinical, radiological and chemical study. *Pediat. Radiol.*, 1973, 108:99-105.

THIEMANN, H. (German physician)

Thiemann syndrome. Synonyms: *Thiemann-Fleischner disease, acrodysplasia epiphysaria, digital osteoarthropathy, epiphyseal acrodysplasia, finger osteochondropathy, phalangeal avascular necrosis.*

A disease of adolescence characterized by painful fusiform swelling of the proximal interphalangeal joints, usually the middle and, less frequently, other fingers. Similar lesions may occur on the great toes and first tarsometatarsal joints. X-ray examination shows an epiphyseal defect with faulty ossification and alternating zones of radiolucency and radiodensity, protuberances on the epiphyses, overriding of the metaphysis laterally, fragmentation of the epiphyses, and dense epiphyses. The syndrome is considered to be a form of avascular osseous necrosis with osteochondritis of the growing bone.

Thiemann, H. Juvenile Epiphysenstörungen. *Fortschr. Röntgen.*, 1909-10, 14:79-87. Fleischner, F. Multiple Epiphysenstörungen an den Händen. Eine bisher unbekannte Localisation der Osteopathia juvenilis. *Fortschr. Röntgen.*, 1923, 31:206-12.

Thiemann-Fleischner disease. See *Thiemann syndrome.*

THIER, CARL JÖRG (German physician)

Weyers-Thier syndrome. See *under Weyers.*

THIERS, JOSEPH (French physician)

Achard-Thiers syndrome. See *under Achard, Emile Charles.*

thin bone osteogenesis imperfecta. See *osteogenesis imperfecta syndrome (dominant form).*

third and fourth pharyngeal pouch syndrome. See *DiGeorge syndrome.*

third diabetic coma. See *Wegierko coma.*

THOMA, K. H.

Sturge-Weber-Thoma syndrome. See *Sturge-Weber syndrome.*

THOMAS

Thomas disease. See *Joseph disease, under Joseph, Antone.*

THOMAS, ANDRE (French physician)

Déjerine-Thomas syndrome. See *olivopontocerebellar atrophy.*

Thomas syndrome. A combination of equilibrium disorders, adiadochokinesia, slow halting speech, writing difficulty, ataxia of extremties, reflex disorders, sensory disorders, and frequent cerebral catalepsy, seen in lamellar atrophy of Purkinje cells. Onset takes place most frequently during the fifth decade.

Thomas, A. Atrophie lamellaire des cellules de Purkinje. *Rev. Neur., Paris,* 1905, 13:917-24.

THOMAS, HENRY M., JR. (American physician)

Thomas syndrome. Hypothyroidism with secondary hypertrophic osteoarthropathy (Marie-Bamberger syndrome) and exophthalmos following partial thyroidectomy for goiter.

Thomas, H. M., Jr. Acropachy. Secondary subperiosteal new bone formation. *Arch. Int. Med., Chicago,* 1933, 51:571-88.

THOMAS, M. (French physician)

Bureau-Barrière-Thomas syndrome. See *under Bureau.*

THOMPSON, A. HUGH (British ophthalmologist)

Thompson syndrome. Synonym: *congenital optic atrophy.*

Familial optic atrophy transmitted as an autosomal dominant trait and characterized by blindness and nystagmus.

Thompson, A. H., & Cashell, G. T. W. A pedigree of congenital optic atrophy embracing sixteen affected cases in six generations. *Proc. Roy. Soc. Med., London,* 1935, 28:1415-26.

THOMPSON, JOHN

Thompson syndrome. See *mucopolysaccharidosis I-H.*

THOMSEN, ASMUS JULIUS THOMAS (Danish physician, 1815-1896)

Thomsen disease. Synonyms: *ataxia muscularis, congenital muscular dystrophy, hereditary myotonia, myotonia congenita.*

A rare hereditary disease, transmitted as an autosomal dominant trait, which begins in early life and is characterized by myotonia, hyperexcitability, and hypertrophy of the volunary muscles, with spasms and an inability to relax the muscles immediately after forceful contraction. The symptoms may become apparent in infants whose eyes are noted to open slowly after crying or sneezing and whose legs are stiff during their first attempts to walk. Blepharoptosis, difficulty in turning the eyes to the side, and an inability to open them rapidly are the ophthalmological symptoms. Muscle biopsy shows enlargement of fibers in hypertrophied muscles.

*Thomsen, J. Tonische Krämpfe in willkürlich bewegliche Muskeln in Folge von ererbter psychischer Disposition (Ataxia muscularis?). *Arch. Psychiat., Berlin,* 1875-76, 6:706-18.

THOMSON, ALLEN (British physician)

Thomson complex. See *mandibulofacial dysostosis.*

THOMSON, MATTHEW SIDNEY (British physician, 1894-1969)

Rothmund-Thomson syndrome (RTS). See *under Rothmund.*

thoracic outlet compression. See *thoracic outlet syndrome.*

thoracic outlet syndrome (TOS). Synonyms: *cervicothoracic outlet compression syndrome, thoracic outlet compression.*

Compression of the nerves and vessels in the outlet of the thorax and the costoclavicular area or between the clavicle and the first rib. It is caused by angulation of the brachial plexus over a fibrous band extending from the transverse process of the seventh cervical vertebra or an abnormal rib (cervical rib), with resulting paresthesia, numbness, skin color changes, claudication, diminished pulse, lowered blood pressure on the affected side, wasting and weakness of muscles of the hand and forearm, and pain involving the chest wall, shoulder, arm, and hand. The syndrome includes the scalenus anticus syndrome and cervical rib syndrome (q.v.).

Murphy, J. B. A Case of cervical rib with symptoms resembling subclavian aneurysm. *Ann. Surg.*, 1905, 41:399.

thoracic-pelvic-phalangeal dystrophy (TPPD). See *Jeune syndrome.*

thoraco-abdominal syndrome (TAS). Synonyms: *Cantrell syndrome, Cantrell-Haller-Ravitch syndrome, abdominothoracic syndrome, thoraco-abdominal wall defect syndrome.*

A congenital syndrome combining midline supraumbilical abdominal defects, defects of the lower sternum, deficiency of the diaphragmatic pericardium, deficiency of the anterior diaphragm, and cardiac defects. Specific abdominal and diaphragmatic anomalies include omphalocele, eventration, diastasis of the rectus abdominis muscle, absence of the umbilicus, and diaphragmatic ventral defect; those of the heart consist of interatrial and interventricular septal defects, superior vena cava abnormalities, aortic stenosis, tetralogy of Fallot, anomalous pulmonary venous return, and bilocular heart. Additional abnormalities may include craniofacial abnormalities, malrotation of the colon, and herniation of the bowel into the pericardial cavity.

Cantrell, J. R., Haller, J. A., & Ravitch, M. M. A syndrome of congenital defects involving the abdominal wall, sternum, diaphragm, pericardium, and heart. *Surg. Gyn. Obst.*, 1958, 107:602-14.

thoraco-abdominal wall defect syndrome. See *thoraco-abdominal syndrome.*

thoracogenous rheumatic syndrome. See *Marie-Bamberger syndrome, under Marie, Pierre.*

thoracolaryngopelvic dysplasia. See *Barnes syndrome.*

THORN, GEORGE WIDMER (American physician, born 1906)

Thorn syndrome. See *renal salt losing syndrome.*

thornwalditis. See *Thornwaldt bursitis.*

THORNWALDT (TORNWALDT), GUSTAV LUDWIG (German physician, 1843-1910)

Thornwaldt bursitis. Synonyms: *Thornwaldt cyst, Thornwaldt disease, Thornwaldt syndrome, Tornwaldt cyst, Tornwaldt disease, Tornwaldt syndrome, nasopharyngeal bursitis, pharyngeal bursitis, thornwalditis, tornwalditis.*

Chronic inflammation of the pharyngeal bursa attended with formation of pus-containing cysts and nasopharyngeal stenosis. It occurs in association with persistent nasopharyngeal drainage, occipital headache, stiffness of the posterior cervical muscles, exacerbation of pain with movement of the head, sore throat, persistent low-grade fever, and halitosis.

*Thornwaldt, G. L. *Über die Bedeutung der Bursa pharyngea für die Erkennung und Behandlung gewisser Nasenrachenkrankheiten.* Wiesbaden, Bergmann, 1885.

Thornwaldt cyst. See *Thornwaldt bursitis.*

Thornwaldt disease. See *Thornwaldt bursitis.*

Thornwaldt syndrome. See *Thornwaldt bursitis.*

THORSON, AKE (Swedish physician)

Biörck-Axén-Thorson syndrome. See *carcinoid syndrome.*

Biörck-Thorson syndrome. See *carcinoid syndrome.*

THOST, ARTHUR (German physician, born 1854)

Unna-Thost syndrome. See *under Unna, Paul Gerson.*

thromboangiitis cutaneo-intestinalis disseminata. See *Degos syndrome.*

thromboangiitis obliterans. See *Buerger syndrome.*

thromboarteritis obliterans subclaviocarotica. See *aortic arch syndrome.*

thrombocytasthenia. See *Glanzmann thrombasthenia.*

thrombocythemia hemorrhagica. See *Mortensen disease.*

thrombocytic acroangiothrombosis. See *Moschcowitz syndrome.*

thrombocytic hemorrhage. See *Mortensen disease.*

thrombocytic thrombocytopenic purpura (TTP). See *Moschcowitz syndrome.*

thrombocytolytic purpura. See *Werlhof disease.*

thrombocytopathic purpura. See *Glanzmann thrombasthenia.*

thrombocytopenia-absent radius (TAR) syndrome. Synonyms: *thrombocytopenia-phocomelia syndrome, thrombocytopenia-radial aplasia syndrome, thrombocytopenia-radial hypoplasia syndrome.*

A familial syndrome of thrombocytopenia and bilateral aplasia or hypoplasia of the radii. Hematological features consist mainly of bone marrow aplasia with transient but recurrent thrombocytopenia and absent or hypoplastic megakaryocytes, bleeding episodes leading to anemia, leukemoid granulocytosis, and eosinophilia. Radius abnormalities are often associated with ulnar hypoplasia and defects of the hands and feet, small stature, nevus flammeus, genu varum, kidney abnormalities, spina bifida, brachycephaly, strabismus, micrognathia, syndactyly, short humerus, hypoplasia of the shoulder girdle, hip dislocation, talipes, Meckell diverticulum, and other abnormalities may also occur. The syndrome is transmitted as an autosomal recessive trait.

Gross, H., *et al.* Kongenitale hypoplastiche Thrombopenie mit Radius-Aplasie, ein Syndrom multipler Abartungen. *Neue Oest. Z. Kinderheilk*, 1969, 1:574.

thrombocytopenia-phocomelia syndrome. See *thrombocytopenia absent radius syndrome.*

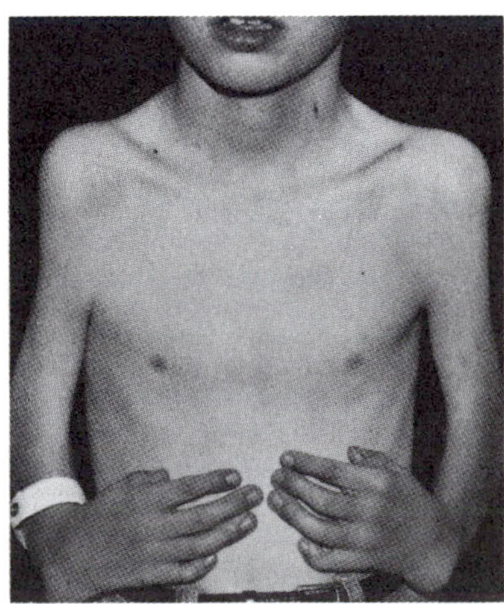

Thrombocytopenia-absent radius syndrome. Courtesy of J. M. Opitz, Helena, MT.

thrombocytopenia-radial aplasia syndrome. See *thrombocytopenia-absent radius syndrome.*

thrombocytopenic purpura-acquired hemolytic anemia syndrome. See *Evans syndrome, under Evans, Robert Sherman.*

thrombocytopenic purpura-disseminated carcinoma syndrome. See *Jarcho synrome.*

thrombocytopenic-radial hypoplasia syndrome. See *thrombocytopenic-absent radius syndrome.*

thrombohemolytic thrombopenic purpura. See *Moschcowitz syndrome.*

thrombopenia-hemangioma syndrome. See *Kasabach-Merritt syndrome.*

thrombophlebitic splenomegaly. See *Frugoni syndrome.*

thrombophlebitis of the thoraco-epigastric veins. See *Mondor disese (1).*

thrombosis of cavernous sinus syndrome. See *cavernous sinus syndrome.*

thrombosis venae axillaris. See *Paget-Schroetter syndrome.*

thrombosis-fibrinolysis-thrombocytopenia syndrome. See *disseminated intravascular coagulation syndrome.*

thrombotic microangiopathic hemolytic anemia. See *Moschcowitz syndrome.*

thrombotic microangiopathy. See *Moschcowitz syndrome.*

thrombotic thrombocytic purpura. See *Moschcowitz syndrome.*

thrombotic thrombocytopenic purpura. See *disseminated intravascular coagulation syndrome.*

THS. See *Tolosa-Hunt syndrome.*

THUCYDIDES (Greek general and historian, c460-400 B.C)

Thucydides syndrome. Synonym: *plague of Athens.*

An infectious disease described by Thucydides on the basis of his observations on the 430-427 B.C. epidemic (the plague of Athens). According to his account, the symptoms consisted of fever, redness and inflammation of the eyes, redness of the tongue and throat, halitosis, sneezing, hoarseness, cough, vomiting, empty retching, open sores, flushed and livid skin, thirst, agitation, sleeplessness, watery diarrhea, amnesia and, frequently, death. The epidemic is believed to have killed tens of thousands of some 300,000 inhabitants of Athens. The nature of the epidemic is unknown, but various conditions, including smallpox, bubonic plague, scarlet fever, measles, typhus, typhoid fever, ergotism, cerebrospinal fever, influenza, dysentery, staphylococcal infection, and toxic shock syndrome, have been proposed as potential causes of the epidemic.

Langmuir, A. D., *et al.* The Thucydides syndrome. A new hypothesis for the cause of the plague of Athens. *N. Engl. J. Med.,* 1985, 313:1027-30. Holladay, A. J. The Thucydides disease: Another view. *N. Engl. J. Med.,* 1986, 315:1170-3.

THYGESON, PHILLIPS (American physician, born 1903)

Thygeson keratitis. Synonym: *superficial punctate keratitis.*

A chronic form of punctate epithelial keratitis that is not associated with conjunctivitis. Typical lesions are small, punctate, and circular or irregular opacities scattered in the superficial layers of the cornea, chiefly in the central zone. The disorder is recurrent, with relapses over a period of 2 to 3 years. A viral etiology is suspected.

Thygeson, P. Superficial punctate keratitis. *JAMA,* 1950, 144:1544-9.

thymic syndrome. See *Pende syndrome.*

thymic alymphoplasia. See *severe mixed immunodeficiency syndrome.*

thymic and parathyroid agenesis syndrome. See *DiGeorge syndrome.*

thymic aplasia syndrome. See *DiGeorge syndrome.*

thymoma with immunodeficiency. See *Good syndrome.*

thymoma-agammaglobulinemia syndrome. See *Good syndrome.*

thyreoiditis nonpurulenta subacuta. See *de Quervain disease (2), under Quervain, Fritz, de.*

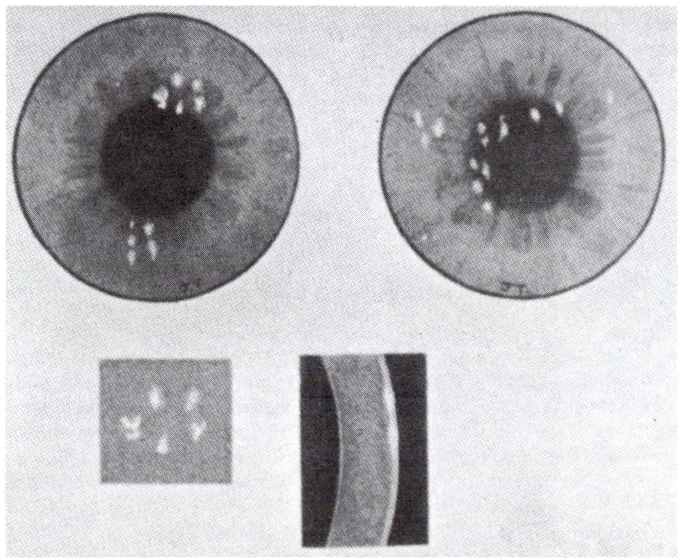

Thygeson Keratitis
Jones, Barrie R., from S. Duke-Elder & A.G. Leigh: Disease of the Outer Eye (Part 2). In Duke-Elder, S.: *System of Ophthalmology* Vol. VIII. London: Henry Kimpton, 1965.

thyro-ovarian insufficiency-acromegaly syndrome. See *Rénon-Delille syndrome.*

thyrocerebrorenal syndrome. A familial syndrome, transmitted as an autosomal recessive trait, characterized by goiter, nephritis, sensorineural deafness, cerebellar ataxia, seizures, slurred speech, muscle wasting, and thrombocytopenia.

Cutler, E. A., *et al.* A familial thyrocerebral-renal syndrome. A newly recognized disorder. *Birth Defects,* 1978, 14(6B):265-74.

thyroid acropachy syndrome. Thickening of the extremities (clubbing of the fingers and soft tissue swelling of the hands and feet) in association with periosteal new bone formation, myxedema, hyperthyroidism, and exophtalmos. The etiology is unknown.

Hoegler, F. Acropachy: Clubbing of the fingers and osteoarthropathy. *Arch. Inn. Med.,* 1920, 1:35-7. Gimlette, T. M. Thyroid acropachy. *Lancet,* 1960, 1:22-4.

thyroid hormone unresponsiveness. See *Refetoff syndrome.*

thyroid steal syndrome. Cerebral ischemia caused by diversion of blood flow from the cerebral circulation to the thyroid gland.

Pont, A., & Risher, L. H. Thyroid steal syndrome? *Clin. Nucl. Med.,* 1982, 7:10-2.

thyroid storm. See *Waldenström disease, under Waldenström, Jan Gösta.*

thyroid-adrenocortical insufficiency syndrome. See *under polyglandular autoimmune syndrome.*

tibia vara. See *Erlacher-Blount syndrome.*

tibial aplasia-ectrodactyly syndrome. A familial syndrome, transmitted as an autosomal dominant trait, characterized by aplasia of the tibiae and split hand/ split foot deformity. Associated defects may include distal hypoplasia or bifurcation of the femora, hypoplasia or aplasia of the ulnae, aplasia of the patellae, hypoplasia of the big toes, polydactyly, and cup-shaped ears.

Majewski, F., *et al.* Aplasia of the tibia with split-hand/split-foot deformity. Report of six families with 35 cases and considerations about variability of penetrance. *Hum. Genet.,* 1985, 70:136-47.

tibial hypoplasia-polydactyly syndrome. Synonym: *tibial hypoplasia-polydactyly-syndactyly syndrome.*

A familial syndrome, transmitted as an autosomal dominant trait, characterized by hypoplasia of the tibia, polydactyly of the hands and feet, and syndactyly. In some cases, the tibia may be completely absent. When present, the tibiae are hypoplastic, thickened, bowed, and dislocated. Triphalangeal thumb is a constant feature. Hypoplastic alar cartilage with depressed tip of the nose may be associated.

Ollerenshaw, R. Congenital defects of the long bones of the lower limbs. A contribution to the study of their causes, effects and treatment. *J. Bone Joint Surg.,* 1925, l7:528. Eaton, G. O., & McKusick, V. A. A seemingly unique polydactyly-syndactyly syndrome in four persons in three generations. *Birth Defects,* 1969, 5(3):221-5.

tibial hypoplasia-polydactyly-syndactyly syndrome. See *tibial hypoplasia-polydactyly syndrome.*

tibial stress syndrome. See *shin splint syndrome.*

tibialis anterior syndrome. See *anterior tibial compartment syndrome.*

tibioperoneal diaphyseal toxopachyostosis. See *Weismann-Netter syndrome.*

tic douloureux. See *trigeminal neuralgia.*

tic douloureux of Jacobson nerve. See *Reichert syndrome, under Reichert, Frederick Leet.*

tic douloureux of the chorda tympani. See *Rosen neuralgia.*

tic douloureux of the glossopharyngeal nerve. See *Reichert syndrome, under Reichert, Frederick Leet.*

TIECHE, MAX (Swiss physician, 1878-1938)

Jadassohn-Tièche nevus. See *under Jadassohn, Josef.*

TIETZ, WALTER (American physician)

Tietz syndrome. Synonym: *albinism-deafness syndrome.*

A syndrome of albinism, blue eyes, deaf-mutism, and hypoplasia of the eyebrows, transmitted as an autosomal dominant trait.

Tietz, W. A syndrome of deaf-mutism associated with albinism showing dominant autosomal inheritance. *Am. J. Hum. Genet.,* 1963, 15:259-64.

TIETZE, ALEXANDER (German physician, 1864-1927)

Tietze disease. See *Tietze syndrome.*

Tietze syndrome. Synonyms: *Tietze disease, chondrodynia costosternalis, chondropathia tuberosa, costal chondritis, costal junction syndrome, costochondral junction syndrome.*

An anterior chest wall disease characterized by painful nonsuppurative fusiform or bulbous swelling of one or more costal cartilages showing on the x-ray picture as medial clavicular hypertrophy, clavicular and costal osteosclerosis, periarticular calcification, and cartilaginous calcification of the ribs. The disease occurs in persons of all ages, with special predilection for the second and third decades. Clinically, it is characterized by upper anterior chest pain that may or may not radiate to the shoulder and arm. It is often aggravated by sneezing, coughing, inspiration, bending, recumbency, or exertion. The terms **Tietze syndrome** and **costochondritis** are often used interchangeably, but the Tietze syndrome is associated with swelling, whereas costochondritis is not.

Tietze, A. Über eine eigenartige Häufung von Fällen mit Dystrophie der Rippenknorpel. *Berlin Klin. Wschr.,* 1921, 58:829-31.

tight building syndrome. See *sick building syndrome.*

tight collar syndrome. See *carotid sinus syndrome.*

tight hamstring syndrome. Tightness, spasm, or contracture of the hamstring muscles (the posterior femoral muscles consisting of the biceps femoris, semitendinosus, and semimembranosus), resulting in spondylolisthesis of the lower spine. It is characterized by severe restriction of straight raising of the legs, inability to bend the trunk forward, and the gait pattern with pelvic waddle. Some patients have a neurologic deficit in the lower extremities. Older children and adolescents are most frequently affected.

Phalen, G. S., & Dickson, J. A. Spondylolisthesis and tigh hamstrings. *J. Bone Joint Surg.,* 1961, 43(A):505-12.

TILLAUX, PAUL JULES (French physician, 1834-1904)

Tillaux-Phocas disease. See *Cheatle disease.*

tilted disk syndrome. An eye disease characterized by myopic astigmatism, situs inversus of the optic disk, congenital conus, lower nasal thinning of retinal pigment epithelium and choroid, and temporal hemianopia in which the field defects often cross the vertical midline.

Young, S. E., *et al.* The tilted disk syndrome. *Am. J. Ophth.,* 1976, 82:16-23.

TIMME, WALTER (American physician, born 1874-1956)

Timme syndrome. A syndrome of thymo-adreno-pituitary insufficiency, characterized by fatigability, hypotension, headache, and growth disorders. The first phase begins before puberty and is marked by disproportionate bone development, delayed fusion of the epiphyses with the bone shafts, hyperexensibility of the joints, sparsity of body hair, muscle cramps, spasmophilia, hemophilic tendency, delayed dentition, enlarged tonsils and adenoids, hypotension, hypoglycemia, epistaxes, cyanosis of the extremities, fatigability, small sella turcica, enuresis, and low carbon dioxide coefficiency of the blood. The second phase, beginning at puberty, is characterized by rapid growth, delayed menstruation, genital infantilism, elicitation of an adrenal line, gastric hyperacidity, and lack of body hair. The third phase, observed during the third decade, is characterized by enlargement of the sella turcica, acromegaly, drowsiness, confusion, headache, epileptiform attacks, and mental deterioration.

Timme, W. A new pluriglandular compensatory syndrome. *Endocrinology,* 1918, 2:209-40.

TIN-uveitis syndrome. See ***t**ubulo**i**nterstitial **n**ephritis-uveitis syndrome.*

tinea decalvans. See *Cazenave vitiligo.*

tinea nososa. See *Beigel disease.*

tinea tonsurans. See *Gruby disease.*

tinnitus-deafness-vertigo syndrome. See *Lermoyez syndrome.*

TINU. See ***t**ubulo**i**nterstitial **n**ephritis-**u**veitis syndrome.*

tired arm. See *Wartenberg disease (1).*

TISDALE, W. K. (American physician)

Sakati-Nyhan-Tisdale syndrome. See *under Sakati.*

TIZZARD, T. (British ophthalmologist)

Tizzard syndrome. Synonym: *microcornea-brachydactyly syndrome.*

A concurrence of short large hands and feet and short fingers with microcorneae.

Tizzard, T. Familial occurrence of microcorneae associated with brachydactyly. *Proc. R. Soc. Med., London,* 1934, 27:151.

TKCR (torticollis-keloids-cryptorchidism-renal dysplasia) syndrome. See *Goeminne syndrome.*

TMJ (temporomandibular joint) dysfunction syndrome. See *temporomandibular joint syndrome.*

TMJ (temporomandibular joint) pain dysfunction syndrome. See *temporomandibular joint syndrome.*

TMJ syndrome. See *temporomandibular joint syndrome.*

TMP. See *Turner-mongolism polysyndrome, under Turner, Henry H.*

TMPDS (temporomandibular pain and dysfunction syndrome). See *temporomandibular joint syndrome.*

TMS (trapezoidocephaly-multiple synostoses) syndrome. See *Antley-Bixler syndrome.*

Tn syndrome. An acquired disorder characterized by polyagglutination of blood cells following an exposure to α-*N*-acetyl-*D*-galactosamine residues (Tn antigen) at the cell surface. The syndrome is sometimes associated with hemolytic anemia and leukemic and preleukemic states.

Nurden, A. T., *et al.* Surface modification in the platelets of a patient with alpha-*N*-acetyl-*D*-galactosamine residues, the Tn-syndrome. *J. Clin. Invest.,* 1982, 70:1281-91.

tobacco withdrawal syndrome. See *under withdrawal syndrome.*

TOBIAS, JOSE W. (Argentine physician)

Pancoast-Tobias syndome. See *Pancoast syndrome.*

Tobias syndrome. See *Pancoast syndrome.*

TODD, J. (Canadian physician)

Todd syndrome. See *Alice in Wonderland syndrome.*

TODD, ROBERT BENTLEY (British physician, 1809-1860)

Todd paralysis. Synonym: *postepileptic paralysis.*

Hemiplegia of an arm or leg, lasting for a few minutes to several days, after an epileptic attack.

Todd, R. B. *Clinical lectures on paralysis, certain diseases of the brain.* 2nd ed. London, Churchill, 1856.

TODV. See *tricho-oculodermovertebral syndrome.*

Tokut-ze disease. See *Kashin-Bek disease.*

TOLKSDORF, M. (German physician)

Wiedemann-Tolksdorf syndrome. See *under Wiedemann.*

TÖLLNER, U. (German physician)

Töllner syndrome. A syndrome of heptacarpo-octatarso-dactyly combined with cheilo-gnatho-palatoschisis, hypertelorism, macroglossia, horseshoe kidney, micropenis, penis palmatus, and cardiovascular abnormalities.

Töllner, U., *et al.* Hepta-octatarso-dactyly combined with multiple malformations. *Eur. J. Pediat.,* 1981, 136:207-10.

TOLOSA, EDUARDO (Spanish physician)

Tolosa-Hunt ophthalmoplegia. See *Tolosa-Hunt syndrome.*

Tolosa-Hunt syndrome (THS). Synonyms: *Tolosa-Hunt ophthalmoplegia, ophthalmoplegia dolorosa, painful ophthalmoplegia, recurrent algetic ophthalmoplegia, recurrent ophthalmoplegia.*

Recurrent unilateral retro-orbital pain with extraocular palsies, usually involving the third, fourth, fifth, and sixth cranial nerves and attributed to inflammation of the cavernous sinus. Scotoma, sluggish pupil reaction to light, and diminished corneal sensitivity are associated. The disease usually lasts several months to several years. Males and females are equally affected, most commonly in their fifth decade. Diabetic ophthalmoplegia, intracavernous carotid aneurysm, and nasopharyngeal tumors are the usual causes.

Tolosa, E. Periarteritic lesions of the carotid siphon with the clinical features of a carotid infraclinoidal aneurysm. *J. Neurol. Neurosurg. Psychiat.,* 1954, 17:300-2. Hunt. W. E., *et al.* Painful ophthalmoplegia. Its relation to indolent inflammation of the cavernous sinus. *Neurology,* 1961, 11:56-62.

toluene sniffing syndrome. A condition caused by toluene-containing vapor sniffing, and characterized by muscle weakness, abdominal pain, hematemesis, mental disorders, cerebellar symptoms, peripheral neuropathy, hypokalemia, hypophosphatemia, hyperchloremia, hypobicarabonatemia, rhabdomyolysis, and hyperchloremic acidosis.

Streicher, H. Z., *et al.* Syndromes of toluene sniffing in adults. *Ann. Intern. Med.,* 1981, 94:758-62.

tomato tumor. See *Brooke epithelioma.*

TOMMASI, M. (French physician)

Jeune-Tommasi syndrome. See *under Jeune.*

tomomania syndrome. See *Munchausen syndrome.*

tonga. See *Charlouis disease.*

tonic pupil. See *Adie syndrome.*

tonic pupil syndrome. See *Adie syndrome.*

tonic pupil plus. See *Ross syndrome.*

TOOD. See *tricho-odonto-onychodermal syndrome.*

TOOMEY, J. (American physician)

Cole-Rauschkolb-Toomey syndrome. See *Zinsser-Engman-Cole syndrome.*

TOOTH, HOWARD HENRY (British physician, 1856-1925)

Charcot-Marie-Tooth disease (CMTD). See *Charcot-Marie-Tooth syndrome.*

Charcot-Marie-Tooth syndrome (CMTS). See *under Charcot.*

Charcot-Marie-Tooth-Hoffmann syndrome. See *Charcot-Marie-Tooth syndrome.*

Tooth muscular atrophy. See *Charcot-Marie-Tooth syndrome.*

tooth-nail syndrome. Synonyms: *Witkop syndrome, Witkop-Weech-Giansanti syndrome, nail dysplasia-hypodontia syndrome.*

An ectodermal dysplasia syndrome, transmitted as an autosomal dominant trait, characterized by fine hair, sparse or absent eyebrows, missing and conical teeth, hypoplasia or koilonychia of the fingernails and especially the toenails in children (adult fingernails may appear normal), and peculiar facies with eversion of the lower lip, large ears, and moderate frontal bossing in some cases.

Witkop, J. C., Jr. Genetic disease of the oral cavity. In: Tiecke, R. W., ed. *Oral pathology*. New York, McGraw-Hill, 1965, pp. 810-4. Giansanti, J. S., *et al.* The "tooth and nail" type of autosomal dominant ectodermal dysplasia. *Oral Surg.*, 1974, 37:576-82. Weech, A. A. Hereditary ectodermal dysplasia (congenital ectodermal defect). A report of two cases. *Am. J. Dis. Child.*, 1929, 37:766-90..

top of the basilar syndrome. Synonyms: *vertebrobasilar insufficiency, vertebrobasilar ischemia.*

An occlusive vascular disease of the rostral basilar artery frequently associated with infarction of the midbrain, thalamus, and parts of the temporal and occipital lobes fed by posterior communicating and posterior cerebral arterial tributaries of the basilar artery. The symptoms include visual, oculomotor, and behavioral disorders, alexia without agraphia, and memory loss. See also *vertebrobasilar syndrome.*

Caplan, L. R. "Top of the basilar" syndrome. *Neurology*, 1980, 30:72-9.

TORCH (**t**oxoplasmosis-**o**ther [congenital syphilis and viruses]-**r**ubella-**c**ytomegalovirus-**h**erpes virus) **syndrome.** Several infections contracted in utero with similar clinical and laboratory findings in newborn infants. Petechiae, purpura, jaundice, chorioretinitis, anemia, thrombocytopenia, hepatomegaly, splenomegaly, and small size for gestational age are the principal clinical symptoms.

Shin, Y. H., *et al.* The "TORCH syndrome." *Pediat. Ann.*, 1976, 5:106-13. Fine, J. D., & Arndt, K. A. The TORCH syndrome: A clinical review. *J. Am. Acad. Derm.*, 1985, 12:697-706.

TORG, JOSEPH S. (American orthopedic surgeon)

Torg syndrome. Synonyms: *hereditary multicentric osteolysis, recessive carpotarsal osteolysis.*

A familial form of multicentric osteolysis, transmitted as an autosomal recessive trait, characterized by progressive resorption involving the hands, wrists, elbows, feet, ankles, and knees, associated with collapse of the carpal and tarsal bones with narrowing of the intercarpal joints, thin cortices, narrowing and subluxation of the metacarpophalangeal and interphalangeal joints, fusion at the intercarpal, metacarpal, and interphalangeal joints, flexion contractures of the knees, hips, and elbows, and fusiform enlargement of the digits. Onset takes place in childhood.

Torg, J. S., *et al.* Hereditary multicentric osteolysis with recessive transmission: A new syndrome. *J. Pediat.*, 1969, 75:243-52.

torn anterior cruciate ligament syndrome. See *anterior cruciate ligament syndrome.*

tornwalditis. See *Thornwaldt bursitis.*

TORNWALDT, GUSTAV LUDWIG. See THORNWALDT, GUSTAV LUDWIG

Tornwaldt cyst. See *Thornwaldt bursitis.*

Tornwaldt disease. See *Thornwaldt bursitis.*

Tornwaldt syndrome. See *Thornwaldt bursitis.*

TORRE, DOUGLAS P. (American physician)

Bloom-Torre-Machacek syndrome. See *Bloom syndrome.*

Muir-Torre (MT) syndrome. See *under Muir.*

Torre syndrome. See *Muir-Torre syndrome.*

TORRICELLI, C. (Italian physician)

Brusa-Torricelli syndrome. See *aniridia-Wilms tumor syndrome.*

torsades de pointes (TP) syndrome. Synonyms: *atypical ventricular tachycardia, cardiac ballet, delayed repolarization arrhythmia, ectopic ventricular tachycardia, paroxysmal ventricular fibrillation, polymorphous ventricular tachycardia, transient recurrent ventricular fibrillation, ventricular fibrilloflutter, repetitive paroxysmal tachycardia.*

Torsades de pointes (twisting of the points) is a form of ventricular tachycardia characterized by a long QT interval, polymorphous QRS complexes with varying RR intervals, and fluctuating QRS axes. It is usually initiated by a ventricular premature contraction occurring late during ventricular repolarization. Syncope is its most serious complication. Quinidine therapy is its principal cause, but other causative factors may include antiarrhythmic and other drugs, long QT syndrome, the Jervell and Lange-Nielsen syndrome, the Romano-Ward syndrome, hypokalemia, hypomagnesemia, myocardial ischemia, myocarditis, bradyarrhythmias, mitral valve prolapse syndrome, liquid protein diets, subarachnoid hemorrhage, and hypothermia.

Chung, E. K. Torsades de pointes. In his: *Electrocardiography. Practical application with vectorial principles.* 3rd ed. Norwalk, Connecticut, Appleton-Century-Crofts, 1985, pp. 273-7.

torsion dystonia. See *Ziehen-Oppenheim syndrome.*

torsion neurosis. See *Ziehen-Oppenheim syndrome.*

torsion spasm. See *Ziehen-Oppenheim syndrome.*

TORSTEN SJÖGREN. See SJÖGREN, KARL GUSTAF TORSTEN

torticollis. See *Cruchet disease.*

torticollis atlantoepistrophealis. See *Grisel syndrome.*

torticollis-keloids-cryptorchidism-renal (TKCR) dysplasia syndrome. See *Goeminne syndrome.*

tortua facies. See *trigeminal neuralgia.*

Torula meningitis. See *Busse-Buschke disease.*

torulopsis. See *Busse-Buschke disease.*

torulosis. See *Busse-Buschke disease.*

TOS. See *thoracic outlet syndrome.*

TOS. See *toxic oil syndrome.*

total allergy syndrome. Synonym: *twentieth century syndrome.*

A psychiatric syndrome of hypersensitivity to one's environment, particularly synthetic items, characterized by a wide variety of mental and physical symptoms.

Stewart, D. E., & Raskin, J. Psychiatric assessment of patients with "20th-century disease" ("total allergy syndrome"). *Canad. Med. Assoc. J.*, 1985, 133:1001-6.

total colonic aganglìosis. See *Jirásek-Zuelzer-Wilson syndrome.*

TOULOUSE-LAUTREC, HENRI MARIE RAYMOND, DE (French painter, 1864-1901)

Toulouse-Lautrec disease. See *pyknodysostosis.*

TOURAINE, ALBERT (French physician, 1883-1961)

Christ-Siemens-Touraine (CST) syndrome. See *hypohidrotic ectodermal dysplasia syndrome.*

Cockayne-Touraine syndrome. See *epidermolysis bullosa syndrome.*

Grönblad-Strandberg-Touraine syndrone. See *pseudoxanthoma elasticum.*

Peutz-Touraine syndrome. See *Peutz-Jeghers syndrome.*

Peutz-Touraine-Jeghers syndrome. See *Peutz-Jeghers syndrome.*

Touraine syndrome. See *Behçet syndrome.*

Touraine-Renault syndrome. Synonym: *benign symmetrical lipomatosis.*

Diffuse, symmetrical, unencapsulated, painless liptomatous lesions of the trunk, occurring chiefly in middle-aged males. Most affected persons are heavy drinkers; some have liver diseases.

Touraine, A., & Renault, P. Lipomatose segmentaire du tronc. *Bull. Soc. Fr. Derm. Syph.*, 1938, 45:924-7.

Touraine-Solente-Golé (TSG) syndrome. See *pachydermoperiostosis syndrome.*

TOURAINE, M. A. (French physician)

Touraine syndrome. Synonyms: *angioid streaks in cardiovascular disorders, systemic elastorrhexia.*

Angioid streaks of the retina in association with with cardiovascular lesions due to elastic degeneration of the middle coat of the arteries, such as aortitis, myocarditis, arteriosclerosis, cerebrovascular disorders, vascular calcification, and hypertension.

Touraine, M. A. L'élastorrhexie systématisée. *Bull. Sc. Fr. Derm., 1940*, 47:255-73.

TOURETTE, GILLES, DE LA. See GILLES DE LA TOURETTE, GEORGES EDMOUND ALBERT BRUTUS

TOURIAN, ARA Y. (American physician)

phenylketonuria, Tourian and Sidbury type. See *under phenylketonuria.*

tourniquet syndrome. The term "tourniquet syndrome" was first used in connection with ischemia due to hair or cloth encircling a toe (*hair strangulation*), thus obstructing its blood supply. It now applies to an ischemic condition caused by any mechanical obstruction of blood vessels supplying the affected part.

Alpert, J. J., *et al.* Strangulations of an appendage by hair wrapping. *N. Engl. J. Med.*, 1965, 273:860.

TOWNES, PHILIP L. (American physician)

Townes syndrome. Synonym: *Townes-Brocks syndrome.*

An autosomal dominant syndrome of imperforate anus, sensorineural deafness, and anomalies of the hands and feet. Hand abnormalities are essentially bifid thumb, triphalangeal thumb, or polydactyly of a triphalangeal thumb and accessory carpal bones related to the supernumerary thumb. Foot abnormalities are absence of a toe, shortening of a foot, small toes, clinodactyly, and flat feet. Ear abnormalities consist mainly of the "satyr" deformity.

Townes, P. L., & Brocks, E. R. Hereditary syndrome of imperforate anus with hand, foot, and ear anomalies. *J. Pediat.*, 1972, 81:321-6.

Townes-Brocks syndrome. See *Towns syndrome.*

TOWNWALDT, GUSTAV LUDWIG. See THORNWALDT, GUSTAV LUDWIG

toxic syndrome (TS). See *toxic oil syndrome.*

toxic allergic syndrome. See *toxic oil syndrome.*

toxic encephalopathy. See *Dupré syndrome.*

toxic epidemic syndrome (TES). See *toxic oil syndrome.*

toxic epidermal necrolysis (TEN). Synonyms: *Brocq-Debré-Lyell syndrome, Debré-Lamy-Lyell syndrome, Lyell syndrome, epidermolysis acuta toxica, epidermolysis combustiformis, epidermolysis necroticans combustiformis, epidemolysis toxica, erythrodermia bullosa with epidermolysis, toxico-allergic epidermal necrolysis.*

A rare but frequently fatal form or exfoliative dermatitis caused by toxic and allergic reactions to a number of factors, e.g., sepsis, lymphoma, graft-versus-host disease, and a variety of drugs, most notably sulfonamides. After the prodromal symptoms (burning sensation of the conjunctiva, skin tenderness, fever, malaise, and arthralgia), there is a morbilliform rash, usually on the face and extremities, which becomes confluent, leading to diffuse erythema. At this stage, traction applied to the skin will cause the epidermis to wrinkle and separate (Nikolsky sign). The rash is followed by vesiculation and confluence of vesicles with formation of large, flaccid, irregular bullae which rupture, exposing red, denuded skin with a burn-like appearance. In some cases, there is a loss of the epidermis from a half or more of the body surface, resembling generalized scalding. The mucous membranes of the lips, mouth, conjunctivae, genitalia, and anus usually show erythema, vesiculation, and erosion. The eyebrows and cilia may be lost with the peeling-off of the epidermis. The fingernails and toenails may be shed. Fever, tracheitis, bronchopneumonia, and gastro-esophageal hemorrhage may occur. Residual scarring of the mucous membranes is common. Hematological and biochemical changes include leukocytosis, albuminuria, increased transaminase levels, and water-electrolyte balance disorders. The *staphylococcal scalded skin syndrome* and *toxic epidermal necrolysis* were once considered the same entity; they are now recognized as separate diseases with different etiologies.

Brocq, A. J. Schème des éruptions bulleuses. Le pemphigus subaigu malin à bulles extensives et faits connexes. *Ann. Derm. Syph., Paris,* 1919, 7:449-61. Debré, R., Lamy, M., & Lamotte, M. Un case d'érythrodermie avec épidermolyse chez un enfant de 12 ans. *Bull. Soc. Pediat., Paris,* 1939, 37:231-8. Lyell, A. Toxic epidermal necrolysis: Eruption resembling scalding of the skin. *Brit. J. Derm.*, 1956, 68:355-61.

toxic hip synovitis. See *observation hip syndrome.*

toxic hydrocephalus. See *pseudotumor cerebri syndrome.*

toxic oil syndrome (TOS). Synonyms: *alimentary toxic oil syndrome, epidemic toxic syndrome, oil-associated pneumonic paralytic eosinophilic syndrome, Spanish oil syndrome, Spanish toxic syndrome, Spanish toxic-allergic syndrome, Spanish toxic oil syndrome, toxic syndrome (TS), toxic allergic syndrome, toxic epidemic syndrome (TES), toxic rapeseed oil syndrome.*

A multisystem toxic syndrome caused by ingestion of olive oil adulterated with rapeseed oil which was denaturated with aniline for industrial purposes and subsequently re-refined. More than 20,000 persons were affected during the 1981 outbreak of mass poisoning in Spain; the mortality rate was 1.7 %. Onset was characterized by fever, acute interstitial pneumonia, pruritus, exanthems, myalgias, and eosinophilia. Fatal respiratory distress syndrome developed in some cases. The principal pulmonary pathological findings were generalized endothelial lesions, septal edema, inflammatory mononuclear infiltrates, and degenerative and desquamative changes. The syndrome evolved in three phases. The acute phase was characterized by symptoms appearing in the following order of frequency: cough, dyspnea, chest pain, cyanosis, wheezing, fever, chills, asthenia, malaise, anorexia, itching, exanthems, myalgia, arthralgia, headache, dizziness, nausea, vomiting, abdominal pain, diarrhea, and hepatosplenomegaly. Blood tests showed eosinophilia, leukocytosis, hypocholesterolemia, and increased levels of LDH, GOT, GPT, and GGT. The subacute phase was characterized mainly by exacerbation of symptoms and the appearance of additional signs, such as skin edema, urticaria, cramps, the sicca syndrome, pulmonary hypertension, and increased eosinophilia. The chronic phase appeared 4 to 6 months after the onset of symptoms, manifested mainly by neuromuscular complications, contractures, muscle atrophy, scleroderma-like skin lesions, and progressive weight loss and cachexia. Immmunoglobulinemia IgE, eosinophilia, and immunologic hypersensitivity suggest possible allergic mechanisms.

Tabuenca, J. M. Toxic-allergic syndrome caused by ingestion of rapeseed oil denaturated with aniline. *Lancet,* 1981, 2:567. Symposium. The toxic oil syndrome. *Eur. J. Resp. Dis.,* 1983, 64(Suppl. 126):409-30.

toxic rapeseed oil syndrome. See *toxic oil syndrome.*

toxic shock syndrone (TSS). Synonyms: *menstrual toxic shock syndrome, staphylococcal toxic shock syndrome.*

An illness caused by penicillin-resistant strains of *Staphylococcus aureus* which produce exotoxin C and enterotoxin F. The symptoms include multisystem dysfunction, erythema, rash with desquamation of the palms and soles, fever, hypotension, and occasional shock. Associated symptoms include pharyngeal redness, strawberry tongue, conjunctival lesions, diarrhea, vomiting, myalgias, rhabdomyolysis, and toxic encephalopathy. Laboratory findings usually show azotemia, elevated serum glutamate oxoloacetate transaminase (SGOT), elevated serum bilirubin, thrombocytopenia, increased serum creatinine kinase levels, myoglobinuria, and hypocalcemia. The syndrome became epidemic in 1980 among young menstruating women at the time when certain brands of superabsorbent tampons were introduced. The syndrome is also associated with some skin infections, vaginal infections, postcesarean wound infections, surgical wound infections, and other infections.

Weinberg, A. N., & Swartz, M. N. General considerations of bacterial diseases. In: Fitzpatrick, T. B., Eisen, A. Z., Wolff, K., Freedberg, I. M., & Austen, K. F., eds. *Dermatology in general medicine.* 3rd ed. New York, McGraw-Hill, 1987, pp. 2089-2100. Locksley, R. M. Staphlylococcal infections. In: Braunwald, E., Isselbacher, K, J., Petersdorf, R. G. Wilson, J. D., Martin, J. B., & Fauci, A. S., eds. *Harrison's principles of internal medicine.* 11th ed. New York, McGraw-Hill, 1987, pp. 537-43.

toxico-allergic epidermal necrolysis. See *toxic epidermal necrolysis.*

toxicomania chirurgica. See *Munchausen syndrome.*

toxigenic osteoperiostitis ossificans. See *Marie-Bamberger syndrome, under Marie, Pierre.*

toxopachy. See *Weismann-Netter syndrome.*

toxopachyostéose diaphysaire tibiopéronière. See *Weismann-Netter syndrome.*

TOYAMA, T. (Japanese physician)

Toyama syndrome. Synonyms: *pityriasis circinata, pityriasis rotunda, pseudoichthyose acuise en taches circulaires.*

A skin disease characterized by well-defined, brown, scaly, perfectly circular patches of various diameters, originally observed in the Far East and, more recently, Egypt and the West Indies. Some writers suggest that it is a form of acquired ichthyosis.

Toyama, I. Isshu no kosshoku enkei rakushosei hifubyo ni tsuite. *Japan. Zschr. Derm.,* 1906, 6:91-105.

TP. See *torsades de pointes syndrome.*

TPPD (thoracic-pelvic-phalangeal dystrophy). See *Jeune syndrome.*

TPS. See *trismus-pseudocamptodactyly syndrome.*

tracheal diverticulosis. See *Mounier-Kuhn syndrome.*

tracheobronchiectasis. See *Mounier-Kuhn syndrome.*

tracheobronchiomegaly (TBM). See *Mounier-Kuhn syndrome.*

tracheobronchiopathic malacia. See *Mounier-Kuhn syndrome.*

trachoma. Synonyms: *Arlt syndrome, chronic follicular keratoconjunctivitis, granular conjunctivitis, Egyptian ophthalmia.*

A contagious *Chlamydia trachomatis* infection of the eyes, characterized by keratoconjunctivitis with pannus, papillary hypertrophy, follicles, and scarring, often leading to blindness. The disease occurs chiefly in Asia, Africa, and the Mediterranean areas, where it is the single greatest cause of blindness.

*Arlt, C. F., von. *Die Krankheiten des Auges.* Prag, Credner & Kleinbub, 1851-6.

trachomatous folliculoma. See *Pascheff folliculoma.*

trachybradycardia syndrome. See *bradycardia-tachycardia syndrome.*

transfusion-associated acquired immunodeficiency syndrome (TA-AIDS). See *under acquired immunodeficiency syndrome.*

transient acantholytic dermatosis (TAD). See *Grover disease.*

transient epiphysitis. See *observation hip syndrome.*

transient erythroblastopenia of childhood (TEC) syndrome. A pure red cell aplasia in infants, characterized by moderate to severe anemia with reticulocytopenia, selective aplasia of the erythroid bone marrow elements, and spontaneous recovery, usually within 1 month after onset.

Ritchey, A. K., *et al.* Variable in vitro erythropoiesis in patients with transient erythroblastopenia of childhood. *Yale J. Biol. Med.*, 1985, 58:1-8.

transient hip synovitis. See *observation hip syndrome.*

transient osteopenia of the hip syndrome. Synonyms: *migratory osteolysis of the lower extremities, partial transitory osteoporosis, transient painful osteoporosis of the lower extremities, transitory demineralization of the femoral head.*

Transient osteopenia of the hip and other joints, characterized by severe pain around a major joint, afflicting most commonly middle-aged or elderly persons. Initial radiographic findings fail to reveal any abnormalities but after 2 to 4 weeks there is a widespread osteopenia around the joint. Recovery follows within 4 to 12 months with remineralization of the affected area.

Lequesne, M., *et al.* Partial transitory osteoporosis. *Skelet. Radiol.*, 1977, 2:1-9.

transient painful osteoporosis of the lower extremities. See *transient osteopenia of the hip syndrome.*

transient recurrent ventricular fibrillation. See *torsades de pointes syndrome.*

transient respiratory distress syndrome of the newborn (TRDN). Synonym: *transient tachypnea of the newborn (TTN).*

Respiratory distress occurring soon after birth in term or near-term infants, characterized chiefly by transient tachypnea, with respiratory rates as high as 120 breaths per minute, which resolves within a few hours to a few days. Common complications include respiratory alkalemia and radiographic signs suggestive of alveolar edema. See also *neonatal respiratory distress syndrome.*

Avesy, M. E., *et al.* Transient tachypnea of the newborn: Possible delayed resorption of fluid at birth. *Am. J. Dis. Child.*, 1966, 111:380-5.

transient tachypnea of the newborn (TTN). See *transient respiratory distress syndrome of the newborn.*

transitory alcoholic hyperlipemia. See *Zieve syndrome.*

transitory coxitis. See *observation hip syndrome.*

transitory demineralization of the femoral head. See *transient osteopenia of the hip syndrome.*

transitory hip arthritis. See *observation hip syndrome.*

transplacental transfusion syndrome. See *twin transfusion syndrome.*

transplant lung. See *adult respiratory distress syndrome.*

transurethral prostatectomy syndrome (TUR, TURP, TURS). A potentially fatal complication of transurethral prostatectomy due to absorption of a surgical irrigant into the vascular system, resulting in hypoosmolar volume overload and secondary hyponatremia and water intoxication. Associated disorders include hypokalemia, hemolysis of the red cells, cardiac arrhythmia, elevated central venous pressure, pulmonary disorders, and cardiac edema. Initially there is a rise in patient's blood pressure, which is associated with decreased pulse rate and, in turn, hypotension. The symptoms include restlessness, confusion, nausea, and visual disorders.

Hagstrom, R. S.. Studies on fluid absorption during transurethral prostatic resection. *J. Urol.*, 1955, 73:852-9. Valk, W. L., & Mebust, W. K. Water intoxication. In: Hinman, F., Jr., ed. *Benign prostatic hypertrophy.* Berlin, Springer, 1983, pp. 851-4.

transverse facial fracture. See *Le Fort fracture III.*

TRANTAS, ALEXIOS (Greek ophthalmologist, born 1867)

Horner-Trantas spots. See *under Horner.*

Trantas dots. See *Horner-Trantas spots.*

trapezoidocephaly-multiple synostoses (TMS) syndrome. See *Antley-Bixler syndrome.*

trapezoidocephaly-synostoses syndrome. See *Antley-Bixler syndrome.*

TRAPME (trichorhino-auriculophalangeal-multiple exostoses) **dysplasia.** See *Langer-Giedion syndrome.*

trapped popliteal artery syndrome. See *popliteal artery entrapment syndrome.*

TRAQUAIR, HARRY MOSS (British physician, born 1876)

Traquair scotoma. Synonym: *junction scotoma.*

Central scotoma seen in bitemporal hemaniopia due to interference with the chiasmal fibers resulting from a variety of disorders, such as chiasmal neuritis or tumors.

Traquair, H. M. Bitemporal hemianopia: The later stages and the special features of the scotoma. With an examination of current theories of the mechanism of production of field defects. *Brit. J. Ophth.*, 1917, 1:216-39; 281-94; 337-52.

TRAUBE, LUDWIG (German physician, 1818-1876)

Traube dyspnea. Difficult breathing marked by slow respiratory movements and full expansion and collapse of the thorax during inspiration and expiration.

Traube, L. *Die Symptome der Krankheiten des Respirationsund Circulation-Apparatas.* Berlin, Hirschwald, 1867.

traumatic amenorrhea. See *Asherman syndrome.*

traumatic appalic syndrome (TAS). See *apallic syndrome.*

traumatic asphyxia syndrome. See *Ollivier syndrome.*

traumatic chondritis of the patella. See *Büdinger-Ludloff-Läwen syndrome.*

traumatic edema of the retina. See *Berlin disease (1), under Berlin, Rudolf.*

traumatic hypomenorrhea-amenorrhea. See *Asherman syndrome.*

traumatic intrauterine synechiae. See *Asherman syndrome.*

traumatic laceration of uterine support. See *Allen-Masters syndrome, under Allen, William Myron.*

traumatic migraine. See *under headache syndrome.*

traumatic retinal angiopathy. See *Purtscher disease.*

traumatic rhabdomyolysis. See *crush syndrome.*

traumatic spreading depression syndrome. Synonyms: *juvenile head truma syndrome, postconcussion seizure syndrome.*

A syndrome of transient neurological disorders following mild head injuries in infants and children. The disorders can be divided into convulsive and nonconvulsive groups. Nonconvulsive symptoms include headache, nausea, vomiting, paleness, somnolence, irritability, restlessness, confusion, stupor, coma, hemiparesis or hemiplegia, and motor aphasia. Convulsions are nearly always preceded by some of the nonconvulsive symptoms. The neurolgical disorders of this syndrome are believed to be manifestations of the spreading depression phenomenon. See also *postconcussive syndrome.*

Okaz, H., *et al.* Traumatic spreading depression syndrome. Review of a particular type of head injury in 37 patients. *Brain*, 1977, 100:287-98. Livingston, K. E., & Mahloudji, M. Delayed focal convulsive seizures after head injury in infants and children. A syndrome that mimics extradural hematoma. *Neurology*, 1961, 11:1017-20. Haas, D. C. *et al.* Juvenile head trauma syndromes and their relationship to migraine. *Arch. Neur., Chicago*, 1975, 32:727-30.

traumatic tension ischemia in muscles. See *compartment syndrome.*

traumatic thrombosis of the axillary vein. See *Paget-Schroetter syndrome.*

traumatic uterine adhesions. See *Asherman syndrome.*

traumatic wet lung. See *adult respiratory distress syndrome.*

TRAUNER, RICHARD (Austrian physician)

Trauner-Rieger syndrome. See *nail-patella syndrome.*

travelers' diarrhea syndrome. A common illness affecting international travelers, usually those who visit less developed, particularly tropical countries with relatively low standards of hygiene. The spectrum of clinical symptoms is most frequently characterized by watery diarrhea, cramps, and nausea. Ingestion of fecally contaminated food or beverages is the usual cause, but some instances of diarrhea may be due to consumption of foods to which travelers are not accustomed. *Escherichia coli* is the most common enteric pathogen in travelers' diarrhea, but other bacteria, viruses, and protozoa have been implicated in some cases.

Gorbach, S. L., & Edelman, R. Travelers' diarrhea: National Institutes of Health consensus development conference. *Rev. Infect. Dis.*, 1986, 8(Suppl. 2):S105-S233.

TRDN. See ***t**ransient **r**espiratory **d**istress syndrome of **n**ewborn.*

TREACHER COLLINS. See COLLINS, EDWARD TREACHER

trefoil skull syndrome. See *Holtermüller-Wiedemann syndrome.*

TREITZ, WENZEL (Austrian physician, 1819-1872)

Treitz hernia. Synonyms: *Treitz-Broesicke hernia, duodenojejunal hernia, hernia retroperitonealis, retroperitoneal hernia.*

A retroperitoneal hernia through the duodenojejunal recess.

Treitz, W. *Hernia retroperitonealis. Ein Beitrag zur Geschichte inner Hernien.* Prague, Credner, 1857. Dorka, G. Magenresektion und Treitz-Broesicke Hernie. *Zbl. Chir.*, 1966, 91:1669-72.

Treitz-Broesicke hernia. See *Treitz hernia.*

TRELAT, U. (French physician)

Trèlat syndrome. See *popliteal pterygium syndrome.*

TRELLES, J. OSCAR (Born 1904)

Lhermitte-Trelles syndrome. See *under Lhermitte.*

TRENAUNAY, PAUL (French physician, born 1875)

Klippel-Trénaunay syndrome. See *Klippel-Trénaunay-Weber syndrome.*

Klippel-Trénaunay-Parkes Weber syndrome. See *Klippel-Trénaunay-Weber syndrome.*

Klippel-Trénaunay-Weber (KTW) syndrome. See *under Klippel.*

Ollier-Klippel-Trénaunay-Weber syndrome. See *Klippel-Trénaunay-Weber syndrome.*

trench fever. See *Werner-His disease, under Werner, Heinrich.*

trench gums. See *Vincent infection.*

trench mouth. See *Vincent infection.*

TRENEL, M. (French physician)

Prieur-Trénel syndrome. See *under Prieur.*

TREVES, NORMAN (American physician)

Stewart-Treves syndrome (STS). See *under Stewart, Fred W.*

TREVOR, DAVID (British orthopedic surgeon)

Trevor syndrome. Synonyms: *Fairbank disease, dysplasia epiphysealis hemimelica, epiphyseal osteochondromatosis, osteochondroma of epiphyses, tarso-epiphyseal aclasis, tarsomegaly.*

A rare congenital bone developmental disorder characterized by unilateral irregular cartilaginous overgrowth, usually involving the lower extremities, the upper ones being rarely affected. The cartilaginous growths histologically resemble osteochondroma. The etiology is unknown.

Trevor, D. Tarso-epiphyseal aclasis: A congenital error of epiphysial development. *J. Bone Joint Surg.*, 1950, 32B:204-13. Fairbank, T. J. Dysplasia epiphysialis hemimelica (tarso-epiphysial aclasis). *J. Bone Joint. Surg.*, 1956, 38B:237-57.

tricho-oculodentomandibular progeroid syndrome. A progeroid syndrome characterized by senile facies, short stature, partial alopecia, bilateral cataract, prominent beaked nose, crowded teeth, microretrognathia, enlarged upper gingiva, joint hypermobility, and dysplasia of the subcutaneous adipose tissue.

Hernández, A., *et al.* Síndrome progeroide tricooculodentomandibular. *Bol. Méd. Hosp. Infant. México*, 1982, 39:41-3.

tricho-oculodermovertebral (TODV) syndrome. An ectodermal dysplasia-multiple abnormalities syndrome, probably transmitted as an autosomal recessive trait, characterized by generalized trichodysplasia, dry skin with scaling, hyperchromic spots on the limbs, hyperkeratosis (particularly intense on the soles), dermatoglyphic abnormalities, onychodysplasia, shortness of stature, kyphoscoliosis, unusual facies, minor limb abnormalities, nuclear cataract, narrow palpebral fissures, entropion, trichiasis, and other deformities.

Alves, A. F. P., *et al.* Brief clinical report: An autosomal recessive ectodermal dysplasia syndrome of hypotrichosis, onychodysplasia, hyperkeratosis, kyphoscoliosis, cataract, and other manifestations. *Am. J. Med. Genet.*, 1981, 10:213-8.

tricho-odonto-onychodermal (TOOD) syndrome. A familial ectodermal dysplasia/multiple malformation syndrome. Hair abnormalities consist of hypotrichosis; dental defects include hypodontia, persistence of deciduous teeth, enamel hypoplasia, delayed eruption, supernumerary teeth, and abnormal tooth shape and size; the nails are dystrophic with onychia on some fingers; and the skin is dry with hypochromic atrophic and poikilodermalike spots, absent nipples, irregular areolae, palmar keratosis, abnormal dermatoglyphics, and aplasia cutis of the scalp. Associated anomalies include peculiar facies (leukoma, long philtrum, cupped ears, microstomia, thin lips, hypoplastic alae nasi, blepharoptosis, and hyperpigmented eyelids and periorbital regions), clinodactyly, syndactyly, hypoplastic and flexionless thumb, manus cava, hypoplastic distal and middle phalanges, and congenital hypertrophy of the frenum linguae.

Pinheiro, M., *et al.* A previously undescribed condition: Tricho-odonto-onycho-dermal syndrome. A review of the tricho-odonto-onychial subgroup of ectodermal dysplasias. *Brit. J. Derm.*, 1981, 105:371-82.

tricho-odontodermal dysplasia. See *odonto-onychodermal dysplasia.*

trichodento-osseous (TDO) syndrome. A syndrome, transmitted as an autosomal dominant trait, characterized by kinky hair at birth; amelogenesis imperfecta, small wide-spaced pitted teeth with poor enamel and taurodontism; osteosclerosis, involving chiefly the skull: and brittle nails. Frontal bossing, dolichocephaly, square jaw, and multiple brown circular lesions on the ankles, pretibial areas, hips, and forearms may be associated. Occasional partial craniosynostosis may occur. The scalp hair is curly and the lashes and eyebrows are long; in some cases the hair tends to straighten with age. The teeth often become abscessed. See also *kinky hair syndrome.*

Lichtenstein, J., *et al.* The tricho-dento-osseous (TDO) syndrome. *Am. J. Hum. Genet.*, 1972, 24:569-82. Robinson, C. C., *et al.* Hereditary enamel hypoplasia; its association with characteristic hair structure. *Pediatrics*, 1966, 37:498-502.

trichoepithelioma papulosum multiplex. See *Brooke epithelioma.*

trichofolliculoma. See *Miescher trichofolliculoma.*

trichomegalia congenita. See *chorioretinopathy-pituitary dysfunction syndrome.*

trichomegaly-tapetoretinal degeneration-growth disturbances syndrome. A syndrome of excessively long eyelashes and eyebrows, tapetochoroidal degeneration, retarded growth, frontal alopecia, sparse implantation of hair, and bulging of the occipital and frontal bones. The syndrome is said to have been first described by Oliver and McFarlane in 1965.

Delleman, J. W., & Valbeek, K., van. The syndrome of trichomegaly, tapetoretinal degeneration, and growth disturbances. *Ophthalmologica, Basel,* 1975, 171:313-5.

trichomycosis nodosa. See *Beigel disease.*

trichomycosis nodularis. See *Beigel disease.*

trichopoliodystrophy. See *kinky hair syndrome.*

trichorhino-auriculophalangeal multiple exostoses (TRAPME) dysplasia. See *Langer-Giedion syndrome.*

trichorhinophalangeal dysplasia type I (TRP I). See *trichorhinophalangeal syndrome.*

trichorhinophalangeal dysplasia type II (TRP II). See *Langer-Giedion syndrome.*

trichorhinophalangeal dysplasia type III (TRP III). Synonym: *Sugio-Kajii syndrome.*

A familial syndrome of multiple abnormalities transmitted as an autosomal dominant trait with variable expressivity and incomplete penetrance. It is characterized by postnatal growth retardation, an oval face with a high forehead, antimongoloid palpebral slant, small beaked nose with hypoplastic alae, small downturned mouth with thin vermilion borders, pointed chin, and short fingers and toes. Less frequently seen are osteochondritis of the lumbar vertebrae, cone-shaped epiphyses of the phalanges, and narrow diaphyses of the metacarpal and metatarsal bones. Additional defects may include sparse hair, narrow maxillae, long upper lip, low-set posteriorly angulated ears, narrow trunk, pectus carinatum, broad hips, scoliosis, short limbs, small hands, incurved fifth fingers, proximal thumb, and small feet. See also *Ruvacalba syndrome (1).*

Sugio, Y., & Kajii, T. Ruvacalba syndrome: Autosomal dominant inheritance. *Am. J. Med. Genet.*, 1984, 19:741-53.

trichorhinophalangeal syndrome (TRPS). Synonyms: *Giedion syndrome, trichorhinophalangeal dysplasia type I (TRP I).*

A syndrome of cone-shaped epiphyses, sparse hypopigmented hair, bulbous nose with tented alae, and mild growth retardation. Orofacial defects may also include a prominent long philtrum, narrow palate, micrognathia, and large ears. Hand x-ray findings show cone-shaped epiphyses, usually in the middle phalanges, the central parts often being fused with the remainder of the shafts. In adults, stigmata of previous cones may be seen by splaying of the distal end or the bone. In infants, before the cones become apparent, the early epiphyses appear to be fused to the metaphyses. Ivory epiphyses are common in the distal phalanges. Brachydactyly may occur. There may be a curvature of the fingers due to abnormal epiphyses. The nails are usually thin. Occasional abnormalities may include dysplasia of the femoral head, scoliosis, kyphosis, pes planus, and mental deficiency. Most

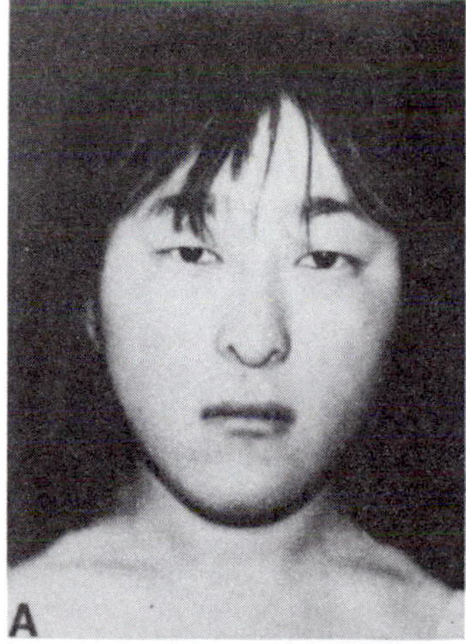

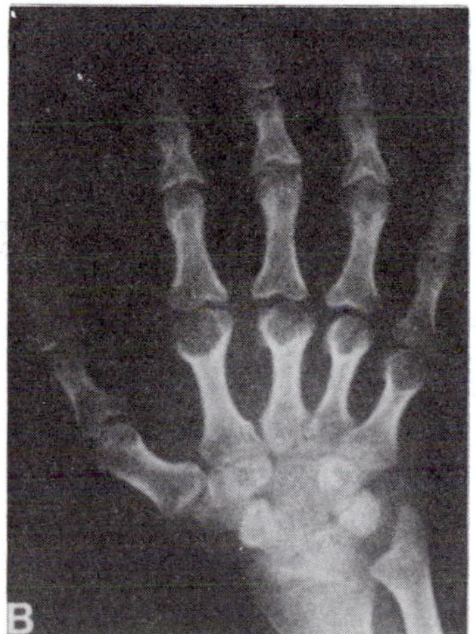

Trichorhinophalangeal dysplasia, type III
Niikawa, Norio & Kamei Tsutomu, *American Journal of Medical Genetics* 24:759-760, 1986. New York: Alan R. Liss, Inc.

cases are inherited as an autosomal dominant trait, but a few instances of recessive transmission have been reported.

Giedion, A. Das tricho-rhino-phalangeale Syndrom. *Helvet. Paediat. Acta*, 1966, 21:141-50.

trichothyodystrophy. See *hair-brain syndrome.*

tricolor syndrome. See *Mondor syndrome (2).*

TRICOT, R. (French physician)

Degos-Delort-Tricot syndrome. See *Degos syndrome.*

tridione syndrome. See *fetal trimethadione syndrome.*

trifacial neuralgia. See *trigeminal neuralgia.*

trigeminal neuralgia. Synonyms: *Fothergill neuralgia, Fothergill syndrome, dolor faciei fothergilli, epileptiform neuralgia, faciei morbus nervorum crucians, neuralgia quinti, neuralgia spasmodica, prosopalgia, tic douloureux, tortua facies, trifacial neuralgia.*

Unilateral, paroxysmal, stabbing pain of high intensity in the area supplied by the second or third division of the trigeminal nerve, usually occurring during middle life. The attacks are sudden, and pain may persist a few seconds to several minutes and then disappear as promptly as they arise. The pain may be associated with spasmodic contraction of the facial muscles, hence the synonym **tic douloureux.** The attacks may precipitated by touching the trigger zones located on the vermilion border of the lips, nasal alae, cheeks, and around the eyes. The condition appears to occur more often on the right side, being more common in women than in men. The etiology is unknown.

*Fothergill, S. *A concise and systematic account of a painful affection of the nerves of the face, commonly called tic douloureux.* London, 1804.

trigeminal sensory neuropathy syndrome. A disorder of the trigeminal nerve, chiefly its second and third division, characterized by numbness, tingling, and impaired taste.

Blau, J. N. Trigeminal sensory neuropathy. *N. Engl. J. Med.*, 1969, 281:873-6.

trigeminal trophic syndrome. Synonyms: *neurotrophic trigeminal ulceration, ulceration en arc.*

Facial ulceration following damage of the sensory root of the trigeminal nerve.

Loveman, A. An unusual dermatosis following section of the fifth cranial nerve. *Arch. Derm. Syph., Chicago,* 1933, 28:369-75. Weintraub, E., *et al.* Trigeminal trophic syndrome. A case and review. *J. Am. Acad. Derm.*, 1982, 6:52-7.

trigemino-encephalo-angiomatosis. See *Sturge-Weber syndrome.*

trigeminosympathetic neuralgia. See *Bonnet syndrome (2), under Bonnet, Paul.*

trigger point syndrome. See *myofascial trigger point syndrome.*

trigonocephaly syndrome. See *Opitz trigonocephaly syndrome.*

trimethadione syndrome. See *fetal trimethadione syndrome.*

trimethadione embryopathy. See *fetal trimethadione syndrome.*

trimethylaminuria. See *fish odor syndrome.*

triphalangeal thumb and brachy-ectrodactyly syndrome. A syndrome of triphalangeal thumbs, short distal phalanges of the index fingers, hypoplastic or absent nails, and shortness of the third toe due to hypoplasia of the phalanges. The syndrome is transmitted as an autosomal dominant trait.

Carnevale, A., *et al.* A new syndrome of triphalangeal thumbs and brachy-ectrodactyly. *Clin. Genet.*, 1980, 18:244-52.

triphalangeal thumb-big toe duplication syndrome. Synonym: *familial opposable triphalangeal thumb-big toe duplication syndrome.*

A familial form of preaxial polydactyly, transmitted as an autosomal dominant trait, characterized by the presence of opposable triphalangeal thumbs associated with duplication of the big toes.

Atwood, E. S., & Pond, C. P. A polydactylous family. *J. Hered.*, 1917, 8:96. Haas, S. L. Tri-phalangeal thumbs. *Am. J. Roentgen.*, 1939, 42:677-82. Merlob, P., *et al.* Familial opposable triphalangeal thumbs associated with duplication of the big toes. *J. Med. Genet.*, 1985, 223:78-80.

triphalangeal thumb-hypoplastic anemia syndrome. See *Aase-Smith syndrome.*

triple edema syndrome. See *Ballantyne syndrome (2).*

triple-X syndrome. See *chromosome XXX syndrome.*

triple-X chromosome syndrome. See *chromosome XXX syndrome.*

triploidy syndrome. See *chromosome triploidy syndrome.*

trismus-pseudocamptodactyly syndrome (TPS). Synonyms: *Hecht syndrome, Hecht-Beals-Wilson syndrome, Dutch-Kentucky syndrome.*

A relatively rare syndrome, with autosomal dominant inheritance, characterized by the inability to open the mouth completely (trismus) and short finger-flexor tendons with wrist extension (pseudocamptodactyly), various foot deformities, and less than normal stature. The syndrome was observed in an Appalachian family of Dutch extraction, hence the synonym *Dutch-Kentucky syndrome.*

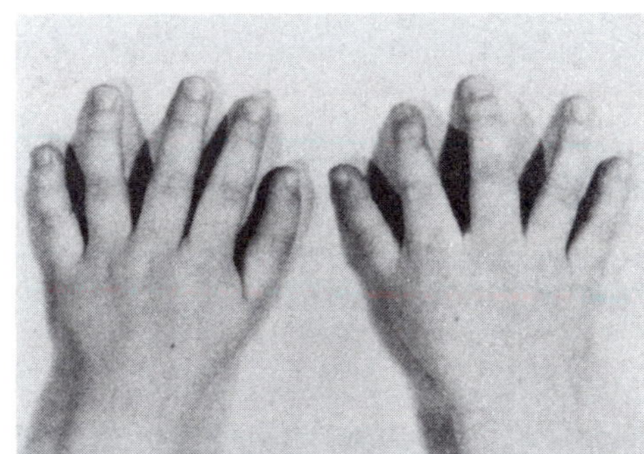

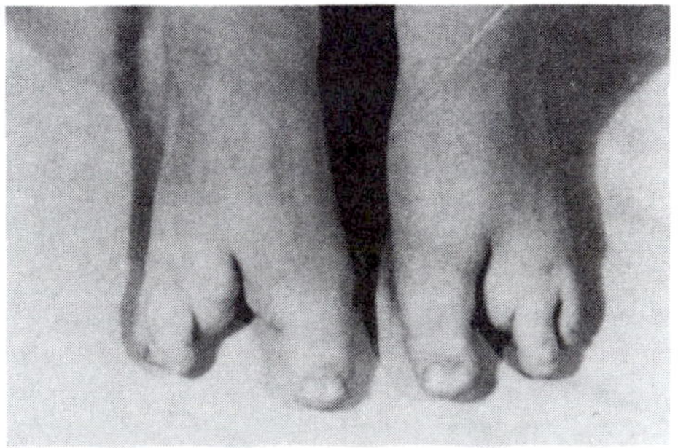

Triphalangeal thumb and brachy-ectrodactyly syndrome
Silengo, M. Cirillo, M. Biagioli, G. Lopez Bell, G. Bona & P. Franceschini, *Clinical Genetics* 31:13-18, 1987. Munksgaard International Publishers, Copenhagen, Denmark.

Hecht, F., & Beals, R. Inability to open the mouth fully: An autosomal dominant phenotype with facultative camptodactyly and short stature. Preliminary note. *Birth Defects*, 1969, 5(3):96-8. Wilson, R. V., *et al.* Autosomal dominant inheritance of shortening of flexor profundus muscle-tendon unit with limitation of jaw excursion. *Birth Defects*, 1969, 5(3):99-102. Mabry, C. C., *et al.* Trismus pseudocamptodactyly syndrome. Dutch-Kentucky syndrome. *J. Pediat.*, 1974, 85:503-8.

trisomy 1q. See *chromosome 1q duplication syndrome.*

trisomy 2p. See *chromosome 2p duplication syndrome.*

trisomy 2q. See *chromosome 2q duplication syndrome.*

trisomy 3p. See *chromosome 3p duplication syndrome.*

trisomy 3q. See *chromosome 3q duplication syndrome.*

trisomy 4p. See *chromosome 4p duplication syndrome.*

trisomy 4q. See *chromosome 4q duplication syndrome.*

trisomy 5p. See *chromosome 5p duplication syndrome.*

trisomy 5q. See *chromosome 5q duplication syndrome.*

trisomy 6p. See *chromosome 6p duplication syndrome.*

trisomy 6q. See *chromosome 6q duplication syndrome.*

trisomy 7. See *chromosome 7 trisomy syndrome.*

trisomy 7p. See *chromosome 7p duplication syndrome.*

trisomy 7q. See *chromosome 7q duplication syndrome.*

trisomy 8. See *chromosome 8 trisomy syndrome.*

trisomy 8p. See *chromosome 8p duplication syndrome.*

trisomy 8q. See *chromosome 8q duplication syndrome.*

trisomy 9. See *chromosome 9 trisomy syndrome.*

trisomy 9p. See *chromosome 9p duplication syndrome.*

trisomy 10 mosaicism. See *chromosome 10 trisomy mosaicism syndrome.*

trisomy 10p. See *chromosome 10p duplication syndrome.*

trisomy 10q. See *chromosome 10q duplication syndrome.*

trisomy 11p. See *chromosome 11p duplication syndrome.*

trisomy 11q. See *chromosome 11q duplication syndrome.*

trisomy 12 mosaicism. See *chromosome 12 trisomy mosaicism.*

trisomy 12p. See *chromosome 12p duplication syndrome.*

trisomy 12q. See *chromosome 12q duplication syndrome.*

trisomy 13. See *chromosome 13 trisomy syndrome.*

trisomy 13-15. See *chromosome 13 trisomy syndrome.*

trisomy 13q. See *chromosome 13q duplication syndrome.*

trisomy 14. See *chromosome 14 trisomy syndrome.*

trisomy 14 mosaicism syndrome. See *chromosome 14 trisomy mosaicism syndrome.*

trisomy 14q. See *chromosome 14q duplication syndrome.*

trisomy 15q. See *chromosome 15q duplication syndrome.*

trisomy 16-18. See *chromosome 18 trisomy syndrome.*

trisomy 16p. See *chromosome 16p duplication syndrome.*

trisomy 16q. See *chromosome 16q duplication syndrome.*

trisomy 17p. See *chromosome 17p duplication syndrome.*

trisomy 17q. See *chromosome 17q duplication syndrome.*

trisomy 18. See *chromosome 18 trisomy syndrome.*

trisomy 18q. See *chromosome 18q duplication syndrome.*

trisomy 19. See *chromosome 19 trisomy syndrome.*

trisomy 19q. See *chromosome 19q duplication syndrome.*

trisomy 20. See *chromosome 20 trisomy syndrome.*

trisomy 20p. See *chromosome 20p duplication syndrome.*

trisomy 20q. See *chromosome 20q duplication syndrome.*

trisomy 21. See *chromosome 21 trisomy syndrome.*

trisomy 22. See *chromosome 22 trisomy syndrome, chromosome 21 trisomy syndrome.*

trisomy C. See *chromosome 8 trisomy syndrome.*

trisomy C mosaicism. See *chromosome 8 trisomy syndrome.*

trisomy D1. See *chromosome 13 trisomy syndrome.*

trisomy D14. See *chromosome 14 trisomy syndrome.*

trisomy E. See *chromosome 18 trisomy syndrome.*

trisomy G. See *chromosome 21 trisomy syndrome.*

trisomy X. See *chromosome XXX syndrome.*

TROELL, NILS ABRAHAM (Swedish physician, 1881-1914)

Troell-Junet syndrome. A combination of acromegaly, toxic (usually nodular) goiter, diabetes mellitus, and hyperostosis of the cranial vault. The disorder occurs predominantly in adult females of all ages. Pathological changes include periosteal and endosteal osteogenic activity and, frequently, spongy transformation of the bone.

Troell, A. "Syndroma Morgagni" hos patienter med samtidig akromegali och tyreotoxikos. *Sven. Lak. Tidn.*, 1938, 35:763-71. Junet, R. Une forme rare d'hypenthyreose: l'hyperostose de la voute cranienne des acromegaliques hyperthyroidiens (syndrome de Troell-Junet). *Helvet. Med. Acta.*, 1955, 22:167-83.

TROISIER, CHARLES EMILE (French physician, 1848-1919)

Troisier syndrome. See *Troisier-Hanot-Chauffard syndrome.*

Troisier-Hanot-Chauffard syndrome. Synonyms: *Hanot-Chauffard syndrome, Troisier syndrome, bronze diabetes, diabetes-hemochromatosis syndrome.*

Diabetes mellitus associated with hypertrophic cirrhosis of the liver and dark-brown skin pigmentation caused by deposition of excess melanin and iron in tissues.

*Troisier, C. E. Diabète sucré. *Bull. Soc. Anat., Paris,* 1871, 16:231. Hanot, V. C., & Chauffard, A. M. Cirrhose hypertrophique pigmentaire dans le diabète sucré. *Rev. Méd., Paris,* 1882, 2:385-403.

trophodermatoneurosis. See *acrodynia.*

trophoneurosis. See *Romberg syndrome (2).*

trophopathia myelodysplastica. See *Marie-Léri syndrome, under Marie, Pierre.*

trophopenic superficial keratitis. See *Petzetakis-Takos syndrome.*

tropical bubo. See *Durand-Nicolas-Favre disease, under Durand, J.*

tropical eosinophilia syndrome. Synonyms: *Frimodt-Möller syndrome, Weingarten syndrome, pseudotuberculosis of lungs with eosinophilia syndrome, spasmodic bronchitis-leukocytosis-eosinophilia syndrome, tropical eosinophilic asthma, tropical pulmonary eosinophilia.*

A tropical disease characterized by eosinophilia and pulmonary infiltrations. The pulmonary lesions are extensive whitish nodules, about 3 to 5 mm in diameter, formed by several alveoli filled with eosinophils and fibrin. Eosinophilic abscesses may develop in some nodules. The symptoms include cough, dyspnea, asthmatic paroxysms, fever, weight loss, and pulmonary shadows seen on the roentgenogram. There is a tendency to relapse over a period of several years. The illness is due to tropical parasites, such as *Necator, Toxocara, Ascaris, Strongyloides, Wuchereria, Ancylostoma braziliensise, Trichuris trichuria,* and *Fasciola hepatica.* Hypersensitivity type I (immunoglobulin E-mediated) may be associated. Some writers use the term loosely to designate any eosinophilia, with or without pulmonary infiltrations, occurring in tropical areas.

Frimodt-Möller, C., & Barton, R. M. A pseudo-tuberculous condition associated with eosinophilia. *Indian Med. Gaz.*, 1940, 75:607-13. Weingarten, R. J. Tropical eosinophilia. *Lancet*, 1943, 1:103-5.

tropical eosinophilic asthma. See *tropical eosinophilia syndrome.*

tropical febrile splenomegaly. See *tropical splenomegaly syndrome.*

tropical pulmonary eosinophilia. See *tropical eosinophilia syndrome.*

tropical splenomegaly syndrome (TSS). Synonyms: *Bengal splenomegaly, idiopathic splenomegaly syndrome, tropical febrile splenomegaly.*

Chronic hepatosplenomegaly, occurring mainly in persons living in endemic malaria areas, characterized by infiltration of the sinusoids by lymphocytes, very high levels of serum immunoglobulin M (IgM), and high malaria antibody titers. Parasitemia is rare. The symptoms may include abdominal swelling, abdominal pain, cough, weakness, leg swelling, epistaxis, pallor, jaundice, and leg ulcers. Normocytic anemia and neutropenia occur in most cases.

Musgrave, W. E., *et al.* Tropical febrile splenomegaly. *Bull. Johns Hopkins Hosp.*, 1906, 17:28. Fakunle, Y. M. Tropical splenomegaly. I. Tropical Africa. *Clinics Haemat.*, 1981, 10:963-75. Crane, G. G. Tropical splenomegaly. II. Oceania. *Clinics Haem.*, 1981, 10:976-82.

TROTTER, WILFRED (British physician, 1872-1939)

Trotter syndrome. Synonym: *sinus of Morgagni syndrome.*

A neurological disease characterized by unilateral neuralgia in the region of the mandible, tongue, and ear due to involvement of the mandibular nerve; ipsilateral middle ear deafness resulting from a lesion of the eustachian tube; preauricular edema caused by neoplastic invasion of the sinus of Morgagni (usually anaplastic carcinoma); ipsilateral akinesia of the soft palate secondary to damage of the levator of the palate; and late trismus.

Trotter, W. On certain clinically obscure malignant tumours of the naso-pharyngeal wall. *Brit. Med. J.*, 1911, 2:1057-9.

TROUSSEAU, ARMAND (French physician, 1801-1867)

Trousseau syndrome. Synonyms: *carcinogenetic thromboplebitis, carcinogenic thrombophlebitis, tumor-associated thromboembolism.*

Venous thrombosis of the upper and lower extremities associated with visceral cancer.

Durham, R. H. Thrombophlebitis migrans and visceral carcinoma. *Arch. Int. Med., Chicago*, 1955, 96:380-6.

TROYER

Troyer syndrome. Synonym: *Cross-McKusick syndrome.*

Spastic paraparesis with distal muscle wasting. The disorder has its onset in childhood with disarthria and muscle wasting (involving mainly the thenar, hypothenar, and dorsal interosseous muscles), followed by spasticity and contractures of the lower limbs (thus making it impossible for the affected persons to walk), drooling, and mild cerebellar signs. The syndrome was named for the surname of the patients in an Amish group in Ohio, in whom the condition was first observed. It is transmitted as an autosomal recessive trait.

Cross, H. E., & McKusick, V. A. The Troyer syndrome. A recessive form of spastic paraplegie with distal muscle wasting. *Arch. Neurol., Chicago*, 1967, 16:473-85.

TRP I (trichorhinophalangeal dysplasia type I). See *trichorhinophalangeal syndrome.*

TRP II (trichorhinophalangeal dysplasia type II). See *Langer-Giedion syndrome.*

TRP III. See *trichorhinophalangeal dysplasia type III.*

TRPS. See *trichorhinophalangeal syndrome.*

truancy syndrome. See *Huckleberry Finn syndrome (1).*

trypanosomiasis. See *Dutton disease.*

TS (Tourette syndrome). See *Gilles de la Tourette syndrome.*

TS (toxic syndrome). See *toxic oil syndrome.*

TS (Turner syndrome). See *chromosome XO syndrome.*

TSCHERNOGUBOW. See CHERNOGUBOV

TSD (Tay-Sachs disease). See *Tay-Sachs syndrome, under Tay, Warren.*

TSS. See *toxic shock syndrome.*

TSS. See *tropical splenomegaly syndrome.*

TSUJI, N. (Japanese physician)

Kawashima-Tsuji syndrome. See *under Kawashima.*

TTN (transient tachypnea of the newborn). See *transient respiratory distress syndrome of the newborn.*

TTP (thrombotic thrombocytopenic purpura). See *Moschcowitz syndrome.*

tubal ligation syndrome. Synonyms: *post-tubal ligation syndrome, tubal sterilization syndrome.*

Dysfunctional uterine bleeding, dysmenorrhea, dyspareunia, pelvic pain, premenstrual tension, and amenorrhea occurring after tubal sterilization. Extensive coagulation of the tube and implantation of the proximal tube into the uterus seem to cause complications more often than other methods.

Hargrove, J. T., & Abraham, G. E. Endocrine profile of patients with post-tubal ligation syndrome. *J. Reprod. Med.*, 1981, 26:359-62.

tubal sterilization syndrome. See *tubal ligation syndrome.*

tuberculosis cutis indurativa. See *Bazin disease.*

tuberculosis cutis papulonecrotica. See *Barthélemy disease.*

tuberculosis indurativa cutanea et subcutanea. See *Bazin disease.*

tuberculosis papulonecrotica. See *Barthélemy disease.*

tuberculous spondylitis. See *Pott disease.*

tuberculum rhombicum medianum glossis. See *Brocq-Pautrier syndrome.*

tuberose (tuberous) sclerosis. See *Bourneville-Pringle syndrome.*

tuberosis cutis pruriginosa. See *Hyde syndrome.*

tubular stenosis-hypocalcemia-convulsions-dwarfism syndrome. See *Kenny syndrome.*

tubular stenosis-periodic hypocalcemia syndrome. See *Kenny syndrome.*

tubulointerstitial nephritis-uveitis (TINU) syndrome. Synonyms: *Kikkawa syndrome, TIN-uveitis syndrome.*

Tubulointerstitial nephritis associated with uveitis. Allergic etiology is suspected.

Kikkawa, Y., *et al.* Interstitial nephritis with concomitant uveitis. Report of two cases. *Contrib. Nephr.*, 1977, 4:1-11.

tubulointerstitial nephropathy-tapetoretinal degeneration syndrome. See *Senior syndrome (1).*

tuftsin deficiency syndrome. A condition manifested mainly by recurrent infections involving primarily the skin, lymph nodes, and lungs. The tetrapeptide tuftsin (Thr-Lys-Pro-Arg) is cleaved off the gamma-globulin molecule as the free active form of two enzymes, one being in the spleen and the other on the outer membrame of the phagocyte. It stimulates phagocytosis by blood neutrophilic granulocytes and tissue macrophages. Its congenital deficiency occurs when the peptide is mutated to an inactive peptide; the acquired type is caused by splenic disorders.

Najjar, V. A. The clinical and physiological aspects of tuftsin deficiency syndromes exhibiting defective phagocytosis. *Klin. Wschr.*, 1979, 57:751-6.

tularemia. See *Francis disease.*

tumor lysis syndrome. Synonym: *tumor overkill syndrome.*

Rapid destruction of sensitive tumor cells by cytoxic drugs, resulting in metabolic complications, such as hyperuricemia, hyperkalemia, hyperphosphatemia, and hypocalcemia, and in life-threatening conditions, including acute renal failure and cardiac arrhythmias. Massive chemotherapy of hematologic malignancies, especially lymphomas (including Burkitt lymphoma) and acute leukemia is the most common cause of this syndrome.

Tsokos, G. C., *et al.* Renal and metabolic complications of undifferentiated and lymphblastic lymphomas. *Medicine*, 1981, 60:218-29. Band, P. R., *et al.* Xanthine nephropathy in a patient with lymphosarcoma treated with allopurinol. *N. Engl. J. Med.*, 1970, 283:354-7.

tumor overkill syndrome. See *tumor lysis syndrome.*

tumor-associated thromboembolism. See *Trousseau syndrome.*

tumoral calcinosis. See *Teutschländer syndrome.*

TUNBRIDGE, R. E. (British physician)

Tunbridge-Paley disease. A syndrome of progressive hearing loss, optic atrophy, and juvenile diabetes mellitus transmitted as an autosomal recessive trait.

Tunbridge, R. E., & Paley, R. G. Primary optic atrophy in diabetes mellitus. *Diabetes*, 1956, 5:295-6.

tunnel anemia. See *Griesinger disease.*

tunnel of Guyon syndrome. See *ulnar tunnel syndrome.*

TUOMAALA, PAAVO (Finnish ophthalmologist)

Tuomaala syndrome. Synonym: *oculo-osteocutaneous syndrome.*

A familial syndrome of brachydactyly, hypopigmentation, hypotrichosis, edentia, broad nasal base, ocular anomalies, and skeletal defects. Shortness of the fingers and toes (especially the third, fourth, and fifth digits), short stature, short skull, small maxilla, and mandibular prognathism are the osseous features of this syndrome. Ocular anomalies consist of antimongoloid palpebral fissures, hypoplastic tarsus, strabismus, nystagmus, distichiasis, lenticular opacities, foveal hypoplasia, and myopia. The syndrome is probably transmitted as an autosomal recessive disorder.

Tuomaala, P., & Haapanen, E. Three siblings with similar anomalies in the eyes, bones, and skin. *Acta Ophth. Copenhagen*, 1968, 46:365-71.

TUR syndrome. See *transurethral prostatectomy syndrome.*

turban tumor. See *Brooke epithelioma.*

TURCOT, JACQUES (Canadian physician, born 1914)

Turcot syndrome. Synonyms: *colonic polyposis-malignant central nervous system tumor syndrome, glioma-polyposis syndrome, intestinal polyposis-glioma syndrome.*

A hereditary disease, transmitted as an autosomal recessive trait, characterized by brain tumors (glioblastoma, astrocytoma, or spongioblastoma) associated with polyposis coli. The symptoms arise most often in the second decade of life, with neurological manifestations of brain tumors and diarrhea secondary to colonic lesions.

Turcot, J., *et al.* Malignant tumors of the central nervous system associated with familial polyposis of the colon. *Dis. Colon Rectum*, 1959, 2465-8.

TÜRK, SIEGMUND (Swiss ophthalmologist)

Stilling-Türk-Duane syndrome. See *under Stilling.*

Türk syndrome. See *Stilling-Türk-Duane syndrome.*

Türk-Stilling syndrome. See *Stilling-Türk-Duane syndrome.*

TÜRK, W. (Austrian physician)

Türk lymphomatosis. See *Filatov disease.*

Turkish sabre syndrome. See *scimitar syndrome.*

TURLER, U. (Swiss physician)

Fanconi-Turler syndrome. See *under Fanconi.*

TURNER, HENRY HUBERT (American endocrinologist, 1892-1970)

familial Turner syndrome. See *Noonan syndrome.*

female pseudo-Turner syndrome. See *Noonan syndrome.*

male Turner syndrome. See *Noonan syndrome.*

Morgagni-Turner syndrome. See *chromosome XO syndrome.*

Morgagni-Turner-Albright syndrome. See *chromosome XO syndrome.*

pseudo-Ullrich-Turner syndrome. See *Noonan syndrome.*

Shereshevskii-Turner syndrome. See *chromosome XO syndrome.*

Turner phenotype with normal karyotype. See *Noonan syndrome.*

Turner syndrome (TS). See *chromosome XO syndrome.*

Turner syndrome in female with normal X chromosomes. See *Noonan syndrome.*

Turner-Albright syndrome. See *chromosome XO syndrome.*

Turner-like syndrome. See *Noonan syndrome.*

Turner-mongolism polysyndrome (TMP). An association of the Turner and Down syndromes, characterized by growth retardation, shield chest, infantile breasts, absent or infantile hair, brachycephaly, low hairline, shork neck, pterygium coli, mongoloid palpebral slant, epicanthus, squat nose, prognathism, mental retardation, cleft or high-arched palate, short hands and feet, frequent cubitus valgus, and mosaic for XO in most instances.

Turner, H. H. A syndrome of infantilism, congenital webbed neck, and cubitus valgus. *Endocrinology*, 1938, 23:566-74. Down, J. L. Marriages of consanguinity in relation to degeneration of race. *London Clin. Lect. Rep.*, 1866, 3:224-36. Villaverde, M. M., & Da Silva, J. A. Turner-mongolism polysyndrome, review of the first eight known cases. *JAMA*, 1975, 234:844-7.

Turner-Noonan syndrome. See *Noonan syndrome.*

Ullrich-Turner syndrome. See *chromosome XO syndrome.*

XX Turner phenotype syndrome. See *Noonan syndrome.*

XY Turner phenotype syndrome. See *Noonan syndrome.*

TURNER, JOHN W. ALDEN (American physician)

Turner syndrome. See *nail-patella syndrome.*

Turner-Kieser syndrome. See *nail-patella syndrome.*

TURP syndrome. See *transurethral prostatectomy syndrome.*

TURPIN, RAYMOND (French physician)

Turpin syndrome. A syndrome combining congenital bronchiectasis, megaesophagus, tracheoesophageal fistula, vertebral deformities, rib malformations, and heterotopic ductus thoracicus.

Turpin, *et al.* Image claire, cervicale, traduction radiographique d'un mégaesophage groupement dysmorphique particulier. *J. Fr. Méd Chir. Thor.*, 19949, 3:436-9.

TURS. See *trausurethral prostatectomy syndrome.*

tussive syncope syndrome. Spasmodic coughing associated with temporary syncope and memory disorders, usually observed in adult males with obstructive respiratory tract diseases and/or pulmonary emphysema. Smoking and alcohol seem to precipitate the attacks.

Haffner, H. T., & Graw, M. Hustensynkope als Unfallursache. *Blutalkohol*, 1990, 27:110-5.

twelfth rib syndrome. See *under slipping rib syndrome.*

twentieth century syndrome. See *total allergy syndrome.*

twidler syndrome. Synonym: *pacemaker twidler syndrome.*

Twidling or manipulation by patients with mechanical therapeutic or diagnostic devices, such as implanted artificial pacemakers, chemotherapy ports, or drip infusion valves, resulting in breakdown or improper operation of these devices.

Gebarski, S. S., & Gebarski, K. S. Chemotherapy port "twidler syndrome." A need for preinjection radiography. *Cancer*, 1984, 54:38-9. Veltri, E. P., *et al.* Twidler's syndrome: A new twist. *PACE*, 1984, 7:1004-9.

twin transfusion syndrome. Synonyms: *fetal transfusion syndrome, fetofetal transfusion, interfetal transfusion syndrome, intrauterine parabiotic syndrome, parabiotic syndrome, parabiotic twin syndrome, transplacental transfusion syndrome, twin-to-twin transfusion syndrome.*

Unbalanced placental circulation in twin pregnancy, whereby the blood is transfused from one fetus to another through an arteriovenous communication or other shunt, resulting in anemia in one twin and polycythemia in the other; the recipient twin being larger than the donor. Most cases of twin transfusion syndrome terminate in stillbirth, but, if both infants are born alive, listnessness or shock is present in the anemic twin, and hypertension, cardiomegaly, hepatosplenomegaly, polyhydramnios, and, later, congestive heart failure occur in the plethoric twin. See also *fetomaternal transfusion syndrome.*

*Schatz, F. Die Gefässverbindung der Placentarkreisläufe eineiiger Zwillinge, ihre Entwicklung und ihre Folgen. *Arch. Gynäk.*, 1884, 24:337.

twin-to-twin transfusion syndrome. See *twin transfusion syndrome.*

twisted limb dwarfism. See *parastremmatic dwarfism syndrome.*

tylosis palmarum et plantarum. See *Unna-Thost syndrome, under Unna, Paul Gerson.*

tympanic plexus neuralgia. See *Reichert syndrome, under Reichert, Frederick Leet.*

tympanites hystericus. See *Roemheld syndrome.*

tympanites in dolichomegacolon. See *Piulachs-Hederich syndrome.*

typhoid fever. See *Eberth disease.*

typhus. See Hildenbrand disease.

typhus abdominalis. See Eberth disease.

typhus fever. See *Hildenbrand disease.*

typus degenerativus amstelodamensis. See *de Lange syndrome (1), under Lange, Cornelia, de.*

typus degenerativus rostockiensis. See *Ullrich-Feichtiger syndrome.*

typus edinburgensis. See *Edinburgh malformation syndrome.*

tyrosinase-negative albinism. See *albinism I syndrome.*

tyrosinase-positive albinism. See *albinism II syndrome.*

tyrosine aminotransferase deficiency. See Richer-Hanhart syndrome.

tyrosine transminase deficiency. See *Richner-Hanhart syndrome.*

tyrosinemia type II. See *Richner-Hanhart syndrome.*

tyrosinosis I. An inborn error of tyrosine metabolism, transmitted as an autosomal recessive trait, characterized by a defect involving liver tyrosine transaminase. Tyrosinemia, tyrosyluria, and hepatorenal disorders are the main features. It presents as an acute progressive illness starting in the neonatal period, marked by hepatic failure, renal tubular dysfunction, and vitamin D-resistant rickets. Most patients die in infancy; those who survive develop severe psychomotor retardation and fatal hepatic and renal failure in the first decade of life. See also *Richner-Hanhart syndrome.*

Medes, G. A new error of tyrosine metabolism: Tyrosinosis. The intermediary metabolism of tyrosine and phenylalanine. *Biochem. J.*, 1932, 26:917-40. Zaleski, W. A., & Hill, A. Tyrosinosis: A new variant. *Canad. Med. Assoc. J.*, 1973, 108:477-84.

tyrosinosis II. See *Richner-Hanhart syndrome.*

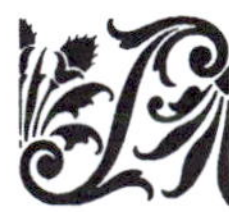

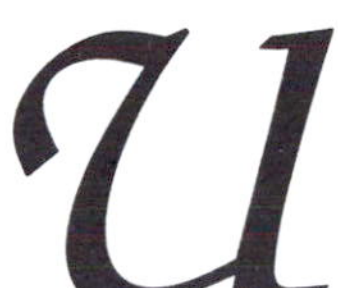

UCHIDA, IRENE (Canadian scientist)

Donohue-Uchida syndrome. See *Donohue syndrome.*

UCS. See *uterine compression syndrome.*

UEHLINGER, ERWIN (Swiss physician, born 1899)

Jaffe-Lichtenstein-Uehlinger syndrome. See *Jaffe-Lichtenstein syndrome.*

Meyenburg-Altherr-Uehlinger syndrome. See *under Meyenburg.*

Uehlinger syndrome. See *pachydermoperiostosis syndrome.*

von Meyenburg-Altherr-Uehlinger syndrome. See *Meyenburg-Altherr-Uehlinger syndrome.*

UGH syndrome. See *uveitis-glaucoma-hyphema syndrome.*

UGH+ syndrome. See *uveitis-glaucoma-hyphema **plus** syndrome.*

UHL, HENRY STEPHEN MAGRAW (American physician, born 1921)

Uhl anomaly. Synonyms: *arrhythmogenic right ventricular dysplasia, hypoplastic right ventricle, parchment heart, parchment right ventricle.*

Congenital hypoplasia or aplasia of the myocardium of the right ventricle. See also *hypoplastic right heart syndrome.*

Uhl, H. S. M. A previously undescribed congenital malformation of the heart. Almost total absence of the myocardium of the right ventricle. *Bull. Johns Hopkins Hosp.,* 1952, 91:197-205.

UHTHOFF, WILHELM (German physician, 1853-1927)

Uhthoff syndrome. Blurring of vision during exercise in patients with multiple sclerosis.

Uhthoff, W. Untersuchungen über die bei der multiplen Herdsklerose vorkommenden Augenstörungen. *Arch. Psychiat. Nervenk.,* 1890, 21:55-116.

UIP (usual interstitial pneumonia). See *Hamman-Rich syndrome.*

ulceration en arc. See *trigeminal trophic syndrome.*

ulcerative gingivitis. See *Vincent infection.*

ulcerative mutilating acropathy. See *Thévenard syndrome.*

ulcero-membranous balanitis. See *Queyrat erythroplasia.*

ulcero-mutilating acropathy. See *Bureau-Barrière syndrome.*

ulcerogenic tumor of the pancreas syndrome. See *Zollinger-Ellison syndrome.*

ulcus callosum recti. See *Hochenegg ulcer.*

ulcus corneae serpens. See *Saemisch ulcer.*

ulcus cruris hypertonicum. See *Martorell syndrome (1).*

ulcus molle. See *Ducrey disease.*

ulcus vulvae acutum. See *Lipschütz ulcer.*

ulerythema centrifugum. See *lupus erythematosus.*

ulerythema ophrogenes. See *Taenzer disease.*

ULLRICH, OTTO (German pediatrician, 1894-1957)

Bonnevie-Ullrich syndrome. See *under Bonnevie.*

Morquio-Ullrich syndrome. See *mucopolysaccharidosis IV-A.*

pseudo-Ullrich-Turner syndrome. See *Noonan syndrome.*

Ullrich and Fremerey-Dohna syndrome. See *Hallermann-Streiff syndrome.*

Ullrich syndrome. Synonym: *congenital atonic sclerotic muscular dystrophy.*

A congenital muscular disorder believed to be a variant of Oppenheim disease. Shortly after birth, the affected children develop kyphoscoliosis, drooping of the head, contractures of large joints and limpness of small joints, and contractures and hardening of the muscles of the neck and trunk. The immobility of the proximal joints and excessive mobility of the distal joints permit children to assume bizarre postures. In contrast to Oppenheim disease, there is excessive excitability of the nervous system. Examination of the muscles shows sclerotic and dystrophic changes.

Ullrich, O. Kongenitale, atonisch-sklerotische Muskeldystrophie. *Mschr. Kinderh.,* 1930, 47:502-10.

Ullrich-Feichtiger syndrome. Synonyms: *dyscraniopygophalangia, micrognathia-polydactyly-genital anomalies syndrome, status degenerativus typus rostockiensis, typus degenerativus rostockiensis.*

A congenital syndrome of ear deformities, deafness, polydactyly, rudimentary toes, clubfoot, partial atresia of the anus, hypospadias, and masklike facies. Vaginal septa, supernumerary phalanges, and a tendency to develop clefts in various structures, especially the palate, may occur.

Ullrich, O. Der Status Bonnevie-Ullrich im Rahmen anderer "Dyscranio-Dysphalangien." *Erg. Inn. Med. Kinderh.* 1951, 2:412-66. *Feichtiger, H. *Ein neuer, typischer, vorwiegend der Akren betreffender Fehlbindungskomplex.* Rostock, 1943. (Thesis).

Ullrich-Nielsen syndrome. See *Nielsen syndrome, under Nielsen, Herman.*

Ullrich-Noonan syndrome. See *Noonan syndrome.*

Ullrich-Scheie syndrome. See *mucopolysaccharidosis I-S.*

Ullrich-Turner syndrome. See *chromosome XO syndrome.*

ulnar aplasia-lobster claw syndrome. A familial syndrome of severe hypoplasia of the ulna and second and fifth fingers, associated with lobster claw deformity of the feet. The syndrome is transmitted as either an X-linked recessive or autosomal dominant sex-influenced trait.

Berghe, H., van den, *et al.* Familial ulnar aplasia and lobster claw syndrome. *Clin. Genet.*, 1978, 13:106-7.

ulnar drift syndrome. See *digitotalar dysmorphism syndrome.*

ulnar hemimelia. See *Weyers oligodactyly syndrome.*

ulnar impingement syndrome. See *ulnar tunnel syndrome.*

ulnar nerve compresion syndrome. See *ulnar tunnel syndrome.*

ulnar nerve entrapment syndrome. See *ulnar tunnel syndrome.*

ulnar tunnel syndrome. Synonyms: *Guyon tunnel syndrome, loge de Guyon syndrome, tunnel of Guyon syndrome, ulnar impingement syndrome, ulnar nerve compression syndrome, ulnar nerve entrapment syndrome.*

Compression of the ulnar nerve within the ulnar tunnel (tunnel of Guyon) caused by the volar carpal ligament anteriorly, the transverse carpal ligament posteriorly, and the pisiform bone with the flexor carpi ulnaris tendon attached to it medially. Lesions or injuries of a fibrotic band running between the pisiform and the hamate bones and anterior pisohamate ligament may cause ulnar nerve compression. Pain, palsy, and atrophy of muscles innervated by the ulnar nerve are the most common symptoms. The syndrome may be associated with bipartite hamulus.

Bakke, I. L., & Wolf, H. G. Occupational pressure neuritis of the deep palmar branch of the ulnar nerve. *Arch. Neur. Psychiat.*, 1948, I50:549. Lotem, M., *et al.* Fibrotic arch around the deep branch of the ulnar nerve in the hand. *Plast. Reconstr. Surg.*, 1973, 52:553-6.

ulnar-mammary syndrome. See *Pallister syndrome (2).*

ulnofibular dysplasia, Reinhardt-Pfeiffer type. See *Reinhardt-Pfeiffer syndrome, under Reinhardt, K.*

ULYSSES (ODYSSEUS) (Greek epic hero, king of Ithaca)

Ulysses syndrome. A complex mental and physical disorder which follows the discovery of false-positive results in the course of routine laboratory tests, leading to additional tests and examinations, some physically, mentally, and financially traumatic, before the patient is found to be healthy. It is attributed to a combination of factors in tests and investigations promoted by mass screening, insurance and pre-employment examinations, application of unnecessary laboratory tests, the physician's hope for a major discovery, the patient's neurotic reactions, uncritical interpretations of results, and retention of outdated records on laboratory forms. The syndrome is named after the Greek epic hero Ulysses (Odysseus), king of Ithaca, who after the Trojan War traveled 20 years, encountering numerus adventures and perils, before returning home.

Rang, M. The Ulysses syndrome. *Canad. Med. Assoc. J.*, 1972, 106:122-3.

UMS. See ***u**rethral **m**anipulation **s**yndrome.*

uncinariasis. See *Griesinger disease.*

uncombable hair syndrome. Synonyms: *pili canaliculi, pili trianguli et canaliculi, spun glass hair syndrome.*

A familial disorder, transmitted as an autosomal dominant trait, characterized by an arrangement of the hair in bundles, whereby individual bundles point in different directions, thus making it difficult to comb the hair. The condition ameliorates with age. Scanning electron microscopy shows triangular cross-sections and longitudinal grooves in the hair.

Dupré, A., *et al.* Cheveux incoiffables: Anomalie congénitale des cheveux. *Bull. Soc. Fr. Derm. Syph.*, 1973, 80:111-2.

unconjugated benign bilirubinemia. See *Gilbert syndrome, under Gilbert, Nicolas Augustin.*

unconjugated idiopathic hyperbilirubinemia. See *Gilbert syndrome, under Gilbert, Nicolas Augustin.*

UNDERWOOD, MICHAEL (British physician, 1737-1820)

Underwood disease. Synonyms: *sclerema adiposum, sclerema neonatorum.*

A disorder of lipid metabolism that is usually present at birth or appears shortly after birth. In the mild form, it is characterized by hardening of the subcutaneous fat and the development of multiple firm nodules on the buttocks, trunk, thighs, cheeks, arms, and feet, which may regress as time passes. In the severe form, the hardening of the fat is generalized and is accompanied by waxiness, coldness, and tightness of the skin. The second type is usually fatal. The chief histological features are an inflammatory reaction of the adipose tissue and dermis; infiltrates consisting of lymphocytes, histiocytes, and foreign body giant cells; fatty acid crystals in the inflamed tissue; and necrotic foci. Olein deficiency in the tissues is believed to be the cause.

Underwood, M. *A treatise on the diseases of children.* London, Mathews, 1784, p. 76.

undescended scapula. See *Sprengel deformity.*

UNDINE. See ONDINE

undulant fever. See *brucellosis.*

unilateral clear lung. See *Swyer-James syndrome, under Swyer, Paul Robert.*

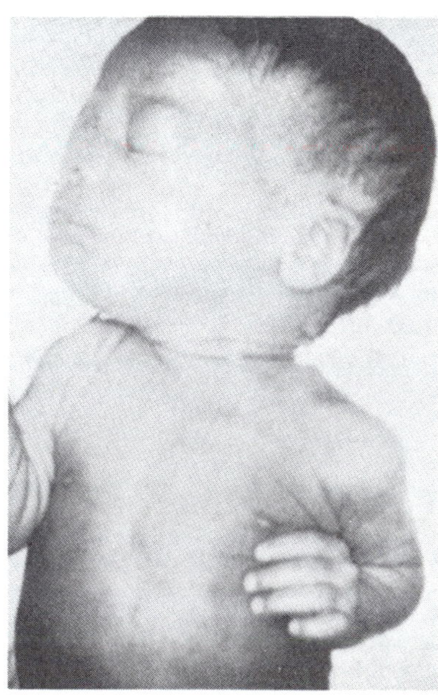

Underwood disease
From the Collection of the American Academy of Pediatrics. Reproduced with permission of the officers of the Academy, Elk Grove, Illinois.

unilateral ectromelia-ichthyosis syndrome. See *ectromelia-ichthyosis syndrome.*

unilateral flush sweat. See *Frey syndrome.*

unilateral gigantism. See *Curtius syndrome (1).*

unilateral global involvement of cranial nerves. See *Garcin syndrome.*

unilateral hyperlucent lung. See *Swyer-James syndrome, under Swyer, Paul Robert.*

unilateral hypertrophy. See *Curtius syndrome (1).*

unilateral mandibulofacial dysostosis. See *Weyers-Thier syndrome.*

unilateral melanosis and hypertrichosis. See *Becker nevus, under Becker, Samuel William.*

unilateral nonfunctioning lung. See *Swyer-James syndrome, under Swyer, Paul Robert.*

unilateral streaked ovary syndrome. See *Slotnick-Goldfarb syndrome.*

unilobar hyperlucency of the lung. See *Swyer-James syndrome, under Swyer, Paul Robert.*

uniocular granulomatous conjunctivitis with preauricular adenopathy. See *Parinaud oculoglandular syndrome.*

universal joint cervix. See *Allen-Masters syndrome, under Allen, William Myron.*

UNNA, MARIE (German physician)

Marie Unna syndrome. See *Unna syndrome.*

Unna hypotrichosis. See *Unna syndrome.*

Unna syndrome. Synonyms: *Marie Unna syndrome, Unna hypotrichosis, Unna trichodysplasia, congenital hereditary hypotrichosis, hereditary trichodysplasia, hypotrichosis congenita hereditaria, hypotrichosis with pili torti.*

A familial form of hypotrichosis transmitted as an autosomal dominant trait. The affected infants are born with short and sparse eyebrows and eyelashes. The hair becomes coarse, wiry, and twisted during adolescence, and there is a gradual development of alopecia. Progressive destruction of hair follicles is believed to be the cause.

Unna, M. Über Hypotrichosis congenita hereditaria. *Derm. Wschr.*, 1925, 81:1167-78.

Unna trichodysplasia. See *Unna syndrome.*

UNNA, PAUL GERSON (German physician, 1850-1929)

Unna disease. Synonyms: *dermatitis seborrhoides, eczema seborrheicum, seborrheic dermatitis, seborrheic eczema.*

A chronic disease of the skin characterized by seborrhea of the scalp and the sebaceous follicle-rich areas of the face and trunk. The affected skin is pink and edematous and is covered with yellowish patches and greasy, moist, or dry scales. Itching is a constant feature. It almost invariably begins on the scalp and sometimes remains limited to this area but, more often, spreads to the ears, eyelids, neck, forehead, temples, nasolabial creases, axillae, and other parts of the body. The cause is unknown.

*Unna, P. G. Das seborrhoische Ekzem. *Mschr. Prakt. Derm.*, 1887, 6:827-46. Plewig, G. Seborrheic dermatitis. In: Fitzpatrick, T. B., Eisen, A. Z., Wolff, K., Freedberg, I. M., & Austen, K. F., eds. *Dermatology in general medicine.* 3rd ed. New York, McGraw-Hill, 1987, pp. 978-81.

Unna-Taenzer disease. See *Taenzer disease.*

Unna-Thost syndrome. Synonyms: *Brauer syndrome, Brünauer syndrome, Greither keratosis, congenital keratoma of the palms and soles, hereditary palmoplantar keratoderma, hyperkeratosis palmaris et plantaris, ichthyosis palmaris et plantaris, ichthyosis palmaris et plantaris corneae, keratoma dissipatum hereditarium palmare et plantare, keratoma palmare et plantare hereditarium, keratosis extremitatum hereditaria progradiens, keratosis palmaris et plantaris, palmoplantar keratoderma, symmetric keratodermia of the extremities, tylosis palmarum et plantarum.*

A rare hereditary skin disease, transmitted as an autosomal dominant trait, with variable involvement of the palms and soles. It is first observed in infancy, but some cases may have their onset in childhood. Typically, the lesions are thick, horny, hard, yellowish plaques with waxy smooth surfaces, although in some cases they may be pitted and verrucous, surrounded by erythematous halos. They are usually symmetrical and may extend to contiguous areas, sometimes involving the knees and elbows. Keratosis pilaris, hyperhidrosis, bromhidrosis, and, less commonly, alopecia and thickening of the nails may be associated. Low blood vitamin A levels have been observed in some cases.

*Unna, P. G. Über das Keratoma palmare et plantare hereditarium. *Vjschr. Derm.*, 1883, 15:231. *Thost. *Über erbliche Ichthyosis palmaris et plantaris corneae.* Heidelberg, 1880. (Thesis). Brauer, A. Über eine besondere Form des hereditären Keratoms (Keratoma dissipatum hereditarium palmare et plantare). *Arch. Derm. Syph., Berlin,* 1912, 114:211-36. Brünauer, S. R. Zur Vererbung des Keratoma hereditarium palmare et plantare. *Acta Derm. Vener., Stockholm,* 1923-24, 4:489-503. Greither, A. Keratosis extremitatum hereditaria progradiens mit dominanten Erbgang. *Hautarzt,* 1952, 3:198-203.

unroofed coronary sinus syndrome. Absence of a part or all of the common wall between the coronary sinus and the left atrium.

Winter, F. S. Persistent left superior vena cava. Survey of world literature and report of thirty additional cases. *Angiology,* 1954, 5:90-132. Kirklin, J. W., & Barrat-Boyes, B. G. Unroofed coronary sinus syndrome. In their: *Cardiac surgery. Morphology, diagnosis, criteria, natural history, techniques, results and indications.* New York, John Wiley, 1986, pp. 533-40.

unstable bladder of childhood. See *Hinman syndrome.*

unstable colon. See *irritable bowel syndrome.*

unstable patella syndrome. Synonyms: *patellar instability syndrome, recurrent patellar dislocation, recurrent patellar subluxation, slipping patella.*

Recurrent dislocation of the patella wherein the bone must be repositioned after each episode. In one form, there is an underlying disorder such as patellar abnormality, a deficient lateral femoral condyle, a high patella, an unduly lateral attachment of the ligamentum patellae, genu valgum, genu recurvatum, or contracture of the lateral retinaculum and capsule; in the second variety acute dislocation is precipitated by an injury.

Hauser, E. D. W. Total tendon transplant for slipping patella: A new operation for recurrent dislocation of the patella. *Surg. Gyn. Obst.*, 1938, 66:199-214. Chen, S. C., & Ramanathan, E. B. S. The treatment of patellar instability by lateral release. *J. Bone Joint Surg.*, 1984, 66B:344-8.

UNVERRICHT, HEINRICH (German physician, 1853-1912)

Lafora-Unverricht disease. See *Lafora disease.*

Lundborg-Unverricht disease. See *Lafora disease.*

Unverricht syndrome. See *Lafora disease.*

Wagner-Unverricht syndrome. See *under Wagner, Ernst Leberecht.*

upper arm type of brachial palsy. See *Duchenne-Erb syndrome.*

upper brachial plexus palsy. See *Duchenne-Erb syndrome.*

upper calyx renovascular obstruction. See *Fraley syndrome.*

upper limb-cardiovascular syndrome. See *Holt-Oram syndrome.*

upper motor neuron syndrome. A neurological disorder characterized by a reduction in the rate of force change associated with generating fine levels of force in the upper lip, lower lip, tongue, and jaw.

Barlow, S. M., & Abbs, J. H. Free force and position control of select orofacial structures in the upper motor nerve syndrome. *Exp. Neur.*, 1986, 94:966-713.

upper quadrant syndrome (UQS). Dull, stabbing, or burning pain in the upper quadrant of the body in association with nonradicular sensory vasomotor or sudomotor disturbances, ranging from extreme vasoconstriction to severe vasodilatation and from hypohidrosis to hyperhidrosis.

Waisbrod, H., & Gerbershagen, H. E. The surgical treatment of the upper quadrant syndrome. A preliminary report. *Arch. Orthop. Traum. Surg., Berlin,* 1983, 102:29-30.

upper radicular syndrome. See *Duchenne-Erb syndrome.*

upper sylvian aqueduct syndrome. See *Koerber-Salus-Elschnig syndrome.*

UPSHAW, JEFFERSON D., JR. (American physician)

Schulman-Upshaw syndrome. See *under Schulman.*

Upshaw factor deficiency. See *Schulman-Upshaw syndrome.*

UQS. See ***u**pper **q**uadrant **s**yndrome.*

URBACH, ERICH (Austrian-born physician in America, 1893-1946)

Oppenheim-Urbach syndrome. See *under Oppenheim, M.*

Rössle-Urbach-Wiethe syndrome. See *Urbach-Wiethe syndrome.*

Urbach lipoproteinosis. See *Urbach-Wiethe syndrome.*

Urbach-Wiethe disease (UWD). See *Urbach-Wiethe syndrome.*

Urbach-Wiethe syndrome. Synonyms: *Rössle-Urbach-Wiethe syndrome, Urbach lipoproteinosis, Urbach-Wiethe disease (UWD), cutaneo-mucous proteinosis, hyalinosis cutis et mucosae, lipoglycoproteinosis, lipoid proteinosis, proteinosis lipoidea.*

A congenital lipid storage disease, transmitted as an autosomal recessive trait, characterized by multiple lipoid infiltrations that produce waxiness and thickening of the skin and mucous membranes of the mouth, pharynx, larynx, and hypopharynx, resulting in hoarseness and an inability to cry, often from birth. Yellowish ivory or waxy nodules from one to several millimeters in size are distributed on the face, neck, hands, and axillary regions, and hyperkeratotic lesions may be found on the knees, elbows, and fingers. Diffuse alopecia is present in some instances. Ulceration may occur in the mouth, with scarring at the sites of healed ulcers. The tongue becomes thickened and woody, and the patient may find it difficult to move it. Intracranial calcifications are common. Dental findings may include maldeveloped teeth and hypoplastic enamel. Associated disorders usually consist of grand mal epilepsy, attacks of rage, and mental retardation. Blood lipids are elevated.

Urbach, E. Über eine familiäre lokale Lipoidose der Haut und der Schleimhaute auf Grundlage einer diabetischen Stoffwechselstörung. *Arch. Derm. Vener., Berlin,* 1929, 159:451-66. Wiethe, C. Kongenitale diffuse Hyalinablagerungen din den oberen Luftwegen Familiärer auftretend. *Zschr. Hals. Nas. Ohrenheilk.*, 1924, 10:359-62. Rössle, R. Beiträge zur Frage der Speicherungskrankheiten. *Verh. Deut. Path. Ges.*, 1939, 31:133-49.

urban cowboy syndrome. An injury received while falling from a mechanical bull, ranging in severity from a minor sprain to thumb fracture and lumbar vertebral fracture.

Seager, S. B., *et al.* The urban cowboy syndrome. *Ann. Emerg. Med.*, 1981, 10:252-3.

uremic-hemolytic syndrome. See *hemolytic-uremic syndrome.*

urethral arthritis. See *Reiter syndrome.*

urethral manipulation syndrome (UMS). Fibrosis and scarring of the corpus cavernosum urethrae following urethral manipulations, including catheterization, urethrocystoscopy, transaurethral resection, and the like.

Kelâmi, A. Urethral manipulation syndrome. Description of a new syndrome. *Urol. Internat.*, 1984, 39:352-4.

urethral rheumatism. See *Reiter syndrome.*

urethral syndrome. Synonyms: *abacterial urethral syndrome, acute urethral syndrome, dysuria-frequency syndrome, female urethral syndrome.*

A feminine urethral disorder characterized by dysuria, frequency, back pressure, suprapubic discomfort, malaise, and occasional dyspareunia. In most instances, there is a history of hematuria. The etiology is not understood, but some organisms in the vagina, vestibule, and urethra are suspected as possible pathogenic agents. *Escherichia coli* and *Chlamydia trachomatis* are most frequently associated with this disorder, and chlamydial infection is usually isolated in women who recently changed sex partners.

Jacobo, E., & Greene, L. F. Diseases of the urethra. In: Buchsbaum, H. J., & Schmidt, J. D., eds. *Gynecology and obstetric urology.* 2nd ed. Philadelphia, Saunders, 1982, pp. 445-67.

urethro-oculosynovial syndrome. See *Reiter syndrome.*

urge incontinence. See *urge incontinence syndrome.*

urge incontinence syndrome. Synonyms: *frequency incontinence, frequency-urgency syndrome, urge syndrome, urgency, urgency incontinence.*

Involuntary loss of urine associated with a strong desire to void. The condition may be subdivided into **motor urge incontinence**, which is associated with uninhibited detrusor contractions, and **sensory urge incontinence**, which is not due to uninhibited detrusor contractions. Interstitial cystitis, neurogenic disturbances from supranuclear lesions, and idiopathic detrusor hyperreflexia are the usual causes.

Moen, M., & Stien, R. Urge incontinence. *Ann. Chir. Gynaec., Helsinki,* 1982, 71:203-7.

urgency. See *urge incontinence syndrome.*

urgency incontinence. See *urge incontinence syndrome.*

urinary bladder immaturity syndrome. See *bladder immaturity syndrome.*

uroarthritis. See *Reiter syndrome.*

urogenital adysplasia. See *Winter syndrome.*
Urov disease. See *Kashin-Bek disease.*
URRETS-ZAVALIA, ALBERTO, JR. (Argentine ophthalmologist)
Urrets-Zavalia syndrome. Synonym: *Castroviejo syndrome.*

A wide, rigid pupil with iris atrophy, multiple posterior synechiae, and occasional late secondary glaucoma occurring after penetrating keratoplasty with postoperative instillation of atropine or other mydriatics. Complications include mydriasis, unresponsiveness to miotics, and photophobia.

Urrets-Zavalía, A., Jr. Fixed, dilated pupils, iris atrophy and secondary glaucoma. A distinct clinical entity following penetrating keratoplasty in keratoconus. *Am. J. Ophth.*, 1963, 56:257-65.

urticaria edematosa. See *Quincke edema.*
urticaria gigantea. See *Quincke edema.*
urticaria perstans verrucosa. See *Hyde syndrome.*
urticaria pigmentosa. See *Nettleship syndrome.*
urticaria xanthelasmatoidea. See *Nettleship syndrome.*
urticarial vasculitis syndrome. Cutaneous necrotizing venulitis with blanching erythematous papules or plaques charcteristic of purpura. Some cases are associated with secondary or collateral vascular diseases, familial complement deficiency, viral infections, serum sickness, and adverse reactions to drugs.

Gammon, W. R. Urticarial vasculitis. *Derm. Clinics*, 1985, 3:97-105.

US. See *Usher syndrome.*
USHER, BARNEY DAVID (Canadian physician, born 1899)
Senear-Usher syndrome. See *under Senear.*

USHER, CHARLES HOWARD (British ophthalmologist, 1865-1942)
Graefe-Usher syndrome. See *Usher syndrome.*
Usher syndrome (US). Synonym: *Graefe-Usher syndrome retinitis pigmentosa-congenital deafness syndrome.*

A hereditary disorder believed to occur in two forms: (1) characterized by congenital deafness and severe retinitis pigmentosa, and (2) in which the inner ear and the retina are less severely affected. Associated disorders may include gait disturbances attributed to labyrinthine lesions, cataracts, mental deficiency, psychoses, and ataxia. Most cases are transmitted as an autosomal recessive trait, but some forms are X-linked.

Usher, C. H. On the inheritance of retinitis pigmentosa. *Roy. Lond. Ophth. Hosp. Rep.*, 1914, 19:130-236.

usual interstitial pneumonia (UIP). See *Hamman-Rich syndrome.*
uterine compression syndrome (UCS). Compression of the pelvic vessels and obstruction of the blood flow by the uterus in the late stages of pregnancy, causing reduction in the stroke volume, increased heart rate, and decreased blood pressure. The condition is most pronounced when the patient is standing up.

Schneider, K. T., *et al.* Premature contractions: Are they caused by maternal standing. *Acta Genet. Med. Gamellol., Roma*, 1985, 34:175-8.

uteroplacental apoplexy. See *Couvelaire syndrome.*
uterus bicornis rudimentarius. See *Mayer-Rokitansky-Küster syndrome.*
uterus bicornis rudimentarius solidus portium excavatum cum vagina solida. See *Mayer-Rokitansky-Küster syndrome.*
uterus bipartitus. See *Mayer-Rokitansky-Küster syndrome.*
uterus bipartitus rudimentarius solidus cum vagina solida. See *Mayer-Rokitansky-Küster syndrome.*
uveal effusion syndrome. Idiopathic serous detachment of the peripheral choroid, ciliary body, and retina, first in one eye and, after a delay of several months or years, in the second eye. The condition is relatively rare, occurring most commonly in apparently healthy middle-aged males.

Schepens, C. L., & Brockhurst, R. J. Uveal effusion. I. Clinical picture. *Arch. Ophth., Chicago*, 1963:189-201.

uveitis-glaucoma-hyphema (UGH) syndrome. Synonym: *Ellingson syndrome.*

Uveitis, glaucoma, and hyphema after anterior chamber lens implant in cataract surgery.

Ellingson, F. T. Complications with the Choyce Mark VIII anterior chamber lens implant (uveitis-glaucoma-hyphema). *Am. Intra-Ocul. Impl. Soc. J.*, 1977, 3:199-201.

uveitis-glaucoma-hyphema plus (UGH+) syndrome. Uveitis, glaucoma, and hyphema plus vitreous hemorrhage after anterior chamber lens implant in cataract surgery.

Hagan, J. C., Jr. A comparative study of the 91Z and other anterior chamber intraocular lenses. *J. Am. Intra-Ocul. Implant Soc.*, 1984, 10:324-8.

uveocencephalitis. See *Harada syndrome.*
uveocutaneomeningo-encephalitic syndrome. See *Harada syndrome.*
uveocutaneous syndrome. See *Vogt-Koyanagi syndrome, under Vogt, Alfred.*
uveomeningeal syndrome. See *Vogt-Koyanagi syndrome, under Vogt, Alfred.*
uveomeningitis syndrome. See *Harada syndrome.*
uveomeningoencephalitis. See *Harada syndrome.*
uveoparotid fever. See *Heerfordt syndrome.*
uveoparotitic paralysis. See *Heerfordt syndrome.*
uveoparotitis. See *Heerfordt syndrome.*
uvula-tongue malposture. See *Cooperman-Miura syndrome.*
UWD (Urbach-Wiethe disease). See *Urbach-Wiethe syndrome.*
UYEMURA, MISAO (Japanese physician)
Uyemura syndrome. Synonym: *fundus albipunctatus-hemeralopia-xerosis syndrome.*

A combination of night blindness, epithelial xerosis, multiple white round spots on the retina, and faulty dark adaptation, probably due to vitamin A deficiency.

Uyemura, M. Über eine merkwürdige Augenhintergrundveränderung bei 2 Fällen von idiopatischer Hemeralopie. *Klin. Mschr. Augenheilk.*, 1928, 81:471-3.
Fuchs, A. White spots in the fundus combined with night blindness and xerosis (Uyemura's syndrome). *Am. J. Ophth.*, 1959, 48:101-3.

UZMAN, L. LAHUT
Farber-Uzman syndrome. See *Farber disease.*

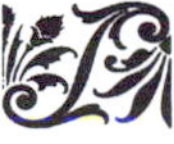

Page #	Term	Observation

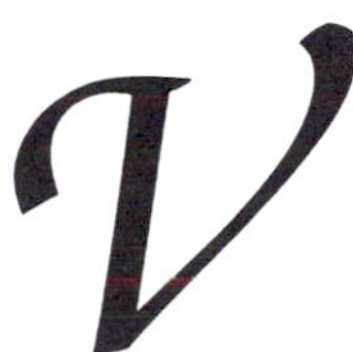

V syndrome. See *AV (A & V) syndrome.*

VAAL, O. M., DE (Dutch physician)

de Vaal-Seynhaeve syndrome. See *Vaal-Seynhaeve syndrome.*

Vaal-Seynhaeve syndrome. Synonyms: *de Vaal-Seynhaeve syndrome, congenital aleukia, congenital panleukia syndrome, generalized hematopoietic hypoplasia, reticular dysgenesia, reticular dysgenesis-congenital aleukia syndrome, severe combined immunodeficiency with leukopenia.*

A form of severe combined immunodeficiency, transmitted as a recessive trait, characterized by congenital agranulocytosis, lymphopenia, lymphoid hypoplasia, thymus hypoplasia, and death in infancy from overwhelming infections.

Vaal, O. M., de, & Seynhaeve, V. Reticular dysgenesis. *Lancet,* 1959, 2:1123-5.

VACTEL (vertebral abnormalities-anal atresia-cardiac abnormalities-tracheo-esophageal atresia-limb defects) association or syndrome. See *VATER association.*

VACTERL (vertebral abnormalities-anal atresia-cardiac abnormalities-tracheo-esophageal fistula-renal agenesis-limb defects) association or syndrome. See *VATER association.*

vacuum headache. See *under headache syndrome.*

vagabonds' disease. See *Greenhow disease.*

vagal syncope. See *carotid sinus syndrome.*

vaginitis ulcerosa. See *Gardner vaginitis, under Gardner, Herman L.*

vago-accessory syndrome. See *Schmidt syndrome, under Schmidt, Adolf.*

vago-accessory-hypoglossal syndrome. See *Jackson-MacKenzie syndrome under Jackson, John Hughlings.*

vagohypoglossal syndrome. See *Tapia syndrome.*

vagovagal syncope after swallowing. See *swallowing syncope syndrome.*

vagrants' disease. See *Greenhow disease.*

VAHLQUIST, BO CONRADSSON (Swedish physician, born 1909)

Vahlquist-Gasser syndrome. Synonyms: *benign essential granulocytopenia, chronic benign infantile granulocytopenia, chronic constitutional granulocytopenia, essential benign granulocytopenia.*

A chronic benign form of granulocytopenia of children, without any serious systemic manifestations.

Vahlquist, B., & Anjou, N. Granulocytopénie chronique bénigne. *Acta Haem., Basel,* 1952, 8:199-208. Gasser, C., & Vrtilek, M. R. Essentielle chronische Granulocytopenie im Kindesalter. *Schweiz. Med. Wschr.,* 1952, 82:122-3.

VAHS. See *virus-associated hemophagocytic syndrome.*

VAIL, H. H. (American physician)

Vail syndrome. Synonym: *vidian neuralgia.*

Attacks of neuralgic pain in the nose, face, eye, ear, head, neck, and shoulder, which are usually unilateral, often nocturnal, and may be associated with subjective symptoms of nasal sinusitis. Irritation or inflammation of the vidian nerve is considered to be the etiologic factor.

Vail, H. H. Vidian neuralgia. *Ann. Otol. Rhinol.,* 1932, 41:837-56.

VAINSEL, M. (Belgian physician)

Guibaud-Vainsel syndrome. See *under Guibaud.*

VALLAT, GEORGES (French physician, born 1918)

Rimbaud-Passouant-Vallat syndrome. See *under Rimbaud.*

VALSUANI, EMILIO (Italian physician)

Valsuani disease. Pernicious anemia in puerperal women.

*Valsuani, E. *Cachessia puerperale racolta nella clinicoginecologica dell'ospetale Maggiore di Milano.* Milano, Bernardoni, 1870.

VALTANCOLI (Italian physician)

Delitale-Valtancoli disease. See *Van Neck disease.*

valvular gallbladder. See *Caroli syndrome (1).*

VAN ALLEN, MAURICE W. (American physician)

Van Allen syndrome. See *amyloid neuropathy type III.*

VAN BOGAERT, LUDO (Belgian neurologist)

Canavan-van Bogaert-Bertrand syndrome. See *Canavan syndrome.*

Nyssen-van Bogaert-Meyer syndrome. See *under Nyssen.*

van Bogaert encephalitis. Synonyms: *Bodechtel-Guttmann disease, Dawson encephalitis, diffuse sclerosing encephalitis, inclusion body encephalitis, lethargic encephalitis, leukoencephalitis subacuta sclerosans, subacute inclusion encephalitis, subacute sclerosing encephalopathy, subacute sclerosing leukoencephalitis, subacute sclerosing panencephalitis (SSPE).*

Subacute progressive encephalitis in children and adolescents, involving the white matter of the cerebrum, brain stem, cerebral cortex, thalamus, and spinal cord. Clinical signs include ataxia, myoclonus, mental deterioration, cachexia, behavior disorders, speech disorders, progressive muscular hypertonia, and decerebrate rigidity. Pathological findings show demyelination, subacute inflammatory reaction with perivascular collections of lymphocytes and plasma cells, and intracellular inclusion bodies indicating the viral etiology. Eosinophilic inclusions are the principal histopathological features of this condition. Typically, there is a history of measles preceding the syndrome. Initial gradual deterioration of proficiency in school and behavioral problems are followed by intellectual deterioration, seizures, myoclonus, ataxia, and occasional visual disorders due to progressive chorioretinitis. In advanced stages, the affected children show Babinski signs, rigidity, hyperactive reflexes, unresponsiveness, autonomic dysfunction, and decorticate rigidity; death usually follows within 1 to 3 years.

van Bogaert L. Une leuco-encéphalite sclérosante subaiguë. *J. Neur., London,* 1945, 8:101-20. Dowson, J. R. Cellular inclusions in cerebral lesions of lethargic encephalitis. *Am. J. Path.,* 1933, 9:7-15. Bodechtel, G., & Guttmann, E. Diffuse Encephalitis mit sklerosierender Entzündung des Hemisphärenmarkes. *Zschr. Ges. Neur. Psychiat.,* 1931, 133:601-19.

van Bogaert-Bertrand syndrome. See *Canavan syndrome.*

van Bogaert-Divry syndrome. Synonyms: *diffuse corticomeningeal angiomatosis, diffuse sclerosis with meningeal angiomatosis, meningeal angiomatosis with diffuse sclerosis.*

A familial syndrome, transmitted as an autosomal recessive trait, characterized by demyelination of the white substance of the centrum ovale, hemianopsia, and cutis marmorata due to telangiectases. The symptoms include epileptic seizures, visual field defects, migraine, focal paresthesia, mental disturbances, and progressive dementia. Pathological findings consist of diffuse capillary and venous leptomeningeal angiomatoses in the sulci, becoming more prominent toward the occipital lobe; fibrotic changes in all abnormally proliferated vessels; anoxic cortical lesions with areas of atrophy and degeneration of the white matter, the changes being most pronounced in the parieto-occipito-temporal area; and fibrillary gliosis of some nuclei and tracts in the brain stem, particularly in the vestibular, reticular, and trigeminal spinal and pyramidal tracts.

van Bogaert, L., & Divry, P. Sur une maladie familiale caractérisée par une angiomatose diffuse cortico-méningée and une démyélinisation de la substance blanche du centre ovale. *Bruxelles Méd.,* 1945, 25:1090-1.

van Bogaert-Hozay syndrome. Synonyms: *Hozay syndrome, acro-osteolysis-facial dysplasia syndrome.*

A familial form of acro-osteolysis associated with a mild mental retardation, skin atrophy, facial dysmorphism, and ocular defects. Facial anomalies consist chiefly of a flat nasal bridge, thickened cheeks, malformed ears, micrognathia, malocclusion, and facial hypotrichosis. Hypertelorism, hypoplastic cilia and eyebrows, blepharoptosis, esotropia, astigmatism, and myopia are the ocular features. The fingers and toes are aplastic, having infantile appearance, and the distal end of the ulna is underdeveloped.

van Bogaert, L. Essai de classement et d'interprétation quelques acro-ostéolyses mutilantes actuellement connues. *Acta Neur. Belg.,* 1953, 53:90-115. Hozay, H. Sur dystrophie familale particulière. Inhibition précoce de la croissance et ostéolyse non-mutilante acrale avec dysmorphie faciale. *Rev. Neur., Paris,* 1953, 89:245-115.

van Bogaert-Nijssen disease. See *metachromatic leukodystrophy.*

van Bogaert-Nijssen-Peiffer syndrome. See *metachromatic leukodystrophy.*

van Bogaert-Nyssen syndrome. See *metachromatic leukodystrophy.*

van Bogaert-Nyssen-Peiffer syndrome. See *metachromatic leukodystrophy.*

van Bogaert-Scherer-Epstein syndrome. Synonyms: *Thiébaut syndrome, cerebral cholesterinosis, cerebrospinal cholesterinosis, cerebrotendinous xanthomamtosis (CTX), cholestanolosis, spinal cholesterolosis.*

A familial disorder of metabolism, probably transmitted as an autosomal recessive trait, characterized by xanthomas of the tendons, lungs, and brain in the presence of normal or nearly normal blood cholesterol and high cholestanol accumulation in the white matter of the brain. The principal histopathological findings include xanthomatous lesions replacing much of the cerebellum; extensive demyelination of the cerebellar white matter, superior cerebellar and cerebral peduncles, and the posterior and lateral columns of the spinal cord; xanthomas in the cerebral peduncles; the presence of large mononuclear cells in areas of demyelination; loss of Purkinje and granule cells; degeneration of the olivocerebellar fibers; a perivascular collection of large mononuclear cells with foamy cytoplasm in the globus pallidus, caudate nucleus, and basal ganglia; gliosis and demyelination in the brain stem; perivascular cuffing by large mononuclear cells in the spinal cord; granulomatous lesions containing birefringent crystalline cells and large foam cells in the lungs and bones; lipid deposits around the pulmonary vessels; and atheromatous plaques in the large vessels. A variant known as **cholesterolosis** is characterized by high blood cholesterol levels associated with spastic paraplegia, bilateral Babinski signs, ankle and patellar clonus, tendinous xanthomas, palmar and plantar xanthomas, xanthelasmas, hepatosplenomegaly, and hyperlipidemia. Cholesterol crystals and free fatty granules are usually found in the spinal cord.

van Bogaert, L., Scherer, H. J., & Epstein, E. *Une forme cérébrale de la cholestérinose généralisée (type particulier de lipidose à cholestérine).* Paris, 1937. Thiébaut, M. F. Paraplégie spasmodique et xanthomes tendineux associés. Des rapports de ce syndrome avec la cholestérinose cérébro-spinale. *Rev. Neur., Paris,* 1942, I74:313-5. Bhattacharyya, A. K., & Connor, W. E. Familial diseases with storage of sterols other than cholesterol. (Cerebrotendinous xanthomatosis and beta-sitosterolemia and xanthomatosis). In: Stanbury, J. B., Wyngaarden, J. B., & Frederickson, D. S., eds. *The metabolic basis of inherited diseases.* 4th ed. New York, McGraw-Hill, 1978, pp. 656-69.

VAN BUCHEM, FRANCIS STEVEN PETER. See BUCHEM, FRANCIS STEVEN PETER, VAN

VAN BUREN, WILLIAM HOLME (American physician, 1819-1883)

Van Buren disease. See *Peyronie disease.*

VAN CREVELD, SIMON. See CREVELD, SIMON, VAN

VAN DEN BERGH, A. A. HIJAMS. See BERGH, A. A. HIJAMS, VAN DEN

VAN DER HOEVE, JAN. See HOEVE, JAN, VAN DER

VAN DER SPIEGHEL, ADRIAAN. See SPIEGHEL, ADRIAAN, VAN DER

VAN DER WOUDE, ANNE (American physician)

van der Woude syndrome (VWS). Synonyms: *Demarquay-Richet syndrome, cleft lip and palate (CLP)-lip pits syndrome, lip pit-cleft lip or palate syndrome.*

A hereditary syndrome, transmitted as an autosomal dominant trait, marked by paramedian pits in the lower lip, cleft lip with or without cleft palate, hypodontia, and missing second premolars.

van der Woude, A. Fistula labii inferioris congenita and its association with cleft lip and palate. *Am. J. Hum. Genet.*, 1954, 6:244-56. Demaraquay, J. N. Quelques considérations sur le bec-de-lièvre. *Gaz. Méd. Paris*, 1845, 13:52-3. Richet, D. D. Bec-de-lièvre double et vice de conformation fort intéressant de la lèvre inférieure. *Bull. Chir. Paris*, 1862, 2:230-2.

VAN GOGH, VINCENT. See GOGH, VINCENT, VAN

VAN LAERE, J. (Belgian physician)

Brown-Vialetto-van Laere syndrome. See *under Brown, C. H.*

VAN LOHUIZEN, CATO, H. J. See LOHUIZEN, CATO H. J.,VAN

VAN MEEKEREN, JOB. See MEEKEREN, JOB, VAN

VAN NECK, M. (Belgian physician)

Van Neck disease. Synonyms: *Delitale-Valtancoli syndrome, Odelberg disease, Van Neck-Odelberg syndrome, chondropathia hypertrophica transitoria ischiopubica, osteochondritis ischiopubica, osteochondropathia ischiopubica.*

Nonspecific ischiopubic osteochondritis seen in children and adolescents of both sexes. The symptoms include pain in the thigh, radiating downward toward the knee, and limping after a long walk or exercise. During the early stages there may be a rise of temperature. Inflammatory etiology is suspected.

*Van Neck, M. Ostéochondrite du pubis. *Arch. Fr. Belg. Chir.*, 1924, 27:238-40. Odelberg, A. Some cases of destruction in the ischium of doubtful etiology. *Acta Chir. Scand.*, 1923-24, 56:273-84.

Van Neck-Odelberg syndrome. See *Van Neck disease.*

VAN WYK, JUDSON J. (American physician)

Van Wyk-Grumbach syndrome. A syndrome of precocious menstruation and galactorrhea in juvenile hypothyroidism. In the original report, three girls had precocious menstruation, galactorrhea, absence of pubic hair, and enlarged sella turcica. One girl was excessively pigmented. The suspected mechanism consists of an overlapping secretion of gonadotropin, mammotropic hormone, and, in some instances, melanocyte-stimulating hormone, along with a presumed high level of thyroid-stimulating hormone.

Van Wyk, J. J., & Grumbach, M. M. syndrome of precocious menstruation and galactorrhea in juvenile hypothyroidism: An example of hormonal overlap in pituitary feedback. *J. Pediat.*, 1960, 57:416-35.

VANDAELE, R. (Belgian physician)

Dupont-Vandaele syndrome. See *Woringer-Kolopp, under Woringer, Frederic.*

vanishing bone disease. See *carpotarsal osteolysis syndrome (dominant and sporadic forms).*

vanishing diabetes mellitus. See *Houssay syndrome.*

vanishing lung. See *Burke syndrome.*

vanishing testes syndrome. A congenital disorder in which affected infants have microphallus, but genital ambiguity, and there are no testes.

Grumbach, M. M., & Van Wyk, J. J. Disorders of sex differentiation. In: Williams, R. H., ed. *Textbook of endocrinology.* 5th ed. Philadelphia, Saunders, 1974, p. 490.

VAQUEZ, LOUIS HENRI (French physician, 1860-1936)

Babinski-Vaquez syndrome. See *Babinski syndrome.*

Vaquez disease. See *Vaquez-Osler syndrome.*

Vaquez polycythemia. See *Vaquez-Osler syndrome.*

Vaquez-Osler erythremia. See *Vaquez-Osler syndrome.*

Vaquez-Osler syndrome. Synonyms: *Osler disease, Vaquez disease, Vaquez polycythemia, Vaquez-Osler erythremia, cryptogenic polycythemia, erythrocytosis megalosplenica, myelopathic polycythemia, polycythemia rubra, polycythemia rubra vera, polycythemia vera, polycythemia with chronic cyanosis, splenomegalic polycythemia.*

A chronic disease, occurring mostly in middle-aged males, in which increased erythrocyte count (reaching sometimes 10,000,000 cells per cmm), blood volume, erythroblastic activity, and blood viscosity is associated with cyanosis and splenomegaly. Headache, gas pain, and belching are the typical presenting symptoms. Other manifestations may include flushing, itching after a bath, ecchymoses, neuralgia, thickening of the phalanges, dyspnea, vertigo, lassitude, weakness, tinnitus, and dyspepsia. Additionally, there may be sweating, weight loss, paresthesia, articular complications, transitory blindness, mesenteric thrombosis, gangrene, and hemorrhage from various organs. Oral manifestations include purplish red coloration of the mucosa, especially of the tongue, and gingivae; ecchymoses, hematomas, and submucosal petechiae are common. Recurrent infection may occur. Leukocytosis, increased blood platelets count, and bone marrow hyperplasia are the other hematological features. When associated with liver cirrhosis, this disorder is known as the *Mosse syndrome.* See also *Gaisböck syndrome (pseudopolycythemia).*

Vaquez, L. H. Sur une forme spéciale de cyanose s'accompagnant d'hyperglobulie excessive et persistante. *C. Rend. Soc. Biol., Paris,* 1892, 44:384-8. Osler, W. Chronic cyanosis, with polycythemia and enlarged spleen. A new clinical entity. *Am. J. Med. Sc.*, 1903, 126:187-201.

VARADI, V. (Hungarian physician)

Váradi-Papp syndrome. A syndrome of large toes, supernumerary fingers, cleft lip or palate, lingual nodules, and psychomotor retardation. Other features sometimes present include absence of the olfactory bulbs and tracts, crypotorchism, inguinal hernia, and congenital heart disease. The syndrome was first observed in an inbred isolate in Hungary.

Váradi, V., Szabó, L., & Papp, Z. Syndrome of polydactyly, cleft lip/palate or lingual lump, and psychomotor retardation in endogamic gypsies. *J. Med. Genet.*, 1980, 17:119-22.

variable erythrokeratoderma. See *Mendes Da Costa syndrome.*

varicella syndrome. See *congenital varicella syndrome.*

varioliform pyoderma. See *Kaposi varicelliform eruption.*

varnished tongue. See *Möller glossitis.*

VARON, HUMBERTO (Colombian physician)

Yunis-Varón syndrome. See *under Yunis, Emilio.*

vascular compartment syndrome. See *compartment syndrome.*

vascular compression of the duodenum. See *cast syndrome.*

vascular hemophilia. See *Willebrand-Jürgens syndrome.*

vascular syphilis of spinal cord. See *Erb-Charcot syndrome, under Erb, Wilhelm Ernst.*

vasculitis superficialis. See *Gougerot-Ruiter syndrome.*
VASILIEV, NIKOLAI PORFIRIEVICH (Russian physician, born 1861)
Vasiliev disease. See *leptospirosis.*
vasoconstriction syncope. See *Gowers syndrome (3).*
vasomotor acroparesthesia. See *Nothnagel acroparesthesia.*
vasomotor ataxia. See *Curtius syndrome (2).*
vasomotor paralysis of the extremities. See *Mitchell syndrome (1).*
vasomotor rhinitis. See *Bostock catarrh.*
vasovagal syndrome. See *carotid sinus syndrome.*
VATER (**v**ertebral defects-**a**nal atresia-**t**racheoesophageal fistula-**e**sophageal atresia-**r**adial and **r**enal dysplasia) **association or syndrome.** Synonyms: *Kaufman syndrome, Say syndrome, Say-Gerald syndrome, polydactyly-imperforate anus-vertebral anomalies syndrome (PIV, PIAVA), VACTERL (vertebral abnormalities-anal atresia-cardiac abnormalities-tracheo-esophageal fistula-renal agenesis-limb defects) association or syndrome, VACTEL (vertebral abnormalities-anal atresia-cardiac abnormalities-tracheo-esophageal fistula-limb defects) association or syndrome.*

A nonrandom association of anomalies consisting of vertebral abnormalities; anal atresia; congenital cardiovascular defects, such as single umbilical artery and interventricular septal defects; tracheoesophageal fistula; esophageal atresia; renal agenesis and dysplasia; and limb abnormalities, including bifid thumbs, polydactyly, radial hypoplasia, and syndactyly of the thumb and index fingers. Other abnormalities occurring in this syndrome may include duodenal atresia, interauricular septal defects, cleft lip, cleft palate, spleen aplasia, lung aplasia, testicular aplasia, female pseudohermaphroditism hypospadias, hip hypoplasia, and common iliac artery. All thus far reported cases have been sporadic.

Quan, L., & Smith, D. W. The VATER association: vertebral defects, anal atresia, treacheoesophageal fistula with esophageal atresia, radial dysplasia. *Birth Defects*, 1972, 8(2):75-78. Kaufman, R. L., *et al.* Family studies in congenital heart disease. II. A syndrome of hydrometrocolpos, postaxial polydactyly and congenital heart disease. *Birth Defects*, 1972, 8(5):85-7. Say, B., & Gerald, P. S. A new polydactyly/imperforate-anus/vertebral-anomalies syndrome? *Lancet*, 1968, 2:688.

VAUGHAN, JANET MARIA (British physician)
Harrison-Vaughan disease. See *Vaughan disease.*
Vaughan disease. Synonyms: *Harrison-Vaughan disease, leukoerythroblastic anemia, leukoerythroblastosis, myelophthisic anemia, osteosclerotic anemia.*

An anemic disease characterized by immature leukocytes of the myeloid series and nucleated red cells in the peripheral blood, usually observed in metastatic carcinoma of the bone marrow and in various neoplastic and non-neoplastic diseases in which the bone marrow is involved in some way.

Vaughan, J. M., & Harrison, C. V. Leuco-erythroblastic anaemia and myelosclerosis. *J. Path. Bact.*, 1939, 48:339-52.

VCF. See *velocardiofacial syndrome.*
VECCHI, V. (Italian physician)
Zanoli-Vecchi syndrome. See *under Zanoli.*
VEENEKLAAS, G. M. H. (Dutch physician)
Veeneklaas syndrome. Synonyms: *dentobronchitis, dentopulmonary syndrome.*

An association of chronic bronchitis and dental caries, believed to be caused by aspiration of material from carious teeth.

Veeneklaas, G. M. H. "Dentobronchitis." *Ann. Paediat., Basel,* 1952, 178:59-63.

vegans syndrome. Synonym: *rastafarianism syndrome.*

Vitamin B_{12} deficiency associated with neurological symptoms (ranging from paresthesia to subacute combined degeneration), gastrointestinal disorders, glossitis, anorexia, epigastric discomfort, vomiting, intermittent claudication, monocytic anemia, and hyperpigmentation of the palms and soles. The syndrome was originally reported among members of the Rastafarian cult, a religious sect that has its origin in Jamaica, living in England.

Campbell, M., *et al.* Rastafarianism and the vegans syndrome. *Brit. Med. J.,* 1982, 285:1617-8.

vegetative pyoderma. See *Hallopeau syndrome (3).*
VEIL, PROSPER (French ophthalmologist, 1892-1941)
Terrien-Veil syndrome. See *Posner-Schlossman syndrome.*
velocardiofacial (VCF) syndrome. A relatively common familial clefting syndrome transmitted as an autosomal dominat trait with variable expression. The most frequent features of this syndrome include cleft palate, learning disability, cardiac defect, retrognathia, prominent nose, hypotonia in infancy, malar flatness, pharyngeal hypotonia, and minor ear malformations. Speech and hearing disorders are usually associated. Less common occurring disorders consist of slender hands and fingers, overabundant scalp hair, microcephaly, mental retardation, small stature, inguinal hernia, umbilical hernia, scoliosis, the Robin anomaly sequence, and hypospadias. Platybasia is a common phenotypic feature.

Shprintzen, R. J., *et al.* A new syndrome involving cleft palate, cardiac anomalies, typical facies, and learning disabilities. Velo-cardio-facial syndrome. *Cleft Palate*, 1978, 15:56-62.

venereal lymphogranuloma. See *Durand-Nicolas-Favre disease, under Durand, J.*
veno-occlusive disease of the liver. See *Stuart-Bras disease, under Stuart, K. L.*
ventricular fibrilloflutter. See *torsades de pointes syndrome.*
verbal aphasia. See *Broca aphasia.*
VERBIEST, H. (Dutch physician)
Verbiest syndrome. Synonym: *claudicatio intermittens spinalis.*

Narrowing of the lumbar vertebral canal characterized by symptoms of compression of the caudal nerve roots, including bilateral radicular pain, sensory disorders, and impaired motor activity of the legs, which are present only when the patient is walking or standing up but not in the recumbent position. All Verbiest's patients were adult males.

Verbiest, H. Primaire stenose van het lumbale wervelkonal bij volwassmen, een nieur ziektebeeld. *Ned. Tschr. Geneesk.,* 1950, 94:2415-33. Verbiest, H. A radicular syndrome from developmental narrowing of the lumbar vertebral canal. *J. Bone Joint Surg.,* 1954, 36B:230-7.

VERBRYCKE, J. RUSSEL, JR. (American physician)
Verbrycke syndrome. Synonym: *cholecystohepatic flexure adhesions.*

A disease characterized by the mechanical pull of localized adhesions between the hepatic flexure of the

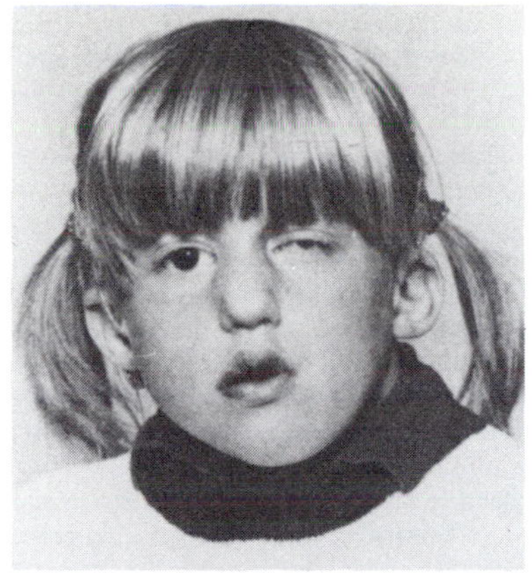

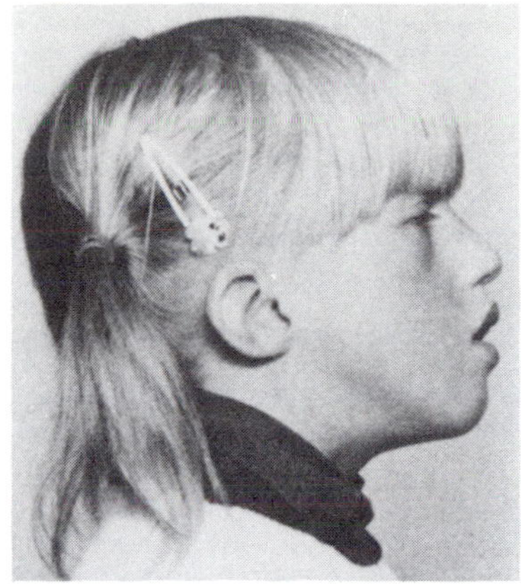

Velocardiofacial syndrome
Beemer, Frits A., J.J.E.M. de Nef, J..W. Delleman, E.M. Bleeker- Wagemakers & Robert J. Shprintzen: *American Journal of Medical Genetics* 24:541-542, 1986. New York: Alan R. Liss, Inc.

colon and the gallbladder, causing epigastric pain, nausea, and tenderness. Downward pull of the gallbladder, when the patient is in the upright position, is responsible for a diurnal increase in the severity of symptoms.

Verbrycke, J. R., Jr. Adhesions of cholelcystohepatic flexure. A new syndrome with specific test. *JAMA,* 1940, 114:314-6.

VERDAN, CLAUDE (French physician)

Verdan syndrome. Limited flexor activity of the uninvolved finger in adhesive tenosynovitis or, in amputation of the little finger, blocking of the extensor tendon and fixation of the deep flexor tendon in the stump.

Verdan, C., & Michon, J. La ténolyse des tendons fléchisseurs. II. Indications dans les blocages cicatriciels. *Rev. Méd., Nancy,* 1957, 82:69-79.

VERGANI, CARLO (Italian physician)

Vergani syndrome. Synonym: *familial hypo-alpha-lipoproteinemia.*

A familial syndrome characterized by low levels of high density lipoprotein-cholesterol and apoliprotein A without other lipoprotein abnormalities. The syndrome is believed to be transmitted as an autosomal dominant trait.

Vergani, C., & Bettale, G. Familial hypo-alpha-lipoproteinemia. *Clin. Chim. Acta,* 1981, 114:45-52.

VERMA, ISHWAR C.

short rib-polydactyly syndrome, Verma-Naumoff type. See *Verma-Naumoff syndrome.*

Verma-Naumoff syndrome. Synonyms: *polydacty with neonatal chondrodystrophy type III; short rib-polydactyly syndrome type III (SRP III); short rib-polydactyly syndrome, Verma-Naumoff type.*

A lethal form of short-limb dwarfism associated with hydropic appearance, narrow thorax, postaxial polydactyly genital anomalies, hypoplastic lungs, saddle nose, and frontal bossing. The syndrome is transmitted as an autosomal recessive trait.

Verma, I. C., *et al.* An autosomal recessive form of lethal chondrodystrophy with severe thoracic narrowing, rhizoacromelic type of micromelia, polydactyly, and genital anomalies. *Birth Defects*, 1975, 11(6)167-74. Naumoff, P. *et al.* Short rib polydactyly syndrome Type 3. *Radiology,* 1977, 122:443-7.

vernal conjunctivitis. See *Angelucci syndrome.*

vernal photodermatosis. See *Buckhardt dermatitis.*

VERNER, JOHN VICTOR (American physician, born 1927)

Verner-Morrison syndrome. Synonyms: *Priest-Alexander syndrome, cholera-like diarrhea, diarrheogenic syndrome, pancreatic carcinoma-hypokalemic watery diarrhea syndrome, pancreatic cholera, VIPoma syndrome, watery diarrhea-hypokalemia-achlorhydria (WDHA), watery diarrhea syndrome (WDS).*

A syndrome of profuse intermittent diarrhea, hypokalemia, dehydration, and achlorhydria (or hypochlorhydria), frequently associated with hyperglycemia, hypercalcemia, hypotension, and episodic flushing. The discharge is rich in electrolytes, especially potassium, leading to hypokalemia with resulting weakness, flaccid paralysis, and hypokalemic nephropathy with renal failure. Diabetes or glucose intolerance are frequently present. Dilation of the gallbladder or small intestine may be seen on x-ray examination. The syndrome has been attributed to a frequently malignant non-beta-cell tumor of the islands of Langerhans (VIPoma) and resulting overproduction of vasoactive intestinal peptide (VIP). In some cases, it is associated with benign hyperplasia of the islet cells of the pancreas or neural crest tumors arising outside of the pancreas, such as bronchogenic carcinoma, ganglioneuroblastoma, or pheochromocytoma. Some tumors may be accompanied by elevated levels of prostaglandin E_2.

Verner, J. V., & Morrison, A. B. Islet cell tumor and a syndrome of refractory watery diarrhea and hypokalemia. *Am. J. Med.,* 1958, 25:374-80. Priest, W. M., & Alexander, M. K. Islet-cell tumor of the pancreas with ulceration, diarrhea, and hypokalemia. *Lancet,* 1957, 2:1145-7.

VERNET, MAURICE ALBIN (French physician, born 1887)

Vernet paralysis. See *Vernet syndrome.*

Vernet syndrome. Synonyms: *Vernet paralysis, jugular foramen syndrome.*

A neurological syndrome in which lesions in the region of the jugular foramen produce paralysis of the areas supplied by the ninth, tenth, and eleventh cranial nerves with secondary ipsilateral paralysis of the soft palate, larynx, pharynx, and the sternocleidomastoid and trapezius muscles. The symptoms include dysphagia, anesthesia of the soft palate, and loss of sensation and taste in the back of the tongue.

Vernet, M. *Les paralysies laryngées associées.* Lyon, 1916. (Thesis).

VERNEUIL, ARISTIDE AUGUSTE STANISLAS (French physician, 1823-1895)

Kümmell-Verneuil disease. See *under Kümmell.*

Verneuil disease. Synonym: *hidratenitis suppurativa.*

A chronic suppurative disease of the apocrine sweat glands of the axilla, areolae, umbilicus, perineum, groin, and buttocks, giving rise to multiple fistulous infected tracts. The condition reportedly was described by Verneuil in 1854.

Gertsch, P., & Mosimann, R. La maladie de Verneuil dans le diagnostic différentiel des suppurations de la région ano-périnéo-fessière. *Helvet. Chir. Acta,* 1980, 47:477-81.

verruca necrogenica. See *Wilks disease.*

verrucosis generalisata et disseminata. See *Lewandowski-Lutz syndrome.*

verrucous carcinoma. See *Ackerman carcinoma.*

verrucous endocarditis. See *Libman-Sacks syndrome.*

verrucous noninfective endocarditis. See *Libman-Sacks syndrome.*

verruga peruana. See *Carrión disease.*

vertebra plana. See *Calvé syndrome.*

vertebra plana osteonecrotica. See *Calvé syndrome.*

vertebral syndrome. See *Putti syndrome.*

vertebral abnormalities-anal atresia-cardiac abnormalities-tracheo-esophageal fistula-limb defects (VACTEL). See *VATER association.*

vertebral ankylosing hyperostosis. See *Forestier syndrome (2).*

vertebral artery compression syndrome. See *Bärtschi-Rochaix syndrome.*

vertebral epiphysitis. See *Scheuermann disease.*

vertebral insufficiency. See *Schanz syndrome.*

vertebral osteochondritis. See *Calvé syndrome.*

vertebral sciatica. See *Putti syndrome.*

vertebrobasilar syndrome. Synonym: *vertebrobasilar arterial syndrome.*

Vertebrobasilar insufficiency caused by atherosclerosis of the vertebral arteries, cervical spondylosis, and, less commonly, congenital malformations and emboli. See also *top of the basilar syndrome.*

Szymchel, J. [Vertebrobasilar arterial syndromes] *Neur. Neurochir. Pol.,* 1982, 16:183-90.

vertebrobasilar arterial syndrome. See *vertebrobasilar syndrome.*

vertebrobasilar insufficiency. See *top of the basilar syndrome.*

vertebrobasilar ischemia. See *top of the basilar syndrome.*

vertical maxillary deficiency. See *short face syndrome.*

vertical retraction syndrome. An ocular motility disorder characterized by restricted elevation associated with retraction of the globe and narrowing of the palpebral fissure.

*Matsumoto, K. [Eye motility disorders] *Chuo Ganka Iho,* 1935, 27:36-46. (Abstr. *Zbl. Ges. Ophth.,* 1935, 34:386).

vertigo of cervical arthrosis. See *Barré-Lieou syndrome.*

VESELL, ELLIOT S. (American physician)

Vesell syndrome. See *symphalangism syndrome.*

vesical-voluntary sphincter dyssynergia. See *Hinman syndrome.*

vesicointestinal fissure. See *OEIS complex.*

vesicular pharyngitis. See *Zahorsky syndrome (2).*

vestibular syndrome. A disease of the vestibular apparatus with asymmetric labyrinthine discharges. The main features include vertigo, nausea, vomiting, nystagmus, and ataxia. The lesions may be peripheral, which are usually caused by infectious diseases or vascular trauma, or central, which are usually vascular, demyelinating, and neoplastic in nature. See also *Ménière syndrome* and *Pedersen syndrome.*

Boghen, D. Vestibular syndrome: Clinical and pathophysiological considerations. *Adv. Otorhinolaryng., Basel,* 1982, 28:33-8.

vestibular aqueduct syndrome. Congenital abnormality of the vestibular aqueduct associated with deafness.

Swartz, J. D., *et al.* The vestibular aqueduct syndrome: Computed tomographic appearance. *Clin. Radiol.,* 1985, 36:241-3.

vestibular neuronitis. See *Ménière syndrome, and see Pedersen syndrome.*

VHF (viral hemorrhagic fever). See *hemorrhagic fever with renal syndrome.*

VHL (von Hippel-Lindau) syndrome. See *Hippel-Lindau syndrome.*

VIALETTO, E. (Italian physician)

Brown-Vialetto-van Laere syndrome. See *under Brown, C. H.*

vibration syndrome (VS). Synonyms: *dead finger disease, digital vibration (DV) syndrome, hand-arm vibration syndrome, occupational Raynaud disease, vibration-induced white finger (VWF), wax finger disease, white finger disease.*

An occupational disease, considered to be a variant of the Raynaud syndrome, caused by adverse effects of vibrations on the human body. In the pre-World War II literature, the condition was believed to consist of various musculoskeletal, neurological, and vascular disorders in tractor and heavy equipment operators. In its current use, the term applies to mainly vascular disorders in workers using hand-held power tools (pneumatic guns, power saws, jackhammers, and the like) and pertains to vascular disorders involving the hands and arms. In its early stages, the condition is characterized by tingling, numbness, or blanching of the finger tips, the symptoms extending to the base of all of the digits. With repeated episodes, there may be nerve damage and infrequent instances of necrosis of the fingers tips. Medial muscular fibrosis, subintimal fibrosis, restriction of blood flow, some loss of touch sensation, and gangrene in severe cases are some of the complications. Peripheral sensory and motor nerve disorders intensify the vasospasm with resulting ischemia and numbness. Cold is a contributing factor.

Taylor, J. S. Vibration syndrome in industry: Dermatological viewpoint. *Am. J. Indust. Med.,* 1985, 8:415-32.

vibration-induced white finger (VWF). See *vibration syndrome.*

VICKERS, ROBERT A. (American oral pathologist)

Gorlin-Vickers syndrome. See *mucosal neuromas syndrome.*

VIDAL, JEAN BAPTISTE EMILE (French physician, 1825-1893)

Vidal disease. See *Brocq disease (1).*

vidian neuralgia. See *Vail syndrome.*
Vietnam syndrome. See *post-traumatic stress syndrome.*
VILANOVA, XAVIER (Spanish physician)
Vilanova-Cañadell syndrome. Synonym: *hypothyroid phrynoderma.*

An association of phrynoderma, hypothyroidism, and vitamin A deficiency.

Vilanova, X., & Cañadell, J. M. Dermopatias, hipotiroidismo y avitaminosis A. *Actas Derm. Sif., Madrid,* 1949, 40:689-95.

Vilanova-Piñol Aguadé syndrome. Synonym: *subacute panniculitis nodosa migrans.*

A dermatological disease characterized by pea-sized, painless, subcutaneous nodules on the anterolateral aspects of the legs, which later become mobilized. The disorder is usually observed 1 to 20 days after an episode of tonsillitis or pharyngitis.

Vilanova, X., & Piñol Aguadé, J. Hypodermite nodulaire subaiguë migratrice. *Ann. Derm. Syph., Paris,* 1956, 83:369-404.

VILLARET, MAURICE (French physician, 1877-1946)
Villaret syndrome. Synonyms: *posterior retroparotid space syndrome, retroparotid space syndrome.*

A syndrome in which lesions of the retroparotid space (bounded posteriorly by the cervical vertebrae, medially by the pharynx, anteriorly by the parotid gland, laterally by the sternocleidomastoid muscle, and superiorly by the skull near the jugular foramen) produce unilateral paralysis of the ninth, tenth, eleventh, twelfth, and occasionally the seventh cranial nerves, resulting in the Horner syndrome (mainly enophthalmos, blepharoptosis, and miosis), and in ipsilateral paralysis of the soft palate, pharynx, larynx, and vocal cords.

Villaret, M. Le syndrome nerveux de l'espace rétroparotidien postérieur. *Rev. Neur., Paris,* 1916, 23:188-90.

villous adenoma depletion syndrome. Synonym: *depletion syndrome.*

A frequently fatal syndrome of villous adenoma of the colon associated with watery diarrhea, which leads to excessive loss of fluid and electrolytes, dehydration, circulatory collapse, prerenal azotemia, and metabolic acidosis.

McKittrick, L. S., & Wheelock, F. C., Jr. *Carcinoma of colon.* Springfield, Illinois, Thomas, 1954, p. 61.

villous gastropathy. See *Ménétrier syndrome.*

VINCENT, JEAN HYACINTHE (French physician, 1862-1950)
Plaut-Vincent infection. See *Vincent infection.*
Plaut-Vincent ulcer. See *Vincent infection.*
Vincent angina. Painful membraneous ulceration with edema and hyperemic patches of the oropharynx and throat, caused by acute necrotizing gingivitis.

Vincent, J. H. Sur l'étiologie et sur les lésions anatomopathologiques de la pourriture d'hôpital. *Ann. Inst. Pasteur,* 1896, 10:488-510.

Vincent gingivitis. See *Vincent infection.*
Vincent infection. Synonyms: *Plaut ulcer, Plaut-Vincent infection, Vincent gingivitis, Vincent stomatitis, acute necrotizing gingivitis, acute infectious gingivostomatitis, acute necrotizing ulcerative gingivitis (ANUG), acute ulcerative gingivitis, acute ulceromembranous gignivitis, fusospirillary marginal gingivitis, fusospirillosis, fusospirochetal gingivitis, necrotizing ulcerative gingivitis, phagodenic gingivitis, putrid sore mouth, putrid stomatitis, trench gums, trench mouth, ulcerative gingivitis.*

A progressive painful infection of the gingiva marked by crateriform lesions of the interdental papillae that are covered by pseudomembranous slough and circumscribed by linear erythema. Fetid breath, hypersalivation, and spontaneous gingival bleeding are associated. It is usually observed in young adults and middle-aged persons. Epidemics may occur in groups in close contact, such as military troops, hence the names **trench gums** and **trench mouth.** A spiral bacterium, *Treponema vincentii,* coexisting in symbiotic relationship with a fusiform bacillus (*Fusobacterium nucleatum*), is considered as a possible etiologic agent, but various other spirochetes, filamentous organisms, vibrios, cocci, and other bacteria have been isolated from infected patients. When lesions spread to the soft palate and oropharaynx, the condition is known as *Vincent angina.*

*Vincent, J. H. Sur l'étiologie et sur les lésions anatomopathologiques de pouriture d'hôpital. *Ann. Inst. Pasteur,* 1896, 10:488-510. Plaut, H. C. Studien zur bacteriellen Diagnostik der Diphtherie und der Anginen. *Deut. Med. Wschr.,* 1894, 20:920-3.

Vincent stomatitis. See *Vincent infection.*
VINSON, PORTER PAISLEY (American surgeon, 1890-1959)
Plummer-Vinson syndrome (PVS). See *under Plummer.*
VIPoma syndrome. See *Verner-Morrison syndrome.*
viral hemorrhagic fever (VHF). See *hemorrhagic fever with renal syndrome.*
VIRCHOW, RUDOLF LUDWIG KARL (German pathologist, 1821-1902)
Virchow-Seckel syndrome. See *Seckel syndrome.*
virilizing adrenocortical hyperplasia. See *congenital adrenal hyperplasia.*
virus A hepatitis. See *Botkin disease.*
virus-associated hemophagocytic syndrome (VAHS). Histiocytic hyperplasia with hemophagocytosis associated with active viral infection. High fever, constitutional symptoms, liver function disorders, blood coagulation abnormalities, and peripheral cytopenias are the characteristic findings. Hepatosplenomegaly, lymphadenopathy, pulmonary infiltrates, and skin rash are often present. Most patients are immunosuppressed. The bone marrow shows decreased granulopoiesis and erythropoiesis with normal to increased numbers of megakaryocytes. In the original report, active infection by the herpes group viruses was documented in fourteen patients and by adenovirus in one.

Risdall, R. J., *et al.* Virus-associated hemophagocytic syndrome. A benign histiocytic proliferation distinct from malignant histiocytosis. *Cancer,* 1979, 44:993-1002. McClain, K., *et al.* Virus-associated histiocytic proliferation in children. Frequent association with Epstein-Barr virus and congenital or acquired immunodefiencies. *Am. J. Pediat. Hemat. Oncol.,* 1988, 10:196-205.

visceral artery ischemia. See *visceral artery syndrome.*
visceral artery syndrome. Synonym: *visceral artery ischemia.*

Occlusive lesions involving the visceral vessels with resulting intestinal ischemia. Acute ischemic disorders are caused by embolic occlusion of a visceral branch of the abdominal aorta, athrombotic occlusion of the diseased visceral artery, and nonocclusive mesenteric vascular insufficiency. Chronic ischemia is usually caused by stenotic or occlusive lesions of one or more of the visceral vessels. Extrinsic compression of the celiac axis by the median arcuate ligament is another cause of ischemia.

Stoney, R. J., & Olcott, C., IV. Visceral artery syndromes and reconstruction. *Surg. Clin. N. America,* 1979, 59:637-47.

viscerocystic retinoangiomatosis syndrome. See *Hippel-Lindau syndrome.*

visceroptosis. See *Glénard syndrome.*

visual anosognosia. See *Anton-Babinski syndrome.*

visual disorientation syndrome. See *Riddoch syndrome.*

vitamin B_6-dependency syndrome. A hereditary disorder, transmitted as an autosomal recessive trait, characterized by neonatal convulsions that respond to large doses of pyridoxine.

Gamstorp, I. Vitamin B_6-afhaengighedssyndromet. *Ugeskr. Laeger,* 1974, 136:2819.

vitamin D-dependent rickets. See *pseudo-vitamin D-deficiency rickets syndrome.*

vitamin D-resistant rickets. See *hypophosphatemic familial rickets.*

vitamin D-resistant rickets-epidermal nevus syndrome. See *hypophosphatemic rickets-osteomalacia-linear nevus sebaceous syndrome.*

vitamin E deficiency syndrome. Dysarthria, cerebellar ataxia, and proprioceptive loss with absent or depressed tendon reflexes associated with vitamin E deficiency in chronic intestinal malabsorption. See also *malabsorption syndrome.*

Rosenbloom, J. L., *et al.* A progressive neurologic syndrome in children with chronic liver disease. *N. Engl. J. Med.,* 1981, 304:503-45. Tomasi, L. G. Reversibility of human myopathy caused by vitamin E deficiency. *Neurology,* 1979, 29:1183-5.

vitelliform macular dystrophy. See *Best macular degeneration.*

vitelloeruptive macular dystrophy. See *Best macular degeneration.*

vitiligoidea plana. See *Addison-Gull syndrome.*

vitreotapetoretinochoroidal degeneration syndrome. A familial eye disease, transmitted as an autosomal dominant trait, characterized by degenerative changes in the macula lutea, peripheral preretinal membranes, and vitreous, associated with optic atrophy.

Wille, H. A family with vitreo-tapeto-retino-choroidal degeneration with dominant transmission. *Acta Ophth., Copenhagen,* 1980, 58:148-57.

vitreous hemorrhage-ruptured cerebral aneurysm syndrome. See *Terson syndrome.*

vitreous wick syndrome. A complication of eye surgery wherein a microperforation or a wound dehiscence may result in vitreous incarceration or vitreous wick.

Ruiz, R. S., & Teeters, V. W. The vitreous wick syndrome. *Am. J. Ophth.,* 1970, 70:483-90.

VKH (Vogt-Koyanagi-Harada) syndrome. See *Vogt-Koyanagi syndrome, under Vogt, Alfred, and see Harada syndrome.*

VOERNER, HANS. See VÕRNER, HANS

VOGT, A. (German physician)

Vogt cephalodactyly. See *Apert-Crouzon syndrome.*

Vogt syndrome. See *Apert-Crouzon syndrome.*

VOGT, ALFRED (Swiss ophthalmologist, 1879-1943)

Vogt cataract. Synonym: *frosted cataract.*

A congenital cataract marked by frostlike whitish scintillating opacities in the superficial layers of the embryonic nucleus, probably transmitted as an autosomal or recessive trait.

Vogt, A. Weitere Ergebnisse der Spaltlampenmikroskopie des vorderen Bulbolsabschnittes. III. Angeborene und früh erwarbene Linsenveränderungen. *Graefes Arch. Ophth.,* 1922, 107:196-240.

Vogt cornea. Synonyms: *cornea farinata, floury cornea.*

A senile or presenile form of corneal opacity characterized by small white punctiform lesions in the deep layers of the corneal parenchyma.

Vogt, A. Neuere Ergebnisse der Spaltlampenmikroskopie. *Schweiz. Med. Wschr.,* 1923, 53:989-95.

Vogt degeneration. Synonyms: *crocodile shagreen, mosaic corneal degeneration.*

A familial form of corneal degeneration, transmitted as an autosomal dominant trait, and primarily affecting the Bowman membrane, in which polygonal or round lesions are arranged in a mosaic pattern, thus giving the affected area the appearance of crocodile skin.

Vogt, A. *Lehrbuch und Atlas der Spaltlampenmikroskopie des lebenden Auges.* Berlin, Springer, 1930.

Vogt disease. Synonym: *cornea guttata.*

A form of corneal dystrophy characterized in its early stages by glints of a golden hue visible under indirect light on the posterior surface of the cornea or by black spheres in the endothelial cells. In advanced stages, the nonreflecting black guttae cover the endothelium in the axial area.

Vogt, A. Weitere Ergebnisse der Spaltlampenmikroskopie des vordern Bulbusabschnittes. (Cornea, Vorderkammer, Iris, Linse, vorderer Glaskörper, Conjunctiva, Lidränder). I. Hornhaut. *Graefes Arch. Ophth.,* 1921, 106:63-103.

Vogt-Koyanagi syndrome. Synonyms: *oculocutaneous syndrome, uveocutaneous syndrome, uveomeningeal syndrome.*

A disease, usually occurring in adult life, characterized by bilateral uveitis with iritis and secondary glaucoma, premature alopecia and graying of the hair, symmetrical vitiligo, hearing disorders, dysacusia, and meningoencephalitis. Mental and growth retardation may occur in some rare familial cases; most cases being sporadic. The symptoms overlap those of Harada disease.

Vogt, A. Frühzeitiges Ergrauen der Zilien und Bemerkungen über den sogenannten plötzlichen Eintritt dieser Veränderung. *Klin. Mbl. Augenh.,* 1906, 44:228-42. Koyanagi, Y. Dysakusis, Alopecie und Poliosis bei schwerer Uveitis nicht traumatischen Ursprungs. *Klin. Mbl. Augenh.,* 1929, 82:194-211.

Vogt-Koyanagi-Harada (VKH) syndrome. See *Vogt-Koyanagi syndrome, and see Harada syndrome.*

VOGT, CECILLE (French physician in Germany, 1875-1962)

Vogt syndrome. Synonyms: *congenital chorea, double athetosis syndrome, état marbré, infantile partial striatal sclerosis, status marmoratus.*

A condition usually associated with birth injury, especially one causing the athetoid form of cerebral palsy. It is characterized by an abnormal aggregation of myelinated nerve fibers in the nervous system, typically in the corpus striatum, which gives it a marblelike appearance. The thalamus, corpus pallidum, and cerebral cortex may also be involved. Clinically, the disorder is manifested by choreiform and athetoid movements that occur during the first year of life and assume the nature of dystonia. Walking difficulty, speech disorders, spasmodic laughing or crying, and mental deficiency may occur.

Vogt, C., & Vogt, O. Zur Lehre der Erkrankungen des striäten Systems. *J. Psychol. Neur., Leipzig,* 1920, 25:627-846.

VOGT, HEINRICH (German physician)

Stock-Spielmeyer-Vogt syndrome. See *under Stock.*

Vogt-Spielmeyer syndrome. See *Stock-Spielmeyer-Vogt syndrome.*

VOHWINKEL, KARL HERMANN (German dermatologist)

Vohwinkel syndrome. Synonyms: *deafness-keratopachyderma-digital constriction syndrome, keratoderma hereditarium mutilans (KHM), keratoma hereditarium mutilans, mutilating keratoderma, mutilating palmoplantar keratoderma.*

A mutilating disease characterized by diffuse hyperkeratosis palmaris et plantaris, hyperhidrosis, stellate keratotic lesions on the dorsal surfaces of the hands and feet, linear keratotic lesions on the knees and elbows, constricted digits that may result in amputation, and deafness. It is a familial disorder transmitted as an autosomal dominant trait, usually affecting white females. Keratotic lesions have their onset in infancy or early childhood; constriction of digits occurs during adolescence.

Vohwinkel, S. H. Keratoma hereditarium mutilans. *Arch. Derm. Syph., Berlin,* 1929, 158:354-64. McKusick, V. A. *Mendelian inheritance in man.* 7th ed. Baltimore, Johns Hopkins Univ. Press, 1986, No. 12450.

VOLAVSEK, W. (Austrian physician)

Volavsek syndrome. An association of keratosis palmaris, involving chiefly the periarticular areas of the fingers; syringomyelia; and nail dystrophy.

Volavsek, W. Zur Klinik der Nagelveränderungen und Palmarkeratosen bei Syringomyelie. *Arch. Derm. Syph., Berlin,* 1941-42, 182:52-7.

VOLHARD, FRANZ (German physician, 1872-1950)

Volhard nephritis. Focal nephritis without elevated blood pressure.

Korcher, G. Die Volhardsche Herdnephritis und ihre Behandlung. *Landarzt,* 1965, 41:133-5.

Volhynia fever. See *Werner-His disease, under Werner, Heinrich.*

VOLKMANN, RICHARD, VON (German physician, 1830-1889)

pseudo-Volkmann syndrome. Traumatic retraction of the fingers in flexion, without ischemia.

Postel, M., & Geneste, R. Traitement des séquelles de la rétraction ischémique des fléchisseurs des doigts. *Rev. Chir. Orthop., Paris,* 1956, 42:514-60.

Volkmann cheilitis. See *Baelz syndrome.*

Volkmann contracture. Synonyms: *Volkmann ischemia, Volkmann syndrome.*

Post-traumatic muscle ischemia and infarction; ischemic contracture of the fingers of the wrist resulting from impaired circulation following an elbow injury or improper application of a turniquet. See also *compartment syndrome.*

Volkmann, R. Die ischämischen Muskellähmungen un Kontrakturen. *Zbl. Chir.,* 1881, 8:801-3.

Volkmann deformity. Synonym: *congenital talus luxation.*

A congenital deformity of the foot due to a tibiotarsal dislocation.

*Volkmann, R., von. Ein Fall von hereditären kongenitaler Luxation beider Sprunggelenke. *Deut. Zschr. Chir.,* 1873, 2:538-42.

Volkmann ischemia. See *Volkmann contracture.*

Volkmann ischemic paralysis. Paralysis caused by ischemia resulting from obstruction or injury of the nutrient vessels of an extrmity.

Volkmann, R. Die ischämischen Muskellähmungen und Kontrakturen. *Zbl. Chir.,* 1881, 8:801-3. Woltman, H. W., Kernahan, J. W., & Goldstein, N. P. Diseases of peripheral nerves. In: Baker, A. B., ed. *Clinical neurology.* 1965. Vol. 4, p. 1860.

Volkmann syndrome. See *Volkmann contracture.*

VOLTOLINI, FREDERICK EDWARD RUDOLF (Breslau physician, 1819-1889)

Voltolini disease. Acute suppurative otitis interna accompanied by severe pain, fever, delirium, and unconsciousness.

Voltolini. Die akute Entzündung des heutigen Labyrinthes, gewöhnlich irrtümlich für Meningitis cerebro-spinalis gehalten. *Mschr. Ohrenh.,* 1867, 1:9-14.

VON ALDER, ALBERT. See ALDER, ALBERT, VON

VON AUTENRIETH, JOHANN HERRMANN FERDINAND. See AUTENRIETH, JOHANN HERRMANN FERDINAND, VON

VON BAMBERGER, HEINRICH. See BAMBERGER, HEINRICH, VON

VON BAUMGARTEN, PAUL CLEMENS. See BAUMGARTEN, PAUL CLEMENS, VON

VON BECHTEREW, VLADIMIR MIKHAILOVICH. See BEKHTEREV, VLADIMIR MIKHAILOVICH

VON BERGMANN, GUSTAV. See BERMANN, GUSTAV, VON

VON BERNUTH, FRITZ. See BERNUTH, FRITZ, VON

VON BUHL, LUDWIG. See BUHL, LUDWIG, VON

VON ECONOMO, CONSTANTIN. See ECONOMO, CONSTANTIN, VON

VON GIERKE, EDGAR OTTO CONRAD. See GIERKE, EDGAR OTTO CONRAD, VON

VON GRAEFE, ALBRECHT FRIEDRICH WILHELM ERNST. See GRAEFE, ALBRECHT FRIEDRICH WILHELM ERNST, VON

VON HANN, F. See HANN, F., VON

VON HEBRA, FERDINAND. See HEBRA, FERDINAND, VON

VON HEINE, JACOB. See HEINE, JACOB, VON

VON HERRENSCHWAND, FRIEDRICH. See HERRENSCHWAND, FRIEDRICH, VON

VON HIPPEL, EUGEN. See HIPPEL, EUGEN, VON

VON HOCHENEGG, JULIUS. See HOCHENEGG, JULIUS, VON

VON JAKSCH, RUDOLF. See JAKSCH, RUDOLF, RITTER VON WARTENHORST

VON JAKSCH-WARTENHORST, RUDOLF See JAKSCH, RUDOLF, RITTER VON WARTERHORST

VON LEYDEN, ERNST VICTOR. See LEYDEN, ERNST VICTOR, VON

VON LUDWIG, WILHELM FRIEDRICH. See LUDWIG, WILHELM FRIEDRICH, VON

VON MEYENBURG, HANS. See MEYENBURG, HANS, VON

VON MONAKOW, CONSTANTIN. See MONAKOW, CONSTANTIN, VON

VON MUNCHAUSEN. See MUNCHAUSEN, BARON, VON

VON MÜNCHHAUSEN. See MUNCHAUSEN, BARON, VON

VON PASSOW, ARNOLD. See PASSOW, ARNOLD, VON

VON RECKLINGHAUSEN, FRIEDRICH DANIEL. See RECKLINGHAUSEN, FRIEDRICH DANIEL, VON

VON ROKITANSKY, CARL FREIHERR. See ROKITANSKY, CARL FREIHERR, VON

VON ROMBERG, MORITZ HEINRICH. See ROMBERG, MORITZ HEINRICH, VON

VON ROTH, MORITZ. See ROTH, MORITZ, VON

VON ROTHMUND, AUGUST, JR. See ROTHMUND, AUGUST, JR., VON

VON RUSTITZKY. See RUSTITSKII

VON SALLMANN, LUDWIG (American physician, born 1892)

Von Sallmann-Paton syndrome. See *Witkop-Von Sallmann syndrome.*

Witkop-Von Sallmann syndrome. See *under Witkop.*

VON SCHROETTER, KRISTELLI LEOPOLD. See SCHROETTER, KRISTELLI LEOPOLD, VON

VON SCHRÖTTER, KRISTELLI LEOPOLD. See SCHROETTER, KRISTELLI LEOPOLD, VON

VON STERNBERG, CARL. See STERNBERG, CARL, VON

VON STRÜMPELL, ERNST ADOLF GUSTAV GOTTFRIED. See STRÜMPELL, ERNST ADOLF GUSTAV GOTTFRIED, VON

VON VOLKMANN, RICHARD. See VOLKMANN, RICHARD, VON

VON WILLEBRAND, ERIK ADOLF. See WILLEBRAND, ERIK ADOLF, VON

VON WINCKEL, FRANZ KARL LUDWIG WILHELM. See WINCKEL, FRANZ KARL LUDWIG WILHELM, VON

VON WINIWARTER, FELIX. See WINIWARTER, FELIX, VON

VON ZAMBUSCH, LEO. See ZAMBUSCH, LEO, VON

VOORHOEVE, NICOLAAS (Dutch physician, 1879-1927)

Voorhoeve disease. See *Voorhoeve syndrome.*

Voorhoeve dyschondroplasia. See *Voorhoeve syndrome.*

Voorhoeve syndrome. Synonyms: *Voorhoeve disease, Voorhoeve dyschondroplasia, osteopathia striata, osteorhabdotosis.*

A bone dysplasia characterized by striations along the axes of the long bones extending from the metaphyses and fan-like striations of the iliac bones which are visible on the roentgenogram, with areas of rarefaction interspersed between dense striations, and occasional multiple small exostoses. There are minimal clinical symptoms.

Voorhoeve, N. L'image radiologique non encore décrite d'une anomalie du squelette. Ses rapports avec la dyschondroplasie et ostéopathia condensans disseminata. *Acta Radiol., Stockholm*, 1924, 3:407-27.

VÖRNER (VOERNER), HANS (German physician)

Steiner-Voerner syndrome. See *carcinoid syndrome.*

Vörner heloderma. A familial form of heloderma (knuckle pads), considered to be a variant of keratosis palmaris et plantaris, in which there is plaquelike fibrous thickening of the extensor surfaces of the proximal interphalangeal articulations of the fingers and toes. Symmetrical thickening of the epidermal horny layers of the palms and soles is associated.

Vörner, H. Zur Kenntniss des Keratoma hereditarium palmare et plantare. *Arch. Derm. Syph., Berlin*, 1901, 56:3-31.

Vörner nevus. Synonym: *nevus anemicus.*

A rare vascular malformation presenting off-white nevi of varying sizes and shapes which appear paler than the surrounding skin. In most instances, lesions are located on the trunk but some are found on the face and extremities. Their shapes are characteristically blotchy or cribriform; larger lesions are surrounded by satellite spots. Pressure on the nevus under a glass slide makes it inapparent. The condition is reported to have been described by Vörner in 1906.

Piotrowski, F. O. Nevus anemicus (Voerner). *Arch. Derm. Syph., Chicago*, 1944, 50:374-7.

vortex corneal dystrophy. See *Fleischer dystrophy (1).*

VOSSIUS, ADOLF (German ophthalmologist, 1855-1925)

Vossius keratitis. Synonym: *keratitis parenchymatosa annularis.*

Interstitial keratitis marked by a hazy ring around the center of the cornea.

Vossius, A. Zur Begründung der Keratitis parenchymatosa annularis. *Graefes Arch. Ophth.*, 1905, 60:116-7.

VRIES, ANDRE, DE. See DE VRIES, ANDRE

VROLIK, WILLEM (Dutch anatomist, 1801-1863)

Vrolik disease. See *osteogenesis imperfecta syndrome (recessive form).*

Vrolik syndrome. See *osteogenesis imperfecta syndrome (recessive form).*

VS. See *vibration syndrome.*

VSR syndrome. A familial syndrome, transmitted as an autosomal dominant trait, characterized by shortness of stature, craniofacial deformity, vertebral abnormalities, and multiple articular disorders. The symptoms include shortness of stature, mesomelic shortness of the arms, rhizomelic shortness of the lower limbs, a craniofacial dysostosis (trigonocephaly, prominent zygomatic bones, broad maxillary and mandibular bones, cleft palate), costovertebral anomalies (scoliosis, sagittal cleft of the vertebral body, broad ribs), and flexion deformities of the elbow, wrist, finger, and ankle joints. The syndrome was first observed in the VSR family, hence its name.

Herrmann, J., & Opitz, J. M. The VSR syndrome. *Birth Defects*, 1974, 10(9):227-39.

VULPIAN, EDMUND FELIX ALFRED (French physician, 1826-1887)

Vulpian-Bernhardt syndrome. A cervicoscapulohumeral form of progressive muscular atrophy, in which weakness and atrophy in the shoulder girdle with early involvement of the neck muscles are the principal symptoms.

*Vulpian, E. F. A. *Maladies du système nerveux.* Paris, 1879. Bernhardt, M. Weiterer Beitrag zur Lehre von den hereditären und familiären Erkrankungen des Nervensystems. Über die spinal-neurotische Form der progressiven Muskelatrophie. *Virchows Arch. Path. Anat.*, 1893, 133:259.

vulvovaginogingival syndrome. An association of a chronic painful erosive vulvitis, an erosive or desquamative vaginitis, and an erosive vestibular gingivitis.

Pelisse, M., *et al.* Un nouveau syndrome vulvo-vagino-gingival. Lichen plan érosif plurimuqueux. *Ann. Derm. Vener., Paris*, 1902, 109:797-8.

vWD (von Willebrand disease). See *Willebrand-Jürgens syndrome, under Willebrand, Erik Adolf, von.*
VWF (vibration-induced white finger). See *vibration syndrome.*
VWS. See *van der Woude syndrome.*

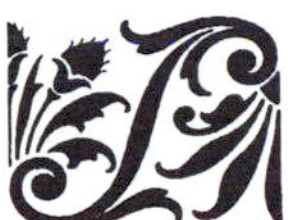

Page #	Term	Observation

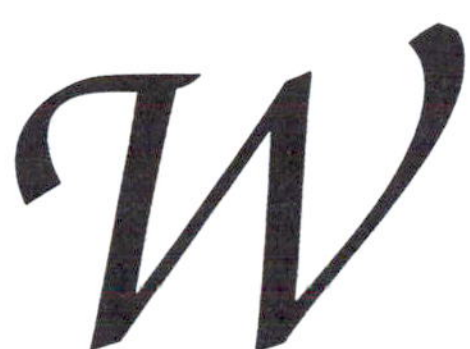

W syndrome. See *Pallister syndrome (I).*

WAARDENBURG, PETRUS JOHANNES (Dutch ophthalmologist, 1886-1979)

Klein-Waardenburg syndrome. See *Waardenburg syndrome (2).*

Shah-Waardenburg syndrome. See *under Shah.*

van der Hoeve-Halbertsma-Waardenburg syndrome. See *Waardenburg syndrome (2).*

Waardenburg anophthalmia syndrome. See *Waardenburg syndrome (3).*

Waardenburg syndrome (1). Synonyms: *acrocephalosyndactyly III (ACS III), acrocephalosyndactyly V (ACS V).*

Acrocephalosyndactyly characterized by the lack of osseous fusion of the short tubular bones, oligodactyly of the feet, and systemic abnormalities, such as short stature, pericardial cysts, rectal prolapse, and deformed ears. Strabismus, hydrophthalmos, elongated nose, contractures of the elbows and knees, and pseudohermaphroditism may occur. It is probably transmitted as an autosomal dominant trait. The syndrome is variously classified as acrocephalosyndactyly III and V.

Waardenburg, P.J. Eine merkwurdige Kombination von angeborenen Missbildungen: doppelseitiger Hydrophthalmus verbunden mit Akrozephalosyndaktylie, Herzfehler, Pseudohermaphroditismus und anderen Abweichungen. *Klin. Mbl. Angenheilk.*, 1934, 92:29-44.

Waardenburg syndrome (2). Synonyms: *Klein syndrome, Klein-Waardenburg syndrome, van der Hoeve-Halbertsma-Waardenburg syndrome, dyschromia iridocutanea et dysplasia auditiva, dystopia canthi medialis lateroversa, ptosis-epicanthus syndrome.*

A hereditary disorder, transmitted as an autosomal dominant trait with complete penetrance and variable expressivity, consisting of lateral displacement of the medial canthi and lacrimal points, hyperplastic broad high nasal root, partial or total heterochromia iridium, hyperplasia of the median portion of the eyebrows, congenital or partial (unilateral) deafness, and circumscribed albinism (white forelock). Vitiligo, pigmentary changes of the fundi, and blue irides in Blacks may also be seen. Oral changes include mandibular prognathism, protruding lower lip, and cleft palate.

Waardenburg, P. J. A new syndrome combining developmental anomalies of the eyelids, eyebrows and nose root with pigmentary defects of the iris and head hair and with congenital deafness. Dystopia canthi medialis et punctorum lacrimalium lateroversa, hyperplasia supercilii medialis et radicis nasi, heterochromia iridum totalis sive partialis, albinismus circumscriptus (surdimutitas). *Am. J. Hum. Genet.*, 1951, 3:195-253. Hoeve, J., van der. Abnorme Länge der Tränenröhrchen mit Ankyloblepharon. *Klin. Mbl. Augenh.*, 1916, 56:232-8. Klein, D. Albinisme partiel (leucisme) avec surdi-mutité, blépharophimosis et dysplasie myo-ostéo-articulaire. *Helvet. Paediat. Acta.*, 1950, 5:38-58.

Waardenburg syndrome (3). Synonyms: *Waardenburg anophthalmia syndrome, anophthalmos-syndactyly syndrome.*

A hereditary syndrome, transmitted as an autosomal recessive trait, characterized by anophthalmia and limb abnormalities, mainly syndactyly.

Waardenburg, P. J. Autosomally-recessive anophthalmia with malformations of the hands and feet. In: Waardenburg, P. J., Franceschetti, A., & Klein, D., eds. *Genetics in ophthalmology.* Assen, Royal Van Gorcum, 1961, v. 1, p. 773.

Waardenburg-Jonkers disease. Progressive corneal dystrophy of young infants, transmitted as a dominant trait and characterized by the appearance after an irritation of minute dots on the parenchyma, resembling snowfakes or hailstones, which tend to occupy the entire surface of the cornea. The dots last a few days and disappear spontaneously without therapy.

Waadenburg, P. J., & Jonkers, G. H. A specific type of dominant progressive dystrophy of the cornea, developing after birth. *Acta Ophth., Copenhagen,* 1961, 39:919,23.

Wildervanck-Waardenburg-Francheschetti-Klein syndrome. See *Wildervanck syndrome (1).*

WACHTEL, S. S.

Gardner-Silengo-Wachtel syndrome. See *under Gardner, L. I.*

wacinko syndrome. A psychological disorder, reported in the Oglala Sioux Indians, characterized by variable symptoms, including excessive anger, pouting, withdrawal, depression, psychomotor retardation, mutism, immobililty, and suicidal tendencies. The disorder is classified as a reactive depressive illness.

Lewis, T. H. A syndrome of depression and mutism in the Oglala Sioux. *Am. J. Psychiat.,* 1975, 132:753-5.

WACKENHEIM, A. (French radiologist)

Wackenheim syndrome. See *cheirolumbar dysostosis.*

WADIA, N. H. (Indian physician)

Wadia-Swami syndrome. Synonym: *cerebellar degeneration-slow eye movement syndrome.*

A familial syndrome, transmitted as an autosomal dominant trait, characterized by spinocerebellar degeneration and slow eye movement, specifically ab-

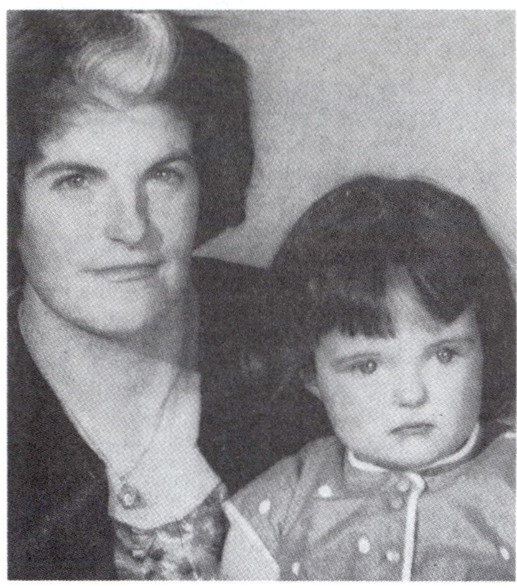

Waardenburg syndrome
Partington, M.W., *Arch. Dis. Child.*, 1959, 34:154. British Medical Association, London, England.

sence of rapid saccades (scanning) and abnormally slow tracking. Mental retardation was present in some patients in the original report.

Wadia, N. H., & Swami, R. K. A new form of heredofamilial spinocerebellar degeneration with slow eye movements (nine families). *Brain*, 1971, 94:359-74.

WAELSCH, LUDWIG (Czech physician, 1867-1924)

Waelsch urethritis. See *Reiter syndrome.*

WAGENER, HENRY PATRICK (American physician, born 1890)

Wagener retinitis. See *Wagener syndrome.*

Wagener syndrome. Synonyms: *Wagener retinitis, Wagener-Keith syndrome.*

An association of severe neuroretinitis, hypertension, moderate arteriosclerosis, and cardiac hypertrophy, in the absence of renal dysfunction. The symptoms may include severe headache, hemiplegia or monoplegia, convulsions, ocular disorders that range from blurring of vision to complete blindness, loss of weight, weakness, cardiac edema, dyspnea, and slight to moderate nocturia. In the original report, the ages of the patients varied from 24 to 49 years.

Wagener, H. P., & Keith, N. M. Cases of marked hypertension, adequate renal function and neuroretinitis. *Arch. Int. Med., Chicago*, 1924, 34:374-87.

Wagener-Keith syndrome. See *Wagener syndrome.*

WAGNER, ERNST LEBERECHT (German physician, 1829-1888)

Wagner polymyositis. See *Wagner-Unverricht syndrome.*

Wagner syndrome. See *Wagner-Unverricht syndrome.*

Wagner-Unverricht syndrome. Synonyms: *Wagner polymyositis, Wagner syndrome, acute parynchymatous myositis, dermatomyositis, dermatomyositis syndrome, myositis universalis acuta infectiosa, polymyositis gregarina, pseudotrichinosis.*

An acute or chronic inflammatory disease of the skin and skeletal muscles of unknown etiology. It is sometimes identified with adult polymyositis, dermatomyositis, myositis with malignancy, childhood myositis, or myositis associated with other connective tissue diseases, such as the overlap syndrome. Pathological findings include lymphocytic infiltration with muscle fiber damage and degeneration. Muscle tissue infiltrates consist of lymphocytes, mononuclear leukocytes, plasma cells, and rare neutrophilic leukocytes. Perivascular and/or interstitial inflammatory cell infiltration is the main feature of polymyositis. Edema and erythema with perivascular lymphocytic and plasma cell infiltrates are the usual pathological skin changes. The symptoms include fever, malaise, edema, tenderness, and weakness of the extremities and about the shoulder girdle, eventually spreading to the intercostal muscles, diaphragm, and muscles of the larynx and pharynx, leading to dysphagia and respiratory failure. Skin lesions are more pronounced in acute cases and include pigmentation and depigmentation, thinning of the epidermis, erythema, desquamation and rash. The face, especially the eyelids, ears, and anterior neck, are most commonly affected. Oral lesions usually consist of stomatitis, pharyngitis, and masticatory muscle disorders.

Wagner, E. Fall einer seltenen Muskelkrankheit. *Arch. Heilk.*, 1863, 4:282-3. Unverricht, H. Über eine eigentümliche Form von akuter Muskelentzündung mit einem der Trichinose ähnelnden Krankheitsbilde. *Münch. Med. Wschr.*, 1887, 34:488-92. Messner, R. P. Dermatomyositis and polymyositis. In: Wyngaarden, J. B., & Smith, L. H., Jr., eds. *Cecil textbook of medicine.* 17th ed. Philadelphia, Saunders, 1985, pp. 1947-50.

WAGNER, H. (Swiss ophthalmologist)

Wagner syndrome. Synonyms: *degeneratio hyaloideoretinalis hereditaria, hereditary hyaloretinal degeneration, hereditary vitreoretinal degeneration.*

A familial eye disease, transmited as an autosomal dominant trait, characterized by changes in the peripheral fundus with narrowed and ensheathed retinal vessels, retinal pigmentation, circular membranes in a liquefied vitreous attached to the equatorial retina, and choroidal atrophy. Retinoschisis, lattice degeneration, and retinal breaks and detachment may be associated.

Wagner, H. Ein bisher unbekanntes Erbleiden des Auges (Degeneratio hyaloideo-retinalis hereditaria), beobachtet im Kanton Zürich. *Klin. Mbl. Augenh.*, 1938, 100:840-57.

WAGNER, SEYMOUR (American physician)

Winter-Kohn-Mellman-Wagner syndrome. See *Winter syndrome.*

WAISMAN

Waisman-Laxová syndrome. A syndrome of X-linked mental retardation and cephalomegaly. The affected males are variably retarded and have frontal bossing and increased head circumference in relation to facial bones. Associated abnormalities may include cogwheel rigidity, Parkinson-like tremors, strabismus, persistent frontal lobe reflexes, seizures, basal ganglion dysfunction, muscle hypotonia, and abnormal gait.

Laxová, R., *et al.* An X-linked recessive basal ganglia disorder with mental retardation. *Am. J. Med. Genet.*, 1985, 21:681-9. Opitz, Reynolds, J. F., Spano, L. M., eds. X-linked mental retardation 2. *Am. J. Med. Genet.*, 1986, 23:16.

waking arm numbness. See *Wartenberg disease (1).*

WALDENSTRÖM, HENNING (Swedish physician, born 1877)

Perthes-Calvé-Legg-Waldenström syndrome. See *Calvé-Legg-Perthes syndrome.*

Waldenström syndrome. See *Calvé-Legg-Perthes syndrome.*

WALDENSTRÖM, JAN (Swedish physician)

Waldenström-Kjellberg syndrome. See *Plummer-Vinson syndrome.*

WALDENSTRÖM, JAN GÖSTA (Swedish physician, born 1906)

Waldenström disease. Synonyms: *acute thyrotoxic encephalopathy, spontaneous thyrotoxic crisis, thyroid storm.*

An acute form of thyrotoxicosis with muscular and cerebral complications, usually observed in elderly patients, and suspected of being due to iodine deficiency. The symptoms are varied and may include exophthalmos, goiter, and thyrotoxic crisis; severe vomiting, diarrhea, and weight loss; increased basal metabolism; slight initial fever in most instances and severe terminal hyperpyrexia in fatal cases; dyspnea; atrial fibrillation and low diastolic pressure; bulbar paralysis and paralysis of the sixth, seventh, and twelfth cranial nerves with resultant deglutition disorders; psychotic behavior and hallucinations; lethargy and general asthenia or agitation and insomnia; coma; profuse perspiration; and frequent apraxia, acalculia, dysarthria, choreiform movements, and amimia.

Waldenström, J. Acute thyrotoxic encephalo- or myopathy, its causes and treatment. *Acta Med. Scand.*, 1945, 121:251-94.

Waldenström hepatitis. Synonyms: *active juvenile cirrhosis, cirrhosis of young women, lupoid hepatitis, plasma-cell hepatitis.*

A chronic liver disease characterized by moderate jaundice, intermittent bilirubinemia, ascites, and amenorrhea. In most cases, there are spider nevi and acne. Biochemical changes include high gamma-globulin and transaminase levels. Histological findings in the liver consist of plasma cell and lymphocytic infiltrations, fibrosis with isolation of cells into small groups, and postnecrotic cirrhosis. L.E. cells are found in some cases. Ulcerative colitis, skin rash, glomerulonephritis, pulmonary infiltrations, diabetes mellitus, and Hashimoto disease frequently occur. This disease and the Bearn-Kunkel syndrome are considered by some writers the same entity.

Sherlock, S. Waldenström's chronic active hepatitis. *Acta Med. Scand.*, 1966, Suppl. 445:426-33.

Waldenström macroglobulinemia. Synonyms: *Waldenström syndrome, macroglobulinemia syndrome, primary macroglobulinemia.*

A progressive immunoproliferative disease with production of large amounts of a monoclonal macroglobulin (IgM), occurring either in a malignant form, which leads to an early death, or in a relatively benign one. Hemorrhagic diathesis is the principal symptom of the disorder, with bleeding from the nose, eyes, and mouth, and, sometimes, the vagina and gastrointestinal tract. Early symptoms include fatigue, loss of weight, anemia, and general malaise. The eyes show retinal and choroidal hemorrhage, clumping of erythrocytes in the conjunctival vessels, and visual disorders. Associated disorders may include swelling of the lymph nodes, hepatosplenomegaly, aphasia, hemiparesis, edema, the Raynaud phenomenon, respiratory tract infections, and osteoporosis. Oral manifestations consist of spontaneous gingival bleeding and continuing oozing of the blood from the mouth. Salivary gland involvement with xerostomia may occur. Prolonged bleeding after tooth extraction is common. Hematological changes include increased erythrocyte sedimentation rate, auto-hemagglutination, rouleau formation, coagulation disorders, peripheral vascular occlusion, and serum hyperviscosity. Sharp peaks in the β and γ-region are found on paper electrophoresis. Ultracentrifugation shows high molecular weight proteins of 15S or more in concentrations greater than 5%. The syndrome occurs twice as often in males as females, seldom before the fifth decade. In some instances, there is a supernumerary marker chromosome originally designated as "W chromosome."

Waldenström, J. Incipient myelomatosis or "essential" hyperglobulinemia with fibrinogenopenia-a new syndrome? *Acta Med. Scand.*, 1944, 117:216-47.

Waldenström syndrome (1). See *Waldenström macroglobulinemia.*

Waldenström syndrome (2). Synonyms: *hyperglobulinemic purpura, hyperglobulinemic purpura syndrome, idiopathic hyperglobulinemia, purpura hyperglobulinemica.*

A chronic blood disease, occurring almost exclusively in women, characterized by high content of γ-globulin, increased 7S G-component, normal levels of blood albumins, and elevated erythrocyte sedimentation rate. The symptoms consist of recurrent episodes of purpura of the lower limbs (precipitated by exertion, irritation by garments, or infection, leaving areas of brown pigmentation), xerophthalmia, and xerostomia. Moderate hepatosplenomegaly may also occur. It is an autoimmune disease that may occur as a primary or secondary condition in conjunction with collagen diseases, granulomatous disorders, hepatopathies, and monoclonal gammopathies. This and the Bearn-Kunkel syndromes are similar in many respects.

Waldenström, J. Zwei interesante Syndrome mit Hyperglobulinämie. (Purpura hyperglobulinaemica und Makroglobulinämie). *Schweiz. Med. Wschr.*, 1948, 78:927-8.

Waldenström syndrome (3). See *acute intermittent porphyria.*

Waldenström uveoparotitis. A disorder related to the Heerfordt syndrome and characterized by bilateral iritis and parotitis. The symptoms vary and may include fever, lethargy, hallucinations, positive Babinski and Oppenheim reflexes, impaired deep sensitivity in the toes, abolished patellar and Achilles reflexes, facial paralysis, increased levels of cerebrospinal albumin, and pleocytosis. In the original report, tuberculosis was the cause.

Waldenström, J. Some observations on uveoparotitis and allied conditions with special reference to the symptoms from the nervous system. *Acta Med. Scand.*, 1937, 91:53-68.

WALKER, ARTHUR EARL (American physician, born 1907)

Dandy-Walker anomaly. See *Dandy-Walker syndrome.*

Dandy-Walker cyst. See *Dandy-Walker syndrome.*

Dandy-Walker syndrome (DWS). See *under Dandy.*

Dandy-Walker-like syndrome. See *under Dandy.*

Walker lissencephaly. See *Walker-Warburg syndrome.*

Walker-Warburg syndrome (WWS). Synonyms: *Walker lissencephaly, Warburg syndrome, cerebro-ocular dysgenesis, HARD ± E syndrome.*

A lethal autosomal recessive disorder of the brain

marked by hydrocephalus, ventriculomegaly, ocular abnormalities, and occcasional occipital encephalocele. Hydrocephalus in the fetus may cause labor complications. Eye abnormalities include microphthalmia and/or anterior and posterior chamber abnormalities, including corneal opacity, cataract, persistent primary vitreous, and retinal dysplasia. Small penis, cryptorchism, hydronephrosis, pelviureteric junction obstruction, anoperineal fistula, and talipes are often associated. Most affected patients die within 1 year.

Walker, A. E. Lissencephaly. *Arch. Neur. Psychiat.*, 1942, 48:13- 29. Warburg, M. The heterogeneity of microphthalmia in the mentally retarded. *Birth Defects*, 1971, 7(3):136-54. Pogon, R. A., *et al.* Hydrocephalus, agyria, retinal dysplasia, encephalocele (HARD ± E) syndrome: An autosomal recessive disorder. *Birth Defects*, 1978, 14(6B):233-41.

WALKER, JOHN C. (American physician)

Walker-Clodius syndrome. See *EEC syndrome.*

WALKER, W. ALLAN (American physician)

Marden-Walker syndrome (MWS). See *under Marden.*

WALLENBERG, ADOLF (German physician, 1862-1949)

Wallenberg syndrome. Synonyms: *dorsolateral medullary syndrome, lateral bulbar syndrome, lateral medullary syndrome, lateral medullary infarction syndrome, posterior inferior cerebellar artery syndrome.*

A disease of the brain stem, usually occurring during the fifth decade, in which thrombosis of the posterior inferior cerebellar artery causes ipsilateral loss of the pain and temperature senses of the face, soft palate, pharynx, and larynx; contralateral pain and temperature hypoesthesia of the extremities and trunk; ipsilateral ataxia; muscle hypotonia; ipsilateral Horner syndrome; nystagmus; vertigo; nausea; difficulty in swallowing and speaking; and ocular disorders, including miosis, enophthalmos, blepharoptosis, and diplopia.

Wallenberg, A. Acute Bulbäraffection (Embolie der Art. cerebellar. post. inf. sinistr.?). *Arch. Psychiat., Berlin*, 1895, 27:504-40.

WALLER, AUGUSTUS VOLNEY (British physician, 1816-1870)

wallerian degeneration. Synonym: *secondary degeneration.*

Degeneration of myelin distal to the most proximal site of axonal inerruption by disease or injury.

Waller, A. V. Experiments on the section of the glossopharyngeal and hypoglossal nerves of the frog and observations of the alterations produced thereby in the structure of their primitive fibers. *Philos. Trans.*, 1850, p. 423-9.

WALLGREN, ARVID JOHAN (Swedish physician, born 1889)

Wallgren disease. Synonym: *pylephlebostenosis splenica.*

Obstruction of the splenic vein resulting in venous stasis of the spleen, followed by splenomegaly and the development of collateral circulation. It is generally observed in children.

Wallgren, A. Contribution à l'étude des splénomégalies de l'enfance. (Pyléphlébo-sténose splénique). *Acta Paediat., Uppsala*, 1926-27, 6(Suppl):1-122.

WALSHE, J. J. (American physician)

Magoss-Walshe syndrome. See *under Magoss.*

WALSHE, J. M.

Summerskill-Walshe syndrome. See *under Summerskill.*

WALT DISNEY. See DISNEY, WALTER ELIAS

WALTER

Walter-Bohmann syndrome. See *postcholecystectomy syndrome.*

WALTERS, T. R. (American physician)

Walters syndrome. Megaloblastic anemia in congenital dihydrofolate reductase deficiency. Mental retardation and sociopathic behavior were associated in the original case. The condition is hereditary and is believed to be transmitted as an autosomal recessive trait.

Walters, T. R. Congenital megaloblastic anemia responsive to N5-formyltetrahydrofolic acid administration. *J. Pediat.*, 1967, 70:686-7. Rowe, P. B. Inherited disorders of folate metabolism. In: Stanbury, J. B., Wyngaarden, J. B., & Frederickson, D. S., eds. *The metabolic basis of inherited disease.* 4th ed. New York, McGraw-Hill, 1978, pp. 431-57.

WALTON, DAVID S. (American physician)

Mirhosseini-Holmes-Walton syndrome. See *under Mirhosseini.*

wandering edema. See *Quincke edema.*

WANDERING JEW. See AHASUERUS

war melanosis. See *Riehl melanosis.*

war neurosis. See *post-traumatic stress syndrome.*

war sailor syndrome. A form of the post-traumatic stress syndrome (q.v.), observed among crew members of merchant ships in World War II, brought about mainly by fear of death and isolation from families, especially among sailors from occupied countries. The symptoms include fatigability, irritability, lack of initiative, emotional instability, dizziness, sweating attacks, gastrointestinal disorders, impotence, pain, nightmares, restlessness, sleep disorders, tendency to withdraw, impaired memory, and concentration difficulty.

Askelvold, F. The war sailor syndrome. *Dan. Med. Bull.*, 1980, 27:220-4.

WARBURG, METTE (Danish ophthalmologist)

Norrie-Warburg syndrome. See *Norrie syndrome.*

Walker-Warburg syndrome (WWS). See *under Walker, Arthur Earl.*

Warburg syndrome. See *Walker-Warburg syndrome.*

WARD, O. C. (Irish physician)

Romano-Ward syndrome. See *under long QT syndrome.*

WARD, W. H. (Australian physician)

Ward syndrome. A syndrome of multiple nevoid basal cell carcinomata associated with dyskeratosis palmaris et plantaris. The carcinomata, which may appear on any part of the body at about the age of puberty, vary in size from less than 1 mm to large tumors of several centimers in diameter. The lesions are painless and cause no trouble until ulceration begins at the onset of the neoplastic phase. Palmar and plantar lesions most commonly appear as if the skin had been pricked with a pin and a complete portion of the epidermis lifted up, leaving punctures about 1 mm in depth, which may be filled with debris. Less frequently, they occur as pinhead-sized macules, suggesting the central point of nevus araneus without the spider leg extensions, and areas of various shapes and sizes that are the color of smoked ham. According to later definitions, the Ward syndrome includes nevoid basal cell carcinoma and dental cysts of the jaw. Bifid ribs and incomplete fusion of the vertebral arches have been associated.

Ward, W. H. Naevoid basal celled carcinoma associated with dyskeratosis of the palms and soles. A new entity. *Austral. J. Derm.*, 1959, 5:204-8. Tobias, C. Zum Basalzellnaevus-Kiefercysten-Syndrom (Ward-Syndrom) mit familiärem Auftreten. *Schweiz. Med. Wschr.*, 1967, 97:949-53.

WARDROP, JAMES (British physician, 1782-1869)

Wardrop disease. Synonym: *onychia maligna.*

Onychia with fetid ulceration and loss of the nail.

Wardrop, J. An account on some diseases of the toes and fingers, with observations on their treatment. *Med. Chir. Tr., London,* 1814, 5:129-43.

warfarin embryopathy. See *fetal warfarin syndrome.*

warfarin syndrome. See *fetal warfarin syndrome.*

WARKANY, JOSEF (Amrican physician)

Warkany syndrome (WS). See *chromosome 8 trisomy syndrome.*

WARTENBERG, ROBERT (American physician, 1887-1956)

Wartenberg disease (1). Synonyms: *Putnam acroparesthesia, Putnam syndrome, Schultze acroparesthesia, Schultze syndrome, brachial paresthesia during sleep, brachialgia paresthetica nocturna, brachialgia statica paresthetica, idiopathic acroparesthesia, neuralgia paresthetica, nocturnal arm dysesthesia, nocturnal arm paresthesia, sleep tetany, tired arm, waking arm numbness.*

A vasomotor disorder characterized by tingling, numbness, stiffness (acroparesthesia), and anesthesia or pain in the upper extremity, observed during sleep while the patient is in the recumbent position. Pressure on the brachial plexus and abnormal relaxation of the muscles are the probable causes. It occurs most commonly in debilitated middle-aged women. See also *sleep shoulder syndrome.*

Wartenberg, R. Brachialgia statica paresthetica (nocturnal arm dysesthesias). *J. Nerv. Ment. Dis.*, 1944, 99:877-87. Schultze, F. Über Akroparästhesie. *Deut. Zschr. Nervenh.*, 1893, 3:300-18. Putnam, J. J. A series of cases of paresthesia, mainly of the hands, of periodical recurrence, and possibly of vaso-motor origin. *Arch. Med., N. Y.*, 1880, 4:147-62.

Wartenberg disease (2). Synonyms: *cheiralgia paresthetica, chiralgia paresthetica, neuritis migrans.*

A neuropathy involving the superficial branch of the radial nerve, manifested by paresthesia, dysesthesia, or hyperesthesia of the ulnar surface of the thumb, occasionally associated with cutaneous discoloration in the area of sensory impairment.

Sprofkin, B. E. Cheiralgia paresthetica-Wartenberg's disease. *Neurology,* 1954, 4:857-62.

WARTHIN, ALFRED SCOTT (American physician, 1866-1931)

Albrecht-Arzt-Warthin tumor. See *Warthin tumor.*

Warthin tumor. Synonyms: *Albrecht-Arzt-Warthin tumor, adenolymphoma, cystic papillary adenoma, oncocytoma, orbital inclusion adenoma, orbital inclusion cyst, papillary cystadenolymphoma, papillary cystadenoma, papillary cystadenoma lymphomatosum.*

A benign salivary gland tumor found almost exclusively in the parotid glands, which occurs bilaterally, and is more common in men than in women. Typically, it is an encapsulated, smooth, round lesion with multiple communicating cysts. It has two components, lymphoid and epithelial, with two layers of cells; the surface row consists of tall columnar cells, and the deep row contains cuboidal, rounded, or polygonal cells.

*Warthin, A. S. Papillary cystadenoma lymphomatosum. A rare teratoid of the parotid region. *J. Cancer Res.*, 1929, 13:116-25.

WAS. See *Wiskott-Aldrich syndrome.*

washboard scalp. See *pachydermoperiostosis syndrome.*

WASSERMANN, AUGUST PAUL, VON (German bacteriologist, 1866-1925)

Wassermann-positive pneumonia. See *Fanconi-Hegglin syndrome.*

Wassermann-positive pulmonary infiltration. See *Fanconi-Hegglin syndrome.*

wasted leg syndrome. Synonym: *compression neuropathy of the lower limb.*

Nonprogressive unilateral atrophy of leg muscles without spinal compression due to compression neuropathy of the sciatic nerve. In the original report, the condition was attributed to prolonged squatting.

*Singh, A., & Jolly, S. S. Wasted leg syndrome: A compressive neuropathy of the lower limb. *J. Assoc. Phys. India*, 1963, 11:1031.

wasting palsy. See *Aran-Duchenne syndrome.*

water-skier colon. Synonyms: *Canadair syndrome, water-skier enema.*

Injuries to the buttocks and abdomen caused by the entry of water into the rectum, occurring in high-speed water-skiing. An observation that the entry of water into the rectum when water-skiing is in some ways similar to the way water is sprayed when fire-fighting with airplane Canadair resulted in naming this condition the "Canadair syndrome".

Kaiser, R. E., Jr., *et al.* Waterskier's enema. *N. Engl. J. Med.*, 1980, 302:1264. Cocheton, J. J.,& Roland, J. Colite aiguë du skier nautique ou le syndrome du Canadair. *Presse Méd.*, 1986, 15:487-8.

water-skier enema. See *water-skier colon.*

WATERHOUSE, RUPERT (British physician, 1873-1958)

Friderichsen-Waterhouse-Bamatter syndrome. See *Waterhouse-Friderichsen syndrome.*

Marchand-Waterhouse-Friderichsen syndrome. See *Waterhouse-Friderichsen syndrome.*

Waterhouse-Friderichsen syndrome. Synonyms: *Friderichsen-Waterhouse-Bamatter syndrome, Marchand-Waterhouse-Friderichsen syndrome, adrenal apoplexy, adrenal hemorrhage syndromes, fulminating meningococcemia, fulminating purpuric meningococcemia, meningococcic adrenal syndrome, sepsis acutissima hyperergica fulminans, suprarenal apoplexy.*

A rapidly fulminating meningococcal septicemia associated with massive purpura, bilateral adrenal hemorrhage, vasomotor collapse, and shock. The symptoms appear suddenly with purpura, dyspnea, and prostration. The initial purpuric lesions and petechiae enlarge rapidly and are accompanied by hemorrhage into the skin. In the preshock stage, patients are alert but pale with coldness and cyanosis of the extremities due to generalized vasoconstriction. Decreased cardiac output, hypotension, and coma are the main features of the shock phase. Collapse and death may follow. Patients who recover may suffer from extensive sloughing of the skin and loss of digits due to gangrene.

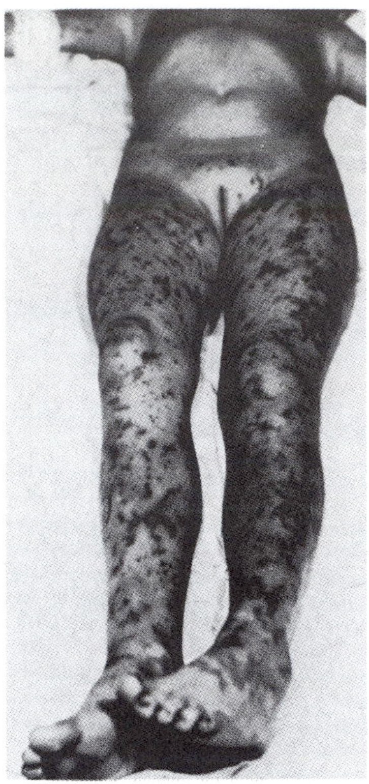

Waterhouse-Friderichsen syndrome
Williams, R.H. (ed.): *Textbook of Endocrinology.* 4th ed. Philadelphia: W.B. Saunders Co., 1968.

Waterhouse, R. A case of suprarenal apoplexy. *Lancet,* 1911, 1:577-8. *Friderichsen, C. Nebennierenapoplexie bei kleinen Kinderh. *Jahrb. Kinderh.,* 1918, 87:109-25. Marchand, F. Über eine eigentümliche Erkrankung des Sympathicus, der Nebennieren, der peripheren Nerven (ohne Broncehaut). *Virchows Arch. Path.,* 1880, 81:477-502.

WATERS, W. REID (Canadian physician)

Elsahy-Waters syndrome. See *under Elsahy.*

watery diarrhea syndrome (WDS). See *Verner-Morrison syndrome.*

watery diarrhea-hypokalemia-achlorhydria syndrome (WDHA). See *Verner-Morrison syndrome.*

WATSON, GEOFFREY H. (British physician)

Watson syndrome. A familial syndrome of café-au-lait spots, pulmonary stenosis, and mental retardation. The syndrome is transmitted as an autosomal dominant trait. Some authors suspect that this and the LEOPARD syndrome are essentially indistinguishable from the Noonan syndrome.

Watson, G. H. Pulmonary stenosis, café-au-lait spots, and dull intelligence. *Arch. Dis. Child.,* 1967, 42:303-7.

Watson-Miller syndrome. See *Alagille syndrome.*

WAUGH, GEORGE ERNEST (British physician)

Waugh syndrome. An intestinal malrotation syndrome with intussusception in infants suffering from primitive fixation of the mesentery.

Waugh, G. E. The morbid consequences of a mobile ascending colon, with a record of operation. *Brit. J. Surg.,*/ 1919-20, 7:343-83.

wax finger disease. See *vibration syndrome.*

waxy disease. See *amyloidosis.*

WBS (Wiedemann-Beckwith syndrome). See *Beckwith-Wiedemann syndrome.*

WCD (Weber-Christian disease). See *Weber-Christian syndrome, under Weber, Frederick Parkes.*

WCS. See *white clot syndrome.*

WDHA (watery diarrhea-hypokalemia-achlorhydria) syndrome. See *Verner-Morrison syndrome.*

WDS (watery diarrhea syndrome). See *Verner-Morrison syndrome.*

weather migraine. See *under headache syndrome.*

WEAVER, DAVID D. (American physician)

accelerated skeletal maturation, Weaver type. See *Weaver-Smith syndrome.*

Weaver syndrome. See *Weaver-Smith syndrome.*

Weaver-like syndrome. A syndrome characterized by symptoms similar to those in the Weaver-Smith syndrome. Its principal features consist of a peculiar facies (hypertelorism, long philtrum, micrognathia, and broad forehead), camptodactyly, limited movement of the elbow and knee, and hirsutism. Accelerated bone maturation and wide distal femora occur in some cases. A possibility of an autosomal dominant or X-linked inheritance is suspected.

Stoll, C., *et al.* A Weaver-like syndrome with endocrinological abnormalities in a boy and his mother. *Clin. Genet.,* 1985, 28:255-9.

Weaver-Smith syndrome. Synonyms: *Weaver syndrome; accelerated skeletal maturation, Weaver type.*

A syndrome of accelerated growth and skeletal maturation, associated with limb, craniofacial, neurological, and other abnormalities. Craniofacial anomalies consist of a broad forehead, flat occiput, large ears, hypertelorism, long philtrum, and relative micrognathia. Limb abnormalities include prominent fingerpads, camptodactyly, broad thumbs, thin and deep-set nails, clinodactyly, limited elbow and knee extension, wide distal long bones, and foot deformities (clubfoot, pes calcaneovalgus, and metatarsus adductus). Hypertonia, hypotonia, psychomotor retardation, and hoarse, low-pitched voice, excess loose skin, umbilical and inguinal hernias, and inverted nipples are associated. The etiology is unknown.

Weaver, D. D., Graham, B., Thomas, I. T., & Smith, D. W. A new overgrowth syndrome with accelerated skeletal maturation, unusual facies, and camptodactyly. *J. Pediat.,* 1974, 84:547-52.

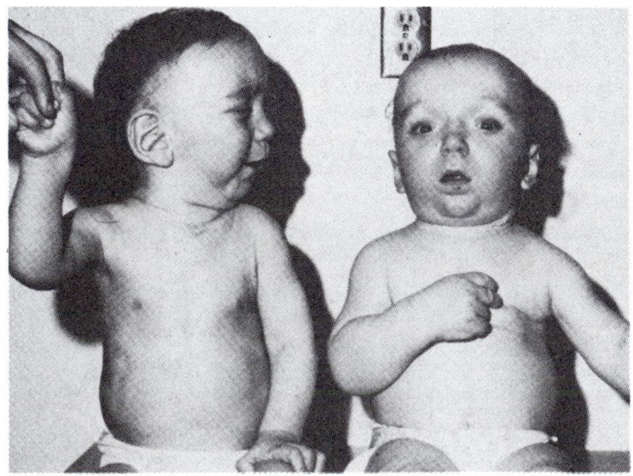

Weaver-Smith syndrome
Weaver, D.D., et al.: *J. Pediatr.* 84:547, 1974. St. Louis: C.V. Mosby Co.

WEBER, FREDERICK PARKES (British physician, 1863-1962)

hemangiectatic hypertrophy of Parkes Weber. See *Klippel-Trénaunay-Weber syndrome.*

Hutchinson-Weber-Peutz syndrome. See *Peutz-Jeghers syndrome.*

Klippel-Trénaunay-Parkes Weber syndrome. See *Klippel-Trénaunay-Weber syndrome.*

Klippel-Trénaunay-Weber (KTW) syndrome. See *under Klippel.*

Ollier-Klippel-Trénaunay-Weber syndrome. See *Klippel-Trénaunay-Weber syndrome.*

Osler-Rendu-Weber syndrome. See *under Osler.*

Parkes Weber syndrome (1). See *Klippel-Trénaunay-Weber syndrome.*

Parkes Weber syndrome (2). See *Sturge-Weber syndrome.*

Parkes Weber-Dimitri syndrome. See *Sturge-Weber syndrome.*

Pfeifer-Weber-Christian disease. See *Weber-Christian syndrome.*

Sturge-Weber anomalad. See *Sturge-Weber syndrome.*

Sturge-Weber syndrome (SWS). See *under Sturge.*

Sturge-Weber-Dimitri syndrome. See *Sturge-Weber syndrome.*

Sturge-Weber-Krabbe syndrome. See *Sturge-Weber syndrome.*

Sturge-Weber-Thoma syndrome. See *Sturge-Weber syndrome.*

Weber syndrome (1). See *Klippel-Trénaunay-Weber syndrome.*

Weber syndrome (2). See *Sturge-Weber syndrome.*

Weber-Christian disease (WCD). See *Weber-Christian syndrome.*

Weber-Christian syndrome. Synonyms: *Pfeifer-Weber-Christian disease, Weber-Christian disease (WCD), panniculitis nodularis febrilis, recurrent febrile nodular panniculitis, relapsing nodular panniculitis, relapsing nonsuppurative nodular panniculitis, spondylopanniculitis.*

A skin disease characterized by recurrent subcutaneous nodules and plaques, resulting in atrophy of the subcutaneous fatty layer of the skin. The trunk and extremities, particularly the thighs and legs, are most frequently affected. The nodules often coalesce to form large lesions, sometimes reaching 10 cm in diameter. The skin over the affected areas is usually normal, but, as the lesions involute, depressions may develop. Liquefying panniculitis is an occasional complication, and malaise, mild fever, tenderness, and redness of the skin followed by pigmentation, hepatomegaly, splenomegaly, and pulmonary, cardiac, and gastrointestinal complications may be present. Radiological findings may show calcification of the nodules, pericardial fibrosis, coronary occlusion, granulomatous pneumonia, enteritis and mesenteritis sometimes complicated by ileus, retroperitoneal fibrosis, liver cirrhosis, and myocardial decompensation. Middle-aged females are most frequently affected.

Pfeifer, V. Über einen Fall von herdweiser Atrophie des subkutanen Fettgewebes. *Deut. Arch. Klin. Med.,* 1892, 50:438-49. Weber, F. P. A case of relapsing non-suppurative nodular panniculitis, showing phagocytosis of subcutaneous fat-cells by macrophages. *Brit. J. Derm. Syph.,* 1925, 37:301-11. Christian, H. A. Relapsing febrile nodular nonsuppurative panniculitis. *Arch. Int. Med.,* 1928, 42:338-51.

Weber-Cockayne syndrome. See *epidermolysis bullosa syndrome.*

Weber-Dimitri syndrome. See *Sturge-Weber syndrome.*

WEBER, G. (German physician)

Hörlein-Weber disease. See *under Hörlein.*

WEBER, HELGA (German physician)

mental retardation, Mietens-Weber type. See *Mietens-Weber syndrome.*

Mietens-Weber syndrome. See *under Mietens.*

WEBER, SIR HERMAN DAVID (British physician, 1823-1918)

Weber paralysis. See *Leyden paralysis (1).*

Weber symptom. See *Leyden paralysis (1).*

Weber-Leyden syndrome. See *Leyden paralysis (1).*

WEDDELL, ALEXANDER GRAHAM MCDONNELL (British physiologist, born 1908)

Falconer-Weddell syndrome. See *costoclavicular compression syndrome.*

WEECH, ALEXANDER ASHLEY (American physician, born 1895)

Christ-Siemens-Weech syndrome. See *hypohidrotic ectodermal dysplasia syndrome.*

Weech syndrome. See *hypohidrotic ectodermal dysplasia syndrome.*

Witkop-Weech-Giansanti syndrome. See *tooth-nail syndrome.*

WEGENER, FRIEDRICH (German pathlogist, born 1907)

Wegener disease. See *Wegener granulomatosis.*

Wegener granulomatosis. Synonyms: *Klinger syndrome, Wegener disease, Wegener syndrome, Wegener-Churg-Klinger syndrome, classical granulomatosis, granuloma-arteritis-glomerulonephritis syndrome, malignant granulomatous angiitis, necrotizing granulomatosis, necrotizing respiratory granulomatosis, rhinogenic polyarteritis.*

A fatal disease in which the principal features consist of acute necrotizing giant cell granuloma of the upper respiratory tract, involving the nose, mouth, paranasal sinuses, larynx, or trachea, followed by necrotizing lesions of the lungs, acute necrotizing vasculitis of the pulmonary and systemic blood vessels, and glomerulonephritis resulting in renal failure and death, often within a month from the onset. The symptoms usually include malaise, weight loss, fever, night sweating, rhinorrhea, dysosmia, ozena, crusting of the nasal passages, dyspnea, hemoptysis, conjunctivitis, purpura, telangiectasia, albuminuria, hematuria, uremia, urinary casts, anemia, leukocytosis, and eosinophilia. The syndrome, thought to be a variant of periarteritis nodosa, is often mistaken for lethal midline granuloma. See also *Stewart syndrome,* under *Stewart, J. P.*

Wegener, F. Über eine eigenartige rhinogene Granulomatose mit besonderer Beteiligung des Arteriensystems und der Nieren. *Beitr. Path. Anat.,* 1939, 102:36-68. Klinger, H. Grenzformen der Periarteriitis nodosa. *Frankf. Zschr. Pathol.,* 1931, 42:455-80. Churg, J., & Strauss, L. Allergic granulomatosis, allergic angiitis, and periarteriitis nodosa. *Am. J. Path.,* 1951, 27:277-94.

Wegener syndrome. See *Wegener granulomatosis.*

Wegener-Churg-Klinger syndrome. See *Wegener granulomatosis.*

WEGIENKA, LAURENCE C. (American physician)

Coffin-Siris-Wegienka syndrome. See *Coffin-Lowry syndrome.*

WEGIERKO, JAKUB (Polish physician)

Wegierko coma. Synonym: *third diabetic coma.*

Diabetic coma without ketonemic acidosis or hypoglycemia. The symptoms include depression, hallucinations, restlessness, insomnia, aversion to food, and vomiting. In the original report, all cases were fatal. Wegierko suspects lesions in the vicinity of the hypothalamus to be the cause.

Wegierko, J. Typowy zespol objawow klinicznych u chorych na cukrzyce zakonczony smercia w spiaczce bez zakwaszenia kotonowego ("trzecia spiaczka"). *Pol. Tyg. Lek.,* 1956, 11:2020-3.

WEGNER, FRIEDRICH RUDOLF GEORG (German physician, born 1843)

Wegner disease. See *Parrot syndrome (1).*

Wegner osteochondritis. See *Parrot syndrome (1).*

WEIL (German physician)

Weil-Albright syndrome. See *McCune-Albright syndrome.*

WEIL, ADOLF (German physician, 1848-1916)

Weil disease. See *leptospirosis.*

Weil icterus. See *leptospirosis.*

Weil syndrome. See *leptospirosis.*

WEILL, GEORGES (French ophthalmologist, 1866-1952)

Weill syndrome. See *Adie syndrome.*

Weill-Marchesani syndrome. Synonyms: *Marchesani syndrome, brachydactyly-spherophakia syndrome, brachymorphism and ectopia lentis syndrome, dysmorpho-dystrophia mesodermalis congenita, dystrophia mesodermalis congenita, dystrophia mesodermalis hypoplastica, inverted Marfan syndrome, spherophakia-brachymorphism syndrome.*

A hereditary syndrome, transmitted as an autosomal recessive trait, characterized by brachydactyly, small posture, broad skull, small shallow orbits, mild maxillary hypoplasia, narrow palate, small spherical crystalline lenses, myopia with or without glaucoma, frequent ectopia lentis, occasional blindness, malformed and malaligned teeth, and cardiac defect. Late ossification of the epiphyses is a constant feature.

Weill, G. Ectopie des cristallins et malformations générales. *Ann. Occul.,* 1932, 169:21-44. Marchesani, O. Brachydaktylie und angeborene Kugellinse als Systemerkrankung. *Klin. Mbl. Augenheilk.,* 1939, 103:392-406.

Weill-Reys syndrome. See *Adie syndrome.*

Weill-Reys-Adie syndrome. See *Adie syndrome.*

WEILL, JEAN A. (French physician, born 1903)

Léri-Weill syndrome. See *under Léri, André.*

WEINBERG, TOBIAS BERNARD (American physician, born 1887)

Weinberg-Himelfarb syndrome. Synonyms: *endocardial dysplasia, endocardial fibroelastosis (EFE), fetal endocardial fibroelastosis, fetal endocarditis.*

Noninflammatory fibrosis with diffuse or patchy thickening of the endocardium, chiefly of the left ventricle, forming a pearly-white lesion with normal endocardium covering the thickened tissue. The disease is usually congenital , but adult cases have also been reported. The symptoms include cyanosis, anorexia, irritability, dyspepsia, and cough. A variety of cardiac defects may be associated, and congestive heart failure is a common complication. Intrauterine anoxia or trauma, vascular lesions, and inflammatory reaction have been suggested as possible causes. Hereditary cases are transmitted as either an autosomal recessive or an X-linked trait.

Weinberg, T., & Himelfarb, A. J. Endocardial fibroelastosis (so-called fetal endocarditis). A report of two cases occurring in siblings. *Bull. Johns Hopkins Hosp.,* 1943, 72:299-306.

WEINGARTEN, R. J. (American physician)

Weingarten syndrome. See *tropical eosinophilia syndrome.*

WEINSTEIN, STEVEN F. (American physician)

Spitzer-Weinstein syndrome. See *under Spitzer.*

WEIR MITCHELL. See MITCHELL, SILAS WEIR

WEISENBURG, T. H. (American physician)

Weisenburg syndrome. See *glossopharyngeal neuralgia syndrome.*

WEISMANN-NETTER, R. (French physician)

Weismann-Netter dysostosis. See *Weismann-Netter syndrome.*

Weismann-Netter syndrome. Synonyms: *Weismann-Netter dysostosis, Weismann-Netter and Stuhl syndrome, dwarfism-congenital anterior bowing of legs, tibioperoneal diaphyseal toxopachyostosis, toxopachy, toxopachyostéose diaphysaire tibiopéronière.*

A congenital syndrome, transmitted as an autosomal recessive trait, characterized by dwarfism, anterior bowing of the tibia and fibula (sabre shin), mental retardation, dural calcification, and mild upper limb involvement, sometimes associated with kyphoscoliosis, rib deformities, dolichophalangy, goiter, anemia, and other disorders.

Weismann-Netter, R., & Stuhl. I. D'une ostéopathie congénitale éventuellement familiale surtout définie par l'incurvation antero-postérieure et l'épaississement des deux os de la jambe (toxopachyostéose diaphysaire tibiopéroniere. *Presse Méd.,* l954, 62:1618-22.

Weismann-Netter and Stuhl syndrome. See *Weismann-Netter syndrome.*

WEISS, KONRAD (Austrian physician)

Müller-Weiss syndrome. See *under Müller, Walther.*

WEISS, L.

Weiss syndrome. An autosomal dominant syndrome consisting of craniosynostosis, medially deviated great toes, and occasional mild syndactyly and various craniofacial anomalies, including oxycephaly.

Gorlin, R. J., Pindborg, J. J., & Cohen, M. M., jr. *Syndromes of the head and neck.* 2nd ed. McGraw-Hill, New York, 1976, p. 232.

WEISS, SOMA (American physician 1898-1942)

Charcot-Weiss-Baker syndrome. See *carotid sinus syndrome.*

Mallory-Weiss syndrome. See *under Mallory.*

Weiss-Baker syndrome. See *carotid sinus syndrome.*

WEISSENBACH, R. J. (French physician)

Thibierge-Weissenbach syndrome. See *under Thibierge.*

WEISSENBACHER, G. (Austrian physician)

Weissenbacher-Zweymüller syndrome. Synonyms: *Insley-Astley syndrome, otospondylofacial dysplasia, otospondylomegaepiphyseal dysplasis (OSMED).*

A congenital syndrome, probably transmitted as an autosomal recessive trait, characterized by sensorineural deafness, short limbs, and abnormal thickness of the joints, especially of the knees and elbows. Cleft palate occurs in most case. The main radiological findings consist of large epiphyses and moderate platyspondyly, especially in the lower thoracic region. The symptoms are usually present at birth and become more apparent in later childhood, consisting mainly of back pain and progressive joint stiffness.

Weissenbacher, G., & Zweymüller, E. Gleichzeitiges Vorkommen eines Syndroms von Pierre Robin und einer fetalen Chondrodysplasie. *Mtschr. Kinderh.*, 1964, 112:315-7. Insley, J., & Astley, R. A bone dysplasia with deafness. *Brit. J. Radiol.*, 1974, 47:244-51.

WELANDER, LISA (Swedish physician, born 1909)

Kugelberg-Welander syndrome. See *Wohlfart-Kugelberg-Welander syndrome.*

Welander syndrome. Synonyms: *late distal hereditary myopathy, myopathia distalis tarda hereditaria.*

A slowly progressive myopathy, transmitted as an autosomal dominant trait, characterized by weakness and wasting, which begin with the small muscles of the hands and feet and the extensors of the fingers and toes, followed by involvement of the extensors of the hands and feet. In the heterozygous (typical) form, the symptoms involve mainly the distal parts of the upper limbs, without incapacitating the patient. In the homozygous (atypical) form, the symptoms predominate in the lower limbs, eventually incapacitating the patient in about 10 to 15 years. Onset usually takes place between the ages of 40 and 60 years.

Welander, L. Myopathia distalis tarda hereditaria. 249 Examined cases in 72 pedigrees. *Acta Med. Scand.*, 1951, 141(Suppl 265):1-124.

Wohlfart-Kugelberg-Welander syndrome. See *under Wohlfart.*

well-water methemoglobinemia. See *Comly syndrome.*

WELLS, G. C. (British physician)

Wells syndrome. Synonyms: *eosinophilic cellulitis, eosinophilic infiltration with flame figures, recurrent granulomatous dermatitis with eosinophilia.*

An acute inflammatory skin disease characterized by an urticarial eruption with infiltrated erythema and annular or circinate patterns, burning sensation, pruritus, redness, local induration, fever, and malaise. An insect bite may be the precipitating factor. Gradually, the eruption spreads out to involve the extremities, while central clearance may develop in some previously affected areas. Eventually, the lesions subside and leave browny bluish or slate colored residual areas which slowly fade away. In the next phase, there may be local morphea-like atrophy which also resolves spontaneously. Eosinophilia, in the early phases, and mild leukocytosis and high erythrocyte sedimentation rate, in the later stages, are the chief hematological findings. Early skin edema, eosinophilic infiltration of the dermis, and histiocytes surrounding collagenous masses (flame figures) are the principal histopathological features of this disorder.

Wells, G. C. Recurrent granulomatous dermatitis with eosinophilia. *Tr. St. Johns Hosp. Derm. Soc.*, 1971, 57:46-56.

WELLS, MICHAEL (British physician)

Muckle-Wells syndrome. See *under Muckle.*

WELLS, R. S. (British physician)

Hay-Wells syndrome. See *AEC syndrome.*

WELTI, JEAN JACQUES (French physician, born 1913)

Lian-Siguier-Welti syndrome. See *under Lian.*

WERDNIG, GUIDO (Austrian physician, 1844-1919)

Werdnig disease. See *Werdnig-Hoffmann syndrome.*

Werdnig-Hoffmann disease (WHD). See *Werdnig-Hoffmann syndrome.*

Werdnig-Hoffmann syndrome. Synonyms: *Hoffmann atrophy, Werdnig disease, Werdnig-Hoffmann diseaee (WHD), familial spinal muscular atrophy, infantile muscular atrophy, infantile spinal muscular atrophy, progressive spinal muscular atrophy, progressive spinal muscular atrophy of infants, spinal muscular atrophy I (SMA I).*

A familial form of progressive spinal muscular atrophy, transmitted as an autosomal recessive trait, associated with hypotonia and wasting of the skeletal muscles, resulting from degeneration of the anterior horn cells of the spinal cord in infants. The clinical picture is that of the floppy infant, with difficulty in holding the head up. The symptoms include sluggish movements, weakness and decreased motion (at first of the pelvic girdle and leg muscles and progressing to large muscles), flaccid and externally rotated lower limbs, diaphragmatic breathing, long and narrow bell-shaped chest, absent tendon reflexes, absence of pain sensation, and fascicular twitching, most readily recognized in the tongue. Additional findings may include bouts of pneumonia, contractures of the large joints, kyphoscoliosis, and fatty infiltrations. Most patients die within the first 3 years of life. See also *Wohlfart-Kugelberg-Welander syndrome.*

Werdnig, G. Zwei frühinfantile hereditäre Falle von progressiver Muskelatrophie unter dem Bilde der Dystrophie, aber auf neurotischer Grundlage. *Arch. Psychiat., Berlin*, 1891, 22:437-80. Hoffmann, J. Weitere Beiträge zur Lehre von der progressiven neurotischen Muskeldystrophie. *Deut. Zschr. Nervenh.*, 1891, 1:95-120.

WERLHOF, PAUL GOTTLIEB (German physician, 1699-1767)

morbus maculosus werlhofii. See *Werlhof disease.*

peliosis werlhoffi. See *Werlhof disease.*

Werlhof disease. Synonyms: *Werlhof purpura, Werlhof-Wichmann syndrome, essential thrombocytopenia, hemogenia, hemogenic syndrome, hemorrhagic purpura, idiopathic thrombocytopenic purpura (ITP), idiopathic thrombopenic purpura, morbus maculosus hemorrhagicus, morbus maculosus werlhofii, peliosis werlhofii, primary splenic thrombocytopenia, primary thrombocytopenia, primary thrombocytopenic purpura, purpura hemorrhagica, purpura thrombocytopenica, splenic thrombocytopenic purpura, thrombocytolytic purpura.*

A hemorrhagic disorder, affecting chiefly adult women, characterized by variable symptoms, including scattered petechiae, minor bleeding tendencies, menorrhagia, epistaxis, and inflammatory purpuric lesions of the skin and mucous membranes, most commonly on the distal upper and lower extremities. Post-traumatic deep ecchymoses may be present, but bleeding into the joints and retina is unusual. In severe cases, there may be hemorrhagic bullae in the oral mucosa. Intracranial hemorrhage occurs in some instances. Enlargement of the spleen is common. The course is marked by remissions and relapses alternating over long periods of time. Blood tests show 5000 to 75,000 platelets per microliter and bizarre giant platelets. Anemia is usually due to blood loss. Clot retraction is diminished, bleeding time is prolonged, and capillary fragility is increased. Immunoglobulin G is believed to be a factor in the autoimmune etiology.

*Werlhof, P. G. *Disquisitio medica et philologica de variolis et anthracibus.* Bruswick, 1735. Aster, R. H. Thrombocytopenia due to enhanced platelet destruction. In: Williams, W. J., Beutler, E., Erslev, A. J., & Lichtman, M. A., eds. *Hematology.* 3rd ed. New York, McGraw-Hill, 1983, pp. 1298-338.

Werlhof purpura. See *Werlhof disease.*

Werlhof-Wichmann syndrome. See *Werlhof disease.*

WERMER, PAUL (American physician)

Wermer syndrome. See *multiple endocrine neoplasia I syndrome.*

WERNER, HEINRICH (German physician, born 1874)

Werner-His disease. Synonyms: *febris quintana, five-day fever, Meuse fever, quintan fever, shin bone fever, trench fever, Volhynia fever.*

A communicable disease caused by infection with *Rickettsia quintana* and transmitted to man by lice. After an incubation period of 10 to 20 days, there is the sudden onset of headache, hyperesthesia of the skin, pain in the back of the legs, and intermittent fever, which recurs every 4 to 5 days. Epidemics were observed in Volhynia and other European battle fronts during World War I.

Werner, H. Über eine besondere Erkrankung, die er als Fünftagefieber bezeichnet. *Berlin. Klin. Wschr.,* 1916, 53:204. His. Über eine neue periodische Fiebererkrankung (Febris Wolhynica). *Berlin. Klin. Wschr.,* 1916, 53:322-3.

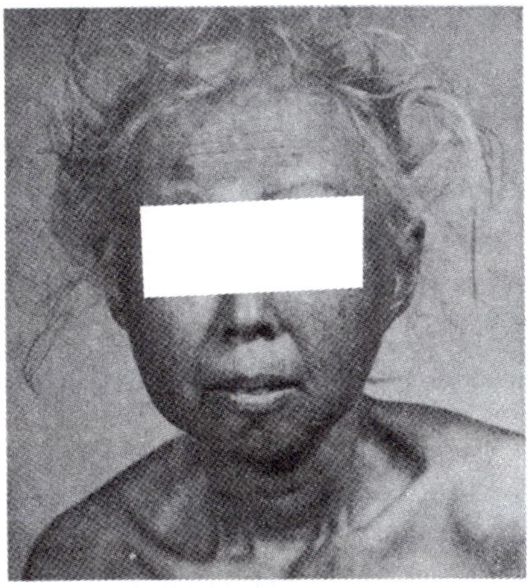

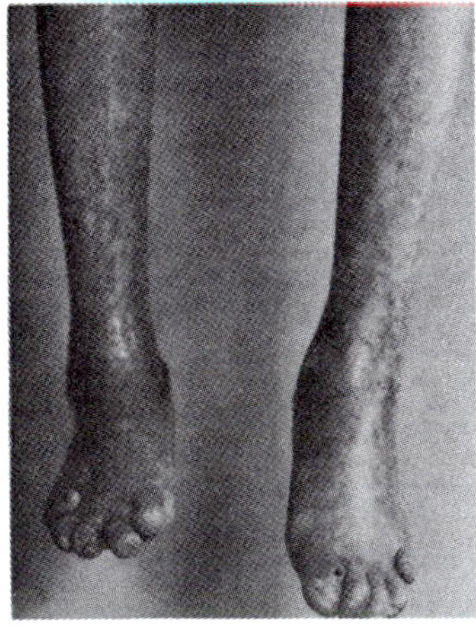

Werner syndrome
Epstein, C.J., et al.: *Medicine* 45:177, 1966. Baltimore: Williams & Wilkins.

WERNER, OTTO (German physician, born 1879)

Werner syndrome (WS). Synonyms: *pangeria, progeria adultorum.*

A hereditary syndrome, transmitted as an autosomal recessive trait, characterized by premature aging, short stature, premature graying of the hair (canities), alopecia, sclerópoikiloderma, trophic leg ulcers, cataracts, hypogonadism, diabetes mellitus, calcification of blood vessels, and osteoporosis. Facial lipoatrophy, a pinched or beaked nose, and protuberant eyes contribute to the progeroid appearance. The skin over bony prominences and the soles may become hyperkeratotic and show ulcerations. Less commonly, there may be hyper- or depigmentation, and telangiectasia. Retinitis pigmentosa, macular degeneration, and chorioretinitis occur in some cases. Wasting of muscles of the legs, feet, and hands and soft tissue calcification may be associated. Poorly developed genitalia and breasts and menstrual disorders are common. The symptoms become apparent during the third or fourth decade. See also *Hutchinson-Gilford syndrome.*

Werner, O. *Über Katarakt in Verbindung mit Sklerodermia.* Kiel, 1904. (Thesis).

WERNICKE, KARL (German physician, 1848-1905)

Gayet-Wernicke syndrome. See *Wernicke syndrome.*

Wernicke aphasia. Synonyms: *Bastian aphasia, auditory receptive aphasia, auditory verbal agnosia, cortical sensory aphasia, cortical word deafness, receptive aphasia, word deafness.*

Loss of comprehension of spoken words in the presence of intact hearing due to cortical lesions in the posterior portion of the left first temporal convolution. The affected persons may speak fluently with a natural language rhythm, but the result has neither understandable meaning nor syntax. Despite the loss of comprehension, the word memory is preserved and words often are chosen correctly. Alexia, agraphia, acalculia, and paraphasia are frequently associated. Some patients are euphoric and/or paranoid.

*Wernicke, K. *Der aphasische Symptomenkomplex. Eine psychologische Studie auf anatomischer Basis.* Breslau, 1874. *Bastian, H. C. On the various forms of loss of speech in cerebral disease. *Brit. For. Med. Chir. Rev.,* 1869, 43:209-36.

Wernicke cramp. Synonym: *cramp neurosis.*

A form of psychogenic muscle cramp precipitated by anxiety or fear.

Wernicke, C. Ein Fall von Crampus-Neurose. *Berlin. Klin. Wschr.,* 1904, 41:1121-4.

Wernicke dementia. Synonym: *presbyophrenia.*

Defective memory, loss of sense of location, and confabulation, seen in old age.

*Nouët, H. Presbyophrenia of Wernicke and psychoneurosis. *Alienist Neur.,* 1913, 34:141-55.

Wernicke disease. See *Wernicke syndrome.*

Wernicke encephalopathy. See *Wernicke syndrome.*

Wernicke syndrome. Synonyms: *Gayet disease, Gayet-Wernicke syndrome, Wernicke disease, Wernicke encephalopathy, alcoholic encephalopathy, cerebral beriberi, polioencephalitis hemorrhagica superioris, pseudoencephalitis acuta hemorrhagica superior, pseudoencephalitis hemorrhagica superior, superior hemorrhagic polioencephalitis.*

A syndrome of mental disorders (listlessness, disorientation, confusion, hallucinations, and other behavioral symptoms), ocular disorders (oculomotor paralysis, chiefly of the external recti, conjugate paralysis, and nystagmus), and ataxia. Nutritional deficiency, skin changes, redness of the tongue, cheilosis, liver diseases, cardiovascular complications (including tachycardia, dyspnea on exertion, postural hypotension, and vascular collapse), and hypothermia are the common features. The symptoms usually have a sudden onset and occur singly or in various combinations. In Wernicke's description, the lesions were bilateral, marked by pinhead-sized petechial hemorrhages, congested capillaries, and proliferation of the capillaries, involving the gray matter around the third and fourth ventricles and the aqueduct of Sylvius. Recent findings show that only a small number of patients have hemorrhage and that lesions are not restricted to the gray matter. Pathological changes include neuronal, axonal, and myelin loss, prominent blood vessels, reactive microglia, gliosis, astrocytosis, occasional small hemorrhages in the brain tissue, and lesions of the thalamus, hypothalamus, midbrain, and medulla oblongata. The term **Gayet disease** applies to the type in which lesions are more extensive than those in the Wernicke type. Nutritional deficiency due to inadequate thiamine intake, which occurs mainly but not exclusively in alcoholics, is a major feature of this syndrome. The Wernicke syndrome is frequently complicated by symptoms of the Korsakoff syndrome (see *Wernicke-Korsakoff syndrome*).

Wernicke, C. Die acute, hämorrhagische Polioencephalitis superior. In his: *Lehrbuch der Gehirnkrankheiten.* Kassel, Fischer, 1881, pp. 229-42. Gayet, M. Affection encéphalique (encéphalite diffuse probable) localisée aux étages superieurs des pédoncles cérébraux et aux couches optiques, ainsi qu'ou plancher due quatrieme ventricule et aux parois laterales du troisieme. Observation recueillie. *Arch. Physiol. Norm. Path., Paris,* 1875, 2:341-51.

Wernicke-Korsakoff complex. See *Wernicke-Korsakoff syndrome.*

Wernicke-Korsakoff syndrome (WKS). Synonyms: *Wernicke-Korsakoff complex, alcohol amnestic syndrome.*

Development of symptoms of the Korsakoff syndrome (mainly amnesia with a tendency to confabulate with or without polyneuropathy) in patients with the Wernicke syndrome.

Wernicke, C. Die acute, hämorrhagische Polioencephalitis superior. In his: *Lehrbuch der Gehirnkrankheiten.* Kassel, Fischer, 1881, pp. 229-42. Korsakov, S. S. Ob alkogol'nom paraliche. *Vestn. Psikhiat.,* 1887, vol. 4.

Wernicke-Mann hemiplegia. Synonym: *Wernicke-Mann paralysis.*

Partial hemiplegia of the extremities characterized by typical posture and gait disorders. It is caused by lesions of the central nervous system which result in contralateral spastic paralysis of the muscles of upper and lower limbs and face.

Wernicke, C. Zur Kenntniss der cerebralen Hemiplegie. *Berlin. Klin. Wschr.,* 1889, 26:9969-70. Mann, L. Klinische und anatomische Beiträge zur Lehre von der spinalen Hemiplegie. *Deut. Zschr. Nervenh.,* 1896-97, 10:1-66.

Wernicke-Mann paralysis. See *Wernicke-Mann hemiplegia.*

WERTER

Werter-Dümling disease. A form of papulonecrotic dermatitis reportedly described by Werter and Dümling in 1910.

Skripkin, Iu. K., *et al.* Sluchai papulonekroticheskogo dermatita Wertera-Dümlinga. *Vestn. Derm. Vener., Moskva,* 1981, No. 11:55-7.

WEST, W. J. (British physician)

West syndrome (WS). Synonyms: *eclampsia nutans, flexion spasm, greeting spasms, infantile salaam, infantile spasms with mental retardation, jackknife spasm, nodding spasm, salaam convulsions.*

Massive myoclonus epilepsy of infancy and early childhood, characterized by seizures involving the muscles of the neck, trunk, and limbs, and manifested by nodding of the head and flexion of the arms. In most cases, the seizures appear during the first year of life. Many patients show EEG abnormalities, consisting of multifocal spikes and slow waves of large amplilitude (hypsarrhythmia). The seizures are frequently associated with developmental or acquired brain abnormalities and mental retardation. The etiology is unknown, but some cases are believed to be transmitted as an X-linked trait.

West, W. J. On a peculiar form of infantile convulsions. *Lancet,* 1840-41, 1:724-5.

WESTBERG, FRIEDRICH (German physician)

Westberg disease. A skin disorder marked by the presence of white spots.

Westberg, F. Ein Fall von mit weissen Flecken einhergehender, bisher nich bekannter Dermatose. *Mschr. Prakt. Derm.,* 1901, 33:355-62.

WESTERHOF, WIETE (Dutch physician)

Westerhof syndrome. A familial syndrome, transmitted as an autosomal dominant trait, characterized by congenital hypomelanotic and hypermelanotic macules. Ultrastructurally, the hypomelanotic skin showed small melanosomes and hypermelanotic skin large melanosomes in keratinocytes. Some affected persons also had growth and mental retardation.

Westerhof, W., *et al.* Hereditary congenital hypopigmented and hyperpigmented macules. *Arch. Derm., Chicago,* 1978, 114:931-6.

WESTPHAL, ALEXANDER KARL OTTO (German physician, 1863-1941)

Westphal ataxia. See *Westphal-Leyden syndrome.*

Westphal-Leyden syndrome. Synonyms: *Leyden ataxia, Westphal ataxia, acute ataxia.*

Acute ataxia of undetermined etiology, usually beginning with vomiting, vertigo, motor disorders, and coma. Later symptoms include slow scanning speech; ataxia with slow jerky movements of the extremities; mental disorders, chiefly excessive excitability, faulty memory, and dementia; equilibrium disorders manifested by swaying of the body; and nystagmus. Motor strength and sensitivity are apparently unaffected.

Leyden, E. Über acute Ataxie. *Zschr. Klin. Med.,* 1890, 18:576-87. *Westphal, A. Eigentümliche mit Einschlafen verbundene Anfälle. *Arch. Psychiat., Berlin,* 1877, 7:631-5.

WESTPHAL, KARL FRIEDRICH OTTO (German neurologist, 1833-1890)

Cavaré-Romberg-Westphal syndrome. See *Westphal syndrome.*

Cavaré-Westphal syndrome. See *Westphal syndrome.*

Westphal neurosis. See *Westphal syndrome.*

Westphal pseudosclerosis. See *Wilson disease, under Wilson, Samuel Alexander Kinnier.*

Westphal syndrome. Synonyms: *Cavaré-Romberg syndrome, Cavaré-Romberg-Westphal syndrome, Cavaré-Westphal syndrome, Westphal neurosis, familial paroxysmal paralysis, family periodic paralysis, hypokalemic periodic paralysis, hypopotassemic periodic paralysis, intermittent myoplegia, paroxysmal paralysis, periodic paralysis.*

A rare form of familial intermittent paralysis, transmitted as an autosomal dominant trait, marked by periodic attacks of flaccid paralysis of the extremities and trunk, in association with complete areflexia and lack of electrical excitability of the muscles and, in some cases, low blood potassium levels. The attacks usually last several hours to several days, beginning with weakness in the back of the thighs and initially spreading to the distal areas of the lower extremities, then to the shoulder girdle and upper extremities, and finally to the neck. Onset is usually observed during childhood or early adolescence. The attacks can be precipitated by infusions of glucose and insulin, eating a large meal, or administration of epinephrine.

Westphal, C. Über einen merkrürdigen Fall von periodischer Lähmung aller 4 Extremitäten mit gleichzeitigem Erlöschensein der elektrischen Erregbarkeit während der Lähmung. *Berlin. Klin. Wschr.*, 1885, 22:489-91; 509-11.

Westphal-Strümpell syndrome. See *Wilson disease, under Wilson, Samuel Alexander Kinnier.*

wet and dry foot syndrome. Synonyms: *atopic winter feet in children, forefoot eczema, juvenile plantar dermatosis (JPD), peridigital dermatosis, recurrent juvenile eczema of the hands and feet.*

A skin disorder in prepuberal children of both sexes, characterized by symmetrical fissuring dermatosis that affects the weight-bearing surfaces of the feet, where the stratum corneum is thick and flexion forces are greatest. It is caused by alernating excessive wetness and dryness of the feet.

Silvers, S. H., & Glickman, F. S. Atopy and eczema of the feet in children. *Am. J. Dis. Child.*, 1968, 116:400-1. Steck, W. D. Juvenile plantar dermatosis: The "wet and dry foot syndrome." *Cleveland Clin. Q.* 1983, 50:145-9.

wet lung syndrome (WLS). Transient tachypnea of the newborn, characterized by increased respiratory rate during the first hours of life, which resolves within a few hours to a few days. Radiographic findings show a pattern of the diffuse bilateral edema with concomitant hyperaeration of the lungs, sternal retraction, and an air bronchogram effect. Delayed resorption of the pulmonary fluid at birth is believed to be the cause. Conditions predisposing to this disorder are believed to be cesarean section, prematurity, maternal diabetes mellitus, and breech delivery. See also *neonatal respiratory distress syndrome.*

Wesenberg, R. L. *et al.* Radiological findings in wet-lung disease. *Radiology*, 1971, 98:69-74.

WEYERS, HELMUT (German pediatrician)

Hertwig-Weyers syndrome. See *Weyers oligodactyly syndrome.*

Meyer-Schwickerath and Weyers syndrome. See *oculodentodigital syndrome.*

Weyers oligodactyly syndrome. Synonyms: *Hertwig-Weyers syndrome, oligodactylia syndrome, ulnar hemimelia.*

A syndrome of deficiency of the fibular and ulnar rays, antecubital pterygia, reduced sternal segments, and congenital malformations of the kidneys and spleen. In the original report, 1 of the 2 cases had cleft lip and cleft palate and the other had maxillary hypoplasia, dental deformities, and hypoplastic acromial end of the clavicle; 1 had 2 fingers on each hand and the other 2 on the right and a single malformed finger on the left hand. The syndrome is transmitted as an autosomal dominant trait.

Weyers, H. Das Oligodactylie-Syndrom des Menschen und seine Parallelmutation bei der Hausmaus. *Ann. Paediat.*, 1957, 189:351-70. Hertwig, P. Sechs neue Mutationen bei Hausmaus in ihrer Bedeutung fur allgemeine Vererbungsfragen. *Zschr. Mensch. Vererh.*, 1942-43, 26:1-21.

Weyers syndrome (1). Synonyms: *atresia multiplex congenita, polyatresia congenita.*

Congenital atresia of various parts of the gastrointestinal system with obstruction of the adjoining vessels, with or without esophageal fistula and in the presence of air in the gastrointestinal system, reportedly described by Weyers.

Weyers syndrome (2). Synonyms: *dysgenesis iridodentalis, dysgenesis mesodermalis corneae et iridis, iridodental dysplasia.*

A familial syndrome characterized by an association of iris abnormalities, corneal disorders, and anomalous tooth development. The abnormalities include dysplasia and minute perforations of the iris, pupillary synechiae, microphthalmos, corneal opacities, microdontia, oligodontia, enamel hypoplasia, and virilization. Dwarfism and myotonic dystrophy may occur.

Weyers, H. *Dysgenesis irido-dentalis. Ein neues Syndrom mit obweichdendem chromosomalen Geschlecht bei weiblichen Merkmalträgern.* (Presented at the meeting of the Deutsche Gesselschaft für Kinderheilkunde, Kassel, 1960).

Weyers syndrome (3). Synonyms: *Curry-Hall syndrome, acrodental dysostosis, acrofacial dysostosis (AFD), acrofacial syndrome.*

A syndrome of postaxial polydactyly of the hands and feet, synostoses of the metacarpal and metatarsal bones, and bony clefts of the mandibular symphysis. Additional defects consist of peg teeth, absence of the teeth, prominent ear anthelices, hypoplastic and dysplastic nails, and mild shortness of stature. The syndrome is inherited as an autosomal dominant trait with variable expression.

Weyers, H. Hexadactylie, Unterkieferspalt und Oligodontie, ein neuer Symptomenkomplex; Dysostosis acrofacialis. *Ann. Paediat., Basel*, 1953, 181:45-60. Weyers, H. Über eine korrelierte Missbildung der Kiefer und Extremitätenakren (Dysostosis acro-facialis). Fortschr. Roentgen., 1952, 77:562-7.

Weyers-Fülling syndrome. Synonyms: *dentofacial dysplasia, dysplasia dentofacialis.*

A syndrome combining multiple oculodentofacial abnormalities, including hypoplasia of the dental root with premature tooth eruption (dentes natales) and an early loss of the teeth; eye anomalies (congenital cataract, microphthalmia, and glaucoma); and peculiar facies, including short philtrum, nasal deformities, relative micrognathia, and incomplete closure of the frontozygomatic suture.

Weyers, H., & Fülling, G. Dysplasia dento-facialis, ein neues Ektodermalsyndrom. *Zahnmed. Bild.*, 1963, 4:25-32.

Weyers-Thier syndrome. Synonyms: *atypical mandibu-*

lofacial dysostosis, dysplasia oculovertebralis, oculovertebral dysplasia, unilateral mandibulofacial dysostosis.

A combination of microphthalmia and colobomas or anophthalmia with small orbit; facial asymmetry, resulting from unilateral maxillary dysplastic soft tissue, macrostomia, alveolar malformations, and dental malocclusion; malformations of the vertebral column consisting of half-developed cleft and wedgelike vertebrae without synostosis, chiefly in the lumbothoracic region; and costal anomalies such as branched and hypoplastic ribs.

Weyers, H., & Thier, C. J. Malformations mandibulo-faciales et délimitation d'un "syndrome oculo-vertébral." *J. Génet. Hum.*, 1958, 7:143-73.

WEYGANDT (German physician)

Weygandt-Heller syndrome. See *Heller syndrome, under Heller, Theodor O.*

WFS (whistling face syndrome). See *Freeman-Sheldon syndrome.*

WHD (Werdnig-Hoffmann disease). See *Werdnig-Hoffmann syndrome.*

WHEELOCK, FRANK CAWTHORNE, JR. (American physician, born 1918)

McKittrick-Wheelock syndrome. See *under McKittrick.*

whiplash syndrome. Synonym: *hyperextension-hyperflexion syndrome.*

Injury of the cervical portion of the spinal cord caused by hyperextension of the neck in rear-end automobile collision or, less frequently, during a fall. As a car is struck, the body of the occupant is propelled forward in relation to the head. At the limit of the stretch of the soft tissue of the neck, the head falls backward and extension strain is applied to the neck and, when the acceleration ceases, the head rebounds forward, the movement being enhanced by contraction of the neck flexor muscles. The symptoms become apparent 1 to 2 days after the accident and include pain radiating from the neck to one or both shoulders and down the arms. In some instances, the pain may be experienced only in the shoulders, in the arm, or in the back of the neck, radiating to the interscapular region and to the chest and into the suboccipital region. Occipital headaches, sometimes associated with retro-ocular pain, extending over the vertex or bitemporally, and subjective numbness in relation to the ulnar border of the hand may occur. Other symptoms include dysphagia (usually due to pharyngeal edema or retropharyngeal hematoma), blurring of vision caused by injury of the vertebral arteries or damage to the cervical sympathetic nerves, the Horner syndrome, tinnitus probably secondary to a temporary spasm caused by injuries of the vertebral arteries or the inner ear. Radiological findings may show an initial loss of the normal cervical lordotic curve followed by an S-shaped curve. The term **late whiplash syndrome** is used when the symptoms become apparent more than 6 months after the injury.

Macnab, I. The "whiplash syndrome." *Orthop. Clin. N. America*, 1971, 2:389-403. Bella, J. I. The late whiplash syndrome. *Austral. NZ J. Surg.*, 1980, 50:610-4. Abbot, K. H. Whiplash injuries. *JAMA*, 1956, 162:917.

whiplash shaken infant syndrome. See *battered child syndrome.*

WHIPPLE, GEORGE HOYT (American physician, born 1878)

Whipple disease. Synonyms: *Whipple intestinal lipodystrophy, Whipple syndrome, idiopathic steatorrhea, intestinal lipodystrophy, intestinal lipogranulomatosis, lipodystrophia intestinalis, lipophagic intestinal granulomatosis, mesenteric chyladenectasis, nontropical sprue, steatorrhea arthropericarditica.*

A disorder characterized by malabsorption, steatorrhea, chills, fever, weakness, weight loss, skin pigmentation, anemia, lymphadenopathy, migratory arthritis with joint pain, pleurisy, pericarditis, valvular endocarditis, and central nervous system complications. Pathological findings include infiltration of the lamina propria of the intestine with PAS-positive macrophages that contain small rod-shaped bacilli. The changes may involve any organ in the body, but the intestine is most frequently affected. In the past, the condition was known to affect chiefly males aged 30 to 40 years, being usually fatal; with the use of antibiotic therapy Whipple disease is now relatively rare and is almost always curable. See also *malabsorption syndrome.*

Whipple, G. H. A hitherto undescribed disease characterized anatomically by deposits of fat and fatty acids in the intestinal and mesenteric lymphatic tissues. *Bull. Johns Hopkins Hosp.*, 1907, 18:382-91.

Whipple intestinal lipodystrophy. See *Whipple disease.*

Whipple syndrome. See *Whipple disease.*

whistling face syndrome (WFS). See *Freeman-Sheldon syndrome.*

whistling face-windmill vane hand syndrome. See *Freeman-Sheldon syndrome.*

WHITAKER, JOANNE (American physician)

Whitaker disease. See *Whitaker syndrome.*

Whitaker syndrome. Synonyms: *Whitaker disease, Whitaker triad.*

A syndrome of familial juvenile hypoadrenocorticism and hypoparathyroidism associated with superficial moniliasis.

Whitaker, J., *et al.* The syndrome of familial juvenile hypoadrenocorticism, hypoparathyroidism and superficial moniliasis. *J. Clin. Endocr. Metab.*, 1956,16:1374-87.

Whitaker triad. See *Whitaker syndrome.*

WHITE, CLEVELAND (American physician)

Marshall-White syndrome. See *under Marshall, Wallace.*

WHITE, HARRY H. (American physician)

May-White syndrome. See *under May, Duane L.*

WHITE, JAMES CLARKE (American physician, 1833-1916)

Darier-White disease. See *Darier disease (1).*

White disease. See *Darier disease (1).*

WHITE, PAUL DUDLEY (American cardiologist, 1886-1973)

Bland-White-Garland syndrome. See *under Bland.*

Wolff-Parkinson-White syndrome (WPW). See *under Wolff.*

WHITE, W. F. (British physician)

Samman-White syndrome. See *yellow nail syndrome.*

white clot syndrome (WCS). Synonym: *heparin-associated thrombocytopenia and thrombosis (HATT).*

A complication of heparin therapy characterized by thrombocytopenia and arterial or venous, multiple, recurrent embolism caused by friable white emboli.

Rhodes, G. R., *et al.* Heparin induced thrombocytopenia

with thrombotic and hemorrhagic manifestations. *Surg. Gyn. Obst.*, 1973, 136:409-16.

white dot syndrome. See *multiple evanescent white dot syndrome.*

white dragon pearl syndrome. A female pattern of drug dependence, named after attractive and well educated Hong Kong women who become addicted as a result of contact with wealthy men in the illegal drug trade.

Smithberg, N., & Westermeyer, J. White dragon pearl syndrome: A female pattern of drug dependence. *Am. J. Drug Alcohol Abuse*, 1985, 11:199-207.

white finger. See *vibration syndrome.*

white folded gingivostomatitis. See *white sponge nevus.*

white liver disease. See *Reye syndrome.*

white lung. See *adult respiratory distress syndrome.*

white sponge nevus. Synonyms: *Cannon nevus, Cannon syndrome, congenital leukokeratosis, familial white folded dysplasia, nevus (naevus) spongiosus albus mucosae, oral epithelial nevus, white folded gingivostomatitis.*

A disease, transmitted as an autosomal dominant trait, characterized by spongy white lesions of the oral and nasal mucosae, in which thickened spongy folded mucosa covers the nasal septum, conchae, cheeks, tongue, palate, gums, and floor of the mouth. The condition, occasionally asymptomatic at first, may have its onset in newborn infants, increasing in severity until adolescence.

Cannon, A. B. White spongy nevus of mucosa (naevus spongiosus albus mucosae). *Arch. Derm., Syph.*, 1935, 31:365-70.

white spots disease. See *Hallopeau syndrome (1).*

WHITMORE, ALFRED (British physician in India, 1876-1946)

Whitmore disease. Synonyms: *Whitmore fever, melioidosis.*

An acute, glanderslike infectious disease, transmitted to man by rodents and caused by the bacterium *Malleomyces pseudomallei (Pseudomonas).* Acute pulmonary and septicemic forms are recognized. The septicemic form is characterized by multiple abscesses, pustules, granulmomas, sinuses, and ulcers of the skin and soft tissues. The disease occurs almost exclusively in the Far East.

Whitmore, A., & Krishnaswami, C. S. An account of the discovery of a hitherto undescribed infective disease among the population of Rangoon. *Indian Med. Gaz.*, 1912, 47:262-7.

Whitmore fever. See *Whitmore disease.*

WHYTT, ROBERT (British physician, 1714-1766)

Whytt disease. Tuberculous meningitis associated with hydrocephalus.

Whytt, R. *Observations on the dropsy of the brain.* Edinburgh, Balfour, 1768.

WICHMANN, JOHANN ERNST (German physician, 1740-1802)

Werlhof-Wichmann syndrome. See *Werlhof disease.*

WIDAL, GEORGES FERNAND ISIDORE (French physician, 1862-1929)

Hayem-Widal syndrome. See *under Hayem.*

Widal disease. See *Hayem-Widal syndrome.*

Widal syndrome. See *Hayem-Widal syndrome.*

Widal-Abrami syndrome. See *Hayem-Widal syndrome.*

WIDAL, M. FERNAND (French physician)

Fernand Widal-Lermoyez syndrome. See *Widal-Lermoyez syndrome.*

Widal syndrome. See *Widal-Lermoyez syndrome.*

Widal-Lermoyez syndrome. Synonyms: *Fernand Widal-Lermoyez syndrome, Widal syndrome, aspirin idiosyncrasy.*

Toxic reaction to aspirin, occurring more frequently in females than males, characterized by rhinitis, polyposis of the paranasal sinuses, cranial sinusitis, bronchitis, and severe asthmatic attacks.

*Widal, M. F., Abrami, P., & Lermoyez, J. Anaphylaxie et idiosyncrasie. *Presse Méd.*, 1922, 30:183. Wayoff, M., *et al.* Polypose naso-sinusienne et maladie à l'aspirine. Syndrome de Fernand Widal et Lermoyez. *Ann. Otolar., Paris*, 1979, 96:229-39.

wide bladder neck syndrome. Relaxation of the sphincter of the bladder, allowing diurnal and at times nocturnal urinary incontinence. Causes include epispadias, single ectopic ureter, urogenital sinus malformations, and trauma.

Williams, D. I., & Lightwood, R. G. Bilateral single ectopic ureters. *Brit. J. Urol.*, 1972, 44:267-73. Williams, D. I., & Morgan, R. C. Wide bladder neck syndrome in children: A review. *J. Roy. Soc. Med., London*, 1978, 71:520-2.

WIDMARK, ERIK JOHAN (Swedish ophthalmologist, 1850-1909)

Widmark conjunctivitis. Synonym: *exfoliative acute catarrhal conjunctivitis.*

An acute inflammation of the conjunctiva marked by a loss of the epithelium.

*Widmark, J. Smärre oftalmologiska iakttagelser. *Hygieia*, 1909, 71:1045-53.

WIEACKER, PETER (German physician)

Wieacker syndrome. See *Wieacker-Wolff syndrome.*

Wieacker-Wolff syndrome. Synonym: *Wieacker syndrome.*

An X-linked mental retardation syndrome associated with contractures of the feet at birth, progressive muscle atrophy, and dyspraxia of the muscles of the eyes, face, and tongue. Other abnormalities may include overlap of the toes, claw toes, kyphoscoliosis, and speech disorders.

Wieacker, P., Wolff, G., *et al.* M. A new X-linked syndrome with muscle atrophy, congenital contractures, and oculomotor apraxia. *Am. J. Med. Genet.*, 1985, 20:597-606. Opitz, J. M., Reynolds, J. F., & Spano. L. M., eds. X-linked mental retardation 2. *Am. J. Med. Genet.*, 1986, 23:15.

WIEDEMANN, HANS RUDOLF (German pediatrician)

Beckwith-Wiedemann syndrome (BW, BWS). See *under Beckwith.*

Genée-Wiedemann syndrome. See *under Genée.*

Holtermüller-Wiedemann syndrome. See *under Holtermüller.*

Maroteaux-Spranger-Wiedemann syndrome. See *metatropic dwarfism syndrome.*

metaphyseal chondrodysplasia, Wiedemann-Spranger type. See *Wiedemann-Spranger metaphyseal chondrodysplasia syndrome.*

Spranger-Wiedemann syndrome. See *spondyloepiphyseal dysplasia congenita.*

Wiedemann syndrome (1). Synonyms: *Lenz syndrome, dysmelia syndrome, fetal thalidomide syndrome, thalidomide embryopathy, thalidomide phocomelia, thalidomide syndrome.*

A syndrome of congenital abnormalities caused by the toxic effects of thalidomide given to pregnant women. Abnormalities are variable and depend on the timing at which the drug was given. Principal features of this syndrome are defects of the limbs, ranging from hypoplasia of the thenar eminences of the thumbs, single digit thumb, triphalangeal thumbs to single limb amelia, phocomelia, and tetraamelia in extreme cases. A variety cf skeletal, neurologic, cardiovascular, urologic, pulmonary, and gastrointestinal deformities may be associated, including anotia or dysotia; deafness; defects of the third, fourth, sixth, and seventh cranial nerves; epiphora; coloboma; microphthalmos; esophageal, anal, and duodenal atresia; pyloric stenosis; choanal atresia; saddle nose; cleft palate; webbed neck; nevus flammeus; defective development of the gallbladder; and other anomalies. The syndrome has become virtually extinct since discontinuation of the use of thalidomide. See also *pseudothalidomide syndrome*.

Wiedemann, H. R. Hinweis auf eine derzeitige Häufung hypo- und aplastischer Fehlbildungen der Gliedmassen. *Med. Welt*, 1961, 2:1863-6. Lenz, W., & Knapp, K. Die Thalidomid-Embryopathie. *Deut. Med. Wschr.*, 1962, 87:1232-42.

Wiedemann syndrome (2). See *Beckwith-Wiedemann syndrome.*

Wiedemann syndrome (3). See *Proteus syndrome.*

Wiedemann-Beckwith syndrome (WBS). See *Beckwith-Wiedemann syndrome.*

Wiedemann-Beckwith-Combs syndrome. See *Beckwith-Wiedemann syndrome.*

Wiedemann-Rautenstrauch syndrome (WRS). Synonyms: *congenital pseudohydrocephalic progeroid syndrome, neonatal progeroid syndrome, neonatal pseudohydrocephalic progeroid syndrome.*

A hereditary progeroid syndrome, transmitted as an autosomal recessive trait, characterized mainly by low birth weight and length, pseudohydrocephalus, small progeroid facies, widely open cranial sutures, and the presence of the incisor teeth at birth. A peculiar facial appearance is characterized by a triangular old-looking face, sparse hair, low-set ears and eyes, scanty eyebrows, facial bone hypoplasia, prominent scalp veins, micromaxilla, beaked nose, relative prognathism, and subcutaneous lipodystrophy. Additional defects include paradoxical accumulation of adipose tissue on the buttocks and flanks or in the anogenital area, open cranial sutures, persistent fontanels, large hands and feet with long fingers and toes, variable mental deficiency, and delayed growth and motor development.

Wiedemann, H. R. Über die Greisenhaftigkeit im Kindesalter, insbesondere die Gilford'sche Progerie: Zugleich ein Beitrag zum Bereich der mesodermalen Dysplasie. *Zschr. Kinderheilk.*, 1948, 65:670. Wiedemann, H. R. Über einige progeroide Krankheitsbilder und deren diagnostische Einordung. *Zschr. Kinderheilk.*, 1969, 107:91-106. Rautenstrauch, T., *et al.* Progeria: Cell culture study and clinical report of familial incidence. *Eur. J. Pediat.*, 1977, 124:101-11.

Wiedemann-Spranger metaphyseal chondrodysplasia syndrome. Synonyms: *metaphyseal chondrodysplasia, Wiedemann-Spranger type.*

A hereditary form of congenital bone dysplasia, of unknown mode of transmission, characterized mainly by pseudorachitic long bone metaphyses and micromelic dwarfism. Associated defects may include

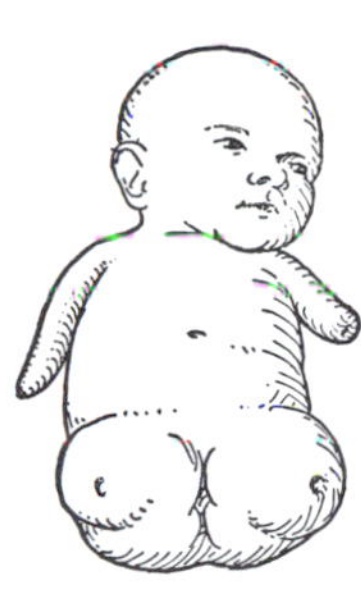
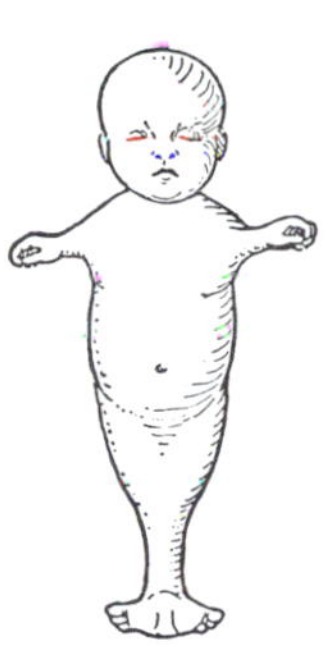

Wiedemann syndrome (1)
Arey, L.B.: *Developmental Anatomy* 7th ed. Philadelphia: W.B. Saunders Co., 1965.

brevicollis, crura vara, limited hip motion, antimongoloid palpebral slant, hourglass appearance of the vertebral bodies on x-rays, slender hands and feet, hypermobility of the shoulders and wrists, frequent lordosis, and swelling around the knees, wrists, and ankles. There is gradual improvement with catch-up growth later in childhood.

Wiedemann, H. R., & Spranger, J. Chondrodysplasia metaphysaria (Dysostosis metaphysaria)-ein neuer Typ? *Zschr. Kinderheilk.*, 1970, 108:171.

Wiedemann-Tolksdorf syndrome. A syndrome of mental retardation, delayed speech development, accelerated growth, peculiar sheep-like facies, and minor deformities of the fingers and toes. Craniofacial abnormalities consist mainly of brachymorphic skull, hypertelorism, large nose with a wide and deeply set root and wide nostrils, long nasal septum, long philtrum, large mouth, high-arched palate, low-set malformed ears, strabismus, exophthalmos, and low posterior hairline. Digital anomalies include thick thumbs, clinodactyly, long distal digits of the fingers, crura valga, pedes excavati, and dorsal flexion of short and wide phalanges of the big toes. The cytogenetic findings show duplication of the long arm of chromosome 2.

Wiedemann, H. R., & Tolksdorf, M. Fehlbildungs-Retardierungs-Syndrom mit "Schafsgesicht" und autosomaler Strukturanomalie. *Klin. Pädiat., Stuttgart,* 1973, 185:346-51.

WIETHE, CAMILLO (Austrian physician, 1888-1949)

Rössle-Urbach-Wiethe syndrome. See *Urbach-Wiethe syndrome.*

Urbach-Wiethe disease (UWD). See *Urbach-Wiethe syndrome.*

Urbach-Wiethe syndrome. See *under Urbach.*

wife abuse. See *battered spouse syndrome.*

wife beating. See *battered spouse syndrome.*

WILDERVANCK, L. S. (Dutch physician)

Franceschetti-Klein-Wildervanck syndrome. See *Wildervanck syndrome (1).*

Wildervanck syndrome (1). Synonyms: *Francheschetti-Klein-Wildervanck syndrome, Wildervanck-Waardenburg-Francheschetti-Klein syndrome, cervico-oculo-acoustic dysplasia, cervico-oculo-acoustic dystrophy, cervico-oculo-acoustic syndrome, cervico-oculo-acusticus syndrome, cervico-oculofacial dysmorphia, cervico-oculofacial syndrome.*

A syndrome of fused cervical vertebrae with torticollis (the Klippel-Feil synd ome), abducens palsy with retractio bulbi (the Duane syndrome), and congenital perceptive deafness. Associated defects may include facial hypoplasia, facial and cranial asymmetry, preauricular tags, subconjunctival lipoma, dental anomalies, micrognathia, narrow palate, cleft palate, mental retardation, epibulbar epidermoids, nystagmus, and heterochromia iridis. The syndrome occurs almost exclusively in females.

Wildervanck, L. S. Een geval van aandoening van Klippel-Feil, gecombineerd med abducensparalyse, retractio bulbi en doofstombeid. *Ned. Tschr. Geneesk.*, 1952, 96:2751-3122. Waardenburg, P. J. Über Retractio bulbi mi Begleiterscheinungen. *Graefes Arch. Ophth.*, 1953, 154:96-109. Francheschetti, A., & Klein, D. Dysmorphie cervico-oculo-faciale avec surdité familiale (Klippel-Feil, retractio bulbi, asymetrie cranio-facialie et autres anomalies congenitales). *J. Genét. Hum.*, 1954, 3:176-83.

Wildervanck syndrome (2). Synonyms: *dysostosis zygomaticomandibulofacialis, zygomaticomandibulofacial dysostosis.*

A congenital syndrome of mental retardation and multiple abnormalities. Craniofacial abnormalities include a small head, large low-set ears, low hairline on the forehead, hooked nose, micrognathia, and malformed teeth. Microphthalmia with only parts of the irides being present, hydrophthalmos (buphthalmos, infantile glaucoma), pale papillae of the optic nerves, and decreased visual acuity are the ocular features. Additional symptoms include small stature, perceptive deafness, hypospadias, and abnormal urethra.

Wildervanck, L. S. A first-arch-syndrome variant? *Lancet*, 1968, 2:350.

Wildervanck syndrome (3). Synonym: *deafness-ear pits syndrome.*

A familial syndrome, transmitted as an autosomal dominant trait, characterized by preauricular sinuses (marginal pits), preauricular appendages, malformed ear auricles, and conductive hearing loss.

Wildervanck, L. S. Hereditary malformatiaons of the ear in three generations. *Acta Otolar.*, 1962, 54:553-60.

Wildervanck syndrome (4). Synonym: *congenital deafness-split hands and feet syndrome.*

A syndrome of congenital deafness and split hands and feet. Some cases are familial and are transmitted as an autosomal recessive trait; others are sporadic.

Wildervanck, L. S. Deafness associated with split hands and feet in two sibliings. A new syndrome. *Proc. 11th Internat. Cong. Genet., Hague*, 1963, pp. 286-7.

Wildervanck-Waardenburg-Francheschetti-Klein syndrome. See *Wildervanck syndrome (1).*

WILDI, ERWIN (Swiss physician)

Morel-Wildi syndrome. See *under Morel, Ferdinand.*

WILKE, F. (German ophthalmologist)

Meesmann-Wilke disease. See *Meesmann dystrophy.*

WILKIE, SIR DAVID PERCIVAL DALBRECK (British physician, 1881-1938)

Wilkie disease. See *superior mesenteric artery syndrome.*

Wilkie syndrome. See *superior mesenteric artery syndrome.*

WILKINS, LAWSON (American physician)

Wilkins disease. See *congenital adrenal hyperplasia.*

WILKINSON, D. S. (British physician)

Duhring-Sneddon-Wilkinson syndrome. See *Sneddon-Wilkinson syndrome.*

Sneddon-Wilkinson syndrome. See *under Sneddon.*

WILKINSON, JOHN FREDERICK (British physician, born 1897)

Israëls-Wilkinson anemia. See *Wilkinson anemia.*

Wilkinson anemia. Synonyms: *Israëls-Wilkinson anemia, achrestic anemia.*

An obscure form of megaloblastic anemia due to folic acid deficiency. It resembles pernicious anemia, except for the lack of gastrointestinal disorders and glossitis and the presence of free hydrochloric acid in the gastric juice.

Israëls, M. C. G., & Wilkinson, J. F. Achrestic anaemia. *Q. J. Med.*, 1936, 5:69-103.

WILKINSON, ROBERT H. (British physician, born 1926)

Moncrieff-Wilkinson syndrome. See *Moncrieff syndrome.*

Wilkinson syndrome. Synonym: *sclerotic pedicle syndrome.*

A spinal disorder characterized by unilateral sclerosis of a lumbar pedicle associated with stress hypertrophy of the pars interarticularis on the contralateral side. Most cases are asymptomatic but back pain and scoliosis may occur in some patients.

Wilkinson, R. H., & Hall, J. E. The sclerotic pedicle: Tumor or pseudotumor? *Radiology*, 1974, 11:683-8.

WILKINSON, SCOTT J. (American physician)

Wilkinson syndrome. Synonym: *cryptogenic infantile cyanosis.*

Cyanosis in otherwise apparently normal infants. Reduced hemoglobin level due to an earlier infection is the suspected cause.

Wilkinson, S. J. Acute cryptogenic cyanosis in early infancy. A clinical report of a unique syndrome of infectious (?) origin. *Ilinois Med. J.*, 1947, 91:29-35.

WILKS, SIR SAMUEL (British physician, 1824-1911)

Wilks disease. Synonym: *verruca necrogenica.*

A form of skin tuberculosis characterized by verrucous or warty lesions of the fingers and caused by inoculation with *Mycobacterium tuberculosis.* It is seen in persons engaged in the handling of infected animals or in dissection of cadavers.

Wilks, S. Disease of the skin produced by post-mortem examinations, or verruca naecrogenica. *Guy's Hosp. Rep., London*, 1862, 8:263-5.

WILLAN, ROBERT (British physician, 1757-1812)

Willan lepra. Synonyms: *Willan-Plumbe syndrome, alphos, lepra alphos, lepra Graecorum, psora, psoriasis vulgaris.*

A chronic, occasionally acute, inflammatory disease of the skin characterized by erythrosquamous lesions which may have annular, circulate, follicular, geographic, guttate, gyrate, nummular pustular, or serpinginous forms. Circular plaques are predominant on the elbows, knees, and the retroauricular areas of the scalp; the guttate form is confined to the trunk and proximal extremities; and the generalized type involves the entire body, presenting erythema. Pitting and thickening of the fingernails with lifting and flaring, and oil droplets under the nails are usually associated. Inflammatory, frequently polyarticular, joint diseases complicate some cases. The condition appears to be transmitted as an autosomal dominant trait.

*Willan, R. *Description and treatment of cutaneous diseases.* London, 1796-1808. Vol. 1, pp. 132-88. *Plumbe, S. *A practical treatise on diseases of the skin.* London, 1824. Christophers, E., & Krueger, G. G. Psoriasis. In:

Fitzpatrick, T. B., Eisen, A. Z., Wolff, K., Freedberg, I. M., & Austen, K. F., eds. *Dermatology in general medicine.* 3rd ed. New York, McGraw-Hill, 1987, pp. 461-91.

Willan-Plumbe syndrome. See *Willan lepra.*

WILLEBRAND, ERIK ADOLF, VON (Finnish physician, 1870-1949)

Minot-von Willebrand syndrome. See *Willebrand-Jürgens syndrome.*

von Willebrand disease (vWD). See *Willebrand-Jürgens syndrome.*

von Willebrand factor deficiency. See *Willebrand-Jürgens syndrome.*

von Willebrand syndrome. See *Willebrand-Jürgens syndrome.*

Willebrand syndrome. See *Willebrand-Jürgens syndrome.*

Willebrand-Jürgens syndrome. Synonyms: *Minot-von Willebrand syndrome, von Willebrand disease (vWD), von Willebrand factor deficiency, von Willebrand syndrome, angiohemophilia, constitutional thrombopathy, hereditary hemorrhagic thrombasthenia, hereditary pseudohemophilia, pseudohemophilia, vascular hemophilia.*

A hemorrhagic disease, inherited as an autosomal dominant, recessive, or X-linked trait, affecting both sexes. It is characterized by prolonged bleeding time in the presence of normal platelet count, associated with epistaxis and bleeding from the gastrointestinal tract, gums, uterus, and at the sites of surgical operations. Most patients have abnormal platelet aggregation in response to the antibiotic ristocetin, low levels of factor VIII procoagulant activity, and decreased amounts of factor VIII-von Willebrand protein. Capillary abnormalities have been reported in most cases. The disease was originally reported in members of three branches of a large family living in the Aland Islands on the Baltic Sea. See also *hemophilia A.*

Willebrand, E. A., von, & Jürgens, R. Über ein neues vererbbares Blutungsübel: Die konstitutionelle Thrombopathie. *Deut. Arch. Klin. Med.*, 1933, 175:453-83. Willebrand, E. A., von. Hereditär pseudohemofili. *Fin. Läkaresäl. Handl.*, 1926, 68:87. Weiss, H. J. Von Willebrand disease. In: Williams, W. J., Beutler, E., Erslev, A. J., & Lichtman, M. A., eds. *Hematology*, 3rd ed. New York, McGraw-Hill, 1983, pp. 1413-20.

WILLI, HEINRICH (Swiss pediatrician, 1900-1971)

Prader-Labhart-Willi syndrome (PLW, PLWS). See *Prader-Willi syndrome.*

Prader-Labhart-Willi-Fanconi syndrome. See *Prader-Willi syndrome.*

Prader-Willi syndrome (PWS). See *under Prader.*

WILLIAMS, E. D. (British physician)

Williams-Pollock syndrome. See *mucosal neuromas syndrome.*

WILLIAMS, HOWARD (Australian physician)

Williams-Campbell syndrome. Congenital bronchiectasis due to a deficiency of bronchial cartilage, of unknown etiology. Early symptoms include persistent cough, wheezing, rhonchi, crepitations and recurrent fever which develop in early infancy after a mild respiratory infection or after measles or pneumonia. Bronchial and bronchiolar obstruction, partial pulmonary collapse, pulmonary fibrosis, and emphysema may result. Death may occur before the age of 5 years; those who survive suffer from frequent respiratory infections and their capacity for physical activity is limited.

Williams, H., & Campbell, P. Generalized bronchiectasis associated with deficiency of cartilage in the bronchial tree. *Arch. Dis. Child., London*, 1960, 35:182-91.

WILLIAMS, J. C. P. (Physician in New Zealand)

Williams syndrome. Synonyms: *Beuren syndrome, Fanconi-Schlesinger syndrome, Williams-Barratt syndrome, Williams-Beuren syndrome, elfin facies, elfin facies syndrome, idiopathic hypercalcemia-supravalvular aortic stenosis syndrome.*

A syndrome of typical (elfinlike) facies, mental retardation, growth deficiency, cardiovascular anomalies, and idiopathic infantile hypercalcemia. Facial characteristics consist of midfacial hypoplasia, depressed nasal bridge, anteverted nostrils, long philtrum, thick lips, wide intercommissural distance, and open mouth. Medial eyebrow flaring, short palpebral fissures, hypotelorism, epicanthus, periorbital fullness, and strabismus are usually associated. Most affected persons are blue-eyed with a stellate iris pattern. Corneal and lenticular opacities and blepharoptosis occur in some instances. Hypercalcemia is a frequent but not constant feature. Craniosynostosis, retarded bone age, and increased density of the metaphyses, epiphyses, and skull are the principal osseous defects. Pes excavatum, hallux valgus, clinodactyly, and onychohypoplasia have been noted in some cases. Microcephaly, mental retardation, and unusual personality, whereby the affected children are overly friendly and loquacious, are the main neurological features. Cardiovascular defects consist mainly of supravalvular or valvular aortic stenosis, aortic hypoplasia, coarctation of the aorta, stenosis of the pulmonary artery, stenosis of peripheral arteries, and other defects. Dental complications include hypodontia, microdontia, small slender tooth roots, and dens invaginatus. Most thus far reported cases have been sporadic.

Williams, J. C., Barratt-Boyes, B. G., & Lowe, J. B. Supravalvular aortic stenosis. *Circulation*, 1961, 24:1311-8. Beuren, A. J. Supravalvular aortic stenosis: A complex

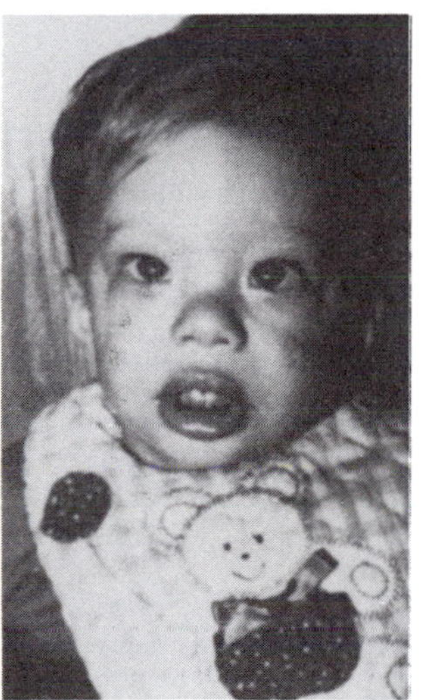

Williams syndrome
Kaplan, Lawrence C., Robert Wharton, Ellen Elias, Frederick Mandell, Timothy Donlon & Samuel A. Latt: *American Journal of Medical Genetics* 28:45-53, 1987. New York: Alan R. Liss, Inc.

syndrome with and without mental retardation. *Birth Defects*, 1972, 8(5):45-56. Fanconi, G., *et al.* Chronische Hyperkalämie, kombiniert mit Osteosklerose, Hyperazotämie, Minderwuchs und kongenitalen Missbildungen. *Helv. Paediat. Acta*, 1952, 7:314-49.

Williams-Barratt syndrome. See *Williams syndrome.*

Williams-Beuren syndrome. See *Williams syndrome.*

WILLIS, THOMAS (British physician, 1621-1675)

Willis disease. Synonym: *asthma.*

An allergic disease characterized by narrowing of the airways due to increased responsiveness of the trachea and bronchi to various stimuli. Wheezing, cough, and dyspnea are the principal symptoms.

Willis, T. On the convulsive cough and asthma. In his: *Practice of physick.* London, Dring, 1684, Pt. e, pp. 92-6. Daniele, R. P. Asthma. In: Wyngaarden, J. B., & Smith, L. H., Jr., eds. *Cecil textbook of medicine.* 17th ed. Philadelphia, Saunders, 1985, pp. 390-6.

WILLS, LUCY (British scientist)

Wills anemia. Synonyms: *nutritional megaloblastic anemia in India, pernicious anemia of pregnancy.*

Megalocytic anemia, often associated with pregnancy and usually occurring in Indian women. The symptoms include weakness, diarrhea, vomiting, glossitis, edema of the ankles and feet, and hypotension. A folic acid deficiency appears to be the cause.

Wills, L., & Mehta, M. M. Studies in "pernicious anemia" of pregnancy. I. Preliminary report. *Indian J. Med. Res.*, 1930, 17:777-92.

WILMS, MAX (German physician, 1867-1918)

Wilms nephroblastoma. See *Wilms tumor.*

Wilms tumor (WT). Synonyms: *Birch-Hirschfeld tumor, Wilms nephroblastoma, embryoma, embryonal adenosarcoma, embryonal carcinosarcoma, embryonal mixed tumor, embryonal nephroma, embryonal sarcoma, nephroblastoma.*

A highly malignant, usually unilateral tumor of the kidney in the form of a large gray or white, solid or cystic mass that may dwarf the kidney. In the early stages some tumors are encapsulated, but they usually rupture and perirenal structures become invaded. Histologically, the tumor consists of embryonic kidney tissue with elongated cells that form abortive glomeruli and tubules. Cartilage, bone, striated muscle, and fibrous tissue may also be found. Infants and children are chiefly affected.

Wilms, M. *Die Mischgeschwülste. I. Die Mischgeschwülste der Niere.* Leipzig, 1899. Birch-Hirschfeld, F. V. Sarkomatöse Drüsengeschwulst der Niere im Kindesalter (Embryonales Adenosarkom). *Beitr. Path. Anat.*, 1898, 24:343-62.

Wilms tumor-aniridia syndrome. See *aniridia-Wilms tumor syndrome.*

WILSON, CLIFFORD (British physician, born 1906)

Kimmelstiel-Wilson syndrome. See *under Kimmelstiel.*

WILSON, JAMES LEROY (American physician, born 1898)

Jirásek-Zuelzer-Wilson syndrome. See *under Jirásek.*

Zuelzer-Wilson syndrome. See *Jirásek-Zuelzer-Wilson syndrome.*

WILSON, KEITH S. (American physician)

Wilson-Alexander syndrome. The triad of periarteritis nodosa, bronchial asthma, and hypereosinophilia.

Wilson, K. S., & Alexander, H. L. The association of periarteritis nodosa, bronchial asthma, and hypereosinophilia. *J. Lab. Clin. Med.*, 1945, 30:361-3.

WILSON, MIRIAM GEISENDORFER (American pediatrician, born 1922)

respiratory distress syndrome of Wilson and Mikity. See *Wilson-Mikity syndrome.*

Wilson-Mikity (WM) syndrome. Synonyms: *bronchopulmonary dysplasia (BPD), bubbly lung syndrome, interstitial pulmonary fibrosis of prematurity, pulmonary anectasis, pulmonary dysmaturity syndrome, respiratory distress syndrome of Wilson and Mikity.*

A type of respiratory distress which occurs primarily in premature infants of less than 32 weeks gestation and weighing less than 1500 g. After a symptomless period of a few days or weeks, there is onset of dyspnea, tachypnea, retraction, cough, cyanotic episodes, fine rales, transient edema, and occasional lung collapse or heart failure. Radiological findings usually show early coarse streaky infiltrates and small cystic areas on the lungs followed by enlargement and coalescence of cystic foci (hence the synonym the *bubbly lung syndrome*) with hyperexpansion of the lower lobes and densities in the upper lobes, heart enlargement, and dilation of the pulmonary artery, resulting in pulmonary hypertension. After a period of several weeks, there is a regression of symptoms, and respiration becomes normal with maturity. See also *neonatal respiratory distress syndrome, sudden infant death syndrome,* and *infant apnea syndrome.*

Wilson, M. G., & Mikity, V. G. A new form of respiratory distress in premature infants. *Am. J. Dis. Child.*, 1960, 99:489-99.

WILSON, RALPH V. (American orthopedic surgeon, born 1938)

Hecht-Beals-Wilson syndrome. See *trismus-pseudocamptodactyly syndrome.*

WILSON, SAMUEL ALEXANDER KINNIER (British neurologist, 1878-1936)

Foville-Wilson syndrome. See *under Foville.*

Kinnier Wilson disease. See *Wilson disease.*

Wilson disease. Synonyms: *Kinnier Wilson disease, Westphal pseudosclerosis, Westphal-Strümpell syndrome, Wilson-Konovalov disease, cerebral pseudosclerosis, hepatocerebral degeneration, hepatocerebral dystrophy, hepatolenticular degeneration, neurohepatic degeneration, progressive lenticular degeneration.*

A hereditary syndrome, transmitted as an autosomal recessive trait, characterized by low ceruloplasmin levels and excessive accumulation of copper in various organs, chiefly the brain, liver, kidneys, and cornea, with faulty biliary copper excretion. The age of onset varies from early childhood to middle age. The symptoms frequently begin with hepatitis or cirrhosis of the liver and are followed by nodular cirrhosis, hepatomegaly (sometimes with splenomegaly), gastrointestinal bleeding, esophageal varices, ascites, anorexia, deglutition disorders, speech difficulties, and lassitude. Intellectual deterioration may be manifested at first by dystonia or abnormal posturing. Extrapyramidal signs may include tremor at rest, rigidity, dysarthria, clumsiness, and a set expression of the face with an open drooling mouth and the teeth exposed in a grimacing smile. Flapping tremor is a late finding. Speech disorders include slurring, high-pitched voice, and intermittent incoherence. As the disease progresses, there are periodic athetoid movements which develop into a fixed dystonic posture. The wrist is frequently held in extreme flexion. Deposition of copper in the Descemet membrane produces Kayser-Fleischer rings with resulting golden brown or grayish-green coloration. Night blindness, sunflower cataract, nystagmus, and extra-ocular muscle palsies are frequently associated.

Wilson, S. A. Progressive lenticular degeneration. A familial nervous disease associated with cirrhosis of the liver. *Brain,* 1912, 34:295-509. Westphal, K. F. Über eine dem Bilde der cerebrospinalen grauen Degeneration ähnliche Erkrankung des zentralen Nervensystems ohne anatomischen Befund, nebst einigen Bemerkungen über paradoxe Kontraktionen. *Arch. Psychiat., Berlin,* 1883, 14:87-134. Strümpell, A., von. Über die Westphalsche Pseudosclerose und über diffuse Hirnsklerose, insbesondere bei Kindern. *Deut. Zschr. Nervenh.,* 1898, 12:114-49. Katsiuba, K. A., & Gzulia, I. I. Gepato-tserebral'naia distrofia u edetei. *Zdravookhr. Kazakhstana,* 1963, No. 4:61. *Konovalov, N. V. *Gepato-tserebral'naia distrofiia.* Moskva, Medgiz, 1960.

Wilson-Konovalov disease. See *Wilson disease.*

WILSON, SIR WILLIAM ERASMUS (British physician, 1809-1884)

Wilson disease (1). Synonyms: *dermatitis exfoliativa generalisata subacuta, eczema exfoliativum, exfoliative dermatitis.*

A form of dermatitis in which the skin is covered with lamellated exfoliating scales, the affected areas varying in color from crimson erysipelatous to purple. The extremities, back, neck, face, and chest are most frequently affected. The scalp may be covered with a crust formed by sebum. Thickening of the nail beds, dystrophy of the nails, and alopecia may develop. Various cutaneous, systemic, and drug-induced diseases may be associated with this disorder.

Wilson, E. On dermatitis exfoliativa. *Med. Times Gaz., London,* 1870, 1:118-20. Freedberg, I. M., & Baden, H. P. Exfoliative dermatitis. In: Fitzpatrick, T. B., Eisen, A. Z., Wolff, K., Freedberg, I. M., & Austen, K. F., eds. *Dermatology in general medicine.* 3rd ed. New York, McGraw-Hill, 1987, pp. 502-5.

Wilson disease (2). Synonyms: *lichen planus, lichen ruber planus, lichen psoriasis.*

A pruritic skin disease marked by the violaceous, scaling, angular patches usually found on the flexor surfaces, mucous membranes, and genitalia. The eruption may be distributed as isolated lesions or in aggregate patterns.

Wilson, E. On lichen planus: The lichen ruber of Hebra. *Brit. Med. J.,* 1866, 2:399-402. Arndt, K. A. Lichen planus. In: Fitzpatrick, T. B., Eisen, A. Z., Wolff, K., Freedberg, I. M., & Austen, K. F., eds. *Dermatology in general medicine.* 3rd ed. New York, McGraw-Hill, 1987, pp. 967-73.

WINCHESTER, PATRICIA (American physician)

Winchester syndrome. See *carpotarsal osteolysis syndrome (recessive form).*

Winchester-Grossman syndrome. See *carpotarsal osteolysis syndrome (recessive form).*

WINCKEL, FRANZ KARL LUDWIG WILHELM, VON (German physician, 1837-1911)

Winckel disease. See *Winckel-Charrin syndrome.*

Winckel-Charrin syndrome. Synonyms: *Winckel disease, bronzed disease of the newborn, neonatal hemoglobinuria.*

Hemoglobinuria in newborn infants, associated with jaundice, bleeding tendency, and cyanosis.

Charrin, S. *Maladie bronzée hematique des enfants nouveau-née (tubulhematie renale de M. Parrot.* Paris, 1873. (Thesis). Winckel, F. Über eine bisher nicht beschriebene endemisch aufgetretene Erkrankung Neugeborener. *Deut. Med. Wschr.,* 1879:303-7; 415-8; 431-6; 447-50.

windblown hip syndrome. The triad of hip dislocation, pelvic obliquity, and scoliosis.

Letts, M., *et al.* The windblown hip syndrome in total body cerebral palsy. *J. Pediat. Orthop.,* 1984, 4:55-62.

windmill-vane camptodactyly/ichthyosis syndrome. A syndrome combining ichthyosis with features of the Freeman-Sheldon syndrome (camptodactyly ulnar deviation of the fingers, talipes equinovarus, and facial immobility). It is transmitted as an autosomal recessive trait.

Baraitser, M., *et al.* A recessively inherited windmill-vane camptodactyly/ichthyosis syndrome. *J. Med. Genet.,* 1983, 20:125-7.

windmill-vane fingers syndrome. See *Freeman-Sheldon syndrome.*

WINIWARTER, FELIX, VON (Austrian physician, 1848-1917)

Winiwarter-Buerger syndrome. See *Buerger syndrome.*

winking jaw syndrome. See *Gunn syndrome.*

WINKLER, C.

Fickler-Winkler syndrome. See *OPCA II, under olivopontocerebellar atrophy.*

olivopontocerebellar atrophy (OPCA), Fickler-Winkler type. See *OPCA II, under olivopontocerebellar atrophy.*

WINKLER, MAX (Swiss physician)

Winkler disease. Synonyms: *chondrodermatitis helicis, chondrodermatitis nodularis chronica helicis.*

A painful disorder of the ear characterized by hard round nodules about 3 to 10 mm in diameter, involving the skin and cartilage. The nodules have depressed cupped surfaces covered by adherent crusty scales and pinhead-sized ulcerations in their centers. Histological findings include inflammatory processes in the corium and cartilage, skin hypertrophy and edema, vascular proliferation, and collagen degeneration.

Winkler, M. Knötchenförmige Erkrankung am Helix (Chondrodermatitis nodularis chronica helicis). *Arch. Derm. Syph., Berlin,* 1915-16, 121:278-85.

WINTER, JEREMY S. D. (American physician)

Winter syndrome. Synonyms: *Winter-Kohn-Mellman-Wagner syndrome, auro-urogenital syndrome, hereditary renal adysplasia, hereditary renal agenesis, hereditary urogenital adysplasia, urogenital adysplasia.*

A familial syndrome, transmitted as an autosomal dominant trait, characterized by renal dysgenesis, ranging from unilateral hypoplasia to bilateral agenesis, in association with internal genital malformations, in particular vaginal atresia, and anomalies in the ossicles of the middle ear.

Winter, J. S. D., Kohn, G., Mellman, W. J., & Wagner, S. A familial syndrome of renal, genital, and middle ear anomalies. *J. Pediat.,* 1968, 72:88-93.

Winter-Kohn-Mellman-Wagner syndrome. See *Winter syndrome.*

winter feet in children. See *wet and dry foot syndrome.*

winter itch. See *Duhring pruritus.*

winter vomiting disease. See *Spencer disease.*

WISE, FRED (American dermatologist, born 1881)
Wise disease. See *Mucha-Habermann syndrome.*
Wise-Rein disease. See *Kaposi disease (1).*
WISEMAN, BRUCE KENNETH (American physician, born 1898)
Wiseman-Doan syndrome. Synonyms: *primary splenic neutropenia, splenic neutropenia syndrome.*

A granulopenic disorder characterized by splenomegaly and peripheral granulopenia in the presence of normal or hyperplastic bone marrow. Histological examination of the spleen shows clasmacytosis and excessive phagocytosis of the granulocytes with excessive lysis of neutrophils by the spleen.

Wiseman, B. K., & Doan, C. A. A newly recognized granulopenic syndrome caused by excessive splenic leukolysis and successfully treated by splenectomy. *J. Clin. Invest.*, 1939, 18:473.

WISHART, J. H. (British physician)
Wishart disease. Synonym: *central neurofibromatosis.*

Multiple tumors of the spinal nerve roots and auditory nerves, usually associated with Recklinghausen disease (1), nervous system abnormalities, and occasional multiple gliomas. The tumors have the features of meningioma and neurilemmoma. Onset is usually observed during early adult life, and the occurrence is familial.

Wishart, J. H. Case of tumours in the skull, dura mater, and brain. *Edinburgh Med. Surg. J.*, 1822, 18:393-7.

WISKOTT, ALFRED (German pediatrician, 1898-1978)
Wiskott-Aldrich syndrome (WAS). Synonyms: *Aldrich syndrome, Witskott-Aldrich-Huntley syndrome, eczema-thrombocytopenia syndrome, eczema-thrombocytopenia-diarrhea syndrome, eczema-thrombocytopenia-immunodeficiency syndrome, X-linked lymphoproliferative (XLP) syndrome.*

An X-linked immunodeficiency syndrome, occurring only in males, consisting of a triad of frequent infections, eczema, and profound thrombocytopenia. Onset is usually in infancy or early childhood and is characterized by thrombocytopenic purpura, eczema, bloody diarrhea, and extreme susceptibility to infection (especially of the skin, middle ear, sinuses, and lungs), in association with antibody deficiency and dysgammaglobulinemia. Low immunoglobulin M, elevated immunoglobulin E, and low isoagglutinins are consistently present. Malignant neoplasms, eosinophilia, leukocytosis, myeloid hyperplasia, anemia, hypoaminoaciduria, joint effusions, and cortical hyperstosis may occur. Without therapy, most affected boys seldom survive past 10 years of age.

Wiskott, A. Familiärer angeborener Morbus Werlhoffi? *Mschr. Kinderh.*, 1937, 68:212-6. Aldrich, R. A., *et al.* Pedigree demonstrating a sex-linked recessive condition characterized by draining ears, eczemataoid dermatitis and bloody diarrhea. *Pediatrics*, 1954, 13:133-9. Huntley, C. C., & Dees, S. C. Eczema associated with thrombocytopenic purpura and purulent otitis media. *Pediatrics*, 1957, 19:351-61.

Wiskott-Aldrich-Huntley syndrome. See *Wiskott-Aldrich syndrome.*
WISSER, P. (German physician)
Schmitt-Wisser disease. See *Schmitt syndrome.*
WISSLER, HANS (Swiss pediatrician, born 1906)
Wissler syndrome. Synonyms: *Wissler-Fanconi syndrome, allergosis sepsiformis, febris periodica hyperergica, pseudosepsis allergica, pseudosepsis allergica erythemato-arthralgica recidivans, pseudosepsis allergogenes, pseudosepticemia syndrome, sepsis allergenica, sepsis hyperergica, subsepsis allergica, subsepsis hyperergica.*

A symptom complex of a high intermittent fever, recurring exanthema, transient arthralgia, carditis, pleurisy, neurotrophil leukocytosis, and increased erythrocyte sedimentation rate. Wissler suggested an allergic reaction to bacteremia as the pathogenic factor. Children and adolescents are most frequently affected.

Wissler, H. Über eine besondere Form sepsisähnlicher Krankheiten (Subsepsis hyperergica). *Mschr. Kinderh.*, 1943, 94:1-15. Fanconi, G. Über einen Fall von Subsepsis allergica Wissler. *Helvet. Paediat. Acta*, 1945-46, 1:532-7.

Wissler-Fanconi syndrome. See *Wissler syndrome.*
withdrawal syndrome. Synonyms: *abstinence syndrome, drug withdrawal disease, substance withdrawal syndrome.*

An organic brain syndrome of neurological and psychological disorders which follow the cessation of or reduction in the intake of addicting substances, the type and severity of disorders varying with individual substances. **Alcohol withdrawal syndrome** or **AWS** (**alcohol abstinence syndrome** or **AAS, ethanol abstinence syndrome**) (see also **Morel disease**) is marked by a coarse tremor of the hands, tongue, and eyelids, nausea, vomiting, malaise or weakness, sweating, tachycardia, anxiety, depression or irritability, and orthostatic hypotension. Associated disorders may include xerostomia, a puffy and blotchy face, mild peripheral edema, sleep disorders, nightmares, hallucinations, and precipitation of pre-existing epileptic seizures. **Amphetamine withdrawal syndrome** is produced by recent cessation or reduction in intake of amphetamines or some sympathomimetic drug, characterized by a depressed mood, fatigue, sleep disorders, and increased dreaming. Associated disorders may include agitated behavior and suicidal tendencies. **Barbiturate withdrawal syndrome** v.i. **opioid withdrawal syndrome. Caffeine withdrawal** is marked by headache, sometimes with drowsiness, lethargy, rhinorrhea, irritability, nervousness, depression, nausea, and occasional yawning. **Opioid withdrawal syndrome** occurrs after the cessation of or reduction of intake of an opioid sedative or hypnotic substances, including barbiturates (**barbiturate withdrawal syndrome**), and includes slurred speech, incoordination, unsteady gait, impaired attention, memory disorders, mood lability, disinhibition of sexual and aggressive impulses, irritability, loquacity, and delirium. **Tobacco withdrawal syndrome** is characterized mainly by irritability, restlessness, dullness, sleep disruptions, gastrointestinal disorders, headache, impaired concentration, memory disorders, anxiety, and, frequently, an increased appetite, EEG changes, decreased heart rate, hypotension, increased muscle contractins, reduced physical performance, and weight gain. See also *steroid withdrawal syndrome.*

Diagnostic and statistical manual of mental disorders. 3rd ed. Washington, D. C., American Psychiatric Association, 1980, p. 480. Kaplan, H. I., & Sadock, B. J., eds. *Comprehensive textbook of psychiatry.* 4th ed. Baltimore, Williams & Wilkins, 1985, 1054 p.

WITKOP, CARL JACOB, JR. (American oral pathologist, born 1920)

Witkop syndrome (1). See *tooth-nail syndrome.*

Witkop syndrome (2). See *amelo-onychohypohidrotic syndrome.*

Witkop syndrome (3). See *hereditary mucoepithelial dysplasia.*

Witkop-Von Sallmann syndrome. Synonyms: *Von Sallmann-Paton syndrome, hereditary benign intraepithelial dyskeratosis.*

A familial syndrome, transmitted as an autosomal dominant trait, originally reported among members of a triracial isolate group of a mixed Caucasian, American Indian, and Negro ancestry in North Carolina. The symptoms include leukoplakialike lesions of the oral mucosa, presenting spongy, macerated lesions varying from delicate opalescent white membranous areas to a rough shaggy mucosa, frequently involving the corners of the mouth. Ocular symptoms include pterygiumlike lesions, presenting superficial, foamy, gelatinous white plaques overlying the cornea, leading to blindness.

Von Sallmann, L., & Paton, D. Hereditary benign intraepithelial dyskeratosis. I. Ocular manifestations. *Arch. Ophth., Chicago,* 1960, 63:421-9. Witkop, C. J., Jr., *et al.* Hereditary benign intraepithelial dyskeratosis. II. Oral manifestations and hereditary transmission. *Arch. Path., Chicago,* 1960, 70:696-711.

Witkop-Weech-Giansanti syndrome. See *tooth-nail syndrome.*

WITTMAACK, THEODOR (German physician)

Wittmaack-Ekbom syndrome. See *restless leg syndrome.*

WITTS, LESLIE JOHN (British physician, born 1898)

Witts anemia. See *Faber syndrome.*

WKS. See *Wernicke-Korsakoff syndrome.*

WL syndrome. See *facio-audio-symphalangism syndrome.*

WL symphalangism-brachydactyly syndrome. See *facio-audio-symphalangism syndrome.*

WLS. See *wet lung syndrome.*

WM syndrome. See *Wilson-Mikity syndrome, under Wilson, Miriam Geisendorfer.*

WOAKES, E. (British physician)

Woakes syndrome. A syndrome of recurrent nasal polyposis with broadening of the nose, frontal sinus aplasia, bronchiectasis, and dyscrinia (production of a high-viscosity mucus). The syndrome appears to be hereditary.

Woakes, E. Necrosing ethmoiditis and mucous polypi. *Lancet,* 1885, 1:619. Kellerhals, B., & de Uthermann, B. Woakes' syndrome: The problem of infantile polyps. *Internat. J. Pediat. Otorhinolar.,* 1979, 1:79-85.

WOHLFART, GUNNAR (Swedish physician)

Gamstorp-Wohlfart syndrome. See *under Gamstorp.*

WOHLFART, KARL GUNNAR VILHELM (Swedish physician, 1910-1961)

Wohlfart-Kugelberg-Welander syndrome. Synonyms: *Kugelberg-Welander syndrome, atrophia musculorum pseudomyopathica, hereditary proximal neurogenic muscular atrophy, hereditary proximal spinal muscular atrophy, juvenile progressive spinal muscular atrophy, juvenile spinal muscular atrophy, progressive muscular dystrophy with fibrillary twitching, progressive myelopathic muscular atrophy, progressive spinal muscular atrophy, proximal spinal muscular atrophy, pseudomyopathic spinal muscular atrophy, spinal muscular atrophy III (SMA III).*

A slowly progressive hereditary form of juvenile muscular atrophy, secondary to anterior horn lesions, with onset between the ages of 2 and 17 years. The early symptoms, consisting of atrophy and weakness of the proximal muscles of the extremities, mainly the legs, are followed by involvement of the muscles of the trunk and distal muscles of the extremities. Fasciculation and electromyographic disorders indicate lesions of the spinal motor neurons. Dominant and recessive forms of inheritance have been reported. See also *Werdnig-Hoffmann syndrome.*

Wohlfart, G. Zwei Fälle von Dystrophia musculorum progressiva mit fibrillären Zuckungen und a typischem Muskelbbefund. *Deut. Zschr. Nervenh.,* 1942, 153:189-204. Kugelberg, E., & Welander, L. Heredofamilial juvenile muscular atrophy simulating muscular dystrophy. *Arch. Neur., Chicago,* 1956, 75:500-9.

WOHLMANN, H. (American physician)

Wohlmann-Caglar syndrome. Synonym: *juxtaglomerular hyperplasia-hyperelectrolytemia syndrome.*

A syndrome of polydipsia and polyuria associated with high serum sodium and chloride levels, normal potassium levels, and high renin content in normotensive infants. Pathological findings consist of hyperplasia and hypergranulation of the juxtaglomerular cells.

Wohlmann, M., & Caglar, M. Juxtaglomerular hyperplasia and elevated renin in normotensive infant with high serum sodium and chloride but normal potassium. *Am. J. Path.,* 1971, 62(2):17a-18a.

WOHLWILL, FRIEDRICH (Physician in Portugal)

Wohlwill-Andrade syndrome. See *amyloid neuropathy type I.*

Wohlwill-Corino Andrade syndrome. See *amyloid neuropathy type I.*

WOILLEZ, EUGENE JOSEPH (French physician, 1811-1882)

Woillez disease. Acute idiopathic pulmonary congestion.

Woillez, De la congestion pulmonaire, considérée comme élément habituel des maladies aiguës. *Arch. Gén. Méd., Paris,* 1854, 3:385-400; 566-79.

WOLCOTT, C. D. (American physician)

Wolcott-Rallison syndrome. Synonyms: *multiple epiphyseal dysplasia with early-onset diabetes mellitus syndrome, infancy-onset diabetes mellitus with multiple epiphyseal dysplasia syndrome, spondylo-epiphyseal dysplasia-diabetes mellitus syndrome.*

A familial syndrome, transmitted as an autosomal recessive trait, characterized by infancy-onset diabetes mellitus and multiple epiphyseal dysplasias. Associated disorders include short-trunk dwarfism, bone demineralization, spontaneous fractures, tooth discoloration, skin abnormalities, hip abduction, arthralgia, hepatomegaly, splenomegaly, and renal failure.

Wolcott, C. D., & Rallison, M. L. Infancy-onset diabetes mellitus and multiple epiphyseal dysplasia. *J. Pediat.,* 1972, 80:292-7.

WOLF, ULRICH (German physician)

Wolf syndrome. See *chromosome 4p deletion syndrome.*

Wolf-Hirschhorn syndrome. See *chromosome 4p deletion syndrome.*

WOLFF, G. (American physician)

Wieacker-Wolff syndrome. See *under Wieacker.*

WOLFF, LOUIS (American cardiologist, born 1898)

Wolff-Parkinson-White syndrome (WPW). A cardiac pre-excitation syndrome in which normal sinoatrial impulses are conducted to the ventricles both by way of the atrioventricular node and by an abnormal pathway (the bundle of Kent), conduction being more rapid through the abnormal pathway with resulting early ventricular activation. Bundle branch block with a short P-R interval and a long QRS interval are the principal feature this syndrome. Supraventricular tachycardia, sometimes causing potentially fatal decreased cardiac output, may occur. See also *preexcitation syndrome.*

Wolff, L., Parkinson, J., & White, P. D. Bundle-branch block with short P-R interval in healthy young people prone to paroxysmal tachycardia. *Am. Heart J.,* 1930, 5:685-704.

WOLFRAM, D. J. (American physician)

Wolfram syndrome. See *diabetes insipidus and mellitus with optic atrophy and deafness.*

WOLMAN, MOSHE (Israeli physician, born 1914)

Wolman disease. See *Wolman syndrome.*

Wolman syndrome. Synonyms: *Wolman disease, familial primary xanthomatosis with adrenal calcification, generalized xanthomatosis with calcified adrenals, primary familial xanthomatosis.*

An inborn lipid metabolism disorder due to lysosomal acid hydrolase deficiency, characterized by onset during the first weeks of life, which include failure to thrive, protuberant abdomen, diarrhea, steatorrhea, hepatomegaly, splenomegaly, anemia, low-grade fever, and death by the age of 3 to 6 months. Xanthomatous changes in the adrenals, liver, spleen, lymph nodes, bone marrow, small intestine, lungs, thymus, and less pronounced modifications in the skin, retina, and central nervous system; disseminated foam cell infiltration in the bone marrow and other organs; vacuolization of lymphocytes; and cholesterol accumulation in the liver and other organs are the chief pathological findings. The syndrome is transmitted as an autosomal recessive trait.

Wolman, M., *et al.* Primary familial xanthomatosis with involvement and calcification of the adrenals. Report of two more cases in siblings of a previously described infant. *Pediatrics,* 1961, 28:742-57.

WOLTERS, MAXIMILIAN (MAX) (German dermatologist 1861-1914)

Wolters nevus. Synonym: *nevus epitheliomatosus sebaceus capitis.*

A congenital epithelial nevus of the scalp, derived from sebaceous glands, hair follicles, and sweat glands. The tumor is slightly elevated, hairless, and yellowish red, with irregular borders surrounded by numerous convex nodules varying in size from that of a pinhead to a millet. Widely dilated follicular openings and enlarged twisted capillaries may be observed on the surface.

Wolters, M. Über einen Fall von Naevus epitheliomatosus sebaceus capitis. *Arch. Derm.. Syph., Berlin,* 1910, 101:197-208.

WOLTMAN, HENRY WILLIAM (American physician, 1889-1964)

Moersch-Woltman syndrome (MWS). See *stiff man syndrome.*

wooden tongue. See *Rivalta disease.*

woody thyroid. See *Riedel disease.*

WOOLF, CHARLES M. (American physician)

Woolf syndrome. Synonyms: *Woolf-Dolowitz-Aldous syndrome, Ziprkowski-Margolis syndrome, albinism-deafmutism syndrome, albinism-deafness syndrome, albinism-piebaldism syndrome, oculocutaneous albinism with deafness syndrome.*

A familial syndrome of deafmutism, heterochromia iridis, and piebaldism transmitted as an X-linked recessive trait.

Margolis, E. A new hereditary syndrome-sex-linked deafmutism associated with total albinism. *Acta Genet. Statist. Med.,* 1962, 12:12-9. Ziprkowski, L., *et al.* Partial albinism and deaf-mutism due to a recessive sex-linked gene. *Arch. Derm.,* 1962, 86:530-9. Woolf, C. M., Dolowitz, D. A., & Aldous, H. E. Congenital deafness associated with piebaldism. *Arch. Otolar., Chicago,* 1965, 82:244-50.

Woolf-Dolowitz-Aldous syndrome. See *Woolf syndrome.*

word deafness. See *Wernicke aphasia.*

WORINGER, FREDERIC (French physician, 1903-1964)

Pautrier-Woringer syndrome. See *under Pautrier.*

Woringer-Kolopp syndrome. Synonyms: *Dupont-Vandaele syndrome, epidermotropic cutaneous reticulosis, pagetoid reticulosis.*

A chronic skin disease presenting scaling erythematous lesions with dense intraepidermal infiltration characteristic of cutaneous T-cell lymphoma. The disorder is classified with mycosis fungoides.

Woringer, F., & Kolopp, P. Lésion érythémato-squameuse polycyclique de l'avant-bras évoluant depuis 6 ans chez un garçonnet de 13 ans. Histologiquement infiltrat intra-épidermique d'apparance tumorale. *Ann. Derm. Syph., Paris,* 1939, 10:945-8. Dupont, A., & Vandaele, R. Réticulose cutanée épidermotrope accompagneé de lésions gastriques et vertebrales. *Arch. Belg. Derm. Syph.,* 1959, 15:267-74.

WORINGER, PIERRE (French physician, 1890-1964)

Woringer syndrome. A disease considered to be a manifestation of faulty fat assimilation that occurs predominantly in children fed fat-rich food. The symptoms include hepatomegaly with attacks of colicky pain, headache, vomiting, nausea, fatigbility, and pallor which are usually precipitated by ingestion of fats.

Woringer, P. Lipidogene Dyshepatie. *Mschr. Kinderh.,* 1943-44, 93:279-96.

WORSTER-DROUGHT, C. V. (British physician)

Worster-Drought syndrome. Synonym: *congenital suprabulbar paresis.*

Congenital suprabulbar paresis transmitted as an autosomal dominant trait with variable expression of penetrance. It is characterized by a selective weakness and impairment of movement of the orbicularis oris muscle, the tongue, and the soft palate, resulting in dysarthria, dribbling, dysphagia, and inability to protrude the tongue. In severe cases there may be involvement of the pharyngeal and laryngeal muscles. Some patients have epilepsy, deafness, and mental retardation. Worster-Drought suggested that a lesion of the motor tract from the motor cortex to the tenth and twelfth nerve nuclei is the cause, but other writers suspect that there may be more generalized lesions.

Worster-Drought, C. Congenital suprabulbar paresis. *J. Laryng. Otol.,* 1956, 70:453-63. Patton, M. A., *et al.* A family with congenital suprabulbar paresis (Worster-Drought syndrome). *Clin. Genet.,* 1986, 29:147-50.

WORTH, H. M. (Canadian physician)

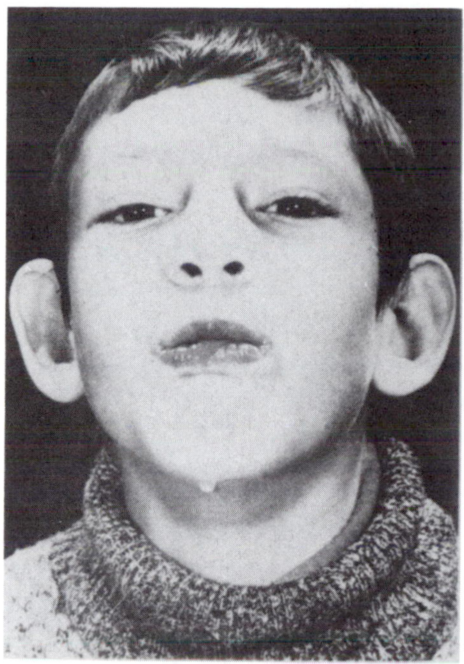

Worster-Drought syndrome
Patton, M.A., M. Baraitser & E.M. Brett, *Clinical Genetics* 29:147-150, 1986. Munksgaard International Publishers, Copenhagen, Denmark.

Worth syndrome. A benign form of congenital hyperostosis corticalis generalisata, transmitted as an autosomal dominant trait, characterized mainly by widened and deepened mandible with increased gonial angle. Endosteal sclerosis of the calvarium with loss of the diploe, osteosclerosis, and hyperostosis of the mandible with absence of the normal antegonial notches, endosteal sclerosis of the diaphyses of long bones, and osteosclerosis of the pelvic bones are the principal radiographic findings. Some involvement of the vertebral bodies, ribs, and clavicles may occur.

Worth, H. M., & Wollin, D. G. Hyperostosis corticalis generalisata congenita. *J.. Canad. Assoc. Radiol.*, 1976, 49:126-32.

WOUDE, ANNE, VAN DER. See VAN DER WOUDE, ANNE

WPW. See *Wolff-Parkinson-White syndrome.*

WRIEDT, C.

Mohr-Wriedt brachydactly. See *brachydactly A-2.*

WRIGHT, IRVING SHERWOOD (American physician, born 1901)

Wright syndrome. See *hyperabduction syndrome.*

wrinkly skin syndrome. A heritable disorder of connective tissue, transmitted as an autosomal recessive trait, characterized by congenital wrinkled skin about the hands and feet, together with an increase of creases on the ventral surfaces. Associated anomalies include poorly developed and hypotonic muscles and winging of the scapulae.

Gazit, E., *et al.* The wrinkly skin syndrome: A new heritable disorder of connective tissue. *Clin. Genet.*, 1973, 4:186-92.

writer's cramps. See *under overuse syndrome.*

WRONG, OLIVER (British physician)

Wrong-Davies syndrome. An incomplete form of the syndrome of renal tubular acidosis with nephrocalcinosis and inability to excrete urine of normal minimum pH in the absence of extracellular acidosis. The affected persons have relatively normal glomerular filtration rate and high levels of ammonium excretion, which prevent them from developing acidosis.

Wrong, O., & Davies, H. E. F. The excretion of acid in renal disease. *Q. J. Med.*, 1959, 28:259-313.

WRS. See *Wiedemann-Rautenstrauch syndrome.*

wryneck. See *Cruchet disease.*

WS. See *Werner syndrome, under Werner, Otto.*

WS. See *West syndrome.*

WS (Warkany syndrome). See *chromosome 8 trisomy syndrome.*

WT. See *Wilms tumor.*

WT syndrome. Synonym: *WT limb-blood syndrome.*

An association of radial or ulnar hypoplasia with panmyelocytopenia, transmitted as an autosomal dominant trait with variable expressivity and complete penetrance. Hand anomalies may include ulnar deviation of the first or third fingers, shortness, clinodactyly, and/or camptodactyly, usually of the fifth fingers, and tapering of the thumb with or without thenar hypoplasia. Easy bruising precedes the development of hematologic complications which may include leukemia. The syndrome was originally observed in two groups, the W and T families, hence its name.

Gonzalez, C. H., *et al.* The WT syndrome-A "new" autosomal dominant pleiotropic trait of radial/ulnar hypoplasia with high risk of bone marrow failure and/or leukemia. *Birth Defects*, 1977, 13(3B):31-8.

WT limb-blood syndrome. See *WT syndrome.*

WUHRMANN, FERDINAND (Swiss physician, born 1906)

Wuhrmann disease. Synonyms: *myocardial fibrosis, myocardosis.*

A primary degenerative parenchymal myocardial disorder characterized by partial atrophy and fatty degeneration of the myocardial fibers, which may develop into myocardial fibrosis and is frequently associated with interstitial edema.

Wuhrmann, F. Myocarditis-Myokardose-Myocardie. *Schweiz. Med. Wschr.*, 1950, 80:715-22.

WUNDERLICH, CARL REINHOLD AUGUST (German physician, 1815-1877)

Wunderlich syndrome. Synonyms: *perirenal apoplexy, perirenal hematoma, perirenal hemorrhage.*

Retroperitoneal hemorrhage in the kidney area.

Wunderlich, C. A. *Grundriss der speziellen Pathologie und Therapie.* Stuttgart, Ebner & Seubert, 1858.

WWS. See *Walker-Warburg syndrome.*

WYATT, JOHN POYNER (Canadian pathologist)

Wyatt disease. Synonyms: *cytomegalia infantum, cytomegalic inclusion disease, generalized salivary gland virus infection, protozoan cell disease, salivary gland virus disease, salivary gland virus inclusion disease.*

A systemic disorder of the neonatal period due to cytomegalovirus (a virus of the herpesvirus group) infection, presumably acquired before birth. Adults are rarely affected. Hepatosplenomegaly, microcephaly, mental retardation, motor dysfunction, hemorrhage, and jaundice are the principal symptoms. Pneumonia, usually involving the lower lobes, may be bilateral or unilateral. Pathological changes may be found in the salivary glands, kidneys, lungs, pancreas, thyroid, adrenals, and brain. The alveolar epithelial cells are enlarged and contain nuclear inclusions surrounded by a clear zone inside the nuclear membrame. Intracytoplasmic inclusions with a strong periodic-acid Schiff reaction are often present.

Wyatt, J. P., *et al.* Generalized cytomegalic inclusion disease. *J. Pediat.*, 1950, 36:271-94.

WYATT, W. (British physician)

Brushfield-Wyatt syndrome. See *under Brushfield.*

WYBURN-MASON, ROGER (British physician)

Wyburn-Mason syndrome. See *Bonnet-Dechaume-Blanc syndrome, under Bonnet, Paul.*

WYERS, HERMAN JOSEPH GERARD (Dutch physician, born 1894)

Ruiter-Pompen-Wyers syndrome. See *Fabry syndrome.*

WYK, JUDSON J., VAN. See VAN WYK, JUDSON J.

X syndrome. Synonyms: *angina pectoris with normal coronary arteriogram, angina pectoris without coronary heart disease, normal coronary angina pectoris.*

Angina pectoris associated with positive exercise test, no evidence of coronary spasm, and angiographically normal coronary arteries. It is usually due to a reduced coronary flow reserve in inappropriate dilation of small resistive vessels.

Kavanagh-Gray, D. Syndrome X: Case report. *Canad. Med. Assoc. J.*, 1977, 116:385-6.

X-linked agammaglobulinemia. See *Bruton syndrome.*

X-linked cataract-dental syndrome. See *Nance-Horan syndrome.*

X-linked congenital cataracts-microcornea syndrome. See *Nance-Horan syndrome.*

X-linked dominant chondrodysplasia punctata syndrome. See *chondrodysplasia punctata, X-linked dominant type.*

X-linked hydrocephalus. See *Bickers-Adams syndrome.*

X-linked hypophosphatemia. See *hypophosphatemic familial rickets.*

X-linked hypophosphatemic rickets. See *hypophosphatemic familial rickets.*

X-linked lymphoproliferative (XLP) syndrome. See *Wiskott-Aldrich syndrome.*

X-linked mental retardation syndrome (XLMR). Mental retardation transmitted as an X-linked gene, usually occurring in association with other disorders. The condition includes chromosome X fragility, Wieacker-Wolff syndrome, Atkin-Flaitz syndrome, and Waisman-Laxova syndromes.

Opitz, J. M., Reynolds, J. F., & Spano, L. M., eds. X-linked mental retardation 2. *Am. J. Med. Genet.*, 1986, 23:1-735.

X-linked spondylo-epiphyseal dysplasia syndrome. See *spondylo-epiphyseal dysplasia tarda.*

X-trisomy. See *chromosome XXX syndrome.*

xanthelasma. See *Addison-Gull syndrome.*

xanthomatous biliary cirrhosis. See *Hanot-MacMahon-Thannhauser syndrome.*

xanthomatous granuloma syndrome. See *Hand-Schüller-Christian syndrome.*

xanthomatous reticuloendotheliosis. See *Hand-Schüller-Christian syndrome.*

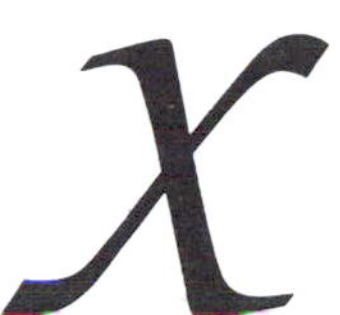

xeroderma pigmentosum (XP) syndrome. Synonyms: *Kaposi dermatosis, angioma pigmentosum et atrophicum, lentigo maligna, lioderma essentialis cum melanosis et telangiectasia, melanosis lenticularis progressiva, pigmented epitheliomatosis.*

A heritable disease, transmitted as an autosomal recessive trait, characterized mainly by sensitivity to sunlight, dry or parched skin, freckling, and neoplastic changes on parts exposed to the sun. Additional cutaneous manifestations in infants include erythema, bullae, freckles, xerosis, scaling, hypopigmentation, telangietasia, atrophy, and keratoses. Basal- and squamous-cell carcinoma, melanoma, and, less commonly, keratoacanthoma, angioma, fibroma, and sarcoma are the common skin neoplasms. Ocular lesions include changes in the eyelids (blepharitis, erythema, pigmentation, keratoses, atrophy with entropion or ectropion, occasional loss of the lid, and neoplasms, such as papillomas, epitheliomas, and basal and squamous-cell carcinomas), lesions in the conjunctivae (conjunctivitis, photophobia, lacrimation, edema, pigmentation, telangiectasia, dryness, symblepharon, inflammatory nodules, and neoplasms, mainly intraepithelial epithelioma and squamous-cell carcinoma), corneal disorders (exposure keratitis, edema, cellular invasion, vascularization, dryness, opacification, ulcers, scarring, and neoplasms), and diseases of the iris (iritis, synechiae, atrophy, and neoplasms). Microcephaly, mental retardation, choreoathetosis, sensorineural deafness, hyporeflexia or areflexia, and electroencephalographic and electromyographic abnormalities are the chief neurological features. The cause of this syndrome is the lack of an enzyme involved in releasing from DNA of thymine dimers formed by ultraviolet radiation, with resulting inability to repair DNA that has been damaged.

Cleaver, J. E. Xeroderma pigmentosum. In: Stanbury, J. B., Wyngaarden, J. B., & Fredrickson, D. S., eds. *The metabolic basis of inherited disease.* 4th ed. New York, McGraw-Hill, 1978, pp. 1072-95. Kraemer, K. H Heritable diseases with increased sensitivity to cellular injury. Fizpatrick, T. B. Eisen, A. Z., Wolff, K., Freedberg, I. M., & Austen, K. F., eds. *Dermatology in general medicine.* 3rd ed. New York, McGraw-Hill, 1987, pp. 1791-811. *Kaposi, M. Xeroderma pigmentosum. *Med. Jahrb.*, 1882, p. 619-33.

xeroderma pigmentosum with neurologic manifestations. See *de Sanctis-Cacchione syndrome.*

xeroderma-talipes-enamel (XTE) defect syndrome. See *Moynahan syndrome (3).*

xerodermic idiocy. See *de Sanctis-Cacchione syndrome.*

xerosis conjunctivae. See *Bitôt spots.*

xerosis corneae. See *Bitôt spots.*

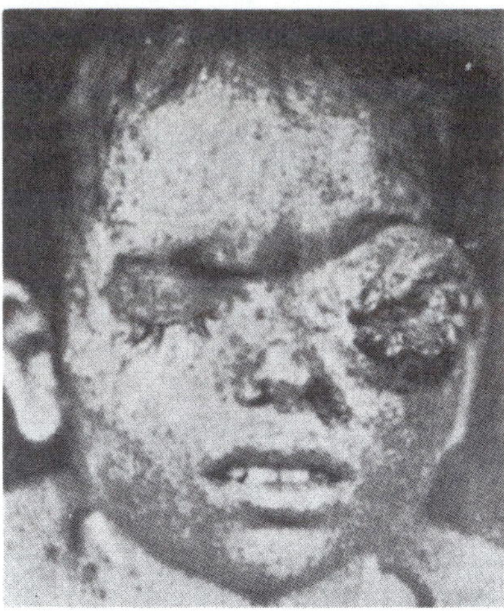

Xeroderma pigmentosum syndrome
Courtesy of Dr. Peter Hansell, Dept. of Medical Illusrations, Institute of Ophthalmology, University of London. From S. Duke-Elder: *Systems of Ophthalmologoy. Vol. VIII, Part 1, Diseases of the Outer Eye.* London: Henry Kimpton, 1965.

xiphoid syndrome. Synonyms: *hypersensitive xiphoid syndrome, xiphoidalgia, xiphoideodynia.*

A painful disorder caused by pressure applied on the hypersensitive xiphoid process, causing discomfort and tenderness in the chest, shoulder, back, and epigastric area. The disorder may occur as a sporadic condition, but in some instances it is associated with diseases or the heart, gallbladder, stomach, esophagus, and bones and joints. Bending, lifting, head turning, or eating heavy meals may precipitate the attacks of pain.

*Linoli, O. Della resezzioni dell'appendice xifoide: Istoria ed osservazioni anatomo-patologico-cliniche. *Ann. Univ. Med. Milano,* 1852, 140:225-35. Lupkin, M., *et al.* The syndrome of the hypersensitive xiphoid. *N. Engl. J. Med.,* 1955, 253:591-7.

xiphoidalgia. See *xiphoid syndrome.*
xiphoideodynia. See *xiphoid syndrome.*

XK syndrome. See *Garcia-Lurie syndrome.*
XK-aprosencephaly syndrome. See *Garcia-Lurie syndrome.*
XLMR. See **X**-*linked* **m**ental **r**etardation *syndrome.*
XLP (X-linked lymphoproliferative) syndrome. See *Wiskott-Alrich syndrome.*
XO syndrome. See *chromosome XO syndrome.*
XO/XY mosaicism. See *chromosome XO/XY syndrome.*
XO/XY syndrome. See *chromosome XO/XY syndrome.*
XP. See **x***eroderma* **p***igmentosum.*
XTE (xeroderma-talipes-enamel defect) syndrome. See *Moynahan syndrome (3).*
XX male syndrome. See *chromosome XX syndrome.*
XX Turner phonotype syndrome. See *Noonan syndrome.*
XX/XXY mosaic. See *chromosome XX/XXY syndrome.*
XX/XXY syndrome. See *chromosome XX/XXY syndrome.*
XXX syndrome. See *chromosome XXX syndrome.*
XXXX syndrome. See *chromosome XXXX syndrome.*
XXXXX syndrome. See *chromosome XXXXX syndrome.*
XXXXY aneuploidy syndrome. See *chromosome XXXXY syndrome.*

XXXXY syndrome. See *chromosome XXXXY syndrome.*
XXXY syndrome. See *chromosome XXXY syndrome.*
XXXYY syndrome. See *chromosome XXXYY syndrome.*
XXY syndrome. See *chromosome XXY syndrome.*
XXYY syndrome. See *chromosome XXYY syndrome.*
XY female syndrome. See *chromosome XY female syndrome.*

XY gonadal dysgenesis (GDXY). See *chromosome XY female syndrome.*
XY Turner phenotype. See *Noonan syndrome.*
XYY syndrome. See *chromosome XYY syndrome.*
XYYY syndrome. See *chromosome XYYY syndrome.*
XYYYY syndrome. See *chromosome XYYYY syndrome.*

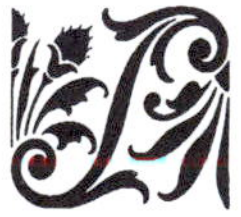

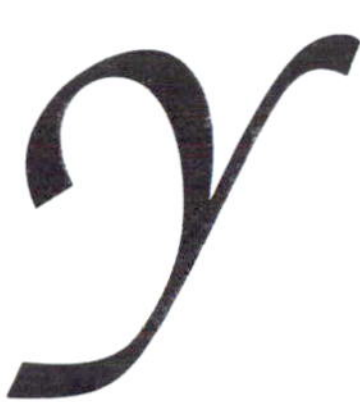

YAGER, JOEL (American physician)

Yager-Young syndrome. Synonyms: *nonhypoglycemia, pseudohypoglycemia syndrome.*

False diagnosis of hypoglycemia on the basis of the patient's own account of symptoms (headache, fatigability, mental dullness, anxiety, phobias, spasms, palpitations, tingling, pains, and sweating), associated with misinterpretation of tests.

Yager, J., & Young, R. T. Non-hypoglycemia is an epidemic condition. *N. Engl. J. Med.*, 1974, 291:907-8.

yato-byo. See *Francis disease.*

yaws. See *Charlouis disease.*

yellow cheese migraine. See *under headache syndrome.*

yellow nail syndrome (YNS). Synonyms: *Samman-White syndrome, bronchiectasis-lymphedema-yellow nail syndrome, yellow nails-bronchiectasis-lymphedema syndrome, yellow nails-lymphedema-pleural effusion syndrome.*

A syndrome, transmitted as an autosomal dominant trait, characterized by yellow, thickened nails with exaggerated lateral curvature and slow rate of growth, associated with lymphedema of the ankles and face, sometimes also involving the genitalia and vocal cords, and respiratory disorders such as chronic bronchitis, sinusitis, and pleural effusions. Both the fingernails and toenails are generally involved. The cuticles are frequently absent. Swelling of the periungual tissues suggests paronychia.

Samman, P. D., & White, W. F. The "yellow nails" syndrome. *Brit. J. Derm.*, 1964, 76:153-7.

yellow nails-brochiectasis-lymphedema syndrome. See *yellow nail syndrome.*

yellow nails-lymphedema-pleural effusion syndrome. See *yellow nail syndrome.*

YNS. See *yellow nail syndrome.*

yo-yo syndrome. A radiological phenomenon wherein the contrast medium flows back and forth like a yo-yo between both pelves in pyelography, indicating the existence of uretero-ureteral outflow in congenital ureteral reduplication (ureter bifidus).

Krzeska, I., *et al.* Uretero-ureteral outflow (yo-yo syndrome) as a cause of abdominal pain. *Internat. Urol. Nephrol.*, 1981, 13:131-6.

YOUNG, DONALD

Barry-Perkins-Young syndrome. See *Young syndrome, under Young, Donald.*

Young syndrome. Synonyms: *Barry-Perkins-Young syndrome, chronic sinopulmonary infection-infertility syndrome, obstructive azospermia-sinopulmonary infection syndrome.*

A hereditary syndrome, transmitted as an autosomal recessive trait, characterized by excretory azospermia in association with sinopulmonary infections (sinusitis, bronchitis, and bronchiectasis).

Young, D. Surgical treatment of male infertility. *J. Reprod. Fertil.*, 1970, 23:541-2.

YOUNG, F. G. (British physician)

Young syndrome. Hyperlactation and rapid weight gain during pregnancy, followed by fetal death or delivery of a large live infant, seen in advanced diabetes mellitus.

Young, F. G. The experimental approach to the problem of diabetes mellitus. *Brit. Med. J.*, 1951, 2:1167-73.

YOUNG, FRIEDA (British scientist)

Dyke-Young syndrome. See *under Dyke.*

YOUNG, I. D. (British physician)

Young-Harper syndrome. A familial form of spinal muscular atrophy, transmitted as an autosomal dominant trait, characterized by progressive distal muscle wasting and weakness, with upper limb changes preceding those in the lower limbs, associated with vocal cord paralysis. Small muscle wasting in the hands, particularly involving the muscles supplied by the median nerve, is the initial disorder. Electrophysiological findings show pathological changes in the anterior horn cells. The disease is most commonly observed in adolescents.

Young, I. D., & Harper, P. S. Hereditary distal spinal muscular atrophy with vocal cord paralysis. *J. Neur. Neurosurg. Psychiat.*, 1980, 43:413-8.

YOUNG, JAMES (British physician)

Young-Paxson syndrome. An obstetric disorder, similar to the crush syndrome (q.v.), caused by retroplacental hemorrhage and trauma of labor. It is characterized by initial tissue damage, shock (that may be severe, moderate, or at times absent), urinary suppression leading to anuria or oliguria with urine containing casts and leukocytes, and uremia reaching its peak between the fifth and the ninth day. Death usually ensues unless there is a substantial increase in the urinary output.

Young, J. Renal failure after utero-placental damage. *Brit. Med. J.*, 1942, 2:715-8. Paxson, N. F., *et al.* The crush syndrome in obstetrics and gynecology. *JAMA*, 1946, 131:500-4.

YOUNG, LIONEL W. (American physician)

Young syndrome. See *craniomandibular dermatodysostosis.*

YOUNG, ROY T. (American physician)

Yager-Young syndrome. See *under Yager.*

young female arteritis syndrome. See *aortic arch syndrome.*

YOUSSEF, ABDEL FATTAH (Egyptian physician)

Youssef syndrome. Synonyms: *menouria syndrome, postcesarean menouria, postcesarean vesicouterine fistula.*

A rare disorder combining urinary incontinence and menstrual hematuria (menouria) due to a vesicouterine fistula which appears after lower-segment cesarean section.

Youssef, A. F. "Hematuria" following lower segment cesarean section. A syndrome. *Am. J. Obst. Gyn.*, 1957, 73:759-67.

YUNIS, EMILIO (Colombian physician)

Yunis-Varón syndrome. A familial syndrome, transmitted as an autosomal recessive trait, characterized by cleidocranial dysostosis, bilateral absence of the thumbs and of the distal phalanges of the fingers, hypoplasia of the first metatarsus, absence of distal phalanx and hypoplasia of the proximal phalanx of the big toe, pelvic dysplasia, bilateral hip dislocation, facial dysmorphism with hypotrichosis, low-set and malformed ears, and retracted and poorly delineated lips. Additional defects include dolichocephaly, depressed temples, microphthalmia, hypoplastic facial bones, anteverted nostrils, diminished nasolabial distance, cystic dental follicles, narrow arched palate, micrognathia, and agenesis of the clavicles. Radiographic findings include skull dysostosis, skull asymmetry, wide fontanels, open cranial sutures, craniofacial disproportion, macrocrania, absence of the ossification center in the sternum, dysplastic pelvis with flattened acetabuli and decreased iliac diameter, and oligosyndactyly.

Yunis, E., & Varón, H. Cleidocranial dysostosis, severe micrognathism, bilateral absence of thumbs and first metatarsal bone, and distal aphalangia. A new genetic syndrome. *Am. J. Dis. Child.*, 1980, 134:649-53.

yuppie (young urban professional) disease. See *chronic fatigue syndrome.*

yusho. See *fetal PCB syndrome.*

YY syndrome. See *chromosome XYY syndrome.*

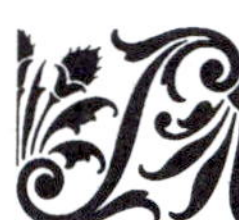

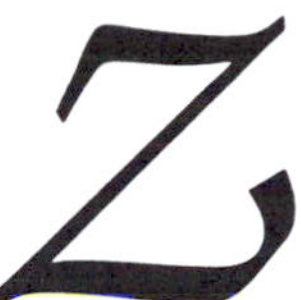

ZACHARY, R. B. (British physician)

Zachary-Morgan syndrome. Synonym: *short colon-imperforate anus syndrome.*

A congenital syndrome characterized by a saccular dilatation of the short colon associated with imperforate anus.

Zachary, R. B., & Morgan, A. Prvostrevo. *Cesk. Pediat.,* 1962, 17:208-10.

ZAHN, FRIEDRICH WILHELM (German physician)

Zahn infarct. Synonym: *atrophic red liver infarct.*

A dark red pseudoinfarct of the portion of the liver supplied by an occluded branch of the portal vein, associated with grossly enlarged capillaries and atrophied liver tissue.

Zahn, F. W. Über die Folgen des Verschlusses der Lungenarterien und Fartaderäste durch Embolie. *Verh. Ges. Deut. Natur. Ärzt.,* 1898, 2(Pt 2):9-11.

ZAHORSKY, JOHN (American physician, 1871-1963)

Zahorsky disease. See *Zahorsky syndrome (1).*

Zahorsky syndrome (1). Synonyms: *Zahorsky disease, exanthema subitum, pseudorubella, rose rash of infants, roseola infantilis, roseola infantum, sixth disease.*

An acute viral disease of infants and young children, characterized by prodromal high fever which disappears after 2 to 5 days and is followed by morbilliform rash. Recovery is complete. See also *congenital rubella syndrome.*

Zahorsky, J. Roseola infantilis. *Pediatrics,* 1810, 22:60-4.

Zahorsky syndrome (2). Synonyms: *angina herpetica, aphthous pharyngitis, herpangina, herpes angina, pharyngitis vesicularis, stomatitis herpetica, vesicular pharyngitis.*

An acute infectious disease caused by Coxsackie viruses group A, seldom lasting more than 3 to 4 days. It usually occurs in young children during the warm months, and is characterized by abrupt fever and the appearance of numerous small vesicles, which are shortly replaced by small painful ulcers, each showing a gray base and an inflamed periphery, on the anterior faucial pillars and sometimes on the palate and tongue. Other manifestations may include anorexia, dysphagia, vomiting, headache, and pain and tenderness in the neck, abdomen, and extremities.

Zahorsky, J. Herpangina (A specific infectious disease). *Arch. Pediat., N. Y.,* 1924, 41:181-4.

ZAK, FREDERICK G. (American physician)

Strauss-Churg-Zak syndrome. See *Churg-Strauss syndrome.*

ZAMBUSCH, LEO, VON (German physician)

von Zambusch disease. See *Hallopeau syndrome (1).*

ZANCA, PETER (American physician)

Zanca syndrome. Hereditary multiple cartilaginous exostoses associated with polyposis of the colon.

Zanca, P. Multiple hereditary cartilaginous exostoses with polyposis of the colon. *U.S. Armed Forces Med. J.,* 1956, 7:116-20.

ZANGE, JOHANNES (German physician, 1880-1969)

Zange-Kindler syndrome. Synonym: *cisternal block syndrome.*

Block of the cerebrospinal fluid in the cisterna magna due to space-occupying lesions of the posterior cranial fossa, such as abscesses, tumors, and inflammatory processes.

Zange, J. Über Subarachnoidalblock, insbesondere den der Cisterna cerebromedullaris ("Zisternenblock"). Entstehungsbedingungen des letzteren, klinische Feststellung und liquordiagnostische Bedeutung, namentlich bei entzündlichen Erkrankungen im Schädel). *Münch. Med. Wschr.,* 1926, l73:1150-2. Kindler, W. Verteile und Gefahren des diagnostischen Zisternenstiches. *Wien. Klin. Wschr.,* 1928, 41:632-4.

ZANIER, J. M.

Zanier-Roubicek syndrome. A syndrome, transmitted as an autosomal dominat trait, marked by hypohidrosis with normal sweating of the palms and soles, hyperthermia, hypotrichosis, hypodontia, yellow discoloration of the teeth, brittle nails, decreased tearing, and occasional mammary hypoplasia.

Zanier, J. M. & Roubicek, M. M. Hypohidrotic ectodermal dysplasia with autosomal dominant transmission. *5th Internat. Cong. Hum. Genet.* Communication 273. Mexico City, 1976.

ZANOLI, R. (Italian physician)

Zanoli-Vecchi syndrome. Postoperative convulsions due to spinal hemorrhage with apnea and loss of consciousness which appear suddenly 2 to 3 hours after spinal surgery. Siphoning of blood to the cerebral ventricles is believed to be the cause.

Zanoli, R., & Vecchi, V. Sindrome convulsiva postoperatoria da emorachide. *Gazz. Sanit., Milano,l* 1956, 27:421-3.

ZAPPERT, JULIUS (Austrian physician, 1867-1938)

Heller-Zappert syndrome. See *under Heller, Theodor O.*

Zappert syndrome. Synonyms: *Zappert tremor, acute cerebellar ataxia, acute cerebral tremor, cerebellar ataxia, hypertonic-dyskinetic syndrome, infantile tremor syndrome.*

A cerebellar disorder characterized by ataxia of station and gait, intention tremor, nystagmus, and slurred speech. Onset occurs suddenly in otherwise apparently normal children or in children recovering from measles, smallplox, or other infectious diseases.

Zappert, J. Über den akuten zerebralen Tremor im frühen Kindesalter. *Mschr. Kinderh.*, 1909, 8:133-49.

Zappert tremor. See *Zappert syndrome.*

ZDS. See ***z**inc **d**eficiency **s**yndrome.*

ZE. See ***Z**ollinger-**E**llison syndrome.*

ZEEK, PEARL M. (American physician)

Zeek disease. Synonym: *hypersensitivity angiitis.*

Periarteritis nodosa-like lesions of different types and distribution, caused by hypersensitivity to various substances, especially to sulfonamides.

Zeek, P. M., *et al.* Studies on periarteritis nodosa. III. The differentiation between the vascular lesions of periarteritis nodosa and of hypersensitivity. *Am.. J. Path.*, 1948, 24:889-917.

ZELIG, SILVIU (Israeli physician)

Feinmesser-Zelig syndrome. See *DOOR syndrome.*

ZELLWEGER, HANS ULRICH (Swiss-born American physician, born 1909)

Fanconi-Albertini-Zellweger syndrome. See *under Fanconi.*

Zellweger syndrome (ZS). Synonyms: *cerebrohepatorenal syndrome (CHR, CHRS).*

A severe, usually fatal, congenital syndrome involving multiple systems. Craniofacial components consist of a high forehead, pear-shaped skull or some degree of turribrachycephaly, flat occiput, flat supraorbital ridges, puffy eyelids, hypertelorism, mild mongoloid palpebral slant, Brushfield spots, cataract, nystagmus, anteverted nostrils, micrognathia, redundant skin on the neck, and posteriorly rotated ears. Hepatomegaly, biliary dysgenesis, and parenchymal lesions are the principal hepatic defects. Renal lesions consist mainly of cysts and foci of dysgenesis. The limbs show camptodactyly of one or more fingers, simian creases, ulnar deviation of the hands, cubitus valgus, flexion disorders of the knees and hips, talipes equinovarus, rocker-bottom feet, and dorsiflexion of the toes. The fontanels and sutures are patent. Growth retardation, muscle hypotonia, respiratory problems, sucking dificulties, and seizures are usually associated. Macrogyria, polymicrogyria, defective myelinization, and white matter lesions are the principal cerebral features. Cardiac complications include patent ductus arteriosus and septal defects. Persons with this syndrome show elevated serum iron and lack of perixisomes and perixisomal enzymes, such as dihydroxyacetone phosphate acetyl transferase. The syndrome is transmitted as an autosomal recessive trait.

Bowen, P., Lee, C. S. N., Zellweger, H., & Lindenburg, R. A familial syndrome of multiple congenital defects. *Bull. Johns Hopkins Hosp.*, 1964, 114:402-14. Opitz, J. M., *et al.* The Zellweger syndrome (cerebro-hepato-renal syndrome). *Birth Defects*, 1969, 5(2):144-60.

ZEMAN, WOLFGANG (American physician)

Zeman-King syndrome. Synonym: *anterior midline syndrome.*

Abnormal affective behavior observed in persons with tumors of the septum pellucidum.

Zeman, W., & King, F. A. Tumors of the septum pellucidum and adjacent structures with abnormal affective behavior: An anterior midline structure syndrome. *J. Nerv. Ment. Dis.*, 1958, 127:490-502.

ZES syndrome. See ***Z**ollinger-**E**llison **s**yndrome.*

ZETTERHOLM, STEN G. (Swedish physician, born 1907)

Myhrman-Zetterholm disease. See *under Myhrman.*

ZETTERSTRÖM, R.

Broberger-Zetterström syndrome. See *under Broberger.*

ZIEHEN, GEORG THEODOR (German physician, 1862-1950)

Schwalbe-Ziehen-Oppenheim syndrome. See *Ziehen-Oppenheim syndrome.*

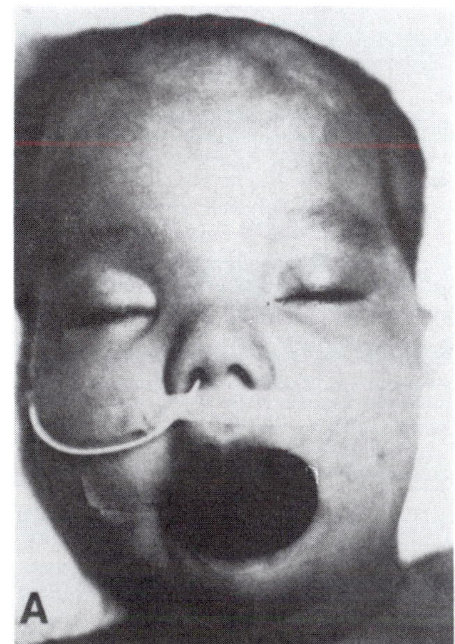

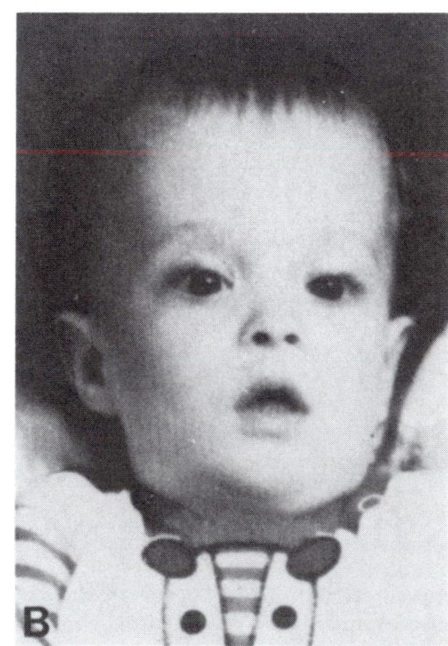

Zellweger syndrome
Wilson, Golder N., Ronald G. Holmes, Joseph Custer, Jeffery L. Lipkowitz, Joan Stover, Nabanita Datta & Amiya Hajra: *American Journal of Medical Genetics* 24:69-82, 1986. New York: Alan R. Liss, Inc.

Ziehen-Oppenheim syndrome. Synonyms: *Schwalbe-Ziehen-Oppenheim syndrome, dysbasia lordotica progressiva, dystonia musculorum deformans, progressive torsion spasm, torsion dystonia, torsion neurosis, torsion spasm.*

A neurological disorder characterized by an overextension or overflexion of the hand, inversion of the foot, latero- or retroflexion of the head, torsion of the spine with arching and twisting of the back, forceful closure of the eyes, and a fixed grimace. Hypertrophy of the muscles of the affected limb and impaired speech are frequently associated. Torsion spasm or dystonia may appear as an independent entity or as a manifestation of some neurological diseases. A variant originally observed in a French-Canadian family is transmitted as an autosomal dominant trait; a form occurring mainly in Jewish children and adolescents is inherited as an autosomal recessive trait; and one reported in the Phillipines is transmitted as an X-linked trait.

*Ziehen, G. T. Demonstrationen im psychiatrischen Verein zu Berlin. *Zbl. Nervenh.*, 1911, 30:109-112. *Oppenheim, H. Über eine eigenartige Krampfkrankheit des kindlichen und jugendlichen Alters (Dysbasia lordotica progressiva, Dystonia musculorum deformans). *Zbl. Nervenh.*, 1911, 30:1090-109.

ZIEVE, LESLIE (American physician, born 1915)

Zieve syndrome. Synonyms: *alcoholic hemolytic anemia-hyperlipemia syndrome, alcoholic hyperlipemia syndrome, hemolytic anemia-hyperlipemic alcoholic syndrome, hepatopancreatic alcoholic syndrome, hyperlipemia-hemolytic anemia-icterus syndrome, pancreaticohepatic syndrome, transitory alcoholic hyperlipemia.*

Jaundice, hyperlipemia or hypercholesterolemia, and hemolytic anemia coexisting with alcoholic fatty liver and mild cirrhosis. The illness usually follows heavy alcohol drinking, and improves once the drinking stops. Scleral lesions, epigastric pain, malaise, and telangiectasia are the the principal clinical symptoms.

Zieve, L. Jaundice, hyperlipemia and hemolytic anemia: A heterofore unrecognized syndrome associated with fatty liver and cirrhosis. *Ann. Int. Med.*, 1958, 48:471-96.

ZIMMERMANN

Zimmermann-Laband syndrome (ZLS). Synonyms: *Laband syndrome, hereditary gingival fibromatosis.*

A hereditary syndrome of gingival fibromatosis, hepatosplenomegaly, and anomalies of the nose, bones, and nails. The nose and pinnas are usually large and poorly structured, giving the affected persons peculiar facial characteristics. Fibromatosis of the gingiva is usually present at birth or appears shortly after. Synophrys and hypertrichosis of the arms, legs, and sacral region are common. Skeletal defects include clubbed tree frog-like fingers and toes, and hyperextensibility of the metacarpophalangeal joints. The nails are usually absent or dysplastic. The syndrome appears to be inherited as an autosomal dominant trait.

Laband, P. F., *et al.* Hereditary gingival fibromatosis. Report of an affected family with associated splenomegaly and skeletal and soft-tissue abnormalities. *Oral Surg.*, 1964; 17:339-51. *Zimmermann. Über Anomalien des Ektoderms. *Vjschr. Zahnheilk.* 1928, 44:419-34.

zinc deficiency syndrome (ZDS). Synonyms: *Prasad syndrome, zinc depletion syndrome, Zn deficiency syndrome.*

Depletion of zinc reserves in the body, generally characterized by skin eruptions, usually involving the face, limbs, perineum, and skin folds; anorexia with changes in the sense of taste and olfactory acuity; neurological disorders, including irritability and depression; growth retardation; depressed wound healing; hypogonadism; immunological disorders; alopecia; impaired vitamin A metabolism with disorders of night vision; diarrhea; and teratogenesis. The syndrome may occur as a genetically determined disorder (see *acrodermatitis enteropathica*) or as a complication of various conditions, including alcoholic liver disease, sickle cell anemia, protein calorie malnutrition, and a variety of intestinal diseases, including the Crohn syndrome, sprue, short bowel syndrome, and other malnutrition syndromes. It may be caused also by geophagia, whereby clay components bind zinc, thus making it unabsorbable. Total parental nutrition can exacerbate zinc deficiency.

Prasad, A. S., *et al.* Syndrome of iron deficiency anemia, hepatosplenomegaly, hypogonadism, dwarfism and geophagia. *Am. J. Med.*, 1961, 31:532-46.

zinc depletion syndrome. See *zinc deficiency syndrome.*

ZINSSER, FERDINAND (American physician, 1865-1952)

Brill-Zinsser disease. See *Brill disease.*

Zinsser syndrome. See *Zinsser-Engman-Cole syndrome.*

Zinsser-Engman-Cole syndrome. Synonyms: *Cole syndrome, Cole-Rauschkolb-Toomey syndrome, Engman syndrome, Zinsser syndrome, congenital dyskeratosis, dyskeratosis congenita (DC).*

Reticular pigmentation, nail dystrophy, and leukoplakia are the principal features of this syndrome. They are associated with skin changes resembling poikiloderma vasculare atrophicans and involving the face, neck, and chest; growth retardation; hyperhidrosis of the palms and soles and occasionally other parts of the body; acrocyanosis; aplastic anemia; hypersplenism; hypotrichosis and/or premature canities; blepharitis; profuse lacrimation; ear malformations; and vesicles and bullae of the tongue and palate. The syndrome occurs mainly in males. X-linked inheritance is suspected.

*Zinsser, F. Atrophia cutis reticularis cum pigmentatione, dystrophia unguium und Leukoplakia oris (Poikilodermia atrophicans vascularis Jacobi). *Ikonograph. Dermat*, 1910(?), p. 219-23. Engman, A. Unique case of reticular pigmentation of the skin with atrophy. *Arch. Derm. Syph., Chicago*, 1926, 13:685-7. Cole, H. N., Rauschkolb, J. E., & Toomey, J. Dyskeratosis congenita with pigmentation, dystrophia unguis and leukokeratosis oris. *Arch. Derm. Syph., Chicago*, 1930, 21:71-95.

Zinsser-Fanconi syndrome. Synonym: *aplastic anemia-dyskeratosis congenita syndrome.*

An association of the Zinsser-Eangman-Cole syndrome with Fanconi aplastic anemia.

Javier, G. Anemia aplástica asociada a desqueratosis congénita (sindrome de Zinsser-Fanconi). *Sangre*, 1981, 26:367-73.

ZIPRKOWSKI, L. (Israeli physician)

Ziprkowski-Margolis syndrome. See *Woolf syndrome.*

ZLS. See *Zimmermann-Laband syndrome.*

Zn deficiency syndrome. See *zinc deficiency syndrome.*

ZOEPFFEL, HEINRICH (German physician, born 1883)

Zoepffel edema. Synonyms: *edematous necrosis of the pancreas, edematous pancreatitis, interstitial pancreatitis.*

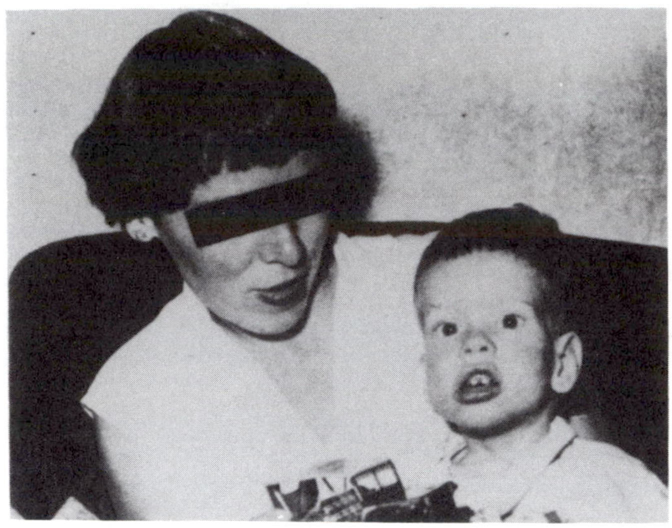

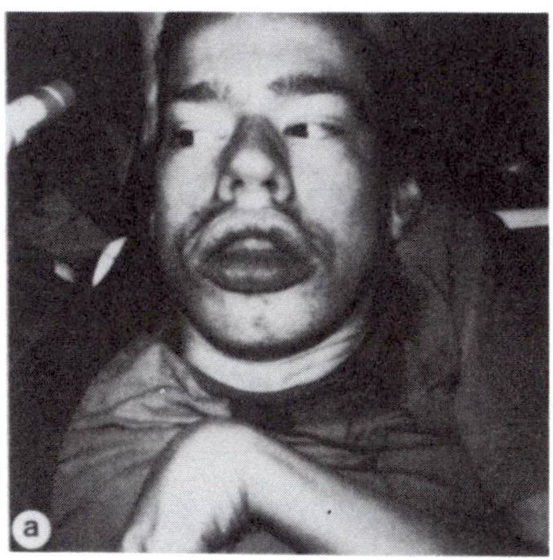

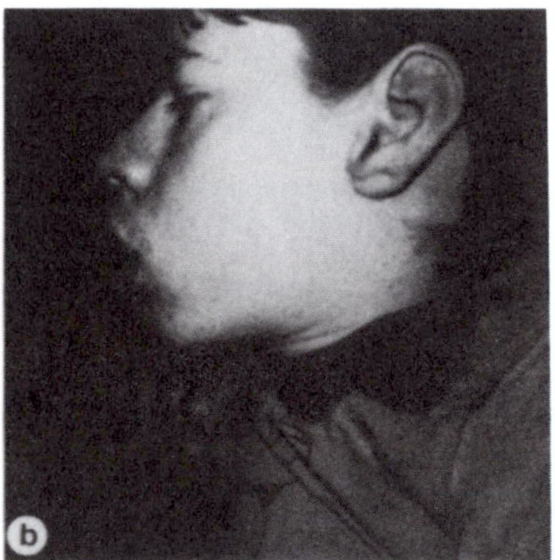

Zimmerman-Laband syndrome
Chodirker, Bernard N., Albert E. Chudley, Milada A. Toffler & Martin H. Reed, *American Journal of Medical Genetics* 25:543-547, 1986. New York: Alan R. Liss, Inc.

A disease of the pancreas marked by edema that may be combined with patches of nonhemorrhagic necrosis, fat necrosis, and mild inflammatory lesions.

Zoepffel, H. Das akute Pankreasödem, eine Vorstufe der akuten Pankreasnekrose. *Deut. Zschr. Chir.*, 1922, 75:301-12.

ZOLLINGER, ROBERT MILTON (American physician, born 1903)

pseudo-Zollinger-Ellison syndrome (Ps-ZES). Synonym: *nontumorous hypergastrinemic hyperchlorhydria (NTHH) syndrome.*

A disease in which peptic ulceration of the duodenum or gastrojejunal stoma is accompanied by gastric hyperacidity due to the humoral effects of hypergastrinemia from hyperplastic antral G cells, without associated neoplasms.

Friesen, S. R., & Tomita, T. Pseudo-Zollinger-Ellison syndrome. Hypergastrinemia, hyperchlorhydria without tumor. *Ann. Surg.*, 1981, 194:481-93. Friesen, S. R., & Tomita, T. Further experience with pseudo-Zollinger-Ellison syndrome: Its place in the management of neuroendocrine duodenal ulceration. *World J. Surg.*, 1984, 8:552-60.

Strom-Zollinger-Ellison syndrome. See *Zollinger-Ellison syndrome.*

Zollinger-Ellison syndrome (ZE, ZES). Synonyms: *Strom-Zollinger-Ellison syndrome, gastric hypersecretion-peptic ulceration-pancreatic tumor syndrome, gastrinoma syndrome, ulcerogenic tumor of the pancreas syndrome.*

A syndrome of non-ß-cell tumors of the islands of Langerhans, or diffuse islet cell hyperplasia, with peptic ulcer due to hypersecretion of gastrin from the tumor and elevated gastric acid concentration. Most tumors are carcinomas but some are benign adenomas. Many cases are complicated by multiple tumor sites. Gastrointestinal hemorrhage, vomiting, gastric perforation, and diarrhea (frequently steatorrhea) are the common clinical features of this syndrome. Radiological findings show rugal hypertrophy, rapid transit through the small intestine, and a cobweblike pattern of tha small intestinal mucosa. High serum gastrin level, decreased pancreatic lipase, and high basal gastric acid output are the principal biochemical findings. When associated with familial multiple endocrine adenomatosis, the syndrome is known as the *multiple endocrine neoplasia I syndrome (MEN I)*.

Zollinger, R. M., & Ellison, E. H. Primary peptic ulcerations of the jejunum associated with islet cell tumors of the pancreas. *Ann. Surg.*, 1955, 142:709-28. Strom, R. A case of peptic ulcer and insuloma. *Acta Chir, Scand.*, 1952-53, 104:252-60.

ZONANA, JONATHAN (American physician)

Bannayan-Zonana syndrome (BZS). See *Bannayan syndrome.*

ZONDEK, BERNHARD (Israeli physician, 1891-1966)

Zondek syndrome. Synonyms: *Zondek-Bromberg-Rozin syndrome, anterior pituitary hyperhormonotropic syndrome.*

A syndrome of excessive production of gonadotropic, lactotropic, thyrotropic, and probably insulinotropic hormones. The condition is manifested by irregularly excessive uterine bleeding, galactorrhea, thyrotoxicosis, and, in some cases, hypoglycemia, anemia, sterility, and neurological symptoms.

Zondek, B., Bromberg, Y. M., & Rozin, S. An anterior pituitary hyperhormonotrophic syndrome (excessive uterine bleeding, galactorrhoea, hyperthyrodism). *J. Obst. Gynaec. Brit. Emp.*, 1951, 58:525-37.

Zondek-Bromberg-Rozin syndrome. See *Zondek syndrome.*

ZONDEK, HERMANN (German physician, born 1887)

Zondek syndrome. Synonym: *myxedema heart.*

Cardiac complications of myxedema.

Zondek, H. Das Myxödemherz. *Münch. Med. Wschr.*, 1918, 65:1180-2.

ZOON, JOHANNES JACOBUS (Dutch physician, born 1902)

Zoon balanitis. See *Zoon erythroplasia.*

Zoon erythroplasia. Synonyms: *Zoon balanitis, balanitis circumscripta chronica, balanitis plasmocellulare, balanoposthitis chronica circumscripta plasmocellularis, plasma-cell balanitis.*

A form of erythroplasia, occurring most commonly in middle-aged or elderly uncircumscribed males, characterized by a solitary glistening, red, persistent plaque on the glans penis or in the preputial sac. A dense bandlike or lichenoid plasma cell infiltrate with vascular proliferation of the dermis is the principal histological feature.

Zoon, J. J. Balanitis circumscripta chronica met plasmacellen-infiltrat. *Ned. Tschr. Geneesk.*, 1950, 94:1529-30.

ZS. See *Zellweger syndrome.*

ZUELZER, WOLF W. (American hematologist, born 1909)

Jirásek-Zuelzer-Wilson syndrome. See *under Jirásek.*

Zuelzer syndrome. Synonym: *familial eosinophilia.*

An association of eosinophilia, leukocytosis, and hypergammaglobulinemia in infants and young children. The symptoms include hepatomegaly, pulmonary infiltrations, asthma, joints lesions, urticaria, and convulsions. The disorder is familial and is transmitted as an autosomal dominant trait.

Zuelzer, W. W., & Apt, L. Disseminated visceral lesions asociated with extreme eosinophilia. Pathologic and clinical observations on a syndrome of young children. *Am. J. Dis. Child.*, 1949, 78:153-81.

Zuelzer-Kaplan syndrome (1). See *Crosby syndrome, under Crosby, William H.*

Zuelzer-Kaplan syndrome (2). Synonyms: *hemoglobin C thalassemia, thalassemia-hemoglobin C disease.*

A hemolytic disease attributed to the interaction of the hemoglobin C gene with the thalassemia gene. In the original report the patient, who was Black, and his father were shown to be a carriers of the hemoglobin trait, and his mother was a carrier of the thalassemia trait. The disorder is usually mild and may be present during pregnancy as a refractory anemia or with folic acid deficiency. Splenomegaly is usually present. See also *thalassemia syndrome.*

Zuelzer, W. W., & Kaplan, E. Thalassemia-hemoglobin C disease. A new syndrome presumably due to the combination of the genes for thalassemia and hemomglobin C. *Blood*, 1954, 9:1047-54. Weatherall, D. J. The thalassemias. In: Williams, W. J., Beutler, E., Erslev, A. J., & Lichtman, M. A., eds. *Hematology.* 3rd ed. New York, McGraw-Hill, 1983, pp. 493-52.

Zuelzer-Ogden syndrome. Synonym: *megaloblastic anemia in infants.*

A hematological disorder in infants characterized by morphological and functional abnormalities in the blood and bone marrow. Erythrocytes show variations in size and shape and, in severe cases, inclusions such as stippling, Howell-Jolly bodies, and Cabot ring, being normochromic and macrocytic. The reticulocyte count is low. Nucleated red cells may appear in the presence of low hematocrit. Hypersegmented neutrophils (macropolycytes) usually indicate megaloblastosis. Chromosomes may be elongated or broken. The bone marrow is cellular and often hyperplastic. Weakness, palpitation, fatigue, shortness of breath, and pallor are the usual symptoms. Congestive heart failure may occur.

Zuelzer, W. W., & Ogden, F. N. Megaloblastic anemia in infancy. A common syndrome responding to folic acid therapy. *Am. J. Dis. Child.*, 1946, 71:211-43. Beck, W. S. The megaloblastic anemias. In: Williams, W. J., Beutler, E., Erslev, A. J., & Lichtman, M. A., eds. *Hematology.* 3rd ed. New York, McGraw-Hill, 1983, pp. 434-65.

Zuelzer-Wilson syndrome. See *Jirásek-Zuelzer-Wilson syndrome.*

ZUGIBE, FREDERICK T. (American physician)

Zugibe disease. See *glycoprotein storage disease.*

ZUNIN, C. (Italian physician)

Durand-Zunin syndrome. See *under Durand, Paul.*

ZURHELLE, EMIL (German physician)

Hoffmann-Zurhelle syndrome. See *under Hoffmann, Erich.*

ZWAHLEN, P. (Swiss physician)

Franceschetti-Zwahlen syndrome. See *mandibulofacial dysostosis.*

Franceschetti-Zwahlen-Klein syndrome. See *mandibulofacial dysostosis.*

Zwahlen syndrome. See *mandibulofacial dysostosis.*

ZWEYMÜLLER, E. (Austrian physician)

Weissenbacher-Zweymüller syndrome. See *under Weissenbacher.*

zygomaticomaxillomandibulofacial dysostosis. See *Wildervanck syndrome (2).*

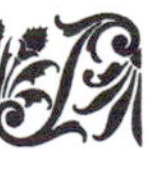

Page #	Term	Observation

Page #	Term	Observation

Page #	Term	Observation

Page #	Term	Observation